NURSING CARE PLANS

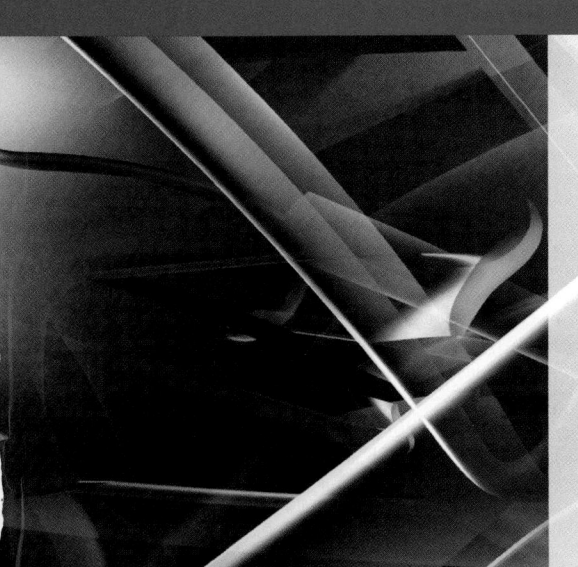

Psychiatric Nursing: Biological & Behavioral Concepts

Second Edition

Deborah Antai-Otong, MS, APRN, BC, FAAN
Veterans Integrated Systems Network (VISN 17)
Program Manager, Care Coordination Home Telehealth
Arlington, Texas
Mental Health Provider, Fort Worth Outpatient Mental Health
Clinic

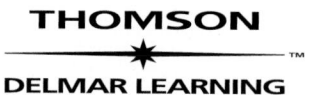

THOMSON
DELMAR LEARNING

Psychiatric Nursing: Biological & Behavioral Concepts, Second Edition
by Deborah Antai-Otong, MS, APRN, BC, FAAN

Vice President, Health Care Business Unit:
William Brottmiller

Editorial Director:
Matthew Kane

Acquisitions Editor, Nursing:
Maureen Rosener

Senior Product Manager:
Patricia Gaworecki

Marketing Director:
Jennifer McAvey

Marketing Channel Manager:
Michele McTighe

Marketing Coordinator:
Chelsey Iaquinta

Content Project Manager:
Jessica McNavich

Technology Product Manager:
Mary Colleen Liburdi

Technology Product Manager:
Ben Knapp

Library of Congress Cataloging-in-Publication Data

Psychiatric nursing : biological & behavioral concepts /
[edited by] Deborah Antai-Otong.— 2nd ed.
  p. ; cm.
  Includes bibliographical references and index.
  ISBN-13: 978-1-4180-3872-4
  ISBN-10: 1-4180-3872-5
1. Psychiatric nursing. 2. Behavior therapy.
I. Antai-Otong, Deborah. II. Title.
  [DNLM: 1. Psychiatric Nursing—methods.
2. Behavior Therapy. WY 160 P97238 2008]
RC440.P7537 2008
616.89'0231—dc22

                                                    2007037941

NOTICE TO THE READER

Publisher does not warrant or guarantee any of the products described herein or perform any independent analysis in connection with any of the product information contained herein. Publisher does not assume, and expressly disclaims, any obligation to obtain and include information other than that provided to it by the manufacturer.

The reader is expressly warned to consider and adopt all safety precautions that might be indicated by the activities described herein and to avoid all potential hazards. By following the instructions contained herein, the reader willingly assumes all risks in connection with such instructions.

The publisher makes no representations or warranties of any kind, including but not limited to, the warranties of fitness for particular purpose or merchantability, nor are any such representations implied with respect to the material set forth herein, and the publisher takes no responsibility with respect to such material. The publisher shall not be liable for any special, consequential, or exemplary damages resulting, in whole or part, from the reader's use of, or reliance upon, this material.

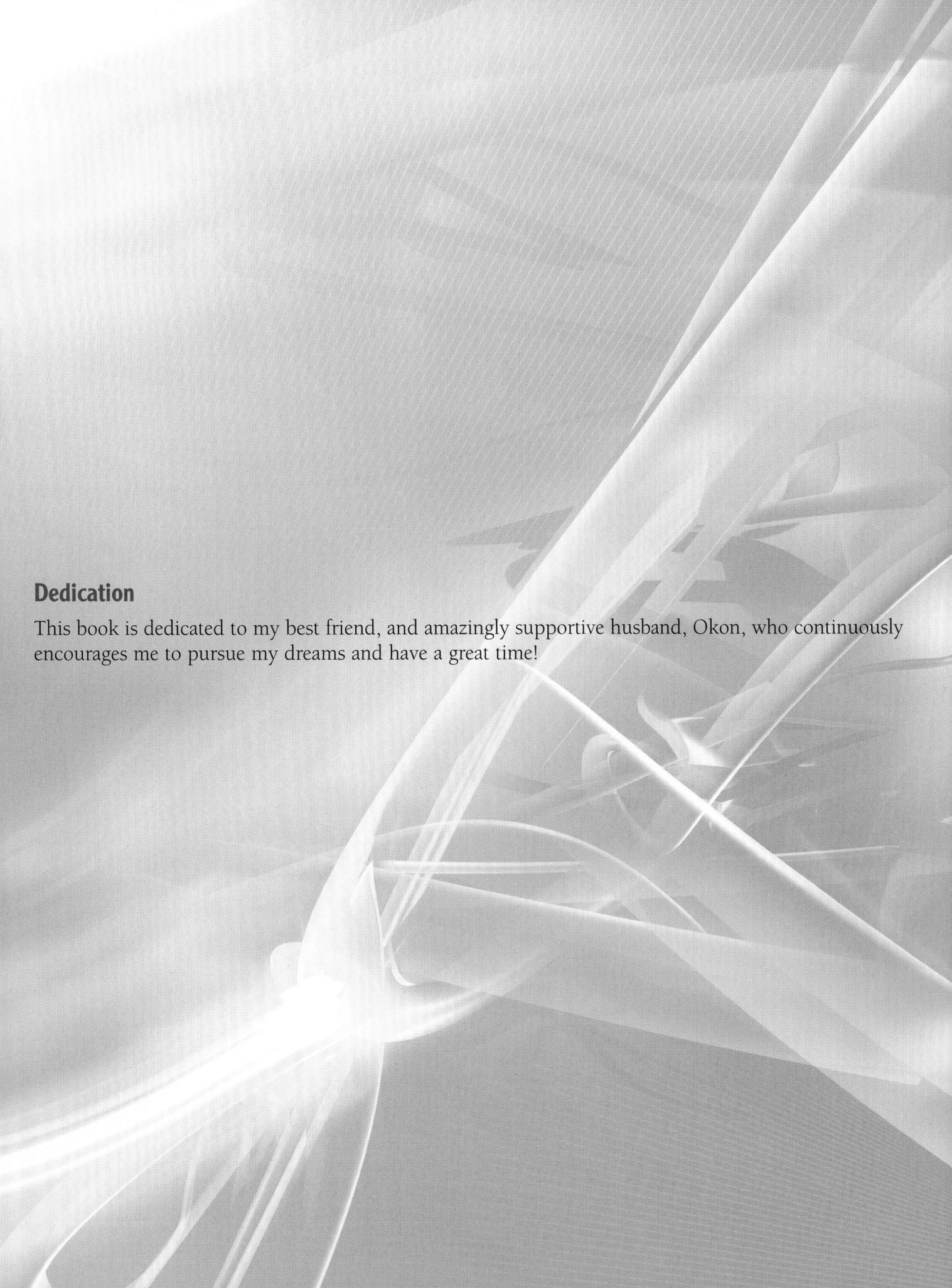

Dedication

This book is dedicated to my best friend, and amazingly supportive husband, Okon, who continuously encourages me to pursue my dreams and have a great time!

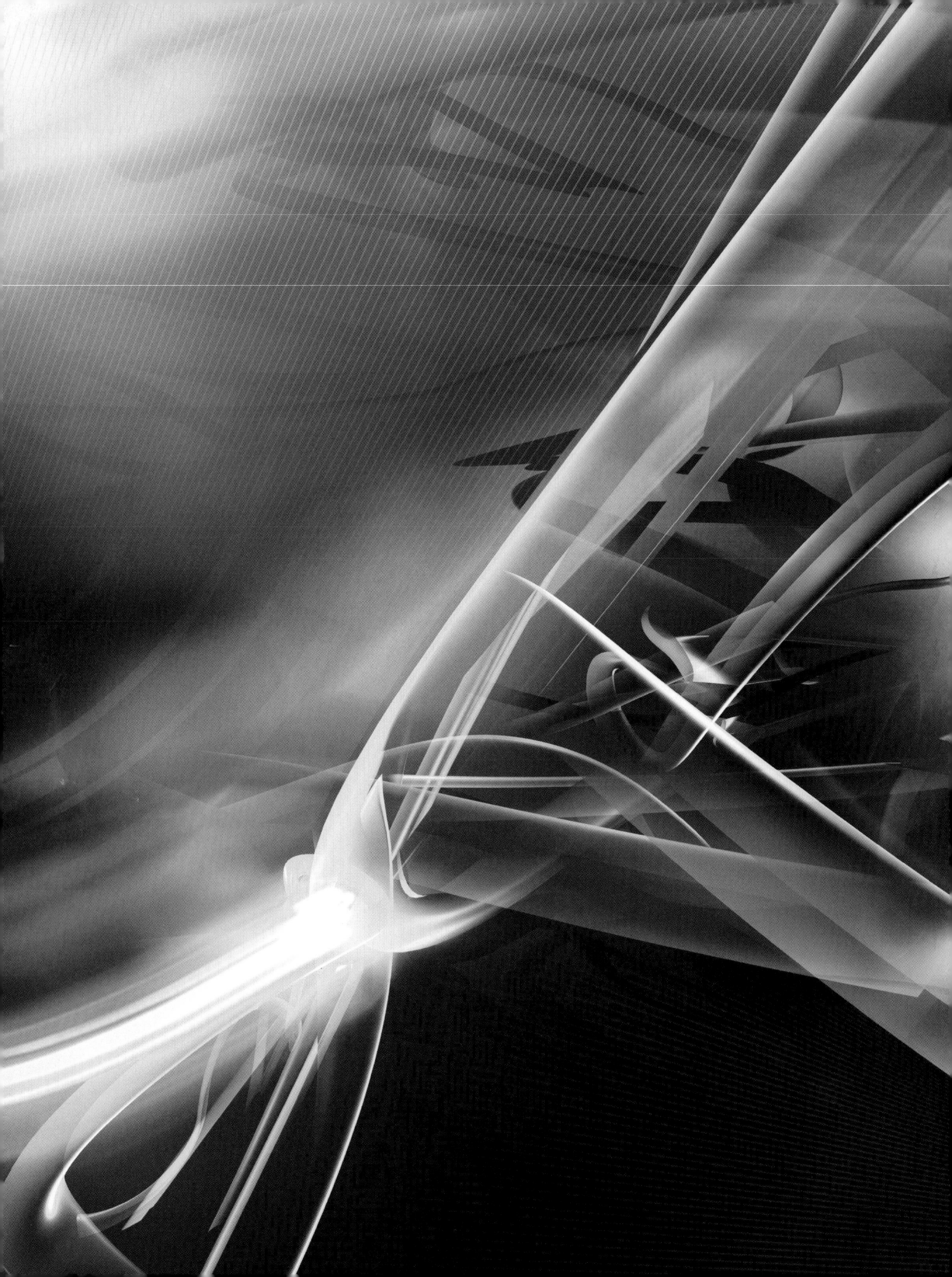

CONTENTS

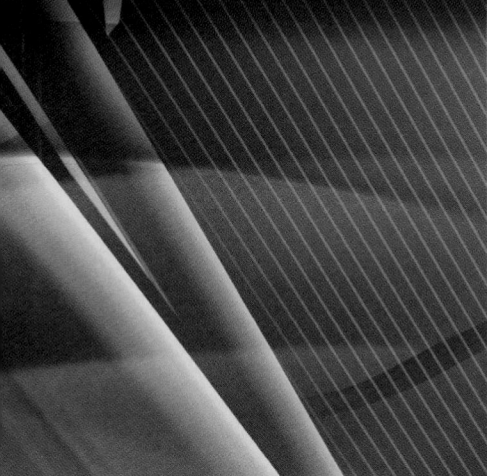

Psychiatric Nursing: Biological & Behavioral Concepts, Second Edition

RESEARCH ABSTRACTS

TABLES

CONTRIBUTORS

Linda Funk Barloon, RN, MS(N), CPNP
Baylor Department of Psychiatry, Research Program,
Houston, Texas
Chapter 8, Legal and Ethical Considerations

Susan Beyer, MSN, APRN, BC, LCDC
Psychiatric Nurse Practitioner, Private Practice of Hadi
Tajani, MD, Bedford, Texas
Chapter 21, The Client with a Substance-Related Disorder

Johnnie Bonner, MS, RNCS
Psychiatric Clinical Nurse Specialist (retired), Rockwall, Texas
Chapter 32, Milieu Therapy/Hospital-Based Care

Margaret Brackley, PhD, RN, CS
The University of Texas Health Science Center at San Antonio
School of Nursing, Department of Family Nursing Care, San
Antonio, Texas
*Chapter 3, Interfacing Biological-Behavioral Concepts
into Psychiatric Nursing Practice*
Chapter 24, The Client with a Sexual Disorder
Chapter 37, The Future of Psychiatric Nursing

Martha Buffum, DNSc, APRN, BC, CS
Associate Chief, Nursing Service for Research, VA Medical
Center, San Francisco, California
Associate Clinical Professor, University of California San
Francisco, School of Nursing, San Francisco,
California
Chapter 27, Group Therapy

Dona H. Caine-Francis, MSN, Psychiatric CNS, PMH-NP
Psychiatric Mental Health Nurse Practitioner, Clinical
Specialist AASECT Certified Sex Therapist
Chapter 24, The Client with a Sexual Disorder

Randy Goodwin, RN, MNSc, CS
Mental Health Provider, Telehealth Coordinator, Central
Texas Veterans Health Care System, Temple, Texas
Chapter 12, The Client with a Somatization Disorder

Christine Grant, PhD, RN
Psychiatric Mental Health Nursing, University of
Pennsylvania, Philadelphia, Pennsylvania
Chapter 25, The Client Who Survives Violence

Ada Lynne Hendricks, RN, CS, FNP-C, MS(N)
Independence, Missouri
Chapter 8, Legal and Ethical Considerations

Vicki Hines-Martin, PhD, RN, APRN, BC
Associate Professor, University of Louisville, Louisville,
Kentucky
Chapter 10, The Client with a Bipolar Disorder

Sheryl A. Innerarity, RN, PhD, FNP, CS
Associate Professor, Clinical Nursing, University of Texas
(Austin), Austin, Texas
Chapter 23, The Client with a Sleep Disorder
Chapter 34, Psychosocial Care in Medical-Surgical Settings

Lisa A. Jensen, MS, APRN, CS
Associate Chief, Nursing Service/Mental Health,
George E. Wahlen Department of Veterans Affairs
Medical Center, VA Salt Lake City Healthcare System,
Salt Lake City, Utah
Chapter 13, The Client with a Stress-Related Disorder
Chapter 18, The Client with a Dissociative Disorder

Susan L. W. Krupnick, MSN, CARN, ANP, CS
Chapter 35, Psychiatric Consultation-Liaison Nursing

Valerie Levi, Pharm D
Daiichi Sankyo, Euless, Texas
Chapter 29, Psychopharmacologic Therapy

Linda Lewin, RN, MSN, CS
Clinical Nurse Specialist, Payne Whitney Manhattan, New
York Presbyterian Hospital, New York, New York
Chapter 9, The Client with a Depressive Disorder

Erika Madrid, DNSc, RN, CS
City of Berkeley, Human and Health Services Department,
Public Health Division, Supervising Public Health Nurse,
Berkeley, California
Chapter 27, Group Therapy

Rose M. Nieswiadomy, PhD, RN
Professor Emerita, Texas Woman's University, Denton, Texas
Chapter 36, Psychiatric Nursing Research

Cindy Parsons, DNP, APRN, BC
Assistant Professor, Nursing, University of Tampa, Tampa,
Florida
Chapter 17, The Client with Attention-Deficit Disorder

Catherine Pawlicki, MSN, RN, CS
Chapter 18, The Client with a Dissociative Disorder

Duane F. Pennebaker, PhD, FNAP, FRCNA
Adjunct Research Fellow, School of Population Health,
University of Western Australia
Chapter 29, Psychopharmacological Therapy

Tracy Poelvoorde, MS, RN
Director of Nursing Programs, Trinity College of Nursing
and Health Sciences, Rock Island, Illinois
*Chapter 16, The Client with Delirium, Dementia, Amnestic, and
Other Cognitive Disorders*

Joy Riley, DNSc, RN, CS
Lecturer, Indiana University School of Nursing,
Indianapolis, Indiana
Schizophrenia Treatment and Rehabilitation (STAR), Inc.,
Indianapolis, Indiana
Chapter 29, Psychopharmacologic Therapy

Martha Sanford, PhD, RN
Former Associate Professor, Baylor, School of Nursing
(retired), Dallas, Texas
Chapter 2, Concepts of Psychiatric Care: Therapeutic Models

Laura Smith-McKenna, RN, MS, DNSc
Walnut Creek, California
Chapter 25, The Client Who Survives Violence

Jacqueline M. Stolley, PhD, RN, CS
Professor, Trinity College of Nursing and Health Sciences,
Moline, Illinois
*Chapter 16, The Client with Delirium, Dementia, Amnestic, and
Other Cognitive Disorders*

Deborah Thomas, EdD, RN, ARNP, BC
Prospect Counseling and Consulting Center, Prospect,
Kentucky
Chapter 10, The Client with a Bipolar Disorder

Barbara Jones Warren, PhD, RN, CNS, CS
Associate Professor of Clinical Nursing, Ohio State
University, Worthington, Ohio
Chapter 7, Cultural and Ethnic Considerations
*Chapter 14, The Client with Schizophrenia and Other Psychotic
Disorders*
Chapter 33, Home- and Community-Based Care

Sylvia A. Whiting, PhD, APRN, BC
North Charleston, South Carolina
Chapter 15, The Client with a Personality Disorder

Michele L. Zimmerman, MA, APRN, BC
Finney Psychotherapy Associates, PLC, Virginia Beach,
Virginia
Chapter 22, The Client with an Eating Disorder

REVIEWERS

Deanah Alexander, RN, MSN, PMHNP, CB
Instructor
West Texas A&M University
Canyon, Texas

Lora Humphrey Beebe, PhD, APRN, BC
Associate Professor
University of Tennessee
Knoxville, Tennessee

Barbara Mathews Blanton, MSN, RN, CARN
Assistant Clinical Professor of Nursing
Texas Women's University
College of Nursing
Dallas, Texas

Jeri L. Brandt, PhD, RN
Professor of Nursing
Nebraska Wesleyan University
Lincoln, Nebraska

Barbara Buchanan Covington, EdD, MSN, FNP
Professor
Tennessee State University

Teresa S. Burckhalter, MSN, RN-C
A.D.N. Faculty
Technical College of the Lowcountry
Beaufort, South Carolina

Leona Dempsey, PhD, RN, APNP, BC
Assistant Professor
University of Wisconsin, College of Nursing
Medication Prescriber
Oshkosh Counseling and Wellness Center

Ginger Evans, MS, MSN, APRN-BC, SANE-A
Assistant Professor
University of Tennessee
Knoxville, Tennessee

Marybeth A. Gillis, MSN, RN
Assistant Professor
Elmira College
Elmira, New York

Jane Goodson, RN, MSN
Associate Nursing Faculty
Gaston College
Dallas, North Carolina

Adelaide Kolb-Selby, MNSc, RN
Instructor, Eleanor Mann School of Nursing
University of Arkansas
College of Education and Health Professions
Fayetteville, Arkansas

Jeanne B. Kozlak, RN, MSN, CNS
Professor of Mental Health Nursing
Humboldt State University
Arcata, California

Yoriko Kozuki, PhD, ARNP
Associate Professor
University of Washington, School of Nursing
Department of Psychosocial & Community Health

Joanne Lavin
Kingsborough Community College

Valerie Levi, Pharm D
Assistant Professor of Pharmacy Practice
Texas Tech School of Pharmacy
Dallas, Texas

Susan McCabe, EdD, APRN, CS
Associate Professor
University of Wyoming
Fay W. Whitney School of Nursing
Laramie, Wyoming

Dana Murphy-Parker, RN, MS, CNS
Coordinator, Acute Psychiatric/Mental Health Nursing
New York University
New York, New York

Ann Peden, ARNP-CS, DSN
Associate Professor
University of Kentucky
College of Nursing
Lexington, Kentucky

Dr. Marita Terese Peppard, RN, ND, MS
Professor of Nursing
Austin Community College
Austin, Texas

Jane Poynter, RN, BSN, MSN
Professor of Nursing
Yuba College
Marysville, California

Anita Rhodes-Kelley, RN, MSN
Dean, Nursing
El Paso Community College
El Paso, Texas

Dawn M. Scheick, MN, RN-CS
Associate Professor, Psychiatric-Mental Health Nursing
Alderson-Broaddus College
Philippi, West Virginia

Linda S. Smith, MS, DSN, RN
Assistant Professor
Oregon Health & Science University
Klamath Falls, Oregon

Melodie Stembridge, ARNP-BC, PhD
Nurse Practitioner, Mental Health Service Line
VA Medical Center–Atlanta
Decatur, Georgia

Linda K. Tuyn, MA, RN, CS, FNP
Clinical Assistant Professor
Binghamton University
Decker School of Nursing
Binghamton, New York

E. Monica Ward-Murray, RN, MA, EdM, EdD
Assistant to the Dean for Research/Assistant Professor
North Carolina A&T State University
Greensboro, North Carolina

Barbara Jones Warren, PhD, RN, CNS, CS
Associate Professor
The Ohio State University, College of Nursing

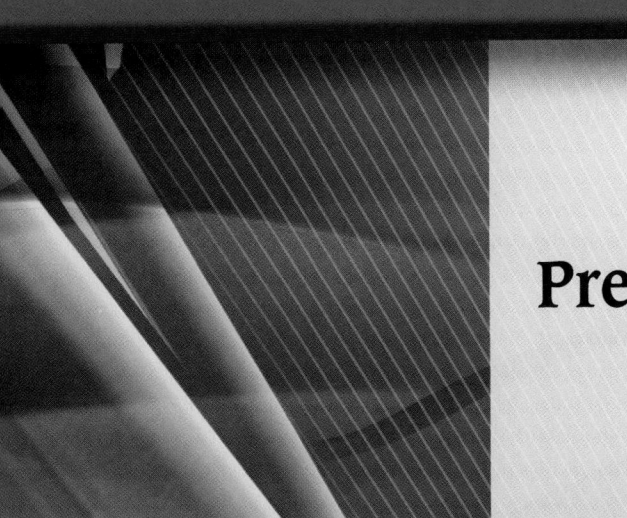

Preface

The plethora of scientific data from technological advances in molecular studies, neurochemistry, neuroimaging of various brain regions and neurocircuitry, and pharmacology provide a plausible explanation for intricate psychiatric brain disorders. In today's world of expanded scientific data, clients and their families have a sense of hope and encouragement concerning optimal functioning that extends beyond symptom management and toward recovery and improved quality of life. Psychiatric mental-health nurses are uniquely poised to comprehend these scientific findings, become a part of scientific inquiry, and integrate findings into holistic, quality, and evidence-based health care. In addition to the wealth of scientific technology and advances in biology, genetics, and psychopharmacology, the publication of the *Surgeon General's 1999 Report on Mental Health* has also revolutionized psychiatric care. Combined with recommendations from the Institute of Medicine's *Crossing the Quality Chasm,* published in 2001—which emphasizes safety, effectiveness, timely health care, client-centered health care, efficiency, quality, and access—the *Surgeon General's 1999 Report on Mental Health* provides a basis for mental health care in the twenty-first century.

The *Surgeon General's 1999 Report on Mental Health* has become one of the most significant contributions to psychiatry in almost 60 years. This extensive report focuses on holistic psychiatric care, parity in mental health services, culture, spirituality, research, theory, and the importance of integrating evidence-based biological and psychotherapeutic interventions into treatment planning. In addition, it emphasizes the importance of mental health care that encompasses the needs of clients, families, communities, and societies. It has become the template for this era in psychiatry, and it is relevant to advancing psychiatric nursing care for clients presenting with various psychiatric disorders.

The conceptual framework of this book integrates a holistic, developmental, and adaptation model that reflects the continuum of health throughout the life span. The continuum of mental health depicts complex and rapid neurobiological development during the prenatal period and the normalcy of aging. Psychiatric-mental health nurses play crucial roles in mental health promotion and maintenance. Advances in neurobiological and genetic research and psychopharmacology offer extensive evidence that supports the importance of holistic health care. The National Institute of Mental Health continues to fund clinical trials in search of the ideal psychotropic drug to treat major psychiatric disorders, including mood disorders, anxiety disorders, substance-use disorders, and schizophrenia, with fewer adverse side effects. Clients and their families benefit from clinical trials but require education about reasons for medications and side effects. Psychoeducation is a critical element of psychiatric nursing care, offering nurses opportunities to form therapeutic relationships; reduce symptoms; and promote safe, quality mental health care. Because mental health is a dynamic process, holistic care requires nursing care that synthesizes biological, psychosocial, cultural, gender, and spiritual concepts. These concepts have profound effects on human behavior and adaptation, primarily by reducing symptoms and promoting restoration and health maintenance of vital processes.

As nurses in vast practice settings face growing populations of persons with diverse mental health problems, understanding their experiences requires astute observational and clinical skills of client symptoms and presentations. Analyzing client symptoms and behaviors begins with a collaborative process that conveys respect, care, genuine interest, and empathy. As the client moves along the mental health continuum and life span, efforts to reduce symptoms, facilitate function, and improve quality of life are high priorities. This challenge and need to synthesize holistic concepts into psychiatric treatment planning underscores the need for a textbook that integrates these nursing concepts. The second edition of *Psychiatric Nursing: Biological & Behavioral Concepts* fulfills this need.

The purpose of this textbook is to help students integrate concepts of holistic nursing, adaptation, and human response across the life span. Moreover, it integrates advances in neurobiology; genetics;

neuroimaging; molecular science; psychosocial, life span, cultural, and spiritual concepts; and principles of complex processes that contribute to psychiatric disorders. Psychiatric nurses and students will find the second edition of this textbook informative and meaningful to the care of the client with a psychiatric disorder.

The second edition of this textbook also provides the nurse with an extensive discussion of adaptive and maladaptive responses to stressors and their impact on the mental health-mental illness continuum. Likewise, the emphasis on holistic nursing care that integrates biological, psychosocial, and cultural influences makes this edition an excellent resource for psychiatric-mental health nurses and students seeking to understand the intricacies of psychiatric disorders and treatment planning.

Additional features of this textbook include its focus on the role of the nurse in various clinical settings, such as hospital-based, medical-surgical, and community-based care. As students explore the diverse roles of psychiatric-mental health nurses they will also discover their roles in providing therapeutic care to their clients and understanding personal responses to individuals presenting with psychiatric disorders. Emphasis on client teaching, research, critical thinking, and myths to overcome will enhance their appreciation of the client experiencing various psychiatric disorders. Overall, the unique features of this textbook provide students and clinicians with a comprehensive and client-centered approach to psychiatric-mental health nursing care.

Organization

Psychiatric Nursing: Biological & Behavioral Concepts consists of 4 units and 37 chapters. Each unit provides a refreshing approach to psychiatric-mental health nursing, beginning with Unit 1, which covers the basic concepts in psychiatric nursing, and ending with Unit 4, which focuses on the unique roles of the psychiatric nurse, including psychiatric consultation-liaison nurse and researcher. Because mental health is dynamic, the role of the psychiatric-mental health nurse must continue to evolve and reflect the needs of clients, families, groups, communities, and societies.

◆ Unit 1, Perspectives and Principles, provides an overview of psychiatric-mental health nursing, encompassing the history and delineation of the discipline. Chapter 3 depicts the interrelationship of the concepts presented and their role in adaptation and maladaptation across the life span. Next, the major principles of psychiatric nursing are discussed. Chapters focus on the nursing process, the nurse-client relationship, cultural attitudes, and legal and ethical considerations involving psychiatric nursing care. Cutting-edge issues such as the Internet and telehealth are also discussed in this section in Chapter 6, Therapeutic Communication.

◆ Unit 2, Response to Stressors across the Life Span, includes the role of the nurse in working with clients

experiencing psychiatric disorders, the developmental considerations involving the condition, and the integration of holistic principles (biological, genetic, psychosocial, cultural, and spiritual influences). Each discussion includes various holistic interventions unique to the needs of clients with diverse psychiatric conditions. This unit also discusses caring for clients who survive violence, experience sexual problems, or attempt suicide and other self-injurious behaviors. Controversial diagnoses such as fibromyalgia and chronic fatigue syndrome are discussed in Chapter 12, The Client with a Somatization Disorder, as related disorders because of their unexplained symptoms similar to somatoform disorders. This unit also contains an extensive discussion dealing with the client who exhibits violence, hostility, and aggressive behaviors. It discusses evidence-based interventions to de-escalate potential and actual violent situations.

◆ Unit 3, Therapeutic Interventions, provides an in-depth discussion of treatment modalities, including individual, family, group, and psychopharmacologic therapies; psychosocial rehabilitation; crisis intervention and management; health education; and electroconvulsive and complementary therapies. The unit also includes an overview of diverse care settings such as hospital-based care, home- and community-based care, and medical-surgical care.

◆ Unit 4, Advancing Psychiatric Nursing Practice, analyzes the specific roles of psychiatric nursing in general practice, as well as specialty areas such as psychiatric consultation-liaison nursing. The pace of research in psychiatric nursing is an integral part of this book. This unit concludes with a general framework for developing psychiatric nursing skills in the context of advances in the specialty and profession.

Special Features

New! CD-ROM—reinforces concepts with 3D animations, an audio glossary, NCLEX-style quizzes, and StudyWare™ activities and games.

New! Brain Scan Images—illustrate the impact of illness and drug therapies on the client.

Competencies—open each chapter and delineate expected learning outcomes.

Key Terms—introduce and define key terms for each chapter. In addition, they guide the learner in understanding key concepts relevant to each chapter.

Critical Thinking—found in each chapter to facilitate analysis and implementation of concepts related to various client situations.

Research Abstracts—provide important scientific studies relevant to each chapter. They also provide implications for psychiatric nursing and application to practice.

Myths—relating to specific mental disorders are included to provide a greater understanding of the misinformation surrounding the disorders. This content also dispels myths that often interfere with objective mental health care.

The More You Know—provide newsworthy items that enhance the learning process. Nurses can learn to focus on articles concerning mental health and gain a greater understanding of the public's view.

My Experience—a feature crucial to understanding the client's experience. Each display offers the client's perspective concerning his or her mental illness as a means of promoting empathy and objective health care.

Clinical Examples—enhance the student's understanding of various mental disorders.

Case Studies and Nursing Care Plans—provide a learning exercise that enables the student to apply the nursing process and relevant concepts to client situations.

Study Questions—in each chapter provide questions that facilitate critical thinking skills.

Suggestions for Clinical Conferences—are activities that promote critical thinking skills and opportunities to enhance understanding of diverse psychiatric disorders and student experiences.

Resources/Web Activities—at the end of each chapter enhance students' awareness of the resources and organizations involved in various psychiatric conditions and professional development for students.

References and Suggested Readings—at the end of each chapter are current and provide a means for students to enhance their understanding of various psychiatric disorders.

Acknowledgments

Completing this edition of this book has been great and at times exhausting! The passion to pursue this great journey comes from the incredible support and encouragement of my husband, family, colleagues, friends, and editors. My appreciation for their support is tremendous.

I also want to acknowledge some extraordinary people. First, I want to express gratitude and a special thanks to my wonderful mother and friend, Gladys, who continues to encourage me to be the best I can.

Second, special thanks go to my colleagues and friends who made writing this edition fun and exciting. Their contributions highlight their commitment, expertise, and contributions to the scholarly integrity of this book.

Third, a very special recognition goes to my granddaughter, Marissa, who inspires my inner child and keeps me focused on the basic things in life.

Finally, a special thanks to my sister, Sharon, whose kindness and compassion keep me humble and grateful for life itself.

About the Author

Deborah Antai-Otong's contributions to psychiatric-mental health nursing and advocacy for quality mental health care are vast and encompass clinical and educational dimensions. She has extensive experience as a psychotherapist, specializing in psychiatric emergencies, medication management, women's issues concerning depression, anxiety disorders, early childhood trauma, personality disorders, and couples and marital therapy. She is an expert in mental issues such as suicide, workplace violence, and quality of care that involve older adults, men, and individuals across the life span. Her clinical and practice experiences are diverse and include being a crisis therapist in a community-based mental health center, a Program Manager of a large medical center Employee Assistance Program, and her current position as a mental health provider, Program Manager for the regional Care Coordination Home Telehealth Program and Continuous Readiness Officer. She is a mental health provider at a community-based outpatient clinic and provides medication management, crisis intervention, brief psychotherapy, and psychiatric evaluation. She is also involved in data analysis, performance measures, quality improvement, and continuous readiness endeavors to ensure preparation for internal and external review and accreditation.

A prolific author and nationally sought speaker and consultant on various mental health and organizational redesign topics, Deborah is a columnist on the art of prescribing in one of the leading psychiatric nursing journals. She has contributed numerous articles to referred nursing and medical journals and is a consultant and content expert with a national educational psychiatric broadcasting company and renowned health care system involved in psychiatric research. She is author and co-author of more than eight books, including textbooks, handbooks, and numerous book chapters ranging from clinical topics to topics of professional development and communication. Deborah is a media consultant and has developed and presented more than 100 educational videos that have been broadcast to more than 2000 health facilities globally. She currently serves on numerous national committees, including a Commission on Certification with the American Nurses Credentialing Center and the Veterans Health Administration's committees involved in nursing practice.

Deborah's contributions extend beyond psychiatric nursing and encompass the entire nursing profession as evidenced by her most prestigious recognition and honor as 2002 Fellow in the American Academy of Nursing. She is a strong advocate for individuals with mental health problems and continuously strives to create environments that promote safe and quality mental health across the life span.

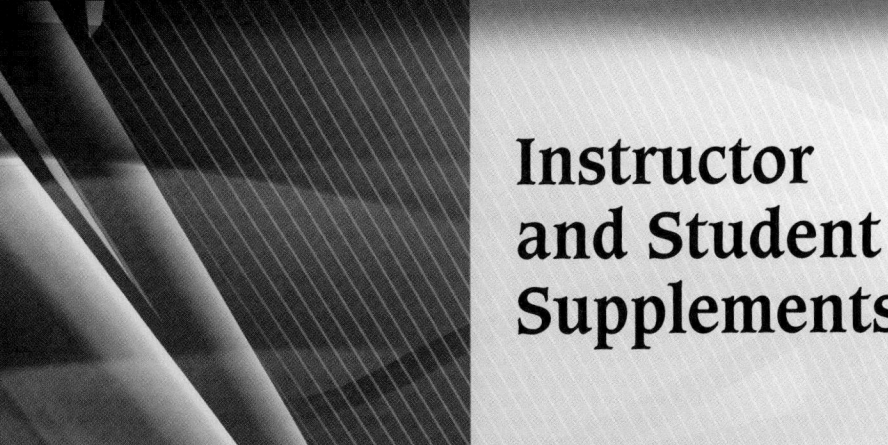

Instructor and Student Supplements

At Delmar Learning, we are committed to providing the nursing instructor with all the appropriate materials necessary to prepare for class, deliver lectures, and evaluate student progress. We also offer students valuable resources to practice and apply their knowledge to succeed in comprehending subject matter. Below are descriptions of both instructor and student tools that accompany *Psychiatric Nursing: Biological & Behavioral Concepts,* second edition.

FOR THE INSTRUCTOR
ELECTRONIC CLASSROOM MANAGER

(1-4180-3873-3)

Instructor's Guide

Organized by chapter, editable, and printable, this standard resource is available on-line as a convenient Microsoft Word® document. Instructional strategies, critical thinking questions with suggested answers, and ideas for integrating 3D animations into classroom teaching are offered here.

PowerPoint Presentation

Focusing on the major themes from the textbook, this created presentation goes beyond key points and provides a solid base for adopters to customize unique lectures. Images may be included in the presentations and can be imported through the use of Delmar's Image Library.

Image Library

Many of the valuable images from this textbook are available as teaching tools, enabling instructors to insert illustrated examples into PowerPoint presentations for classroom lecture or to create transparencies.

Computerized Test Bank

The creation of quizzes and tests is a breeze with the most intuitive Computerized Test Bank available. A variety of question types that number in the thousands can be found in each one of these resources, including challenging multiple choice and true-false. Instructors can codify questions based on difficulty level, scramble question order so no two students have the same test, and create electronic "take-home" quizzes with Internet-based examination capability. The program even allows instructors to create their own questions to expand the memory bank.

WEBTUTOR ADVANTAGE ON WEBCT (ISBN 1-4283-5939-7) AND BLACKBOARD (ISBN 1-4283-5940-0)

New! WebTutor Advantage (both **WebCT** and **Blackboard** formats) accompanies the second edition of *Psychiatric Nursing: Biological & Behavioral Concepts.* These online supplemental courses offer must-have classroom management tools such as chats and calendars, as well as additional content resources, including FAQs, PowerPoint slides, 3D animations, an audio glossary, and more.

ONLINE COMPANION

(http://www.delmarhealthcare.com)

(1-4180-3876-8)

The Online Companion gives you access to all the components of the Electronic Classroom Manager and StudyWare™ resources to reinforce the content in each chapter and enhance classroom teaching. 3D animations, an audio library, NCLEX-style quizzes, and case studies are just some of the resources found here.

Conversion Grids

Delmar Learning recognizes how busy life can be for a nursing instructor. To make life a little easier, Conversion Grids have been formulated that demonstrate how to adjust one's syllabus and course notes from the instructor's current textbook to *Psychiatric Nursing: Biological & Behavioral Concepts*. Grids can be accessed via link from the Electronic Classroom Manager or through http://www.delmarhealthcare.com.

Curriculum Guides

Learn about the latest and greatest print and electronic nursing education materials with Delmar Learning's Curriculum Guides. This tool offers brief descriptions of our products and order information for our growing suite of popular resources.

FOR THE STUDENT

STUDENT STUDY GUIDE

(1-4180-3875-x)

Reinforcing the major concepts presented in the textbook, each chapter of the Student Study Guide includes a Reading Assignment, Exercises and Activities, and a Self-Assessment Quiz. Resources are provided for further investigation.

PSYCHIATRIC NURSING CLINICAL COMPANION

(1-4180-3874-1)

Key information regarding major disorders comprises the *Psychiatric Nursing Clinical Companion*. The reader will find symptoms, causes, and treatment for each category of disorders found in the text chapters, and each entry is specially designed for appropriate nursing care.

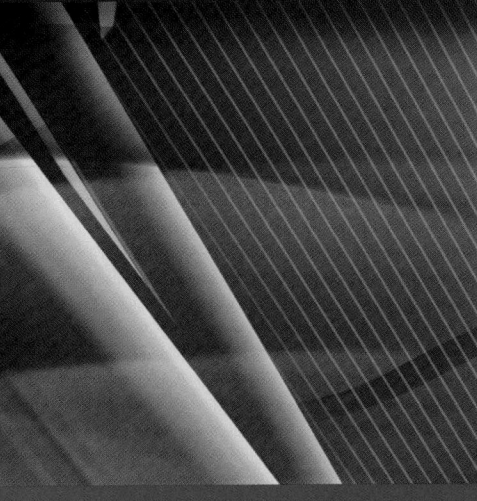

How to Use

The content presentation is designed to engage the reader on a variety of levels. The following suggests how you can maximize the numerous features of the text to gain a broad understanding of psychiatric nursing and competence in its practice.

CLIENT TEACHING

Anxiolytic Agent for the Client with an Anxiety Disorder (Sertraline [Zoloft] a Selective Serotonin Reuptake Inhibitor (SSRI))

- Take the medication during the morning or afternoon to reduce insomnia and restlessness (bedtime only if it produces sedation during the day).
- Administer or take the medication as prescribed. For instance, if you miss a morning dose, take it as soon as you remember (preferably during the morning or afternoon, because taking it at bedtime may interfere with your sleep).
- You may experience dry mouth: drink plenty of water or use sugarless candy. Constipation may occur, but do not rely on laxatives: increase dietary roughage or discuss taking a stool softener with your health care provider.
- Major side effects of this medication include: insomnia, diarrhea, nervousness, and nausea. This medication may also cause sexual dysfunction and decrease lib

◀ CLIENT TEACHING

Effective communication is a key nursing responsibility. This feature provides the tools for you to inform clients about their care, understand their condition, weigh treatment options, and promote health. Use this as a guide to advise clients in a clinical setting.

CRITICAL THINKING

You are working the evening shift on a medical unit and one of your clients states, "I just can't deal with this pain anymore. I wish I were dead!" Based on your understanding of this situation, what is the most appropriate response?

1. Do nothing because most people who kill themselves don't give a warning.
2. Ask, "What do you mean you wish you were dead?"
3. Go immediately to the charge nurse and report that he is going to kill himself.
4. Ask him about his religious beliefs.

◀ CRITICAL THINKING

This feature was created to foster analytical thought in clinical situations and promote active problem solving. As you read through the chapters, consider the questions posed and provide responses. Discuss your responses with other students and faculty to promote the exchange of ideas.

▼ CLINICAL EXAMPLE

Exposure to practical situations accelerates the learning process. This feature offers you the opportunity to observe a typical clinical example, with assessment and treatment information.

CLINICAL EXAMPLE

The Client at Risk for Suicide

Mr. Jones is a 46-year-old man who recently had a massive heart attack. His business is failing and his wife of 20 years has decided that she does not want to be married to an "invalid." He has few social supports. He is referred to a mental health professional on a psychiatric consultation. His mood is sad and depressed and he is expressing feelings of hopelessness about his situation and thoughts of dying. He reports a poor appetite, concentration difficulties, loss of interest in things that were once pleasurable (anhedonia), and extreme fatigue since the heart attack.

What places Mr. Jones at risk for suicide? He is depressed and has feelings of hopelessness, a major physical health problem, an impending divorce, and he is preoccupied with dying.

Myths to Overcome: Psychobiological Disorders

- It is often thought that so-called psychosomatic illnesses are imaginary, or "all in their head." For example, a person complaining of headaches may be thought by others not to be experiencing any pain. In reality, these are physical disorders in which both emotions and thinking play a role. In addition, persons with the disorder are unable to deal effectively with stress in their life.

- Some people believe that having negative or "bad thoughts" can lead to disorders such as cancer. Another popular belief is that having a positive attitude will allow a person to overcome a chronic illness. In reality, although there is a close relationship between the body and the mind, and having a negative attitude may increase one's stress level, people are not able to completely control physical symptoms through their thought processes.

▲ COMMON MYTHS

Because there are many common misconceptions surrounding mental health, it is important to identify and dispel them. Pay close attention to the myths and corresponding facts surrounding disorders. You may be surprised by what you learn.

▼ CONSIDERATIONS FOR THE CAREGIVER

Mental illness often affects the families of those afflicted in a serious way. Listening, empathizing, and providing encouragement to family members and caregivers is all part of professional nursing care. Use this feature as a reminder to care for families, as well as to understand the proper techniques for doing so.

Considerations for the Caregiver: The Child with Separation Anxiety

Parents or caregivers of a preschool or school-age child often find it frustrating and distressful when the child cries and refuses to go to school. These children often experience intense anxiety and fears. Separation anxiety disorder refers to excessive anxiety concerning separation from home or parents. These children often express fears of something happening to their parents and complain of physical symptoms, such as headaches and stomachaches. It is the most common prepubertal anxiety disorder. Typical anxiety-producing situations include:

- When they are walking out of the house to attend school
- Riding the bus
- Provide health education about separation anxiety and teach cognitive-behavioral approaches to their child's care.
- Make referrals to various community support groups for parents of children with anxiety disorders.

The following interventions are useful in reducing the child's anxiety:

- Recognize that attending school all day is overwhelming to the child.
- Avoid colluding with the child—the child must attend school.

▼ THE MORE YOU KNOW

National events, legislation, and research findings are continually changing the environment in which you will practice. Digest newsworthy stories and think about how they might impact nursing care. Have you read or viewed any other media item that would fall under this category?

THE MORE YOU KNOW

Depression Simmers in Japan's Culture of Stoicism

A report in the *New York Times* International section indicates that Japan has more suicides than the United States, however, less than half the population. "Thirty thousand people commit suicide in Japan annually, but if we could diagnose them and treat them in time, that number would go down dramatically," said Tadashi Onda, a Tokyo psychiatrist. There is a prevailing feeling that no one wants to think they have a mental problem, such as depression. Many experts say the greatest barrier to treatment is the sense of shame about mental conditions, which some compare to the way depression was whispered about darkly in the United States during the 1950s, during the era of electroconvulsive therapy. When Japanese experience depression, physicians report, they prefer to imagine something is wrong with their character rather than their minds, and a cultural impulse known as "gaman," or the will to endure, takes precedence over seeking mental health care. "In a culture of shame, the only thing to do about illnesses of the mind is to hide them," Dr. Onda reported. "They carry a stigma here that can haunt a family down through the generations. The perception is that dying is preferred in hopeless situations rather than surrendering because of the power of shame."

RESEARCH ABSTRACT

Pediatric Autoimmune Neuropsychiatric Disorders Associated with Streptococcal Infections: Clinical Description of the First 50 Cases

Swedo, S. E., Leonard, H. L., Garvey, M., Mittleman, B., Allen, A. J., Perlmutter, S., et al. (1998). *American Journal of Psychiatry, 155,* 264–271.

Study Problem/Purpose
To describe the clinical characteristics of a novel group of clients with OCD and tic disorders, designated as pediatric autoimmune neuropsychiatric disorders associated with streptococcal group A beta-hemolytic streptococcal (GABHS) infections (PANDAS).

Methods
The investigators conducted a systematic clinical workup of 50 children who met all of the following diagnostic criteria: presence of OCD or tic disorder, prepubertal onset, episodic symptoms, association with GABHS infections, and neurological deficits. Children with an acute onset or severe exacerbations of OCD or tics were sought through mailings to various child psychiatrists, physicians, pediatric neurologists, and the Tourette's Syndrome Association's national newsletter. More than 270 telephone interviews were conducted, of whom 109 were invited to the NIMH for a face-to-face screening evaluation. Depending on the seriousness of the symptoms, the children were placed in one or two protocols—a placebo-controlled study of penicillin prophylaxis or a randomized-control study of various immunotherapies. Several instruments were used to assess the children's mood, intelligence, and cognitive deficits. Data were gathered from both children and their parents.

Findings
Clinical findings showed that many of these subjects' symptoms had an acute onset and early onset (n = 6.3 years for tics and 7.4 years for OCD) typically triggered by GABHS infections. The clinical course of these episodes was relapsing and remitting with dramatic comorbidity with other mental disorders, such as separation anxiety, nightmares and fears, emotional lability, cognitive deficits, and oppositional behaviors.

These data clearly indicate a homogenous client group whose symptom exacerbations are precipitated by GABHS exposure.

Implications for Psychiatric Nurses
These findings suggest the early influence and course of OCD and other anxiety states in young children exposed to GABHS infections. Nurses need to assess young children presenting with these symptoms for infections to facilitate early identification and reduce the potential risk of serious physical and mental consequences of untreated infections. This also reinforces the need to assess each client's current and past health status to assess a pattern of symptoms that implicates a more serious medical condition.

▲ RESEARCH ABSTRACT

Evidence-based findings help define nursing practice and mold nursing behavior. This feature emphasizes the significance of clinical research to the profession and illustrates the correct format to write an abstract for a research project. Take particular note of the implications included within each study.

▶ CASE STUDIES AND NURSING CARE PLANS

These real-world scenarios provide a valuable learning experience that allows the student to apply relevant concepts and the nursing process to various client situations.

▼ SUGGESTIONS FOR CLINICAL CONFERENCES

Nurses must practice their skills to become adept professionals. Following each chapter are suggestions for you to gain experience in the field. You will be called upon to assess clients and plan interventions. Work with your instructor to identify those opportunities.

SUGGESTIONS FOR CLINICAL CONFERENCES

1. Present several case histories of clients with attention-deficit hyperactivity disorder (ADHD); the cases should be representative of clients across the life span. For each case, identify (a) biological, environmental, and hereditary factors, (b) life span and developmental issues, (c) psychosocial issues, (d) diverse treatment modalities, (e) client and family education needs.
2. Discuss several treatment modalities for the treatment of clients with ADHD, such as pharmacologic options, social skills training, classroom modifications, and behavioral management plans.

▼ MY EXPERIENCE

It is important for the nurse not to become disconnected from the thoughts and feelings of their patients and clients. People experiencing mental illness speak about their conditions within this feature. Take the opportunity to read through these vignettes as a reminder of the clients within your care.

My Experience with Heart Disease

I was diagnosed with heart disease 5 years ago. I was working in sales, a high-stress occupation. I felt pressured to sell more and produce more all the time. I worked many hours, often putting in 60 to 70 hours a week. After my heart attack, I had to make a number of changes in my life. My family and I reassessed our goals in life. I discovered that some of the things I thought were important to me didn't matter at all.

I had to change jobs, finding a position that was much less stressful. My eating and exercise habits have also changed dramatically. Fried foods are pretty much taboo from my diet, as are rich, high-fat desserts. I also have limited my alcohol intake significantly. I exercise every day now. All this has led to quite a weight loss for me. I no longer keep my feelings bottled up inside. When I'm upset with my wife, she and I sit down and talk about it calmly. I write in a journal nearly every day, writing about my feelings and my experiences. I spend more time with my family, just doing fun things like playing with the kids in the park, going for walks, and playing board games at home.

I still worry about my heart, but I know I'm doing the things I need to do to take care of myself. Overall, I feel much better about my life, my future, and myself than I ever have in the past.

CASE STUDY

The Client with Attention-Deficit Hyperactivity Disorder (Joe C.)

Joe C. is an 8-year-old male referred by his pediatrician for evaluation of academic and behavioral problems of at least 1-year duration. His parents accompany him. He has two siblings, both girls, ages 10 and 6. His parents are married and there has been no history of marital discord. The parents are concerned about Joe's grades, his behavior at home, school, and with his soccer team. They comment that "he seems a lot more immature than the other boys his age."

Joe is currently in the second grade after failing reading and language arts (writing skills) last year. Currently he is continuing to perform very poorly in these areas. He is currently in a class of 24 children. Joe has few friends and his classmates identify him as one of the least-liked children in the class. His teacher notes the following problem areas:

- Is frequently out of his seat
- Appears to be daydreaming when he is supposed to be working on an assignment
- Has difficulty getting along with peers during recess or free time
- Has trouble following the rules of games
- Becomes easily angered and can be aggressive with other children

NURSING CARE PLAN 17–1

The Client with Attention-Deficit Hyperactivity Disorder (Joe C. [Age 8])

Nursing Diagnosis: Impaired Social Interaction

Outcome Identification	Nursing Actions	Rationales	Evaluation
1. By [date], Joe C. will complete assignments in class in allotted time.	1. With Joe's teacher, identify distracters in the classroom and modify the environment to decrease stimulation (e.g., move desk close to teacher, do not place desk near doors or windows).	1. By decreasing stimuli the child with ADHD can more easily focus on tasks, assignments, or projects and become distracted less easily or frequently.	*Goals met:* By the end of the first month, Joe, his parents, and teachers report a marked improvement in task completion.

NEW to this edition: Engaging student CD-ROM software is available **FREE** to each user of *Psychiatric Nursing: Biological & Behavioral Concepts,* second edition. The StudyWare™ packaged within the text features:

Case Studies—Foster critical thinking and analytical skills by reviewing real-world client scenarios that promote the application of concepts and theories.

Animations—Full-color 3D animations visually enhance comprehension of difficult concepts.

Audio Glossary—Definition and pronunciation of all key terms used in the text.

NCLEX-Style Quizzes—Take NCLEX-style quizzes in both practice and quiz modes. Use the practice mode to improve mastery of the material with instant feedback. Use quiz mode for self-testing and keep a record of your scores.

Scores—View the last quiz scores and print your results.

Activities—Include games such as concentration, flashcards, and hangman using the key terms from the text. Have fun while you learn!

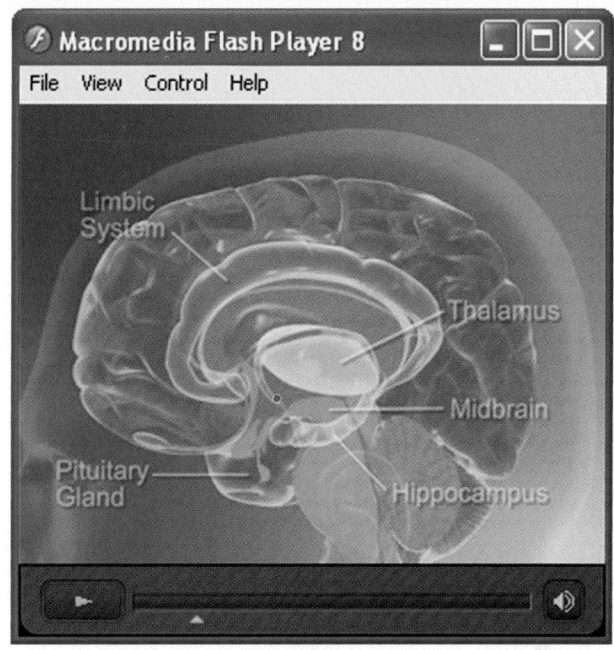

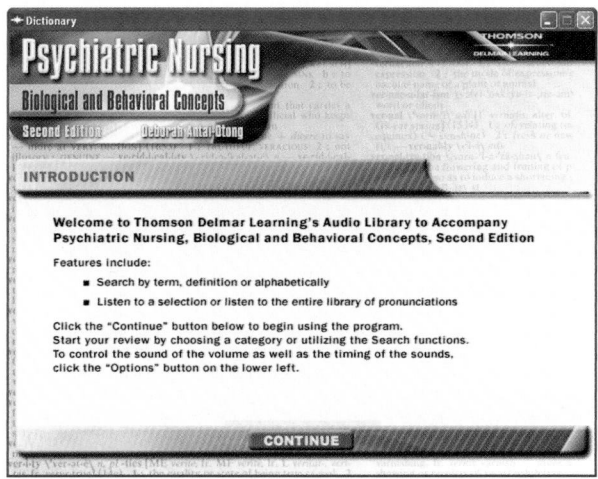

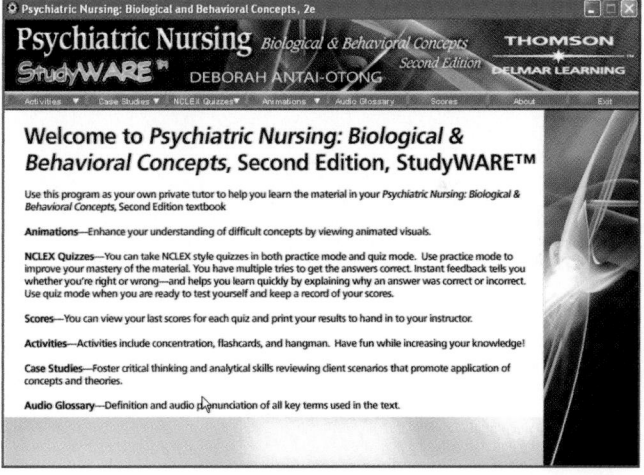

UNIT 1

Perspectives and Principles

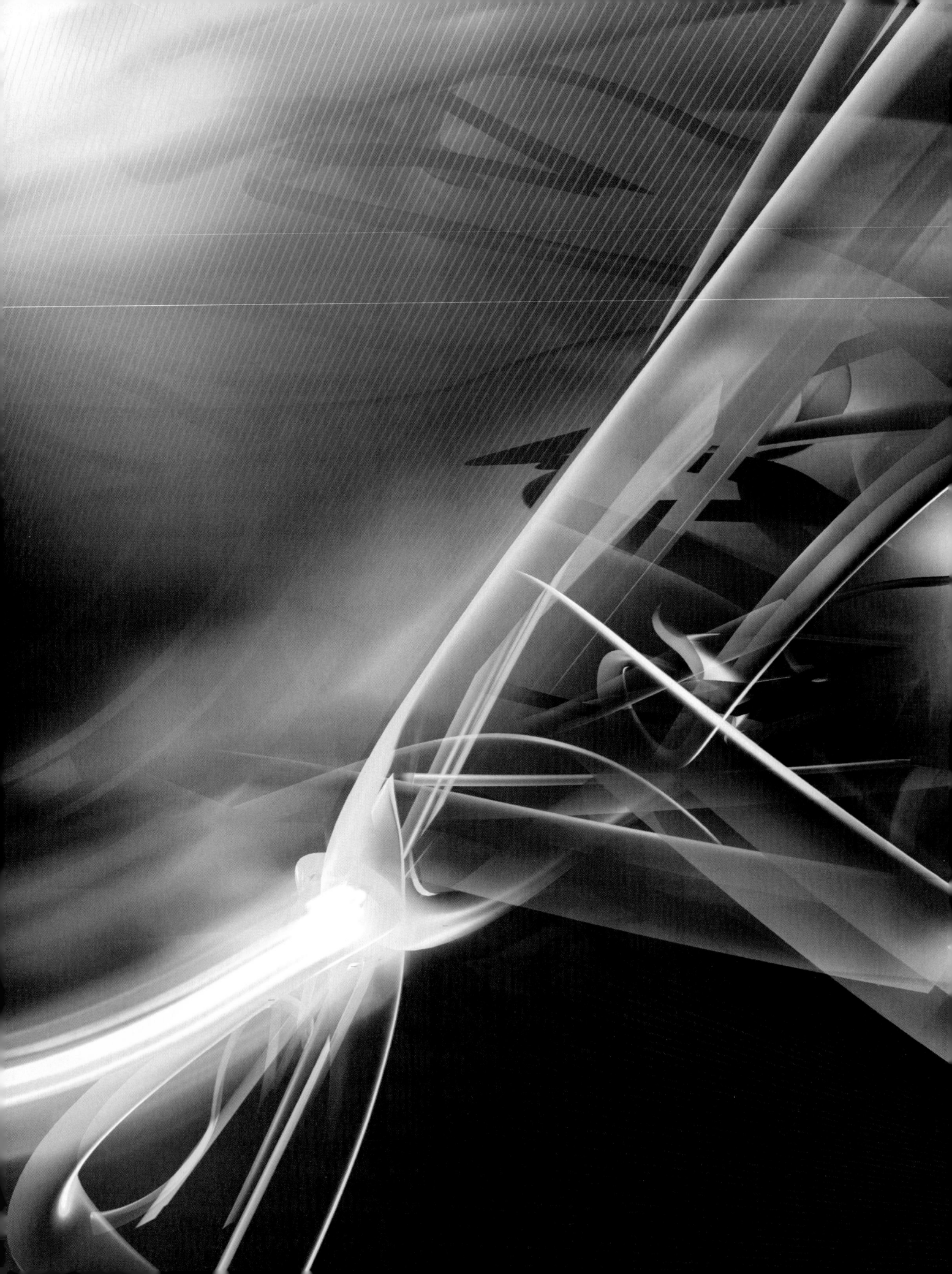

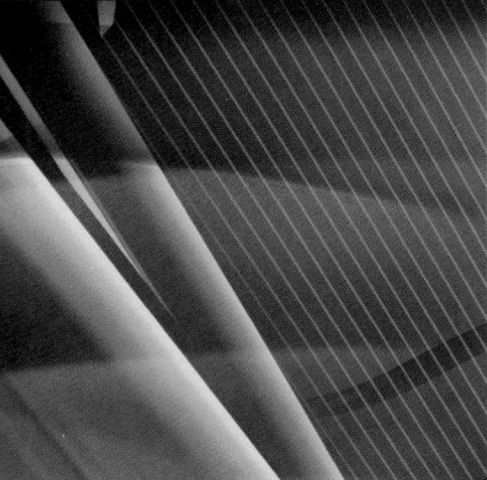

CHAPTER 1

History of Psychiatric Nursing

Deborah Antai-Otong, MS, APRN, BC, FAAN

KEY TERMS

Complementary Therapies: Refer to unconventional therapies that encompass a spectrum of practices and beliefs, including herbs, visual imagery, acupuncture, and massage therapy.

Decade of the Brain: Proclamation by the United States Congress that explains mental illness as a disease of the brain. It underscores the significance of technological advances in neurobiology and genetics and their impact on understanding mental illness.

Deinstitutionalization: Caring for people outside the hospital who have been previously hospitalized for an extended period; caring for people in the community rather than in a state facility. A humanizing recommendation made by the Joint Commission on Mental Illness and Mental Health (1961) that moved the care of the mentally ill from large state institutions to community mental health centers.

Mental Health Movement: A movement that began more than 50 years ago that focuses on humane treatment of the mentally ill, initially advocating their release from state institutions to community mental health centers.

Moral Treatment: Humane treatment of the mentally ill; for example, releasing clients from mechanical restraints and improving physical care. Phillippe Pinel, a French physician, and Benjamin Rush, an American physician, were instrumental in promoting this movement.

National Institute of Mental Health: A federally funded agency whose goals include developing and helping various states to identify and use the most effective methods of prevention, diagnosis, and intervention of mental illnesses through research funding and staff development and education of mental health professionals to provide mental health treatment.

Neurobiology: Biology of the nervous system, particularly the brain.

Neuroscience: The science and study of the central nervous system.

Psychotropics: Various pharmacologic agents, such as antidepressants and antipsychotic, antimanic, and antianxiety agents used to affect behavior, mood, cognition, and feelings.

COMPETENCIES

Upon completion of this chapter, the learner should be able to:

1. Discuss the impact of society, culture, economics, and religion on attitudes toward mental illness.

2. Describe the evolution of psychiatry and its influence on psychiatric-mental health nursing.

3. Describe the role and purpose of professional organizations such as the American Nurses Association and the National League for Nursing in relation to nursing.

4. Discuss the future of psychiatric-mental health nursing.

5. List the influence of technological advances in neurobiology and the information system on psychiatric-mental health nursing.

6. Identify major issues confronting psychiatric-mental health nursing in the twenty-first century.

CHAPTER OUTLINE

The Evolution of Psychiatric-Mental Health Care

Early History

The history of psychiatric-mental health nursing is rich and reflects the evolution of societal, economic, legislative and cultural influences, and technological advances. Despite their conservative beginnings as custodians of care, the role of psychiatric-mental health nurses continues to reflect contemporary socioeconomic and legislative trends and the explosion of technological advances in neuroscience and cyberspace. As these technological advances make an impact on lifestyles and health, cultural factors remain an integral part of society and influence individual health practices and response to life span stressors. Today, the psychiatric-mental health nurse faces the challenge of integrating the intricacies of scientific studies, societal norms, and cultural factors and their effects on human behavior into evidence-based interventions.

This chapter focuses on the evolution of psychiatry and psychiatric-mental health nursing. It also analyzes major socioeconomic, cultural, and legislative trends and their effects on the treatment of the mentally ill. It provides a glimpse of this evolution whose origins stem from inhumane and appalling treatment of individuals suffering from mental illnesses to contemporary client-centered treatment. Understandably, these changes parallel the advent of biological therapies, including psychotropics, and other biological treatment, such as complementary therapies.

As psychiatric nursing progresses into the twenty-first century, efforts to promote its survival in a changing health care system are paramount. The historical influences of professional organizations, nurse researchers, and educators continue to affect psychiatric-mental health nursing. Nurse educators, nurse researchers, and professional nursing organizations are challenged to play quintessential roles in the future of psychiatric nursing. Their roles are likely to involve integrating psychiatric-mental health nursing concepts into nursing curricula and developing and offering innovative clinical and classroom experiences to nursing students.

THE EVOLUTION OF PSYCHIATRIC-MENTAL HEALTH CARE

The evolution of mental health care over the past century has varied from driving out evil spirits to confinement and to the present community-based and primary mental health care. Before 1985, mental health services were likely to occur in acute, inpatient, or private practice settings. The provision of these services was linked to insurance reimbursement. Alleged client abuse and insurance fraud ultimately led to dramatic changes in health care delivery in the nation. Growing concerns for cost containment and accountability forced mental health providers to develop appropriate, cost-effective, and evidence-based care to meet the growing needs of their clients at a lower cost (Galambos, Rocha, McCarter, & Chansuthus, 2004). Contemporary mental health care parallels these sweeping economic changes governed by managed care concepts that continue to overturn conventional assumptions and mental practice models.

Managed care principles continue to be the driving force behind today's mental health treatment models. Brief, focused interventions, particularly for those clients with severe and persistent mental illnesses, are replacing traditional long-term and intensive treatment strategies. Because of the dramatic influence of managed care on health care delivery systems, acutely ill clients are most likely diverted from hospitalization, or receive shorter lengths of stay. They are more likely to receive care in community-based and primary care settings. This trend challenges psychiatric nurses to be innovative and responsive to the needs of clients in vast practice settings. As a result of shorter hospital stays, nurses and other mental health care providers are developing innovative strategies that facilitate rehabilitation and champion client-centered care. Client-centered mental health care encompasses cultural, biological, psychosocial, and individual preference and interdisciplinary approaches that facilitate health promotion. The success of these programs emanates from their focus on personal development, adaptive behavioral skills building, and independence for persons with severe and persistent mental illnesses (International Association of Psychosocial Rehabilitation Services Publication Committee, 1997). The prevailing trends in mental health care reflect the realization that quality of life is an integral part of mental health care. This evolution is partly a reflection of profound changes in the philosophical and theoretical foundations of treatment, impact of managed care principles, technological advances, and societal factors.

Scientific and technological advances continue to influence treatment of psychiatric clients by advancing our knowledge of the brain's structure and function, and through the influence of biochemical agents, endocrinology and genetic origins of psychiatric disorders. Clinical findings from these data contribute to the development of safer and more effective medications that target specific brain regions and affect intricate neurobiological process and subsequent behavioral changes. The new-generation atypical antipsychotic agents are examples of these discoveries. These agents have fewer side effects, reduce negative symptoms of schizophrenia, improve mood and cognitive function, and significantly improve one's quality of life and functional status. These discoveries are providing hope for clients, their families, and advocates for the mentally ill.

As our society struggles with health care issues, other stressors continue to place tremendous strain on individuals, families, communities, and diverse cultures. The influence of cyberspace and intricate informational systems; advances in technology, particularly in neuroscience and genetics; a growing population of people over the age of 65 and the risk of chronic illness and disability and resultant mental illness; and an alarming rate of societal and workplace violence, all are placing enormous strain on societal and human resources. Consequently, there has been a simultaneous increase in demand for mental health services. Presently, approximately 19 percent of the general population have some form of mental illness, about one-third of whom seek treatment (Kessler et al., 2005; Narrow, Rae, Robins, & Regier, 2002).

Additional societal changes include a growing population of infants surviving premature births because of technological advances in neonatology and the resultant increase in developmental disorders. These advances are enabling individuals to survive serious illnesses, thus increasing the prevalence of older adults and those with chronic mental and physical illnesses. The global epidemic of acquired immunodeficiency syndrome (AIDS), particularly in Third World countries, with women and children increasingly at risk, is yet another factor that increases the demand for services. Women's health concerns, including abuse and violence, and a growing cultural transition from minority to majority populations are among expansive societal trends. Recent studies indicate that one in three people use complementary therapies. These trends, coupled with shorter hospital stays, dwindling health care resources, growing societal violence, in tandem with shrinking health care resources are overtaxing an already overwhelmed health care system (American Nurses Association, 1991). Although vast advances in research, technology, and treatment have occurred during the past 40 to 50 years, societal problems persist and contribute to fragmented mental health care, poor access to care, and health disparities. Solutions to complex societal challenges require an overhaul of health care systems to reduce stigma associated with mental illness, and to facilitate recovery and resilience among individuals and families experiencing mental illness. Resources and efforts must focus on a national move to fund programs to promote mental health across the life span, implement evidence-based care, and access to technologies and treatment that promote an optimal level of health care to all individuals regardless of race, gender, age, culture, socioeconomic status, English proficiency, and ethnicity. These contemporary socioeconomic and cultural transitions add new dimensions to psychiatric nursing practice.

Psychiatric-mental health nurses are likely to play pivotal roles in identifying clients at risk, in assessing client responses to stress across the life span, and in developing innovative therapeutic interventions. Predictably, as the health care delivery system evolves and poises itself for dramatic economic and societal changes, nurses must be at the forefront of client advocacy encouraging clients and families to be active partners in their health care. Moreover, psychiatric nurses must understand the relationship between technological advances in neurobiology and neuroscience, etiology, symptoms, and the treatment of mental illness. They must also be able to integrate neurobiological and psychosocial concepts into psychiatric-mental health nursing practice. In essence, nurses must seize opportunities to develop innovative measures and meet the needs of their clients by developing evidence-based outcome measures and redefining their practice through research and education.

Throughout history the plight of the mentally ill has often depended on the cultural and religious beliefs of the civilization in which they lived. Normally, mental health care parallels existing health care delivery systems and socioeconomic and cultural trends. The plethora of scientific and technological advances and current health care trends suggest that caring for people with mental illnesses requires an understanding of its historic origins and diverse factors that govern its future.

EARLY HISTORY

During ancient times insanity was associated with sin and demonic possession. Healers were summoned to extract these unseen spirits through rituals and by using herbs, ointments, and precious stones. Mental illness was often perceived as incurable, and treatment of the insane was sometimes inhumane and brutal.

THE MIDDLE AGES

Throughout the Middle Ages, mentally ill people who were not cared for within their families were often imprisoned or forced to live on the streets and beg for food. For more humane treatment they depended on the charity of religious groups, who dispensed alms or food or other donations to the needy or poor and ran almshouses and general hospitals where the insane were admitted.

The first mental asylum was the Hospital of St. Mary of Bethlehem, from which the term *bedlam* was coined. Built in London, England, during the fourteenth century, Bethlehem was conceived as a sanctuary or refuge for the destitute and afflicted, and the model for similar institutions elsewhere.

THE FIFTEENTH THROUGH SEVENTEENTH CENTURIES

Skepticism about the curability of mental illness, rampant during the Middle Ages, continued in this period. Asylums became repositories for prolonged enclosure of the chronic mentally ill. Conditions were deplorable. Because they were thought to have no feelings and were believed to lack understanding, the insane were treated more like animals than human beings. Men and women were not given separate quarters, and violent inmates were placed with those who were convalescing or tranquil. The inhabitants were poorly clothed and fed, often chained and caged, and deprived of heat and sunlight (Conolly, 1968; Ellenberger, 1974).

Care in these institutions was custodial and was administered by attendants who were also ill treated. Their wages were meager, less than the amount paid to domestic workers and laundresses. They had to sleep on wards and rarely received respite from continual care responsibilities. These working conditions made it difficult to attract and keep attendants (Scull, 1982).

During the latter part of the seventeenth century, American colonists of European origin carried their perceptions and superstitions about the mentally ill from their mother countries. Deeply rooted ideas about the mentally ill and witchcraft culminated in witch-hunts and executions, such as those that occurred in Salem, Massachusetts. The Salem hysteria persisted for many years and interfered with the transition to humane treatment of those suffering from mental illness.

THE EIGHTEENTH CENTURY

The French and American Revolutions, inspired by the desire to broaden the rights of mankind and bring freedom and fair treatment, provided the catalyst for transforming society's attitudes toward the mentally ill and poor. A myriad of today's social concerns originated during this century, with campaigns for the abolition of slavery through the championing of equal rights for women and care for the impoverished.

Benjamin Rush (1745–1813)

American physician Benjamin Rush was a forerunner in bringing attention to the plight of those suffering from mental disorders. He emphasized the need for pleasant surroundings and diversional and moral treatment for the mentally ill.

Some of Rush's treatments, such as bloodletting and the administration of cold and hot baths, harsh purgatives, and emetics, were considered controversial. He felt that the inducement of fright or *shock* would cause the mentally ill to regain their sanity. He was credited with inventing the tranquilizer chair and the Gyrator. The principle behind the *tranquilizer chair,* in which the mentally ill person's extremities were strapped down, was that a reduction in motor activity and pulse rates produced calming effects. The *Gyrator* was a form of shock therapy consisting of a rotating, swinging platform onto which the person was strapped and moved at a high speed. The idea was to increase cerebral circulation, the major focus of Rush's theories and therapies.

Rush's advocacy for humane treatment and his concerns for the mentally ill became the basis for his work, *Medical Inquiries and Observations upon the Disease of the Mind,* published in 1812, the first American treatise on psychiatry. This document was considered the authoritative work on the topic for several decades. Rush later came to be known as the *father of American psychiatry.*

Phillippe Pinel (1745–1826)

Another concerned physician and advocate for humane treatment of the mentally ill during this era was the Frenchman,

Phillippe Pinel, who advocated kindness and moral treatment. His perceptions and concerns about the dire living conditions and brutal treatment of the mentally ill influenced the new social consciousness of his era.

Pinel's greatest impact came after he was placed in charge of a large hospital for the insane, the Bicerte. He proved that releasing the insane from chains and providing moral treatment improved their prospect. He earned fame for championing moral treatment by emphasizing an atmosphere of kindness and understanding. His compassionate endeavors brought about sweeping changes in French institutions for the mentally ill and reformation of societal attitudes toward those suffering from mental illness, creating optimism about its curability.

William Tuke (1732–1822)

Another pioneer during the eighteenth century was William Tuke, an English merchant and devout member of the Society of Friends. He began a 4-year dynasty that advocated humane treatment of the mentally ill. He abhorred the deplorable conditions of several asylums, including Bethlehem, and his services were often sought in developing humane conditions in mental institutions. Tuke's descendants played major roles in increasing public awareness of the vile living conditions and treatment of those suffering from mental illness. His efforts were instrumental in raising money to establish homes, including the York Retreat, which provided comfort, security, and safety for the mentally ill.

Franz Anton Mesner (1734–1815)

Another approach to treatment of the mentally ill was mesmerism, named after the Austrian physician, Franz Anton Mesner. He renewed the art of suggestive healing that stemmed from the ancient use of trances, which later became the basis of hypnosis. Mesner and his followers used a form of hypnotism, a dreamlike trance, to explore the basis of neurosis. His techniques, which he attributed to "animal magnetism," were used to effect cures.

THE NINETEENTH CENTURY: THE EVOLUTION OF THE PSYCHIATRIC NURSE

During the nineteenth century, European countries and the United States began a movement that championed reformation of ideas in establishing state hospitals. The evolution of psychiatric-mental health nursing (Table 1–1) marks its beginning with the building of the first psychiatric hospital in America at Williamsburg, Virginia, in 1773. In 1817, the McLean Asylum (Figure 1–1), located in Massachusetts, became the first U.S. institution to provide humane treatment for the mentally ill. Humane treatment emphasized an environment of understanding and promoted a sense of contentment and mental and physical health. Daily exercise and activities involving useful tasks were part of the daily rituals, which offered opportunities for learning and spiritual growth.

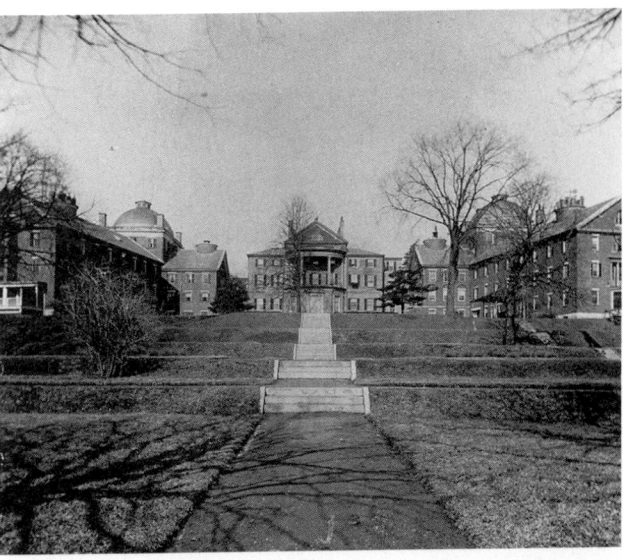

(A)

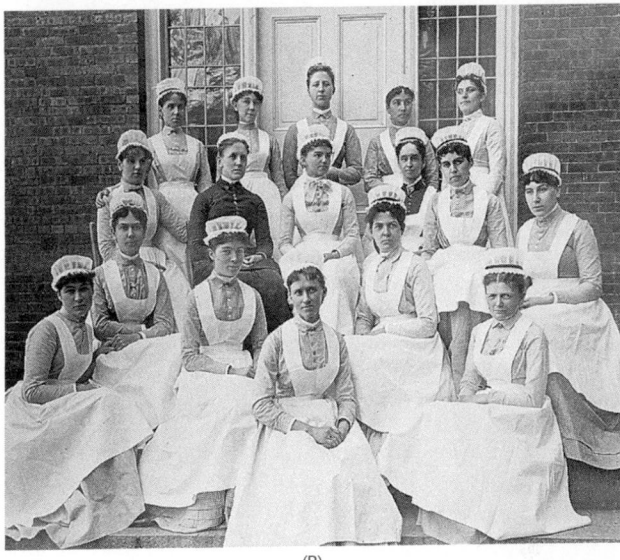

(B)

Figure 1–1 (A) Rear view of McLean Hospital, Belmont, Massachusetts, circa 1980. *(Photo courtesy of McLean Hospital, Belmont, Massachusetts.)* **(B)** America's first trained psychiatric nurses: The first class of 15 women graduated from the McLean Asylum Training School for Nurses in 1886. *(Photo courtesy of McLean Hospital, Belmont, Massachusetts.)*

Before this period, care was primarily administered by attendants because the psychiatric nursing role had not yet been established. Increased concerns and sensitivity to the needs of the mentally ill generated a need for better-educated attendants to care for severely disturbed clients.

Shattuck (1948), a noted physician, wrote in his *Report of the Sanitary Commission of Massachusetts of 1850* that nurses, rather than physicians, play a greater role in caring, preventing disease, and promoting health.

This progressive attitude waned with the decline in public resources and the influx of poor European immigrants, which compounded social stress and poor living conditions. These factors placed individuals at risk for mental illness. The increased incidence of mental illness was met with little public concern for humanitarian care, apathy coupled with poor

TABLE 1-1
The Evolution of Psychiatric Nursing

Dates and Events	Type of Mental Health Treatment	Role of Psychiatric Nurse	Historical Figures	Significant Contributions
1773: First psychiatric hospital in America at Williamsburg, Virginia.	Custodial care provided by nonnursing attendants.	Essentially nonexistent.	Florence Nightingale stressed the significance of emotional support.	Nightingale's *Notes on Nursing* was published in 1859.
1882: First training school for nursing of the mentally ill established at McLean Asylum, Waverly, Massachusetts (first humane treatment established).	Primarily consisted of custodial care.	Nurses attempted to create a safe, kind, clean environment.	Linda Richards was the first graduate psychiatric nurse in the United States.	Richards was instrumental in establishing nursing education in psychiatric and general hospitals.
1920s–1940s, including World War II (1943): Postwar casualties (including increased mental illness) increased funding for advanced training in psychiatry. National Mental Health Act of 1946 increased funding and stimulated advanced training and research preparation of psychiatric nurses. NIMH began offering "integration grants" to promote integration of mental health and behavioral concepts into clinical practice.	Care focused on a disease model rather than the client. Primarily "curative care."	Nursing care paralleled the medical or disease model. Primarily "maternal" and companion role with custodial care. Some nurses were involved in advanced practice and worked in community mental health centers, inpatient settings, academic institutions, and private practice.	Harriet Bailey published the first psychiatric nursing textbook, *Nursing Mental Disease* (1920), which focused on the disease rather than the client.	Peplau's (1952) book, *Interpersonal Relations in Nursing*, delineated the role of psychiatric nursing. Mellow (1967) and Tudor (1952) published clinical studies of nursing and interpersonal relationships. ANA Division on Psychiatric and Mental Health Nursing Practice published the *Statement on Psychiatric Nursing Practice* (1967). Aguilera & Messick published the first edition of *Crisis Intervention: Theory and Methodology* (1970). Shirley Smoyak's book,
1950s–1960s: NLN-ANA coalition recommended sanctioned integration of psychiatric nursing into clinical experience in generic curricula. Advent of psychotropic drugs (1950s). Comprehensive Mental Health Act of 1960 increased federal funding to build community mental health centers, which led to the development of community psychiatry.	Psychotropics replaced restraints and seclusion. Decentralization began, with a focus on improved client care. Deinstitutionalization began with a move of clients from state and long-term facilities to community-based services. Focus was on primary prevention. Major treatment involved inpatient partial hospitalization and day hospitals.	Emphasis on therapeutic relationship, nursing process, and research. In the 1960s, psychiatric nurses continued to have an undifferentiated role and were involved in creating a therapeutic environment (milieu therapy). Major focus was on primary prevention and community-based treatment • interdisciplinary collaboration • use of various treatment modalities, such as crisis intervention, supportive therapy, and psychotherapies	Major nursing contributions were made by Hildegard Peplau, Gwen Tudor, June Mellow, and Ida Orlando, who stressed the importance of the interpersonal or therapeutic relationship. Additionally, Theresa Muller focused on the significance of coping with everyday stresses. Madeline Leininger (1969) stressed the importance of community-based care within various cultures and societies. Aguilera & Messick (1970) integrated Caplan's crisis	

Deinstitutionalization began in 1963; chronically ill clients were released to community mental health centers.

1970s–1980s: A decrease in federal funding for advanced psychiatric-mental health nursing training, education, and research led to decreased psychiatric clinical experiences. Late 1980s experienced increased inpatient psychiatric treatment with evidence of abuse within private psychiatric settings, which led to increases in health care costs.

1990s–2000: Continued advances in technology and understanding of mental illness within domains of neurobiology (genetics, brain mapping, neurotransmitters, and psychopharmacology). Health care reform focuses on primary health care, prevention, and community-based treatment and services.

U.S. Public Health Service, Department of Human and Health Services (DHHS), 1999. *Mental Health: A Report of the Surgeon General.* Compilation of noteworthy advances in mental disorders, the brain, and mental health.

The role of psychiatric nursing in community-based settings continued to be unclear.

Focus continued on community-based services and increased on technological advances and neurobiology in the study of mental illness. Late 1980s experienced increased inpatient psychiatric treatment with evidence of abuse within private psychiatric settings, which led to increases in health care costs.

Present focus on prevention, community-based services, and primary prevention using various approaches such as mental health centers, partial hospitalization, day care centers, home health, and hospice care.

---

intervention concepts into nursing practice.

Psychiatric nurses in advanced practice began using an array of psychotherapeutic approaches, including various psychotherapies, behavior modification, cognitive therapy, and prescriptive authority and performing research. Treatment focused on psychogeriatric and pediatric nursing; trauma throughout the life span; and severe personality disorders.

Advanced nurse practitioners continue to provide various psychotherapeutic interventions. Increased emphasis on researching client outcomes and improving the quality of cost-effective client care.

The *Psychiatric Nurse as a Family Therapist* (1975), stressed the significance of treating clients within their social contexts.

Major nursing leaders continued to define nursing practice within a changing health care system. Major focus included various age groups, prevention and health promotion, and outcome identification. Other areas of concern included researching outcomes and the effectiveness of nursing interventions.

Various nursing organizations are uniting to present a strong and cohesive posture to maximize benefits from proposed health care reforms in the 1990s and beyond.

The 1976 ANA *Statement on Psychiatric and Mental Health Nursing Practice* defined the standards of psychiatric nursing practice. The 1982 ANA *Standards of Psychiatric and Mental Health Nursing Practice* delineated specific outcome criteria for clinical practice in the specialty.

The 1994 ANA Statement on Psychiatric-Mental Health Clinical Practice and Standards of Psychiatric-Mental Health Clinical Practice was the first revision in the 1990s.

ANA recently revised its *Scope and Standards of Psychiatric-Mental Health Nursing Practice* (2000).

(continues)

TABLE 1–1

The Evolution of Psychiatric Nursing (continued)

Dates and Events	Type of Mental Health Treatment	Role of Psychiatric Nurse	Historical Figures	Significant Contributions
2001–2008: In 2002 the President's New Freedom Commission on Mental Health was established. The commission submitted an executive summary to the President in 2003. As of 2007 recommendations have not been implemented. Recommendations reflected those from the 1999 Mental Health: A Report of the Surgeon General. 2005: Growing concerns concerning implementation of these recommendations continue to be expressed and addressed by mental health professionals and advocates for persons with mental illness.	Integration of various treatment models with emphasis on chronic self-care management, use of diverse communication venues, including Telemental Health, Care Coordination Home Telehealth that integrates medical and mental health treatment management in the client's home. Internet dialogues and Interactive, online treatment algorithms. Self-care management involving the client and family in shared-decision making .	Movement toward one Advanced Practice Psychiatric Registered Nurse role Increased focus on the client's physical needs and integration with mental health care and continued collaborative relationships with primary care providers and other specialty care providers.		
2005–2008: Preliminary data from research funded NIMH large randomized studies of medication efficacy, including: • Clinical Antipsychotic Trials of Intervention Effectiveness (CATIE) • Sequenced Treatment Alternatives to Relieve Depression (STAR*D) • Systematic Treatment Enhancement Program for Bipolar Disorder (STEP-BD) The projects provide guidance to health care providers and consumers evidence to guide treatment options to enhance clinical outcomes and quality of life.	Treatment focus extends beyond symptom management and involves higher quality of life and functional status.	Psychiatric nurses must stay abreast of clinical trials, results of large clinical trials; practice guidelines and integrate these data into clinical practice to improve symptom management, quality of life, and help clients reach an optimal level of functioning.		

Note. From "The Role of the Federal Government in Development of Psychiatric Nursing," by J. G. Chamberlain, 1983, Journal of Psychosocial Nursing, 21, pp. 11–18. Adapted with permission; "Future Directions in Psychiatric Nursing From the Perspective of History," by H. E. Peplau, 1989, Journal of Psychosocial Nursing, 2, pp. 18–28. Adapted with permission; "Historical Developments and Issues in Psychiatric-Mental Health Nursing," by G. M. Sills, 1973, in M. L. Leininger (Ed.), Contemporary Issues in Mental Health Nursing, pp. 125–136. Boston: Little, Brown. Adapted with permission. NIMH Longitudinal Studies on Medication Efficacy (e.g., CATIE, STAR*D).

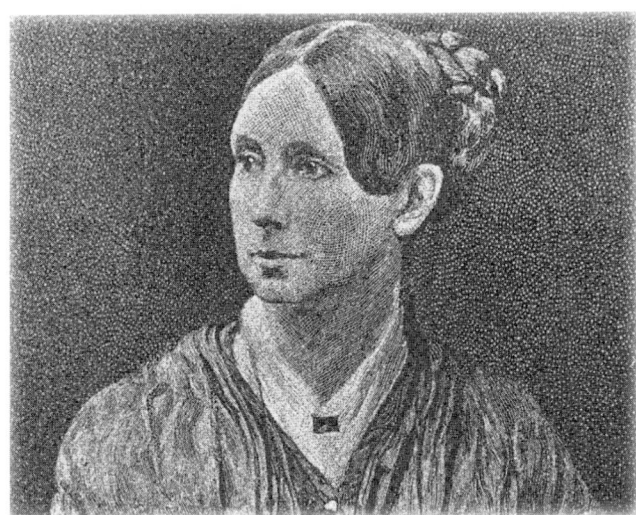

Figure 1–2 Dorothea Lynde Dix. *(Courtesy of the American Nurses Association.)*

public funding, and increased brutality and malevolence toward the mentally ill. Conditions in jails and mental institutions became deplorable and the need for reform was urgent.

Dorothea Lynde Dix (1802–1887)

Dorothea Lynde Dix (Figure 1–2), a retired schoolteacher from Massachusetts, led the crusade that brought attention of these conditions to the public and legislature. She discovered the deplorable inhumane treatment of the jailed mentally ill while substituting for a theology student. She was appalled by the miserable conditions of prisoners, who were chained, caged, and deprived of heat. The frigid Massachusetts weather made the lack of heat and sunlight deadly and heartless. Her undertakings revitalized humane treatment of the mentally ill.

Renewed public and legislative concern improved standards of care for the mentally ill, which led to proliferation of state hospitals. Unfortunately, the number of state hospitals was unable to meet the tremendous needs of the mentally ill, and care remained primarily custodial and inadequate at the end of the nineteenth century.

THE TWENTIETH CENTURY: THE ERA OF PSYCHIATRY

The dawning of the twentieth century in the United States found that improved social attitudes promoted sensitivity toward the mentally ill. These changes endured and reflected society's increasing concerns for others. The progressive era and burgeoning role of community health nurses in the 1900s as social activists played a role in advancing these changes. Likewise, legislators ultimately responded to these changes by developing widespread measures for welfare reform and enactment of child labor laws. These moving transformations encouraged medicine to take the lead and explore the basis of mental illness through scientific and clinical studies.

Several major breakthroughs in the evolution of psychiatric care emerged during the twentieth century. Exploration of the reasons for mental disease accelerated with contributions from numerous theorists and researchers who laid the foundation for understanding and demystifying mental illness.

Adolph Meyer (1866–1950)

In 1902, Adolph Meyer, a psychiatrist from Sweden, initiated the psychobiological theory and dynamic concept of psychiatric care. He focused on physical and emotional maturational changes. He emphasized the need to study the person's *whole* environment to determine its effects on the total personality. His psychobiological theory centered on treatment rather than disease and integrated biochemical, genetic, psychosocial, and environmental stresses on mental illness. He accepted the concept that mental disease resulted from the individual's maladaptation to his/her environment. Meyer introduced the concept of commonsense psychiatry, which was based on ways that clients could realistically improve life situations (Lewis, 1974).

Clifford Beers (1876–1943)

Clifford Beers, who himself had been treated for mental illness, contributed to preventive care through his classic work, *A Mind That Found Itself,* which was published in 1908. His work provided a descriptive account of his tormenting experiences in mental institutions. He played a major role in establishing the Mental Hygiene Movement in New Haven, Connecticut, in 1908 and promoting the early detection of mental illness. National recognition and adoption of this movement began within a year.

Emil Kraepelin (1856–1926)

Emil Kraepelin, a noted psychiatrist from Munich, devised a classification of mental disorders, which gave momentum to the advancement of psychiatry. His work shifted from an emphasis on research in the pathobiological laboratory to the observation and research in conditions known as praecox dementia and mania.

Eugen Bleuler (1857–1939)

At the end of the century, Eugen Bleuler, one of Kraepelin's students, coined the term *schizophrenia* and included among its characteristics the four As: apathy, associative looseness, autism, and ambivalence. His noted treatise, "Dementia Praecox or Group of Schizophrenias," delineated the complexity of schizophrenia.

Sigmund Freud (1856–1939)

During this period, a Viennese neurologist named Sigmund Freud was credited with the development of psychoanalysis, psychosexual theories, and neurosis. He revolutionized psychiatry through his use of psychoanalysis, a method that serves as the basis for treatment and a theory for personality development. He popularized the term *catharsis*, dream interpretations, and explanations for hysteria. His contributions stimulated the development and rationale for research and established the basis of modern psychoanalytical technique. This technique focused on increasing awareness of the unconscious aspects of the client's personality.

Carl Gustav Jung (1875–1961)

Carl Gustav Jung, a Swiss psychiatrist, broke away from Freud and developed his own theory of the origins of neurosis. He was one of the earliest neo-Freudians who later founded *analytic psychology*. Jung proposed and originated the concepts of extroverted and introverted personality. He integrated spiritual concepts, reasoning, ancestral emotional trends, and mysticism, and the creative notion of human beings. Eventually, he forged his own group to pursue these beliefs and his work focused on the creative impulse and spirituality of the individual.

Karen Horney (1885–1952)

Karen Horney, a prominent psychoanalyst, another neo-Freudian, objected to Freud's notion that neurosis and personality development were based on biological drives. Her theory suggested that neuroses stem from cultural factors and impaired interpersonal relationships. Overall, neo-Freudian theorists broadened the psychodynamic concepts and stressed the impact of disturbed interpersonal relationships in maladaptive responses. Furthermore, they minimized the biological factors of mental illness.

Numerous studies examining the relationship between biochemical, genetic, and psychosocial reactions took place in the early-twentieth century. These included clinical studies in psychiatry and neurology, such as Hans Seyle's (1956) stress syndrome and general adaptation syndrome. Psychosomatic medicine also emerged and gained prominence during the mid-twentieth century (Alexander, 1950).

Harry Stack Sullivan (1892–1949)

Harry Stack Sullivan (1940, 1953) postulated the hypothesis of interpersonal theory and stimulated the development of multidisciplinary approaches to psychiatric and milieu therapy. He believed that anxiety interfered with the ability to cope and communicate effectively, resulting in mental illness. He surmised that anxiety could be reduced through a meaningful interpersonal relationship that stresses the process of effective communication. His interpersonal theory influenced psychiatric-mental health nursing practice and has become an integral part of nursing education.

Other Contributions

In 1952, the American Psychiatric Association published the *Diagnostic and Statistical Manual of Mental Disorders*. This manual provided a new and comprehensive classification of mental disorders.

The importance of the nurse's "therapeutic use of self" was advanced in 1952 by Hildegard Peplau's text, *Interpersonal Relations in Nursing: A Conceptual Framework for Psychodynamic Nursing*. Peplau's theory stemmed primarily from the interpersonal theory of Harry Stack Sullivan, but she expanded it with her own concepts and applied them to nursing. Her work provided the first theoretical framework for psychiatric-mental health nurses and defined nursing as an interactive, exploratory, caring, and health-promoting process. Peplau delineated four overlapping phases of the nurse-client relationship: orientation, identification, exploration, and resolution. Peplau asserted that all nurse-client interactions are opportunities to build a mutual understanding and to identify goals that have an impact on client outcomes and responses.

The Advent of Somatic Therapies

Somatic therapy is synonymous to *biological* therapies. These therapies were introduced in the late 1930s and included the advent of hypoglycemic shock to treat schizophrenia. Other treatment modalities included metrazol shock, electroshock, and psychosurgery, which was mainly frontal lobotomy. This radical treatment was used to manage anxiety in clients suffering from agitated and psychotic disorders. Somatic therapies brought optimism to psychiatry and revolutionized psychiatric nursing, because these therapies required physical and custodial nursing care. Optimism stemmed from the advent of somatic treatment, such as psychotropic agents, that reduced psychiatric symptoms and improved quality of life for the mentally ill.

Psychotropics emerged in the 1950s with the advent of Thorazine (chlorpromazine) and Tofranil (imipramine). These agents revolutionized the treatment of mental illness and generated a tremendous change in the role of psychiatric-mental health nursing. These medications calmed clients and reduced the need for other somatic therapies such as insulin and electroconvulsive shock. The optimism generated by new psychodynamic approaches and these major tranquilizers led to the Community Mental Health Movement of the 1960s.

The Mental Health Movement

During the mid-twentieth century numerous strides were made to improve services for the mentally ill. The mental health movement gained support and progressed in the form of federal provisions, which gave authority to the United States Public Health Service to address mental health. These impelling changes gained momentum from experiences in treating soldiers following World War II. The result was the passage of the National Mental Health Act of 1946.

The mental health movement gained momentum during the World War II period; psychiatry finally progressed from its primitive stage of confinement and brutality to one that emphasized the need for interpersonal relations. The role of nursing evolved at the same time and transformed from that of custodial care to a more active role on the mental health team. This new role broadened the scope of nursing practice. After World War II increased public acceptance, awareness, and understanding provided a climate that fostered restoration of the psychological wartime casualties. World War II served as a pivotal point in the transition of nursing practice. Because of their increased visibility associated with caring for the wounded, nurses attained respect for their innovative contributions to nursing care (Stevens & Henrie, 1966).

The nation's attitude toward the mentally ill began to change, exhibiting increased sensitivity and optimism in support of mental health professions, such as psychiatry, nursing, social work, and psychology. The basis of legislative efforts, such as the 1961 President's Commission on Mental Illness and Health, established by President Eisenhower, and later the Federal Community Mental Health Centers Legislation, during the Kennedy and Johnson administrations, emphasized prevention, primary care, and rehabilitation. Proponents of this legislation hoped to reduce long-term hospitalization or institutionalization and developed comprehensive community-based services. Refer to Table 1–2 for a summary of the major developments in the mental health movement.

Deinstitutionalization and Community-Based Care

Deinstitutionalization of the mentally ill followed the legislative initiatives discussed earlier, fueled by the notion that institutions were unhealthy for the mentally ill. The Community Mental Health Centers Act of 1963 was an attempt to release chronically ill clients from institutions and place them back into community rehabilitation settings (Bassuk & Gerson, 1978). The emphases of community mental health were in part a result of the deinstitutionalization of clients from long-term residential hospitals that began in the 1960s and expanded in the 1970s. The mental health movement also heralded in federal financing programs in the 1960s that depicted new perspectives on the civil rights of people, including those with mental illnesses. These federal initiatives also propelled a dramatic trend in the mental health delivery systems (Parades, 1979).

Gerald Caplan's (1961) contributions in identifying primary, secondary, and tertiary prevention had an impact on psychiatric nursing as it emerged from the back wards of institutions to community-based settings. He believed that using preventive measures, such as early case findings, diagnosis, and crisis intervention, could minimize the incidence and severity of mental illness. Caplan's work was consistent with the intent of the mental health movement, which sought to provide comprehensive psychiatric services to clients, families, communities, and various cultures.

Historically, psychiatric nursing interventions centered on illness rather than prevention and health promotion. Leininger (1969, 1973) described the shift from hospital-based to community-based care as one of the "most significant trends" (p. 2) in the care and treatment of the mentally ill. Leininger noted that primary prevention is critical to minimizing and reducing the prevalence of mental illness. She added that this process involves understanding and researching unique individual needs and responses to stress within diverse cultures and societies.

How would psychiatric nursing be integrated into the community mental health movement? Three key issues had an impact on this process: (1) nursing education and experience, (2) nursing role and function, and (3) the relationship of nursing with other mental health disciplines (Glittenberg, 1963; Leininger, 1969).

Several research groups attempted to identify these dilemmas along with possible solutions. The first was a national survey of the psychiatric nurse's role in outpatient clinics, which discovered that fewer than 10 percent of nurses were included as part of the mental health team (Glittenberg, 1963). Inconsistent educational preparation, which varied among associate to doctoral preparation, complicated the perception of the nurse in community-based facilities. Additionally, other disciplines did not respect the advanced training of nurses with a master's degree or a PhD. However, the study found that more than half of nurses participated in the initial assessment, cotherapy, and home visits (Glittenberg, 1963). Another nursing study, conducted at Maimonides Medical Center from 1963 to 1968, concluded that most psychiatric nurses functioned as generalists, and many believed their role on the mental health team was underrated or ancillary (Stokes, Williams, Davidites, Bulbulyen, & Ullman, 1969). More significantly, data from these two studies suggested that the psychiatric nurse was an invaluable resource and member of the mental health team, regardless of educational preparation. These findings also implicated a need to increase dialogue and collaboration with other disciplines to promote understanding and comprehensive mental health services.

New Psychotherapies

Sweeping changes in the 1960s also created opportunities for innovative psychotherapies that centered on self-actualization (Abraham Maslow), transactional analysis (Eric Berne), and Gestalt therapy (Fritz Perls). These therapies overshadowed strategies associated with pure psychoanalysis. They broke away from traditional long-term psychotherapy and evolved in a decade in which people wanted variety and quick solutions to old problems. These therapies provided seemingly quick solutions that put people "in touch with themselves" and focused on the "here and now" rather than on early life experiences proposed by pure psychoanalytic theory. This decade reflected an era of theorists who asserted the relevance of mental health and self-actualization and responsibility for life choices.

Biological Aspects of Mental Illness

The 1970s and 1980s produced an explosion of interest in the biological aspects of mental illness. Researchers focused on neurobiology, biological markers, and genetic bases for mental illness, and on changing treatment modalities. The new generation of antidepressants and anxiolytics emerged during the latter decade. The early 1980s also ushered in a decade of reduced federal allocations for community mental health services and decreased the mandated services from 12 to 5. (See Chapter 33.) By 1984 the government no longer funded mental health centers. Reduction in funding has had far-reaching effects on the mental health movement. It has contributed to the widening gap between those who can afford health care and those who cannot. Lack of adequate funding has led to fragmentation of community mental health services, poor access to care, health disparities, a lack of coordination in aftercare or rehabilitation, and duplication of services caused by a lack of coordinated services.

TABLE 1–2
The Mental Health Movement—The Mid-Twentieth Century

Date	Event	Changes
1946	Passage of the Mental Health Act	Authorized formation of the National Institute of Mental Health (NIMH) Supported research of: • crisis intervention • psychiatric diagnoses • prevention and treatment of mental illness • education of psychiatric specialties, including many nurses
1961	President's Commission on Mental Illness and Health	Legislative support for educating mental health professional (i.e., nurses, social workers, psychiatrists, psychologists)
1963	The Community Mental Health Act Movement	Deinstitutionalization (chronically mentally ill released from institutions to community rehabilitation centers): • increased access to care in own community
1970–1980	Explosion of interest in biological markers/neurobiological basis of mental illness and treatment	Advent of third-generation psychotropics; increased popularity of biological therapies
1990s	Decade of the Brain Human Genome Project	Advances in technology and neurobiology; identification of innovative diagnostic studies, especially for schizophrenia and mood disorders; genetic basis of mental disorders
1990s–twenty-first century	Impelling social and economic changes. Health care reforms	Soaring rate of homelessness; lack of legislative funding; primary, secondary, tertiary prevention; global AIDS epidemic; recognition of the need for systematized health care delivery; growing high risk of mental illness among pregnant women, children, the aged, substance abusers, and victims of violence
2001–2008	Societal and economic issues remain constant; greater emphasis on resolving health disparities, increasing cultural competence to address the needs of a diverse population; mounting concerns about the emotional impact of war and disaster-related trauma and international terrorism. • Pharmacological efficacy studies that offer persons with mental health problems additional treatment options to facilitate symptom management, improve quality of life and overall functional status, recovery and self-care management	

Note. From U.S. Congress (1989). *Decade of the Brain Proclamation.* Pub. L. N. 101-58 [HJ Res. 174], 130 Stat. 152–154 (July 25, 1989).

The 1990s: The Decade of the Brain

In 1989, the U.S. Congress declared the 1990s the "decade of the brain." This declaration was based on the fact that 50 million Americans are affected by disorders that involve the brain, ranging from familial illnesses to prenatal trauma to affective and addictive disorders. The need for knowledge and expertise in biological and psychological sciences continues to be essential because they are the source of new psychopharmacologic agents and comprehensive psychotherapeutic interventions. Since the late 1980s, the expansion of technological advances, such as brain imaging, has provided direct examination of the living brain. These techniques, which assess brain structure and some aspects of brain function, include computed tomography, positron emission tomography, magnetic resonance imaging, magnetic resonance spectroscopy, diffusion-tensor imaging, and single-photon emission computerized tomography.

Perhaps the future of psychiatry is contingent on research opportunities that focus on the role of molecular biology, neuroscience, genetics, and behavior in mental illnesses. Likewise, its future will stem from researchers and clinicians developing evidence-based interventions and practice guidelines that target these intricate structures and processes and produce positive treatment outcomes (Cowan, Kopnisky, & Hyman, 2002).

THE TWENTY-FIRST CENTURY: NEUROSCIENCE AND GENETICS

Psychiatry faces vast challenges and opportunities in the twenty-first century. Neuroscience and genetics constitute the most momentous research opportunities in modern science history (Cowan et al., 2002). These unique opportunities afford a greater understanding of the link between behavior and emotions, brain, and genes. The 1990s offered a greater understanding of the complexity of human behaviors and underlying neurobiological processes. Contemporary mental health care integrates neuroscience, genetic research, and environmental factors. These factors appear to increase the risk of mental illness in vulnerable populations, such as those with schizophrenia, bipolar disorder, Alzheimer's disease, and pervasive developmental disorders. Understandably, the complexities of mental illnesses will also govern specific treatment modalities that meet the client's individual needs. The plethora of pharmacologic agents, complementary therapies, and diverse psychotherapies offer new approaches to research and evidence-based mental health care (Yellowlees, 2005).

Information Systems: The Internet and Cyberspace

More and more consumers are using the Internet and other informational systems to learn about their health concerns (Yellowlees, 2005). These issues include mental and physical health and complementary therapies. As consumers familiarize themselves with health care choices via the Internet and other informational systems, psychiatric nurses must be able to talk with their clients regarding their health concerns and treatment options. These auspicious nurse-client collaborative opportunities indicate the importance of creative communication skills, which involve computer literacy, access to E-mail, and the Internet.

Obviously, the advent of vast informational systems presents psychiatric nurses with new avenues to assess human experiences and form therapeutic relationships. In addition to the Internet, other nurse-client interactions exist. Telemedicine is an example of technological advances being used in vast clinical areas, including psychiatry. This technology provides a forum for interviewing the client via a telemedicine setup or conversing with the video camera, home monitoring, cell phones, and interactive online treatment. This method of interviewing is especially helpful in assessing the client during a psychiatric emergency and provides a venue for mental and physical assessment and triage. Psychiatrists and psychiatric nurses may also use this psychiatric-liaison-consultation when called by other health care providers. This forum offers a cost-effective approach to evaluation and treatment that curtails transportation expenses, and increases and provides access to clinical experts and health care services. Major disadvantages of telemedicine include high investment cost, privacy and confidentiality issues (lacks visual or face-to-face contact), presently a lack of protocol standardization, and uncertainty about reimbursement (Meltzer, 1997; Yellowlees, 2005).

Despite barriers to telemedicine or telemental health care major advantages of these services include increasing access to clients and their families living in rural and remote areas where driving may be less cost-effective and more burdensome. It also brings care to the client in their homes and enables the psychiatric mental health nurse to establish therapeutic relationships while employing client-centered nursing interventions and quality health care similar to a face-to-face visit. As more and more clients learn about various treatment options and technologies that improve access and quality across the health care continuum, psychiatric nurses must be prepared to address their needs, preferences, and wishes while maintaining therapeutic interactions that promote self-care management and self-efficacy.

Another uncertainty inherent in the technological informational systems is its potential impact on establishing and maintaining healthy interpersonal relationships. Despite the advantages of telemedicine and other informational systems, they are likely to interfere with forming trusting interactions with the client and family. This concern extends beyond this approach and also includes dealing with society and a younger generation that has been brought up on the Internet and expects immediate gratification due to the instantaneous feedback of cell phones, video games, E-mails, text messaging, and facsimiles. These factors are likely to make an impact on how psychiatric nurses communicate and establish healthy nurse-client interactions with this age group. A sharp decline in personal interactions because of E-mail systems and increased access to health information on the Internet challenge psychiatric nurses to be creative and proactive. Proactive responses, such as developing innovative communication skills and remaining apprised of the latest treatment strategies, including complementary therapies, are likely to bolster consumer confidence, enhance the nurse-client relationship, impart health education, and generate diverse treatment options.

Complementary Therapies

The noteworthy research of Eisenberg and colleagues (1993) revealed that in 1990, the American consumer made approximately 425 million visits to providers offering complementary therapies. These data suggest that one in three clients seeking conventional health care was also using complementary therapies. Remarkably, today's consumers use various complementary therapies, such as aromatherapy, acupuncture, biofeedback, massage therapy, herbs, and nutritional approaches (Ernst & Fugh-Berman, 2002; Kim, Kverno, Lee, Park, Lee, & Kim, 2006; Werneke, Turner, & Priebe, 2006) to promote a sense of well-being and health. These therapies offer clients choices and independent decision making regarding their mental and physical health. The growing number of consumers using complementary therapies suggests that psychiatric nurses must familiarize themselves with the advantages and potential risks of these approaches. Interestingly enough, the advent of complementary therapies has not replaced conventional therapies. Despite the proliferation of these therapies, psychiatric nurses can support their clients' choices, encourage client autonomy, and promote trusting and therapeutic interactions with their clients.

Cultural Considerations

Culture reflects one's individuality and personal expression of self and influences one's perception of health and illness. Psychiatric nurses, like other health care providers, bring beliefs and values concerning health and illness from both their culture and those of their profession. Ultimately, they must recognize and appreciate cultural differences and understand all facets of the health-illness continuum and make them the basis of nurse-client interactions, assessment, and interventions. (See Chapter 7 for an in-depth discussion of cultural and ethnic considerations.)

More importantly, efforts to respond to individual client needs require cultural competency skills. As the face of our society continues to change and become more culturally and ethnically diverse, psychiatric-mental health nurses are challenged to meet the global health needs of diverse client populations. Meeting the needs of a changing society requires cultural competence. Cultural competence is a process that entails cultural awareness and knowledge and application in all facets of health care (Warren, 2000). Ideally, culturally competent mental health care is individualized to meet the client's holistic needs. This century challenges psychiatric nurses to integrate cultural factors with technological advances in neurobiology and informational systems and develop quality and holistic health care.

Mounting concerns among health care leaders and some lawmakers are health disparities and poor access to quality care among distinct populations (Mayberry, Mili, Ofili, 2000).

Healthy People 2010 defines health disparities as differences in disease prevalence or access to treatment based on gender, race, language, ethnicity, socioeconomic status, sexual orientation, geographic locale, and education (U.S. Department of Health and Human Services, 1999). Whilst there is no consensus concerning the bases of health disparities, most researchers have identified several factors including client preferences, poor communication with clinicians, alienation, mistrust, and access difficulties to physicians (Carrasquillo, Orva, Brennan, & Burstin, 1999). An estimated 3.5 million U.S. school-aged children have limited English proficiency (Flores, Abreu, & Tomany-Korman, 2005). Limited English proficiency impedes equitable health across the life span. Reducing health disparities requires cultural competence in which the psychiatric nurse uses effective communication to understand the client and family's experience and unique cultural and gender needs to ensure client-centered and holistic care across the life span.

The Future

As psychiatry evolves in the twenty-first century, nurses and other mental health professionals are challenged to deal with enormous technological, socioeconomic, and scientific discoveries. Such changes require expanded knowledge and skills in neuroscience and genetics from a developmental perspective and intricate informational systems. It behooves psychiatric nurses to recognize the impact of the Internet and other informational technology on health care and respond proactively by developing innovative communication strategies and staying abreast of varied treatment approaches. These advances also challenge psychiatric nurses to recognize the impact of scientific discoveries on mental and physical health and cyberspace on consumer needs and communication patterns. Technological and psychological adaptations to these developments are transitions into the future.

The impact of wars in various parts of the world along with national concerns about terrorism and natural and manmade disaster continue to be researched. Preliminary data indicate short- and long-term traumatic sequel. Addressing these issues and discerning implications for mental health is a global concern. Psychiatric nurses and other clinicians are in key positions to work with various organizations and health care systems to address and mitigate actual and potential adverse effects of traumatic events.

Numerous social changes continue to evolve, such as those in Europe, the Middle East, and Eastern block countries. Major changes include increased violence in certain regions that are contributing to growing injuries and deaths among ethnic populations. Poverty and illnesses are rampant among many of the war-torn countries. These social conditions affect human relations and coping patterns and place tremendous demands on individuals, families, communities, and countries. Similarly, overwhelming societal demands often compromise individual coping skills, consequently increasing the risk of personal and societal violence. Lifestyle changes and transforming attitudes toward the mentally ill continue to parallel society's participation in economic, social, and legislative issues. The soaring cost and poor access to health care continue to coincide with an increased risk of chronic debilitating illnesses, particularly in vulnerable populations, and a decline in primary prevention. Nurses must remain proactive and play quintessential roles in health promotion and prevention (Parse, 1992; Pender, 1996) and in the evolution of psychiatric nursing.

PSYCHIATRIC NURSING EDUCATION: EVOLUTION OF A SPECIALTY

Looking to the future of psychiatric-mental health nursing involves reviewing the evolution of societal issues that affect individual responses to stress and the treatment of the mentally ill. Psychiatric nursing has evolved from a role in which the primary concern was providing a clean, humane environment to one in which assessing stress responses and establishing, prescribing, and implementing treatment, and evaluating interventions that deal with these responses are paramount. Nurses play pivotal roles in determining and promoting developmental progression and personal needs of clients toward the establishment and maintenance of mental health.

The unique contributions of the nurse in caring for the mentally ill have been well documented throughout the ages. Before the eighteenth century, the attitude and nature of servants or attendants were recognized to be important in creating relaxed, calm surroundings for those with mental illness. The advent of moral treatment involved recognizing and treating the mentally ill as human beings.

Nursing care of the mentally ill was extremely limited during the early part of the nineteenth century partly because nurses lacked formal training and education. Custodial care remained the primary mode of treatment within institutions. Because of the work of Linda Richards, the first graduate nurse in America (1873) who collaborated with Dr. Edward Cowles of McLean Asylum, several schools in general and mental hospitals were established. Their efforts were instrumental in organizing the first formal training for nursing of the mentally ill in the United States in 1882. This was a 2-year training program that focused primarily on custodial care and placed little emphasis on developing psychosocial skills. Custodial care centered on providing for safety and physical needs. Using male attendants to control clients and protect nurses continued. Richards (1911) stressed the need for students to take courses in state hospitals and develop prudence and compassion, which, she emphasized, were essential nursing qualities. Although her efforts did not focus directly on the psychosocial aspects of these clients, they laid the early foundations of psychiatric nursing. By modifying the physical environment, clients were likely to have felt emotionally comfortable and secure because their basic needs were being met. She also made notes concerning the seriously ill and gave reports, which were reviewed by other workers and eventually physicians who requested to see them. Her brief notes gave rise to the current system of medical records. In addition, she sought to develop a scientific or theoretical base for the practice of nursing.

These early accomplishments laid the foundation of psychiatric nursing and provided men with their first opportunity to become trained nurses. Until then, men were not allowed to enter nursing because there was concern that they were not as nurturing as women (Mericle, 1983).

Training for mental health nurses was significant because it provided care, rather than incarceration, for treatment of mental illness. The role of nursing until 1937 remained custodial and was under the auspices of medicine rather than nursing. Nurses, like other women, were not revered as were their male counterpart physicians during this era.

Before the National Mental Health Act of 1946, there was no systematic effort to address the needs of the mentally ill. This legislation supported increased funding for training of mental health professionals to reduce the prevalence of mental disorders through understanding and prevention. Increased funding and societal efforts to support humane treatment for the mentally ill allowed university nursing schools to strengthen their curricula. These endeavors increased the number of available trained psychiatric-mental health nurses to promote the quality of psychiatric nursing education in undergraduate schools (baccalaureate level), and integrate concepts throughout the nursing curricula. Nursing schools began to transform their modified "maternal" or custodial role to therapeutic and preventive perspectives.

Another milestone in the evolution of psychiatric nursing was the formation of the National League for Nursing (NLN) in 1952. This organization was also concerned with the education and training of nurses in the mental health area, and as a result, the Mental Health and Psychiatric Advisory service was formed. Kathleen Black, a registered nurse, was its first director. Representatives from this service acted as educational consultants for nursing schools nationwide. More importantly, the NLN required that the schools they accredited have an identifiable psychiatric-mental health nursing course. This requirement supported and advanced the significance of psychiatric-mental health nursing practice to the nursing profession.

NURSING THEORISTS
Hildegard Peplau

In 1952, Hildegard Peplau's publication, *Interpersonal Relations in Nursing: A Conceptual Framework for Psychodynamic Nursing,* influenced nursing practice (see earlier discussions of Peplau's contribution to psychiatric nursing). The foundation of her theory came from Harry Stack Sullivan's postulates. Her concepts and perspectives were developed into nursing theory, which became the basis of interpersonal processes in nursing. These were related to the promotion of healthy adaptation to life stressors.

June Mellow and Gwen Tudor

Other theorists during the 1950s included June Mellow, who developed concepts in nursing theory that were based on work with clients suffering from schizophrenia. She stressed the influence of the nurse-client relationship and the nursing process on client outcomes. Furthermore, Gwen Tudor (1952) defined psychiatric nursing as an interpersonal process of observation, intervention, and evaluation. Tudor described three major functions of the nurse: as a facilitator of communication, social interaction, and self-care. Additionally, she stressed the significance of social context and its impact on the nurses' attitude and response to their clients' needs and subsequent mental health. Contributions from these nurses were instrumental in legitimizing the role of psychiatric nursing and establishing the foundation for current therapeutic interventions.

NATIONAL INSTITUTE OF MENTAL HEALTH

In 1954, the National Institute of Mental Health (NIMH) supported a pilot program to integrate behavioral concepts and psychiatric content into undergraduate curricula. It also identified the shortage of psychiatric-mental health nurses trained to care for emotionally disturbed children and the need for primary prevention of mental illness. Opportunities for trained psychiatric-mental health nurses flourished during the 1950s and 1960s, evolving within nursing and becoming an integral part of the profession. The role of the psychiatric clinical specialist during this era focused on the need for advanced preparation built on the foundation of behavioral and nursing concepts. Additionally, nursing leaders expressed the need for doctoral training and research. The federal government's role has been critical in identifying and supporting the preparation of nurses in psychiatric-mental health nursing (Chamberlain, 1983).

AMERICAN NURSES ASSOCIATION

The American Nurses Association (ANA) was established in 1893. The ANA has also had a major impact on the evolution of psychiatric-mental health nursing. These origins reflect the contributions of early leaders in psychiatric-mental health nursing who played an important role in advancing the nursing profession. This organization later stressed the importance of including clinical preparation in psychiatric nursing as part of training for nursing students. McLean and several hospitals in Boston provided clinical settings for this training.

The ANA has been instrumental in providing the foundation of psychiatric-mental health nursing practice as we know it today. The initial efforts to delineate the levels and standards of practice in psychiatric nursing began in 1961. Renowned leaders in psychiatric nursing who participated in this task force were Hildegard Peplau and Grayce Sills. As a result of these efforts the ANA's Division on Psychiatric and Mental Health Nursing Practice published the *Statement on Psychiatric Nursing Practice* in 1967. It validated the significance and impact of psychiatric nursing education and the diversity of this specialty in meeting the needs of the mentally ill. These 1967 standards advocated that nurses needed to define and develop nursing practice based on theory, experience, research, and prevention, and use of the nursing

process. Additionally, the *Statement* played a vital role in the historical development of psychiatric-mental health nursing education and practice.

In the fall of 1974, the Executive Committee of the Division on Psychiatric Mental Health Nursing appointed an ad hoc committee to revise the *Statement* to meet ANA's commitment to maintain high standards of nursing practice and improve the quality of nursing care. Furthermore, the ad hoc committee decided to increase the consumer's understanding of the psychiatric-mental health nurse by clarifying the relationship between education, experience, and specialties. The following major themes evolved from this committee's efforts (ANA, 1976):

- ◆ The strong trend toward community-based, short-term treatment models, with a concomitant emphasis on deinstitutionalization
- ◆ Emphasis on the assurance of quality care
- ◆ Significant development in the arena of litigation and mental services

The ANA established the first certification program in 1973 to provide an objective and tangible means of recognizing professional expertise in the specialty for both functional and clinical domains of nursing. More than 150,000 registered nurses throughout the United States and its territories in more than 50 specialties since 1975 have been certified in two broad categories as generalist or advanced practice through the American Nurses Credentialing Center (ANCC). Certification has allowed nurses to compete within the health care delivery system as distinguished health care providers (ANCC, 2005).

In 1976, the ANA established two levels of professional nurses: baccalaureate and advanced practice. In psychiatry, the advanced level was initially established as the clinical specialist for adult psychiatric-mental health nursing. This was later followed by the clinical specialist practice for child and adolescent mental health nursing and most recently another advanced practice registered nurse (APRN), notably, the psychiatric-mental health nurse practitioner (PMHNP). Refer to Table 1–3 for a summary of the development in child and adolescent psychotherapy.

In 1989, the American Nurses Commission on Organizational Assessment and Renewal recommended that the ANCC be considered as a distinct agency used by the ANA for credentialing purposes. Credentialing programs are based on the ANA's Congress for Nursing Practice. The goals of ANCC entail "promoting and enhancing health by certifying nurses and accrediting organizations using ANA standards of practice, nursing services and continuing education" (ANCC, 1993, p. 3).

The 1994 publication, *A Statement of Psychiatric-Mental Health Clinical Nursing Practice and Standards of Psychiatric-Mental Health Clinical Nursing Practice,* represented a collaboration of various psychiatric nursing organizations that delineates the role of the generalist and the advanced-practice nurse (ANA, 1994).

Over the years, ANA's publications of psychiatric-mental health nursing standards reflect the format of the original

TABLE 1–3
Milestones in Child and Adolescent Psychiatry

1890: Psychology

- interest in the nervous child
- school phobias
- residential care for the poor (asylum, workhouse reformatory)

1895: Adolph Meyer

- stressed preventive care and the need for formal training in child psychiatry
- he initiated Kanner's research of childhood psychiatry
- stressed appraisal of psychobiological and social factors that increase understanding of mental illness in children and families (Kanner, 1935)

1906: Psychoanalysis/Psychodynamic Focus on Assessment and Treatment

- impact of family on child
- play therapy (Isaacs, 1961)
- child psychotherapy
- White House Conference on Children (1909) announced goals of developing strong, innovative program to care for emotionally disturbed children

1920s–1930s: The Child Guidance Movement (Social Reforms: Development of Community Services for Children)

- focused on prevention of juvenile delinquency
- first child guidance clinic
- development of teaching department on child psychiatry in hospitals
- White House Conference on Child Health and Protection proclaimed that the emotionally ill child has a right to live in a world that does not separate him/her from others (Kanner, 1935)

1940s–1960s: Post World War II Reforms

- identification of large numbers of severely disturbed children and increased institutionalization in punitive establishments, homes, and special schools (interdisciplinary approach)

1970s: Family Therapy

- educational opportunities flourished

Late 1970s to Present

- decreased federal funding for children
- reduction in support of childhood nutritional programs, education, and day care

1980s: Child and Adolescent Psychiatric-Mental Health Nursing Came of Age

- certification
- advocates for child and adolescents

1990s–Twenty-First Century: Decade of the Brain

- surge in family studies of mood disorders, schizophrenia, and other mental disorders
- DHHS (1999). Mental Health: A Report of the Surgeon General

2000–2005

- explosion of neuroscience and genetic research and advances that continue to link genetic and neurobiological factors to individualized pharmacologic interventions and improving the quality of life for individuals and families experiencing serious and chronic mental disorders
- explosion in psychotropic use in children and adolescents; issues concerning suicide risk secondary to novel antidepressant use in this population and older age groups emerged prompting the U.S. Food and Drug Administration to enact a "black box" warning to consumers and health care providers; greater focus on quality of life and functional status rather than just symptom management
- increased focus on violence and treatment of substance use disorders

(continues)

TABLE 1–3
Milestones in Child and Adolescent Psychiatry *(continued)*

2007–Future

- increased psychotropic use in children and adolescents; issues concerning suicide risk secondary to novel antidepressant use emerged; trends toward prescribing antidepressants declined as a result
- focus on violence, substance use disorders
- demographic changes associated with growing minority populations—particularly Hispanics—and need to address cultural needs, improve communication and decrease health disparities among diverse populations
- juvenile detention centers have spent more than $4,200 million "warehousing" youth instead of providing mental health services

document published in 1967. Recently, a task force of experts along with input from nurses in the field developed the 2000 version of this publication. This version is entitled *Scope and Standards of Psychiatric-Mental Health Nursing Practice* (ANA, 2000). Its contents offer nurses, other health care professionals, policy makers, insurers, and consumers information about vast levels and standards of psychiatric-mental health nursing (Billings, 2000).

Other milestones in 2000 include the first examination for the psychiatric-mental health nurse practitioner, marking a new national recognition of the advanced-practice psychiatric nurse. The ANA publication on psychiatric-mental health nursing (ANA, 2000) includes an in-depth discussion of the APRN in this specialty.

PSYCHIATRIC NURSING JOURNALS

Other landmarks from the 1960s to the 1990s included the advent of psychiatric nursing journals: *Perspectives in Psychiatric Care* (1963), *Journal of Psychosocial Nursing and Mental Health Services* (1963); *Issues in Mental Health Nursing* (1979); *Archives of Psychiatric Nursing* (1987); *Journal of the American Psychiatric Nurses Association* (1995); *Journal of Child and Adolescent Psychiatric Mental Health Nursing* [*JCAPMH Nursing*] (1988–1993); *Journal of Child and Adolescent Psychiatric Nursing* [formerly *JCAPMH Nursing*] (1994).

International journals include *The International Journal of Psychiatric and Mental Health Nursing* (1994) (England); *International Journal of Psychiatric and Mental Health Research* (1994) (England); and *International Journal of Mental Health Nursing* (2002) Australia.

FEDERAL FUNDING OF PSYCHIATRIC NURSING EDUCATION

Chamberlain (1983) described the impact of federal spending on the evolution of psychiatric-mental health nursing as having the following results:

- ◆ More master's degree–level psychiatric nursing programs
- ◆ More practicing nurses with a master's degree

- ◆ Greater interest in the integration of mental health concepts in baccalaureate nursing program curricula
- ◆ Development of continuing education programs that focused on psychiatric nursing concepts
- ◆ Diversity of NIMH master's and doctoral program graduates in service delivery settings (i.e., administrators, faculty, practitioners, and research)

Legislative allocations of funds for psychiatric-mental health education peaked in 1969, when a major setback occurred in appropriating financial support for both undergraduate and graduate psychiatric nursing programs. This trend has continued through the 1970s into 2008 despite increased community demands to treat the mentally ill.

AMENDMENTS TO THE COMMUNITY MENTAL HEALTH CENTERS ACT

The 1975 amendments to the Community Mental Health Centers Act of 1963 addressed the needs of the least restrictive care, changes in the commitment process, and deinstitutionalization of the mentally ill. The amendments were adopted by the passage of the Mental Health Act of 1980 and the National Plan for the Chronically Ill in 1981. This legislation centered on increasing remission and decreasing exacerbation of symptoms by providing continuity of care in U.S. communities and health care organizations. The legislation resulted in nurses being replaced with other health care professionals and attendants to run units and direct client care. The trend toward replacing registered nurses with paraprofessionals has reflected rising health care costs and lack of access to that care.

Presidents New Freedom Commission on Mental Health was designated in 2002 as part of an effort to eliminate inequities among persons with disabilities and expand hope and care of vulnerable populations. Major goals of the commission include:

1. Educate consumers about the importance of mental health within the scope of overall health
2. Provide client- and family-centered mental health care

3. Eliminate disparities in mental health services

4. Use primary prevention principles through early mental health screening, assessment, and referrals

5. Accelerate the use of research as a guide to excellent mental health services

6. Increase access to mental health care using technologies and other forms of communication (visit website for further information about the President's New Freedom Commission on Mental Health) http://www.mentalhealthcommission. gov/reports/reports.htm (Accessed October 15, 2006)

Despite these ambitious goals, critics report few changes have occurred since the report was submitted in 2003. Today, inadequate housing and gainful employment among persons with psychiatric disorders along with continued disparities and poor access to health care across the health care continuum remain a challenge. This is evidenced by the growing number of persons with mental illness who continue to make up a large part of the homeless population and penal system. The NIMH has launched and sponsored large controlled randomized studies exploring the efficacy of medication in the treatment of psychiatric disorders. Nurses play key roles in early identification and screening and are poised to decrease the stigma associated with mental illness. They also play key roles in working with various health care providers, clients, and families to ensure client-centered mental health care. Challenges continue to plague most societies seeking to improve mental health services and the stigma of mental illness. Psychiatric nurses must take the lead and advocate for equitable mental health care, improve access to various treatments, participate in research to ensure adherence to ethical, legal, and safety issues involved in clinical trials. Technological advances provide diverse opportunities to improve access, develop quality nurse-client relationships, and understand the client's experience, wishes, and preferences needed to maintain overall health.

TRENDS IN PSYCHIATRIC-MENTAL HEALTH NURSING

Psychiatric health care systems are influenced by the social and economic climate of the times. Before and during the nineteenth century these systems were predominantly paternal and closed to nurses (Peplau, 1989). During the 1960s and 1970s changes within health facilities paralleled the deinstitutionalization of mental health care. Social concerns for the mentally ill and legislative support for preventive interventions were the basis of funding and training for advanced-practice psychiatric-mental health nurses. Before the 1980s, mental health facilities were comprised primarily of clients with chronic mental illness.

The 1980s drastically changed psychiatric nursing in several ways. Initially, there was a noticeable drop in funding and traineeships from the NIMH. A lack of funding led to a decrease in the number of advanced-level psychiatric-mental health nurses. Second, there was an enormous growth in freestanding

psychiatric facilities that resulted in client abuse and misuse of health care to fill empty beds. Finally, an outcry from clients, their families, and client advocacy groups led to numerous investigations and a subsequent decrease in the number of psychiatric admissions and eventual closure of psychiatric units and hospitals. These changes affected job security and increased job loss of nurses working in the private sector. Managed care continues to have a profound impact on mental health care and offers psychiatric nurses opportunities to carve out innovative roles that meet the holistic needs of clients. Evidence-based health care is the driving force behind treatment approaches, client responses, and treatment efficacy. Understanding the emphases of these strategies and integrating holistic health care concepts into practice are crucial to the survival of the psychiatric-mental health specialty.

Future trends of psychiatric nursing will be determined by a number of factors. As psychiatric-mental health nursing moves into the next century, it is challenged to meet the complex demands of advanced technology; client advocacy groups; payors, telecommunications; and cultural, societal, and economic transitions. Research continues to direct and provide the basis for understanding mental illness in such areas as neurobiology, molecular and cellular neuroscience, genetics, psychodynamics, psychosocial rehabilitation, and exploration of life span and cultural issues. New lifestyle patterns will continue to affect societal, economic, cultural, and legislative agendas, and health care delivery systems.

CONCEPTS OF PRACTICE

Other solutions include integrating complex concepts into nursing practice. Expanding neurobiological technological advances and psychosocial factors are major issues that presently confront psychiatric nurses. During the 1990s Angela McBride (1990) supported this notion and urged psychiatric-mental health nurses to reexamine their future roles in meeting societal needs. She advocated integrating evidence-based practice with revaluing biological knowledge and becoming fundamentally reacquainted with care and caring.

McBride (1990) also suggested that the research agenda for psychiatric nurses is an important component of integrating biological concepts into practice. Areas that need change include the following:

◆ Closing the gap of nursing knowledge regarding the relevance of neurobiology of mental illness

◆ Implementing the NIMH agenda

◆ Revamping nursing curricula to interface psychiatric-mental health nursing with the biological and behavioral sciences

McBride further stressed the importance of nurses reassociating themselves with caring, described as the following:

◆ Being responsive to clients rather than being judgmental

◆ Using the concept of nurturing as one that encompasses the protection of client rights

- Having a health care system that fosters effective communication at all levels
- Exploring ethical issues and values associated with professional commitment of working with mentally ill clients

Other nursing leaders support these concepts and advocate increased collaboration within psychiatric nursing practice, academia, specialties, and organizations to confront complex issues and factors affecting nursing in the next decade (Pothier, Stuart, Puskar, & Babich, 1990). As health care systems place a greater priority on evidence-based practice, psychiatric nurses must respond proactively by providing quality and holistic health care to clients with complex needs (Gilliss & Mundinger, 1998). As payors and legislatures continue to govern health care delivery systems and mental health care, psychiatric-mental health nurse leaders, nurses, and nurse educators must play key roles in redefining the role and significance of this specialty.

DIRECTIONS FOR NURSING EDUCATION

The twenty-first century finds psychiatric nursing education in a dilemma arising from the peril of losing its distinctiveness and status in the nursing profession (McCabe, 2000). McCabe asserts that the core of current psychiatric nursing textbooks reflects two broad bodies of knowledge that focus on psychosocial content and neurobiology, genetics, and immunology. Moreover, she notes concern about the addition of new knowledge without deleting the old knowledge and that this dichotomy runs the risk of blurring "professional boundaries" (p. 112). Her comments also reflect the crisis in psychiatric nursing that constitutes a lack of specialty identity and a decline in graduate school enrollment (Center for Mental Health Services, 1996; Delaney, Chisholm, Clement, & Merwin, 1999). Other nursing leaders express dismay about the sharp reduction in the content and clinical experiences in psychiatric-mental health nursing (Dumas, 1994; Olson, 1996; Taylor, 1997).

Unfortunately, this trend also reveals a decline or limited exposure to psychiatric nursing in baccalaureate nursing curricula and a lack of interest in pursuing graduate studies in this specialty. Conceivably, the standing debate about Clinical Nurse Specialist and PMHNP has also contributed to the decline in graduate enrollment. Growing concerns about the lack of identity and decrease in clinical and classroom exposure in Bachelors of Science in Nursing programs suggest that nurse educators need to develop strategies that address these concerns by developing curricula that reaffirm the relevance of psychiatric nursing education. McCabe (2000) has several recommendations that address the current psychiatric nursing crisis and they include the following:

- Reconceptualize what constitutes the core psychiatric nursing content (generalist and advanced)
- Identify critical clinical competencies that reflect the core content, role, and scope of psychiatric-mental health nursing

- Identify and standardize measurable clinical outcomes based on content and competencies
- Establish a national research agenda that expands and builds on the psychiatric nurse's unique knowledge base

McCabe (2000) also suggests that changes in nursing curricula can be made by incorporating core concepts, such as relatedness, adaptation, regulation, vulnerability, integrity, and efficacy and integrating them in the care of clients who are mentally ill. These core concepts provide a theoretical framework that encompasses the educational needs of generalist and advanced-practice psychiatric nurses. Topics of course work, include sleep cycles, circadian rhythms, stress-related responses, neurological assessment, psychosocial and neurobiological factors that contribute to client compliance, early signs and symptoms of violence, and the neurobiological basis of mental illness (McBride, 1990).

Other variables affecting nursing education include growing changes in the health care system. Based on the Pew Health Care Professions Commission report, all professions, including nursing, need to meet the challenges of the year 2005 (O'Neil, 1993). The commission's report projected a changing health care system that will have limited resources, client-centered health care and treatment outcomes, and health provider accountability. Client-centered health care must integrate gender and developmental, cultural, and societal factors that influence treatment outcomes. These projections offered considerations for contemporary and future nursing education.

Emphasis on quality care across the continuum has become the cornerstone of health care delivery systems. The Committee on the Quality of Health Care in America and National Institute of Medicine (IOM)'s, *Crossing the Quality Chasm* (2001) and previous publication *To Err is Human: Building a Safer Health System* have revolutionized health care. The IOM determined a need for quintessential changes in the health care delivery systems. Chief emphasis was placed on the transforming or redesigning of health with evidence-based processes and technologies, chronic disease management, client-centric care, and implementation by interdisciplinary teams. Six recommendations focus on safety, evidence-based care, client-centered approaches, timeliness, efficiency, and equitable care to all populations (IOM, 2001).

SOCIETAL CHANGES

As the health care system strives to improve access to care for populations at risk, such as women, children, low-income groups, the homeless, and the elderly, psychiatric nurses will be confronted with redefining their role. Health disparities also jeopardize and decrease access to quality mental health services. A pivotal role of psychiatric nurses is identifying vulnerable populations; developing cultural competence to address the needs of diverse individuals; and collaborating with clients, families, and other clinicians to better provide client-centered care. Mental illness is increasing, especially among the chronically ill and those misusing substances. Society is faced with vast challenges that must address deteriorating social structures, global epidemic of AIDS, increased personal and workplace violence, inadequate access to health care, and rising poverty levels. Low salaries and unemployment continue to increase and family breakdown affects all levels of society. These situations increase the incidence of crisis and mental illness among individuals across the life span. Other societal changes include the technological advances in cyberspace and the Internet, which provide consumers with an array of information regarding conventional and complementary therapies. The precise effects of the information systems remain obscure, but they are likely to motivate psychiatric nurses to remain abreast of client-centered health care approaches and develop novel communication skills. In brief, societal changes continue to influence the health of its citizens, particularly vulnerable populations. Psychiatric nurses must be visionaries and take the lead and advocate and promote health across the life span in vast venues.

Health promotion across the life span requires nurses to be primary advocates for health promotion and prevention from the time clients enter the health care system until their treatment ends. Complex client needs require psychiatric-mental health nurses to integrate neurobiological, psychosocial, developmental, cultural, and holistic concepts into their practice so they can effectively assess, direct, and evaluate health care. Survival of psychiatric-mental health nursing will be contingent on the nurses' ability to work effectively with others to navigate complex health care systems and identify and develop evidence-based interventions. These factors are critical to health promotion and disease prevention and evidence-based nursing practice.

HEALTH CARE TRENDS

The health care continuum of mental health care encompasses vast services with a focus on preventive principles, primary care, holistic and client-centered health care delivery models. These concepts provide a wealth of opportunities for psychiatric-mental health nurses to redefine their roles as major providers in a changing health care system (ANA, 1994; Billings, 1993b). Many clients with psychiatric disorders receive their mental health care from non mental health providers in diverse practice settings. Psychiatric-mental health nurses need to be in these clinics providing this care. Nursing interventions that promote health and prevention are critical to expanded acute-, primary-, and community-based care. Many clients are being treated in community facilities such as day hospitals, private practice, day treatment centers, hospices, crisis stabilization units, partial hospitals or day hospitals, homes, and community-based and primary care mental health centers. Other mental health care services include assertive community treatment programs, home health, mobile crisis units, therapeutic foster care, telemental health, and respite care. Nursing interventions include interdisciplinary mental health care that uses case management, telemedicine, psychoeducation, prescriptive authority, psychotherapy, medication clinics, and dual diagnosis groups. A continued lack of funding impels nurses and other health care professionals to maximize resources and develop evidence-based treatment to meet the present and future needs of a society under tremendous stress.

COLLABORATION OF NURSING ORGANIZATIONS

As psychiatric-mental health nursing continues its path in the present century, other significant changes are occurring. A new partnership within a number of major psychiatric organizations reflects the bid of these organizations to collaborate and revolutionize the scope and standards of psychiatric-mental health nursing practice with the ANA. Major nursing organizations engaging in this endeavor include the Coalition of Psychiatric Nursing, the American Psychiatric Nurses Association, and the International Society of Psychiatric-Mental Health Nurses, which represents the Alliance of Psychiatric Mental Health Nurses. The Alliance of Psychiatric-Mental Health Nurses represents the previous Society for Education and Research in Psychiatric-Mental Health Nursing, the Association of Child and Adolescent Psychiatric Nurses, and the International Society of Psychiatric Consultation-Liaison Nurses. This concerted unifying effort of psychiatric-mental health nurses enables them to form a powerful and collaborative partnership among organizations. These organizations play key roles in addressing legislative issues that affect nursing practice and the care of the mentally ill. This collaborative tone is crucial to making successful advances and changes within a transforming society and health care system and responding proactively and effectively to the needs of the psychiatric-mental health nurse and the consumer (Billings, 1993a).

SUMMARY

◆ Historically, the treatment and perception of the mentally ill have been influenced by religious and social norms. Treatment has varied from brutal, inhumane torture in asylums to community-based residential settings.

◆ Psychiatric nurses did not exist before 1882, at which time the McLean hospital in Massachusetts began the first formal training for psychiatric nurses.

◆ As psychiatric-mental health nursing practice continues to evolve, it is a far cry from the roles of custodian and controller.

◆ The 1990s heralded in the decade of the brain, and psychiatric nursing emerged as a specialty that required integration of neurobiological and behavioral concepts.

◆ The twenty-first century is placing greater emphasis on neuroscience, genetics, psychosocial rehabilitation, and the integration of client-centered mental health care. Even though these prevailing issues are important, psychiatric nurses face a more daunting challenge—the survival of their specialty.

◆ During the twenty-first century, psychiatric nurses are facing a crisis stemming from a lack of identity, failing stature in the nursing profession, and declining psychiatric nursing clinical experiences and content.

- Nurse educators must respond to this crisis by developing curricula that reconceptualize core content and provide classroom and clinical experiences that enable nurses to apply theoretically sound and evidence-based therapeutics to the care of the mentally ill.

- The challenges of the twenty-first century continue to mirror societal, economic, and legislative factors on individuals throughout the life span.

- Psychiatric-mental health nurses can rise to the occasion by identifying clients at risk, and standardizing measurable clinical outcomes (McCabe, 2000), and participating in research endeavors that enable them to advance and build on their unique knowledge base. This process also involves redefining the role of psychiatric-mental health nursing within a health care system in crisis, and psychiatric-mental health nurses positioning themselves in key positions to direct client care and navigate complex health care systems.

STUDY QUESTIONS

The following three questions apply to this case history.

You are caring for Ms. Jones, a 75-year-old retiree, who has been diagnosed with major depressive episode and is being treated in her home. She insists on taking her antidepressant in the evening although the medication bottle says one capsule in the morning because side effects may interfere with sleep. She reports taking this medication every evening and has not had problems sleeping.

1. What is the most appropriate nursing action?
   a. Allow her to take the medication as she wishes.
   b. Insist that she take the medication at the recommended time.
   c. Report her actions to her primary care provider.
   d. Educate her about the medication's side effects that will interfere with sleep.

2. The best explanation for the nurse's action in this case reflects which of the following?
   a. Culturally sensitive considerations
   b. Client-centered health care
   c. Client safety
   d. Cost containment

3. Besides medications, what types of care is Ms. Jones likely to be receiving under managed care?
   a. Partial hospitalization
   b. Intensive psychotherapy
   c. Long-term inpatient treatment
   d. Occupational therapy

4. During the early history era, healers were often sought to treat the mentally ill. Major treatment consisted of herbs, ointments, and precious stones. Which of the following best describes the basis of this treatment during the early history era?
   a. Mental illness was associated with sin and demonic possession.
   b. Mental illness was curable when these special measures were used.

   c. Mental illness was associated with special powers.
   d. Mental illness was often treated humanely.

5. You are caring for Mr. Murray who is experiencing high anxiety. Which of the following interventions has its roots in interpersonal theory?
   a. Forming a nurse-client relationship to facilitate expression of the client's feelings
   b. Explaining the adaptive nature of stress management
   c. Discussing the client's ambivalence and effects associated with his symptoms
   d. Providing health education about the role of stress and anxiety

6. The most significant contributions of somatic therapies to psychiatric nursing practice is best described by which of the following?
   a. Miss Lily is more agitated after electroshock therapy and requires more nursing care.
   b. Mr. Barnes' symptoms improve and offer nurses opportunities to use psychosocial interventions.
   c. Mr. King is more sedated and less agitated and requires less nursing care.
   d. Mrs. Moore is calmer post lobotomy and requires more nursing care.

7. World War II played a pivotal role in the practice of psychiatric-mental health nursing. Which statement best describes the reasons for these changes?
   a. Clients were likely to be seen in community-based clinics after the war.
   b. Nurses were visible in caring for the wounded and restoring psychological care.
   c. Nurses were seen as the lone health care providers during the postwar era.
   d. The role of nurses was no longer custodial, although they were not part of the mental health team.

8. Major legislation that transformed psychiatric nursing included all of the following *except:*
   a. the National Mental Health Act of 1946
   b. U.S. Congress Proclamation "Decade of the Brain"
   c. the Community Mental Health Act of 1963
   d. the Deinstitutionalization Act of 1961

9. Gerald Caplan's contributions to psychiatric nursing are significant and underlie community-based mental health care. Which of the following is the best description of primary prevention?
   a. Discussing options to a family whose child has just overdosed on medications
   b. Administering medication to a client exhibiting psychotic symptoms
   c. Admitting a client to an acute inpatient unit to manage his suicidal behaviors
   d. Providing crisis intervention to a man who has just lost his job

10. Advances in psychiatry over the past decade have made a great impact on psychiatric nursing. Efforts to integrate neurobiology and psychosocial concepts remain a

priority. Which of the following situations best emanates this concept?
a. Establishing rapport and administering a medication to an anxious client
b. Using crisis intervention and deep breathing exercises to reduce anxiety
c. Administering an antidepressant and teaching skills to reduce negative thoughts
d. All of the above

11. Telemedicine has numerous benefits for clients being treated in their homes. Which of the following depicts a *major disadvantage* of telemedicine?
a. The client reports that his insurance is willing to pay for services despite cost.
b. The nurse has difficulty forming a trusting relationship with the client.
c. The nurse encourages the family to take the client to the nearest emergency room.
d. The client calls seeking assistance in dealing with his anger.

12. Mr. Effiong reports that he is using an herb that controls his anxiety and wonders if it is safe. What is the *most important* consideration when answering this question?
a. Concerns about the actual benefits of this therapy
b. Established protocols regarding herbal therapy
c. The nurse's personal beliefs about such therapy
d. Cultural and individual preferences

13. The American Nurses Association played a key role in legitimizing the significance of psychiatric-mental health nursing in the nursing profession with its 1967 publication, *Statement on Psychiatric Nursing Practice*. Which of the following had the most significant influence on these efforts?
a. Influence by renowned leaders in psychiatric nursing, namely, Peplau and Sills
b. Recognition of the impact of psychiatric nursing education and meeting the needs of the mentally ill
c. Validation of the significance of clinical preparation of psychiatric nursing in nursing curricula
d. All of the above

14. Which of the following organizations played a critical role in the advancement of graduate-prepared psychiatric-mental health nursing?
a. American Nurses Association
b. American Nurses Credentialing Center
c. National Institute of Mental Health (NIMH)
d. National League of Nursing

15. Which of the following trends is most likely to have the most influence on the future of psychiatric nursing?
a. Increased graduate school enrollments
b. Advances and research in neurobiology, neuroscience, and genetics
c. A plethora of studies focusing on psychodynamic mental health care
d. Increased inpatient admissions and decreased community-based care

16. Survival of the psychiatric-mental health specialty requires nurse educators to make all of the following curricula changes *except:*
a. reconceptualize what constitutes psychiatric nursing content
b. integrate neurobiological rather than psychosocial concepts into mental health care
c. standardize clinical outcomes based on content and competencies
d. develop client-centered and evidence-based interventions

17. Historically psychiatric nursing has focused on symptom management. The current trend in mental health care is best described by:
a. Mr. C's symptoms are under control and he no longer hears voices.
b. Mr. C is gainfully employed and lives in a residential housing unit.
c. Mr. C participates in an outpatient substance abuse program.
d. Mr. C takes his medication as ordered and lives with his parents.

18. Mr. Lean is a 27-year-old client recently diagnosed with schizophrenia and his current medication is an atypical antipsychotic medication. Based on your understanding about his illness and treatment it is imperative for psychiatric nurses to:
a. Maintain competency in physical assessment skills to reduce health-related problems
b. Assess for major side effects associated with pharmacological interventions
c. Collaborate with the client and family to ensure client-centered health care
d. All of the above

RESOURCES

Please note that because Internet resources are of a time-sensitive nature and URL addresses may change or be deleted, searches should also be conducted by association or topic.

Internet Resources
Professional Organizations and Advocacy Groups Concerned with Mental Health Issues

www.nimh.nih.gov   National Institute of Mental Health

www.healthfinder.gov   Department of Health and Human Services

www.nami.org   NAMI national Web page

nursingworld.org/anp/pcatalog.cfm   American Nurses Association Web site

www.nursingworld.org/ancc/   American Nurses Credentialing Center (2002)

www.apna.org   Journal of the American Psychiatric Nurses Association

ANCC@ana.org   American Nurses Credentialing Center
www.surgeongeneral.gov/library/mentalhealth/summary.
html Surgeon General
http://www.tcns.org/   Leininger, M (1998). What is transcultural nursing? (Accessed September 17, 2005)
http://gucchd.georgetown.edu/nccc/selfassessment.html
National Center for Cultural Competence—Georgetown
Center for Child and Human Development (Accessed
September 6, 2005)
http://gucchd.georgetown.edu/nccc/orgselfassess.html#
benefits Self-Assessment: An essential component of
Cultural Competence (Accessed September 6, 2005)
http://www.hcqualitycommission.gov/final Advisory
Commission Protection and Quality in the Health Care
Industry (1998). Quality first: Better health care for all
Americans. (Accessed August 23, 2005)

REFERENCES

Aguilera, D., & Messick, J. (1970). *Crisis intervention: Theory and methodology.* St. Louis, MO: Mosby.

Alexander, F. (1950). *Psychosomatic medicine, its principles and applications.* New York: Norton.

American Nurses Association. (1967). *Statement on psychiatric nursing practice.* Kansas City, MO: Author.

American Nurses Association. (1976). *Statement on psychiatric and mental health nursing practice.* Kansas City, MO: Author.

American Nurses Association. (1982). *Standards of psychiatric and mental health nursing practice.* Kansas City, MO: Author.

American Nurses Association. (1991). *Nursing agenda for health care reform.* Kansas City, MO: Author.

American Nurses Association. (1994). *Statement on psychiatric-mental health clinical nursing practice and standards of psychiatric-mental health clinical nursing practice.* Washington, DC: American Publishing.

American Nurses Association. (2000). *Scope and Standards of psychiatric-mental health nursing practice.* Washington, DC: American Nurses Publishing.

American Nurses Cedentialing Center. (1993). *American nurses cedentialing catalog* (p.3). Washington, DC: Author.

American Nurses Credentialing Center. (2005). *American nurses credentialing center catalog,* (p. 3). Washington, DC: Author.

Bassuk, E. L., & Gerson, S. (1978). Deinstitutionalization and mental health services. *Scientific American, 238,* 46–53.

Beers, C. (1908). *A mind that found itself.* New York: Doubleday.

Billings, C. V. (1993a). Forging professional partnerships. *American Nurses Association Council Perspectives, 2,* 46–53.

Billings, C. V. (1993b). The "possible" dream of mental health reform. *The American Nurse, 25(2),* 5–9.

Billings, C. (2000). Scope and standards of psychiatric-mental health clinical nursing practice—2000 edition. *APNA News, 12,* 6.

Caplan, G. (1961). *An approach to community mental health.* New York: Basic Books.

Carrasquillo, O., Orva, E. J., Brennan, T. A., & Burstin, H. R. (1999). Impact of language barriers on patient satisfaction in an emergency department. *Journal of General Internal Medicine, 14,* 82–87.

Center for Mental Health Services. (1996). An update on human resources in mental health. In R. W. Manderscheild & M. A. Sonnenschien (Eds.), *Mental health, United States* (DHHS Publication No. 96-3098). Washington, DC: U.S. Government Printing Office.

Chamberlain, J. G. (1983). The role of the federal government in development of psychiatric nursing. *Journal of Psychosocial Nursing, 21,* 11–18.

Conolly, J. (1968). *The construction and government of lunatic asylums.* London: Dawsons of Pall Mall.

Cowan, W. M., Kopnisky, K. L., & Hyman, S. E. (2002). The human genome project and its impact on psychiatry. *Annual Review of Neuroscience, 25,* 1–50.

Delaney, K. R., Chisholm, M., Clement, J., & Merwin, E. I. (1999). Trends in mental health nursing education. *Archives of Psychiatric Nursing, 13(2),* 67–73.

Dumas, R. G. (1994). Psychiatric nursing in an era of change. *Journal of Psychosocial Nursing, 32(1),* 11–14.

Eisenberg, D. M., Kessler, R. C., Foster, C., Norlock, F. E., Calkins, D. R., & Delbanco, T. L. (1993). Unconventional medicine in the United States. *New England Journal of Medicine, 328,* 246–252.

Ellenberger, H. F. (1974). Psychiatry from ancient to modern times. In S. Areti (Ed.), *American handbook of psychiatry* (2nd ed., pp. 3–27). New York: Basic Books.

Ernst, E., & Fugh-Berman, A. (2002). Complementary and alternative medicine: What is it all about? *Occupational and Environmental Medicine, 59,* 140–144.

Flores, G., Abreu, M., & Tomany-Korman, S. C. (2005). Limited English proficiency, primary language at home, and disparities in children's health care: How language barriers are measured matters. *Public Health Report, 120,* 418–430.

Galambos, C., Rocha, C., McCarter, A. K., & Chansuthus, D. (2004). Managed care and mental health: Personal realities. *Journal of Health and Social Policy, 20,* 1–22.

Gilliss, C., & Mundinger, M. (1998). How is the role of the advanced practice nurse changing? In E. O'Neil & J. Coffman (Eds.), *Strategies for the future of nursing: Changing roles, responsibilities, and employment patterns of registered nurses* (pp. 171–191). San Francisco: Jossey-Bass.

Glittenberg, J. A. (1963). The role of the nurse in outpatient psychiatric clinics. *The American Journal of Orthopsychiatry, 33,* 713–716.

Institute of Medicine. (2001). *Crossing the quality chasm. A new health system for the 21st century.* Washington, DC: National Academy Press.

International Association of Psychosocial Rehabilitation Services Publication Committee (Eds.). (1997). *Practice guidelines for the psychiatric rehabilitation of persons with severe and persistent mental illness in a managed care environment.* Columbia, MD: Author.

Isaacs, S. (1961). Obituary: Melanie Klein 1882–1960. *Journal of Child Psychology and Psychiatry, 2,* 1–4.

Joint Commission on Mental Illness and Health. (1961). *Action for mental health.* New York: Basic Books.

Kanner, I. (1935). *Child psychiatry.* Springfield, IL: Charles C. Thomas.

Kessler, R. C., Demler, O., Frank, R. G., Olfson, M., Pincus, H. A., Walters, E. E., Wang, P., Wells, K. B., & Zaslavsky, A. M. (2005). Prevalence and treatment of mental disorders, 1990–2003. *New England Journal of Medicine, 352,* 2515–2523.

Kessler, R. C., Zhao, S., Katz, S. J., Kouzis, A. C., Frank, R. G., Edlund, M., & Leaf, P. (2005). Past-year use of outpatient services for psychiatric problems in the national comorbidity survey. *American Journal of Psychiatry, 156,* 115–123.

Kim, S., Kverno, K., Lee, E. M., Park, J. H., Lee, H. H., & Kim, H. L. (2006). Development of a music group psychotherapy intervention for the primary prevention of adjustment difficulties in adolescent girls. *Journal of Child and Adolescent Nursing, 19,* 103–111.

Leininger, M. (1969). Community psychiatric nursing: Trends, issues, and problems. *Perspectives in Psychiatric Care, 71,* 10–20.

Leininger, M. (1973). *Contemporary issues in mental health nursing.* Boston: Little, Brown.

Lewis, N. C. D. (1974). American psychiatry from its beginnings to World War II. In S. Areti (Ed.), *American handbook of psychiatry* (2nd ed., pp. 28–42). New York: Basic Books.

Mayberry, R. M., Mili, F., & Ofili, E. (2000). Racial and ethnic differences in access to medical care. *Medical Care Research Review, 57* (suppl. 1), 108–145.

McBride, A. B. (1990). Psychiatric nursing in the 1990s. *Archives of Psychiatric Nursing, 4,* 21–28.

McCabe, S. (2000). Bring psychiatric nursing into the twenty-first century. *Archives of Psychiatric Nursing, 14*(3), 109–116.

Mellow, J. (1967). Evolution of nursing therapy through research. *Psychiatric Opinion, 4,* 15–21.

Meltzer, B. (1997). Telemedicine in emergency psychiatry. *Psychiatric Services, 48*(9), 1141–1142.

Mericle, B. P. (1983). The male psychiatric nurse. *Journal of Psychosocial Nursing, 21,* 28–34.

Narrow, W. E., Rae, D. S., Robins, L. N., Regier, D. A. (2002). Revised prevalence estimates of mental disorders in the United States. *Archives of General Psychiatry, 59,* 115–123.

Nightingale, F. (1859). *Notes on nursing.* London: Harrison & Sons.

Olson, T. (1996). Fundamental and special: The dilemma of psychiatric-mental health nursing. *Archives of Psychiatric Nursing, 10*(1), 3–10.

O'Neil, E. (1993). *Health professions education for the future: Schools in service to the nation.* San Francisco: PEW Health Professions Commission.

Parades, H. (1979). Future needs for psychiatrists and other mental health personnel. *Archives of General Psychiatry, 36*(12), 1401–1408.

Parse, R. R. (1992). Nursing knowledge for the 21st century: An international commitment. *Nursing Science Quarterly, 5*(9), 8–12.

Pender, N. J. (1996). *Health promotion in nursing practice* (3rd ed.). Stamford, CT: Appleton & Lange.

Peplau, H. E. (1952). *Interpersonal relations in nursing: A conceptual framework for psychodynamic nursing.* New York: GP Putnam & Sons.

Peplau, H. E. (1989). Future directions in psychiatric nursing from the perspective of history. *Journal of Psychosocial Nursing, 2,* 18–28.

Pothier, P. C., Stuart, G. W., Puskar, K., & Babich, K. (1990). Dilemmas and direction for psychiatric nursing in the 1990s. *Archives of Psychiatric Nursing, 5,* 284–291.

Richards, L. A. (1911). *Reminiscences of Linda Richards.* Boston: M. Barrows.

Scull, A. T. (1982). *Museums of madness.* Hammondsworth, Middlesex, London: Penguin Education.

Seyle, H. (1956). *The stress of life.* New York: McGraw-Hill.

Shattuck, L. (1948). *Report of the sanitary commission of mental health 1850.* Cambridge, MA: Harvard University Press.

Sills, G. M. (1973). Historical developments and issues in psychiatric-mental health nursing. In M. L. Leininger (Ed.), *Contemporary issues in mental health nursing* (pp. 125–136). Boston: Little, Brown.

Smoyak, S. (1975). *The psychiatric nurse as a family therapist.* New York: John Wiley & Sons, Inc.

Stevens, L. F., & Henrie, D. D. (1966). A history of psychiatric nursing. *Bulletin of the Menninger Clinic, 30,* 32–38.

Stokes, G. A., Williams, F. A. S., Davidites, R. M., Bulbulyen, A., & Ullman, M. (1969). *The roles of psychiatric nurses in community mental health practice: A giant step.* New York: Faculty Press.

Sullivan, H. S. (1940). *Conceptions in modern psychiatry.* New York: WW Norton.

Sullivan, H. S. (1953). *The interpersonal theory of psychiatry.* New York: Norton.

Taylor, C. M. (1997). Finite resources—finite demands. *Archives of Psychiatric Nursing, 11*(3), 105–106.

Tudor, G. E. (1952). A sociopsychiatric nursing approach to intervention in a problem of mutual withdrawal on a mental hospital ward. *Psychiatry: Journal of the Study of Interpersonal Processes, 15*(2), 193–217.

Tudor, G. E. (1970). A sociopsychiatric nursing approach to intervention in a problem of mutual withdrawal on a mental hospital ward. *Perspectives in Psychiatric Care, 8*(1), 11–35. (Reprinted from *Psychiatry: Journal for the Study of Interpersonal Processes, 15*[2], 1952.)

U.S. Congress. (1989). *Decade of the brain proclamation.* Pub. L. No. 101-58 [HJ Res. 174], 130 Stat. 152-154 (July 25, 1989).

U.S. Department of Health and Human Services. (1999). *Mental health: A report of the surgeon general —executive summary.* Rockville, MD: U.S. Department of Health and Human Services Administration, Center for Mental Health Services, National Institutes of Health, National Institute of Mental Health. Retrieved June 12, 2007, from http://www.surgeongeneral.gov/library/mentalhealth/summary.html

U.S. Department of Health and Human Services. *Healthy people 2010: Understanding and improving health.* 2nd ed. Washington, DC: U.S. Government Printing Office, 23–28.

Warren, B. J. (2000). Cultural competence: A best practice process for psychiatric-mental health nursing. *Journal of American Psychiatric Association, 6,* 135–138.

Werneke, U., Turner, T., & Priebe, S. (2006). Complementary medicines in psychiatry: Review of effectiveness and safety. *British Journal of Psychiatry, 188,* 109–121.

Yellowlees, P. M. (2005). Successful developing a telemedicine system. *Journal of Telemedicine and Telecare, 11,* 331–335.

SUGGESTED READINGS

Antai-Otong, D. (2007). *Nurse-client communication: A life span approach.* Sudbury, MA: Jones and Bartlett.

Leininger, M. (1995).Transcultural nursing. Development, focus, importance, and historical development. In M. Leininger (Ed.), *Transcultural Nursing: Concepts, theories, research, & practices,* 2nd ed (pp. 3–57). New York, NY: McGraw-Hill.

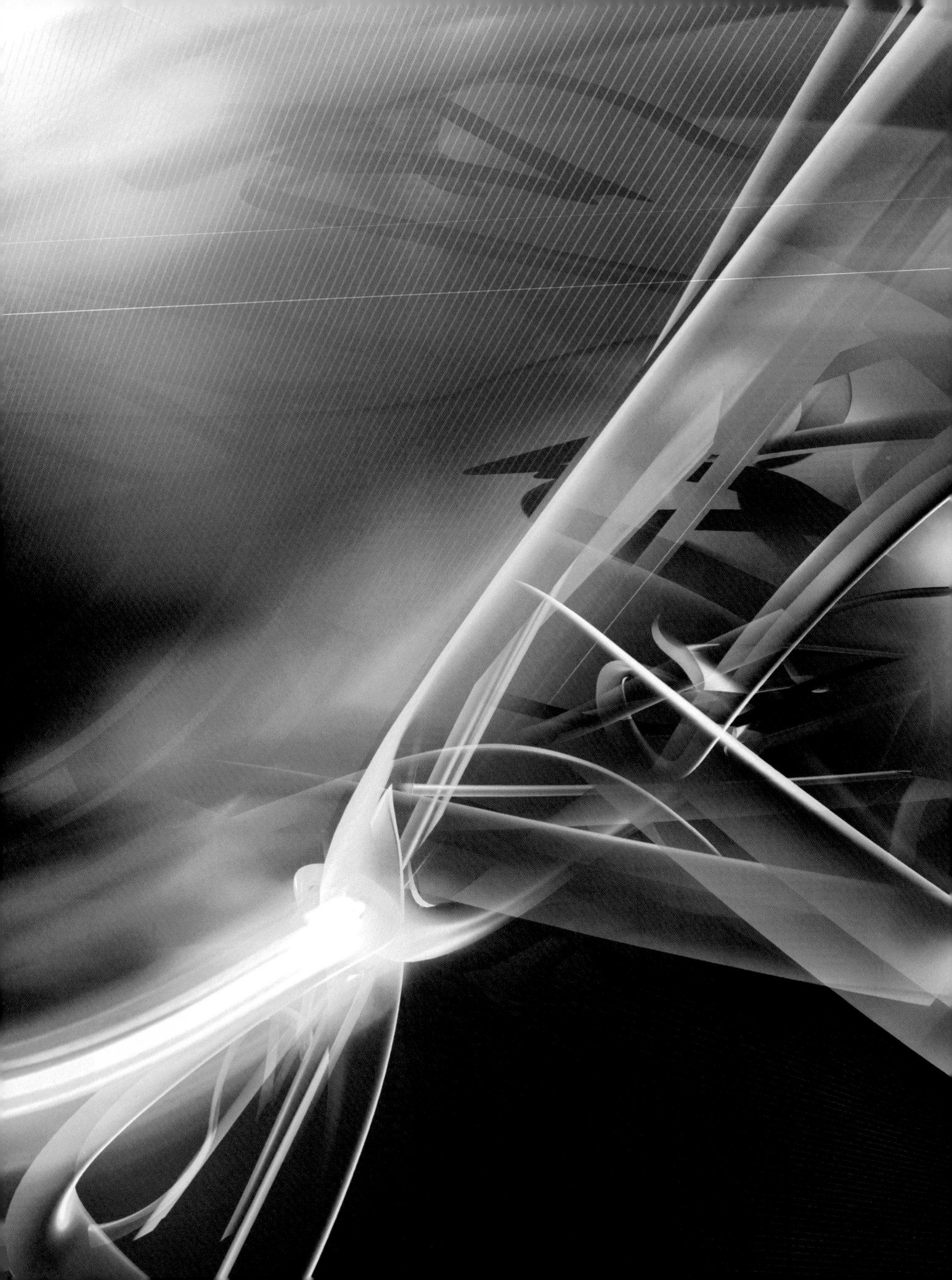

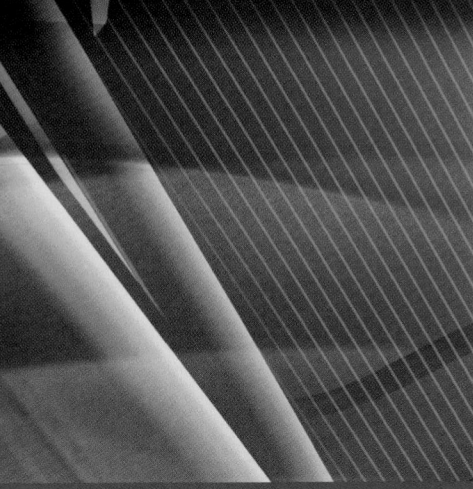

CHAPTER 2

Concepts of Psychiatric Care: Therapeutic Models

Deborah Antai-Otong, MS, APRN, BC, FAAN
Martha Sanford, PhD, RN

KEY TERMS

Anima: The female aspect of the male personality.

Animus: The masculine aspect of the female personality.

Archetypes: Primordial images that serve as the building blocks of collective unconscious.

Attachment: A classic term for the primary tie between a child and her caregiver and a process seen as evolving and biologically adaptive and critical to emotional and physiological development and survival.

Attachment System: A system that is instinctual or motivational and, like hunger and thirst, integrates the infant's memory processes, prompting the child to satisfy them by interacting with the caregiver.

Chronobiology: Field of science and medicine that explores the many bodily changes governed by the hours and the seasons; includes studies of cellular rhythms all the way through those of populations and ecosystems.

Circadian Rhythms: Biological cycles occurring over an approximate 24-hour period and influencing biochemical, biological, and behavioral processes.

Classic Conditioning: A form of learning in which existing responses are attached to new stimuli by pairing those stimuli with those that naturally elicit the response; also referred to as respondent conditioning.

Cognitive Processes: Higher cortical mental processes, including perception, memory, abstraction, and reasoning, by which one acquires knowledge, solves problems, employs judgment, and makes plans.

Defense Mechanisms: Unconscious self-protective processes that seek to protect the ego from intense and overwhelming feelings of affect and impulses.

Dialectical behavior therapy (DBT): A psychosocial cognitive behavioral therapy approach used in the treatment of borderline personality disorder. It is an adaptation of behavioral therapy using skills training to help the client with borderline personality disorder and other impulsivity disorders effectively control or manage intense emotional states and associated self-harm or self-injurious behaviors.

Drive: Instinctual urges and impulses arising from biological and psychological needs.

Ego: The part of the mind that mediates between external reality and inner wishes and impulses.

Entropy: The tendency to increase randomness by the degradation of energy; the running-down of a system.

Equifinality: The sameness of the end result starting from various points.

Eros: The instinct or drive for love.

Id: The sum total of biological instincts, including sexual and aggressive impulses.

Inferiority Complex: An exaggeration of feelings of inadequacy and insecurity resulting in defensiveness and anxiety.

Infradian Rhythms: Biological variations with a frequency lower than circadian (rhythms that have longer, slower cycles than circadian rhythms).

Libido: The basic driving force of personality in Freud's system; it includes sexual energy but is not restricted to it.

Modeling: A form of learning in which a person observes another person perform a desired response.

Negentropy: The counterforce to entropy; the evolving or more complete organization, complexity, and ability to convert resources.

Operant Conditioning: A type of learning in which responses are modified by their consequences. Reinforcement increases the likelihood of future occurrences of the reinforced response; punishment and extinction decrease the likelihood of future occurrences of the responses they follow.

Persona: A disguised or masked attitude useful in interacting with one's environment but frequently at variance with one's true identity.

Recovery: Refers to a state of wellness or function characterized by symptom management and attaining an optimal level of function and quality of life. It is client-centered and based on principles of hope, healing, and optimism.

Reinforcement: In classical conditioning, the process following the conditioned stimuli with the unconditioned stimulus; in operant conditioning, the rewarding of desired responses.

Repression: An unconscious process that removes anxiety-producing thoughts, desires, or memories from the conscious awareness.

Resilience: The capacity to recover from or adapt to distress, overwhelming change, or potentially harmful risk factors.

Schemata: Cognitive structures, or patterns, that consist of the person's beliefs, values, and assumptions.

Self-efficacy: Refers to the expectation that one can effectively cope with and master situations, such as addictions, achieving desired outcomes through one's own personal efforts.

Shadow: Carl Jung's term that refers to the unconscious.

Superego: The part of the personality structure that evolves out of the ego and reflects early moral training and parental injunctions.

Thanatos: The instinct toward death and self-destruction.

Theory: An organized and systematic set of statements related to significant questions in a discipline. Theories describe, explain, predict, or prescribe responses, events, situations, conditions, or relationships. Theories consist of concepts that are related to each other.

Untradian Rhythms: Biological variations with a frequency higher (less than 24 hours) than circadian (rhythms that have shorter, faster cycles than circadian rhythms). Biological rhythms refer to cyclic variations in biological and biochemical function, activity, and emotional state.

Zeitgeber: A synchronizer or periodic environmental stimulus that is the dominant factor in determining a rhythm.

COMPETENCIES

Upon completion of this chapter, the learner should be able to:

1. Identify the basic concepts of each theory discussed in the chapter.
2. Discuss the assumptions concerning the contributing factors that lead to mental disorders.
3. Understand the importance of using theories in practice.
4. Discuss how each theory suggests a person can be helped.
5. Identify the stages of growth and development in various theories.
6. Compare and contrast the developmental stages according to various theorists.
7. Describe the implications of theories for nurses.
8. Discuss the assumptions about people derived from each theory.
9. Use concepts from the theories to design interventions.
10. Assess cognitive distortions used by the psychiatric nurse and by clients.
11. Describe the client outcomes suggested by each theory.

CHAPTER OUTLINE

Psychoanalytical Theory

Drives

Structure of Personality

Defense Mechanisms

Psychosexual Theory of Development

Application to Nursing

Social Theories

Erik Erikson

Application to Nursing

Carl Jung

Application to Nursing

Interpersonal Social Theory

Alfred Adler

Harry Stack Sullivan

Karen Horney

Application to Nursing

Attachment Theory

John Bowlby

Mary Ainsworth

Application to Nursing

Behavioral Theories

B. F. Skinner

A. Bandura and R. H. Walters

What are therapeutic models, and why do we need to study them? Models give us structures that we can use to visualize phenomena. Therapeutic models guide our thinking about phenomena. When we care for clients with complex mental and physical disorders, we need some framework for organizing our thinking about the manifestations, the development, and the treatment of the disorders. Once we have structure for observing these disorders, we can begin to develop theories about how they evolve and how they can be treated.

Nurses use theories to direct assessment and to suggest interventions and causes. Theories from a variety of professional fields have implications on nursing care. Although nurses may not find a single theory that is adequate for practice, they find useful concepts and principles from various theories. Each theory developed attempts to establish a scientific method for studying an individual as a living, social being, and contributes to a language with which to examine and communicate human action. This chapter briefly examines major concepts of the most commonly used theories.

PSYCHOANALYTICAL THEORY

Freud's psychoanalytical theory addresses the relationship among inner experiences, behavior, social roles, and functioning (Arlow, 1989). This theory proposes that conflicts among unconscious motivating forces affect behavior. People usually do not like conflicts and therefore develop certain structures in their mind, or ways of responding, to maintain equilibrium and to keep conflicts from causing too much discomfort. This defensive process is called repression. It is an unconscious process that requires energy to keep conflicts out of the realm of awareness, thus avoiding discomfort and pain.

DRIVES

Sigmund Freud (1952), often called the *father of psychoanalysis,* viewed human beings as stimulus driven, who respond to both internal and external stimuli. The perceived stimulus produces a state of excitation known as drive or instinct. These drives are instinctual urges and impulses arising from biological and psychological needs. They produce mental activity that seeks gratification, or discharge, that results in a decrease in tension.

The psychoanalytical theory assumes that humans have two primary drives or forces: the drive toward life (eros) and the drive toward death (thanatos). Eros includes instincts concerned with self-preservation and survival of the species. Thanatos is expressed as aggression or hate, which can be directed inwardly (as in suicide) or outwardly (as in murder).

STRUCTURE OF PERSONALITY

Freud proposed hypothetical structures—the id, the ego, and the superego—to explain his observation that behaviors are a result of conflicts among the needs of the individual, the restrictions of the environment, and internalized moral values (Figure 2–1).

The id represents psychological energy, or libido. According to Freud, this energy is primarily a sexual and aggressive drive. The id is the first structure to develop in the personality, and it operates on the pleasure principle to reduce tension. For example, a hungry infant reflexively sucks to receive nourishment, thus reducing her hunger. Id is also characterized by primary process thinking, a mode of thought that is primarily imagery. It is irrational and not based on reality. Hallucinations of psychotic clients are examples of primary thinking.

The ego is the chief executive officer of the mind. It mediates between the drives, forces, or conflicts of the id and the superego, maintaining a reality orientation for the person. It keeps the strong forces of the superego from being extremely inhibitive, and the id from causing the person to become overly exhibitionistic. The ego operates on the reality principle and is characterized by secondary process thinking, which is logically oriented in time and distinguishes between reality and unreality. As much, it provides a means of delaying gratification of needs. The ego is partially under conscious control, whereas the id is unconscious.

The superego has two main functions: reward and punishment. It is the superego that rewards moral behavior and punishes actions that are not acceptable by creating guilt. The superego is our conscience, a residue of internalized values and moral training of early childhood. An overly strict superego may lead to extremes of guilt and anxiety.

The ego manages the sexual and aggressive drives of the id, keeping it from being destructive. When the ego cannot mediate against the unconscious drives, anxiety results. Anxiety is a warning to the ego of an emerging danger. Repression is the first line of defense against unacceptable, painful, and unwanted memories. Repression is an unconscious process that keeps unacceptable impulses out of awareness and prevents these impulses from becoming conscious. The energy associated with these impulses, or drives, is not changed or sublimated into something else but into extra energy to keep the drive out of the awareness. Some repressed conflicts break through awareness and are defended against in other ways.

DEFENSE MECHANISMS

Anna Freud (1937), Sigmund Freud's daughter, further explicated the defense mechanisms. She asserted that defense mechanisms evolve during specified developmental stages and are more likely to result in maladaptive behaviors when they are used too early or too long. For instance, immature defense mechanisms, such as projection or repression, are adaptive when used during early childhood in contrast to being maladaptive during adolescence or adulthood. Vaillant (1977), in his analysis of data from a 30-year-old cohort study of healthy male college students, classified the defense mechanisms in a hierarchy from psychotic to healthy (Table 2–1). The defense mechanisms have two aspects. First, they keep unwanted thoughts out of the awareness and use energy to do this. Second, energy cannot be contained indefinitely; therefore, some defense mechanisms allow the energy to be discharged, as

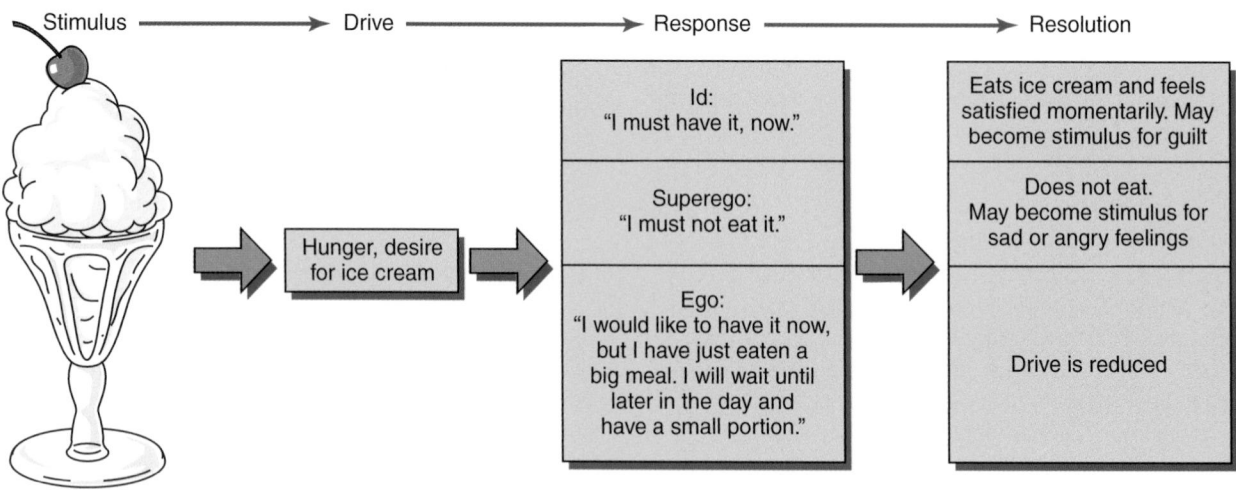

Figure 2–1 Example of the operation of id, ego, and superego in resolving conflicts. The resolution depends on which force predominates.

TABLE 2–1
Vaillant's Four Levels of Defense Mechanisms

Level	Defense	Example
Level I Psychotic mechanisms: these mechanisms are common in healthy individuals before age 5	Delusional projection: frank delusions about external reality, usually of a persecutory type	Example: "The Devil is devouring my heart"
	Denial: denial of external reality, including the use of fantasy as a substitute for other people	Example: "I will make a new him in my own mind"
	Distortion: grossly reshaping external reality to suit inner needs	Example: hallucinations, wish-fulfilling, delusions, and megalomaniacal beliefs
Level II Immature mechanisms: common in healthy individuals ages 3 to 15, in character disorder, and in adults in psychotherapy. They may change with improved interpersonal relationships or with repeated and forceful interpretation during long therapy	Projection: attributing one's own unacknowledged feeling to others	Example: prejudice, rejections of intimacy and suspicion
	Schizoid fantasy: tendency to use fantasy and to indulge in autistic retreat for the purpose of conflict resolution and gratification	Example: avoidance of intimacy and use of eccentricity to repel others
	Hypochondriasis: the transformation of reproach toward others arising from bereavement, loneliness, or unacceptable aggressive impulses into, first, self-reproach and then complaints of pain, somatic illness, and neurasthenia	Example: chronic pain syndromes
	Passive-aggressive behavior: aggression toward others expressed indirectly and ineffectively through passivity or directed against the self	Example: procrastinations, failures, illnesses that affect others more than self
	Acting out: direct expression of an unconscious wish or impulse in order to avoid being conscious of the effect that accompanies it. Acting out involves chronically giving in to impulses in order to avoid the tension that would result were there any postponement of instinctual expressions	Example: using behavior or delinquent or impulsive acts to avoid being aware of one's feelings. Chronic use of drugs, perversion, self-inflicted injury to relieve tension
Level III Neurotic defenses: these mechanisms are common in healthy individuals aged 3 to 90, in neurotic disorder, and in mastering acute adult stress. These defenses can be changed by brief therapy	Intellectualization: thinking about instinctual wishes in formal, affectively bland terms and not acting on them. The idea is in consciousness, but the feeling is missing. Vaillant believes intellectualization includes mechanisms of isolation, rationalization, ritual, undoing, restitution, and magical thinking	Example: paying attention to the inanimate to avoid intimacy with people, or paying attention to external reality to avoid expression of inner feelings
	Repression: seemingly inexplicable naivete, memory lapse, or failure to acknowledge input from a selected sense organ. The feeling is in consciousness, but the idea is missing. It blocks conscious perception of instinct feelings	Example: a man who weeps, but does not know for whom he weeps

(continues)

TABLE 2–1
Vaillant's Four Levels of Defense Mechanisms (continued)

Level	Defense	Example
Level III (*continued*)	Displacement: the redirection of feelings toward an object relatively less cared for than the person or situation arousing the feelings	Example: practical jokes with hidden hostile intent, phobias, hysterical conversion reactions, and some prejudice
	Reaction formation: behavior in a fashion diametrically opposed to an unacceptable instinctual impulse	Example: overtly caring for someone else when one wishes to be cared for oneself
	Dissociation: temporary but drastic modification of one's character or of one's sense of personal identity to avoid emotional distress	Example: fugues, hysterical conversion reactions, a sudden unwarranted sense of superiority, counterphobic behavior in order to block out anxiety
Level IV Mature mechanisms: these mechanisms are common in healthy individuals ages 12 to 90	Altruism: vicarious but constructive and instinctually gratifying service to others	Example: philanthropy and well-repaid service to others
	Humor: overt expression of ideas and feelings without individual discomfort or immobilization and without unpleasant effect on others	Example: jokes and games
	Sublimation: indirect or attenuated expression of instincts without either adverse consequences or marked loss of pleasure	Example: expressing aggression through pleasurable games, sports, and hobbies

Note. From *Adaptation to Life*, by G. E. Vaillant, 1977, Boston: Little, Brown. Reprinted with permission.

in reaction formation, projection, and sublimation. Defense mechanisms are the methods used by the ego to fight instinctual outbursts of the id and superego.

PSYCHOSEXUAL THEORY OF DEVELOPMENT

The psychoanalytical theory proposes that adult character traits, behaviors, and thinking processes are a result of crucial events in the developmental years. The personality is almost completely formed by 5 years of age. During the various stages, the child is motivated by the need for pleasure and derives that pleasure by stimulating the various erogenous zones of the body or by being stimulated by parents in their handling. Each stage is localized in specific body zones (Table 2–2).

The *oral stage* of development begins at birth, extending about 18 months. During this stage, stimulation of the mouth, such as in sucking, biting, and swallowing, is the primary source of satisfaction. Not getting needs met at this stage may produce problems with eating and habits such as smoking and biting nails. A wide range of adult behaviors, from excessive optimism to sarcasm, cynicism, and pessimism, has been attributed to problems during this stage. Fixation at this stage is characterized by narcissism and incorporation of loved objects (the instinctual behavior that motivates the person to receive gratification by symbolically swallowing the important other) (Fenichel, 1945).

During the *anal stage* (18 months to 3 years of age), sexual gratification shifts to the anus. This occurs during the period of toilet training. The child is concerned with retaining and letting go of feces. Problems occurring in resolution of this phase may result in rebelliousness and an exaggerated need to be in control across the life span. If the fixation is with retention or holding in, the adult may be excessively neat, clean, and compulsive. If, however, expulsion is the problem, the adult may be dirty, wasteful, and extravagant.

During the *phallic stage*, which occurs at the end of the third or fourth year, erotic gratification shifts to the genital region. The child becomes sexually attracted to the parent of the opposite sex and fears the parent of the same sex, who is now perceived as the rival. The child overcomes this conflict

TABLE 2–2

Freud's Stages of Psychosexual Growth and Development

Stage of Development	Critical Experiences	Developmental Task	Major Characteristics	Other Possible Personality Traits
Oral (birth–18 months)	Weaning	Establishing trust	Autoeroticism, narcissism, omnipotence, pleasure principle, frustration, dependence	Fixation at the oral stage is associated with passivity, gullibility, and dependence, the use of sarcasm, and the development of orally focused habits (e.g., smoking, nail biting)
Anal (18 months–3 years)	Toilet training	Developing sphincter control, self-control, feeling of autonomy	Reality principle, fear of loss of object love, approval and disapproval, beginning superego development	Fixation associated with anal retentiveness (stinginess, rigid thought patterns, obsessive-compulsive disorder), or anal expulsive character (messiness, destructiveness, cruelty)
Phallic (3–5 years)	Oedipal conflict, castration anxiety	Establishing sexual identity; beginning socialization	Differentiation between the sexes, superego more internalized	Unresolved outcomes may result in difficulties with sexual identity and with authority figures
Latency* (6–12 years)	Peer group experience, intellectual growth	Group identification	Superego influence in erotic interests, immense intellectual development	Fixations can result in difficulty in identifying with others and in developing social skills, resulting in a sense of inadequacy and inferiority
Prepuberty and adolescence (12–15 years)	Established heterosexual relationships	Developing social control over instincts	Identity, turmoil, consideration of needs of others	Inability to negotiate this stage could result in difficulties in becoming emotionally and financially independent, lack of strong personal identity and future goals, and inability to form satisfying intimate relationships
Genital (15 years–adult)	Sexual maturity	Resolving dependence–independence conflict	Heterosexual relations	

*The latency and prepuberty and adolescence stages of psychosexual development were not included in Freud's original description of development. Anna Freud (1946) extended Freud's works when she described developments in these periods of life.

by identifying with the parent of the same sex. Object love at this stage is ambivalent and may affect object relations in adult life.

The early school-age years (6 to 12 years) constitute a period of quiescence Freud called *latency*. The child begins to submit to the demands of the superego and sublimate instincts. The way the person handles the internal and external demands, for better or for worse, becomes consolidated during this time.

At the start of adolescence, the final stage, called the *genital stage*, begins. Heterosexual behavior is evident, and the person undertakes various activities in preparation for marriage and family.

APPLICATION TO NURSING

It is important for nurses to understand that the role of unconscious conflict is the motivation of behavior. When we are tempted to ask, "Why did you . . . ?" we are reminded that often the person cannot identify the motivation because it is unconscious.

Psychoanalytical theory has demonstrated the central role of anxiety in maladaptive behavior. Nurses must be aware of the client's defense mechanisms against instinctual demands and anxiety. When we recognize that a client is using a defense mechanism, we know that the anxiety may need to be reduced before the defenses can be disengaged.

SOCIAL THEORIES

Social theories reflect significant social interactions that govern developmental milestones that influence adaptation across the life span. These theories also focus on challenges and achievements of each developmental stage and their impact on resolving the next stage. By understanding various human responses across the life span and the whole personality, nurses can collaborate with their clients and develop interventions that can enhance adaptation to each developmental stage.

ERIK ERIKSON

Erik Erikson was a student of Anna Freud. Unlike Freud, however, Erikson (1963) believed that a person's social view of self is more important than libidinal urges, and unlike Freud he believed that personality development continues over the life span. He also identified psychosocial stages of ego development in which individuals establish new understandings of themselves in their relationship to others. According to Erikson's eight stages of psychosocial development, the early four stages involve socialization of the child, whereas the succeeding four to socialization of the adult.

Erikson's optimistic outlook on human growth and development speak to new opportunities for particular strengths to develop at each stage. These strengths emerge when each crisis is met and must be continuously upheld throughout the life span to be useful. The task of identity is seen as the major task of life. All previous tasks are fundamental to self-discovery, and all adult tasks are predicated on comfortable resolution of identity.

Erikson believed that human institutions evolved along with the human species and that a particular institutional form can be related to each developmental stage (Table 2–3). He also asserted that there are distinct psychosocial crises or tasks that must be mastered or resolved by the ego to advance through various developmental stages. Failure to resolve each developmental task, particularly trust, leads to maladaptation or mental illness. Although resolution of each developmental task is a goal, realistically they are never completely mastered. Despite a complete mastery of each stage, Erikson asserted that each needs to be mastered enough to effectively cope with conflicts of later stages.

In conclusion, Erikson did not identify an institution for the last stage. Perhaps he believed that no society had progressed far enough to produce such an institution.

Application to Nursing

Clients with mental illnesses usually exhibit some degree of developmental delays or incomplete resolution of developmental tasks that parallel their chronological age. A major strength of Erikson's developmental model is its potential to facilitate adaptive mastery of each developmental crisis or task. That is, sufficient mastery to help the client cope effectively with present developmental crisis in preparation of later stages. In addition, his theory provides a comparison of adaptive versus maladaptive behavioral responses to each life span crisis or task. Psychiatric nurses can facilitate adaptive resolution of various developmental crises or tasks by using the nursing process to assess the client's level functioning and subsequent treatment planning. The nursing process involves assessing developmental crises and synthesizing data concerning the client's symptoms and behavioral patterns to determine mastery of each stage. Issues such as trust or difficulty forming interpersonal relationships often reflect unresolved issues during the earliest developmental stage.

Erikson's theory also provides a basis for client-centered nursing interventions. Nursing interventions include providing a therapeutic environment that enables the client to master crises unique to various developmental stages. In addition, interventions must focus on mobilizing internal and external resources that strengthen the client's repertoire of coping skills. (See Chapter 31 for an in-depth discussion of Crisis Theory.)

By developing and using client-centered interventions, psychiatric nurses provide supportive environments that facilitate the development, mobilization, and use of adaptive coping responses. Ultimately, psychiatric nursing interventions can assist the client in resolving demands unique to each developmental stage and attaining an optimal level of emotional maturity resilience and adaptation. Resilience is the capacity to adapt to distressful and overwhelming change or stressors across the life span.

TABLE 2–3
Erikson's Eight Stages of Ego Development

Stages	Nuclear Conflict	Strengths	Institution
1. Oral-sensory (birth–1 year)	1. Trust–mistrust	1. Drive and hope	1. Religion
2. Muscular–anal (1–3 years)	2. Autonomy–doubt, shame	2. Self-control and willpower	2. Law and order
3. Locomotor–genital (3–5 years)	3. Initiative–guilt	3. Direction and purpose	3. Education and economic
4. Latency (6–11 years)	4. Industry–inferiority	4. Method and competence	4. Technology
5. Adolescence (12–18 years)	5. Identity–role confusion	5. Devotion and fidelity	5. Ideology
6. Young adulthood (19–35 years)	6. Intimacy–isolation	6. Affiliation and love	6. Ethics
7. Adulthood (35–50 years)	7. Generativity–stagnation	7. Production and care	7. Generative succession
8. Maturity (50+ years)	8. Ego integrity–despair		8. Unnamed

CARL JUNG

Carl Jung (1967) differed from Freud on the nature of the unconscious. He postulated a collective unconscious containing the universal memories and history of all humans. The collective unconscious is that part of unconscious material that is universal in humans, in contrast with the personal unconscious that is determined by individual personal experience. From his study of international myths, folklore, and art, Jung discovered common, repeated images that he called archetypes. The collective unconscious contains symbolic access to archetypes, which serve as its building blocks. An archetype can be a mythical figure, such as the Hero, the Nurturing Mother, the Powerful Father, or the Wicked Witch. Other powerful archetypes are the persona and the shadow. The persona is the public personality, the aspects of self that one reveals to others, the role that society expects one to play. The persona is frequently at variance with true identity. The shadow archetype reflects the prehistoric fear of wild animals and represents the animal side of human nature. The shadow contains the opposite of what we feel ourselves to be.

Two of the most popular archetypes are those of men and women themselves. Jung recognized that humans are psychologically bisexual, that is, that "masculine" and "feminine" qualities are found in both sexes. The anima represents the feminine archetype in men, and the animus, the masculine archetype in women. A man understands the nature of women by virtue of his anima, and a woman understands a man by virtue of her animus. Problems can arise, though, if a member of either gender projects an idealized archetype onto the other and does not accept the real personality of the individual.

In Jung's view, motivation comes not only from past conflicts but also from future goals and the need for self-fulfillment. There are two basic personality orientations: *introversion*, which describes the person who is focused inward, cautious, shy, timid, and reflective; and *extroversion*, which describes the person who is outgoing, sociable, assertive, and energetic. Jung believed that the healthy personalty maintains a balance in all spheres—male and female, introversion and extroversion, conscious and unconscious—and has the ability to accept the past and strive for the future.

Application to Nursing

Most nursing theories have a developmental perspective derived from Erikson and other such theorists. Assessing the developmental stage of clients gives us direction in designing interventions (Table 2–4). If the client is distant and suspicious, we know that we are going to work on developing a sense of trust in the nurse-client relationship. We know that interventions for a 16-year-old girl with a newborn will be different from interventions for a 30-year-old woman with a newborn. The 16-year-old girl is faced with having to construct an identity as a mother before she has consolidated her identity as a woman.

Jung emphasized the importance of symbolism, rituals, and spirituality. When we enter a client's environment, we see symbols of importance to that person. We become aware

TABLE 2–4
Stages of Development:
Comparison of Freud's, Erikson's, and Piaget's Theories

	Freud	Erikson	Piaget
Old age		Integrity vs. despair	
Middle age		Generativity vs. self-absorption	
Early adulthood		Intimacy vs. isolation	
17 yrs	Genital		Formal operations
16 yrs		Identity vs. role confusion	
9 yrs			Concrete operations
8 yrs	Latency	Industry vs. inferiority	
4 yrs	Phallic	Initiative vs. guilt	
2 yrs	Anal	Autonomy vs. shame and doubt	Preoperational thought
1 yr	Oral	Trust vs. mistrust	Sensorimotor

Courtesy of Chris McCormick Pries, ARNP.

of the client's rituals of self-care. When clients' rituals interfere with growth and health, we look for the conflicts and anxiety behind the behaviors.

INTERPERSONAL SOCIAL THEORY

Interpersonal theorists emphasize the importance of social forces or what one does in relation to others rather than internal or biological factors. Theorists assert that the adult mental disorders stem from impaired interpersonal relationships of childhood. Because of the dynamics of interpersonal relationships, understanding these concepts enables nurses to form healthy relationships with their clients at various developmental stages and have an impact on the client's ability to adapt to environmental stressors.

ALFRED ADLER

Alfred Adler (Ansbacher & Ansbacher, 1956), another psychoanalyst, departed from Freudian theory by emphasizing the conscious as the core of personality. He believed that one's social environments shape personality and interactions and that people actively guide their own growth and development.

Adler proposed that inferiority feelings are the stimulus for growth, but that inferiority complex prevents people from solving life's problems. An inferiority complex is an exaggeration of feelings of inadequacy and insecurity resulting in defensiveness and neurotic behavior. Feelings of inferiority arise from being biologically inferior, by being spoiled and then rejected, or by being neglected. When people strive for improvement, superiority, or perfection, tension increases, and more energy is expended. Each person creates a unique pattern of striving for superiority that is learned from early parent-child interactions.

According to Adler, all people must solve three categories of problems during their lifetime: problems involving behavior toward others, problems of occupation, and problems of love. He described four basic styles that people use in working through these problems: avoiding, expecting to get everything from others, dominating others, and cooperating with others. Healthy people are characterized by self-reliance and cooperatively working with others within the culture.

HARRY STACK SULLIVAN

Harry Stack Sullivan (1940) studied traditional psychoanalysis but focused on interpersonal relationships instead of on the unconscious. He believed that cultural environment greatly shapes personality and that personality development does not end at 5 years of age but continues until young adulthood. Sullivan extended the description of personality development through stages. He emphasized the importance of the development of the self-concept and discussed how this progresses through adolescence. He called this development of the self-system *personification*. Personification includes all related attitudes, feelings, and concepts about oneself or another acquired from extensive experience. The persona is what one is talking about when one refers to "I" or "me." The development of the persona begins in infancy with perceiving the mother as good or bad. As the self begins to differentiate, the infant comes to perceive the mother as both good and bad.

The persona, or self-concept, begins with the idea of "good me," "bad me," and "not me." The good me is perceived when the mother is rewarding the infant. The bad me arises in response to the negative experiences with the mother. The "not me" arises out of extreme anxiety that the child rejects as part of the self. As development proceeds, the child integrates these personas into a realistic view of self.

Sullivan emphasized the importance of peers and reciprocal relationships to the developing child and adolescent. When a child learns patterns of responding that hinder interpersonal relationships and cause others to respond negatively, she experiences intense anxiety that further interferes with social relationships (Table 2–5). These ways of responding are primarily communication patterns. Sullivan (1971) believed that if communication patterns between individuals, groups, and nations could be changed, then each of those entities could be changed.

KAREN HORNEY

Karen Horney's (1937) key concept was that of basic anxiety, the feeling of isolation and helplessness in a potentially hostile world. Because people are dependent on each other, she believed, they often find themselves in a state of anxious conflict when others do not treat them well. Insecure, anxious children develop personality patterns to help them cope with their feelings of isolation and helplessness. They may become aggressive as a way of protecting what little security they do have. They may become too submissive, or they may become selfish and self-pitying as a way of gaining attention or sympathy.

In general, people relate to each other in one of three ways: (1) they can move toward others, seeking love, support, and cooperation; (2) they can move away from others, trying to be independent and self-sufficient; or (3) they can move against others, being competitive, critical, and domineering. Ideally, the healthy personality balances all three orientations. Problems arise when people become locked into only one mode; too weak-willed and self-denying, afraid to

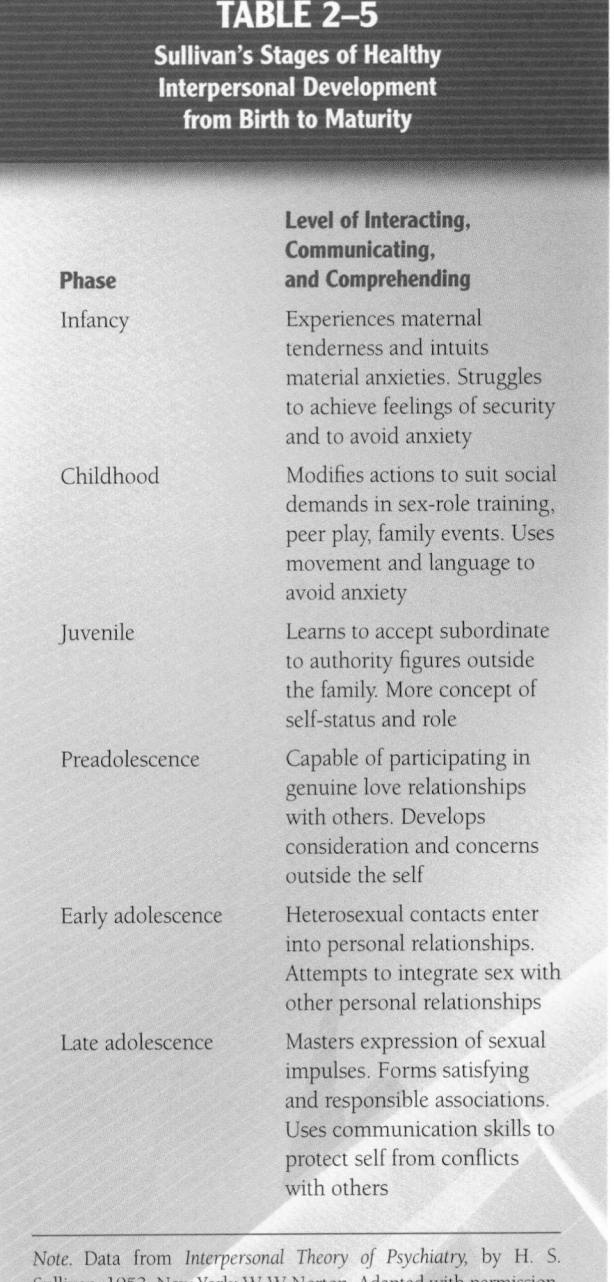

TABLE 2–5
Sullivan's Stages of Healthy Interpersonal Development from Birth to Maturity

Phase	Level of Interacting, Communicating, and Comprehending
Infancy	Experiences maternal tenderness and intuits material anxieties. Struggles to achieve feelings of security and to avoid anxiety
Childhood	Modifies actions to suit social demands in sex-role training, peer play, family events. Uses movement and language to avoid anxiety
Juvenile	Learns to accept subordinate to authority figures outside the family. More concept of self-status and role
Preadolescence	Capable of participating in genuine love relationships with others. Develops consideration and concerns outside the self
Early adolescence	Heterosexual contacts enter into personal relationships. Attempts to integrate sex with other personal relationships
Late adolescence	Masters expression of sexual impulses. Forms satisfying and responsible associations. Uses communication skills to protect self from conflicts with others

Note. Data from *Interpersonal Theory of Psychiatry*, by H. S. Sullivan, 1953. New York: W. W. Norton. Adapted with permission.

offend another; too independent, afraid to admit dependency; or too hostile, afraid to express affection.

Application to Nursing

Interpersonal theories provide important foundations to psychiatric nursing practice. Psychiatric nurses can use interpersonal relationships to strengthen support systems; foster interpersonal relationships; strengthen the client's belief system; and facilitate faith, hope, and life. Interpersonal theory focuses on the importance of distinct social interactions during various developmental stages. For example, important social interactions during childhood may be with parents, whereas during adolescence, peers may be significant. These relationships lay the foundation of self-systems, notably one's perception of self in relationships with families, others, and society. Psychiatric nurses must identify important relationships during distinct developmental stages and implement client-centered interventions that foster new patterns of interpersonal relationships and adaptive behavioral changes.

The nursing process can be used to gather data that influence the client's present symptoms and behaviors and assess them within the context of the nurse-client relationship. In addition, nurses need to assess the client's strengths, quality of interpersonal relationships, and coping patterns. These data are crucial to establishing healthy nurse-client interactions, understanding the client's present symptoms and behaviors, and developing client-centered interventions.

Through healthy and encouraging relationships, psychiatric nurses can help the client understand situational stressors about relationships and related symptoms and maladaptive behaviors. Inherent in the nurse-client relationship is an environment of acceptance that instills hope; improves self-esteem, self-worth, and dignity; promotes social interactions; and facilitates healthy interpersonal skills. Similarly, the client can learn to separate past learning from the present and gain a realistic and hopeful perspective of self in relationships with others and society.

ATTACHMENT THEORY

Attachment has become a classic term for the primary tie between a child and his or her caregiver and a process seen as evolving and biologically adaptive and critical to emotional and physiological development and survival (Ainsworth & Bell, 1970; Ainsworth, Blehar, Waters, & Wall, 1978; Bowlby, 1969, 1973). Attachment is readily observable when an infant is separated from the primary caregiver because the child protests and tries to reestablish contact with this individual.

John Bowlby and Mary Ainsworth have made significant contributions to the study and definition of attachment theory. Findings from contemporary studies continue to support their earlier findings. These data validate the significance of early caregiving and its lifelong impact on one's perception of self and others (Bartholomew & Horowitz, 1991; Ognibene & Collins, 1998; Schieche & Spangler, 2005; Pauli-Pott, Mertesacker, & Beckman, 2004).

JOHN BOWLBY

John Bowlby expanded the works of Anna Freud and others from a study involving a hospitalized 2-year-old and documentation of the child's separation reactions from caregivers. Bowlby's (1969) later work delineated the predictable patterns of behaviors of infants and young children during and following their stay for designated periods in nurseries or hospital units. He postulated that children who experience healthy and protected relationships with their mothers exhibit predictable phases of behaviors during normal separations.

As a result of his early work, Bowlby (1969, 1973) believed that the interaction between the infant and caregiver evolved from the infant's helplessness. He postulated that the helpless infant maintains intimacy with the primary caregiver by means of emotional and behavioral responses referred to as the attachment system. Theoretically, the attachment system is instinctual or motivational and, like hunger and thirst, integrates the infant's memory processes, prompting the child to satisfy them by interacting with the mother. Infant behaviors, such as crying, anger, and pain, usually signal distress, whereas smiling, vocalizing, reaching, and looking, strengthen attachment. These behaviors elicit various responses in the caregiver, including a calming voice, rocking and holding and comforting, and further reinforce the child-parent attachment. The attachment system plays a vital role in survival by allowing the infant's undeveloped brain to use the caregiver's developed or mature functions to regulate her life process. The caregiver's emotional responsiveness to the infant's emotional and behavioral demands or signals governs the maturity of the attachment system. The amount of time spent with early caregivers is less significant than the quality of time and interactions between child and caregiver. The level of distress, manifested as anxiety, arising from separations parallels the child's developmental stage and distinct attachment phase (Bowlby, Robertson, & Rosenbluth, 1952, 1969).

Bowlby (1969) described separation anxiety as a predictable process involving several stages: *protest, despair,* and *detachment*. Situations that interfere with the closeness of the attachment (mother or other caregiver) produce anxiety, anger, and protest. Protest behaviors are thought to have adaptive properties and reflect the infant's attempt to restore closeness with the caregiver. Examples of protest behaviors include increasing anxiety, crying, clinging, throwing self down, and searching. The child's ability to modulate anxiety depends on the mother or caregiver's ability to modulate anxiety or fear. Normally, when the mother calms the child through holding, smiling, rocking, or other comforting behaviors, the child gains a sense of comfort and security. In contrast, prolonged separation produces despair, and the infant's response moves from anxiety and anger to despondency. If the child's anxiety or fears persist because of the caregiver's inability to provide comfort and reduce anxiety and fear, attachment disturbances are likely to ensue. Common manifestations of despair include sadness, helplessness, and a sense of hopelessness, which the caregiver will return. In addition, the infant's energy declines and she becomes socially isolative. Unlike the adaptive qualities of protest, despair is thought to play a role in passive survival by conserving energy and resulting in withdrawal from danger. Detachment behaviors are similar to despair in that the child appears listless, is apathetic, and socially isolates and withdraws from the caregiver even when she returns. The latter two contribute to attachment disturbances, including various anxiety disorders, difficulty forming trusting relationships, and low self-esteem.

Bowlby's (1969) theory indicates that early interactions play key roles in how an individual perceives herself and others, and how she modulates or copes with anxiety throughout the life span. The infant internalizes early child-caregiver experiences and forms cognitive models or schemata that resolve if the person deserves care (self-perception) and whether others are reliable providers of care (perception of others). Early child-caregiver interactions or attachments shape one's perceptions of self and others and the quality of relationships throughout the life span (Bowlby, 1969, 1973).

Emerging data from animal and clinical functional MRI studies also demonstrate the neurobiological effects of early attachment and a distinct correlation between the quality of early attachments and infant brain development (Schore, 2005). Schore (2005) submitted that neurons fire and develop when infants interact with parents or caregivers. He asserts that Bowlby's attachment theory is an interactive congruous biological and regulatory process between the child and primary caregiver. Inference from this concept indicates the significance of early child-parent interactions. Major benefits of early quality attachments include strengthening the child's capacity for resilience in managing stress, developing ego function, and feeling emotionally secure. In summary, findings from attachment theorists (Crockenberg & Leerkes, 2004; Dix, Gershoff, Meunier, & Miller, 2004) continue to strengthen the premise that early relationships between positive parent-child interactions promote emotional and mental health across the life span. (See Chapter 11 for a comprehensive discussion of anxiety disorders.)

MARY AINSWORTH

Mary Ainsworth's research extended and clarified Bowlby's theory and revolutionized developmental research. Her systematic study of infant-caregiver attachment behaviors by means of the Strange Situation protocol (Ainsworth & Bell, 1970) has provided an empirical template for delineating and measuring Bowlby's attachment theory. This template spurred a plethora of clinical and scholarly contributions that transformed researchers' and clinicians' perception of early child-parent interactions. These first relationships make a greater impact on an individual than was once thought and reflect the continuous need and capacity of infants for secure attachment.

The *strange situation* protocol focused on assessing the quality and security of the infant's attachment. It involved a series of brief stress-inducing laboratory sequences that began with the mother and infant in a strange room with toys, and evolved through a series of diverse situations, each lasting less than 3 minutes. A series involved the stranger joining the pair, the mother leaving the child with the stranger, and the mother eventually returning. The infant's behavior was then rated as a function of her avoidant, enthusiastic, or varied responses to the mother's return. Ainsworth's findings revealed diverse reactions from the infant and confirmed that attachment modulates anxiety and serves as a secure base. Overall, Ainsworth's theory supports the importance of attachment and its anxiety-reducing qualities in helping children separate effectively from

primary caregivers and subsequent self-regulation of internal and external stressors across the life span.

Application to Nursing

Bowlby and Ainsworth's contributions to the attachment theory offer invaluable information about the importance of early infant-caregiver relationships and their impact on interpersonal skills, self-esteem, and trust across the life span. Most clients with mental disorders, particularly anxiety disorders, are likely to have some disturbances in their attachment systems. Psychiatric nurses must assess the client's levels of functioning and anxiety. The assessment process must also include questions about early relationships with primary caregivers and determine their impact on the client's ability to form healthy interpersonal relationships. This process begins by providing an accepting and empathetic environment that promotes trust and eventually therapeutic relationships. The nurse can improve trust, self-esteem, and coping behaviors through client-based interventions, and self-regulatory activities that reduce anxiety. For example, an infant who is hospitalized and left alone by primary caregivers is likely to be at risk of developing attachment disturbances. Efforts to ensure that the child is held, rocked, and talked to during feedings and other activities are crucial to health promotion. Psychiatric nurses need to provide health education to parents, other primary caregivers, and other health providers concerning the importance of physical and emotional responsiveness to a hospitalized child. Development of age-specific activities for hospitalized children also offers them an opportunity to form positive interactions and cope with their fears.

An adolescent who has difficulty forming interpersonal relationships with primary providers, schoolmates, or peers can learn to do so through health nurse-client interactions. The psychiatric nurse needs to identify high-risk groups, such as infants, children, and adolescents by their behavioral responses, which may range from social withdrawal to intense or inappropriate anxiety or fears when caregivers or the nurse leaves the room, and a lack of trust.

Adults and older adults can also learn to manage their anxiety and improve their self-esteem by forming therapeutic interactions with the nurse. Efforts to improve self-esteem include assessing the nature of the client's distress, mobilizing resources based on individual needs, and providing opportunities to succeed.

BEHAVIORAL THEORIES

Behavioral theories do not address the unconscious or the self-concept as do the psychosocial theories of personality. In behavioral theories the emphasis is on the behaviors of the person. These theories assume a learning model of human behavior that differs from the intrapsychic or disease model of mental disorders. Behaviors, both adaptive and maladaptive, are most likely learned.

Differences in human behavior are accounted for by the experiences in the person's life that initiate a response. The

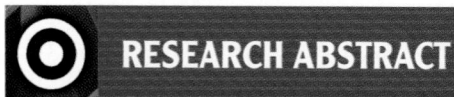

The Affective Structure of Supportive Parenting: Depressive Symptoms, Immediate Emotions, and Child-Oriented Motivation

Dix, T., Gershoff, E. T., Meunier, L. N. & Miller, P. S. (2004). *Developmental Psychology, 40,* 1212–1227.

Study Problem/Purpose

To investigate the association between maternal concerns and emotional state to one form of sensitive parenting, ability to meet child's emotional needs and intentions.

Methods

The study consisted of 128 mothers and their 4- to 27-month-old children. The average age of the children was 20 months and the average age of the mothers was 31 years of age. The initial session involved observing interactions between the mothers in a university playroom with their children for 20 minutes. Researchers divided the interactions into three parts. Interactions were designed to elicit emotional reactions in mothers. The initial 5 minutes consisted of mothers completing questionnaires while waiting for the researcher to return with toys. The next 10 minutes involved the mother and child interacting with age-appropriate toys without further demands made on mothers. During the completion of the 20-minute interactions, various demands were placed on mothers, including keeping children from playing with several attractive toys. Parent-child interactions were videotaped behind a one-way mirror to capture mother-child interactions. Following the 20-minute interactions, mothers were asked to review the videos and discuss their emotional reactions to each encounter with their children and their children's reactions. Fifty percent of the mothers were randomly asked to report their own emotions first.

The mother's explanations for their emotions were coded to ascertain if each emotion had occurred because of new events impacting the mothers' concerns for their children (child-oriented concerns) or how the encounters had affected the mothers directly (parent-oriented concerns).

Several tools were used to evaluate mother-child interactions and included the Center for Epidemiological Study Depression Scale (CES-D); measures to evaluate supportive maternal behavior; and the Toddler Behavior Assessment Questionnaire (TBAQ).

Findings

These data are consistent with previous findings that infer that supportive parental behaviors are governed in part by the intentions and intention-related processes that are aroused when parents experience distressed or emotional states. Furthermore, findings indicate that parents' concerns or orientation, either child- or parent-oriented, are continuously and automatically activated during stressful interactions with their children. The research also implies that child- and parent-oriented motivation may play a role in modulating parental behavior. Children-oriented motivation predicted more autonomy in the child and disharmony between the child and parent. Whereas, parent-oriented motivation predicted more constraints and control and increased parental detachment and disharmony between the parent and child.

Implications for Psychiatric Nurses

Nurses working with parents and children are poised to assess high-risk and stressful situations that have potentially harmful effects on the developing child. They can use proactive approaches, such as stress management, supportive parenting, and anger management classes to help parents develop appropriate coping and communication skills with their children to strengthen parent-child relationships and promote mental health in the child and parents.

---

human being is like a machine that operates according to fixed laws. Behavior can be controlled by the kind and extent of reinforcement that follows a particular behavior. A behavior that is reinforced will likely be repeated. A person is best understood by observing what he or she does in a particular situation.

B. F. SKINNER

B. F. Skinner (1953), a prominent behavioral theorist in America, identified two types of behavior: respondent and operant. Respondent behaviors occur when a known and specific stimulus elicits a response. They can be simple, as in a reflex action, or learned, such as those behaviors involved in conditioning. Operant behaviors are those that obtain a response or reinforcement from the environment or from another person.

All aspects of behavior are controlled through reinforcement; therefore, a person is a product of past reinforcements. Past experiences are important only to the degree that they are still active in directly contributing to the client's present distress. For example, a toddler who falls down the steps may

have a lifelong fear of going up a flight of stairs or may develop a fear of heights.

Some psychologists trained in the behavioral school began to believe that behavior was not merely the product of environmental stimuli. In the social learning approach, **cognitive processes** mediate the influence of environmental events on behavior by determining what stimuli are attended to, perceived, and interpreted. Rotter (1954) added the belief that the likelihood of a particular behavior occurring is influenced by the person's expectancy that the behavior will lead to goal attainment and the values attached to these goals. In other words, people generally choose actions that they expect will lead to valued goals. For instance, the toddler who fell down the steps, may choose not to go when confronted with a flight of stairs because she does not want to feel anxious.

A. BANDURA AND R. H. WALTERS

Bandura and Walters (1963) placed emphasis on the role of **modeling** in learning behaviors. Many social responses and personality characteristics are acquired simply by imitating or coping with the behavior of the models one observes. Modeling typically involves a social situation and a social relationship (the model and the imitator). The model can be an actual person, a film, or a cartoon representation. Modeling, or imitation, can produce rapid acquisition of social behaviors. Learning does not require direct, or external, reinforcement of imitated behavior. The person merely "tries on" the behavior.

Bandura (1977) also emphasized the importance of internal reinforcement. A person is able to reinforce his or her own behaviors that have a sense of self-efficacy. Self-efficacy refers to the expectation that one can effectively cope with and master situations such as addictions, and achieve the desired outcomes through one's own personal efforts. This model offers high-risk groups a range of coping responses that often lead to relapse. Although this theory has been used primarily for the treatment of addiction, it can also be applied to other mental disorders and reduce the incidence of relapse. The major appeal of this model is its emphasis on the client's self-efficacy, hope, and optimism.

The primary goal of self-efficacy is to encourage or persuade the client that he or she has the capacity to make adaptive behavioral changes in an identified problem area. For example, the client with schizophrenia who has just found out that he is going to lose his job may experience overwhelming anxiety and subsequently give up and stop taking prescribed medications and have a relapse. The nurse can use the self-efficacy model to encourage the client to explore options to manage his or her anxiety, through either supportive therapy or anxiety-reducing activities, to reinforce current coping skills, thereby reducing relapse. The success of this model stems from the client's motivation to change maladaptive coping behaviors and develop adaptive coping skills. This behavior can be positively reinforced with each successful resolution of a crisis or overwhelming situation and be used to facilitate adaptive behavioral changes.

CONDITIONING

Basic concepts of behavioral theories derive from stimulus, response, and reinforcement. In classic conditioning, the reinforcement is the presenting stimulus that causes the response. If a neutral stimulus is paired with the reinforcing stimulus repeatedly, the neutral stimulus will become a reinforcing stimulus producing the same response. The original stimulus is called the *unconditioned stimulus*, and the original response becomes the *unconditioned response*. The neutral stimulus becomes the conditioned response, and the response then becomes the conditioned response. An example of classic conditioning is Pavlov's experiment with dogs. The dogs learned to salivate at the sound of a tone that had been previously presented at the same time as meat powder on the tongue.

Operant conditioning occurs when behavior is produced without an observable external stimulus. The person's response

is seemingly spontaneous in that it is not related to any unknown observable stimulus. Operant behavior operates on the person's environment, resulting in a reward. An example is the bell that rings when a person fails to buckle the seat belt. The person puts on the seat belt, and the bell stops ringing. The operant behavior is the act of putting on the seat belt in expectation of a reward. The reinforcement occurs when the bell stops ringing. This is also an example of negative reinforcement. The response in classic conditioning does not operate on the environment, and the reinforcement comes before instead of after the response.

When a person's behavior is rewarded, the behavior will likely be repeated. Behavior is strengthened by positive and negative reinforcement; it is weakened by punishment. *Positive reinforcement* refers to an increase in the frequency of a response followed by a favorable event. *Negative reinforcement* refers to an increase in behavior as a result of avoiding or escaping from an aversive event that one would have expected to occur had the escape behavior not been emitted. *Punishment* is an aversive event contingent on a response. The result is a decrease in the frequency of that response. *Extinction* refers to the cessation or removal of a response.

To learn new behaviors, reinforcement of animal studies may be presented in several ways. The behavior can be rewarded each time the behavior occurs, at fixed intervals, or at a fixed ratio. None of these is what actually happens. Realistically, rewards are random and are the most potent form of reinforcement. The shorter the interval between reinforcement, the more rapidly animals will respond. Conversely, as the interval between reinforcement gets longer, the rate of animal response decreases.

The frequency of reinforcement affects the extinguishing of a response. Behaviors are extinguished more frequently when they are reinforced continuously and the reinforcement is then stopped when reinforced intermittently. Animals of a fixed-ratio schedule respond much faster than those on a fixed-interval schedule. Responding faster on fixed-interval reinforcement does not make any difference; for example, the animal presses the bar for food 5 times or 50 times and it will still be reinforced only when the predetermined interval has passed.

A fixed-ratio schedule of payment is used in industry in situations when a worker's pay depends on the number of units produced, or the salesperson's commission depends on the number of items sold. This reinforcement schedule is effective as long as the ratio is not set too high and the reinforcement is worth the effort.

Other reinforcement schedules include variable ratios, variable intervals, and mixed schedules (Skinner, 1963).

MARSHA LINEHAN'S DIALECTICAL BEHAVIORAL THERAPY

Marsha Linehan introduced dialectical behavioral therapy (DBT), a unique adaptation of behavior therapy in 1987.

A basic postulation of DBT is that individuals with borderline personality disorder have a pervasive deficit in their ability to effectively modulate intense emotional states and mobilize adaptive coping behaviors. Individuals with borderline personality disorder tend to maintain this deficit through insidious interface between the person's emotional vulnerability and continuous invalidation through the use of maladaptive behaviors and negative encounters with others. Targeting these behaviors facilitates acceptance, compassion, and validation in the client with borderline personality disorder. The DBT model helps the client modify a common tendency to lack insight into his or her behavior and blame others for emotional states and subsequent use of maladaptive coping behaviors (Linehan, Heard, & Armstrong, 1993; Linehan, 1999; Verheual, Van Den Bosch, Koeter, De Ridder, Stijnen, Van Den Brink et al., 2003). In comparison to other cognitive behavior therapies, DBT is also used to challenge distorted cognitions or schemata that produce enormous anxiety and distress in clients with borderline personality. Skills training is the core feature of DBT in which the psychotherapist focuses on behavioral control and master skills to resolve trauma issues; integrate positive concept and self-respect, develop adaptive behavioral changes, experience sustained joy, and attain client-centered goals. Five essential features of DBT include:

◆ Weekly skills training group

◆ Weekly individual psychotherapy

◆ Encouraging and coaching skills via telephone interactions between sessions

◆ Consultation with the client rather than consultation with those in the client's environment about the client

◆ Treatment environments are developed by DBT program directors and case managers to help client structure his or her environment (Linehan, 1999).

The success of DBT necessitates considerable commitment and accountability from the client. It also requires a shift from a "crisis" mode to one in which the client learns how to cope with negative and distressful emotions to one in which the client works with the psychotherapist and treatment team to develop a contingency plan that mitigates maladaptive behaviors, including suicide attempts, substance misuse, and self-injury and facilitates adaptive coping responses. Linehan uses several approaches to address problems associated with the client's environment (Table 2–6).

Application to Nursing

Nurses can use classic conditioning to initiate a behavior and operant conditioning to ensure that the behavior is repeated, but there is no guarantee that behavioral changes will occur. In classic conditioning, the reward comes before the behavior; in operant conditioning, the reward comes after the behavior. The difficulty with applying behavior modification to humans is finding the appropriate reinforcement. In nursing, we seldom know our clients well enough to discern reinforcement or how to initiate a response that can be reinforced. This theory sounds simple and straightforward, but it

---

TABLE 2–6
Linehan's Approach to Helping the Client Structure His or Her Environment

Behavioral Chain Analyses (active and directive to analyze and modify target maladaptive behaviors)

- Helps the client understand targeted (adaptive) behaviors

Problem Solving (focus on distorted cognitions)

- Cognitive restructuring
- Exposure therapy
- Self-efficacy skills training
- Psychoeducation to resolve trauma issue
- Contingency plan

Daily Monitoring

- Daily diary entries for review with psychotherapist

---

requires ingenuity, imagination, and perceptual skill to implement.

One of the best reinforcements nurses can use is the "placebo effect"—an attitude of optimistic concern and belief in the efficacy of the intervention.

COGNITIVE THEORIES

The foundations of cognitive theories involve mental processes, such as thinking, remembering, attending, planning, wishing, and fantasizing in relation to self, others, and the future. The person's perceptions and interpretations influence subsequent biological and behavioral responses. Predictably, if the person consistently misinterprets or overgeneralizes an event, emotional and physiological distress and maladaptation are likely to occur and require interventions that restore homeostasis.

AARON BECK

Aaron Beck (1991) is one of the foremost proponents of cognitive psychology. Cognitive theories emphasize the mental processes involved in knowing. The field looks at how people direct their attention, perceive, think, remember, solve problems, form mental images, and arrive at beliefs. Cognitive researchers study how people explain their own behavior, understand a sentence, do arithmetic, solve intellectual problems, reason, form opinions, and remember events. These mental processes determine, to a great extent, emotional, behavioral, and physiological responses.

A basic assumption of cognitive theories is that schemata shape personality. Schemata are cognitive structures, or patterns, that consist of a person's beliefs, values, and assumptions.

Schemata develop early in life from personal experiences, and become active in response to stressful situations. Schemata influence people to interpret certain life situations in a biased or distorted way. The content of cognitive processing is determined starting with preferential selection of data to which the person attends, through the evaluation, interpretation, and recall from short-term memory, activated by schemata, or biases. These schemata even influence retrieval from long-term memory. According to this theory, these cognitive distortions produce the symptoms of various psychological disturbances and mediate physiological responses that contribute to anxiety disorders and mood disorders. Clients with cognition themes of loss or defeat are likely to be depressed. A client with an anxiety disorder interprets situations as dangerous. In paranoid conditions, the person selectively interprets themes of abuse or interference. Exaggerated interpretations of personal gain characterize the client with mania (Beck, 1991). Beck identifies six common cognitive distortions that result in maladaptive behaviors (Table 2–7).

ALBERT ELLIS

Albert Ellis (1984, 1985) called his cognitive theory *rational emotive therapy* (RET). He believed that irrational thoughts cause maladaptive behavior and emotional distress. He explained his theory using the acronym ABC. An activating event or situation (A) arises that is threatening to the person. Because the person has a certain belief (B), an emotional response or consequence (C) occurs (Figure 2–2). RET modifies the underlying irrational beliefs (D) to change the emotional consequence.

Beck and Ellis disagree on certain issues. Beck views the cognition as maladaptive rather than irrational. Ellis believes that irrational belief causes the maladaptive behaviors, whereas Beck believes that cognitions are symptoms of, rather than the cause of, the disorder. The activation of the schemata is the mechanism, and not the cause, by which the depression or anxiety or aggression develops. Biological, genetic, stress, and personality factors combine to predispose people to various mental disorders.

Therapy helps the person recognize the connections among cognition, affect, and behavior. Reality-oriented interpretations for the distorted cognition are substituted for the distorted thoughts. This requires identifying and altering the maladaptive beliefs that predispose one to distorted experiences and distress. Excessive maladaptive behavior and distressing emotions found in diverse mental disorders are exaggerations of normal adaptive processes (Beck, 1991).

COGNITIVE THERAPY

Cognitive therapy addresses the person's cognitive organization and structure, which are biologically and socially influenced. Therapy helps modify assumptions that maintain maladaptive behaviors, distortion in logic, and systematic distortions in thinking. The therapist and the client together

TABLE 2–7
Beck's Common Cognitive Distortions

- Arbitrary inference: the process of drawing a specific conclusion in the absence of evidence to support the conclusion. The evidence may be contrary to the conclusion
- Selective abstraction: focusing on a detail taken out of context, ignoring more salient features of the situation, and conceptualizing the whole experience on the one detail
- Overgeneralization: the pattern of drawing a general rule or conclusion from one or more isolated incidents and applying the concept across the board to related and unrelated situations
- Magnification and minimization: errors in evaluating the significance or magnitude of an event that are so gross as to constitute a distortion
- Personalization: the proclivity to relate external events to oneself when there is no basis for making such a connection
- Absolutist (dichotomous) thinking: places all experiences in one of two opposite categories; for example, flawless or defective, immaculate or filthy, saint or sinner. In describing himself, the patient selects the extreme negative categorization

Note. From *Cognitive Therapy of Depression* (p. 14), by A. T. Beck, A. J. Rush, B. F. Shaw, & G. Emery, 1979, New York: Guilford Press. Reprinted with permission.

construct "counters," to the cognitive distortions. A counter is a statement that counteracts or negates the thought. Clients are often asked to challenge these distortions by questioning their bases and practicality. This theory does not yet identify the factors that produce a shift in information processing to the negative and what factors maintain the shift.

Research over the past 40 years supports certain aspects of the theory (Beck, 1991). Studies' outcomes support the effectiveness of the therapy in the outpatient treatment of unipolar depression, anxiety disorders, and panic disorder (Bryant & Harvey, 2000). In the past two decades, the efficacy of cognitive therapy for the treatment of major depression has been extensively studied in more than 80 controlled trials. Some meta-analytical studies have quantified the effectiveness of cognitive therapy (Dobson, 1989; Gaffan, Tsaousis, & Kemp-Wheeler, 1995; DeRubeis, Gelfand, Tang, & Simons, 1999). The National Institute of Mental Health's collaborative study of the treatment of depression has shown the superiority of cognitive therapy in comparison to antidepressant drugs and interpersonal therapy (Elkin et al., 1989; Shea et al., 1990). Other

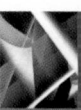

CASE STUDY (Cognitive Distortions)

Mr. G is a 55-year-old who has been employed as a national salesman for the past 22 years. Several months ago a manager from one account asked that he be removed because they were having difficulties with the account. Mr. G denies having problems with the account and expresses concerns that he is being removed because the manager wants someone else to handle the account. He presents today complaining of difficulty sleeping, concentrating, and losing interest in things he once found pleasurable and fun. He also mentions that his friends are probably saying he is "over the hill" and unable to do his job. He also mentions that he feels helpless and inadequate since losing the account.

Which of his statements reflects distorted cognitions?

1. "My co-workers feel like I'm over the hill since I lost the account."

2. "I am useless and inadequate."

3. "I just can't do the job I used to do. Maybe I should retire."

4. "I can't sleep or concentrate anymore."

Answer: All of the above except #4 are examples of distorted cognitions.

The significance of understanding cognitive distortions, particularly in depression and anxiety disorder is the role they play in generating anxiety and depression and sustaining negative self-talk and thinking. Interesting, these thoughts or distortions are also the focus of cognitive behavioral therapy, which encourages the client to provide the proof of these beliefs or cognitive distortions. Oftentimes negative thoughts that are assumed to generate from others reflect the client's own negative thoughts.

How to Challenge Distorted Thoughts (Cognitions)

When challenging distorted cognitions it is imperative to remember that the client truly believes his thinking is rational. It is imperative to ask the client where is the proof that his friends think he is over the hill or "just because you lost the account does not mean you are a failure or no longer an effective salesman." This latter assumption is referred to as overgeneralizaton or "all or none thinking" and when questioned, the client is forced or encouraged to provide a rational basis for this assumption or distorted cognition. Using homework assignments to monitor thoughts, feelings, and behaviors are an integral part of cognitive behavioral therapy. Homework assignments offer an opportunity to monitor the impact of negative or distorted cognitions on feelings such as "I am over the hill or a failure" [thoughts] (generates depression or anxiety [feelings]) which may result in isolation from others, and show a lack of confidence to pursue positive experiences [behavior]. Cognitive behavioral techniques engender a sense of power, confidence, and clarity about a given situation. Resolution of cognitive distortions also decrease feelings of helplessness, hopelessness, and inadequacy—major cognitive themes associated with depression and anxiety. Nurses need to know about cognitive behavioral therapy when working with anxious or depressed clients. These techniques offer another approach that complements antidepressant medications commonly used to treat these disorders.

Answer #4 is incorrect—it reflects signs of depression that can be sustained by negative self-talk, assumptions, and distorted cognitions.

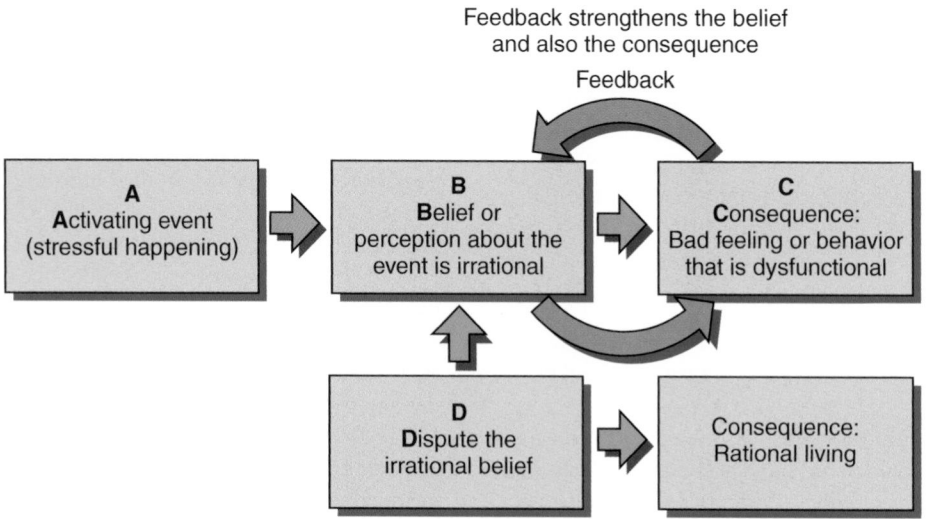

Figure 2–2 Ellis's ABCs of rational emotive therapy.

studies showed the efficacy of the therapy in treating anxiety disorders (Beck, 1976; Bryant & Harvey, 2000; Simpson & Kozak, 2000).

JEAN PIAGET

Cognitive theories also address human development. Whereas the psychoanalytical theorists addressed psychosexual development and Erikson described social development, Jean Piaget (Inhelder & Piaget, 1958) proposed a sequence of cognitive development that emphasized the relationship between action and thought (see Table 2–4). Piaget began his research on children in the early 1920s. He studied the responses of children and young people to various tasks concerning physical phenomena. Piaget and his coworkers developed a theory of reasoning based on these responses. They identified stages that are characterized by distinctive features in the patterns of a person's reasoning (Table 2–8). Piaget proposed that each stage serves as a precursor to all succeeding stages so that reasoning develops sequentially, always from the less effective to the more effective stage. This progression is not necessarily at the same rate for every person, and people do not progress through the stages exhibiting all the reasoning characteristics of a particular stage. Reasoning develops gradually, at a particular time showing the features of stage 1 on some problems, while exhibiting certain features of stage 2 on others. The stage concept is more useful in classifying reasoning patterns than for describing the overall intellectual behavior of a particular person at a given time.

The first stage is called *sensorimotor*. This stage is characteristic of children's thinking from birth to about 2 years of age. The young infant appears to think that the only objects that exist are the objects that can be seen. As the child grows in experience, she develops an awareness of the permanence of material objects. Information is obtained through the senses and motor action.

The preoperational stage moves through three periods between the ages of 2 and 7 years. In the first period, children can differentiate an image or a word from what it stands for (e.g., a chair) and can name an object not in sight. As children begin to speak, they develop representational thought and can grasp several events as a whole, whereas at the level of sensorimotor intelligence, successive actions and perceptual states are linked one by one. Children can differentiate image and language from action and reality, but they lack casual reasoning. Interactions with the physical world are essential to intellectual development in the first two periods.

Between the ages of 4 and 5½, children are more able to examine and set about a specific task, adapt their intelligence to it, and reason about more difficult everyday problems. However, a distinct characteristic of thought at this stage is their tendency to center on some striking feature of the object they are reasoning about to the exclusion of other relevant aspects, resulting in distorted reasoning. Each situation is viewed egotistically from a personal point of view. Between the ages of 5 and 6 years, the rigid and irreversible intellectual structures begin to become more flexible, and children begin the transition to the third stage of thought.

Concrete operational thought extends from about 7 years of age to pubescence (see Table 2–8). Operations are mental actions that have a definite and strong structure. At this stage, children's logical thoughts extend only to objects and events of first-hand reality. Children are able to consider two contrasting features, for example, height and width, that may balance and compensate for any distortion brought about by concentrating on one aspect of the situation. As children approach 7 or 8 years of age, they begin to look at their own thinking and monitor it. They can look at alternative actions that will achieve the same outcome.

The fourth stage, formal operational, is characterized by formal reasoning (see Table 2–8). Children become better at organizing and structuring data with the methods of concrete operational thought. They become aware that such methods do not lead to a logically exhaustive solution to their problems. These children can use hypothesis, are able to deduce its consequences in the light of other known information, and then verify empirically whether, in fact, those consequences occur. They can reflect on their own reasoning to look for inconsistencies. They can check their results in numerical calculations against order-of-magnitude estimates. Piaget called these abilities combinatorial reasoning, control of variables, functional relationships, and probabilistic correlations.

Development theories suggest that all facets of development follow a predictable pattern (Maier, 1969) that is orderly and can be described readily by criteria, making distinct developmental phases. Childhood is distinctly different from adulthood in all areas of human functioning. Cognitive, behavioral, psychosocial, cultural, and spiritual development are interrelated and interdependent, leading toward integration and maturity. When the needs of children are compromised, development may not progress. Examples of these situations include significant losses or other traumatic events, such as the death of a parent or child abuse. Clients with borderline personality disorders often have abusive and traumatic childhood histories. They grow physically, but other development is impaired.

Application to Nursing

Cognitive theories are a rich source for nursing intervention. Strategies detailed in the writings of the practitioners are practical and useful. Basic cognitive distortions are easy to recognize and learn. The difficult part is helping the client develop effective counters, or statements, that counteract negative and destructive self-talk.

Piaget's theory of cognitive development helps nurses recognize impaired development and prove a relationship that facilitates the person's accomplishment of developmental tasks. Early childhood interventions also enable nurses to develop and implement preventive measures that facilitate specific developmental tasks. It is not uncommon that medical treatment cannot proceed because psychosociocultural and spiritual needs are not being met. Developmental stage based

TABLE 2–8
Piaget's Stages of Cognitive Development

Period	Characteristics of the Period	Major Change of the Period
Sensorimotor (0–2 years)	—	
Stage 1 (0–1 month)	Reflex activity only; no differentiation	Development proceeds from reflex activity to representation and sensorimotor solutions to problems
Stage 2 (1–4 months)	Hand–mouth coordination: differentiation via sucking reflex	
Stage 3 (4–8 months)	Hand–eye coordination: repeats unusual events	
Stage 4 (8–12 months)	Coordination of two schemata; object permanence attained	
Stage 5 (12–18 months)	New means through experimentation—follows sequential displacements	
Stage 6 (18–24 months)	Internal representation: new means through mental combinations	
Preoperational (2–7 years)	Problems solved through representation: language development (2–4 years); thought and language both egocentric: cannot solve conservation problems	Development proceeds from sensorimotor representation to prelogical thought and solutions to problems
Concrete operational (7–11 years)	Reversibility attained; can solve conservation problems—logical operations developed and applied to concrete problems; cannot solve complex verbal problems	Development proceeds from prelogical thought to logical solutions to concrete problems
Formal operational (11 years–adulthood)	Logically solves all types of problems—thinks scientifically; solves complex verbal problems; cognitive structures mature	Development proceeds from logical solutions to concrete problems to logical solutions to all classes of problems

Note. From "Extending Piaget's approach to intellectual functioning," by S. I. Greenspan & J. F. Curry, 2000, in B. J. Sadock & V. A. Sadock (Eds.), *Kaplan & Sadock's Comprehensive Textbook of Psychiatry* (7th ed., pp. 402–413). Philadelphia: Lippincott Williams & Wilkins. Copyright © 2000 by Lippincott Williams & Wilkins. Reprinted with permission.

on an assessment of behavior, cognition, and belief patterns must be identified if the nurse is to plan holistic interventions to achieve positive client outcome. Cognitive development is not emphasized as much as social development, but it is equally important. Assessing knowledge level and client and family education needs is an integral part of nursing care, and cognitive theory can guide in treatment planning.

NEUROBIOLOGICAL THEORIES

An important theory of modern psychiatric therapy is that all behaviors are a reflection of brain function, and all thought processes represent a range of functions mediated by nerve cells (neurons) in the brain. Just as the brain controls complex behaviors as normal feeling, learning, thinking, and speaking, it is the origin of disorders of affect (emotion), perception, and cognition (thought) that characterizes diverse mental disorders.

Neurons and glial cells are the two most abundant cell types in the brain. Neurons consist of a cell body; specialized appendages called *dendrites*; and an *axon* (Figure 2–3). Neurons respond to an internal or external stimulus by generating chemical or electrical signals (impulses) that collectively create thought and action. Dendrites are the receptor filaments of impulse transmission from other neurons. The axon extends to the adjacent neurons to carry on the information in a manner similar to electrical conduction. At the end of the axon, the impulse jumps across the gap to the next dendrite. This region between the axon and dendrite of two neurons is the *synapse* (Figure 2–4). (See Chapter 29 for detailed discussion of neuronal anatomy and physiology.)

Brain regions are specialized for different functions (see Figure 2–4). Multiple layers of neurons make the cortex, or brain surface, and their axons reach into the subcortical brain to form a connection between related but separate parts of the cortex. These dense numbers of neurons in the cortex

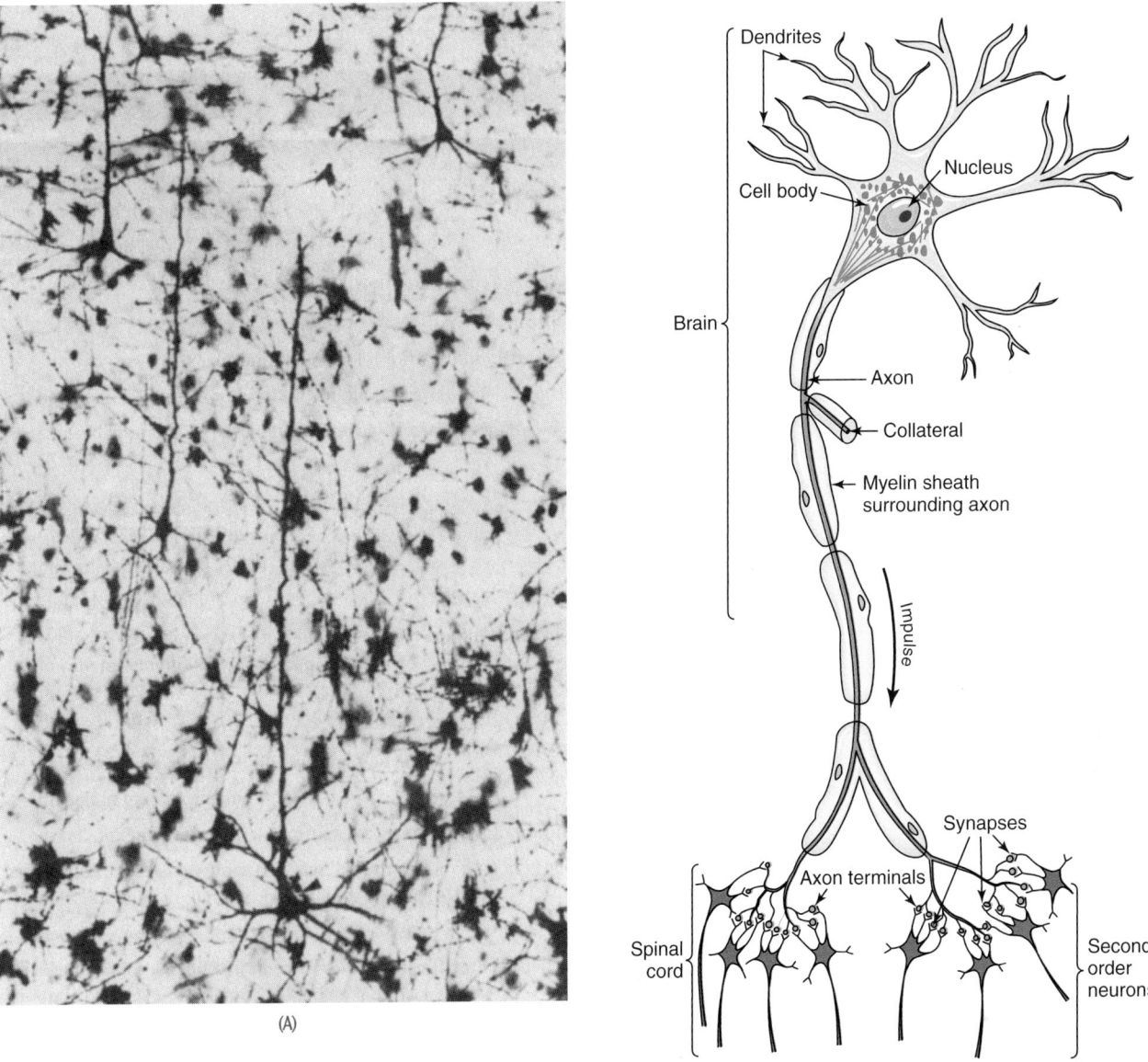

(A)

(B)

Figure 2–3 (A) Medium-sized pyramidal neuron from the human cerebral cortex. The bar represents 100 μm. **(B)** Structure of a large neuron of the brain, showing its important functional parts. *(Note. A, from* Textbook of Neuroanatomy *[p. 34] by A. M. Burt, 1993, Philadelphia: W. B. Saunders. Reprinted with permission.)*

contribute to the gray appearance and are called *gray matter*, whereas the axons travel in bundles or "tracts" in the subcortical *white matter*.

Clusters of specialized neurons are organized spatially within the brain. Cognitive function is primarily located in the frontal lobe cortex, motor and sensory function in the parietal lobes, and affective processes in the temporal lobe and limbic system. Receiving and responding to stimuli require integration of the activity of many of these specialized areas, some of which are isolated from each other but connected by an elaborate system of tracts that carry impulses between the functional areas. The specific nature of the information and response is a function of the cells recruited to carry the impulse and the type of chemical signal, or neurotransmitter, produced at the synapse. Dysregulation in these chemical signals, or neurotransmitters, appears to play pivotal roles in the primary origins of mental disorders.

Neurobiological theory of mental disorders suggests that cognitive and emotional dysregulation result from multiple causes, such as genetic vulnerability, nutrition, infectious processes, exposure to trauma, and other pathological conditions that cause neurotransmitter disturbances in the brain. These neurochemical disruptions may contribute to maladaptive cognitive and emotive responses that characterize mental illness.

NEUROSCIENCE

Studies of brain function in persons with mental disorders indicate that there are abnormalities in the amount of neurotransmitters produced or that are available to the receptor sites. Normally, neurons communicate through neurotransmitters synthesized at the end of the axon. As the electrical impulse moves to the terminal plate of the axon, the transmitter substance is released into the synaptic cleft (see Figures 2–3 and 2–4). Receptor sites on the receiving neuron (postsynaptic neuron) pick up the neurotransmitter substance that, in turn, causes the receiving neuron to activate. Once enzymes deactivate the neurotransmitter, it is taken back (reuptake) into the cytoplasm of the presynaptic neuron. This process and the transmitter chemicals involved are key elements in understanding the medications used to treat mental illnesses and their effect on the transmitters at receptor sites to alleviate symptoms.

Five important neurotransmitters are dopamine (DA), norepinephrine (NE), serotonin (5-HT), gamma-aminobutyric acid (GABA), and glutamate and N-methyl-D-asparate (NMDA) (Table 2–9). These neurochemicals are synthesized in the axon terminals, where they are released.

Dopamine

Dopamine (DA) is primarily responsible for fine motor movement, sensory integration, cognition, memory, and emotional behavior. Dopamine is metabolized by monoamine oxidase

CEREBRAL CORTEX (LATERAL VIEW)

The **cerebral cortex** consists of several layers of billions of nerve cells called *neurons* (see Figure 2–3). These neurons are specialized for functions such as movement and sensation (parietal cortex), vision (occipital cortex), speech and hearing (temporal cortex), and mentation (frontal cortex). Axons extend from the neurons and merge into bundles (nerve fibers) to make up the white matter. These fibers connect the neurons of specialized cortical areas to related and complementary areas of the brain, facilitating integrated processing of information and complex responses.

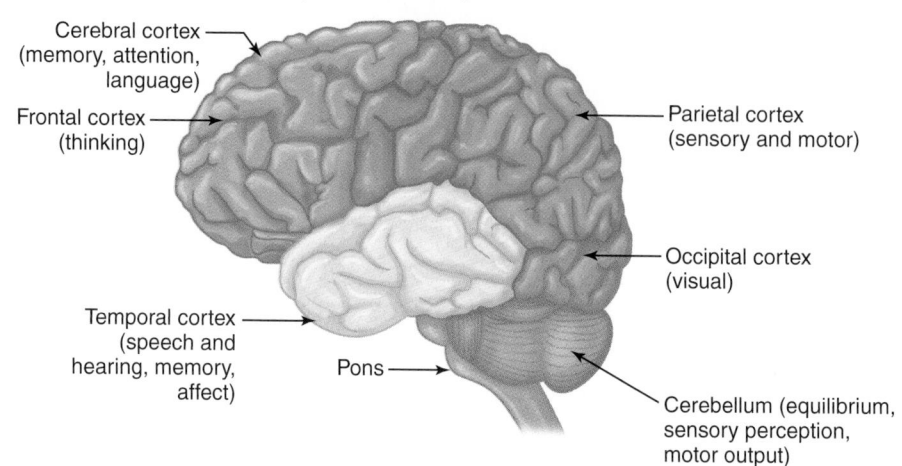

LIMBIC SYSTEM AND BRAIN STEM

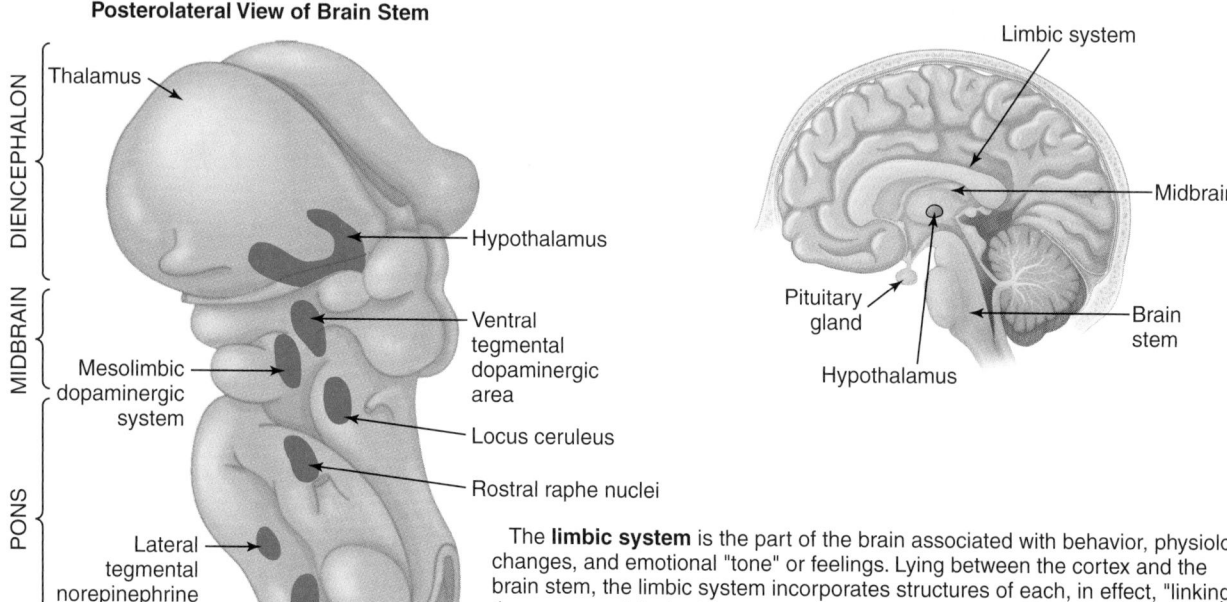

The **limbic system** is the part of the brain associated with behavior, physiologic changes, and emotional "tone" or feelings. Lying between the cortex and the brain stem, the limbic system incorporates structures of each, in effect, "linking" these areas of the brain. The brain stem (midbrain, pons, and medulla) is a central nerve pathway that receives and sends impulses between the brain and the rest of the body. Motor and sensory tracts meet and diverge here. Cardiac, vasomotor, and respiratory centers are also nearby. The **hypothalamus** influences these vital tracts and centers for normal physiologic maintenance, and also plays a role, along with the *pituitary gland*, in producing stress and anxiety responses. The *locus ceruleus*, the *dopaminergic* and *norepinephrine* systems, and the *raphe nuclei* are groupings of neurons that produce neurotransmitters important in brain function.

Figure 2–4 Neurobiological concepts basic to the understanding of psychiatric disorders.

(MAO). A plethora of dopamine receptors exist, including at least five with pharmacologic significance including (D_1, D_2, D_3, D_4, and D_5). Each D receptor carries out different degrees of stimulation or inhibition of the postsynaptic response. D_4 receptors have a greater affinity for "atypical antipsychotic agents." Hyperactivity of the dopaminergic system is impli-cated in schizophrenia and mania, whereas hypoactive dopamine systems are believed to contribute to depression and Parkinson's disease (Stahl, 2000). Likewise, dopamine plays a major role in addiction because drugs, such as cocaine, opi-ates, and alcohol, increase the amount of dopamine to act on D_2 receptors and stimulate the reward system in the brain

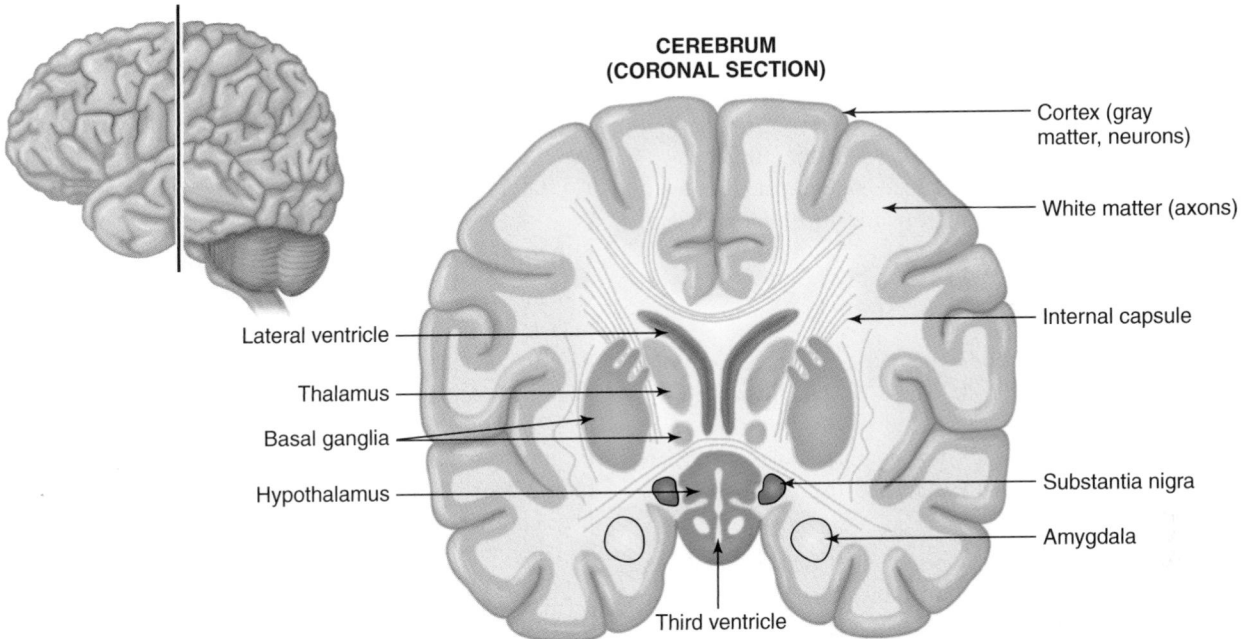

CEREBRUM (CORONAL SECTION)

Cortex (gray matter, neurons)

White matter (axons)

Internal capsule

Lateral ventricle

Thalamus

Basal ganglia

Hypothalamus

Substantia nigra

Amygdala

Third ventricle

The basal ganglia are nests of neurons located deep in the subcortical white matter. They control fine motor activity, particularly of the arms and legs. Bundles of nerve fibers from the motor cortex pass through tracts in the internal capsule and deliver impulses to the midbrain, thalamus, hypothalamus, pituitary gland (hypophysis), and limbic system located nearby. Abnormal information processing in these areas results in the characteristic behav-iors of anxiety disorders, mood disorders, ab-normal stress responses, endocrine disorders, and symptoms associated with schizophrenia.

SYNAPSES AND NEUROTRANSMITTERS

The **synapse** is the junction between one neuron and the next. Impulses (electrical or chemical) begin in the cell body of one neuron in response to stimuli and travel along the axon to an adjacent neuron.

Neurotransmitters are the chemical substances that transfer an impulse from one neuron to another. Each neuron can secrete several different transmitter substances at its synapse. The synaptic vesicles which store the neurotransmitters, migrate to the presynaptic membrane of the transmitting neuron, where they release the neurotransmitter into the synaptic space (synaptic cleft). The neurotransmitter diffuses across the synaptic space to the postsynaptic membrane of the target neuron. Receptor sites on the postsynaptic membrane take up the neurotransmitters, and in this way the impulse is transferred to the next neuron.

Neurotransmitter dysfunction plays a role in a number of psychiatric disorders, including mood disorders, anxiety states, and schizophrenia.

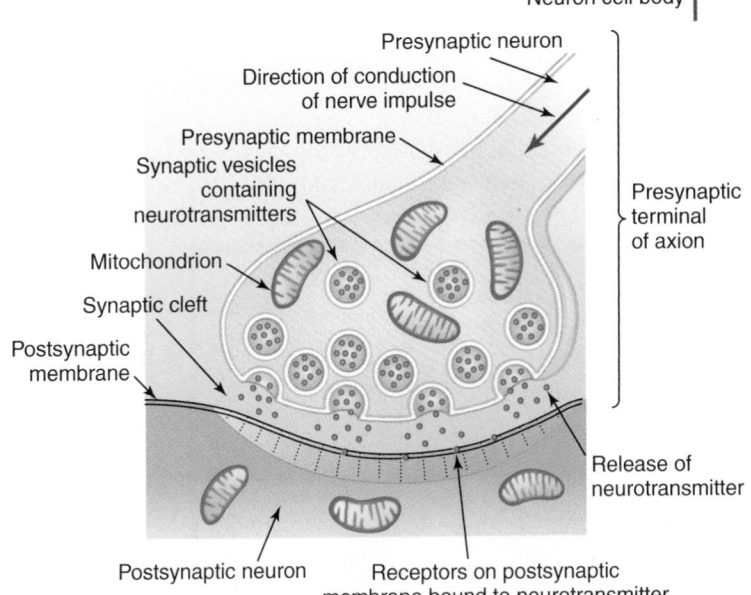

Neuron cell body

Presynaptic neuron

Direction of conduction of nerve impulse

Presynaptic membrane

Synaptic vesicles containing neurotransmitters

Presynaptic terminal of axon

Mitochondrion

Synaptic cleft

Postsynaptic membrane

Release of neurotransmitter

Postsynaptic neuron

Receptors on postsynaptic membrane bound to neurotransmitter

Figure 2–4 *(continued)*

(Ganong, 2005). Dopamine action is discussed in Chapters 14 and 28.

Norepinephrine

Norepinephrine (NE) is also known as noradrenaline. It is closely related to its precursor DA and is secreted primarily by noradrenergic neurons in the locus ceruleus in the pons, but also in scattered neuron bundles in the cerebral cortex, limbic system, amygdala, thalamus, and hypothalamus (Antai-Otong, 2000) (see Chapter 10 and Figure 10–1). NE is the precursor to adrenaline, the main ingredient in the sympathetic "fight or flight" response to a real or perceived threat. Two classes of noradrenergic receptors (alpha and beta) exist to mediate different postsynaptic responses to NE release. NE transmission and reuptake are impaired in a variety of mental illnesses, but primarily in the anxiety and substance-related disorders.

Serotonin

Serotonergic neuron cell bodies are located in the upper pons raphe nuclei (see Figure 2–5). These neurons project to the basal ganglia, the limbic system, and the cerebral cortex (see Chapter 9 and Figure 9–1). They modulate wakefulness and alertness and are known to influence the transmission of sensory pain.

Alterations to the serotonergic system or serotonin (5-hydroytryptamine, 5-HT) function along with NE have been implicated in the pathogenesis of depressive syndromes. Restoration of normal function of 5-HT and NE neural pathways has been the target of antidepressant medications. Deficit serotonergic transmission is postulated as a contributing factor to the vulnerability diathesis for major depression. Explanations for lower serotonin neurotransmission may include various mechanisms such as a decrease or depletion in the precursor L-tryptophan necessary for serotonin synthesis and a subsequent decline in the conversion of plasma tryptophan into brain serotonin. Additional mechanisms involving the pathogenesis of serotonin include dysregulation or reduced metabolism, release, or reuptake and reduced brain serotonin transporter availability (Booij, Van der Kloot, Benkelfat, Bremner, Cowen, et al., 2002; Willeit, Praschak-Rieder, Neumeister, Pirker, Asenbaum, et al., 2000).

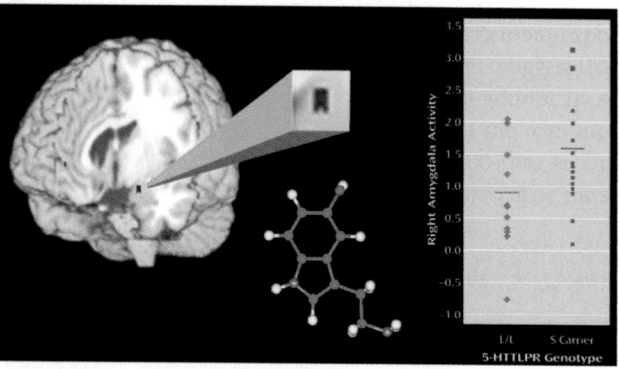

Figure 2–5 Serotonin. *(From Serotonin in* American Journal of Psychiatry, 163, *by A. R. Harriri & S. A. Brown, p. 12 [2006]).*

Gamma-aminobutyric Acid

Gamma-aminobutyric acid (GABA) is an inhibitory neurotransmitter that serves as the brain's modulator. GABA receptors throughout the brain counteract the effects of the excitatory neurotransmitter NE and DA, preventing disorganized and frenzied responses to stimuli and dampening emotional arousal. A person with low levels of GABA or fewer GABA receptors is more vulnerable to anxiety disorders or panic symptoms. Previous studies implicated dysregulation of GABA in the pathogenesis of anxiety disorders. More recent data involving animal and human subjects also implicate GABA deficits in the occipital cortex to a subtype of major depression (Sanacora, Gueroguieva, Epperson, Wu, Appel, et al., 2004; Sanacora, Mason, Rothman, & Krystal, 2002).

Glutamate and N-methyl-D-asparate

Glutamate is the main excitatory neurotransmitter in the mammalian central nervous system. It plays an important role not only in synaptic transmission but also in acute and chronic neuropathologies. It activates three classes of ionotropic receptors, including N-methyl-D-asparate (NMDA). Hypofunction in glutamatergic function, specifically involving the neurotransmission of NMDA-type glutamate receptors is believed to play a pivotal role in the pathogenesis of negative symptoms of schizophrenia and anxiety. This assumption evolved from data in which phencyclidine (PCP) and ketamine induced psychosis in animals, perhaps by blocking NMDA-type glutamate receptors on GABA neurons and subsequent increased release of glutamate and subsequent hyperstimulation of non-NMDA glutamate receptors (Konradi & Heckers, 2003). Glutamatergic dysregulation is associated with NMDA-type glutamate receptors and pathogenesis of schizophrenia may be associated with dysregulation of the dopamine-glutamate interface involving the prefrontal cortex. Specifically, cortical and subcortical glutamate release seems to be modulated by dopaminergic and, to a less significant degree, serotoninergic pathways. Pharmacological, anatomical, and biochemical studies have demonstrated hope in the future treatment of schizophrenia and other neurodegenerative disorders, through the development of novel compounds that modulate the activity of NMDA-type glutamate receptors (de Bartolomeis, Fiore, & Iasevoli, 2005; Laruelle, Frankle, Narendran, Kegeles, & Abi-Dargham, 2005).

Psychopharmacologic Agents and Neurotransmitters

Psychopharmacologic agents are prescribed to manipulate the processes of neurotransmitter production and absorption to reestablish "normal" neurochemical balance. For instance, antidepressants increase the amount of NE and serotonin in the synaptic cleft. The selective serotonin reuptake inhibitors (SSRIs) prevent the reuptake of serotonin, thus leaving more transmitter substance in the synaptic cleft to activate other neurons. Major side effects of SSRIs include restlessness, sexual disturbances, GI distress, and insomnia. The selective

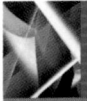

CASE STUDY

Ms. L is a 43-year-old client who recently filed for divorce from her husband of 20 years. You suspect that she is depressed. Based on your understanding of the neurobiology of depression, which symptoms is she likely to experience?

1. Elevated mood

2. Few complaints of concentration difficulties

3. Increased anxiety and energy

4. Poor concentration and sleep disturbances

Answers

1. Incorrect. Elevated mood is incorrect because due to low levels of serotonin and norepinephrine the client is most likely to present with depressed or "low mood."

2. Incorrect. Low levels of serotonin and norepinephrine are also associated with poor concentration or forgetfulness.

3. Incorrect. Elevated mood and energy are not associated with low levels of serotonin and norepinephrine. These symptoms are more likely to occur with mania or bipolar disorders.

4. Correct. Poor concentration and fatigue or low energy are associated with low serotonin and norepinephrine levels and are hallmark symptoms of depression.

Linking underlying theories to psychiatric symptoms helps the nurse understand the basis of interventions and their efficacy. In this case, which medications would you administer to treat Ms. L?

1. A medication that increases gamma-amino-butyric acid (GABA)

2. An agent that increases dopamine

3. A medication that increases serotonin and norepinephrine reuptake

4. A medication that reduces dopamine

Answers

1. Incorrect. Medication that increases GABA is most likely to be used to treat anxiety.

2. Incorrect. An agent that increases dopamine is more likely to be used to reverse muscle rigidity associated with dopamine reducing agents.

3. Correct. Based on the depression theory, reduced levels of serotonin and norepinephrine contribute to depression.

4. Incorrect. Medication that decreases dopamine levels is often used to treat psychotic symptoms.

serotonin norepinephrine reuptake inhibitor (SNRI), venlafaxine, is used in major depressive disorders and generalized anxiety disorder. Interestingly, this drug acts as a serotonin inhibitor in low doses; NE reuptake inhibitor in moderate doses, and inhibitor of DA reuptake at high doses. These newer agents have complex properties and are likely to selectively target symptoms of major depression and anxiety than older antidepressant medication (see Chapter 29).

A discussion of pharmacologic agents would be incomplete without some mention of the age of the genome and its potential impact on revolutionizing the treatment of mental illness. Recent discoveries of the Human Genome Project promise to have a profound impact on gene therapy and its potential to treat inherited illnesses. Although molecular biology is in its infancy and faces numerous challenges, it promises to assist scientists in the discovery of abnormal function at the cellular level, identify target molecules affecting this state, and discover custom-made drugs that act on various receptors or enzymes that up-regulate or down-regulate cellular processes (Drews, 2000; Etkins, 2000).

Mental disorders are simply not the result of too little or too much neurotransmitter substance, but they stem from complex and multidimensional etiologies. Levels and combinations fluctuate with important brain function, individual responses, and processes of growth and aging. Many questions remain regarding the complexity and role of neurotransmitters in mental illnesses. Increased knowledge of the therapeutic actions of psychopharmacologic agents has contributed to much of the understanding of neurotransmitter involvement.

NEUROANATOMICAL AND OTHER DIAGNOSTIC TECHNOLOGY

Recent advancement in brain imaging technology has provided information to improve our understanding of the actual and electrical and chemical processes in brain function and metabolism. Discoveries of the molecular and cellular activities of neurons clarify the role of the brain and neurotransmitters in translating neurophysiological events into behavior, thought, and emotion. Radiological and metabolic measurements have demonstrated structural abnormalities in persons with abnormal behavior, thought, and expressed emotion patterns of mental illness. For example, data from

TABLE 2–9
Important Neurotransmitters in Mental Illness

Neurotransmitters	Control, Effect, or Response	Sites of Secretion	Important in These Disorders
Biogenic Amines			
Dopamine	Fine movement, sensory integration, emotional behavior, cognition, and memory	• Nigrostriatum (substantia nigra) • Mesolimbic and limbic systems • Posterior pituitary	• Bipolar disorder • Schizophrenia
Norepinephrine	"Fight or flight" response (sympathetic system)	• Locus ceruleus • Adrenal medulla • Amygdaloid body	• Certain mood disorders • Addictions
Serotonin	Temperature, sleep, hunger, consciousness, behavior	• Raphe nuclei • Hypothalamus	• Certain mood disorders • Anxiety • Personality disorders • Schizoaffective disorders
Amino Acids			
Gamma-aminobutyric acid	Inhibitory	• Throughout cerebral cortex	• Anxiety states
Glutamate	Excitatory	• Brain, spinal cord	• Depression • Schizophrenia • Anxiety states
Neuropeptides			
Hypothalmic hormones: epinephrine, histamine	Alertness; inflammatory response	• Hypothalamus • Adrenal medulla	• Stress response • Anxiety states
Pituitary hormones: vasopressin, growth hormone, thyroid-stimulating hormone, corticotropin	Blood pressure regulation, cellular renewal, healing, stimulation of thyroxine secretion to control metabolism; corticosteroid release	• Pituitary gland	• Endocrine disorder with associated depressed mood

positron emission tomography (PET) have revealed reduced blood flow in the frontal lobe, temporal lobe, and basal ganglia during cognitive testing in some persons with schizophrenia.

Perfusion weighted magnetic resonance imaging (PW-MRI) is a newer brain mapping technique that quantifies brain perfusion. Imaging data from PW-MRI reveal the functional status of cerebral tissue with a high spatial resolution of morphology and various hemodynamics, including cerebral blood volume (CBV), cerebral blood flow (CRF), and mean transit time (MTT). Three-dimensional (3D) whole-brain perfusion technique based on echo-shifting (PRESTO) as well as multisliced mapping and quantification of brain perfusion are primarily used as diagnostic procedures to evaluate brain structures associated with symptoms and behaviors associated with schizophrenia and other mental disorders

(Antonova et al, 2005; Farrow, Hunter, Wilkinson, Green, & Spence, 2005; Hesse et al., 2005); degenerative brain disorders, such as Alzheimer's disease; and cerebral hemodynamics of central nervous system disorder, including brain tumors and strokes (Wong, Provenzale, & Petrella, 2000).

There is growing evidence of structural and functioning neuroimaging studies, specifically magnetic resonance imaging (MRI) and clinical trials, that link mental illnesses, such as obsessive-compulsive disorders, with abnormalities. Abnormalities exist primarily in the ventral prefrontal cortex and subcortical regions. Alterations in these brain regions often reflect widespread synaptic dysregulation or faulty wiring that ultimately affects higher cortical functioning (Antai-Otong, 2000; Rosenberg & Keshavan, 1998). Temporal lobe atrophy and dysfunction of the limbic system are implicated in panic disorder. Emerging data from magnetic resonance imaging studies also indicate the impact of mental disorders, such as depression—specifically untreated depression—on hippocampal volume and subsequent cognitive deficits, such as memory difficulties. Implications from these data suggest the importance of early recognition and timely and appropriate treatment of major depression (Saylam, Ucerler, Kitis, Ozand, & Gonul, 2006; Videbech & Ravnkilde, 2004). Although these findings provide strong evidence of a possible cause and are used in diagnostic evidence for the diagnosis, they are not established diagnostic criteria and require further study.

PRENATAL AND OBSTETRIC RESEARCH

Structural specialization in the brain occurs early in fetal development of the neural system. At about 4½ months' gestation, large numbers of specialized neurons migrate toward their specific destinations. Organized cell arrays of cell bodies are achieved before birth in the cortex and islands (nuclei) within the deeper regions of the brain. It is possible that these neurons migrate erratically or become disorganized in persons with mental illness, specifically schizophrenia (Conrad, Abebe, Austin, Forsythe, & Schechel, 1991). Torrey and Kaufman (1986) suggested that this damage might be due to an in utero infectious process. After the 1957 pandemic of Asian flu, studies in Finland (Mednick, Machon, & Huttunen, 1988) and another in England (O'Callaghan, Sham, Takei, Glover, & Murray, 1991) showed a significant increase in the number of births of people who later developed schizophrenia. Another study in the United States demonstrated that persons with schizophrenia were more likely to have been born in the late winter or early spring months, suggesting an infectious process. More recent studies support these findings (Cannon et al., 2003; Brown et al., 2004).

The notion that schizophrenia is a neurodevelopmental disorder has been substantiated by literature indicating that (Cannon et al., 2003; Brown et al., 2004) anomalies and other structural changes in the brain appear to have a gestational origin (Cannon et al., 2003). Obstetrical complications, particularly those involving fetal hypoxia and subsequent neurotoxic effects, may lead to an earlier onset of psychotic symptoms owing to premature pruning of cortical synapses (Cannon et al., 2000). Current data suggest that genetic and prenatal influences increase the risk of schizophrenia and are most likely to be linked to an aggregation of complications, rather than sole causes such as hypoxia and viral infections. This posit also suggests that prenatal complications interact with postnatal brain development in the pathogenesis of schizophrenia (Brown et al., 2004; Cannon et al., 2003; van Erp et al., 2002). Historically, pregnancy was perceived as "protective" against mental illness in both the mother and child. There is mounting evidence to challenge the assumption that pregnancy is protective. In fact, rates of depression are substantially high, up to 25 percent, during the second and third trimesters of pregnancy (Zlotnick, Miller, Pearlstein, Howard, & Sweeney, 2006; Bennett, Einarson, Taddio et al., 2004; Heron, O'Connor, Evans, Golding, Glover, et al., 2004). Pregnancy is a high-risk period for new onset or recurrent depression and if left untreated persists throughout the postpartum period. Recent data indicate that mood and anxiety disorders are common during the prenatal and postpartum period and adversely impact the health of women and unborn child (O'Connor, Heron, Glover, & Alspac Study Team, 2004; Ross & McLean, 2006). Neuroendocrine, neuroanatomical, and biochemistry is impacted by these conditions. Apart from biological alterations, mental illness also has a negative impact on the mother-child bonding and subsequent relationships. Nurses are poised to do early screening during the prenatal and postpartum period. Evidence of depression must be evaluated and treated based on the client and family's choices. The decision to initiate antidepressants is a strong argument, but risks and benefits of treatment versus nontreatment must be discussed with the patient and family. Mounting data indicate the efficacy and safety of antidepressants during gestation and the postpartum period (Ryan, Milis, & Misri, 2005).

GENETICS

Mental illness may be transferred genetically, just as other familial traits. Twin studies and family histories reveal a genetic vulnerability toward the development of mood disorders, anxiety disorders, schizophrenia, and other mental disorders (Cheng et al., 2006).

Twin studies have shown that certain personality traits are genetically transmitted, such as temperament, introversion, and extroversion. Researchers have produced evidence that brain pathways determining behavior patterns in men and women differ because of the different hormones produced by each sex (de Weerth, van Hess, & Buitelaar, 2003; Tsuang, 2000).

Several physiological studies have suggested that persons experiencing recurrent panic attacks may have genetically determined carbon dioxide hypersensitivity in brain stem–mediated autonomic nervous system control. This is based on the discovery that hyperventilation occurs first, followed by an increase in heart rate (Papp et al., 1989). Temporal lobe abnormality has also been implicated in panic disorders, causing people to experience psychosensory symptoms similar to those seen in temporal lobe epilepsy (Boulenger, Bierer, Uhde, Silberman, & Post, 1986). These findings have supported the efforts to determine genetic or structural origins for many of the other mental disorders.

Twin studies in schizophrenia suggest that not everyone who inherits a tendency for schizophrenia will become ill. Only those subjected to physical stress—such as a virus, head injury, and birth complications—are at risk of developing schizophrenia. Gottesman and Bertelsen (1989) traced 150 offsprings of Danish twins. In some sets of twins studied, only one had schizophrenia. These researchers found that the risk of schizophrenia was about the same—one in six—in the children of people with the disease and in children of unaffected genetically identical twins. In children of unaffected fraternal twins of schizophrenic clients, only 1 in 50 had the disease. Similar findings occur in bipolar disorders.

The incidence of schizophrenia and the age of onset of the disorder are similar throughout the world and across a variety of cultures and geographic areas that have wide differences in prenatal mortality rates and prevalence of serious infectious illness, lending credence to the genetic theory. Gender differences exist in the incidence and severity of mental illness as well. Men with schizophrenia have a far worse outcome than do women and more frequently exhibit classic and negative symptoms of the disorder (Salokangas & Stengard, 1990). Researchers are investigating a group of genes, rather than just one, that may predispose people to major mental disorders (Cheng et al., 2006; Delisi & Bertisch, 2006).

IMMUNE SYSTEM STUDIES

Increasing physiological evidence proves that the brain and the immune system communicate directly and indirectly through a complex array of hormones and neurotransmitters. Pituitary hormones affect the cells of the immune system, and the sympathetic nerves penetrate into the lymph nodes and spleen (Aguis, Glasg, & Arnason, 1991). Many studies show that stress may predispose persons to illness via an immune system effect (Irwin & Strausbaugh, 1991). Stress-related disorders are associated with either a decrease in immunologic competence or an alteration in the regulation of the immune system (Eutamene et al., 2003) (see Chapter 14).

Many of the immune system disorders such as systemic lupus erythematosus and multiple sclerosis include depression, emotional lability, nervousness, and confusion in the symptomatology, giving rise to the hypothesis that certain psychiatric symptoms arise from abnormal immune processes. Studies of the immune system functioning in schizophrenia and mood have shown increases in certain immune cells and products (Raison, Capuron, & Miller, 2006). This was especially true in research done before the administration of antipsychotic medication. Antipsychotic agents inhibit the binding of anti-human leukocyte antigen (HLA) antibodies to lymphocytes. HLAs are part of the system used by lymphocytes to recognize and process foreign material. HLAs are associated with autoimmune disorders, such as ankylosing spondylitis, rheumatoid arthritis, narcolepsy, multiple sclerosis, diabetes mellitus, and systemic lupus erythematosus.

Apart from medical conditions previously discussed, mood disorders have also been implicated in the activation of the immune system. Although there is a lack of consensus concerning the role of depression and activation of the immune system, growing research implicates increased levels of pro-inflammatory cytokines in individuals with major depression (Luby, Heffelfinger, Mrakotsky, Brown, Hessler, & Spitznagel 2003). Pro-inflammatory cytokines are potent modulators of corticotropin-releasing hormone (CRH) and contribute to alterations in reactivity of the hypothalamic-pituitary-adrenal (HPA) axis which is manifested by elevated ACTH and corti-

sol levels, both of which are implicated in the pathogenesis of major depression. Elevated concentrations of serum cortisol and pro-inflammatory cytokines suggest a state or biological marker in these individuals and might contribute to prolonged neuroendocrine dysregulation that are also associated with depression (Luby et al., 2003). Despite these findings, it is evident that additional research is needed to examine the cytokine link in mood disorder.

NEUROENDOCRINE STUDIES

Endocrine studies of depressed persons have shown functional differences in the hypothalamic-pituitary-thyroid axis compared with healthy subjects and clients with dysthymia. Changes occur in thyroid-stimulating hormone (TSH) and thyroid hormones subsequent to dexamethasone administration (Watson, Gallagher, Ritchie et al., 2004).

This is demonstrated in the fact that persons with endocrine disorders often have symptoms of mental disorders as well. Depression is common in persons with hyperadrenalism (Cushing's syndrome) and hypodrenalism (Addison's disease). Hyperthyroidism causes anxiety, and hypothyroidism often results in depression. Both hypoparathyroidism and hyperparathyroidism are associated with anxiety and depression. Hypomania and depression often follow administration of corticotropin. (See Chapter 9 for further discussion.)

Cortisol dysregulation is also indicated in various anxiety disorders, such as acute stress disorder and post-traumatic stress disorder. Individuals with these disorders tend to have significantly lower cortisol levels, particularly those with previous exposure to trauma. (See Chapter 11 for an extensive discussion.)

Alternative therapies, such as phototherapy, have an antidepressant effect in the treatment of seasonal affective disorder, suggesting that neuroendocrine dysregulation plays a role in depressive disorders arising from changes in the external environment (Wileman et al., 2001; Terman & Terman, 2005).

CHRONOBIOLOGY

Often what affects one body system can affect another system directly or indirectly. This is particularly true of the interaction of the nervous, endocrine, and immune systems.

Many mental disorders, especially the mood disorders, are accompanied by problems in biological rhythms. Chronobiology is the field of science that studies the rhythms of life. Biological phenomena fluctuate over time in response to internal and external factors. Internal rhythms in humans are believed to be controlled by the suprachiasmatic nucleus within the hypothalamus (Bernard, Gonze, Cajavec, Herzel, & Krumer, 2007). Individual factors such as genetic vulnerability, arrangement of neural pathways, and age and gender of the person affect the rhythmic patterns.

Rhythms external to humans influence the internal rhythms as well. The external rhythms that set, or synchronize, the internal rhythm is called a zeitgeber. The process by which these zeitgebers synchronize the internal clock is called *entrainment*. An example of entrainment is the sleep-wake cycle. People have regular times for sleeping and waking based on external factors such as school and work. Processes that alter some aspect of a biological rhythm, with the exception of the rhythm's period, are called maskers. Drinking coffee to stay awake to study for an examination is an example of *masking*. The coffee can mask the rhythm of mental alertness by creating a brief period of alertness at a time when the person is normally ready for sleep.

The interrelationships among the many rhythms of life are quite complex. Many biological activities rise and fall in rhythm patterns. Biological rhythms that repeat approximately every 24 hours are called circadian rhythms. Body temperature, hormone secretion, the immune system, sleep and wakefulness, and the cardiovascular and other body systems all exhibit circadian rhythms. Infradian rhythms refer to biological variations with a frequency lower than circadian (rhythms that have longer, slower cycles than circadian rhythms). In contrast, untradian rhythms are defined as biological variations with a frequency higher (less than 24 hours) than circadian (rhythms that have shorter, faster cycles than circadian rhythms).

Disturbances in these rhythms of life are exhibited in mood disorders. Depression is often characterized by marked disturbances in the daily sleep-wake cycle and disturbances in rapid eye movement (REM) and non-REM sleep. (See Chapter 23 for a discussion of sleep disorders.)

Recent research indicates that light, especially bright light, is effective in shifting human circadian rhythms and can alleviate some depression in seasonal affective disorder (Terman & Terman, 2005). Changes in amplitudes of temperature and TSH circadian rhythms also occur in depression. The most consistent abnormal finding is an advance in the timing of the nadir of the cortisol secretion in depression. All these events are influenced by the pituitary-thyroid-adrenal axis. (See Chapter 30 for a detailed discussion of biological therapies.)

Some scientists are investigating the implications circadian rhythms have for the timing of surgery and the administration of drugs in an effort to optimize their therapeutic effects.

Application to Nursing

Advances in technology expand the concept and theories of neurobiology and implications for psychiatric nurses. Neurobiological studies provide the basis of target sites for pharmacological and psychotherapeutic interventions that mitigate symptoms of various psychiatric disorders. By linking complex and multidimensional brain regions, molecular and biochemical processes to specific psychiatric symptoms and behaviors, the psychiatric nurse is poised to understand the client's experience through caring and healing nurse-client relationships. Healing nurse-client relationships provide a venue that enables the nurse to understand the relationship between neurobiological processes, client symptoms, and goal-setting along with implementation of client-centered interventions. Through shared decision making the client learns to cope with and effectively self-manage his illness, grasp the meaning of his or her illness, and experience hope and recovery through empathy, health education, and adherence to holistic treatment planning across the life span.

SUMMARY

Mental disorders are most likely caused by a variety of factors, including intrinsic external environmental conditions. The difficulty in forming conclusions about the causes of mental disorders relates to the nature of the research itself. Brain studies are performed on animals or on humans post mortem. There is no way to tell what the brain was like before the disorder developed. With the newer technological advances in neuroimaging, researchers can view what is occurring in the brain at the time of the scan. The scans are performed on people who have a particular disorder as well as on normal control subjects, but the number of persons who can be studied is limited because of time and cost. At some point, research studies must include people before and after the disorder becomes apparent. The question remains about which comes first, the structural multidimensional problems or the learned ways of behaving, thinking, feeling, and believing. Do the neuroendocrine problems in depression or post-traumatic stress disorder come before the illness, or does the sense of helplessness, hopelessness, or fear cause the neuroendocrine problems? Is the propensity of anxiety inherited, or is it learned? Each theory offers a convincing argument when studied in depth and a piece of the truth emerges. However, to understand the etiology of mental disorders, one must consider the valid points from all the theories.

Nursing is caring in which the nurse is guided by the unique health care needs of clients and their families. It involves shared decision making with clients and their families and is guided by healing relationships that instill hope, facilitate recovery and resilience, and enable the client to cope with treating responses to health problems. Based on previously discussed theories, responses to health problems impact cognitive functioning, thought processes, memory, sleeping and eating patterns, ability to experience pleasure, adapt to stressful life events, and attain a sense of well-being and overall mental and physical health.

SYSTEMS THEORY

Systems theory is a way of viewing a person, families, groups, and society. Several theories of nursing are based on systems theory, warranting a brief overview of its concepts.

BASIC CONCEPTS

General systems theory was introduced in 1928 by Ludwig von Bertalanffy (1968). Although it began as a theory for explaining biological systems, other scientific disciplines found it useful as well.

In general systems theory, a system is a set of components or units interacting with each other within a boundary that filters the kind and rate of flow of inputs and outputs to and from the system. For example, the body is the structure, but the body also has a multitude of functions. Systems can be open or closed. Open systems are open to the exchange of matter, energy, and information about their environment. Biological and social systems are open systems. Open systems move in the direction of greater differentiation, elaboration, and a higher level of organization. The system can be explained only as a totality, or whole. Holism, or synergism, is the concept that the whole is not just the sum of the parts but is something different from its parts.

Systems have boundaries that separate them from their environments. The open system has permeable boundaries between itself and a broader suprasystem. The closed system has rigid, impenetrable boundaries. Boundaries are easily defined in physical and biological systems but are difficult to delineate in social systems such as organizations. Boundaries keep out what is not necessary or desirable to the system and bring in the necessary and desirable resources.

In a dynamic relationship with the environment, the open system receives various inputs. Inputs are the resources needed by the system. Inputs are transformed in a process called throughput and are exported as output.

Closed systems engender entropy. As entropy increases, the system fails. Entropy is a movement toward disorder, lack of resource transformation, and death. An example is when the body fails to function, the person can no longer use inputs and therefore dies.

Negentropy, or negative entropy, is a process of more complete organization and ability to transform resources, and of increasing complexity and higher organization. It is the process of building up, whereas, entropy is the process of running down. An example of negentropy is the learning process. Information is an input, learning is the throughput, or the higher organizational complexity. The result can be referred to as negentropy. In terms of the nursing process, entropy can be equated with health problems, and negentropy, with healthful outcomes or a state of greater organization.

Open systems seek equilibrium and homeostasis through the continuous inflow of materials, energy, and information. The concept of feedback is important in understanding how a system maintains a healthy steady state. Information concerning the outputs or process of the system is fed back as an input into the system, perhaps leading to changes in the transformation process and future outputs. Feedback can be both positive and negative. Negative input is information that suggests the system is deviating from a steady state. An example of this is fever.

Systems are arranged in hierarchies. A system is composed of subsystems of a lower order and is also part of a suprasystem. Open systems are further characterized by equifinality, which indicates that goals or purposes may be achieved with different initial conditions and in different ways. Individuals and social systems can accomplish goals with diverse inputs and with adaptable internal activities. Closed systems are repetitious, with a direct cause-and-effect relationship between the initial condition and the final state.

Application to Nursing

Each client is viewed holistically as a system functioning within a system. The client cannot be treated in isolation. Family involvement is a critical and essential component to client-centered care. Nurses must enlist the family's input into treatment planning; identify their needs, strengths, preferences, health practices, and understanding of the client's experience and illness. This process helps the nurse evaluate the quality of support systems and glean insight into the client's and family's strengths and challenges. If the client is to achieve a steady state, or optimal level of functioning, then boundaries, input, output, and throughput must be addressed. Throughput is what happens to the input before it is exported. In humans, throughput is what happens to food between ingestion and elimination. It is what happens between sensation and observable behavior. The goal of treatment is to achieve equilibrium; to manage resources effectively; and to change the throughput processes, such as changing perception.

A general systems theory perspective offers a model that reflects and fosters change, growth, learning, and the interrelatedness of all living systems. Humans are viewed as holistic, goal-directed, self-maintaining, and self-creating persons of intrinsic worth, capable of self-reflection on their own uniqueness. This healthy perspective also provides an ecological view of persons as interrelated, interdependent, interacting, validating, and complex organisms constantly influencing and being influenced by the environment. In systems theory, mental illness is viewed as multidimensional and involves inadequate resources and social systems to sustain homeostasis and neurobiological processes and systems gone awry.

HUMAN NEEDS THEORY

All theories about human development and behavior address human needs, but Abraham Maslow's (1943, 1970) explication of human needs fits well into a model of personhood and nursing.

Need motivates the behavior of a person. According to Maslow, a basic need is inactive or functionally absent in the healthy person. If basic needs are not met, illness is likely to occur. When basic needs are met, health occurs.

According to Maslow, needs are hierarchical, with the lower level needs being critical to survival. The needs at the lower levels must be met before the needs at the higher level can be met (Figure 2–6).

Maslow also specified cognitive and aesthetic needs. Cognitive needs include the need to know and understand, to be curious, to explain, to organize, to analyze, and to look for relations and meanings. The aesthetic needs include the need for order, symmetry, closure, and beauty.

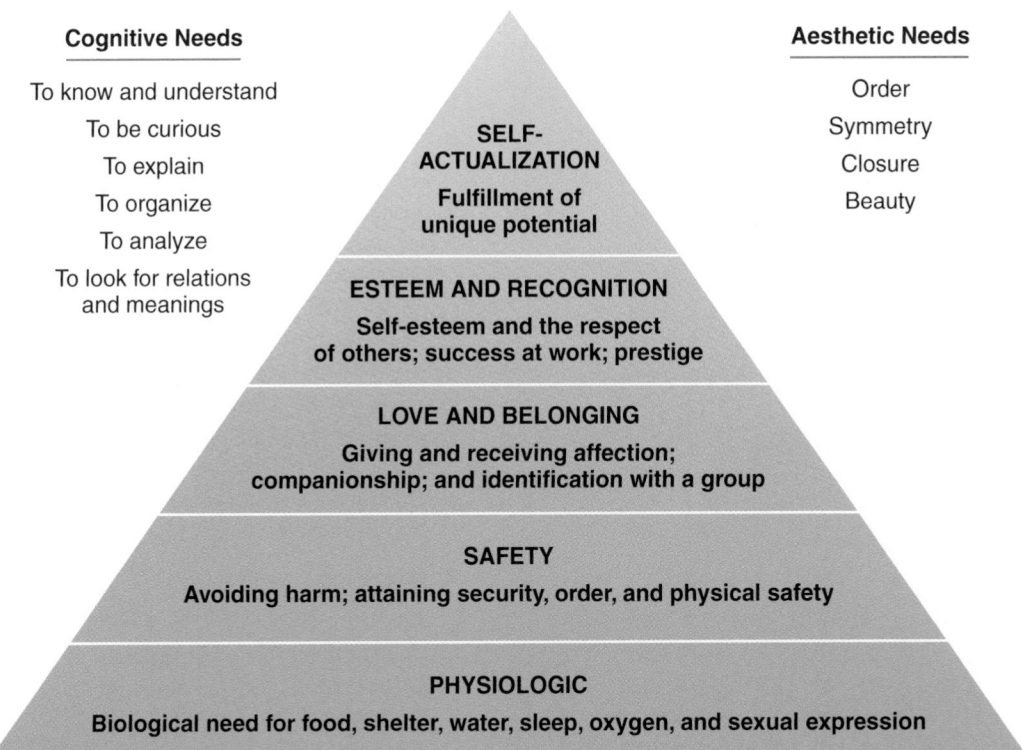

Cognitive Needs

To know and understand

To be curious

To explain

To organize

To analyze

To look for relations
and meanings

Aesthetic Needs

Order

Symmetry

Closure

Beauty

SELF-ACTUALIZATION

Fulfillment of
unique potential

ESTEEM AND RECOGNITION

Self-esteem and the respect
of others; success at work; prestige

LOVE AND BELONGING

Giving and receiving affection;
companionship; and identification with a group

SAFETY

Avoiding harm; attaining security, order, and physical safety

PHYSIOLOGIC

Biological need for food, shelter, water, sleep, oxygen, and sexual expression

Figure 2–6 Maslow's Hierarchy of Needs. Maslow postulated that if basic needs are not met, illness is likely to occur. Maslow also specified cognitive and aesthetic needs.

APPLICATION TO NURSING

Recognition of human needs is crucial to nursing care. The behavior of the client will give clues to needs. The nurse must then coordinate interventions to promote need attainment.

Human needs theory has been useful to nursing in organizing curricula and in assessing and giving care, but it may have contributed to the emphasis on the physiological needs. The need to maintain life and physical integrity is the first priority when life and physical integrity are in jeopardy. Nonetheless, the nurse's role does not end by meeting only physiological needs. Psychiatric nurses must also integrate the client's physiological needs with a greater understanding and focus on complex underlying processes that govern symptoms and behavioral responses.

THE WELLNESS-ILLNESS CONTINUUM

Before the 1960s, one common definition subscribed to by nursing to define health was provided by the World Health Organization ([WHO], 1947), stating that health is a state of complete physical, mental, and social well-being and not merely the absence of disease or infirmity. In 1961, Halbert Dunn first published his classic text, *High-Level Wellness*, and changed the focus to levels of wellness rather than disease. He viewed health and illness as dynamic and moving along a continuum rather than circumscribed states.

High-level wellness is an integrated method of functioning oriented toward maximizing the client's optimal level of functioning. High-level wellness occurs when the physical

and psychosocial needs are met in ways that support maximum functioning, leaving the person with an energy reserve from which to draw. Low-level wellness or severe illness is the inability of people to meet their needs in a way that allows them to function and that depletes their energy reserve.

The concepts germane to Dunn's model are totality, uniqueness, energy, inner and outer worlds, and self-integration and energy use (Table 2–10).

For a person to use energy in maintaining high-level wellness, she must function in an integrated way. When the person faces change, she must make changes that use energy efficiently. For example, when a person develops a sore elbow after a golf game, she will take measures to conserve energy so that the physical resources needed to reduce swelling and pain are accessible. The person may seek psychosocial support to conserve energy but will not, if functioning in an integrating manner, play another round of golf.

Wellness is often viewed as synonymous to health or function. Illness is often associated with disease and disability. Many national and international organizations define health as a worldwide concern and focus on health promotion across the life span and diverse cultures and populations. For example, the World Health Organization is the United Nations specialized agency for health. This renowned organization was established in 1948 and its primary aim centers on the "attainment by all peoples of the highest level of health." The WHO defines health "as a state of complete physical, mental and social well-being" and not just the absence of disease or ill-health.

TABLE 2–10
Basic Concepts of Dunn's Model of Wellness–Illness

- **Totality:** integration of the physical and psychosocial components into a unified whole. The person must be viewed as a whole. Each aspect of a person is interdependent on all other aspects

- **Uniqueness:** each person's life experiences, genetic make-up, and developmental processes come together to make an individual unlike any other

- **Energy:** the environment must provide people with a constant source of energy to meet their physical and psychosocial needs

- **Self-integration:** all parts of the personality must be balanced and linked

- **Energy use:** How a person uses energy affects the level of wellness and illness

- **Inner and outer worlds:** a person's experiences, both inner and outer and past and present, influence the person's behavior

Note. From *High-Level Wellness* (7th ed.), by H. L. Dunn, 1972, Arlington, VA: Beatty. Adapted with permission.

Other organizations committed to funding initiatives that promote and advance the health of all Americans include the Robert Wood Johnson Foundation (RWJF) and the Centers for Disease Control and Prevention (CDC). Funding initiatives from the RWJF focus on:

- Assuring that all Americans have access to quality health care at a reasonable cost

- Improving the quality of care and supporting persons with chronic health problems

- Promoting healthy communities and lifestyles

- Reducing the personal, social, and economic consequences of substance-related disorders

Similar to the WHO and RWJF, the CDC seeks to protect the health and safety of individuals and provide essential human services to individuals who are least able to help themselves. The CDC was founded in 1946 to control malaria. It remains at the leading edge of public health initiatives to prevent and control infectious and chronic diseases, injuries, disabilities, and environmental health threats. Because health problems and disease control are global concerns, the organizations' efforts are tailored to meet and address them from a national and worldwide perspective. The CDC, like other agencies and organizations concerned with health promotion, is committed to improve peoples' health across the life span, world, and mitigate emerging health threats. (See sites for these organizations' in the Internet Resources section at the end of this chapter.) As previously discussed, the global defin-

ition of health extends beyond the absence of disease or symptom management and refers to a state of mental, physical, and social well-being. Increasingly, the goal of mental health extends to recovery and hope that are guided by psychosocial rehabilitation and recovery.

Recovery refers to a paradigm shift that constitutes remission of symptoms; client choices and preferences; and instills hope, resilience, and mainstream employment (Kelly & Gamble, 2005; Rosenheck, Struop, Keefe, et al., 2005; Cutcliffe & Herth, 2002). Historically, the goal of psychiatric treatment involved symptom reduction. Today's focus in treating persons with psychiatric conditions extends beyond symptoms management, social disabilities, and high resource utilization (Harrison et al., 2001) and goes a step further to include recovery. The present recovery movement constitutes a new paradigm in mental health care. Major characteristics of the recovery model include:

- Focusing on client-centered care that includes preferences, choices, culture, and ethnicity

- Identifying behaviors and strategies needed to control symptoms and maintain mental, physical, and psychosocial health

- Sustaining hope and guarding against despair

- Promoting resilience

- Focusing on client and family strengths

- Valuing personal experiences

- Being humanistic

- Facilitating self-efficacy and self-management

- Expecting the client to take personal responsibility

- Accepting relapses and setbacks as part of the recovery process

- Validating and respecting the meaning of the client's experience

Recovery is every client and family's right. Correlates of recovery include symptom management, attaining an optimal level of functioning, and quality of life. As mental health treatment paradigms shift, nurses must work with clients, families, and other health care professionals to facilitate and implement recovery-based interventions. Recovery begins with the initial nurse-client interaction that engenders hope and optimism and a willingness to help. Problem solving and other interventions promote resilience in clients as they struggle with stressors or challenges of daily living. Sustained recovery requires comprehensive, coordinated, consistent, competent, compassionate, and client-centered treatments for the advance delivery and clinical outcomes of pharmacotherapy and psychosocial interventions (Kopelowicz & Liberman, 2003).

APPLICATION TO NURSING

The wellness-illness model highlights a holistic view of health. Mental health and illness also exist on a continuum and are not separate from physical health and illness.

The role of the nurse in the wellness-illness continuum involves integration of various health promotion interventions that improve health and wellness across the life span. Health promoting interventions involves identifying high-risk behaviors; vulnerable populations, such as frail older adults and infants; and collaborating with clients, families, caregivers, and health care providers to reduce risk factors and promote healthier lifestyles. Health education, parenting classes, adequate nutrition, balanced diet, stress management, regular exercise are just a few interventions nurses can use to work with clients, families, and communities to promote overall mental, physical, and social health.

Nurses work with people experiencing varying levels of wellness and illness, with the goal of helping others achieve an optimal level of functioning or wellness. The nurse distinguishes positive and negative aspects of wellness, builds on positive attributes, and reduces negative influences. Nurses help people conserve energy and make the most efficient use of available energy. Together, the nurse and client work to resolve conflicts between the person and the environment and within the self to maintain integrity. This theory underscores the need for nurses to be attentive in treating the whole person and not merely addressing the physiological needs.

HEALTH RECOVERY

A health promotion and recovery-based paradigm requires understanding and embracing the concept of recovery as an integral aspect of care for clients and their families. They must move from the traditional disease-illness model to the wellness-health model that involves helping clients achieve symptom management, achieve optimal functioning and quality of life as evidenced by gainful employment, integration into their communities, and psychosocial skills that enable them to cope with stressors before they become crises. Through empathy, collaboration, mutual respect, and acceptance of the client's uniqueness and strengths nurses can instill these qualities in clients and facilitate optimal functioning and state of well-being.

STRESS-ADAPTATION MODELS

The concept of stress provides a means of understanding holistic responses to external and internal demands that unfold into important complex neurobiological or psychosocial processes. A person's perception of a stressor ultimately determines the outcome of neurobiological responses: appraisal and response. This response is further influenced by the level of ego function, developmental stage, available resources, previous experiences, and the number and severity of stressors. Adaptive emotional and biological responses are pivotal to regulation of human behavior (Lazarus & Folkman, 1984; Lazarus, 1991; Seyle, 1976). Seyle's classic stress-adaptation theory describes stress as an inevitable physiological response; whereas Lazarus's interactional theory explains stress in terms of the person's cognitive appraisal systems.

Seyle's (1976) important contribution to defining health was his explanation of stress relative to adaptation. He asserted that a stress response occurs whenever a person encounters continuous stress. He described this phenomenon as generalized stress syndrome. The following process explains this stress reaction:

◆ Alarm reaction (first phase)—mobilizes the body's defenses and homeostatic responses against the stressor—"fight or flight response"

◆ Stage of resistance (second phase)—the body attempts to reduce damage from the stressor

◆ Stage of exhaustion (third phase)—evolves after the body's attempts to adapt to change fail to manage the stressors if appropriate interventions to reduce the stress are unsuccessful (see Chapter 4)

In comparison to Seyle's theory, Lazarus's theory focuses on the person's cognitive appraisal of the life event that ultimately determines the response as expressed by emotions (Lazarus & Launier, 1978; Lazarus, 1991). Appraisal of an event gives it value or recognition, and relative to coping it refers to the meaning of internal and external events. Events may be perceived as irrelevant, benign or nonthreatening, or threatening or harmful. Lazarus (1966) identified two forms of appraisal: primary and secondary. Primary appraisal is the initial response to a stressor. Lazarus (1966) described three types of primary appraisal: irrelevant, benign positive, and stressful. *Irrelevant appraisals* occur when the person confronts external occurrences that do not pose a threat to his or her livelihood. *Positive benign appraisals* are events that have a genuinely positive appraisal, or they enhance adaptation or stimulate a sense of well-being. These events generate feelings of pleasure, joy, and happiness and may also be accompanied by guilt or anxiety.

Stressful appraisals are regarded as injurious, hazardous, and demanding or challenging (Lazarus, 1966). Encounters that have negative connotations or cause damage, such as physical illness, injury to quality of life, and loss of normal functioning, are defined as *injurious*. *Hazardous threats* are foreseen occurrences that spur people to mobilize coping responses to reduce likely risks. This form of appraisal normally arouses negative thoughts and feelings, such as anger, helplessness, anxiety, and fear. The capacity for adaptive as well as maladaptive responses exists with hazards. *Demanding* or *challenging* situations also provide opportunities for using and enhancing coping and adaptive responses, but these responses differ from the hazardous form because they generate positive feelings such as zeal, motivation, and excitement. A challenge form of appraisal normally produces positive thoughts, such as "Anything is possible." The implication is that challenge appraisals depict healthier adaptive coping responses that promote a sense of well-being.

Secondary appraisals arise from a perceived threat or harm if primary appraisals are ineffective in managing the stressful event, and they enhance or promote a positive outcome of primary appraisals (Lazarus, 1966).

Apart from the nature and perception of stress, the individual's ability to mobilize internal and external biological and behavior responses are an integral part of these processes. Resilience is the capacity to recover or adjust to a stressful or life-threatening situation in which the individual employs adaptive physiological and psychosocial responses to maintain homeostasis. The concept of resilience offers an explanation of individual coping mechanisms, both internal and external, being able to ameliorate potentially harmful or deleterious effects of a life-threatening event by mobilizing complex adaptive coping behaviors that allow the individual to maintain mental and physical homeostasis. (Further discussion of adaptive coping responses is discussed in Chapter 4.)

APPLICATION TO NURSING

Stress theories offer psychiatric nurses a framework to assess their clients' response to life events, and to develop appropriate interventions that promote adaptive coping behaviors and positive outcomes. Assessing the client's cognitive appraisal of life events and subsequent biological aspects of stressful events enables the nurse to work with the client to reduce stress using stress management techniques, such as meditation and deep abdominal breathing exercises, cognitive therapy, and other stress-reducing interventions. This process involves helping the client assess the meaning of stressors and mobilizing resources that promote adaptive coping behaviors. By helping the client gain control over physiological and cognitive appraisals, she gains a sense of competence, control, self-efficacy, resilience, and health, thus improving self-esteem.

NURSING THEORIES AND MODELS

A theory is an organized set of statements related to significant questions in a discipline communicated into a meaningful whole. It is the picture of reality that describes, explains, predicts, or prescribes responses, events, situations, conditions, or relationships. Theories have concepts relating to the discipline's phenomena. These concepts relate to each other to form theoretical statements. Theoretical statements are based on repeated observations over time.

Theories are made up of assumptions, concepts, propositions, and exemplars that form the foundation for a discipline or profession. Theories provide goals for practice, define the boundaries of practice, and describe behaviors for members of the profession (Riehl-Sisca, 1989). Nursing theory provides the nurse with goals for assessment, diagnosis, and intervention, and as a result makes practice more efficient and effective. The language of nursing theory provides a common ground for communication. It describes scientific principles to accurately predict the consequences of care and the range of client responses or outcomes.

The major concepts in nursing theory have been identified as human beings, nursing, health, and the environment. Generally, *human beings* are described as holistic and interactive, a developing system in interaction with the environment.

The description of *nursing* includes the nursing process, the recipient of care, and the role of the nurse. The goal of nursing takes some form of assisting, restoring, maintaining, enhancing, or promoting optimal health. The *environment* includes various aspects of society: events, conditions, and elements that make up the client's surroundings. The health care system is part of the environment. Most theories address the internal environment as well. *Health* is depicted as a state of wellness or optimal functioning. Internal and external environments are determinants of the health state.

In the following theories, you will notice how each describes the four concepts. This is merely a brief overview of the conceptual framework of nursing.

NEUMAN'S SYSTEMS MODEL

Person. People are a unique composite of characteristics within a normal given range of response. Each person in a state of wellness or illness is a dynamic composite of the interrelationship of physiological, psychological, sociocultural, and developmental variables. People maintain harmony and balance with their environment by a process of interaction and adjustment.

Each person has a basic structure or central core of survival factors unique to the individual but in a range common to other humans, such as temperature, genetic, response pattern, ego structure, and strengths and weaknesses of body organs. The central core is protected from stressors by concentric rings. The outside ring is the normal line of defense—a normal range of response that evolves over time. An inner ring consists of a flexible line of defense—a dynamic, rapidly changing protective buffer that prevents stressors from breaking through the normal line of defense.

Nursing. Nursing is a unique profession concerned with all the variables affecting a person's response to stressors. The nurse seeks the highest potential level of stability for each client and assesses the client's response to stressors and the relationship of the environment to the client's reactions. The nurse assists individuals, families, and groups to attain or maintain a maximum level of wellness by interventions directed toward reducing stress, strengthening the line of defense, and maintaining a reasonable degree of adaptation.

Health. Wellness is the ability of the person's flexible line of defense to maintain equilibrium against any stressor. Any variances in wellness occur when stressors are able to penetrate the flexible line of defense. Health is seen on a continuum, depending on the degree of need fulfillment. Failing to meet one's needs results in a diminished state of wellness. A stressor is anything that attempts to penetrate a person's normal line of defense to cause disequilibrium.

Environment. The environment includes all internal and external factors. The *internal* environment is the flexible line of defense against stressors, such as ego functioning or cognitive abilities. The *external* environment is the normal line of defense and consists of coping abilities, lifestyle, and developmental stage (Neuman, 1989).

OREM'S SELF-CARE MODEL

Person. The person is a total being with universal developmental needs and is capable of continuous self-care. The person is a unity that can function biologically, symbolically, and socially. People have the ability to perform self-care activities they initiate and perform independently to maintain life, health, and well-being. The ability to care for oneself is self-care agency; the ability to care for others is dependent-care agency. Agency means action. Self-care is undertaken to meet three types of self-care requisites: universal, developmental, and health deviation.

Nursing. Nursing consists of deliberate and purposeful actions to provide assistance to those who are unable to meet health-related self-care needs. The nurse is required to design, create, provide, and manage systems or therapeutic care to a person with self-care deficits until the person can care for himself or herself. In chronic poor health or disability, the nurse seeks to stabilize or minimize the effects.

Health. Health is a state of being whole, sound, and fully integrated. It includes physiological and psychobiological mechanisms in relation to and in interaction with other human beings.

Environment. Orem presented a limited view of the environment that comprises the factors and conditions that can be regulated in caring for clients. The individual and the environment form an integrated functional whole or system (Orem, 1980).

ORLANDO'S NEEDS-ORIENTED THEORY

Person. People are developmental beings with needs and are distinct in their responses, thoughts, and feelings.

Nursing. Nursing consists of understanding and providing the client's immediate need for help to avoid, relieve, diminish, or cure her sense of helplessness, until she experiences an increased sense of well-being and an improvement of behavior. The nurse assesses behavior and its meaning, shares these perceptions, and explores the client's experiences.

Health. Health is a sense of adequacy or well-being, comfort, and fulfilled needs (Orlando, 1961).

Environment. Orlando did not define the environment.

ROY'S ADAPTATION MODEL

Person. Roy describes the person as a biopsychosocial being in constant interaction with a changing environment. To cope with a changing world, the person uses both innate and acquired mechanisms that are biopsychosocial in nature. Health and illness are one inevitable dimension of the person's life. To respond positively to environmental changes, the person must adapt. Adaptation is a result of the stimulus one is exposed to, and the adaptation level. The person has four modes of adaptation: physiological needs, self-concept, role function, and interdependence.

Nursing. The goal of nursing is to contribute to the person's health, quality of life, and dying with dignity by promoting adaptation in each of the four modes. Nurses assess behavior and the stimuli that influence adaptation. Interventions manage these stimuli and enhance the interaction of the person and the environment.

Health. Health is a state and a process of being and becoming an integrated, whole person. It is a reflection of the level of adaptation. Lack of integration represents a lack of health.

Environment. The environment includes conditions, circumstances, and influences that surround and affect the development and behavior of the person. These influencing factors are categorized as focal, contextual, and residual stimuli. The changing environment stimulates the person to make adaptive responses (Roy, 1984).

PARSE'S THEORY OF HUMAN BECOMING

Person. People are intentional beings and by nature live a seamless symphony throughout the life span. People are involved with the universe in directing their personal becoming through relationships with others. Individuals live in the moment within the presence of mutual processes with the universe structures which are multidimensional. Mutual processes enable the person to manage her life and health through the freedom and right to make choices and live their lives as they choose (Parse, 1998, 2002).

Nursing. The goal of nursing is being with or in the presence within mutual nurse-client processes to understand and value the meaning of the client's lived experience, assimilate preferences and beliefs that influence health care choices and preferences (Parse, 1998). The nurse also uses a nonjudgmental approach and reveres the client's expertise in knowing what is best for him or her within the nurse-client relationship. The nurse uses her true presence with the client to establish mutual processes and ensure shared decision making with the client to assess behavior, identify treatment choices, develop a client-centered treatment plan, and observe changing health patterns. True presence in the nurse involves mindfulness to the client.

Health. Health is an individual commitment to mutual processes created with others and by being in the true presence with the nurse. People may modify their health patterns or behaviors in response to parallel their health care expectations or concerns.

Environment. The environment includes the universe and mutual processes. Humans are in mutual process with the universe structure or with others who are with the individual.

ROGERS' UNITARY HUMAN THEORY

Person. The person is a unified whole with unique attributes and who manifests behaviors or characteristics that extend beyond the sum of his or her parts.

Nursing. Nursing consists of compassion and value of each person's individuality. Its primary goal is to strengthen the integrity of the human field and promote optimal health potential (Rogers, 1970). The nurse ensures individuality by using client-centered and a holistic approach in which she assesses preferences, beliefs, and values unique to the client; assimilates and synthesizes relevant data; monitors and trends patterns of events; and initiates health care that facilitates well-being, optimal functioning, and health.

Health. Health is an attainment of wholeness and openness, safety, and overall human functioning.

Environment. The person continuously interacts with the environment through mutual exchange of matter and energy.

PEPLAU'S INTERPERSONAL THEORY

In psychiatric nursing, perhaps the most influential theorist has been Hildegard Peplau (1952). A survey of psychiatric-mental health nurses (Hirschmann, 1989) indicated that one half used this theory as a foundation for practice. Peplau's work has influenced every aspect of nursing so that her work is now considered "public domain." She introduced nursing to the importance of interpersonal relationship and communication strategies, the nursing process, the concept of nursing diagnosis, and more. The concepts that are important to her theory are also important concepts in other psychosocial theories; therefore, they may serve as a summary of how nurses can help clients. Table 2–11 identifies the concepts and shows how these concepts are interrelated.

Person. Persons are described as unique in experiences, beliefs, expectations, and patterns of relation to others. The client is viewed "as a person responding in the situation and in relation to whatever or whoever is in it with him or her—illusionary or real" (Peplau, 1952, p. 270). The client includes individuals, groups, families, and communities.

Nursing. "Nursing is a significant, therapeutic, interpersonal process. It functions co-operatively with other human processes that make health possible for individuals in the community. . . . Nursing is an educative instrument, a maturing force, that aims to promote forward movement of personality in the direction of creative, constructive, productive, personal and community living" (Peplau, 1952, p. 16). The focus of nursing is the "reactions of the client to the circumstances of illness or health problems, thus overlapping medicine only when dealing with disease processes directly" (Peplau, 1969, p. 37).

Health. Health "is a word symbol that implies forward movement of personality and other ongoing human processes in the direction of creative, constructive, productive, personal and community living" (Peplau, 1952, p. 12).

Environment. The environment includes the physiological, psychological, and social fluidity that is the context of the nurse-client relationship (Peplau, 1952). Peplau recognized the positive contribution that a therapeutic milieu and a supportive environment make to health.

Application to Nursing

Therapeutic relationships are the keystone of psychiatric nursing. Peplau's (1952) interpersonal theory provides a template that delineates the evolution of the nurse-client relationship and its role in problem solving or resolution. The nurse's ability to approach a client and form a nurse-client relationship requires a therapeutic process that begins with orientation or the time when the client seeks help. An empathetic and accepting attitude promotes trust as the nurse assesses or *identifies* the client's strengths, needs, stressors, and coping patterns and collaborates to develop client-based interventions. Active listening and collaboration with the client promotes growth and self-confidence. Throughout this process the nurse assesses or *explores* the client's understanding of her symptoms or distress, and potential treatment options that facilitate problem solving or crisis resolution. Healthy *resolution* of the client's presenting symptoms also involves evaluating specific treatment outcomes with a focus on the nature of the nurse-client relationship. Overall, Peplau's theory enables the nurse to form a therapeutic environment that empowers the client to understand and manage stressful situations and opportunities to develop adaptive behavioral changes.

SUMMARY

◆ Nurses provide care to individuals, clients, their families, and to groups. This is an expansive mandate that requires an array of skills. Nurses develop expertise in caring for unique persons in unique circumstances.

◆ Centuries of observations of human functioning provide the bases on which nurses can establish their practice. Each theory discussed provides a unique field of study unto itself, and nurses can feel confident that the concepts are based on repeated observations over time.

◆ Nursing is an applied science that uses concepts from the study of humans in a variety of disciplines, including medicine, psychology, sociology, anthropology, ecology, political science, mathematics, and philosophy.

◆ Nurses use the concept of wholeness from Dunn's (1972) concept of high-level wellness, and systems theory to organize data to show relationships and suggest ways to manage interventions and manage the environment.

◆ Nurses also use theories of personality development to understand behavior and thinking and provide strategies for interventions.

◆ Ideas about how people think and behave and what nurses can do to foster homeostasis, self-efficacy, resilience, integrity, adaptation, and recovery were addressed differently by various theories.

◆ Psychoanalytical theory provides a language and structure for thinking about thought and behavior.

TABLE 2–11
Peplau's Model of Interpersonal Theory: Basic Concepts and Their Interrelationships

	Nursing is related to:	Person is related to:	Health is related to:	Environment is related to:	Interpersonal Relationships (I.P.R.'s) are related to:
Person	Nursing is a process between persons (nurse and patient).				
Health	Health is the goal of nursing.	Health is within the person.			
Environment	Environment provides the context of nursing.	The person is within the environment.	The environment can be health promoting or illness maintaining.		
Interpersonal Relationships (I.P.R.'s) (Nurse–Patient + Other)	I.P.R.'s are the crux of essential processes of nursing.	Persons develop through I.P.R.'s	I.P.R.'s contribute to a person's health and a person's health will in turn influence ongoing I.P.R.'s.	The environment forms the context of I.P.R.'s.	
Communication (Verbal & Nonverbal)	Communication is an essential component of nursing.	Communication is a transaction between persons.	Communication facilitates health by contributing to I.P.R.'s.	Communication occurs within the context of the environment and is part of the environment.	Communication occurs within interpersonal relationships.
Pattern Integration	Pattern integration occurs in nursing to create change.	Pattern integration occurs between persons as an interaction of individual patterns.	Pattern integration can facilitate health by contributing to ongoing I.P.R.'s.	Pattern integration is a part of the environment.	Pattern integration occurs within interpersonal relationships.
Roles	Roles are the means for conducting nursing.	Roles are used by the nurse to promote health within the client.	Roles are used by the nurse to promote health.	Roles are used in the context of the environment.	Roles are used within interpersonal relationships.

TABLE 2-11

Peplau's Model of Interpersonal Theory:
Basic Concepts and Their Interrelationships *(continued)*

	Nursing is related to:	Person is related to:	Health is related to:	Environment is related to:	Interpersonal Relationships (I.P.R.'s) are related to:
Thinking (Includes Self-Understanding & Preconceptions)	Thinking occurs in nursing as a prerequisite.	Thinking is used by persons to process experience.	Self-understanding can promote health. Preconceptions can impede or promote health depending on their impact on interpersonal relationships.	Thinking occurs in the person within the environment.	Self-understanding can promote I.P.R.'s. Preconceptions can promote or hinder I.P.R.'s & vice versa.
Learning	Learning occurs in nursing as a consequence.	Learning is an interpersonal process used for growth.	Learning promotes health.	Learning occurs in the person within the environment.	Learning occurs within the context of I.P.R.'s. The interactions between learning and I.P.R.'s can enhance or hinder each other.
Competencies	Competencies develop as a consequence of nursing.	Competencies are skills developed within persons.	The development of competencies promotes health.	Competencies occur in the person within the environment.	Competencies can assist in the development of I.P.R.'s.
Anxiety	Anxiety occurs in nursing.	Anxiety occurs as a result of perceived personal threat.	Anxiety impedes health at severe or panic levels.	Anxiety occurs in the person within the environment.	Anxiety impedes the development of relationships at severe or panic levels.

Note. From "Peplau's theory: Concepts and their relations," by C. Forchuk, 1990, *Nursing Science Quarterly, 4*(2), 58–59. Reprinted with permission.

Interpersonal theory emphasizes the importance of social and environmental relationships. Behavioral theories provide potent methods for changing behavior. Cognitive theories provide ways to change thinking processes. All theories propose to foster a higher level of wellness, integrity, adaptation, and negentropy.

◆ New and developing knowledge can be structured within a theory that, in turn, provides the basis for lifelong learning. Each nurse's practice is based on a particular theory, whether it is implicit or explicit.

STUDY QUESTIONS

1. The structure of personality that maintains reality orientation and mediates conflict is the:
   a. id
   b. ego
   c. eros
   d. superego

2. According to psychoanalytical theory, the personality's first line of defense to keep unwanted thoughts out of awareness is:
   a. sublimation
   b. anxiety
   c. suppression
   d. repression

3. According to psychoanalytical theory, problems with excessive orderliness and neatness arise in which of the following developmental stages?
   a. Oral
   b. Anal
   c. Phallic
   d. Genital

4. Carl Jung termed the public personality, or the aspects of the self that one reveals to others, the:
   a. persona
   b. anima
   c. animus
   d. shadow

5. The concept of "good me," "bad me," and "not me" was explicated by which of the following theorists?
   a. Freud
   b. Horney
   c. Sullivan
   d. Adler

6. Reinforcement occurs before the response in which of the following behavioral theories?
   a. Operant conditioning
   b. Classic conditioning
   c. Modeling
   d. Respondent conditioning

7. The concept from cognitive theory that refers to applying a rule, drawn from one or more isolated incidents, across the board to unrelated situations is:
   a. arbitrary inference
   b. selective abstraction

c. overgeneralization
d. personalization

8. Distorting the significance of an event is:
   a. magnification
   b. dichotomous thinking
   c. selective abstraction
   d. overgeneralization

9. The theorist who defined nursing as a significant, therapeutic, interpersonal process is:
   a. Roy
   b. Neuman
   c. Orem
   d. Peplau

10. Attributing one's own unacknowledged thoughts and feelings to others is:
    a. intellectualization
    b. displacement
    c. denial
    d. projection

11. Which of the following did Vaillant call a mature defense?
    a. Sublimation
    b. Denial
    c. Repression
    d. Reaction formation

12. Which of the following best describes how nurses can assess the client's resilience?
    a. "Mr. Loew, how did you get to the clinic today? Did your family bring you in?"
    b. "Mr. Loew, what are your current stressors and what kind of support system to you have?"
    c. "Mr. Loew, tell me about your strengths and how you have coped with this problem in the past."
    d. "Mr. Loew, I noticed this is your second visit to the clinic in 2 months. How are things going?"

13. Which of the following statements is the *least accurate* description of the recovery model in psychiatric mental health nursing?
    a. It focuses primarily on symptom management and avoidance of hospitalization.
    b. It integrates client preferences, wishes, and needs to ensure client-centered care.
    c. It instills hope and uses client strengths to facilitate self-management.
    d. It enables the nurse to collaborate with the client and family in shared decision making.

14. Which of the following nursing interventions best describes how the psychiatric nurse integrates neurobiological and psychosocial nursing interventions to manage a psychiatric disorder?
    a. Administering an IM medication to manage an adverse drug reaction associated with haloperidol
    b. Demonstrating deep breathing exercises to the client having a panic attack
    c. Teaching parenting classes to an anxious couple expecting their first child
    d. Administering risperidone concentrate to an agitated client

15. Neurotransmitters are important target sites for pharmacological interventions. When caring for the client who presents with an anxiety disorder, such as Panic Disorder, which neurotransmitter is the primary target site(s) for pharmacotherapy?
    a. Serotonin
    b. Gamma aminobutyric acid (GABA)
    c. Dopamine
    d. a and b

16. The efficacy of cognitive behavioral therapy is based on which of the following interventions?
    a. Challenging negative self-talk and distorted cognitions
    b. Teaching the client ways to form meaningful interpersonal relationships
    c. Challenging negative statements from others
    d. Understanding the relationship between mental and physical states

17. Linehan's dialectical behavior therapy model has demonstrated efficacy in the treatment of borderline personality disorder. Which of the following best describes how this intervention works?
    a. It helps the client gain insight into maladaptive behaviors, modulate negative emotions, and improve coping skills.
    b. It helps the client stay out of the hospital by taking medications as ordered to manage maladaptive behaviors.
    c. It reduces suicidal ideations, intent, and gestures by helping the client manage strong emotions.
    d. It uses confrontation and challenges the client to take responsibility for maladaptive behaviors.

RESOURCES

Please note that because Internet resources are of a time-sensitive nature and URL addresses may change or be deleted, searches should also be conducted by association or topic.

Internet Resources

http://www.cdc.gov/about/default.htm;

http://www.cdc.gov/about/goals/goals.htm   Centers for Disease Control and Prevention (CDC): Retrieved January 28, 2006.

http://www.nimh.nih.gov/   National Institute of Mental Health (NIMH): Retrieved January 28, 2006.

http://www.rwjf.org   Robert Wood Johnson Foundation (RWJF): Retrieved January 28, 2006.

www.surgeongeneral.gov/library/mentalhealth/.html Review "Mental Health: A Report of the Surgeon General," Rockville, MD

http://www.who.int/about/en/   World Health Organization (WHO): Retrieved January 28, 2006.

Other Resources

Jacox, A., Suppe, F., Campbell, J., & Stashinko, E. E. (1999). Diversity in philosophical approaches. In A. S. Hinshaw, S. L. Feetham, & J. L. F. Shaver (Eds.), *Handbook of clinical research* (pp. 3–17). Thousand Oaks: Sage.

Mental health: A report of the surgeon general. (1999). Rockville, MD: U.S. Department of Health and Human Services, Substance Abuse and Mental Health Services Administration, Center for Mental Health.

REFERENCES

Aguis, M. A., Glasg, F. R., & Arnason, B. G. (1991). Autoimmune neurological diseases and their potential relevance to psychiatric diseases. In J. Gorman & R. Kertzner (Eds.), *Psychoimmunology update* (pp. 9–29). Washington, DC: American Psychiatric Press.

Ainsworth, M. D., & Bell, S. M. (1970). Attachment, exploration, and separation: Illustrated by the behavior of one-year-olds in a strange situation. *Child Development, 41,* 49–67.

Ainsworth, M. D., Blehar, M. C., Waters, E., & Wall, S. (1978). *Attachment: A psychological study of the Strange Situation.* Hillsdale, NJ: Erlbaum Associates.

Ansbacher, H. L., & Ansbacher, R. R. (1956). *The individual psychology of Alfred Adler: A systematic presentation in selections from his writing.* New York: Basic Books.

Antai-Otong, D. (2000). The neurobiology of anxiety disorders: Implications for psychiatric nursing practice. *Issues in Mental Health Nursing, 21,* 71–89.

Antonova, E., Kumari, V., Morris, R., Halari, R., Anilkumar, A., Mehrotra, R., & Sharma, T. (2005). The relationship of structural alterations to cognitive deficits in schizophrenia: A voxel-based morphometry study. *Biological Psychiatry, 58,* 457–467.

Arlow, J. A. (1989). Psychoanalysis. In R. J. Corsini & D. Wedding (Eds.), *Current psychotherapies (4th ed.).* Itasca, IL: F.E. Peacock.

Bandura, A. (1977). *Social learning theory.* Englewood Cliffs, NJ: Prentice-Hall.

Bandura, A., & Walters, R. H. (1963). *Social learning and personality development.* New York: Holt.

Bartholomew, K., & Horowitz, L. M. (1991). Attachment styles among young adults: A test of a four-category model. *Journal of Perspectives in Social Psychology, 61,* 226–244.

Beck, A. T. (1976). *Cognitive therapy and the emotional disorders.* New York: International Universities Press.

Beck, A. T. (1991). Cognitive therapy: A 30-year retrospective. *American Psychologist, 46,* 368–375.

Beck, A. T., Rush, A. J., Shaw, B. F., & Emery, G. (1979). *Cognitive therapy of depression.* New York: Guilford Press.

Bennett, H. A., Einarson, A., Taddio, A., Koren, G., & Einarson, T. R. (2004). Prevalence of depression during pregnancy: Systematic review. *Obstetrics and Gynecology, 103*, 698–709.

Bernard, S., Gonze, D., Cajavec, B., Herzel, H., & Kramer, A. (2007). Synchronization-induced rhythmicity of circadian oscillators in the suprachiasmatic nucleus. *PLoS Computational Biology, 3*, e68. Retrieved June 7, 2007, from http://compbiol.plosjournals.org/perlserv/?request-get-document&doi-10.1371/journal.pcbi.0030068

Booij, L., Van der Kloot, W. A., Benkelfat, C., Bremner, J. D., Cowen, P. J., Fava, M., Gillin, C., Leyton, M., Moore, P., Smith, K. A., Van der Does, W. (2002). Predictors of mood response to tryptophan depletion: A reanalysis. *Neuropsychopharmacology, 27*, 852–861.

Boulenger, J. P., Bierer, L. M., Uhde, T. W., Silberman, E. K., & Post, R. M. (1986). Psychosensory phenomena in panic and affective disorder. In C. Shagass, R. C. Joiassen, W. H. Bridger, W. J. Weiss, D. Stoff, & G. H. Simpson (Eds.), *Biological psychiatry* (pp. 462–465). New York: Elsevier.

Bowlby, J. (1969). *Attachment and loss Vol. I: Attachment.* London: Hogarth (New York: Basic Books).

Bowlby, J. (1973). *Attachment and loss Vol. II: Separation: Anxiety and anger.* New York: Basic Books.

Bowlby, J., Robertson, J., & Rosenbluth, D. (1952, 1969). A two-year-old goes to the hospital. *The Psychoanalytic Study of the Child, 7*, 82–94.

Brown, A. S., Begg, M. D., Gravenstein, S., Schaefer, C. A., Wyatt, R. J., Bresnahan, M., Babulas, V. P., & Susser, E. S. (2004). Serologic evidence of prenatal influenza in the etiology of schizophrenia. *Archives of General Psychiatry, 61*, 774–780.

Bryant, R. E., & Harvey, A. G. (2000). Acute stress disorder: *A handbook of theory, assessment, and treatment.* Washington, DC: American Psychological Association.

Cannon, T. D., Rosso, I. M., Hollister, J. M., Bearden, C. E., Sanchez, L. E., & Hadley, T. (2000). A prospective cohort study of genetic and perinatal influences in the etiology of schizophrenia, *Schizophrenia Bulletin, 26*, 351–366.

Cannon, T. D., van Erp, Bearden, C. E., Loewy, R., Thompson, P., Toga, A. W., Huttunen, M. O., Keshaven, M. S., Seidman, L. J., & Tsuang, M. T. (2003). Early and late neurodevelopmental influences in the prodrome to schizophrenia: Contributions of genes, environment, and their interactions. *Schizophrenia Bulletin, 29*, 653–669.

Cheng, R., Juo, S. H., Loth, J. E., Nee, J., Iossifov, I., Blumenthal, R., Sharpe, L., Kanyas, K., Lerer, B., Lilliston, B., Smith, M., Trautman, K., Gillman, T. C., Endicott, J., & Baron, M. (2006). Genome-wide linkage scan in a large bipolar disorder sample from the National Institute of Mental Health genetics initiative suggests putative loci for bipolar disorder, psychosis, suicide, and panic disorder. *Molecular Psychiatry*, 1–9 (online publication: doi:10.1038/sj.mp.4001778.

Conrad, A. J., Abebe, T., Austin, R., Forsythe, S., & Schechel, A. B. (1991). Hippocampal pyramidal cell disarray in schizophrenia as a bilateral phenomenon. *Archives of General Psychiatry, 40*, 413–417.

Crockenberg, S. C., & Leerkes, E. M. (2004). Infant and maternal behaviors regulate infant reactivity to novelty at 6 months. *Developmental Psychology, 40*, 1123–1132.

Cutcliffe, J., & Herth, K. (2002). The concept of hope in nursing 2: Hope and mental health nursing. *British Journal of Nursing, 11*, 891–893.

de Bartolomeis, A., Fiore, G., & Iasevoli, F. (2005). Dopamine-glutamate interaction and antipsychotics mechanism of action: Implication for new pharmacological strategies in psychosis. *Current Pharmaceutical Design, 11*, 3561–3594.

Delisi, L. E., & Bertisch, H. (2006). A preliminary comparison of the hopes of researchers, clinicians, and families for the future ethical use of genetic findings on schizophrenia. *American Journal of Medical Genetics. Part B, Neuropsychiatric Genetics, 141*, 110–115.

De Rubeis, R. J., Gelfand, L. A., Tang, T. Z., & Simons, A. D. (1999). Medications versus cognitive behavior therapy for severely depressed outpatients: A meta-analysis of four randomized comparisons. *American Journal of Psychiatry, 156*, 1007–1013.

de Weerth, C., van Hess, Y., & Buitelaar, J. K. (2003). Prenatal maternal cortisol levels and infant behavior during the first 5 months. *Early Human Development, 74*, 139–151.

Dix, T., Gershoff, E. T., Meunier, L. N., & Miller, P. C. (2004). The affective structure of supportive parenting: Depressive symptoms, immediate emotions, and child-oriented motivation. *Developmental Psychology, 40*, 1212-1227.

Dobson, K. S. (1989). A meta-analysis of the efficacy of cognitive therapy for depression. *Journal of Clinical Psychology, 57*, 414–419.

Drews, J. (2000). Drug discovery: A historical perspective. *Science, 287*, 1960–1964.

Dunn, H. L. (1972). *High-level wellness* (7th edition). Arlington, VA: Beatty.

Elkin, I., Shea, M. T., Watkins, J. T., Imber, S. D., Sotsky, S. M., Collins, J. F., Glass, D. R., Pilkonis, P. A., Leber, W. R., Docherty, J. P. (1989). National Institute of Mental Health treatment of depression collaborative research program: General effectiveness of treatments. *Archives of General Psychiatry, 46*, 971–982.

Ellis, A. (1984). Rational-emotive therapy. In R. J. Corsini (Ed.), *Current psychotherapies* (3rd ed., pp. 196–238). Itasca, IL: Peacock.

Ellis, A. (1985). *Overcoming resistance: Rational-emotive therapy with difficult clients.* New York: Springer.

Erikson, E. H. (1963). *Childhood and society* (3rd ed.). New York: W.W. Norton.

Etkins, A. (2000). Drugs and therapeutics in the age of the genome. *Journal of the American Medical Association, 284*, 2786–2787.

Eutamene, H., Theodorou, V., Fioramonti, J., & Bueno, L. (2003). Acute stress modulates the histamine content of mast cells in the gastrointestinal tract through interleukin-1 and corticotrophin-releasing factor release in rats. *The Journal of Physiology, 553,* 959–966.

Farrow, T. F., Hunter, M. D., Wilkinson, I. D., Green, R. D., & Spence, S. A. (2005). Structural correlates of unconstrained motor activity in people with schizophrenia. *British Journal of Psychiatry, 187,* 481–482.

Fenichel, O. (1945). *The psychoanalytic theory of neurosis.* New York: W.W. Norton.

Forchuk, C. (1990). Peplau's theory: Concepts and their relations. *Nursing Science Quarterly, 4,* 54–60.

Freud, A. (1937). *The ego and mechanisms of defense.* London: Hogarth Press.

Freud, A. (1946). *The ego and mechanisms of defense* (C. Baines, Trans.). New York: International Universities Press.

Freud, S. (1952). New introductory lectures on psychoanalysis. In M. J. Adler (Ed.), *Great books of the western world, vol. 54. Freud* (W. J. H. Sprott, Trans.). Chicago: William Benton. Encyclopedia Britannica. (Original work published 1932.)

Gaffan, E. A., Tsaousis, I., & Kemp-Wheeler, S. M. (1995). Researcher allegiance and meta-analysis: The case of cognitive therapy for depression. *Journal of Consulting Clinical Psychology, 63,* 966–980.

Ganong, W. F. (1999). *Review of medical physiology* (19th ed.). Stamford, CT: Appleton & Lange.

Ganong, W. F. (2005). *Review of medical physiology* (22nd ed.). Upper Norwalk, CT: McGraw-Hill.

Gilmore, J. H., Lin, W., & Gerig, G. (2006). Fetal and neonatal brain development. *American Journal of Psychiatry, 163,* 2046

Gottesman, I. I., & Bertelsen, A. (1989). Confirming expressed genotypes for schizophrenia: Risks in the offspring of Fischer's Danish identical and fraternal discordant twins. *Archives of General Psychiatry, 46,* 478–480.

Greenspan, S. I., & Curry, J. F. (2000). Extending Piaget's approach to intellectual functioning. In B. J. Sadock & V. A. Sadock (Eds.), *Kaplan & Sadock's comprehensive textbook of psychiatry* (7th ed., pp. 402–413). Philadelphia: Lippincott Williams & Wilkins.

Harrison, G., Hopper, K., Craig, K., Laska, E., Seigel, C., Wanderling, J., et al. (2001). Recovery from psychotic illness: A 15 and 25 year international follow-up study. *British Journal of Psychiatry, 178,* 506–517.

Heron, J., O'Connor, T. G., Evans, J., Golding, J., Glover, V., & The ALSPAC Study Team. (2004). The course of anxiety and depression and the postpartum in a community sample. *Journal of Affective Disorders, 80,* 65–71.

Hesse, S., Muller, U., Lincke, T., Barthel, H., Villman, T., Angermeyer, M. C., Sabri, O., & Strengler-Wenzke, K. (2005). Serotonin and dopamine transporter imaging in patients with obsessive-compulsive disorder. *Psychiatry Research, 140,* 63–72.

Hirschmann, M. (1989). Psychiatric and mental health nurses' beliefs about therapeutic paradox. *Journal of Child and Adolescent Psychiatric-Mental Health Nursing, 2,* 7–13.

Horney, K. (1937). *The neurotic personality of our time.* New York: W.W. Norton.

Inhelder, B., & Piaget, J. (1958). *The growth of logical thinking from childhood to adolescence.* New York: Basic Books.

Irwin, M. R., & Strausbaugh, H. (1991). Stress and immune changes in humans: A biopsychosocial model. In J. Gorman & R. Kertzner (Eds.), *Psychoimmunology Update* (pp. 55–79). Washington, DC: American Psychiatric Press.

Jung, C. (1967). *Collected works.* Princeton, NJ: Princeton University Press.

Kelly, M., & Gamble, C. (2005). Exploring the concept of recovery in schizophrenia. *Journal of Psychiatric and Mental Health Nursing, 12,* 245–251.

Konradi, C., & Heckers, S. (2003). Molecular aspects of glutamate dysregulation: Implication for schizophrenia and its treatment. *Pharmacological Therapies, 97,* 153–179.

Kopelowicz, A., & Liberman, R. P. (2003). Integrating treatment with rehabilitation for persons with major mental illnesses. *Psychiatric Services, 54,* 1491–1498.

Laruelle, M., Frankle, W. G., Narendran, R., Kegeles, L. S., & Abi-Dargham, A. (2005). Mechanism of action on antipsychotic drugs: From dopamine (D2) receptor antagonism to glutamate NMDA facilitation. *Clinical Therapies, 27,* (Suppl A), S16–S24.

Lazarus, R. S. (1966). *Psychological stress and the coping process.* New York: McGraw-Hill.

Lazarus, R. S. (1991). *Emotion and adaptation.* New York: Oxford University Press.

Lazarus, R. S., & Folkman, S. (1984). *Stress, appraisal, and coping.* New York: Springer.

Lazarus, R. S., & Launier, R. (1978). Stress-related transactions between personality and environment. In L. A. Pervin & M. Lewis (Eds.), *Perspectives in international psychology* (pp. 287–327). New York: Plenum.

Linehan, M. M. (1999). *Understanding borderline personality disorder: The dialectical approach.* New York: Guilford.

Linehan, M. M., Heard, H. L., & Armstrong, H. E. (1993). Naturalistic follow-up of a behavioral treatment for chronically parasuicidal borderline patients. *Archives of General Psychiatry, 50,* 971–974.

Luby, J. L., Heffelfinger, A., Mrakotsky, C., Brown, K., Hessler, M., Spitznagel, E. (2003). Alterations in stress cortisol reactivity in depressed preschoolers relative to psychiatric and no-disorder comparison groups. *Archives of General Psychiatry, 60,* 1248–1255.

Maier, H. W. (1969). *Three stories of child development.* New York: Harper & Row.

Maslow, A. H. (1943). A theory of human motivation. *Psychological Review, 50,* 370.

Maslow, A. H. (1970). *Motivation and personality* (2nd ed.). New York: Harper & Row.

Mednick, S., Machon, R. A., Huttunen, M. O. (1988). Adult schizophrenia following prenatal influenza epidemic. *Archives of General Psychiatry, 45,* 189–192.

Neuman, B. (1989). *The Neuman systems model.* East Norwalk, CT: Appleton-Century-Crofts.

O'Callaghan, E., Sham, P., Takei, N., Glover, G., & Murray, R. M. (1991). Schizophrenia after prenatal exposure to 1957 A2 influenza epidemic. *Lancet, 1,* 1248–1250.

O'Connor, T. G., Heron, J., Glover, V., & ALSPAC Study Team. (2004). Antenatal anxiety predicts child behavioral/emotional problems independently of postnatal depression. *Journal of the American Academy of Child and Adolescent Psychiatry, 41,* 1470–1477.

Ognibene, T. C., & Collins, N. L. (1998). Adult attachment styles, perceived social support and coping strategies. *Journal of Social and Personal Relationships, 15,* 323–345.

Orem, D. E. (1980). *Nursing: Concepts of practice* (2nd ed.). New York: McGraw-Hill.

Orlando, I. J. (1961). *The dynamic nurse-patient relationship.* New York: G. P. Putnam.

Papp, L. A., Goetz, R. R., Cole, R., Klein, D. F., Jordon, F., Liebowitz, M. R., Flyer, A. J., Hollander, E., & Gorman, J. M. (1989). Hypersensitivity to carbon dioxide in panic disorder. *American Journal of Psychiatry, 146,* 779–781.

Parse, R. R. (1998). *The human becoming school of thought: A perspective for nursing and other professionals.* Thousand Oaks, CA: Sage.

Parse, R. R. (2002). Transforming healthcare with a unitary view of the human. *Nursing Science Quarterly, 15,* 46–50.

Pauli-Pott, U., Mertesacker, B., Beckman, D. (2004). Predicting the development of infant emotionality from maternal characteristics. *Developmental Psychobiology, 16,* 19–42.

Peplau, H. (1952). *Interpersonal relations in nursing.* New York: Putnam.

Peplau, H. (1969). Theory: The professional dimension. In C. M. Norris (Ed.), *Proceedings from the First Nursing Theory Conference* (pp. 33–46). Kansas City: University of Kansas Medical Center.

Raison, C. L., Capuron, L., & Miller, A. H. (2006). Cytokines sing the blues: Inflammation and the pathogenesis of depression. *Trends in Immunology, 2006,* 24–31.

Riehl-Sisca, J. (1989). *Conceptual models for nursing practice* (3rd ed.). Norwalk, CT: Appleton & Lange.

Rogers, M. (1970). *An introduction to the theoretical basis of nursing.* Philadelphia, PA: FA Davis.

Rosenberg, D. R., & Keshavan, M. S. (1998). Toward a neurodevelopmental model of obsessive-compulsive disorder. *Society of Biological Psychiatry, 43,* 623–640.

Rosenheck, R., Stroup, S., Keefe, R. S. E., McEvoy, J., Swartz, M., Perkins, D., Hsiao, J., Shumway, M., & Lieberman, J. (2005). Measuring priorities and preferences in people with schizophrenia. *British Journal of Psychiatry, 187,* 529–536.

Ross, L. E., & McLean, L. M., (2006). Anxiety disorders during pregnancy and the postpartum period: A systematic review. *Journal of Clinical Psychiatry, 67,* 1285–1298.

Rotter, J. B. (1954). *Social learning and clinical psychology.* Englewood Cliffs, NJ: Prentice-Hall.

Roy, C. (1984). *An introduction to nursing: An adaptation model* (2nd ed.). Englewood Cliffs, NJ: Prentice-Hall.

Ryan, D. Milis, L., & Misri, N. (2005). Depression during pregnancy. *Canadian Family Physician, 51,* 1087–1093.

Salokangas, R. K., & Stengard, E. (1990). Gender and short-term outcome in schizophrenia. *Schizophrenia Research, 3,* 333–345.

Sanacora, G., Gueroguieva, R., Epperson, N., Wu, Y-T., Appel, M., Rothman, D. L., Krystal, J. H., & Mason, G. F. (2004). Sub-type specific alterations of γ-aminobutyric acid and glutamate in patients with major depression. *Archives of General Psychiatry, 61,* 705–713.

Sanacora, G., Mason, G. F., Rothman, D. L., & Krystal, J. H. (2002). Increased occipital cortex GABA concentrations in depressed patients after therapy with selective serotonin reuptake inhibitors. *American Journal of Psychiatry, 159,* 663–665.

Saylam, C., Ucerler, H., Kitis, O., Ozand, E., & Gonul, A. S. (2006). Reduced hippocampal volume in drug-free depressed patients. *Surgical and Radiologic Anatomy,* 1–6.

Schieche, M., & Spangler, G. (2005). Individual differences in biobehavioral organization during problem-solving in toddlers: The influence of maternal behaviors, infant-mother attachment, and behavioral inhibition on the attachment-exploration balance. *Developmental Psychobiology, 46,* 293–306.

Schore, A. N. (2005). Back to basics: Attachment, affect regulation, and the developing right brain: Linking developmental neuroscience to pediatrics. *Pediatrics in Review, 26,* 204–217.

Seyle, H. (1976). *The stress of life.* New York: McGraw-Hill.

Shea, M. T., Pilokonis, P. A., Beckham, E., Collins, J. F., Elkin, I., Sotsky, S. M, & Docherty, J. P. (1990). Personality disorders and treatment outcome in the NIMH Treatment of Depression Collaborative Research Program. *American Journal of Psychiatry, 147,* 711–718.

Simpson, H. B., & Kozak, M. (2000). Cognitive-behavioral therapy for obsessive-compulsive disorder. *Journal of Psychiatric Practice, 6,* 59–69.

Skinner, B. F. (1953). *Science and human behavior.* New York: MacMillan.

Skinner, B. F. (1963). Operant behavior. *American Psychologist, 18,* 503–515.

Stahl, S. M. (2000). *Essential psychopharmacology: Neuroscientific basis and practical application* (2nd ed.). Cambridge, UK: Cambridge University Press.

Sullivan, H. S. (1940). *Conceptions in modern psychiatry.* New York: W.W. Norton.

Sullivan, H. S. (1953). *Interpersonal theory of psychiatry.* New York: W.W. Norton.

Sullivan, H. S. (1971). *The fusion of psychiatry and social science*. New York: W.W. Norton.

Terman, M., & Terman, J. S. (2005). Light therapy for seasonal and nonseasonal depression: Efficacy, protocol, safety, and side effects. *CNS Spectrum, 10,* 647–663.

Torrey, E. F., & Kaufman, C. A. (1986). Schizophrenia and neurovirus. In H. A. Nasarallah & D. R. Weinberger (Eds.), *Handbook of schizophrenia: Vol. 1: The neurology of schizophrenia* (pp. 361–376). Amsterdam: Elsevier.

Tsuang, M. (2000). Schizophrenia: Genes and environment. *Biological Psychiatry, 47,* 210–220.

Vaillant, G. E. (1977). *Adaptation to life.* Boston: Little, Brown.

van Erp, T. G. M., Saleh, P. A., Rosso, I. M., Huttunen, M, Lönnqvist, J., Pirkola, T., Salonen, O., Valanne, L., Poutanen, V-P., Standertskjöld-Nordenstam, C-G., & Cannpn, T. D. (2002). Contributions of genetic risk and fetal hypoxia to hippocampal volume in patients with schizophrenia or schizoaffective disorder, their unaffected siblings, and health unrelated volunteers. *American Journal of Psychiatry, 159,* 1514–1520.

von Bertalanffy, L. (1968). *General systems theory.* New York: Braziller.

Verheul, R., Van Den Bosch, L. M., Koeter, M. W., De Ridder, M. A., Stijnen, T., Van Den Brink, W. et al. (2003). Dialectical behaviour therapy for women with borderline personality disorder: 12-month, randomised clinical trial in The Netherlands. *British Journal of Psychiatry, 182,* 135–140.

Videbech, P., & Ravnkilde, B. (2004). Hippocampal volume and depression: A meta-analysis of MRI studies. *American Journal of Psychiatry, 161,* 1957–1966.

Watson, S., Gallagher, P., Ritchie, J. C., Ferrier, I. N., & Young, A. H. (2004). Hypothalamic-pituitary-adrenal axis function in patients with bipolar disorder. *British Journal of Psychiatry, 184,* 496–502.

Wehr, T. A. (2000). Chronobiology. In B. J. Sadock & V. A. Sadock (Eds.), *Comprehensive textbook of Psychiatry/VI* (Vol. 1., 7th ed., pp. 133–142). Philadelphia: Lippincott Williams & Wilkins.

Wileman, S. M., Eagles, J. M., Andrew, J. E., Howie, F. L., Cameron, I. M., McCormack, K., & Naji, S. A. (2001). Light therapy for seasonal affective disorder in primary care: Randomised controlled trial. *British Journal of Psychiatry, 178,* 311-316.

Willeit, M., Praschak-Rieder. N., Neumeister, A., Pirker, W., Asenbaum, S., Vitouch, O., Tauscher, J., Hilger, E., Stastny, J., Brucke, T., & Kasper, S. (2000). [^{123}I]-Beta-CIT SPECT imaging shows reduced brain serotonin transporter availability in drug-free depressants patients with seasonal affective disorder. *Biological Psychiatry, 47,* 482–489.

Wong, J. C., Provenzale, J. M., & Petrella, J. R. (2000). Perfusion MR imaging of brain neoplasms. *American Journal of Roentgenology, 174,* 1147–1157.

World Health Organization. (1947). *Constitution.* Geneva: Author.

Zlotnick, C., Miller, I. W., Pearlstein, T., Howard, M., & Sweeney, P. (2006). A preventive intervention for pregnant women on public assistance at risk for postpartum depression. *American Journal of Psychiatry, 163,* 1443–1445.

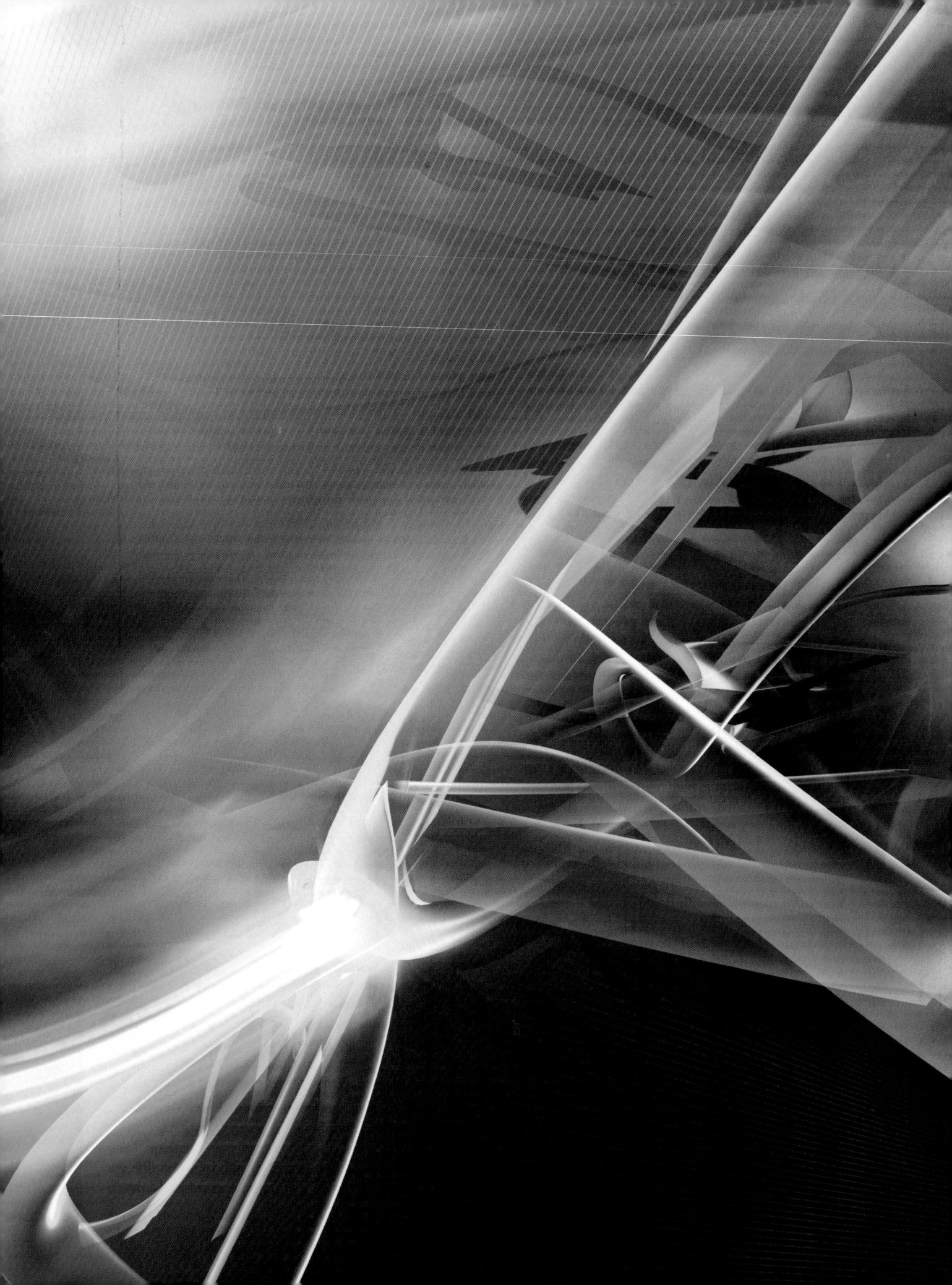

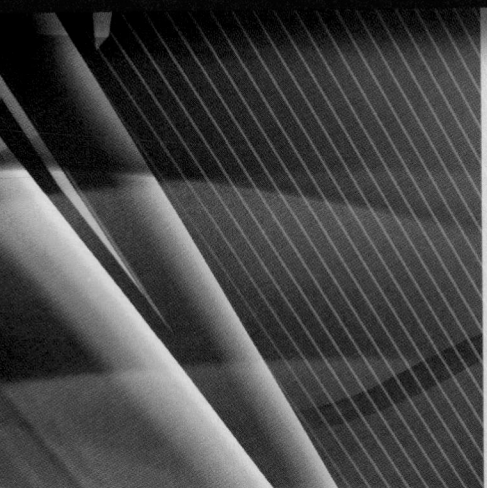

CHAPTER 3

Interfacing Biological-Behavioral Concepts into Psychiatric Nursing Practice

Deborah Antai-Otong, MS, APRN, BC, FAAN
Margaret Brackley, PhD, RN, CS

KEY TERMS

Amygdala: A nucleus in the limbic system or medial temporal lobe that affects neuroendocrine and behavioral functions. It also plays a role in behaviors, including eating, drinking, and sexuality, and the emotions linked to these behaviors. It plays a role in the emotional significance of events or memories and governs the level of hippocampal activity accordingly. Consequently, a traumatic or overwhelming event is permanently etched into the memory, whereas irrelevant events are immediately ignored.

Genetic Vulnerability: The relationship between genetic and enzymatic defects and vulnerability to mental illness. Genetic function is influenced by prenatal and environmental factors that activate intricate biochemical processes and affect behavior. A number of researchers have attempted to explore the relationship between genetic factors and mental disorders using twin, adoption, and family studies.

G-proteins: Part of the cell's second messenger system in the plasma involved in sending signals from regulatory chemicals such as hormones and neurotransmitters to target cells.

Hippocampus: Located in the medial temporal lobe, it is an important site for the formation and storage of immediate and recent memories, and it is influenced by the amygdala emotional rating of an event. This part of the brain is damaged by Alzheimer's disease.

Hypothalamus: Combined with the pituitary gland, thyroid gland, adrenal glands, gonads, and the pancreas, the hypothalamus forms the major regulatory system and is involved in the biological aspects of behavior. The hypothalamus-pituitary-adrenal axis (HPA) is important in understanding certain mental disorders. The hypothalamus regulates autonomic, endocrine, and visceral integration and is surmised to be the foundation of the limbic system and the brain center for emotions and certain behaviors

such as eating, drinking, aggression, and sexuality. Information in the hypothalamus is modulated by ascending sensory pathways, hormones, and descending pathways of the cerebral cortex.

Kindling: The electrophysiological process that over time produces an action potential after repetitive subthreshold stimulation or progressive sensitization of a neuron. This concept is thought to play a role in recurrent mood disorders.

Neuroendocrinology: The study of how the neural and endocrine systems work together to maintain homeostasis. Communication between these systems is involved in biological and behavioral responses. Major organs of the neuroendocrine system are the hypothalamus, the pituitary, thyroid, and adrenal glands; the gonads; and the pancreas.

Protein Kinase C (PKC): A group of enzymes that activate other enzymes.

Psychoneuroimmunology: The study of the role of the immune system in health and illness in the face of biological and psychosocial stress. This field is a developing knowledge about the interconnectedness of the nervous system and the immune system.

Reinforcers: Personal, complex, learned, and biochemical rewards that are used to modify maladaptive behavior. Reinforcers can be positive, negative, or punishing, and are personally determined.

Twin Studies: Researchers attempt to explore the relationship between genetic factors and mental disorders using these studies that usually include monozygotic or single ovum and dizygotic or two ova twins. Twin studies are helpful in isolating genetic and environmental influences and determining preventive and precipitating factors.

COMPETENCIES

Upon completion of this chapter, the learner should be able to:

1. Identify major paradigms of mental disorders.

2. List major aspects of the central nervous system and its relationship to mental disorders.

3. Describe the role of genetics in the predisposition of mental disorders.

4. Discuss brain function and its impact on human behavior.

5. Understand the human response to acute and chronic stress.

6. Explain the interrelationships between mind, brain, and hormones.

7. Develop a plan of care using biological and behavioral interventions.

CHAPTER OUTLINE

When the U.S. Congress proclaimed the 1990s to be the "Decade of the Brain," the families of mentally ill clients welcomed this new perspective of mental disorders. In the past, parents and siblings were thought to be responsible for many mental illnesses, during which time clinicians sought to explain these disorders solely in a behavioral context. As a consequence, family members felt demoralized and were blamed for their loved one's illnesses. Recently, however, neurobiological and genetic research findings have helped clinicians and researchers begin to understand the biological component of mental illness, particularly in terms of brain function and dysfunction, genetics, immunology, and endocrinology. Clients, families, and mental health professionals are hopeful about the potential impact of neurobiological studies on mental illnesses. These studies are also likely to improve quality of life and provide possible cures for serious mental disorders (U.S. Congress, 1989).

Advances in neurobiology and neuroendocrinology reflect the sweeping biotechnological findings of brain mapping, imaging, and scanning. Studies have demonstrated the underlying biological bases of schizophrenia, bipolar disorder and other mood disorders, anxiety disorders, dementia, and the aging process. Likewise, the use of psychopharmacologic agents has produced remarkable results, such as decreased

side effects, decreased exacerbation of symptoms, improved quality of life, and increased treatment adherence in clients with severe schizophrenia, bipolar disorder, pervasive developmental disorder, depression, and anxiety disorders.

More importantly, advances in neurobiology and neuroscience offer unprecedented opportunities for the expansion and strengthening of the scientific underpinnings of mental health research. Presently, researchers are using molecular and genetic mechanisms to identify genes and proteins that give rise to mental illness. They are also discovering that they can modify these neurobiological alterations by using psychopharmacologic and environmental interventions. These data provide novel targets for the development of pharmacologic agents and psychotherapies for mental disorders. They also afford clients with a plethora of interventions (Kelsoe, 2004; NIMH, 1998).

Many symptoms or behaviors observed in people with mental illness are linked to underlying biological factors. Disturbances in mood, cognitions, sensory-perceptual responses, aggression and other impulse control, and social interactions are examples of behaviors that have been linked to biological abnormalities or disruption.

The purpose of this chapter is to explore major concepts of the biological-behavioral interface and its impact on psychiatric nursing practice. The chapter also identifies client outcomes from nursing interventions that meet the complex needs of the mentally ill.

HISTORY OF THE BIOLOGICAL-BEHAVIORAL DICHOTOMY

Novel expansion of neurobiological technology emphasizes the need to explain the biological-behavioral phenomena and its relationship to mental illness. The interrelatedness of biology and behavior is not a new concept. It has its beginnings as far back as the fourteenth century stemming from the works of Hippocrates, who explained the concept of mental illness as a process of the brain rather than a spiritual event. He surmised that the brain gave rise to pleasure, joy, sorrow, pain, and grief and contributed to disturbances in affect or mood. Although his early description of the tenuous balance of four humors (blood, phlegm, and yellow and black bile) and their relationship to mood disorders proved inaccurate, his premise that maladaptive behaviors arise from complex biological processes was accurate.

In more recent times, Sigmund Freud contributed to neurobiology in the late 1800s through the phase of his work known as the *neurological phase*. Freud sought to establish a relationship between neural mechanisms, behavior patterns, and cognitive distortions. Freud and others sought to understand psychopathology in relation to disturbances of specific areas of brain dysfunction. Ultimately, this work has led to the recent plethora of neurobiological research and discoveries.

The search for the ideal treatment for mental illness found a major breakthrough in the discovery of tranquilizers in the 1950s. These agents relieved clients with varied symptoms of mental illness such as intense anxiety, agitation, delusions, and hallucinations. Some of the tranquilizing agents uncovered during this era included the phenothiazines, such as chlorpromazine (Thorazine), the first of the medications that was effective in treating behavioral manifestations of schizophrenia. Other tranquilizers induced major behavioral and biological changes in the mentally ill, thus generating further clues to the biological aspects of mental illness.

Newer psychotropics have emerged since the 1950s that have proven effective in the treatment of various mental disorders, such as schizophrenia and mood, anxiety, and addictive disorders (see Chapter 29, Psychopharmacologic Therapy). Over the past decade the effectiveness of these agents has increased because of improvements made in their ability to target behavioral manifestations of the complex neurobiological processes, such as those located in the hypothalamus and other regions in the limbic system. Psychotropics appear to act on neurochemical mechanisms that modify or alter or interfere with behavioral patterns. Examples include selective serotonergic reuptake blocking agents such as fluoxetine (Prozac) and sertraline (Zoloft), and serotonin norepinephrine reuptake inhibitors such as venlafaxine (Effexor) and duloxetine (Cymbalta) which are used to treat major depression, eating, impulsivity, and anxiety disorders, and atypical neuroleptics such as clozapine (Clozaril), quetiapine (Seroquel), and aripiprazole (Abilify) which are used to treat schizophrenia. Research and clinical trials have drastically reduced the disabling side effects of some of these agents and have improved the quality of life and provided hope and relief for clients and their families. Genetic and genome research offer even greater hope for clients by identifying the phenotypes for mental disorders and further linking behavior, brain, and genetics and providing molecular targets for more effective therapies (Cowan, Kopnisky, & Hyman, 2002).

MAJOR NEUROBIOLOGICAL MODELS

To understand the neurobiological models of mental illnesses and their implications for nursing, one must be familiar with the structure and function of the central nervous system (CNS) and its neurochemical processes (Figure 3–1). One also needs some basic knowledge of neuroendocrinology, psychoneuroimmunology, and genetics. Each of these models has widespread implications for behavioral and psychopharmacologic and non-pharmacologic interventions relevant to nursing practice.

THE CENTRAL NERVOUS SYSTEM

The central nervous system acts as the body's primary information processing system, gathering data about the internal and external environments. It is the most complex of human systems, governing emotional and behavioral as well as biological processes. It consists of the brain, the spinal cord, and the peripheral nervous system. Highly developed networks of specialized cells work together to integrate a variety of stimuli to respond appropriately to internal and external needs.

Diverse conditions, such as mental illness, trauma, aging, and degenerative processes, influence brain function. Abnormalities in neurotransmitter production or absorption, neuroendocrine response, immunology responses, and genetic predisposition all appear to contribute to mental disorders. It has not been clearly established whether neurotransmitter or neuroendocrine abnormalities cause mental illness or vice versa; that is, underlying functional or structural disorders contributing to mental illness may cause neurotransmitter and neuroendocrine abnormalities.

Neurodegenerative Processes

Degenerating processes may occur at any age, leading to cognitive and affective impairment. More importantly, these processes may arise from underlying general medical conditions or their treatments. For example, many medications used to treat medical conditions contribute to a depressed mood. Also, for years health providers have recognized that cognitive impairment may be linked to depressive disorders, particularly among older adults. Researchers also submit that cognitive impairment is strongly associated after left hemispheric stroke and intellectual impairment (Downhill & Robinson, 1994; Kase et al., 1998). Finally, the link between

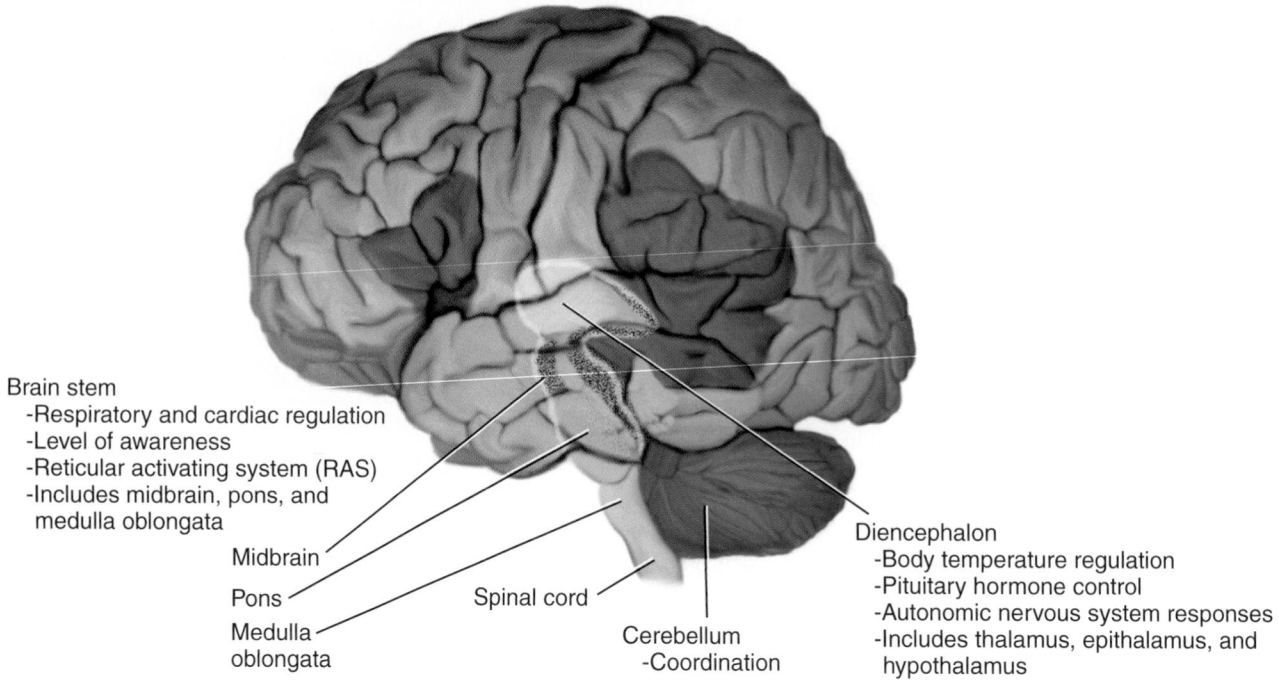

Brain stem
-Respiratory and cardiac regulation
-Level of awareness
-Reticular activating system (RAS)
-Includes midbrain, pons, and
 medulla oblongata

Midbrain

Pons

Medulla
oblongata

Spinal cord

Cerebellum
-Coordination

Diencephalon
-Body temperature regulation
-Pituitary hormone control
-Autonomic nervous system responses
-Includes thalamus, epithalamus, and
 hypothalamus

Figure 3–1 Locations and functions of the cerebral lobes, brain stem, and cerebellum.

mood disturbances, such as depression and adverse outcomes in heart disease, specifically myocardial infarction, is well documented and accounts for half of the cases in those recovering from myocardial infarctions (Glassman & Shapiro, 1998; Ziegelstein, 2001).

The brain shrinks with age and loses a considerable number of neurons after the fifth decade of life. Aging may also be connected with decline in learning and memory. Age-related memory impairment may be related to altered synaptic plasticity mechanisms in the hippocampus, including long-term potentiation. Long-term potentiation (LTP) is associated with learning across the life span. Based on the underpinning of LTP it may be conceivable for nurses to develop therapeutic interventions to enhance memory in normal ageing. Despite these neuronal changes, there is no definitive evidence of mental or cognitive decline associated with aging. Some researchers suggest that the brain adapts to aging by preserving an abundance of nerve cells rich in acetylcholine in neurotransmitter pathways between the hippocampus and the cerebral cortex. These maturational changes are linked with higher cortical function (e.g., "wisdom"). Deterioration of these neurons is linked with degenerative processes such as those found in dementia associated with Alzheimer's disease (AD) (Erickson & Barnes, 2003; Mesulam & Geula, 1991; Pickering-Brown et al., 2002).

Contemporary data suggest that these neurons die more rapidly than normal neurons and become sensitive to biochemical stress, which often leads to proteins that adhere together and form damaging clumps called fibrils and free radicals. Eventually, the concentration of fibrils and free radicals—the cumulative theory—increases and destroys the cells (Heintz, 2000). Recently, researchers exploring the cause of neurodegenerative diseases, such as Alzheimer's disease, questioned the cumulative death or "one-hit" or single-event hypothesis and submit that neuronal death occurs randomly. The "one-hit" model or theory suggests that a single event activates a mutant steady on the neuron that results in cellular death. Random cell death supposedly arises from genetic mutations that alter proteins. These proteins have not been identified at this time (Clarke et al., 2000; Huang, 2006).

Other researchers have explained Alzheimer's disease and other frontal lobe dementia as a degeneration of cholinergic fibers that arise from the nucleus basalis of structures innervating the cortex and hippocampus and ultimately causing neuronal death. Death of cortical neurons in the hippocampus, cortex, and parietal and temporal lobes interrupts pathways and loss of information storage and retrieval. Eventually, these structural alterations correlate with cognitive decline and produce classic symptoms of AD. Prominent behavioral changes and symptoms of AD include executive deficits, language difficulties, and inattentiveness.

Although AD is probably the most well-described neurodegenerative disease, other non-Alzheimer's forms of dementia are associated with progressive degenerative processes of the frontal and temporal lobes. Frontotemporal dementia (FTD) is characterized by personality and behavioral changes. Major symptoms are similar to AD and include impaired word comprehension and naming; recognition disorders, including facial and object; progressive speech difficulties (aphasia), particularly when it affects the left frontotemporal lobe primarily (Pickering-Brown et al., 2002; Snowden, Neary, & Mann, 1996) (See Chapter 16).

Managing and searching for a cure for AD and other neurodegenerative disorders is complex owing to a lack of knowledge about their exact etiology. Recent data (de la Torre, 2002) indicate that it should be classified as a vascular disorder rather than a neurodegenerative disorder. More data are needed to understand the etiology of these complex conditions. No drug on the market is totally effective in the treatment of AD or in altering its progressive course. Drugs that prolong the life of existing cholinergic neurons, such as donepezil (Aricept) or galantamine hydrobromide (Reminyl) may delay clinical decline in clients who suffer from AD (Othmer, Othmer, & Othmer, 1998; Wahlund, 1996).

A newer agent, memantine (Namenda) is the only approved agent in the United States for the treatment of moderate-to-severe Alzheimer's disease. Memantine may facilitate neuroprotection against excess glutamate by partially blocking N-methyl-D-aspartate (NMDA) receptors. Memantine has demonstrated efficacy in slowing the progression of cognitive symptoms in clients with moderate to severe AD (Tariot, 2006).

Neurochemical Processes

Neural regulation is based on a complex network of transmitter pathways that are sensitive to fluctuation of transmitter and hormonal balance. Neurotransmitters initially interact with receptor terminals of the postsynaptic cell membrane, resulting in either inhibitory or excitatory response. The type of neurotransmitter and receptors determine the nature of the response. Norepinephrine, dopamine, acetylcholine, and serotonin are examples of excitatory transmitters, whereas amino acids, such as gamma-aminobutyric acid, are examples of inhibitory transmitters. Abnormal concentrations of these substances are associated with impulsivity and mental disorders such as depression, anxiety, addictive disorders, and schizophrenia (Figure 3–2). Antidepressants, antipsychotics, anxiolytics, and other pharmacologic agents act on the neurotransmitters to increase or decrease their release, ultimately modifying relative concentration to improve the symptoms of mental disorders (see Chapter 29, Psychopharmacologic Therapy). Nurses must understand the neurochemical and systemic impact of the medication they administer whether treating mental or concurrent medical illnesses. In this way, optimal responses will more often be achieved.

NEUROENDOCRINOLOGY

Neuroendocrinology, the study of neural and endocrine systems, indicates that these systems work together to maintain normal body function or homeostasis. These systems communicate through biofeedback mechanisms to establish a basis for all biological and behavioral responses. The neuroendocrine system contains the hypothalamus, pituitary gland, thyroid gland, adrenal glands, gonads, and pancreas. The hypothalamic-pituitary-adrenal (HPA) axis is particularly important in the response to threat or stress. The HPA axis provides a cascade of processes governing positive and negative control at various areas, consequently modulating energy and cellular activity throughout the body (Campeau, Day, Helmreich, Kollack-Walker, & Watson, 1998). Abnormalities in the HPA axis are known to contribute to, and are diagnostic of, functional psychosis, phobias, bipolar disorder, and depressive and anxiety disorders (Abelsen, Liberzon, Young, & Khan, 2005; Nemeroff & Vale, 2005; Watson, et al., 2004; Wolkowitz & Reus, 1999) (see Chapter 11 and Figure 11–1).

Emerging research implicate the activation of the pro-inflammatory cytokine system have been associated with alterations in the HPA axis in major depression and interplay with the immune systems although with inconsistent results (Kaestner, et al., 2005). Newer studies also implicate immunological *deficiencies* in the neurobiology of autism (Cohly & Panja, 2005). It is important for nurses to be aware of the endocrine-neural influences of mental disorders to better assess for and understand underlying pathology and potential treatment.

PSYCHONEUROIMMUNOLOGY

The immune system plays a key role in the development of infections and tumors when it is underactive, and in the development of allergies and autoimmune diseases when it is overactive (Borysenko, 1987; Solomon, 1987). It is now becoming clear that the immune system plays a role in health and illness in the face of biological and psychosocial stress as well. This relatively new field of psychoneuroimmunology is a developing knowledge concerned with the interconnections between the nervous system and the immune system.

Each cell in a human body contains a marker that identifies the cell as part of "self." Any material that does not contain this marker is identified as foreign antigen. The immune system serves the body by first detecting and protecting it from invasion of antigens. One way in which it may do this is through humoral immunity by producing antibodies to destroy or neutralize the foreign body. The character of the

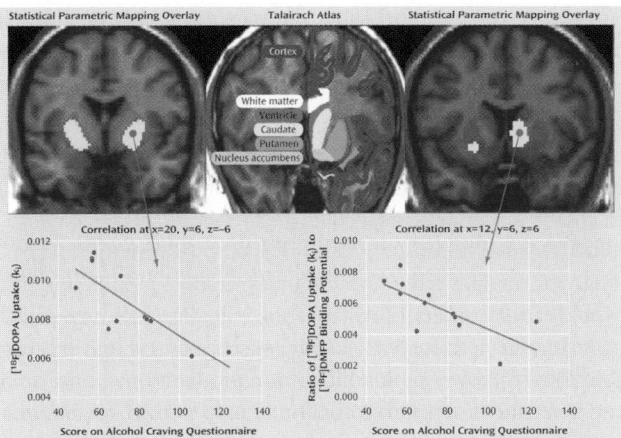

Figure 3–2 Correlation of alcohol craving with striatal dopamine production. *(Heinz, A., Siessmeir, T., Wruse, J., Buchholtz, H.G., Grunder, H. et al., [2005]. Correlation of alcohol craving with stiatal dopamine production [F18] DOPA influx normalized to local D2/3 receptor availability.* American Journal of Psychiatry, 162, *1515–1520. Used with permission.)*

antigen and the specific antibody are stored in the memory of the immune cells, so that response to another attack is more rapid and rigorous.

The immune system may be chronically activated as occurs in a stress response, or it may fail to recognize the self-marker and attack itself such as in autoimmune diseases. An attack is mounted against "non-self" material, and when the immune system fails to differentiate self from non-self, it can attack itself such as in autoimmune diseases like systemic lupus erythematosus (SLE).

The manner in which the immune system works has many implications for psychiatric nurses. Research has long shown that negative life events and stress affect health (Cazzullo, Trabattoni, Saresella, Annoni, et al., 2003; Cohly & Panja, 2005). Recently, psychiatric illnesses, notably affective disorders, panic disorders, and autism have been linked to immune dysfunction. Continued research in this area is critical. The National Institute of Nursing Research has called for research development in the area of immunoincompetence as well as for interventions that bolster appropriate immune response.

GENETICS

Numerous research studies confirm the relationship between genetic and enzymatic defects and genetic vulnerability to mental illness. For most mental disorders— schizophrenia, bipolar disorder, and pervasive developmental disorder—the site involving genes, acting at distinct times in brain development in vast regions of the brain, interfaces with epigenetic and environmental influences. Clearly, genetic function is influenced by prenatal and environmental factors that activate intricate biochemical processes, which may, in turn, affect behavior and increase the likelihood of mental disorders (Cowan, Kopnisky, & Hyman, 2002; Kelsoe, 2004). These patterns are often apparent in families with positive histories of various mental disorders, such as depression and suicidal behavior. For example, children whose parents are depressed are genetically vulnerable to depression and may also experience compromised parental caregiving by the depressed parent. Consequently, the child is more vulnerable to depression because of both genetic and environmental modes of transmission (Field, 1998; Francis, Caldji, Champagne, Plotsky, & Meaney, 1999; Gorwood, Batel, Ades, Hamon, & Boni, 2000).

Twin, Adoption, and Family Studies

A number of researchers have attempted to explore the relationship between genetic factors and mental disorders using twin, adoption, and family studies. Twin studies are helpful in isolating genetic and environmental influences and in determining preventive and precipitating factors. These studies usually include monozygotic (MZ) or single-ovum and dizygotic (DZ) or two-ova twins. Adoption studies try to determine the impact of environmental factors on genetic expression. These studies generally examine and compare biological and adoptive parents of affected subjects and those of healthy biological and adoptive control subjects. Family studies contrast the occurrence of mental disorder among relatives of affected subjects and assess the relevance of heredity (Sadock & Sadock, 2005; Lohr & Bracha, 1992).

Genetic theories regarding the cause of schizophrenia date back to Kraepelin in the early 1900s, who observed that bizarre behavior was commonly found in families of clients with schizophrenia. Twin, adoption, and family studies consistently link genetic, individual vulnerability, and psychosocial stressors with manifestations of schizophrenia; pervasive developmental disorders; mental retardation; dementias; and affective, addictive, and other disorders (Amir et al., 1999; Kendler & Prescott, 1999; Lyons et al., 1998; Sullivan, Neale, & Kendler, 2000; Tsuang, Stone, & Faraone, 2000).

Environmental Factors

Genetic factors do not account for all variances between heredity and mental illness. Such studies suggest that environmental factors are just as relevant as molecular-based genetic processes. Twin, adoption, and family studies tend to support this premise. Environmental factors include parental treatment or caregiving patterns, family structures, age spacing, and gender. These factors may buffer or protect genetically vulnerable clients (Berretini, 2000; Field, 1998; Kendler, Kessler, Neale, Heath, & Eaves, 1993), so that people with a predisposition to a particular mental illness may not develop it because of exposure to protective environmental factors.

Genetics and Addiction

A leading area of concern for nurses is identifying clients at risk for alcoholism and other addictions. One possible explanation for substance abuse perhaps lies in the mesolimbic-mesocortical areas in the brain, which enhance dopamine and generate reward and reinforcement behaviors. A blend of biological and psychosocial factors places certain individuals at risk for addictive behaviors.

The role of genetic factors and alcoholism has generally been well supported by twin, family, and adoption studies. Biological or gene markers are found in dopamine and mu-opioid receptors (Persico, Bird, Gabbay, & Uhl, 1996; Barr et al., 2007). More recent studies also implicate dysfunction of serotonergic transmission as a risk factor for excessive alcohol consumption and dependence (Gorwood et al., 2000; Heinz et al., 1998). In addition, certain behaviors are commonly seen in clients who abuse substances (Hill, Shen, Lowers, & Locke, 2000). Many people who have genetic predisposition for substance abuse may adhere to cultural or religious principles, or both, that never allow substance use; therefore, addiction will not occur even though the person has a vulnerability marker. Religious groups, such as Muslims and Mormons that forbid use of alcohol are believed to have fewer alcoholics than other religious groups. However, this finding does not mean that predisposition for addiction is not present in their genetic makeup. Researchers continue to explore the impact of genetics on mental illness and human behavior. The implications for finding clinical markers and detecting biological and psychosocial factors include searching for the cause of mental illness, identifying clients at risk, developing effective treatment, and preventing exposure to noxious factors that produce illness.

Genetic Research

Scientific studies involve identifying genes and proteins that appear to cause mental disorders and are clearly altered by psychopharmacologic agents and the environment. A key purpose of this clinical evidence is the development of novel pharmacologic agents. Efforts to hasten the development of novel treatment have necessitated the establishment of partnerships between biotechnology and pharmaceutical industries. The National Institute of Mental Health's Mammalian Genetics and Genome studies are already making great strides in genetic research, and studies are being conducted that manipulate the mouse genome. These studies are allowing scientists opportunities to take genes out, alter them, and replace them, and through brain probing, understand brain function relevant to behaviors, cognition, and emotions with precision (Hyman, 1999; NIMH, 1998). Researchers are currently ambitiously involved in discovering "vulnerability genes" and in identifying the neural pathways that regulate mood, emotion, energy, and other mechanisms that are affected by bipolar disorder and other mental disorders. They also propose that these discoveries will be the bases of novel and clinical trials that integrate pharmacologic and psychosocial interventions that improve the quality of care and provide clients and insurers with evidence-based outcomes (Hyman, 2000).

Newer technological advances in stem cell research that involve culturing brainstem cells have the potential for replacing any cell in the body. The great hope of medicine is that stem cells will one day be used as universal donor cells and offer cures to incurable diseases such as childhood diabetes, Alzheimer's disease, and spinal cord injury. Of course, these studies are controversial, but in the near future will offer cures for clients, families, and communities suffering from mental and physical disorders.

Finally, for more than three decades research has succinctly demonstrated the significance of neurobiological factors in the pathogenesis of psychiatric conditions. Data implicate environmental, developmental, and genetic influences as powerful mediators of neurobiological processes and subsequently mental health. Psychiatric mental health nurses along with other mental health providers are challenged to integrate the complexities of the neurobiological process to assess and make sense of the client's subjective experiences and behavior and develop a holistic plan of care that addresses the client's health care needs over the health continuum.

MAJOR BEHAVIORAL MODELS

Behavior represents an array of responses to internal and external stimuli. The behavioral approach to human activity assumes that behavior is influenced by specific interconnections between complex neural processes, heredity, environment, instinct, conditioning, and reinforcement. Behavior is directed toward meeting basic human needs. Most human behavior is voluntary and related to avoiding negative experiences—behavior is not simply stimulus-response interactions. Behaviors are generally reinforced by rewards for doing the right thing or punishment for doing the wrong thing. Human responses are directed either at goal attainment, such as asking for another piece of cake, or object avoidance, such as avoiding crowds or elevators. These responses are labeled either *approach* or *avoidance* of stimuli.

Reinforcers are used to modify maladaptive behavior and can be positive or negative. Reinforcers are personally determined. For example, it may be difficult to predict whether two people at a party where alcohol is served will drink: One may drink beer after beer regardless of the morning-after consequences, whereas the other may avoid alcohol altogether. Reinforcers account for the difference. One student may have a biochemical predisposition to alcohol and thus will gain reinforcement directly from it. Another student may avoid alcohol because parental drunkenness resulted in his taking an oath not to drink. Or perhaps one of the people agreed to serve as the designated driver at this party and will be rewarded by drinking at the next. Perhaps both have a heavy workload the next day and cannot face the consequences of drinking. Good job performance is the reinforcer in this example. Evidently, reinforcers are personal, complex, learned, and may be biochemical.

Behavior is observable and offers clues about the brain's functioning in relation to internal and external stimuli. Internal stimuli include complex biological changes or disturbances, personality traits, perception, or temperament. Examples of external stimuli include developmental transitions, seasonal or circadian cycle changes, or other psychosocial stressors. Major behavioral theorists include Skinner, Bandura, and Walters (see Chapter 2, Concepts of Psychiatric Nursing).

INTEGRATION OF BRAIN AND BEHAVIOR

The interrelatedness of human behavior and brain function is complex. Neural processes that govern thirst, hunger, sex drive, aggression, and motivation are located in the hypothalamus and other areas in the limbic system. The brain analyzes internal and external stimuli as either irrelevant or threats, and this process is the basis of perception. Perceptions generate neural signals that either inhibit or arouse cellular innervations. Motor commands arise from these signals. Complex nerve cell activity along the spinal cord governs motor and behavioral patterns. Lesions or alterations in the limbic system or sensory-perceptual mechanisms generate maladaptive behavioral patterns, such as those seen in psychosis. Psychosis is believed to arise from biochemical and anatomical abnormalities that are manifested by vast behavioral responses, such as agitation, sensory-perceptual alterations, and social withdrawal.

Determining the origins and influences of behavior is difficult, but researchers continue to demonstrate more conclusive evidence of biological bases for mental illness. Determinants of various behavioral responses include psychosocial stress and neurobiological, genetic, and cultural factors. Appreciating the intricate link between psychosocial and neurobiological factors as causes of mental illness is critical to developing effective interventions, participating in research that integrates these concepts, and understanding the magnitude of technological advances.

KINDLING

Neurochemical changes are surmised to be associated with psychosocial stressors. Kindling is an example of a neurobiological response that is activated by significant early stress and losses. Kindling is the electrophysiological process that over time produces an action potential after repetitive subthreshold stimulation or progressive sensitization of a neuron. Clinical studies over the past 40 years have sought to discover the underpinnings of unipolar and bipolar disorders. Most findings suggest that monamine signaling and HPA axis dysregulation play integral roles in the pathophysiology of both mania and depression. Kindling and progressive sensitization to seizures come from the epilepsy literature and is a useful premise that explains neurobiological processes at the molecular and cellular levels and the genetic predisposition of mood dysregulation. Kindling appears to produce dramatic increases in membrane-associated protein kinase C and certain G-proteins (Kendler, Thornton, & Gardner, 2000; Post & Weiss, 1999).

Protein kinase C (PKC) is a group of enzymes that activate other enzymes. G-proteins are part of the cell's plasma membrane and are involved in sending signals from regulatory chemicals such as hormones and neurotransmitters to target cells. Collectively, PKC and G-proteins trigger a cascade of chemical reactions that produce target cells' responses, and play roles in cellular proliferation, enzymatic reactions, and regulation of certain genes. Lithium and valproate acid regulate PKC activities and have efficacy in the treatment of acute mania (Berretini, 2000; Kendler et al., 2000; Manji & Lenox, 2000; Post & Weiss, 1999). Early losses and trauma are examples of stressors that result in mood dysregulation and its chronic and recurrent course.

Early losses and traumas are thought to increase sensitivity at some receptor sites by activating biochemicals that impair responsiveness and increase vulnerability to future mood disorders. In other words, in early life, a psychosocial stressor, like the death of a parent, may precipitate a depressive episode. The next time a major psychosocial stressor occurs, depression is experienced again. At some point, after repeated recurrences, depressive episodes begin to occur without a precipitating stressor. The basis of this premise is encoding of a "long-standing trait marker" to affective illness that increases susceptibility to stress (Post, 1992). Feelings of helplessness are marked in people who have experienced repeated trauma (Maier & Seligman, 1976).

TRAUMA

Traumatic events across the life span are also tied to neurobiological and behavioral changes, frequently seen in clients with borderline personality, post-traumatic stress disorder, depression, and dissociative identity disorder. Responses to trauma are generally behavioral and biological. Clients experiencing trauma often experience flashbacks, intrusive thoughts, "being in a daze" numbing, anxiety, startle reactions, nightmares, and fatigue (American Psychiatric Association [APA], 2000).

Traumatic events involve activation of brain regions related to perceiving and responding to a threat in which the HPA axis has a principal role. The HPA axis is primarily responsible for the secretion of the two main stress hormones, cortisol and norepinephrine (NE). These mechanisms orchestrate a cascade of complex responses that include brain nuclei determining facial expression and the rate and depth of cardiac and respiratory patterns. These neurobiological and behavioral responses are modulated by the principal nucleus of the amygdala, which also acts as a powerful modulator of fear responses. Together the amygdala and hippocampus play "crucial roles" in the encoding and retrieval of memories, eventually activating neurochemicals that give rise to dissociative amnesia (Grillon, Southwick, & Charney, 1996). The brain circuits involved in fear parallel a rapid and transitory response to environmental stimuli. The identification of neural substrates of fear have made it possible to appreciate the underpinnings of anxiety disorders (Fanselow & LeDoux, 1999; Shekhar, Truitt, Rainnie, & Sajdyk, 2005). This premise also underscores the biological and behavioral responses to trauma that are likely to be intense and goal-directed social isolation or withdrawal, startle response, alienation, irritability, and agitation.

In addition, trauma interferes with modulation of anxiety and aggression because of hyperarousal of the autonomic nervous system and heightened sensitivity to feelings or environmental stimuli. Persistent, severe distress is associated with increased risk for certain cancers and immunosuppressive disorders, such as autoimmune deficiency syndrome, biochemical changes in neurotransmitters, and endogenous opioid (endorphin) production and release. Presumably, during sustained stressful periods, immense quantities of neurotransmitters such as norepinephrine and dopamine are secreted, increasing the risk of chronic stress-related illnesses. With prolonged stimulation, repletion of neurotransmitters occurs, leading to receptor hyperstimulation and depletion of cortisol, consequently increasing the risk of post-traumatic stress disorder (O'Donnell et al., 2004; Shalev, 2000; Yehuda, McFarlane, & Shalev, 1998). In other words, when the stress response is turned on too long or too often, it cannot be turned off. This area of research has potential for nursing practice in the area of preventive health care. See Table 3–1 for the bioneurochemical and behavioral responses to severe stress.

Acute trauma or stress increases dopamine release and metabolism in certain brain centers, particularly the prefrontal cortex. Moreover, activated dopaminergic systems appear to be directly involved in mobilizing coping responses and play a

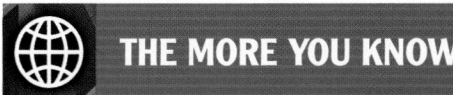
Will Complementary Therapies Threaten the Use of Conventional Psychotherapeutic Biological and Behavioral Treatment Approaches?

From Fugh-Berman, A., & Cott, J. M. (1999). Dietary supplements and natural products as psychotherapeutic agents. *Psychosomatic Medicine, 61,* 712–728.

Complementary and alternative therapies are challenging nurses and other health care providers to gain an appreciation for unconventional treatment of psychiatric disorders. Studies show that consumer interest in complementary therapies was up 34 percent in 1997 from 1991 and continues to climb. Herbal medicine use has risen sharply over the past decade from 3 to 12 percent, and the majority of consumers use these therapies for chronic, rather than life-threatening, conditions. Many consumers may not inform their health care providers of such use. A number of herbs and nutritional supplements have observable effects on mood, memory, and sleep disturbances.

The surge of complementary therapies crosses all socioeconomic, age, culture, gender, and ethnic groups. The most cited health problems are chronic pain, anxiety, arthritis, chronic fatigue syndrome, and headaches. Psychiatric treatment appears to be a target of treatment, particularly anxiety and depression. The skyrocketing use of these therapies among the mentally ill has prompted the National Institute of Health Office of Alternative Medicine and the National Institute of Mental Health to fund a $4.3 million study to determine the efficacy of these therapies on major depression, biological, and behavioral therapies. Many clients consume these agents and use various complementary therapies because they are readily accessible on the Internet, pharmacies, and health food stores. Critics worry that consumers will abandon conventional therapies and experience deleterious consequences. Do these consumer patterns reflect the need for people to take charge of their lives in a seemingly out-of-control society, or does it reflect consumers' need for immediate gratification?

Regardless of the bases of this lucrative market of complementary therapies, psychiatric nurses must apprise themselves of these diverse treatments. It is important for nurses to be aware of data available on herbs and dietary supplements that consumers are likely to be using. Likewise, although these agents have demonstrable effects on clients' mood, memory, and energy levels, they are not regulated. Health education is an integral part of psychiatric nursing care. Controversies prevail about the safety of drug and herbal interactions and the lack of regulation of complementary therapies. The reality is that consumers will continue to take control over their lives by using complementary and conventional treatment. Understanding the effects of diverse herbs, dietary supplements, and other complementary therapies provides opportunities to assess, educate the consumer, and integrate various therapies with conventional interventions to promote health.

major role in the development of post-traumatic stress disorder (Layton & Krikorian, 2002). This may explain why trauma leads to lifelong consequences in susceptible persons. It also validates the consideration of both psychosocial stressors and neurobiological and behavioral responses in a holistic view of nursing.

Behavioral responses to dysregulation of certain neurotransmitters include social isolation, startle reactions, irritability, paranoia, distrust, and agitation. Serotonin is thought to modulate the activity of other neurotransmitters, resulting in behavioral and emotional responses (Sadock, Sadock, & Sussman, 2006).

TABLE 3–1
Biochemical and Behavioral Responses to Stress

Biochemical Responses	Cognitive Appraisal	Possible Behavioral Responses
Forebrain		
Screens emotional responses to internal and external stimuli.	Irrelevant stimuli	Ignored, no responses
Links hypothalamus to environment to activate proper neurochemical responses (i.e., autonomic nervous system, neuroendocrine)	Perceived danger, threat	Anxiety, sweating, restlessness, agitation, avoidance/social isolation, anger, aggression
Hypothalamus		
Acts as principal ganglion	Reappraisal of threat or danger	Calmness, decreased anxiety, fear, restlessness
Activates proper neurochemical responses (e.g., anterior pituitary to adrenal coA1ex)		

Adaptation to trauma is related to a number of factors (van de Kolk, 1987a), including:

a. severity of stressor
b. genetic vulnerability
c. developmental stage
d. available support system
e. history of trauma
f. ego function (personality traits)

Similarly, adaptation to stress is generally related to a person's repertoire of coping behaviors. The severity of a stressor is determined by individual perception of the event.

The developmental stage during which the trauma is experienced influences the impact of the trauma. For instance, adults with adequate coping behaviors and support systems are likely to be less vulnerable to trauma than a child would be. Social systems during traumatic or stressful events act as buffers to sustain trust, security, and safety (Davidson et al., 2005; Kangas, Henry, & Bryant, 2005; van der Kolk, 1987b). The emotionally abused 1-year-old child is more likely to experience difficulty forming trusting and healthy interpersonal relationships throughout the remainder of the life span than the battered housewife. Besides the developmental stage, other factors influence a child's response to trauma. Early traumatic experiences also interfere with normal growth and development tasks such as learning trust, self-esteem, and autonomy; influence adaptive responses throughout the life span; and increase the risk for biological and behavioral morbidity. These risk factors include being a female, being in close proximity or exposure to the event, the degree of personal injury, injury or death of a family member, parental psychopathology, lack of quality support system, and the degree of life threat (Chemtob, Nakashima, & Hamada, 2002; Lipschitz, Rasmusson, & Southwick, 1998).

Neurological damage has also been detected in a number of abused children who have no symptoms of traumatic brain injury. Psychosocial factors such as chaotic and abusive environments are tied with delayed impaired CNS maturation such as attention deficit disorder (ADD) (Fish-Murray, Koby, van der Kolk, 1987).

Bowlby (1973) believed that early attachments and relationships with primary caregivers mediate maturation of the CNS, and that abuse impairs emotional and intellectual development. He noted the effect of early emotional bonding and formation of endorphins or endogenous opiates. Endorphins play a major role in managing severe stress, producing calmness, and buffering one from emotional pain (Molina, 2002). See Table 3–2 for biological-behavioral client outcomes, as incorporated into a nursing care plan. Understanding human response to trauma and other psychosocial stressors is critical to health maintenance. Pseudoseizures, abnormal electroencephalograms (EEGs), and clients with dissociative identity disorder have been associated with neurological trauma (Bailles, Pinto, Fernandez-Egea et al., 2004). Interventions that provide emotional support and empathy, modulate feelings, create trust, reduce anxiety, and promote a sense of control and power include various psychotherapies, cognitive-behavioral therapy, crisis intervention, stress management, and psychotropics. (See Chapter 11, Chapter 29, and Chapter 31 for in-depth discussions of these interventions.)

MAJOR PARADIGMS OF PSYCHIATRIC-MENTAL HEALTH NURSING

The recent explosion of research and knowledge in the area of neurobiology—involving advances in genetics brain mapping, imaging, and scanning—has opened up a fascinating world

CASE STUDY

Ms. M is a 30 year old who was verbally attacked by a co-worker while standing at the printer. The attack results from an earlier discussion of work assignment. After the frightening altercation she excuses herself and seeks assistance from the company's Employee Assistance Program (EAP). Based on your understanding of normal stress reactions and underlying neurobiological processes, which of the following best describe how she may behave during the meeting with the EAP counselor?

1. Reduced concentration and fearfulness that the incident will recur
2. Calm demeanor and provide a clear description of the incident
3. Increased heart rate, sweating, and shortness of breath
4. Provide explanation of incident with mild to moderate anxiety depending upon her perception of safety

Answer(s)

1. All of these answers are correct. How one responds to a stressful or traumatic event varies among individuals and is governed by numerous factors including past history of trauma, quality of coping skills and support systems, severity of stress, and developmental stage. A calm demeanor as noted in answer 2 does not parallel severity of stressors especially if the client is still in a state of shock or one who minimizes the incident. Recent studies also indicate the potentially deleterious effects of stress debriefing in a post-traumatic or stressful event, suggesting that it may actually increase the risk of post-traumatic stress disorder due to its impact on memory consolidation or emotional encoding of memory.

TABLE 3–2

Nursing Care Plan: The Client Experiencing Sensory–Perceptual Disturbances (Psychosis): Biological–Behavioral Client Outcomes

Nursing Diagnosis: Disturbed Sensory Perception (Visual, Auditory)

Outcome Identification	Nursing Actions	Rationales	Evaluations
1. By [date], responds appropriately to internal/external stimuli.	1a. Establish rapport.	1a. Facilitates a trusting alliance and reduces anxiety and agitation.	Goal met:
	1b. Assess the presence of hallucinations and/or delusions (i.e., smiling or nodding head inappropriately).	1b. Enables nurse to assess basis of client behavior and responses.	Client initially has difficulty trusting staff because of auditory hallucinations and persecutory delusions.
	1c. Decrease environmental stimuli.	1c. Reduces anxiety and risk of aggression.	Client experiences decreased hallucinations and delusions and agitation—no adverse responses noted except excessive sedation, which was decreased with dose reduction.
2. By [date], verbalizes coherently to others.	2a. Give direct and concrete explanations.	2a. Decreases anxiety and increases coherence.	Client's thoughts are coherent and anxiety is minimized.
	2b. Collaborate with client and family to establish a plan of care.	2b. Essential part of self-care/health promotion.	Client able to perform self-care needs with minimal assistance.
	2c. Assist in self-care.	2c. Disturbed thought processes interfere with self-care.	
3. By [date], exhibits decreased agitation.	3. Administer antipsychotic and observe for desired and adverse responses.	3. Neuroleptics are important to reduce hallucinations/delusions and agitation and improve thought process.	

Nursing Diagnosis: Impaired Social Interaction

Outcome Identification	Nursing Actions	Rationales	Evaluations
1. Initiates and interacts with others appropriately.	1. Designate staff for one-to-one relationships.	1. Decrease environmental stimuli and establish trusting relationships.	Goal met:
2. Verbalizes coherently with others.	2. Reinforce and validate clear communication.	2. Enables client to learn effective communication skills.	Client is able to establish one-to-one alliance with several staff.
			Client continues to have difficulty interacting with some group members.

concerning the human brain and behavior. Psychiatric nursing educators and clinicians are challenged in their ability to integrate traditional psychiatric nursing and neurobiological concepts into nursing curricula and practice. Psychiatric nursing continues to struggle with integrating biological concepts into undergraduate and graduate curricula despite advances in neurobiology, neuroscience, and genetics. Overall, technological advances in neurobiological discoveries and other psychiatric nursing challenges offer vast opportunities to integrate biological and behavioral concepts into holistic interventions and improve the quality of life for the mentally ill.

CLINICAL AND PRACTICE ISSUES

Recent discoveries in the field of neurobiology continue to revolutionize the understanding and treatment of mental illness. Because psychiatric nurses work collaboratively with other disciplines for the most part, they cannot help but to be influenced by these advances and must continually stay abreast of new findings to communicate knowledgeably with other mental health professionals. Likewise, evidence-based research should guide nursing practice. Obviously, nursing must not lose sight of its holistic tradition, taking all aspects of the client into consideration, including the spiritual, cultural, psychosocial, as well as the biological.

Historically, in spite of technological advances in neurobiology in understanding and treating mental illness, there has been some controversy and doubt over its relevance to psychiatric nurses. Peplau (1989) noted that specific mental disorders are difficult to explain as a "global or single entity" (p. 26) and determined that psychiatric nurses need to explore the basis of impaired behavioral patterns rather than the biological aspects, and focus on human responses to stress and societal changes. At the same time, Peplau strongly encouraged psychiatric nurses to value and appreciate the biological components of mental illness, as well as the psychosocial concepts such as caring. Application of biological interventions does not negate the effectiveness of other treatment modalities. Besides, psychosocial interventions such as psychoeducation, psychotherapy, stress management, relaxation, and cognitive therapy continue to be viable treatment options.

NURSING INTERVENTIONS

Historically, one of the major biological interventions used by psychiatric nurses involved assessing the need for prescribing and administering psychotropics to calm agitated clients experiencing hallucinations and delusions. Recent neurobiological findings have promoted the creation of new psychopharmacologic agents that target specific areas of the brain to reduce symptoms and modify behaviors. Other research findings link gender, culture, and genetic and familial factors to the efficacy of these agents. Selective serotonin reuptake inhibitors such as sertraline (Zoloft) and serotonin-norepinephrine reuptake inhibitors such as venlafaxine and duloxetine (Cymbalta) and combination olanzapine/fluoxetine (Symbyax) for mania. The use of electroconvulsive therapy (ECT) is gaining renewed acceptance as an effective treatment modality for severe depression and various schizophrenic disorders. Other examples of biological therapies include complementary therapies, such as St. John's Wort for mild depression, rest-sleep manipulation for bipolar disorder, music or touch therapy in dementia, administration of full-spectrum lighting for seasonal affective disorder, and nutritional alterations in alcoholism.

Health promotion and primary prevention remain major nursing goals. These goals parallel managed health care concepts that emphasize cost-effective and evidence-based health care. Prevention minimizes maladaptive behaviors and chronicity in high-risk clients and groups. The domain of psychiatric nurses lies in recognizing and assessing age-appropriate responses to developmental tasks, biological dysregulation, and changes that define health and illness across the life span. Understanding the realm of normal or adaptive responses to stress helps nurses identify abnormal or maladaptive responses and formulate evidence-based outcomes and interventions that incorporate biological and behavioral concepts.

Client symptoms or behaviors allow the nurse to discern the client's inner world that comprises biological and behavioral processes activated by internal and external stressors. Active listening and astute observation of verbal and nonverbal cues are key aspects of assessing client responses. For instance, the psychotic client may smile or talk inappropriately and have a disheveled appearance. These nonverbal cues link the nurse with complex neurobiological processes that affect the client's behavior and effective treatment modalities.

Major treatment modalities include providing psychotherapy, behavioral modification, cognitive therapy; assessing the need for medications; administering, prescribing, and monitoring client responses to psychotropics; and facilitating sleep-rest, light-dark, exercise-relaxation, and nutritional aspects of care. These interventions integrate the biological and behavioral aspects of mental illness.

PSYCHIATRIC NURSING EDUCATION

The National League of Nursing has long stipulated that schools provide psychiatric nursing experiences for accreditation. Core areas of curricula focused on holistic concepts and health promotion and prevention, and major concepts have included caring and psychosocial needs of clients (American Nurses Association [ANA], 2000; McBride, 1990; McCabe, 2000; Perrand et al., 2006). A wealth of psychiatric nursing literature has permitted faculty to define the scope and character of this specialty. Over the years educators have become leaders in directing psychiatric nursing practice and generating specialization. These changes have paralleled with the ANA specialization and scope of practice.

During the 1990s psychiatric nurses began to define major biological and behavioral concepts, integrating them into nursing practice. McBride (1990) suggested that balancing these concepts with care and caring to collaborate with other disciplines to develop effective client outcomes might accomplish this.

Some educators and clinicians have already defined outcomes that integrate biological and behavioral concepts into nursing practice. Additionally, undergraduate baccalaureate students were expected to gain knowledge of studies regarding the brain and neuroscience and their impact on human adaptation to stress. Vast advances of the twenty-first century in neurobiology and the information system provide even greater opportunities for educators and clinicians to gain a greater understanding of neurobiological research and its impact on human behavior and the treatment of mental illness. These efforts are likely to help nurses further define their roles and individualize mental health care more precisely than ever before.

McCabe (2000) also suggests that changes in nursing curricula can be made by integrating core concepts, such as relatedness, adaptation, regulation, vulnerability, integrity, and efficacy and integrating them in the care of clients who are mentally ill. These core concepts provide a theoretical framework that encompasses the educational needs of generalist and advanced-practice psychiatric nurses. Integrating biological-behavioral concepts with present nursing education trends affords opportunities for novel approaches to psychiatric-mental health nursing education and clinical practice.

The ANA continues to support psychiatric nurses and advocates the integration of biological and behavioral concepts into nursing practice. The newest edition of *A Statement on Psychiatric-Mental Health Nursing Practice* (ANA, 2000) addresses enormous changes in psychiatric nursing and the health care delivery system. The ANA stresses the impact of rapid evolution of biological sciences and advances in technology on psychiatric nursing practice. This statement establishes that neurobiological advances and development of interventions promise more effective response for the mentally ill. Moreover, the ANA confirms the need for psychosocial interventions, such as psychotherapy, cognitive therapy, psychoeducation, crisis intervention, and administration and prescribing of psychotropics to help clients develop effective coping patterns. Finally, this publication provides an in-depth discussion of the Advanced-Practice Psychiatric Registered Nurse, which is useful in helping the public, legislators, and other professionals understand the role of the generalist and the advanced-practice role in psychiatric-mental health nursing.

THE ROLE OF THE NURSE

The generalist and advanced-practice registered nurse can use an array of biological and behavioral interventions to facilitate adaptive responses to internal and external stressors. Psychiatric nurses are faced with providing complex care that meets the holistic needs of clients in inpatient, ambulatory, primary care, and home health and community settings. These needs include psychosocial and biological factors that affect client behavior. Aggression, suicide, irritability, noncompliance, sleep–wake cycle disturbances, and social withdrawal are common behavioral responses to stress, which often arise from psychosocial and biological alterations.

THE GENERALIST NURSE

The generalist or psychiatric-mental health nurse works with clients, families, groups, and communities and uses the nursing process to assess adaptive and maladaptive responses. This nurse understands the relationship between underlying biological processes, facilitates and reinforces adaptive coping patterns, and assesses and prevents further disability. Specific interventions encouraging health promotion and maintenance include psychoeducation, administration of psychotropic medications and monitoring client response, milieu therapy, and crisis intervention. These interventions occur during activities such as intake and screening, telecare, case management, and in diverse settings such as community and mental health centers, day hospitals, home health settings, and homeless shelters (ANA, 2000). Biological and psychosocial interventions enable the generalist psychiatric-mental health nurse to alter or modify maladaptive responses seen in various mental disorders, such as attention deficit disorders, psychosis, and depression.

A combination of biological and psychosocial interventions can be used in caring for a client who is experiencing psychosis. The psychotic client experiences perceptual disturbances, such as auditory hallucinations that lead to suspiciousness, and may result in irritability, social reclusiveness, and refusal to eat. Perceptual disturbances represent neurobiological phenomenon that results in behavior in response to this internal and external stimuli. The client may act on the command of the hallucinations and step in front of a car or refuse to eat because "someone poisoned the food." Assessing the nature of hallucinations is crucial to the client and staff's safety. Administering a typical antipsychotic such as haloperidol (Haldol) or an atypical agent such as olanzapine (Zyprexa) are biological interventions that target certain neurotransmitters, specifically dopamine, also serotonin in the latter case, that give rise to psychotic symptoms. The psychosocial intervention is a calm, firm approach that conveys empathy and provides the client with structure and limit setting. These interventions can work together to decrease hallucinations, delusions, and anxiety, and increase the client's impulse control, thus reducing the risk of violent, aggressive behaviors (see Table 3–2 for the nursing care plan).

Behavioral patterns can be adaptive or maladaptive. The depressed adolescent may use maladaptive behavioral patterns such as alcohol, stealing, or quarreling, to manage internal emotional pain and to deal with psychosocial stressors of family pressures and school. Conversely, another adolescent may use adaptive responses and seek out family, friends, or clergy to verbalize feelings about a stressful situation. The nurse must operate on the premise that all behavior has meaning and can be clarified. Therefore, assessing behavioral responses to internal and external stimuli is a major nursing responsibility and involves collaborating with the client and other mental health professionals to develop effective interventions and evidence-based outcomes.

THE ADVANCED-PRACTICE PSYCHIATRIC REGISTERED NURSE

The role of the advanced-practice psychiatric registered nurse encompasses that of the generalist in addition to providing direct clinical care, such as psychotherapy and prescriptive authority. Advanced educational and clinical preparation enables the advanced-practice psychiatric registered nurse to assess complex problems and employ knowledge, skills, and clinical experience to alter or modify maladaptive responses in various clinical settings (ANA, 2000).

Specific advanced-practice psychiatric registered nurse interventions include prescribing, administrating psychotropics, and evaluating client responses to various biological therapies such as psychotropics, electroconvulsive therapy, complementary therapies, phototherapy, and integrating them with behavioral strategies. Furthermore, conducting research study to assess client responses to behavioral and biological interventions is critical to evaluating and developing evidenced-based care.

Behavioral interventions offered by the advanced-practice psychiatric registered nurse include cognitive-behavioral therapy, progressive relaxation, guided imagery, psychotherapy, and psychoeducation. Various interventions depend on nurse-client collaboration that allows nurses to empower clients in understanding the basis of mental illness and create interventions that can alleviate symptoms and promote health maintenance.

RELATED RESEARCH

Psychiatric nurses are in the midst of a neurobiological explosion that provides vast opportunities to define and investigate client outcomes that integrate biological and behavioral concepts. Studies that compare the effectiveness of biological and behavioral interventions can also assist nurses in developing evidence-based outcomes that meet the complex needs of the mentally ill (refer to the Research Abstract). Survival of psychiatric nurses depends on the ability of educators, clinicians, and researchers to integrate biological and behavioral concepts into academic curricula and scope of practices. Evaluating student experiences that incorporate these concepts can generate data that direct students and practicing nurses.

SUMMARY

◆ Advances in neurobiological research offer clinicians and researchers a greater understanding of the complexity of mental health and illness.

RESEARCH ABSTRACT

Foot Acupressure and Massage for Patients with Alzheimer's Disease and Related Dementias
Sutherland, J. A., Reakes, J., & Bridges, C. (1999). *Image: Journal of Nursing Scholarship, 31,* 347–348.

Study Problem/Purpose
To determine the effects of foot acupressure and massage on wandering, pulse, respirations, and quiet time behaviors in patients with AD and other dementias.

Methods
The researchers used a quasi-experimental design with purpose sampling and random assignment of patients to experimental (n = 5) and control (n = 5) groups. The patients resided in an AD specialty care center. Subjects met the following criteria for inclusion: (a) required assistance with activities of daily living; (b) exhibited varying degrees of behavioral problems; (c) had disruptive verbal behaviors; (d) were independent with locomotion; (e) exhibited various wandering behaviors or other disruptive behaviors; and (f) had resided in the center for at least 3 months. A Behavioral Documentation Instrument (BDI) was used to collect narrative; data were logged in immediately before and during the experiment by a nurse-massage therapist.

Foot acupressure and massage therapy was applied to the experimental group for 5 minutes on each foot during a 10-day treatment period. Treatment consisted of massage with long, smooth, rhythmic strokes of the entire foot and ankle, using clockwise movement of four acupressure points. Independent variables such as wandering, pulse, respirations, and quiet time for both groups were taken every 2 hours and recorded for the 10-day treatment period and 3 days after treatment. Scores were calculated for each variable to discern differences between treatment and baseline data with t-tests performed on the groups' mean change scores.

Findings
The experimental group post treatment means decreased wandering, pulse, and respirations and an increase in quiet-time post treatment. However, these scores were not statistically significant by t-test.

Implications for Psychiatric Nurses
Despite the major limitation of a small sample size, psychiatric nurses can use acupressure and massage therapy, combining therapeutic touch and nursing presence to promote calmness and emotional support of clients experiencing AD and other dementias.

- The expansion of biological knowledge gives clients, families, communities, and psychiatric nurses hope for more effective treatment to improve their quality of life.

- The human experience arises from the complex interaction of the person's neurobiological mechanism and the individual's environment.

- The biological-behavioral interface of mental health and illness is complex and challenges nurses to integrate these concepts into practice, education, and research.

STUDY QUESTIONS

1. Mary, a 28-year-old college student, encounters a situation during her class that reminds her of a previous traumatic predicament. Her immediate reaction involves intense fear and immediately getting out of the situation. The most accurate description of her reactions reflects which neurobiological processes?
   a. The hypothalamus-pituitary-adrenal axis and amygdala
   b. Kindling, neurotransmitters
   c. Genetic predisposition
   d. Hippocampus

2. Mr. Murray presents in the mental health center complaining of "hearing voices," and he is smiling and talking to himself during the assessment. The most appropriate explanation for his behavior involves which of the following?
   a. Dysregulation of a neurotransmitter such as dopamine
   b. Stressful home situation caused by frequent arguments with his mother
   c. Dopamine dysregulation and interpersonal conflicts
   d. Overmedication with antipsychotic and related side effects

3. You are assessing the new client who is brought in by her father, who reports that he is concerned about her behavior. As her nurse, which of the following is *critical* in making an appropriate assessment of this client?
   a. What kind of pressure has she been under lately?
   b. Describe her relationship with family members.
   c. How long has she lived with you?
   d. Is there a family history of mental illness?

4. Mikie, a 7-year-old boy, is brought in by his parents who report that he has been irritable and fearful since he witnessed his friend being viciously attacked by a dog several days ago. Which of the following is the most appropriate immediate response to the parents and child?
   a. Reassure the child and parents about the normalcy of his behavior.
   b. Encourage the parents to consider an antidepressant for their child.
   c. Refer them to a trauma counselor so the child can explain the impact on his life.
   d. Educate them about normal stress reactions.

5. Health maintenance is an integral part of psychiatric nursing practice. Which of the following interventions *most accurately* depicts health maintenance?
   a. The client who loses his job is seen in a crisis center.
   b. The anxious pregnant client who is referred for stress management.
   c. The client with acute psychosis is offered an injection of haloperidol.
   d. The client experiencing an acute panic attack is taught deep breathing exercises.

6. Mrs. Nelson, an 86-year-old woman who has been recently diagnosed with Alzheimer's disease, is seen during a home health visit and is very confused. Her daughter explains that she does not recognize family members, and this has been very difficult to handle. Which of the following behaviors might you expect from Mrs. Nelson during this visit?
   a. She will respond appropriately after the nurse reorients her.
   b. She is likely to become calm and cooperative.
   c. She is likely to be aggressive and verbally abusive.
   d. She is likely to remember things that happened years ago, but not recent events.

7. Kindling is an important concept in psychiatric-mental health nursing. Which of the following nursing interventions reflect kindling?
   a. Administering an antimanic agent to a client with bipolar disorder
   b. Providing client education about the importance of taking medications as prescribed
   c. Monitoring client response to antidepressant medication
   d. All of the above

8. Several days ago Mary was recently seriously injured in a motor vehicle accident. Her injuries are not life-threatening nor did she sustain head trauma or injury. During your interview with her on the orthopedic unit you notice she is easily startled and mildly agitated and complains of difficulty concentrating and sleep disturbances. What is the best explanation for her symptoms?
   a. She is exhibiting symptoms of post-traumatic stress disorder (PTSD).
   b. Her symptoms reflect normal stress reactions.
   c. She needs medications to promote rest.
   d. Her symptoms are serious and will worsen over time.

9. Your client, John, complains of hearing voices and fears people can read his thoughts. He also shouts, "don't you hear my cousin talking in the corner?" What is the most appropriate response to the client?
   a. "Yes, I hear your cousin talking."
   b. "John, I understand that you hear your cousin talking, but I don't hear him."
   c. "John, your mind is playing tricks on you again. You don't hear anyone talking."
   d. "Lets go for a walk to get your mind off the voices."

10. In addition to responding to John's query about hearing his cousin talking in the above question, additional nursing interventions may include:
    a. Administering a typical antipsychotic medication
    b. Assessing John's level of danger to self and others
    c. Reducing John's anxiety through empathy and using nonthreatening behavior
    d. All of the above

RESOURCES

Please note that because Internet resources are of a time-sensitive nature and URL addresses may change or be deleted, searches should also be conducted by association or topic.

Internet Resources

1. National Association of Clinical Nurse Specialists (NACNS)
   3969 Green Street
   Harrisburg, PA 17110
   (717) 234-6799
   http://www.nacns.org

2. American Nurses Association
   600 Maryland Ave, SW
   Suite 100 W
   Washington, DC 20024
   (202) 651-7000
   (800) 274-4262
   http://www.ana.org

3. The *American Nurse* Online Journal of Issues in Nursing
   (800) 274-4262
   www.nursingworld.org

4. American Psychiatric Nurses Association
   Colonial Place Three
   2107 Wilson Boulevard, Suite 300A
   Arlington, VA 22201
   (703) 243-2443
   http://www.apna.org/

5. The American Heart Association
   National Center
   7272 Greenville Avenue
   Dallas, TX 75231
   (800) 242-8721
   www.americanheart.org

6. Alzheimer's Association
   919 North Michigan Ave., Ste 1000
   Chicago, IL 60611-1676
   (800) 272-3900
   http://www.alz.org

7. International Society of Psychiatric-Mental Health Nurses (ISPN)
   810 Crossroads Dr. Suite 3800
   Madison, WI 53718
   (866) 330-7227
   http://www.ispn-psych.org

Professional Organizations Involved in Brain and Genetic Research

www.nimh.nih.gov   National Institute of Mental Health

www.nature.com   Nature

www.sciencemag.org/misc/e-perspectives.shtml   Science on line

http://www.grb.nimh.nih.gov/gi.html   Department of Health and Human Services NIMH, Human Genetics Initiative

http://www.edc.gsph.pitt.edu/stepbd   Epidemiology Data Center. STEP-BD. Systematic Treatment Enhancement Program for Bipolar Disorder

http://www.hapmap.org/   Map of the human genome (International Hap Map Project) (Accessed May 14, 2006)

REFERENCES

Abelson, J. L., Liberzon, I., Young, E. A., & Khan, S. (2005). Cognitive modulation of the endocrine stress response to a pharmacological challenge in normal and panic disorder subjects. *Archives of General Psychiatry, 62,* 668–675.

American Nurses Association. (2000). *A Statement on psychiatric-mental health nursing practice.* Washington, DC: Author.

American Psychiatric Association. (2000). *Diagnostic and statistical manual of mental disorders,* 4th edition, Text Revision (*DMS-IV-TR*). Washington, DC: Author.

Amir, R. E., Van den Veyver, I. B., Wan, M., Tran, C. Q., Francke, U., & Zoghbi, H. Y. (1999). Rett syndrome is caused by mutations in X-lined MECP2, encoding methyl-CpG-binding protein 2. *Nature and Genetics, 23,* 185–188.

Bailles, E., Pinto, L., Fernandez-Egea, E., Torres, X., Matrai, S., De Pablo, J., & Arroyo, S. (2004). Psychiatric disorders, trauma, and MMPI profile in a Spanish sample of nonepileptic seizure patients. *General Hospital of Psychiatry, 26,* 310–315.

Barnes, C. A. (2003). Long-term potentiation and the ageing brain. *Philosophical Transactions of the Royal Society B: Biological Sciences, 358,* 765–772.

Barr, C. S., Schwandt, M., Lindell, S. G., Chen, S. A., Goldman, D., Suomi, S. J., et al. (2007). Association of a functional polymorphism in the mu-opioid receptor gene with alcohol response and consumption in male rhesus macaques. *Archives of General Psychiatry, 64,* 369–376.

Berretini, W. H. (2000). Are schizophrenic and bipolar disorders related? A review of family and molecular studies. *Biological Psychiatry, 48,* 531–538.

Borysenko, M. (1987). Area review: Psychoneuroimmunology. *Annals of Behavioral Medicine, 9*(2), 3–10.

Bowlby, J. (1973). *Attachment and loss, Vol. II, Separation.* New York: Basic Books.

Campeau, S., Day, H. E. W., Helmreich, D. L., Kollack-Walker, S., & Watson, S. J. (1998). Principles of psychoneuroendocrinology. *The Psychiatric Clinics of North America, 21,* 259–276.

Cazzullo, C. L., Trabattoni, D., Saresella, M., Annoni, G., Arosio, B., & Clerici, M. (2003). Research on psychoimmunology. *World Journal of Biological Psychiatry, 4,* 119–123.

Chemtob, C. M., Nakashima, J. P., Hamada, R. S. (2002). Psychosocial intervention for postdisaster trauma symptoms in elementary school children: A controlled community field study. *Archives of Pediatric and Adolescent Medicine, 156,* 211–216.

Clarke, G., Collins, R. A., Leavitt, B. R., Andrews, D. F., Hayden, M. R., Lumsden, C. J., & McInnes, R. R. (2000). A one-hit model of cell death in inherited neuronal degenerations. *Nature, 406,* 195–199.

Cohly, H. H., & Panja, A. (2005). Immunological findings in autism. *International Review of Neurobiology, 71,* 317–341.

Cowan, W. M., Kopnisky, K. L., & Hyman, S. E. (2002). The human genome project and its impact on psychiatry. *Annual Review of Neuroscience, 25,* 1–50.

Davidson, J. R., Payne, V. M., Connor, K. M., Foa, E. B., Rothbaum, B. O., Hertzberg, M. A., & Weisler, R. H. (2005). Trauma, resilience and saliostasis: Effects of treatment in post-traumatic stress disorder. *International Clinical Psychopharmacology, 20,* 43–48.

Downhill, J. E., Jr., & Robinson, R. G. (1994). Longitudinal assessment of depression and cognitive impairment following stroke. *Journal of Nervous and Mental Disorders, 182,* 425–431.

Erickson, C. A., & Barnes, C. A. (2003). The neurobiology of memory changes in normal aging. *Experimental Gerontology, 38,* 61–69.

Fanselow, M. S., & LeDoux, J. E. (1999). Why we think plasticity underlying Pavlovian fear conditioning occurs in the basolateral amygdala. *Neuron, 23,* 229–232.

Field, T. (1998). Maternal depression affects infants and early interventions. *Preventive Medicine, 27,* 200–203.

Fish-Murray, C. C., Koby, E. V., & van der Kolk, B. A. (1987). Evolving ideas: The effects on children's thoughts. In B. A. van der Kolk (Ed.), *Psychological trauma* (pp. 89–126). Washington, DC: American Psychiatric Press.

Francis, D. D., Caldji, C., Champagne, F., Plotsky, P. M., & Meaney, M. J. (1999). The role of corticotropin-releasing factor-norepinephrine systems in mediating the effects of early experience on the development and endocrine responses to stress. *Society of Biological Psychiatry, 46,* 1153–1166.

Glassman, A. H., & Shapiro, P. A. (1998). Depression and the course of coronary artery disease. *American Journal of Psychiatry, 155,* 4–11.

Gorwood, P., Batel, P., Ades, J., Hamon, M., & Boni, C. (2000). Serotonin transporter gene polymorphisms, alcoholism, and suicidal behavior. *Society of Biological Psychiatry, 48,* 259–264.

Grillon, C., Southwick, S. M., & Charney, D. S. (1996). The psychobiological basis of posttraumatic stress disorder. *Molecular Psychiatry, 1,* 278–297.

Heinz, A., Ragan, P., Jones, D. W., Homner, D., Williams, W., Knable, M. B., Gorey, J. G., Doty, L., Geyer, C., Lee, K. S., Coppola, R., Weinberger, D. R., & Linnoila, M. (1998). Reduced central serotonin transporters in alcoholism. *American Journal of Psychiatry, 155,* 1544–1549.

Heintz, N. (2000). One-hit neuronal death. *Nature, 406,* 137, 139.

Hill, S. Y., Shen, S., Lowers, L., & Locke, J. (2000). Factors predicting the onset of adolescent drinking in families at high risk of developing alcoholism. *Society of Biological Psychiatry, 48,* 265–275.

Huang, Y. (2006). Apolipoprotein E and Alzheimer disease. *Neurology, 66* (2 Suppl.), S79–S85.

Hyman, S. E. (1999). Introduction to the complex genetics of mental disorders. *Biological Psychiatry, 45,* 518–521.

Hyman, S. E. (2000). Goals for research on bipolar disorder: The view from NIMH. *Biological Psychiatry, 48,* 436–441.

Kaestner, F., Hettich, M., Peters, M., Sibrowski, W., Hetzel, G., Ponath, G., Arolt, V., et al. (2005). Different activation patterns of proinflammatory cytokines in melancholic and nonmelancholic major depression are associated with HPA axis activity. *Journal of Affective Disorders, 87,* 305–311.

Kangas, M., Henry, J. L., & Bryant, R. A. (2005). Predictors of posttraumatic stress disorder following cancer. *British Journal of Health Psychology, 24,* 579–585.

Kase, C. S., Wolf, P. A., Kelly-Hayes, M., Kannel, W. B., Beiser, A., & D'Agostino, R. B. (1998). Intellectual decline after stroke: The Farmington Study. *Stroke, 25,* 805–812.

Kelsoe, J. R. (2004). Genomics and the human genome project: Implications for psychiatry. *International Review of Psychiatry, 16,* 294–300.

Kendler, K. S., Kessler, R. C., Neale, M. C., Heath, A. C., & Eaves, L. J. (1993). The prediction of major depression in women: Toward an integrated etiologic model. *American Journal of Psychiatry, 150,* 1139–1145.

Kendler, K. S., & Prescott, C. A. (1999). A population-based twin study of lifetime major depression in men and women. *Archives of General Psychiatry, 56,* 39–44.

Kendler, K. S., Thornton, L. M., & Gardner, C. O. (2000). Stressful life events and previous episodes in the etiology of major depression in women: An evaluation of the "kindling" hypothesis. *American Journal of Psychiatry, 157,* 1243–1251.

Layton, B., & Krikorian, R. (2002). Memory mechanisms in posttraumatic stress disorder. *Journal of Neuropsychiatry and Clinical Neuroscience, 14,* 254–261.

Lipschitz, D. S., Rasmusson, A. M., & Southwick, S. M. (1998). Childhood posttraumatic stress disorder: A review of neurobiologic sequella. *Psychiatric Annals, 28,* 452–457.

Lohr, J. B., & Bracha, H. S. (1992). A monozygotic mirror-image twin pair with discordant psychiatric illness: A neuropsychiatric and neurodevelopmental evolution. *American Journal of Psychiatry,* 1091–1095.

Lyons, M. J., Eisen, S. A., Goldberg, J., True, W., Lin, N., Meyer, J. M., Toomey, R., Faraone, S. V., Merren, J., &

Tsuang, M. T. (1998). A registry-based twin study in males. *Archives of General Psychiatry, 55,* 468–472.

Maier, S. F., & Seligman, M. E. P. (1976). Learned helplessness: Theory and evidence. *Journal of Experimental Psychology: General, 105,* 3–46.

Manji, H. K., & Lenox, R. H. (2000). Signaling: Cellular insight into the pathophysiology of bipolar disorder. *Society of Biological Psychiatry, 48,* 518–530.

McBride, A. B. (1990). Psychiatric nursing in the 1990s. *Archives of Psychiatric Nursing, 4,* 21–28.

McCabe, N. (2000). Bring psychiatric nursing into the twenty-first century. *Archives of Psychiatric Nursing, 14,* 109–116.

Mesulam, M. M., & Geula, C. (1991). Acetylcholinesterase-rich neurons of the human: Cytoarchitectonic and ontogenetic patterns of distribution. *Journal of Comprehensive Neurology, 306,* 193–220.

Molina, P. E. (2002). Stress-specific opioid modulation of haemodynamic counter-regulation. *Clinical Experimental Pharmacology and Physiology, 29,* 248–253.

National Institute of Mental Health. (1998). *Genetics and mental disorders: Report of the National Institute of Mental Health genetics workgroup* (NIH Publication No. 98-4268). Bethesda, MD: NIMH.

Nemeroff, C. B., & Vale, W. W. (2005). The neurobiology of depression: Inroads to treatment and new drug discovery. *Journal of Clinical Psychiatry, 66* (Suppl. 7), 5–13.

O'Donnell, T., Hegadoren, K. M., & Coupland, N. C. (2004). Noradrenergic mechanisms in the pathophysiology of post-traumatic stress disorder. *Neuropsychobiology, 50,* 273–283.

Othmer, E., Othmer, J. P., & Othmer, S. C. (1998). Brain functions and psychiatric disorders: A clinical view. *The Psychiatric Clinics of North America, 21,* 517–566.

Peplau, H. E. (1989). Future direction in psychiatric nursing from the perspective of history. *Journal of Psychosocial Nursing, 27,* 18–28.

Perrand, S., Delaney, K. R., Carlson-Sabelli, L., Johnson, M. E., Shephard, R., & Paun, O. (2006). Advanced practice psychiatric mental health nursing, finding our care: The therapeutic relationship in the 21st century. *Perspectives in Psychiatric Care, 42,* 215–226.

Persico, A. M., Bird, G., Gabbay, F. H., & Uhl, G. R. (1996). D_2 dopamine receptor gene TaqI and B1 restriction fragment length polymorphisms: Enhanced frequencies in psychostimulant-preferring polysubstance abusers. *Biological Psychiatry, 15,* 776–784.

Pickering-Brown, S. M., Richardson, A. M., Snowden, J. S., McDonagh, A. M., Burns, A., Braude, W., Baker, M., Liu, W. K., Yen, S. H., Hardy, J., Hutton, M., Davies, Y., Allsop, D., Craufurd, D., Neary, D., & Mann, D. M. (2002). Inherited frontotemporal dementia in nine British families associated with intronic mutations in the tau gene. *Brain, 125* (Pt. 4), 732–751.

Post, R. M. (1992). Transduction of psychosocial stress in the neurobiology of recurrent affective disorder. *American Journal of Psychiatry, 149,* 999–1010.

Post, R. M., & Weiss, S. R. B. (1999). Neurobiological models of recurrent mood disorder. In D. S. Charney, E. J. Nester, & B. S. Bunney (Eds.), *Neurobiology of Mental Illness* (pp. 365–384). New York: Oxford University Press.

Pothier, P. C., Stuart, G. W., Puskar, K., & Babich, K. (1990). Dilemmas and direction for psychiatric nursing in the 1990s. *Archives of Psychiatric Nursing, 4,* 284–291.

Sadock, B. J., & Sadock, V. A. (2005). *Kaplan & Sadock's Pocket Handbook of Clinical Psychiatry* (4th ed.). Philadelphia: Lippincott Williams & Wilkins.

Sadock, J., Sadock, V. A., & Sussman, N. (2006). *Kaplan & Sadock pocket handbook of psychiatric drug treatment* (4th ed.). Philadelphia, PA: Lippincott Williams & Wilkins.

Shalev, A. Y. (2000). Biological responses to disasters. *Psychiatric Quarterly, 17,* 277–288.

Shekhar, A., Truitt, W., Rainnie, D., & Sajdyk, T. (2005). Role of stress, corticotrophin releasing factor (CRF) and amygdala plasticity in chronic anxiety. *Stress, 8,* 209–219.

Snowden, J. S., Neary, D., & Mann, M. N. A. (1996). *Frontotemporal lobar degeneration: Frontotemporal dementia, progressive aphasia, semantic dementia.* New York: Churchill-Livingstone.

Solomon, G. F. (1987). Psychoneuroimmunology: Interaction between central nervous system and immune system. *Journal of Neuroscience, 18,* 1–9.

Sullivan, P. F., Neale, M. C., & Kendler, K. S. (2000). Genetic epidemiology of major depression: Review and meta-analysis. *American Journal of Psychiatry, 157,* 1552–1562.

Tariot, P. N. (2006). Contemporary issues in the treatment of Alzheimer's disease: Tangible benefits of current therapies. *Journal of Clinical Psychiatry, 67,* (Suppl. 3), 15–22.

de la Torre, J. C. (2002). Alzheimer disease as a vascular disorder. *Stroke, 33,* 1152–1174.

Tsuang, M. T., Stone, W. S., & Faraone, S. V. (2000). Toward reformulating the diagnosis of schizophrenia. *American Journal of Psychiatry, 157,* 1041–1050.

U.S. Congress. (1989). *Decade of the Brain-Proclamation.* Pub. L. No. 101-58 [HJ Res. 174], 130 Stat. 152–154 (July 25, 1989).

van der Kolk, B. A. (1987a). *Psychological trauma.* New York: American Psychiatric Press.

van der Kolk, B. (1987b). The trauma spectrum: The interaction of biological and social events in the genesis of trauma response. *Journal Traumatic Stress, 1,* 273–290.

Wahlund, L. O. (1996). Magnetic resonance imaging and computed tomography in Alzheimer's disease. *Acta Neurologica Scandinavica (Supplementation), 168,* 50–53.

Watson, S., Gallagher, P., Ritchie, J. C., Ferrier, I. N., & Young, A. H. (2004). Hypothalamic-pituitary-adrenal axis function in patients with bipolar disorder. *British Journal of Psychiatry, 184,* 496–502.

Wolkowitz, O. M., Reus, V. I. (1999). Treatment of depression with antiglucocorticoid drugs. *Psychosomatic Medicine, 61,* 698–711.

Yehuda, R., McFarlane, A. C., & Shalev, A. Y. (1998). Predicting the development of post-traumatic stress disorder from acute response to a traumatic event. *Biological Psychiatry, 44,* 1305–1313.

Ziegelstein, R. C. (2001). Depression after myocardial infarction. *Cardiolology Review, 1,* 45–51.

SUGGESTED READINGS

Antai-Otong, D. (2000). The neurobiology of anxiety disorders: Implications for psychiatric nursing practice. *Issues in Mental Health Nursing, 21,* 71–89.

Faraone, S. V., Tsuang, M. T., & Tsuang, D. V. (1999). *Genetics of mental disorders: A guide for students, clinicians, and researchers.* New York: Guilford Publications, Inc.

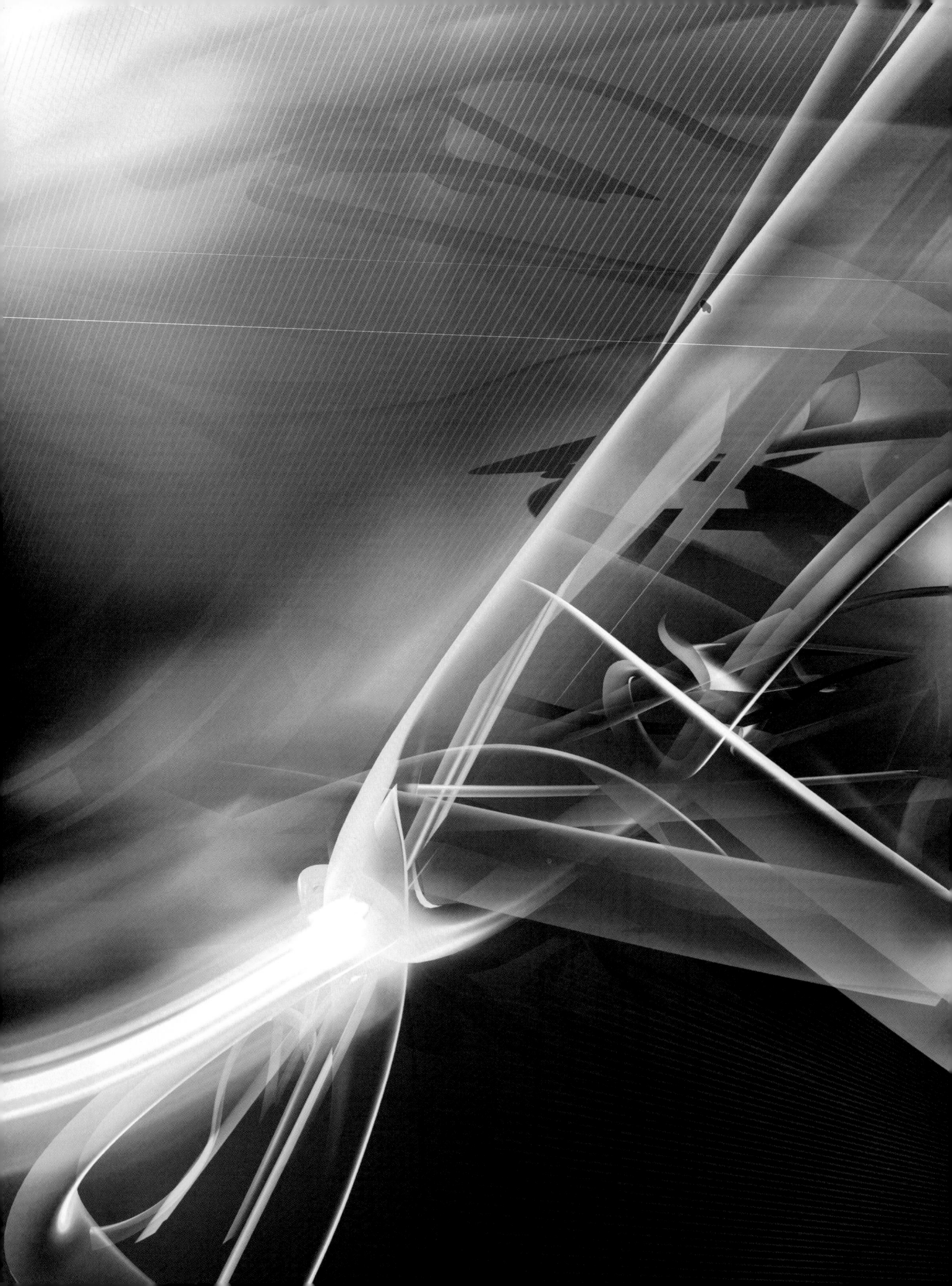

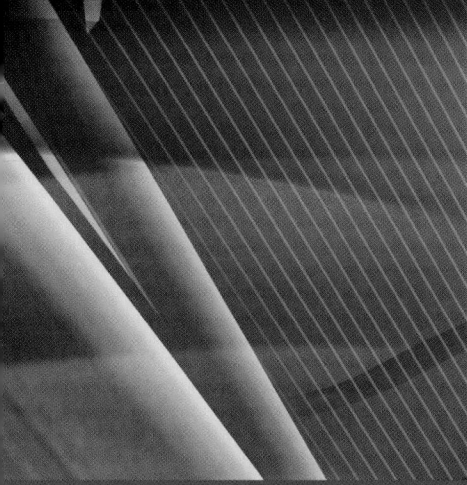

CHAPTER 4

Foundations of Psychiatric Nursing

Deborah Antai-Otong, MS, APRN, BC, FAAN

KEY TERMS

Adaptation: Sustaining homeostasis; the ability to mobilize resources and adjust to demands of internal and external environments.

Coping: An effort to reduce tension by minimizing, replacing, and resolving uncomfortable feelings such as anxiety, anger, frustration, and guilt.

Defense Mechanisms: Unconscious self-protective processes that seek to protect the ego from intense feelings or affect and impulses.

Ego Function: Intrapsychic processes that enable people to mediate stress and adaptation using various defense mechanisms.

Empathy: Refers to putting oneself into the psychological frame of reference of another. It conveys an understanding of the client's situation without becoming emerged or overwhelmed by the experience.

Mental Health: A relative state of well-being that enables persons, couples, families, and communities to adaptively respond to external and internal stressors.

Mental Health Team: An interdisciplinary group of mental health staff who collaborate to assess, intervene, and evaluate client responses to treatment.

Mental Illness: A mental disorder or condition manifested by disorganization and impairment of function that arises from various causes such as psychological, neurobiological, and genetic factors.

Primary Appraisal: Refers to initial responses to a stressor and the ultimate goal of prevailing over or effectively managing a given situation.

Primary Prevention: Refers to measures or interventions to counteract circumstances or conditions that are potentially harmful. Additionally, these measures generate coping skills and reduce vulnerability to illness and promote health.

Secondary Appraisal: Emerges with any form of perceived threat or harm if primary appraisals are ineffective or maladaptive. The rationale for secondary appraisal is to assess coping resources, options, and choices.

Secondary Prevention: Refers to measures or interventions used to curtail disease processes.

Stress: A stimulus or demand that has the potential to generate disruption in homeostasis or produce a reaction.

Tertiary Prevention: Refers to measures that minimize relapse and chronic disability, and restore the client to an optimal level of functioning.

COMPETENCIES

Upon completion of this chapter, the learner should be able to:

1. Discuss the role of the psychiatric-mental health nurse in primary, secondary, and tertiary prevention.

2. Analyze the relationship between adaptive responses and stress throughout the life span.

3. Identify internal and external factors that influence coping ability.

4. Define primary and secondary appraisals.

5. Understand the impact of stress on mental illness.

6. Identify essential qualities of psychiatric-mental health nurses.

7. Discuss the role of the psychiatric-mental health nurse as a member of the mental health team.

CHAPTER OUTLINE

The first surgeon general's report on mental health was issued in 1999 after 50 years of data collection focusing on noteworthy advances in the understanding of mental disorders, the brain, and the importance of health and well-being. This report also stresses the urgency of preventing and treating mental disorders and promoting mental health in our society. It provides a contemporary review of scientific advances in mental health and mental illness, which affect at least one in five Americans. Several conclusions from this report indicate an array of mental disorders that occur throughout the life span and evidence-based treatments for a vast number of mental disorders. Despite advances in technology and genetic discoveries, however, the stigmatization of people with mental disorders that has endured throughout history continues today. Manifestations of persistent stigmatization of people with mental disorders include to avoid hiring, renting to, or working with this population. Societal biases toward these clients limit their access to basic needs, including housing, services, and opportunities to participate in society. More distressing is that societal biases result in isolation, despair, and low self-esteem (Corrigan & Penn, 1999).

Accordingly, the stigma and prevalence of mental illness endure as psychiatric-mental health nurses confront challenges of the twenty-first century. Numerous forces affect social reactions to mental illness, including the media, which continue to portray people with mental illness as violent, unpredictable, and disruptive. The increased visibility of the homeless and incarcerated mentally ill people also reinforces these stereotypes and beliefs.

Psychiatric nursing has evolved over the past decade in tandem with socioeconomic changes and neurobiological and genetic discoveries. Nurses are actively involved in integrating these changes into their practice and research endeavors. Linking mental illness with brain function, genetic vulnerability, socioeconomic, and psychosocial factors is complex and requires a basic understanding of human responses. The complexity of mental illness challenges psychiatric nurses to understand and integrate neurobiological processes into interventions that restore and maintain health.

Health promotion is a major domain of psychiatric nursing and includes assessment of client strengths, preferences, and reinforcement of adaptive responses and self-care management. Activities that facilitate this process include health education, identification of high-risk groups, stress management, and crisis intervention.

This chapter discusses the major concepts of psychiatric nursing that include mental health promotion, stress and adaptation, life span factors, therapeutic use of self, and collaboration.

MENTAL HEALTH PROMOTION: AN INTEGRAL ASPECT OF PSYCHIATRIC-MENTAL HEALTH NURSING

The twenty-first century offers psychiatric nurses enormous opportunities to identify and care for clients at risk for mental illness. High-risk groups include older adults who are poor; those with acquired immune deficiency syndrome (AIDS)-related illnesses; those with a family history of dementia, anxiety, and mood disorders; substance abusers; and victims and perpetrators of violence. Unemployment, homelessness, and disintegration of families and communities also increase vulnerability to mental illness. Societal stressors, coupled with a lack of adequate access to health care, further compromise and increase the risk of mental illness (ANA, 1991). Psychiatric nurses are challenged to form collaborative and shared decision making with clients, families, other health care providers, and communities to mobilize and strengthen resources that facilitate health promotion, disease management, and ensure access to quality health

care. Identifying clients at risk (Table 4–1) and providing early intervention are major nursing goals.

Changes in health care delivery systems has resulted in an explosion of sicker mentally ill clients being prematurely discharged into the community as a result of cost-cutting measures, which shorten the length of hospital stays. Reduced lengths of stay compromise treatment stabilization and usually involve heavy reliance on medication management. In addition, dwindling and inadequate community resources are resulting in an appalling number of mentally ill clients to be incarcerated. A number of these clients are also homeless, substance abusers, and victims of crime. Treatment often consists of "Band Aid" approaches provided in emergency departments and community shelters. Emergency psychiatric treatment is becoming an increasingly important aspect of mental health care systems, and for many clients, a major point of entry to acute psychiatric services (Buraff, Janowicz, & Asarnow, 2006).

Psychiatric nurses can respond to these changes by collaborating with clients, mental health professionals, and community service workers to create innovative treatment modalities and facilitate positive outcomes. Caring for persons with psychiatric conditions requires skills and knowledge to initiate holistic approaches that enlist shared decision making to establish client-centered care. Preventive measures must be a major aspect of outcomes and interventions. Three areas of prevention are advocated in caring for mentally ill clients: primary, secondary, and tertiary.

PRIMARY PREVENTION

Primary prevention is the first stage of care that involves using measures that prevent or reduce the risk of mental illness and provide quality and cost-effective interventions. These interventions are used to counteract circumstances or conditions that are potentially harmful. They generate coping

TABLE 4–1
Populations at Risk for Mental Illness

- Those with familial or genetic predisposition to mental illness, such as clients with a family history of affective or mood disorders and schizophrenia
- Those with poor access to health care
- Those disadvantaged, i.e., homeless and poor
- Those undergoing significant lifestyle changes, i.e, pregnant adolescent
- Those misusing substances
- Victims of violence
- Elderly poor

skills and other measures that reduce vulnerability to illness and promote health (Caplan, 1964). Coping stems from the Latin word *colpus*, which means to alter. It is an effort to reduce tension by minimizing, replacing, and resolving uncomfortable feelings such as anxiety, anger, frustration, fear, and guilt. Additional examples of primary prevention include bereavement counseling and stress management.

During the past decade, there has been a resurgence of interest in the prevention of mental health disorders by the World Health Organization (WHO, 2001). This organization identified an agenda of "Mental Health: New Understanding, New Hope," (Geneva: WHO) which calls for measures to prevent mental illness, neurological, and psychosocial disorders. Areas of interest include protecting the developing brain, minimizing predisposition to illness, and increasing resistance to disease (WHO, 2001).

Psychiatric nurses can incorporate primary prevention measures into practice initially by identifying persons at risk and, later, by reinforcing existing adaptive coping responses. Interventions that protect the developing brain include genetic counseling, education about substance abuse, maternal immunization against rubella, and prenatal and parenting classes. Parenting classes need to focus on child rearing, normal growth and development, anger management, the importance of immunization, and proper nutrition for nursing mothers and children.

Education is a key component of primary prevention, and it can be used to minimize predisposition to illness and increase resistance to disease. Teaching prospective parents to avoid prolonged separation, child abuse, and battering is an example of primary prevention. Other teaching measures include educating families about the acute and long-term effects of substance abuse, and the risks of sexually transmitted diseases, problem-solving and conflict resolution skills, and the importance of wearing protective gear (when riding bicycles) using age-specific car seats and seat belts (in vehicles) to minimize head trauma and other serious physical injuries. Bereavement counseling and stress management also offer relief and strengthen coping and problem-solving skills.

Overall, nurses can use primary preventive measures to collaborate with clients and families to promote adaptive coping measures that minimize the risk of mental illness. Furthermore, these measures must be culturally sensitive and congruent with the client's value and belief system. When clients do not respond to primary interventions, symptoms of mental illness are likely to evolve and require aggressive treatment. An integral part of this process involves assessing coping patterns and behaviors unique to the client. Recognizing behaviors and responses unique to the client promotes a greater understanding of his or her experience.

SECONDARY PREVENTION

Secondary prevention is the second stage in which measures are used to curtail the disease processes. They focus on early detection, case finding, and priority interventions

(WHO, 1980). Psychiatric nurses participate in this process by assessing the nature and degree of client response, identifying available resources, and implementing measures that reduce symptoms and mobilize adaptive coping responses. Collaboration with clients, families, and health care professionals is also a crucial part of secondary prevention.

Case management is a good example of secondary prevention. Psychiatric-mental health nurses can use this comprehensive approach to support client strengths, *facilitate* the highest level of functioning, and facilitate growth and an optimal level of health. Additionally, it can be used to provide supportive therapy and to monitor client responses to medication and other interventions. Case management can be used in both inpatient and outpatient settings to provide a continuity of care (ANA, 2000).

The following interventions are also examples of how case management can be used to establish secondary prevention:

◆ Medication maintenance

◆ Health education

◆ Crisis intervention

◆ Telemental health

◆ Care Coordination Home Telehealth

◆ Mobile crisis services

◆ Screening for early detection of developmental and emotional disturbances in childhood and adolescent populations

◆ Screening for cognitive and affective disorders in older adult populations

Once client symptoms are identified and interventions are initiated, treatment focuses on minimizing long-term disability.

TERTIARY PREVENTION

Tertiary prevention is the third stage of prevention. Measures are used to minimize relapse and chronic disability and to restore clients to their optimal level of functioning. Adaptation, restoration, reintegration, and aftercare are major components of tertiary prevention. Adaptation refers to mobilizing resources and sustaining homeostasis. Nursing intervention involves promoting an understanding of the impact of stress, medication adherence, and maladaptive responses on mental illness. These measures include stress management, health education, mobile crisis services, emergency supportive housing, relapse prevention, crisis intervention, fostering of adaptive coping behaviors, and reinforcement of client strengths.

In summary, primary, secondary, and tertiary prevention are the foundation of health promotion. The processes involve identifying high-risk groups, intervening when maladaptive responses are identified, and minimizing the deleterious effects of mental illness.

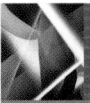

CASE STUDY

Ms. M is a 32-year-old insulin-dependent diabetic who recently was told she was pregnant. She and her husband are very excited about the upcoming pregnancy. During your interview with Ms. M in the diabetic clinic you gather data about past depression when she was initially diagnosed with diabetes several years ago. Based on the importance of mental health during pregnancy and the postpartum period, which of the following is the most important to the mental health of Ms. M and her unborn child?

1. Screen her for depression.
2. Encourage her to discuss concerns about pregnancy and diabetes.
3. Discuss ways to take care of the newborn when she gets home.
4. Provide parenting classes.

Answer(s)

1. Correct. This is the most important primary prevention intervention. The incidence of depression in diabetes is present in 1 in 4 clients and a past history of depression increases the risk in this population. Detecting depression early and educating the client and spouse is an important primary prevention intervention.
2. Incorrect. Although this is an important intervention it is not the most important.
3. Incorrect. Like No. 2, this is important, but not the most important primary prevention intervention.
4. Incorrect. Although parenting classes are important, this client is at risk for depression and screening for depression is critical to mental health in both the mother and unborn child.

CRITICAL THINKING

Primary Prevention

1. Mr. J, a 76-year-old man, presents in the primary care clinic with complaints of concerns about his wife's of 50 years recent diagnosis of Alzheimer's disease. Major complaints include difficulty sleeping and concentrating, and poor appetite. Which of the following is the most important appropriate intervention?

    a. Reassure him that his wife will not suffer as long as he does not leave her alone.
    b. Assess his current support systems for quality and access.
    c. Ask him if he is having thoughts about killing himself.
    d. Refer him to a counselor to deal with his depression.

Answers

a. Incorrect because you do not have enough information to make this assumption.
b. Correct. Coping skills can be buffered by quality and accessible support systems. Nurses can use this information to help the patient strengthen coping skills.
c. Incorrect. Although this is an important question, it is imperative to establish rapport with the patient and look for clues that may indicate signs of depression or risk of danger to self or others. Asking this question during the initial interaction with this patient increases defensiveness.
d. Incorrect. It is important to gather more information and formulate a basis for the referral rather than assuming the referral is necessary.

CRITICAL THINKING

Tertiary Prevention

Mr. B is a 46-year-old patient who has just been discharged from the inpatient substance abuse unit with a diagnosis of alcohol dependence. This is his second admission within the past 12 months. Which of the following is a tertiary nursing intervention?

a. "Mr. B, here is a list of AA groups in your community."
b. "I noticed that this is your second admission during the past 12 months. Please list the number of meetings you attended the last time."
c. "Let's review ways to manage your triggers to avoid relapse."
d. "Let's talk to your wife to make sure she knows how important it is for both of you to attend these meetings."

Answers

a. Incorrect. Although this is an intervention it does not address ways for the patient to maintain his sobriety.
b. Incorrect. This intervention sounds judgmental and nontherapeutic.
c. Correct. This intervention is part of relapse prevention and is necessary to assess during hospitalization and discharge planning.
d. Incorrect. Although family involvement is important, it does not address the patient's responsibility in maintaining his own sobriety.

THE MENTAL HEALTH-MENTAL ILLNESS CONTINUUM

Throughout history, the plight and perception of the mentally ill have been influenced by social, economic, and legislative conditions. Psychiatric-mental health nurses must continue to advocate for the rights of mentally ill clients and transform the negative image of mental illness while promoting mental health throughout the life span. This process begins by defining mental health and mental illness. Mental health and mental illness are dynamic and subject to change. At any given time, a person's mental status represents the person's genetic characteristics, biological underpinnings, and life experiences. No single gene has been detected as the cause of mental illness. Instead, researchers submit that alterations in various genes contribute to the disturbance in healthy brain function, when exposure to overwhelming internal and external demands results in mental illness. The brain interacts with and responds in function and structure to continuous complex internal and external influences across the life span. The brain's ability to mediate complex neurobiological and genetic mechanisms are the bases of coping responses that can either bolster mental health or result in mental illness (*Mental Health: A Report of the Surgeon General,* 1999).

It is difficult to define health, but most researchers describe it is as physical, psychological, and social well-being. Healthy People 2000 (U.S. Department of Health and Human Services, 1990), a statement of the National Health Promotion and Disease Prevention objectives, parallels health with people's sense of well-being. Additionally, it suggests that health results from "reducing unnecessary suffering, illness, and disability, . . . and improved quality of life" (p. 6).

Mental health refers to the ability of people—couples, families, and communities—to respond adaptively to internal and external stressors. Complex factors including neurobiological, genetic, psychosocial, and cultural influences are key determinants of mental health.

NEUROBIOLOGICAL FACTORS

Seyle's (1976) major contribution to defining mental health was his explanation of stress in terms of adaptation. He believed that **stress** compromises health when adaptive and coping patterns are unable to master the condition. Additionally, he concluded that stress responses occur whenever an organism encounters persistent stress. He described this phenomenon as generalized adaptation syndrome. Reactions that occur with generalized adaptation syndrome include the following:

♦ *Alarm reaction* (first phase): mobilizes the body's defenses and protective responses against stressors; as the autonomic nervous system reacts to stress, large amounts of adrenaline and cortisone are activated, preparing the person for "fight or flight."

♦ *Stage of resistance* (second phase): adaptive responses attempt to lessen damage from the stressor by limiting its effects and resisting change.

♦ *Stage of exhaustion* (third phase): final stage, which evolves after the body's attempts to adapt to change fail; in essence, the stressor overwhelms existing adaptive reservoirs of interventions to relieve the stress.

Others depict mental health as successful adaptation that maintains homeostasis or equilibrium and the physiochemical state (Cannon, 1914; 1939; Menninger, 1963). Mental health has many definitions, but there is broad agreement that its key biological components include the following:

♦ The ability to respond to stress effectively

♦ The capacity to tolerate anxiety, stress, and frustration, and to delay gratification of needs (impulse control)

♦ The capacity to realistically and objectively appraise events and situations in one's world

CULTURAL FACTORS

The U.S. Census Bureau (2000) predicts more than 30 percent of the population will comprise a plurality of ethnic minorities other than non-Hispanic whites. According to this prediction, about one in every three individuals in this country considers him- or herself as a "minority." Based on this assumption this minority group will comprise about 50 percent of the entire U.S. population by 2050 (U.S. Census, 2000). As societies become more pluralistic, nurses will have daily encounters with clients from various cultures, and ethnic and socioeconomic backgrounds. Growing concerns about health disparities and changing demographics must be a prioty to ensure cultural competence to address each client's unique needs, wishes, preferences, and health care practices. Psychiatric nurses are poised to establish quality nurse-client interactions to address the needs of each client. Chapter 7 provides an in-depth discussion of culture and its impact on the client experience and implications for the psychiatric nurse.

PSYCHOSOCIAL FACTORS

Psychosocial factors play pivotal roles in a person's ability to mobilize adaptive coping processes. *Ego* maturity and function, along with the person's defense mechanisms are crucial to healthy adaptation and mental health. Efforts to assess and enhance ego function and adaptive defense mechanisms facilitate healthy resolution of life experiences.

Ego Function and Health

Caplan (1961) believed that the most essential factor that predicts mental health is ego function. *Ego* is defined as the major personality mechanism that mediates between the person and the environment. Major ego functions include adaptation to reality, modulation of anxiety, and problem solving. Menninger (1963) described the ego as the guardian of vital balance, "which recognizes, receives, stores, discriminates, integrates, and acts by restraining, modifying, and directing impulses" (p. 104).

Ego function refers to the inherent ability to adapt to internal and external demands or stress of environments (Hartman, 1958). Its foundation arises from early significant relationships that established trust and meaningful interactions. Ego function evolves over time and varies with personality structure and developmental stage.

Defense Mechanisms

The term defense mechanism refers to a predominantly unconscious self-protective process that seeks to shield the ego from intense feelings or affect and impulses. Additionally, these intrapsychic processes modify, nullify, or convey painful affects or tendencies so they can be tolerated consciously. (See Table 4–2 for a list of common defense mechanisms.)

STRESS AND ILLNESS

A number of studies have shown a relationship between stress and disequilibrium or illness (Brewin, Andrews, Rose, & Kirk, 1999; Davis, Matthews, & McGrath, 2000; Koren, Arnon, & Klein, 1999; Russak & Schwartz, 1997; Sapolsky, Romero, & Munck, 2000). Holmes and Rahe (1967) developed a system for determining the degree of life stressors and predicting illness by placing a value on various life events that require change and adaptive responses. Their Readjustment Rating

TABLE 4–2
Major Defense Mechanisms

Defense Mechanism	Definition	Example
Displacement	Redirection of negative urges or feelings from an original object to a safer or neutral substitute	The man who is angry with his boss and returns home and becomes angry instead with his wife or children
Denial	Refusal to admit to a painful reality, which is treated as if it does not exist	The woman who miscarries denies that she has lost the baby and continues to wear maternity clothes
Intellectualization	Use of excessive reasoning rather than reacting or changing	A woman attending an Alcoholics Anonymous meeting reports that she is a nurse and has conducted many 12-step sessions
Introjection	Engulfment or incorporation of specific traits, behaviors, or qualities into self or ego structure	A depressed man who incorporates the negative feelings and hatred of his estranged wife, who recently filed for divorce
Projection	Blame of others or things for one's own feelings or thoughts	The client experiencing paranoia blames others for disliking him
Rationalization	An effort to replace or justify acceptable reasons for feelings, beliefs, thoughts, or behaviors for real ones	A woman with overextended credit cards rationalizes that she can use her savings to pay for a new dress she recently purchased
Reaction formation	Repression of painful or offensive attitudes or traits with unconscious opposite ones	The college student who feels angry and hostile toward her professor is overtly friendly and agreeable in class
Regression	Retreat to an earlier developmental stage	The 3-year-old child who begins wetting his pants after the birth of a new sibling
Repression	Unconscious, purposeful forgetting of painful or dangerous thoughts (the most basic defense mechanism)	The married woman who expresses hostility toward a male co-worker to avoid dealing with her sexual attraction to him
Sublimation	Normal form of dealing with undesirable feelings or thoughts by keeping them in an acceptable context	The woman who is unable to bear children begins working in a preschool
Suppression	Conscious and deliberate forgetfulness of painful or undesirable thoughts and ideas	A rape victim attempts to forget the incident and fails to report it to the proper authorities

Scale was developed to measure a number of stressful events over a 12-month period. They found that vulnerability to medical and psychiatric illness increased with an increasing number of events during this period. If scores reached 300 on this scale, the chance of illness increased 80 percent. The Readjustment Rating Scale has been criticized because it lacks relevancy to many ethnic groups and developmental stages.

Criticism of this scale has led to the development of other tools that determine how people handle daily hassles. One such tool is the Jalowiec Coping Scale (Jalowiec, 1979; Table 4–3), which determines how people cope with various life stressors. It consists of 40 coping behaviors that are rated on a scale of 1 to 5 and indicate the magnitude of use, with 1 indicating "never" and 5, "always." A checklist format is used to indicate the frequency that each response is used to handle certain situations (Jalowiec, 1988; Jalowiec & Powers, 1983). See Chapter 13 for an in-depth discussion of stress-related illnesses. (Refer to the Research Abstract.)

In brief, mental health and adaptation are relative and lie on a continuum with mental illness and maladaptation. Although stress responses are primarily biological, psychosocial factors influence the perception of and the number of stressors. Disorganization or mental illness occurs as available coping and adaptive mechanisms, including complex biological processes, fail to handle stress. Mental illness may be manifested in various ways, such as ineffective problem solving, poor reality testing, and impaired cognitive functioning.

TABLE 4–3
Examples of Coping Behaviors from the Jalowiec Coping Scale

1. Hope for improvement	13. Handle problem in steps	25. Sleep
2. Maintain control	14. Seek comfort/help from others	26. Don't worry
3. Information seeking	15. Set goals	27. Withdraw from situation
4. Think through solutions	16. Accept situation	28. Activity/exercise
5. View problem objectively	17. Want to be alone	29. Compromise
6. Eat/smoke	18. Laugh it off	30. Take tensions out on others
7. Try out solutions	19. Put problem aside	31. Resign because it's hopeless
8. Make use of past experience	20. Daydream	32. Try anything
9. Find purpose/meaning	21. Expect the worst	33. Blame others
10. Pray	22. Discuss problem	34. Let someone else solve the problem
11. Get nervous	23. Try to change situation	
12. Worry	24. Get mad	

Note. From "Stress and Coping in Hypertensive and Emergency Room Patients," by A. Jalowiec and M. J. Powers, 1983, *Nursing Research, 30*(1), pp. 10–15. Reprinted with permission.

 RESEARCH ABSTRACT

Coping Profile Differences in the Biopsychological Functioning of Patients with Temporomandibular Disorder

Epker, J., & Gatchel, R. J. (2000). *Psychososomatic Medicine, 65,* 69–75.

Study Problem/Purpose

To determine if there were differences in the biopsychosocial functioning between groups of clients with temporomandibular disorder (TMD) whose coping profiles differed on the Multidimensional Pain Inventory.

Methods

A population of 322 clients who presented with TMD were administered a comprehensive biopsychosocial assessment battery, and researchers assessed their state of the disorder as either acute or chronic. Subjects were contacted by telephone for 3- to 6-month follow-up evaluation to

(continues)

Research Abstract *(continued)*

evaluate the status of their pain. At the end of the 6-month interval, clients whose CPI score was <15 were determined to have nonchronic TMD, and those whose scores were >15 were determined to have chronic TMD.

A comparison of the dysfunctional and interpersonally distressed groups, using analysis of variance, *t* tests, and X^2 analyses, showed that the two groups had similarities across demographic, physiological, and psychosocial indices. The final group sizes were 156 for subjects exhibiting maladaptive coping profile and the adaptier coper sample.

Findings

Data from the study showed that the group exhibiting maladaptive coping profiles had more acute and chronic psychosocial disturbances than the adaptier coper group. The authors also inferred that having a maladaptive coping profile may be a predictive value in developing chronicity in the absence of treatment.

Implications for Psychiatric Nurses

The presence of maladaptive coping behaviors is likely to increase chronicity in clients with TMD. Preventive measures that promote health education and provide holistic nursing interventions, such as stress management, medication management, and cognitive behavioral therapy, can be used to manage pain and reduce disability.

CLASSIFICATION OF MENTAL ILLNESS AND DISORDERS

Classification of mental disorders flourished during the nineteenth century. Many symptoms were reported during earlier writings, but there was a lack of formal classification of mental disorders until the twentieth century.

EMIL KRAEPELIN

Emil Kraepelin, a German psychiatrist, was a pioneer in the classification of mental disorders. His description of dementia praecox was later referred to as schizophrenia; however, his description of manic depression fell short because he focused primarily on the course of the mental illness rather than its etiology. In spite of major shortcomings, his work inspired others to create a formal classification of mental disorders (Deutsch, 1937).

EUGEN BLEULER

Eugen Bleuler (1950), a Swiss psychiatrist, followed in Kraepelin's footsteps, but he ventured further than merely describing symptoms and the syndrome. He explored specific responses generated by symptoms and presented the term *schizophrenia*, which replaced Kraepelin's *dementia praecox*. A major flaw in Bleuler's description of schizophrenia was its lack of precision, which led to numerous misdiagnoses. Bleuler's work also encouraged psychiatry to explore the underlying processes of mental illness.

SIGMUND FREUD, ADOLF MEYER, AND FRANZ ALEXANDER

Other contributions to the systematization of mental disorders include the works of Freud (1953), who linked mental disorders with unconscious conflicts or neurosis. Meyer (1957) believed in the holistic personality theory, which comprised biological, psychosocial, and cultural factors; he also believed that mental disorders had psychobiological origins. Alexander (1939) also emphasized the interrelationship between emotions and biological processes, which suggested the influence of external and internal causes of disease.

DIAGNOSTIC AND STATISTICAL MANUAL OF MENTAL DISORDERS (DSM)

DSM-I (1952) and *DSM-II* (1968)

In 1934, the American Psychiatric Association (APA) attempted to classify mental illnesses and identified 24 main groups with 82 subdivisions. This format produced upheaval within the profession and questionable treatment practices. Efforts to provide a useful and consistent classification were made in 1952, when the APA published the *DSM-I*; *DSM-II* was published in 1968. *DSM-I* and *DSM-II* presented a classification based on a hierarchical system with the following categories: organic mental disorders, followed by psychotic, neurotic, and personality disorders. This system lacked consistency and clarity in defining psychosis and neurosis, which led to a continued need to improve the differentiation of mental disorders.

DSM-III (1980) and *DSM-III-Revised* (*DSM-III-R*) (1987)

DSM-III (1980) and *DSM-III-R* (1987) differed from previous editions in that they formulated childhood mental disorder categories. Additionally, *DSM-III* deleted the psychosis and neurosis categories and replaced them with a new section that classified disorders based on psychopathology, such as mood, anxiety, and dissociative disorders. This new format allowed for multiple diagnoses on several axes (Table 4–4 and Table 4–5) and placed less emphasis on hierarchical exclusions and advanced experimental research.

TABLE 4–4
Organizational Framework for *DSM-IV-TR*

Axis	Explanation
Axis I	Clinical syndromes and V codes Conditions not attributable to a mental disorder that are a focus of attention or treatment, e.g., marital problems or other family circumstances
Axis II	Personality disorders Specific developmental disorders
Axis III	Physical disorders and conditions
Axis IV	Severity of psychosocial stressors
Axis V	Highest level of adaptive functioning in the past year

The first three axes constitute the official diagnostic assessment. Axes IV and V are available for use in special clinical and research settings.

Note. From *Diagnostic and Statistical Manual of Mental Disorders* (4th edition, Text Revision) (*DSM-IV-TR*), by the American Psychiatric Association, 2000, Washington, DC: Author. Reprinted with permission.

There had been discussion among nursing educators and practitioners regarding the overall usefulness of the *DSM-III-R* because it did not address issues associated with self-care or nursing's unique contribution to 24-hour care. Furthermore, around-the-clock monitoring had been described as one of the most significant efforts to meet basic human needs, which include comfort, hygiene, nutrition, and social interaction. However, there was a consensus among other psychiatric-mental health nurses who contend that *DSM-III-R* was useful in many ways. First, it permitted nurses to share roles and communicate effectively with other members of the interdisciplinary mental health team. Second, it provided opportunities to assess the client's biopsychosocial needs, identifying diagnostic data, current stressors, and overall level of functioning (APA, 1987). Third, it provided financial opportunities for third-party and Medicare reimbursement. Finally, *DSM-III-R* was used with nursing models integrating major concepts with nursing diagnoses to identify the complex needs of clients when planning nursing care.

DSM-IV (1994)

DSM-IV (APA, 1994) was a welcomed attempt to increase the proficiency of diagnosis and differential diagnosis among clinicians. This edition was distinct from previous editions in several ways. First, diagnostic criteria were not bound by specific categories or mental disorders. This simply meant that a set of symptoms may have been listed under several categories, such as "Disorders Due to a General Medical Condition." It took into account general medical conditions that may have contributed to or may have been the sole sources of presenting psychiatric symptoms (i.e., anxiety disorder caused by alcohol withdrawal or hyperthyroidism).

A second noticeable change in the *DSM-IV* was its strong emphasis on using clinical judgment and various measures to assess the client's condition other than the diagnosis. A third change was the description of mental disorders as serious behavioral and psychological manifestations triggered by a stressful event that affects the level of function and increases the risk of disability (APA, 1994).

An outcry from various groups for cultural sensitivity and awareness contributed to the fourth major change in the *DSM-IV*. The importance of diversity, specifically ethnic and cultural considerations, was underscored as an integral part of client care. Amazingly, previous editions of the *DSM* regarded certain cultural practices, rituals, and beliefs as manifestations of mental illness. An appreciation of these behaviors as culture bound contributed to changes in the *DSM-IV*. Another interesting feature of this edition was its description of culture-bound syndromes that were not classified as mental disorders, but were listed in the *DSM-IV* Appendix I, along with a template of cultural frame of reference and a glossary. The section had been useful in helping clinicians value and systematically assess their clients' cultural needs.

The last major feature of the *DSM-IV* was its well-defined diagnostic criteria. Well-defined criteria improve communication between mental health professionals and help them identify patterns, individuality, and diversity among various populations. These data can be used to promote quality care through research endeavors.

DSM-IV-Text Revision (DSM-IV-TR) (2000)

Historically, the *DSM-IV* has been useful as a teaching tool, particularly concerning diagnostic criteria sets for mental disorders. Because of the long interval between *DSM-IV* and the proposed *DSM-V*, authors of the *DSM-IV* submitted that because of the magnitude of research data from 1992 to a proposed publication date, the latter edition would be outdated before it was published. Thus, the publication of the text revision was adopted. The APA (2000) delineated the major goals of the *DSM-IV-TR* as follows:

1. To resolve errors found in the *DSM-IV*
2. To appraise the *DSM-IV* to ensure a state-of-the-art text
3. To make revisions that reflect empirical or evidence-based data available since 1992
4. To strengthen the educational value of the *DSM-IV*
5. To update those ICD-9-CM codes that have changed since the *DSM-IV 1996 Coding Update* (APA, 2000)

All of these changes were limited to text sections, such as Associated Features and Prevalence. The authors did not make noteworthy changes in the criteria, nor were new disorders, subtypes, or changes made in the status of the

TABLE 4–5
Comparison of *DSM-III-R* and *DSM-IV*

Major Features of the *DSM-III-R* (APA, 1987)	Major Features of the *DSM-IV* (APA, 1994)
1. Focuses on past improvement from previous diagnoses.	1. Focuses on presenting manifestations of biological behaviors and psychological patterns generated by a stressful event that interfere with optimal level of function (includes severity and specific course of mental disorders).
2. Diagnostic categories provide more criteria than previous editions, but there is still a need to use empirical research to improve the credibility of clinical judgment.	2. Minimal labeling is used, and more factual descriptions are used to define a condition, such as "the client experiencing delirium" rather than "the delirious client."
3. Diagnostic categories are not applicable to diverse populations (culture, gender, or age).	3. Distinct clarification of diagnostic criteria is based on considerable empirical research.
4. Axis III is the only category that considers the impact of a general medical condition on mental disorder.	4. Acknowledges the significance of diversity and provides a section on culture-bound syndromes (Appendix I: Outline for Cultural Formulation and Glossary of Culture-Bound Syndromes). Each diagnostic category suggests using clinical judgment to include the influence of the culture, age, and sex of the client.
5. Categorizes cognitive disorders under "organic mental syndromes and disorders."	5. Delineates the contrast between mental disorder and general medical condition and includes new criteria under major mental disorders and labeled "indicate general medical condition" (e.g., anxiety disorder due to: *indicate general medical condition*).
6. The Psychoactive Substance Use Disorders is described primarily in terms of a separate entity.	6. New category for cognitive disorders is "Delirium, Dementia, and Amnestic and Other Cognitive Disorders" (including dementia due to HIV disease and head trauma).
7. No discussion of medication-induced movement or adverse drug reactions. Abuse is not included in diagnostic categories.	7. "Substance-induced . . . disorder" is listed under major mental disorders/conditions, such as anxiety and delirium.
8. Appendix A lists several diagnostic criteria (limited number of cases) for research study.	8. New category labeled "Other Conditions that may be a Focus of Clinical Attention" includes a section on Medication-Induced Movement Disorders (e.g., neuroleptic malignant syndrome, neuroleptic-induced acute akathisia and tardive dyskinesia, and adverse effects of medication not otherwise specified). This section also includes "Problems Related to Abuse or Neglect" across the life span (e.g., physical abuse of a child, sexual abuse of a child, sexual abuse or rape of an adult).
	9. Appendix B list criteria sets and axes provided for further study: this section includes numerous diagnostic categories ranging from postconcussional disorder and medication-induced movement disorders. It also includes several research tools.

DSM, Diagnostic and Statistical Manual of Mental Disorders.
Note. From *Diagnostic and Statistical Manual of Mental Disorders, Third Edition, Revised,* by the American Psychiatric Association, 1987, Washington, DC: Author; and from *Diagnostic and Statistical Manual of Mental Disorders* (4th edition, Text Revision) (*DSM-IV-TR*), by the American Psychiatric Association, 2000, Washington, DC: Author. Reprinted with permission.

TABLE 4–6
Diagnostic and Statistical Manual of Mental Disorders, 4th edition, Text Revision (DSM-IV-TR) Multiaxial Format

Axis I:	Clinical Disorders and Other Conditions That May Be a Clinical Focus
Axis II:	Personality Disorders and Mental Retardation
Axis III:	ICD-9-CM General Medical Condition
Axis IV:	Psychosocial and Environmental Problems
Axis V:	Global Assessment of Functioning (GAF) Scale

DSM-IV appendix sections (APA, 2000). (See Table 4–6 for an example of a multiaxial *DSM IV-TR*.)

Overall, the *DSM-IV* is strikingly different and more useful than previous editions. However, it is very similar to the newer *DSM-IV-TR*, except for changes made in the text criteria, including prevalence and associated features, which reflect recent empirical data available since 1992. Nurses can use it confidently alone or as an adjunct to other assessment tools to improve quality care.

COPING MECHANISMS

Using coping mechanisms refers to overcoming or managing stress effectively by mobilizing internal and external resources. Internal resources include one's repertoire of mechanisms, such as ego function (intrapsychic) and neurobiological factors and genetic vulnerability, whereas external resources include social support and cultural factors. Coping mechanisms serve to do the following:

- Influence overall morale, health, and well-being
- Promote growth and maturity
- Assist in problem solving
- Influence adaptation to stress

The concept of stress provides a means of understanding holistic responses to external and internal demands that unfold into important complex neurobiological or psychosocial processes. Examples of stressful events include a major motor vehicle accident, reaction to a spider bite, and the death of a loved one. When a stressor is encountered, it is perceived as a challenge or threat, triggering the fight-or-flight response. Responses to stress are influenced by an appraisal of the event. A person's perception of a stressor is decisive in determining the outcome of neurobiological responses. Neurobiological responses resulting from acute stress reactions activate a cascade of processes that protect the individual during these events. In contrast, prolonged stress reactions, such as those seen in unresolved trauma (e.g., a rape or witness of a murder) are likely to result in

stress-related medical conditions such as hypertension or coronary artery disease, or mental disorders such as post-traumatic stress disorder. Appraisal and response generally reflect the client's level of ego function, developmental stage, available resources, previous experiences, and the number and severity of stressors. Additionally, adaptive emotional and biological responses are effective and pivotal to the regulation of human behavior (Lazarus, 1991; Lazarus & Folkman, 1984; Seligman, 1975; Seyle, 1976).

Empirical studies suggest that cognitive appraisal of life events determines the response as expressed by emotions (Lazarus, 1991; Lazarus & Launier, 1978). Appraisal of events pertains to the value or appreciation, and in terms of coping refers to the significance of internal and external events that are linked with health and adaptation. Events may be perceived as irrelevant, benign or nonthreatening, or threatening or harmful. Lazarus (1966) identified two forms of appraisal: primary and secondary.

PRIMARY APPRAISALS

Lazarus (1966) described the initial response to a stressor as primary appraisal and the ultimate goal of prevailing over the situation. Furthermore, he delineated three types of primary appraisal: irrelevant, benign positive, and stressful. *Irrelevant appraisals* take place when the person confronts external occurrences that do not pose a threat to her livelihood. *Benign appraisals* are events that have a genuinely positive appraisal, or they enhance adaptation or stimulate a sense of well-being. These events generate feelings of pleasure, joy, and happiness and may also be accompanied by guilt or anxiety.

Stress appraisals are regarded as injurious, hazardous, and demanding or challenging (Lazarus, 1966). Life events that have negative connotations or cause damage, such as physical illness, injury to self-esteem, and loss of normal functioning, are defined as *injurious*. *Hazardous threats* are anticipated occurrences that encourage people to mobilize coping skills to reduce anticipated risks. This form of appraisal normally arouses negative thoughts and feelings such as anger, helplessness, anxiety, and fear. The potential for adaptive as well as maladaptive responses exists with hazards. For example, the man who discovers that his wife is having an affair perceives this situation as a threat to his marriage. The wife is determined to keep her marriage together by seeking marital therapy. Initially, her husband is reluctant to seek treatment, but later agrees and discovers the basis of marital discord and attempts to work things out. *Demanding* or *challenging* situations also provide opportunities for using and enhancing coping and adaptive responses, but responses differ from the hazardous form because they generate positive feelings such as enthusiasm, motivation, and excitement. The couple anticipating the birth of triplets is challenged to manage multiple births with enormous parental responsibilities. A challenge form of appraisal normally produces positive thoughts such as "We've been through worse times. We can make it on one income." The implication is that challenge appraisals represent healthier adaptive coping skills that promote a sense of well-being.

SECONDARY APPRAISALS

Secondary appraisal emerges with any form of perceived threat or harm if primary appraisals are ineffective or maladaptive. The rationale for secondary appraisal is to assess coping resources, options, and choices. Lazarus (1966) emphasized the significance of secondary appraisals as follows:

◆ They are the basis of coping mechanisms.

◆ They enhance or promote a positive outcome of primary appraisals.

◆ They strengthen coping resources and options.

The outcome of the coping process depends on individual efforts to alter threatening events and attempts to change the person's appraisal of the stress to minimize the threat (Hansen & Johnson, 1979).

The impact of psychosocial factors and neurobiological processes has been demonstrated in illnesses, such as posttraumatic stress disorder, that produce biochemical and morphological and structural changes in the brain. These changes are generated by recurring stimulation from the client's environment that exceeds the cortex's ability to process events, such as a rape or act of violence, causing permanent synaptic and biochemical changes. Even with this disorder, the client's perception of the event determines the extent of synaptic and biochemical alterations (Gabbard, 2005; Griffin, Resick, & Yehuda, 2005).

Managing stress is a complex process that involves mobilizing internal and external resources. Overall, the impact of stressors on human behavior is determined by a person's ability to use a repertoire of adaptive coping responses to maintain homeostasis or equilibrium. The following clinical examples demonstrate cognitive appraisal and biological responses.

All in all, responses to stress throughout the life span consist of coping, both action and action oriented and intrapsychic, to master, tolerate, curtail, and lessen environmental and

CLINICAL EXAMPLE

The Client with Agoraphobia

John is afraid of open spaces and crowds. His psychological appraisal of these situations is that they are frightening and threatening. His biological responses include increased heart rate, shortness of breath, diaphoresis, dry mouth, lightheadedness, and bouts of confusion. Behavioral responses are avoidance of crowds, social isolation, and possibly suicidal gestures. John seeks psychiatric therapy for agoraphobia. Treatment strategies include biological interventions with a benzodiazepine, such as lorazepam (Ativan), and psychotherapeutic interventions, such as cognitive-behavioral therapy and desensitization.

CLINICAL EXAMPLE

The Client with an Adjustment Disorder with Depressed Mood

Marsha's cognitive appraisal of the event of divorce is failure and uncertainty about the future and her family's reaction to it. Her biological responses include depressed mood, loss of appetite, and decreased energy and motivation, and her behavioral responses include social isolation, irritability, and agitation. She seeks crisis intervention at a local women's center. She strengthens her support systems by her professional contacts and by talking to friends and family who validate, support, and accept her feelings and decisions. She focuses on her strengths, and her self-esteem increases. This clinical example shows the importance of social systems during stressful events.

internal demands. Coping focuses on altering behaviors and cognitions or appraisal to promote a sense of well-being through neurobiological, genetic, and psychosocial processes. Response to stress depends on the direct attempts to alter the threatening conditions.

COPING AND ADAPTATION ACROSS THE LIFE SPAN

Roy (1976) conceptualized that people are open and dynamic systems interchanging with their environments to sustain adaptation (Table 4–7). Furthermore, she surmised that instinctual and learned coping skills enable people to adapt to constant environmental changes. Coping skills are determined by biological, psychosocial, and cultural influences. These concepts can be applied throughout the life span based on the premise that people are adaptive systems. Goals for adaptation include survival, growth, reproduction, and mastery (Roy & McLeod, 1981). (Refer to the Research Abstract.)

TABLE 4–7

Roy's Adaptation Model: Assumptions and Beliefs about the Human Organism

- Human beings are dynamic; they constanty interact with their environment.
- Human behavior has meaning and purpose.
- Emotions activate, orient, and organize adaptive processes.
- Human beings are whole persons in action.
- Human beings are biologically rooted but socially interactive.
- The human body is sensitive to change and automatically adjusts to maintain homeostasis.
- Human beings need to be free of overwhelming anxiety.
- Foundations of adaptation and coping evolve and change throughout the life span.
- Stress is part of life, and response to it varies from individual to individual, based on neurobiological, psychosocial, and cultural factors.
- Self-care must be supported and maintained.

Note. Data from Dix, 1991; Nightingale, 1860; and Roy, 1976.

The human organism is complex, and understanding the role of stress, coping, and adaptation throughout the life span involves appreciating the premise that all behaviors have meaning and purpose. Accordingly, neurobiological and psychosocial factors affect the appraisal of these encounters and determine the outcomes.

Stress plays a crucial role in the developmental process, because each stage requires adequate coping skills to master age-specific challenges that prepare for subsequent stages. A repertoire of adaptive coping behaviors is vital to mastering developmental tasks, and failure to achieve it usually triggers or precipitates illness or maladaptive responses. Numerous studies suggest that individual coping and adaptive patterns begin forming prenatally or during gestation and evolve throughout the life span. These patterns may change or adjust to given circumstances based on one's appraisal of stressors, access to resources, developmental stages, and level of vulnerability.

Health promotion and prevention must begin as early as the prenatal period and continue through older adulthood. Preventive measures need to foster a sense of well-being and self-actualization throughout the·life span. Specific interventions include education, stress management in children and adolescents, parenting classes, and assisting older adults in adjusting to retirement (WHO, 2001).

PRENATAL PERIOD

Dramatic changes in the knowledge of neuroscience have emerged over the past 25 years. Earlier research conducted by Patterson, Potter, and Furshpan (1978) and Gabella (1976) associated genetics with maternal stress during the first 6 weeks of gestation, at which time the autonomic nervous system is undergoing differentiation. Additionally, these studies inferred that stress affects the chemical environment that regulates the development of the sympathetic nervous system and nerve growth and lays the foundation for adaptive coping processes. The major site of production of nerve growth is the placenta. The chemical composition is determined by disease and stress (Sroufe & Rutter, 1984). Increasingly, research is showing that anomalies that occur during early gestation may result in dysregulation in the neural circuitry and eventually produce enduring neurodevelopmental abnormalities. Modern studies concerning the impact of stress during gestation point to its potential role in the loss or neurons, particularly in the hypothalamus and subsequent cognitive disturbances and memory (Cannon, 1999; Harvey, Naciti, Brand, & Stein, 2003). These data indicate that early exposure to prolonged stress may affect neurodevelopmental processes and result in the genesis of mental illness across the life span.

Recent studies support these inferences and link defects and anomalies to the mother's coping mechanisms, which include using alcohol and other drugs. For example, the use of alcohol and other drugs can produce well-documented defects and anomalies such as fetal alcohol syndrome, mental retardation, and disturbances in intrauterine growth. Additionally, exposure to a toxic prenatal environment is likely to contribute to poor social functioning and other developmental problems throughout the life span (Yehuda et al., 2005). Implications from these findings emphasize the importance of promoting mental health in prospective parents through innovative interventions such as a gender-based substance abuse rehabilitation program, stress management, health education about drug use, adequate rest and nutrition, and healthy parenting skills.

INFANCY

Other important processes are begun during infancy, including neurobiological and perceptual growth of the central nervous system in the first few months of life. Infancy represents the most vulnerable stage of development because resources and coping abilities have not yet evolved. External environments and primary caregivers influence vulnerability to trauma and disruption. During this developmental stage, infants learn about the world and themselves through early interactions with primary caregivers. The infant receives pleasure through fulfillment of basic needs such as feeding, attachment or bonding, and nurturing (Dreyfus-Brisac, 1979).

Bowlby (1969) believed attachment or bonding to be an essential aspect of development that prepared the infant for defending against negative environmental stressors. He delineated four critical stages of early childhood as the following:

1. *First stage* (2 to 3 months): the infant has ambiguous social responsiveness; the infant has not bonded with primary caregivers and can only distinguish people from inanimate objects in the environment.

2. *Second stage* (2 to 6 months): the infant learns to discern primary caregivers from others.

3. *Third stage* (6 to 35 months): the infant begins to develop neuromuscular abilities that facilitate mobility and independence.

4. *Fourth stage* (3 years): final stage of attachment, at which time the child understands the relationship with caregivers.

Furthermore, Bowlby considered these stages of attachment as a source of stress for the infant and the child.

Early influences, such as the infant's responses to discomfort and pain associated with hunger and a wet diaper, also produce stress. Reactions to these stressors include crying, fretfulness, and disturbances in sleeping and eating patterns. Lipsitt (1983) considered crying as a human response to distress and an adaptive mechanism that gets attention, produces comfort, and eases pain. Additionally, crying is considered the primary coping mechanism for responding to stress. Other coping mechanisms found during infancy include the startle reflex response to loud noises such as the Moro reflex. These early coping and defense mechanisms reflect basic underdeveloped neurobiological and adaptive processes. Overall, early developmental changes and experiences are related to complex processes, both psychosocial and neurobiological, and at any given stage of development, adaptive or maladaptive responses may be used.

Caregiver's Influence on Coping and Adaptation in Infancy

The capacity of parents or early primary caregivers to effectively manage stress is vital to the developmental responses in the infant. The perception of stressors and the level of coping and adaptation govern the quality of parenting. High stress levels in the parents usually parallel inconsistent or harsh discipline. Likewise, chronic and intense effects of stress in parents indicate dysfunction and distress and increase the risk of abuse and maladaptive developmental outcomes in children (Davies, Cummings, & Winter, 2004; Griffin, Resick, & Yehuda, 2005; Grych, Raynor, & Fosco, 2004; McFarlane, et al., 2003).

In comparison, parents who handle stressful situations effectively are more likely to enhance adaptive coping skills in their children. Parents who are able to solve problems and resolve conflicts and who are caring and nurturing exhibit healthy coping skills. Overall, parental competence and vulnerability to stress are influenced by early developmental experiences and genetic, psychosocial, and neurobiological factors, which are the bases of coping and adaptive mecha-

nisms. The importance of parental competency and nurturing parallels optimal childhood functioning by fostering the child's ability to interact with peers, which determines adult responses to stress later in life. These processes are the bases of child development and adaptation (Melnyk, et al., 2000; Swindle, Cronkite, & Moos, 1998).

As the child becomes mobile and autonomous, stress arises from limit setting, early discipline, and prolonged separation from primary caregivers. Stress reactions include temper tantrums, withdrawal, anxiety, and depression. The encounters allow the toddler to experience successes and failures, further producing a sense of self-worth that is reinforced through primary caregivers. Major parental stressors include toilet training and learning how to maintain consistent limit setting with the mobile toddler.

CHILDHOOD

The child's temperament; behavioral style; neurobiological, genetic, and cultural factors; and psychosocial environment affect early and late childhood responses to stress. As children mature, their coping and adaptive skills also change. Major stressors associated with exploration of self and others vary with social interactions. Specific determinants for social interactions include school, the community, and religious affiliations, which facilitate learning how to compete and interact with peers, skills for sharing, and problem solving. Early social interactions with parents and later interactions with peers and other adults enhance coping and adaptive skills (Caplan, 1961; Erikson, 1963, 1968).

Caregiver's Influence on Coping and Adaptation in Childhood

Major parental tasks during this developmental stage include praising the child's efforts and accomplishments while preparing for the event of puberty. Parents' interest in the child's academic and sports activities enhances the youth's self-worth and acceptance.

In summary, early and late childhood developmental tasks include achieving trust, attachment or bonding, autonomy, initiative, mastery, and self-esteem. As the person emerges from childhood, her life experiences become the foundation for adult responses. Understanding the adaptive level of parental function enables one to predict adaptation in children. Moreover, the emotional and behavioral states of the parents and the child are interdependent and influence adaptation throughout the life span.

ADOLESCENCE

Adolescence is a time of profound neurobiological and psychosocial changes; the major developmental tasks are role and sexual identity and neurobiological adaptation and demands associated with cultural and academic expectations. Each area represents turmoil, increased psychosocial stress, and the struggle to adapt to changes in body image, control of the environment, movement from dependence to independence within social contexts, and the formation of meaningful interpersonal relationships. Roles are tested with the need to integrate ideals, values, and norms with internal and external demand (Blos, 1962; Erikson, 1968; Mishne, 1986).

Stress in the adolescent is normally manifested by disagreements with authority figures, anxiety, suicide, homicide, and depression. Some adolescents may experience stress reactions and exhibit them through acting-out behaviors, such as misusing substances (alcohol, nicotine, or illicit drugs), practicing unsafe sex and promiscuity, and carrying out antisocial behaviors (such as shoplifting). These latter behaviors may also be symptoms of psychiatric illnesses. Twenty percent of adolescents experience psychiatric disorders or mental illness, the most common diagnoses including personality, anxiety, mood, and conduct disorders (Portzky, et al., 2005; Klein, Lewinsohn, Rohde, Seeley, & Durbin, 2002; Kovacs, Goldston, & Gatsonis, 1993; Zohar, 1999).

Healthy interpersonal relationships with family and peers reduce vulnerability to stress and promote high self-esteem and positive self-worth. Accomplishment of developmental tasks allows adolescents to deal with life experiences and stressors effectively, producing healthy separation from families and increasing independence. Additionally, healthy separation and independence allow the adolescent to make the transition into adulthood with adaptive coping skills.

EARLY AND MIDDLE ADULTHOOD

The young adult enters life experiences with a sense of identity and integration of values and health personality traits. The major commitments during early adulthood include career goals and interpersonal relationships or intimacy. Stressors are often associated with relationship problems, job changes or pressures, unemployment, and parenthood.

As adults establish stable relationships and move into marriage or other long-term relationships, and later, parenthood, the major developmental tasks include generativity versus stagnation (Erikson, 1963). During this period adults begin to examine their contributions to society, which arise from creativity and productivity. The basis of these endeavors is making contributions to or influencing the next generation and may include activities such as rearing children, producing works of art, writing, or participating in projects that protect the environment.

Other stressors generated by middle adulthood include neurobiological and psychosocial changes such as menopause, retirement, and the "empty nest syndrome." Because of the growing number of aging parents, middle-aged adults are also likely to spend many years caring for their parents, which is a major stressor. Adults using healthy coping mechanisms normally mobilize resources and adapt to these changes. Others using maladaptive coping skills may experience stagnation and feel they have not made any significant contributions in life and perceive the aging process as threatening and empty. Major stressors in adulthood manifest in many ways, including anger, hostility, substance abuse, dysfunctional family interactions, and poor social and occupational performance. Other symptoms of stress may include mood or anxiety disorders.

OLDER ADULTHOOD

Adaptation in the older adult depends on defense mechanisms used throughout the life span. The major developmental task of older adults is integrity versus despair (Erikson, 1963). Adaptive coping mechanisms help older adults maintain mental and physical health. Loss is the predominant theme that characterizes stress in older adults. Major losses include close relatives and friends, physical abilities and stamina, and financial status. The ability to resolve grief taxes the older adult's coping skills.

Nursing interventions during this last stage of development include crisis intervention, grief counseling, and support of adaptive coping mechanisms. Older adults are at risk for suicide if there are significant losses, especially in males, due to the death of a spouse or loss of health. Additional losses include the stress of caregiving of an aging spouse or significant other. Nurses can assess these clients for signs of depression, level of dangerousness, and ineffective coping patterns.

In summary, development is a dynamic process that places enormous stress on people throughout the life span. Adaptive resources that foster mastery of age-specific tasks determine the potential for growth and maturity and resolution of stressful situations.

ESSENTIAL QUALITIES OF THE PSYCHIATRIC-MENTAL HEALTH NURSE

Psychiatric nurses have the unique role of helping clients in distress. Continuous care and monitoring of client responses during acute hospitalization and episodic assessment in community-based settings provide distinct opportunities for psychiatric interventions. This unique role allows the nurse to assess client response to stressful situations. Distressed clients may use adaptive or maladaptive behaviors to reduce tension. Assessing their needs compels nurses to understand the role of neurobiological, genetic, psychosocial, and behavioral variables on human response. This knowledge helps psychiatric nurses develop effective interventions, outcomes, and evaluations that facilitate adaptive behaviors in the mentally ill.

The foundation of client interventions, outcomes, and evaluations are based on the therapeutic relationship between the nurse and the client. The unique nature of the therapeutic relationship requires certain qualities in the nurse. The seven essential qualities include therapeutic use of self, genuineness, warmth, empathy, acceptance, maturity, and self-awareness (Table 4–8). These qualities enable nurses to assess the complex needs of the mentally ill through therapeutic relationships.

TABLE 4–8
Essential Qualities of Psychiatric Nurses

- Therapeutic use of self
- Acceptance
- Genuineness
- Maturity
- Warmth
- Self-awareness
- Empathy

THERAPEUTIC USE OF SELF

The heart of psychiatric nursing is the therapeutic use of self. *Therapeutic use of self* refers to forming a trusting relationship that provides comfort, safety, and acceptance of the client. Active listening, self-awareness, mutuality, and effective communication are elements of this concept. This relationship begins when the nurse approaches the client with genuine interest and concern and continues throughout treatment. As the relationship evolves, the client feels less threatened and frequently seeks out the nurse for reassurance and support. Therapeutic relationships help clients recognize their strengths, resources, and maladaptive responses.

GENUINENESS AND WARMTH

The second and third essential qualities of psychiatric nurses are genuineness and warmth. Genuineness implies a sense of openness, realness, and a lack of defensiveness (Truax & Carkhuff, 1967), and it conveys congruence between verbal and nonverbal behaviors in nurses and clients.

Freud (1912) stressed the curative properties of warmth, associating it with respect, acceptance, and positive regard for clients in distress. Warmth imparts consistency, kindness, patience, and caring for the client (Menninger, 1947). It can be conveyed only if it is genuine. Psychiatric nurses must convey genuineness and warmth as major aspects of the therapeutic use of self. These qualities are tools that foster the expression of feelings and thoughts in distressed clients. Sharing of feelings allows nurses to accurately interpret the client's experiences and responses.

EMPATHY

The fourth nursing quality is empathy. A number of theorists have defined empathy as a crucial aspect of therapeutic relationships. The first ones were Truax and Carkhuff (1967), who asserted that empathy occurs when the nurse successfully assumes the "internal frame of reference of the client" (p. 285) and "experiences client feelings as though they were his own" (p. 313). In other words, the nurse "walks a mile in the client's shoes" and experiences the world from her emotional perspective without being emerged or overwhelmed by the experience. Empathy allows nurses to perceive and communicate more accurately with the client.

The second theorist was Ehmann (1971), who defined empathy "as a means to share and experience the feelings of the patient" (pp. 75–76). Empathy is a powerful communication tool that conveys "I am with you, and I have a sense of what you are experiencing." During the empathic process, the nurse never totally loses her identity. The therapeutic use of empathy facilitates a deeper understanding of the client's situation while it helps the client move toward self-awareness, feelings, and their meaning (Table 4–9).

The following situation demonstrates empathy.

Nurse-Client Dialogue

CLIENT: I cannot talk about the rape (client begins to cry).

NURSE: I know this must be very difficult for you to talk about.

CLIENT: I shouldn't have gone out with Jimmy because I've never trusted him.

NURSE: Sounds like you are blaming yourself.

CLIENT: Well, who else can I blame?

NURSE: You are not responsible for what happened.

The nurse's response conveys caring and genuine concern for the client's distress. The nurse understands what she must be going through without allowing the client's overwhelming sadness to affect her.

Empathy is often confused with sympathy. Sympathy differs from empathy because it interferes with formation of therapeutic relationships. Sympathy blurs boundaries between the nurse and the client, making it difficult for each of them to distinguish her feelings from those of the other (Katz, 1963). Sympathy is feeling or sharing the identical concerns of another. Empathy fosters autonomy and self-care, whereas sympathy encourages dependency.

ACCEPTANCE

The fifth nursing quality is acceptance. Acceptance suggests neither approval nor disapproval but tolerance and appreciation of the client as a human being regardless of gender, culture, religion, or socioeconomic status. Client attributes are received without judgment. Therapeutic relationships use acceptance to create environments that encourage expression of feelings, thoughts, and behaviors. Acceptance and tolerance of differences in others require maturity and self-awareness, which are the sixth and seventh qualities of psychiatric nurses.

MATURITY AND SELF-AWARENESS

Maturity plays a major role in the nurse's ability to tolerate differences and be responsive to client needs. It also denotes that the nurse is aware of personal responses to given or potentially uncomfortable situations, or clients who interfere with objectivity. Self-awareness of certain feelings or reactions, such as anger, protectiveness, dependency, and anxiety,

TABLE 4–9
Ehmann's Empathy Process:
The Client Who Has Experienced Trauma (Rape)

Phases	Characteristics	Nurse's Behavior
Identification	Absorption in client's situation (temporary) Allows nurse to establish a sense of similarity	Attentive to client's expression of shame and guilt after rape
Incorporation	The act of merging the client's experience with the nurse's	Imagines what the client must be going through
Reverberation	Interaction of the nurse and client experiences	Feels sadness for client, reaches out and touches client when she cries (when appropriate)
Detachment	Separation or withdrawal of subjective involvement and resumption of one's own identity	Hands client a tissue, stating "This must be very difficult for you to talk about"

Note. From "Empathy: Its Origins, Characteristics, and Process," by V. E. Ehmann, 1971, *Perspectives in Psychiatric Care, 9,* pp. 72–80. Reprinted with permission.

helps the nurse assist clients with similar issues. Maturity and self-awareness are crucial to the promotion of client safety, comfort, and appreciation of individual attributes, capacities, and limitations.

Psychiatric-mental health nurses are confronted with the daily and episodic responsibilities of assessing, intervening, and evaluating client responses to stress. Client interactions, especially those exhibiting maladaptive responses such as a demanding behavior, verbal abuse, and uncooperativeness, generate various reactions in nurses. Client responses to stress vary and include vast treatment modalities and hospitalization.

Psychiatric nurses need to identify the meaning of their own stress and develop strategies that increase personal and professional growth. Increased client demands and workplace violence, coupled with the persistent nursing shortage and uncertainty about health care delivery systems, increase stress in psychiatric nurses. Increased stress often generates feelings of powerlessness and apathy. Suggested strategies include nurse support or supervision groups that create climates of empathy, caring, and opportunities to explore the meaning of specific reactions to clients and various clinical situations.

Support groups can assist nurses in the following tasks:

◆ Exploring the meaning of negative or overly protective reactions to specific client behaviors

◆ Learning how to take care of themselves by attending to their biological and psychosocial needs, both personal and professional

◆ Using stress reduction and progressive relaxation techniques

◆ Enhancing altruism among colleagues

◆ Developing effective problem-solving, conflict resolution, and communication skills

Self-awareness is the foundation of exploring nurses' reactions to specific clients and clinical situations. Nurses need to be aware of themselves in relation to others. Support or supervision groups offer opportunities for personal and professional growth. The complexity of mental illness and the human response to others compel psychiatric nurses to create workplace environments that help them manage their stress effectively (Antai-Otong, 2001).

LEADERSHIP

Too often nurses forget about the importance of leadership skills when caring for clients in vast practice settings. On inpatient units, psychiatric nurses provide 24-hour care for clients, but they and other staff tend to minimize their contributions and power. In community-based settings, psychiatric nurses also provide direct and indirect care of clients. Leadership skills are essential in these settings because astute problem solving and decision making have immediate impact on the well-being of clients. Management and administration must provide a climate that fosters the development and maintenance of leadership skills. Work environments that promote leadership skills engender a sense of power and pride in their contributions to the health care system. All nurses are leaders, regardless of their responsibilities. Leadership behaviors include empowerment, directing and managing client care, monitoring client outcomes, and collaborating with clients and other mental health professionals.

The role of psychiatric nurses is greatly influenced by their ability to integrate leadership skills into their practice. Developing leadership skills must be an integral aspect of professional development, beginning with the student experience, and nurtured in practice settings through mentoring, role modeling, and other professional growth endeavors.

THE PSYCHIATRIC-MENTAL HEALTH NURSE AS A MEMBER OF THE MENTAL HEALTH TEAM

The concept of nursing has always existed in association with the role of caretaker, surrogate, and nurturer. Psychiatric nursing has come of age and emerged from the primary role of custodian or attendant from the back wards of asylums and state institutions to a role that is theory based and includes evaluating, managing, directing, and collaborating in the care of the mentally ill.

THE ROLE OF THE PSYCHIATRIC NURSE TODAY

Psychiatric nurses are vital members of the mental health team. They actively direct, manage, and evaluate client responses to stress across the life span. The mental health team is an interdisciplinary group of mental health staff who collaborates to assess, intervene, and evaluate client responses to treatment. Their continuous monitoring of clients experiencing crises further employs the nurses' input to intervene and create environments that minimize maladaptive responses and promote mental health. The impact of these interventions on client outcomes is often minimized by psychiatric nurses and members of the mental health team.

Psychiatric nurses need to appreciate their roles in vast mental health settings. This process can initially be accomplished by

recognizing the importance of daily or episodic interventions and client responses. The agitated client who calms down when the nurse establishes trust and explains that the oral lorazepam (Ativan) will reduce irritability is an example of a frequently used psychiatric nursing intervention. Understanding the effects of benzodiazepines on complex biochemical processes helps the nurse recognize the impact of the medication on client behavior. Student nurses observing this nurse-client interaction can learn about therapeutic interactions.

Student supervision is another mechanism that establishes the significance of psychiatric nurses by helping students appreciate the specialty of psychiatric nursing while integrating certain skills into their educational process. As students recognize the importance of the nurse's role on the mental health team, they can emulate basic therapeutic interactions, such as active listening and effective communication, and understand the complexity of mental illness.

A major role of the psychiatric nurse involves advancing safe and quality care that restores the client's level of functioning to a higher one. Primary prevention can be used to identify high-risk groups and provide health education. The nurse can intervene at this stage by using secondary prevention to halt the disease process or deterioration.

Secondary prevention can be initiated during an acute phase in inpatient settings, emergency departments, or homeless shelters. As clients respond to interventions and health is restored, the psychiatric nurse is concerned with preventing the deleterious effects of mental illness. This stage is referred to as tertiary prevention.

The role of the nurse in tertiary prevention is to prevent disability and promote rehabilitation and health maintenance. Aftercare programs such as social skills training or relapse prevention are examples of tertiary care. Other examples of tertiary prevention include Alcoholics Anonymous, Narcotics Anonymous, and Gamblers Anonymous. Nurses may also be involved in education programs for the mentally ill and focus on social skills training, medication management and adherence, dual diagnoses, stress management, and coping skills training.

THE MENTAL HEALTH TEAM

As previously discussed, the role of the psychiatric nurse has varied over the years, evolving from a custodial role to one that directs, manages, and collaborates with members of the mental health team to promote health. However, in spite of this evolution, the role of the psychiatric nurse remains unclear to many consumers, lawmakers, payers, and mental health professionals. Nurses must continue to educate through active dialogue, emphasizing their strength and diversity as health care providers.

Educating mental health professionals and consumers begins with psychiatric nurses actively participating in client care as members or leaders of the mental health team. Mental health teams are interdisciplinary groups usually led by a psychiatrist or other mental health professionals, such as a psychiatric nurse.

The mental health team provides a collaborative approach to client care. Collaboration maximizes and provides enormous opportunities to assess clients as the members reduce fragmentation and dehumanization. The team generates treatment planning that incorporates input from various disciplines, such as nursing, psychiatry, psychology, social work, and occupational therapy, and from mental health aides to meet the complex needs of the mentally ill and their families. Some mental health teams also have other disciplines including chaplains, registered dieticians, internists or primary care providers, and physical therapists.

Psychiatrist

Psychiatrists are physicians who have specialized in psychiatry. These mental health practitioners are usually certified by the American Board of Psychiatry and Neurology and are responsible for making psychiatric diagnoses and prescribing treatment. Additional responsibilities include prescribing psychotropic or other medications and providing medical treatment such as electroconvulsive therapy. Psychiatrists are also responsible for directing research, such as drug trials, and for providing psychotherapy and supervision of medical students and residents.

Clinical Psychologist

Clinical psychologists have a doctorate in psychology and are generally involved in administering and interpreting psychological or neuropsychological testing that assists the mental health team in diagnosing psychiatric conditions. Psychologists also provide psychotherapy and behavioral modification.

Psychiatric Social Worker

Psychiatric social workers are graduates of a master's or doctoral social worker program and are nationally certified. They are primarily involved in identifying and dealing with social issues that affect clients and their families, and mobilizing community resources. They also gather psychosocial data on admission and provide crisis intervention and psychotherapy.

Occupational Therapist

Occupational therapists are graduates of a master's or doctoral program in occupational therapy. They are primarily involved in providing an array of activities that enable clients to gain skills needed to perform activities of daily living such as hand-to-eye coordination and vocational skills. Activities focus on altering the course of illness, including arts and crafts, which enable clients to express intrapsychic and interpersonal responses. Often, the client's relationship with the occupational therapist is more therapeutic than the activity itself.

Mental Health Worker or Psychiatric Aide

Mental health workers or psychiatric aides provide direct care to clients. There are no formal mental health requirements for this position. These providers are important members of the mental health team, and they play a vital role in maintaining a therapeutic milieu under the supervision of the professional registered nurse.

Internist or Primary Care Provider

The high co-occurrence of medical problems and conditions necessitates collaboration with internists or primary care providers to ensure continuity of care across the health continuum. As more and more clients experience co-occurring medical conditions, such as obesity, diabetes mellitus, hypertension, and engage in high-risk behaviors, including smoking, psychiatric nurses and other members of the mental health team must provide holistic health care to ensure appropriate and consistent levels of mental and physical health involving treatment in acute inpatient and community and home-based settings. The internist brings medical expertise to manage medical conditions as part of an interdisciplinary approach.

The Collaborative Process

Overall, the mental health team identifies complex client needs based on input from various team members. The collaborative process involves an active participation by members of the mental health team and the consumer or client. These endeavors foster health care environments that promote safety, holistic approaches to client care through communication; sharing of innovative ideas; impacting continuous quality improvement; and promoting creativity, autonomy, and accountability. The mental health team establishes the tone, foundations, and milieus that promote a sense of trust and respect for similarities and differences among professionals to assess client needs, develop outcomes, and evaluate the consumers' response to treatment (ANA, 1982). In brief, the collaborative process provides quality, comprehensive, and outcome-based care.

THE ROLE OF THE NURSE

Prevention and health promotion are major domains of psychiatric-mental health nursing. Understanding the effects of stress, coping, and adaptation is crucial to health promotion. Accordingly, appreciating the impact of stress on human behavior enhances the assessment process and helps the nurse identify client strengths, resources, and interventions that can reduce the deleterious effects of stress across the life span. Assessing present and past coping behaviors and developmental and behavioral competencies is a vital component of the nursing process.

Psychiatric-mental health nurses are challenged to integrate major neurobiological, genetic, and psychosocial concepts to grasp the meaning of their clients' global responses to stress. Nursing implications for understanding these concepts involve understanding the meaning of the client's perception of stress, identifying available resources, and providing education that fosters adaptive health practices. The nurse can identify clients at risk for mental illness or exacerbation and develop interventions that encourage a sense of well-being, mastery, and mental health.

THE GENERALIST NURSE

Changes in the role of the psychiatric nurse parallel the changes in psychiatry and, presently, the neurobiological and advances in genetics continue to receive increasing attention. The American Nurses Association (ANA, 2000) has delineated two levels of psychiatric-mental health nursing practice: basic (or generalist) and advanced practice. Roles concur with specific educational preparation, clinical experiences, specialty, and certification. The generalist nurse is clinically prepared to care for clients with mental illness. Certification as a mental health nurse validates clinical competence.

THE ADVANCED-PRACTICE PSYCHIATRIC REGISTERED NURSE

The advanced-practice registered nurse has a master's or doctoral degree in psychiatric-mental health nursing, commands the advanced knowledge and theory of mental illness needed to resolve complex mental health problems, and academically supervises graduate students (ANA, 2000). Prescriptive authority enables the advanced-practice nurse to work within state regulation and support clients on maintenance medications and evaluate their response over time and through direct observation and drug levels. Medication management and various psychotherapies enable the advanced-practice nurse to provide holistic mental health care. (See Chapter 29 for a detailed description of prescriptive authority.)

A subspecialty of advanced-nursing practice is the psychiatric consultation-liaison nurse (PCLN). The scope of the PCLN is vast and integrates concepts of primary, secondary, and tertiary prevention. The primary emphasis of the PCLN role includes assessment, diagnosis, and treatment of clients in diverse settings experiencing diverse responses to stress. Advanced-practice psychiatric nurses in this role also provide consultation and liaison activities (Krupnick & Antai-Otong, 2003).

Consultation refers to a dynamic process between the consultant and the consultee. The expert consultant provides an interpersonal educational process with the person seeking advice (consultee) and participates in health planning and treatment (Blake & Mouton, 1983). Liaison is defined as the linkage of health care providers to facilitate communication, collaboration, and establishing partnerships between clients and the consultant (Hackett, Cassem, Stern, & Murray, 1997). The core of the liaison process involves education and health education.

Historically, psychiatric nurses have incorporated holistic concepts in the nursing process. An increased emphasis on the brain function and genetics and their impact on client global responses suggest that psychiatric nurses need to redefine their roles and understand and meet the complex needs of the mentally ill. Integrating biological concepts into nursing practice does not negate the significance of psychosocial concepts, but it provides a comprehensive appreciation of the client as whole systems with complex needs. (See Chapter 34 for an in-depth discussion of the PCLN practice and role.)

THE NURSING PROCESS

The nursing process is defined as diagnosis and treatment of human responses to actual and potential problems (ANA, 1980). It is a deliberate and interactive problem-solving approach to effect change in the client. (The major phases of the nursing process are described in Chapter 5.) The nurse's understanding, synthesis, and application of broad behavioral and neurobiological concepts of adaptation influence the effectiveness of the nursing process across the life span. Moreover, effective communication and therapeutic use of self are necessary to interact with clients, families, and other members of the interdisciplinary mental health team.

During this interactive process the client and the nurse mutually determine a plan of care. Assessing the client's responses to internal and external demands, such as neurobiological and psychosocial factors, can be accomplished during this initial phase of the nursing process.

ASSESSMENT

Mood disorders are linked to chemical dysregulation or have some neurobiological basis. Psychosocial factors and cognitive appraisals also play a major role in precipitating mood disorders. Mr. L.'s present psychosocial stressors include a recent job loss associated with low self-esteem, hazard appraisal—using negative self-talk and thoughts, including a sense of loss and helplessness regarding the prospect of finding employment because of his age and mental illness.

NURSING DIAGNOSES

- ◆ Risk for Self-Directed Violence
- ◆ Ineffective Coping
- ◆ Situational Low Self-Esteem
- ◆ Disturbed Sleep Pattern
- ◆ Imbalanced Nutrition: Less than Body Requirements

See Table 4–10 for a comparison of the nursing diagnosis with *DSM-IV-TR* diagnosis

OUTCOME IDENTIFICATION

Major planning and nursing interventions include enhancing Mr. L.'s present strengths and promoting adaptive and lasting coping skills that will enable him to appraise

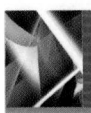

CASE STUDY

The Client with a Bipolar Disorder, Type 1, Manic Episode (Mr. L.)

Mr. L is a 56-year-old man with a history of bipolar disorder Type I, depressed episode. His wife is very supportive, and he has been compliant with treatment for the past 3 years. He was recently laid off from his job in sales in which he had worked for the past 15 years. Accompanied by his wife, Mr. L presented with complaints of increased social withdrawal and depression during the past few weeks. He is psychomotorly "slowed down" and withdrawn and has poor eye contact. His appearance is unkempt, and his mood is depressed; his speech is monotone and clear; and he is alert and oriented to time, place, and person. Additionally, his thoughts are relevant, logical, and coherent. He denies having suicidal or homicidal ideations or making gestures in the past, but he admits feeling that his family would be better off if he were dead. His appetite is poor, and he reports a weight loss of 15 pounds over the past 3 to 4 weeks. He sleeps at least 10 hours a day and he still feels tired. He is presently taking valproic acid, which has stabilized his mood during the past 3 years. This is his first experience with major depression, but he has had several manic episodes (see Nursing Care Plan 4–1).

NURSING CARE PLAN 4–1

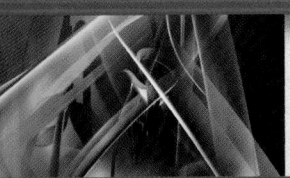

The Client with a Bipolar Disorder, Type 1, Manic Episode (Mr. L)

Nursing Diagnosis: Ineffective Coping

Outcome Identification	Nursing Actions	Rationales	Evaluation
1. By [date], client will develop adaptive and lasting coping skills.	1a. Establish and maintain a caring, nonjudgmental, and supportive attitude.	1a. Helps client feel less defensive and more comfortable sharing feelings.	*Goal met:* Client returns to a precrisis level of functioning. Client develops adaptive coping skills (i.e., improved problem solving). Client resumes meaningful relationships.
	1b. Assist client in identifying meaning of current stressors.	1b. Helps client understand self and present responses.	
	1c. Collaborate with client and wife to identify strengths and past and present coping skills.	1c. Places focus on positive attributes and increases self-esteem.	

Nursing Diagnosis: Disturbed Sleep Pattern

Outcome Identification	Nursing Actions	Rationales	Evaluation
1. By [date], client will resume normal sleeping patterns.	1a. Assess normal sleeping patterns.	1a. Determines baseline sleeping patterns.	*Goal met:* Client resumes normal sleeping patterns.

(continues)

Nursing Diagnosis: Imbalanced Nutrition: Less than Body Requirements

Outcome Identification	Nursing Actions	Rationales	Evaluation
1. By [date], client will maintain nutritional status to sustain body requirements.	1a. Assess client's nutritional status.	1a. Determines nutritional needs status.	*Goal met:* Client's normal eating patterns are reestablished and, before leaving the hospital, client is within 4 lb of normal weight.
	1b. Weigh as needed. Monitor intake and output.	1b. Assesses nutritional and hydration status.	
	1c. Encourage selection of favorite, appealing foods.	1c. Improves appetite and establishes eating patterns.	
	1d. Provide pleasant eating environment.	1d. Improves appetite.	
	1e. Encourage mouth care.	1e. Improves taste sensations and appetite.	

present and future crises realistically. Adaptive coping skills facilitate resumption of self-care, maintenance of adequate nutritional status, and restore past interests and responsibilities. Normal sleeping patterns and mood stabilization generally return with interventions that facilitate restoration of neurobiological processes and resolution of present crisis (see the accompanying Nursing Care Plan).

IMPLEMENTATION

Establishing and maintaining caring, nonjudgmental, and supportive attitude (essential nursing qualities) enables the nurse to assist the client and his wife in identifying the meaning of current stressors and recent lifestyle changes as well as present and past coping patterns. Maladaptive responses interfere with successful resolution of a crisis. Nurses must assess the client's level of dangerousness to self and others, current nutritional status, self-care, and sleeping patterns to minimize the deleterious effects of the present crisis and maladaptive responses. Other nursing interventions include measures to reduce stress, stabilize his mood, enhance coping skills, and increase knowledge. Administering or prescribing psychotropics, monitoring client responses and serum drug levels, and collaborating with the client and family members in treatment planning can facilitate successful resolution of the crisis situation.

EVALUATION

To evaluate the client's response to treatment, the nurse needs to determine whether the client has returned to a precrisis level of functioning. Indications of successful crisis resolution and formation of adaptive coping skills include minimal or absent depression; expression of hope and a will

---

TABLE 4–10

The Client with Bipolar I Disorder (Most Recent Episode Depressed): Comparison of Nursing Diagnosis with *DSM-IV-TR* Diagnosis

Axis I:	296.53 Bipolar I Disorder, Most Recent Episode Depressed
Axis II:	No diagnosis
Axis III:	Weight loss (15 lb over 3 weeks)
Axis IV:	Recent job loss
Axis V:	51 (current) Global Assessment of Functioning (GAF) Scale

to live; a realistic, positive outlook on life; increased self-esteem; and resumption of meaningful relationships.

In the case study, Mr. L's chief stressors are identified, such as losing his job, and mood disturbance and poor self-esteem generated by the loss. His general appearance and mood and information from his wife facilitate problem identification or nursing diagnoses as alterations in perception, nutrition, and mood. Outcome identification provides opportunities to implement both medical and nursing interventions, such as administering psychotropics, maintaining adequate nutrition, monitoring his responses (both desired and adverse), and providing emotional support that encourages restoration to previous level of functioning. Additionally, facilitating the wife's participation is an important nursing intervention in health promotion and disease prevention.

In addition to helping clients meet their basic needs, nurses continue to play pivotal roles in prevention and client advocacy.

SUMMARY

◆ Today psychiatric nurses are facing enormous challenges. Major challenges include changes in the health care system, a staggering increase in violence, family disintegration, and increases in the number of vulnerable populations, such as substance abusers, the aging poor, and the homeless.

◆ Mental health and adaptation are relative and lie on a continuum with mental illness and maladaptation.

◆ Stress and coping are natural aspects of developmental stages.

◆ One's ability to manage stress and cope effectively is influenced by a myriad of highly complex internal and external processes that begin prenatally and evolve throughout the life span.

◆ Integrating neurobiological and behavioral concepts into nursing interventions enables nurses to assist their clients in developing adaptive coping responses.

◆ As members of the mental health team, psychiatric nurses continue to play a crucial role in advancing the needs of clients experiencing distress.

STUDY QUESTIONS

Abbey, a 10-year-old girl, is brought to the mental health clinic by her parents, who report that she has become isolative and severely depressed since the death of her close friend several weeks ago. They have attempted to engage her in various family activities, but her depression has worsened over the past week.

1. What is the most important determinant of the child's coping patterns?
   a. Her early social interactions with parents
   b. The quality of the child-peer relationships
   c. The child's problem-solving capacity
   d. The child's sense of self

2. A major nursing intervention for Abbey would be to:
   a. encourage her to verbalize her feelings
   b. reinforce her peer relationships
   c. teach her parents how to talk to her
   d. encourage her to depend on her parents

3. During the morning mental health team meeting, the social worker criticizes the night nurse because the client complained of receiving his medication late. The most effective way for the nurse to deal with this situation is to:
   a. tell the social worker she is out of line
   b. leave the meeting and look at the medication chart
   c. talk to the social worker after the meeting
   d. express anger over the social worker's criticism

4. Overall, adaptation and coping are influenced by a number of factors. Which of the following factors has the least influence on adaptation and coping?
   a. Developmental level
   b. Neurobiological factors
   c. Cultural background
   d. Social development

5. The chief role of the mental health team is to:
   a. provide continuous and comprehensive care
   b. reduce conflict between various disciplines
   c. help clients understand the role of the mental health staff
   d. provide a forum for health care providers to deal with their feelings

6. Mr. Jones calls the crisis hotline and reports that his wife of 23 years has just asked him for a divorce and that she has already moved out of the home. He calls the crisis hotline and states that he is a failure and does not believe he can go on without his wife. What type of appraisal has Mr. Jones made of his present stressors?
   a. Primary appraisal-stress-injurious
   b. Primary appraisal-stress-challenging
   c. Primary appraisal-irrelevant-challenging
   d. Secondary appraisal-stress-hazardous

7. Primary prevention is an important nursing intervention in which the nurse identifies high-risk behaviors and implements preventive measures to promote health. Which of the following is an example of primary prevention?
   a. Administering an atypical antipsychotic agent to reduce psychosis and agitation
   b. Setting up a health fair at a local shopping mall to educate families about prodromal symptoms of schizophrenia
   c. Teaching parenting classes to a young couple whose child has been placed in a foster home
   d. Teaching deep breathing and relaxation therapy techniques to a client having a panic attack

8. One of your clients expresses anger toward her father who left her when she was three and she will never forgive him

for the hardship this placed on her mother and the family. During the discussion you recognize that you are angry and you too feel anger toward the client's father. What is the best explanation for your reactions?

a. You feel sorry for the client and wish her father had been more responsible.

b. The client's father should have provided for his family.

c. A lack of self-awareness and appropriate responsiveness to the client's situation

d. You are over-identifying with the client's feelings and situation

9. Paul is a-30-year old client with a diagnosis of schizophrenia and currently takes an atypical antipsychotic medication. As his nurse it is imperative to monitor for desired and adverse side effects. An *important* nursing intervention involving his care is which of the following?

a. Monitoring his abdominal circumference and weight

b. Inquiring about his daily exercise program

c. Educating him about the importance of employment

d. Helping him find adequate housing

10. Mary has just lost her job and is stressed about paying her bills. Her husband reassures her that this is a temporary setback and they will be able to manage their bills. Her husband's response to her distress describes which stress appraisal?

a. Hazardous threats

b. Challenging situations

c. Irrelevant appraisal

d. Benign appraisal

RESOURCES

Please note that because Internet resources are of a time-sensitive nature and URL addresses may change or be deleted, searches should also be conducted by association or topic.

Internet Resources

www.ncptsd.org/facts/disasters/fs_riskfactors.html
National Center for PTSD, (802) 296-5132

www.ncptsd.org/facts/disasters/fs_treatment_disaster.html
National Center for PTSD, (802) 296-5132

www.mentalhealth.org/specials/surgeongeneral.gov
Review Mental Health: A Report of the Surgeon General

REFERENCES

Alexander, F. (1939). Psychological aspects of medicine. *Psychosomatic Medicine, 1,* 7–18.

American Nurses Association. (1980). *A social policy statement.* Kansas City, MO: Author.

American Nurses Association. (1982). *Standards of psychiatric and mental health nursing practice.* Kansas City MO: Author.

American Nurses Association. (1991). *Nursing agenda for health reform.* Kansas City, MO: Author.

American Nurses Association. (2000). *Scope and standards of psychiatric-mental health nursing practice.* Washington, DC: Author.

American Psychiatric Association. (1952). *Diagnostic and statistical manual of mental disorders.* Washington, DC: Author.

American Psychiatric Association. (1968). *Diagnostic and statistical manual of mental disorders* (2nd ed.). Washington, DC: Author.

American Psychiatric Association. (1980). *Diagnostic and statistical manual of mental disorders* (3rd ed.). Washington, DC: Author.

American Psychiatric Association. (1987). *Diagnostic and statistical manual of mental disorders,* (3rd ed., revised). Washington, DC: Author.

American Psychiatric Association. (1994). *Diagnostic and statistical manual of mental disorders* (4th ed.). Washington, DC: Author.

American Psychiatric Association. (2000). *Diagnostic and statistical manual of mental disorders,* 4th edition, Text Revision (*DSM-IV-TR*). Washington, DC: Author.

Antai-Otong, D. (2001). Creative stress-management techniques for self-renewal. *Dermatology Nursing, 13,* 31–32, 35–39.

Blake, R. R., & Mouton, J. S. (1983). *Consultation: A handbook for individual and organizational development* (2nd ed.). Reading, MA: Addison Wesley.

Bleuler, E. (1950). *Dementia praecox or the group of schizophrenias* (J. Zinkin, Trans.). New York: International Press. (Original work published in 1911.)

Blos, P. (1962). *On adolescence.* New York: Free Press.

Bowlby, J. (1969). *Attachment and loss* (Vol. 1). New York: Basic Books.

Buraff, L. J., Janowicz, N., & Asarnow, J. R. (2006). Survey of California emergency departments about practices for management of suicidal patients and resource available for their care. *Annals of Emergency Medicine, 48,* 452–458.

Brewin, C. R., Andrews, B., Rose, S., & Kirk, M. (1999). Acute stress disorder and posttraumatic stress disorder in victims of violent crime. *American Journal of Psychiatry, 156,* 360–366.

Cannon, C. D. (1999). Neurodevelopmental processes in the ontogenesis and epigenesis of psychopathology. *Developmental Psychopathology, 11,* 375–393.

Cannon, W. B. (1914). The emergency function of the adrenal medulla in pain and the major emotions. *American Journal of Physiology, 33,* 356–372.

Cannon, W. B. (1939). *The wisdom of the body* (2nd ed.). New York: W.W. Norton.

Caplan, G. (1961). *An approach to community mental health.* New York: Grune & Stratton.

Caplan, G. (1964). *Principles of preventive psychiatry.* New York: Basic Books.

Corrigan, P. W., & Penn, D. L. (1999). Lessons from social psychology on discrediting psychiatric stigma. *American Psychologist, 54,* 765–776.

Davies, P. T., Cummings, E. M., Winter, M. A. (2004). Pathways between profiles of family functioning, child security in the interparental subsystem, and child psychological problems. *Developmental Psychopathology, 16,* 525–550.

Davis, M. C., Matthews, K. A., & McGrath, C. E. (2000). Hostile attitudes predict elevated vascular resistance during interpersonal stress in men and women. *Psychosomatic Medicine, 62,* 17–25.

Deutsch, A. (1937). *Mental illness in America.* New York: Doubleday.

Dix, T. (1991). The affective organization of parenting: Adaptive and maladaptive processes. *Psychological Bulletin, 110,* 3–25.

Dreyfus-Brisac, C. (1979). Ontogenesis of brain bio-electrical activity and sleep organization in neonates and infants. In F. Faulkner & J. M. Tanner (Eds.), *Human growth* (Vol. 3; pp. 157–182). New York: Plenum Press.

Ehmann, V. E. (1971). Empathy: Its origins, characteristics, and process. *Perspectives in Psychiatric Care, 9,* 72–80.

Erikson, E. (1963). *Childhood and society.* New York: W.W. Norton.

Erikson, E. (1968). *Identity: Youth and crisis.* New: York: W.W. Norton.

Freud, S. (1912). *The dynamics of transference* (Standard ed., 12; pp. 97–108). London: Hogarth Press.

Freud, S. (1953). *The standard edition of the complete psychological works of Sigmund Freud.* New York: MacMillan.

Gabbard, G. O. (2005). Mind, brain, and personality disorders. *American Journal of Psychiatry, 162,* 648–655.

Gabella, G. (1976). *Structure of the autonomic nervous system.* London: Chapman & Hall.

Griffin, M. G., Resick, P. A., & Yehuda, R. (2005). Enhanced cortisol suppression following dexamethasone administration in domestic violence survivors. *American Journal of Psychiatry, 162,* 1192–1199.

Grych, J. H., Raynor, S. R, Fosco, G. M. (2004). Family processes that shape the impact of interparental conflict on adolescents. *Developmental Psychopathology, 16,* 649–665.

Hackett, T. P., Cassem, N. H., Stern, T. A., & Murray, G. B. (1997). Beginnings: Consultation psychiatry in a general hospital. In N. H. Cassem, T. A. Stern, J. F. Rosenbaum, & M. S. Jellinek (Eds.), *Massachussetts General Hospital: Handbook of general hospital psychiatry* (4th ed., pp. 1–9). St. Louis, MO: Mosby.

Hansen, D. A., & Johnson, V. A. (1979). Rethinking family stress theory: Definitional aspects. In W. R. Burr, R. Hill, F. I. Nye, & I. L. Reiss (Eds.), *Contemporary theories about the family: Researched-based theories* (Vol. 1; pp. 582–603). New York: Free Press.

Hartman, J. (1958). *Ego psychology and the problem of adaptation.* New York: International Universities Press.

Harvey, B. H., Naciti, C., Brand, L., & Stein, D. J. (2003). Endocrine, cognitive, and hippocampal/cortical 5HT1A/2A receptor changes evoked by a time-dependent sensitization (TDS) stress model in rats. *Brain Research, 983,* 97–107.

Holmes, T. H., & Rahe, R. H. (1967). The social readjustment rating scale. *Journal of Psychosomatic Research, 11,* 213–218.

Jalowiec, A. (1979). *Stress and coping in hypertensive and emergency room patients.* Unpublished master's thesis, University of Illinois, Chicago.

Jalowiec, A. (1988). Confirmatory factor analysis of the Jalowiec Coping Scale. In C. F. Waltz & O. L. Strickland (Eds.), *Measurement of nursing outcomes, vol. I. measuring client outcomes* (pp. 287–308). New York: Springer.

Jalowiec, A., & Powers, M. J. (1983). Stress and coping in hypertensive and emergency room patients. *Nursing Research, 30,* 10–15.

Katz, R. L. (1963). *Empathy: Its nature and uses.* London: Free Press of Glencoe.

Klein, D. N., Lewinsohn, P. M., Rohde, P., Seeley, J. R., & Durbin, C. E. (2002). Clinical features of major depressive disorder in adolescents and their relatives: Impact on familial aggregation, implications for phenotype definition, and specificity of transmission. *Journal of Abnormal Psychology, 111*(1), 98–106.

Koren, D., Arnon, I., & Klein, E. (1999). Acute stress response and posttraumatic stress disorder in traffic accident victims: A one-year prospective, follow-up study. *American Journal of Psychiatry, 156,* 367–373.

Kovacs, M., Goldston, D., & Gatsonis, C. (1993). Suicidal behaviors and childhood onset depressive disorders: A longitudinal investigation. *Journal of Academy of Child and Adolescent Psychiatry, 32,* 1–8.

Krupnick, S. L., & Antai-Otong, D. (2003). Psychiatric consultation-liaison nursing. In D. Antai-Otong (Ed.), *Psychiatric nursing: Biological and behavioral concepts* (pp. 923–948). Clifton Park, NY: Thomson Delmar Learning.

Lazarus, R. S. (1966). *Psychological stress and the coping process.* New York: McGraw-Hill.

Lazarus, R. S. (1991). *Emotion and adaptation.* New York: Oxford University Press.

Lazarus, R. S., & Folkman, S. (1984). *Stress, appraisal, and coping.* New York: Springer.

Lazarus, R. S., & Launier, R. (1978). Stress-related transactions between personality and environment. In L. A. Pervin & M. Lewis (Eds.), *Perspectives in interactional psychology* (pp. 287–327). New York: Plenum.

Lipsitt, L. R. (1983). Stress in infancy: Towards understanding the origins of coping behaviors. In N. Garmezy & M. Rutter (Eds.), *Stress coping, and development in children* (pp. 161–190). New York: McGraw-Hill.

McFarlane, J. M., Groff, J. Y., O'Brien, J. A., & Watson, K. (2003). Behaviors of children who are exposed and not exposed to intimate partner violence: An analysis of 330 black, white, and Hispanic children. *Pediatrics, 112,* (3Pt1), 202–207.

Melnyk, B. M., Feinstein , N. F., Alpert-Gillis, L., Fairbanks, E., Crean, H. F., Sinkin, R. A., Stone, P. W., Small, L., Tu., X., & Gross S. J. (2006). Reducing premature infants' length of stay and improving parents' mental health outcomes with the Creating Opportunities for Parent Empowerment (COPE) neonatal intensive care unit program: A randomized, controlled trial. *Pediatrics, 118,* e1414–1427

Menninger, K. A. (1947). *The human mind* (3rd ed.). New York: Alfred A. Knopf.

Menninger, K. A. (1963). *The vital balance.* New York: Viking Press.

Mental Health: A Report of the Surgeon General. (1999). Rockville, MD: U.S. Department of Health and Human Services, Substance Abuse and Mental Health Services Administration, Center for Mental Health Services, National Institutes of Health, National Institute of Mental Health.

Meyer, A. (1957). *Psychobiology: A science of man.* Springfield, IL: Charles C Thomas.

Mishne, J. M. (1986). *Clinical work with adolescents.* New York: Free Press.

Nightingale, F. (1860). *Notes on nursing: What it is and is not.* London: Harrison.

Patterson, P. H., Potter, D. D., & Furshpan, E. J. (1978). The chemical differentiation of nerve cells. *Scientific American, 239,* 50–59.

Portzky, G., Audenaert, K., & van Heeringen, K. (2005). Suicide among adolescents: A psychological autopsy study of psychiatric, psychosocial, and personality-related risk factors. *Social Psychiatry and Psychiatric Epidemiology, 40,* 922–930.

Roy, C. (1976). *Introduction to nursing: An adaptation model.* Englewood Cliffs, NJ: Prentice-Hall.

Roy, C., & McLeod, D. (1981). Theory of person as an adaptive person. In C. Roy & S. L. Roberts (Eds.), *Theory construction in nursing: An adaptation model.* Englewood Cliffs, NJ: Prentice-Hall.

Russak, L. G., & Schwartz, G. E. (1997). Feeling of parental care predict health status in midlife: A 35-year follow-up of the Harvard Mastery of Stress Study. *Journal of Behavioral Medicine, 20,* 11.

Sapolsky, R. M., Romero, L. M., & Munck, A. U. (2000). How do glucocorticoids influence stress responses? Integrating permissive supressive, stimulatory, & preparative actions. *Endocrinology Review, 21,* 55–89.

Seligman, M. E. D. (1975). *Learned helplessness: On depression and development.* San Francisco: W.H. Freeman.

Seyle, H. (1976). *The stress of life.* New York: McGraw-Hill.

Sroufe, L. A., & Rutter, M. (1984). The domain of developmental psychopathology. *Child Development, 55,* 17–29.

Swindle, R. W. Jr., Cronkite, R. C., & Moos, R. H. (1998). Risk factors for sustained nonremission of depressive symptoms: A 4-year follow-up. *Journal of Nervous and Mental Disorders, 186,* 462–469.

Truax, C. B., & Carkhuff, R. R. (1967). *Towards effective counseling and psychotherapy.* Chicago: Aldine.

http://www.census.gov/prod/cen2000/dp1/2kh00.pdf U.S. Census Bureau (2000). Profile of general demographics characteristics. Accessed September 17, 2005.

U.S. Department of Health and Human Services. (1990). *Healthy people 2000: National health promotion and disease prevention* (DHHS Publication No. PHS 91-50212). Washington, DC: U.S. Government Printing Office.

World Health Organization. (1980). Changing patterns in mental health care: Copenhagen reports on a working group. *EURO Reports and Studies, 25.*

World Health Organization. (1985). *Targets for health for all.* WHO Regional Office for Europe, Copenhagen, Denmark: Author.

World Health Organization. (2001). *The world health report 2001.* Mental Health: New Understanding, New Hope. Geneva: WHO.

Yehuda, R., Engel, S. M., Brand, S. R., Seckl, J., Marcus, S. M., & Berkowitz, C. S. (2005). Transgenerational effects of posttraumatic stress disorder in babies of mothers exposed to the World Trade Center attacks during pregnancy. *Journal of Clinical Endocrinology and Metabolism, 90,* 4115–4118.

Zohar, A. (1999). The epidemiology of obsessive-compulsive disorder in children and adolescents. *Psychiatric Clinics of North America, 8,* 445–460.

SUGGESTED READINGS

American Nurses Association. (2003). *Nursing: Scope and standards of practice.* Washington, DC: Author. Amer. Nurses Association.

Lachman, V. (2006). *Applied ethics in nursing.* New York: Springer Publishing Company.

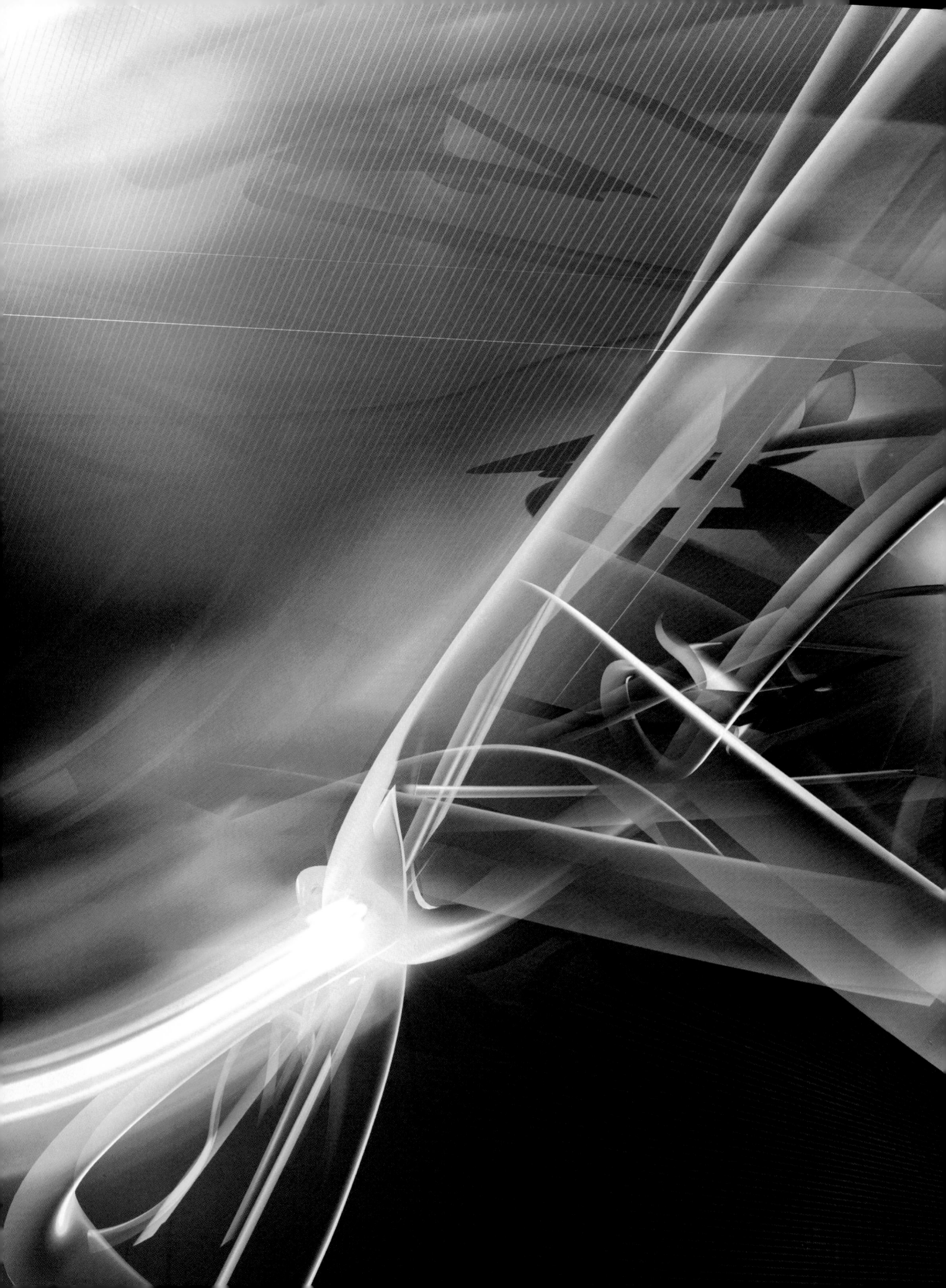

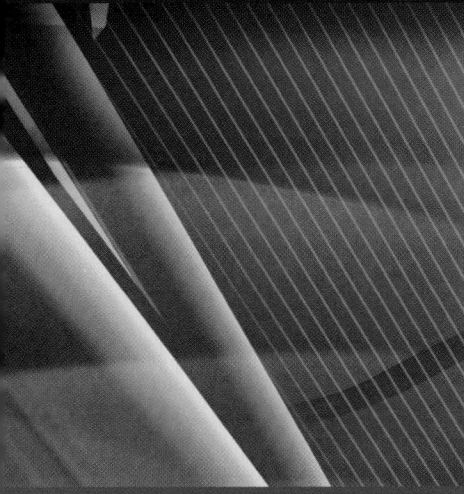

CHAPTER 5

The Nursing Process

Deborah Antai-Otong, MS, APRN, BC, FAAN

KEY TERMS

Affect: The visible and overt manifestations of the person's feeling or mood. Examples of affect are appropriate or congruent with mood and thought content, blunted, flat, labile, restricted, or constricted.

Client-centered care: An approach that conveys empathy and compassion, a willingness to understand the client's experience of illness and health and respect for the client's preferences, wishes, expressed needs, and values.

Clinical practice guidelines: Evidence-based statements that facilitate implementation of quality and client-centered health care established by syntheses of the evidence.

Compulsion: Repetitive, ritualistic, unrealistic behaviors used to neutralize or prevent discomfort of stressful events, circumstances, or recurring thoughts, images, or impulses such as obsessions.

Delusion: False, rigid belief that is incongruent with the client's cultural background. Examples of delusions include thought insertion, paranoid, somatic, and jealousy.

Flight of Ideas: Manifests as rapid thinking or ideas that have a common theme and that are likely to be seen in clients with major psychotic disorders such as a manic episode of bipolar disorder.

Hallucination: False sensory perception of internal stimuli. Examples of hallucinations include auditory, visual, olfactory, and tactile.

Illusion: Refers to a misinterpretation of an external stimulus such as a shadow for a person.

Loose Association: Manifests as a flow of thoughts or ideas unrelated to each other and shift from one subject to another. They are often seen in clients with schizophrenia and other major psychotic disorders.

Memory: A complex brain function that involves storing and retrieving information that is later recalled to consciousness.

Mental Status Examination (MSE): Refers to the part of the clinical assessment that compiles nursing observations and impressions of the client during the interview. Data from this exam include general appearance, mood and affect, speech patterns, perception, thought content and processes, level of consciousness and cognition, impulsivity, ability to abstract, judgment and insight, and reliability.

Mood: Refers to the client's sustained emotional state that reflects the client's perception of the world—depressed, sad, labile, elated, expansive, or anxious.

Nurse-Client Relationship: A dynamic, collaborative, therapeutic, interactive process between the nurse and the client.

Nursing Diagnosis: A statement of the client's nursing problem that includes both the adaptive or maladaptive health response and contributing stressors.

Nursing Process: An interactive, problem-solving process; a systematic and individualized problem-solving approach for administering nursing care that meets the client's needs comprehensively and effectively.

Obsession: Intrusive, recurrent, and persistent thoughts, images, or feelings that generate intense anxiety. Anxiety is usually temporarily dampened by ritualistic behaviors, known as compulsions, such as excessive hand washing associated with intense fears at contamination.

Orientation: Refers to one's sense of time, person, or place.

Preoccupation: Refers to recurrent thoughts or centers on a particular idea or thought with an intense emotional component.

Psychosocial Assessment: Refers to the data collection process that includes major elements such as psychosocial, biological, cultural, and spiritual data collections.

Speech: The process of expressing ideas, thoughts, and feelings through words and language.

Thought Content: Refers to the content of the client's thoughts that may include preoccupations, obsessions, compulsions, suicidal or homicidal ideations, and delusions.

Thought Process: Refers to what the client is actually thinking about, which may include preoccupations, obsessions, compulsions, suicidal or homicidal ideations, and delusions.

Visuospatial Ability: Refers to time and space.

COMPETENCIES

Upon completion of this chapter, the learner should be able to:

1. Review major components of the nursing process.

2. Discuss major components of a psychosocial assessment.

3. Perform a mental status examination.

4. Delineate potential barriers to the nursing process.

5. Develop an individualized plan of care for the client with a mental illness.

CHAPTER OUTLINE

Foundations of the Nursing Process

Psychiatric-Mental Health Nursing Standards

American Nurses Association

North American Nursing Diagnosis Association (NANDA)

Therapeutic Nurse-Client Relationship

The Nursing Process

Assessment

Standard I: Assessment (Data Collection Process)

Nursing Diagnosis

Standard II: Diagnosis

Diagnostic and Statistical Manual of Mental Disorders, 4th edition, Text Revision (DSM-IV-TR) Diagnoses

Outcome Identification and Planning

Standard III: Outcome Identification and
Standard IV: Planning

Implementation

Standard V: Implementation

Evaluation

Standard VI: Evaluation

Sweeping changes in technological, genetic, and biological discoveries and health care challenge psychiatric nurses to assess complex client responses and to implement effective approaches that strengthen nursing and interdisciplinary contributions to client outcomes. In addition to relying on the nurse's clinical expertise and understanding of the underpinnings of mental disorders, psychiatric nurses must be able to appraise and synthesize data and discern the most appropriate treatment for their clients (Goode & Piedalue, 1999; Institute of Medicine (IOM), 2001; Kohn, Corrigan, & Donaldson, 2000; Rosswurm & Larrabee, 1999). Furthermore, they must be able to link these data to practice models that facilitate positive treatment outcomes and ensure client participation and cost-effective quality health care. Invariably, the method of delivering this evidence-based practice is the *nursing process*.

Current trends in health care place greater emphasis on quality and safe care that reflects evidence-based care and practice guidelines. **Clinical practice guidelines** are defined as evidence-based statements that facilitate implementation of quality and client-centered health care established by syntheses of the evidence. Clinical practice guidelines offer nurses and other clinicians formal conclusions and recommendations that enable them to make clinical decisions and health care appropriate for psychiatric and other client populations (Lohr,

Eleazer, & Mauskopf, 1998; Lohr, 2004). Apart from the growing emphasis on evidence-based health care, client-centered strategies that ensure individual needs are met and client satisfaction is attained are critical to positive clinical outcomes.

Client-centered care refers to an approach that conveys empathy and compassion, a willingness to understand the client's experience of illness and health and sensitivity to each client's needs and uniqueness (IOM, 2001). Client-centered care also advocates client and family participation in the decision-making process. Clearly, quality and client-centered care require psychiatric nurses to employ empirically based data to establish quality nurse-client relationships to promote an optimal level of functioning. The nursing process offers nurses diverse opportunities to integrate these principles into health care and provide quality and client-centered treatment across the health care continuum (Antai-Otong, 2007).

FOUNDATIONS OF THE NURSING PROCESS

The **nursing process** is a systematic and cyclic problem-solving model for planning and delivering nursing care to clients, their families, and groups in diverse practice settings. This interactive and dynamic process helps ensure quality, individualized, and holistic care. Entry into the health care system puts the nursing process in motion, during which time the nurse collects and analyzes data, identifies the client's needs or problems (nursing diagnoses), constructs goals or outcome identification, and determines nursing interventions to facilitate the client in meeting these goals or outcomes. Once these interventions are implemented, the nurse evaluates treatment planning based on designated client responses or outcomes.

The concept of the nursing process originated in the 1950s initially as a three-step process of assessment, planning, and evaluating client needs based on the empirically based approach of observation, data collection, and analysis of the findings. During this period, leaders described the nursing process as an interactive and interpersonal approach with a problem-solving process (King, 1971; Peplau, 1952; Travelbee, 1971). It has evolved over the past 5 decades to provide a viable empirically based nursing tool. As psychiatric nurses confront the challenges of technological and neurobiological advances, assessing and anticipating complex client needs continue to rise (Doenges, Moorehouse, & Burley, 2000).

PSYCHIATRIC-MENTAL HEALTH NURSING STANDARDS

The American Nurses Association (2000) and the North American Nursing Diagnosis Association (NANDA, 2007) have made vast contributions to the evolution of the nursing process and provide the bases of standards of care, professional performance, and nursing diagnoses, respectively.

American Nurses Association

The American Nurses Association (2000) delineates standards of care as those professional activities in which psychiatric nurses use the nursing process to assess, diagnose, plan, implement, and evaluate various forms of care. Table 5–1 lists the ANA standards and the nursing behaviors that define them as applied to psychiatric-mental health nursing. The contemporary six-step nursing process model helps the nurse accurately analyze client assessment data and use critical thinking skills to synthesize, evaluate, and construct a diagnosis, which is crucial to individualized treatment planning (ANA, 2000; Doenges, Moorehouse, & Burley, 2000).

North American Nursing Diagnosis Association (NANDA)

According to the NANDA's (2007) and ANA's publication *Scope and Standards of Psychiatric-Mental Health Nursing Practice* (ANA, 2000), aspects of the nursing process are interrelated, cyclic, and dynamic. This scientific method of problem solving involves six steps that guide nurses in using the nursing process (Figure 5–1):

◆ Standard I: (Re-) Assessment
◆ Standard II: Diagnosis
◆ Standard III: Outcome Identification
◆ Standard IV: Planning

TABLE 5–1
ANA Standards of Psychiatric-Mental Health Nursing Practice

STANDARD I. ASSESSMENT

The psychiatric-mental health nurse collects client health data.

STANDARD II. DIAGNOSIS

The psychiatric-mental health nurse analyzes the assessment data in determining diagnosis.

STANDARD III. OUTCOME IDENTIFICATION

The psychiatric-mental health nurse identifies expected outcomes individualized to the client.

STANDARD IV. PLANNING

The psychiatric-mental health nurse develops a plan of care that is negotiated among the patient, family, and health care team and prescribes interventions to attain expected outcomes.

STANDARD V. IMPLEMENTATION

The psychiatric-mental health nurse implements the interventions identified in the plan of care.

STANDARD Va. COUNSELING

The psychiatric-mental health nurse uses counseling interventions to assist patients in improving or regaining their previous coping abilities, fostering mental health, and preventing mental illness and disability.

STANDARD Vb. MILIEU THERAPY

The psychiatric-mental health nurse provides, structures, and maintains a therapeutic environment in collaboration with the patient and other health care clinicians.

(continues)

STANDARD Vc. SELF-CARE ACTIVITIES

The psychiatric-mental health nurse structures interventions around the patient's activities of daily living to foster self-care and mental and physical well-being.

STANDARD Vd. PSYCHOBIOLOGICAL INTERVENTIONS

The psychiatric-mental health nurse uses knowledge of psychobiological interventions and applies clinical skills to restore the patient's health and prevent further disability.

STANDARD Ve. HEALTH TEACHING

The psychiatric-mental health nurse, through health teaching, assists patients in achieving satisfying, productive, and healthy patterns of living.

STANDARD Vf. CASE MANAGEMENT

The psychiatric-mental health nurse provides case management to coordinate comprehensive health services and ensure continuity of care.

STANDARD Vg. HEALTH PROMOTION AND HEALTH MAINTENANCE

The psychiatric-mental health nurse employs strategies and interventions to promote and maintain mental health and prevent mental illness.

The certified advanced practice registered psychiatric-mental health nurse uses individual, group, and family psychotherapy, child psychotherapy, and other therapeutic treatment to assist clients in fostering mental health, preventing mental illness and disability, and improving or regaining previous health status and functional abilities.

The following interventions (Vh-Vj) may be performed only by the APRN-PMH.

Advanced-Practice Interventions—Vh–Vj

STANDARD Vh. PSYCHOTHERAPY

The APRN-PMH uses individual, group, and family psychotherapy, and other therapeutic treatment to assist patients in preventing mental illness and disability, treating mental health disorders, and improving mental health status and functional abilities.

STANDARD Vi. PRESCRIPTION OF PHARMACOLOGICAL AGENTS

The APRN-PMH uses prescriptive authority, procedures, and treatments in accordance with state and federal laws and regulations to treat symptoms of psychiatric illness and improve functional health status.

STANDARD Vj. CONSULTATION

The APRN-PMH provides consultation to enhance the abilities of other clinicians to provide services for patients and effect change in the system.

STANDARD VI. EVALUATION

The APRN-PMH evaluates the patient's progress in attaining expected outcomes.

Note. From *Scope and Standards of Psychiatric-Mental Health Nursing Practice* by the American Nurses Association, 2000, Washington, DC: Author.

◆ Standard V: Implementation
◆ Standard VI: Evaluations (ANA, 2000)

THERAPEUTIC NURSE-CLIENT RELATIONSHIP

Effective data collection or assessment begins by establishing rapport and developing a therapeutic **nurse-client relationship** (Figure 5-2). This relationship requires self-awareness of the nurse's personal feelings, values, beliefs, and perceptions that may interfere with objective data collection. Nurses must identify and reduce potential barriers to effective communication throughout the nursing process.

Initially, the nurse must introduce himself and use supportive body language (i.e., eye contact, normal tone voice, and physical distance) and active listening skills. Active listening skills and supportive body language convey empathy and facilitate the nursing process. Active listening requires an unhurried approach and paying close attention to what the client says. Of particular relevance to active listening is the client's

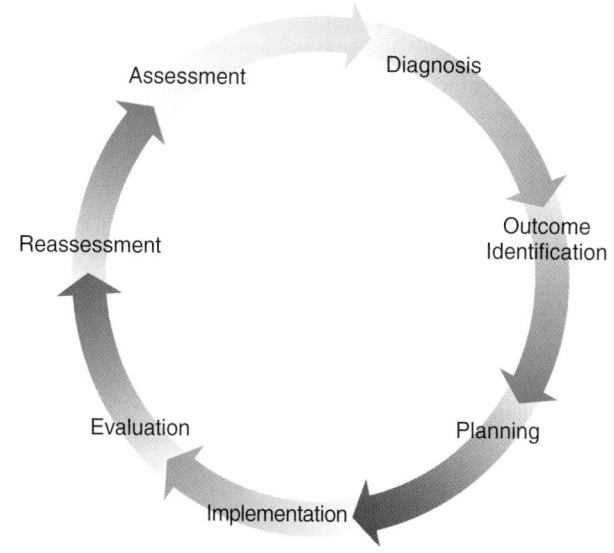

Figure 5–1 The dynamic nursing process

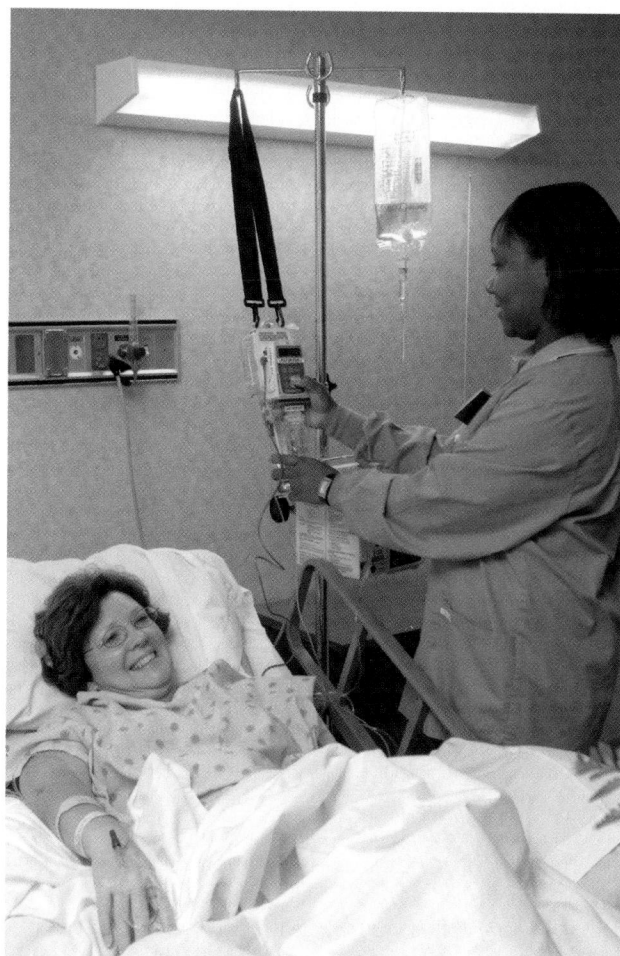

Figure 5–2 A therapeutic nurse-client relationship can help put a client at ease.

ability to communicate. Clients seeking psychiatric treatment often experience high levels of anxiety and distress, making it difficult for them to relax and communicate effectively. The nurse can put the client at ease by talking in a normal tone of voice, using good eye contact, and conveying warmth and understanding. If the client has a language barrier or an underlying medical condition that interferes with the communication process, efforts to understand the client's experiences and needs may require other strategies such as using an interpreter, asking the client to write or list concerns and needs, or asking family members to assist. (See Chapter 6 for a discussion of therapeutic communication.)

Additional issues that influence the nursing process include the client's developmental stage, culture, and religion and spirituality. Failing to recognize these issues may interfere with the nurse's perception of the client's present condition and result in an inaccurate assessment of the client's symptoms, which ultimately may have an impact on treatment planning. Self-awareness and appreciation of the client's unique attributes facilitate a greater understanding of the client's behavior, thus promoting a greater understanding of the client's experiences and needs. (See Chapter 7 for a full discussion of cultural factors.)

THE NURSING PROCESS

The following case study of Ms. Adiaha demonstrates how the nursing process and standards of care can be used to identify client responses and develop a plan of care.

ASSESSMENT

Assessment data concerning this client reveal a recent episode of:

◆ Decreased appetite

◆ Sleep disturbances

◆ Irritable and agitated mood

◆ Social withdrawal

The data collection process involves gathering data from the client, family members, and others and is the initial part of the nursing process.

Standard I: Assessment (Data Collection Process)

The psychiatric-mental health nurse collects health data.

Data collection and analysis are the bases of nursing interventions that are unique to the client's health needs. This

CASE STUDY

The Depressed Client (Ms. Adiaha)

Ms. Adiaha, a 52-year-old woman, presents with symptoms of decreased appetite and sleep, increased irritability and agitation, and social withdrawal. She is seeking evaluation in a community mental health clinic and is accompanied by her husband of 23 years.

process encompasses engaging the client in an interview to allow the nurse to observe verbal and nonverbal communication. Factors that make an impact on data collection include the quality of the nurse-client relationship and the client's developmental stage, culture, educational level, communication skills and language, mental status, and cognitive function. The young child is more likely to have difficulty expressing feelings than the young adult. Additionally, clients with cognitive impairment, such as those with schizophrenia and dementia, also have difficulty organizing their thoughts, expressing feelings, and responding effectively during assessments.

Data collection is based on various theoretical models that enable the nurse to interpret, validate and organize findings, and set up a plan of care. Various data collection tools may be used. Additional data, relevant to the care of the client with psychiatric disorders, come from the mental status examination (MSE), psychosocial and spiritual assessments, and physical examination. When indicated, psychometric examinations offer additional clinical data. Data also are collected from various sources such as clients, significant others, other health care providers, and medical records. Refer to Table 5–2, Psychosocial Assessment Tool, and Table 5–3, Major Components of the Mental Status Examination.

Mental Status Examination

The mental status examination (MSE) is a crucial part of the data collection process and provides an overall description of the client's mental status, including general appearance, mood and affect, quality of speech, thought content and processes, level of consciousness and cognition, impulsivity, ability to abstract, judgment and insight, and reliability. Major goals of the MSE are to:

1. Gather baseline data about the client's level of functioning
2. Identify actual and potential problems
3. Facilitate making accurate psychiatric and medical diagnoses

Major components of the MSE are described next.

General Appearance

The nurse observes and gathers data concerning the client's level of consciousness, dress, facial expressions, posture, level of understanding, gait, grooming, psychomotor behavior or activity level, eye contact, age, and attitude toward the nurse, as well as with whom and how the client arrived (i.e., alone, family member or significant other, police officer, parent, or counselor). For example, clients experiencing depression may present with psychomotor retardation (very slowed down) or agitation in the form of restlessness and pacing.

Mood and Affect

Mood refers to a pervasive and sustained emotional state that depicts the client's perception of the world. Examples of mood presentations include depressed, sad, labile, elated, expansive, or anxious. Affect reflects the client's present state of emotional responsiveness and is observable with body language.

The range of affect includes blunted, flat, restricted, depressed, expansive, and angry. A major point is whether the thought content is *congruent, appropriate,* or both, with the *mood* and *affect.* For instance, if the client complains of sadness and despair owing to the recent death of his father, the nurse can expect the client's mood to be sad or depressed and his affect to be sad or depressed or congruent with his thoughts.

Quality of Speech

Speech is the process of expressing ideas, thoughts, and feelings through language. It is the use of words and language. The quality of speech involves physical descriptions of the client's speech. When assessing speech, the nurse must note its quality or articulation (e.g., older adults with dementia, such as Alzheimer's disease, have difficulty generating speech), quantity, and rate (e.g., pressured speech seen in clients in a manic episode). Other descriptors of speech include spontaneous, talkative, rapid, whispered, loud, stuttered, or with any accents. Clients who have been traumatized often have difficulty responding spontaneously, whereas clients who are suspicious and distrustful may whisper.

Perceptual-Sensory Disturbances

Hallucinations and illusions are examples of perceptual-sensory disturbances and include visual, olfactory, auditory, or tactile. Hallucinations are false sensory perceptions of internal stimuli. The client who reports "hearing the voice of his dead sister" is an example of an auditory hallucination. In contrast, illusions refer to a misinterpretation of an external stimulus such as a shadow for a person. Nurses must inquire about the content of hallucinations and illusions and the circumstances in which they occur. Many clients complain of hallucinations when they feel "stressed or anxious." The nurse must also consider cultural factors when assessing perceptual-sensory aspects of the MSE. Inquiring about the presence of hallucinations or illusions helps the nurse enlist this information. (See Chapter 14 for an in-depth discussion of schizophrenia and other psychotic disorders.)

Thought Content and Processes

Thought content refers to what the client is actually thinking about, including preoccupations, obsessions, compulsions, suicidal or homicidal ideations, and beliefs, delusions, and ideas of reference. Preoccupations refer to recurrent thoughts or center on a particular idea or thought with an intense emotional component. Obsessions are maladaptive persistent patterns of thoughts, images, or feelings that generate anxiety. Compulsions are maladaptive urges to act on an impulse and involve ritualistic behaviors such as excessive handwashing. Delusions are defined as false beliefs and include persecutory, somatic, or jealous types. During the data collection process, the nurse must assess whether the client has suicidal or homicidal ideations to determine the client's risk of danger to self or others. Thought processes refer to the form in which the client thinks and includes loose associations, flight of ideas, phobias, tangentiality, circumstantiality, and racing thoughts. Loose associations manifest as a flow of thoughts

TABLE 5–2
Psychosocial Assessment Tool

Client's Name: _____   Date of Birth: _____

Sex: M   F   Marital Status: _____

Source of Information (client, relative, other—please specify):

1. **Recent stressor(s)**   (e.g., loss, lifestyle changes, hospitalization)

> *Assess* the client's perception of the stressor(s).
>
> *Hospitalization* is a major source of stress for most clients because it places them in positions of powerlessness and loss of control. Hospitals have scheduled times to eat, bathe, and sleep.
>
> *Fears of the unknown,* such as tests, surgical procedures, pain, and separation from significant others, also increase anxiety and stress in clients.
>
> *Others areas of stress* (e.g., financial and familial) must be identified because they play pivotal roles in determining the client's responses to the present situation.
>
> *History of present signs and symptoms,* both emotional and physical, must be assessed because they are often chronic in nature. If a client complains of feeling depressed and this has persisted for many years, it is imperative to ask the client, "What made you decide to seek treatment at this time?"

2. **Current strengths** (individual, family, and community) **and resources** (e.g., spiritual beliefs, culture, or religious affiliation; past problem/crisis resolution; financial)

3. **History of psychiatric treatment or counseling/psychotherapy**

Have you sought psychiatric treatment?   No_____ Yes_____

What made you seek treatment?

Explain your response to treatment:

History of family psychiatric treatment or counseling: No_____ Yes_____

Explain:

(continues)

TABLE 5–2
Psychosocial Assessment Tool *(continued)*

4. ***Support systems*** (i.e., marital status, job, and relationships)

5. ***Suicidal or homicidal potential***

Are you having thoughts of killing yourself or others at this time?   No_____ Yes_____

If yes, describe:

How long have you had these thoughts?_____

What has stopped you from acting on them?

History of attempt(s):   No_____ Yes_____

Explain:

Dates:_____

Circumstances:

Were you abusing drugs or alcohol during the time of attempt(s)?   No_____ Yes_____

Explain:

What kind of treatment did you receive?

Family history of suicide or attempts: No_____ Yes_____

Explain:

Relationship: _____

(continues)

TABLE 5–2
Psychosocial Assessment Tool *(continued)*

Question for family member:

What is your understanding of the reason(s) for the client's attempt(s)?:

> **Factors that increase the risk of suicidal behaviors:**
>
> - Age (adolescents and males >65 years of age; older adults usually see a provider 1 month or less before suicide)
> - Race
> - Previous attempts
> - Family history
> - Death or debilitating illness in spouse
> - Substance abuse
> - Lack of adequate support systems
> - History of psychiatric disorders (i.e., psychosis, personality disorders, and substance misuse)
> - Family turmoil, divorce, separation, death of a parent (adolescents)
> - Depression
> - Feelings of hopelessness, helplessness, or despair ("no options")

6. *History of substance abuse:* No_____ Yes_____

   Type:

   Frequency:

   Amount:

   Last consumption:

   Family history:

   Treatment history:

   Length of sobriety:

   Legal history:

   Blackouts: No_____ Yes_____

   Explain:

   Withdrawal seizures: No_____ Yes_____

   Explain:

   Hallucinosis or delusions: No_____ Yes_____

   Explain:

(continues)

TABLE 5–2
Psychosocial Assessment Tool *(continued)*

History of severe withdrawal requiring immediate medical attention or hospitalization: No _____ Yes _____

Consequences of substance misuse: No _____ Yes _____

Explain:

Health/Medical_____ _____

Psychiatric_____

Legal_____

Occupational_____

Interpersonal____

7. *Mental status examination*

Purpose:

1. To gather baseline information about the patient's level of functioning, i.e., memory, appearance, behavior, and capacity for logical thought

2. To assess individual and family strengths and coping patterns

3. To identify actual and potential problems

4. To assist the treatment team in making a medical diagnosis

The mental status examination must be done in an unhurried manner and in an environment that provides patients with privacy, safety, and acceptance.

Level of consciousness: Alert_____ Drowsy_____ Other (describe): _____

Cooperative: No _____ Yes _____

Mode of arrival: Accompanied by:

Describe:

General appearance

Orientation: Person_____ Place_____ Date/Time_____

Dress: Appropriate_____ Neat_____ Disheveled_____ Other_____

Eye contact (consider cultural aspects): Good_____ Poor_____

Affect: Congruent/appropriate_____ Flat_____ Blunted_____

Hallucinations: No_____ Yes_____ Auditory_____ Visual_____ Other_____

Describe:

(continues)

TABLE 5–2
Psychosocial Assessment Tool (continued)

Delusions: No_____   Yes_____   Persecutory_____   Grandiose_____

Describe:

Illusions: No_____   Yes_____

Describe:

Obsessions: No_____   Yes_____

Describe (Do you have habits that *bother* you?):

Compulsions: No_____   Yes_____

Describe (Do you have special ways that you do things?):

Phobias: No_____   Yes_____

Describe:

Speech: Clear_____   Rapid_____   Slurred_____   Pressured_____   Aphasic_____   Mute_____

Mood: Appropriate_____   Anxious_____   Agitated_____   Elated_____   Depressed_____

Activity level: Appropriate_____   Restless_____   Psychomotor retarded_____   Lethargic_____   Agitation_____

Tremulous_____   Changes positions often_____

Explain:

Ability to Abstract

Memory: Intact_____;   Difficulty with: Recent events_____   Remote events_____

Test recent memory with three objects in a 5-minute exercise (when needed)

Thought processes: Logical_____   Relevant_____   Coherent_____

Does patient look stated age?   Yes_____   No_____;   Older_____   Younger_____

8. **Medical history**

During the past 6 to 12 months, have you had changes in the following:

Sleeping patterns?   No_____   Yes_____

Describe:

Appetite?   No_____   Yes_____

Describe:

Weight?   No_____   Yes_____

Describe:

(continues)

TABLE 5–2
Psychosocial Assessment Tool *(continued)*

Concentration patterns?   No_____ Yes_____

Describe: _____

Energy level?   No_____ Yes_____

Describe: _____

Libido?   No_____ Yes_____

Describe:

Mood?   No_____ Yes_____

Describe:

Current medical treatment: No_____ Yes_____

Explain:

Current medication(s):   No_____ Yes_____ List_____

How long have you taken this medication?

Directions for taking:

What is your understanding of the reason(s) for taking this medication?

Are you taking your medications as ordered by your physician or provider?   No_____ Yes_____

Explain:

List all over-the-counter medication

List all herbal medications (e.g., St. John's Wort, Kava Kava) or complementary therapies (e.g., acupuncture)

Surgical procedures during the past 12 months: No_____ Yes_____

Explain:

Allergies: No_____ Yes_____

Describe reaction:

TABLE 5–3
Major Components of the Mental Status Examination

- General Appearance
- Mood and Affect
- Speech
- Perceptual-Sensory Function
- Thought Content and Processes
- Higher Brain Function
  - Level of consciousness and orientation
  - Memory
  - Concentration and attention
  - Reading and writing
  - Cognition and intellectual functioning
  - Visuospatial ability
  - Impulsivity
  - Judgment and insight
  - Reliability

or ideas unrelated to each other and shift from one subject to another. In contrast, flights of ideas are rapid thinking or ideas that have a common theme. Sometimes clients are overwhelmed by many ideas, whereas others experience impoverished or paucity of ideas. Clients in a manic episode often have racing, tangential, and circumstantial thoughts, which are reflected in their rapid and pressured speech.

Higher Brain Function

Assessing higher brain function involves several areas, including level of consciousness and orientation (refers to one's sense of time, person, or place), memory, concentration and attention, reading and writing, cognition and intellectual performance, visuospatial ability, ability to abstract, impulsivity, judgment and insight, and reliability. Questions include "Is the client alert and oriented to person, place, and time?" "Is the client comatose or lucid one minute and drowsy the next?" A change or fluctuation in sensorium strongly suggests that the client has an underlying medical condition, such as delirium, drug (licit or illicit) intoxication or withdrawal, or fluid and electrolyte imbalance.

- Memory is a complex brain function that involves storing and retrieving information that is later recalled to consciousness. Assessing the client's memory includes remote (long-term), recent (what the client had for dinner or breakfast), recent past (current events), immediate memory (short-term), and immediate recall. Questions such as asking the client to name three objects in 5 minutes is one way to assess the client's immediate recall and memory. It is also important to note the client's responses to memory disturbances.

- Various conditions produce concentration and attention disturbances, including delirium or other medical conditions and anxiety or depression. A simple test using serials of 7s offers invaluable information concerning concentration and attention. The client is asked to begin with 100 and subtract 7s. Other activities include asking the client to spell W-O-R-L-D backwards or asking the client to name five things that begin with a specific letter such as "Ms. Jones, please list five things that begin with the letter 'M.'"

- The client's educational level and ability to read and write can be assessed throughout the assessment process. Cultural factors, educational preparation, and a previous level of functioning must be considered during this process. Sometimes clients are asked to write a sentence as part of this assessment.

- A screening tool can be used to assess for cognition or the client's ability to think and know. Some screening tools such as the Mini Mental State Exam (MMSE) (Folstein, Folstein, & McHugh, 1975) can be used to assess cognitive and intellectual performance. See Table 5–4 for major components of the MMSE.

- Visuospatial ability refers to time and space. The MMSE can also be used to test for this characteristic by asking clients to draw clocks with designated times or a geometrical figure to test this higher brain function. Questions can be asked such as "Has your loved one been getting lost more often?" (This is significant if the client has lived in the same neighborhood for many years.)

- Ability to abstract involves testing for concrete thinking. Proverbs can be used to test the client's ability to abstract. An example of a proverb is "It's raining cats and dogs outside." If the client has never heard this proverb, it cannot be used to test abstraction. If the client responds by saying, "It means there is torrential rain outside" it is likely that the client retains this ability. In contrast, if the client says, "Cats and dogs are falling from the sky" it is likely that the client has problems abstracting and is using concrete thinking or the literal meaning of the proverb. Clients with various dementias (such as Alzheimer's disease) and various mental disorders (such as schizophrenia) often have difficulty abstracting.

- Impulsivity refers to the ability to control or manage various urges appropriately. Certain clients who present with cognitive impairment, drug intoxication or withdrawal, brain injury and other dementias, and personality disorders, tend to have difficulty controlling impulses. Inquiring about the client's past history and circumstances of violence or aggression is helpful in assessing for impulsivity.

- The nurse can assess for judgment by asking "what if questions" such as "What if you were babysitting and the house caught afire, what would you do first?" or asking the client about past situations. Insight involves the client's understanding about being ill and the need for treatment when warranted.

TABLE 5–4
Mini-Mental State Examination (MMSE)

Maximum Score	Score	
		Orientation
5	( )	What is the (year) (season) (date) (month)?
5	( )	Where are we: (state) (county) (town or city) (hospital) (floor)
		Registration
5	( )	Name 3 common objects (e.g., *apple, table, penny*): Take 1 second to say each. Then ask patient to repeat all 3 after you have said them. Give 1 point for each correct answer. Then repeat them until he/she learns all 3. Count trials and record. Trials:
		Attention and Calculation
5	( )	Spell "world" backwards. The score is the number of letters in correct order (D_L_R_O_W_).
		Recall
3	( )	Ask for the 3 objects repeated above. Give 1 point for each correct answer. (Note: recall cannot be tested if all 3 objects were not remembered during registration.)
		Language
2	( )	Name a "pencil," and "watch."
1	( )	Repeat the following "no ifs, or buts."
3	( )	Follow a 3-stage command: "Take a paper in your right hand, Fold it in half, and Put it on the floor."
		Read and obey the following:
1	( )	Close your eyes.
1	( )	Write a sentence.
1	( )	Copy the following design.

Total Score _____

Note. From "Mini-mental State: A Practical Method for Grading the Cognitive State of Patients for the Clinician, by M. E. Folstein, S. E. Folstein, & P. R. McHugh, 1975, *Journal of Psychiatric Research, 12,* p. 189. Reprinted with permission.

♦ *Reliability* refers to whether the client's perception of a presenting problem and its history are credible.

The MSE, combined with the psychosocial assessment and physical examination, provide relevant client data that help the nurse and other members of the mental health team make an accurate diagnosis and individual plan of care.

Psychosocial Assessment

The psychosocial assessment focuses on the client's holistic needs and includes psychosocial and physical data collection. Areas of interest include:

1. Recent stressors: *"What brought you in today?" "Tell me about recent lifestyle or personal changes you have experienced over the past 6 to 12 months." "Have you felt this way in the past?" "If so, what was helpful?" or "What was not helpful?"*

2. Strengths: *Tell me about your strengths and things you do well.*

3. Present medications, including over-the-counter and herbal medications: *"How long have you been on this/these medication(s)?" "Who prescribed them?" "When was the last time you saw your health care provider?" "Tell me your reasons for taking medication(s)."*

4. History of psychiatric treatment or counseling/psychotherapy: *"How helpful were they?" "How long were you in treatment?" "What is your preference?"*

5. Substance abuse history, including type, duration, frequency, last use, and present and past treatment.

6. Quality of support systems and strengths.

7. Presence and history of suicidal or homicidal ideations, gestures, and risk assessment: *"Are you having thoughts of killing yourself or anyone else?" "Do you have a plan, the means?" "What has made suicide an option at this time?"* (recent stressors). *"Do you have a history of suicide and treatment?" "What means were used under what circumstances?"* (See Chapter 19 for a discussion of the client who is suicidal or homicidal.)

8. Present and past coping patterns/skills.

9. Self-concept, self-esteem, and strengths.

10. Spiritual and cultural needs.

11. Legal and occupational history (including history of domestic violence).

Life Span Considerations
Children and Adolescents

An in-depth evaluation of children and adolescents requires an understanding of normal growth and development, family dynamics and the impact of stress, coping, and parenting styles. Normally, children and adolescents are often accompanied by an adult who is a parent, caregiver, grandparent, family member, friend, neighbor, teacher, nurse, or other health care provider. Similar to the psychosocial assessment of an adult establishing rapport with both the child and parent(s) is critical to establishing trust. Ideally, the child or adolescent is interviewed alone; followed by interviewing

the parent(s) and finally, seeing the child or adolescent with the family. Major questions to ask include reasons for the current appointment; family strengths, spiritual, or religious needs (Tanyi, 2006) and preferences, academic and social performance; behaviors that got the child or adolescent in trouble. Younger children have difficulty articulating reasons for the appointment—other assessment tools, such as art or painting or play therapy may provide important data. The 3-year-old child who is grieving with her parents about the recent loss of a younger sibling may exhibit regressive behavior, such as sucking her thumb or wetting her pants after being potty trained. Other children may cry a lot, become apathetic or irritable. Information from parents or caregivers provides additional information that balances the child's explanation or behavior. Extensive evaluation of children and adolescents, particularly for trauma-related and child abuse issues, requires advanced educational preparation and clinical expertise in trauma, particularly when the legal system requests a psychiatric evaluation.

The adolescent who is acting out as reflected by apathy, frequent arguments, and isolation may be depressed or abusing substances. Due to the sensitivity and sometimes distrust of adults, the nurse must discuss confidentiality issues during the beginning of the interview. Specifically, it is important to ensure confidentiality except when the youth is at risk for harming self or others. Compared with boys, girls have evaluated a higher amount of perceived interpersonal stress and have used more social support. Gender-related issues must also be considered during the evaluation process. Researchers submit that girls tend to score higher than boys on maladaptive coping styles and emotional distress and score lower on distraction than boys (Hampel & Petermann, 2006). It is imperative to assess the youth's perception of their coping style, which may include suicide attempts, impulsivity, or sexually acting out. The nursing process requires data collection from both youth and parent(s) that includes facilitating active participation in the decision-making process—based on the youth's developmental state. (See Table 5–5, Key Points for Assessing the Child and Adolescent.)

Older Adults

Working with older adults, like other age groups, requires an empathetic and respectful approach that allays anxiety and fears, engenders trust, and encourages the client to share their experience about mental and physical concerns. Enlisting the client in the decision-making process engenders a sense of mastery and confidence. Of particular importance is to determine how the client wants to be addressed (e.g., surname). Ageism interferes with objective nursing process and ability to determine the client's values, beliefs, and health practices, and generational and cultural needs. Nurses must initially and continuously assess the client's strengths and spiritual and religious needs to ensure client-centered and holistic health care. Due to high co-existing medical and psychiatric conditions in the older adult, a differential diagnosis is imperative to ensure an accurate diagnosis is made and appropriate interventions are initiated. (See Table 5–6, Key Points for Assessing the Older Adult.)

TABLE 5–5
Key Points for Assessing the Child and Adolescent

- Be familiar with normal growth and development and behaviors unique to each age group
- Identify reasons for referral
- Establish rapport with the child and caregiver
- Assess reasons for appointment
- Ask parents who made the referral
- What is the parent's understanding of causes and the nature of the child's/adolescent's problem?
- What are the parent's expectations about the assessment and treatment options?
- Ask questions about academic and behavioral functioning
- Identify hobbies, normal daily activities
- Discuss confidentiality and privacy issues based on child's or adolescent's age
- Inform child/adolescent of issues in which confidentiality cannot be maintained (i.e., thoughts of suicide or homicide, danger to self or others)
- Inquire about fears

Assess

- Developmental history and milestones
- Psychiatric or medical problems and treatment
- Family social history
- Peer relationship history
- Quality of parent–child interaction; relationships with siblings, close associates
- Peers
- Safety; suicidal and homicidal risk
- Dress and general appearance (i.e., hygiene, grooming, appropriateness)
- Language, level of English proficiency

See Table 5–2 for additional Mental Status Examination information.

Spiritual Assessment

An essential component of data collection is the spiritual assessment. There is a resurgence of interest in the spiritual domain of care. This renewed interest and integration of spirituality into the nursing process is consistent with nursing's commitment to holistic and individualized health care (Kylma & Venvilainen-Julkunen, 1997; Latorre, 2000; Longo & Peterson, 2002). Integrating spirituality into the nursing process helps reduce symptoms and distress, strengthens integrity, fosters interpersonal relationships, and validates and enhances the nurse and client's personal quest for meaning (Weaver, Flannelly, Flannelly, Koenig, & Larson, 1998). In addition, the spiritual assessment helps the nurse recognize his own spirituality and religious beliefs and gain a greater understanding of the client's. The following can assist in the spiritual assessment:

- Determine the meaning and significance of spirituality or religious practices.
- Assess and understand spiritual and religious values that are different from the nurse's.
- Assess the client's sources of faith and strength and the relationship between spirituality and health (Coleman, 2006; Dalmida, 2006; Tanyi, 2006).

Understanding the meaning of the client's experiences, strengths, and coping behaviors provides a solid foundation for individualized holistic treatment planning.

Although data concerning clients' mental status and psychosocial issues are crucial to health planning for clients with psychiatric disorders, it is vital, if not life-saving, to assess their physical needs. Ruling out medical conditions and ensuring that the client's "psychiatric" symptoms do not arise from underlying medical conditions (i.e., diabetes, hypothyroidism) must be an integral part of the nursing process.

TABLE 5–6
Key Points for Assessing the Older Adult

- Recognize age-related changes unique to older adults, including sensory deficits, such as hearing loss and potential and actual impact on level of functioning
- Assess degree of loneliness and isolation and sense of hope
- Use MMSE in Table 5–4 to assess memory and cognitive function

Assess capacity and functional status that may include:

- Capacity to maintain independence
- Perform activities of daily living (e.g., bathing, grooming, hygiene, eating, shopping, driving)
- Gait and mobility
- Hobbies and recreational activities
- Quality of life and support system

Physical Examination

Major aspects of the physical examination include a review of systems and questions about the last physical examination and results of diagnostic tests. Major diagnostic tests, can be used to assist in assessing the client's physical status and ruling out medical conditions. These tests include a complete blood count, with differential thyroid function tests, chemistry profile, toxicology screens, renal and liver function studies, blood tests for sexually transmitted diseases (STDs), electrocardiogram (ECG), pregnancy tests for women of childbearing age, and a thyroid profile. Additional data are obtained from the physical examination, including vital signs, neurological status (i.e., gait, pupil size or response to light, tremors), laboratory findings, sleep patterns, change in libido, appetite and concentration patterns, and overall level of functioning.

In summary, the assessment or data collection process is the first step in the nursing process. On completion of the initial database or assessment, the nurse must synthesize and analyze relevant client data and discern actual and potential problems or diagnoses.

Data collection from Ms. Adiaha includes changes in sleeping, eating, and concentration patterns over the past 6 weeks. She reports losing her job several months ago after being employed 20 years as an engineer. She fears that she will be unable to find employment because of her age. Her husband corroborates her history and expresses concerns about her present behavioral changes.

NURSING DIAGNOSIS

Diagnoses are synonymous with client problems. **Nursing diagnosis** is a statement of the client's nursing problem that includes both the adaptive or maladaptive health response and contributing stressors.

Standard II: Diagnosis

The psychiatric-mental health nurse analyzes assessment data in determining diagnoses.

The criteria for psychiatric nursing diagnoses include recognizing *defining characteristics* and identifying patterns or *related factors* of response or actual or potential mental illness and mental health defined within the scope of psychiatric-mental health nursing practice (NANDA, 2007). These data depict the client's present condition and continuous progression through various stages of illness or maladaptation until the resolution of the actual problem(s). Furthermore, diagnosing involves making inferences and using sound clinical judgment regarding client problems.

Diagnoses comply with accepted classification systems developed by the NANDA (2007), which are used in clinical settings to identify the client's actual and potential adaptive and maladaptive responses. After the nurse makes a diagnosis, it needs to be further validated by the client, significant others, and other health care providers. These findings are documented to promote identification of client outcomes, care plans, and research (ANA, 2000). Nursing diagnoses provide the basis of nursing interventions necessary to achieve outcomes for which the nurse is accountable (Doenges, Moorehouse, & Burley, 2000). Refer to the Research Abstract.

Diagnostic and Statistical Manual of Mental Disorders, 4th edition, Text Revision (DSM-IV-TR) Diagnoses

The *DSM-IV-TR* (APA, 2000) is an approved psychiatric coding system. Specific criteria are listed for specific mental disorders. These criteria must be present before a diagnosis is

RESEARCH ABSTRACT

A Taxonomy of Passive Behaviors in People with Alzheimer's Disease

Colling, K. B (2000). *Image: Journal of Nursing Scholarship, 32,* 239–244.

Study Problem/Purpose

To construct a taxonomy of passive behaviors for understanding people with Alzheimer's disease (AD). Passive behaviors were defined as those associated with a decline in motor movements, decrease in social interactions, and feelings of apathy and listlessness.

Methods

The taxonomy was constructed using extensive reviews of fifteen empirical studies published from 1985 through 1998. Research data were collected using key words: AD, apathy, and passive and negative symptoms. Major data sources included Medline, PsychLit, and Cumulative Index of Nursing and Allied Health Literature (CINAHL). Criteria for selection included (a) data-based research; (b) focus on passivity of AD; (c) referred journals. Concept analysis was formulated into a coding system or taxonomy.

Findings

Five categories of behaviors were delineated and comprised categories of behaviors associated with passivity in AD: diminutive cognition, psychomotor activity, emotions, interactions with people, and interactions with the environment. These data added to the midrange theoretical propositions of the Need-Driven Dementia-Compromised Behavior (NDB) model that indicates that behaviors of clients with AD arise from pursuit of goals or expression of needs.

Implications for Psychiatric Nurses

Psychiatric nursing can use these data to further delineate a taxonomy of passive behaviors in people with cognitive impairment. These data can assist in the nursing process and identify apathy and passivity behaviors as distinct patterns of personality changes that occur in clients with AD.

made. The *DSM-IV-TR* is an interdisciplinary tool used by all members of the mental health care team. Nursing and medical diagnoses may complement each other, but each is a unique and separate entity. See Chapter 4 for a comprehensive discussion of the *DSM-IV-TR*.

Data from the case example suggest that Ms. Adiaha is depressed. The findings include the following nursing diagnoses:

◆ Violence, Risk for Self-Directed

◆ Ineffective Coping

◆ Sleep Pattern, Disturbed

◆ Self-esteem, Low

See Nursing Care Plan 5–1.

OUTCOME IDENTIFICATION AND PLANNING

Standard III: Outcome Identification and Standard IV: Planning

Standard III: The psychiatric-mental health nurse identifies expected outcomes individualized to the client.

Standard IV: The psychiatric-mental health nurse develops a plan of care that prescribes interventions to attain expected outcomes.

Planning guides the nurse and helps to ensure that therapeutic interventions are used in a systematic manner to achieve planned outcomes for the client. The major treatment intent of identification of client outcomes is health promotion and restoration, that is, what the client can expect from nursing interventions or treatment. Client outcomes must be realistic, attainable, therapeutic, individualized, measurable, and cost-effective.

An individualized plan of care directs therapeutic interventions that facilitate successful resolution of client problems by restoring physical and mental health, preventing illness, and effecting rehabilitation. It is a blueprint that guides nurses and mental health professionals in identifying client outcomes, effective treatment options, and client activities, and that delegates specific functions to the mental health team. The nurse's role is determined by educational level, clinical experience, and certification.

For instance, all nurses are trained to use the nursing process, but specific interventions require specialized training, certification, and educational preparation. The generalist nurse is a baccalaureate-prepared registered nurse who is primarily involved in promoting health restoration, assessing maladaptive responses, improving coping behaviors, and preventing further maladaptation. This is accomplished by managing the client's basic needs such as activities of daily living, maintaining a therapeutic milieu, practicing case management, administering psychotropics, and assessing client response and milieu therapy. Community functions may include home visits, case management, and joining the crisis team of a mental health center or homeless shelter.

In contrast, the advanced-practice registered nurse (APRN) has a master's degree, PhD or DNP, who has acquired an in-depth knowledge of human behaviors and complex causal factors. This nurse is able to apply this knowledge and

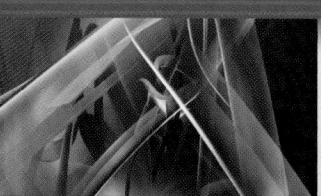

NURSING CARE PLAN 5–1

The Depressed Client (Ms. Adiaha)

Nursing Diagnosis: Risk for Self-Directed Violence

Outcome Identification	Nursing Actions	Rationales	Evaluation
1. By [date], client verbalizes feelings rather than acting on them.	1a. Establish rapport. Encourage expression of feelings.	1a. Establishes therapeutic interaction. Conveys empathy, caring, and interest.	*Goal met:* Nurse forms therapeutic relationship. Client expresses feelings. Client does not express suicidal ideations or act on thoughts.
	1b. Maintain a safe environment. Assess level of dangerousness.	1b. Provides safety and control and decreases acting-out behaviors.	
	1c. Observe for mood changes. Notify physician of changes in behavior.	1c. Change in mood increases risk of dangerousness.	

Nursing Diagnosis: Ineffective Coping

Outcome Identification	Nursing Actions	Rationales	Evaluation
1. By [date], client develops realistic perception of present stressor(s).	1a. Explore meaning of recent job loss and other stressors.	1a. Helps the client understand self and present responses.	*Goal met:* Client returns to precrisis level of functioning. Client develops adaptive coping skills. Client's self-esteem increases.
	1b. Understand meaning of present stressors.	1b. Validates understanding of meaning of present symptoms.	
2. By [date], client develops enduring adaptive coping skills.	2. Assist in identifying strengths, resources, and coping skills.	2. Places focus on positive attributes and increases self-esteem.	

Nursing Diagnosis: Disturbed Sleep Pattern

Outcome Identification	Nursing Actions	Rationales	Evaluation
1. By [date], client's normal sleeping patterns return to optimal level.	1a. Assess normal sleeping patterns.	1a. Helps nurse identify normal sleeping patterns.	*Goal met:* Client's normal sleeping patterns return and are maintained.
	1b. Maintain quiet environment.	1b. and c. Promotes rest, sleep.	
	1c. Provide comfort measures.		

Nursing Diagnosis: Self-esteem, Low

Outcome Identification	Nursing Actions	Rationales	Evaluation
1. By [date], client verbalizes 2–3 positive attributes and increased self-esteem.	1a. Provide successful experiences.	1a–c. Positive experiences increase confidence and self-esteem.	*Goal met:* Client's self-esteem increases. Client is able to explore options to deal with present stressors.
	1b. Convey acceptance and empathy.		
	1c. Encourage active participation in treatment.		

solve complex problems involved in mental health and mental illness. Specific interventions often consist of an array of psychotherapy, unit management, private practice, consultation and liaison functions, and prescriptive authority. Regardless of the nurse's role, collaboration with clients, families, and other mental health professionals broadens the scope of practice, the efficaciousness of treatment, and the evaluation of client responses.

IMPLEMENTATION

After the nurse assesses the client, identifies problems or nursing diagnoses, establishes client outcomes, and develops a plan of care, how will he implement the plan? Application of knowledge and testing hypotheses are critical components of implementation and intervention. An array of interventions can be used to promote health and minimize the deleterious effects of mental illness. Specific interventions are determined by the identified client needs and may include milieu therapy, stress management, health education, behavior modification, psychotropic medications, and various psychotherapies.

Standard V: Implementation

The psychiatric-mental health nurse implements the interventions identified in the plan of care.

Implementation is an open, dynamic process, and interventions are continuously being monitored by client responses. This process enhances nurse-client collaboration, maximizes resources, and provides seamless health care services.

EVALUATION

Criterion-focused evaluations are standards by which nursing interventions are measured. The decision to continue

interventions and continuously monitor client responses is a major nursing role in caring for persons with mental illness.

Standard VI: Evaluation

The psychiatric-mental health nurse evaluates the client's progress in attaining expected outcomes.

As the client's health status changes, so does the nursing care. The complexity of mental illness and client responses challenges nurses to use sophisticated evaluation measures to assess client needs. The acutely ill client experiencing hallucinations, delusions, and agitation requires immediate relief of these symptoms. Major nursing interventions include establishing trust, administering or prescribing medication to reduce anxiety and agitation, maintaining nutrition, and promoting self-care. Acutely ill clients have numerous needs and require ample nursing care. In contrast, when acute symptoms are alleviated, nursing care decreases and often involves decreased monitoring. Specific interventions may include individual or marital therapies, discharge planning, stress management, intensive case management, and health education. Overall, nursing care is a dynamic process that varies with client needs, cost-effectiveness, available resources, and the preparedness of the nurse.

SUMMARY

- The nursing process is the foundation of nursing.
- The nursing process provides a systematic and scientific approach to identifying client needs and potential outcomes.
- Opportunities to promote health reduce deleterious effects of mental illness.
- Psychiatric-mental health nurses can maximize the effects of the nursing process by collaborating with members of the mental health team and client and family members to identify and respond to clients in distress.

STUDY QUESTIONS

1. Mr. Jones presents in the emergency room complaining of a tight neck and difficulty turning his head. He reports a history of taking haloperidol (Haldol) over a period of 2 weeks. Haldol is an antipsychotic agent used to treat schizophrenia and other psychotic disorders. What is the most appropriate nursing action?
   a. Attempt to develop a therapeutic relationship with him.
   b. Gather more information about his medication.
   c. Inquire if he has had these symptoms before.
   d. All of the above.

2. During the interview the nurse asks the client questions about delusions, preoccupations, and obsessions. These

 **CRITICAL THINKING**

Mr. Curry is seen in the emergency department (ED) complaining of a stiff neck and difficulty moving it shortly after taking his morning dose of haloperidol (Haldol). He also reports a history of bipolar disorder and that he has been on this medication for about a week along with his mood stabilizer. Based on this scenario and data collection process, what is the most appropriate nursing action?

a. Establish rapport and reassure the client that help is available.

b. Establish rapport and ask the client if he is taking his medication as ordered.

c. Reassure that his symptoms are minor and non-life-threatening.

d. Tell the client that his symptoms are rare but manageable.

questions are likely to elicit data concerning which of the following?

   a. Thought content

   b. Orientation

   c. Thought processes

   d. Cognition

3. Mary, an 18-year-old girl, is seen in a community mental health clinic. She has a history of bipolar disorder, and today she is complaining of stomach pain. What is the *most* appropriate nursing action?

   a. Disregard her "stomach pain" because she is probably delusional.

   b. Inquire about the duration and progression of pain.

   c. Offer her medication to manage her thoughts.

   d. Document her complaints and ask her to call if it persists.

4. Michael is a 25-year-old client with a diagnosis of depression. He presents with persistent complaints of sleep disturbances. All of the following are appropriate nursing interventions *except:*

   a. inquiring about present medications

   b. documenting his complaints

   c. assessing for suicide risk

   d. instructing him to take an over-the-counter sleep medication

5. Ms. Marry, a 59-year-old married woman, is seen in primary care clinic by the nurse who looks hurried and busy. The client immediately accuses the nurse of being unconcerned. What is the *most appropriate* nursing action?

   a. Acknowledge the client's concerns and take time to listen.

   b. Take time to listen, but let her know that there are more clients waiting.

   c. Ask another nurse to talk to the client.

   d. Apologize and reschedule her for a less busy time.

6. Mark is a 21-year-old who has just been diagnosed with first episode schizophrenia. During your interview with him he talks about the wind whispering and being able to communicate with the television. Based on your understanding of schizophrenia, what is the most accurate explanation for his symptoms?

   a. He is having sensory-perceptual disturbances.

   b. He is unable to sleep due to the voices and has sleep deprivation.

   c. He has disorganized thought processes.

   d. His speech is incoherent.

7. When performing a mental status examination and assessing the client's mood, what is the most important data to document in the client's record?

   a. Congruency or incongruency between thought content, affect, and mood.

   b. Congruency between thought processes and mood.

   c. The presence or absence of delusions and mood changes.

   d. Congruency between thought processes, affect, and mood.

8. What of the following questions is most likely to help the nurse assess visuospatial ability?

   a. "How often does your loved one get lost?"

   b. "What would be the first thing you would do if you lost your wallet in a busy airport?"

   c. "Subtract serials of 7s from 100."

   d. "What does 'a rolling stone gathers no moss mean'?"

9. Mrs. King has been recently admitted to the psychiatric emergency room with a diagnosis of acute psychosis. During the interview her speech is rapid, pressured, and circumstantial. These symptoms are typically seen in persons with which of the following conditions?

   a. Schizophrenia

   b. Bipolar disorder, manic episode

   c. Major depression

   d. Panic disorder

10. During your nursing assessment you want to test the client's ability to abstract a proverb. What is the most important information needed before testing the client's ability to abstract?

   a. Is the client familiar with the proverb?

   b. What is the client's educational level?

   c. Is the client cooperative enough to respond to the question?

   d. Is the proverb consistent with the client's culture?

RESOURCES

Please note that because Internet resources are of a time-sensitive nature and URL addresses may change or be deleted, searches should also be conducted by association or topic.

Internet Resource

www.NANDA.org   North American Nursing Diagnosis Association

Other Resources

Sadock, B. J., & Sadock, V. A. (2005). *Kaplan and Sadock's Comprehensive textbook of psychiatry,* 8th edition. Philadelphia: Lippincott, Williams & Wilkins.

REFERENCES

American Nurses Association. (2000). *Scope and standards of psychiatric-mental health nursing practice.* Washington, DC: American Nurses Publishing.

American Psychiatric Association. (2000). *Diagnostic and statistical manual of mental disorders, 4th edition, Text Revision (DSM-IV-TR).* Washington, DC: Author.

Antai-Otong, D. (2007). Nurse client communication: A lifespan approach. Sudsbury, MA: Jones-Bartlett Publishers.

Coleman, C. L. (2006). Spirituality: An ongoing search for meaning: Implications for mental and physical health, *Issues in Mental Health Nursing, 27,* 113–115.

Colling, K. B. (2000). A taxonomy of passive behaviors in people with Alzheimer's disease. *Image: Journal of Nursing Scholarship, 32,* 239–244.

Dalmida, S. G. (2006). Spirituality, mental health, physical health, and health related to quality of life among women with HIV/AIDS: Integrating spirituality into mental health care. *Issues in Mental Health Nursing, 27,* 185–198.

Doenges, M. E., Moorehouse, M. F., & Burley, J. T. (2000). *Application of nursing process and nursing diagnosis* (3rd ed.). Philadelphia: F.A. Davis.

Folstein, M. E., Folstein, S. E., & McHugh, P. R. (1975). Mini-mental state: A practical method for grading the cognitive state of patients for the clinician. *Journal of Psychiatric Research, 12,* 189–198.

Goode, C. J., & Piedalue, F. (1999). Evidence-based clinical practice. *Journal of Nursing Administration, 29,* 15–21.

Hampel, P. & Petermann, F. (2006). Perceived stress, coping, and adjustment in adolescents. *Journal of Adolescent Health, 38,* 409–415.

Institute of Medicine. (2001). *Crossing the quality chasm: A new health system for the 21st century.* Washington, DC: National Academy Press.

North American Nursing Diagnosis Association. (2007). *Nursing diagnoses: Definition & classifications, 2007–2008 (nursing diagnoses).* Philadelphia: Author.

King, I. (1971). *A theory for nursing: Systems, concepts, process.* New York: John Wiley & Sons.

Kohn L. T., Corrigan J., & Donaldson M. S., (eds) for the Committee on Quality Health Care in America, Institute of Medicine. (2000). *To err is human: Building a safer health system.* Washington, DC: National Academy Press.

Kylma, J., & Venvilainen-Julkunen, K. (1997). Hope in nursing research: A meta-analysis of the ontological and epistemological foundations of research on hope. *Journal of Advanced Nursing, 25,* 364–371.

Latorre, M. A. (2000). A holistic view of psychotherapy: Connecting mind, body, and spirit. *Perspectives in Psychiatric Care, 36,* 67–68.

Lohr, K. N. (2004). Rating the strength of scientific evidence: Relevance for quality improvement programs. *International Journal of Quality Health Care, 16,* 9–18.

Lohr, K. N., Eleazer, K., & Mauskopf, J. (1998). Health policy issues and applications for evidence-based medicine and clinical practice guidelines. *Health Policy,. 46,* 1–19.

Longo, D. A., & Peterson, S. M. (2002). The role of spirituality in psychosocial rehabilitation. *Psychiatric Rehabilitation Journal, 25,* 333–340.

North American Nursing Diagnosis Association. (2005). *Nursing diagnoses: Definitions & classification 2005–2006.* Philadelphia: Author.

Peplau, H. E. (1952). *Interpersonal relations in nursing: A conceptual frame of reference for psychodynamic nursing.* New York: Putnam.

Rosswurm, M. A., & Larrabee, J. H. (1999). A model to change evidence-based practice. *Image: Journal of Nursing Scholarship, 31,* 317–322.

Tanyi, R. A. (2006). Spirituality and family nursing: Spiritual assessment and interventions for families. *Journal of Advanced Nursing, 53,* 287–297.

Travelbee, J. (1971). *Interpersonal aspects of nursing* (2nd ed.). Philadelphia: F.A. Davis.

Weaver, A. J., Flannelly, L. R., Flannelly, K. J., Koenig, H. G., & Larson, D. B. (1998). An analysis of research on religious and spiritual variables in three major mental health journals, 1991–1995. *Issues in Mental Health, 19,* 263–276.

SUGGESTED READINGS

Alfaro-Lefevre (2005). *Applying the nursing process: A tool for critical thinking* (6th ed.). Philadelphia: Lippincott-Williams & Wilkins.

Atkinson L. D. & Murray, M. E. (2000). *Understanding the nursing process: In a changing health care environment.* McGraw-Hill.

ANA. (2004). *Nursing scope and standards of practice,* Washington, DC: Author.

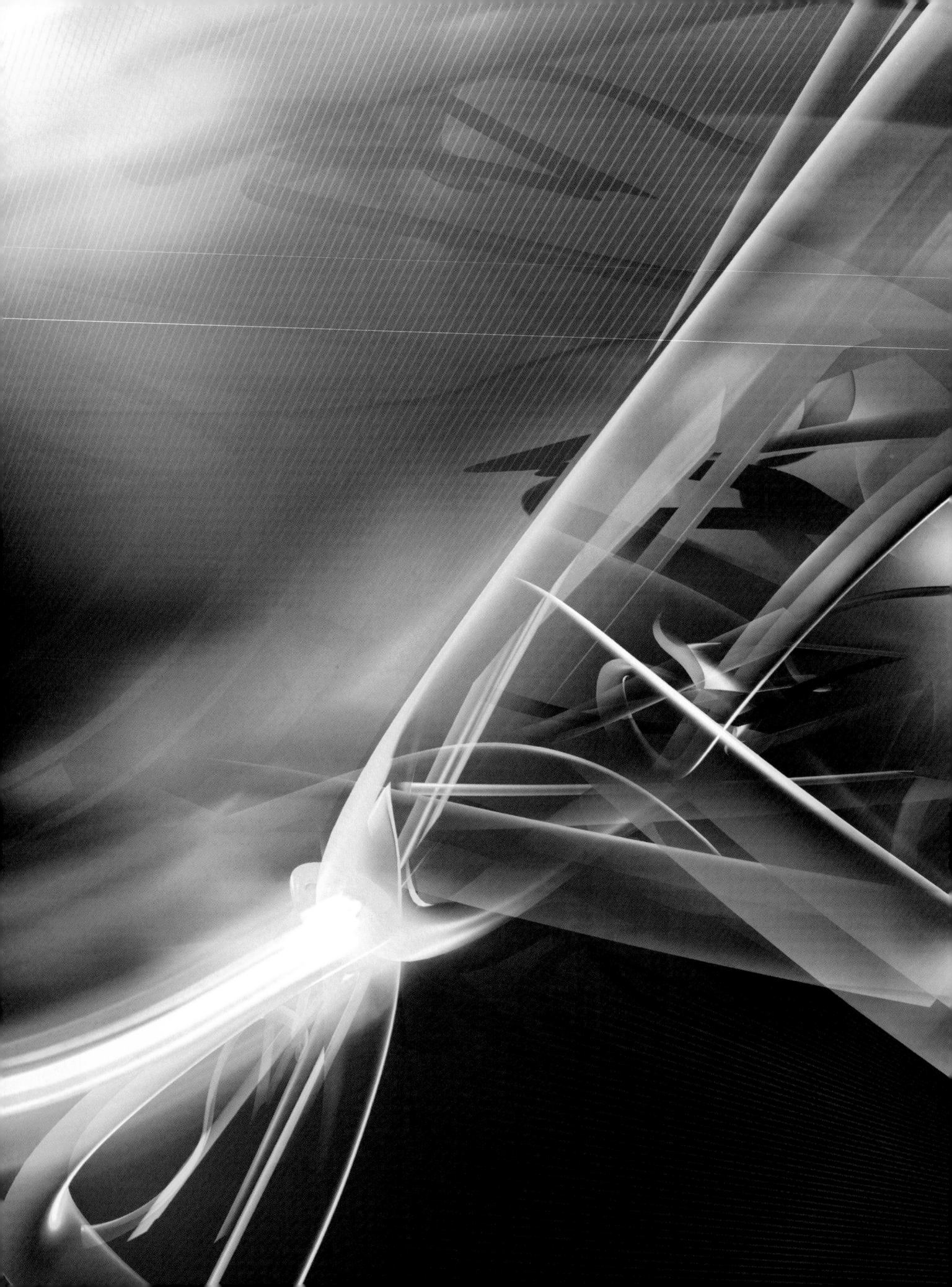

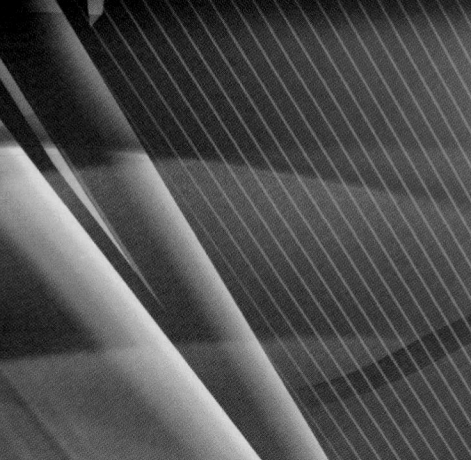

CHAPTER 6

Therapeutic Communication

Deborah Antai-Otong, MS, APRN, BC, FAAN

KEY TERMS

Active Listening: A dynamic process that requires using all senses to assess verbal and nonverbal messages.

Body Language: Nonverbal communication or transmission of messages by way of physical gestures.

Clarifying Technique: Act of clearing or making a message understandable.

Communication: The act of transmitting feelings, attitudes, ideas, and behaviors from one person to another.

Confrontation: The act of pointing out contradictions or incongruencies between feelings, thoughts, and behaviors; specifically, pointing out parts of an assessment or treatment process that are contradictory or confusing.

Empathy: Refers to putting oneself into the psychological frame of reference of another. It conveys an understanding of the client's situation without becoming emerged or overwhelmed by the experience.

Focusing: The act of clarifying a perception or spotlighting a specific aspect of communication.

Language: A complex phenomenon and tool used to communicate.

Nonverbal Communication: Refers to body language or transmission of messages without the use of words.

Personal Space: A subjective definition of comfortable space between one person and another.

Rapport: Refers to harmony or accord between people.

Telemental Health: The use of technologies such as videoconferencing to provide mental health and psychiatric services.

Therapeutic Communication: A healing or curative dialogue between people.

COMPETENCIES

Upon completion of this chapter, the learner should be able to:

1. Understand the neurobiological, psychosocial, and developmental factors of communication.
2. Discuss major communication theories.
3. Assess verbal and nonverbal communication.
4. List the major principles of therapeutic communication.
5. Recognize developmental factors that interfere with communication patterns.
6. Describe the concepts of the nurse-client relationship.
7. Integrate Peplau's theory into the nursing process.

CHAPTER OUTLINE

Causative Factors of Communication Patterns

Neurobiological Issues

Psychosocial Issues

Developmental Issues

Communication Theories

Dyadic Interpersonal Communication Model

Behavior and Communication

Communication Competency

Transactional Analysis and Communication

People are social beings who use communication as the basis of all interactions. They convey feelings, attitudes, and emotions through speech, touch, facial expression, and various other modes. Communication is a dynamic and complex process between people used to influence, gain mutual support, and gather from others the essentials needed for well-being, growth, and survival (Howells, 1975).

Human beings depend on verbal and nonverbal communication to master their world. The infant learns to differentiate and relate to caregivers through feeding, crying, and touching. Early experiences lay the foundation of lifelong communication patterns and interpersonal relationships.

Establishing interpersonal relationships is an integral part of psychiatric-mental health nursing. It enables the nurse to appreciate the uniqueness of human behavior and establish healthy nurse-client interactions. *Interpersonal* refers to relations between persons. Clients experiencing distress benefit from therapeutic interactions with nurses.

Communication refers to the transmission of feelings, attitudes, ideas, and behaviors from one person to another. This process is generally classified as therapeutic or nontherapeutic.

Therapeutic communication refers to a healing or curative dialogue between people. This is particularly significant to the nurse because it is the basis of therapeutic relationships. Therapeutic communication fosters an active collaborative process that facilitates problem solving, change, learning, and growth. The nurse-client relationship is a dynamic partnership that defines, directs, and evaluates treatment outcomes.

The purpose of this chapter is to discuss and integrate the major communication theories into psychiatric-mental health nursing practices.

CAUSATIVE FACTORS OF COMMUNICATION PATTERNS

Therapeutic communication is the matrix of psychiatric-mental health nursing. It involves an exchange of information between clients and nurses. Communication is conveyed through feelings, attitude, or thoughts. This reciprocal process enables the nurse to effect adaptive changes in the client (Travelbee, 1971).

The foundation of therapeutic communication is rapport. Rapport refers to harmony or accord between people. This initial alliance is vital to the formation of trust. As the therapeutic relationship evolves, so does the client's willingness to trust and share information. This relationship affords psychiatric-mental health nurses with opportunities to assess complex client needs, develop mutual outcome identification, and evaluate client responses. Evaluation is determined by the client's verbal and nonverbal communication patterns.

The nature of communication patterns is complex and involves several components. The major components of communication patterns relate to an array of neurobiological, psychosocial, and developmental issues.

NEUROBIOLOGICAL ISSUES

Information exchange occurs within the brain and central nervous system. This process arises from biochemical processes that alter emotional and behavioral responses to higher brain levels, such as the cortex. Mediation of information throughout the nervous system is crucial to human survival and adaptation.

Historically, technological advances provided clearer depictions of the neurobiological processes that govern communication. Promising studies on emotional body language are gaining acceptance as a new arena in cognitive and affective neurobiology. Neuroimaging via brain mapping illustrates neural systems involved in cognitive process and more recently limbic activation to emotional and physiologic stimuli. Gläscher and her colleagues (2004) assert that human faces provide significant signals during social interactions by positing two primary forms of communication, individual uniqueness and emotional expression. The ability to readily assess both the variance and consistency among emotional expressions in diverse people is central to the individual interpretation of the immediate environment. Researchers assert that the basis of body language, including facial expression and distance are governed by cognitive processing or cortical input and subsequent limbic activation. This premise indicates the pivotal role of the amygdala in emotional and cognitive processing, and infers its receptivity to the task relevance or irrelevance of the emotional expression (Gur, Schroeder, Turner, McGrath, Chan, Turetsky, et al., 2002). The amygdala and anterior cingulated gyrus are implicated in the network involved in distinguishing and ascribing affective information presented below the normal threshold of conscious or executive function visual perception (Kilgore & Yurgelun-Todd, 2004). Studies also demonstrate alterations in emotional and cognitive processing and subsequent facial expressions with age. Typically, during neuroimaging studies involving emotional discrimination tasks, younger adults activated visual, frontal, and temporal-limbic and amygdala neural pathways, while older adults activated parietal, temporal, and left-frontal cortices (Gunning-Dixon, Gur, Perkins, Schroeder, Turner, et al., 2003). Alterations in these brain regions result in impaired processing of facial expressions relating to certain negative emotions, such as fear, anxiety, and anger and often underlie clinical symptoms of psychiatric disorders, such as post-traumatic stress disorder and other anxiety disorders and schizophrenia. Common behavioral responses

and communication patterns associated with these neurobiological underpinnings include intense fear, worrying, anxiety and hyperarousal along with sensory–perceptual disturbances.

Adaptation models suggest that people constantly interact with internal and external environments. Appraisal of one's environment is determined by higher brain centers and mediated by neuroendocrine processes. Stress activates the hypothalamus directly or indirectly through the limbic system (see Figure 13–1). The cerebrum, the hypothalamus, and the surrounding structures constitute the limbic system. The cerebrum is responsible for cognitive function, creativity, and intentional information, whereas the hypothalamus is the core of the limbic system. This area is only the size of a thumb tip, but its blood supply is one of the most abundant in the whole body. The hypothalamus is the locus of feelings of pleasure, rage, anger, sexual arousal, hunger, and thirst. The neural links of the cerebrum and the hypothalamus allow a constant circulation of biochemical processes that modulate human instinct and emotions. Emotional responses are located in these areas, and they evoke distress and other adaptive responses to internal and external stimuli (Gur, Schroeder, et al., 2002).

Sensations and perceptions are used to experience internal and external stimuli. The senses enable people to acquire information through neural pathways and organs. What one hears, sees, feels, smells, and tastes influences one's perception of the world. *Perception* refers to the dynamic process of assimilating and organizing sensations.

People who are unable to communicate effectively for neurobiological or psychosocial reasons experience feelings of frustration, shame, and despair. Clients with aphasia or sensory deficits are vulnerable to psychological distress. Older adults in extended or long-term care facilities are particularly at risk for maladaptive responses to impaired communication. Assessing the needs of this population is vital to its socialization, self-care, and independence (Raymer et al., 2007).

Buckwalter, Cusack, Beaver, Sidles, and Wadle (1988) described behavioral changes generated by a collaborative nursing and speech-language pathology intervention. Their subjects were elderly aphasic and dysarthric clients in a long-term care facility. Findings from this study suggested several interventions that minimize maladaptive responses in aphasic and dysarthric elderly clients, including the following:

◆ Develop client-based treatment planning.
◆ Provide therapeutic environments that enhance social interactions.
◆ Establish one-to-one therapeutic relationships.

Another study (Irish, 1997) described how selected encoding (facial expressions, expression of pain, speech-related gestures, gaze, and touch) and decoding (pain expression, hearing and vocal affect, and sensory impairment barriers) characteristics have relevant outcomes in terms of satisfaction with care, quality of life, and health status. Data from this study indicate that improved nonverbal communication between the health care provider and older adults improved the quality of care.

Findings from these studies reinforce the need for nurses to appreciate sensory and perceptual deficits in various age groups and the mentally ill. The client experiencing auditory hallucinations and persecutory delusions is an example of how impaired sensory and perceptual processes affect communication. This client often communicates impaired verbal and nonverbal cues, such as incoherent speech, agitation, and aggressiveness. These behaviors suggest that neurobiological processes are largely responsible for impaired communication patterns.

Nurses need to assess impaired communication patterns and formulate interventions that reduce client distress. Establishing rapport and providing biological interventions, such as medication, can calm and reduce impaired sensory and perceptual responses. Accurate assessment and appropriate interventions reduce distress and restore health. Psychiatric-mental health nurses can optimize this process by exploring the psychosocial and developmental factors that affect adaptation and communication.

PSYCHOSOCIAL ISSUES

People are social beings. Emotional ties foster a sense of identity, comfort, security, and support. From birth to death, relationships with others are central to human existence.

Early attachments lay the foundation of healthy relationships. Attachment theorists, Bowlby (1969) and Ainsworth (1985), purport that early relationships are essential to growth and development, and they govern a person's ability to relate to others and manage anxiety. The quality of early attachments is influenced by the cultural, socioeconomic, and mental health status of the caregivers. Through various parental gestures and communication patterns, the infant learns about the world. Ideally, attentive parents convey safe and secure environments that nurture growth and facilitate congruent communication development. (See Chapter 2 for an in-depth discussion of attachment theory.)

In contrast, the person who grows up in an environment that lacks clear communication and uncertainty about the world is likely to have difficulty relating to others. Difficulty forming meaningful relationships interferes with expression of feelings, thoughts, and needs, further compromising optimal functioning.

Communication is critical to healthy human interactions. Integrating neurobiological and psychosocial factors into the communication process enhances the nurse-client relationship. Overall, it enables the psychiatric-mental health nurse to respond to complex client needs and facilitate health restoration.

DEVELOPMENTAL ISSUES

The third major factor that influences communication is developmental stage. Four stages have been identified in language development and communication:

1. The first stage and initial communication begins with the birth cry, which evolves into gurgles and variations in sounds and sucking rates that convey different needs.

2. The second stage involves cry vocalizations and variations in sounds and pitches.

3. The third stage consists of babbling, which varies with culture and is influenced by the intonation patterns and language of the primary caregivers.

4. The evolution of "true speech" begins in the fourth stage, which ends the first year, and is described as prelinguistic vocabulary. These stages parallel cognitive and neurobiological development, which influence refinement of schemata and systematic growth of logical operations or understanding of self and the world. In applying Piaget's theory, nurses can interpret a child's behaviors (both verbal and nonverbal), depending on the stage of cognitive functioning, that is, sensory-motor, preoperational, concrete operational, or formal operational stage of reasoning. Sociological factors also play a major role in language and communication development. Learning takes place in the context of reciprocating motor gestures between the infant and the primary caregivers (Condon & Sander, 1974; Piaget, 1970).

Communication processes begin prenatally, at which time the stress level and coping abilities of parents influence neurobiological maturity. The fetus is also vulnerable to conditions that affect neurobiological development, such as genetics, rubella, and other teratogenic influences.

As the fetus moves from intrauterine life to the newborn stage, parents continue to provide basic survival needs. Bonding and attachment are essential aspects of infancy. Tactile stimulation promotes psychological and neurobiological growth. Early attachments and interactions with caregivers depend on how emotions, warmth, trust, and safety are conveyed. The sound and tone of the caregivers' voices, stroking, and facial expressions symbolize early messages about the world. Parents who transmit warmth and love foster trust and safety in the child (Ainsworth, 1985; Bowlby, 1969).

In comparison, parents who are unresponsive to the child's basic needs convey anger, distrust, and uncertainty about the world. A negative or indifferent portrayal of the world compromises neurobiological and psychosocial development. Delayed cognitive and motor development and, in severe cases, failure to thrive and death are potential outcomes for the neglected child. Delayed or impaired cognitive and motor development interferes with the child's ability to express feelings, thoughts, and ideas. Inability to communicate effectively affects the child's self-esteem, social skills, and growth. As the child moves into adolescence, these factors become more pronounced. The child who fails to develop trust, self-esteem, and autonomy is at risk for mental illness, particularly in adolescence.

Adolescence is a stage that exemplifies early childhood frustrations. The adolescent who fails to master previous developmental tasks is at risk for maladaptive responses such as depression, substance abuse, and suicide. Several developmental issues that interfere with establishing therapeutic interactions in this age group include the following:

◆ Difficulty developing trust

◆ Frequent limit testing and acting out

◆ Need for immediate gratification

◆ Expressed hostility toward authority figures such as parents and teachers

◆ Low tolerance to stress and frustration

The family who instills trust, self-esteem, and autonomy in the adolescent fosters growth, effective coping, and communication skills. Thus, the adolescent can form meaningful and lasting relationships and master future developmental tasks.

The relationship between early childhood interactions and adult behaviors is well documented. Adults can use competent communication skills to solve problems, meet basic needs, and form stable interpersonal relationships. Major adult developmental tasks are intimacy, generativity, and integrity.

Developmental issues are pertinent to understanding human behavior. Trust is crucial to human development because it influences how people relate to others. The complexity of therapeutic communication challenges nurses to understand factors that affect client behavior. In working with younger children in particular, the message conveyed may exist beyond the spoken language. Nurses must listen for children's voices in a variety of dimensions, including audible sounds and words, artwork, facial expressions, body language, music, and silence. It is the nurse's responsibility as advocate to attend to expressions outside the normal realm and try to understand their meaning (McPherson & Thorne, 2000). Factors such as the client's ability to establish trust and the effects of neurobiological, psychosocial, and developmental issues are relevant to human responses. Refer to Table 6–1.

TABLE 6–1
Communication with Clients across the Life Span

	Developmental Influences	Age-Specific Behaviors	Age-Specific Communication
Prenatal	Genetics, maternal mental health, particularly during the 2nd and 3rd trimesters affects the fetuse's HPA axis regulation, damage during birth process		
Infancy	Mental retardation, fetal alcohol syndrome, sensory deprivation (aloof caregivers), impaired nutrition	Crying, cooing, poor eating, fretfulness, touching, eye contact, babbling (beginning of language at 6 months; putting sounds together)	Stroking; holding; feeding; eye contact (mirroring); soft, warm voice from caregivers
Childhood	Autism, mental retardation, sensory deprivation	Limited vocabulary that evolves using tones, inflections, tense	Concrete explanations; drawing a picture; warm, accepting approach
Adolescence	Psychosis, substance abuse, depression	Abstract thinking evolves, increased comprehension	Encourage participation in decision-making process; accepting and supportive approach; active listening
Adulthood	Medical conditions, substance abuse, psychosis, impaired nutrition	Cognitive function and abstract capabilities, adequate interpersonal skills	Establish rapport, genuine interest, empathy, active listening
Late adulthood	Medical conditions, aphasia, impaired cognitive/sensory function	Cognitive function intact, impaired hearing/vision, slowed thinking processes	Active listening, assess ability to speak, read, write; develop alternate way to communicate as needed; allow time to express feelings and respond to questions

COMMUNICATION THEORIES

What is communication? The word *communicate* means to share, impart, and participate. Several theorists have defined communication.

DYADIC INTERPERSONAL COMMUNICATION MODEL

According to the dyadic interpersonal communication model described by Berlo in 1960, communication is a dynamic interaction that consists of a source, who has a purpose that is understandable to another person, and an encoder, who is able to understand the meaning of the message. The message is processed and decoded and understood by the recipient, or decoder (Figure 6–1). In essence, people must convey clear messages if they expect the information to be understood.

BEHAVIOR AND COMMUNICATION

Walzlawick, Beavin, and Jackson (1967) contended that behavior is a form of communication and that messages convey information. They described this process as the message is the basic communication unit; a series of messages is called an *interaction;* and levels of communication are associated with specific patterns of interactions.

COMMUNICATION COMPETENCY

Virginia Satir (1967) surmised that the degree of communication competency represents how well people interact with others. The client who is suffering from hallucinations or delusions is an example of how impaired communication affects social interactions. This client is distracted by internal and external stimuli that compromise interactions with the nurse.

In contrast, the politician who campaigns across the state uses effective communication skills to convey the political message to potential voters. This person's communication skills enable her to interact with constituents with little effort.

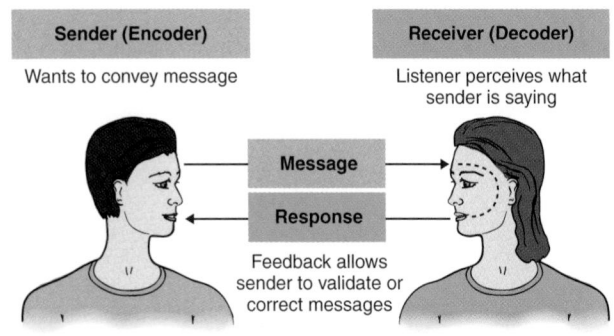

Figure 6–1 Berlo's (1960) dyadic interpersonal communication model.

TRANSACTIONAL ANALYSIS AND COMMUNICATION

Eric Berne (1964) coined the term *transactional analysis* (TA). This theory incorporates four major themes necessary to understand human behavior: structural analysis, to assess what people are experiencing; TA, to assess what is going on between two people; racket and game analysis, to assess specific interactions that have negative payoffs; and script analysis, to assess individual life plans. TA is discussed for purposes of describing communication patterns.

TA is based on games people play to act out life scripts. A game is a set of behaviors and attitudes exhibited by a person interacting with another person. Berne (1964, 1973) asserted that everyone has three functional parts called *ego states.* Ego states depict feelings and relate sets of behavioral patterns. The three major ego states are known as PAC:

Parent: comprises attitudes and behaviors from parental figures. This ego state is further subdivided into critical, or controlling parent and nurturing parent.

Adult: comprises rational and logical processes that appraise reality; the main sources are information from internal and external environments.

Child: comprises feelings or emotions and impulses that represent the natural or spontaneous part of the person. This is further subdivided into the "free child," "adapted child," or "little professor."

The fundamental element of TA is appraising interactions between people. The healthy individual puts the Adult in charge but allows the Child to emerge during fun times and dismisses early critical messages from the Parent ego stage. TA may be especially helpful in working with the difficult client or in communicating with subordinates from a nursing leadership perspective (Bailey & Baillie, 1996).

THERAPEUTIC COMMUNICATION

Reusch (1961) described communication as a universal function that occurs everywhere. He enumerated the following major components of therapeutic communication:

◆ It can occur anywhere.

◆ It can be used to promote independence and improve interactions with others.

◆ It is a natural part of human beings.

◆ It relies on spontaneous expression of feelings and thoughts.

◆ It enables clients to accept past experiences and integrate them into present-day perceptions.

To summarize, communication is a complex, dynamic process that involves a sender and a receiver. Messages are conveyed through various symbols and clues within a social context. The value of communication lies in the ability to use various symbols or ideas to convey a common understanding of the message (Peplau, 1952). Psychiatric-mental health nurses are confronted with having to decipher verbal and nonverbal messages regarding client responses.

TYPES OF COMMUNICATION

Major mechanisms of communication are diverse and often influenced by culture, ethnicity, biological, and developmental and psychosocial factors. However, information is generally imparted by nonverbal and verbal communication.

NONVERBAL COMMUNICATION

Nonverbal communication refers to body language or transmission of messages without using words. It comprises behaviors such as facial expression, tears, laughter, affect, physical appearance, posture, touch, eye contact, body movement, gestures, and speech rate and volume. Nonverbal communication is a natural and spontaneous process that often occurs with verbal communication. Nonverbal behavior is a potent form of communication, especially in terms of building rapport and conveying empathy and support. Assessing the meaning of various client responses is an integral aspect of psychiatric-mental health nursing.

Nurse-client interactions consist of both verbal and nonverbal communication. *Nonverbal* communication refers to the process or feeling, whereas *verbal* refers to the content (Birdwhitsell, 1970). The goal of therapeutic interactions is congruency between nonverbal and verbal communication. The nursing student who tells the client that he is feeling well today, and his thoughts, mood, and facial expression reflect this message, conveys to the client that he indeed feels good today. In contrast, the client who tells the nursing student that she is not upset, but her facial expression is grimaced and her fists are clenched, conveys that she is upset. The client's verbal and nonverbal communications are incongruent.

Nonverbal communication has greater impact than verbal communication and yet not enough attention in nursing is focused on this area in communication training programs (Kruijver, Kerkstra, Francke, Bensing, & van de Wiel, 2000). The old adage, "action speaks louder than words," is relevant to understanding communication in any society. Birdwhitsell (1970) believed that 65 to 70 percent of communication is based on nonverbal cues and that 30 percent is spoken, or verbal. The impact of nonverbal communication on nurse-client interactions is noteworthy because it affects one's perception of clinical situations. For example, individuals who are highly suspicious and paranoid are extremely sensitive to environmental stimuli and nonverbal communication such as sudden movements, touching, or raising one's voice. It is imperative for the nurse to approach these individuals cautiously using a normal voice tone, maintaining a safe distance, and avoiding physical contact.

A major limitation of nonverbal communication is the inability to validate the meaning of feelings. Nonverbal expression such as screaming or shouting is easy to assess as anger. However, the meaning of a sad expression or inappropriate smiling is more difficult to assess unless the client validates its meaning. Nurses can validate perceptions through observations and verbal interactions with clients. Observing body language is a critical aspect of validating nonverbal communication.

Body language refers to manifestation of feelings or thoughts by way of body gestures. The nurse's body language is just as significant as the client's. Clients observe nurses' behaviors and can readily identify incongruent verbal and nonverbal communication. Gladstein (1987) and Egan (1994) described several of a nurse's nonverbal behaviors that convey warmth, caring, and calmness to clients. They are:

◆ Facing the client directly

◆ Turning and leaning the face and body to the client

◆ Maintaining eye contact (avoid staring)

◆ Nodding to convey validation, acceptance, and understanding

◆ Positioning the body to imply an open and natural behavior

◆ Presenting a natural, soft smile to communicate warmth

Body language is a powerful nonverbal communication tool. Recognizing its usefulness helps nurses understand their own behaviors and those of the client. Body language includes the following:

◆ Facial expressions

◆ Physical appearance

◆ Eye contact

◆ Posture and gait

◆ Hand movements and gestures

◆ Tone of voice and rate of speech

Facial Expressions

Facial expressions reveal internal feelings and emotions. They convey a number of feelings that are reflected in the client's forehead, lips, mouth, and eyes. Intense messages are easier to assess than subtle responses. Expression of a flat, blunted, or incongruent affect often masks feelings and emotions.

Physical Appearance

Physical appearance, such as personal hygiene, posture, dress, and appropriateness of clothes for season and weather; and coordination of color, patterns, and accessories, reveals the client's level of functioning, confidence, and self-worth. Clients with psychosis may present in a disheveled manner, suggesting that their ability to manage self-care is impaired. In addition to a disheveled appearance, these clients' clothes may be soiled, wrinkled, and smell of body odor. Mental status, emotional state, and current employment must be considered when assessing physical appearance.

Eye Contact

Eye contact provides a channel for nurses to connect with clients in a manner that conveys genuine concern and care. Inner feelings are often reflected through one's eyes. Eyes disclose important messages and communicate important information about the nurse and the client. Direct eye contact suggests involvement. In contrast, limited eye contact communicates a lack of interest or low self-esteem. Cultural and ethnic considerations must be made because the significance of eye contact varies among specific populations. Other factors that may influence the client's eye contact are alterations in mood or thought processes. The client with depression or schizophrenia may have poor eye contact, whereas the client with mania may be overly direct and intrusive.

Posture and Gait

Posture and gait communicate several nonverbal cues. Authority is communicated by the height from which one interacts with others. This can be seen when one person stands and the other sits; the former unconsciously places the self in a position of power. The client in a group session who jumps up to confront another client establishes power by this behavior.

The manner in which clients carry themselves often reflects self-concept, mood, and health. An erect posture and an active, purposeful stride reflect high self-esteem. Low self-esteem or physical discomfort is exhibited by a slouched, slow, shuffling stride. Rigid, tense, or rapid posture and gait usually convey anxiety or anger. Pacing is indicative of agitation and restlessness in clients with psychotic disorders or those with a potential for violence toward themselves or others.

Hand Movements and Gestures

Hand movements and gestures, like other body movements, are expressive. These gestures and others, such as pacing or speaking loudly, may indicate agitation and potential violence. Nursing interventions include recognizing the meaning of these behaviors and reducing the risk of further escalation of the client's anger and agitation. Specific nonverbal communications that may be used in this situation include approaching the client from the side in a calm, firm, and cautious manner; responding to eye contact; and maintaining a comfortable distance.

Clients with schizophrenia or paranoia tend to distance themselves and remain on guard. Guardedness and social withdrawal are shown when clients turn away from the nurse and present an invisible wall that shields them from external stimuli generated by interactions. In comparison, clients with a manic type of bipolar disorder are often intrusive and invade the personal space of others.

Tone of Voice and Rate of Speech

Voice tone and rate of speech are other nonverbal cues that mirror the client's emotional state. Manic or anxious clients often speak at a pressured or rapid rate, angry or agitated clients may speak loudly, and depressed clients may speak in a low, passive tone.

VERBAL COMMUNICATION

Verbal communication, like nonverbal behavior, transmits feelings such as anger and happiness. This process involves an exchange of words, both spoken and written, between people. Nurses cannot assume that what is spoken means

RESEARCH ABSTRACT

Expressing Health Experience through Embodied Language

Liehr, P., Takahashi, R., Nishimura, C., Frazier, L., Kuwajima, I., & Pennebaker, J. W. (2002). *Image: Journal of Nursing Scholarship, 34*, 27–32.

Study Problem/Purpose

The purpose of this study was to describe embodied language for Japanese older adults who suffered a stroke or cardiac disease within the previous 12 months.

Method

Blood pressure measurements and spoken words were recorded simultaneously when 17 subjects with cardiac disease and 20 subjects with strokes were asked to describe their personal health experiences for 4 minutes. Language data (life stories or descriptors of health expression) were analyzed with word analysis software, which was tape recorded and transcribed and translated from Japanese to English by a single interpreter. A second interpreter, also fluent in Japanese and English, also reviewed these data.

Findings

Data from the Japanese older adults (n = 37) ranging in ages from 60 to 89 years of age, average age of 75.1 years, showed that those with strokes retained higher blood pressure after talking than those with cardiac disease. The two groups showed contrasting relationships between word use and blood pressure readings, especially for temporal words. These findings also demonstrated the unity and pursuit of meaning when bodily and linguistic descriptors overlap.

Implications

These data from this collaborative research study between Japanese and American researchers, suggest the importance of cultural influences and promote a greater understanding of life-threatening experiences on older adults. It also indicates the power of communication, both in terms of body language or descriptors (blood pressure) and verbal communication. It offers psychiatric nurses opportunities to work with diverse populations in promoting mental and physical health.

what is said. The effective use of verbal communication varies among individuals. It is influenced by developmental stage, neurobiological components such as stress, cognitive function, and psychosocial and cultural factors.

What are the major principles of effective verbal communication? Rapport is the foundation of effective communication. It evolves as the client feels safe and at ease with the nurse. Specific techniques that encourage rapport are:

◆ A warm, caring approach

◆ Good eye contact

◆ A clear, firm voice

◆ Assertive, but not aggressive posture

◆ Quiet, comfortable environment

◆ Simple, clear explanations based on education, developmental stage, and cognitive function

◆ Active listening

These techniques allay client anxiety, foster expression of feelings, resolve miscommunication, and provide a model for effective communication patterns.

Verbal communication is an integral part of nurse-client interactions. Nurses can use it to share thoughts, encourage expression of feelings, enhance problem-solving skills, and clarify miscommunication. A study by Elliott and Wright (1999) showed that verbal communication even with unconscious or sedated clients allows for an exchange of information, provides emotional support during stress, and may improve outcome measures depending on the level and degree of interaction and training.

FACTORS THAT DIRECT COMMUNICATION PATTERNS

Therapeutic communication is a complex process, and its effectiveness is influenced by various factors that direct the communication process, including:

◆ Attitude

◆ Trust

◆ Empathy

◆ Language

◆ Culture

◆ Perception and observation

◆ Self-concept and self-esteem

◆ Anxiety and stress

◆ Personal space

ATTITUDE

The nurse's interest, acceptance, and attitude toward the client play major roles in therapeutic interactions. The nurse's *attitude* sets the mood of the nurse-client relationship. Clients need to feel valued and respected. The nurse conveys trust and empathy through verbal and nonverbal communication. The client needs to be approached in an unhurried manner, avoiding abrupt or indifferent responses. The client is more likely to be cooperative and participate in treatment when the nurse uses a calm, concerned approach. In one study examining the evolving nurse-client relationship, helping influences included consistency, pacing, listening, positive initial impressions, and attention to comfort and control. Relationships were hampered by inconsistency, unavailability, client factors related to trust, nurses' feelings about the client, confrontation of delusions, and unrealistic expectations (Hanson & Taylor, 2000).

TRUST

The concerned and caring nurse generates trust. The client feels confident and safe in these environments. Building trust involves a number of conditions such as the following:

◆ Keeping promises

◆ Exhibiting consistency and reliability

◆ Expressing genuine interest and concern

◆ Accepting the client's feelings and concerns

◆ Providing safe client care

◆ Encouraging active participation in care

◆ Encouraging independence and growth through positive experiences

◆ Providing ongoing feedback regarding response to treatment

Four common themes of competence in nursing practice include trusting, caring, communication skills, and knowledge and adaptability (Locsin, 1998). Therapeutic interactions foster feelings of closeness as each person maintains a sense of self, or separateness.

EMPATHY

Empathy communicates understanding and concern. Interestingly enough, a review of the literature reveals a lack of clarity and consensus on what exactly is meant by "empathy" (Reynolds, Scott, & Austin, 2000), yet it is always viewed as a critical aspect of therapeutic relationships. La Monica (1981) defined it as follows: "Empathy signifies a central focus and feeling with and in the client's world. It involves accurate perception of the client's world by the helper, communication of this understanding to the client, and the client's perception of the helper's understanding." (p. 398).

Similarly, Peplau (1987) described empathy as an ability to feel in oneself the feelings being experienced by another person. This powerful communication tool conveys "I am with you and I have a sense of what you are experiencing," without totally losing one's identity. More specifically though, empathy involves the sensitivity to current feelings and the ability to communicate this understanding in language attuned to the client's feelings (Truax, 1961), thus promoting change, growth, and health restoration. This temporary sharing enables the nurse to appreciate the client's feelings and thoughts. Empathy is an interpersonal skill that is dependent on the attitudes and behaviors of the nurse. The client can more easily develop trust when the nurse conveys warmth and empathy. This can be communicated by nonverbal and verbal cues. Eye contact, an unhurried manner, and a simple touch are examples of nonverbal cues. Reynolds (1994) developed an empathy scale to teach the skill in a more structured educational program. Unfortunately, the findings indicate major clinical barriers, including staffing levels, workload, rapid discharge, negative attitude of colleagues, and a lack of understanding of the therapeutic value of empathy. Another staff-patient interaction response scale (SPIRS) used in a study of pain management in an acute care setting indicated that empathic responses were not associated with patients' perceptions of less pain or being given adequate analgesia (Watt-Watson Garfinkel, Gallop, Stevens, & Streiner, 2000). Without adequate support and clinical supervision, emotional involvement can lead to stress and burnout. To practice empathy is to maintain one's own identity *while feeling with another;* it is to be objective while at the same time offering support and understanding (Antai-Otong, 2007).

LANGUAGE

Verbal cues consist of using words to communicate ideas, thoughts, and feelings. The basis of verbal communication is language. Language is a complex phenomenon and the tool we use to communicate with each other. It activates higher cognitive processes such as understanding, thinking, remembering, and reasoning. Through language we learn, educate, socialize, create, and validate perceptions of the world and ourselves by sharing feelings and thoughts. Effective communication through language is linked with mental health.

Language is mainly transmitted through speech and received through the senses. Communication relies on recognizable codes. Words are the central part of codes, and their meanings vary among people, cultures, states, and countries. Words alone do not convey feelings or thoughts. The interpretation of words is influenced by the recipient's perception of the message. The key to effective therapeutic communication is congruency between what the client says and the nurse's interpretation of the message. Effective communication is a reciprocal process. What the nurse says has an impact on this process along with the client's response. Unclear messages need to be validated through discussions with the client.

CULTURE

Culturally sensitive care is crucial to therapeutic communication. Whereas it may not be possible to know all cultural nuances, being attentive to understanding various influences may facilitate the delivery and quality of health care. Communication is difficult at best, but when the sender and receiver are from different cultures, the difficulty becomes even more pronounced. Psychiatric-mental health nurses must assess cultural congruency to minimize misunderstanding. Cultural influences may occur indirectly during client interactions and affect perception of client responses. When cultural incongruence is identified, the nurse needs to accept her limitations and seek ways to appreciate the client's uniqueness (Antai-Otong, 2007; Baumann, 2005). Cultural relativism refers to the notion that "behaviors of individuals should be judged only from the context of their cultural system" (Baker, 1997). Clients need to feel accepted and be treated with respect even though they are culturally different. Edward Hall (1966, 1989), a renowned anthropologist, recognized the significance of diversity and ethnicity as sources of strength. He described diversity as an invaluable asset to learn from others. Learning about others increases self-awareness. But why is intercultural communication so difficult? Taylor (2000) identified these reactions to explain the lack of receptivity: assumed similarity, ethnocentrism or denigration of differences, anxiety or tension, prejudice, stereotyping, and comfort with the familiar. She further advised six steps to overcoming these difficulties:

- ◆ Gain cultural knowledge.
- ◆ Look into your own cultural heritage.
- ◆ Confront prejudices.
- ◆ Get out of your comfort zone.
- ◆ Resist judgmental reactions.
- ◆ Improve communication skills.

In a culturally and ethnically diverse health care system, cultural competence promotes quality care and enhances excellence in nursing education, practice, and research (Warren, 2000). These processes and differences are cornerstones of therapeutic interaction and are crucial to the enrichment of nursing practice. (See Chapter 7 for an in-depth discussion of cultural influences.)

PERCEPTION AND OBSERVATION

Perception is the way events are interpreted through sensory stimulation. Past and present experiences and innate traits that validate or correct the receiver's interpretation determine perception. Thoughts are stimulated by perceptions, and feelings respond to thoughts. In the following example, the nurse's perception interferes with objective client care.

Nurse Brown may perceive clients who drink excessively as "bums." Her father was abusive when he drank excessively. Thoughts of her father generate negative feelings and anger toward the client abusing alcohol. Her ability to work with this client is compromised by her distorted perception of clients abusing alcohol.

Perceptions contribute to stereotyping and labeling of client responses. Historically, studies have shown that certain populations are more likely be diagnosed with chronic debilitating illnesses such as schizophrenia. Other groups are more likely to be diagnosed with less debilitating illnesses when their values and cultural and socioeconomic status are similar to those of the nurse.

Self-awareness is the key to understanding inaccurate perceptions and observations of client responses. Orlando (1961) asserted the importance of nurses developing skills that enable them to explore the meaning of their perceptions of clients rather than making assumptions. Additionally, she surmised that this process is "crucial in understanding more fully what the patient is trying to communicate" (p. 45).

Accurate interpretation of data is crucial to therapeutic communication. It affects data collection, care planning, interventions, and the evaluation of client responses. Psychiatric-mental health nurses must strive to provide quality care using accurate perceptions and assessments of client needs.

SELF-CONCEPT AND SELF-ESTEEM

Self-concept refers to one's beliefs and feelings about self. It serves as a frame of reference for life experiences and perceptions of the world. It evolves over time and arises from interactions with others. Self-concept plays a major role in adaptation and the maturational process. Successful resolution of developmental tasks or stressors shapes a positive self-concept.

Smits and Kee (1992) investigated the relationship between self-concept and self-care among older adults residing in the community. The findings showed a significant relationship between self-care and self-concept scores.

Similar assertions were made in a recent study in which researchers compared health-promoting behaviors and their relationship to self-esteem in institutionalized and non-institutionalized older adults in Korea (Kim, Jeon, Sok, & Kim, 2006). Researchers found that non-institutionalized older adults scored significantly higher on the Health Promoting Lifestyle Profile (HPLP), the Rosenberg Self-Esteem Scale (RSES), and the General Self-Efficacy Scale than institutionalized older adults and implicated the role of self-esteem on self-efficacy and self-care. Implications for psychiatric nurses include working with institutionalized older adults and developing client-centered interventions to increase their self-esteem and improve self-care.

Self-concept is relevant to psychiatric-mental health nurses because it determines how clients experience and manage stress. It affects the client's willingness to ask for and accept help. Clients with a poor self-concept are likely to feel unworthy of their needs being met. Their hesitancy to seek help often hinders the building of adaptive coping skills.

Self-esteem refers to self-worth and personal value. Maslow (1968, 1970) asserted that self-esteem is associated with having basic needs met. Basic needs are defined as physiological well-being, love, and safety. Self-esteem is closely related to self-concept.

Positive regard for self is comparable to high self-esteem. In contrast, negative self-regard suggests low self-esteem and associated feelings of worthlessness and inadequacy. These feelings can generate mood disorders such as depression and anxiety. These clients are also likely to use self-destructive behaviors such as substance abuse and suicide attempts to resolve stress.

Self-esteem and self-concept are dynamic and largely shaped by interactions with significant others. Psychiatric-mental health nurses can use these concepts to understand certain communication patterns in clients experiencing distress. Clients with high self-esteem express and share their feelings with others. Conversely, those with low self-esteem are likely to be passive and hesitant to share feelings. Assessing these behaviors helps nurses establish therapeutic interactions that increase self-worth.

ANXIETY AND STRESS

Client interactions normally produce anxiety in both the client and the nurse. *Anxiety* is described as a vague, uncomfortable feeling that manifests itself psychologically and biologically. Response to anxiety varies among people and can be both motivating and distressful. Lower levels of anxiety increase alertness and enhance problem-solving abilities. However, heightened levels of anxiety decrease cognitive processing, causing disruption and distress.

Sullivan (1954) described anxiety as the chief barrier to effective communication because it threatens self-esteem and self-respect. He also admitted that it is an inherent part of the human experience. As a natural part of human experiences, nurses need to take steps to help clients handle anxiety. Attempts to put the client at ease can be facilitated by using a calm, caring approach. A quiet, safe environment reduces distractions and facilitates expression of feelings and problem solving. Clients can manage their feelings constructively by using relaxation and stress-reducing exercises. Reducing anxiety and redirecting it into useful channels enhances communication.

PERSONAL SPACE

Hall (1966) introduced the concept of personal space in interpersonal relationships. He believed that human beings are constantly changing positions and that social interactions are affected by space. He defined space or zone norms from a Western cultural perspective as the following:

1. Intimate distance: 6 to 18 inches (between people touching)

2. Personal distance: 1½ to 4 feet (arm's length)

3. Social distance: 4 to 12 feet (most frequently used in business activities)

4. Public distance: 12 to 25 feet (entertainer, public speaker)

Hall stressed the need to appreciate cultural differences as the basis of space and individual differences when interpreting the meaning of space. The role of space in the nurse-client interaction is significant because it is difficult to assess another's comfort zones. As a rule of thumb, personal distance is usually considered comfortable. However, some cultures define comfort zones as close as 6 to 8 inches (Hall, 1966). It is important for the nurse to respect comfort zones and be aware of any boundary violations that may threaten one's safety.

THERAPEUTIC COMMUNICATION TECHNIQUES

A question often posed by students and nurses is, "What are therapeutic communication techniques?" A simple definition is that a therapeutic communication technique is one that facilitates therapeutic communication. In reality, the ability to communicate effectively is an art that uses basic listening and communication skills. The nurse can use this collaborative interaction to assess the client's needs, formulate client outcomes, and evaluate the effectiveness of interventions. Therapeutic techniques include the following:

◆ Active listening
◆ Questioning
◆ Clarifying techniques
◆ Therapeutic use of touch
◆ Therapeutic use of silence
◆ Humor
◆ Focusing
◆ Confrontation
◆ Summarizing

ACTIVE LISTENING

Active listening is the basis of all nurse-client interactions. Listening is more than just hearing. It is a dynamic and active process that requires enormous concentration and energy. It literally means using all the senses to assess verbal and nonverbal messages. The nurse listens for content as well as how the message is stated and what feelings are expressed. Active listening encourages clients to express feelings and thoughts.

Ceccio and Ceccio (1982) described qualities of a good listener as the following:

◆ Maintains eye contact
◆ Gives the client full attention, both mentally and physically, that is, makes a conscious effort to inhibit sounds and screen distractions
◆ Minimizes or eliminates barriers (see the following)
◆ Avoids interruptions and interpretations

◆ Responds to the content and feeling components of the message
◆ Listens for ideas, an essential aspect of interaction
◆ Provides the client with evidence that one is listening, (that is, reviews and restates in own words and reflects or plays back the message)
◆ Responds only to the content of the client's verbal message

Active listening conveys concern and respect for the client. It fosters a trusting relationship that encourages the client to express feelings and share thoughts. "Knowing the patient" and encouraging her to "tell their story" (Chambers-Evans, Stelling, & Godin, 1999) is essential in providing individualized and quality nursing care. However, recognizing nursing behaviors that interfere with active listening is just as important as appreciating those that promote it.

Barriers to Active Listening

Barriers to active listening (Table 6–2) exist in all clinical situations. The psychiatric-mental health nurse plays an active role in reducing or eliminating them. Pluckman (1978) noted that most barriers are psychological rather than physical. Additional barriers include the following:

◆ Lack of privacy
◆ Noises
◆ Seating arrangements
◆ Use of jargon
◆ Perceptual and sensory distortions in clients

TABLE 6–2
Major Barriers to Active Listening

1. Judgmental attitude (perception)
2. Blaming
3. Rigidity, dogmatic thinking (closed mindedness)
4. Providing solutions rather than facilitating this process in clients
5. Wrong vocabulary, clichés
6. Introducing unrelated information
7. Expressing disapproval
8. Giving advice rather than options
9. Discounting the client's feelings, e.g., asking questions such as "How can you be upset over something like that?"
10. Interrupting or changing the subject

- Countertransference
- Anxiety in the nurse
- Pain in the client

Other barriers include stereotyping the client by race, ethnic background, gender, age, class, religion, or illness.

Students and nurse clinicians can enhance their communication skills by identifying barriers to active listening. The art of active listening requires perseverance and patience. Initially, the nurse enters the relationship with a genuine interest and concern for the client. This puts the client at ease and enables the nurse to provide a safe, quiet, and private environment. Finally, the client experiences a sense of calmness, acceptance, and security and is able to verbalize feelings and thoughts.

QUESTIONING

Questioning is a valuable tool that nurses use to encourage the expression of feelings and self-disclosure and to gain insight into the meaning of present stressors. The basis of the client's response depends on her level of trust and security or in the comfort with the questions. Nurses can put their clients at ease by introducing themselves and calling them by name; making eye contact and shaking hands at the same time helps nurses connect with clients both verbally and nonverbally. This establishes a safe environment that promotes trust, care, and empathy. The nurse can use questioning as a tool to elicit pertinent information from the client.

Some examples of questions that elicit the most information from clients include the following:

- What major changes have you had during the past 6 months?
- How have they affected you or your lifestyle?
- What made you come in today?

Questions that begin with what, which, when, how, or who allow nurses to gather factual information and are defined as *open-ended questions*. They are direct, that is, they encourage clients to discuss and clarify their thoughts and feelings while passing the responsibility to the client to explore and understand these issues.

In contrast, *closed-ended questions* are less effective in collecting data than are open-ended ones. Closed-ended questions such as, "Would you like help with your problem today?" limit the client's response to yes or no, thus minimizing the quality of information. A more efficient way to assess what the client wants may be asked in a question such as, "What can I help you with today, Mrs. Read?" This question allows the client to explain her needs while taking responsibility for problem identification. Closed-ended sentences are relevant at times when specific factual information is needed, such as marital or employment status.

Questions should be generated by client responses, both verbal and nonverbal. A raised eyebrow, nodding, and increased voice tone are examples of nonverbal cues to the client's thoughts or feelings.

As the relationship evolves, clients may feel comfortable or entitled to know about the nurse. Nurse clinicians or students may wonder how to respond to personal questions. It is essential to keep clients directed and focused on their own issues. Questioning the nurse may mean that the client is anxious, curious, or distracted. The nurse can use these situations to clarify what the questioning means to the client.

CLARIFYING TECHNIQUE

Clarifying technique refers to the use of certain methods to clear up or make messages understandable. Communication is a complex, dynamic process that involves interaction between people. The likelihood of confusion exists in all human interactions. Clarifying communication patterns and exploring client responses are basic psychiatric-mental health nursing tools that reduce miscommunication and misunderstanding.

Specific clarifying techniques are paraphrasing or restatements. Paraphrasing involves listening to the client's basic messages and repeating them using similar words. This technique focuses on the content of the message. It affords the nurse with a clearer understanding of the client's distress. Client responses to paraphrasing validate or invalidate the nurse's perception of the client's message. Overall, the nurse's perception and observational skills are enhanced by clarifying techniques.

The following dialogue is an example of a nurse using clarifying techniques. The nurse begins the process by using a question to verify the meaning of a message. Note the use of this technique in the following situation:

Nurse-Client Dialogue 1

NURSE (clarifying question): Mr. Key, what do you mean when you say your mind feels like scrambled eggs? (Puzzled look on nurse's face)

CLIENT: I don't know!

NURSE (paraphrasing statement): It sounds like you are confused.

CLIENT: I am confused! Yes, I am very confused.

NURSE: What do mean "very confused?"

CLIENT: Well, my mind is playing tricks on me, and I feel like someone is watching me all the time.

NURSE: How long have you felt like this?

CLIENT: About 3 weeks.

NURSE (paraphrasing statement): You have been feeling confused and afraid for the past 3 weeks.

CLIENT: Yes, that's it, I feel like I'm going out of my mind.

In this example, the nurse was unsure of what the client meant by saying his "mind felt like scrambled eggs." The nurse could have made assumptions about the meaning of these words, but the nurse chose to ask him to explain it. His explanation gave the nurse a clearer understanding of his distress. In addition to seeking clarification, the nurse communicated empathy and concern.

THERAPEUTIC USE OF TOUCH

Touching is another powerful, sometimes controversial, nonverbal communication. It is a critical aspect of human relationships throughout the life span. Touching is key to survival, particularly during infancy, because it conveys trust, safety, and love, and it nurtures neurobiological and psychosocial development. As the child develops, touching becomes less important than other communication processes. Children tend to respond more favorably to touch than do adults.

Therapeutic use of *touch* refers to the healing powers of touch. Therapeutic touch enables the client to experience trust, reassurance, and acceptance (Figure 6–2). A trusting relationship is a prerequisite to the effective use of touch. Clients who are tearful and feeling sad usually find comfort from a touch on the shoulder or hand. One study by Peck (1998) indicated that therapeutic touch and progressive relaxation might be beneficial and improve functional ability of older adults with arthritis. The most improved functional abilities were mobility and hand function. Pain, tension, mood, and client satisfaction also improved after these interventions. Touching is both mentally and physically comforting, especially to clients with hearing and visual impairments. Confused and regressed clients also value human contact.

Prior to using therapeutic touch the nurse must assess each clinical situation for appropriateness and safety. The use of therapeutic touch must also be guided by the type and role

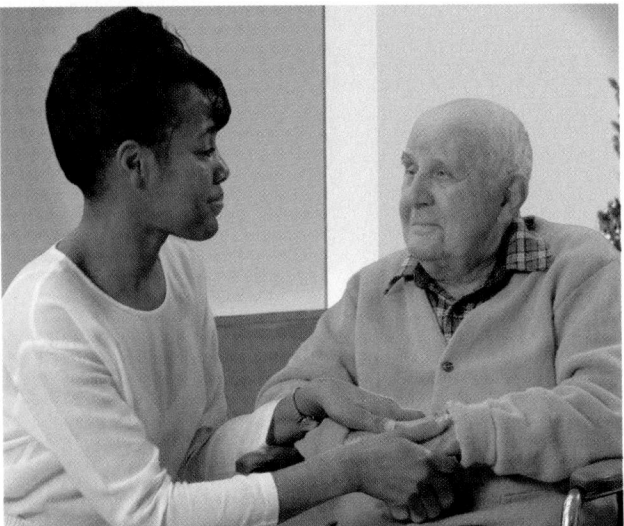

Figure 6–2 Clasping the client's hand is one way to communicate through touch.

of touch, developmental and cultural considerations, gender, the client's perception or expectations of touch, history of abuse in the client and family, and ethical considerations (McNeil-Haber, 2004). The nurse's personal safety, including boundary issues, history of abuse, and treatment goals must also be part of the decision to use therapeutic touch.

Some clients have difficulty responding to touch favorably. The client may perceive this as an invasion of her personal space and react defensively. Clients who have difficulty trusting, such as children or adults who have been abused, may be highly agitated and perceive touch as traumatic, invasive, frightening, or threatening. Clients with a history of abuse or violence may also misinterpret "good" touch as aggression. An inability to express feelings and warmth toward others undermines forming meaningful relationships. Some caution is typically advised in touching clients in a psychiatric setting but should not preclude its use. Much depends on the nurse's comfort level, correct interpretation of the situation, the client's cultural background, and the appropriate use of touch.

Therapeutic use of touch, like other communication techniques, enables nurses to establish meaningful interactions with clients in distress. Its healing qualities foster growth, vitality, and health.

THERAPEUTIC USE OF SILENCE

Silence is a natural phenomenon; it is a deliberate restraint from verbal expression. Therapeutic use of silence is another effective communication technique, but it requires practice and skill to master. Generally, novice nurses are uncomfortable with prolonged periods of silence.

Silence can be used to help clients explore the meaning of feelings and thoughts. An accepting, safe environment fosters self-awareness in both the nurse and the client. The depressed and tearful client needs silence to explore feelings and thoughts related to sorrow and loss. Silence may be uncomfortable to the nurse or the client, but it allows the nurse to collect thoughts and formulate responses until the client resumes the interaction. Silence can convey concern, interest, or acceptance of the client. The nurse needs to explore the meaning of feelings generated by silence, including the evaluation of the client's and the nurse's own level of anxiety or relief from emotionally charged content.

HUMOR

Humor is an important but underutilized therapeutic communication technique. Its value includes physiological, psychological, social, and cognitive benefits. Physiologically, it stimulates the circulatory and respiratory systems, relaxes the muscles, and increases production of endorphins. Humor helps clients express feelings, thereby reducing anxiety and tension or stress (Bennett, 2003; Wild, Rodden, Grodd, & Ruch, 2003), particularly during intense situations. Humor also reduces anxiety and promotes psychological adjustment and sense of well-being, particularly in clients with major medical and psychiatric illnesses (Dowling, Hockenberry, & Gregory, 2003). In addition, humor is culture-bound and must be used with caution in cross-cultural settings. Socially and clinically, humor has the capability of facilitating and enhancing interpersonal relationships and maintaining a sense of perspective (Dean & Gregory, 2004). Palliative care studies also demonstrate the importance of humor in humanizing various dimensions of care for the dying client and family (Adamle & Ludwick, 2005; Dean & Gregory, 2004). It enables the hospice or palliative care client to form genuine connectedness with caregivers and nursing staff while maintaining a sense of dignity and quality of life (Dean & Gregory, 2005). Cohen (1990) has said that laughter is the shortest distance between people. It can cut through barriers, provide opportunities to feel comfortable talking about things, and open the lines of communication, thus enhancing feelings of closeness, togetherness, warmth, and friendliness (Parse, 1993). Nurses can also use humor to normalize the abnormal and minimize the intensity of whatever is occurring, especially in difficult or stressful situations. Everyone loves to laugh, but inappropriate and untimely humor or laughter may be offensive. Although laughter evokes positive feelings, humor may generate unpredictable emotional responses. When used in a respective and sensitive manner, humor can facilitate quality and meaningful interactions between the nurse and client, caregiver and family (Penson, Partridge, Rudd, Seiden, Nelson, et al., 2005). Considerations, such as developmental stage, coping behaviors, culture and ethnicity, and timing must guide the nurse in the decision to use humor. Cognitively, humor facilitates learning by capturing attention and increasing memory (Astedt-Kurki, Isola, Tammentie, & Kervidenen, 2001).

Nurses can use humor to generate adaptive coping skills and to build self-esteem (Figure 6–3). In a study by Beck (1997), humor was found to:

◆ Help nurses deal with difficult situations and patients

◆ Foster a cohesiveness between nurses and their clients and also among nurses themselves

◆ Be an effective communication technique helping to decrease anxiety, depression, and embarrassment and foster a positive nurse-client relationship

◆ Be planned and routine but also unexpected and spontaneous

◆ Create lasting effects beyond the immediate situation

Humor, like other communication techniques, offers nurses and clients innovative strategies that enhance trust and acceptance. When used, its focus should be on an idea or situation or something other than the client. Successful use of humor also requires appropriate timing. Nurses should avoid humor during situations when the client is fatigued or feels unprotected or overly sensitive. In contrast, when the situation is tense, a humorous remark can reduce tension. Nurses can also benefit from humor by keeping a humor journal, sharing cartoons, using imagery, and conducting a humor

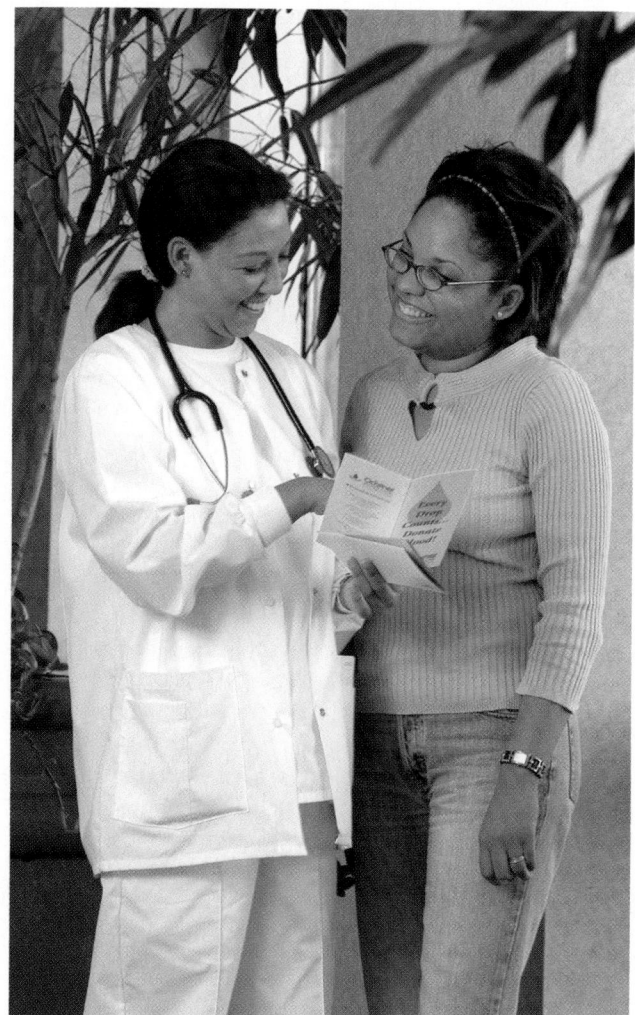

Figure 6–3 Nurses can use humor as a therapeutic communication technique.

self-appraisal (Antai-Otong, 2007). When nursing burnout is high and staff morale is low, laughter and humor should be valued and encouraged. Ultimately, humor seems to be closely tied to quality of life and health promotion.

FOCUSING

Focusing refers to clarifying a perception or spotlighting certain aspects of communication. This technique is useful when clients are vague and need assistance with goal-directed communication. Focusing is useful when clients do not express their feelings and thoughts clearly, when they ramble, or when they discuss several issues at one time. Nurses can use it to assess relevant client needs by selecting certain aspects of the client's discussion. The following dialogue is an example of focusing.

Nurse-Client Dialogue 2

NURSE: You have looked concerned since returning from your leave.

CLIENT: My wife says she cannot pay the bills and take care of the children while I am looking for a job.

> NURSE: It sounds like you are concerned about how she will manage things.
>
> CLIENT: I am unsure. We have always had two incomes.
>
> NURSE: It seems like you need to talk to her about your concerns.

This last statement asks for a specific response to a situation and provides a structure that helps the client organize his ideas and thoughts. The statement, "It sounds like you are concerned about how she will manage things," is an effort by the nurse to help the client focus on his feelings and concerns about his financial situation.

Focusing, like other communications, is used with other techniques to establish therapeutic interactions. Nurses use them to clarify and understand the meaning of client responses.

CONFRONTATION

Confrontation refers to an encounter or face-to-face meeting. Nurses often associate this term with conflict or angry discussions between opposing bodies. In reality, confrontation is a necessary aspect of nurse-client interactions. Like other techniques, it is an art that involves pointing out contradictions or incongruities between feelings, thoughts, and behaviors. These discrepancies interfere with insight and self-exploration regarding specific conflicts.

Confrontation is a useful tool that enables clients to examine maladaptive behaviors. Nurses must employ patience, tact, and support rather than a punitive approach to pointing out contradictory behaviors. The following is an example of confrontation:

> ### Nurse-Client Dialogue 3
>
> CLIENT: This is my third hospitalization, and I am still drinking.
>
> NURSE: Mr. Lett, what does this mean to you?
>
> CLIENT: You are the nurse, you tell me!
>
> NURSE: Mr. Lett, I have worked with you for the past year and I've notice that when you are discharged from the hospital, you do not attend Alcohol Anonymous meetings. It is difficult for you to stay sober if you do not participate in your 12-step program.

The nurse approaches the client in a warm but firm manner. This interaction encourages the client to appreciate certain behaviors, such as refusal to attend Alcoholics Anonymous meetings, which contribute to frequent relapses.

Confrontation is a dynamic, powerful interaction. Active empathetic listening is crucial to confrontation. Assessing verbal and nonverbal cues during this interaction enables the nurse to explore client strengths and maladaptive behaviors and to promote self-examination. Clients often respond in an angry or defensive manner when confronted.

Acceptance and tolerance of this behavior is essential to confrontation. Additionally, nurses must refrain from reacting in an angry or rejecting manner. These behaviors undermine the effectiveness of confrontation and interfere with objective client care.

SUMMARIZING

Summarizing is a communication tool that helps clients explore key points of a nurse-client interaction. This dynamic and collaborative process integrates perceptions from the nurse and client. Major points are reviewed and used to generate future client outcomes.

The following interaction is an example of summarizing:

> ### Nurse-Client Dialogue 4
>
> NURSE: Mr. Effiong, I noticed that you have been stressed since you were diagnosed with diabetes 2 months ago.
>
> CLIENT: You are right. I have been unable to sleep and concentrate because I have never been sick before.
>
> NURSE: What does it mean to have diabetes?
>
> CLIENT: I don't know, but my uncle also had diabetes, and he eventually lost one of his legs.
>
> NURSE: Tell me what you know about diabetes.
>
> CLIENT: Well, I know that I have to take pills because my pancreas doesn't put out enough insulin. I am also on a special diet.
>
> NURSE: How has this regimen affected your lifestyle?
>
> CLIENT: Not bad, because I have always watched my diet, and taking one more pill in the morning doesn't bother me. Besides, my uncle had to take insulin shots. (The client sighs with relief, and his facial expression is more relaxed.)
>
> NURSE: You look more relaxed. What does that mean?
>
> CLIENT: I guess I am not as sick as my uncle, and as long as I watch my diet and take my medication, I will be fine.
>
> NURSE: You were concerned about losing your leg.
>
> CLIENT: You are right, and I realize that if I do as I'm told, the chances of this happening to me are slim.
>
> NURSE: Well, now you know what was stressing you, which had to do with losing your leg. It sounds like you have decided that if you take your medication and stay on your diet, the chance of losing your leg is slim.
>
> CLIENT: That's right.

The nurse and client summarized major components of this interaction, and the nurse's comments reflected perceptions of the client's feelings, thoughts, and behaviors. The client validated these perceptions and helped the nurse understand his response to the situation. The client was an active participant in this process and was able to perceive his situation realistically. Verbalization of feelings and thoughts reduced his anxiety and helped him solve his problems more effectively.

TECHNOLOGIES AND COMMUNICATION

The concept of telepsychiatry and telemental health has existed for at least 40 years, but not until recently has the concept become more popular in an effort to provide mental health services to individuals living in rural areas and those with little or poor access to health care. Telemental health is the provision of consultation or training activities using diverse telecommunication systems to facilitate two-way interactive "real-time" communication to meet mental health needs. Recent advances in telepsychiatry or telemental health offer an array of cost-effective mental health services to clients in their homes and other community settings. Telemedicine increases access to mental health interventions by linking the client and the nurse using videoconferencing (VC) (see Figure 6–4). Individuals residing in rural areas have gained better access to services ranging from consulta-

tion, psychiatric evaluations and assessment, health education, and psychotherapy. A review of the literature involving telemedicine supported the premise that assessments can produce reliable results and psychiatric services involving this approach can facilitate improved clinical status, and clients and clinicians are satisfied with treatment delivered via telepsychiatry (Monnier, Knapp, & Frueh, 2003). Data from this study also demonstrated telemental health service as a cost-effective means of providing mental health care despite a limited number of studies that revealed economic models of telemental health. (See Table 6–3, Types of Telemental Health Services.)

Apart from telemental health care using videoconferencing, other technologies including telephone care, the Internet, and electronic messaging can be used to provide diverse mental health services. For example, in a randomized control study of 600 participants using a care coordination telephone program integrating care management and structured cognitive-behavioral therapy, researchers found a significant improvement in client satisfaction and clinical outcomes to clients on antidepressant medications. This approach reduces disparities in mental health services and offers care to lower-income clients and individuals living in rural communities (Simon, Ludman, Tutty, Operskalski, & von Korff, 2004). Similar results have been demonstrated, when other distancing

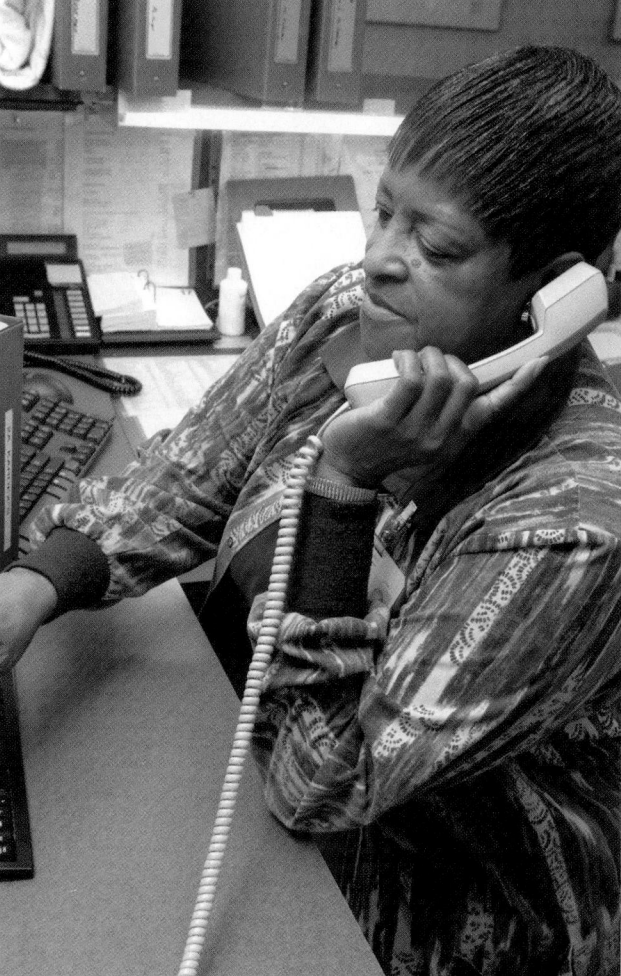

Figure 6–4 Videoconferencing is an example of Telemental Health Technology.

| TABLE 6–3 |
| Types of Telemental Health Services |

- Psychiatric evaluations
- Case management
- Medication management
- Crisis response
- Pre-admission and pre-discharge planning
- Treatment planning
- Individual and group therapy
- Family therapy
- Mental status evaluations
- Court commitment hearings
- Case conferences
- Family visits
- Family and consumer support groups
- Staff training
- Administrative activities
- Consultative services

Data from: Smith, H. A. & Allison, R. A. (1998). *Delivering mental health care at a distance. A summary report.* Rockville, MD: U.S. Department of Health and Human Services, Substance Abuse and Mental Health Services (1998). Health Resources and Services Administration Office for the Advancement of Telehealth, Rockville, MD (with permission), http://telehealth.hrsa.gov/pubs/mental/mental.pdf

technologies such as telemental consultation (Hunkeler et al., 2000) and computer programs using the telephone and Internet were used, to impart psychoeducation and other psychiatric interventions (Patten, 2003). Collaboration with primary care nurses and other clinicians using telemental health is growing in popularity as a cost-effective and quality approach to treating clients with depression, anxiety, and other psychiatric conditions. Psychiatric nurses are poised to provide mental health services using diverse approaches, including telemental health and other distancing technologies. As we approach the end of the next 5 years, it is imperative to meet the growing needs of clients in rural areas, provide health education and other resources to the Internet savvy consumer, and collaborate with clinicians in primary care and specialty clinics to facilitate holistic treatment and continuum of health across the life span.

NURSE-CLIENT RELATIONSHIPS: THE BASIS OF THE NURSING PROCESS

The nurse-client relationship is the basis of the nursing process. Therapeutic communication techniques are tools that are used to build and maintain these relationships. The effectiveness of these skills requires considerable thought and an understanding of the complexity of human behavior across the life span (see the Research Study display). According to Fortinash and Holoday-Worrat (1996), therapeutic relationships differ from social relationships in focusing on helping clients do the following:

◆ Solve problems
◆ Achieve growth
◆ Learn coping strategies
◆ Let go of unwanted behavior
◆ Reinforce self-worth
◆ Enhance self-concepts and confidence
◆ Examine relationships

The importance of the nurse-client relationship was recognized as early as 1946 by a number of nurse theorists. Major contributors to the evolution of the one-on-one or nurse-client relationship are Peplau (1952), Mellow (1967), and Orlando (1961). These theorists established the foundation of psychiatric-mental health nursing. The heart of this specialty is therapeutic communication.

The communication process is complex and dynamic. Its breadth extends beyond talking and listening to clients. This nurse-client interaction is a powerful process that uncovers issues within the nurse and client. These discoveries lay the foundation of adaptation and resolution of distress. Emphasis on this relationship is crucial to the psychiatric-mental health nurse and understanding complex human responses. Peplau (1994) has argued that the stimuli for constructive changes that clients need to make in their thinking and behavior take place in the interpersonal relationships between the nurse and client.

This discussion of the nurse-client interaction arises from the extensive contributions of Peplau. Her work has had profound impact on psychiatric-mental health nursing and the nurse-client relationship. Peplau's theory integrates major concepts from Sullivan's interpersonal theory. She delineated ways that the nurse uses in the nurse-client relationship to appraise and formulate effective interventions. Interventions are used to reduce maladaptive responses and enhance interpersonal interactions.

NURSE-CLIENT RELATIONSHIP PHASES

Peplau's (1952, 1991) classic work, *Interpersonal Relations in Nursing*, describe four phases of the nurse-client relationship. These phases are overlapping and interlocking, each outlining the task and role of the nurse and the client. The four phases are the following:

◆ Orientation
◆ Identification
◆ Exploitation
◆ Resolution

Orientation Phase

During the beginning, or orientation phase, the client recognizes a need and seeks help. The orientation phase is the foundation of the nurse-client relationship. It establishes the basis of subsequent phases. Major nursing roles are "resource person, counseling relationship, surrogate for mother, and technical expert" (Peplau, 1952, p. 21). The resource person provides pertinent information that helps the client understand her personal problems. In the counseling relationship, the nurse uses active listening skills to assess the reasons for the client's present distress and the client's perception of it. The surrogate role allows the nurse to deal with transference issues. Finally, in the technical expert role, the nurse uses various health-promoting interventions to facilitate adaptation. Overall, this phase affords the client with a caring and accepting environment that fosters expression of feelings and thoughts. Client responses are assessed, and outcomes are identified. Client outcomes need to be written in measurable and behavioral terms. Refer to Table 5–2 for an example of a psychosocial assessment tool.

The following dialogue uses the nursing process to facilitate therapeutic interactions:

Nurse-Client Dialogue 5

NURSE: Mr. Lynn, I am Ms. Marshall, your nurse today. I understand that you were admitted several hours ago. I would like to know about your reasons for coming in today. (The nurse sits next to the client and on the same level. She has good eye contact, and her voice is clear and soft.)

> **CLIENT:** My wife and kids say that I'm nuts! (The client's arms are folded, and he has poor eye contact.)
>
> **NURSE:** Nuts? What do you mean?
>
> **CLIENT:** Well, I have been sleeping 12 hours a day and I can't function at work. I am so depressed and feel like giving up.
>
> **NURSE:** What do you mean by "giving up?"
>
> **Client:** I am not sure, but I do not want to die.
>
> **NURSE:** How long has this been going on?
>
> **CLIENT:** Well, about a month this time.
>
> **NURSE:** What made you come in today rather than one or two weeks ago?
>
> **CLIENT:** Well, my boss is threatening to fire me. She's been through this too many times.

The nurse maintains a calm demeanor and uses good eye contact; her speech tone is unchanged. As a result, the client sees the nurse as genuinely concerned about his well-being. He relaxes his arms and increases eye contact. He is less agitated and more cooperative and begins to trust the nurse.

The major nursing diagnoses (see Nursing Care Plan 6–1) based on this nurse-client interaction are:

- ◆ Risk for Self-Directed Violence
- ◆ Ineffective Coping
- ◆ Disturbed Sleep Pattern
- ◆ Self-Esteem Low

Identification Phase

The second phase, identification, emerges after the client clarifies and recognizes interventions that facilitate adaptive changes. This is the beginning of the working phase of the relationship. The client becomes optimistic and ready for problem solving as the nurse-client relationship evolves. Exploration of distressful feelings and thoughts, such as powerlessness, inadequacy, and helplessness, begins. The nurse-client relationship nurtures initiative and learning (Peplau, 1952). This process encourages growth and adaptive coping patterns.

During the next few meetings, the client in the previous case begins to focus on his responsibilities in the treatment process. He discusses his feelings and thoughts and identifies

---

NURSING CARE PLAN 6–1

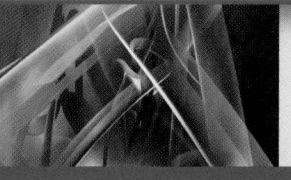

The Role of Therapeutic Communication in Therapy

Nursing Diagnosis: Risk for Self-Directed Violence

Outcome Identification	Nursing Actions	Rationales	Evaluation
1. By [date], client verbalizes feelings rather than acting on them.	1a. Establish rapport. Encourage expression of feelings.	1a. Establishes therapeutic interaction. Conveys empathy, caring, and interest.	*Goal met:* Nurse forms therapeutic relationship. Client expresses feelings. Client does not express suicidal ideations or act on thoughts.
	1b. Maintain a safe environment. Assess level of dangerousness.	1b. Provides safety and control and decreases acting-out behaviors.	
	1c. Observe for mood changes. Ask significant other to notify staff if mood changes.	1c. Change in mood or anxiety level increase risk of dangerousness.	

(continues)

Nursing Diagnosis: Ineffective Coping

Outcome Identification	Nursing Actions	Rationales	Evaluation
1. By [date], client develops realistic perception of present stressor(s).	1a. Identify and explore meaning of present stressors involving fear of losing job.	1a. Helps the client understand self and present responses.	*Goal met:* Client returns to pre-hospitalization level of functioning. Client develops adaptive coping skills. Client's self-esteem increases.
	1b. Understand meaning of present stressors. (recurrent depression and insecurity about job situation).	1b. Validates understanding of meaning of present symptoms.	
2. By [date], client develops enduring adaptive coping skills.	2. Assist in identifying strengths, resources, and coping skills.	2. Places focus on positive attributes and increases self-esteem.	

Nursing Diagnosis: Disturbed Sleep Pattern

Outcome Identification	Nursing Actions	Rationales	Evaluation
1. By [date], client's normal sleeping patterns return to optimal level.	1a. Assess normal sleeping patterns.	1a. Helps nurse identify normal sleeping patterns.	*Goal met:* Client's normal sleeping patterns return and are maintained.
	1b. Maintain quiet environment.	1b–d. Promotes restful and refreshing sleep.	
	1c. Provide health education about sleep hygiene.		
	1d. Encourage to keep a sleep diary.		

Nursing Diagnosis: Self-esteem, Low

Outcome Identification	Nursing Actions	Rationales	Evaluation
1. By [date], client verbalizes 2–3 positive attributes and increased self-esteem.	1a. Provide successful experiences.	1a–c. Positive experiences increase confidence and self-esteem.	*Goal met:* Client's self-esteem increases. Client is able to explore options to deal with present stressors.
	1b. Convey acceptance and empathy.		
	1c. Encourage active participation in treatment		

maladaptive behaviors. This process generates behavioral changes and growth.

Nurse-Client Dialogue 6

NURSE: Mr. Lynn, what do you expect from this hospitalization?

CLIENT: I want to feel better about myself. I feel depressed all the time, and sometimes I wish I were never born.

NURSE: What do you mean, you wish you were never born?

CLIENT: I have disappointed my family, my boss, and myself. I just think they would be better off if I were dead.

NURSE: Mr. Lynn, are you saying that you want to kill yourself?

CLIENT: Not really, but there are times I wish I didn't wake up.

NURSE: I am concerned about your thoughts of dying and death. Have you ever tried to kill yourself?

CLIENT: No! I would never kill myself, but I feel very depressed at times.

NURSE: Have you had these thoughts before?

CLIENT: Yes, but not this bad.

NURSE: What was going on in your life when you had these thoughts in the past?

CLIENT: I was having marital problems, but we worked them out.

NURSE: How did you work things out?

CLIENT: We talked to a marriage counselor for about 6 months.

NURSE: What's your relationship like at this time?

CLIENT: It's fine. She just worries about me a lot.

NURSE: Tell me about recent changes or stressors in your life.

CLIENT: I really don't know of any, but I am concerned about my job. I feel worthless and helpless all the time.

NURSE: Tell me about these feelings, particularly about their duration.

CLIENT: I feel old. A young college boy was promoted to supervisor 2 months ago, and it didn't bother me at first. Then I began to think about it, and I realized that I have been an accountant for 25 years and I have reached my peak in promotions. This depresses me.

The nurse continues to encourage expression of feelings and provide an empathic response to the client's distress. She also recognizes that the client is experiencing a developmental crisis related to his career and concerns about his age.

Outcome Identification
The nurse and client identify several client outcomes:

◆ The client verbalizes his feelings rather than acting on them.

◆ The client makes a no-suicide contract with the nurse and other staff.

◆ The client identifies several positive self-attributes.

◆ The client develops enduring adaptive coping skills.

Exploitation Phase
The phase of exploitation emerges as the client appreciates the importance of the nurse-client relationship. The client learns how to get his needs met through these interactions. Anxiety emerges as the client struggles with dependence and independence factors in the relationship. The nurse must assess the client's responses and formulate interactions that encourage self-care and independence.

Resolution Phase
The final phase of the nurse-client relationship is the resolution or termination phase. Previous ones determine the success of this mutually planned stage. Resolution is influenced by the client's ability to use the nurse-client relationship to develop adaptive coping behaviors. Major themes in this phase include the exploration of feelings about termination and the summarization of major aspects of the relationship, including accomplishments and growth.

Peplau (1952) refers to this phase as a *freeing process*. Ideally, the client maintains independence and develops adaptive coping patterns. Appreciating the client's experience enhances the collaborative process and encourages empathy and likelihood of education and growth.

The resolution phase is illustrated in the final part of the previous dialogue.

Nurse-Client Dialogue 7

NURSE: Mr. Lynn, how are you feeling today?

CLIENT: I am feeling a lot better, thanks to you and the others. I suddenly realized that there are more things in life than my job. My wife seems to think that we need a vacation.

NURSE: When was the last time you had a vacation?

CLIENT: It's been at least 10 years. I have always been too busy to do anything with my family.

NURSE: It sounds like you are long overdue for a vacation.

> CLIENT: You are right. I have always looked at the negative side of things. I have to stop myself from thinking negative thoughts and focus on the brighter side of life. I am going home in two days. I am going to miss you and the other nurses.
>
> NURSE: Mr. Lynn, it has been my pleasure to work with you too. You have made a lot of progress over the past few weeks.

This phase of the relationship allowed the client and nurse to discuss areas of accomplishments and feedback regarding his progress. He developed adaptive coping skills and did not attempt to harm himself during hospitalization (see Nursing Care Plan 6–1 for an evaluation).

The nurse-client relationship is an invaluable process that integrates various theories to assess maladaptive behaviors and develop therapeutic interventions. Therapeutic interventions enable clients to assess maladaptive behaviors and replace them with adaptive ones that restore health.

EVALUATING COMMUNICATION USING PROCESS RECORDING

The nurse-client interaction can be evaluated using feedback from clients, other health care providers, and the process *recording*. Process recordings are a method of supervising the development of effective interpersonal communication and counseling skills. This process involves choosing a part of the nurse-client interaction, approximately 5 minutes, and recording a verbatim (word-for-word) account of the entire interaction, including verbal and nonverbal communication (Table 6–4). The process and the content influence the analysis of process recording.

TABLE 6–4
Instructions for Process Recordings

1. Establish rapport with the client.
2. Determine the appropriateness of client and the situation.
3. Select a portion of the nurse-client interaction.
4. Write reports immediately after contact.
5. Answer the following questions:
   a. Were verbal and nonverbal cues identified?
   b. Were the student's/nurse's verbal and nonverbal responses congruent?
   c. Were they therapeutic or nontherapeutic?
6. Discuss the evaluation with the instructor, peers, and nurses.

Since the early 1980s, there has been a need to incorporate specific communication and interpersonal skills into the nursing curriculum. The process recording is an in-depth evaluation of communication skills that provides an opportunity to link theory to practice in the clinical setting. Audio- or video-based material can also be used to help students identify their strengths and weaknesses through structured reflective activity and self-evaluation. The major shortcomings of this learning method are that it requires students to focus more on a passive recording of the interaction versus the needs of the client, that the potential exists to alter the record to conceal difficulties, and that there's no valid criteria to measure the quality and value of the communication skills. The nature of the supervision often determines the benefit of this exercise.

DEVELOPING SELF-AWARENESS OF COMMUNICATION PATTERNS

Self-awareness helps nurses recognize their strengths and limitations and adds dimension to the nurse-client relationship. According to Rawlinson (1990), "it is the use of the self as a tool which may be seen as the contribution of self-awareness to effective nursing care." This process is pertinent to understanding client responses and enables nurses to explore these issues in their clients. This growth-producing phenomenon involves recognition of anxiety-provoking circumstances. Understanding and exploring these issues are vital aspects of personal and professional growth. Nurses can learn to develop greater cognitive self-awareness and self-acceptance and, in turn, promote understanding and acceptance of others (Antai-Otong, 2007). Experiential learning methods such as therapeutic writing in the form of journal keeping or logs (Hayes, 2005; Kok & Chabeli, 2002; Yonge, 2000) and interactive computer videodisc tutorials contribute to self-awareness development.

Circumstances that generate anxiety or strong emotions interfere with objective, logical decision making. Personal characteristics such as values, attitudes, prejudices, personal motives and needs, competencies, skills, and limitations affect self-awareness. Nurses must recognize and explore the source of negative reactions, biases, and stereotyping (Antai-Otong, 2007; Baker, 1997).

Self-awareness helps nurses identify verbal and nonverbal communication patterns. Clients sense positive and negative reactions in nurses. Some clients may confront nurses to clarify their perception of a negative reaction. Frowns, abruptness, or unwarranted expression of fears are examples of negative nonverbal communication cues. The client's reactions and feedback must be explored because they may reflect the nurse's nonverbal communication cues.

Self-awareness encourages nurses and clients to analyze their reactions using therapeutic interactions. Healthy nurse-client interactions can use reality checks to maintain congruency. The capacity for total self-scrutiny is impossible, so nurses have to depend on others for validation or peer supervision.

Furthermore, everyone has "blind spots" and unresolved issues from past experiences. Specific clients, situations, and issues arouse intense anxiety and defensiveness. These feelings usually interfere with objectivity and impede healthy client interactions. The term for these reactions is *countertransference*.

Countertransference is a psychoanalytical term that denotes unconscious conflict resulting from unresolved developmental issues (Freud, 1958). Basch (1988) asserted that countertransference affects the nurse's capacity to assess client responses.

Clients diagnosed with borderline personality disorder stir up intense reactions in nurses. These clients are experts in evoking anger and negative responses in nurses. Maladaptive patterns of manipulation and acting out help them re-create their own chaotic family dynamics. Chaotic relationships with nurses and other caregivers interfere with therapeutic interactions and formation of effective interventions. Countertransference is monitored by the constant internal vigilance of the nurse, who notes the emergence of both positive and negative feelings toward the client and reflects on their possible origin. This monitoring process is a deliberate attempt to avoid reenactment of past conflictual relationships (Gabbard, 2001). (For an in-depth discussion of countertransference, refer to Chapter 15.)

Nurse-client relationships require enormous stamina, ingenuity, and commitment. Complex client problems challenge the nurse to explore her own personal issues. Recognizing one's abilities and strengths also means assessing one's limitations and weaknesses. Self-awareness means growing personally and professionally. (See the Critical Thinking question concerning self-awareness.)

DOCUMENTATION SYSTEMS

Communication among nurses and other health care providers is critical to quality client care. The client's progress is generally conveyed orally in morning rounds, shift changes, informal meetings, or it is provided in documentation.

Documentation is the written form of communication that serves as a legal record with numerous purposes, including the following:

◆ Provides information needed for continuity of care

◆ Maximizes resources by using input from various health care providers to evaluate the treatment plan

◆ Indicates reimbursement needs

◆ Provides data for peer review

◆ Provides data for total quality improvement

◆ Prevents an opportunity for research

◆ Offers opportunities for education and teaching

Documentation communicates information about the client's ongoing health status and current responses to interventions. Specific data may include medication administration, client interactions, mental status, and changes in

CRITICAL THINKING

1. During a discussion with Mary, a 21-year-old client, the nurse notices that she blames everyone but herself for present and past difficulties, including the nurse. She confronts the nurse and tells her that she is just like all the others who dislike her. Which of the following indicates that the nurse has self-awareness concerning responses to the client?

   a. "The client lacks insight into her illness, and this is not a personal attack on me."

   b. "The client is blaming me, and I need to defend myself and others."

   c. "There is little hope for this client, and I will distance myself from her in the future."

   d. "The client reminds me of my younger sister, and I need to let her know who is in charge."

2. Which of the following response to this situation does not reflect self-awareness?

   a. "Although I have strong feelings about this client, I need to maintain a nurse-client relationship."

   b. "I must defend myself, because she needs to know that I really care."

   c. "I am having a difficult time dealing with my feelings and discussing my feelings with my co-workers."

   d. "I am very upset and I know that I am responsible for my own feelings."

behavioral patterns. Documentation is an account of the client's participation and response to treatment. Data are documented in progress notes, nursing care plans, and interdisciplinary treatment plans. The client's record can be used in a legal setting to elicit information that supports or disputes certain claims, such as a malpractice. Clients' records belong to the respective facilities, but clients can obtain copies because of the Patient Bill of Rights.

Clients are usually concerned about accuracy, reliability, and confidentiality of their records. The advent of computers threatens the security of client records, but institutions are responsible for maintaining confidentiality. As a new medium of communication, the Internet offers potential risks, including the loss of visual and auditory cues, confidentiality, competence, crisis management, and legal and jurisdictional issues. Potential benefits of online therapeutic interventions include screening, treatment of nonclinical problems, unique advantages available to online communication, support groups, and adjunctive Internet use (Childress, 2000).

Documentation, like oral reporting, is a form of communication that involves clients, nurses, and other health care providers. Accurate accounts of client interventions, response, and behavioral patterns are vital elements of quality care.

SUMMARY

◆ Communication is a complex, dynamic process that evolves throughout the life span. Primary caregivers provide the basis of socialization and communication.

◆ Early interactions, as well as neurobiological, psychosocial, and cultural factors, affect the quality of social interactions.

◆ Communication is the foundation of survival and social interactions.

◆ Basic needs are met through communication that conveys information from one person to another.

◆ Therapeutic nurse-client interactions are built on trust, empathy, and understanding human responses.

◆ Clients can get their needs met when they feel safe and secure. Therapeutic interactions afford the client with opportunities to express feelings and thoughts. Accurate assessment of client needs is the basis of effective interventions.

◆ The psychiatric-mental health nurse is often challenged to form interpersonal relationships with clients who are using maladaptive coping patterns.

◆ Nurses can use the nursing process to identify maladaptive behaviors and formulate interventions that promote health.

◆ Effective communication enables the nurse to form therapeutic nurse-client relationships and to communicate with other health care providers through written documentation. Communication maximizes resources and facilitates health promotion.

STUDY QUESTIONS

1. R.L. is suspicious and paranoid. Which of the following techniques should be avoided?
   a. Therapeutic touch
   b. Silence
   c. Direct eye contact
   d. Encouragement of expression of feelings

2. R.L. begins to pace and clench his fist. What should the nurse do in this instance?
   a. Leave the room.
   b. Offer an injection of haloperidol (Haldol).
   c. Explore the meaning of the behavior.
   d. Call security services.

3. The major purpose of the process recording is to
   a. Evaluate the client's responses
   b. Evaluate the nurse's response
   c. Evaluate the nurse-client interaction
   d. Evaluate the client's verbal cues

4. Which of the following statements reflects self-awareness?
   a. "I am very angry at A.J. because she is so irritable."
   b. "J.T., you can stay up later than the other clients tonight."
   c. "The client in Room 10 is an alcoholic."
   d. "I do not want to be assigned to Mr. B.P. tonight."

5. Which of the following statements indicates active listening?
   a. "Mr. Jones, it sounds like you are depressed because of your recent job loss."
   b. "Mr. Jones, there is no reason to feel upset because your family loves you."
   c. "Mr. Jones, I find it difficult to believe that losing your job makes you depressed."
   d. "Mr. Jones, you must be feeling pretty low because you are so quiet."

6. Which is the *most* appropriate reason for using humor?
   a. Make light of an otherwise serious situation.
   b. Promote trust by reducing tension and frustration.
   c. Reduce anxiety in the nurse.
   d. Reduce tension in the too "serious" client.

7. The advent of technologies increases access to clients in their communities and homes. What is the most important responsibility of the psychiatric mental health nurse using technologies, such as telemental health, the Internet, and e-mails?
   a. Involving the family in the treatment plan
   b. Maintaining confidentiality and privacy and timely documentation
   c. Providing the client with 24/7 access to mental health services
   d. Monitoring the client for adherence to treatment through timely documentation

8. Therapeutic touch is an important nursing intervention, however, when working with clients it is important for the nurse to use it prudently. Marty is a 25-year-old who is admitted to an acute psychiatric unit for evaluation and treatment of bipolar disorder, manic episode. She is very intrusive and talkative. Which of the following depicts appropriate use of touch in this situation?
   a. Using a handshake to greet the client during your assessment
   b. Touching the client on the shoulder to demonstrate concern
   c. Allowing the client close proximity in case she gets upset
   d. Embracing the client when she begins to cry

9. During your assessment, Mr. Lunden begins to laugh and smile when asked how long he has been married and he says, "I really don't know for sure. My wife is going to get on me about this." What is the *best* explanation for the client's laughter?
   a. His laughter means he is hearing voices and is possibly psychotic.
   b. He is probably anxious about the interview and laughter "breaks the ice."

c. He is evasive and doesn't want to answer the question.

d. He is uncooperative and sarcastic.

10. Interviewing adolescents requires astute communication and listening skills. What is the most appropriate response to a 15-year-old who asks you to promise to keep everything she discusses confidential?

a. "I am unwilling to make that promise."

b. "I have to discuss what you say with your parents because they are worried about you."

c. "Everything you share is confidential except information that indicates you are a danger to yourself or others."

d. "I promise I will keep everything you share with me confidential."

RESOURCES

Please note that because Internet resources are of a time-sensitive nature and URL addresses may change or be deleted, searches should also be conducted by association or topic.

Internet Resources

La Mendola, W. (1997). *Telemental health services in U.S. frontier areas* (Frontier Mental Health Services Resource Network, Letter to the Field, No. 3). Retrieved from http://www.du.edu/frontier-mh/letter3.html

http://www.va.gov/occ/toolkits/telementalhealth/

Telemental Health Toolkit (Veterans Health Administration), (Accessed May 14, 2006)

Other Resources

The National Institute of Mental Health
Office of Communications and Public Liaison
6001 Executive Boulevard, Room 8184, MSC 9663
Bethesda, MD 20892-9663
Voice (301) 443-4513
Fax (301) 443-4279

http://www.surgeongeneral.gov/topics/cmh/default.htm

More information on the mental health of children and adolescents is available at

http://www.nimh.nih.gov/publicat/childmenu.cfm and http://www.mentalhealth.org

REFERENCES

Adamle, K. N. & Ludwick, R. (2005). Humor in hospice care: Who, where, and how much? *American Journal of Hospital and Palliative Care, 22,* 287–290.

Ainsworth, M. D. S. (1985). Attachments across the life span. *Bulletin of the New York Academy of Medicine, 61,* 792–812.

Antai-Otong, D. (2007). Nurse-client interactions: Strengthening care partnerships. In D. Antai-Otong (Ed.), *Nurse-client communication: A life span approach* (pp. 99–152), Sudsbury, MA: Jones and Bartlett Publishers.

Astedt-Kurki, P., Isola, A., Tammentie, T., & Kervidenen, U. (2001). Importance of humor to client-nurse relationships and clients' well-being. *International Journal of Nursing Practice, 7,* 119–125.

Bailey, J., & Baillie, L. (1996). Transactional analysis: How to improve communication skills. *Nursing Standard, 35,* 39–42.

Baker, C. (1997). Cultural relativism and cultural diversity: Implications for nursing practice. *Advanced Nursing Science, 20,* 3–11.

Basch, M. F. (1988). *Understanding psychotherapy.* New York: Basic Books.

Baumann, S. L. (2005). Standing at the doorway looking in. *Nursing Science Quarterly, 18,* 258.

Beck, C. T. (1997). Humor in nursing practice: A phenomenological study. *International Journal of Nursing Studies, 34,* 346–352.

Bennett H. J. (2003). Humor in medicine. *Southern Medical Journal, 96,*1257–1261.

Berlo, D. K. (1960). *The process of communication.* New York: Holt, Rinehart, & Winston.

Berne, E. (1964). *Games people play.* New York: Grove Press.

Berne, E. (1973). *What do you say after you say hello?* London: Corgi.

Birdwhitsell, R. (1970). *Kinesics and content.* Philadelphia: University of Pennsylvania Press.

Bowlby, J. (1969). *Attachment and loss: Vol. 1. Attachment.* New York: Basic Books.

Buckwalter, K. C., Cusack, D., Beaver, M., Sidles, E., & Wadle, K. (1988). The behavioral consequences of a communication intervention on institutionalized residents with aphasia and dysarthria. *Archives of Psychiatric Nursing, 2,* 289–295.

Ceccio, J. F., & Ceccio, C. M. (1982). *Effective communication in nursing: Theory and practice.* New York: John Wiley & Sons.

Chambers-Evans, J., Stelling, J., & Godin, M. (1999). Learning to listen: Serendipitous outcomes of a research training experience. *Journal of Advanced Nursing, 29,* 1421–1426.

Childress, C. A. (2000). Ethical issues in providing psychotherapeutic interventions. *Journal of Medical Internet Research, 2,* E5.

Clarke, D. J. (1998). Process recording: Of what value is examining nursing. *Nurse Education Today, 18,* 138–143.

Cohen, M. (1990). Caring for ourselves can be funny business. *Holistic Nursing Practice, 4,* 1–11.

Condon, W. S., & Sander, L. W. (1974). Neonate movement is synchronized with adult speech: Interactional participation and language acquisition. *Science, 183,* 99–101.

Dean, R. A. & Gregory, D. M. (2004). Humor and laughter in palliative care: An ethnographic investigation. *Palliative Supportive Care, 2,* 139–148.

Dean, R. A. & Gregory, D. M. (2005). More than trivial: Strategies for using humor in palliative care. *Cancer Nursing, 28,* 292-300.

Dowling, J. S., Hockenberry, M., & Gregory, R. L. 2003). Sense of humor, childhood cancer stressors, and outcomes of psychosocial adjustment, immune function, and infection. *Journal of Pediatric Oncology Nursing, 20,* 271–292.

Egan, G. (1994). *The skilled helper* (5th ed.). Pacific Grove, CA: Brooks/Cole.

Elliott, R., & Wright, L. W. (1999). Verbal communication: What do critical care nurses say to their unconscious or sedated patients? *Journal of Advanced Nursing, 29,* 1412–1420.

Fortinash, K. M., & Holoday-Worrat, P. A. (1996). *Psychiatric mental health nursing.* St Louis, MO: Mosby.

Freud, S. (1958). *The dynamics of transference.* In J. Strachey (Ed. and Trans.), *The standard edition of the complete psychological works of Sigmund Freud* (Vol. 19, pp. 97–108). London: Hogarth Press. (Original work published 1923.)

Gabbard G. O. (2001). Psychoanalysis and psychoanalytic psychotherapy. in W. J. Livesey (Ed.), *A handbook of personality disorders: Theory, research, and treatment* (pp. 359–376). New York: Guilford.

Gladstein, G. A. (1987). *Empathy and counseling.* New York: Springer-Verlag.

Gläscher, J., Tüscher, O., Weiller, C., & Büchel, C. (2004). Elevated responses to constant facial emotions in different faces in the human amygdala: An fMRI study of facial identity and expression. *BMC Neuroscience,* doi: 10.1186/1471-2202-5-45.

Gunning-Dixon, F. M., Gur, R. C., Perkins, A. C., Schroeder, L., Turner, T., Turetsky, B. I., Chan, R. M., Loughead, J. W., et al. (2003). Age-related differences in brain activation during emotional face processing. *Neurobiology of Aging, 24,* 285–295.

Gur, R. C., Schroeder, L., Turner, T., McGrath, C., Chan, R. M., Turetsky, B. I., Alsop, D., et al. (2002). Brain activation during facial emotion processing. *Neuroimaging, 16,* 651–662.

Hall, E. T. (1966). *The hidden dimension.* Garden City, NJ: Doubleday.

Hall, E. T. (1989). Beyond culture. New York: Doubleday.

Hanson, B., & Taylor, M. F. (2000). Being-with, doing with: A model of the nurse-client relationship in mental health nursing. *Journal of Psychiatric Mental Health Nursing, 7,* 417–423.

Hayes, A. (2005). A mental health nursing clinical experience with hospice patients. *Nurse Educator, 30,* 85–88.

Howells, J. G. (1975). *Principles of family psychotherapy.* New York: Brunnel/Mazel.

Hunkeler, E. M., Meresman, J. F., Hargreaves, W. A., Fireman, B., Berman, W. H., Kirsch, A. J., et al. (2000). Efficacy of nurse telehealth care and peer support in augmenting treatment of depression in primary care. *Archives of Family Medicine, 9,* 700-708.

Irish, J. T. (1997). Deciphering the physician-older patient interaction. *International Journal of Psychiatric Medicine, 27,* 251–267.

Kilgore, W. D. & Yurgelun-Todd, D. A. (2004). Activation of the amygdala and anterior cingulate during nonconscious processing of sad versus happy faces. *Neuroimaging, 21,* 1215–1223.

Kim, S. Y., Jeon, E. Y., Sok, S. R., & Kim, K. B. (2006). Comparison of health-promoting behaviors of noninstitutionalized and institutionalized older adults in Korea. *Journal of Nursing Scholarship, 38,* 31-35.

Kok, J. & Chabeli, M. M. (2002). Reflective journal writing: How it promotes reflective thinking in clinical nursing education: A students' perspective. *Curationis, 25,* 35-42.

Kruijver, I. P., Kerkstra, A., Francke, A. L., Bensing, J. M., & van de Wiel, H. B. (2000). Evaluation of communication training programs in nursing care: A review of the literature. *Patient Education and Counseling, 39,* 129–145.

La Monica, E. (1981). Construct validity of an empathy instrument. *Research in Nursing and Health, 4,* 389–400.

Liehr, P., Takahashi, R., Nishimura, C., Frazier, L., Kuwajima, I., & Pennebaker, J. W. (2002). Expressing health experience through embodied language. *Image: Journal of Nursing Scholarship, 34,* 27–32.

Locsin, R. C. (1998). Technologic competence as caring in critical care nursing. *Holistic Nursing Practice, 12,* 50–56.

Maslow, A. H. (1968). *Toward a psychology of being* (2nd ed.). New York: Van Nostrand Reinhold.

Maslow, A. H. (1970). *Motivation and personality* (2nd ed.). New York: Harper & Row.

McNeil-Haber, F. M. (2004). Ethical considerations in the use of nonerotic touch in psychotherapy with children. *Ethics and Behavior, 14,* 123–140.

McPherson, G., & Thorne, S. (2000). Children's voices: Can we hear them? *Journal of Pediatric Nursing, 15,* 22–29.

Mellow, J. (1967). Evolution of nursing therapy through research. *Psychiatric Opinion, 4,* 15–21.

Monnier, J., Knapp, R. G., & Frueh, B. C. (2003). Recent advances in telepsychiatry: An updated review. *Psychiatric Services, 54,* 1604–1609.

Orlando, I. J. (1961). *The dynamic nurse-patient relationship.* New York: G.P. Putnam.

Parse, R. (1993). The experience of laughter: A phenomenological study. *Nursing Science Quarterly, 6,* 39–43.

Patten, S. B. (2003). Prevention of depressive symptoms through the use of distance technologies. *Psychiatric Services, 54,* 396–398.

Peck, S. D. (1998). The efficacy of therapeutic touch for improving functional ability in elders with degenerative arthritis. *Nursing Science Quarterly, 11,* 123–132.

Penson, R. T., Partridge, R. A., Rudd, P., Seiden, M.V., Nelson, J. E., Chabner, B. A., & Lynch, T. J. Jr. (2005). Laughter: The best medicine? *Oncologist, 10,* 651–660.

Peplau, H. E. (1952). *Interpersonal relations in nursing.* New York: G.P. Putnam.

Peplau, H. E. (1987). Interpersonal constructs for nursing practice. *Nurse Education Today, 7,* 201–208.

Peplau, H. E. (1991). *Interpersonal relations in nursing: A conceptual framework of reference for psychodynamic nursing.* New York: Springer.

Peplau, H. E. (1994). Psychiatric mental health nursing: Challenge and change. *Journal of Psychiatric and Mental Health Nursing, 1,* 3–7.

Piaget, J. (1970). Piaget's theory. In P. H. Mussen (Ed.), *Carmichael's manual of child psychology* (pp. 703–732). New York: John Wiley & Sons.

Pluckman, M. L. (1978). *Human communication: The matrix of nursing.* New York: McGraw-Hill.

Rawlinson, J. W. (1990). Self-awareness: Conceptual influences, contribution to nursing, and approaches to attainment. *Nurse Education Today, 10,* 111–117.

Raymer, A. M., Ciampitti, M., Holliway, B., Singletary, F., Blonder, L. X., Ketterson, T., et al. (2007). Semantic-phonologic treatment for noun and verb retrieval impairments in aphasia. *Neuropsychological Rehabilitation, 17,* 244–270.

Reusch, J. (1961). *Therapeutic communication.* New York: W.W. Norton.

Reynolds, W. (1994). The influence of clients' perceptions of the helping relationship in the development of an empathy scale. *Journal of Psychiatric and Mental Health Nursing, 1,* 23–30.

Reynolds, W., Scott, P. A., & Austin, W. (2000). Nursing, empathy and perception of the moral. *Journal of Advanced Nursing, 32,* 235–242.

Satir, V. (1967). *Conjoint family therapy* (Rev. ed.). Palo Alto, CA: Science and Behavior Books.

Simon, G. E., Ludman, E. J., Tutty, S., Operskalski, B., & von Korff, M. (2004). Telephone psychotherapy and telephone care management for primary care patients starting antidepressant treatment: A randomized controlled trial. *Journal of the American Medical Association, 292,* 935–942.

Smits, M. W., & Kee, C. C. (1992). Correlates of self-care among the independent elderly. *Journal of Gerontological Nursing, 18,* 13–18.

Sullivan, H. S. (1954). *Psychiatric interview.* New York: W.W. Norton.

Taylor, R. (2000). Check your cultural competence. *Critical Care Choices,* 60–66.

Travelbee, J. (1971). Interpersonal aspects of nursing. Philadelphia: F.A. Davis.

Truax, C. (1961). A scale for the measurement of accurate empathy. *Discussion Paper 20,* Madison: Wisconsin Institute Press.

Walzlawick, P., Beavin, J. H., & Jackson, C. D. (1967). *Pragmatics of human communication: A study of interactional patterns, pathologies, and paradoxes.* New York: W.W. Norton.

Warren, B. J. (2000). Cultural competence: A best practice process for psychiatric-mental health nursing. *Journal of the American Psychiatric Nurses Association, 6,* 135–138.

Watt-Watson, J., Garfinkel, P., Gallop, R., Stevens, B., & Streiner, D. (2000). The impact of nurses' empathic responses on patients' pain management in acute care. *Nursing Research, 49,* 191–200.

Wild B., Rodden F. A., Grodd W., Ruch, W. (2003). Neural correlates of laughter and humour. *Brain, 126,* 2121–2138.

Yonge, O. (2000). Logs as adjuncts to therapy for adolescents in a residential psychiatric program. *Journal of Psychosocial Nursing, 38,* 33–39.

SUGGESTED READINGS

Langs, R. (1978). *The listening process.* New York: Jason Aronson.

Mahler, M. S. (1979). *Selected papers of Margaret S. Mahler, vol. II: Separation-individuation.* New York: Jason Aronson.

Pennebacker, J. W. (1997). *Opening up: The healing power of expressing emotion.* New York: Guilford.

Thorson, J. A., Powell, F. C., Sarmany-Schuller, I., & Hampes, W. P. (1997). Psychological health and sense of humor. *Journal of Clinical Psychology, 53,* 605–619.

U.S. Public Health Service. (2000). *Report of the surgeon general's conference on children's mental health: A national action agenda.* Washington, DC: Department of Health and Human Services.

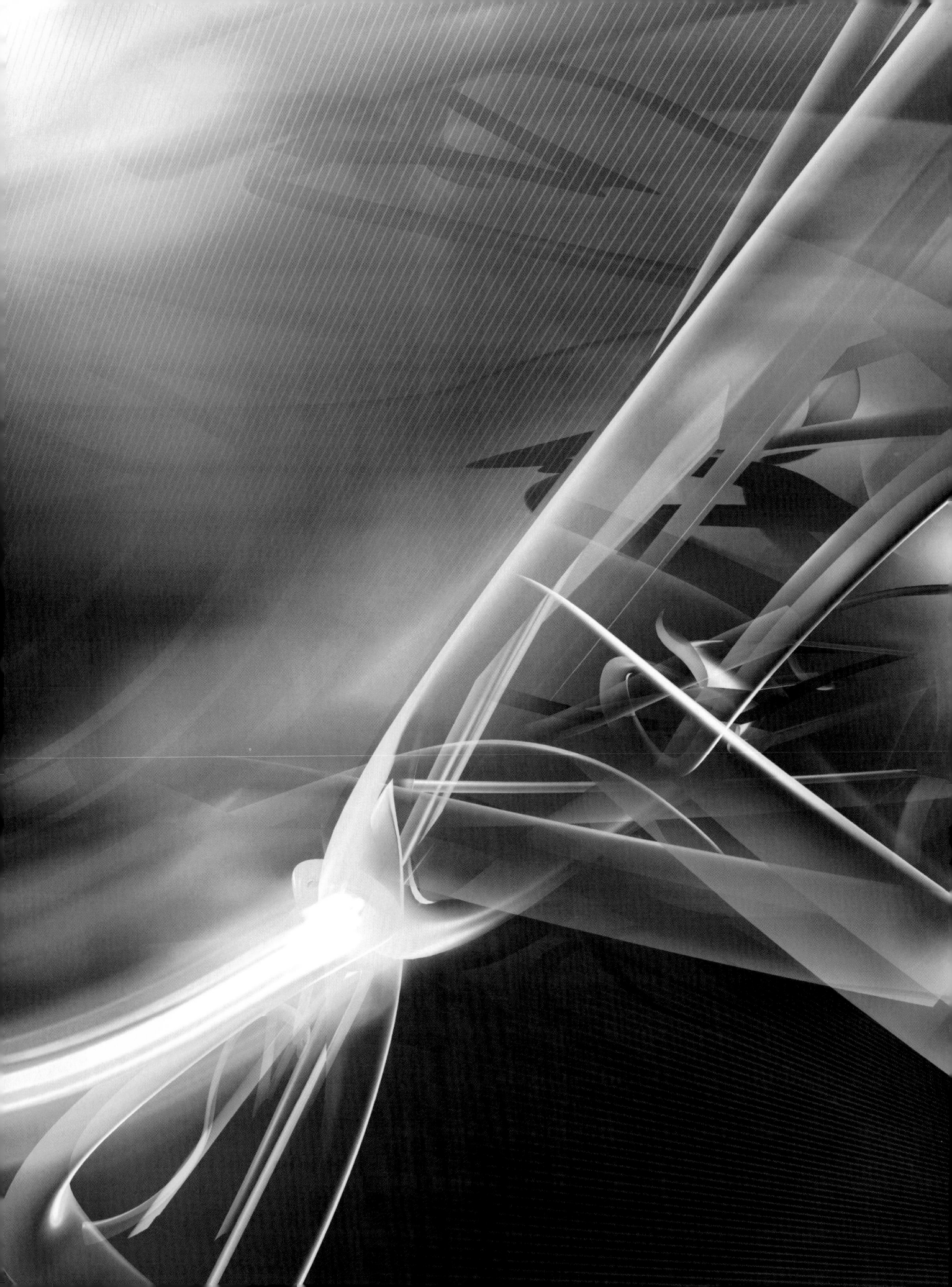

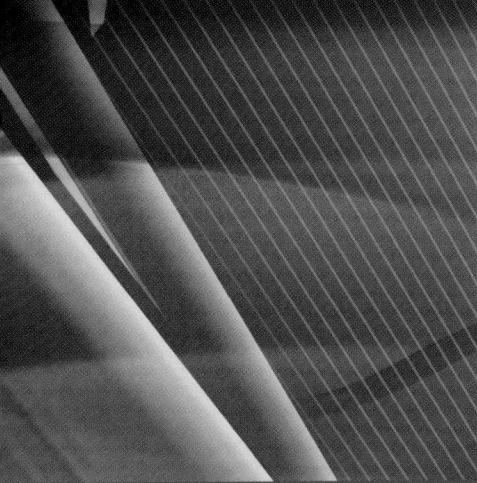

CHAPTER 7

Cultural and Ethnic Considerations

Barbara Jones Warren, PhD, RN, CNS, CS

KEY TERMS

Analytic Worldview: Worldview perspective that espouses and values specific detail to time, calculation, individuality, and acquiring material objects as being important in life.

Community Worldview: Worldview perspective that espouses and values the importance and needs of the community over the individual in the context of transcendence and meditation in life.

Critical Thinking: Systematic and purposeful process of reasoning.

Cultural Competence: Circular process whereby a person develops an understanding and valuing of different worldview perspectives and then enculturates the understanding and valuing into interactions with clients and other health care professionals.

Culturally Bound Factors: Health ideas and behaviors that a person exhibits in relationship to his environment and everyday life functioning.

Culture: A person, group, or community's internal and external daily expression of their beliefs, values, and norms.

Culture of Nursing: The nursing profession's body of values, knowledge, beliefs, and practices, which form the bases of how individual nurses delineate their nursing roles and functions within health care environments.

Drug Polymorphism: Contextual chemical factors involved in individuals' genetic responses to pharmacologic agents.

Ecological Worldview: Worldview perspective that a person espouses, values, and accepts in his role of interconnectedness and responsibility for the world and its habitants in the context of peace and tranquility.

Enculturates: A person's internalization and adoption of another worldview perspective into his existing worldview perspective.

Enculturation: Process by which a person accepts and internalizes another person's or group's worldview into or in place of his existing worldview.

Ethnicity: Categorical determination of a group whose members have a common social and cultural heritage that is passed from generation to generation.

Ethnopsychopharmacology: The study of intensity and duration (e.g., absorption, distribution, metabolism, and elimination) of psychotropic medications for different racial groups of individuals.

Intracultural Variations: Alterations in cultural ideation and psychological or physical characteristics between persons from different racial and ethnic groups.

Mental Disorder or Illness: Any health condition that is identified by a change in thinking, mood, or behavior and one that creates distress or problems with everyday functioning.

Metabolic Pathways: Chemical sites (e.g., acetylation, debrisoquine-ds, mephenytoin) that are involved in the conversion of pharmacologic agents within a person's biological system.

Race: Taxonomy of a group's identity based on genetic factors that produce physical characteristics and distinguish the persons within that group from persons within another group.

Relational Worldview: Worldview perspective that espouses and values the development of interactions, relationships, and spirituality as a contextual importance in life.

Worldview Perspective: A person's belief regarding what he considers to be true and valued.

COMPETENCIES

Upon completion of this chapter, the learner should be able to:

1. Describe and define culture from a broad perspective.

2. Identify worldwide perspectives of different cultural groups.

3. Explain the relationship between culture, mental health, wellness, and psychopathology.

4. Discuss the role of cultural competence in relationship to nursing process.

5. Recognize the components of the nursing process and critical thinking as they relate to the development of evidence-based culturally competent nursing strategies and interventions.

6. Develop a culturally competent nursing care plan using the components of a cultural assessment as the basis of the nursing assessment process to address the levels of mental health, wellness, and illness in a specific case exemplar.

CHAPTER OUTLINE

Overview of Culture and Behavior

Worldview Perspectives of Culture
Cultural Competence

Culture Issues across the Life Span

Infancy, Childhood, and Adolescence
Adulthood and Older Adulthood

Components of the Cultural Assessment

Culturally Bound, Mental Health, and Psychosocial Issues

Barriers to Culturally Competent Care
Life Span and Gender Issues

Culture and Psychopathology
Symptomatology in Children and Adults
Older Adulthood

Incidence and Prevalence of Mental Disorders across Cultural Groups
Issues of Gender and Sexual Orientation

Ethnopsychopharmacology

Neurobiological Factors

Critical Thinking and Cultural Competence

Nursing Process as a Culturally Competent Tool

The Role of the Nurse

The Generalist Nurse

The Advanced-Practice Psychiatric Registered Nurse

The past decade of the brain promoted an intense examination regarding individuals' genetic and physiological status on the development and manifestation of psychopathology. Mental health education, practice, and research approaches were grounded in biological theories. The first surgeon general's report on mental health, issued at the end of 1999, acknowledged the importance of biological influences on the maintenance of mental health and wellness (U.S. DHHS, 1999). However, it also states that there is much to be learned regarding the prevention, etiology, and treatment of mental disorders. National health indicators and goals were also developed during the decade of the brain and are delineated in the *Healthy People 2010* report (U.S. DHHS, 2000). The primary goals of this report are to increase the quality and years of life for persons as well as eliminate health disparities. The surgeon general's report defines a mental disorder or illness as any health condition that is identified by a change in thinking, mood, or behavior and one that creates distress or problems with everyday functioning (U.S. DHHS, 1999, 2000). Both the surgeon general's report and *Healthy People 2010* indicate that there is disparity associated with the prevention and treatment of mental illness for persons from diverse cultural groups. In addition, the United States census tract data and population studies indicate that there is a continuing increase in the numbers of diverse ethnic and racial populations. It is estimated that

almost 13 percent of the population consists of persons from African American, 11 percent from Latino(a) or Hispanic, 4 percent from Asian and Pacific Islander, and 0.9 percent from Indigenous or Native American cultures (DHHS, 2000). Since these individuals often present a different clinical picture of mental health, wellness, and illness, they have a variety of mental health care needs that need to be addressed by nurses (Carter, 1995; Muñoz & Luckmann, 2005; IOM, 2003; Warren, 2000). The purpose of this chapter is to provide a nursing perspective and introductory examination regarding the role of culture as it applies to issues of mental health, wellness, and illness. Acquisition of this knowledge is important for nurses because cultural patterns and influences affect how clients function on a daily basis and cope with mental health challenges. In addition, it is imperative that nurses understand their values and beliefs as these affect how they interact with their peers, other health care providers, and clients.

OVERVIEW OF CULTURE AND BEHAVIOR

The state and perception of an individual's mental health and wellness are determined by holistic (e.g., the unification of mind, body, and spirit) and cultural factors. Culture represents a person, group, or community's internal and external daily expression of their beliefs, values, and norms (Bell, 1994; Campinha-Bacote, 2003 2005; Tylor, 1871). The concept of culture is much broader than the traditionally thought of cultural issues such as race (e.g., taxonomy of a group's identity based on genetic factors that produce physical characteristics and distinguish the persons within that group from persons within another group), ethnicity (e.g., categorical determination of a group whose members have a common social and cultural heritage that is passed from generation to generation), and religion (Warren & Alley, 2005). It also entails age, class, gender, sexual orientation, work status, race, and ethnicity. Individuals hold on to their cultural beliefs and values because they provide the essence of meaning in life. The cultural perspective influences health care practices and perceptions of the mental health care system and providers within that system. Current national mental health and wellness protocols and goals indicate that prevention and treatment protocols and strategies need to be adaptable for persons from different cultural groups. This adaptability can maximize health care quality and create successful outcomes. Nurses are often the initial health care providers whom persons encounter when entering the health care system. Consequently, it is important that nurses understand different value and belief systems in order to adapt prevention and treatment protocols and strategies to meet the needs of the diverse persons they may encounter and to support their recovery process (Andrews & Boyle, 2002; Anthony, 1993; Giger & Davidhizar, 2004; Lutz & Warren, 2001; Spector, 2004).

WORLDVIEW PERSPECTIVES OF CULTURE

A worldview perspective is a person's belief regarding what he considers to be true and of value, and it represents the person's thoughts about values, knowledge development, interactions with others, and role in the universe (Nichols, 1987; Warren, 2002). Each person may function using a variety of worldview perspectives. However, when someone is seeking health advice or becomes ill, he often operates under the initial or primary worldview perspective that was culturally learned because it is more comfortable, familiar, and healing. Nurses also need to be aware of their perspective(s) when they are providing care to a client because their perspective(s) may affect how they develop and provide mental health care services. In fact, nurses who understand and use the process of cultural competence have more successful outcomes with clients.

Cultural Competence

Cultural competence is a circular process whereby a person develops an understanding and valuing of different worldview perspectives and then enculturates the understanding and valuing into interactions with other persons (Campinha-Bacote, 2003; Purnell & Paulanka, 2003). A nurse continues to develop culturally competence knowledge and techniques as he enculturates (learns and adopts another worldview perspective into his internal worldview perspective) other worldview perspectives into interactions with clients and other

health care professionals (Leininger & McFarland, 2006). Misinterpretation and miscommunication may occur if the nurse is culturally incompetent, because the client and the nurse operate under different or divergent worldview perspectives. This misinterpretation can lead to feelings of confusion, frustration, or anger that interfere with successful implementation of nursing process approaches and appropriate delivery of mental health care services. Ultimately, clients may ignore or refuse health care services that may intensify their level of psychopathology. Finally, it is important for nurses to understand there is no one worldview perspective that is valued or devalued. Each perspective is unique and contributes to the contextual framework of an individual.

According to Nichols (1987), worldviews evolve from racial groups' cultural beliefs and values. However, as previously mentioned, a person often enculturates and uses a variety of perspectives based on one's situation or environment. For example, a nurse may have developed his original value system in one culture (e.g., female, male, Asian, Indigenous, African, or European American). The culture of nursing (e.g., the nursing profession's body of values, knowledge, beliefs, and practices, which form the bases of how individual nurses delineate their nursing roles and functions within health care environments) is also superimposed on a nurse's initial worldview perspective. Perspectives may develop, emerge, or be extended as the nurse evolves. The nurse's professional expertise and experience, age, class, and religious preference may affect how a nurse practices, educates others, or participates in or conducts research. Using cultural literature, data from Nichols' (1987) initial conceptual model and professional nursing experience, four expanded perspectives can be devised: analytic, relational, community, and ecological. Nichols' conceptual model correlates these latter four worldviews to the following racial cultural groups: European; African; Latino(a) and Hispanic; Asian; and Native American groups (Table 7–1).

Nichols' (1987) worldview explanations may often match persons from specific racial groups. However, racial blending and cultural enculturation strongly influence the development and alteration of a person's worldview. It is also important to recognize that there is no higher value, importance, or correctness to any one of the views. Each characteristic of a worldview perspective contributes to the uniqueness and value of any individual. The nurse needs to exercise caution in subscribing certain worldviews to *only* one racial culture as opposed to another. As previously mentioned, most persons are "blends" of different cultures, either genetically, psychologically, or spiritually. In addition, persons may work in one environment that is defined by one worldview perspective and live and socialize in another environment that is defined by an entirely different worldview. Hence, persons may use different worldviews as needed. Of course, the use of an alternating worldview may also contribute to increased stress and strain for persons if the worldviews represent very opposite perspectives. This increased stress may then predispose certain persons to mental distress or exacerbation of mental illness symptoms. Consequently, nurses need to

TABLE 7–1
Worldview Perspectives

Warren Worldview Perspectives	Nichols Worldview Perspectives
Analytic:	
• Detail to time, calculations.	European American Cultural Groups
• Values individuality and acquiring material goods.	
• Prefers learning through visual and written sources.	
Relational:	
• Spirituality is an important concept in life.	African, Latino(a)/Hispanic American Cultural Groups
• Values the development of relationships and interactions with others as a means of everyday functioning.	
• Verbal communication is valued as a learning style.	
Community:	
• Community needs are more important than individual needs.	Asian American Cultural Groups
• Meditation and transcendence are a learning method.	
• Quiet, respectful approach in interactions.	
Ecological:	
• Sees interconnectedness with the world and its inhabitants.	Native American Cultural Groups
• Feels a sense of responsibility to "take care" of the world and environment.	
• Learns through "taking in" and quiet contemplation.	
• Conversation is quiet and kept to a minimum.	

assess the enculturation and level of every person's worldview when providing mental health care services.

For example, a client or nurse using an analytic worldview perspective might espouse specific detail to time, calculations, individuality, and acquiring of material objects as being the important beliefs in life, such as being on time for appointments, getting immediately to the purpose of a health visit, and valuing printed pamphlets and books for health education. Nurses and other health care professionals need to be quite accurate and precise when providing care to clients and developing strategies, interventions, and protocols. The example of individuality and valuing material goods are often embodied in traditional American society's values, beliefs, and actions.

The relational worldview values the development of interactions and relationships, may prefer learning through verbal communication, and views spirituality as an important context for living life. A client or nurse who proposes the relational worldview places an importance on interaction and communication in the context of being spiritual (e.g., directed purpose in life). These individuals may want to "chat" a while before getting to the heart of the health visit. The client may desire the involvement of relatives, friends, or spiritual and religious advisors during the health visit and the nurse's development of nursing process, or both. The relational worldview may be seen in certain persons from African, Latino(a), or Hispanic American cultures.

The community worldview espouses the importance and needs of the community over the individual. A client with this view may need to elevate himself to a higher level of thought through the use of meditation and contemplation techniques. A client with this view is respectful and polite regarding health care advice and may not want to question a nurse or physician. This may occur even if the client does not understand what is being recommended. According to Nichols (1987), persons from some of the Asian cultural groups often embody these philosophies.

Finally, a client or nurse with an ecological worldview perspective may illustrate the following characteristics or values: an interconnectedness with other persons and the universe, a responsibility for taking care of others and the world in which he lives, and a need to maintain peace and tranquility within oneself, others, and the world. For example, a client with this perspective would feel a responsibility to safeguard the world and its inhabitants. He would also prefer a quiet restful approach in interactions with others (e.g., "take in" more of what is being said than commenting on every aspect of a conversation). Conversation is often kept to a minimum, being respectfully and concisely delivered. Nichols (1987) indicates that persons from some of the Indigenous or Native American cultures may embrace this worldview.

CULTURE ISSUES ACROSS THE LIFE SPAN

The impact of culture on client responses and health practices is well documented. Understanding the significance of culture on the client who presents with a mental illness is critical to accurately assess the meaning of the client's experiences. The following discussion depicts the evolution of culture across the life span and implications for the psychiatric nurse.

Infancy, Childhood, and Adolescence

Infants and children are enculturated into the cultural environment in which they grow and develop. This process begins when a woman becomes pregnant. For example, persons from Latino culture believe that mothers should receive additional attention, eat well, and rest frequently (Chong, 2002; Muñoz & Luckmann, 2005). The entire process of pregnancy and labor is a very female experience, with prospective mothers being pampered by other women in the family. Families are close, and everyone is involved in the rearing of children and adolescents. Discipline is more relaxed. Finally, all of the previously discussed beliefs are enculturated into children and adolescent upbringing, and they are taught to value very traditional female and male roles (Juarbe, 1996).

Many Asian American cultural groups also think mothers are special and need to get a great deal of rest during pregnancy. Male children may be more valued in certain Asian

populations. Children are taught to be obedient and dutiful to their elders (Shiba & Oka, 1996).

In many African American homes, children are expected to complete household tasks. Discipline and good behavior are encouraged. In addition, children are expected to "give back to the community" (e.g., make something of themselves and help other members of the community) and to respect their elders.

Adulthood and Older Adulthood

Adults, especially older individuals, are greatly revered in persons from Native American culture (Kramer, 1996). They participate in various roles such as counseling, teaching, parenting, and grandparenting within the community. Adults within the community are expected to exercise self-discipline, control, and positive attitudes.

COMPONENTS OF THE CULTURAL ASSESSMENT

The nurse should not view cultural components as isolated assessment factors because a client's cultural perspective cannot be separated out any more than his brain or body can be. The nurse needs to include the components of a cultural assessment in every assessment he conducts. As previously mentioned, this is important because an individual's cultural reference and worldview perspective affect health care beliefs and practices. Cultural components for every nursing assessment need to include examination of the following factors: communication patterns and styles; overview and identified cultural heritage; living environment and length of time in this environment or location; nutritional patterns and practices during times of wellness and illness; identified significant others or family members, or both; view of health, wellness, and illness; education and learning style preferences; presence of any spiritual or religious beliefs; and the person's physical status and biological and genetic factors affecting his status (Baker, 2001; Kelly, Kopac, & Rosselli, 2007; Mahoney, Carlson, & Engebretson, 2006; Siantz & Meleis, 2007).

Performing a cross-cultural assessment requires an understanding of individual needs, wishes, and preferences that may reflect cultural health practices. Some gender issues stem from how women are valued and treated in various societies.

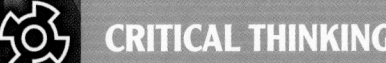

CRITICAL THINKING

How could a nurse incorporate various psychosocial issues into a nursing care plan for different age persons from Latino, Asian, or African American culture?

INTERNET ACTIVITY

Go to the Web and look for issues affecting the mental health and wellness of persons from European, African, Asian, and Native American cultural groups. Incorporate this information into the development of a nursing care plan.

Hint: The National Institutes of Mental Health, the Department of Health and Human Services, and Closing the Gap are excellent sources to pursue.

For instance, women who live in strong patriarchal societies where they are devalued, discouraged from self-expression and choices in life, and are emotionally and financially dependent on their spouses often feel disempowered and suffer depression and other psychiatric conditions. Assessing the client's sense of control, self-choices and self-expression within various cultural groups and ethnicities increases the nurse's understanding of the client's experience and level of distress and coping patterns.

Questions about the preceding cultural components may be directly asked, or the nurse may just observe a client's response to and interactions with him, the environment, or others. For example, the nurse can ascertain whether the person speaks English and to what level when he conducts the initial introduction. However, he would still need to ask if the client speaks any other languages and which language is the preferred one. Other questions such as, "Is there anyone you would like me to notify or have here during the assessment?" "How may I, as a nurse, help you?" "What do you generally eat in a day?" "Are there foods or medications you prefer or avoid?" "What does being healthy mean for you?" provide the client with an opportunity to express his ideas, values, and beliefs. In addition, these questions may provide the nurse with the chance to continue probing for additional information. Cultural clinical guidelines also may facilitate assessment of clients. These guidelines are listed in Table 7–2.

CULTURALLY BOUND, MENTAL HEALTH, AND PSYCHOSOCIAL ISSUES

Experts in the area of culture have been able to define certain culturally bound factors (e.g., health ideas and behaviors that a person exhibits in relationship to his environment and everyday life functioning) that may be mis-

interpreted as or mask psychopathology. One of the most recent additions to the *Diagnostic and Statistical Manual of Mental Disorders-IV (DSM-IV-TR)* (APA, 2000) includes some of the cultural variations in each of the sections on mental disorders. In addition, Appendix I in the manual delineates many of the culturally bound syndromes for persons from diverse cultural groups. However, it is prudent for nurses to exercise caution in the interpretation of these cultural variations because not all of them represent mental illness symptomatology. Often these symptoms are "normal" cultural reactions to naturally occurring life situations. However, when symptoms persist, intensify, or interfere with daily functioning, it may be an indication of the presence of psychopathological conditions such as dysthymic, major depressive, anxiety, dissociative, somatoform, or panic disorders.

Persons from diverse populations may also use different terminology for symptoms of mental health distress. For example, persons from some Latino(a) populations may say they are experiencing "ataque de nervios" (literally translated as an attack of the nerves) when they incur depressive, anxiety, tension, insomnia, anhedonia, or panic symptoms. Individuals from some of the Asian cultures may speak of someone running "amok." Psychopathologic symptoms that mirror this disorder include paranoia, dissociative thinking, confusion, agitation, impending death, and violent behavior. Some persons from the Nations or Indigenous American populations may describe similar symptomatology that they term "ghost behavior." Mental distress among children or women from certain Latino(a), Hispanic, or Mediterranean cultures may be expressed as the "mal de ojo" or evil eye. Symptoms may include feelings of anxiety, insomnia, and digestive irregularities. "Susto" symptomatology mirrors that of depressive disorders because it involves fatigue, insomnia, and lack of self-esteem and work. Persons from African American or Caribbean cultures may speak of mental distress in terms of someone "falling out," "being stressed," or having "spells" when individuals from these groups have symptoms similar to depressive, dissociative, conversion, or psychotic disorders (Delahanty et al., 2001; Diala et al., 2001; Neighbors et al., 2007; Ross, 2001).

BARRIERS TO CULTURALLY COMPETENT CARE

Diverse persons receiving mental health treatment may encounter barriers to treatment. These barriers are generally grounded in cultural differences between health care providers and receivers of care, organizations, or diagnostic and monetary factors. Nurses, other health care providers, or systems of care may be culturally incompetent. In fact, the 1999 surgeon general's report indicates that the mental health system is not always ready or designed to meet the needs of persons from diverse populations. This lack of preparedness on the part of the system is particularly apparent in outpatient mental health settings where persons from diverse populations are greatly underserved. On the other hand, greater numbers of diverse persons may often use emergency rooms in an attempt to manage the level of their symptomatology. However, even

---

TABLE 7–2
Cultural Competence Clinical Guidelines

The nurse needs to:

1. Explore the meaning of the aberrant behavior from the client's point of view, avoid projection of the nurse's worldview onto the client.

2. Be aware of the cultural context of help-seeking behavior. The nurse should not assume that the client wants what he would want under the same situation.

3. Recognize that mental health disorders are complex and are influenced by culture.

4. Be aware of the nurse's worldview and level of cultural competence because this influences the therapeutic relationship.

when they gain access into the mental health system, diverse persons are often under- or misdiagnosed regarding mental health disorders (Fontaine, 2000; Giger & Davidhizar, 2004; Vega, Sribney, Miskimen, Escobar, & Aguilar-Gaxiola, 2006).

Life Span and Gender Issues

For example, African American men with psychotic symptoms are frequently diagnosed with schizophrenia versus psychotic mood disorders (e.g., bipolar disorders) or physiologically based disorders (Minsky, Vega, Miskimen, Gara, & Escobar, 2003). Similarly, women are overdiagnosed with anxiety or panic disorders versus actual physiological problems, depressive disorders or schizophrenia. Mental illness disorders are often not diagnosed in children or persons from Asian cultures because the symptomatology from the disorders may be expressed in the form of physical complaints such as head, stomach, or muscle aches and pains. And certain physical problems or illnesses may be intertwined with mental illness symptomatology. Chronic fatigue syndrome and endocrinology disorders symptomatology is often vague and similar to depressive and anxiety symptomatology (Schuster, 2000; Taylor, 2003).

Diverse persons face even more challenges receiving appropriate treatment in these situations because their cultural patterns and nurses and other health care providers who lack culturally competent knowledge may misinterpret symptomatology. Finally, issues of medication, alcohol, and substance use and abuse contribute to the complexity of treatment for diverse persons because of the genetic differences in the metabolism of these substances (Antai-Otong, 2006).

Other issues contributing to barriers for mental health treatment include diverse persons' suspicion regarding the mental health system, their lack of access to insurance coverage, lack of ethnically and culturally diverse nurses within the health care system, health care provider bias and lack of cultural knowledge and the presence of societal stigma associated with mental illness (Leininger & McFarland, 2006; Muñoz & Luckmann, 2005; Pouissaint & Alexander, 2002; Barrett, 2006). All of these factors intensify the stigma and stress that diverse persons may encounter, which also create a climate conducive to diverse persons' lack of appropriate mental health treatment or premature withdrawal from treatment.

CULTURE AND PSYCHOPATHOLOGY

Symptomatology of mental health disorders is similar across cultures. However, the clinical picture or presentation of symptoms may be expressed differently based on cultural variations (APA, 2000; Tseng & Streltzer, 2004). As already stated, the verbal descriptions and manifestations of symptoms may vary based on culturally bound factors.

Symptomatology in Children and Adults

Children may have difficulty pinpointing where they "hurt" when mental distress occurs. In fact, they may cite physical symptoms as the cause of their "sickness" (e.g., stomachaches or headaches, "feeling sick to their tummies," or undefined pain

throughout the body), or their activity patterns may become altered. Children may exhibit hyperactivity, withdrawal, or nonresponsiveness (APA, 2000). Some may even attempt to hurt themselves or others when their symptomatology exacerbates. Individuals over the age of 70 years may experience muscle aches and pains as well as digestive and sleep disturbances when they incur depressive symptomatology (U.S. DHHS, 1999).

Finally, treatment issues may be confounded when nurses and other health care professionals lack knowledge regarding cultural variations in the cause of mental distress (Lutz & Warren, 2001; Warren, 2005; Tseng & Streltzer, 2004). For example, persons from some Latino(a), Hispanic, or Asian cultures may believe that any illness is caused by an imbalance within the body between the mind, body, and spirit or hot and cold forces. Consequently, any treatment approaches need to restore the ying and yang (e.g., mental, physical, and spiritual) or hot and cold balance (e.g., temperature, color, and spiritual) within an individual.

Older Adulthood

Working with older adults requires sensitivity and appreciation of various factors to this age group. Cultural, socioeconomic, and generational issues and concurrent health problems influence the quality of nurse-client relationships (Antai-Otong, 2007). Cultural and ethnic beliefs also frame the perception of aging. The nurse's perception of aging further influences how older clients are treated. Regardless of one's perception of aging it is imperative to treat all clients, including older adults with respect and dignity. This may be as simple as addressing the client by his or her surname. Psychiatric-mental health nurses must use a patient and unhurried approach in which the nurse speaks slowly and clearly. An additional generational issue associated with older adulthood is how emotional states are expressed. Stoicism and the need to "be strong" often interfere with the ability to express fear, anxiety, or depression. Working with this age group requires asking questions in a manner that enables the client to "tell his or her story" rather than making assumptions without validation. Storytelling provides a venue that older adults may find comfortable and safe to express feelings about their inner experiences (Antai-Otong, 2007). See Critical Thinking Questions.

INCIDENCE AND PREVALENCE OF MENTAL DISORDERS ACROSS CULTURAL GROUPS

Literature regarding cultural variations in mental health, wellness, and illness is sparse but continuing to grow based on recommendations, goals, and priorities from *Healthy People 2010* and the 1999 surgeon general's report on mental health and wellness as well as the report on culture, mental health, and wellness (U.S. DHHS, 1999, 2000). There are an estimated 51 million persons who incur mental illness annually in the United States. However, persons from diverse cultural groups often incur mental distress and illness at disproportionate rates. Contributing to the higher rates are issues of societal stigma and bias regarding diverse ethnic and cultural

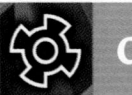

CRITICAL THINKING

1. Mr. L is an 80-year-old who has just been admitted for day surgery procedure. During a conversation he reports that his wife of 60 years was recently diagnosed with Alzheimer's disease. Which of the following statements reflects your understanding about client-centered health care?

    a. "John, when was your wife diagnosed with Alzheimer's disease?"

    b. "Would you like to talk about how depressed you are?"

    c. "How has your life been since your wife was diagnosed with Alzheimer's disease?"

    d. "Mr. L, you had a lot of productive years together and you were lucky to be married to the same woman for so many years."

Answer

a. Incorrect. Calling the client by his first name conveys a lack of respect and positive regard for an older adult.

b. Incorrect. This statement infers the client is depressed. He may be depressed and grieving about his wife's condition, but it is important to encourage him to express his feelings to validate this assumption.

c. Correct. Obviously this is a difficult time for the client. This question actually encourages him to tell "his story."

d. Incorrect. This question minimizes the client's experience and suggests that he should be grateful for the productive years.

---

groups as well as lower socioeconomic status for persons from many of these groups.

Issues of Gender and Sexual Orientation

Older adults and women between the ages of 25 and 44 years have higher rates of depression than do members from other cultural groups (U.S. DHHS, 1999, 2000). Persons from Indigenous or Native American cultures between 5 and

24 years of age incur a suicide rate three times as great as persons from other cultural groups in the same age range (U.S. DHHS, 1999, 2000). Current literature indicates that this increase is caused by socioeconomic differences, not internal differences, between these racial groups. It is difficult to estimate the incidence and prevalence of mental illness in persons from various cultural groups due to vast causes including cultural, religious, and social issues, especially when

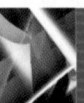

CASE STUDY

Mrs. Kelly is a 90-year-old client who was admitted several days ago for a left hip replacement. Her spouse died 10 years ago and she has lived alone since his death and has been very independent. Several days ago she slipped on ice while getting into her car and fractured her hip. You are making rounds and notice she is still asleep.

Nurse: Good morning Mrs. Kelly, I am your nurse today. How was your night?

Client: You woke me up. I am okay. I would really like to sleep a little more.

Nurse: I really need to help you prepare for breakfast.

Client: I am not ready to get up. I usually get up about 9 a.m. at home. Why do you wake us up so early in the morning?

Nurse: We have a pretty tight schedule and routine and we want to make sure your meal doesn't get cold.

Client: I don't know why I have to get on your schedule. I have always gotten up around 9 a.m. and this is just too early!

Nurse: I understand that the hospital schedule is different than yours, but we have to keep you on a schedule.

Client: Suppose I don't want to get up this early?

Nurse: I understand. Can we negotiate getting up at 8 a.m. rather than 7 a.m.?

Client: I guess so. I just hate coming to the hospital.

Discussion. In this scenario the nurse recognizes that the client feels pretty helpless and powerless in the hospital. She has lived alone for years and has established daily routines that meet her needs. Although it is important to maintain a schedule on the unit, it is equally important to respect the client's wishes and negotiate a time that both can live with.

women are in subordinate positions. History of mistrust of mental health providers to make accurate diagnosis and provide appropriate treatment and failure to explore the meaning of the individual's experience continue to impede mental health services to cultural groups (Choi & Lee, 2007; Neighbors et al., 2007). Current epidemiological statistics indicate that women from Latina or Hispanic cultures incur depressive symptoms at a rate of 46 percent as opposed to the 20 percent occurrence of these symptoms in Latino or Hispanic men (U.S. DHHS, 1999).

It is also estimated that gay males are three times as likely to commit suicide than males from other cultural groups (D'Augelle, Grossman, Salter, Vasey, Starks, et al., 2005; U.S. DHHS, 2000). Being gay is a risk factor for adolescent suicide. Due to the high risk of suicide among gay adolescents, psychiatric nurses are poised to assess past and current reactions to childhood gender behavior including level of openness about the youth's sexual orientation and any verbal abuse associated with sexual orientation. A small body of literature indicates that lesbian women may incur stress at a higher rate than heterosexual women (Diala et al., 2001). As many as 4 million children and adolescents experience and are disabled by a severe mental illness. It is also estimated that 10 million children under the age of 7 are in homes with a mentally distressed parent.

ETHNOPSYCHOPHARMACOLOGY

The growing body of literature on ethnopsychopharmacology (the study of intensity and duration of psychotropic medication responses for different racial groups of persons) indicates that drug polymorphism is the interaction of chemical factors and individuals' genetic responses to pharmacologic agents (Harty, Johnson, & Power, 2006). The reaction of chemical factors is affected by a person's age, gender, physical size, and genetic patterns in the absorption, distribution, metabolism, and elimination of pharmacologic agents (Muñoz & Hildenberg, 2006; Spector, 2004). Nurses need to be aware of these possible differences because they may prescribe or dispense medications to clients. In addition, nurses are most often the health care professionals who assess clients' responses to pharmacologic agents (see Chapter 9).

CRITICAL THINKING

What symptoms would you look for that would be indicative of lithium toxicity for a person from African or Asian American descent? What other medication could be used instead of lithium?

NEUROBIOLOGICAL FACTORS

Persons from diverse racial and ethnic cultures may also have variations in the pharmacologic responses within the three primary metabolic pathways (chemical sites involved in the conversion of pharmacologic agents within a person's biological system). Names of the metabolic pathways are acetylation, debrisoquine-ds, mephenytoin. Genetic variations within the metabolic pathways create different conversion responses within persons' systems. Persons may be slow or poor metabolizers of a particular class or type of medication owing to an insufficient conversion of medications within the pathways (Liou, Lin, Wu, & Wu, 2006). These persons may then have a greater risk of toxic reactions to certain pharmacologic agents. Other persons may be rapid or extensive metabolizers, which cause pharmacologic agents to be metabolized at a faster or more therapeutic rate.

For example, persons from Indigenous or Native American, African American, and Asian American populations are more susceptible to toxic reactions from the benzodiazepine anxiolytics and tricyclic antidepressants. Anxiolytics are metabolized through the acetylation and mephenytoin pathways, whereas antidepressants are metabolized through the debrisoquineds and mephenytoin pathways (Lin, Smith, & Ortiz, 2001). Some persons from Asian culture metabolize the anxiolytics, antidepressants, and lithium at a slower rate. Hence, they may respond more appropriately to smaller doses. Some persons from Native or Asian cultural groups may have a toxic reaction to the ingestion of alcohol because they are deficient in one of the metabolic precursors for enzyme production. This deficiency results in the occurrence of a "flushing syndrome," which causes them to experience sudden increased heartbeat, palpitations, sweating, and intense heat and redness of the neck and face (Bell, 1994). The nurse needs to assess persons from these cultural groups regarding their prudent use or avoidance of medications with alcohol or the ingestion of alcohol in social situations because of this toxic possibility. In addition, nurses need to carefully assess the level of pharmacologic dosing in women, children, senior persons, and men with smaller muscle mass because these individuals may also be susceptible to pharmacologic polymorphism.

Persons from African American cultures may have a different response to lithium than do other racial and ethnic persons because of their reaction to salt ingestion. Research indicates that African Americans tend to be more sensitive to salt and more readily hold greater concentration of salt within their cells than other racial populations (Lawson, 1996). Consequently, lithium may not be the best pharmacologic agent for the management of bipolar symptoms in African Americans. Because lithium is a salt, it may build up in the cells and not be metabolized or distributed efficiently. This increases the risk of toxicity and nonabatement or exacerbation of manic symptoms. Tegretol seems to be a better alternative for the treatment of bipolar symptomatology (Lawson, 1996).

Finally, nurses need to be aware that intracultural variations (alterations in cultural ideation and psychological or physical characteristics) regarding pharmacologic responses may exist in persons from diverse cultures. These differences are a result of the genetic blending of racial and ethnic cultures that affects or changes the genetic patterns and enculturation (process by which a person accepts and internalizes another person's or group's worldview into or in place of his own perspective) within persons. In addition, nurses need to be aware of the increase in the numbers of persons who use natural herbs or herbal supplements in order to treat mental distress. Nurses need to include this information as part of their assessment of clients in order to avoid toxic or nontherapeutic reactions to medications. Particularly problematic are the tricyclic antidepressants and antipsychotics because certain herbs and herbal supplements have the same therapeutic action as the synthetically made medications. Among these are swertia japonica, kamikihi-to, datura candida, Nigerian root extract, and the South American holly.

CRITICAL THINKING AND CULTURAL COMPETENCE

Critical thinking is a systematic and purposeful process of reasoning (Alfaro-LeFevre, 2004; Pesut & Herman, 1999). Cultural competence is an extension of critical thinking because it is a process that entails a systematic examination of clients' cultural influences on their mental, physical, and spiritual well-being. The psychiatric-mental health nurse artfully and logically uses nursing process in order to provide culturally competent care for clients. In fact, the role of the psychiatric-mental health nurse (PMH) is pivotal to the development of culturally competent mental health care for clients, because the nurse is often the gatekeeper to the mental health system and often coordinates care within the mental health system and other care systems that clients use (Peplau, 1991; Purnell & Paulanka, 2003; Spector, 2004). Nursing process provides a complementary approach to the development of culturally competent mental health care because it combines the use of nursing knowledge, art, and logic.

NURSING PROCESS AS A CULTURALLY COMPETENT TOOL

Nursing process is a circular process of assessment, determination of client needs, development of interventions, strategies and outcomes, outcomes measurements, and evaluation. The process is subject to reevaluation and adjustment at any point in order to adapt and meet the needs of the client. Cultural competence is also a circular process based on knowledge regarding assessment of cultural immersion of persons in the context and level of their mental health, wellness, or illness. Cultural assessments need to be enculturated into every nursing assessment process (Ryan, Carlton, & Ali, 2000; Warren, 2001). Cultural components for assessment include overview and heritage, communication patterns and preferences, significant other or family roles, nutritional practices, health beliefs and practices, learning preferences and educational level, spirituality or religious patterns, and genetic and physiological status. Answers to questions regarding cultural issues may be obtained by the nurses' overall observations of clients' reaction and behavior to the environment and persons within it as well as asking direct questions regarding their physical status. It is also advisable to begin any assessment with a question similar to the following, "How may I help you today?" or "What do you expect of me today?" or "How may I as a nurse help you today?" All of these questions may make the client more comfortable by providing him with the opportunity to give the nurse his cultural perspective and define his health care needs.

THE ROLE OF THE NURSE

The role of the psychiatric nurse in providing culturally sensitive mental health care requires self-awareness of one's own culture and its potential impact on the perception of symptoms in diverse populations. Self-awareness enhances sensitivity to the client's needs and preferences. The cornerstone of therapeutic interactions requires an environment that conveys acceptance and respect regardless of ethnicity and culture.

THE GENERALIST NURSE

The scope and depth of practice in the implementation of culture into client care is different for the generalist and the advanced-practice psychiatric-mental health nurse (Leininger, & McFarland, 2006). The generalist nurse knows and understands the role of culture in persons' lives. In

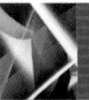

CASE STUDY

A Client with Depression (Mrs. Lee)

Mrs. Lee, a 30-year-old woman from Chinese heritage, comes into the emergency room crying and expressing multiple physical complaints. Her husband, mother, and acupuncturist also accompany her. They have copies of her most recent physical examination, which was completed last week. Mrs. Lee reports, "I have always been well, but recently I have trouble sleeping and have frequent stomachaches and headaches. The fatigue and aches make me so tearful. I can't seem to stop crying. Perhaps I have something wrong within my brain. I don't want to let the others around me down." The nurse also ascertains that Mrs. Lee is currently employed as a teacher in a local public school system. In addition, she is married and has two children, aged 10 and 13 years, at home. Her mother also lives with Mrs. Lee and her husband. Mr. Lee reports that Mrs. Lee has "not been herself" during the last 3 months. He also reports that she sometimes has periods of crying, is not sleeping well, and seems to have lost interest in her usual activities. Her mother states, "She often just sits by herself and stares into space. This is not my daughter. I have prepared some

(continues)

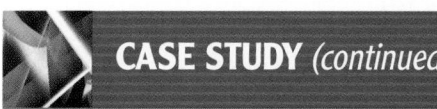
herbs for her but they have not worked. She also had a complete physical just last week at a general physician's office. Nothing was found. In fact, she has gotten worse. We also had her go to Mr. Liau, an acupuncturist, but this did not work either. Her stomachaches and headaches returned. Mr. Liau stated she might need some additional Western medication because her pulses were still not balanced. How can we help her now?"

Cultural Issues to Consider During the Nursing Process

1. Mrs. Lee is of Chinese heritage. However, the nurse needs to assess for the type, immersion, and level of Mrs. Lee's worldview perspective. The nurse ascertains that Mrs. Lee is a second-generation Chinese American born woman. In addition, English is Mrs. Lee's first language but she also speaks Chinese. Mrs. Lee also states, "My mother has taught me a great deal about our Chinese culture and I value her beliefs and perspectives. We often speak Chinese at home and celebrate many of the Chinese holidays." The fact that her mother lives with her and helps with household decisions is an indication that Mrs. Lee is grounded in the thought that elders are an important part of the family. All of this assessment information indicates that Mrs. Lee is deeply grounded in a community worldview perspective. It is important for the nurse to understand this perspective as she conducts additional assessment areas and develops the nursing plan for Mrs. Lee.

2. It is also important for the nurse to acknowledge the importance of the alternative medicine approaches (e.g., herbs, pulse regulation, acupuncture) that have been tried and to find out if herbs are still being used because they may be similar to any psychiatric medications that might be considered in Mrs. Lee's treatment.

3. Her husband, mother, and acupuncturist accompany Mrs. Lee. This indicates the importance of these significant others within her life. Development of the plan needs to include the involvement of these individuals.

4. A review of the previous physical examination and a current updated one indicates no apparent physical problem. Mrs. Lee also indicates she eats a diet high in fruits, vegetables, and rice. "I eat no beef, just some chicken and fish. But I have eaten very little lately. My appetite just isn't there."

5. In addition, the nurse needs to conduct a depression screen to ascertain the level of any depressive symptomatology. This is based on the physical examination being negative and the symptoms Mrs. Lee exhibits and talks about indicating the strong possibility of Mrs. Lee having a depressive disorder.

Next Step after the Assessment:

The nurse determined no other physical issues. The depression screen indicated that Mrs. Lee was severely depressed with some occasional thoughts of "not wanting to be around." Further questioning by the nurse indicated that Mrs. Lee had no plans for suicide. In fact, she stated "doing any harm to myself would shame my family and cause them great embarrassment." It is decided that Mrs. Lee will not need hospitalization. However, she will be coming in to see the nurse for therapy. Mrs. Lee has expressed a desire that her husband, mother, and Mr. Liau attend the sessions as well. Culturally important issues for Mrs. Lee include the inclusion of her family and Mr. Liau in her treatment process. Meditation, yoga, and acupuncture also are identified as important to her. These ideas are all incorporated into the nursing care plan. The nurse develops the following nursing plan with the involvement of Mr. and Mrs. Lee, her mother, and Mr. Liau.

addition, he or she can use aspects of cultural knowledge into the nursing process and clinical work with clients. The generalist nurse also knows the different cultural worldviews and perspectives. He understands the concept of cultural competence and uses it as an evidence-based practice in interactions with clients.

THE ADVANCED-PRACTICE PSYCHIATRIC REGISTERED NURSE

The advanced-practice PMH nurse has a greater depth and understanding about cultural issues. This level of nurse is quite proficient and knowledgeable about specific cultural populations and practices. The advanced-practice PMH nurse has had in-depth, numerous experiences with members from a wide variety of cultural groups (Leininger, & McFarland, 2006). Leininger states that the advanced practice PMH nurse has a master's degree or PhD and is a clinical expert who may also participate in cultural research and development of protocols within education, practice, or research settings. Refer to Nursing Care Plan 7–1.

SUMMARY

◆ Culture is one of the most important parts of an individual's life.

◆ A person's worldview perspective is the foundation for how persons think, react, and develop their mental health care beliefs and practices.

◆ Culture is broader than the traditionally thought of race, ethnicity, and religion because it extends to age, class, socioeconomic status, gender, sexual orientation, profession or work status, and so on.

◆ Culture may be defined as any way in which a person, group, or community defines itself or is defined by others.

◆ Nurses need to become familiar with aspects of culture because it affects how they interact with clients, their peers, and other health care professionals as well as how they provide care to and develop strategies and protocols with their clients.

◆ The foundation of appropriate mental health care is grounded in the elements of critical thinking, nursing process, and cultural competence.

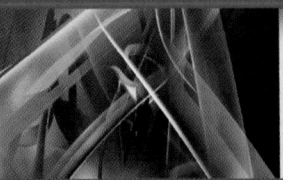

A Client with Depression (Mrs. Lee)

Nursing Diagnosis: Risk for Self-Directed Violence

Outcome Identification	Nursing Actions	Rationales	Evaluation
1. By [date], client verbalizes feelings rather than acting on them.	1a. Establish rapport. Encourage expression of feelings and somatic complaints.	1a. Establishes therapeutic interaction. Conveys empathy, caring, and interest. Anxiety and depression are sometimes conveyed by somatic complaints in some cultures.	*Goal met:* Nurse forms therapeutic relationship. Client expresses feelings. Client does not express suicidal ideations or act on thoughts.
	1b. Maintain a safe environment. Assess level of dangerousness including change in mood.	1b. Provides safety and control and decreases acting-out behaviors. 1c. Change in mood or anxiety level increases risk of dangerousness.	

Nursing Diagnosis: Ineffective Coping
due to the presence of depressive symptoms, including crying, lack of appetite, sleep disturbances, anhedonia, desire not to be around, failure to respond to Western and cultural treatments

Outcome Identification	Nursing Actions	Rationales	Evaluation
1. By [date], client develops realistic perception of present stressor(s).	1a. Explore meaning of present stressors associated with adaptation to Western and cultural treatments.	1a. Helps the client understand self and present responses.	*Goal met:* Client returns to prehospitalization level of functioning.
	1b. Understand meaning of present stressors.	1b. Validates understanding of meaning of present symptoms.	
2. By [date], client develops enduring adaptive coping skills.	2. Assist in identifying strengths, resources, and coping skills. Encourage the use of cultural stress management techniques (e.g., meditation, yoga).	2. Places focus on positive attributes and increases self-esteem.	Client develops adaptive coping skills. Client's self-esteem increases.

(continues)

Nursing Care Plan 7–1 *(continued)*

Outcome Identification	Nursing Actions	Rationales	Evaluation
	3. Provide information about medications and consider cultural factors associated with metabolism of medication. 3a. Assess for adverse side effects.	3/3a. Awareness of ethnopharmacological factors assist in providing a safe dose of medication and reduce adverse side effects.	Client tolerates medications and does not experience adverse drug reactions.

Nursing Diagnosis: Self-esteem, Low

Outcome Identification	Nursing Actions	Rationales	Evaluation
1. By [date], client verbalizes two to three positive attributes and increased self-esteem.	1a. Provide successful experiences. 1b. Convey acceptance and empathy. 1c. Encourage active participation in treatment. 1d. Encourage participation in culturally based stress reduction.	1a–d. Positive experiences increase confidence and self-esteem.	*Goal met:* Client's self-esteem increases. Client is able to explore options to deal with present stressors.

RESEARCH ABSTRACT

A Cross-Cultural Comparison of Family Resiliency in Hemodialysis Patients

White, N., Richter, J., Koeckeritz, J., Lee, Y. A., & Munch, K. L. (2002). *Journal of Transcultural Nursing, 13,* 218–227.

Study Problem/Purpose

The purpose of this descriptive comparative survey was to examine differences in family resilience between Endstage hemodialysis patients and caregivers among three ethically diverse populations that involved Anglo-Americans (n = 35), Mexican Americans (n = 20), and South Koreans (n = 13).

Methods

A descriptive comparative survey was used to collect data from subjects who were initially contacted during their dialysis treatment and had informed consent to participate. The two American groups were assessed through two, 25-bed private, freestanding dialysis centers, whereas the South Korean subjects were recruited from a 3-bed dialysis center. Questionnaires were administered on-site or taken home and returned during their next treatment. The study was based on the Family Resilience Model developed by McCubbin, Thompson, and McCubbin. Multivariate analysis of variance (MANOVA) was used to compare patient and caregiver perceptions of stressors (Demands of Illness), family resources and Resiliency across all 3 groups. A total sample of all patients (n = 68) and caregivers (n = 58) completed the surveys.

Findings

A comparison of chronic illness stressors revealed that the South Korean patient group perceived their illness stressors to impact them in moderately to quite a bit range, whereas the Anglo-American patient group rated the same stressors in the little to moderately range. The Mexican-American patient group perception of stressors was similar to the Anglo-Americans, except for the Appearance/Function subscale that was similar to the South Korean patients.

A comparison of family resources among the three groups demonstrated that their perceptions were similar. When the 3 groups were compared on Resiliency (Family Well-Being), the Anglo-American and Mexican American patients were similar and rated themselves higher (mean = 5.2) than South Koreans (mean = 3.7).

(continues)

Research Abstract *(continued)*

Caregiver comparison analysis showed no significant differences among the 3 groups on Provider Problems, but significant differences between the groups on Personal Meaning and Economic Impact of the Illness. The South Korean caregivers reported the most illness demands in these areas and Anglo-Americans the least. An important posit from this study indicates that none of the group means showed resiliency levels beyond the moderate range and suggest that these patients were not as resilient as one might desire.

Implications for Psychiatric Nurses

The role of the family and its ability to recover from significant stressors such as chronic illness requires resilience and ability to maintain integrity. The long-term impact of dialysis requires an ability to mobilize resources and support systems that enhance resilience and adaptation. Working with the client with a chronic physical or mental illness requires a comprehensive assessment of the client and family's strengths, resources and coping skills. Nursing interventions that strengthen resources and enhance family integrity are likely to facilitate an optimal level of functioning and quality of life.

SUGGESTIONS FOR CLINICAL CONFERENCES

1. Discuss the way that culture affects nurses and other persons' health care beliefs and practices. Provide specific examples to illustrate.

2. Discuss the variations in worldview perspectives in conjunction with how those views affect persons' responses to mental health, wellness, and illness. Cite relevant examples.

3. Review how culturally bound syndromes affect the clinical picture of mental health, wellness, and illness. Provide specific literature sources for discussion of these syndromes. Provide clinical examples if possible.

4. Discuss the relationship between culture and psychopathology. Cite relevant literature.

5. Discuss the connection between development of critical thinking, nursing process, and cultural competence. Develop case studies that are representative of this development.

STUDY QUESTIONS

1. Psychiatric nurses who are unclear about their own values and beliefs tend to be
   a. assertive
   b. inconsistent
   c. apathetic
   d. reliable

2. An adaptive response to some clients from non-Western cultures is
   a. extended future perspective
   b. fatalistic perspective
   c. individualism
   d. egalitarianism

3. Ms. Lincoln is an 82-year-old client who is seen in the adult community center for a grief reaction associated with the recent death of her husband of 55 years. The most important aspects of the nursing assessment include which of the following?
   a. Questions about her preferences, health practices, wishes, and expectations
   b. Questions about her husband and their relationship
   c. Questions about her relationship with her adult children
   d. Questions about her expectations from grief counseling

4. During the interview, Ms. Lincoln responds to your queries and mentions that she is uncomfortable doing grief counseling because she was raised to believe everyone should be able to take care of themselves and people who seek counseling are "weak." Her concerns are an example of which of the following?
   a. Worldview perspective
   b. Gender gap
   c. Stoicism
   d. Lack of knowledge about mental health services

5. You are working with a client whose culture and ethnicity differ from yours. In an effort to understand the client's experience you inquire about the meaning of his illness and what he feels will help him cope with present stressors. Through questioning you begin to understand the meaning of his experiences, needs, and expectations and can collaborate with the client to develop a plan of care. This is an example of which of the following?
   a. Cultural awareness
   b. Cultural competence
   c. Cultural understanding
   d. Worldview connectivity

6. Which of the following statements best describes *enculturation*?
   a. "What is the most difficult part of your illness?"
   b. "It sounds like this is a very difficult time for you and your family."
   c. "How can we work together to help you manage your symptoms more effectively?"
   d. All of the above

7. Mr. Lesser is a 45-year-old client who is brought to the outpatient psychiatric department with several relatives. It is imperative to understand their reasons for the visit. To minimize distractions during the interview, which of the following statements reflects sensitivity to the client and family's needs?
   a. "Mr. Lesser, which two relatives would you like to have with you during today's visit?"
   b. "Mr. Lesser, you have to attend this visit alone."
   c. "I'm sorry, but you will need to stay in the waiting room during his visit?"
   d. "Mr. Lesser will share what we discussed today. Everything is confidential."

8. One of your clients, Mr. P, asks, "What is your religion?" You answer Protestant. He expresses disbelief in your religion and states he wants to see someone of his own faith and religious beliefs. What is the most *appropriate response* to his request?
   a. "Mr. P, I can assure you that I am just as capable as anyone else on staff."
   b. "Mr. P, I really don't appreciate your criticism of my religion."
   c. Mr. P, I understand you are uncomfortable. I will ask someone else to see you."
   d. "Mr. P, I am really offended by your comments."

9. Mary's female partner accompanies her during today's visit. You have strong feelings about their relationship. What is the *most appropriate* way to work with this couple?
   a. Although you may not agree with their lifestyle, treat them the same as other clients.
   b. Discuss your discomfort to staff and ask someone else to see the client.
   c. Tell the client and her partner you are uncomfortable with their lifestyle.
   d. Ask a colleague to see the client without sharing your discomfort.

10. Mr. Chuma has recently been diagnosed with bipolar disorder, manic episode. His family reports he has been taking his antimanic agent, lithium, as ordered and they don't understand recurrent mania. What is an important question to ask concerning his current symptoms?
    a. "Has he modified his salt intake the past few weeks?"
    b. "Has he ever taken other medications for bipolar disorder, such as carbamazepine?"
    c. "Has he had similar reactions to other medications used to treat bipolar disorder?"
    d. All of the above

11. Increased susceptibility to side effects associated with pharmacological agents may be explained by *all but* which of the following?
    a. Genetics
    b. Age
    c. Gender
    d. Psychiatric disorder

REFERENCES

Alfaro-Levre, R. (2004). *Critical thinking and clinical judgment: A practical approach* (3rd ed.). Philadelphia: Elsevier.

American Psychiatric Association. (2000). *Diagnostic and statistical manual of mental disorders,* 4th edition, Text Revision *[DSM-IV-TR]*. Washington, DC: Author.

Andrews, M. M., & Boyle, J. S. (2002). *Transcultural concepts in nursing care* (2nd ed.). Philadelphia: J.B. Lippincott.

Antai-Otong, D. (2006). Women and alcoholism and gender-related medical complications: Treatment considerations. *Journal of Addictions Nursing, 17,* 33–42.

Antai-Otong, D. (2007). *Nurse-client communication: A life span approach.* Sudbury, MA: Jones and Bartlett Publishers.

Baker, F. M. (2001). Diagnosing depression in African Americans. *Community Mental Health Journal, 37*(1), 31–38.

Barrett, S. (2006). Interviewing techniques for the Asian-American population. *Journal of Psychosocial Nursing, 44*(5), 29–34.

Bell, R. (1994). Prominence of women in Navajo healing beliefs and values. *Nursing Health Care, 15*(1), 232–242.

Campinha-Bacote, J. (2003). *The process of cultural competence in health care: A culturally competent model of care* (3rd ed.). Wyoming, OH: Transcultural C.A.R.E. Associates, Perfect Printing Press.

Campinha-Bacote, J. (2005). *A Biblically-based model of cultural competence in the delivery of healthcare services.* (4th ed.). Wyoming, Ohio: Transcultural C.A.R.E. Associates.

Carter, R. T. (1995). *The influence of race and racial identity in psychotherapy: Toward a racially inclusive model.* New York: Wiley & Sons.

Choi, Y. J., & Lee, K. J. (2007). Evidence-based nursing: Effects of a structured program for the health of Korean women with hwa-hyung. *Archives of Psychiatric Nursing, 21,* 12–16.

Chong, N. (2002). *The Latino patient: A cultural guide for health care providers.* ME: Intercultural Press.

D'Augelle, A. R., Grossman, A. H., Salter, N. P., Vasey, J. J., Starks, M. T., & Sinclair, K. (2005). Predicting the suicide attempts of lesbian, gay and bisexual youth. *Suicide and Life Threatening Behaviors, 35,* 646–660.

Delahanty, J. et al. (2001). Differences in rates of depression in schizophrenia by race. *Schizophrenia Bulletin, 27*(1), 29.

Diala, C. C., Muntaner, C., Walrath, C., Nickerson, K., LaVeist, T., & Leaf, P. (2001). Racial/ethnic differences in attitudes toward professional mental health care and the use of services. *American Journal of Public Health. 91*(5), 805.

Douki, S., Ben Zineb, S., Nacef, F., & Halbreich, U. (2007). Women's mental health in the muslim world: Cultural, religious and social issues. *Journal of Affective Disorder* [Epub ahead of print].

Fontaine, K. L. (2000). *Healing practices: Alternative therapies for nursing.* Upper Saddle, River, NJ: Prentice-Hall.

Giger, J. N., & Davidhizar, R. E. (2004). *Transcultural nursing: Assessment and intervention* (4th ed.).

Harty, L., Johnson, K., & Power, A. (2006). Race and ethnicity in the era of emerging pharmacogenomics. *Journal of Pharmacology, 46,* 405–407.

Health Resources and Services Administration (HRSA), Bureau of Health Professions, Division of Nursing. (2004). *Moving toward elimination of health disparities in the United States.* Retrieved May 12, 2006, from http://www.hrsa.gov/OMH/OMH/disparities/. St. Louis, MO: Mosby.

Juarbe, T. (1996). Puerto Ricans. In J. G. Lipson, S. L. Dible, & P. A. Minarik (Eds.), *Culture and nursing care: A pocket guide* (pp. 222–238). San Francisco: University of California, San Francisco Nursing Press.

Kelley, F. J., Kopac, C. A., & Rosselli, J. (2007). Advanced health assessment in nurse practitioner programs: Follow-up study. *Journal of Professional Nursing, 23,* 137–143.

Kramer, J. (1996). American Indians. In J. G. Lipson, S. L. Dible, & P. A. Minarik (Eds.), *Culture and nursing care: A pocket guide* (pp. 11–22). San Francisco: University of California, San Francisco Nursing Press.

Lawson, W. B. (1996). The art and science of the psychopharmacotherapy of African Americans. *Mt. Sinai Journal of Medicine, 63,* 301–305.

Leininger, M., & McFarland, M. R. (2006). *Cultural care diversity and universality: A worldwide nursing theory* (2nd ed.). Boston: Jones and Bartlett Publishers.

Liou, Y. H., Lin, C. T., Wu, Y. J., & Wu, L.S. (2006). The high prevalence of the poor and ultrarapid metabolite alleles of CYP2D6, CYP2C9, CYP2C19, CYP3A4, and CYP3A5 in Taiwanese population. *Journal of Human Genetics, 51,* 857–863.

Lutz, W. J., & Warren, B. J. (2001). Symptomatology and Medication monitoring for public mental health consumers: A cultural perspective. *Journal of the American Psychiatric Nurses Association, 7(4),* 115–124.

Mahoney, J. S., Carlson, E., & Engebretson, J. C. (2006). A framework for cultural competence in advanced practice psychiatric and mental health education. *Perspectives in Psychiatric Care, 42,* 227–237.

Minsky, S., Vega, W., Miskimen, T., Gara, M., & Escobar, J. (2003). Diagnostic patterns in Latino, African American, and European American psychiatric patients. *Archives of General Psychiatry, 60,* 637–644.

Muñoz, C., & Hildenberg, C. (2006). Ethnopharmacology: Understanding how ethnicity can affect drug response is essential in providing culturally competent care. *Holistic Nursing Practice, 20,* 227–234.

Muñoz, C., & Luckmann, J. (2005). *Transcultural communication in nursing.* New York: Thomson Delmar.

National Academy of Sciences, Institute of Medicine (IOM). (2003). *Unequal treatment: Confronting racial and ethnic disparities in health care.* Washington, DC: National Academies Press.

Neighbors, H. W., Caldwell, C., Williams, D. R., Nesse, R., Taylor, R. J., Bullard, K. M., et al. (2007). Race, ethnicity, and the use of services for mental disorders: Results from the National Survey of American Life. *Archives of General Psychiatry, 64,* 485–494.

Nichols, E. (1987, June). *Nichols' model of the philosophical aspects of cultural difference.* Paper presented at the meeting of the faculty, The Ohio State University, Columbus.

Peplau, H. (1991). *Interpersonal relations in nursing.* New York: Putnam.

Pesut, D. J., & Herman, J. (1999). *Clinical reasoning: The art and science of critical & creative thinking.* Clifton Park, NY: Delmar Learning.

Pouissaint, A. F., & Alexander, A. (2000). *Lay my burden down: Unraveling suicide and the mental health crisis among African Americans.* Boston: Beacon Press.

Purnell, L. D., & Paulanka, B. J. (2003). The Purnell model for cultural competence. In Purnell, L. D., & Paulanka, B. J. (Eds.). *Transcultural health care: A culturally competent approach,* Philadelphia: F. A. Davis.

Ross, H. (2001). Office of Minority Health publishes final standards for cultural and linguistic competence, *Closing the Gap* 1, February/March.

Ryan, M., Carlton, K. H., & Ali, N. (2000). Transcultural nursing concepts and experiences in nursing curricula. *Journal of Transcultural Nursing, 11,* 300–307.

Schuster, P. M. (2000). *Communication: The key to the therapeutic relationship.* Philadelphia: F. A. Davis.

Shiba, G., & Oka, R. (1996). Japanese Americans. In J. G. Lipson, S. L. Dible, & P. A. Minarik (Eds.), *Culture and nursing care: A pocket guide* (pp. 180–190). San Francisco: University of California, San Francisco Nursing Press.

Siantz, M. L., & Meleis, A. I. (2007). Integrating cultural competence into nursing education and practice: 21st century action steps. *Journal of Transcultural Nursing, 18,* 1 Suppl, 86S–90S.

Spector, R. (2004). *Cultural diversity in health & illness.* (6th ed.). Upper Saddle River, NJ: Prentice-Hall Health.

Taylor, J. S. (2003). The story catches you and you fall down: Tragedy, ethnography, and "cultural competence." *Medical Anthropology Quarterly, 17,* 159–181.

Tseng, W-S., & Streltzer, J. (2004). *Cultural competence in clinical psychiatry.* Washington, DC: American Psychiatric Publishing.

Tylor, E. (1871). *Primitive culture* (Vol. I). London: Bradbury, Evans, & Co.

U.S. Department of Health & Human Services (U.S. DHHS). (2000 January). *Healthy people* 2010. Understanding and improving health. Retrieved from http://www.health.gov/healthypeople/DOCUMENT/HTML/volume1/opening.html.

U.S. Department of Health & Human Services (U.S. DHHS). (2002). *Healthy people* 2010. McLean, VA: International Medical Publications. Retrieved May 12, 2006, from http://www.healthypeople.gov.

U.S. Public Health Service, Department of Health and Human Services [DHHS]. (1999). *Mental health: A report of the surgeon general.* Retrieved July 16, 2002, from http://www.surgeongeneral.gov/library/mentalhealth.html

Vega, W. A., Sribney, W. M., Miskimen, T. M., Escobar, J. I., & Aguilar-Gaxiola, S. (2006). Putative psychotic symptoms in the Mexican American population: Prevalence and co-occurrence with psychiatric disorders. *Journal of Nervous and Mental Disorders, 194,* 471–477.

Warren, B. J. (2000). Point of view: A best practice process for psychiatric mental health nursing. *Journal of the American Psychiatric Nurses Association, 6*(4), 135–138.

Warren, B. J. (2001, September/October). The rainbow approach for culturally competent care of people of African-American heritage. *The Case Manager,* 52–55.

Warren, B. J. (2002). Interlocking paradigm of cultural competence: A model for psychiatric mental-health nursing practice. *Journal of the American Psychiatric Nurses Association, 8*(6), 209–213.

Warren, B. J. (2005). The cultural expression of dying. *The Case Manager, 16*(1), 44–47.

Warren, B. J. (in press). Cultural competence in psychiatric nursing. In N. L. Keltner, L. H. Schwecke, & C. E. Bostrom (Eds.), *Psychiatric Nursing* (Ch. 28, pp. 382–421). St. Louis: Mosby.

Warren, B. J., & Alley, S. (2005). Innovative educational aspects: Culture and genetics: Critical aspects within nursing education. *Journal of Nursing Education, March/April,* 2–3.

Warren, B. J., & Lutz, W. J. (2000). A consumer-oriented practice model for psychiatric mental health nursing. *Archives of Psychiatric Nursing, 14*(3), 117–126.

SUGGESTED READINGS

Barrio, C. (2000). Cultural relevance of community support programs. *Psychiatric Services, 51,* 879–888.

Carter, J. H. (2002). Religion/spirituality in African-American culture: An essential aspect of psychiatric care. *Journal of the National Medical Association, 94,* 371–375.

Carter, R. T. (1995). *The influence of race and racial identity in psychotherapy: Toward a racially inclusive model.* Toronto, Canada: John Wiley & Sons.

Harden, J. T., & McFarland, G. (2000). Avoiding gender and minority barriers to NIH funding. *Image: Journal of Nursing Scholarship, 32,* 83–86.

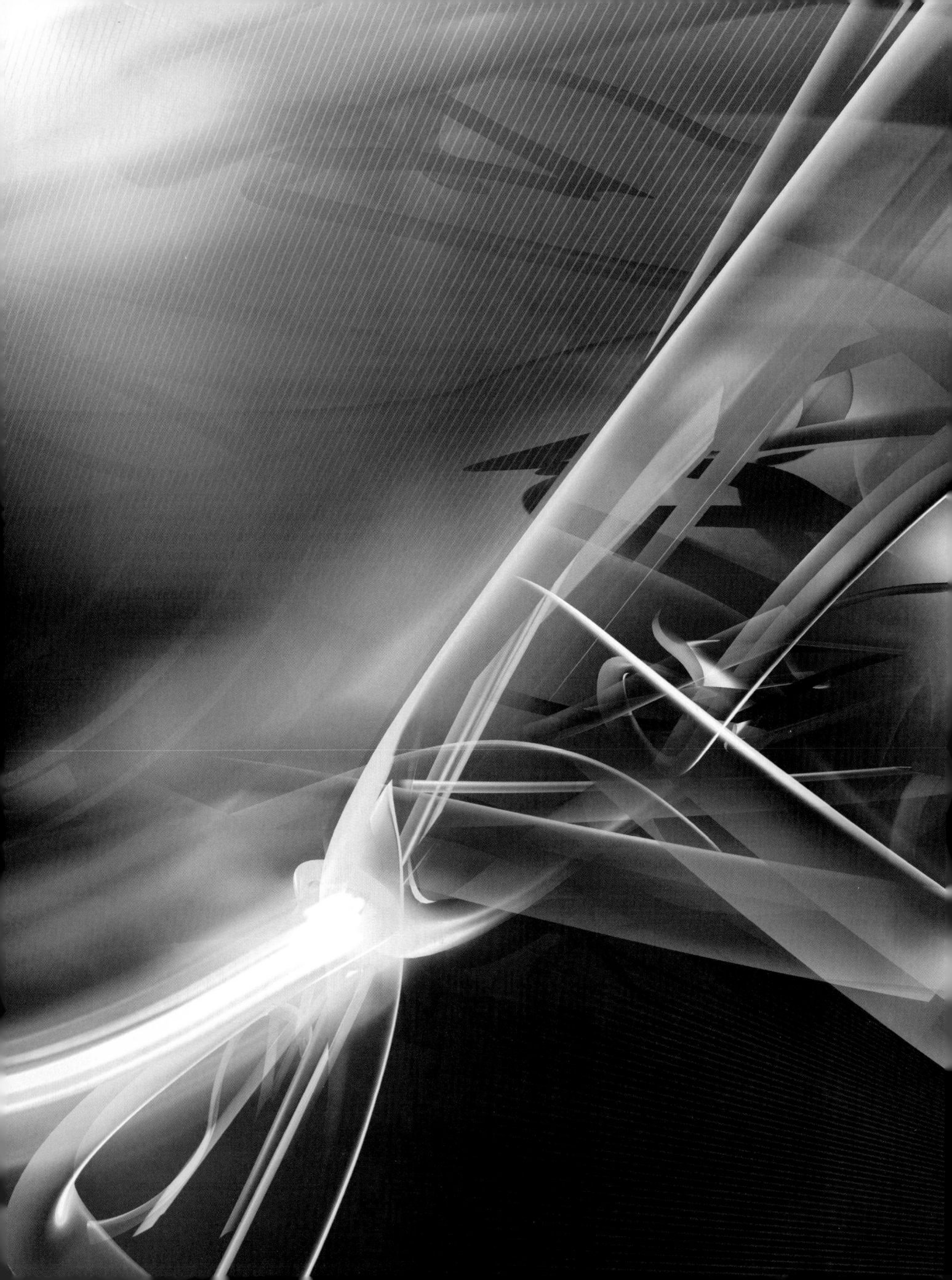

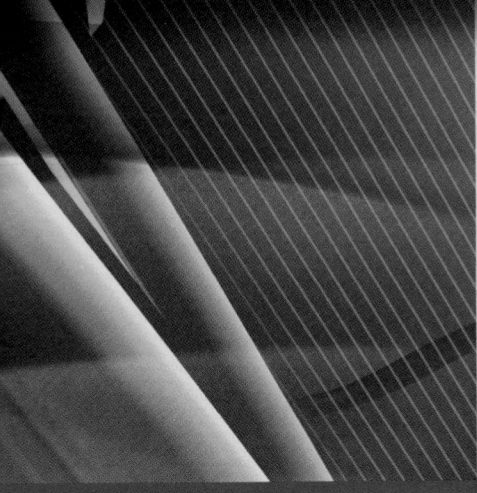

CHAPTER 8

Legal and Ethical Considerations

Linda Funk Barloon, RN, MS(N), CPNP
Ada Lynne Hendricks, RN, CS, FNP-C, MS(N)

KEY TERMS

Advocacy: Defending a cause or pleading a case in another's behalf (Bloom & Asher, 1982); putting the interest of the client before the interest of the nurse.

Autonomy: The ability of individuals to make independent personal decisions and act in their own behalf, recognizing the inherent value of each individual.

Beneficence: Doing good and avoiding doing harm.

Bioethics: Ethics applied to health care.

Civil Commitment: The ability of the state to hospitalize a person without consent.

Competency: The ability of a person to perform certain tasks; to be able to understand legal proceedings and assist in that process.

Deinstitutionalization: The systematic process of moving mentally ill clients from long-term, inpatient institutions to less structured settings such as group homes and community mental health centers.

Distributive Justice: The concept that resources should be distributed equitably across society or a collective group.

Fidelity: Keeping promises and obligations.

Justice: Treating all people fairly and equitably.

Malpractice: Intentional professional misconduct that fails to comply with professional standards and results in injury.

Mental Illness: A disability involving loss of contact with reality and nonpsychotic disorders that causes impairment in functioning or emotional distress.

Negligence: Unintentional injury that results from failure to act as a reasonable person would.

Psychiatric Genetics: The science of heritable factors related to psychiatric disorders.

Tort: Unintentional or intentional injury.

Veracity: Telling the truth; honesty.

COMPETENCIES

Upon completion of this chapter, the learner should be able to:

1. Discuss the history of legal and ethical changes in mental health treatment.
2. Define commonly held ethical principles.
3. Discuss a systematic approach to ethical decision making.
4. Explain how major U.S. mental health laws apply to psychiatric clients.
5. Discuss client rights and the application of rights in the clinical setting.
6. Identify legal and ethical issues affecting the psychiatric nurse today and in the future.

CHAPTER OUTLINE

Legal Issues in Psychiatric Care: Historical Perspectives

Ethics and Psychiatric Nursing

Ethical Concepts

Professional Ethics in Nursing

Ethical Dilemmas and a Decision-Making Model

Topics of Ethical Concern in Psychiatric Nursing Practice

Professional Boundaries

Psychiatric nurses are routinely involved in the complex life events of clients. These clients' lives are often complicated by legal and ethical issues. The application of clinical knowledge to legal questions while at the same time being sensitive to ethical issues is increasingly demanded of health care providers (Young, Spitz, Hillbrand, & Daneri, 1999). Fitzgerald (1999, p. 60) states, "The law defines the minimum expected level of conduct for a health care professional and where the law ends, ethics begins." In making these judgments one must decide the protective measures that are consistent with good clinical care (Felthous, 1999). Not only must nurses make legal and ethical decisions for themselves, they also must guide and support clients as they struggle with these same issues (Wilkinson, 1987). It is critical, therefore, that nurses have the necessary tools to accomplish these objectives. In adapting to the frequent changes in the health care system and the world around them, clients depend on nurses to assist them in finding access to the most effective care possible. An understanding of the legal and ethical issues and the ability to address them influence the care provided by psychiatric nurses.

LEGAL ISSUES IN PSYCHIATRIC CARE: HISTORICAL PERSPECTIVES

Both clients and health care providers are aware of their legal rights now more than ever (Kim, et al., 2007). Nurses have a responsibility to be aware of the legal and ethical rights of their clients because consumers depend on nurses to understand the system and aid in their care. Many changes in psychiatric care have occurred throughout history, and changes continue to occur as knowledge, technology, social and political forces, and other dynamics influence the mental health care system. See Table 8–1 for a historical overview.

In colonial times, Americans used English common law to decide how to handle the mentally ill. Methods of treatment included arrests, beatings, and placement in prisons, poor houses, or cages. In 1751, the Pennsylvania Colonial Assembly passed a law establishing a hospital for the poor who were sick and for the mentally ill. It was the first hospital known to have a philosophy of curing the mentally ill rather than simply housing them. Even so, clients were restrained and beatings were frequent. The insane were believed not to feel heat or cold and therefore were unprotected from the weather. There

TABLE 8–1
Historical Overview of Legal Events in Psychiatric Care

1751	The first mental hospital was established in the American colonies with a philosophy for curing the mentally ill.
Early 1800s	A few states made laws that the mentally ill could be kept in prison only for a short time or in an emergency.
1840s	Dorothea Dix traveled and conducted public hearings about conditions for the insane.
1843	The M'Naghten case in Britain established the legal basis for "not guilty by reason of insanity."
1860s	Efforts of Mrs. E. P. W. Packard, a victim of involuntary commitment, resulted in new commitment laws.
1908	Ex-patient Clifford Beers helped found the Committee for Mental Hygiene.
1946	The National Mental Health Act of 1946 was passed, and the National Institute of Mental Health was created.
1960s	Client rights movement protecting restrictions on liberty for the mentally ill evolved from the Civil Rights movement.
1963	The Community Mental Health Centers Act was passed.
1970s	The U.S. Supreme Court ruled that the right to legal counsel applies to the mentally ill.
1976	The Tarasoff ruling established that mental health professionals have the "duty to warn" potential victims of violence by clients.
1980s	Medication administration policies in most states and territorial jurisdictions establish clients' right to refuse medication.
1990s	Proliferation of health maintenance organizations managing mental health expenditures.
2000	Genetics and Genomics. Increased use of prescription psychotropics in children and adolescents. Issuance of "black warnings" for suicide risk involving antidepressant use among children and adolescents.
2000–2007	Advance directives.

were no laws protecting the liberty of the mentally ill. To initiate hospitalization, a relative or friend could obtain an order for admission from a hospital manager or physician, resulting in the client being forcibly detained in the hospital. The hospital could earn extra revenue by displaying clients and charging a fee for the public's entertainment (Dice, 1987).

At that time, mental health caregivers thought it necessary to attempt to domesticate the spirits of the mentally ill. Dr. Benjamin Rush, known as the Father of Psychiatry, invented two mechanical restraint devices. He believed in physical punishment; however, he was humane by the standards of the time. Rush required attendants to pay attention to personal hygiene and show respect for clients. He succeeded in separating the men and women into different buildings (Dice, 1987).

During the 1840s, Dorothea Dix traveled around Massachusetts and Rhode Island, visiting the mentally ill who were living in jails and almshouses because of inadequate space in asylums. She found conditions in which the insane were tied, chained, or placed in iron collars in dirty, dark, unheated cells. Some victims froze to death, and caretakers maimed others. Dix brought her findings to lawmakers and the public, who were horrified at the inadequate living conditions. Considered the most influential reformer of her era, Dix advocated for and assisted in the expansion of state hospitals and public institutions (Gamwell & Tomes, 1995; Sanders & DuPlessis, 1985).

During the last half of the nineteenth century, the population of clients chronically cared for in institutions continued to grow. During this period, mental hospitals were seen as a necessity to protect both society and the mentally ill, but they were not viewed as treatment (Dain, 1994).

In the 1860s, Mrs. E. P. W. Packard was committed by her husband, Rev. Theophilus Packard, to psychiatric hospitalization because of accusations that she was mentally ill. After her discharge, Mrs. Packard traveled nationally, accusing her husband of conspiring to have her locked up unnecessarily and contending that incarceration should not be based solely on the opinions of others but on the behavior of the individual (Dain, 1994).

In 1908, former psychiatric client Clifford Beers helped found the National Committee for Mental Hygiene, which campaigned for hospital reform and public education regarding mental illness. The committee later played a role in improving the training of psychiatrists in the 1920s and 1930s. Beers is considered the founder of the modern mental health movement (Dain, 1994).

Following both world wars, interest in mental health care grew because of the large number of returning veterans with emotional problems. The National Mental Health Act of 1946 was passed, the National Institute of Mental Health was created, and mental health goals for the nation were set as the public became more aware of its citizens with psychiatric problems (Betrus & Hoffman, 1992).

The terms *psychiatric* and *mental health* first came into use during the 1950s (Betrus & Hoffman, 1992). Also during the postwar years, the psychoanalytic community led by Dr. Karl Menninger championed the development of therapeutic communities rather than state-operated institutions, and during this same period, new medications such as chlorpromazine (Thorazine) were developed, which allowed clients better control of their symptoms in less structured settings.

These new developments in mental health care resulted in the proliferation of community mental health centers during the 1950s and 1960s (Dain, 1994). The Community Mental Health Centers Act of 1963 further provided an opportunity for outpatient treatment or short-term hospitalization in community mental health centers close to clients' homes (Dice, 1987). This act also resulted in modifying the education of nurses to include community mental health (Betrus & Hoffman, 1992).

Between 1955 and 1980, the number of clients in state mental hospitals decreased by more than 75 percent, partly because states were no longer required to provide the funding to care for the mentally ill outside the hospital setting in an effort to encourage the use of community mental health resources. If clients were discharged from the hospital, federal Medicaid funds would provide financial support for their care. Clients who were discharged into the community had difficulty adjusting outside the hospital because of poor continuity of care and often ended up in other institutionalized settings, in poor living conditions, or even on the streets (Dice, 1987).

During the 1960s, increasing concern with the rights of psychiatric clients was a by-product of the Civil Rights movement, the availability of legal services, public disgust with the conditions in mental institutions, and an assertion by the mentally ill of their legal rights. The 1960s' liberal philosophy of equality, self-determinism, and liberty provided the framework that influenced developments such as client rights, confidentiality, informed consent, and deinstitutionalization.

Other changes in the 1970s and 1980s affected the rights of the mentally ill. After the U.S. Supreme Court ruled that a person accused of a capital offense has a right to legal counsel and acknowledged that the Constitution emphasizes the right to liberty, the right to legal counsel was successfully applied to the mentally ill (McFadyen, 1989). The psychiatric client has constitutional rights explicitly protected by the Constitution that are not relinquished because of psychiatric status. These rights include freedom of speech, the right to due process, freedom from cruel and unusual punishment, and the right to equal protection under the law. The psychiatric client also has rights that are considered fundamental rights; for example, the right to marry, the right to choose one's own fate, and entitlements that are provided by state and federal statutes, such as civil commitment procedures (Bloom & Asher, 1982). These legal rights set the foundation from which decisions are made.

The 1980s and 1990s marked an era of the proliferation of managed health care organizations (MCOs). In an attempt to contain health care costs, MCOs serve as both the insurer and provider of access to health care. The purpose of MCOs is to decrease health care costs by assessing symptomatology, finding health care options, and determining choices that result in using the least restrictive environment at the minimal cost that will meet the needs of the client. Often companies contract with health maintenance organizations (HMOs) to obtain benefits for the employees in which the HMO sets up a network of providers that must be used, and determines the level of treatment chosen and the length of time or visits necessary for care. Some states have made decisions to allow clients to file medical malpractice claims against HMOs for damages. New York has required that MCOs provide information regarding the number of grievances received, including the number of decisions made in favor of clients' accusations (Slovenko, 1999). Legal issues surrounding MCOs include malpractice charges if cost containment decisions restrict the quality and availability of care (Burkhardt & Nathaniel, 1998). The rights of psychiatric clients are explored further in this chapter.

ETHICS AND PSYCHIATRIC NURSING

Along with legal parameters, psychiatric nurses have ethical obligations that affect their practice. In many instances, laws reflect the popular moral values of a society and interface closely with ethical positions. However, that which is legal is not always considered ethical and vice versa (Burkhardt & Nathaniel, 1998). Nurses use professional judgment in determining what actions are right and best in the care of clients, and they often face ethical dilemmas. An understanding of basic ethical principles, guidelines for analyzing issues, and knowledge of professional standards are valuable resources in ethical decision making.

ETHICAL CONCEPTS

The branch of philosophy called ethics is concerned with the examination of moral judgments and decisions about conduct. The term *ethics* is derived from the Greek word *ethos*, which means conduct or character. The terms *ethics* and *morals* are often used interchangeably. Bioethics, formerly called medical ethics, is ethics applied to health care (Davis & Aroskar, 1991).

There are two traditional ethical positions: (1) deontology and (2) utilitarianism, or teleology. In the deontological approach an act has an inherent moral significance, and decisions are based on adherence to certain principles without regard to consequences. An example of using this method is never telling a lie, regardless of the consequences. The utilitarian approach focuses on the consequences of actions and is concerned with maximizing the greatest good and least harm for the most people. With this reasoning, telling a lie is justified if the outcome results in the most good (Davis & Aroskar, 1991). An example of applying the utilitarian approach is a nurse who administers p.r.n. lorazepam (Ativan) to a client earlier than the order indicates because the client is severely agitated and threatening to harm other clients. The nurse then falsifies the medication administration record so that it appears that the medication was given at the correct time. The nurse reasons that although the medication is not prescribed at this time, the outcome of protecting the client and others justifies the actions taken. Although the nurse may believe that administering the medication to the client earlier than ordered and then falsifying the record is ethically appropriate, these actions are not legal and perhaps not clinically indicated. This example illustrates the importance of considering clinical and legal issues in addition to ethical principles in decision making.

Principles are general rules that guide conduct and decision making. Commonly accepted ethical principles include autonomy, beneficence, justice, veracity, and fidelity (Figure 8–1). Although ethical principles are thought to be universal, in fact, acceptance of principles is dependent on the culture and society (Hall, 1997). In addition, the application of principles may vary from person to person or among cultures. For example, basing an action on the principle of beneficence, two nurses may decide on two different actions to take in a situation, both based on the goal of being beneficent. Likewise an individual nurse may have to choose between two morally defensible positions; for example, deciding that veracity or truth telling with a client is the more compelling action to take than withholding information, which may seem more beneficent.

PROFESSIONAL ETHICS IN NURSING

In applying ethical reasoning, nurses may use moral principles in decision making. In addition, nursing, like other health professions, has codes of ethics to guide its practice. Originally, nurses followed ethical standards associated with the religious orders with which they were allied. In the late 1800s, the Florence Nightingale Pledge was created to reflect the ethical principles of the nurses trained by Nightingale. Its tenets included treating the client rather than the disease and loyalty to the profession (Davis & Aroskar, 1991). Since that time, nurses have continued to develop statements of standards to guide professional practice and to symbolize the values of the profession. The American Nurses Association (ANA) has published a Code of Ethics for nurses. The most recent published revision of the code, which was originally adopted in 1950, was in 2001 (Table 8–2). The ANA code also establishes standards of practice to which nurses are held accountable.

Autonomy: Individuals have the right to make decisions that affect their personal life; each person is worthy of respect and unique yet interdependent with others.

Beneficence (Nonmaleficence): People should promote good, do no harm, and prevent harm.

Justice: People should be treated fairly, and resources should be equitably distributed.

Veracity (Truth telling): People should be honest and open.

Fidelity: People should be faithful to their promises and obligations.

Figure 8–1 Examples of ethical principles. *(Data from Ethics and Issues in Contemporary Nursing, by M. A. Burkhardt and A. K. Nathaniel, 2002, Clifton Park, NY: Delmar Learning.)*

In addition to the ANA Code for Nurses, the American Association of Colleges of Nursing (1986) has set forth the following professional values for nursing: altruism, equality, esthetics, freedom, human dignity, justice, and truth.

ETHICAL DILEMMAS AND A DECISION-MAKING MODEL

Despite principles and standards of conduct, nurses still face ethical dilemmas. An ethical dilemma is a situation that involves deciding between equally unsatisfactory alternatives based on a moral claim, often with conflicting principles. For example, a nurse may support the autonomy of a mentally ill client to make decisions, but the client's refusal of treatment may be harmful. Standards of conduct and principles are useful tools for nurses to help justify moral actions taken. See Figure 8–2 for strategies for improving ethical decision-making abilities.

The use of a decision-making model may be helpful in analyzing a situation; however, nurses should be cautioned not to expect simplistic solutions to ethical dilemmas. There are a number of models that can be used as a framework to dissect ethical dilemmas, and most address similar issues and concepts. The following model is a guide to ethical decision making (Burkhardt & Nathaniel, 1998; Eriksen, 1989):

a. *Gather facts:*
   What are the facts of the situation? What information is fact, and what is an assumption or emotional reaction? What are the gaps in information, and what is the best source of information?

b. *Identify the conflicting moral positions:*
   Is this truly an ethical dilemma or just a difficult clinical situation? What, if any, ethical issues are involved? What ethical aspects are in conflict?

Familiarize yourself with ethical principles, professional codes, position statements, and institutional policies. Use this knowledge confidently in your discussions with others about ethical concerns.

a. Attend educational programs about ethical and legal issues.

b. Know the chain of command in your setting and follow it.

c. Discuss ethical dilemmas with co-workers and supervisors. Ask seasoned and respected nurses how they might handle a given situation.

d. Become involved in your institution's ethics committee or nursing ethics committee and use the committee as a resource.

e. Develop greater awareness about your own personal, cultural, and professional values through self-exploration and discussions with others.

f. Work in a setting that promotes and supports nursing practice that is congruent with your values and ethics.

Figure 8–2 Strategies for improving the ethical decision-making abilities of nurses.

TABLE 8–2
American Nurses Association Code of Ethics for Nurses

- **Provision 1:** The nurse, in all professional relationships, practices with compassion and respect for the inherent dignity, worth, and uniqueness of every individual, unrestricted by considerations of social or economic status, personal attributes, or the nature of the health problems.
- **Provision 2:** The nurse's primary commitment is to the patient, whether an individual, family, group, or community.
- **Provision 3:** The nurse promotes, advocates for, and strives to protect the health, safety, and rights of the patient.
- **Provision 4:** The nurse is responsible and accountable for individual nursing practice and determines the appropriate delegation of tasks consistent with the nurse's obligation to provide optimum patient care.
- **Provision 5:** The nurse owes the same duties to self as to others, including the responsibility to preserve integrity and safety and to maintain competence, and to continue personal and professional growth.
- **Provision 6:** The nurse participates in establishing, maintaining, and improving health care environments and conditions of employment conducive to the provision of quality health care and consistent with the values of the profession through individual and collective action.
- **Provision 7:** The nurse participates in the advancement of the profession through contributions to practice, education, administration, and knowledge development.
- **Provision 8:** The nurse collaborates with other health professionals and the public in promoting community, national, and international efforts to meet health needs.
- **Provision 9:** The profession of nursing, as represented by associations and their members, is responsible for articulating nursing values, for maintaining the integrity of the profession and its practice, and for shaping social policy.

From *Code of Ethics for Nurses*, by the American Nurses Association, 2001, Silver Spring, MD: Author. Reprinted with permission.

c. *Identify key participants:*
Who should make this decision? Who will be affected? What are the rights, duties, and capabilities of the participants?

d. *Consider possible options and act:*
What are the consequences of each option and what is the moral justification for each? Which choice is most desirable, which are unacceptable? Are the decision makers willing to act on the choices?

e. *Evaluate the outcome:*
How well was the case examined? Were the consequences of the action accurately predicted?

The following clinical example illustrates the application of this model.

TOPICS OF ETHICAL CONCERN IN PSYCHIATRIC NURSING PRACTICE

Figure 8–3 outlines some topics of ethical concern in psychiatric nursing practice.

PROFESSIONAL BOUNDARIES

Psychiatric nurses become involved in ethical decision making with clients because of the intimate nature of the nurse-

client relationship. For example, a nurse may struggle with the need to obtain parental consent for an adolescent to be treated for substance abuse, while realizing that the client may refuse to participate if it means telling the parents. Similarly, a nurse may wonder if a client who consents to the use of antipsychotic agents truly understands the risks and is competent to make that decision. The intimate nature of the psychiatric nurse-client relationship makes maintaining

- Stigma associated with mental illness
- Impact of labeling clients with psychiatric diagnoses
- Accuracy with which clients are diagnosed
- Factors that impact delivery of treatment such as source of payment, cost of treatment, access to care, etc.
- Clients who may be considered less desirable (i.e., violent, chemically dependent, indigent, incarcerated) which may impact care
- Faddish vs. known effective treatment
- Genetic vulnerability
- Balancing individual rights with the protection of others
- Providing culturally competent care
- Balancing the benefits of treatment with risks

Figure 8–3 Topics of ethical concern in psychiatric nursing.

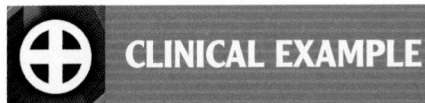

Applying an Ethical Decision-Making Model

A 32-year-old man with a history of alcohol and cocaine dependence requests admission to a chemical-dependence treatment unit at a private facility. The client had been treated at this facility three times in the past year and had been discharged against medical advice on all three occasions. The facility has a policy that a client who has left against medical advice on more than two occasions will not be readmitted. The man contacted the treatment team leader regarding his request and stated that in the past he had not been motivated for treatment because he had been court ordered to enter treatment due to domestic violence charges. He expressed remorse about his past behavior toward his wife and toward the staff during his previous treatment. The client was recently treated for ulcers and hypertension and his doctor warned him that he will kill himself if he does not stop drinking and using cocaine. The man stated that he did not want to leave his wife a widow and his two young sons without a father. He and his wife have just started marital therapy. He was concerned because there was no other substance abuse treatment center within a 60-mile radius from where he lives. The treatment team leader spoke with the client initially about his request and has asked the treatment team to meet along with the client to discuss whether or not to readmit him. The client has also asked his wife and marriage/family therapist to attend the meeting. Although this is not an exhaustive list, the following issues are raised.

a. *Gather facts:*
   Why does the client want to be readmitted? What was the course of previous treatments? What were the circumstances of previous discharges against medical advice? What is different at this time? Is there a waiting list for clients to enter this program? What are the client's supports? What is the client's motivation for treatment? How have we differentiated between fact and assumption? What other information can the client provide? What information can others (such as family members and Alcoholics Anonymous sponsors) provide?

b. *Identify the conflicting moral positions:*
   How do ethical principles such as beneficence, autonomy, and fidelity relate to this case? What is our responsibility to this client? What personal values of team members come into play? How do the relationships of team members with the client relate to this case? Are there other issues that might influence the decision, such as the client's position in the community and his financial status? Is it just to set aside the institution's policy to admit this client? What are the conflicting ethical principles?

c. *Identify key participants:*
   Who will decide whether the client is admitted? Who else has a stake in the decision? Is there anyone else who should speak with the team and the client?

d. *Consider possible options and act:*
   What are the possible choices of action? What treatment alternatives are available in the community? What changes in the treatment plan could be made if the client is admitted (such as having the client work with the team to develop a daily contract and anticipatory planning for substance withdrawal)? What immediate and long-term consequences can we predict for each option? What legal and institutional constraints affect the decision? Should the hospital ethics committee be consulted?

e. *Evaluate the outcome:*
   After carefully analyzing the case, the team, in conjunction with the client, will choose a course of action that seems most "right."

professional boundaries an important obligation of psychiatric nurses. It is important for nurses not to exploit the dependency of clients on the nurse in whom they put their trust and the power nurses have due to their knowledge and position. In the therapeutic relationship, nurses put aside their own needs to address the needs of clients. Some violations of professional boundaries may be made explicit in institutional policies or laws; however, many are not. Much emphasis has been placed on sexual transgressions such as dating or having a sexual relationship with clients, but there are more subtle examples of lack of professional boundaries. For example, accepting gifts or services, hugging clients, using unprofessional language or excessive self-disclosure by the nurse may be viewed as violations of professional boundaries. Confusion in the roles between the nurse and client can impair the nurse's judgment and ability to remain objective with clients (Antai-Otong, 2006).

CULTURAL FACTORS

To be able to work well with psychiatric clients, the nurse must not only be sensitive to the needs of clients, she should also be able to communicate, assess, and intervene, keeping in mind the cultural background of the client. Cultural sensitivity may mean the difference between a client and family accepting or rejecting the proposed intervention. One must be respectful of the culture's beliefs and practices and use acceptable concepts to explain problems and interventions. Being a psychiatric nurse does not necessarily mean that these professionals are without prejudice, even subconsciously; however, this is an influence of which the nurse must always be sensitive. Living in a world where everyone is equal, with differences being accepted by everyone, would be wonderful, but racism is alive and well in America (Garyali, 1999). Butts (1999, p. 635) states that it is amazing that people would think that knowledge of "psychopathology and psychodynamics of white individuals equips them to evaluate and treat black individuals; almost as if there was no difference between blacks and whites or as if there was nothing to know about blacks." There is a need for mental health education to enhance cultural sensitivity and awareness and to explicitly focus on unconscious effects of behavior such as nonverbal communication. Training may not only include didactic information but possibly also involve videos and role-playing experiences. Increasing one's knowledge and sensitivity to cultures while applying this knowledge to working with clients of all cultures will improve communication and, in doing so, improve outcomes.

DISTRIBUTIVE JUSTICE (ALLOCATION OF RESOURCES)

Traditionally, bioethics has been concerned with the ethics of the cases of individual clients and providers with its foundation in the principle of autonomy. From this ethical position, the best medical care that can be provided for individuals should be provided regardless of the cost. But a broader ethical perspective founded in the principle of justice is concerned with distributive justice, or the allocation of resources, and the collective rather than the individual rights of society. The principle of distributive justice implies that it is ethical for providers and society to consider efficiency and the cost of care and to determine how resources should best be used. To do otherwise would be unjust to those persons who do not have adequate health insurance or individual resources and would further the inequities in access to care. Providers, lawmakers, insurance companies, employers, and society in general will continue to address issues of distributive justice as medical technology expands and the costs of health care rise (Hall, 1997).

RESEARCH ABSTRACT

Compliance and Coercion in Psychiatric Care

Sjöström, S. (2006). Invocation of coercion context in compliance communication—Power dynamics in psychiatric care, *International Journal of Law and Psychiatry, 29,* 36–47.

The investigator conducted ethnographic fieldwork by working as a mental health worker in an inpatient psychiatric clinic over the course of 18 months, to study the relationship between compliance and coercion by the staff in caring for clients. The researcher found that staff members, including nurses, exercised dominant influence over activities on the unit in order to maintain reasonable order, meet treatment goals, and to help control the cost of care. Compliance may be coerced through subtle means such as keeping the unit locked at all times, restricting grounds privileges, conducting body searches, and by staff suggesting that the client has no alternative option but to comply with requests. In the psychiatric setting, staff has greater power than clients, which originates from the client's need for help, the staff's clinical expertise, the traditional paternalistic design of the health care system, and the staff's superior knowledge of the system. The researcher concluded that this power dynamic may contribute to the ability of staff to use coercion to gain compliance.

Implications for Psychiatric Nurses

Psychiatric nurses are poised to offer clients structure and guidance in motivating them to adhere to treatment. They must be sensitive and mindful of the clients' need to adhere to treatment while creating a safe and healing environment.

MORAL DISTRESS

The nurse may examine an ethical dilemma and use a systematic approach to come to a moral decision, but it is not always in the nurse's power to carry out that decision. Wilkinson (1987) defined this inner turmoil of not being able to act on an ethical decision as moral distress: "Because of their conflicting loyalties and responsibilities—to licensing bodies, employing institutions, physicians, other nurses, patients, and patients' families—nurses are especially prone to suffer moral distress" (p. 16). Carpenter (1991) suggested, based on research findings, that problems with ethical decision making may be an important factor in the stress associated with nursing. It may also affect the nurse's self-concept and attitude toward the nursing profession and whether the nurse changes to a different career.

CLIENT ADVOCACY

Nurses are obligated to act on their values rather than simply internalizing them as beliefs or principles. It is commonly understood that a nurse should be an advocate for individual clients by ensuring that the client's voice is heard and by educating clients about the health care system and their rights within the system (Long, 1996). Client advocacy refers to the nurse defending a cause or pleading a case on the client's behalf. Advocacy is an integral aspect of nursing care and reflects the nurse's concerns about appropriate, quality, safe, and culturally sensitive care. Fully protecting the client's rights requires a high degree of professional autonomy in practice to empower the nurse to put the client first (Bernal, 1992). As an advocate, the nurse holds the interests of the client above the interests of others, and at times the nurse may have divided loyalties; for example, having loyalty to uphold professional standards but also institutional philosophies and policies that may be in conflict.

Legal advocacy is concerned with changing the way society responds to the mentally ill through the legal system. The field of mental health disability law developed in the 1960s, and since that time there has been a proliferation of litigation aimed at defining and protecting the rights of the mentally disabled (Carty, 1992). In addition to individual client cases, professional values should also be applied to organizational and broader social issues. Nurses can influence the development of this type of change through political action, leadership in professional nursing organizations and public service groups, and research (Long, 1996).

Many health care organizations have adopted statements regarding client rights. The Joint Commission, a private accrediting agency, outlines standards for client rights, which include respect and dignity, privacy, safety, and the right of the client to know the identity of caregivers. The American Hospital Association and many individual health institutions have adopted policies concerned with client rights (Annas, 1992) (see the section on client rights later in this chapter).

Health care continues to move away from a paternalistic model, in which the health care team knows what is best for the client, to a model that views clients as consumers and emphasizes client rights and decision making (Valentine, Verhey, Hundert, & Kayne, 1990). An understanding of the law and an ability to communicate with clients, physicians, lawyers, and administrators are basic qualifications for the nurse who is an effective client advocate (Annas, 1992).

GENETIC VULNERABILITY

The field of genetics in psychiatry is in its infancy. Researchers have recently identified the serotonin transporter protein, a form of which may predispose people to depression, and there will be many more discoveries to come. Most psychiatric disorders are complicated and have multiple genes as well as the environment which influence their development (Appelbaum, 2004a). Perhaps one day, a saliva sample will identify which persons may be predisposed to develop depression, schizophrenia, and bipolar disorder.

Ethical questions arise as we consider how genetic information will be used. How might genetic testing affect individuals and society? What would be the impact of prenatal genetic testing and the testing of children for adult onset disorders? There are many different uses of genetic information including the potential development of more individualized and effective treatments and preventative interventions. But who would have access to this information? Would insurers and employers have access? Such questions will demand continued discussion and development of public policies in the area of psychiatric genetics in the coming years.

DEFINING MENTAL ILLNESS

In the general population the term mental illness is used indiscriminately, but legally, the term has more specific yet difficult-to-define criteria. Although most states have statutes that attempt to define mental illness, there is some variation from state to state (Weiner & Wettstein, 1993). A mental illness may be defined as "a disability severe enough to warrant hospitalization, continued treatment, or monitoring" (Weiner, 1990, p. 153). Mental illnesses may involve a loss of contact with reality and nonpsychotic disorders that cause significant impairment in functioning and emotional distress (Bennett, 1986). Some states specifically exclude diagnoses such as mental retardation, alcoholism, and substance abuse from the legal definition of mental illness (Weiner & Wettstein, 1993).

UNITED STATES MENTAL HEALTH LAWS

There are a number of sources of law with which the psychiatric nurse must be familiar that mandate the treatment of the mentally ill. Among them are constitutional and statutory laws that are enacted by federal or state legislative bodies. Also, federal and state agencies such as the United States Department of Health and Human Services and state mental health agencies mandate rules and regulations that have the same authority as law. It is important for the nurse to be aware that many laws affecting the mentally ill vary from state to state (Reid, 2003a). Other accrediting agencies such as the Joint Commission also influence the care of mentally ill clients. This section outlines the various admission criteria for psychiatric hospitalization and reviews the laws that pertain to the rights of the mentally ill client.

ADMISSION CRITERIA

Criteria for psychiatric inpatient admission varies from state to state, but typically rests on severity of symptoms, risk of danger to self and others, client and family preferences, and financial situations. There are two general types of psychiatric admissions: voluntary and involuntary hospitalization (commitment).

Voluntary Hospitalization

Voluntary commitment to a psychiatric hospital occurs when persons meeting admission criteria freely choose to be hospitalized. Approximately half of the admissions to state mental health facilities are voluntary (Weiner & Wettstein, 1993). A client may feel pressured into treatment by family members or health care professionals because of the threat of involuntary commitment. For an admission to be considered voluntary, the client must be informed of the physical conditions and the expectations of the institution, the admission process, and alternatives to hospitalization (Bloom & Asher, 1982). Persons who are incapable of giving informed consent might not be admitted on a voluntary basis (*Zinermon v. Burch*, 1990). A voluntary client may leave the hospital at will; however, many states have laws that allow the client to be detained if the client meets the criteria for involuntary commitment, namely, danger to self or others or grave disability (Cushing, 1988) (see the section on discharge later in this chapter).

Involuntary Hospitalization (Commitment)

Voluntary hospitalization is always preferred, but when someone who is mentally ill is potentially dangerous to self or others and refuses hospitalization or is incompetent to consent, involuntary hospitalization may be necessary. The client should also be assessed for dangerousness to self, clients, and staff. If dangerousness is judged to be present, further precautions should be taken to help ensure safety (Felthous, 1999). The state has the authority to require the hospitalization of an unwilling person when that person meets the requirements of the civil commitment standards. The ability of the state to hospitalize a person without consent is at the center of legal and ethical debates regarding the rights of the mentally ill. The goal of the civil commitment process is to balance the individual right to freedom with the protection of mentally ill people who are unable to care for themselves and the protection of society (Weiner & Wettstein, 1993) (Figure 8–4). For a client to be involuntarily committed for psychiatric treatment, there must be "clear

and convincing" evidence of imminent danger to the client or others (*Addington v. Texas*, 1979). The "clear and convincing standard is a lower standard of evidence than in criminal cases, which require evidence "beyond a reasonable doubt" (Reid, 2003a). Table 8–3 lists criteria that states use for involuntary commitment.

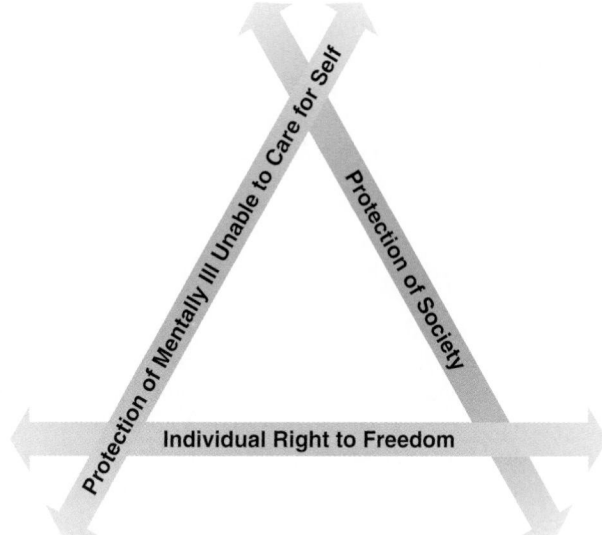

Figure 8–4 Balancing rights in civil commitment.

TABLE 8–3
Criteria for Involuntary Commitment

Each state has specific statutes establishing criteria for involuntary commitment that usually contain the following elements:

a. A person who is mentally ill, and because of that mental illness is in imminent danger of physically hurting himself or someone else based on something they did or a significant threat, or

b. A person who is mentally ill, and because of that mental illness has demonstrated an inability to attend to basic physical needs such as food, clothing, and shelter that are needed to prevent serious harm, and

c. A person who is mentally ill and considered gravely disabled, whose judgment is so impaired that he or she is unable to understand the need for treatment and whose behavior can reasonably be expected to result in significant physical harm to himself or someone else.

Note. Data from *Legal Issues in Mental Health Care* by B. A. Weiner and P. M. Wettstein, 1993, New York: Plenum Press.

Often, it is a family member or mental health professional who identifies when a person is in need of hospitalization. If the person is unwilling to be hospitalized, a petition must be filed with the state's attorney in the county in which the person resides explaining why she should be involuntarily committed. A civil commitment hearing must take place to determine if the person meets civil commitment standards (Figure 8–5). See also the section on due process. The conditions of senility, epilepsy, alcoholism, or drug dependence in themselves are not sufficient grounds for commitment—the person must also meet civil commitment requirements (Bloom, 2004).

As involuntary clients are hospitalized and then are stabilized by medication or other therapies, they no longer meet the standards for commitment and may be released or given the option of voluntary hospitalization. These persons are often part of the "revolving door" of mental health care, where they move in and out of hospitals. Some states now have outpatient commitment in an effort to stabilize persons with acute symptoms in the community. The person must have the capacity to function safely in the community with adequate supervision, often provided by family or friends. If the client fails to comply with outpatient treatment, a law enforcement officer may bring the client to the treatment center, or a new civil commitment petition may be initiated (Hiday & Scheid-Cook, 1989). Current civil commitment procedures may not address the needs of persons with severe and chronic mental illness with a history of dangerousness to self or others who are not imminently a danger but may become dangerous if untreated.

Emergency Hospitalization

In addition to the general commitment process, all states also have the authority to detain a person in an emergency situation for a limited time until a probable cause hearing is held. The same criterion of imminent danger to self or others or an inability to meet physical needs because of mental illness is used. The amount of time a person can be held varies from state to state, but it is usually 3 to 5 days. This allows time to provide lifesaving treatment, determine the diagnosis, and evaluate, and to decide if commitment will be sought (Weiner & Wettstein, 1993). The following clinical example illustrates the application of the criterion for emergency hospitalization.

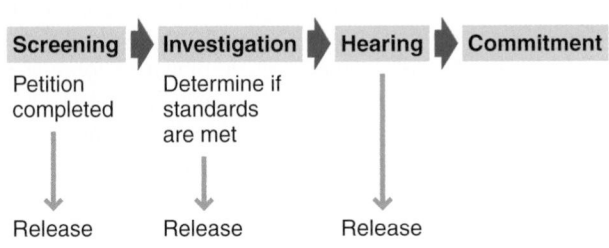

Figure 8–5 The civil commitment process.

Temporary Involuntary Hospitalization (Observational Commitment)

Following the emergency treatment period, the court will find that a small number of clients remain seriously mentally ill, and in some states, additional treatment following emergency commitment may be sought. Some clients agree to voluntary treatment, others are discharged, because they no longer meet the criteria to be held involuntarily, and still others may be categorized as incompetent and guardianship may be sought. Temporary involuntary hospitalization is generally 2 to 6 weeks in length, and treatment focuses on stabilizing symptoms (Bloom & Asher, 1982: Weiner & Wettstein, 1993).

Extended Involuntary Hospitalization

Most people who are committed to treatment return quickly to the community. However, a few are mandated to extended hospitalization and are subjected to periodic review at least annually. The focus of treatment is to improve the ability of clients to live in the community (Bloom & Asher, 1982).

TRANSFER

Transfer may occur within an institution, such as between units or rooms, or it may be accomplished from institution to institution. The client or the institution within the guidelines of the law may initiate the transfer. The Consolidated Omnibus Budget Reconciliation Act (COBRA) of 1985 was revised in 1991. This act states that if a facility has the needed services, the client may not be transferred to a different hospital unless she requests transfer. The client may be transferred to another hospital if the original facility does not provide the needed services or if there are no available beds (Simon & Goetz, 1999). Often the client will request a transfer to a different facility if the hospital is out of network for the health care insurance and the client will be held responsible for the entire bill or pay a higher deductible or percentage of the cost of hospitalization. The transfer requires documentation, which remains at the first facility, and also documentation on the

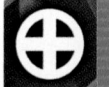

CLINICAL EXAMPLE

Emergency Hospitalization

A 57-year-old woman with a history of bipolar disorder told her daughter over the phone that she wanted to kill herself. The daughter went to her mother's house and found her mother incoherent, with slurred speech, and locked in her bedroom. The mother threatened to take her whole bottle of lithium, and the daughter realized the lithium was missing from the bathroom medicine cabinet. The mother stated, "I don't see any reason to go on, and I'm not coming out of here alive." The daughter called the police for assistance with emergency hospitalization.

transfer form, which goes to the accepting facility including information verifying that the reason for the transfer meets the acceptable standards. The client can be transferred to another institution if the physician certifies that she is stable and that there is no foreseeable risk to health (Annas, 1992).

ELOPEMENT (ESCAPE)

Elopement, absconding, and absent without official leave are terms used for hospitalized clients who are absent from a psychiatric facility without complying with the proper procedures for absence. Departure from the institution under these circumstances constitutes leaving against medical advice (AMA). Institutions have removed restrictions on client's liberties, which often include having unlocked units, and this may add to the risk of elopement. Elopement can cause great anxiety to staff members, who must assess the client's legal status and the risks involved with the client being out in the community. Clients often return to the hospital on their own or by having been brought back by the police or by relatives (Falkowski, Watts, Falkowski, & Dean, 1990).

DISCHARGE

Discharge from a psychiatric hospital ideally occurs when the client has successfully met the treatment goals for that hospitalization, is no longer a danger to self or others, and is sufficiently stabilized to return to the community. Discharge requires a written order from a physician who is familiar with the client's condition. The nurse should communicate with the treatment team and document using objective information regarding the client's readiness for discharge. A person who is legally competent and does not meet the state's criteria for involuntary commitment may leave the hospital, and any attempt to restrict the person from leaving would be considered false imprisonment in a court of law. In the absence of a physician's order, a client may be asked to sign a form indicating that the discharge is AMA (Annas, 1992). Many states require that requests for discharge be in writing. By law, discharge is not required to occur at the moment of the request but within a short period of time, which varies from state to state. This allows the providers to determine whether or not the client meets civil commitment criteria (Weiner & Wettstein, 1993).

Over the past two decades, hospital lengths of stay have decreased dramatically, and admission and continued hospitalization are based on "medical necessity" of inpatient treatment (Freishtat, 1991). Many third-party payers of psychiatric treatment (such as insurance companies) employ utilization review practices to monitor the appropriateness of hospitalization for their subscribers. This review is concurrent with hospitalization and it is conducted with the treating physician or a designee (often a nurse) from the hospital by discussing the case on an ongoing basis with the third-party payer. Based on the review and the "medical necessity"

criteria, the third-party payer will determine whether to certify the use of insurance benefits for continued treatment. The hospitalized client faced with no longer receiving insurance benefits for hospitalization may choose to be discharged despite the treatment team's objections (Freishtat, 1991).

Until recently, the physician bore sole legal responsibility for any improper or premature discharge when an untoward event occurred subsequently; for example, when a client committed suicide shortly after discharge. Legislation ruled that third-party payers are not immune from liability related to utilization review activities if their actions are a "substantial factor" in improper discharge (Freishtat, 1991). It is important for the company that manages the mental health benefits to be aware of the status of the client, who is considered the company's "member," and to act in response to the specific needs of the individual.

Conditional Discharge

A person who has been civilly committed to treatment may be discharged with conditional requirements in most states. The conditions of release may include stipulations such as where the client will live, follow-up treatment requirements, or behavior that must be avoided. If a client violates the conditions of the release within a set period, inpatient hospitalization may be mandated. If a client disagrees with a revocation of discharge, a hearing may be requested (Weiner & Wettstein, 1993).

Outpatient Discharge

Most states reserve the right to mandate outpatient commitment as a treatment option (with and without specific procedures for enforcement) or at least do not prohibit this type of commitment.

Absolute Discharge

An absolute or unconditional discharge often takes place after a hospitalized client has successfully completed a conditional release. Absolute discharge means that no further treatment is legally required after discharge, and the client is no longer under court jurisdiction.

COMPETENCY VERSUS INCOMPETENCY

Competency refers to the ability to perform a specific act or decision; it may vary over time and between particular tasks (Davis & Underwood, 1989). Legal incompetency refers to the status of persons who have been declared incompetent in a court of law and to minors. The legal criteria for competency include the ability to understand the proceedings of due process and to assist an attorney in preparing for a hearing. The competency evaluation is a separate process that involves persons who have already been determined to be mentally ill (Bloom & Faulkner, 1987). Mental illness does not necessarily mean incompetence. Even a civilly committed client is assumed competent, and only when the court has declared the client incompetent may the nurse assume incompetence (Szasz, 2005).

FORENSIC PSYCHIATRY

Forensic psychiatry involves mental health issues that relate to the legal system. This includes both civil procedures, such as determining when a mentally ill person requires legal guardianship, and determining when a defendant is competent to stand trial (National Institute of Mental Health, 1991) and criminal matters involving crimes. Although some mental health units and clinics are specifically designated for individuals with forensic needs, these clients may be treated with the general population of psychiatric clients (Reid, 2003a).

INSANITY DEFENSE

For a person to be held legally accountable for a crime, the physical act of the crime and the mental state of intention at the time of the crime are both necessary elements (Weiner & Wettstein, 1993). The insanity defense argues that a person by virtue of mental illness cannot know and appreciate the nature of a criminal act and cannot control her behavior because of the mental illness. The criterion for the insanity defense is the client's knowledge that the action was against the law or was wrong. This principle is based on the idea that when in certain mental states, the client would not be held responsible for her actions. Ultimately, insanity is not decided by the psychiatrist but by a jury who represents society. This results in the insanity issue becoming a moral or social issue. This may also result in the severely emotionally ill to be found legally sane. The specific insanity standard varies across the country so that the criterion is based on the local standard (Gutheil, 1999). Antisocial personality disorder and "voluntary insanity" produced by substance abuse are excluded (Vandenberg, 1993). The insanity defense is used in fewer than 1 percent of U.S. criminal cases (Missouri Department of Mental Health, 1993; Weiner & Wettstein, 1993).

DUTY TO WARN

Mental health care is not an exact science. A health care professional who is counseling a client is expected to use reasonable judgment when assessing, planning, and intervening. It is important to assess and inquire about signs and symptoms as well as to use available information to make sound treatment judgments (Knapp & Vandercreek, 1983). It is not always possible to know whether or not a client has serious intentions to hurt others, however clinicians can attempt to assess risk (Reid, 2003b).

The duty to warn and the duty to protect are closely related. They are legal obligations based on the case of *Vitaly Tarasoff v. the Regents of the University of California,* which was brought to the California Supreme Court in 1976. In this case, the university and its psychotherapists were accused of being responsible for the murder of Tatiana Tarasoff by a psychiatric client (Vitaly Tarasoff, 1976). The death was reportedly due in part to Tatiana Tarasoff and her parents' not having been informed of the client's plan to murder her when she returned from vacation (Smith, 1990). The court determined that if a professional believes that a client is a danger to others, the professional has a legal responsibility to take the necessary steps to protect the potential victim (Vitaly Tarasoff, 1976). Figure 8–6 provides guidelines for assessing a client's intent to harm.

The Tarasoff case has been used to approve laws regarding breaking client confidentiality and protecting others (by warning possible victims). As a result of the Tarasoff decision, the nurse may be held liable if the victim is not warned and if there is lack of reasonable judgment in confining the client and using the commitment laws for that state (Slovenko, 1999). Although many states have laws similar to those based on the decision of the Tarasoff case, each individual state has its own laws, and these laws may vary from the Tarasoff decision (Knapp & Vandercreek, 1983). At this time, the duty to warn is mandated in almost every state; two exceptions are Florida and Virginia (Slovenko, 1999). It is the nurse's responsibility to know the law and variations in her state. Based on reasonable judgment, failure to warn the victim usually gains approval by the court, whereas lack of knowledge of the law is an unacceptable defense (Yorker, 1988). Nurses are expected to assess clients regarding dangerousness but this is very difficult to accomplish accurately. The availability of more sophisticated weapons further complicates assessment because individuals may act impulsively in an unplanned response when in crisis (Goldzband, 1998).

DOCUMENTATION

Documentation is a record of occurrences, observations, and planning related to client care. Documentation includes not only charting on both the progress notes and medication sheets but also ongoing nursing care plans and multidisciplinary treatment plans (Sanders & DuPlessis, 1985). It is important that all significant situations, actions, and interventions, including any resolutions and treatment outcomes, be written in a factual, nonbiased manner because they inform and guide other nursing shifts and other health care workers outside the inpatient unit or clinic (such as outpatient therapists who are working with the client and family). Documentation also provides important information that will

When assessing for serious intention to harm others, it is necessary to look for the characteristics that would increase the likelihood of harm, such as the following:

1. A definite plan to harm

2. Resources to carry out the plan

3. Ability to carry out the plan (e.g., does the client know how to use a gun?)

4. History of violence

5. Impulsivity

6. Extreme emotional changes

7. Depression

Figure 8–6 Assessing intent to harm.

RESEARCH ABSTRACT

Are the Mentally Ill Dangerous?

Binder, R. L. (1999). *The Journal of the American Academy of Psychiatry and the Law, 27*(2), 189–201.

Study Problem/Purpose

To review the charts of all clients who had been violent and had been admitted to a psychiatric unit over the past 15 years, and to determine the ability of staff to assess potential for violence.

Methods

Clients who were involuntarily admitted because of dangerousness to others were compared with clients who were voluntarily admitted for reasons other than violence. It was found that when clinicians predicted violence on admission, there was a high probability of accuracy if the prediction was limited to only a 2-day period. Longer periods of time from the day of admission were much more inaccurate for forecasting violence, with both groups having about the same probability of predicted violence.

Findings

Clinicians were found to underpredict violence in women and overpredict violence in nonwhite clients. Clusters of symptoms were more helpful in predicting violence compared to diagnosis alone. Another interesting finding was that clients were rarely dangerous to the public. Usually violence was directed toward those with whom clients were living who confronted their behavior and beliefs. The minority of psychotic clients who did become violent directed violence toward people with whom they were living.

Implications for Psychiatric Nurses

Psychiatric nurses need to identify risk factors associated with violence. Assessing past violence during the initial assessment and throughout treatment afford opportunities for the nurse to initiate interventions that reduce its occurrence.

aid in providing the rationale for treatment given. The following clinical example illustrates proper documentation.

Key elements of the documentation in the clinical example include the use of quotations, specific interventions attempted to decrease agitation, specific nonverbal responses of the client, and steps taken to ensure the safety of everyone. Only facts were documented. Other sources of documentation include the medication administration record, suicide/homicide assessment, and restraint documentation. While a client is in restraints, documentation must continue to indicate the ongoing need for control in this manner with no other available option to ensure the safety of the client and others. The nurse must document that the client is observed constantly while in leather restraints and describe the client's behavior during this time.

Careless or partial documentation can make good care appear delinquent (Morgan, 1987). Objective documentation such as describing behavior and using direct quotes must be present to show evidence of the use of proper procedures and to demonstrate that adequate professional care was given. This evidence may include items such as observations, assessments, treatments, and medications given. If the nurse delegates documentation to other members of the health care team, the documentation should still reflect whether care that would be expected was completed. It can be assumed in court that only those things documented were done. Jakacki and Payson (1985) advised the following:

> Document enough information to prove that you acted as any reasonable, prudent nurse would act under the same or similar circumstance. If, in your judgment, an emergency exists, document all observable facts plus the thinking you used in determining that immediate intervention was necessary. (p. 1336)

Adequate documentation is a responsibility that nurses have for all clients in their care.

CONFIDENTIALITY

Confidentiality is an obligation that is necessary of nurses to foster a professional, trusting relationship with clients (Melrose, 1990). Information that is shared verbally or in writing between the health team members should be kept confidential from those outside the health care team. Specific laws pertaining to confidentiality may vary; therefore, nurses must be aware of the laws in the state in which they practice. A nurse is challenged when the police, the family who plans to care for the client, the outpatient therapist, the employer, and others insist on obtaining confidential information related to the client. It is important to always elicit the client's preference in handling these situations and to request a release of information form. The client must sign the release of information form when necessary for treatment (Puskar & Obus, 1989).

Even though information is not shared outside the hospital by the staff, the client's medical record may be subpoenaed by the court and used by the judicial system (Bender, Murphy, & Mark, 1989; Smith, 1990). Nurses should know the requirements of the law to avoid litigation and to protect themselves if accused of breaking a client's confidentiality (Stern, 1990). Figure 8–7 shows a list of situations in which the nurse may break a client's confidentiality.

The availability of personal medical records sparks a number of ethical dilemmas regarding client confidentiality and privacy. Often clients who receive health insurance benefits or join an HMO are required to sign forms that authorize

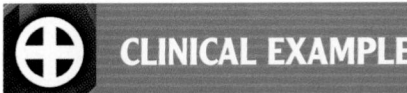

CLINICAL EXAMPLE

Applying Proper Documentation

A 15-year-old male was admitted yesterday to the adolescent psychiatric unit for depression. His admission orders include Suicide Awareness due to a recent suicide attempt. He has no prior hospitalizations and no prior history of violence. Consider the use of objective information and the details provided by the nurse. How can this information be helpful to other members of the team in providing this client's care? The nurse made the following entry into the medical record:

The client had been attending group therapy when he came out of the group and stated loudly to the RN, "You need to let me leave the unit right now! This place is making me crazy. I can't control myself!" The RN listened to the client's concerns and asked staff to move other clients from the immediate area. The client continued to pace in the day area and was able to lower his voice with encouragement. The nurse explained the current status of the client's admission and offered alternatives to leaving such as writing a letter or using the phone after group therapy was over. The client was able to speak calmly after about ten minutes and stated, "I just don't know if I can stay here, my girlfriend doesn't even know that I am here." The client was encouraged to return to group therapy which he did and was able to remain in group without incident. The client was placed on Elopement Awareness and his physician was contacted about the client's behavior and concerns about his girlfriend.

---

1. During an emergency involving an immediate danger of serious physical harm; for example, notifying a relative without consent about a client's suicide attempt

2. Protecting others from potential violence by client, for example, notifying an ex-spouse that a client has threatened bodily harm to the ex-spouse

3. Conforming to child abuse reporting requirements; for example, notifying the proper authorities of suspected sexual abuse of a minor

4. Conforming to other statutory reporting requirements; for example, notifying the proper authorities of reportable sexually transmitted diseases

5. Discussing the client with supervisors and other providers directly participating in care

6. Situations in which civil commitment is being sought; for example, providing information without consent explaining why civil commitment is warranted

Figure 8–7 Situations in which the nurse may legally breach confidentiality. *(Data from Legal Issues in Mental Health Care, by B. A. Weiner and R. M. Wettstein, 1993, New York: Plenum Press.)*

blanket release of all health information needed in order to receive benefits. This information is requested to help ensure quality control and cost control, but many clients may feel an "economic compulsion" to sign such releases because they are unsure about what information might be in the record in the future and what specifically will be released or to whom.

In addition, according to Etzioni (1999), through unauthorized and sometimes legal means, other non-health care parties such as employers and marketers may have access to information. The use of electronic records also adds another element to the privacy dilemma with records; however, ultimately, electronic records may actually help to improve the privacy of records. Electronic records can be "layered" whereby certain information is only accessible to certain providers. Additionally, electronic records leave audit trails that identify who are accessing the record. In the future, electronic records may allow the client to be the holder of the medical record and therefore have more control over who accesses the record information (Etzioni, 1999). Still, nurses should be cautious in the use of E-mail and fax, which is often unsecured, for relaying confidential information. Finally, the nurse cannot verify that the client is in the hospital, even to family members, unless consent is given.

The deadline for compliance with the privacy rule of the Health Insurance Portability and Accountability Act of 1996 (HIPAA) occurred in 2003. HIPAA privacy rules apply to psychiatric care as well as all other areas of health care. Among the goals of HIPAA was to provide a minimum standard of privacy for protected health information (PHI). Essentially, these rules state that written consent must accompany the disclosure of PHI except in limited situations outlined by law such as in an emergency. State and federal laws (such as abuse reporting) take precedence over HIPAA rules (Touchet et al., 2004).

REPORTING OF ABUSE

Child abuse is any action by a caretaker that purposefully injures the child physically or emotionally. Types of abuse include physical, emotional, and sexual, or neglect of a child younger than 18 years of age. Nurses and physicians in all states are required to report child abuse (Fiesta, 1992). Nurses report child abuse to various agencies, depending on the state in which the abuse occurs. The nurse has no responsibility to keep that information confidential, and the child's right to be protected takes precedence over laws of confidentiality (D. P. Smith, 1989; J. Smith, 1990). Most states provide immunity for the health care worker who acts in good faith. Failure to report child abuse may result in the health care worker being liable for abuse that occurs later, owing to lack of previous intervention (Fiesta, 1992). These laws have contributed to an increasing number of reported child abuse cases (D. P. Smith, 1989). (See Chapter 25 for a discussion on abuse throughout the life span.)

Elder Abuse

Most states have some type of reporting system that mandates reporting elder abuse. It is important to know the particular laws associated with elder abuse in the state in which the nurse works. Interventions vary and range from criminal prosecution of the abuser to guardianship of the victim (Haviland & O'Brien, 1989).

Hospitals or other health care institutions caring for older clients need explicit policies in compliance with state and nursing standards regarding abuse. Nurses must assess, document, and take actions associated with the requirements of the laws of the state. It is both a legal and an ethical duty to intervene when abuse occurs ("Nursing Practice," 1992). Janing (1992) stated, "It is not enough to be angered by the specific cases of abuse we see. . . . We must speak out as individuals and as a profession to both our state and federal legislatures. It is time to be an advocate" (p. 58).

PRINCIPLES OF TORT LAWS

Few would argue about the growing numbers of mental health professionals, including nurses, who find themselves involved in the legal system. Issues inherent in caring for clients with mental disorders, such as suicide, involuntary commitment and other treatment issues suggest the importance of laws that govern and guide standards of care and practice.

Negligence and Malpractice

A tort is an injury that someone incurs as the result of another either intentional or unintentional. Christoffel and Teret (1991) define negligence as injury that is unintentional due to failure to take the usual precautions expected in that instance, for example, cleaning up broken glass or spills. Often there are no laws or standards surrounding the conduct. Malpractice is negligence reserved for professionals resulting from misconduct, lack of skills, or failure to follow set standards (Burkhardt & Nathaniel, 1998). The legal standard of care determines the obligations of the nurse to the client. The requirements for proving malpractice are more stringent than negligence. For malpractice to be determined it must be proven that there was a duty, that the duty was not fulfilled because of error or omission, that the unfulfilled duty caused actual injury, and that the injury was foreseeable. The standard of care is what a nurse with similar experience and education with sound judgment would have done in a similar situation. For example, a psychiatric nurse in charge of an inpatient unit assesses that a client's restraints are improperly applied but chooses not to act because of time constraints, resulting in the client being injured by the restraints. This nurse may be found liable of malpractice. One should review and be familiar with standards of care set forth by state and national professional bodies (Fitzgerald, 1999). Figure 8–8 outlines the components of malpractice.

a. The nurse has a duty to the client.

b. The nurse fails to follow the set standard.

c. Actual harm or injury occurs.

d. The failure to act according to the standards has caused the injury.

Figure 8–8 Components of malpractice. (*Data from* Ethics and Issues in Contemporary Nursing, *p. 115, by M. A. Burkhardt and A. K. Nathaniel, 2002, Clifton Park, NY: Delmar Learning.*)

- Promote an atmosphere of respect and concern for clients.
- Listen carefully and assess client's understanding.
- Keep up to date in knowledge and skills.
- Maintain complete, objective, and timely records and do not make alterations.
- Carefully guard the confidentiality of records and other forms of communication.
- Be familiar with and follow professional standards and institutional policies.
- Do not attempt tasks or give medications with which you are not familiar.
- Challenge questionable orders.

Figure 8–9 Decreasing the risk of malpractice. (*Data from* Ethics and Issues in Contemporary Nursing, *p. 115, by M. A. Burkhardt and A. K. Nathaniel, 2002, Clifton Park, NY: Delmar Learning; and from "Malpractice Liability of Mental Health Professionals and Institutions," by S. R. Smith, 1996, in* Law, Mental Health, and Mental Disorders, *pp. 91–92, by B. D. Sales and D. W. Shuman (Eds.), Pacific Grove, CA: Brooks/Cole Publishing.*)

Nurses may also be found liable for intentional torts or actions that violate another's rights. One such tort is fraud; that is, intentionally providing false information for some gain. For example, a nurse may embellish the documentation about a client's mental status and functional ability in order to secure further authorization of treatment. Another example of an intentional tort is invasion of privacy, such as a nurse informing one client about another client's diagnosis (Burkhardt & Nathaniel, 1998). Figure 8–9 outlines steps that nurses can take to decrease the risk of malpractice.

The Nurse in Court

If a nurse is called into court to testify, for example, in an abuse case, there are several issues. A nurse may be called on as an expert witness or to give a clinical judgment. Assessment based on direct observation will provide the foundation for interpretation of the data. The nurse should be prepared to explain the method used to determine an opinion. Opinions will have more validity if they are based on what the nurse directly saw, heard, or physically experienced (Grudzinskas, 1999).

CLIENTS' RIGHTS

The 1970 case *Wyatt v. Stickney* sparked the proliferation of laws establishing the rights of hospitalized mentally ill clients. This case established a precedent in psychiatric facilities for staff-client ratios, nutritional requirements of hospital meals, and physical requirements such as the minimum number of showers, among other standards. Hospitalized mentally ill clients today maintain a number of rights that are mandated by law (Weiner & Wettstein, 1993). Client rights, however, are not self-executing, and the psychiatric nurse plays a significant role in defending them.

RIGHTS OF CHILDREN OR MINORS

During the 1970s there was a movement to protect the right to liberty of minors regarding hospitalization as had been accomplished previously for adults. In *Parham v. J. L. & J. R.* (1979), the U.S. Supreme Court's majority decision was that the court would support the family unit as it had historically, and therefore the right to due process in matters of psychiatric hospitalization did not apply to minors. The court stated that parents make decisions for the child when the child has not developed adequate cognitive ability. They further stated that the affection parents have for their children results in parents making the best decision for the child with regard to psychiatric treatment, and parents may consent to treatment on behalf of their children.

During the 1980s, there was a dramatic increase in the psychiatric hospitalization of often disruptive adolescents who did not necessarily have mental disabilities. Parents, often well intended, rightly judged that they needed help, but hospitalization in psychiatric settings may not have been the best solution. Parents assume that providers and institutions give objective recommendations regarding treatment for adolescents, but psychiatric hospitals may have direct financial interest in admitting clients. Despite the still existing legal standard that parents consent for their minor children, inappropriate use of treatment raises ethical concerns (Ellis, 1996).

The nurse's relationship regarding the child's rights includes using interventions that protect the child, supporting the family's decision-making ability while supporting the child's best interests, and ensuring that the child is treated fairly (deLeon Siantz, 1988). Although minors may not legally refuse treatment, a method by which the nurse can acknowledge a minor's need to have control is the ethical means of asking the child to give informal assent or agreement to treatment. Information regarding treatment should be given to children on a level they can understand. Giving minors the opportunity for assent and choices when possible provides empowerment and results in fewer power struggles between the nursing staff and the client. This sets the stage for positive relationships with the nursing staff by providing the child with an opportunity to develop decision-making skills and may result in increasing *his or her* openness to treatment (Erlen, 1987). Adolescents may be developmentally able to give consent to treatment and, if interested, should be given the opportunity to sign a consent form along with the parent or guardian.

DISABILITY RIGHTS

According to the federal government Web site summarizing the federal law of Title 1 of the Americans with Disabilities Act (ADA), individuals with a "mental impairment that substantially limits one or more life activities, has a record of such impairment, or is regarded as having such an impairment" are qualified to be protected against discrimination in employment. One must have a disability that the federal government deems to be permanent in order to be legally protected. Although polysubstance abuse and alcohol dependence are *DSM-IV-TR* diagnoses, if one is currently

CRITICAL THINKING

A dilemma for psychiatric nurses when working with adolescents is the issue of confidentiality and trust and specifically what to share and not share with the adolescent's parents or legal guardian.

You are working with Marty, a 16-year-old female who has been brought to the outpatient mental health clinic by her parents seeking an evaluation for her recent outbursts in school. During your assessment, Marty is distant and asks, "Will everything I say to you be kept in confidence?" Which of the following statements is the best response to Marty's queries?

1. "Marty, I promise to keep everything you share with me in confidence."
2. "Marty, I understand your concerns, but I have to share our discussion with your parents."
3. "Marty, I will maintain confidentiality on matters that do not pose a threat to you and/or others."
4. "Marty, don't you think you have caused enough problems for your family? It is important for them to know what's troubling you."

1. *Incorrect.* Promising to keep everything in confidence is a false promise because if the youth threatens to harm self or others, the nurse is legally and ethically obligated to report this information. False promises jeopardize the nurse-client relationship.

2. *Incorrect.* Adolescents have a right to confidentiality unless they pose a threat to self and/or others. Telling an adolescent you will share all information with parents prevents the adolescent from sharing inner feelings and thoughts and threatens the integrity of the nurse-client relationship. It also impedes the adolescent's legal and ethical rights to confidentiality.

3. *Correct.* Adolescents have a right to discuss their concerns and feelings in a safe and confidential environment. It is imperative to be honest about matters you will keep confidential and those you must share with parents. This honest response fosters trust and confidence and conveys understanding and empathy.

4. *Incorrect.* This response is derogatory and judgmental. It conveys a lack of understanding about the legal and ethical rights of adolescents and displays a lack of respect and unprofessional behavior.

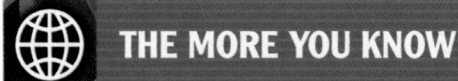
Erosion of Parental Rights

Thomas, K. (2000, August 8). Parents pressured to put kids on drugs: Courts, schools force Ritalin use, *USA Today*.

The courts have historically sided with parents in their decision-making capacity regarding treatment of their children in non-emergencies; however, a recent legal trend pits the courts against parents by ruling that the children must be medicated against the parents' wishes. Cases in which divorced parents disagree over treatment are not new and have been brought before the courts. Yet in two recent cases in New York State, parents acting in agreement were ordered by the court to give their children medication for attention deficit hyperactivity disorder. In one of the cases both parents agreed to take their child off medication because of side effects. The other is the first known case in which teachers sought and were granted a court ruling to force a child on medication despite both parents' objections.

involved in using illegal drugs or actively involved in alcoholism, this law does not protect the individual.

DUE PROCESS

The right to due process is a constitutional right based on the Fourteenth Amendment, which states that no citizen may be denied life, liberty, or property without an impartial hearing and the same rights as all citizens. Although due process was first applied to criminal law, it also applies to noncriminal matters such as mental health disability commitments. The right to due process specifies that in commitment cases, there is a procedural process about which the client must be informed, the decision maker will be impartial, and the client has the right to be heard and represented by counsel (Costello, 1996).

RIGHT TO TREATMENT

Although the constitution is the basis for civil commitment for inpatient treatment, no such constitutional link exists for out-

patient treatment mandating that community mental health services be provided; however, many states do have statutes that mandate publicly funded outpatient community treatment. Clients using private insurance or paying for their own treatment enter into contractual agreements for treatment that are subject to contractual or tort law (Kapp, 1996). In the 1999 United States Supreme Court case of *Olmstead v. L.C.*, Justice Ginsburg stated that a waiting list for community mental health facilities that moves at a reasonable rate is acceptable. Justice Kennedy added that, "A state cannot be forced to create a community treatment program where none exists." This serves to support decisions of individual states regarding mental health center availability (Appelbaum, 1999).

LEAST RESTRICTIVE ALTERNATIVES

Psychiatric care may consist of various alternatives, including hospitalization, outpatient treatment, and other community-based options. The goal of treatment is to move the client to a productive life in the community as soon as possible. The level of treatment is determined by the client's particular needs, providing the maximum amount of liberty while protecting the client from danger (*Dixon v. Weinberger*, 1975). States are mandated to provide the least restrictive programs and services available; however, states do not always have a wide continuum of services (Cushing, 1988).

SECLUSION AND RESTRAINT

The principle of least restrictive alternative encompasses the use of seclusion and restraint for psychiatric clients. In managing the therapeutic milieu, the psychiatric nurse employs a host of strategies in maintaining a safe environment. The use of seclusion and restraint (S/R) are options that should be used only in situations of imminent danger when other options have failed or are not viable. *Seclusion* refers to physically confining a client to an area such as placing a client in a locked seclusion room and *restraint* refers to physically restricting a client's movements by physically holding the client or with the use of a mechanical device such as leather belts. S/R should not be used for purposes of discipline, coercion, or convenience. The use of S/R cannot be used to

RESEARCH ABSTRACT

Termination of Social Security Benefits among Los Angeles Recipients Disabled by Substance Abuse

Watkins, K. E., Wells, K. B., & McLellan, A. T. (1999). *Psychiatric Services, 50*(7), 914–918.

This study examined the effect of Public Law 104-121 on persons with chemical dependence in 2001 who previously had received disability benefits but were later denied benefits after the passing of PL 104-121 in 1996. It was expected that many of these individuals would reapply and be recertified for benefits based on their scores for the Addiction Severity Index. Of the 2001 subjects, only 67 percent appealed the denial and of those, only half were recertified. This raises concerns for the welfare of these clients as well as possible resultant shifting of costs to care for these clients from the federal to local governments.

compensate for inadequate staffing or lack of treatment (Huckshorn, 2005). The use of seclusion and restraint is carefully governed by institutional policies, oversight organizations (such as the Joint Commission), and by laws and rules (which carry the same weight as law) such as those established by the Federal Centers for Medicare and Medicaid Services (CMS, formerly HCFA) (Huckshorn, 2005).

Nurses are often the member of the treatment team who initiates the use of seclusion and restraint and participates in and supervises unlicensed staff who carry out the procedure. The risks of S/R include physical and psychological injury to staff, and trauma, psychological damage, physical injury, and even death for clients (Weiss et al., 1998; Frueh et al., 2005). Therefore, it is incumbent upon all psychiatric nurses to know, demonstrate, and supervise the proper use of seclusion and restraint.

INFORMED CONSENT

Informed consent is based on the fundamental belief that clients should be able to have control over their own bodies (Grove, 1990). This not only legally provides autonomy for the client (in which no one should touch or treat the client without permission from the client) but also encourages the ethical aspect of the client's decision-making ability (Weiss, 1990).

There are four elements necessary for legal consent (Kjervik & Grove, 1988):

1. A person must be capable of consenting.

2. A person must have the ability to refuse consent.

3. A person must have adequate information for consent or have agreed to waive the right to information.

4. The consent must not be illegal.

The nurse has a vital role in aiding the client to understand the information (including risks) in any case requiring informed consent (Slovenko, 2000). The nurse or physician should witness the client's or legal guardian's verbalization of understanding and observe the signature being placed on the consent form or, in an emergency, hear the telephone consent given (Davis & Underwood, 1989).

Informed consent for medications and other treatment is an important responsibility in psychiatric nursing that involves informing the client about the indications and side effects before initiating medication. Often written material is included in the information provided. When a crisis occurs, informed consent may be waived at the discretion of the nurses and physicians if a true life-threatening emergency exists and medications may be administered (Fitzgerald, 1999). An ethical dilemma may emerge for the nurse if consent is needed for treatment for which the client is reluctant to sign. For instance, a client who has been unresponsive to treatment of depression may be hesitant to sign for electroconvulsive therapy (ECT). The nurse is faced with the dilemma of encouraging (not coercing) the client, providing further information, or choosing to say little and respecting her decision (Loubardias, 1991). The nurse may encourage a client to look at options, but if the client's decision is different from what the nurse believes to be best, the final decision should still be that of the client.

If a client is not competent, then a substitute must give consent for treatment. The process to obtain a petition for treatment varies from state to state. When a substitute is designated, then that individual must be provided information for consent in the same way that the competent individual would be provided that information (Simon & Goetz, 1999). If a client is believed to be permanently unable to make treatment decisions because of mental illness, the court may appoint a guardian. The powers of that guardian vary from state to state (Miller, 1999).

RIGHT TO REFUSE TREATMENT

A client has the right to refuse treatment when she is considered competent (Carroll & Maher, 1990) or not imminently dangerous to self or others. If treatment is given without consent, it may be considered battery. If consent is given without adequate information, it may be considered malpractice. Methods to assist the client in understanding the meaning of treatment refusal include for the nurse to:

a. Solicit information regarding the basis for the client's refusal

b. Provide information that addresses the client's concerns

c. Assist in management of side effects if this is a concern

d. Consult with the physician regarding treatment options

e. Involve caring family members or significant friends (with consent of the client) in the treatment team (as well as the client)

f. Continue to develop a therapeutic relationship with the client

Treatment refusal is a complex situation, and it is therefore important that the nurse accurately document the treatment proposed, the client's refusal, the interventions attempted in working through this process, as well as the risks and alternatives offered to the client (Wettstein, 1999). This documentation will provide the nurse with information to refer to in the future if needed.

The judicial system has the right to make a final clinical decision in circumstances in which there is a conflict of opinion between health care providers and the client. The legal system considers the autonomy of the client to be paramount without considering that the mental illness may have already robbed the client of autonomy (Schwartz, Vingiano, & Perez, 1988). Thus, if unresolved conflict arises, the intervention must be postponed until the court decides the outcome.

The client's desire or refusal to follow the treatment plan is a legal and ethical right, unless otherwise ordered by the judicial system. It is the nurse's responsibility to be an advocate and to protect client rights by being aware of the laws of the state (and eventually working to change those laws if necessary), discussing with other professionals involved in the care and the hospital legal counsel to focus attention on questionable ethical and legal issues.

RIGHT TO REFUSE MEDICATION

The legal right to refuse antipsychotic medication was established more than 25 years ago, with differing interpretations and methods of enforcement, depending on the jurisdiction. Weiss (1990) noted that "by the early 1980s, 45 of 51 state and territorial jurisdictions in the United States had implemented a variety of medication administration policies in their public treatment facilities" (p. 25). Even involuntarily committed clients have been allowed to refuse medication, although refusal may further delay discharge by prolonging symptoms and extending the length of hospitalization. The interesting aspect of this is that most clients who initially refuse medication eventually receive it anyway because of a court decision (Appelbaum, 1988). A therapeutic alliance, which is the responsibility of the treaters, as well as monitoring of adverse side effects and medication blood levels when appropriate can promote voluntary client compliance to the medication regimen and thus reduce confrontation between the treatment team and the client (Young et al., 1999). This provides more opportunity for the client to access the benefits of needed medications.

The nurse may not forcibly give medication unless the client is seen as an imminent danger to self or others. If the nurse does not give p.r.n. medication as ordered, owing to client refusal, and the client hurts herself or others, the nurse's actions will be reviewed by the hospital and possibly by a court to see if the incident could have been prevented. If the nurse forcibly gives medication, her actions will also be reviewed to see if she had the right to administer the medication. How does the nurse get out of this "double bind"? The nurse must document observations of the details surrounding the events and the interventions attempted during the incident to indicate the basis for judgments made. The decision of the nurse must be supported in the documentation to substantiate that she acted as any professional nurse would according to the legal standards of the state (Jakacki & Payson, 1985).

PSYCHIATRIC ADVANCE DIRECTIVES

Psychiatric advance directives are an extension of medical advanced directives which are recognized in all states. Some states have recently developed statutes that allow the development of special provisions for psychiatric care. In this way, for example, clients with chronic mental illnesses might while competent, indicate their preferences for treatment for such time when they might become incompetent due to their mental illness. In the 2003 case of *Hargrave v. Vermont*, a woman with a history of paranoid schizophrenia had completed an advance directive stating that she did not want to receive antipsychotics in the event that she became incompetent. The state decided to override the advance directive

and allow clinicians to treat the client against her will. This case found that there may be situations where the interests of the state outweigh the individual interests of the client and therefore other existing laws, such as court-ordered treatment, may supersede advance directives. The outcome of *Hargrave v. Vermont* may undermine the original purpose of advance psychiatric directives and may discourage clients from developing them and clinicians from promoting them to clients knowing that advance directives may not be followed (Appelbaum, 2004b; Van Dorn, et al., 2005).

OTHER CLIENT RIGHTS

All states have statutes that mandate the right of hospitalized clients to communicate with others outside the facility. Contact may include visitation, mail, and telephone contact. Most states allow institutions to employ reasonable restrictions, such as designated visitation hours. Some states require unrestricted access to clients' attorneys. These rights may be restricted if communication is harassing or harmful to someone. For example, if the nurse overhears a client using the phone to make threatening statements, the phone privileges may be suspended with a physician's order. The restriction as well as the rationale for the restriction must be documented in the client's record (Weiner & Wettstein, 1993).

Until the 1970s, hospitalized psychiatric clients frequently worked for the institution without compensation providing services such as housekeeping and grounds maintenance. The work was often of little therapeutic value. Today, about half of the states guarantee compensation for work such as employment in sheltered workshop programs that teach necessary skills. Even so, clients may still be expected to perform chores such as making their own beds and doing their own laundry (Weiner & Wettstein, 1993).

About half of the states have laws guaranteeing clients the right to personal possessions while hospitalized. This includes the right to wear their own clothes and have grooming items. These rights may be restricted if the personal items are potentially harmful (such as razors and belts), stolen or damaged, expensive, or disruptive to the unit. For example, the nurse may restrict a client from bringing an expensive stereo to the unit. On admission to the hospital, psychiatric clients may be searched, including their clothing, belongings, and rooms. Clients may be searched at other times with reasonable cause for suspicion of the presence of contraband or disallowed items that could potentially harm clients or others (Weiner & Wettstein, 1993).

SOMATIC THERAPIES

The mere nature of somatic therapies suggests that they are invasive and potentially harmful. The decision to consent to such treatment requires an informed consent, a basic client right. As a client advocate, the psychiatric nurse plays a pivotal role in informing the client of somatic treatment options, benefits, and potential adverse effects.

Electroconvulsive therapy (ECT) or Vagus Nerve Stimulation (VNS) may be recommended for persons with psychiatric disorders such as treatment resistant depression who do not respond to other treatments. ECT involves the use of anesthesia and VNS involves surgery for implantation of a pulse generator (Nahas et al., 2005; Reisner, 2003). (See Chapter 30.) Clients need to have adequate information about the risks and benefits of these procedures as a competent person has the right to agree to or refuse ECT or VNS.

Psychosurgery, such as lobotomy conducted on sections of the brain, used as therapy for psychiatric disorders may be considered effective in eliminating symptoms such as aggression. The use of this treatment has declined since the mid-1950s with the advent of other less-invasive treatments (Lesse, 1984). To prevent possible abuses, the practice of psychosurgery, although not banned, is subject to strict regulations. See Chapter 30 for a discussion on elecroconvulsive and complementary therapies.

FUTURE ISSUES CHALLENGING PSYCHIATRIC NURSES

Psychiatric nursing is at a crossroads as it faces the future. Increased knowledge of the biological aspects of the brain and behavioral science needs to be incorporated into psychiatric nursing as it becomes available. Advances in the field of psychiatric care bring the potential for further ethical quandaries and additional changes in the law.

The United States faces difficult financial questions related to health care now and in the future, and it faces the challenge of changing with the trends and needs of the nation. Psychiatric nursing has been a pacesetter historically, and psychiatric nurses are called to move into the community to create and direct preventive as well as other inventive treatment programs. It is time for psychiatric nursing to be proactive in meeting the legal and ethical challenges facing the citizens of our country, including opportunities related to:

a. Continued changes in the delivery method of health care as new treatments and technology develops and the cost of health care continues to affect treatment

b. Psychiatric nursing adapting from a traditionally inpatient setting to the outpatient setting

c. The needs of the aging population, such as coping with the aging process, multiple grief issues, changes in living situations, and organic disorders

d. Issues related to dysfunctional families, violence, addiction, and the impact of intrafamily and extrafamily relationships

e. Ethical and legal issues related to psychiatric genetics

f. Improving the quality of life for clients with medical illnesses

g. Access and availability of mental health services in a time of rising health care costs

h. Educating culturally competent nurses to provide culturally competent care

i. The evolving role of the advanced-practice psychiatric nurse

These needs must be met by a variety of creative means in a diversity of settings. Psychiatric nurses will continue to develop new roles and methods of providing care as they evaluate and shape the mental health system of the future. The methods, knowledge base, and clinical settings used in teaching psychiatric nursing are being reshaped in response to the changing health care system. This is an exciting era to be at the forefront of psychiatric nursing. The future of psychiatric nursing depends in large part on active participation in decision making regarding legal and ethical issues that shape the roles that nursing will play and affect clients' treatment.

SUMMARY

◆ This chapter has addressed the complex legal and ethical issues that nurses are compelled to consider when intervening with clients.

◆ In cases requiring ethical or moral judgments, there are many subjective factors that influence nurses' decisions, and although nurses have tools and standards to guide them, there are few clear-cut answers.

◆ In legal matters, nurses must often rely on judgment that is grounded in the law but is often subject to interpretation.

◆ Persons with psychiatric disorders are protected by a number of rights; some are based on the U.S. Constitution (such as the right to due process), and others stem from statutory law and case law (such as confidentiality). Still other more informal rights have been developed from a sense of ethical obligation to clients.

◆ Nurses play a key role in educating clients about these rights and protecting them from having their rights violated.

◆ Nurses are held accountable to adhere to the standards and laws that govern their practice. They must be able to explain and defend the actions they take. Having a solid foundation in ethical and legal concepts, along with keeping abreast of changes in the law, can protect nurses from liability as well as enhance their ability to be advocates for their clients and safeguard their rights.

SUGGESTIONS FOR CLINICAL CONFERENCES

1. Using the ethical decision-making model provided in this chapter, discuss how you would analyze the following situations:

   a. A 16-year-old adolescent is scheduled for discharge at the end of the week. His parents are frustrated by his multiple hospitalizations and say they do not want him at home. The insurance company has stated that they will not certify any further hospital days. The client says that he will run away if he is sent home. What are the ethical issues involved in this case? What are the alternatives available, and what would the consequences of each be?

b. A 25-year-old woman with anorexia nervosa has been hospitalized for a week. She is refusing to eat, and she continues to lose weight. The mental health team is concerned that the client is becoming dehydrated, so the physician orders tube feedings. The client states that she does not want the tube feedings. Using ethical principles, describe what actions the nurse should take.

c. Someone you work with has had many stresses in his life during the last 6 months, including divorce, the death of his mother, and the hospitalization of his child with depression. You smell an odor that resembles alcohol on his breath. The co-worker is not stumbling or having any apparent difficulty functioning. What should you do?

2. What changes would you like to see take place in your community that would affect mental health care? What could you do directly or indirectly to influence or support these innovations?

3. If a neighbor called to ask your help in admitting a relative to a psychiatric facility:
   a. What information would you need?
   b. Where would you refer them for further assistance?

4. You are working on an inpatient unit and a client comes to you to ask for a prn medication for anxiety. The order indicates the client can have the medicine every 6 hours and the last dose was given 4 hours ago. How might you handle this situation? How would the following information affect your decision?
   a. The client's mental state?
   b. The client's history?
   c. The medication being requested?
   d. Other medications the client is taking?
   e. The client's health status?
   f. The availability of other nurses or team members to consult?
   g. The availability of the physician?
   h. Other considerations?

STUDY QUESTIONS

1. Which of the following is *true* regarding the history of mental health laws?
   a. The only reform in mental health laws in the United States took place in the 1960s.
   b. Changes in the delivery of health care and technology make ongoing review of mental health laws necessary.
   c. Lawyers initiated all of the important changes in mental health laws in the United States.
   d. Mental health laws are all based on the United States Constitution.

2. Which *one* of the following statements regarding ethical principles is true?
   a. All cultures believe in the same ethical principles.
   b. Nurses who base their practice on ethical principles will always be acting within the law.
   c. Ethical principles can be used to help guide nursing actions.
   d. If health care providers disagree, one of them is not basing her view on ethical principles.

3. A student nurse is working in a community mental health setting. All of the following may represent a violation of professional boundaries *except*:
   a. the student nurse informs a client that she is a nursing student during introductions
   b. the student nurse gives a backrub to a client who is stressed
   c. the student nurse gives a client a ride home
   d. the student nurse describes having been abused as a child to a client

4. Nurses who work with clients of other cultures or races should:
   a. be aware of their own stereotypes or prejudices about other cultures or races
   b. attempt to learn more about the cultures and races of the clients they serve
   c. be aware of how cultural issues may affect the nursing process
   d. all of the above

5. Which of the following statements about mental health laws is *true*?
   a. No one in the United States can be hospitalized against her will.
   b. Minors have the same legal rights as adults regarding mental health issues.
   c. A client who is civilly committed to treatment still has the right to refuse treatment.
   d. All Americans have the legal right to the same mental health care.

6. The legal "duty to warn" refers to:
   a. the obligation of nurses to tell fellow staff when a client has a history of violence
   b. the obligation of mental health providers to warn potential victims of violence by clients
   c. the obligation of nurses to report substance abuse by fellow nurses
   d. the obligation of clients to warn staff about other violent clients

7. Which of the following statements is true about confidentiality?
   a. A nurse should keep private all information shared by clients.

b. A nurse may provide information about clients to any other nurses at the same institution because they all have the same obligation to keep the information private.

c. Reporting suspected child abuse is one situation in which the nurse may breach confidentiality.

d. Spouses have the same right to the record as the client.

8. Of the options listed, the best way for a nurse to avoid malpractice allegations is to:

a. carry malpractice insurance

b. keep abreast of professional and clinical standards and follow them

c. keep personal documentation of every situation with a negative outcome

d. attend at least ten continuing education programs a year

9. A client is brought to the emergency room by the local police department exhibiting psychotic symptoms due to poor adherence to medications. His mood is agitated and he exhibits florid psychotic symptoms. You are ordered to administer IM haloperidol. The client refuses to take the medication. What is the most appropriate response to the client?

a. Explain reasons for the medication and administer it as ordered.

b. Refuse to administer the medication until the client agrees to take it.

c. Explain reasons for the medication and wait until the client agrees to take it.

d. Ask the physician to administer the medication against the client's will.

10. Mr. Mann is brought in by his adult daughter. During the assessment you notice several bruises on the client's arm. What is the most immediate and appropriate nursing action?

a. Call protective services and report elder abuse.

b. "Tell me how you got those bruises on your arms."

c. Ask the client if his daughter injured her father.

d. Discuss your concerns with your supervisor.

RESOURCES

Please note that because Internet resources are of a time-sensitive nature and URL addresses may change or be deleted, searches should also be conducted by association or topic.

Internet Resources

1. Over the past decade, bioethics centers have proliferated, including those associated with universities and medical schools as well as freestanding centers. Do an Internet search of bioethics centers and:

a. Locate any bioethics centers in your area.

b. Explore the types of ethical issues they discuss on their Web site.

c. Investigate the types of graduate programs that are available in the field of bioethics.

2. Search the Internet to find a listing of your state and federal representatives and senators. See what, if any, bills are being introduced that relate to mental health issues.

http://www.ncbi.nih.gov/entrez/query.fcgi   Bioethicsline—a PubMed database for reviewing the literature for bioethical literature available online through the National Library of Medicine

http://www.imhl.com   Institute of Mental Health Law

http://www.jointcommission.org/AccreditationPrograms/BehavioralHealthCare/Standards/FAQs/Provision+of+Care+Treatment+and+Services/Restraint+and+Seclusion/Restraint_Seclusion.htm   The Joint Commission—frequently asked questions about restraints and seclusion

Other Resources

Kennedy Institute of Ethics
37th and O Streets, NW
Washington, DC 20057
(202) 687-8099
E-mail: medethx@georgetown.edu

The Hastings Center
21 Malcom Gordon Road
Garrison, NY 10524-5555
(914) 424-4040
E-mail: mail@thehastingscenter.org

Midwest Bioethics Center
1021-1025 Jefferson Street
Kansas City, MO 64105
(800) 344-3829
E-mail: bioethic@midbio.org

The Judge David L. Bazelon Center for Mental Health Law
1101 15th Street, NW
Suite 1212
Washington, DC 20005
Voice: (202) 467–5730
Email: www.brazelton.org

Treatment Advocacy Center (TAC)
200 N. Glebe Road
Suite 730
Arlington, VA 22203
(703) 294–6001/6002
Email: info@psychlaws.org

REFERENCES

Addington v. Texas, 441 U.S. 418 (Clearinghouse No. 17, 736, 1979).

American Association of Colleges of Nursing. (1986). *Essentials of college and university education for professional nursing.* Washington, DC: Author.

Annas, G. (1992). *The rights of patients.* Totowa, NJ: Humana Press.

Antai-Otong, D. (2006). Psychiatric patients and ethical issues. In V. D. Lachman (Ed.), *Applied ethics in nursing* (pp. 133–144). New York: Springer Publishing Company.

Appelbaum, P. S. (1988). The right to refuse treatment with antipsychotic medications: Retrospect and prospect. *American Journal of Psychiatry, 145*(4), 413–419.

Appelbaum, P. S. (1999). Least restrictive alternative revisited: Olmstead's uncertain mandate for community-based care. *Psychiatric Services, 50*(10), 1271–1272.

Appelbaum, P. S. (2004a). Ethical issues in psychiatric genetics. *Journal of Psychiatric Practice, 10*(6), 343–351.

Appelbaum, P. S. (2004b). Psychiatric advanced directives and the treatment of committed patients. *Psychiatric Services, 55*(7), 751–752, 763.

Bender, B. M., Murphy, D. K., & Mark, B. A. (1989). Caring for clients with legal charges on a voluntary psychiatric unit. *Journal of Psychosocial Nursing and Mental Health Services, 27*(3), 16–20.

Bennett, P. E. (1986). The meaning of "mental illness" under the Michigan mental health code. *Cooley Law Review, 4*(65), 65–100.

Bernal, E. W. (1992). The nurse as patient advocate. *Hasting Center Report, 22*(4), 18–23.

Betrus, P. A., & Hoffman, A. (1992). Psychiatric-mental health nursing: Career characteristics, professional activities, and client attributes of members of the American Nurses Association Council of Psychiatric Nurses. *Issues in Mental Health Nursing, 13*(1), 39–50.

Binder, R. L. (1999). Are the mentally ill dangerous? *The Journal of the American Academy of Psychiatry and the Law, 27*(2), 189–201.

Bloom, B. L., & Asher, S. J. (Eds.). (1982). *Psychiatric patient rights and patient advocacy*. New York: Human Sciences Press.

Bloom, J. D. (2004). Thirty-five years of working with civil commitment statutes. *The Journal of the American Academy of Psychiatry and the Law, 32*, 430–439.

Bloom, J. D., & Faulkner, L. R. (1987). Competency determinations in civil commitment. *American Journal of Psychiatry, 144*(2), 193–196.

Burkhardt, M. A., & Nathaniel, A. K. (1998). *Ethics and issues in contemporary nursing*. Clifton Park, NY: Delmar Learning.

Butts, H. F. (1999). Psychoanalytic perspectives on racial profiling. *The Journal of the American Academy of Psychiatry and the Law, 27*(4), 633–635.

Carpenter, M. A. (1991). The process of ethical decision making in psychiatric nursing practice. *Issues in Mental Health Nursing, 28*(10), 19–25.

Carroll, P., & Maher, V. F. (1990). Legal considerations for psychiatric patients. *Advancing Clinical Care, 5*(6), 16–17.

Carty, L. A. (1992). The mental health law project's 20 years. *Clearinghouse Review, 26*(1), 57–65.

Christoffel, T., & Teret, S. P. (1991). Epidemiology and the law: Courts and confidence intervals. *American Journal of Public Health, 81*(12), 1661–1666.

Costello, J. C. (1996). Why would I need a lawyer? Legal counsel and advocacy for people with mental disabilities. In B. D. Sales & D. W. Shuman (Eds.), *Law, mental health, and mental disorders*. Pacific Grove, CA: Brooks/Cole Publishing.

Cushing, M. (1988). *Nursing jurisprudence*. Norwalk, CT: Appleton & Lange.

Dain, N. (1994). Psychiatry and anti–psychiatry in the United States. In M. S. Micale & R. Porter (Eds.), *Discovering the history of psychiatry*. New York: Oxford University Press.

Davis, A. J., & Aroskar, M. A. (1991). *Ethical dilemmas and nursing practice* (3rd ed.). Norwalk, CT: Appleton & Lange.

Davis, A. J., & Underwood, P. R. (1989). The competency quagmire: Clarification of the nursing perspective concerning the issues of competence and informed consent. *International Journal of Nursing Studies, 26*(3), 271–279.

deLeon Siantz, M. L. (1988). Children's rights and parental rights. *Journal of Child and Adolescent Psychiatric and Mental Health Nursing, 1*(1), 14–17.

Dice, M. R. (1987). The emerging constitutional rights of the mentally ill: 1787–1987. *Colorado Lawyer, 16*(9), 1619–1623.

Dixon v. Weinberger, 405 F. Supp. 974 (D.D.C.) (Clearinghouse No. 17. 175, 1975).

Ellis, J. W. (1996). Voluntary admission and involuntary hospitalization of minors. In B. D. Sales & D. W. Shuman (Eds.), *Law, mental health, and mental disorders*. Pacific Grove, CA: Brooks/Cole Publishing.

Erlen, J. A. (1987). The child's choice: An essential component in treatment decisions. *Children's Healthcare, 15*(3), 156–160.

Eriksen, J. (1989). Steps to ethical reasoning. *Canadian Nurse, 85*(7), 23–24.

Etzioni, A. (1999). Medical records: Enhancing privacy, preserving the common good. *Hastings Center Report, 29*(2), 14–23.

Falkowski, J., Watts, V., Falkowski, W., & Dean. T. (1990). Patients leaving hospital without knowledge or permission of staff—absconding. *British Journal of Psychiatry, 156*, 488–490.

Felthous, A. R. (1999). The clinician's duty to protect third parties. *Psychiatric Clinics of North America, 22*(1), 49–60.

Fiesta, J. (1992). Protecting children: A public duty to report. *Nursing Management, 23*(7), 14–15, 17.

Fitzgerald, W. L. (1999). Legal and ethical considerations in the treatment of psychosis. *The Journal of Clinical Psychiatry, 60*(Suppl. 19), 59–65.

Freishtat, H. W. (1991). View from the nation's courts: Premature discharge due to utilization review—an emerging area of liability. *Journal of Clinical Psychopharmacology, 11*(2), 133–134.

Frueh, B. C., Knapp, R. G., Cusack, K. J., Grubaugh, A. L., Sauvageot, J. A., Cousins, V. C., Yim, E., Robins, C. S., Monnier, J., & Hiers, T. G. (2005). Patients' reports of traumatic or harmful experiences within the psychiatric setting. *Psychiatric Services, 56*(9), 1123–1132.

Gamwell, L., & Tomes, N. (1995). *Madness in America: Cultural and medical perceptions of mental illness before 1914.* Ithaca, NY: Cornell University Press.

Garyali, V. (1999). "The color of suspicion": Race profiling or racism? *The Journal of the American Academy of Psychiatry and the Law, 27*(4), 630–632.

Goldzband, J. G. (1998). Dangerousness: A mutating concept passes through the literature. *The Journal of the American Academy of Psychiatry and the Law, 26*(4), 649–654.

Grove, K. (1990). Tardive dyskinesia: A key issue facing the psychiatric-mental health nurse. *Perspectives in Psychiatric Care, 26*(3), 29–32.

Grudzinskas, A. J. (1999). Kumho Tire Co., Inc. v. Carmichael. *The Journal of American Psychiatry Law, 27*(3), 482–488.

Gutheil, T. G. (1999). A confusion of tongues: Competence, insanity, psychiatry, and the law. *Psychiatric Services, 50*(6), 767–773.

Hall, M. A. (1997). *Making medical spending decisions: The law, ethics, and economics of rationing mechanisms.* New York: Oxford University Press.

Hargrave v. Vermont, 340 F. 3d 27 (2nd cir. 2003)

Haviland, S., & O'Brien, J. (1989). Physical abuse and neglect of the elderly: Assessment and intervention. *Orthopaedic Nursing, 8*(4), 11–18.

Hiday, V. A., & Scheid-Cook, T. L. (1989). A follow-up of chronic patients committed to outpatient treatment. *Hospital and Community Psychiatry, 40*(1), 52–59.

Huckshorn, K. A. (2005). Re-designing state mental health policy to prevent the use of seclusion and restraint. *Administration and Policy in Mental Health,* Oct. 22, 1–10.

Jakacki, M., & Payson, A. L. (1985). Out of control. *American Journal of Nursing, 85*(12), 1335–1336.

Janing, J. (1992). Tarnis . . . the golden. *Emergency, 24*(9), 40–43, 58.

Kapp, M. B. (1996). Treatment and refusal rights in mental health: Therapeutic justice and clinical accommodation. In B. D. Sales & D. W. Shuman (Eds.), *Law, mental health, and mental disorder.* Pacific Grove, CA: Brooks/Cole Publishing.

Kim, M. M., Van Dorn, R. A., Scheyett, A. M., Elbogen, E. E., Swanson, J. W., Swartz, M. S., et al. (2007). Understanding the personal and clinical utility of psychiatric advance directives: A qualitative perspective. *Psychiatry, 70,* 19–29.

Kjervik, D. K., & Grove, S. J. (1988). The legal meaning of consent in unequal power relationships. *Journal of Professional Nursing, 4*(3), 192–204.

Knapp, S., & Vandercreek, L. (1983). Malpractice risks with suicidal patients. *Psychotherapy: Theory, Research, and Practice, 20*(3), 274–280.

Lesse, S. (1984). Psychosurgery. *American Journal of Psychotherapy, 38*(2), 224–228.

Long, K. A. (1996). Ethical responsibility for the community's mental health: A professional nursing role. *Journal of Child and Adolescent Psychiatric Nursing, 9*(3), 39–44.

Loubardias, S. (1991). Ethics of electroconvulsive therapy consent. *Rehabilitation Nursing, 16*(2), 98–100.

McFadyen, J. A. (1989). Who will speak for me? *Nursing Times, 8*(85), 45–48.

Melrose, N. H. (1990). "Duty to warn" vs. "patient confidentiality": The ethical dilemmas in caring for HIV-infected clients. *Nurse Practitioner, 15*(2), 58–69.

Miller, R. D. (1999). Coerced treatment in the community. *Psychiatric Clinics of North America, 22*(1), 183–195.

Missouri Department of Mental Health. (1993). *Your rights and expectations as a forensic client.* Jefferson City, MO: Author.

Morgan, N. E. (1987). The current litigation crisis and tort reform. *Journal of American Medical Record Association, 58*(1), 19–21.

Nahas, Z., Marangell, L. B., Husain, M. M., Rush A. J., Sackeim H. A., Lisanby S. H., Martinez J. M., & George M. S. (2005). Two-year outcome of vagus nerve stimulation (VNS) for treatment of major depressive episodes. *Journal of Clinical Psychiatry, 66*(9), 1097–1104.

National Institute of Mental Health. (1991). *Law and mental health: Major developments and research needs* (DHHS Publication No. ADM 91-1875). Washington, DC: U.S. Government Printing Office.

Nursing practice: Issues and answers. (1992). *Ohio Nurses Review, 67*(2), 16.

Parham v. J. L. & J. R., 442 U.S. 584 (1979).

Puskar, K. R., & Obus. N. L. (1989). Management of the psychiatric emergency. *Nurse Practitioner, 14*(7),9–24.

Reid, W. H. (2003a). Back to basics: Law and mental health. *Journal of Psychiatric Practice, 9*(3), 240–244.

Reid, W. H. (2003b). Risk assessment, prediction, and foreseeability. *Journal of Psychiatric Practice, 9*(1), 82–86.

Reisner, A. D. (2003). The electroconvulsive therapy controversy: Evidence and ethics. *Neurophsychology Review, 13*(4), 199–219.

Sanders, J. B., & DuPlessis, D. (1985). An historical view of right to treatment. *Journal of Psychosocial Nursing and Mental Health Services, 23*(9), 12–17.

Schwartz, H. I., Vingiano, W., & Perez, C. B. (1988). Autonomy and the right to refuse treatment: Patients' attitudes after involuntary medication. *Hospital and Community Psychiatry, 39*(10), 1049–1054.

Simon, R. L., & Goetz, S. (1999). Forensic issues in the psychiatric emergency department. *Psychiatric Clinics of North America, 22*(4), 851–864.

Sjöström, S. (2006). Invocation of coercion context in compliance communication—power dynamics in psychiatric care. *International Journal of Law and Psychiatry, 29,* 36–47.

Slovenko, R. (1999). Malpractice in psychotherapy: An overview. *Psychiatric Clinics of North America, 22*(1), 1–15.

Slovenko, R. (2000). Update on legal issues associated with tardive dyskinesia. *The Journal of Clinical Psychiatry, 61*(Suppl. 4), 45–57.

Smith, D. P. (1989). Child abuse and neglect: Legal and clinical implications for school nursing practice. *School Nurse, 5*(4), 17–20, 25–26, 28.

Smith, J. (1990). Privileged communication: Psychiatric-mental health nurses and the law. *Perspectives in Psychiatric Care, 26*(4), 26–29.

Smith, S. R. (1996). Malpractice liability of mental health professionals and institutions. In B. D. Sales & D. W. Shuman (Eds.), *Law, mental health, and mental disorders.* Pacific Grove, CA: Brooks/Cole Publishing.

Stern, S. B. (1990). Privileged communication: An ethical and legal right of psychiatric clients. *Perspectives in Psychiatric Care, 26*(4), 22–25.

Szasz, T. (2005). "Idiots, infants, and the insane": Mental illness and legal incompetence. *Journal of Medical Ethics, (31),* 78–81.

Tarasoff, V. (1976). Plaintiffs and appellants v. the regents of the University of California et al., defendants and respondent. SF 23042. *Pacific Reporter, 551*p.2d, 334–362.

Thomas, K. (2000, August 8). Parents pressured to put kids on drugs. *USA Today,* D1.

Touchet, B. K., Drummond, S. R., & Yates, W. R. (2004). The impact of fear of HIPAA violation on patient care. *Psychiatric Services, 55*(5), 575–576.

Valentine, N. M., Verhey, M., Hundert, E., & Kayne, P. (1990). A collaborative approach to clinical standards development. Psychiatry and psychiatric nursing in a changing world. *Psychiatric Clinics of North America, 13*(1), 171–185.

Van Dorn, R. A., Swartz, M. S., Elbogen, E. B., Swanson, J. W., Kim, M., Ferron, J., McDaniel, L. A., & Scheyett (2005). Clinicians' attitudes regarding barriers to the implementation of psychiatric advanced directives,"Administration and Policy in Mental Health and Mental Health Services Research," October 2005 (published online), 1–12.

Vandenberg, G. H. (1993). *Court testimony in mental health: A guide for mental health professionals and attorneys.* Springfield. IL: Thomas Press.

Watkins, K. E., Wells, K. B., & McLellan, A. T. (1999). Termination of social security benefits among Los Angeles recipients disabled by substance abuse. *Psychiatric Services, 50*(7), 914–918.

Weiner, B. A. (1990). A general practitioner's guide to mental health law. *Illinois Bar Journal, 78*(3), 153–155.

Weiner, B. A., & Wettstein, R. M. (1993). Legal issues in mental health care. New York: Plenum Press.

Weiss, E. M., Altimari, D., Blint, D. F., & Megan, K. (1998, October). Deadly restraints: A nationwide pattern of death. *The Hartford Courant,* 1–16.

Weiss, J. (1990). The right to refuse: Informed consent and the psychosocial nurse. *Journal of Psychosocial Nursing and Mental Health Services, 28*(8), 25–30.

Wettstein, R. M. (1999). The right to refuse psychiatric treatment. *Psychiatric Clinics of North America, 22*(1), 173–182.

Wilkinson, J. M. (1987). Moral distress in nursing practice: Experience and effect. *Nursing Forum, 23*(1), 16–29.

Wyatt v. Stickney, 344 F. Suppl. 373, 375 (1970).

Yorker, B. C. (1988). Confidentiality—an ethical dilemma. Balancing the "duty to warn" against the right to privacy. *AAOHN J, 36*, 346–347.

Young, J. L., Spitz, R. T., Hillbrand, J., & Daneri, G. (1999). Medication adherence, failure in schizophrenia: A forensic review of rates, reasons, treatments, and prospects. *Journal of American Academy of Psychiatry and the Law, 27*(3), 426–444.

Zinermon v. Burch, 108 L. Ed. 2d 115, 117 (1990).

SUGGESTED READINGS

Appelbaum, P. S. (2001). *Informed consent: Legal theory and clinical practice.* New York: Oxford University Press.

Burkhardt, M. A., & Nathaniel, A. K. (2002). *Ethics and issues in contemporary nursing.* Australia, Albany: Delmar/Thomson Learning.

Crigger, B. (Ed.). (1998). *Cases in bioethics.* New York: St. Martin's Press.

Fry, S. T., & Johnstone, M. (2002). *Ethics in nursing practice: A guide to ethical decision making.* Malden, MA, Blackwell Science.

Howell, J. H., & Sale, W. F. (Eds.). (1995). *A Hastings Center introduction to bioethics.* Washington, DC: Georgetown University Press.

O'Keefe, M. E. (2000). *Nursing practice and the law: Avoiding malpractice and other legal risks.* Philadelphia: F. A. Davis.

UNIT 2

Response to Stressors across the Life Span

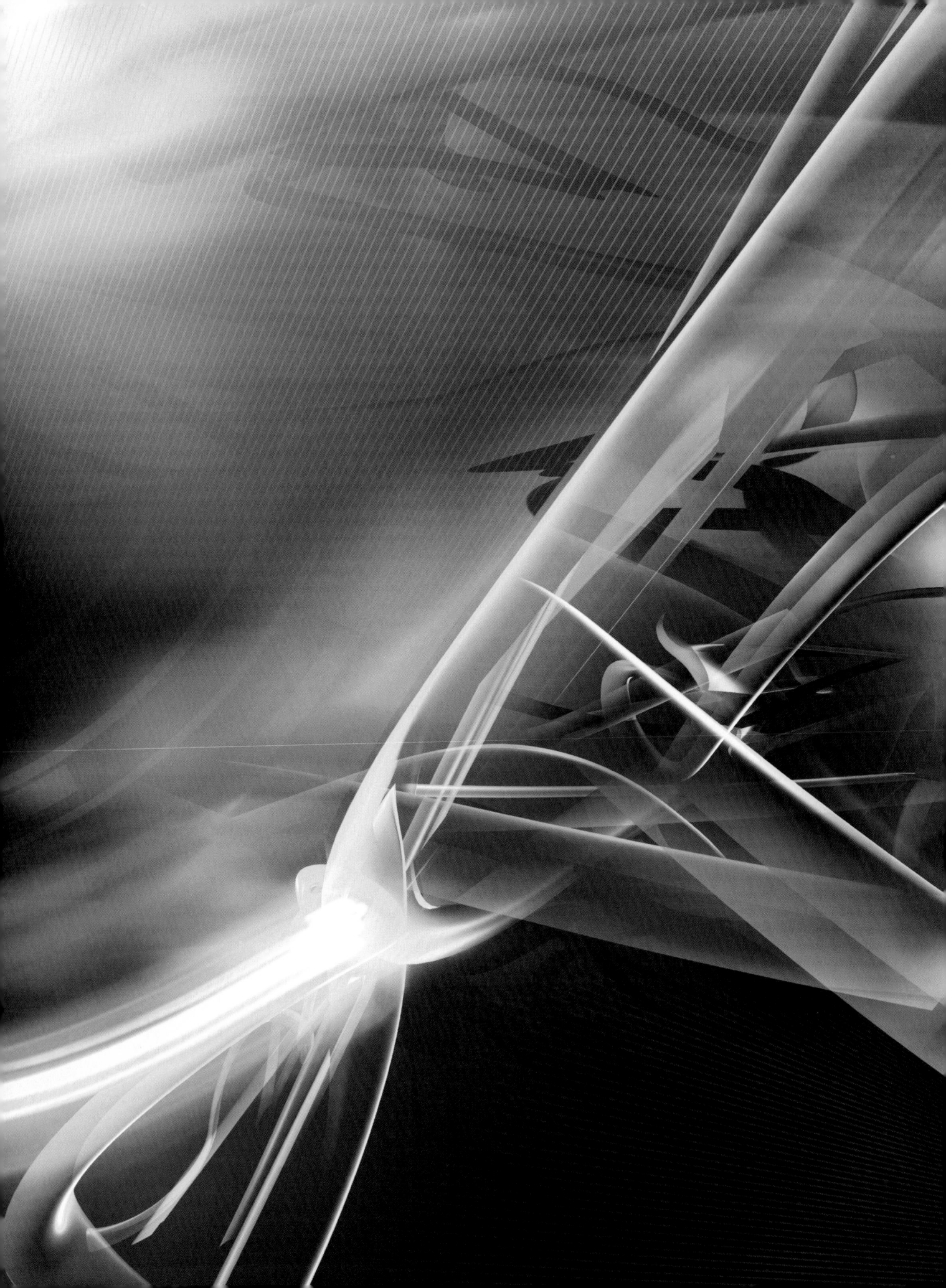

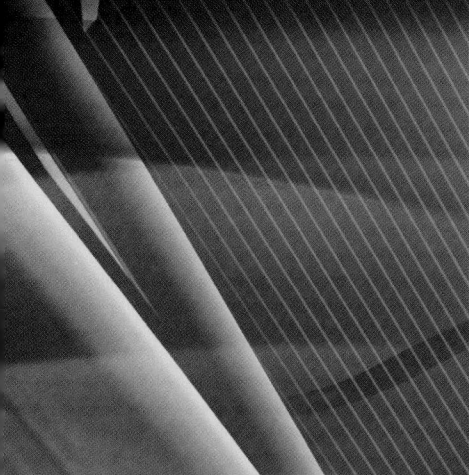

CHAPTER 9

The Client with a Depressive Disorder

Linda Lewin, RN, MSN, CS

KEY TERMS

Anhedonia: The inability to experience pleasure from activities that usually produce pleasurable feelings.

Dysphoria: Marked feelings of sadness.

Hyperphagia: Excessive amount of eating.

Hypersomnia: Excessive amount of sleep.

Insomnia: Inability to fall asleep, difficulty staying asleep, or early morning awakening.

Libido: Urge or desire for sexual activity.

Mood: An emotional state.

Neurovegetative: Refers to biological functions such as sleep pattern, eating pattern, energy level, sexual functioning, and bowel functioning.

Psychomotor Retardation: A slowing of physical and emotional reactions, including speech, affect, and movement.

Ruminations: Repetitive or continuous thinking about a particular subject that then interferes with other thought processes.

Self-Deprecatory Ideas: Negative thoughts about the self.

Somatic Preoccupation: Excessively focused on one's own body functioning.

COMPETENCIES

Upon completion of this chapter, the learner should be able to:

1. Differentiate major depressive episodes according to *DSM-IV-TR* diagnostic criteria.

2. Analyze the neurobiological, genetic, and psychosocial theories relevant to depression.

3. Describe actual or potential complications of depression across the life span.

4. Differentiate between depression and dementia in the older adult.

5. Distinguish normal grief from pathological grief.

6. Discuss major evidence-based treatment modalities of depression.

7. Implement a plan of care for a client with major depression.

8. Apply the nursing process to the care of the depressed client.

CHAPTER OUTLINE

Epidemiology

Causative Factors

Neurobiological Theories

Genetic Factors

Neurotransmitter Dysregulation Theory

Neuroendocrinology Theories

Neuroanatomical Theories

Hypothalamic-Pituitary-Adrenal (HPA) Axis

Psychoanalytic Theories

Cultural Factors

Psychosocial Factors

Cognitive-Behavioral Theories

EPIDEMIOLOGY

Major depressive disorders (MDDs) are highly prevalent in the general population and clinical settings. Major depression is considered a mood disorder. Mood refers to an emotional state such as depressed or irritable. Epidemiological studies consistently demonstrate that about 10 to 12 percent of primary care clients experience significant depressive disorders (Runkewitz, Kirchmann, & Strauss, 2006). Depression is the fourth most significant cause of global disability and by the year 2020, it is projected to become the second (Murray & Lopez, 1997a, 1997b). The prognosis of MDD is poor in older adults with a chronic course or recurrent course (Cole & Dendukuri, 2003).

According to the *Diagnostic and Statistical Manual of Mental Disorders, 4th edition, Text Revision (DSM-IV-TR)* (American Psychiatric Association [APA], 2000) the lifetime risk for MDD in community samples varies from 10 to 25 percent for women and from 5 to 12 percent in men. The point prevalence for MDD varies from 5 to 9 percent for women and 2 to 3 percent for men and appears to be unrelated to culture, education, socioeconomic status, or marital status.

MDD is one and one-half to three times more likely to occur in a first-degree biological relative (e.g., mother, sister, or father) affected with the disorder than among the general population. Oftentimes, a psychosocial stressor, especially the death of a loved one, divorce, or childbirth may precipitate a major depressive episode (Pincus et al., 1999).

The lifetime prevalence of dysthymic disorder (DD) with or without comorbid MDD is about 6 percent and the point prevalence is 3 percent. Mood disorders due to general medical conditions range from 25 to 40 percent of people with neurological conditions (e.g., Alzheimer's disease, multiple sclerosis). Non-neurological general medical condition rates are difficult to determine and more variable, ranging from 8 percent in end-stage renal disease to 60 percent in Cushing's disease (American Psychiatric Association [APA], 2000).

Other depressive disorders included under Mood Disorders in the *DSM-IV-TR* (APA, 2000) are substance-induced disorders and those that meet the criteria for Atypical Features Specifiers, such as postpartum depression and seasonal affective disorder (SAD). Although bipolar disorders are mood disorders with depressive episodes, they are not discussed in this chapter. See Chapter 10.

Gender factors appear to play a role in the epidemiology of MDD (APA, 2000; Ustun, 2000). Cross-cultural community surveys consistently show a female preponderance of depressive disorders (Brommelhoff, Conway, Merikangas, & Levy, 2004).

A number of studies also show a high prevalence of concomitant anxiety disorder and other psychiatric disorders with major depressive illness (Kessler et al., 2005; Moffitt et al., 2007).

The course of MDD varies, but the average onset is the late 20s, although it may occur during childhood, adolescence, or older adulthood. A prodromal period may include anxiety symptoms and mild depression several weeks before the onset of full MDD. The onset of symptoms ranges from days to months to sudden, particularly when precipitated by a psychosocial stressor. The duration of MDD also varies but when left untreated, the episode typically lasts 6 months or longer (APA, 2000). Others may develop other mood disorders, such as bipolar disorder. Additionally, because of its recurrent and potentially debilitating course, MDDs are associated with significant functional impairment, reduced productivity, and high utilization of health care services (Stewart, Ricci, Chee, Hahn, & Morganstein, 2004). Furthermore, depressive illnesses may produce extensive grief and pain, disrupt the family's functioning, and contribute to premature death or suicide (Mann, Apter, Bertolote, et al., 2005; Oquendo et al., 2007).

The prevalence of depressive disorders in practice settings requires astute assessment skills that enable the nurse to make an accurate diagnosis and initiate interventions that shorten the course and reduce recurrence and chronicity. Nurses also face the responsibility of identifying other psychiatric and medical conditions that mimic depressive illnesses and initiate appropriate treatment to manage them. Because the risk of suicide across the life span is significant, nurses need to assess all clients for depression and suicide and facilitate adaptive resolution of causative factors to restore clients to an optimal level of functioning.

This chapter focuses on depressive disorders across the life span and integrates major theories into the treatment planning. The role and practice of the generalist and advance-practice nurses caring for the client with a depressive illness are the central focus. Lastly, this chapter provides an overview of major nursing interventions that focus on or integrate pharmacologic and psychotherapeutic interventions such as antidepressant medication and cognitive behavioral therapy.

CAUSATIVE FACTORS

Contemporary researchers suggest that the cause of depressive disorders is complex and that a combination of neurobiological, cultural, and psychosocial factors are likely to be involved in the etiology of depressive disorders. In addition, genetic or familial patterns are also indicated as causative factors of depression.

NEUROBIOLOGICAL THEORIES

The primary areas of neurobiological research into mood disorders include genetics, neurotransmitters, neuroendocrine studies, circadian rhythms, and neuroanatomical abnormalities. Findings related to depressive disorders are reviewed here.

GENETIC FACTORS

Studies of unipolar and bipolar disorders in families consistently show that these illnesses are highly familial. In a widely documented investigation of female-female twin pairs (n = 2,164), Kendler and colleagues (1995) found that both genetic factors and psychosocial stressors were involved in the prediction of major depression. The study found that the most powerful stressors were the death of a loved one, assault, serious marital discord, and divorce or marital separation. They also concluded that the nature of the stressor was mediated by genetic factors and in part by modifying the vulnerability of individuals to depression-inducing effects of psychosocial stressors. These data have recently been replicated and confirm earlier assertions concerning the depressogenic effects associated with the interaction between depression and stressful events and adversities (Kendler, Kuhn, Vittum, Prescott, & Riley, 2005). Researchers also submit that individual coping skills and genetic vulnerability govern how people modulate stressful life events and adversities. Based on genetic studies involving serotonin transporter polymorphism or genetic influences some people are *stress-sensitive* and at high-risk for depression in response to moderate stressors, while others are *stress-resistant* and depression free (Kendler et al., 2005). Kendler and his colleagues (2006) explored developmental models of depression in men and women and submit that similarities exist between genders. Results from this study indicated that major depression stems from internalizing symptoms, externalizing symptoms, and stressful events or adversities and that childhood parental loss and low self-esteem were compelling variables in both sexes (Kendler, Gardner, & Prescott, 2006).

Together these data posit female gender, childhood sexual abuse, genetic predisposition, early parental loss, low parental warmth, stressful life events, low self-esteem, and early-onset anxiety are the most salient predictors of depression and recurrent depression.

Implications from these data suggest that identification of genetic or familial patterns are risk factors for depression, particularly when they experience pronounced psychosocial stress. By identifying these risk factors, the nurse can develop primary preventive measures that help clients at risk for recurrent depression, using interventions that reduce stress and strengthen coping and problem-solving skills to reduce the impact of environmental stressors.

NEUROTRANSMITTER DYSREGULATION THEORY

Neurobiological theories involving neurotransmitters in depressed persons are complex and generally based on the therapeutic effects of antidepressant medications (see Fig. 9–1). Supposedly these medications are effective because of their role in regulating specific neurotransmitters in the brain. The precise mechanism that neurotransmitters play in the etiology and treatment of depression is unclear and other mechanisms may also be involved in these processes. Antidepressants appear to change the level of neurotransmitters in the brain to help regulate depression, but their therapeutic effects are not immediate and a significant number of clients respond poorly. Studies consistently demonstrate that, although people take antidepressants, full therapeutic responses may not occur for weeks or even several months. Further research is necessary to determine the precise correlation between specific neurotransmitters and depression.

Dysregulation of either noradrenergic (norepinephrine [NE]) or serotonergic neurotransmitter systems and mechanism of action of antidepressant drugs is the most widely accepted explanation for depression. Major theories concerning the role of NE is that there is a reduction in release or production from presynaptic neurons and an increase in presynaptic alpha 2-adrenergic activities that results in reduced NE. In addition, people with depressive disorders have dysregulation in this system (Leonard, 2005; Nemeroff et al., 2006).

Early work by Coppen, Eccleston, and Peet (1973) implicated low levels of tryptophan (the key precursor of serotonin) in depressed clients. Presently, there is a plethora of evidence indicating an abnormality in presynaptic serotonin function in depression. Specifically, most research points to a decrease in transport or release and synthesis of serotonin, or reduced efficacy of serotonergic transmission (Charney, 1998). These transporters are the *sites of action* for serotonin selective reuptake inhibitors (SSRIs). Additionally, people who are depressed have reduced levels of serotonin in platelet transporters (Nelson, Portera, & Leon, 2005; Nemeroff et al., 2006). Researchers further submit that the relationship between reduced levels of the metabolite of serotonin (5-hydroxyindoleacetic [5-HIAA]) in cerebrospinal fluid and suicide is well documented (Sullivan, Mann, Oquendo, et al., 2006). The major neurotransmitters that have been studied in relation to mood disorders are outlined in Table 9–1. A schematic representation of these processes is provided in Figure 9–1.

Although neurobiological theories of depression have focused on two monoamine systems—noradrenergic (norepinephrine) and serotonin—most believe that these systems fail to provide a full explanation for the pathogenesis of depression. The hypothalamic-pituitary-adrenal (HPA) axis, including the effects of corticotropin-releasing hormone (CRH) and cortisol, also play significant roles in the etiology of depressive disorders along with second and third messenger systems (Flores, Kenna, Keller, Solvason, & Schatzberg, 2006). Growing evidence implicates the glutamatergic system in the etiology and treatment of mood disorders. Compared to the efficacy of conventional antidepressants the onset of treatment may take as long as weeks to several months for a single intravenous dose of an N-methyl-D-aspartate antagonist; onset occurred within 2 hours after infusions and remained significant for 1 week. These preliminary results indicate the role of the glutamatergic system (Norman & Burrows, 2007; Pittenger, Sanacora, & Krystal, 2007; Zarate, Singh, Carlson, Brutsche, Ameli et al., 2006).

Understanding underlying dysregulation of neurotransmitter systems provides a basis for actions of various antidepressant

TABLE 9–1
Neurotransmitters Theoretically Involved in Mood Disorders

Monoamine neurotransmitters
  Catecholamines
    Epinephrine
    Norepinephrine (noradrenergic)
    Dopamine
  Indoleamines
    Serotonin
Cholinergic neurotransmitter
  Acetylcholine
Amino acid neurotransmitter
  Gamma-aminobutyric acid
  Glutamatergic System
  N-methyl-D-aspartate (NMDA)

agents. For instance, SSRIs such as Prozac (fluoxetine) increase serotonin in the brain, thus increasing the client's mood. By having a basic understanding of these processes, the nurse can use this information to teach clients with depression the reasons for taking antidepressant medications. See Chapter 29.

NEUROENDOCRINOLOGY THEORIES

Neuroendocrinology theories further explain the origins of depression and the role of the brain and complex endocrine systems. There is growing evidence that indicates dysregulation of the hypothalamic-pituitary-adrenal axis in depression and other psychiatric disorders.

NEUROANATOMICAL THEORIES

Abnormalities of the hippocampus appear to contribute to the biological underpinnings of depression and other mood disorders. Researchers submit that increased cortisol secretion associated with major depressive disorder may cause atrophy and reduced hippocampal volume (Videbech & Ravnkilde, 2004). (See Figure 9–2.) Apart from hippocampal reduction, data also demonstrate additional evidence of cerebral atrophy of the prefrontal cortex, cingulate gyrus, caudate nucleus, and cerebellum (Kanner, 2004; Siegle, Thompson, Carter, Steinhauer, & Thase, 2007; Wagner et al., 2006). Understanding the neurobiological causes of depression provide a basis for nursing interventions, such as medication administration and prescription and psychotherapeutic approaches.

HYPOTHALAMIC-PITUITARY-ADRENAL (HPA) AXIS

Research has consistently shown that clients with major depression (especially severe or psychotic type) secrete abnormally large amounts of cortisol. Activation of the HPA axis, ultimately leading to the secretion of cortisol, occurs when an individual experiences psychological or physiological stress. Specifically, the hypothalamus in the brain secretes CRH, which stimulates the anterior pituitary gland to release adreno-corticotropic hormone (ACTH). ACTH acts as a messenger to the adrenal glands to secrete cortisol. Normally, cortisol then shuts off the stress response by acting on the hypothalamus to stop its secretion of CRH (Flores, Kenna, Keller, et al., 2006). In the depressed person this process goes awry. The body's response to stress in effect does not shut off, resulting in hypercortisolemia. Numerous studies also link high cortisol level to pronounced cognitive deficits in depressed clients, especially those with psychotic features (Belanoff, Kalehzan, Sund, Ficek, & Schatzberg, 2001; Gomez et al., 2006).

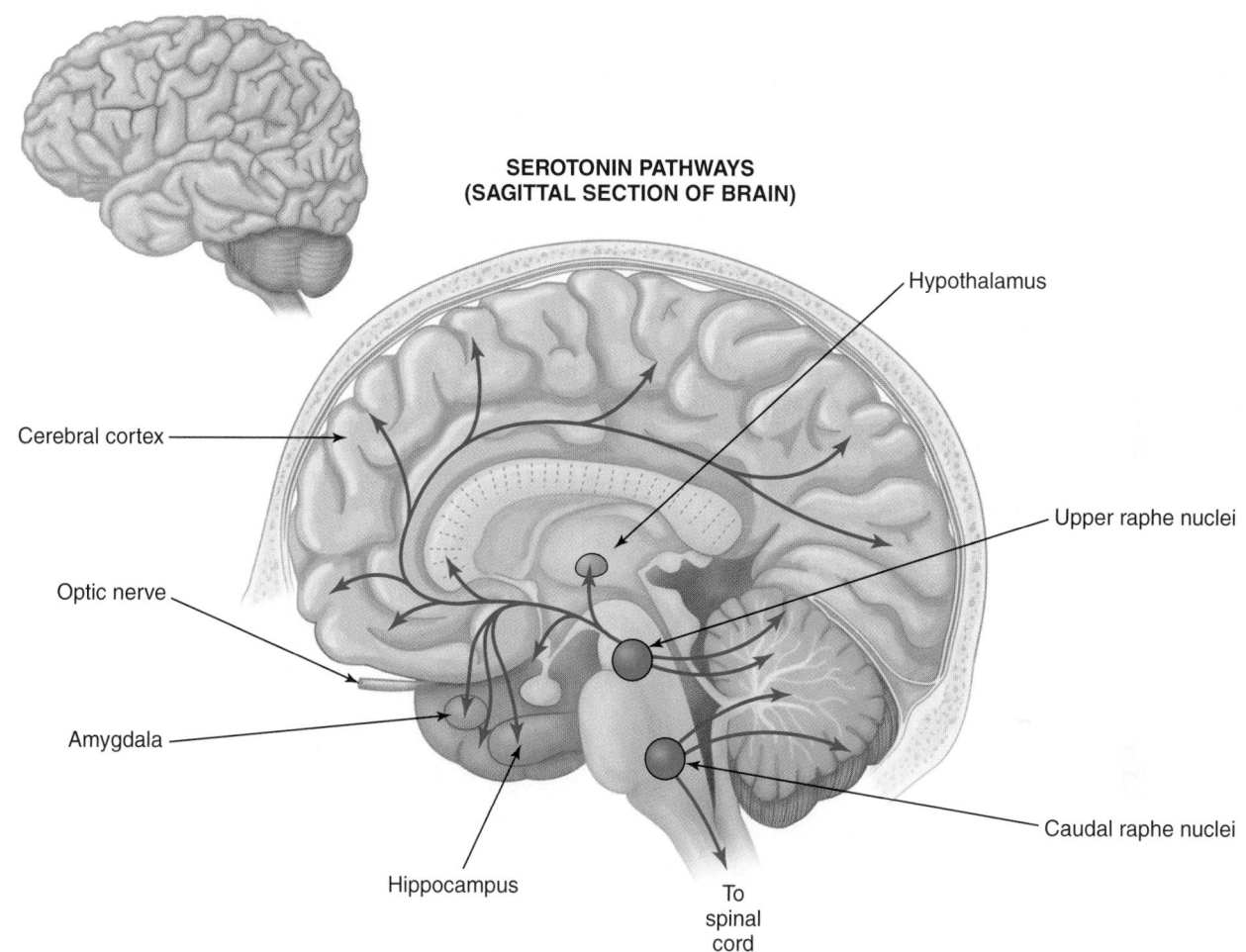

SEROTONIN PATHWAYS (SAGITTAL SECTION OF BRAIN)

Hypothalamus

Cerebral cortex

Upper raphe nuclei

Optic nerve

Amygdala

Caudal raphe nuclei

Hippocampus

To spinal cord

The neurotransmitter serotonin is produced in the upper and caudal raphe nuclei and travels to other areas of the brain and to the spinal cord along serotonergic pathways. Serotonin normally regulates mood and the sleep-wake cycle. There is physiologic evidence that serotonin receptor sites are sparse in the serotonin pathways of depressed persons. As a result, less serotonin is available to regulate mood and contribute to a sense of well-being. The neurotransmitter norepinephrine may also play a role in mood disorders (see text).

Figure 9–1 The serotonin hypothesis in relation to mood disorders. *(continues)*

SEROTONIN AND THE LIMBIC SYSTEM

The limbic system is a network of neuronal clusters connected by neurotransmitter pathways. This subdivision of the cortex overlying the brain stem plays a primary role in behavioral responses, mood, memory, and learning.

A deficit in the amount of serotonin available to the limbic system has a number of physiologic and emotional effects. A decrease in serotonin available to the **amygdala,** the emotional center of the brain, can cause sadness, a decreased libido, and a general lack of motivation. A serotonin deficit also affects the **hypothalamus,** which is responsible for appetite control; the depressed person may have little appetite or may overeat. The **pituitary gland** may react to serotonin deficit by releasing an excess of pituitary hormones that can cause gastric distress, menstrual irregularities, and sleep disturbances.

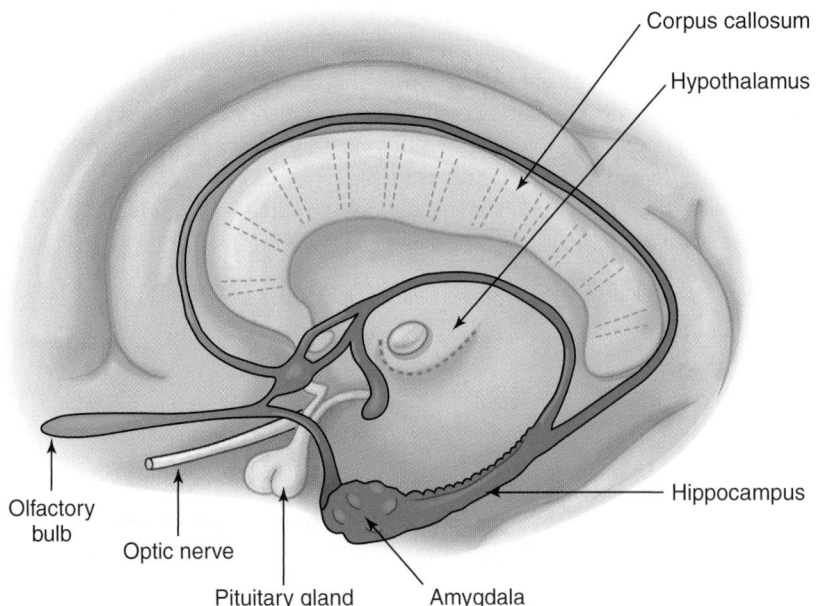

Corpus callosum

Hypothalamus

Hippocampus

Olfactory bulb

Optic nerve

Pituitary gland

Amygdala

HOW MEDICATIONS AFFECT THE SEROTONERGIC SYNAPSES

Some depressed clients are treated with medications that affect the breakdown of serotonin or block or inhibit its reuptake. These drugs act to increase the amount of serotonin available for transmission. On the other hand, drugs used to treat certain medical conditions can cause or exacerbate depression as a side effect because they decrease the level of serotonin at the serotonergic synapses. *(See Fig. 2–4 for an explanation of synaptic structures.)*

1. Serotonin is synthesized from tryptophan, a basic amino acid.
2. Serotonin is stored in synaptic vesicles. *Some antihypertensive drugs can cause depression because they interfere with the uptake and storage of serotonin.*
3. Vesicles migrate to the presynaptic membrane and release serotonin.
4. Stimulation of the postsynaptic receptor sites initiates an impulse in the dendrite of the next neuron. *Most antidepressants work by prolonging exposure of the postsynaptic membrane to serotonin.*

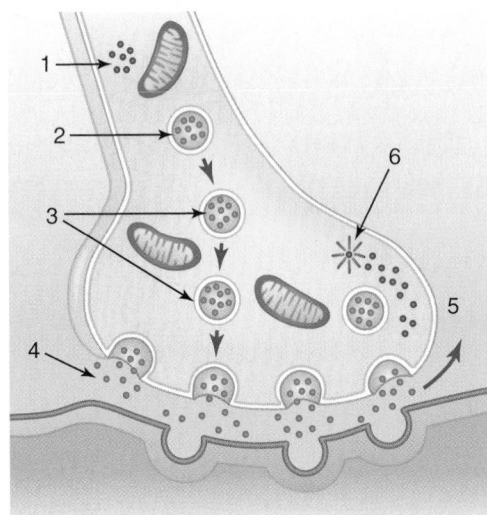

5. Serotonin action is stopped by resorption into the presynaptic terminal. *Fluoxetine (Prozac) and most tricyclic anti-depressants probably work by acutely blocking serotonin reuptake. Serotonin reuptake inhibitors (SRIs) work in a similar way.*
6. Serotonin present in a free state within the presynaptic terminal can be broken down by the enzyme monoamine oxidase (MAO). *MAO inhibitors (MAOIs), used to treat some forms of depression, prevent the breakdown of serotonin.*

Figure 9–1 *(continued)*

The clinical picture of depression supports the notion of hypothalamic dysfunction. Hypothalamic centers govern food intake, libido, and circadian rhythms. Depressed clients can exhibit anorexia or hyperphagia (overeating), hypersomnia or insomnia, decreased libido, and disturbances in rapid eye movement sleep and body temperature rhythms (Ganong, 2005). Findings that the neurohormones, which are responsive to stress, play a prominent role in the pathophysiology of depression are also consistent with clinical observations that the onset and natural history of major depression is influenced by psychological conflict, counterproductive methods of coping, and external stressors. Another neuroendocrine theory

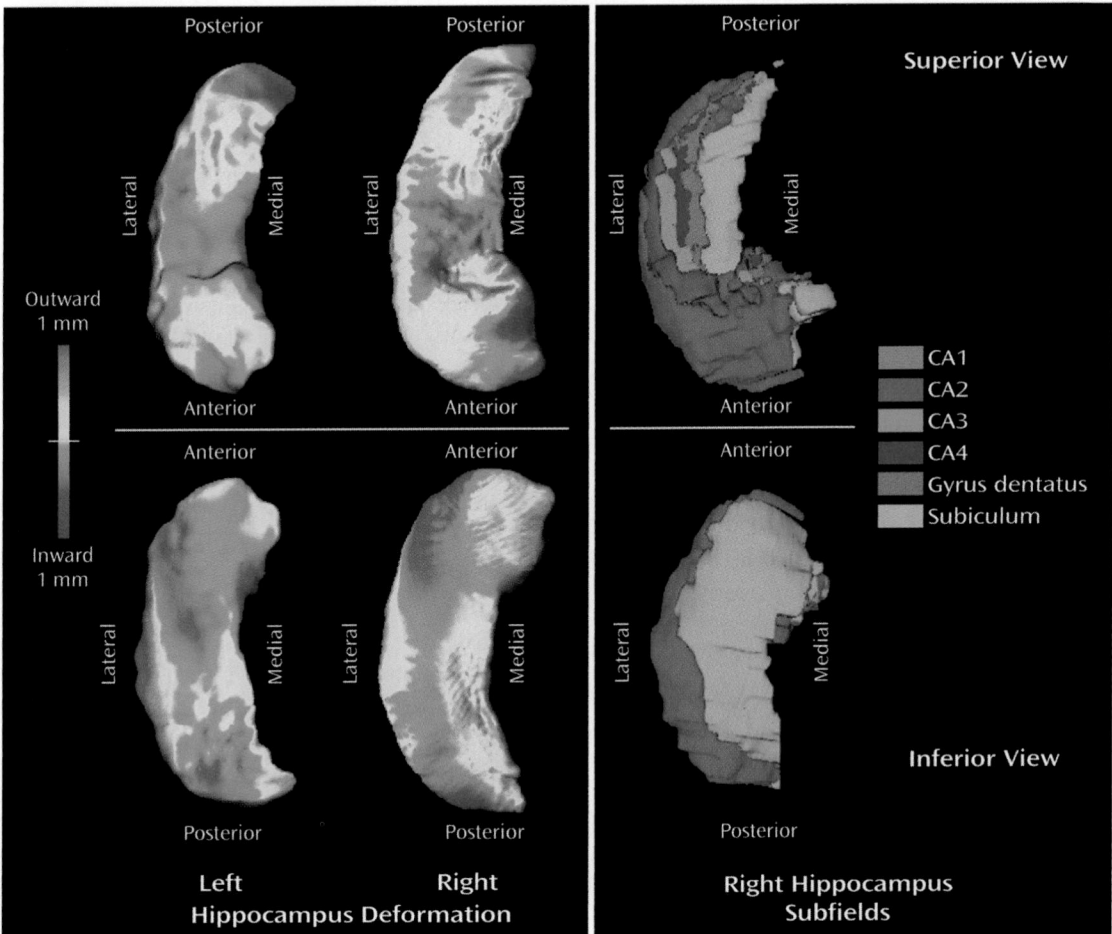

Figure 9–2 Hippocampal abnormalities in individuals with major depressive disorder compared to the hippocampus healthy subjects. (*From Posener, J. A., Wang L., Price, J. L., Gado. M. K. Province, M. A., Miller, M.I., et al., (2003). High-dimensional mapping of the hippocampus in depression. American Journal of Psychiatry, 160, 83–89. Used with permission.*)

concerning depression involves the thyroid-stimulating hormone (TSH), which is dampened on thyrotropin stimulation.

Researchers submit that abnormalities of the timing of the oscillations of the circadian pacemaker may play a role in depressive disorders. The timing of the sleep-wake cycle appears to shift later as in delayed sleep phase syndrome. The client experiencing delayed sleep phases is likely to complain of having difficulty falling asleep and difficulty awakening the next morning. Seasonal affective disorder (SAD) is associated with alterations in melatonin secretion associated with winter months and reduced light (Lewy, Emens, Jackman, & Yuhas, 2006; Terman & Terman, 2006).

Psychiatric nurses play key roles in administering, prescribing, and monitoring the effects of somatic treatments, such as antidepressant medications, sleep manipulation, and light therapy. The efficacy of these treatment modalities suggests the link between complex neurobiological processes and depression.

PSYCHOANALYTIC THEORIES

Early psychoanalytic theorists sought to understand pathological depression by comparing it with grief and mourning. Karl Abraham (1911, 1924) submitted that mourning represented the grief of a lost loved one. In addition, he linked depression to feelings of loss, guilt, and inadequacy resulting from unconscious hostility toward the lost person. Abraham also posited that depression arose from withdrawal of maternal love and support during the oral phase of psychosexual development and later experiences of loss—either real, threatened, or perceived—result in depression.

Sigmund Freud (1957) expanded on the work of Abraham in his 1917 paper, *Mourning* and *Melancholia*. Freud described

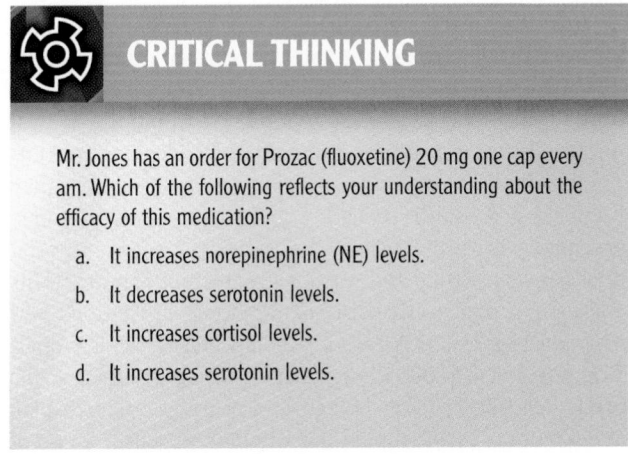

CRITICAL THINKING

Mr. Jones has an order for Prozac (fluoxetine) 20 mg one cap every am. Which of the following reflects your understanding about the efficacy of this medication?

a. It increases norepinephrine (NE) levels.

b. It decreases serotonin levels.

c. It increases cortisol levels.

d. It increases serotonin levels.

that the normal grieving process following a loss involves the working through of ambivalent feelings and anger toward the lost person through recalling and expressing past experiences and feelings related to this person. Instead, anger toward the lost person is turned inward, leading to dysphoria, guilt, and loss of self-esteem. **Dysphoria** refers to marked feelings of sadness. His theory suggests that anger toward the lost person is turned inward. Like his predecessor Abraham, Freud believed that traumatic experiences, such as loss, in early childhood increased vulnerability to depression when future losses occur. In essence, the psychoanalytic view of depression stems from disturbances in interpersonal relations in early childhood, usually involving a loss or disappointment that interfere with forming meaningful relationships across the life span.

CULTURAL FACTORS

Depression exists worldwide, and rates of depression have increased globally. An individual's culture colors the experience of depression; however, a core of symptoms is found to exist across cultures (Beals et al., 2005). There is a growing body of evidence of cross-cultural variation in the identification and meaning of diagnostic criteria for mood disorders. This is partly associated with the client's symptomatology and mental health professional's interpretation of symptoms. The debate between culture and diagnostic parameters has to do with a tendency of various cultures to present with somatic or physical symptoms that may actually represent emotional issues such as depression and anxiety.

Some cultures that are described as stoic (Midwestern farmers, Amish, Central Europeans) often avoid reporting symptoms of depression. They resist reporting emotional symptoms and rely more on family members and religion or spiritual rituals rather than seeking professional help. Other cultures, namely, Asian, often view the mind and body holistically and often report their symptoms using somatic terms. Because they see the mind and body as unitary rather than dualistic, they tend to focus on physical distress rather than on emotional symptoms, such as depression, resulting in an overdepiction of somatic complaints (Bhuri, Bhugra, et al., 2004; Conrad & Pacquiao, 2005; Harris, 2004).

Ethnic minorities are typically centered on the family and community, whereas Western European cultures have focused on and encouraged individualism and independence. This approach, or with some cultural groups, often produces negative treatment outcomes (Betancourt, 2006; Vega et al., 2007). Traditional health practices also vary among cultures, and they are used to alleviate distress before seeking conventional mental health services. Families and communities play a critical role in the client's experiences and symptoms. Acceptance of treatment increases when the client's cultural values are considered and varies with different cultures. This might be related to distrust of traditional institutions and past negative experiences with mental health professionals (Trierweiler et al., 2006). For example, Koreans, who have difficulty believing in mental illness and consider public display of emotion a sign of immaturity, might experience "a loss of face" in openly expressing their depressive symptoms (Bryant & Njenga, 2006; Jang, Kim, Hansen, & Chiriboga, 2007). Because families and communities play a significant role in accepting or rejecting mental illness and mental health services, it behooves the nurse to enlist them in the client treatment planning process (Bryant & Njenga, 2006; Kanazawa, White, & Hampson, 2007; Kim, Han, Shin, Kim, & Lee, 2005). It is important for the nurse to use interventions that integrate the family and other support groups and convey a prosocial approach that facilitates symptom management and return to an optimal level of functioning.

Other cultural considerations pertain to ethnopharmacology. This science involves the influence of culture and ethnicity on pharmacologic processes. Previous studies have demonstrated cross-cultural variance in how medications are metabolized and distributed throughout the body (Chen, 2006). A discussion of these issues is too extensive for this chapter to fully cover. See Chapters 7 and 29 for an in-depth discussion.

Finally, the nurse's own culture and ethnicity may affect the perception of the client's cultural expression of distress. It is imperative for the nurse to assess the client's cultural needs and preferences, recognize the role of families and communities in defining these symptoms, and gather data that determine an accurate diagnosis and plan of care. Considerations for the client as an individual living within a social context enables the nurse to accurately assess the level of distress and initiate appropriate treatment planning.

PSYCHOSOCIAL FACTORS

As previously discussed, psychosocial factors associated with stressful events increase the risk of depressive episodes. This is particularly evident in clients with a positive history of depression. Significant losses, such as the death of a loved one, divorce, job or financial problems, or traumatic events are examples of various psychosocial stressors. Other factors, such as genetic vulnerability, cognitive distortions, and learned helplessness also play a role in depressive disorders.

COGNITIVE-BEHAVIORAL THEORIES

In the early 1970s, a concerted effort to apply learning models to the phenomena of depression began. Behavioral models (e.g., reinforcement theory) were the first learning approaches to be applied. Later, the psychology of learning went through a cognitive revolution. The earlier behavioral theories of depression have evolved in a cognitive perspective (e.g., learned helplessness theory), and new theories were developed from a cognitive perspective (e.g., Beck's cognitive theory).

Reinforcement Theory

The extensive work of Peter M. Lewinsohn (1974) on depression and the behavioral model is well documented. He associated depression with significant losses of important sources of positive reinforcement in a person's life or a high rate of aversive experiences. In addition to depressed mood, a reduction in behavior occurs. Other symptoms such as low self-esteem and hopelessness are believed to stem from the reduced level of functioning. For example, a man experiences depressed mood following a breakup with his girlfriend (an important source of reinforcement). Much of his behavior was likely organized around his relationship with her; for example, going to the movies with her was a pleasurable activity, thus reinforcing. Reinforcement theory proposes that if as part of his depression this man no longer goes to the movies, it is because he had gone with his girlfriend in the past and that source of reinforcement is no longer present.

According to this theory there are two other ways in which insufficient reinforcement may occur. In addition to the loss of reinforcement as in the example above, the person may (a) lack the necessary skills to obtain reinforcement even though this is potentially available; for example, poor interpersonal skills could preclude the development of satisfying social relationships; or (b) lack of ability to enjoy available reinforcers secondary to interfering anxiety.

Reinforcement theory asserts that once a depressive syndrome has occurred, it is maintained through the reinforcing concern and sympathy as well as the negative responses that depressive behaviors elicit from others (Coyne, 1976).

Learned Helplessness Theory

Seligman (1975) and his colleagues coined the phrase, *learned helplessness*. It was used to describe the helpless behavior developed by dogs exposed to uncontrollable shocks in the laboratory. Many analogies to human depression were seen in the behavior of these animals, leading to the adoption of the learned helplessness paradigm as an explanation of human helplessness and depression. The inescapable shock was viewed as analogous to the traumatic loss that may precipitate depression. Other symptom parallels included passivity, weight loss, and lack of appetite (Rehm, 1990).

Subsequent revisions to the model have been important in attempting to explain key symptoms of depression, such as guilt and loss of self-esteem, that were not addressed in the original formulation. In its revised form, the theory suggests that the individual's attributions, or interpretation of negative events, determine whether the occurrence of such events will result in depression. Specifically, three types of attributions or causal explanations are hypothesized to result in depression following negative events (Beck, Rush, Shaw, & Emery, 1979):

1. That the cause of the event is perceived as internal (oneself is to blame) rather than external (cause is due to something about the situation).

2. That the cause is a factor perceived to be stable (persistent or unchangeable) rather than unstable (transitory, able to be changed).

3. That the cause is perceived to be global (affecting a wide range of areas of living) rather than specific (limited to a particular event).

The learned helplessness model of depression can be summarized as follows: Individuals develop consistent attributional styles or ways of understanding the causes of events in their lives. A particular attributional style consists of habitually attributing negative outcomes to internal, stable, global causes and ascribing positive events to external, unstable, specific causes. Mild to severe depression results when this attributional style is coupled with uncontrollable, aversive events (Rehm, 1990). The following example of a depressed woman illustrates this process:

Ms. M. is a 27-year-old woman who was admitted to the psychiatric inpatient unit for depression and suicidal ideation. Her boyfriend of 5 years had recently left her and was dating another woman. Ms. M. viewed herself as completely to blame for the breakup even in the face of evidence to the contrary (internal attribution). She described herself as pitiful and worthless and believed that this would always be so (stable attribution). Furthermore, Ms. M. saw herself as a failure not only in her relationship with her boyfriend but also in her job and at school (global attribution).

Cognitive Theory

Cognitive behavioral theories of depression stem from the early works of Aaron T. Beck (1963, 1964, 1967) and his colleagues (Beck et al., 1979). The basis of the cognitive-behavioral theory is that depression, in its various forms (major, melancholic, dysthymic, and bipolar), consists of a negative cognitive triad, specific schemas, and cognitive errors, or faulty information processing.

The *cognitive triad* is made up of (1) a negative view of self (e.g., seeing oneself as defective, inadequate, worthless, and undesirable), (2) a negative view of the world (e.g., the world is experienced as a demanding and defeating place) in which failure and punishment are to be expected, and (3) a negative view of the future (e.g., an expectation of ongoing hardship, suffering, deprivation, and failure).

Schemas are stable cognitive patterns through which a person interprets or understands his experience. In depression, schemas are analogous to viewing the world through dark glasses. The theory proposes that schemas are activated by negative life events (e.g., a loss) that are psychologically similar to the early life experiences in which the schemata developed (Beck et al., 1979).

Cognitive errors, or distortions, are automatic errors in thinking that stem from the activation of negative schemas. They are designated "automatic" because they occur rapidly and are not subjected to systematic, logical analysis. Although depressed persons are usually not aware that these thoughts are occurring, they are conscious thoughts and can be retrieved with careful questioning (Wright & Beck, 1983).

Several types of cognitive distortions have been identified in depressed persons. Selective abstraction involves coming to a conclusion based on a single detail while other more important aspects of a situation are ignored. For example, while congratulating an employee on a promotion an employer says, "don't underestimate your future with this company."

The depressive employee concludes, "she thinks I have no self-confidence." *Maximization* and *minimization* are cognitive distortions in which negatives are overemphasized and positives are underemphasized. Applying a distorted label to an event and then reacting to the label rather than the event is termed "inexact labeling." The conversation with the boss described earlier is labeled a "criticism session," and the employee expects to be fired (Rehm, 1990).

Clients who use negative automatic thoughts or distorted cognitions tend to dwell on data that confirms their conclusions or assumptions. Homework assignments are used to record or monitor situations that generate anxiety, depression, or anger, which are commonly found in depressed clients. Situations, thoughts, mood, and automatic thoughts are recorded along with challenges to demonstrate evidence that supports or does not support the "emotionally" charged thought. In addition, the client is asked to document an alternative or neutral thought and rerate the mood that was documented earlier. Nurses can use these logs to educate the client about the role his or her thoughts and feelings contribute to negative self-talk and thinking associated with depression and anxiety.

Teaching the client how to explore alternative ways of looking at a situation can be facilitated by asking the following questions:

- *Think back.* "What would you have thought before you were depressed or anxious?"
- *Consider from another's perspective.* "How would you explain the validity of your thoughts to a friend or family member?"
- *Look for alternative interpretations.* "What other ways can you look at this situation more realistically?"
- *Identify alternative solutions.* "Are there alternative solutions to the situation?"

Cognitive behavioral techniques are important nursing interventions that facilitate competency and mastery of negative self-talk and help the client grasp a realistic understanding of emotions and thoughts and their impact on mood. By replacing negative themes with realistic and positive thoughts the client is able to mitigate anxiety and depression and develop a sense of hopefulness and empowerment.

The cognitive theory of depression suggests that disturbances in thinking are the core of depression and that other

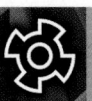

CRITICAL THINKING

Mary is a 21-year-old who is seeking evaluation and treatment for depression. She reports a recent breakup with boyfriend of 2 years and states she always ends up with losers saying, "I am a failure." Based on your understanding of how thoughts and emotions contribute to anxiety and depression what is the *most appropriate* response to this client?

1. "Sounds like you are feeling pretty down right now. Stop calling yourself a failure."
2. "Just because you broke up with your boyfriend does not mean you are a failure."
3. "What does it mean to be a failure?"
4. "How many times have you broken up with someone?"

symptoms associated with depression (e.g., sad mood, an inability to experience pleasure, decreased motivation) are reinforced by the cognitive disturbances. The cognitive model does not posit a cause-and-effect relationship between cognitive dysfunction and depression; rather, the cognitive distortions are viewed as but one component of the depressive syndrome (Beck, Rush, Shaw, & Emery, 1979).

THE ROLE OF COPING AND ADAPTATION

Coping has been defined as "constantly changing cognitive and behavioral efforts to manage specific external and/or internal demands that are appraised as taxing or exceeding the resources of the person" (Lazarus & Folkman, 1984, p. 141). The possible role of coping style in the etiology of clinical depression has only recently been the focus of empirical research. Depressed individuals have been found to show different coping styles compared with nondepressed persons.

Depressed people use more emotion-focused coping strategies (e.g., emotional release, seeking emotional support, hostile confrontation, and wishful thinking) compared with nondepressed individuals (Folkman & Lazarus, 1986). Depression has also been associated with the use of fewer adaptive coping strategies (e.g., problem solving) and the use of avoidance (APA, 2000). It remains unclear, however, whether these coping strategies contribute to the development of depression or are the result of the illness.

CRITICAL THINKING

Whether the nurse is experienced or novice, principles of cognitive behavioral therapy can be used in various situations to reduce depression and anxiety and enhance antidepressant effects of depression. As previously discussed, cognitive-distorted information processes or systems-distorted cognitions perpetuate negative self-talk through unrealistic negative perceptions and beliefs of self, the world, and the future. Negative thoughts seem to be the predominant theme of depressed clients and they occur "automatically" or spontaneously. See Table 9–2 for examples of Cognitive Distortions and Nursing Interventions.

TABLE 9–2
Cognitive Distortions and Nursing Interventions

Cognitive Distortion	Example	Intervention
Overgeneralization (if it's true in one situation it's true in all situations)	"My girlfriend cheated on me so you can't trust women."	Ask the client to list supportive evidence of this assumption. Where is the evidence that does not support this assumption? (Encourage the client to evaluate similarities and differences.)
Mental filter (focus on negative details rather than on positive or neutral ones— "the glass is half empty vs. half full")	"Everything seems to be going down hill since we broke up."	"I understand you are feeling pretty bad, but what is going well in your life?" (Look for alternative sources of responsibility.)
Emotional reasoning (emotions are equivalent to reality or what is perceived as factual and true; it "feels true so it must be true")	"I will never find anyone like Mary. I will never be able to find another girlfriend."	"What proof do you have that it will be difficult to find another girlfriend?" (It's important to separate objective facts from emotional beliefs.)
"Should" statements (*shoulds* or *musts* represent what ought to be—the individual feels guilty when things are different; often leads to unreasonably high expectations)	"I should have done what she asked and maybe we would still be together. It's my entire fault."	"I understand that you feel you should have done what she asked. However, it sounds like you felt you needed to do what she asked, but what proof do you have that this would have saved your relationship?" (Represent preferences instead of vital needs.)
All or nothing or "none thinking" (tendency to see things as black or white; good or bad; perfect or failure)	"I must be a failure since my girlfriend broke up with me."	"Breaking up is a painful experience. Help me understand how breaking up means you are a failure. What are you basing this on?" (It is important to use a continuum for evaluating each situation.)
Catastrophizing (the worse thing that can happen will occur; exaggeration of a minor mistake or problem)	"Breaking up with Mary was the worst day of my life. I will never be happy again."	"As hurt as you feel right now, it's easy to see how this may be a difficult time. However, there is no guarantee that you won't find happiness in future relationships." (Calculate the probability that the worse will happen.)

DEPRESSIVE DISORDERS ACROSS THE LIFE SPAN

Although there are certain characteristics of depression that are consistently seen across the life span, developmental stage is important in influencing how these disorders are manifested. Table 9–3 outlines characteristics that distinguish depression in various age groups.

Prognosis: About 50 percent of people experiencing a first episode of MDD experience recurrent symptoms within 10 years. Varying degrees of severity govern the client's prognosis and treatment. For example:

Mild to moderate depression—characterized by depression and moderate functional impairment. Some people recover from the short term, but 50 percent have recurrent symptoms.

CRITICAL THINKING

Mark, a 40-year-old accountant, is seen in the primary care clinic complaining of sleep disturbances, fatigue, and difficulty concentrating. During the initial nursing assessment he mentions that he is having marital problems due to extensive traveling on his job. He mentions that his parents have been married for 38 years and he wants his marriage to work out, but his wife of 20 years wants a separation. He mentions that everything is his fault and he should have spent more time with his family rather than spending so much time working. "I just don't know what I am going to do if my wife asks for a divorce." What is the best explanation for Mark's presenting symptoms?

1. He is using negative self-talk and "shoulds" and "all or none thinking" to explain his current situation.

2. He has a medical problem that contributes to sleep disturbances and fatigue.

3. He is responsible for his present marital problems.

4. He needs a complete physical examination to rule out depression.

CRITICAL THINKING

Depression in children and adolescents is likely to present as an irritable mood rather than a depressed mood. A major treatment consideration when working with these age groups is asking the right questions to gather important data. Which of the following statements is true about working with depressed children and adolescents?

1. Interview the child alone.

2. Interview the parents alone.

3. Interview the child and family together.

4. All of the above

Severe depression—characterized by agitation or psychomotor retardation with profound neurovegetative (biological) symptoms (sleep, concentration, appetite, and energy disturbances).

Psychotic depression—characterized by depression or delusions and hallucinations (APA, 2000).

CHILDHOOD

Depression is relatively uncommon in preschoolers, but estimates among children and adolescents in the community range from 2 to 6 percent, which tends to increase with age (Birmaher, et al., 2004; Luby, Belden, & Spitznagel, 2006). Chronic physical conditions; physical abuse; homelessness; poverty; parental separation, divorce, or death; and parental psychiatric illness all increase the risk of depression during childhood (Biederman et al., 2001; Kendler et al., 2006; Pilowsky et al., 2006).

Caring for children at risk for depression requires astute nursing observations, including recognition that depression in children may vary and manifest significantly different than in adults. Younger children may exhibit behavioral problems, such as aggression, apathy, sleep disturbances, and weight loss. Children may also have an irritable versus sad or depressed mood. Nurses need to elicit information from the child, parents or guardians, and teachers. Children, like other age groups, must be assessed for suicide. This includes gathering information about past attempts, family history, and present family stressors. In addition to assessing the child, the family's coping skills, level of stress, history of violence, substance abuse, past history of mental and physical disorders, and suicidal behaviors must also be assessed. These data assist in making decisions about disposition; referrals and the parents or guardians ability ensure the child's safety.

ADOLESCENCE

The prevalence of depression in adolescents has been mentioned previously and suggests that it increases with age and is more common in girls than boys (Birmaher et al., 2004). Depressed adolescents may express somatic complaints and

Myths to Overcome about Depression	
MYTH	FACT
Depression is a personal weakness.	Depression is the result of a chemical imbalance in the brain often medicated by psychosocial stressors.
Recovery from depression is a matter of will power.	Depression is a medical disorder that requires treatment.
Depression is very difficult to treat.	Depression is treated successfully in over 80 percent of sufferers who recognize the symptoms and get help.
Children do not get depression.	Depression can occur at any age.

TABLE 9–3
Characteristics of Depression across the Life Span

Childhood

Infants and Preschoolers

Insidious onset

Apathy, fatigue, withdrawal

Poor appetite, weight loss

Few spontaneously describe feeling sad

Prepubertal Children

May report sadness, suicidal thoughts

Irritability, self-criticism, weepiness

Decreased initiative and responsiveness to stimulation, apathy

Fatigue, sleep disturbance, enuresis, encopresis, weight loss, anorexia, somatic complaints

Poor school performance

Social withdrawal, increased aggressiveness

Adolescence

Feelings of sadness less frequent

Unhappy restlessness, boredom, irritability

Affects are intense and labile

Low self-esteem, hopelessness, worthlessness

Feelings of loneliness and being unloved

Pessimism about the future

Loss of interest in friends and activities, apathy

Low frustration tolerance

Thoughts of suicide

Poor school performance

Argumentativeness

Increased conflict with peers

Acting out behavior, e.g., running away, stealing, physical violence

Sexual activity (promiscuity)

Substance abuse

Complaints of headaches, abdominal pain

Hypersomnia

Isolation

Early and Middle Adulthood

Depressed mood

Anhedonia

Feelings of worthlessness, hopelessness, guilt

Reduced energy, fatigue

Sleep disturbance, especially early morning awakening and multiple nighttime awakenings

Thoughts of death

Decreased sexual interest and activity

Psychomotor retardation

Anxiety

Decreased appetite and weight loss or increased appetite and weight gain

Decreased concentration, forgetfulness, indecisiveness

Later Adulthood

Frequently do not complain of depressed mood or present with tearful affect

Feelings of helplessness

Pessimism about the future

Rumination about problems

Critical and envious of others

Loss of self-esteem

Guilt feelings

Depressions tend to last longer and are more severe

Perceived cognitive deficits

Somatic complaints

Constipation

Social withdrawal

Loss of motivation

Change of appetite

Fixed, Core Symptoms across Age Groups

Suicidal ideation, diminished concentration, sleep disturbance

Note. Data from Alexopoulos, G. S. (2005). Geriatric Psychiatry. Mood Disorders. In Sadock, B. J., & Sadock, V. A. (eds). *Kaplan & Sadock's Comprehensive Textbook of Psychiatry*, 8th ed. (pp. 3677–3687). Philadelphia: Lippincott Williams & Wilkins; Liu, X., Gentzler, A. L., Tepper, P., Kiss, E., Kothencne, V. O., Tamas, Z., Vetro, A., Kovacs, M. (2006). Clinical features of depressed children and adolescents with various forms of suicidality. *Journal of Clinical Psychiatry, 67*, 1442–1450; Stewart, C., Spicer, M., & Babl, F. E. (2006). Caring for adolescents with mental health problems: Challenges in the emergency department. *Journal of Paediatric and Child Health, 42*, 726–730.

have an irritable mood. Similar to children, they tend to exhibit behavioral problems such as poor academic and social performance, suicidal ideations, apathy, social withdrawal, rebelliousness, low self-esteem, and aggressive behaviors. They also tend to engage in risky behaviors such as promiscuity and substance abuse. Family stressors may play a role in the youths' behaviors along with a physical or mental condition. The depressed adolescent must also be assessed for suicide throughout treatment, and appropriate measures must be taken to protect the youth from harm. See Chapter 19.

Nurses need to gather relevant physical data and perform a mental status examination to rule out underlying medical and psychiatric conditions such as substance-induced mood disorder. This often requires interviewing the youth alone, then the parents or guardians and, later, the entire family. Depressed adolescents may be distrustful of adults initially, but efforts to engage the youth are crucial to the assessment process.

ADULTHOOD

Major adulthood issues concerning depression have been discussed previously. The *DSM-IV-TR* (APA, 2000) criteria for major depressive disorders include: a period of 2 weeks during which there is depressed mood or loss of interest in things that were once pleasurable (anhedonia) and the following:

◆ Alterations in appetite and weight

◆ Sleep disturbances, usually insomnia

◆ Psychomotor retardation or agitation

◆ Fatigue

◆ Concentration disturbances—forgetfulness, memory difficulties, difficulty making decisions

◆ Feelings of worthlessness, inadequacy, guilt

◆ Recurrent thoughts of death or suicidal ideations, plans or attempts

Anhedonia, or a loss of interest or pleasure, is usually present and the client feels apathetic or has little interest in hobbies or other pleasant activities. Family members often report that the client is socially isolative and shows less interest in sexual activity or desire. All in all, the level of impairment produced by MDD varies. Some clients may experience significant impairment and have difficulty performing normal daily responsibilities, whereas others may not. Atypical depressive symptoms are more common in adults and may include increased appetite, weight gain, or increased sleep and cravings for high carbohydrate foods (APA, 2000).

The depressed client may feel worthless and question the nurse's interest in knowing about present symptoms, preferences, and other assessment data. Nurses need to use empathy and patience to establish a therapeutic relationship. In addition, a thorough examination must be performed to rule out medical and mental conditions. Gathering information about mood changes during the woman's menstrual cycle and postpartum and menopause offer important information about hormonal influences.

Table 9–4, Table 9–5, and Table 9–6 list the diagnostic criteria for some depressive disorders found in adulthood.

DEPRESSION IN WOMEN

The myth that pregnancy offers *protection* against depression has been dispelled by growing evidence that suggests pregnancy does not mitigate the risk of relapse of major depression (Cohen, Altshuler, Harlow, et al., 2006). Women at risk of depression, such as those with previous histories of depression, who are considering discontinuing antidepressants during pregnancy, should be educated about the propensity for relapse during pregnancy when this occurs. Researchers submit that women are at a greater risk of developing depression, particularly during reproductive or childbearing years and the transition into menopause. Pregnancy and the birth of a child are biologically and emotionally arduous. Multiple factors contribute to depression in women and include alterations in endocrine and neurotransmitter processes, stressful events, trauma, cultural factors, childhood losses, divorce, and low self-esteem. The following section focuses on postpartum depression and transitional or perimenopausal and menopausal depression.

Postpartum Depression

Postpartum depression (PPD) is a serious illness that impedes infant-mother bonding and their overall mental and physical well-being. Epidemiological studies generally demonstrate that 10 to 15 percent of recently delivered women are affected by postpartum depression (Dindar & Erdogan, 2007; Howell, Mora, Horowitz, & Leventhal, 2005). Emerging data from epidemiological studies indicate that prevalence may be almost twice as high in South Asian mothers (Dindar & Erdogan, 2007; Howell et al., 2005). Risk factors associated with PPD include:

◆ Marital discord

◆ Poor or inadequate social support or perceived social isolation during pregnancy

◆ History of depression or psychiatric disorder(s)

◆ Personality vulnerability (e.g., ineffective coping skills)

◆ Stressful life events during pregnancy or near delivery

◆ Poverty

◆ Sociocultural factors (Howell et al., 2005; Verkerk, Denollet, Van Heck, Van Son, & Pop, 2005)

There is compelling evidence that postpartum depression adversely affects the psychological and intellectual development of the newborn and other children (Halligan, Murray, Martins, & Cooper, 2007; Swartz, Shear, Wren, & Greeno, 2005). Postpartum depression increases the risk of infanticide, marital and family discord, and impacts the neurodevelopment of the infant. Therefore, timely and appropriate interventions are important for women and their babies' mental health. Depressive mood in the postpartum period is

TABLE 9–4
Diagnostic Criteria for Major Depressive Episode

Note: A "Major Depressive Syndrome" is defined as criterion A below.

A. At least five of the following symptoms have been present during the same two-week period and represent a change from previous functioning; at least one of the symptoms is either (1) depressed mood, or (2) loss of interest or pleasure. (Do not include symptoms that are clearly due to a physical condition, mood-incongruent delusions or hallucinations, incoherence, or marked loosening of associations.)

  (1) depressed mood (or can be irritable mood in children and adolescents) most of the day, nearly every day, as indicated either by subjective account or observation by others

  (2) markedly diminished interest or pleasure in all, or almost all, activities most of the day, nearly every day, (as indicated either by subjective account or observation by others of apathy most of the time)

  (3) significant weight loss or weight gain when not dieting (e.g., more than 5% of body weight in a month), or decrease or increase in appetite nearly every day (in children, consider failure to make expected weight gains)

  (4) insomnia or hypersomnia nearly every day

  (5) psychomotor agitation or retardation nearly every day (observable by others, not merely subjective feelings of restlessness or being slowed down)

  (6) fatigue or loss of energy nearly every day

  (7) feelings of worthlessness or excessive or inappropriate guilt (which may be delusional) nearly every day (not merely self-reproach or guilt about being sick)

  (8) diminished ability to think or concentrate, or indecisiveness, nearly every day (either by subjective account or as observed by others)

  (9) recurrent thoughts of death (not just fear of dying), recurrent suicidal ideation without a specific plan, or a suicide attempt or a specific plan for committing suicide

B. (1) It cannot be established that an underlying medical condition (i.e., hypothyroidism) initiated and maintained the disturbance.

  (2) The disturbance is not a normal reaction to the death of a loved one (Uncomplicated Bereavement).

  Note: Morbid preoccupation with worthlessness, suicidal ideation, marked functional impairment or psychomotor retardation, or prolonged duration suggest bereavement complicated by Major Depression.

C. At no time during the disturbance have there been delusions or hallucinations for as long as two weeks in the absence of prominent mood symptoms (i.e., before the mood symptoms developed or after they have remitted).

D. Not superimposed on Schizophrenia, Schizophreniform Disorder, Delusional Disorder, or Psychotic Disorder NOS.

NOS, not otherwise specified.

Note. From *Diagnostic and Statistical Manual of Mental Disorders* (4th edition text Revision) *(DSM-IV-TR)*, by the American Psychiatric Association, 2000, Washington, DC: Author. Reprinted with permission.

delineated into three categories according to levels of severity: postpartum "blues" (the most common and relatively benign type); nonpsychotic postpartum depression (less common than the former) and manifests as depressed mood, lack of interest in normally enjoyed activities, and suicidal ideations (APA, 2000; Cohen, Altshuler, Harlow, et al., 2006). Self-report rating instruments, such as the Edinburgh Postnatal Depression Scale (EPDS), have been developed and administered to postpartum women to promote early detection. Nonpsychotic postpartum depression can be treated with antidepressants and cognitive behavioral therapy. (See the following Research Abstract.) The third category, postpartum psychosis, is the rarest of the three and requires immediate inpatient psychiatric treatment and management. Symptoms can emerge within 48 to 72 hours postnatal, with most women developing within the first 2 to 4 weeks postdelivery and include severe insomnia, hallucinations, suicidal and homicidal ideations, delusions about the baby may exist, irritability, agitation, manic or depressed mood, and disorganized thoughts (APA, 2000). Treatment includes antipsychotic agents, mood stabilizers with manic episodes, or ECT (Cohen, Altshuler, Harlow, et al., 2006). The infant must not be left alone with the mother during this period. Early recognition and prevention can facilitate accurate diagnosis and implementation of appropriate treatment for women at risk and experiencing postpartum depression.

TABLE 9–5
Diagnostic Criteria for Dysthymia

A. Depressed mood (or can be irritable mood in children and adolescents) for most of the day, more days than not, as indicated either by subjective account or observation by others, for at least two years (one year for children and adolescents).

B. Presence, while depressed, of at least two of the following:

   (1) poor appetite or overeating

   (2) insomnia or hypersomnia

   (3) low energy or fatigue

   (4) low self-esteem

   (5) poor concentration or difficulty making decisions

   (6) feelings of hopelessness

C. During a two-year period (one year for children and adolescents) of the disturbance, never without the symptoms in A for more than two months at a time.

D. No evidence of an unequivocal Major Depressive Episode during the first two years (one year for children and adolescents) of the disturbance.

Note: There may have been a previous Major Depressive Episode, provided there was a full remission (no significant signs or symptoms for six months) before development of the Dysthymia. In addition, after these two years (one year in children or adolescents) of Dysthymia, there may be superimposed episodes of Major Depression, in which case both diagnoses are given.

E. Has never had a Manic Episode or an unequivocal Hypomanic Episode.

F. Not superimposed on a chronic psychotic disorder, such as Schizophrenia or Delusional Disorder.

G. It cannot be established that an organic factor initiated and maintained the disturbance, e.g., prolonged administration of an antihypertensive medication.

Specify primary or secondary type:

   Primary type: the mood disturbance is not related to a preexisting, chronic, nonmood, Axis I or Axis III disorder, e.g., Anorexia Nervosa, Somatization Disorder, a Psychoactive Substance Dependence Disorder, an Anxiety Disorder, or rheumatoid arthritis.

   Secondary type: the mood disturbance is apparently related to a preexisting chronic, non-mood Axis I or Axis III disorder.

Specify early onset or late onset:

   Early onset: onset of the disturbance before age 21.

   Late onset: onset of the disturbance at age 21 or later.

Note. From *Diagnostic and Statistical Manual of Mental Disorders* (4th edition Revision) *(DSM-IV-TR)*, by the American Psychiatric Association, 2000, Washington, DC: Author. Reprinted with permission.

Perimenopausal and Menopausal Depression

Historically, transition to menopause has long been believed a time of heightened risk for depressive symptoms. It is unclear if the emergence of depressed mood is independently linked to alteration in ovarian function or secondary to vasomotor symptoms (Morgan, Cook, Rapkin, & Leuchter, 2005). Data from community-based studies exploring depressive symptoms in women in midlife indicate depression is not a natural part of menopause and that stress, relationship discord, or previous depressive episodes contribute (Bromberger, Harlow, Avis, Kravitz, & Cordal, 2004; Cohen, Soares, Vitonis, Otto, & Harlow, 2006). However, when perimenopausal women were compared to menopausal women, the researchers found higher levels of depression in the former group (Cohen, Soares, Vitonis, et al., 2006). Women with a history of depression and self-report vasomotor symptoms may be at a greater risk of depression during this transitional period than those with no previous history. Women in early transition to menopause were also found to be three times more likely to report depressive symptoms than premenopausal women (Cohen, Soares, Vitonis, et al., 2006; Freeman, Sammuel, Liu, et al., 2004). Women experiencing

TABLE 9–6
Diagnostic Criteria for Seasonal Pattern

A. There has been a regular temporal relationship between the onset of an episode of Bipolar Disorder (including Bipolar Disorder NOS) or Recurrent Major Depression (including Depressive Disorder NOS) and a particular 60-day period of the year (e.g., regular appearance of depression between the beginning of October and the end of November).

Note: Do not include cases in which there is an obvious effect of seasonally related psychosocial stressors, e.g., regularly being unemployed every winter.

B. Full remissions (or a change from depression to mania or hypomania) also occurred within a particular 60-day period of the year (e.g., depression disappears from mid-February to mid-April).

C. There have been at least three episodes of mood disturbance in three separate years that demonstrated the temporal seasonal relationship defined in A and B; at least two of the years were consecutive.

D. Seasonal episodes of mood disturbance, as described above, outnumbered any nonseasonal episodes of such disturbance that may have occurred by more than three to one.

NOS, not otherwise specified.

Note. From *Diagnostic and Statistical Manual of Mental Disorders* (4th edition text Revision) *(DSM-IV-TR)*, by the American Psychiatric Association, 2000, Washington, DC: Author. Reprinted with permission.

 RESEARCH ABSTRACT

Physical Activity in Low-Income Postpartum Women
Wilkinson, S., Huang, C.-M., Walker, L. O., Sterling, B. S., & Kim, M. (2004). *Journal of Nursing Scholarship, 36,* 109–114.

Purpose
The aim of this study was to validate the 7-day physical activity recall (PAR), using pedometer readings with low-income postpartum women and describe physical activity patterns of low-income women.

Methods
Researchers conducted a longitudinal study of postpartum women using a 7-day PAR. Data were gathered at the 3-month postpartum assessment. During the 20-minute semi-structured interview the participants were guided through the recall process to assess frequency, duration, and intensity of physical activities. Each participant received the Yamax-Digi-Walker pedometer (attached to the belt or waistband) and was instructed to wear it upon arising in the morning until going to bed at night, except during swimming or bathing for three separate days. Participants were also asked to record the step counts on forms and include the time worn. The recording forms were returned by mail.

Findings
Data analysis revealed the largest amount of active time was spent in light activity (384.4 minutes per day) and the average time spent per day was 16 minutes in moderate and high-intensity activities. Based on these data, the women in this study failed to meet recommendations to attain moderate or high-intensity physical exercise.

Implications for Psychiatric Nurses
Although the subjects failed to participate in moderate or high-intensity physical exercise, psychiatric nurses can explore strategies that ensure adequate exercise and overall healthy lifestyle changes in women during the postpartum period to ensure mental and physical health and reduce obesity.

perimenopause and menopause must be assessed for mood changes, particularly depression.

Diagnostic studies used to diagnose perimenopause and menopause include hormonal assays—estradiol, follicle stimulating hormone (FSH), and luteinizing hormone (LH). Selective serotonin reuptake inhibitors (SSRIs) and selective norepinephrine reuptake inhibitors (SNRI), antidepressants, and hormone therapy have demonstrated efficacy in the treatment of perimenopausal and menopausal minor and major depression, although the role of the latter remains unclear (Cohen, Soares, Poitras, Prouty, et al., 2003). When considering the treatment of perimenopause and menopausal depression it is imperative to consider the phase of the woman's cycle or use of oral contraceptives or estrogen replacement therapy, which may influence response to anti-depressant treatment. Research is inconclusive about the impact of age on response to antidepressants due to variability in response (Cohen et al., 2003). Performing a comprehensive biopsychosocial history that includes a history of menstrual cycles, cyclic-related mood changes, postpartum, and peri-menopause are important questions to ask. Apart from questions during hormonal stages it is equally important to determine past history of mood changes, including mania and depression. Inquiring about past history of depression or mood changes, including with menses, is critical to making accurate diagnoses and initiating appropriate treatment.

OLDER ADULTHOOD

In contrast to other age groups, depressed older adults may present with more atypical features such as low mood may be masked and anxiety and cognitive impairments may be prominent features (Cohen, Soares, Vitonis, et al., 2006). A differential diagnosis of dementia and other underlying medical and mental conditions should be considered in this age group. An estimated 10 to 15 percent of older adults have significant depressive symptoms, although MDDs are uncommon (Penninx et al., 2007). Biological, psychological, and social variables appear to increase the risk for depression in older adults. Among some clients with late-onset depression, there is evidence of neurological brain disorders associated with cerebrovascular disorders, resulting in more neurovegetative states. Behavioral manifestations of these underlying neurological conditions include memory difficulties, forgetfulness, and complaints of dysphoria (marked feelings of sadness). Older adults are also more likely to focus on somatic preoccupation, such as an ache here or there and ruminations. Somatic preoccupation involves an excessive focus on one's body function and distress. Ruminations manifest as repetitive or continuous thinking about a particular matter that eventually interferes with other thought processes. The client may ruminate about not going to an outing with the family for several days and have difficulty thinking about more important matters.

Psychosocial factors increasing the risk of depression in older adults include significant loss, loneliness, and debilitating medical conditions. Older adults often feel isolated and inadequate and are at risk for depression. Because older adults residing in nursing homes are at risk of feeling alone and isolated and vulnerable to for depression, nurses need to identify these groups and initiate interventions that increase their self-worth and value as older adults. Examples of interventions include reminiscence groups, music and pet therapy, and other activities that increase self-esteem and value to reduce the incidence of depression. Another implication from this study is the need to assess for depression in this age group and treat it accordingly.

It is imperative for the psychiatric nurse to understand age-related changes in older adults and distinguish them from dementia and depression. Often, depressive symptoms are misdiagnosed as dementia in older clients. Efforts to accurately assess these symptoms can be life-threatening if mistaken for dementia. Because depression is a treatable disorder, psychiatric nurses must initiate appropriate interventions that promote resolution. (See Table 9–7, Differentiating Characteristics of Depression and Dementia.)

It is well documented that older men experiencing late-onset depression are less likely to seek mental health services and are at a higher risk of suicide than women. Older adults often present in primary care settings complaining of somatic or physical problems rather than seeking mental health treatment (Menchetti et al., 2006). Typically, a thorough physical work reveals unexplained somatic symptoms. For these reasons all older adults complaining of physical problems and other stressors must be assessed for depression and suicide. Nurses must also assess the cultural and social context in which physical complaints occur to rule out culture bound disorders.

Suicide is a significant risk in the depressed older adult. Suicide rates are the highest among older adults (50 percent higher than the young), and the majority of these suicides occur within the context of a depressive disorder (Centers for Disease Control and Prevention [CDC], 2005; Duberstein, Conwell, Conner, Eberly, & Caine, 2004). White males and the very old (75+) are at highest risk. Feelings of hopelessness and helplessness are especially characteristic of depression and suicide in the older adult, and the period following the loss of a spouse, especially in men, is a time of high risk.

CRITICAL THINKING

Mrs. N is an 80-year-old who is seen in the adult care center and reports her husband of 56 years recently died from complications of diabetes. She spends a lot of time alone and is sometimes argumentative and mildly agitated. One of the staff asks her questions about her deceased spouse and she seems forgetful. During your assessment concerning forgetfulness, Mrs. N responds by saying, "I don't know why you are asking these questions. I don't know and don't care." Based on your understanding of memory problems in older adults, which of the following best explains her response to your query?

1. This is a typical response in depressed older adults when questioned about forgetfulness and memory disturbances.

2. This is a typical response in older adults with dementia when questioned about memory disturbances.

3. This response is common in older adults with depression and dementia.

4. This is an uncommon response to both depressed and older adults.

TABLE 9–7
Differentiating Characteristics of Depression and Dementia

Clinical Features	Depression	Dementia
Onset	Relatively rapid	Insidious
Precursors	Many have recent history of stressful event	No clear precursor
Psychiatric History	History of depression	No history of depression
Cognitive Impairment	Fluctuates (e.g., forgetfulness)	Constant
Orientation	Oriented in all spheres	Orientation impaired
Memory	Equal or no impairment of recent and remote memory	Greater impairment in recent compared with remote memory
Learning Capacity	Usually intact	Impaired
Mental Status Results	"Don't know" answers typical Emphasizes impairments	Frequent errors Minimizes or conceals impairments
Sense of Distress (Feels Depressed)	Yes	No
Affect	Irritable, constricted	Shallow and labile
Behavior	Little effort expended to perform even simple tasks	Often struggles to perform tasks
Response to Treatment	Improvement with antidepressants or ECT	Lack of response

ECT, electroconvulsive therapy.

Note. From *Diagnostic and Statistical Manual of Mental Disorders* (4th edition text Revision) *(DSM-IV-TR)*, by the American Psychiatric Association, 2000, Washington, DC: Author. Adapted with permission; from *Practice Guidelines for the Treatment of Patients With Major Depressive Disorder* (Rev. ed.), by American Psychiatric Association Work Group, 2000, Washington, DC: Author; and from Beekman, Geerling, Deeg, Smit et al., 2002.

LOSS AND GRIEF ISSUES

Loss and grief issues often place tremendous burdens on clients and their families. Normal responses to loss include bereavement and mourning. Psychiatric nurses are often challenged to distinguish between normal and maladaptive grief responses across the life span.

BEREAVEMENT

Every year an estimated eight million Americans experience the death of an immediate family member. Numerous others grieve the loss of significant people in their lives (Wakefield, Schmitz, First, & Horwitz, 2007). Bereavement is an extreme stressor with physiological, psychological, and social consequences. As with other stressors, the consequences of bereavement are variable and will be influenced by the constitutional makeup and personality of the bereaved, nature of the relationship with the deceased, and the circumstances of the death.

Certain facts about bereavement are clear. Grief is associated with measurable distress in virtually everyone. Second, although the intensity of the distress and its effect on functioning will vary, it is long lasting—anywhere from 1 to 3 years. Furthermore, although patterns of bereavement have been identified, reactions to the death of another are highly individualistic and do not fit neatly into well-defined stages. Finally, some bereaved individuals are at increased risk for illness as well as death (Jones, Marcantonio, & Rabinowitz, 2002; Stroebe, Stroebe, & Abakoumkin, 2005).

Research related to the potential complications of bereavement has revealed the following:

◆ Young and middle-aged widowed men are about one and one-half times more likely to die than their married counterparts. This risk is greatest during the first year, unless the men remarry, and continues for many years (Stimpson, Kuo, Ray, Raji, & Peek, 2007).

- Higher mortality rates in men are related to death by suicide, accidents, cardiovascular disease, and some infectious diseases (Boelen & van den Bout, 2005).

- Women have an increased mortality rate in the second year following the death of a spouse (Jaffe, Eisenbach, Neumark, & Manor, 2006).

- Clinically diagnosable depressions have been found in 10 to 20 percent of widows and widowers a year or more after their loss (Stroebe, Stroebe, & Abakoumkin, 2005). The rates of depression following other types of bereavement—death of a child, sibling, or parent—is unknown.

- The risk for suicide is relatively high for older widowed men and for single men who have lost their mothers (Stroebe, Stroebe, & Abakoumkin, 2005).

- Bereaved children are at greater risk for depression and suicide in adult life although this is not as widespread or inevitable as previously thought (Cerel, Fristad, Verducci, Weller, & Weller, 2006).

- A perceived lack of social support is one of the most significant predictors of poor outcome among the bereaved (Phillips et al., 2006). The presence of a consistent, dependable caretaker appears to be especially important in determining outcome in children who have lost a parent or sibling (Kirwin & Hamrin, 2005).

Culture plays a critical role in how individuals grieve and cope with terminal illness and death. Studies indicate diverse cultural responses to death and dying issues and the importance of recognizing coping patterns, health practices, preferences, and beliefs associated with bereavement and grief (Lalande & Bonnano, 2006). Distinguishing culturally based beliefs about death, such as communicating with the dead and symbolic images of dead loved ones, and pathological grief and bereavement is essential to quality care (Hsu, Khan, Yee, & Lee, 2004).

MOURNING

Disequilibrium occurs following a loss, and certain tasks need to be accomplished in order to work through the loss and regain equilibrium. These four tasks of mourning are outlined as follows:

1. To accept the reality of the loss. This first task involves accepting the fact on both an intellectual and emotional level that the person is dead and will not return. Rituals, such as the funeral, are often helpful in this process. Although disbelief and denial are common early on and then intermittently while working through the loss, ongoing denial indicates maladaptation.

2. To work through to the pain of grief. Physical and emotional pain is experienced with loss and it is important for the grieving person to allow himself to feel this. Cutting off or denying feelings can be done through avoiding painful thoughts or any reminders of the deceased as well as through the use of alcohol or drugs. Avoiding painful feelings at the time of loss increases the risk of emotional problems such as a depressive disorder at some point in the future.

3. To adjust to an environment in which the deceased is missing. The various roles filled by the deceased (e.g., household manager, child caretaker, finance handler) will influence the extent to which the bereaved needs to develop new skills and take on new roles. One's sense of the world may also require adjustment because loss through death often challenges one's fundamental life values and philosophical beliefs.

4. To emotionally relocate the deceased and move on with life. This last task can be the most difficult to accomplish because it involves letting go of one's attachment to the deceased and forming new ones. This does not mean giving up thoughts and memories of the lost loved one but rather relocating these in one's emotional life in a way that allows for going on with life (Worden, 2003).

UNCOMPLICATED GRIEF

A wide range of feelings and behaviors are commonly experienced after a loss. Table 9–8 outlines how these are manifested during different periods of a person's life.

Although children have many of the same feelings of grief experienced by adults, their reactions are at the same time unique. This is because of their immaturity and lack of well-developed coping skills. Rather than directly expressing feelings of sadness, anger, and fear, they may be manifested in misbehavior or temper tantrums that can last for many years after the loss. Because a child's capacity to experience intense emotions is more limited compared to the adult, emotional and behavioral manifestations of grief are intermittent rather than continuous (Kirwin & Hamrin, 2005).

Manifestations in each stage are not exclusive and may occur during any developmental stage. Young children are more likely to express their grief through feelings and behaviors such as those listed in Table 9–9, depending on their developmental stage and ability to verbally express their grief. Adolescents may express their grief physically, although many will verbally express feelings and exhibit similar behaviors to children and adults. Because of age-related sensory changes arising in older adulthood, they may exhibit behaviors that reflect these changes.

"What did I do to cause this to happen?" "Will this happen to me too?" and "Who will take care of me now?" are three common concerns of children who have lost a parent. Children should be repeatedly reassured as to the answers to these questions even if they remain unasked. A more favorable outcome can be expected for the child who is able to talk freely about the dead parent in either positive or negative terms (Kirwin & Hamrin, 2005).

Factors that may increase a child's risk of psychological or behavioral problems following the death of a parent or sibling include a troubled relationship with the deceased before the

TABLE 9–8
Manifestations of Uncomplicated Grief across the Life Span

Children	Adolescents	Adults	Older Adults
Feelings	**Physical Sensations**	**Behaviors**	**Cognitions**
Sadness	Hollowness in stomach	Sleep disturbance	Disbelief
Fearfulness	Chest & throat tightness	Appetite disturbance	Confusion
Angry outbursts	Oversensitivity to noise	Absent-mindedness	Preoccupation
Eating disturbance	Depersonalization	Social withdrawal	Sense of presence
Bowel & bladder disturbance	Breathlessness	Dreams of deceased	Hallucinations
Speech disturbances	Muscle weakness	Searching and calling out	
Withdrawn or excessively caregiving	Lack of energy	Sighing	
Deterioration of school behavior & academic achievement	Dry mouth	Restlessness	
	Sexual promiscuity	Crying	
Guilt	Similar to adult except for following:		
Tendency to grieve silently	Physical sensations more pronounced & may take on pattern similar to one present in deceased		
Denial			
Alcohol & drug use	Marked irritability		
Worry about future, preservation of family and new responsibilities	Negativistic thinking		

Note. Data from *Clinical Management of Bereavement: A Handbook for Healthcare Professionals,* by G. M. Burnell and A. L. Burnell, 1989, New York: Human Sciences Press, 1989; "Bereavement Reactions, Consequences, and Care," in *Biopsychosocial Aspects of Bereavement,* by S. Zisook (Ed.), 1987, Washington, DC: American Psychiatric Press; and from *Grief Counseling and Grief Therapy: A Handbook for the Mental Health Practitioner* (3rd ed.), by J. W. Worden, 2003, New York: Springer.

death; unstable, inconsistent caregiving; and a troubled surviving parent who depends excessively on the bereaved child and a family member's homicide. A study conducted by Clements and Burgess (2002) of 13 children, ages 9 to 11 years of age, 1 to 3 months after a family homicide, found that the witnessing of a murder or hearing the news of a family member's murder has a powerful association for childhood trauma related disorders and complicated grief. Despite developmental issues that may interfere with processing grief, children of all ages must be given an opportunity to grieve (Antai-Otong, 2007; Stuber & Mesrkhani, 2001).

A literature review conducted by Stuber & Mesrkhani (2001) delineate salient points that are helpful in promoting health in grieving children:

◆ Children have the same tasks as other age groups in the grieving process, but their developmental stage,

relationship to the deceased, and circumstances of the death govern their responses.

◆ Bereaved children may experience abandonment issues and that other loved ones will also die.

◆ They may experience guilt for actual or real misbehavior; have academic and social impairments.

◆ Very young children understand that something very terrible has occurred after the loss of a parent or guardian, even when they are not directly told (caregivers should avoid withholding information because it is not protective and reduces support for the grieving child).

◆ Ideally, children should be allowed to participate in the decision to attend the funeral of their loved one (if allowed to attend, adults need to provide emotional support as needed).

TABLE 9–9
Risk Factors for Pathological Grief Reactions

Circumstances Surrounding the Loss

Uncertainty over the loss, e.g., a soldier missing in action during war

Multiple losses, e.g., resulting from fires, airplane crashes

Relationship to the Deceased

Ambivalent relationship with unexpressed hostility

Highly dependent relationship

History of deceased having been sexually abusive to mourner

Social Variables

Absence of social support network

Death not socially accepted as a loss, e.g., abortion

Socially unacceptable death, e.g., suicide

Personal Variables

Personal history of depressive illness

Self-concept includes assuming the role of the "strong one's" personality such that unable to tolerate severe emotional distress

Note. Data from *Grief Counseling and Grief Therapy: A Handbook for the Mental Health Practitioner* (3rd ed.), by J. W. Worden, 2003, New York: Springer.

◆ Children need to be encouraged to return to "normal" daily activities after the loss (provides consistency and a sense of security) (Stuber & Mesrkhani, 2001).

Psychiatric nurses can facilitate the grief process in children by educating caregivers and assessing the child's developmental needs. Ultimately, the responsibility of sharing information about death and dying issues lies with family members and other caregivers. Nurses can help families respond to the child's needs, considering their developmental stage, relationship to the deceased, and events surrounding the death (Stuber & Mesrkhani, 2001).

Helpful strategies that help children cope with grief:

1. Read stories to children that enable them to project or talk about their feelings onto story characters (e.g., Dora).

2. Encourage the child to visualize their hurt, fear, and pain; use crayons, finger paints, or clay to express feelings.

3. Invite the child to make a loss timeline, filling it in with people and dates according to when they died.

4. Help the child create a family tree using various symbols to represent people still living and those who have passed away in their life.

5. When the child mentions the deceased sibling or parent, listen for themes and recognize their pain and sadness are real.

6. Model thoughts and behavior for children.

7. Allow the child to attend a funeral to observe how the deceased are respected and how loved ones comfort each other.

Adolescents tend to show less outward manifestation of their grief compared to other age groups. This may stem from a fear of appearing different or abnormal during an already turbulent developmental period (Antai-Otong, 2007; Cohen, Mannarino, & Staron, 2006; Davies et al., 2007).

Manifestations of grief have been most extensively described for the adult and all are normal following the loss of a loved one. Sadness is the most common feeling. A sense of relief is typical following a lengthy or painful illness. Anxiety, ranging from a sense of insecurity to panic, stems from a heightened sense of the survivor's own mortality and a fear of being unable to manage without the deceased. A preoccupation with the deceased is common and often includes obsessive thoughts about how to recover the lost person. The grieving adult frequently senses that the deceased is still present and will describe seeing or hearing the voice of his loved one (Worden, 2003).

The relationship of the bereaved to the deceased influences how grief is manifested as well as subsequent adjustment. The loss of a spouse through death is typically associated with later adulthood, so it is particularly stressful at a younger age when it requires major lifestyle adjustments. The loss of a child is likely the most traumatic experience a parent can undergo. Feelings of guilt, self-blame, and anger are more prominent and intense than in other types of losses. The course of grief is lengthy, lasting from 2 to 5 years. Marital stress is common, with estimates of subsequent divorce at 50 to 70 percent. The ability of parents to meet the needs of surviving siblings may also be impaired. Because it is generally accepted that as people age they will die, the loss of a parent during adulthood is comparatively less traumatic (Kirwin & Hamrin, 2005).

Manifestations of grief normally diminish in frequency and intensity over time. It is not uncommon or abnormal, however, for the characteristic feelings and behaviors associated with mourning to recur at various points throughout a person's life. Anniversary dates of the death, birthdays of the deceased, holidays or other occasions that remind the survivor of the deceased are typical periods when this occurs.

DISTINGUISHING BETWEEN GRIEF AND DEPRESSION

Grief is often indistinguishable from depression and so when assessing a person with symptoms of depression it is always important to question the presence of recent losses. Certain characteristics of the two states do differ, however. The bereaved regard their feelings of depression as normal rather than abnormal. There is usually not a loss of self-esteem in the depressed grieving individual, and feelings of guilt are typically associated with some specific aspect of the loss rather than being more pervasive. Freud described that the world looks poor and empty to the bereaved, whereas the depressed person feels poor and empty (Worden, 2003).

COMPLICATED BEREAVEMENT

Complicated bereavement and unresolved grief may be manifested in several ways. Worden (2003) categorizes these under four headings: (1) chronic grief reactions, (2) delayed grief reactions, (3) exaggerated grief reactions, and (4) masked grief reactions.

Chronic grief is excessive in duration and never comes to a satisfactory conclusion. The person with this reaction is generally aware of the problem and may describe his distress as "I'm not getting back to living," or "This thing is not ending for me."

In delayed grief the person did not sufficiently experience his emotional reactions at the time of the loss. Subsequently, when another loss occurs, he may experience intense symptoms of grief that seem excessive.

Exaggerated grief responses refer to situations where there is an intensification of a normal grief reaction that becomes disabling. Although a depressive syndrome is a normal reaction to the loss of a loved one, when this is associated with suicidal ideation, severe functional impairment, and morbid preoccupation with a sense of worthlessness, bereavement may be complicated by an MDD (APA, 2000). Severe alcoholism or other substance abuse that develops or is exacerbated by a death is another example of exaggerated grief (Worden, 2003).

The person with a masked grief reaction does not recognize that his symptoms are related to a loss. Grief may be masked as a physical symptom or through some type of maladaptive behavior. Physical symptoms that develop may be similar to those of the deceased.

Factors that may predispose an individual to a pathological grief reaction include circumstances surrounding the loss, relationship to the deceased, and social and personal variables. Table 9–9 provides an outline of these risk factors.

TREATMENT MODALITIES

Technological advances in neurobiology have increased the understanding of brain chemistry, genetics, neuroanatomy, and neuroendocrinology and their link to behavior. Furthermore, they have spawned a plethora of research that confirms the efficacy of somatic and psychotherapeutic interventions in the treatment of depression.

SOMATIC TREATMENTS

Somatic therapies are intertwined in the history of mental disorders. Contemporary approaches using somatic therapies to manage depression usually include pharmacotherapy, electroconvulsive therapy VNS, and light therapy.

Medication treatment options for depression are antidepressants, mood stabilizers, neurostimulants. and antipsychotics.

Antidepressants are thought to increase levels of norepinephrine, serotonin, or dopamine at the synapse to restore equilibrium to neurotransmitter activity. Antidepressant agents' primary mechanisms of action are as a serotonin and norepinephrine reuptake inhibitor, a monoamine oxidase inhibitor, a norepinephrine/dopamine reuptake inhibitor, a selective serotonin reuptake inhibitor, a selective serotonin antagonist, and a presynaptic alpha-2 adrenergic/serotonin antagonist.

The most used antidepressants are selective serotonin reuptake inhibitors (SSRIs) such as citalopram (Celexa), escitalopram (Lexapro), paroxetine (Paxil CR), fluoxetine (Prozac) and sertraline (Zoloft); and selective norepinephrine reuptake inhibitors (SNRIs) or dual-action antidepressants venlafaxine (Effexor) XR, duloxetine (Cymbalta). Novel antidepressants, such as mitrazipine (Remeron) and bupropion (Wellbutrin) SR/XL have also proven efficacy in the treatment of depression. Abrupt discontinuation of an SSRI may result in discontinuation syndrome characterized by vivid dreams, nightmares, tremor, dizziness, crying spells, nausea, disorientation, and poor concentration. To minimize this syndrome, avoid abrupt withdrawal and gradually taper the dose over 7 to 10 days. This is more likely to occur with SSRIs with a short half-life such as paroxetine, and is less likely to occur with drugs with a long half-life. However, this may not be necessary with fluoxetine because of its extended half-life. Older adults and children generally require smaller doses but show a similar time course of response to antidepressants with SSRIs. Low doses of trazodone (Desyrel) are used to help the depressed person with sleep problems and reduce sleeplessness associated with SSRIs and SNRIs.

Pharmacologic Treatment

According to the American Psychiatric Association (2000) practice guidelines for the treatment of MDD, treatment involves the following phases:

1. **Acute Phase:** Treatment options are considered, including psychopharmacology, psychotherapy, a combination of medications, and psychotherapy or electroconvulsive therapy (ECT). Potential benefits and side effects are discussed with the client and family along with treatment options and preferences. First-line antidepressants include SSRIs, Duloxetine (Cymbalta), bupropion (Wellbutrin), or venlafaxine (Effexor) (see Table 9–10). During this phase the client's response to treatment is monitored along with assessment of side effects and suicide risk throughout treatment phases. See Chapter 29.

2. **Continuation Phase:** During 16 to 20 weeks following remission of symptoms.

3. **Maintenance Phase:** Because of the high risk of relapse or recurrent symptoms, this phase is suggested to prevent recurrence.

TABLE 9–10
Health Education—Information on Venlafaxine (EFFEXOR)

1. Venlafaxine is a serotonin reuptake inhibitor and norepinephrine reuptake inhibitor (considered a dual action antidepressant).

2. Take the medication as prescribed. If you miss a dose, take it as soon as you remember. However, if it is almost time for your next dose, skip the missed dose and continue your usual dosing schedule.

3. This medication comes in two forms: an immediate release pill, venlafaxine; and a long-acting capsule, venlafaxine XR.

4. Venlafaxine should not be stopped suddenly. Your dose needs to be reduced gradually before it is discontinued.

5. Avoid taking other antidepressants or other medications, including over-the-counter or herbal (e.g., St. John's Wort), without discussing it with your health care provider.

6. Avoid taking alcohol or other central nervous system depressants while on this medication.

7. Avoid performing activities that require mental and physical alertness, such as driving or operating heavy machinery.

8. Major side effects of this medication include sweating, loss of appetite, dry mouth, anxiety, tremor, blurred vision, constipation, change in sexual ability, and hypertension. Contact your health care provider if these side effects continue or are severe.

9. If one or any of the following occur, report them immediately to your provider:

Rapid, pounding or irregular heartbeat	Chest pain
Severe headache	Trouble breathing
Painful or difficult urination	Seizures
Depression	Skin rash (see Chapter 29)

Home Care for the Depressed Client

Home care is becoming increasingly important. Clients are being discharged earlier with many depressive symptoms present. Therefore, community resources for treating depression are critically important.

The major goals of community treatment are to support the recovery process, to maintain a sense of hopefulness, and to maintain confidence in the abilities of the individual. Additionally, the nurse needs to recognize the stressors the family experiences living with the depressed individual. How the family copes with these stressors is a crucial factor in the client's recovery process. The client and family both require education about the illness and medication (Antai-Otong, 2007). The family members view education as an important intervention.

Besides being knowledgeable about psychopathology and psychopharmacology, the psychiatric home health nurse must pos-

sess psychosocial behavioral assessment skills and the ability to work autonomously. She must also be able to foster trust in his client and work collaboratively with other health givers.

The nurse's tasks are varied—from identifying a need for hospitalization to coordinating laboratory follow-up of blood levels necessary for medication treatment to working with clinicians to change medications based on the response of the depressed client. Additionally, a holistic approach to the client's treatment helps the nurse develop an individualized care plan for him, (e.g., cultural, spiritual, and social needs). Because of the high co-occurrence of medical conditions in the client with a mental clinicians disorder, the nurse needs to have skills that enable him to assess the client's physical, and mental status (Marek, Popejoy, Petroski, & Rantz, 2006).

---

4. **Discontinuation Phase:** Discontinuation of active treatment—the precise timing of discontinuation of treatment both somatic and psychotherapeutic, varies and often parallels the client's response and preferences. Discontinuation of pharmacologic agents requires tapering the medication over several weeks to reduce recurrence and medication discontinuation syndrome. Health education during this period also focuses on early symptoms of recurrent depressions and the importance of reporting them to their health care provider. See Chapter 29.

Electroconvulsive Therapy

Electroconvulsive therapy (ECT) is the electrical induction of modified grand mal seizures for the purpose of inducing therapeutic change. It is an accepted, safe, and efficacious form of treatment for major depression although the exact mechanism of action remains unclear. Generally, ECT is used only after a trial of antidepressant medication has failed to work, although in certain situations, it might be chosen as an initial treatment; for example, a history of poor antidepressant drug response or good ECT response, or a high risk of suicidal behavior (Dannon, Lowengrub, Gonopolski, & Kotler, 2005). The nursing care of the client undergoing ECT and additional somatic therapies, including sleep manipulation and light therapy, is discussed in Chapter 30.

Of particular importance when working with the depressed client is the risk of suicide. It is imperative for the nurse to assess the client's level of danger to self and others throughout treatment and educate family members about reporting ideations, threats, gestures, and attempts regardless of how trivial they are.

Major responsibilities of the nurse concerning somatic interventions include administration, prescribing, and monitoring drug levels and adverse side effects. Documenting the client's response is crucial along with health education about various treatment options and potential risk factors.

Repetitive Transcranial Magnetic Stimulation (rTMS)

Despite recent advances in the pharmacotherapy of depression, major challenges remain unresolved. Major challenges include the treatment-resistant or nonresponse rate of about 30 percent to conventional antidepressant pharmacotherapy, negative side-effect profile, and the lag time of several weeks until clinical improvement (Fava, 2003). Nonpharmacological interventions such as ECT appear to produce rapid antidepressant effects. Advances in technology show promise in other somatic therapies, such as repetitive transcranial magnetic stimulation (rTMS) and vagal nerve stimulation. Modest to substantial antidepressant effects have been demonstrated in the majority of clinical trials (Fitzgerald et al., 2006; Padberg et al., 2002). In TMS, treatment generally involves a special electromagnet that delivers a brief burst of energy to stimulate nerve cells in the brain. Although the precise mode of efficacy continues to be studied, most researchers submit that its antidepressant effects result from altering brain chemistry. Major advantages include its positive side-effect profile; it can be performed in outpatient settings, and is noninvasive. Duration of treatment is normally 5 times a week for 2 to 4 weeks. Common complaints among clients include muscle contractions on the scalp, mild headaches or lightheadedness, mild nausea, all of which abate postprocedure. The most significant risk is that the device could precipitate a seizure (rare). Unlike ECT, no memory loss or cognitive changes have been reported.

Vagus Nerve Stimulation (VNS)

The vagus nerve is an important source of afferent information about physical states and its effects stem from activation of neurons in the nucleus locus coeruleus (LC) resulting in the release of norepinephrine (NE) throughout the brain, notably in the cortex and hippocampus. Stimulation of the vagus nerve has demonstrated improved mood, learning, and memory storage processes in animal studies and human subjects (Roosevelt, Smith, Clough, Jensen, & Browning, 2006). Based on these findings, vagal nerve stimulation (VNS) exerts at least some of its antidepressant effects through its capacity to increase noradrenergic and serotonergic transmission and efficacy in treatment-resistant depression (Roosevelt et al., 2006). VNS has been approved by the Food and Drug Administration (FDA) for individuals 18 years or older with chronic or recurrent treatment-resistant depression. This treatment has demonstrated efficacy equivalent to unipolar depression and bipolar disorder. Recent data suggest that clients with chronic or treatment-resistant depression may experience long-term benefits from VNS (Nahas et al., 2005).

The normal procedure for VNS requires two small incisions in the upper arm area (pulse generator site) and left neck for insertion of thin flexible wires connected to the pulse generator to the vagal nerve near the carotid artery. The procedure takes about one hour and is performed under general anesthesia. The physician can control the intensity and rate of generator firing by holding a device over the chest wall/generator. Side effects from VNS include transitory hoarseness or alterations in voice tone, vomiting, coughing during stimulation, tickling in throat, infection, and dyspnea during exertion. Healing at insertion sites occurs in 1 to 2 weeks. Similar to rTMS, no cognitive, sedative, or coordination side effects have been reported.

Nonpharmacological therapies offer additional treatment options to clients with treatment-resistant depression (failure to two antidepressants in the current episode). Health education is critical to the success of all treatment and psychiatric nurses must be prepared to discuss these options with a general focus on reasons for treatment, estimated response time, side effects, and signs and symptoms to report.

TREATMENT RESISTANT DEPRESSION: THE NIMH STAR*D PROJECT

A discussion of the client with depression would be incomplete without a brief mention of treatment resistant depression and research trends. Only 25 to 45 percent of clients with major depression attain remission after an acute trial of an antidepressant (Trivedi, Fava, Wisniewski, Thase, Quitkin, et al., 2006). As a result of growing concerns for the low remittance of depression after an adequate trial of antidepressants, the National Institute of Mental Health (NIMH) funded a 6-year, $35 million project, titled Sequenced Treatment Alternatives to Relieve Depression (STAR*D), to determine "next steps" for persons with major depression who failed to respond from initial and sequential treatments. The principal goal of this study was remission. The STAR*D project used a different approach to study persons with treatment-resistant depression and it is hailed as the largest ecologically valid "real world" trial of outpatients with nonpsychotic major depression. This multistep, 41-site study began with 2,876 subjects. Those whose symptoms failed to remit after Levels 1 and 2 went on to treatment Levels 3 and 4. The project was conducted in a "real world" setting, mainly in primary and specialty care settings to assess efficacy of treatments in generalizable samples and implement adequate treatment. Data from this study extended beyond evaluating safety and efficacy; it also measured practical outcomes, such as subsequent phases of the study and the level of functioning to include a year later. A more in-depth discussion of the STAR*D NIMH project including definitions of Levels 1 to 4 can be found at the websites listed under Internet Resources at the end of this chapter.

PSYCHOTHERAPEUTIC INTERVENTIONS

Several forms of psychotherapy are available for the treatment of depression that may or may not be used in conjunction with somatic interventions. The advanced-practice psychiatric mental health nurse is educationally (e.g., master's degree or PhD) and clinically prepared to provide various psychotherapies.

Psychotherapy

The primary goal of psychoanalytic psychotherapy is to effect change in personality structure rather than to simply alleviate symptoms. Therapy is aimed at improving a person's capacity for interpersonal trust and intimacy, strengthening coping mechanisms, developing the ability to experience a wide range of emotions, and enhancing the capacity to grieve. Therapy often continues for many years, although in recent decades several short-term psychoanalytic approaches have been developed.

Individuals most suitable for this form of treatment include those who are highly motivated to change; have the capacity for introspection and the ability to see a connection between thoughts, feelings, and behavior; as well as the capacity to tolerate anxiety and frustration. A psychodynamic treatment approach is most commonly used in depressions that are chronic and of mild severity. Because of cost constraints associated with managed care, brief and focused psychotherapies are most likely to be used.

Interpersonal Therapy

Interpersonal therapy was developed by Gerald Klerman and Myrna Weissman and colleagues (1984), and based on the theoretical work of Adolf Meyer (1948–1952) and Harry Stack Sullivan (1953). The primary goals of interpersonal therapy are the alleviation of depressive symptoms, improvement of self-esteem, and the development of more effective skills for dealing with social and interpersonal relationships. The therapeutic focus is on current situations in the person's life, and the course

of treatment is relatively short (e.g., 12 to 16 weekly sessions). This approach was specifically developed to treat MDDs.

In interpersonal therapy the client is educated about depression, with emphasis placed on the fact of its good prognosis. One or two major problem areas are then defined and become the focus of treatment. Problem areas commonly addressed include abnormal grief reactions, interpersonal role disputes (e.g., marital conflict), role transitions (e.g., divorce), and interpersonal deficits (e.g., lack of social skills). Medications are often used as an adjunct in reducing depressive symptoms

Behavioral Therapy

The behavioral theories of depression guide the treatment approach in behavioral therapy. Which behavioral theory of depression is followed guides the treatment approach used. Regardless of the interventions used, the primary goals of therapy are to increase the number of positively reinforcing interactions with the environment and to decrease the number of negative interactions in the depressed person's life. Treatment is usually short term (4 to 12 weeks) and highly structured.

Strategies used in behavioral therapy include having the client keep a daily record of his moods and activities. Based on these records the therapist encourages increased involvement in activities associated with positive moods and avoidance of situations that trigger feelings of depression. In addition, the client is taught how to better manage reactions to negative events, that is, through preparation for such events as well as substituting positive for negative thoughts in relation to them. Time management is used to increase participation in enjoyable events. Assertiveness training and role playing may be used to address social skills deficits and problematic interaction patterns. Relaxation training is used to produce a mood state incompatible with depression. Detailed manuals that outline specific behavioral treatment approaches for unipolar, nonpsychotic depression have been developed (Sadovy, 2000).

Cognitive-Behavioral Therapy

As previously discussed, cognitive-behavioral therapy (CBT) was developed by Beck and his colleagues (1979). Typically, CBT lasts from 12 to 20 sessions and its primary goals are to alleviate depression and decrease the likelihood of its recurrence by helping the individual change his way of thinking.

The following are the three overall components to cognitive-behavioral therapy:

◆ Didactic teaching, in which the cognitive-behavior view of depression is explained

◆ Cognitive techniques, involving the eliciting and testing of negative automatic thoughts and identifying and analyzing the maladaptive assumptions on which they are based

◆ Behavioral techniques, such as scheduling pleasurable activities, role playing, and graded task assignments

The major principle behind these techniques is that identifying and changing maladaptive cognitions and relevant behaviors will reverse the symptoms of depression (Beck, 1963, 1967; Beck et al., 1979). See Chapters 26 and 27.

Family Therapy

Although family therapy is not viewed as a primary treatment for depression, it is indicated for situations in which a client's depression appears to be maintained by marital and family interactions or when the depression is negatively influencing the individual's family functioning. Episodes of depression have been associated with family dysfunction. Furthermore, children with a depressed parent are at increased risk of psychiatric disorder. Although the advanced-practice psychiatric mental health nurse is best prepared to provide family therapy, the psychiatric staff nurse can fulfill the important role of educating family members about mood disorders and their treatment. Such education can serve to improve the clients' adherence to treatment as well as the family's ability to provide a supportive environment. See Chapter 27.

THE ROLE OF THE NURSE

Because of the complexity of major depressive episodes and grief reactions, psychiatric nurses must understand integral processes and treatment modalities that facilitate mental health. Individualized treatment planning often includes pharmacological interventions to manage neurobiological processes and nonpharmacological interventions, such as cognitive behavioral therapy to challenge thoughts that contribute to depression. Holistic health care enables the client to understand depression, reduce symptoms, and reach an optimal level of functioning. Various roles of the nurse facilitate recovery and reduce relapse in clients experiencing depression and various mood disturbances.

THE GENERALIST NURSE

The generalist is most likely to see depressed clients in all practice settings. The major roles of the generalist nurse include performing a thorough psychosocial assessment and participating in the physical examination that involves taking vital and neurological signs. The nurse uses observational skill and data collection guided by knowledge of various theories and uses principles of the psychiatric interviewing process. The nurse considers the client's holistic needs that include spiritual, cultural, psychosocial, and environmental (American Nurses Association [ANA], 2000). The nurse asks questions about current medications, treatment, past and present surgeries, and functional status. Important questions to ask include:

- ◆ Reasons for seeking treatment at this time
- ◆ Duration and frequency of mood changes and what has worked in the past
- ◆ Family history of symptoms and treatment
- ◆ Questions about appetite and weight changes
- ◆ Sleeping patterns

Nursing Interventions for the Significant Others

If a family member is depressed, encourage him or her to get an accurate diagnosis and appropriate treatment.

Learn as much as you can about depression and how it influences a person's thoughts, behavior, and mood.

Learn how to communicate with the depressed person in a helpful way. Avoid comments like "Cheer up," "Snap out of it," "Oh, it's not so bad," or "I know—I've felt the same way myself." Don't give advice like "Just try a little harder," "What you need is a vacation," "What you need is regular exercise."

Focus on being a good listener and convey empathy and understanding. "I can see you are really suffering. I wish there was something I could say to make you feel better." It's okay that you can't do everything you used to. One day you will again. But for now take some time and concentrate on your health. If there is anything you need just ask."

Don't respond to his/her irritability with bad temper. The irritability is part of the illness and responds better to brief withdrawal on your part.

Engage in neutral conversation as much as possible and avoid constant talking about depression.

Allow the depressed person to be alone if he wishes. Only if you believe him to be suicidal should you insist he not be alone.

If you feel the person is suicidal, or if he states he is, ask about it in detail, inquiring about his feelings, his plans, his access to a means for suicide. If you feel there is a risk, contact his health care provider and stay with him/her.

Continue with your own life. You'll be in much better shape to help if you stay physically and emotionally healthy. Make time to get away and do things you enjoy.

Talk to others who can help you cope: friends, family, clergy, a therapist. Families need to talk about the problems of living with someone who is ill.

National Foundation for Depressive Illness, Inc. (NAFDI) has resources for family members and referrals to local support groups and professionals who specialize in the treatment of depression. Contact the National Alliance for the Mentally Ill (NAMI) at http://www.nami.org

Helpline: (800) 950-NAMI

Advocate, 200 N Glebe Road Suite 1015

Arlington, VA 22203-3754

(Used with permission from National Alliance for the Mentally Ill [NAMI].)

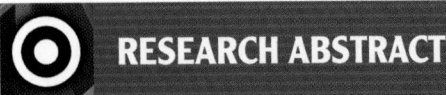

RESEARCH ABSTRACT

The Relationship among Health Functioning Indicators and Depression in Older Adults with Diabetes

Hu, J., Amoako, E. P., Gruber, K. J., & Rossen, E. K. (2007). *Issues in Mental Health Nursing, 28,* 133–150.

Study/Problem
Researchers examined the relationship among gender, race, coexisting conditions, symptom distress, and function status with depression.

Method
A convenience sample of older adults with diabetes was collected from individuals living in three subsidized housing units for older adults. Subjects were recruited through nursing centers operated by a local university. Flyers in which the study was described were posted in nursing centers and housing units to recruit older adults. Several tools were used to measure variables, including the Symptom Distress Scale, Instrumental Activities Daily Living Scale, and short form Geriatric Depression Scale.

Findings
Findings revealed that gender, symptom distress, and functional status were positively correlated with depression, whereas the coexisting conditions were not significantly correlated with depression scores.

Implications for Psychiatric Nurses
Older adults with moderate levels of symptom distress must be assessed for depression to determine appropriate interventions. Screening for symptom distress affords opportunities to educate clients about symptom management and initiate nursing intervention to prevent depression or to mitigate distress.

◆ Concentration difficulties

◆ Social support systems

◆ History of suicide and circumstances

◆ Substance abuse history and treatment (last use)

◆ Legal, occupational, or interpersonal problems (see Chapter 5)

Additional responsibilities of the generalist nurse include a continuous assessment of the client level of safety to self and others. During intake and screening the nurse makes triage decisions and facilitates movement into appropriate referrals and dispositions. Working with the depressed client also involves administering prescribed medications, family and heath education groups, and initiating various health promoting activities that increase self-esteem, ensure safety, and facilitate adaptive coping skills and resolution of present stressors and depression (see Research Abstract).

THE ADVANCED-PRACTICE PSYCHIATRIC REGISTERED NURSE

The advanced-practice psychiatric mental health nurse performs a comprehensive mental, physical, and psychiatric evaluation, including ordering appropriate diagnostic studies to rule out medical conditions, substance misuse, and monitoring drug levels. Based on clinical findings, the APN determines a diagnosis, collaborates with the client or family, develops a holistic treatment plan, and implements various treatments, such as prescribing, monitoring, managing, and evaluating the client's response to pharmacologic interventions. (See Table 9–11, Rating Scales for Depression.) Other responsibilities include providing psychotherapy and psychoeducation about the client's illness, medications, symptoms to report, and treatment options. An integral part of the treatment plan involves assessing the client for suicide and homicide risk. Ultimately, the APN facilitates psychosocial rehabilitation.

THE NURSING PROCESS

The nursing process enables the nurse to collect data concerning the client's reasons for seeking treatment, duration and course of symptoms, level of functioning, support systems, spiritual and cultural needs, and risk of danger to self and others. Baseline data assists in making an accurate diagnosis and guides treatment planning, interventions, and evaluation of client responses.

ASSESSMENT

The nursing process involves the Case Study: "The Client with Major Depression (Mary M.)."

DIAGNOSIS

The following nursing diagnoses for Mary M. are derived from the assessment data gathered:

◆ Dysfunctional Grieving

◆ Risk for Suicide

◆ Chronic Low Self-Esteem

◆ Self-Care Deficits

◆ Social Isolation

◆ Imbalanced Nutrition: Less than Body Requirements

PLANNING

Nursing Care Plan 9–1 for Mary M. illustrates how nursing diagnoses guide the development of goals and therapeutic inter-

TABLE 9–11
Rating Scales for Depression

Rating scales for depression are an objective way to measure depression at the initial visit and during subsequent visits to measure the effectiveness of treatment. The table below lists the various rating scales. The rating scales have been adapted to suit children, adolescents, and older adults. A health care practitioner needs special training to administer the Clinician Interview Rating Scales. Self-administered rating scales are the tools most likely to be used by nursing practitioners.

Self-Rating Scales for Depression

These scales are self-report questionnaires that contain less than 30 items and take 15 to 30 minutes for a client to complete. A self-reported rating gives a score that is the sum of the weighted item ratings. The scores range from normal to depressed.

Self-Report Instruments

Beck Depression Inventory (BDI)—13-item scale designed to measure the depth of depression as well as to quickly screen depressed clients

Center for Epidemiological Studies Depression Scale (CES-D)—20-item scale that was originally used to measure depression for epidemiological research

Geriatric Depression Scale (GDS)—15-item scale to rate depression in the elderly

Hopelessness Scale for Children—17-item scale measures cognition of hopelessness in children age 7 and older

Zung Scale—20-item self-report questionnaire that is widely used as a screening tool, covering affective, psychological, and somatic symptoms associated with depression. The questionnaire takes about 10 minutes to complete

Clinician-Rated Self-Report Instruments

Hamilton Rating Scale for Depression—a clinician-administered 21-item scale for assessing the severity of an adult patient's depression and for showing changes in depressive symptoms

CASE STUDY

Case Study: The Client with Major Depression (Mary M.)

Mary M. is a 61-year-old married woman referred to the inpatient psychiatric unit by her internist. She is a practicing Roman Catholic and has worked as a secretary for 18 years at a school for emotionally disturbed children. Mary lives with her husband, Ron, and her 24-year-old daughter, Gail, in their own home. Mary states, "My husband is tired of me crying all the time, and so am I." Mary states that over the past 3 months, she has experienced increasing dysphoria, anhedonia, feelings of guilt and worthlessness, intense crying, social isolation, and inadequate work performance. Mary sleeps 10 to 15 hours per night, experiencing no difficulty falling asleep or middle-of-the-night or early-morning awakening. Her appetite has diminished during the past month, with a reported weight loss of 12 pounds. She eats erratically, usually snacks, and her husband and daughter prepare meals. She has not been able to work, cook, sew, or do household chores and generally spends the day in bed. She has no sexual interest or activity for the past year. Mary describes no interest or involvement outside the home, except for weekly attendance at church. Mornings are the most difficult for Mary—she feels increased anxiety, has difficulty breathing, and cries a lot. She admits to occasional suicidal ideation in the form of a passive wish to be dead in hopes of relieving her emotional pain. She denies a history of suicide or drug abuse.

ventions. Ideally, the nurse collaborates with the client in planning care. This can be difficult to do with the depressed person who is feeling hopeless, helpless, and unmotivated. The nurse's communication of the firm belief that the client will feel better with time can often be enough to engage her in at least "going along" with the care plan. Setting realistic short-term goals that the client can accomplish are important in fostering a sense of hope and improved self-esteem. The nurse should expect that with the immobilized, depressed client early interventions may need to be aimed at "doing for" the client with the gradual expectation that the client take on more independent functioning.

IMPLEMENTATION

Nursing interventions are guided by the nursing care plan. For the depressed client, priority needs to be given to preventing self-harm through ongoing assessment of suicide potential and maintenance of a safe environment. Improving

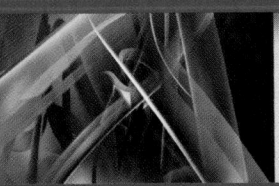

The Client with Major Depression (Mary M.)

Nursing Diagnosis: Risk for Suicide

Outcome Identification	Nursing Actions	Rationales	Evaluation
1. Mary will not harm herself.	1a. Maintain a safe environment.	1a. Easy access to means of harming themselves increases clients' likelihood of acting on suicidal ideation.	*Goal met:* Mary has been able to discuss her wish to be dead, rather than act on it. Her wish to be dead is no longer present.
	1b. Assess risk of suicide on an ongoing basis.	1b. Ongoing assessment is crucial, because clients with depression are at higher risk of acting on suicidal ideation when their energy level increases in response to treatment.	
2. By [date], Mary will discuss her wishes to be dead, rather than act on them.	2. Encourage therapeutic expression of feelings.	2. Describing and analyzing thoughts and feelings reduces the potential for acting on them destructively.	

Nursing Diagnosis: Imbalanced Nutrition: Less Than Body Requirements

Outcome Identification	Nursing Actions	Rationales	Evaluation
1. By [date], Mary will achieve adequate nutritional status, and this will be maintained.	1a. Obtain Mary's diet history to determine her food preferences and eating habits.	1a. Allows nursing staff to ensure adequate nutrition that integrates the client's food preferences.	*Goal met:* Mary has achieved adequate nutritional status through eating regular meals, as evidenced by return to her baseline weight.
	1b. Consult with the nutritionist.	1b. The nutritionist can determine the client's nutritional needs and recommend how they can best be met.	
	1c. Monitor Mary's intake and weight.	1c. Information on the client's progress is important for ongoing planning.	

(continues)

Nursing Care Plan 9–1 (continued)

Outcome Identification	Nursing Actions	Rationales	Evaluation
	1d. Physically feed Mary, if necessary.	1d. Severe depression can leave clients unable to feed themselves. As the illness improves with treatment, clients are actively encouraged to take responsibility for feeding.	
	1e. Sit with Mary during meals and encourage eating and drinking.	1e. Because eating tends to be a social experience, it can be helpful to be with the client during meals.	

Nursing Diagnosis: Disturbed Sleeping Pattern

Outcome Identification	Nursing Actions	Rationales	Evaluation
1. By [date] Mary's sleeping patterns will return to normal	1. Assess client's normal sleeping patterns.	1. Baseline data provides data about normal sleep patterns and strategies to improve or return to normal.	1. Based on comprehensive sleep assessment, the nurse and client can develop a realistic plan of care to establish criteria to determine if her sleeping patterns return to normal, such as 8 hours of sleep, waking up feeling rested, improved mood and improved concentration.
	2. Gather data from significant other about client's sleeping patterns.	2. Significant others provide important information the client may not know, such as frequent tossing and turning or snoring.	
	3. Ask when sleep disturbances began and how they have been resolved in the past.	3. Linking certain stressors to sleeping disturbances offers insight to cause.	
	4. Ask how many hours do "you normally sleep"? "When you wake up do you feel rested?"	4. Again, this helps the nurse assess normal sleeping patterns. Restful or restorative sleep results in waking up feeling rested (quality sleep).	
	5. Administer antidepressant and monitor for sleep improvement or worsening sleep disturbances.	5. Many antidepressants, such as SSRIs, may cause additional sleep disturbances or improve sleep. Monitoring for these effects reflects improved mood.	
	6. Teach sleep hygiene techniques • Avoid caffeine and strenuous exercise before sleep • Use bed for sleep and intimacy only • Take antidepressant as ordered • Use deep breathing exercises to promote relaxation	6. Sleep hygiene promotes restorative sleep.	

(continues)

Nursing Diagnosis: Self-Care Deficit

Outcome Identification	Nursing Actions	Rationales	Evaluation
1. By [date], Mary will resume self-care behaviors.	1a. Gradually increase the expectation that Mary will assume responsibility for hygiene and grooming. 1b. Provide Mary with positive feedback on her self-care behaviors.	1a. The expectations of those in a person's environment can significantly influence the person's behavior. 1b. Positive feedback increases the likelihood that desired behavior will recur.	*Goal met:* Mary has resumed self-care activities; her hygiene is good, and her appearance is no longer disheveled.

Nursing Diagnosis: Low Self-Esteem

Outcome Identification	Nursing Actions	Rationales	Evaluation
1. By [date], Mary will evidence a decrease in verbalizations of self-deprecatory ideas and will verbalize feelings of self-worth.	1a. Encourage Mary to get involved in tasks that can be accomplished with success. 1b. Provide praise for Mary's accomplishments. 1c. Assist Mary in identifying her strengths.	1a. Experiences of success lead to feelings of self-worth. 1b. Praise from others reinforces sense of self-worth. 1c. Clients with depression have a distorted cognitive view of themselves and need help identifying their strengths.	*Goal met:* Mary is able to express feelings of self-worth in relation to tasks accomplished and expresses fewer negative comments about herself.

Nursing Diagnosis: Social Isolation

Outcome Identification	Nursing Actions	Rationales	Evaluation
1. By [date], Mary will become integrated into the unit milieu.	1. Encourage Mary to participate in groups, meetings, and social activities.	1. Participation with others on the unit decreases clients' social isolation, which not only stems from, but contributes to, depression.	*Goal met:* Mary has become an active participant within the unit milieu. She has taken on a leadership role in groups, encouraging the involvement of others.
2. By [date], Mary will initiate interactions with others.	2. Provide Mary with constructive feedback on her style of interactions with staff and others.	2. Depressed clients are often unaware that they tend to push others away through their negative style of interacting.	

(continues)

Nursing Diagnosis: Dysfunctional Grieving

Outcome Identification	Nursing Actions	Rationales	Evaluation
1. By [date], Mary will identify recent and impending losses.	1. Assist Mary in the identification of losses.	1. Clients often do not identify certain events as losses. Being aware of losses facilitates the grieving process.	*Goal met:* Mary is able to identify her recent and impending losses.
2. By [date], Mary will express her thoughts and feelings related to her multiple losses.	2a. Encourage Mary to verbalize her thoughts and feelings and be available simply to listen.	2a. Verbalizing thoughts and feelings related to losses serves to decrease the client's sense of isolation, allows for unrealistic blame and guilt to be challenged, and permits an exploration of the meaning of the losses to the client.	Mary is able to express her thoughts and feelings related to these losses with her nurse and family members.
	2b. Foster communication between Mary and her family related to developmental life changes (e.g., daughter's marriage, Mary's retirement).	2b. Open communication among family members can lead to individual members' supporting each other and thus can strengthen the unit as a whole.	

and maintaining physical health is an important focus of care for the depressed client who often has an altered nutritional status and disturbed sleeping pattern. Monitoring for side effects of somatic treatments for depression is equally important in maintaining physical and mental integrity.

The depressed client has often become socially isolated and withdrawn. Involving the client in individual and group interactions in the hospital unit milieu will decrease isolation and can foster a sense of self-worth.

As the client's symptoms of depression respond to the psychotherapeutic and somatic interventions implemented, psychoeducation becomes feasible. Clients should be educated about the type of depression they have as well as its possible causes. Specifically, the contribution of both neurobiological and psychosocial factors to the onset of depressive illness should be discussed. Education about specific signs and symptoms of depression are important so that these can be identified early if they recur. Education regarding maintenance of medication regimes should be conducted and supplemented with written materials.

EVALUATION

Evaluation of client responses to nursing interventions should be done in an ongoing manner. Questions the nurse might ask in this phase of the nursing process with the depressed client include the following:

◆ Does the client describe an improvement in mood and energy level?

◆ Is there any evidence of suicidal ideation present?

◆ Has the client learned new, more effective ways of expressing feelings?

◆ Has the verbalization of self-deprecatory ideas diminished?

◆ Is the client initiating interactions with others?

◆ Is there an improvement in appetite? Has the client gained or lost weight?

In asking these and other questions the nurse reflects his own observations, the observations of other team members and the client's family, and very importantly seeks the client's description of his own experience.

SUMMARY

◆ Depressive disorders are characterized by persistent sad or depressed mood, loss of interest in things that were once pleasurable, and sleep, appetite, weight, energy, and concentration disturbances.

- The prevalence of depression is two times more in females than in males.

- Older adults have a poorer prognosis than other age groups.

- Suicide risks must be assessed throughout treatment planning.

- Major causes of depressive disorders include neurobiological, psychosocial stressors, cognitive-behavioral distortions, and genetic or familial patterns.

- Depression is one of the most treatable mental disorders.

- Research demonstrates an array of evidence-based treatment modalities.

- Grief and bereavement are associated with loss and differ from major depressive disorders.

SUGGESTIONS FOR CLINICAL CONFERENCES

1. As an empathy-enhancing exercise, read William Styron's (1990) book about his own depression: *Darkness Visible*. Discuss your reactions to the book with your group.

2. Role-play an interview between a nurse and a grieving person who recently lost a loved one. Using the section on loss and grief, discuss and evaluate the findings of the interview, taking into account the client's phase in the life span.

3. Obtain case studies that portray examples of the several types of depression described in this chapter.

STUDY QUESTIONS

1. Misty is a 34-year-old receptionist who is seeking treatment in the mental health clinic complaining of crying spells, poor appetite, sleep and concentration disturbances, and depression. She reports a history of these symptoms since losing her job several weeks ago. A primary concern for this client includes which of the following?
   a. Suicide risk
   b. Weight loss
   c. Financial concerns
   d. Low self esteem

2. Psychiatric nurses must distinguish between normal and abnormal grief. Which of the following represents an abnormal grief reaction?
   a. "I have not changed the linen on the bed since my father's death 3 months ago."
   b. "I feel so sad and really miss my father and the good times we used to have."
   c. "I am so angry at God for letting my father die!"
   d. "Why did he have to die? He said he would never leave me."

3. Risk factor(s) for abnormal or pathological grief include which of the following?
   a. Dependent relationship with the deceased
   b. Adequate social support
   c. Limited losses
   d. A lack of preoccupation with deceased

4. One of the major benefits of the new generation antidepressants is their safety profile. Which of the following situations poses the greatest concern when administering or ordering antidepressants?
   a. Mary, a 55-year-old mother of two, who just lost her job.
   b. Judy, an 18-year-old, has a history of suicide attempts and self-mutilation.
   c. John, a 43-year-old with a history of cocaine use, but he has been "clean" 1 year.
   d. Mikhail reports a history of a positive response to antidepressant treatment.

5. Marty, a 16-year-old, has just lost his best friend in a motor vehicle accident. His parents report that he is isolating from the family, has irritable mood, and his grades are slipping in school. What is the *most* important nursing assessment data concerning this adolescent?
   a. Has he expressed thoughts of suicide?
   b. Has he been emotionally abused?
   c. Does he have close friends?
   d. What is his appetite like?

6. Mary is a 24-year-old who recently gave birth to a daughter 2 to 3 months ago. During one of the well baby visits you notice she is tearful and her mood is sad. What is the most important response to this client?
   a. "How long have you been depressed?"
   b. "How is your baby doing?"
   c. "I am concerned about your mood and need to make a mental health referral."
   d. "Are you thinking about killing yourself?"

7. Which of the following statements is true about complicated grief?
   a. It is unrecognized and undertreated.
   b. It, along with bereavement, has been associated with increased morbidity and mortality.
   c. More research is needed to guide clinical care.
   d. All of the above

8. Mr. Link is an 89-year-old whose wife of 60 years died 2 months ago. He complains of difficulty sleeping, eating, concentrating, and is isolating himself from friends and family. He states he misses his wife very much. What is the most appropriate nursing intervention during this visit?
   a. Reassure him that his reactions are normal parts of the grief process.
   b. Ask him if he has thoughts of joining his wife.
   c. Refer him to a mental health professional for antidepressant medication.
   d. Reassure him that his wife is in a much better place.

9. Ms. Vendor is in for a follow-up appointment after being on an antidepressant for several weeks. During the visit she reports she still feels depressed. Which of the following is the most appropriate response to her comment?
   a. "Normally it takes about 6 to 8 weeks to respond to your medication."
   b. "Tell me more about your depression and how it's affecting your life."
   c. "Your medication needs to be increased so I will refer you to your provider."
   d. Both a and b

10. Which of the following statements best describes symptoms of depression in children and adolescents?
    a. "He has been very irritable and agitated the past few months and is doing poorly in school."
    b. "He has new friends and doesn't want to do his chores or homework."
    c. "He mouths off a lot and refuses to do his homework."
    d. "He spends lots of time on his Ipod and seems distant from the family."

11. Which of the following would best indicate to the nurse that a depressed client is improving?
    a. Has fewer complaints about anxiety
    b. Changes in sleep, concentration, energy, and appetite
    c. Adheres to medication regimen
    d. Requests to talk to the nurse

12. The nurse performing a mental status examination of a 45-year-old woman with seasonal affective disorder can expect to find which of the following?
    a. A pattern of depression that occurs during winter months and remits during spring and summer months
    b. Depression that worsens during spring and summer months and remits during fall and winter months
    c. A pattern of depression that occurs during pregnancy and worsens in postpartum
    d. Mania that occurs during winter months and remits during spring and summer months

13. When assessing the client with dysthymia the nurse should expect to find which of the following?
    a. Chronic and mild depression
    b. Episodic cycles of low and high moods
    c. Chronic anxiety superimposed with severe depression
    d. Sleep disturbances associated with daytime sleepiness

RESOURCES

Please note that because Internet resources are of a time-sensitive nature and URL addresses may change or be deleted, searches should also be conducted by association or topic.

Internet Resources

http://www.bereavedfamilies.net/   Bereaved Families Online Support (Accessed September 19, 2006)

http://www.cancer.gov/cancer-information   National Cancer Institute (a resource for patients, families, caregivers, and professionals)

http://www.nimh.nih.gov/publicat/nimhdepression.pdf NIMH Publication on Depression (Handbook for Professionals, Clients, and Families)

http://www.nami.org   National Alliance for the Mentally Ill (NAMI)

http://www.drada.org   Depression and Related Affective Disorders Association (DRADA)

http://www.mentalhealth.org   The Knowledge Exchange Network (KEN)

http://nimh.nih.gov   The National Institute of Mental Health (NIMH), provides information services, publications, and the Depression/Awareness, Recognition, and Treatment Program (D/ART)

Several websites provide educational materials for clients, families, and professionals that include alternative treatment for depression, fact sheets on depression and medications, support groups for clients and families dealing with depression, as well as current research on depression and its treatment. Also provided is information on access to care, interactive chat rooms, discussion forums, and opinion polls.

http://www.nimh.nih.gov/healthinformation/stard_qa_general.cfm   NIMH STAR*D (background information and results)

http://www.nimh.nih.gov/healthinformation/stard.cfm Primary Results for Sequenced Treatment Alternatives to Relieve Depression (STAR*D) Study

http://www.phrma.org   Pharmaceutical Research and Manufacturers of America (PhRMA). Information on new mental health medications. Identifies companies that may offer assistance programs through physicians for patients who cannot afford certain medications.

http://www.who.int/mental_health/management/depression/definition/en/   Depression. Geneva: World Health Organization, 2006 (Accessed May 15, 2006)

Other Resources

National Alliance for the Mentally Ill (NAMI)
Advocate
200 N Glebe Road, Suite 1015
Arlington, VA 22203-3754
Helpline: (800) 950-NAMI
http://www.nami.org

National Institute of Mental Health
5600 Fishers Lane, Room 15C-05
Rockville, MD 20857

National Depressive and Manic-Depressive Association (NDMDA)
Merchandise Mart
Box 3395
Chicago, IL 60654
(312) 446-9009

National Foundation for Depressive Illness
20 Charles Street
New York, NY 10014

REFERENCES

Abraham, K. (1960). A short study on the development of the libido. In *Selected papers on psychoanalysis* (pp. 418–501). New York: Basic Books. (Original work published 1924.)

Abraham, K. (1960). Notes on the psychoanalytic investigation and treatment of manic-depressive insanity and allied conditions. In *Selected papers on psychoanalysis* (pp. 137–156). New York: Basic Books. (Original work published 1911.)

American Nurses Association. (2000). *Scope and standards of psychiatric-mental health nursing practice.* Washington, DC: American Nurses Publishing.

American Psychiatric Association. (2000). *Diagnostic and statistical manual of mental disorders* (4th edition, Text Revision) (*DSM-IV-TR*). Washington, DC: Author.

American Psychiatric Association Work Group. (2000). *Practice guideline for the treatment of patients with major depressive disorder* (Rev. ed.). Washington, DC: American Psychiatric Association.

Antai-Otong, D. (2007). Nurse-client interactions: Strengthening care partnerships. In D. Antai-Otong (Ed.). *Nurse-client communication: A life span approach* (pp. 99–152). Sudbury, MA: Jones and Bartlett Publishers.

Beals, J., Manson, S. M., Whitesell, N. R., Spicer, P., Novins, D. K., Mitchell, C. M. (2005). Prevalence of DSM-IV disorders and attendant help-seeking in 2 American Indian reservation populations. *Archives of General Psychiatry, 62,* 99–108.

Beck, A. T. (1963). Thinking and depression, I: Idiosyncratic content and cognitive distortions. *Archives of General Psychiatry, 2,* 36–45.

Beck, A. T. (1964). Thinking and depression, II: Theory and therapy. *Archives of General Psychiatry, 10,* 561–571.

Beck, A. T. (1967). *Depression: Clinical, experimental, and theoretical aspects.* New York: Harper & Row.

Beck, A. T., Rush, A. J., Shaw, B. F., & Emery, G. (1979). *Cognitive theory of depression.* New York: Guilford.

Beekman, A. T., Penninx, B. W., Deeg, D. J., de Beurs, E., Geerling, S. W., & van Tilburg, W. (2002). The impact of depression on the well-being, disability and use of services in older adults: A longitudinal perpective. *Acta Psychiatrica Scandinavica, 105,* 20–27.

Beekman, A. T., F., Geerling, S. W., Deeg, D. J. H., Smit, J. H., Schoevers, R. S., de Beurs, E., Braam, A. W. et al., (2002). The natural history of late life depression: A 6-year prospective study in the community. *Archives of General Psychiatry, 59,* 605–611.

Belanoff, J. K., Kalehzan, M., Sund, B., Ficek, S. K. F., & Schatzberg, A. F. (2001). Cortisol activity and cognitive changes in psychotic major depression. *American Journal of Psychiatry, 158,* 1612–1616.

Betancourt, J. R. (2006). Cultural competency: Providing quality care to diverse populations. *The Consulting Pharmacist, 21,* 988–995.

Bhuri, K., Bhugra, D., Goldberg, D., Sauer, J., & Tylee, A. (2004). Assessing the prevalence of depression in Punjabi and English primary care attenders: The role of culture, physical illness and somatic symptoms. *Transcultural Psychiatry, 41,* 307-322.

Biederman, J., Faraone, S. V., Hirshfeld-Becker, D. R., Friedman, D., Robin, J. A., & Rosenbaum, J. F. (2001). Patterns of psychopathology and dysfunction in high-risk children of parents with panic disorder and major depression. *American Journal of Psychiatry, 158,* 49–57.

Birmaher, B., Bridge, J. A., Williamson, D. E., Brent, D. A., Dahl, R. E., Axelson, D. A., et al. (2004). Psychosocial functioning in youths at high risk to develop major depressive disorder. *Journal of the American Academy of Child and Adolescent Psychiatry, 43,* 839–846.

Boelen, P. A., & van den Bout, J. (2005). Complicated grief, depression, and anxiety as distinct postloss syndromes: A confirmatory factor analysis study. *American Journal of Psychiatry, 162,* 2175–2177.

Bromberger, J. T., Harlow, S., Avis, N., Kravitz, H. M., Cordal, A. (2004). Racial/ethnic differences in the prevalence of depressive symptoms among middle-aged women: The Study of Women's Health Across the Nation (SWAN). *American Journal of Public Health, 94,* 1378–1385.

Brommelhoff, J. A., Conway, K., Merikangas, K., & Levy, B. R. (2004). Higher rates of depression in women: Role of gender bias within the family. *Journal of Women's Health, 13,* 69–76.

Bryant, R. A., & Njenga, F. G. (2006). Cultural sensitivity: Making trauma assessment and treatment plans culturally relevant. *Journal of Clinical Psychiatry, 67,* Suppl 2, 74–79.

Centers for Disease Control and Prevention, National Center for Injury Prevention and Control. (2005). *Web-based Injury Statistics Query and Reporting System* (WISQARS) [online]. http://www.cdc.gov/ncipc/wisqars.

Cerel, J., Fristad, M. A., Verducci, J., Weller, R. A., & Weller, E. B. (2006). Childhood bereavement: Psychopathology in the 2 years postparental death. *Journal of the American Academy of Child and Adolescent Psychiatry, 45,* 681–690.

Charney, D. S. (1998). Monamine dysfunction and the pathophysiology of depression. *Journal of Clinical Psychiatry, 59*(Suppl. 14), 11–14.

Chen, M. L. (2006). Ethnic or racial differences revisited: Impact of dosage regimen and dosage form on pharmacokinetics and pharmacodynamics. *Clinical Pharmacokinetics, 45,* 957–964.

Clements, P. T., & Burgess, A. W. (2002). Children's responses to family member homicide. *Family and Community Health, 25,* 32–42.

Cohen, L. S., Altshuler, L. L., Harlow, B. L., Nonacs, R., Newport, D. J., Viguera, A. C., Suri, R., Burt, V. K. et al., (2006). Relapse of major depression during pregnancy in women who maintain or discontinue antidepressant treatment. *Journal of the American Medical Association, 295,* 499–507.

Cohen, J. A., Mannarino, A. P., & Staron, V. R. (2006). A pilot study of modified cognitive-behavioral therapy for childhood traumatic grief (CBT-CTG). *Journal of the American Academy of Child and Adolescent Psychiatry, 45,* 1465–1473.

Cohen, L. S., Soares, C. N., Vitonis, A. F., Otto, M. W., & Harlow, B. L. (2006). Risk for new onset of depression during the menopausal transition: The Harvard study of moods and cycles. *Archives of General Psychiatry, 63,* 385–390.

Cohen, L. S., Soares, C. N. N., Poitras. J., Prouty, J., Alexander, A. B., & Shifren, J. L. (2003). Short term use of estradiol for depression in perimenopause and postmenopausal women: A preliminary report. *American Journal of Psychiatry, 160,* 1519–1522.

Cole, M. G., & Dendukuri, N. (2003). Risk factors for depression among elderly community subjects: A systematic review and meta-analysis. *American Journal of Psychiatry, 160,* 1147–1156.

Conrad, M. M., & Pacquiao, D. F. (2005). Manifestation, attribution, and coping with depression among Asian Indians from the perspectives of health care practitioners. *Journal of Transcultural Nursing, 16,* 32–40.

Coppen, A., Eccleston, E. G., & Peet, M. (1973). Total and free tryptophan concentration in the plasma of depressed patients. *Lancet, 2,* 60–62.

Coyne, J. C. (1976). Toward an interactional description of depression. *Psychiatry, 39,* 28–40.

Dannon, P. N., Lowengrub, K., Gonopolski, Y., & Kotler, M. (2005). Current and emerging somatic treatment strategies in psychotic major depression. *Expert Review of Neurotherapeutics, 6,* 73–80.

Davies, B., Collins, J., Steele, R., Cook, K., Distler, V., & Brenner, A. (2007). Parents' and children's perspectives of a children's hospice bereavement program. *Journal of Palliative Care, 23,* 14–23.

Dindar, I., & Erdogan, S. (2007). Screening of Turkish women for postpartum depression within the first postpartum year: The risk profile of a community sample. *Public Health Nursing, 24,* 176–183.

Duberstein, P. R., Conwell, Y., Conner, K. R., Eberly, S., & Caine, E. D. (2004). Suicide at 50 years of age and older: Perceived physical illness, family discord and financial strain. *Psychological Medicine, 34,* 137–146.

Fava, M. (2003). Diagnosis and definition of treatment-resistant depression. *Biological Psychiatry, 53,* 649–659.

Fitzgerald, P. B., Benitez, J., de Castella, A., Daskalakis, Z. J., Brown, T. L., & Kulkarni, J. (2006). A randomized, controlled trial of sequential bilateral repetitive transcranial magnetic stimulation for treatment resistant depression. *American Journal of Psychiatry, 163,* 88–94.

Flores, B. H., Kenna, H., Keller, J., Solvason, H. B., & Schatzberg, A. F. (2006). Clinical and biological effects of mifepristone treatment for psychotic depression. *Neuropsychopharmacology, 31,* 628–636.

Folkman, S., & Lazarus, R. S. (1986). Stress processes and depressive symptomatology. *Journal of Abnormal Psychology, 95,* 107–113.

Freeman, E. W., Sammuel, M. D., Liu, L., Gracia, C. R., 1Nelson, D. B., Hollander, L. (2004). Hormones and menopausal status as predictors of depression in women in transition to menopause. *Archives of General Psychiatry, 61,* 62–70.

Freud, S. (1957). Mourning and melancholia. In J. Strachey (Ed. & Trans.), *The standard edition of the complete psychological works of Sigmund Freud* (Vol. 14, pp. 243–258). London: Hogarth Press. (Original work published 1917.)

Ganong, W. F. (2005). *Review of medical physiology,* 22nd ed., New York: The McGraw-Hill Companies.

Gomez, R. G., Fleming, S. H., Keller, J., Flores, B., Kenna, H., Debattista, C., Solvason, B., & Schatzberg, A. F. (2006). The neuropsychological profile of psychotic major depression and its relation to Cortisol. *Biological Psychiatry, 60,* 472–478.

Halligan, S. L., Murray, L., Martins, C., & Cooper, P. J. (2007). Maternal depression and psychiatric outcomes in adolescent offspring: A 13-year longitudinal study. *Journal of Affective Disorders, 97,* 145–154.

Harris, P. A. (2004). The impact of age, gender, race, and ethnicity on the diagnosis and treatment of depression. *Journal of Managed Care Pharmacy, 10,* 2 Suppl P, S2–S7.

Howell, E. A., Mora, P. A., Horowitz, C. R., & Leventhal, H. (2005). Racial and ethnic differences in factors associated with early postpartum depressive symptoms. *Obstetrics and Gynecology, 105,* 1442–1450.

Hsu, M. T., Kahn, D. L., Yee, D. H., & Lee, W. L. (2004). Recovery through reconnection: A cultural design for family bereavement in Taiwan. *Death Studies, 28,* 761–786.

Jaffe, D. H., Eisenbach, Z., Neumark, Y. D., & Manor, O. (2006). Effects of husbands' and wives' education on each other's mortality. *Social Science Medicine, 62,* 2014–2023.

Jang, Y., Kim, G., Hansen, L., & Chiriboga, D. A. (2007). Attitudes of older Korean Americans toward mental health services. *Journal of American Geriatrics Society, 55,* 616–620.

Jones, R. N., Marcantonio, E. R., Rabinowitz, T. (2002). Prevalence and correlates of unrecognized depression in U.S. nursing homes. *Journal of the American Geriatric Psychiatry, 51,* 1404–1409.

Kanner, A. M. (2004). Structural MRI changes of the brain in depression. *Clinical EEG Neuroscience, 35,* 46–52.

Kanazawa, A., White, P. M., & Hampson, S. E. (2007). Ethnic variation in depressive symptoms in a community sample in Hawaii. *Cultural Diversity and Ethnic Minority Psychology, 13,* 35–44.

Kendler, K. S., Gardner, C. O., & Prescott, C. A. (2006). Toward a comprehensive developmental model for major depression in men. *American Journal of Psychiatry, 163,* 115–124.

Kendler, K. S., Kessler, R. C., Walters, E. E., MacLean, C., Neale, M. C., Heath, A. C., & Eaves, L. J. (1995). Stressful life events, genetic liability, and onset of an episode of major depression in women. *American Journal of Psychiatry, 152,* 833–842.

Kendler, K. S., Kuhn, J. W., Vittum, J., Prescott, C. A., & Riley, B. (2005). The interaction of Stressful Life Events and a Serotonin Transporter Polymorphism in the Prediction of Episodes of Major Depression: A Replication. *Archives of General Psychiatry, 62*:529–535.

Kessler, R. C., Berglund, P., Demler, O., Jin, R., Merikangas, K. R., & Walters E. E. (2005). Lifetime prevalence and age onset of distributions of DSM-IV disorders in the National Comorbidity Survey Replication. *Archives of General Psychiatry, 62,* 593–602.

Kim, M. T., Han, H. R., Shin, H. S., Kim, K. B., & Lee, H. B. (2005). Factors associated with depression experience of populations: A study of Korean immigrants. *Archives of Psychiatric Nursing, 19,* 217–225.

Kirwin, K. M., & Hamrin, V. (2005). Decreasing the risk of complicated bereavement and future psychiatric disorders in children. *Journal of Child and Adolescent Psychiatric Nursing, 18,* 62–78.

Klerman, G. L., Weissman, M. M., Rounsaville, B. J., & Chevron, S. (1984). *Interpersonal psychotherapy of depression.* New York: Basic Books.

Lalande, K. M., & Bonnano, G. A. (2006). Culture and continuing bonds: A prospective comparison of bereavement in the United States and the People's Republic of China. *Death Studies, 30,* 303–324.

Lazarus, R., & Folkman, S. (1984). *Stress, appraisal, and coping.* New York: Springer.

Leonard, B. E. (2005). The HPA and immune axes in stress: The involvement of the serotonergic system. *European Psychiatry, Suppl 3,* S302–306.

Lewinsohn, P. M. (1974). A behavioral approach to depression. In R. Friedman & M. Katz (Eds.), *The Psychology of depression: Contemporary theory and research* (pp. 157–185). New York: John Wiley & Sons.

Lewy, A. J., Emens, J., Jackman, A., & Yuhas, K. (2006). Circadian uses of melatonin in humans. *Chronobiology International, 23,* 403–412.

Luby, J. L., Belden, A. C., & Spitznagel, E. (2006). Risk factors for preschool depression: The mediating role of early stressful life events. *Journal of Child Psychology and Psychiatry, 47,* 1292–1298.

Mann, J. J., Apter, A., Bertolote, J., Beautrais, A., Currier, D., Haas, A., Hegerl, U., Lonnqvist, J., et al. (2005). Suicide prevention strategies: A systematic review. *Journal of the American Medical Association, 294,* 2064–2074.

Marek, K. D., Popejoy, L., Petroski, G., & Rantz, M. (2006). Nurse care coordination in community-based long-term care. *Journal of Nursing Scholarship, 38,* 80–86.

Menchetti, M., Cevenini, N., De Ronchi, D., Quartesan, R., & Berardi, D. (2006). Depression and frequent atten-

dance in elderly primary care patients. *General Hospital of Psychiatry, 28,* 119–128.

Meyer, A. (1948–1952). *Collected papers of Adolf Meyer* (Vols. 1–4). Baltimore: Johns Hopkins University Press.

Mitchell, E. S., Wood, N. F. (1996). Symptom experiences of midlife women: Observations from the Seattle Midlife Women's Health Study. *Maturitas, 25,* 1–10.

Moffitt, T. E., Harrington, H., Caspi, A., Kim-Cohen, J., Goldberg, D., Gregory, A. M., et al. (2007). Depression and generalized anxiety disorder: Cumulative and sequential comorbidity in a birth cohort followed prospectively to age 32 years. *Archives of General Psychiatry, 64,* 651–660.

Morgan, M. L., Cook, I. A., Rapkin, A. J., & Leuchter, A. F. (2005). Estrogen augmentation of antidepressants in perimenopausal depression: A pilot study. *Journal of Clinical Psychiatry, 66,* 774–780.

Murray, C. J., & Lopez, A. D. (1997a). Regional patterns of disability-free life expectancy and disability-adjusted life expectancy: Global burden of disease study. *Lancet, 349,* 1347–1352.

Murray, C. J., & Lopez, A. D. (1997b). Alternative projections of mortality and disability by cause 1990–2020: Global burden of disease study. *Lancet, 349,* 1498–1504.

Nahas, Z., Marangell, L. B., Husain, M. M., Rush, A. J., Sackheim, H. A., Lisanby, S. H., et al. (2005). Two-year outcome of vagus nerve stimulation (VNS) for treatment of major depressive episodes. *Journal of Clinical Biology, 66,* 1097–1104.

Nelson, J. C., Portera, L., & Leon, A. C. (2005). Are there differences in the symptoms that respond to a selective serotonin or norepinephrine reuptake inhibitor? *Biological Psychiatry, 57,* 1535–1542.

Nemeroff, C. B., Mayberg, H. S., Krahl, S. E., McNamara, J., Frazer, A., Henry, T. R., et al. (2006). VNS therapy in treatment-resistant depression: Clinical evidence and putative neurobiological mechanisms. *Neuropsychopharmacology, 31,* 1345–1355.

Norman, T. R., & Burrows, G. D. (2007). Emerging treatments for major depression. *Expert Review of Neurotherapeutics, 7,* 203–213.

Oquendo, M. A., Bongiovi-Garcia, M. E., Galfalvy, H., Goldberg, P. H., Grunebaum, M. F., Burke, A. K., et al. (2007). Sex differences in clinical predictors of suicidal acts after major depression: A prospective study. *American Journal of Psychiatry, 164,* 134–141.

Padberg, F., Zwanzger, P., Keck, M. E., Kathmann, N., Mikhaiel, P., Ella, R., et al. (2002). Repetitive transcranial magnetic stimulation (rTMS) in major depression: Relation between efficacy and stimulation intensity. *Neuropharmacology, 27,* 638–645.

Penninx, B. W., Beekman, A. T., Bandinelli, S., Corsi, A. M., Bremmer, M., Hoogendijk, W. J., et al. (2007). Late-life depressive symptoms are associated with both hyperactivity and hypoactivity of the hypothalamo-pituitary-adrenal axis. *American Journal of Psychiatry, 15,* 522–529.

Phillips, A. C., Carroll, D., Burns, V. E., Ring, C., Macleod, J., & Drayson, M. (2006). Bereavement and marriage are associated with antibody response to influenza vaccination in the elderly. *Brain, Behavior and Immunity, 20,* 279–289.

Pilowsky, D. J., Wickramaratne, P. J., Rush, A. J., Hughes, C. W., Garber, J., Malloy, E., King, C. A., et al. (2006). Children of currently depressed mothers: A STAR*D ancillary study. *Journal of Clinical Psychiatry, 67,* 126–136.

Pincus, H. A., Zarin, D. A., Tanielian, T. L., Johnson, J. L., West, J. C., Pettit, A. R., Marcus, S. C., Kessler R. C., & McIntyre, J. S. (1999). Psychiatric patients and treatment in 1997: Findings from the American Psychiatric Practice Research Project. *Archives of General Psychiatry, 56,* 441–449.

Pittenger, C., Sanacora, G., & Krystal, J. H. (2007). The NMDA receptor as a therapeutic target in major depressive disorder. *CNS Neurological Disorders and Drug Targets, 6,* 101–115.

Rehm, L. P. (1990). Cognitive and behavioral theories. In B. B. Wolman & G. Stricker (Eds.), *Depressive disorders: Facts, theories, and treatment methods* (pp. 64–91). New York: John Wiley & Sons.

Roosevelt, R. W., Smith, D. C., Clough, R. W., Jensen, R. A., & Browning, R. A. (2006). Increased extracellular concentrations of norepinephrine in cortex and hippocampus following vagus nerve stimulation in the rat. *Brain Research, 1119,* 124–132.

Rosenstein, L. D. (1998). Differential diagnosis of the major progressive dementias and depression and late adulthood: A summary of the literature of the early 1990s. *Neuropsychological Review, 8,* 109–167.

Runkewitz, K., Kirchmann, H., & Strauss, B. (2006). Anxiety and depression in primary care patients: Predictors of symptom severity and developmental correlates. *Journal of Psychosomatic Research, 60,* 445–453.

Sadovy, J. (2000). Psychosocial treatments: General principles. In B. J. Sadock & V. A. Sadock (Eds.), *Comprehensive textbook of psychiatry/VI* (Vol. 1, 7th ed., pp. 3112–3114). Philadelphia: Lippincott Williams & Wilkins.

Seligman, M. E. P. (1975). *Helplessness: On depression, development, and death.* San Francisco: Freeman.

Siegle, G. J., Thompson, W., Carter, C. S., Steinhauer, S. R., & Thase, M. E. (2007). Increased amygdala and decreased dorsolateral prefrontal BOLD responses in unipolar depression: Related and independent features. *Biological Psychiatry, 61,* 198–209.

Stewart, W. F., Ricci, J. A., Chee, E., Hahn, S. R., & Morganstein, D. (2004). Cost of lost productive work time among U.S. workers with depression. *Journal of the American Medical Association, 289,* 3135–3144.

Stimpson, J. P., Kuo, Y. F., Ray, L. A., Raji, M. A., & Peek, M. K. (2007). Risk of mortality related to widowhood in older Mexican Americans. *Annals of Epidemiology, 17,* 313–319.

Stroebe, M., Stroebe, W., & Abakoumkin, G. (2005). The broken heart: Suicidal ideation in bereavement. *American Journal of Psychiatry, 162,* 2178–2180.

Stuber, M. L., & Mesrkhani, V. H. (2001). "What do we tell the children?" *Western Journal of Medicine, 174,* 187–191.

Sullivan, G. M., Mann, J. J., Oquendo, M. A., Lo, E. S., Cooper, T. B., & Gorman, J. M. (2006). Low cerebrospinal fluid transthyretin levels in depression: Correlations with suicidal ideation and low serotonin function. *Biological Psychiatry, 60,* 500–506.

Sullivan, H. S. (1953). *The interpersonal theory of psychiatry.* New York: W. W. Norton.

Swartz, H. A., Shear, M. K., Wren, F. J., Greeno, C. G., Sales, E., Sullivan, B. K., et al. (2005). Depression and anxiety among mothers who bring their children to a pediatric mental health clinic. *Psychiatric Services, 56,* 1077–1083.

Terman, M., & Terman, J. S. (2006). Controlled trial of naturalistic dawn simulation and negative air ionization for seasonal affective disorder. *American Journal of Psychiatry, 163,* 2126–2133.

Trierweiler, S. J., Neighbors, H. W., Munday, C., Thompson, E. E., Jackson, J. S., & Binion, V. J. (2006). Differences in patterns of symptom attribution in diagnosing schizophrenia between African American and non-African American clinicians. *American Journal of Orthopsychiatry, 76,* 154–160.

Trivedi, M. H., Fava, M., Wisniewski, S. R., Thase, M. E., Quitkin, F., Warden, D., Ritz, L., Nierenberg, A. A., Lebowitz, B. D., Biggs, M. M., et al. (2006). Medication augmentation after the failure of SSRIs for depression. *New England Journal of Medicine, 354,* 1243–1252.

Ustun, T. B. (2000). Cross national epidemiology of depression and gender. *Journal of Gender Specific Medicine, 3,* 54–58.

Vega, W. A., Karno, M., Alegria, M., Alvidrez, J., Bernal, G., Escamilla, M., et al. (2007). Research issues for improving treatment of U.S. Hispanics with persistent mental disorders. *Psychiatric Services, 58,* 385–394.

Verkerk, G. J. M., Denollet, J., Van Heck, G. L., Van Son, M. J. M., & Pop, V. J. M. (2005). Personality factors as determinants of depression in postpartum women: A prospective 1-year follow-up. *Psychosomatic Medicine, 67,* 632–637.

Videbech, P., & Ravnkilde, B. (2004). Hippocampal volume and depression: A meta-analysis of MRI studies. *American Journal of Psychiatry, 161,* 1957–1966.

Wagner, G., Sinsel, E., Sobanski, T., Köhler, S., Marinou, V., Mentzel, H. J., et al. (2006). Cortical inefficiency in patients with unipolar depression: An event-related FMRI study with the Stroop task. *Biological Psychiatry, 59,* 958–965.

Wakefield, J. C., Schmitz, M. F., First, M. B., & Horwitz, A. V. (2007). Extending the bereavement exclusion for major depression to other losses: Evidence from the National Comorbidity Survey. *Archives of General Psychiatry, 64,* 433–440.

Worden, J. W. (2003). *Grief counseling and grief therapy: A handbook for the mental health practitioner* (3rd ed.). New York: Springer.

Wright, J. H., & Beck, A. T. (1983). Cognitive therapy for depression: Theory and practice. *Hospital & Community Psychiatry, 34,* 1119–1127.

Zarate C. A. Jr., Singh, J. B., Carlson, P. J., Brutsche, N. E., Ameli, R., Luckenbaugh, D. A., Charney, D. S., & Manji, H. K. (2006). A randomized trial of an N-methyl-D-aspartate in treatment-resistant major depression. *Archives of General Psychiatry, 63,* 856–864.

SUGGESTED READINGS

Younger Children

Kohlenberg, S. (1993). *Sammy's mother has cancer.* New York: Magination Press.

Older Children

Simon, N. (1986). *The saddest time.* Morton Grove, IL: Albert Whitman.

Adults

Beck, A. T. (1995). *Cognitive therapy: Basics and beyond.* New York: Guilford Press.

Scott, J., & Derubeis, R. J. (2001). Cognitive therapy and psychosocial interventions in chronic and treatment resistant mood disorders. In J. Amsterdam & N. Neirberg (Eds.), *Treatment of refractory mood disorders.* Cambridge, UK: Cambridge University Press.

Silverman, P. R. (2000). *Never too young to know: Death in children's lives.* New York: Oxford University Press.

Sood, A. B., Razdan, A., Weller, E. B., & Weller R. A. (2006). Children's reactions to parental and sibling death. *Current Psychiatry Reports 8,* 115–120.

Styron, W. (1990). *Darkness visible: A memoir of madness.* New York, NY: Random House.

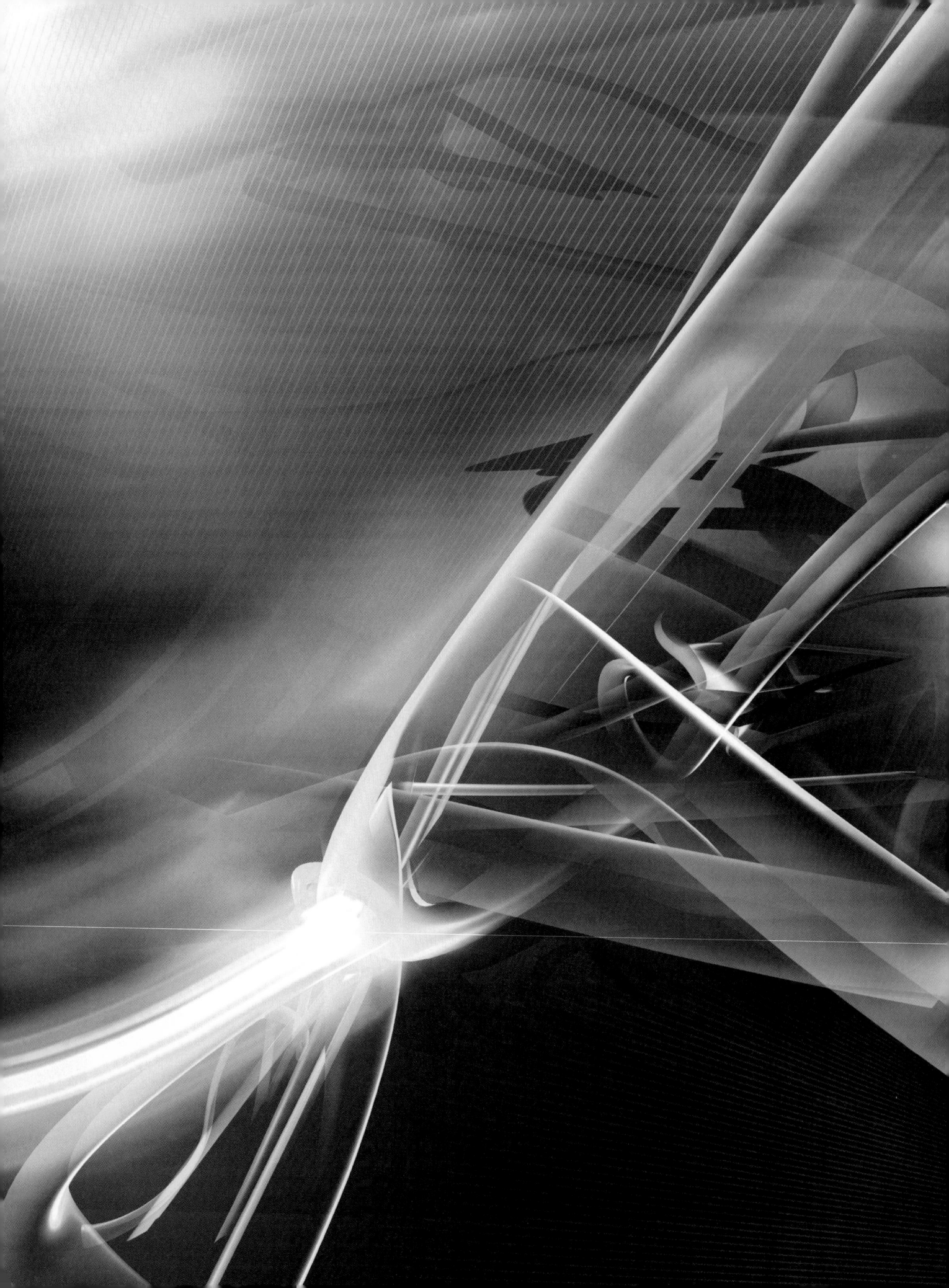

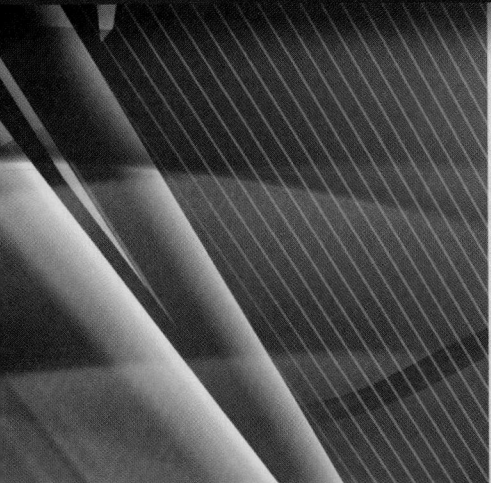

CHAPTER 10

The Client with a Bipolar Disorder

Vicki Hines-Martin, PhD, RN, APRN, BC
Deborah Thomas, EdD, RN, ARNP, BC

KEY TERMS

Affect: The visible and over mainfestations of the person's feeling or mood. Examples of affect are appropriate or congruent with mood and thought content, blunted, flat, labile, restricted, or constricted.

Bipolar: The two extreme mood states of mania and depression illustrated in bipolar disorder.

Circumstantiality: A thought and speech process in which an individual digresses into unnecessary details and inappropriate unrelated thoughts while trying to express a central idea.

Cyclothymia: A condition in which numerous periods of abnormally elevated, expansive, or irritable moods are experienced interspersed with periods of depressed mood. Neither mood state reaches the height nor depth to qualify as bipolar disorder.

Depression: A mental disorder marked by sustained alteration in mood in which there is loss of interest and pleasure, altered weight, concentration, and sleep disturbance.

Distractibility: The inability to maintain attention, shifting from one area or topic to another with minimal provocation, or attention being drawn too frequently to unimportant or irrelevant external stimuli.

Dysphoria: Marked feelings of sadness.

Euphoria: An exaggerated feeling of well-being or elation.

Flight of Ideas: Manifests as rapid thinking or ideas that have a common theme and that are likely to be seen in clients with major psychotic disorders such as a manic episode of bipolar disorder.

Grandiosity: An inflated appraisal of one's worth, power, knowledge, importance, or identity and may include delusional thinking.

Hypomania: A clinical syndrome that indicates an elated mood state similar but less severe than that described by the term *mania* or manic episode; it generally does not cause social or occupational impairment and has a duration of more than 4 days.

Kindling: The electrophysiological process that overtime produces an action potential after repetitive subthreshold stimulation or progressive sensitization of a neuron. This concept is thought to play a role in recurrent mood disorders.

Mania: A disorder characterized by exalted feelings, delusions of grandeur, elevated mood, psychomotor overactivity, and overproduction of ideas.

Mixed State: A behavioral condition displayed for a period of at least 1 week in which manic and major depressive mood states are exhibited every day. Symptoms are sufficiently severe to cause impairment in social and occupational functioning.

Mood: Refers to the client's sustained emotional state that reflects the client's perception of the world—depressed, sad, labile, elated, expansive, or anxious.

Pressured Speech: Disturbance in verbal expression of thought characterized by an overproduction of rapid speech that is frequently loud, unsolicited by social interaction, and difficult to interrupt.

Racing Thoughts: A rapid series of ideas that occur during manic episodes.

Rapid Cycling: A pattern of bipolar disorder characterized by at least four distinct episodes of depression, mania, or mixed states each year.

Tangentiality: A speech pattern that illustrates an inability to respond completely in a focused manner. Individuals may begin to respond appropriately but progress to related topics, never completing the originally desired response.

COMPETENCIES

Upon completion of this chapter, the learner should be able to:

1. Identify causes and symptoms of bipolar disorder.

2. Explain the cognitive changes as they occur in various bipolar disorders.

3. Discuss the role of neurobiological and psychosocial factors in bipolar disorder.

4. Recognize symptoms that may vary across the life span.

5. Identify strategies to support family adaptation.

6. Develop a plan of care for the client experiencing a bipolar episode.

7. Identify three major classifications of pharmacological agents used for acute stabilization and maintenance of bipolar disorders.

Life for someone with bipolar disorder, or manic-depressive illness, is often described as living on a continuous roller coaster ride. Sometimes the ride is big and scary, other times it is exciting and pleasurable. However, regardless of the experience, there is always some degree of ups, downs, and dips in equilibrium.

Human beings experience a variety of moods, from happiness to sadness to anger. Usually these can be experienced on a daily basis and can be linked to a specific precipitating event. However, in people with mood disorders, mood changes are often extreme and disproportionate to the event or not linked to any causative event at all. Often these severe changes in mood affect the individual's family, social, or work life. If these mood changes are severe enough, they can impair the individual's ability to function and care for herself on a daily basis.

Mood disorders are biological illnesses that affect our ability to experience normal mood states. The two general mood disorders are unipolar depressive disorders (which were discussed in Chapter 9) and bipolar disorders. In bipolar disorder there is some abnormal elevation of mood at various times. In any instance, individuals with a mood disorder are not weak in character nor are they unable to cope with life's normal stressors. Mood disorders are medical illnesses, not unlike diabetes, for which there are specific medications and treatments available. Current research suggests a strong biological or genetic component to mood disorders, including bipolar disorder.

According to the *Diagnostic and Statistical Manual of Mental Disorders*, 4th edition, Text Revision (*DSM-IV-TR*), **bipolar** disorder is a recurrent mood disorder featuring one or more episodes of mania or mixed episodes of mania and depression (American Psychiatric Association [APA], 2000). Bipolar disorder differs from major depressive disorder in that there is a history of manic or hypomanic (milder and not psychotic) episodes. *Mental Health: A Report of the Surgeon General* (U.S. Department of Health and Human Services [U.S. DHHS], 1999) reports that other differences are related to the nature of **depression** (an alteration in mood usually with feelings of sadness or feeling down) in bipolar disorder. Its depressive episodes are typically associated with an earlier age at onset, a greater likelihood of reversed vegetative symptoms, more frequent episodes or recurrences, and a higher familial prevalence (APA, 2000).

A key difference between bipolar and unipolar major depression is the differential therapeutic effect of lithium salts, which are more helpful for bipolar disorder. The word **mania** is derived from a French word that means crazed or frenzied. In bipolar disorder, the mood disturbance ranges from pure **euphoria**, or elation, to irritability to a labile admixture that also includes **dysphoria** (unpleasant mood). There are basically four different kinds of mood episodes that occur in bipolar disorder. These include episodes of *mania, hypomania, depression,* and *mixed episodes* (symptoms of both mania and depression at the same time or alternating frequently during the day).

In the manic phase of bipolar disorder, thought content is often grandiose but can also be paranoid. **Grandiosity** usually takes the form both of overvalued ideas (e.g., "My computer program is the best one ever written") and of frank delusions (e.g., "I can control others in the room just by looking at them"). Auditory and visual hallucinations can complicate more severe episodes. **Racing thoughts, flight of ideas,** and **tangential** and **circumstantial** speech are common symptoms of bipolar disorder during a manic episode. However, problems with **distractibility** and poor concentration often prohibit the implementation of new creative ideas.

Judgment is often compromised to varying degrees. This can be experienced as spending sprees, offensive or disinhibited behavior, drug or alcohol binges, promiscuity, or other objectively reckless behaviors. Individuals with bipolar disorder typically experience an increase in energy, libido, and activity. However, a perceived reduced need for sleep can deplete physical reserves and complicate the course of the disorder.

Sleep deprivation can also exacerbate cognitive difficulties and contribute to development of catatonia or a florid, confusional state known as delirious mania. If the client with mania is delirious, paranoid, or catatonic, the behavior is difficult to distinguish from that of a client with schizophrenia. Most people with bipolar disorder have a history of

remission and return to optimal level of functioning before onset of the index episode of illness.

THE BIPOLAR SPECTRUM

According to the *DSM-IV-TR* (APA, 2000), bipolar depression includes type I (prior mania) and type II (prior hypomanic episodes only). About 1.1 percent of the adult population suffers from the type I form, and 0.6 percent suffers from the type II form. Recent findings from a lifetime and 12-month prevalence of bipolar spectrum disorder from the National Comorbidity Survey Replication demonstrated that subsyndromal BPD is prevalent, clinically significant, and often goes undetected and inadequately treated (Kessler, Berglund, et al., 2005; Merikangas et al., 2007). More than 2 million American adults are affected by bipolar disorder. It also includes cyclothymia and bipolar disorder not otherwise specified. Tables 10–1 through 10–5 describe the particular criteria sets used to specify the nature of the current or most recent episode in individuals who have had recurrent mood episodes. In addition to these particular variations of bipolar disorder there also are mood disorders caused by general medical conditions or by substances.

According to *Mental Health: A Report of the Surgeon General* (U.S. DHHS, 1999), manic episodes occur, on average, every 2 to 4 years, although accelerated mood cycles can occur annually or even more frequently. Bipolar type I disorder is about equally common in men and women, unlike major depressive disorder, which is more common in women.

Hypomania is the subsyndromal counterpart of mania (APA, 2000; Kessler, Berglund, et al., 2005; Merikangas et al., 2007). An episode of hypomania is never psychotic nor are hypomanic episodes associated with marked impairments in judgment or performance. In fact, some people with bipolar disorder long for the productive energy and heightened creativity of the hypomanic phase.

Hypomania can be a transitional state (i.e., early in an episode of mania), although at least 50 percent of those who have hypomanic episodes never become manic (Kessler, Berglund, et al., 2005; Merikangas et al., 2007). Whereas a majority have a history of major depressive episodes (bipolar II disorder), others become hypomanic only during antidepressant treatment (Kessler, Berglund, et al., 2005; Merikangas et al., 2007). Despite the relatively mild nature of hypomania, the prognosis for clients with bipolar type II disorder is poorer than that for recurrent (unipolar) major depression, and there is some evidence that the risk of **rapid cycling** (four or more episodes each year) is greater than with bipolar type I.

The spectrum of bipolar disorder is a clinical reality that spans from core symptoms to temperamental traits (Angst & Cassano, 2005). Both clinicians and researchers recognize a need for better diagnostic criteria and assessment methodology. Classical (Kraepelin, 1921) and contemporary (Perlis et al., 2006; Nierenberg et al., 2006) observations support the thesis that bipolarity is expressed along a severity spectrum. The past

TABLE 10–1
Diagnostic Criteria for 296.0x Bipolar I Disorder, Single Manic Episode

A. Presence of only one Manic Episode and no last Major Depressive Episodes.

   Note: Recurrence is defined as either a change in polarity from depression or an interval of at least 2 months without manic symptoms.

B. The Manic Episode is not better accounted for by Schizoaffective Disorder and is not superimposed on Schizophrenia, Schizophreniform Disorder, Delusional Disorder, or Psychotic Disorder Not Otherwise Specified.

Specify if:

   Mixed: If symptoms meet criteria for a Mixed Episode

If the full criteria are currently met for a Manic, Mixed, or Major Depressive Episode, specify its current clinical status and/or features:

   Mild, Moderate, Severe Without Psychotic Features/Severe With Psychotic Features

   With Catatonic Features

   With Postpartum Onset

If the full criteria are not currently met for a Manic, Mixed, or Major Depressive Episode, specify the current clinical status of the Bipolar I Disorder or features of the most recent episode:

   In Partial Remission, In Full Remission

   With Catatonic Features

   With Postpartum Onset

Note. From *Diagnostic and Statistical Manual of Mental Disorders* (4th edition text Revision) (*DSM-IV-TR*), by American Psychiatric Association, 2000, Washington, DC: Author. Reprinted with permission.

TABLE 10–2
Diagnostic Criteria for 296.40 Bipolar I Disorder, Most Recent Episode Hypomanic

A. Currently (or most recently) in a Hypomanic Episode.

B. There has previously been at least one Manic Episode or Mixed Episode.

C. The mood symptoms cause clinically significant distress or impairment in social, occupational, or other important areas of functioning.

D. The mood episodes in Criteria A and B are not better accounted for by Schizoaffective Disorder and are not superimposed on Schizophrenia, Schizophreniform Disorder, Delusional Disorder, or Psychotic Disorder Not Otherwise Specified.

Specify:

   Longitudinal Course Specifiers (With and Without Interepisode Recovery)

   With Seasonal Pattern

   With Rapid Cycling

Note. From *Diagnostic and Statistical Manual of Mental Disorders* (4th edition text Revision) (*DSM-IV-TR*), by American Psychiatric Association, 2000, Washington, DC: Author. Reprinted with permission.

TABLE 10–3
Diagnostic Criteria for 296.4x Bipolar I Disorder, Most Recent Episode Manic

A. Currently (or most recently) in a Manic Episode.

B. There has previously been at least one Major Depressive Episode, Manic Episode, or Mixed Episode.

C. The mood episodes in Criteria A and B are not better accounted for by Schizoaffective Disorder and are not superimposed on Schizophrenia, Schizophreniform Disorder, Delusional Disorder, or Psychotic Disorder Not Otherwise Specified.

If the full criteria are currently met for a Manic Episode, specify its current clinical status and/or features:

Mild, Moderate, Severe Without Psychotic Features/Severe With Psychotic Features

With Catatonic Features

With Postpartum Onset

If the full criteria are not currently met for a Manic Episode, specify the current clinical status of the Bipolar I Disorder and/or features of the most recent Manic Episode:

In Partial Remission, In Full Remission

With Catatonic Features

With Postpartum Onset

Specify:

Longitudinal Course Specifiers (With and Without Interepisode Recovery)

With Seasonal Pattern (applies only to the pattern of Major Depressive Episodes)

With Rapid Cycling

Note. From *Diagnostic and Statistical Manual of Mental Disorders* (4th edition text Revision) *(DSM-IV-TR)*, by American Psychiatric Association, 2000, Washington, DC: Author. Reprinted with permission.

TABLE 10–4
Diagnostic Criteria for 296.89 Bipolar II Disorder

A. Presence (or history) of one or more Major Depressive Episodes.

B. Presence (or history) of at least one Hypomanic Episode.

C. There has never been a Manic Episode or a Mixed Episode.

D. The mood symptoms in Criteria A and B are not better accounted for by Schizoaffective Disorder and are not superimposed on Schizophrenia, Schizophreniform Disorder, Delusional Disorder, or Psychotic Disorder Not Otherwise Specified.

E. The symptoms cause clinically significant distress or impairment in social, occupational, or other important areas of functioning.

Specify current or most recent episode:

Hypomanic: if currently (or most recently) in a Hypomanic Episode

Depressed: if currently (or most recently) in a Major Depressive Episode.

If the full criteria are currently met for a Major Depressive Episode, specify its current clinical status and/or features:

Mild, Moderate, Severe Without Psychotic Features/Severe With Psychotic Features

Chronic

(continues)

TABLE 10–4
Diagnostic Criteria for 296.89 Bipolar II Disorder *(continued)*

    With Catatonic Features

    With Melancholic Features

    With Atypical Features

    With Postpartum Onset

If the full criteria are not currently met for a Hypomanic or Major Depressive Episode, specify the current clinical status of the Bipolar II Disorder and/or features of the most recent Major Depressive Episode (only if it is the most recent type of mood episode):

    In Partial Remission, In Full Remission

    Chronic

    With Catatonic Features

    With Melancholic Features

    With Atypical Features

    With Postpartum Onset

Specify:

    Longitudinal Course Specifiers (With and Without Interepisode Recovery)

    With Seasonal Pattern (applies only to the pattern of Major Depressive Episodes)

    With Rapid Cycling

Note. From *Diagnostic and Statistical Manual of Mental Disorders* (4th edition text Revision) *(DSM-IV-TR)*, by American Psychiatric Association, 2000, Washington, DC: Author. Reprinted with permission.

TABLE 10–5
Diagnostic Criteria for 301.13 Cyclothymic Disorder

A. For at least 2 years, the presence of numerous periods with hypomanic symptoms and numerous periods with depressive symptoms that do not meet criteria for a Major Depressive Episode.

    Note: In children and adolescents, the duration must be at least 1 year.

B. During the above 2-year period (1 year in children and adolescents), the person has not been without the symptoms in Criterion A for more than 2 months at a time.

C. No Major Depressive Episode, Manic Episode, or Mixed Episode has been present during the first 2 years of the disturbance.

    Note: After the initial 2 years (1 year in children and adolescents) of Cyclothymic Disorder, there may be superimposed Manic or Mixed Episodes (in which case both Bipolar I Disorder and Cyclothymic Disorder may be diagnosed) or Major Depressive Episodes (in which case both Bipolar II Disorder and Cyclothymic Disorder may be diagnosed).

D. The symptoms in Criterion A are not better accounted for by Schizoaffective Disorder and are not superimposed on Schizophrenia, Schizophreniform Disorder, Delusional Disorder, or Psychotic Disorder Not Otherwise Specified.

E. The symptoms are not due to the direct physiological effects of a substance (e.g., a drug of abuse, a medication) or a general medical condition (e.g., hyperthyroidism).

F. The symptoms cause clinically significant distress or impairment in social, occupational, or other important areas of functioning.

Note. From *Diagnostic and Statistical Manual of Mental Disorders* (4th edition text Revision) *(DSM-IV-TR)*, by American Psychiatric Association, 2000, Washington, DC: Author. Reprinted with permission.

two decades have provided considerable evidence related to varied phenomenology and epidemiology. There has been significant interest in identifying subclinical or subthreshold expressions of bipolar disorder.

Failure to recognize the subclinical symptoms or expressions of mania contributes to frequent underdiagnosis of bipolar disorder. There is also a need to better delineate the manic/hypomanic component of bipolar disorder (Angst & Cassano, 2005). Rapid cycling can be experienced in both bipolar I and bipolar II disorder, thus resembling cyclothymic disorder by virtue of the frequent shifts in mood (APA, 2000). However, the specific diagnostic criteria sets will help the nurse make the appropriate differential diagnosis.

RISK FACTORS FOR WOMEN

Gender differences between men and women with BPD remain unclear, but most data indicate little difference. Research also indicates that women are less likely than men to have co-occurring impulse-control and substance-use disorders. Women with bipolar disorder are more likely to report concomitant anxiety disorders than men (Benedetti et al., 2007). They are also more likely to endorse the depressive spectrum of bipolar disorder (Cassano et al., 2004). Implications for psychiatric nurses include assessing mood changes in women across the reproductive continuum and implementing appropriate gender-specific interventions to address the needs of women with BPD.

BIPOLAR I DISORDER

There are six separate criteria sets for bipolar I disorder: single manic episode, most recent episode hypomanic, most recent episode manic, most recent episode mixed, most recent episode depressed, and most recent episode unspecified. Other than the category of single manic episode, the criteria sets are used to specify the nature of the current or most recent episode in individuals who have had recurrent episodes of depression, mania, or both (APA, 2000).

BIPOLAR II DISORDER

Bipolar II disorder, as currently defined in the *DSM-IV-TR* (APA, 2000), shows diagnostic stability, a greater risk of the same disorder among relatives, a high frequency of episodes, increased risk of suicidality (usually during the depressed phase; 10 to 15 percent of those with bipolar II), and comorbidity. The diagnosis remains underused because hypomania is frequently not recognized, especially when occurring in the context of atypical depression. According to the current *DSM-IV-TR* classification system, the diagnosis of bipolar II disorder requires the presence of a full hypomanic and a major depressive episode. A diagnosis of bipolar II disorder cannot be made in individuals who experience fewer than four characteristics of hypomania, do not manifest the first criterion (elevated, expansive, or irritable mood), or have symptoms apparent only to themselves, as well as individuals whose hypomania is not preceded by a major depressive episode.

CYCLOTHYMIA

Cyclothymia, sometimes categorized as bipolar III, is marked by manic and depressive states, yet neither is of sufficient intensity nor duration to merit a diagnosis of bipolar disorder or major depressive disorder. The diagnosis of cyclothymia is appropriate if there is a history of hypomania but no prior episodes of mania or major depression. Longitudinal follow-up studies indicate that the risk of bipolar disorder developing in clients with cyclothymia is about 33 percent; although 33 times greater than that for the general population, this rate of risk still is too low to justify viewing cyclothymia as merely an early manifestation of bipolar type I disorder.

DIFFERENTIAL DIAGNOSIS

Mood disorders are sometimes caused by general medical conditions or medications. Classic examples include the depressive syndromes associated with dominant hemispheric strokes, hypothyroidism, Cushing's disease, and pancreatic cancer (APA, 2000). Antihypertensives and oral contraceptives are the most frequent examples of medications that may cause depression.

Transient depressive syndromes are also common during withdrawal from alcohol and various other drugs of abuse. Mania is not uncommon during high-dose systemic therapy with glucocorticoids and has been associated with intoxication by stimulant and sympathomimetic drugs and with central nervous system (CNS) lupus, CNS human immunodeficiency viral (HIV) infections, and nondominant hemispheric strokes or tumors. Together, mood disorders due to known physiological or medical causes may account for as many as 5 to 15 percent of all treated cases. They often go unrecognized until after standard therapies have failed. A challenge to clinicians is to balance their search for relatively uncommon disorders with their sensitivity to aspects of the medical history or review of symptoms that might have etiologic significance.

MIXED PRESENTATIONS

Mixed states can be described as the coexistence of depressive and manic symptoms. Mixed states have not received extensive research evaluation. They can be expressed on a continuum ranging from psychotic features to milder and subclinical states. Frequently, the entire episode presents with severe depression with agitated features and acceleration of thought suggestive of a depressive mixed state.

EPIDEMIOLOGY

Bipolar disorders are a major public health concern. Bipolar disorder I affects 1 to 1.5 percent of the general population of the United States affecting equal numbers of males and females

> Genetic studies implicate a shared genetic risk among individuals with schizophrenia and mood disorders. Family studies provide further supporting evidence of a genetic susceptibility factor for both bipolar disorder and schizophrenia.

Figure 10–1 Epidemiological risk factors. *(From Blackwood, D. H., Pickard, B. J., Thomson, P. A., Evans, K. L., Porteous, D. J., & Muir, W. J. [2007]. Are some genetic risk factors common to schizophrenia, bipolar disorder and depression? Evidence from DISC1, GRIK4 and NRG1. Neurotoxicity Research, 11, 73–83.)*

(Kessler, Berglund, et al., 2005; Merikangas et al., 2007). Bipolar II has been identified as affecting 0.5 to 0.6 percent of the population, with females being more affected than males (Kessler, Berglund, et al., 2005; Merikangas et al., 2007). Bipolar disorder is a severe and often chronic disorder with lifetime incidence of bipolar spectrum disorders of up to 6.5 percent in the general population. Younger subjects are mainly affected by bipolar disorder and associated with alcohol and substance abuse or dependence. Clients with bipolar disorder often report co-occurring substance-related disorders. Co-occurring substance-related disorders and bipolar disorders represent a serious public health problem and challenge the efficacy of conventional treatment (Albanese & Pies, 2004). Overall economic costs of bipolar disorder in the United States is estimated at $45 billion per year. Research indicates that there are gender differences in bipolar disorder. Males have more manic episodes, are more likely to be hospitalized with a manic episode, and are likely to have a concomitant substance abuse or dependence. In the initial episode of mania, males display more hyperactivity, grandiosity, and risky behavior, and females more often display racing thoughts and distractibility. Of individuals hospitalized for mania, 30 percent remain unemployed for 6 months and 23 percent for 1 year. Across physical and psychiatric disorders, bipolar disorder is ranked as the sixth leading cause of disability. The personal costs of this disorder are that as many as 19 percent of bipolar individuals die from suicide. Figure 10–1 describes one risk factor for bipolar disorder.

CULTURAL CONSIDERATIONS

There are few cross-cultural studies of bipolar disorder. However, the Cross-National Collaborative Group study found a lifetime prevalence of bipolar disorder that varied from 3 per 1,000 in Taiwan, 4 per 1,000 in Korea, 5 per 1,000 in Germany, and 6 per 1,000 in Canada and Puerto Rico, to 9 per 1,000 in the United States Epidemiologic Catchment Area (ECA data), and 15 per 1,000 in New Zealand (Weissman et al., 1996). Data are still limited about comparative rates of psychiatric disorders in minority populations in the United States. However, a study of the prevalence and treatment of mental disorders from 1990 to 2003 found little variation in rates of disorders by race or ethnicity (Kessler, Demler, et al., 2005). Findings from this study also revealed that most individuals with psychiatric conditions did not receive treatment, particularly among ethnic minority populations. In 2005, Kessler, Berglund, and colleagues, in their National CoMorbidity Survey Replication, found that blacks had lower rates of mood disorders and there were no psychiatric disorders that were consistently higher in the population than for whites. These data support earlier findings from the 1999 *Mental Health: A Report of the Surgeon General* in which several studies were cited that provided comparative analysis of disorder prevalence based on race or ethnicity alone, but significant difference in mental health service access and use between the majority population and minority populations (U.S. DHHS, 1999).

Figure 10–2 indicates that misdiagnosis of disorder by race occurs.

CAUSATIVE FACTORS: THEORIES AND PERSPECTIVES

Major theories of bipolar disorders are well documented and include psychodynamic, existential, cognitive-behavioral and developmental, and complex biologic and genetic factors. A plethora of neurobiological advances add to the complexity of these disorders and offer hope and quality treatment to clients and their families.

PSYCHODYNAMIC, EXISTENTIAL, COGNITIVE-BEHAVIORAL, AND DEVELOPMENTAL THEORIES

Descriptions of bipolar disorder and its etiology can be traced back to the early second century, when Aretaeus of Cappadocia recognized the association between melancholia and mania. It was not until the end of the 1800s that another major contribution to our understanding of this mood disorder was developed. In 1896, Kraepelin separated the functional psychosis into two groups, dementia praecox and manic-depressive psychosis. Since that time there have been many schools of thought about the classification and origins of bipolar disorder as well as other mood disorders. Psychodynamic, existential, cognitive-behavioral, and developmental theories have all been postulated as the underlying cause of the illness. Parenting, grief, or dysfunctional defense mechanisms were once seen as underlying causes for the onset of bipolar disorder. However, current research indicates that biological and genetic factors may be the most significant etiological factors. Bipolar disorder is seen as a complex disorder that has many contributors to onset. The above-mentioned theories all play an important role in understanding the interplay of etiological and precipitating or contributing

> There have been disparities in diagnosis of disorders based on race. Research has shown that clinicians are prone to misdiagnose mania as schizophrenia in African Americans (U.S. DHHS, 2001).

Figure 10–2 Disparities in diagnosis. *(From Mental Health: Culture, Race, and Ethnicity—a Supplement to Mental Health: A Report of the Surgeon General, by U.S. Department of Health and Human Services Administration, Center for Mental Health Services.)*

factors, and the development of nonpharmacologic treatment modalities. For example, psychosocial stressors can precipitate the onset of illness episodes (when biologic or genetic factors are present). Precipitating and contributing factors more commonly play a part in earlier episodes of depression and mania than in later ones.

BIOLOGICAL THEORIES

The evidence of biological and genetic factors associated with bipolar disorders is well documented. Psychiatric nurses need to understand these underpinnings and develop treatment planning that integrates various theories, including biological that help the client manage symptoms and attain an optmal level of functioning.

Neurochemical and Neuroendocrine Factors

Because individuals with bipolar disorders may exhibit two extremely divergent sets of moods and behaviors, the neurochemical theories underlying each must be understood to successfully treat the illness. Research has more clearly delineated the mechanisms underlying the depressive aspect of the disorder, and as a result, the understanding of the neurochemical processes. Neurochemical processes underlying depression have been identified as the Biogenic Amine theory. The Biogenic Amine theory of depression essentially implies that an imbalance or relative deficiency exists in relation to certain neurotransmitters or biogenic amines such as norepinephrine and serotonin. Deficiencies of these substances result in neurochemical imbalance. For more detail, see Chapter 9, The Client with a Depressive Disorder.

Psychopharmacologic treatment is based on the restoration of neurotransmitter systems (Sadock, Sadock, & Sussman, 2006). Psychopharmacologic treatment and neurotransmitter effects in bipolar disorder are discussed more fully in the pharmacologic intervention section of this chapter.

The mechanisms that underlie the development of mania are much less understood. Limited data are available regarding specific neurochemical processes as they relate to alterations experienced with mania. It has been suggested that the symptoms of bipolar disorder result from an inability to modulate neuronal excitation. This regulatory inability in the brain affects sleep-wake cycles and other daily rhythms. For example, researchers have discovered that lithium stabilizes a brain receptor that serves as a pivotal link in the regulatory process by synchronizing rhythmic feedback loops and modulating daily rhythms (Yin, Wang, Klein, & Lazar, 2006). It is also suggested that divalproex (Depakote) increases gamma-aminobutyric acid GABAergic inhibitory activity (among other actions), thereby dampening aberrant neuronal excitation through a different physiological mechanism. Research is ongoing to support these hypotheses and to develop a more complete understanding of the neurochemical processes involved in mania (Ganong, 2005).

Thyroid Function

Frequently, individuals with bipolar disorder also have abnormal thyroid gland function. Because too much or too little thyroid hormone can lead to mood and energy changes it is important that thyroid levels are monitored by the health care provider. Individuals with rapid cycling tend to have co-occurring thyroid problems and may need to take thyroid medication in addition to their regular bipolar medications. Lithium treatment may cause decreased thyroid levels in some individuals resulting in the need for thyroid supplement.

Neuroanatomical Factors

Scientific knowledge about the neuroanatomical component of bipolar disorder is just beginning and will act as a foundation

CRITICAL THINKING

Medications are an important part of treating bipolar disorders. Based on your understanding about medications used to treat bipolar disorders, which of the following tests is *critical* prior to the safe administration of antimanic agents to a 25-year-old woman?

1. B12 and folate level
2. Pregnancy test
3. Lipid and cholesterol levels
4. Hearing exam

Answers

1. *Incorrect.* B12 and folate levels are unnecessary when administering antimanic agents.
2. *Correct.* Due to the harmful teratogenic effects of most antimanic agents and reduced efficacy of birth control pills, a pregnancy test is imperative to ensure the 25-year-old is not pregnant.
3. *Incorrect.* Lipid and cholesterol levels are not affected by antimanic agents and hence are unnecessary.
4. *Incorrect.* Hearing problems are not associated with antimanic agents and thus are not a critical diagnostic study.

TABLE 10–6
Variations in Brain Structure and Impaired Functioning in Clients with Bipolar Disorder

Structural Variation/Abnormality*	Functional Impairment (all decreased)
Diencephalon (thalamus, mamillothalamic tract, and internal medullary lamina)	Memory performance
Prefrontal cortex	Verbal memory (recall of a story or single word)
Frontal subcortical	Attention dysfunction
Brain lesions	Verbal learning
Midsagittal areas reduction	Verbal fluency
Abnormal white brain matter (increase with age)	Psychomotor speed
Medial temporal lobe (hippocampus, parahippocampal and perirhinal cortices—episodes of depression and mania may result in hypercortisolemia, producing damage)	Declarative memory (conscious recollection of facts and events)
Basal ganglia	

*The functional impairments do not necessarily correspond with the identified structural variation.

for further neurochemical discovery. Findings indicate that individuals with bipolar disorder exhibit the following variations in brain structure and impaired functioning. See Table 10–6.

Of all the findings mentioned, the most consistent findings to date have been the appearance of specific abnormalities, or lesions in the white matter of the brain in people with bipolar disorder. White matter consists of groups of nerve cell fibers surrounded by fatty sheaths that appear white in color. These sheaths help the transmission of electrical signals within the brain. Although the white matter abnormalities appear in many parts of the brain in individuals with bipolar disorder, they tend to be concentrated in areas that are responsible for emotional processing. These brain changes appear more often than expected in young people with bipolar disorder. This finding suggests that the white matter abnormalities seen in MRI are related to the presence of the disorder.

The indicated neuroanatomical changes and functional impairments have been identified in individuals who are euthymic and stable in their disease as well as those who are acutely ill. Cognitive dysfunction seems to be associated with severity and chronicity of the illness and with increasing age although research with adolescents has indicated similar findings (Birmaher et al., 2006; Malhi, Ivanovski, Hadzi-Pavlovic, Mitchell, & Sachdev, 2007). It is still unclear what role the side effects of psychopharmacologic treatment for bipolar disorder have on cognitive functioning impairment. New areas of investigation have begun to understand the relationship between the condition of hypothyroidism and stabilizing rapid cycling bipolar disorder. A number of studies have found that among people with bipolar disorder, women are more

likely than men to have a thyroid disorder. Anecdotal evidence indicates that there may be some therapeutic benefit from the understanding of the relationship between the two disorders.

Genetic Factors

Findings from more than 40 family, twin, and adoption studies spanning six decades consistently show that the risk to relatives of those individuals with bipolar disorder is significantly greater than the risk for those individuals without bipolar disorder in the family history (see Figure 10–3). The risk of developing bipolar disorder is greatest when the disorder is present in first-degree family members (i.e., mother, father, or siblings). One or more genes that could contribute to as many as one in four cases of bipolar disorder may be located on a region of chromosome 18. Of the genes identified, one codes for a protein that plays a specific part in chemical signal reception; the other is involved in stress hormone production, a physiological function that has been shown to be hyperexcitable in both depression and bipolar disorder. Other genetic findings include identification of

A genetic study conducted by Pauls, Bailey, Carter, Allen, and Egeland (1995) with 42 old order Amish families, which included 689 relatives, identified that an autosomal dominant inheritance model was found to be consistent with the transmission of bipolar type I disorder within close relatives. This strongly supports the genetic transmission theory of bipolar disorder.

Figure 10–3 Cultural considerations. *(From Complex Segregation Analyses of Old Order Amish Families Ascertained Through Bipolar I Individuals, by D. L. Pauls, J. N. Bailey, A. S. Carter, C. R. Allen, & J. A. Egeland, 1995, American Journal of Medical Genetics, 60[4], pp. 290–297.)*

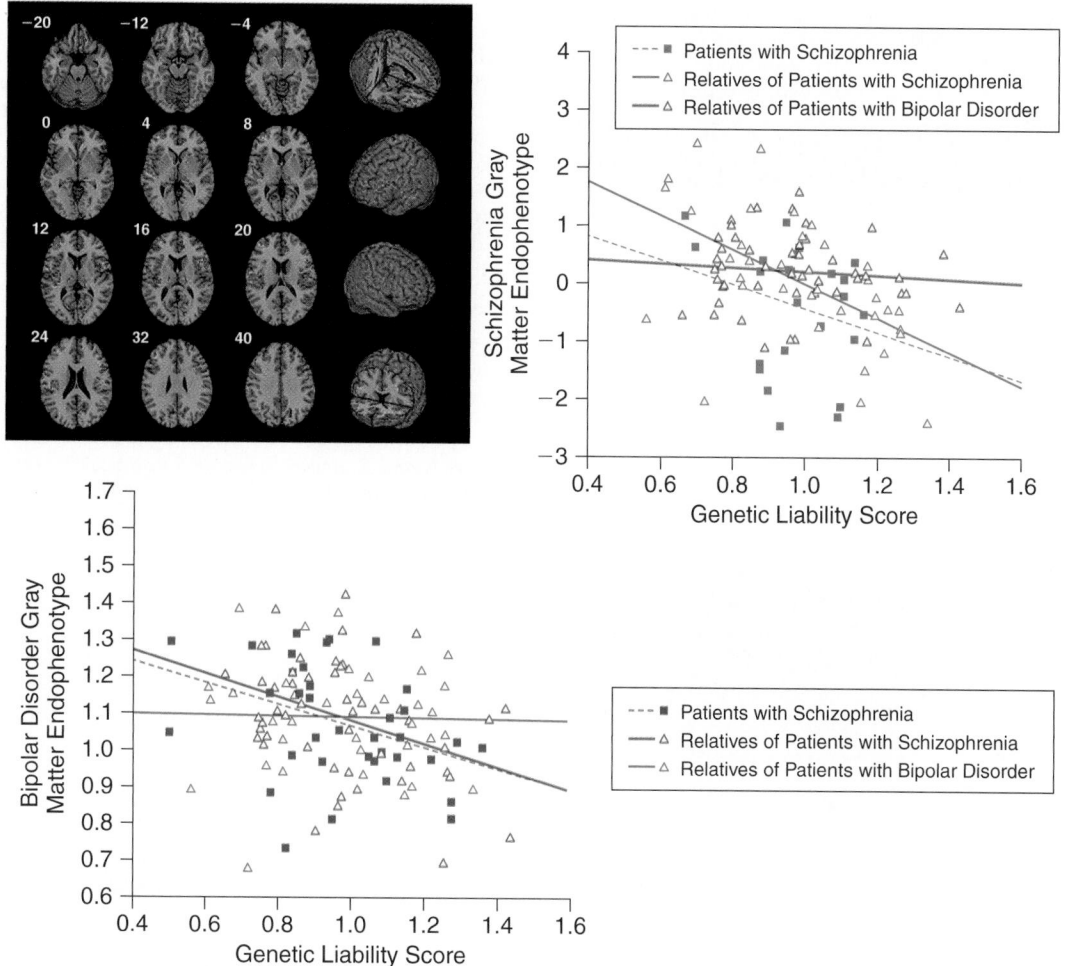

Figure 10–4 Brain imaging study implicating similar genetic vulnerabilities in subjects with bipolar disorder and schizophrenia. *(From McDonald, C., Bullmore, E. T., Sham, P. C., Chitnis, X., Wickham, H., Bramon, E., & Murray, R. M. [2004]. Association of genetic risk factors for schizophrenia and bipolar disorder with specific and generic brain structural endophenotypes. Archives of General Psychiatry, 61, 974–984. Used with permission.)*

region 22.3 of chromosome 21 and chromosome 11 and a possible relation with bipolar illness. Growing research indicates similar genetic vulnerability to bipolar and schizophrenia as evidenced by brain imaging studies (see Figure 10–4).

Circadian Rhythms Theory

Another important factor that plays a significant role in the development of bipolar disorder is the study of chronobiology. This study focuses on the circadian rhythm, or sleep-wake cycle. Several studies support the hypothesis that chronobiologic mechanisms are involved in the pathogenesis of bipolar disorder (Yin et al., 2006). For example, the clustering of affective episodes in spring and fall, and the high prevalence of bipolar type II disorder among individuals with winter depression (or seasonal affective disorder) suggest that seasonal variations in circadian rhythms (internal clock mechanisms related to the seasons) may precipitate affective episodes. In addition, the strong association between sleep deprivation and the development of manic symptoms suggests that disruption of circadian rhythms may precipitate affective relapse. As a result of this research, it also appears that social routine patterns (sleeping, eating,

exercise, daily activity) can cause disruption of circadian rhythms and thereby precipitate manic episodes.

Kindling Theory

The kindling theory may explain the continuum of bipolar disorder from the initial episode and how it is maintained over time. Supposedly, bipolar disorder evolves as a result of biologic and genetic predisposition mediated by environment factors. This process often results in less severe episodes of mood disturbances that initially occur infrequently and escalate over time. Repeated mood episodes result in neural sensitization to genetic and stress factors, resulting in progressive vulnerability to future bipolar episodes (Papadimitriou, Calabrese, Dikeos, & Christodoulou, 2005).

BIPOLAR DISORDERS ACROSS THE LIFE SPAN

Although some individuals may experience only a single episode of mania and depression in their lifetimes, over 95 percent of people with bipolar disorder have recurrent

TABLE 10–7
Co-occurring—Anxiety

	Bipolar type I	Bipolar type II
Obsessive-Compulsive Disorder	14–30%	28%
Panic Disorder	18–33%	5%
General Anxiety Disorder	42%	
Phobias	42–66%	

TABLE 10–8
Co-occurring—Substance Abuse

	Bipolar	Unipolar
Alcohol	46%	21%
Drugs	41%	18%

episodes of depression and mania throughout their lives. The probability of experiencing new episodes of depression or mania increases with each subsequent episode despite treatment. There is also evidence that the time between episodes decreases during the course of the illness. The marked changes in mood, personality, thinking, and behavior that are part of the disorder often have significant effects on interpersonal relationships across the life span. In addition to the direct effects of the disorder on the life of the diagnosed individual and her family, there are increased co-occurring disorders for this population (Tables 10–7 and 10–8).

Because of the vulnerability of individuals with this disorder, it is imperative that nurses understand the course, presentation, and opportunities for intervention from a life span perspective. Some factors are unique according to age categories, whereas other issues apply regardless of age group. The following information will identify unique characteristics of bipolar disorder according to age group.

CHILDHOOD AND ADOLESCENCE

Bipolar disorder was once thought to be rare in children. However, researchers are discovering that not only can it begin very early in life, it is much more common than previously believed (see Figure 10–5). Bipolar disorder is often misdiagnosed or overlooked in children because it manifests differently than in adults. Too often children are inaccurately diagnosed and

A study examined neuropsychological deficits in children with concomitant attention-deficit/hyperactivity disorder (ADHD). The study involved 102 unmedicated children with ADHD without bipolar disorder, and 120 children without bipolar disorder or ADHD were studied. Most of the subjects were Caucasian; 58% were boys, and 42% were girls from mostly middle to upper socioeconomic status. A series of comprehensive neuropsychological battery and measures used academic achievement, school failure, and special education placement to measure function.

The following information was demonstrated:

The co-occurrence of bipolar disorder and ADHD are highly prevalent. Youths with these co-occurring disorders are likely to perform poorly on neuropsychological tests.

Figure 10–5 Research and bipolar disorder in children. *(From Henin, A., Mick, E., Biederman, J., Fried, R., Wozniak, J., Faraone, S. V., et al. [2007]. Can bipolar disorder-specific neuropsychological impairments in children be identified?* Journal of Consulting and Clinical Psychology, 75, *210-220.)*

CRITICAL THINKING

During your visit at a local elementary school, the teacher asks you to talk to Lisa, an 8-year-old. As you talk to her, she is very energetic, mildly irritable, but much focused on a classroom assignment. She is cooperative when questioned and expresses an interest in becoming a nurse. Her teacher reports she seems to be overly energetic, but is easily redirected. Based on your preliminary nursing assessment, what is the most *appropriate* question to ask her teacher?

1. "Do you like Lisa?"
2. "Is she taking any medications?"
3. "Tell me your reasons for asking me to talk to Lisa today."
4. "Do you think she has a mental problem?"

Answers

1. *Incorrect.* This is an irrelevant question and has little to do with her reasons for asking you to talk to Lisa. Obviously she cares about this student or she would not have asked you to talk to her.
2. *Incorrect.* There is little evidence that this child is taking medication. Her behavior is normal for an 8-year-old.
3. *Correct.* Based on the presentation, Lisa's behavior is normal for an 8-year-old. It is imperative for the nurse to understand the teacher's reasons for asking her to see the child. Maybe other things have occurred that made her feel a referral was necessary.
4. *Incorrect.* This answer is based on an assumption that Lisa's behavior is abnormal or that she has a psychiatric problem. There is no evidence to support this assumption.

treated with stimulants or certain antidepressants, which can worsen the bipolar condition. Long-term effects of mood disorders in children can have a negative influence on the accomplishment of the normal developmental tasks of childhood. Peer and family relationships as well as academic progress often suffer when a child experiences bipolar disorder (Wozniak, 2007).

Children and adolescents with bipolar disorder often experience very fast mood swings between depression and mania many times within a day. Children with mania are more likely to be irritable and prone to destructive tantrums rather than overly happy and elated. Mixed symptoms are also common in youths with bipolar disorder. Older adolescents who develop the illness may have more classic, adult type episodes and symptoms which are more clearly defined and thus easier to diagnose. Effective treatment depends on appropriate and accurate diagnosis with attention to the more common differential diagnoses and potential co-morbid diagnoses.

Henin and colleagues (2007) reported many parents describing their children with bipolar disorder as being different from early infancy. Frequently, parents described their infants as sleeping erratically; not sleeping long; being irritable, fussy, and difficult to settle; temperamental; and extremely anxious, often experiencing great difficulty with separation from the mother. Night terrors, rages, fear of death, and behaviors that fit into the diagnostic category of oppositional defiant disorder are often an aspect of bipolar disorder.

Currently, the assessment, diagnosis, and treatment of children with bipolar disorder in children and adolescents present a number of unique risks and challenges. It is noteworthy that the diagnosis in children and adolescents is established using the same *DSM-IV-TR* (APA, 2000) criteria as are used with adults. The differential diagnosis between bipolar disorder, attention-deficit hyperactivity disorder, oppositional defiant disorder, conduct disorder, and other anxiety disorders requires special consideration (Luby, Tandon, & Nicol, 2007). (See Chapters 15 and 17.)

Bipolar disorders in children and adolescents have been far less studied than adult-onset bipolar illness. Particularly in prepubertal children, the incidence and validity of the diagnosis remain unsettled. The epidemiology of juvenile-onset bipolar disorder continues to be an open topic for research. The course of bipolar disorder in children and adolescents has also received limited systematic study. However, research to date supports a clinical picture of a relapsing, recurrent illness with substantial morbidity (Birmaher et al., 2006).

Systematic studies of pharmacologic intervention of acute mania in children and adolescents are limited in number and scope. Clinical justification for the use of acute antimanic agents such as lithium and divalproex sodium (Depakote) continues to be based on studies conducted in adults. There remains an immediate and significant need for additional research into all aspects of early-onset bipolar disorder.

OLDER ADULTHOOD

Bipolar disorder is frequently missed or misdiagnosed in the older adult. Depression is beginning to be more readily diagnosed both in primary care settings and in community settings. However, the mood elevation, increase in energy and activity, and other subtle manifestations of bipolar disorder are often left unrecognized. Bipolar disorder in the older adult increases the risk of suicide. Complicating the assessment and diagnosis of bipolar disorder in the geriatric population is that the client may present with various medical conditions, such as dementia. Twenty percent of the older adult population will have their first episode of the illness after the age of 50 (Aziz, Lorberg, & Tampi, 2006). Mixed state bipolar disorder is more common in adolescents and individuals over the age of 60.

TREATMENT MODALITIES

The treatment of bipolar disorders requires a holistic approach that involves pharmacologic and psychotherapeutic interventions. Acute symptoms require pharmacologic interventions that reduce symptoms and facilitate a higher level of function and quality of life. First-line treatment of bipolar disorders depends upon the clinical presentation, but involves administering atypical antipsychotic medications; lithium and prescribing novel mood stabilizers have proven efficacy in the acute stabilization and maintenance treatment of bipolar disorder. Psychiatric nurses play key roles in administering these agents and monitoring client responses.

PHARMACOLOGIC

Three major categories of psychotropic medications are used in the successful treatment of bipolar disorder: lithium, mood stabilizers, and antipsychotics. In the American Psychiatric Association's (2002) Practice Guidelines for the Treatment of Patients with Bipolar Disorder in the *American Journal of Psychiatry*, there is a high level of consensus on key steps in treating bipolar disorder. These can best be understood by reviewing Table 10–9.

Myths to Overcome

MYTH	FACT
1. Bipolar disorder occurs only in adults.	1. Bipolar disorder is most commonly diagnosed in adults. However, bipolar traits or characteristics are frequently identified in the pre-adolescent and adolescent population (Sachs, Baldassano, Truman, Christine, & Guille, 2000; Geller et al., 2001; Birmaher et al., 2006).
2. Bipolar disorder is easily diagnosed and treated.	2. Bipolar disorder is frequently misdiagnosed as schizophrenia, ADHD, or other mood or anxiety disorders (Goodwin, 1999; Torrey, 1999; Cassano et al., 1999; U.S. DHHS, 2001).

TABLE 10–9
Acute Psychopharmacological Treatment

Manic or Mixed Episodes—First-line treatment for more severe mixed episodes is either lithium plus an antipsychotic or valproate plus an antipsychotic. (Alternatives include carbamazapine or oxcarbazepine instead of lithium or valproate.)

- First-line treatment for breakthrough episodes should be to optimize the medication dose. Introduction or resumption of antipsychotic medication may be necessary. Acutely ill clients may also require a combination of an antipsychotic medication and benzodiazepine to manage agitation, anxiety, and psychosis.

Depressive Episodes—First-line treatment is initiation of lithium or lamotrigine. Antidepressant monotherapy is not recommended. In severely suicidal or psychotic clients, ECT may be a reasonable alternative (especially during pregnancy).

Rapid Cycling—Initial intervention is to identify and treat hypothyroidism or drug and/or alcohol use that may contribute to cycling. Initial treatment should be carbamazepine (Tegretol) or valproate. Alternative treatment is lamotrigine (Lamictal) and may include a combination of medications.

MOOD STABILIZERS

There are two properties that define mood stabilizers: (1) they provide relief from acute episodes of mania or depression or prevent them from occurring, and (2) they do not worsen depression or mania or lead to increases in cycling. Pharmacologic treatment of bipolar disorder often requires a combined pharmacologic approach. This often involves an antidepressant and a mood stabilizer (Tables 10–10 and 10–11). Before administering mood stabilizers, nurses need to check basic laboratory studies, including electrolytes, complete blood count (CBC), chemistries, thyroid function test, and pregnancy tests in women of childbearing age. Because these agents are harmful to the developing fetus, nurses also need to ask questions about birth control methods. Health education is an integral part of caring for the client with bipolar disorder.

Lithium carbonate was the first psychotropic agent shown to prevent recurrent episodes of illness. The three major indications for lithium are relapse prevention, management of

mania, and suicide prevention. Lithium has provided a major pharmacologic leap in the treatment of bipolar disorder. Studies indicate that Lithium turns off the enzyme GSK-3β causing the receptor REV-erba to degrade, leading to rhythmic turning on of the protein Bmal 1 which starts the clock cycle that acts to restore daily rhythms in bipolar disorder (Yin et al., 2006). Before lithium, the primary psychotropic agents used to treat bipolar disorder were antipsychotics.

Several anticonvulsants have been found effective in the treatment of bipolar disorder. The most frequently used are valproic acid (Depakene), also known as divalproex (Depakote), and carbamazepine (Tegretol). Consensus and practice guidelines concerning the treatment of bipolar disorders indicate the efficacy of newer agents such as lamotrigine (Lamictal), oxcarbazepine (Trileptal), and topiramate (Topamax) (Sadock et al., 2006). The most common side effects of lamotrigine (Lamictal) include dizziness, headaches, somnolence, and a dangerous allergic rash. Major side effects associated with topiramate include ataxia, dizziness, and kidney stones. Major benefits of

TABLE 10–10
Commonly Used Mood Stabilizers, Usual Adult Doses and Therapeutic Serum Levels

Mood Stabilizer	Adult Dose Range	Therapeutic Serum Levels
Lithium (Eskalith, Lithobid, Lithonate)	600–1800 mg/d	0.6–1.2 mEq/L
Divalproex (Depakote)	750–4200 mg/d	50–100 µ/ml
Other anticonvulsants used as mood stabilizers		
Carbamazepine (Tegretol, Carbatrol)	400–1600 gm/d	4–12 µ/ml
Lamotrigine (Lamictal)	300–500 mg/d	N/A
Topiramate (Topamax)	400–1600 mg/d	N/A

TABLE 10–11
Antidepressants Used in Bipolar Disorder (Not Used as Monotherapy)

Buproprion (Wellbutrin)

Selective Serotonin Reuptake Inhibitors (SSRIs):

　Citalopram (Celexa)

　Escitalopram (Lexapro)

　Fluoxetine (Prozac)

　Fluvoxamine (Luvox)

　Paroxetine (Paxil)

　Sertraline (Zoloft)

Venlafaxine (Effexor)

Duloxetine (Cymbalta)

If these are ineffective or cause undesirable side effects, other
　choices include:

　Mirtazapine (Remeron)

*Monoamine oxidase inhibitors:

　Phenelzine (Nardil)

　Tranylcypromine (Parnate)

　Selegiline transdermal (Emsaim)

†Trycyclic antidepressants:

　Amitriptyline (Elavil)

　Desipramine (Norpramine, Pertofrane)

　Imipramine (Tofranil)

　Nortriptyline (Pamelor)

---

*These are effective but require the client to stay on a special diet to
avoid dangerous side effects.
†Tricyclics are more likely to cause side effects or set off manic
episodes or rapid cycling than newer ADP agents.

---

these agents include neutral weight gain and weight loss
(Sadock et al., 2006). (See Chapter 29.)

Several of these newer anticonvulsant medications, including lamotrigine (Lamictal), have demonstrated efficacy in the treatment of these disorders. Anticonvulsant medications may be combined with lithium, or with each other, for maximum effect (www.nimh.nih.gov/public/bipolar.cfm).

CONTROVERSIES ABOUT ANTIDEPRESSANTS

Bipolar disorder is a chronic and recurrent psychiatric condition. Mood stabilizers, such as lithium, valproate, and novel agents, such as lamotrigine are used to control and manage symptoms and reduce relapse. The mainstay treatment of manic episodes is a combination of an atypical antipsychotic medication and mood stabilizer (Keck, 2006;

Lin, Mok, & Yatham, 2006). A brief mention of antidepressants is important because they are not mainstay treatment for bipolar disorder, but they continue to be prescribed for persons with bipolar disorder. The risk-benefits of using antidepressants as monotherapy or adjuncts to mood stabilizers continue to be debated among experts (Post et al., 2006). Sometimes clients are misdiagnosed with unipolar disorder until they fail to respond to monotherapy antidepressants or switch from depressive episode to hypomania or mania. It is usually during these periods that a differential diagnosis of bipolar disorder needs to be confirmed. Finally, monotherapy use of antidepressants has not demonstrated efficacy in the treatment of bipolar depression and is discouraged due to the risk of "switching" from a depressive episode to a manic or hypomanic episode especially with novel antidepressants, such as selective serotonin reuptake inhibitors (SSRIs) and selective norepinephrine reuptake inhibitors (SNRIs) (Post et al., 2006).

ANTIPSYCHOTICS

Antipsychotics are often used as an adjunct to benzodiazepines to acute psychosis and agitation (Sadock, 2006) until the mood stabilizer becomes effective. There are two kinds of antipsychotics used today: the "older," or "conventional," types and the "newer," or "atypical," types. Serious problems can occur with the use of older, or conventional, antipsychotics such as the potential to develop extrapyramidal symptoms (EPS) and tardive dyskinesia. The primary mode of antipsychotic action is still likely dopamine blockade although there is controversy about the precise mechanism at the receptor level (Sadock et al., 2006). The emergence of data supporting the use of olanzapine for mania has resulted in its inclusion in the revised APA guidelines. Lithium, valproate, and the antipsychotic olanzapine are now the first-line recommended treatment for mania (APA, 2002). Today the atypical antipsychotics are usually the first choice for clinicians. See Table 10–12 for a list of atypical antipsychotics, and see Chapter 29 for a discussion of psychopharmacologic therapy.

Children and adolescents with bipolar disorder are generally treated with lithium, but valproate and carbamazepine are also used. Researchers are evaluating the safety and efficacy of these and other psychotropic medications in children and adolescents. There is some evidence that valproate may lead to adverse hormone changes in teenage girls and polycystic ovary syndrome in women who began taking the medication before the age of 20. Thus, young female clients should be closely monitored using periodic pregnancy tests and for signs of polycystic ovaries syndrome (e.g., irregular menses, lower abdominal pain).

Women with bipolar disorder who want to become pregnant face special challenges due to the possible harmful effects of existing mood stabilizing medications on the developing fetus and the nursing infant. Thus, risks and benefits of all possible treatment options should be discussed fully with a clinician with expertise in this area. Controversy about

TABLE 10–12 Current Atypical Antipsychotics
Olanzapine (Zyprexa)
Quetiapine (Seroquel)
Risperidone (Risperdal)
Clozapine (Clozaril)
Ziprasidone (Geodon)
Aripiprazole (Abilify)
*Olanzapine & Fluoxetine (Symbyax)
*Used to treat bipolar mania

TABLE 10–13 Goals for the Client— Inpatient Setting
• Provide a safe environment
• Decrease environmental stimuli
• Eliminate danger to self and others
• Provide avenues for safe energy expenditure
• Stabilize and facilitate adherence to treatment
• Thought processes intact
• Eliminate perceptual disturbances
• Encourage social interactions/decrease isolation
• Improve self-esteem
• Restore normal sleep and eating patterns
• Understand psychoeducation about medications and psychotherapeutic interventions

using these agents during antepartal, pregnancy, and lactation continue to be debated. An in-depth discussion between the client, her significant other, and the obstetrician concerning the risk-benefits is a critical part of treatment planning. New treatments with reduced risks during pregnancy and lactation continue to be studied.

ELECTROCONVULSIVE THERAPY

Electroconvulsive therapy (ECT) is an effective and often life-saving treatment for mania or depression if pharmacologic interventions fail or if symptom severity requires immediate relief (APA, 2000). ECT continues to be criticized by some but remains a safe and effective treatment with minimal side effects. Clients receiving ECT are anesthetized in a closely monitored medical setting and typically receive 6 to 10 treatments over a few weeks. Some of the most common side effects include headaches and temporary memory loss, which returns usually after the course of treatment.

PSYCHOSOCIAL AND BEHAVIORAL INTERVENTIONS

Psychotherapeutic interventions, such as psychosocial and behavioral interventions, combined with pharmacologic approaches, are crucial to positive treatment outcomes. During the acute phase of treatment, psychiatric nurses must maintain a safe and therapeutic milieu that facilitates resolution of symptoms and minimizes complications. Through various psychosocial interventions, the nurse also educates the client and family about medications, treatment options, and other psychotherapies.

TREATMENT CONSIDERATIONS

The most important consideration, whether in an acute (inpatient) or community (outpatient) setting, is safety. The consideration of safety is best addressed if viewed in the

context of appropriate client, family, and milieu management. Also important are issues such as confidentiality and supportive resources for the individual and the family. Clinical management is generally based on pharmacologic intervention and psychotherapy designed to improve client functioning. Treatment considerations must always be based on identification and use of the available resources for the client and the family. It is imperative that every client (and the family, if available) be assisted in the design of a crisis intervention plan. Learning to live with bipolar disorder requires that the client be educated about the disorder and receive specific instructions (Table 10–13) on how best to manage life on a daily basis.

Milieu Management in the Acute Setting

Milieu management is important if the client requires hospitalization in order to be stabilized. Stabilization can be viewed in terms of medications, moods, and behaviors. Clients can be hospitalized for stabilization of either mania or severe depression. Regardless of the reason for admission, environmental stimuli must be controlled and managed appropriately to meet the individual needs of the client and others on the unit. Disruptive behaviors are often prevalent if the client is in the manic phase of bipolar. These behaviors must be managed in a timely and appropriate manner with a predictable plan for the client and staff to follow. Awareness and prevention of suicidal and homicidal intent may necessitate that the client be managed one-on-one with a psychiatric professional. It is imperative that the nurses understand that suicidal or homicidal intent can be expressed in many ways. Aggressive behaviors can quickly escalate and be directed internally or externally (toward the self or others). Once the client is stabilized, psychoeducational classes are helpful in maintaining biological and psychological equilibrium. This will be followed up in the community or outpatient setting. In summary, effective milieu management requires three essential elements: safety, limit setting, and stabilization (see Chapter 32).

Community Setting

Equally important as management in the acute care setting is management in the community setting. During the acute phase of illness and intervention, the focus is on *stabilization* of medications, moods, and behaviors. Once the client has achieved stabilization and returns to the community, the focus is on *maintenance* and *monitoring* of medications, moods, and behaviors. During the *acute phase* of illness and treatment, the client and nurse develop a healthy plan of daily living (see Table 10–14). As the client regains status as an active and productive member of the community, she will be able to develop and maintain the supportive resources needed to maintain mental health and well-being. It is important for the nurse to assist the client in understanding the importance of continuing to take the prescribed medications and participating in any prescribed psychotherapy. A review of the research literature on bipolar relapse prevention identifies that individuals receiving psychotherapy treatment in addition to medication had significantly fewer relapses (Gutierrez & Scott, 2004).

In order to identify best practice in the treatment of bipolar disorder, the Systematic Treatment Enhancement Program (STEP-BD) research study was undertaken from 1998 to 2005. This multisite study included 4,360 community-based participants with bipolar disorder. Findings from this study are currently being published and initial results indicate that 58 percent of this client group achieved recovery as a result of participation. Treatment consisted of a standardized

treatment protocol used by trained health care providers. The STEP-BD protocol included the use of mood stabilizing medication, both newer and older classes of antidepressants, atypical antipsychotics, and psychosocial interventions (Sadock, 2006). Additional outcomes from the research are forthcoming and have potential to improve evidence-based practice strategies for persons with this diagnosis. When psychotherapy is part of the comprehensive approach to care it should involve individual, family, and group therapy as appropriate to the client's needs (see Chapter 33).

TABLE 10–14
Learning to Live with Bipolar Disorder

- Maintain a stable sleep pattern
- Maintain a regular pattern of activity
- Avoid alcohol and/or other substances (both licit and illicit drugs)
- Ask for and use the support of family and friends
- Reduce stress at home and at work
- Be aware of your own early warning signs (often the first clue is change in sleep needs)
- Develop a repertoire of effective coping and problem-solving skills
- Develop emotional tolerance/regulation skills
- Recognize automatic negative thinking and mitigate them appropriately

---

CASE STUDY

Mark is a 23-year-old client admitted to the acute psychiatric unit with a diagnosis of bipolar disorder, most recent episode manic. His speech is rapid and pressured; his thoughts are disorganized as evidenced by flight of ideas, and irritable and agitated mood. During your interview with him he states, "I am the President of Nigeria."

The following scenario depicts the nurse-client interaction. Prior to interviewing the client, which of the following is the *most* important nursing intervention?

a. Ensuring personal and staff safety by making sure there is a clear exit and not seeing the client alone

b. Administering an antipsychotic medication to manage his agitation and psychotic symptoms (e.g., grandiose delusions, disorganized thoughts)

c. Correcting the client's delusion that he is the President of Nigeria

d. Both a and b

Answers

a. *Correct.* It is paramount that the nurse ensure personal and staff safety prior to interviewing a client with psychotic symptoms. Under these circumstances, it is difficult to reason with the client and predict his behavior.

b. *Correct.* Administering an antipsychotic medication reduces psychotic symptoms, agitation, fearfulness, and anxiety.

c. *Incorrect.* Correcting the client's delusion is counterproductive and serves to increase agitation and risk of violence.

d. *Correct.* Both a and b are correct.

Family Focused

Unstable mood swings, financial extravagance, impaired social skills, sexual indiscretions, and violent behaviors are clearly a source of turmoil, conflict, and concern to the significant others of individuals who have bipolar disorder. During the acute phase of the disorder, family members will have many questions about the symptoms of mania and depression, the treatment, and the prognosis for the future. Education of the family is paramount at this time. Educating family members about bipolar disorder serves two functions. First, it helps the family members cope with their own pain and suffering and prepares them for difficult times to come. Second, it encourages them to become active partners in the treatment process.

Those who live with, have regular contact with, or who may be in a position to assist clients with treatment should be involved in the education process. Spouses, children, and parents are possibilities for inclusion. Of particular importance when dealing with diverse cultures is the consideration of individuals who are *designated*, or *extended*, family for involvement in the education process. For each nurse the real question should be, "Who does the client want involved in the treatment?" It is necessary to tailor the involvement of significant others to the special needs of each individual. Maintaining client confidentiality by seeking permission before communicating clinical information to significant others is of particular importance.

Because of the genetic component of bipolar disorder, couples frequently need information about the effect of this disorder on future children. Questions such as medication management during pregnancy are common as well as the effect of illness episodes on the psychological development of current children. None of these questions have answers that apply to all client situations, however. Assessing each situation and seeking appropriate expert referrals in the areas of reproductive counseling, pharmacologic consultation, or family therapy best serve the needs of clients and their families.

Nursing interventions that involve treatment of the client with bipolar disorder within the context of the family must address two important areas: (1) stabilizing the client and (2) supporting the family as a functional, adaptive unit. Both have equal importance, and interventions and resources must be identified and targeted toward both. Clients with this disorder precipitate levels of family discord during and following episodes of illness that lead to poor short-term outcomes and

vulnerability to social isolation. Social isolation or lack of social support places the individual with the disorder at higher risk for future episodes. Studies have found that family-focused interventions along with mood stabilizing medications lead to improved long-term adherence among married clients where one spouse has a bipolar disorder, especially female clients.

Family-focused, psychoeducational programs have gained prominence because of their multifaceted approach to client and family needs. Psychoeducational programs consist of lectures and information about the disorder, its treatment, and prognosis; communication-enhancement training; and problem-solving skills training. Clients with families who participate in this therapeutic approach remained stable for longer periods in the community without relapsing. They also showed greater reductions in mood disorder symptoms over a 1-year period. The limitation of the family approach is that it appears to be more effective in mediating the onset of depressive episodes than those of manic episodes. Family-focused psychoeducational (FFP) approaches can be used in inpatient or outpatient settings and can be adapted to brief family interventions with positive outcomes. Regardless of the theory (e.g., psychodynamic, cognitive-behavioral) supporting the FFP program, all have been demonstrated as more beneficial than using medication alone. Consistency and constancy of the treatment approach contribute to wellness and enhanced stability when the program is well matched to the needs of clients and their families.

One final consideration for the nurse when discussing family needs is *adequately* matching the family's identified needs with compatible resources. In mental health care, congruence between perceived need and service provision is critical to recovery. In the area of mental health, evidence suggests that services have not been sufficiently responsive to the needs of ethnic minority clients. When compared with the white majority, ethnic minority populations are less likely to use mental health services, are more likely to drop out of treatment prematurely, and are less likely to discuss their problems openly. One common explanation for these reactions is that ethnic minority clients' values conflict with the process of traditional mental health treatment. Many individuals of ethnic groups associate stigma and shame with using mental health service or hold beliefs about mental illness that bring them to seek medical or spiritual care rather than

---

TABLE 10–15
Minority Clients and Barriers to Mental Health Care Use

- Misinterpretation of culturally based behaviors by health professionals
- Lack of a client and health professional racial or ethnic match
- Unrecognized characteristics of family structure of minority groups

- Unrecognized socioeconomic pressures on, and isolation of, the client/family (especially with immigrant populations)
- Client mistrust of the providers and the systems providing services

mental health care for their problems. On the other hand, traditional mental health services have been criticized for insufficiently addressing cultural factors important to these clients and for their inaccessibility resulting from inconvenient appointment times and locations. Such difficulties are exacerbated by the fact that the majority of health care providers (including nurses) come from nonminority groups and have been trained to provide care using approaches largely developed by nonminorities. Problems for clients of minority groups generally arise from one or more of the situations listed in Table 10–15.

THE ROLE OF THE NURSE

Nursing care of the client with bipolar disorders is likely to occur in both inpatient and outpatient practice settings. Normally, during the acute manic episode, the client requires a structured milieu that provides safety and a therapeutic environment that promotes symptoms management and adaptive behavioral changes. The role of the nurse is also likely to include pharmacologic and psychotherapeutic interventions. The following section describes the role of the generalist and advanced-practice psychiatric-mental health nurse in caring for the client with biopolar disorder.

THE GENERALIST NURSE

The generalist nurse working in a mental health care setting has a critical role in the provision of care to clients and their families. In the inpatient setting, the nurse must be aware of the specific goals for each client and modify the environment to assist the client in achieving those goals. Addressing the

essential elements of safety, limit setting, and stabilization requires critical thinking and problem solving on the part of the nurse. Communication with the client during the manic phase is a challenge that requires patience and assertive communication skills. Attending to tone, verbal, and nonverbal messages to and from the client is important. Creativity is required to identify avenues for safe energy expenditure, adequate nutrition, and sleep. Collaboration among all inpatient team members is necessary to avoid or minimize potential conflict resulting from manic behaviors and impulsivity. The nurse needs to be keenly aware of escalating thoughts and behaviors, and when to decrease the client's exposure to environmental stimuli. Consistency among all staff in the application of rules and therapeutic decisions is key to building trust.

The nurse is frequently one of the first recognizable professionals encountered by the individual seeking services, whether the setting is an inpatient or outpatient one. In outpatient care of the client, the generalist nurse continues to be responsible for assessing basic physical and mental status, maintaining the client's safety, monitoring medication response and side effects, educating the client and significant others about the client's condition and its treatment, identifying community resources, and coordinating the plan of care with the multidisciplinary team. In the broader arena, the generalist nurse frequently functions as community educator and advocate for clients with mental health concerns. These roles are essential in relation to clients who have a persistent illness that is poorly understood by the community at large. Undertaking the role of educator and advocate helps to counteract stigma and makes it easier for others with bipolar disorder to seek services early. Lastly, the generalist nurse has the obligation to keep abreast of scientific knowledge that

RESEARCH ABSTRACT

The Association of Comorbid Anxiety Disorders with Suicide Attempts and Suicidal Ideation in Outpatients with Bipolar Disorder

Simon, N. M., Zalta, A. K., Otto, M. W., Ostacher, M. J., Fischmann, D., Chow, C. W., et al. (2007). *Journal of Psychiatric Research, 41,* 255–264.

Study/Problem

Researchers examined the association between concomitant anxiety disorders with suicide attempts and suicidal ideations in clients with bipolar disorder in outpatient clinics.

Method

Researchers used the ancillary to the Systematic Treatment Enhancement Program for Bipolar Disorder (STEP-BD) to explore this relationship. The study comprised 120 subjects in outpatient settings who were asked to complete a comprehensive assessment of suicidal ideation and behaviors. Data were used to determine the relationship between current and lifetime concomitant anxiety disorders with suicidal ideation and behaviors with adjustment for potential extraneous variables in regression models; bipolar severity, including an earlier age at bipolar onset; and a lack of current bipolar recovery.

Findings

Findings revealed that although concomitant anxiety disorders and bipolar disorder may increase the risk of suicidal behaviors, other factors, such as severity of symptoms, early age onset, and persistent symptoms, may also increase the risk of these behaviors. Additional studies are needed to determine the precise relationship between these variables and suicide risk. Gender, symptom distress, and functional status were positively correlated with depression, whereas the coexisting conditions were not significantly correlated with depression scores.

Implications for Psychiatric Nurses

Individuals with bipolar disorder are at high risk for suicidal behaviors and completed suicide. As with other psychiatric disorders, suicide risk requires an in-depth nursing and psychiatric assessment initially and throughout treatment. High-risk behaviors and individuals at risk are crucial nursing interventions that mitigate suicide risk in clients with bipolar disorder.

supports professional development, cultural competence, and a high level of evidence-based care for these clients.

THE ADVANCED-PRACTICE PSYCHIATRIC REGISTERED NURSE

Roles and responsibilities of the advanced-practice nurse include all of those previously discussed under the generalist nurse. For the APN, however, there is an expanded expectation of participating in research. The importance of participating in psychiatric-mental health nursing research lies in the need to add to the knowledge base and establish best practice standards for psychiatric nursing.

Additionally, functions of the APN will vary according to the situation and APN's particular role. Factors influencing the role of the APN include whether the continuum of care is an inpatient or an outpatient one and the legal parameters of practice. All APNs are guided by their particular state's nurse practice act. This determines whether or not nurses are allowed to prescribe medications and if they are required to have a collaborative agreement with a physician.

If the client is being seen by the APN in a private practice site, the nurse may provide individual psychotherapy, family psychotherapy, group therapy, psychoeducational information, medication evaluation and management, and referral to other health care providers if needed. One overriding role of the APN is to coordinate the care among the network of providers, thus maintaining a clear picture of the overall plan of care.

THE NURSING PROCESS

The nursing process should be viewed as a mechanism through which nurses develop their contribution to the plan of care established by a multidisciplinary team in collaboration with the client. As such, the first step before developing a care plan is to identify desired outcomes based on team input and client and family needs. As the nurse develops a perspective of the independent and interdependent roles that can be played in attaining the desired therapeutic outcome, the nursing interventions can be formulated in a manner that reflects an understanding of the nursing role.

ASSESSMENT

Appropriate identification of nursing focused problems or diagnoses must be a result of an ongoing thorough assessment. Areas of assessment that provide the most specific data related to bipolar disorder include mood, motor activity-energy, sexual interest, sleep, irritability, speech (rate and amount), language-thought processes, content of speech, disruptive-aggressive behavior, appearance, and insight regarding the current situation. In today's mental health care system, clients are only admitted to inpatient settings when they exhibit the most severe symptoms. Assessment (and treatment) is performed within a restricted period; therefore, the nurse must be efficient

and precise in accomplishing these activities. One standardized instrument that can assist the nurse in systematic assessment in these areas is the *Young Rating Scale for Mania* (Young, Biggs, Ziegler, & Meyer, 1978). Clients can be evaluated through observation, and use of the instrument can provide objective data regarding the client's current status. Observational assessment is particularly useful during the acute stages of mania. As the individual stabilizes and is better able to focus and interact, other methods of assessment are available for use by the nurse, including client self-rating scales, symptom tracking by the client and the nurse, and client mood charting (Figure 10-6). These methods are particularly useful in outpatient settings where most clients receive their care.

NURSING DIAGNOSIS

Nursing diagnoses are identified based on the client's subjective and objective data gathered during a bipolar episode. Table 10-16 includes a list of common nursing diagnoses when developing a plan of care for an individual with bipolar disorder. According to the type of the disorder, and the stage of illness (acute, intermediate, or long term), variations are expected in the priority given each identified diagnoses and the interventions chosen to address them.

OUTCOME IDENTIFICATION

The nurse caring for an individual with bipolar disorder, as with all psychiatric disorders, must identify incremental goals

TABLE 10–16
Common Nursing Diagnoses

Risk for activity intolerance	Deficit knowledge
Impaired adjustment	Imbalanced nutrition: less than body requirements
Impaired verbal communication	Impaired parenting
	Risk for powerlessness
Compromised family coping	Self-care deficit
Interrupted family processes	Risk for situational low self-esteem
Dysfunctional grieving	
Ineffective health maintenance	Social isolation
Hopelessness	Disturbed thought processes
Ineffective coping	Risk for self-directed violence
Risk for injury	Risk for other-directed violence

Note. From *Nursing Diagnosis: Definitions and Classification* 2007–2008, by North American Nursing Diagnosis Association (NANDA), 2007, Philadelphia: Author. Adapted with permission.

MOOD LOG

Name: _____   Month: _____   Year: _____

Rate mood

```
0 --------- 50 --------- 100
Dep      Normal      Mania
```

Days of Month →	1	2	3	4	5	6	7	8	9	10	11	12	13	14	15	16	17	18	19	20	21	22	23	24	25	26	27	28	29	30	31
Mania																															
Depression																															
Anxiety (1–10)																															

Medication

	1	2	3	4	5	6	7	8	9	10	11	12	13	14	15	16	17	18	19	20	21	22	23	24	25	26	27	28	29	30	31

Menses

Sleep

Figure 10–6 Mood log

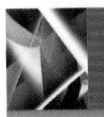

CASE STUDY

A Client with Bipolar Disorder (Mary)

The client, "Mary," was a 43-year-old divorced African American female, referred to the college mental health clinic by the faculty in her program of study. She was a graduate student in religious studies. Her professors mandated her evaluation and treatment in the clinic in order for her to remain in their program. They cited behavioral problems, especially chaotic interactions and inappropriate anger while on community assignments, as the reason for the referral. When Mary called to schedule her appointment with the nurse, she sounded very angry and voiced her belief that the faculty was discriminating against her because of her race. She also requested a therapist who was Christian and willing to discuss theological issues. As a psychiatric-mental health advanced-practice nurse at the clinic, I assumed the role as Mary's therapist.

During presentation for her evaluation, Mary was clean, well-groomed, and dressed appropriately for the weather. Her **affect** was angry and hypomanic as evidenced by loose associations, **pressured speech,** paranoid ideation about her teachers, and an intense level of energy. Pressured speech refers to a disturbance in verbal expression of thought characterized by an overproduction of rapid speech that is often loud, unsolicited by social interaction, and difficult to interrupt. However, she was able to complete her interview and follow directions. The assessment revealed other symptoms, including decreased need for sleep, restlessness, increased productivity, and racing thoughts. There was evidence of possible grandiosity as she repeatedly discussed her need to help minority people overcome oppression by the dominant culture.

Her pediatric history was highly significant. She was the fifth of seven children born to a working-class, married African American couple. The family resided in a rural southern state. Mary was the only child in the family to be singled out for sexual abuse by her alcoholic father. Her mother and siblings abused and blamed her for her father's abuse. She reported verbal abuse by her mother in the form of sexualized names and insults that the client at the time was too young to understand. Both parents physically abused her. She further reported attempted sexual abuse by two of her brothers and molestation by a paternal uncle. Her father was killed in a motor vehicle accident when Mary was 10 years old. This loss resulted in her first episode of reactive depression. Mary recalls crying uncontrollably, which resulted in her family verbally abusing her for this reaction. She again suffered depression at ages 12 and 14.

At 16, she became pregnant but was able to finish high school that year. She gave birth to a son and suffered a severe postpartum depression that resulted in a suicide attempt by overdose. The family physician gave her a trial of lithium carbonate, but she did not continue taking it because it made her feel fatigued. She married a year after her son's birth. Mary again became pregnant and bore a daughter. She divorced her husband after 4 years because he was physically and emotionally abusive.

Her second marriage came a year after the divorce. Mary gave birth to another daughter that year and 2 years later she gave birth to her fourth child, a son. Her second marriage lasted 14 years. She divorced the second husband because of his alcoholism, physical abuse, infidelity, and alleged molestation of their two youngest children. A friend of her second husband also raped Mary.

Despite her difficulties during this time, Mary was able to earn an associate's degree in information technology and a bachelor's degree in special education. She suffered her first onset of mania at age 20, and has had hypomania interspersed with occasional depression episodes ever since. Mary credited her hypomania with helping her to achieve her academic goals while caring for her family. Her credentials also included ordination in the ministry through her church. During the intake interview, it was unclear how effective her parenting was with her children. However, it became increasingly evident that contact with her children was minimal at the initiation of treatment.

Mary was eventually able to accept her diagnosis, as evidenced by her continued participation in treatment, mental health support groups, and conferences. She remained alienated from her family of origin but maintained contact with her children and grandchildren. Her oldest son, in particular, was very supportive of his mother's recovery. She was seen in the clinic for a total of 3 years until she finished her master's degree. At completion of her degree, she accepted a job in another state working as a hospital chaplain.

Mary was diagnosed according to the following *DSM-IV-TR* (APA, 2000):

Axis I:	296.89 Bipolar II Disorder, With Psychotic Features
	309.81 Post-traumatic Stress Disorder
	V62.89 Phase of Life Problem
Axis II:	No Diagnosis
Axis III:	Hypertension
Axis IV:	Severe Stressors Related to Symptom Management, Academic Courseload, Family Dysfunction, Decreased Social Support
Axis V:	GAF Current: 50
Year to Date:	60

A plan of care was developed and implemented over a period of 3 years. See Nursing Care Plan 10–1. Care strategies included those directed toward the client, and her support systems.

through which the client makes measurable, attainable (realistic) steps toward improvement. These incremental goals or outcomes in bipolar disorder are prioritized according to (1) safety and physiological functioning, (2) improved coping, and (3) return to preillness level of functioning. The nurse must be sure to identify outcomes directed at both the individual and the family or significant others to support the client's successful transition and growth.

PLANNING

Planning of any therapeutic activity involves determining the ability of the client to be involved in the planned intervention. Initially, expectations should be low for clients with acute presentations of mania. However, nurses must be creative in identifying areas in which a person can be involved in even the smallest aspect of the planning process.

Newly admitted inpatient clients should be informed of the identified plan of care, which may include limit setting of disruptive behaviors, strategies to provide nutrition during a manic episode, and safety measures versus potentially injurious activities. As the client's condition stabilizes, the nurse must incorporate the client and family's priorities into plans that eventually lead to preparation for discharge. Planning should include areas such as education and resources.

IMPLEMENTATION AND EVALUATION

These two aspects of care must be considered jointly when working collaboratively with clients and their families. Successful reintegration of the client into the family and the community is a long-term goal that hinges on successful coordination of interventions and evaluation of their effectiveness. Instillation of hope into the client's life is best facilitated by the development of interventions and methods of evaluation that are valued by the client and family. An example of this may be implementing a medication regimen that includes a dietary education program that will minimize weight gain resulting from the mood stabilizing medication. The evaluative component would not only examine medication effectiveness and compliance but also prevention of weight gain and client satisfaction.

The following case study illustrates one individual experiencing bipolar disorder. The case provides an example of characteristics of the diagnosis and the effects of the illness on interpersonal relationships, such as the family and the nurse as an integral part in the client's recovery. A nursing care plan follows that is based on this case study.

SUMMARY

◆ Bipolar disorder is a recurrent mood disorder featuring one or more episodes of mania or mixed episodes of mania and depression.

◆ Bipolar disorder manic episode is characterized by impulsivity, racing thoughts, and hyperthymia.

◆ Bipolar disorder affects 1 to 1.5 percent of the general population in the United States, affecting equal numbers of males and females.

◆ There are many theories related to the etiology of this disorder, including psychological, developmental, and neurobiological theories. Research findings indicate that individuals with bipolar disorder exhibit variations in brain structure, neurochemistry, and impaired brain function.

◆ Figure 10–7 is a summary of factors influential in the development of bipolar disorder. Bipolar disorder occurs in children and the elderly and is frequently misdiagnosed in both populations.

◆ There are three major categories of psychotropic medications used in the treatment of this disorder: lithium, mood stabilizers, and antipsychotics.

◆ In the acute phase of the disorder, the focus of treatment is safety, limit setting, and stabilization.

◆ For most people, bipolar disorder is lifelong; therefore treatment considerations must always be based on identification and use of available resources for the client and the family.

◆ In caring for the client with bipolar disorder, the generalist nurse is responsible for assessing basic physical and mental status, maintaining the client's safety, monitoring medication response and side effects, educating the client and significant others about the client's condition and its treatment, identifying culturally appropriate community resources, and coordinating the plan of care with the multidisciplinary team.

◆ The advanced-practice psychiatric nursing roles most often employed with clients with bipolar (or other) disorders include psychiatric evaluation, diagnosis, treatment (including various modes of psychotherapy), and medication management.

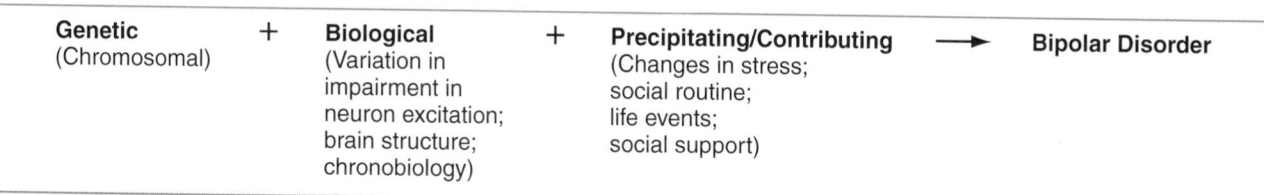

Figure 10–7 Summary of known factors influential in the development of bipolar disorder.

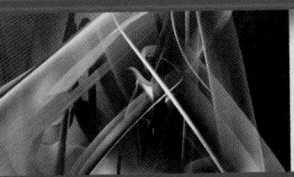

A Client with Bipolar Disorder (Mary)

Nursing Diagnosis: Disturbed Thought Processes as evidenced by paranoid ideation anger, loose associations, pressured speech, racing thoughts, restlessness, decreased sleep, and possible grandiosity

Outcome Identification	Nursing Actions	Rationales	Evaluation
1. By [date], Mary will no longer experience altered cognition and mood will be stabilized.	1a. Assess Mary for safety concerns.	1a–b. Determining client's basic safety and care needs must be priority.	*Goal met:* Mary reports that she is no longer experiencing racing thoughts, and that sleep has improved. The nurse notes that Mary no longer exhibits loose associations, pressured speech, or expresses paranoid ideation.
	1b. Assess Mary's thought processes and level of hyperactivity.		
	1c. Administer prescribed mood stabilizer and/or antipsychotic medication.	1c. Medications are calming and restore brain chemistry, reduce agitation, reduce suicide risk, and help behavioral control.	
	1d. Decrease environmental stimuli.	1d. Reduces stimuli and mitigates anxiety and agitation.	
	1e. Communicate with Mary in a calm voice, using brief direct statements and refocus interaction as needed.	1e. Allows the client the best opportunity to focus and process information.	
	1f. Identify mutual perspectives that can be used to begin a therapeutic alliance.	1f–g. Forming a therapeutic relationship with a client experiencing any level of mania must begin with assessing and using reality based data for therapeutic agreement.	
	1g. Develop a contract with Mary regarding safety and treatment.		
	1h. Collaboratively evaluate effectiveness of prescribed medications.		
	1i. Educate Mary about her medications.	1h–i. Assists the client in managing thoughts and facilitates adequate self care.	

(continues)

Nursing Care Plan 10–1 (continued)

Nursing Diagnosis: Ineffective Coping

as evidenced by patterns of chaotic interpersonal interaction with family, peers, teachers, and history of suicidal attempts

Outcome Identification	Nursing Actions	Rationales	Evaluation
1. By [date], Mary will be able to use adaptive strategies for interpersonal interaction and problem solving.	1a. Assess Mary's perceptions of her current situation. 1b. Provide positive feedback on Mary's accomplishments to date.	1a–b. Understanding and addressing Mary's pattern of behavior fosters self awareness and her willingness and ability to assume adaptive approaches to ongoing situations and lifelong illness.	*Goal met:* Through a lengthy treatment process (2 years), Mary was active in the treatment process. She was able to identify areas for needed change, and developed and practiced new ways of coping.
	1c. Assist Mary in identifying educational and career goals that are important to her, and evaluate the effect of her behavior on those goals.	1c. Identifying and verbalizing her accomplishments throughout the therapeutic process assists her in focusing and building on her strengths. A positive rather than negative self-image is supported.	Mary is currently able to manage interactions and problem solving with her family and others.
	1d. Collaboratively develop a plan to address crisis management and interpersonal problems. 1e. Develop and rehearse strategies with Mary to facilitate adaptive interaction. 1f. Discuss with Mary feelings associated with problem behaviors and recognition of warning signs of mania. 1g. Explore with Mary the outcome of adaptive strategies put into practice.	1d–g. Strategies for behavioral change must include the collaboration and evaluation of the client throughout the process to ensure investment in and appropriateness of the interventions.	
	1h. Provide positive feedback on each improvement.	1h. Positive feedback is reinforcement and motivation for sustained change.	
	1i. With Mary's approval, identify strategies to incorporate the family into the treatment process.	1i. Because bipolar disorder is a lifelong illness, involvement of the family for support and collaboration enhances the success of the client.	

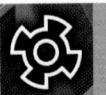

CRITICAL THINKING

1. As a result of managed care, many inpatient mental health settings have only 3 to 4 days to stabilize and care for the client with bipolar disorder. If a client enters your unit in the acute manic phase, identify the approach you would take to make that brief stay as therapeutic as possible and prepare the client for ongoing treatment.

2. Many generalist nurses work within medical settings. As part of the general population, clients with bipolar disorder are frequently seen for medical conditions. What would be the nurse's role when a client diagnosed with bipolar disorder comes in for another condition? What might be the approach for providing comprehensive assessment and holistic care for such a client?

3. As a nurse, the role of community educator is an important one. While functioning in that capacity, nurses frequently identify opportunities to act as advocates. During a presentation on stress and physical health, a comment is made by someone in the audience about how a relative has becama stressed, started acting "hyper" and "crazy," and had to be hospitalized. How might those comments be addressed?

SUGGESTIONS FOR CLINICAL CONFERENCES

1. Select an adolescent or older adult client with bipolar disorder. Identify the mood disturbance and behavioral changes that were present during the episode of bipolar disorder. Identify which signs and symptoms were typical and which ones were not according to the age group.

2. Discuss the history of a client with bipolar disorder. Identify if any family members of that client have experienced depression or mania and how many family members could be identified.

3. Select a client with bipolar disorder who has significant others with whom the client routinely interacts. Identify communication issues that might be improved by psychoeducation. Plan an intervention that might be appropriate and how the intervention might be evaluated.

STUDY QUESTIONS

1. Current knowledge indicates that bipolar disorder is caused by:
   a. biological factors
   b. genetic factors
   c. psychosocial stressors
   d. all of the above

2. Across all types of bipolar disorder, common symptoms of mania include:
   a. labile affect and paranoia
   b. distractibility and dysthymia
   c. hyperthymia and racing thoughts
   d. dysphoria and rapid cycling

3. Older adults may develop bipolar disorder for the first time during their senior years. What differences may be observed when assessing these individuals' histories?
   a. Greater degree of circulatory disease
   b. Less social support
   c. More stressful life events
   d. More depression

4. The nurse uses many techniques to assist in the client's recovery. All of the following interventions are appropriate for the generalist to perform *except*:
   a. psychoeducation about the disorder
   b. psychotherapy work with the client
   c. identification of resources in collaboration with the client
   d. monitoring of medication effects

Mary has successfully completed her education and has obtained a position in another town. She has come to your setting to maintain her care and medication regimen.

5. What techniques could be used by the nurse and Mary to assist in ongoing evaluation of her mood?
   a. Self-rating scales
   b. Symptom tracking
   c. Mood charting
   d. All of the above

6. Mary tells you that she would like to receive family counseling to improve interpersonal relationships and family coping. All of the following strategies are appropriate toward this goal *except*:
   a. enrolling Mary and her oldest son into family therapy
   b. identifying the client's designated family
   c. validating client and family needs
   d. assessing own perceptions about minority family structure

7. Marco is a 17-year-old adolescent seen in the community mental health clinic for the first time. He is accompanied by his parents who report he has problems sleeping, talks all the time, and is doing poorly in school. In the interview his speech is rapid, pressured, and tangential. His mood is irritable and elated. Which statement is the *most* accurate about his behavior?
   a. Normally, initial symptoms of bipolar disorder in males are a manic episode.
   b. As a rule, the initial presentation of bipolar disorder in males is depression.

c. Adolescents are usually agitated when stressed and he is just having a "bad" day.

d. As a rule, the initial presentation of bipolar symptoms in males is mixed.

8. Mr. M is a new client in the mental health clinic. He complains that he sleeps 10 hours a day, is depressed, and has been unable to concentrate at work and subsequently has lost his job as an administrative assistant. The most important question to ask this client is which of the following?

a. "How often do you feel hopeless and want to end your life?"

b. "How often do you have mood swings?"

c. "Describe your most important relationships."

d. "How long have you been depressed?"

9. When assessing a client with bipolar disorder II in a hypomanic episode, the nurse should expect to find which of the following?

a. Talkativeness, easily distracted, and impaired academic and job performance

b. Depressed mood, sleep disturbances, and irritability

c. Grandiose delusions, excessive sleep, and appetite changes

d. Mild elation or depression episode that lasts two days

10. The nurse is teaching a client about side effects associated with lithium, an antimanic agent. Which of the following would not be included?

a. Polyuria and glycosuria

b. Hypothyroidism

c. Increased liver enzymes

d. Sedation

11. A 23-year-old has been recently diagnosed with bipolar disorder. She asks the nurse which medications would be safe during pregnancy. The nurse's best response is which of the following?

a. Lithium

b. Divalproex

c. Carbamazepine

d. None of the above

12. The anticonvulsant most associated with polycystic ovaries and neural tubal birth defects is which of the following?

a. Carbamazepine

b. Lamotrigine

c. Divalproex

d. Topiramate

RESOURCES

Please note that because Internet resources are of a time-sensitive nature and URL addresses may change or be deleted, searches should also be conducted by association or topic.

Internet Resources

Go to the National Mental Health Association Web site (http://www.nmha.org)

http://www.surgeongeneral.com   Mental Health: A Report of the Surgeon General, U.S. DHHS

http://www.bipolarchild.com

http://www.BPSO.org

http://www.pendulum.org Online Support Group

www.mhsource.com

www.DBSalliance.org

www.BPchildresearch.org

www.nimh.nih.gov/public/bipolar.cfm

Other Resources

National Alliance for the Mentally Ill (NAMI)
  200 N. Glebe Rd., Suite 1015
  Arlington, VA 22203
  (703) 524-7600
  Fax (703) 524-9094
  Helpline: (800) 950-NAMI
  http://www.nami.org

Child and Adolescent Bipolar Foundation
  1000 Skokie Blvd., Suite 425
  Willmette, IL 60091
  (847) 256-8525
  E-mail: www.bpkids.org

National Alliance for Research on Schizophrenia and Depression (NARSAD)
  60 Cutter Mill Road, Suite 404
  Great Neck, NY 11021
  (516) 829-0091
  http://www.mhsource.com

National Mental Health Association
  1021 Prince St.
  Alexandria, VA 22314
  (800) 969-NMHA
  http://www.nmha.org

Federation of Families for Children's Mental Health
  9605 Medical Center Drive, Suite 280
  Rockville, MD 20850
  (240) 403-1901
  http://www.ffcmh.org

International Society of Psychiatric-Mental Health Nurses
  2810 Crossroads Drive, Suite 3800
  Madison, WI 53718
  1-866-330-7227
  http://www.ispn-psych.org

REFERENCES

Albanese, M. J., & Pies, R. (2004). The bipolar patient with comorbid substance use disorder: Recognition and management. *CNS Drugs, 18,* 585–596.

American Psychiatric Association. (2000). *Diagnostic and statistical manual of mental disorders* (4th edition Revision) (*DSM-IV-TR*). Washington, DC: Author.

American Psychiatric Association (2000). *Practice guidelines for the treatment of psychiatric disorders.* Washington, DC: Author.

American Psychiatric Association. (2002). Practice guidelines for the treatment of patients with bipolar disorder (revision). *American Journal of Psychiatry, 150,* (4 Suppl): 1, 50.

Angst, J., & Cassano, G. (2005). The mood spectrum: Improving the diagnosis of bipolar disorder. *Bipolar Disorder, 7,* Suppl 4, 4–12.

Aziz, R., Lorberg, B., & Tampi, R. R. (2006). Treatments for late-life bipolar disorder. *American Journal of Geriatrics Pharmocotherapeutics, 4,* 347–364.

Benedetti, A., Fagiolini, A., Casamassima, F., Mian, M. S., Adamovit, A., Musetti, L., et al. (2007). Gender differences in bipolar disorder type 1: A 48-week prospective follow-up of 72 patients treated in an Italian tertiary care center. *Journal of Nervous and Mental Disorders, 195,* 93–96.

Birmaher, B., Axelson, D., Strobe, M., Gill, M. K., Valeri, S., Chiapetta, L., Neal, R., Leonard, H., Hunt, J., Iyengar, S., & Keller, M. (2006). Clinical course of children & adolescents with bipolar spectrum disorders. *Archives of General Psychiatry, 63,*(2), 175–183.

Cassano, G. B., Dell'Osso, L., Frank, E., Miniati, M., Fagiolini, A., Shear, K., Pini, S., & Maser, J. (1999). The bipolar spectrum: A clinical reality in search of diagnostic criteria and an assessment methodology. *Journal of Affective Disorders, 54*(3), 319–328.

Cassano, G. B., Rucci, P., Frank, E., Fagiolini, A., Dell'Osso, L., Shear, M. K., et al. (2004). The mood spectrum in unipolar and bipolar disorder: Arguments for a unitary approach. *American Journal of Psychiatry, 161,* 1264–1269.

Ganong, W. F. (2005). *Review of medical physiology* (22nd ed.). New York: The MacGraw-Hill Companies.

Geller, B., Craney, J., Bolhofner, K., DelBello, M., Williams, M., & Zimmerman, B. (2001). One-year recovery and relapse rates of children with a prepubertal and early adolescent bipolar disorder phenotype. *The American Journal of Psychiatry, 158*(2), 303–305.

Goodwin, G. M. (1999). Prophylaxis of bipolar disorder: How and who should we treat in the long term? *European Neuropsychopharmacology, 9*(Suppl. 4), S125–S129.

Gutierrez, M. J., & Scott, J. (2004). The current status of psychological treatments in bipolar disorders: A systematic review of relapse prevention. *Bipolar Disorders, 6,* 498–503.

Henin, A., Mick, E., Biederman, J., Fried, R., Wozniak, J., Faraone, S. V., et al. (2007). Can bipolar disorder-specific neuropsychological impairments in children be identified? *Journal of Consulting and Clinical Psychology, 75,* 210–220.

Keck, P. E. Jr. (2006). Long-term management strategies to achieve optimal function in patients with bipolar disorder. *Journal of Clinical Psychiatry, 67,* (Suppl. 9), 19–24.

Kessler, R. C., Berglund, P., Demler, O., Jin, R., Merikangas, K. R., & Walters, E. E. (2005). Lifetime prevalence and age-of-onset distributions of DSM-IV disorders in the National Comorbidity Survey Replication. *Archives of General Psychiatry, 62,* 593–602.

Kessler, R. C., Demler, O., Frank, R. G., Olfson, M., Pincus, H. A., Walters, E. E., et al. (2005). Prevalence and treatment of mental disorders, 1990 to 2003. *NEJM, 352,* 2515–2523.

Kraepelin, E. (1921). *Manic-depressive insanity and paranoia.* Edinburgh: Livingston.

Lin, D., Mok, H., & Yatham, L. N. (2006). Polytherapy in bipolar disorder. *CNS Drugs, 20,* 29–42.

Luby, J., Tandon, M., & Nicol, G. (2007). Three clinical cases of DSM-IV mania symptoms in preschoolers. *Journal of Child and Adolescent Psychopharmacology, 17,* 273–243.

Malhi, G. S., Ivanovski, B., Hadzi-Pavlovic, D., Mitchell, P. B., & Sachdev, P. (2007). Neuropsychological deficits and functional impairment in bipolar depression, hypomania and euthymia. *Bipolar Disorder, 9,* 114–125.

Merikangas, K. R., Akiskal, H. S., Angst, J., Greenberg, P. E., Hirschfeld, R. M., Petukhova, M., et al. (2007). Lifetime and 12-month prevalence of bipolar spectrum disorder in the national comorbidity survey replication. *Archives of General Psychiatry, 64,* 543–552.

Nierenberg, A. A., Ostacher, M. J., Calabrese, J. R., Ketter, T. A., Marangell, L. B., Miklowitz, D. J., Miyahara, S., Bauer, M. S., Thase, M. E., Wisniewski, S. R., & Sachs, G. S. (2006). Treatment-resistant bipolar depression: A STEP-BD equipoise randomized effectiveness trial of antidepressant augmentation with lamotrigine, Inositol, or Risperidone. *The American Journal of Psychiatry, 163,* 2, 210–216.

Papadimitriou, G. N., Calabrese, J. R., Dikeos, D. G., & Christodoulou, G. N. (2005). Rapid cycling bipolar disorder: Biology and pathogenesis. *International Journal of Neuropsychopharmacology, 8,* 281–292.

Pauls, D. L., Bailey, J. N., Carter, A. S., Allen, C. R., & Egeland, J. A. (1995). Complex segregation analyses of old order Amish families ascertained through bipolar I individuals. *American Journal of Medical Genetics, 60*(4), 290–297.

Perlis, R. H., Ostacher, M. J., Patel, J., Marangell, L. B., Zhang, H., Wisniewski, S. R., Ketter, T. A., Miklowitz, D. J., Otto, M., Gyulai, L., Reilly-Harrington, N., Nierenberg, A., Sachs, G. S., & Thase, M. (2006). Predictors of recurrence in bipolar disorder: Primary outcomes from the Systematic Treatment Enhancement Program for Bipolar Disorder (STEP-BD). *The American Journal of Psychiatry, 163,* 2, 217–224.

Post, R. M., Altshuler, L. L., Leverich, G. S., Frye, M. A., Nolen, W. A., Kupka, R. W., Suppes, T., McElroy, S. et al. (2006). Mood switch in bipolar depression: Comparison of adjunctive venlafaxine, bupropion and sertraline. *British Journal of Psychiatry, 189,* 124–131.

Sachs, G., Baldassano, C., Truman, C., Christine, J., & Guille, C. (2000). Comorbidity of attention deficit disorder with early- and late-onset bipolar disorder. *The American Journal of Psychiatry, 157*(3), 466–468.

Sadock, J., Sadock, V. A., & Sussman, N. (2006). *Kaplan & Sadock pocket handbook of psychiatric drug treatment* (4th ed.). Philadelphia: Lippincott Williams & Wilkins.

Torrey, E. F. (1999). Epidemiological comparison of schizophrenia and bipolar disorder. *Schizophrenia Research, 39,* 101–106.

Torrey, E. F., Rawlings, R. R., Ennis, J. M., Merrill, D. D., & Flores, D. S. (1996). Birth seasonality in bipolar disorder, schizophrenia, schizoaffective disorder and stillbirths. *Schizophrenia Research, 21,* 141–149.

U.S. Department of Health and Human Services (U.S. DHHS). (1999). *Mental health: A report of the surgeon general.* Rockville, MD: U.S. Department of Health and Human Services Administration, Center for Mental Health Services, National Institutes of Health, National Institute of Mental Health.

U.S. Department of Health and Human Services (U.S. DHHS). (2001). *Mental health: Culture, race, and ethnicity—a supplement to mental health: A report of the surgeon general.* Rockville, MD: U.S. Department of Health and Human Services Administration, Center for Mental Health Services.

Weissman, M. M., Bland, R. C., Camino, O. J., Faravelli, C., Greenwald, S., Hwu, H. G., et al. (1996). Cross-national epidemiology of major depression and bipolar disorder. *Journal of American Medical Association, 276,* 293–299.

Wozniak, J. (2007). Recognizing and managing bipolar disorder in children. *Journal of Clinical Psychiatry, 66,* Suppl 1, 18–23.

Yin, I., Wang, J., Klein, P. S., Lazar, M. A. (2006). Nuclear receptor rev-erba is a critical lithium-sensitive component of the circadian clock. *Science, 311,* (5763), 1002–1005.

Young, R. C., Biggs, J. T., Ziegler, W., & Meyer, D. A. (1978). A rating scale for mania: Reliability, validity, and sensitivity. *British Journal of Psychiatry, 133,* 429–435.

SUGGESTED READINGS

Birmaher, B. (2004). *New hope for children and teens with bipolar disorder.* New York: Three Rivers Press.

Carlson, T. (2004). *The life of a bipolar child: What every parent and professional needs to know.* Minnesota: Benline Press.

Castle, L. R. (2003). *Bipolar disorder demystified.* New York: Marlowe and Company.

Fieve, R. R. (1989). *Moodswing.* New York: Bantam Books.

Isaac, G. (2001). *Bipolar not ADHD: Unrecognized epidemic of manic depressive illness in children.* New York Writers Club Press.

Jamison, K. R. (1995). *An unquiet mind.* New York: Alfred A. Knopf.

Miklowitz, D. J. (2002). *The bipolar disorder survival guide: What you and your family need to know.* New York: The Guilford Press.

Mondimore, F. M. (1999). *Bipolar disorder: A guide for patients and families.* Baltimore: The Johns Hopkins University Press.

NIMH. A Story of Bipolar Disorder. Bethesda (MD): National Institute of Mental Health, National Institutes of Health, U.S. Department of Health and Human Services; 2002. (NIH Publication Number 5124). 20 pages. Available from: http://www.nimh.nih.gov

Oliwenstein, L. (2004). *Psychology today here to help: Taming bipolar disorder.* New York: Alpha: The Penguin Group.

Waltz, M. (2000). *Bipolar disorders: A guide to helping children & adolescents.* California: O'Reilly & Associates, lnc.

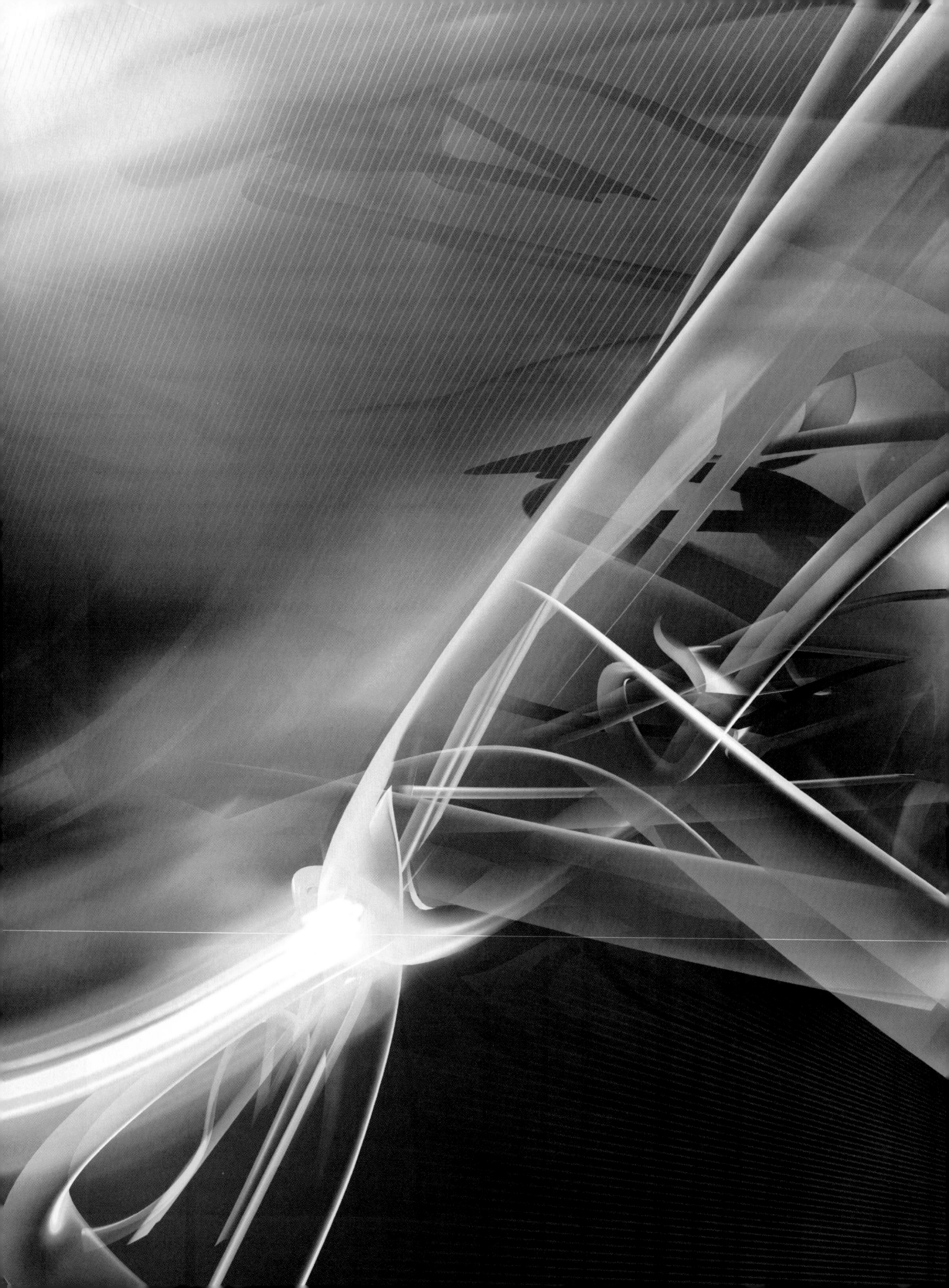

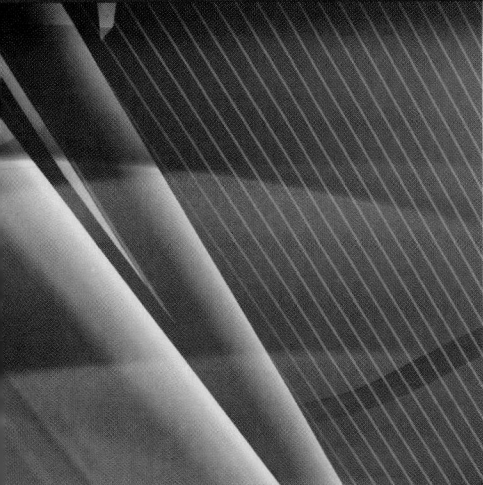

CHAPTER 11

The Client with an Anxiety Disorder

Deborah Antai-Otong, MS, APRN, BC, FAAN

KEY TERMS

Adaptation: Sustaining homeostasis; the ability to mobilize resources and adjust to demands of internal and external environments.

Anxiety: An affect or emotion arising from stress or change accompanied by biological arousal, behavioral responses, and elements of apprehension, impending doom, and tension.

Anxiolytic Agent: A drug used for the relief of anxiety; also called antianxiety agent or mild tranquilizer.

Attachment Theory: Theory based on the classic works of Bowlby and Ainsworth that define attachment or bonding as an evolutionary and biological process of eliciting and maintaining physical closeness between a child and a parent or primary caregiver. This theory also infers that the infant's relationships with early caregivers are responsible for influencing future interactions and relationships.

Avoidant Behavior: Refers to constricted social interaction with unfamiliar people or situations that activate intense anxiety reactions, resulting in excessive social impairment and interactions with others.

Cognitive Processes: Higher cortical mental processes, including perception, memory, and reasoning, by which one acquires knowledge, solves problems, employs judgment, and makes plans.

Compulsion: Repetitive, ritualistic, unrealistic behaviors used to neutralize or prevent discomfort of stressful events, circumstances or recurring thoughts, images, or impulses such as obsessions.

Co-occurring: Coexistence of more than one psychiatric disorder.

Depersonalization: A person's subjective sense of feeling unreal, strange, unfamiliar, or emotionally numb.

Derealization: A subjective sense that one's environment is unreal or unfamiliar.

Desensitization: A cognitive-behavioral therapy technique developed by Joseph Wolpe that involves three steps: relaxation training, gradual or hierarchy exposure (using visual imagery or real situations) to an anxiety-provoking or fearful situation or object, and desensitization to the stimulus. This technique is useful in the treatment of phobias.

Dissociation: An unconscious defense mechanism that refers to a detachment or alteration in one's sense of reality, psychogenic amnesia, and perception of self and environment; used by a person to protect self from being overwhelmed by anxiety, usually from a traumatic experience. Memory and feeling related to an event are sealed off from the conscious awareness.

Eye Movement Desensitization and Reprocessing (EMDR): Involves asking the client to imagine an anxiety-provoking or traumatic memory. This technique is used to treat post-traumatic stress disorder by processing a traumatic experience in a non-threatening manner.

Homeostasis: Refers to a state of adaptation or ability to effectively manage internal and external environmental demands.

Neurotransmitter: A central nervous system biochemical involved in facilitating the transmission of impulses across synapses between neurons. Examples include serotonin, dopamine, and norepinephrine.

Obsession: Intrusive, recurrent, and persistent thoughts, impulses, or images.

Paresthesia: Unnatural tactile sensations manifested by tingling, tickling, or creeping sensations that have no physical basis. This sensation often results from activation of the hypothalamic-pituitary-adrenal axis.

Phobia: An exaggerated or irrational fear of an event or object, such as a presentation or spider, respectively.

Progressive Relaxation: A form of relaxation training that involves visualizing and sequentially relaxing specific muscle groups, starting with the scalp to the tips of the toes. This technique involves teaching the client to tense and relax various muscle groups in an effort to reduce tension and stress.

Separation Anxiety: Refers to a common childhood and adolescent anxiety disorder whose symptoms involve panic or intense fear of losing one's primary caregivers.

Visual Imagery: Refers to a stress or anxiety-reducing cognitive exercise that involves creating relaxing thoughts or visual images or place of serenity and calmness.

COMPETENCIES

Upon completion of this chapter, the learner should be able to:

1. Identify causes and symptoms of the most prevalent anxiety disorders.
2. Explain the relationship between cognitive processes and anxiety.
3. Discuss the role of neurobiological cultural and psychosocial factors in anxiety disorder.
4. Develop a plan of care for the client experiencing an anxiety disorder.
5. Recognize symptoms of anxiety disorders across the life span.

CHAPTER OUTLINE

Levels of Anxiety: Normal versus Abnormal Anxiety

Epidemiology

Cultural Factors

Causative Factors: Perspectives and Theories

Psychodynamic Theories

Existential Theories

Cognitive-Behavioral Theories

Developmental Theories

Biological Theories

Neurotransmitter and Neuroendocrinology Theories

Neuroanatomical Theories

Genetic Factors

Anxiety across the Life Span

Childhood and Adolescent Anxiety Disorders

Separation Anxiety Disorder

Social Phobia

Overanxious Disorder

Post-traumatic Stress Disorder

Obsessive-Compulsive Disorder

Co-occurring Issues

Summary of Childhood and Adolescent Disorders

Adulthood Disorders

Generalized Anxiety Disorder

Panic Disorder

Agoraphobia

Social Anxiety Disorder and Specific Phobia

Obsessive-Compulsive Disorder

Acute Stress Disorder

Post-traumatic Stress Disorder

Summary of Adulthood Disorders

Older Adulthood Disorders

Specific Age-Related Issues

Summary of Older Adulthood Disorders

Treatment Considerations for the Client in Community and Home Settings

The Role of the Nurse

The Generalist Nurse

The Advanced-Practice Psychiatric Registered Nurse

The Nursing Process

Assessment

Nursing Diagnoses

Outcome Identification

Planning

Implementation

Psychopharmacology

Complementary Treatment of Anxiety Disorders

Evaluation

The term anxiety stems from the Latin word *anxietus*, which means "to vex or trouble." Anxiety represents uneasiness, and it is an integral aspect of human nature because it plays a crucial role in adaptation and homeostasis (the ability to mobilize resources and adjust to demands of internal and external environments). It often extends beyond adaptive importance for the individual. Anxiety is a state arising from stress or change and frequently emanates from fear. However, anxiety differs from fear in that it is a diffuse, internal, and anticipatory reaction to danger that may be ambiguous or nonspecific, and the reaction may be disproportionate to the degree of danger. In comparison, fear stems from real and external or potential threats of danger. The continuum of anxiety ranges from a mild form, which produces little physiological effect, to a severe form, which disrupts homeostasis by activating neuroendocrine processes that culminate in maladaptive responses such as avoidant behaviors or phobias (American Psychiatric Association [APA], 2000).

The aim of this chapter is to discuss major anxiety disorders as they evolve over a developmental continuum stemming from infancy to older adulthood. It delineates anxiety disorders in the the *Diagnostic and Statistical Manual of Mental Disorders* (4th edition, Text Revision) (*DSM-IV-TR*) (APA, 2000). It also focuses on various factors that contribute to normal and abnormal, or anxiety, disorders; the role of psychiatric nursing in the evaluation of clients with anxiety disorders; and the prevention and treatment of these complex disorders.

LEVELS OF ANXIETY: NORMAL VERSUS ABNORMAL ANXIETY

Normal anxiety is a protective response and an innate form of communication that the body uses to mobilize its coping resources to maintain homeostasis. Likewise, everyone experiences fear in response to the threat of injury, and the production of adrenaline accompanies the "flight or fight" response.

Anxiety normally accompanies developmental changes and life span issues. Anticipating an examination or new clinical experience is an example of normal anxiety. By acting as a protective response to various situations, anxiety enables individuals to use behaviors such as studying or getting enough sleep before a big exam to reduce their sense of helplessness and frustration. These responses minimize the long-term sequelae of anxiety and promote a state of health. Conversely, maladaptive responses or failure to mobilize homeostatic processes often culminate and contribute to formation of anxiety disorders. Overwhelming and enduring anxiety often produces maladaptive responses that globally affect one's level of functioning.

The *DSM-IV-TR* (APA, 2000) describes anxiety disorders as one of the most common psychiatric conditions (Table 11–1). APA delineates major anxiety disorders as panic disorder with or without agoraphobia, specific phobia and social phobia, obsessive-compulsive disorder, post-traumatic stress disorder, acute stress disorder, and generalized anxiety disorder. Major

TABLE 11–1
Specific Anxiety Disorders

Anxiety Disorder/Condition	*DSM-IV-TR* Criteria
Acute Stress Disorder	A. Person exposed to a traumatic event that posed threat to self or others' physical integrity; impact on person involves profound fear, powerlessness, or terror
	B. During exposure or after exposure to trauma event, *three* or more of the following dissociative manifestations are present: • numbness, void of emotional responsiveness • "being in a daze" • derealization • depersonalization • dissociative amnesia
	C. The traumatic event is persistently reexperienced in one of the following: recurrent vivid memories, nightmares, flashbacks, and distress (neurobiological arousal) arising from memory of the event
	D. Marked avoidance of stimuli behaviors
	E. Profound anxiety or autonomic arousal
	F. Interference with optimal level of function
	G. Duration of symptoms persists for at least 2 days and no longer than a month and occurs within a month of traumatic exposure

(continues)

TABLE 11–1
Specific Anxiety Disorders *(continued)*

	H. Not due to a substance or medical condition • Differs from post-traumatic stress disorder because manifestations of this disorder must evolve within 1 month and resolve within this 1-month period
Anxiety due to a General Medical Condition	A. Pronounced anxiety, specific anxiety disorder (e.g., panic attacks) is chief complaint B. Physiological symptoms directly parallel a general medical condition (e.g., hypoglycemia, hyperthyroidism) C. Symptoms are not associated with another mental disorder D. Symptoms are not part of the course of delirium E. Symptoms interfere with optimal level of functioning
Substance-Induced Anxiety Disorder	A. Pronounced anxiety, specific anxiety disorder (e.g., panic attacks) is chief complaint B. Anxiety symptoms evolved during or within the past month of substance intoxication or withdrawal; medication use is directly associated with presenting symptoms C. Symptoms are not directly caused by a specific anxiety disorder D. Manifestations are not part of the course of delirium E. Symptoms interfere with optimal level of function

Note. From *Diagnostic and Statistical Manual of Mental Disorders* (4th edition, Text Revision) *(DSM-IV-TR)*, by American Psychiatric Association, 2000, Washington, DC: Author. Adapted with permission.

symptoms of these disorders include autonomic nervous arousal, a sense of doom, fear, depersonalization, **paresthesias**, and avoidant behaviors. Naturally, the severity of abnormal anxiety or anxiety disorders varies, but most arise from distinct causes, such as traumatic exposure and exaggerated fears or phobias, and require holistic interventions to reduce their potentially debilitating effects.

Regardless of its nature, anxiety generates an array of biological, behavioral, motor, and cognitive responses. Biological responses arise from activation of complex neuroendocrine processes that modulate the autonomic nervous systems. Manifestations of biological responses include increased respirations and blood pressure, tachycardia, paresthesias, headache, tightness in the chest, diaphoresis, and lightheadedness. Behavioral responses include rituals, social isolation, avoidance behaviors, help seeking, self-care deficits, and increased dependency. Motor reaction often presents as muscle tension, tremors, shakiness, stuttering, pacing, compulsions, and restlessness. Cognitive, or psychological, symptoms include a sense of doom or powerlessness and "going crazy or dying," helplessness, vigilance, rumination, preoccupations, obsessions, dissociation, distortions, and confusion. Table 11–2 lists global manifestations of anxiety responses.

 CRITICAL THINKING

Which of the following most accurately defines normal anxiety?

a. John's heart races and he feels uneasy about an upcoming meeting with his boss about his quarterly financial reports.

b. Mary has tremendous fears about going outside and turns down an offer to go for a ride with a friend.

c. Susan experiences an intense urge and obsession to wash her hands after shaking hands with her boss.

d. Marty is driving in her car and out of the blue has palpitations and muscle tension and feels dizzy.

EPIDEMIOLOGY

Anxiety disorders are among the oldest, most recognizable, and prevalent mental disorders, affecting approximately 15 percent of the general population at some point during their lifetime. Longitudinal studies of anxiety disorders indicate that they evolve over time, with an early onset, high morbidity, chronicity, and recurrence. More significantly, anxiety is

TABLE 11–2
Global Manifestations of Anxiety Responses

Autonomic/Biological
- Increased respirations
- Shortness of breath
- Tachycardia
- Diaphoresis
- Dizziness
- Paresthesias

Behavioral
- Rituals
- Avoidance
- Increased dependence
- Clinging
- Following (infant)
- Crying (infant or school-age child)

Motor
- Tension
- Pacing
- Tremors
- Stuttering
- Restlessness

Cognitive/Psychological
- Sense of doom
- Powerlessness
- Intense fear
- Vigilance
- Rumination
- Helplessness
- Dissociation
- Distortions
- Confusion
- Overgeneralization

one of the most common reasons for seeking medical and psychiatric treatment (Kessler, Chiu, Demier, Merikangas, & Walters, 2005; Weissman et al., 1997). Results from the 2005 National Comorbidity Survey Replication demonstrated that one in four people has met the criteria for at least one anxiety disorder and that there is a 12-month prevalence rate of 17.7 percent. There is a higher prevalence of anxiety disorders among women (30.5 percent) than men (9.2 percent) (Kessler et al., 2005). Another epidemiologic study demonstrates the prevalence of social phobia, an often overlooked anxiety disorder, ranges from 7 to 8 percent—a rate that far exceeds the rate of detection by health care providers (Magee, Eaton, Wittchen, McGonagle, & Kessler, 1996; Stein, Torgrud, & Walker, 2000). More importantly, anxiety disorders are the most prevalent mental disorders in older adults, although the incidence is slightly less than in younger age groups (Flint, 2005; Le Roux, Gatz, & Wetherell, 2005). Several studies also link cultural factors to the universality of anxiety disorders.

CULTURAL FACTORS

Although anxiety is a normal emotion, the manner in which people interpret and respond to it stems from cultural beliefs, health practices, and rituals. More importantly, cultural beliefs and practices mediate cognitive, biological, and behavioral responses to danger and fear and determine specific coping and avoidance responses. Cultural beliefs also influ-

ence parenting and socialization and are the basis of attachment, separation, sense of security, and one's perception of danger. Ultimately, these factors play key roles in anxiety disorders (Feldman, 2007; Grover, Ginsburg, & Ialongo, 2005; Palapattu, Kingery, & Ginsburg, 2006).

Anxiety disorders are also prevalent in children. Data from various community surveys demonstrate that girls are more likely to experience anxiety symptoms than are boys; African American children more than Caucasian American children. The incidence of anxiety disorders extends beyond various age groups and also involves ethnic and cultural influences.

Findings from a large National Epidemiologic survey (n = 43,093) of nativity and psychiatric conditions, including anxiety disorders among island-born Puerto-Ricans, foreign-born Cuban-Americans, and foreign non-Latino whites and their American-born counterparts, demonstrated cultural and ethnic protective effects among foreign-born subjects. Moreover, these researchers emphasized the importance of assessing variation among groups and unique cultural and protective factors to reduce the risk of psychiatric disorders (Alegria, Canino, Stinson, & Grant, 2006). A clinical implication for psychiatric nurses is assessment of client strengths and resilience among various cultures to understand their experience and reduce anxiety and other psychiatric disorders across the life span.

Cultural variations in the presentation and epidemiology of anxiety disorders are diverse. Emerging findings also indicate the need for cultural and gender-sensitive evaluation and assessment tools to ensure accurate diagnosis of clinical presentations and implementation of appropriate treatment (Alegria et al., 2006; Johnson et al., 2007). In summary, research on socioeconomic deprivation, violence, and trauma in many battle-torn countries and inner-city neighborhoods contributes to the endemic of anxiety disorders among various cultures, especially post-traumatic stress disorder (Adams & Boscarino, 2005; Alegria, Canino, Stinson, & Grant, 2006).

Cultural factors, like individual differences, contribute to anxiety disorders and treatment planning. Psychiatric nurses, like other health care providers, face the daily challenge of understanding the meaning of unusual symptoms and responding to various situations in a sociocultural context. An accurate interpretation of the client's experience can only occur when the nurse examines anxiety disorders within the system and sociocultural context in which they occur.

The prevalence of anxiety makes it a serious worldwide health problem that requires early identification, greater understanding of causative factors, and more research to explore innovative treatment approaches. This process begins by exploring individual responses to stress and origins of anxiety states. Individual and sociocultural responses to anxiety states are contingent on one's interpretation of danger or a threat and the ability to mobilize adaptive coping skills and understand underlying causative factors. When these resources fail, anxiety and disorganization often ensue, with the potential for anxiety to become overwhelming and chronic. Gaining control over anxiety reactions requires understanding of the causative factors that precipitated them.

CAUSATIVE FACTORS: PERSPECTIVES AND THEORIES

Various theories explain the cause of anxiety disorders in terms of their complexity and relationship to adaptation and homeostasis. Adaptation to stress and subsequent anxiety depend on the nature of the circumstance, accessible internal and external resources, psychological defenses or ego functioning, and repertoire of coping mechanisms. Psychodynamic, existential, cognitive-behavioral, developmental, and biological theories strengthen the premise that anxiety is an integral aspect of human nature. These theories provide conceptual and practical value in the understanding and management of anxiety disorders.

PSYCHODYNAMIC THEORIES

The foundation of psychoanalytic theory is the premise that various factors, such as conflict, pleasure, morality, and fantasies, are the bases of symptoms and neurosis. Biological, behavioral, and psychosocial expansions have been replaced or added to psychodynamic theories as the primary bases of mental illness. Despite these expansions, an appreciation of the major psychodynamic concepts of anxiety is vital to understanding the significance of anxiety and human responses.

Sigmund Freud (1936) believed that anxiety occurs when the ego attempts to deal with psychic conflict or emotional tension. He defined anxiety as "the reaction to danger," and that the birth process is the initial response to danger that varies over time, beginning with infancy. This initial trauma originates from separation from the mother, and the severity of anxiety parallels the infant's ability to overcome it. Lifelong adaptive responses to anxiety arise from this early developmental task. As the ego matures, the person becomes more adept at managing internal and external stress (S. Freud, 1936). Thus a child is less able than an adult to cope with traumatic experiences.

Freud's daughter, Anna Freud (1936), produced a classic work, *The Ego and the Mechanisms of Defense*, which also contributes to the understanding of the psychodynamics of anxiety. She contended that everyone uses various defense mechanisms to defend against and reduce discomfort that arises from internal and external demands. Major coping processes include unconscious defense mechanisms such as repression, sublimation, denial, projection, and reaction formation, the purposes of which are to control, reduce, and protect the ego from intense anxiety reactions. In addition, psychodynamic theories suggest that if repression fails to protect the ego from overwhelming anxiety, other primitive or immature defense mechanisms, such as dissociation, displacement, or regression may evolve, thus increasing the risk of mental illness (Breuer & Freud, 1957). (See Chapter 2, Concepts of Psychiatric Care: Therapeutic Models, for an explanation of defense mechanisms.) Normally, the integrity of defense mechanisms parallels chronological development and reflects a capacity to cope with internal and external environmental demands. The more immature or primitive the defense mechanism, the less likely the individual will cope or manage anxiety.

EXISTENTIAL THEORIES

Jean-Paul Sartre, a German prisoner of war, coined the term *existentialism*. This term is of European origin and refers to human existence and its relationship to one's perception of life and despair from which God does not exist. Major themes of this theory include impotence, fragility, the threat of nothingness, and isolation. A lack of competency, or sense of nothingness, predictably results in inadequate coping skills and generates empty feelings that result in people viewing their lives as meaningless, aimless, and worthless and having ineffective coping skills. Consequently, maladaptive coping skills produce anxiety, which interferes with the individual's ability to preserve his existence.

Similarly, Rollo May (1977), another existentialist, further defines maladaptive anxiety as a reaction to a threat to survival. He and other existentialists believe that treatment involves looking beyond anxiety symptoms. This process involves moving the client from a maladaptive level of existence or functioning to one that fosters adaptive coping skills, competency and realistic perceptions of self.

COGNITIVE-BEHAVIORAL THEORIES

Beck, Emery, & Greenberg (1985) defined anxiety from a cognitive processes perspective and asserted that it occurs when a threat or danger is perceived. (*Cognitive* refers to thought processes related to judgment, reasoning, comprehension, attitude, and perception of self, the world, and future.) Anxious persons often exaggerate the threat of danger by using faulty cognitions. For instance, a secretary with an excellent work history makes a mistake on a report and as a result fears that he will lose his job. This exaggerated fear of losing one's job because of a mistake represents how one's unrealistic or distorted cognitions can produce intense anxiety and fears.

Faulty or distorted cognitions are characterized by overgeneralization, "awfulizing," and "all or none" perceptions of self, others, and the world. These thoughts often generate intense anxiety and impaired social functioning (e.g., avoidant behaviors), which cause the individual to feel powerless and helpless. Public speaking is an example of an event that often produces anxiety or social phobia. The businessperson preparing a talk may experience severe anxiety arising from the fear of "losing it" and looking foolish during the presentation. If this lack of confidence is sensed by the audience, its negative reaction may increase the person's anxiety about public speaking.

Behaviorists propose that intense or disabling anxiety is a learned maladaptive response to stress (Eysenck 1990; Wolpe, 1961; Wolpe & Lazarus, 1966). They also believe that if behavior originates from lifelong maladaptive learning experiences or conditioning, the individual can also "unlearn" them by developing new and adaptive behaviors. The basis of "unlearning" maladaptive responses to stress and ineffective management of anxiety stems from the learning theory, specifically operant or classical conditioning. Operant or classical conditioning refers to a type of learning that evolves from *reinforcement*, which predicts the likelihood of future occurrence, and *punishment*, which predicts a decrease or extinction of future occurrence. Individual learning experiences resulting from reinforcement and punishment contribute to maladaptive coping responses and anxiety throughout the life span.

Life span learning experiences evolve over time, from infancy to older adulthood, and involve diverse environmental factors and influences that shape coping and personality development. Families and other psychosocial factors shape various personality traits and one's ability to cope and respond to stress effectively. Specific family qualities, such as a lack of warmth and nurturance or overprotectiveness, increase the likelihood of maladaptive responses in children (Andrews & Crino, 1991; Leon & Leon, 1990).

Throughout the life span, varied learning experiences, negative and positive reinforcers, and internal and external demands become the underpinning of adaptation to anxiety and coping behaviors.

DEVELOPMENTAL THEORIES

Bowlby's (1969) attachment theory asserted that anxiety initially occurs with separation from early primary caregivers. He described separation anxiety as a predictable process involving several stages:

1. Protest (separation anxiety): the child cries and often looks and calls for caregiver(s).

2. Despair (grief and mourning): the child fears that the caregiver will not return.

3. Detachment (coping/defense mechanism): the child emotionally separates from caregivers.

Separation anxiety refers to anxiety that occurs when a child exhibits symptoms of panic or extreme fear of losing primary caregiver(s). The infant's attachment behaviors, such as smiling, clinging, crying, and following, activate a response from the primary caregivers and facilitate closeness or bonding. The infant often uses these behaviors during the first 4 months of life and continues to do so until age 3. Throughout infancy and childhood, behavioral patterns change from clinging and sucking to using words and playing alone. By the age of 3, the child is able to tolerate the short-term absence of the primary caregivers and feel secure with surrogate attachment figures, such as a relative or babysitter. Bowlby believed that the child's ability to cope successfully with separation anxiety depends on the quality of attachment or bonding during early infancy.

Ainsworth (1985, 1990) supported and clarified Bowlby's attachment theory, emphasizing the importance of attachment and its anxiety-reducing qualities in helping children to separate successfully from primary caregivers and adapt to external and internal stressors. Specifically, parents who respond to the infant's verbal and nonverbal cues or communication foster a sense of control and predictability over the environment. Moreover, these early developmental stages offer the child a sense of security and development of adaptive coping skills. She also asserts that mastery of this developmental task is the basis of lifelong adaptive coping skills, ego development, self-esteem, and modulation of anxiety and other intense feelings.

On the other hand, children who leave infancy with disturbed or inadequate attachment or bonding tend to experience developmental incompetency manifested by impaired socialization and problem solving, low self-esteem, and a lack of emotional stability. A failure to master these early developmental milestones are likely to result in *high-intensity-attachment*-seeking behaviors that usually manifest as dependency or "neediness" of others or external means to modulate anxiety.

The ability to form normal social attachments therefore contributes to one's ability to modulate anxiety and adapt to separation. In contrast, a failure to form early social attachments predictably results in maladaptive coping responses and inability to modulate anxiety and stress.

BIOLOGICAL THEORIES

Biological theories of anxiety disorders historically focused on the role of the hypothalmic-pituitary-adrenal (HPA) axis and other neuroendocrine systems that contribute to the physiological and behavioral manifestations of anxiety disorders. Contemporary studies continue to demonstrate the role of neuroendocrinology in the genesis and treatment of anxiety disorders. Technological advances, neurochemistry, neuroendocrinology, and neuroimaging studies continue to provide vast clinical data about the origins and treatment of anxiety disorders.

Neurotransmitter and Neuroendocrinology Theories

Many of the biological theories of anxiety disorders have come from examination of behavior and adaptation to internal and external stimuli that may result in a positive or negative response (Cannon, 1914; Eysenck, 1981; Pavlov, 1927). A combination of neurochemicals and neuroendocrine systems affects the network of brain regions whenever a person experiences anxiety. Data from animal studies and drug trials posit that dysregulation of three major neurotransmitters, specifically, norepinephrine (NE), serotonin (5-HT), gamma-aminobutyric acid (GABA), and glutamate, contribute to the genesis of diverse anxiety disorders. Overall, vast neurotransmitters and their receptors appear to play complex roles in the genesis of anxiety.

A landmark study conducted by Hans Eysenck (1981) revealed that anxiety results from activation of the autonomic nervous system (ANS) and arousal of the limbic system to prepare for increased mental and physical demands to confront the threat. Two clusters of specialized neurons of the ANS in the brainstem—the locus ceruleus (LC) and the lateral tegmental NE cell system—receive the stimuli of impending danger or sensory pain and secrete norepinephrine, a stimulating neurotransmitter, which floods the limbic system and HPA axis (Simeon et al., 2007; Yehuda, 2006). Manifestations of physiological arousal include increased heart rate, increased breathing rate, and hyperalertness that arise from the hormone corticotropin-releasing factor (CRF) from the hypothalamus and the adrenocorticotropic hormone (ACTH) from the pituitary and adrenalin glands. In concert, these processes maintain a state of adaptation or homeostasis. Understanding the relationship between stress and homeostasis requires a further discussion of maladaptive responses to stress and subsequent anxiety disorders.

A number of neuroendocrine studies suggest that increased cortisol levels in acute stress and related symptoms are comparable to what happens in anxiety disorders. Suppression of cortisol through administration of dexamethasone has been associated with post-traumatic stress disorder (PTSD), suggesting an underlying heightened glucocorticoid feedback sensitivity of the HPA axis in these clients (Griffin,

Resick, & Yehuda, 2005). However, investigations have failed to support the notion that anxiety disorders consistently result from activation of the HPA, and that stress and anxiety are generally considered separate phenomena (Abelson, Curtis, & Uhde, 2005).

Rosenbaum (1990) referred to autonomic nervous system arousal as "limbic alert." The limbic system, an area of the forebrain encircling the brainstem, plays a major role in the formation of abnormal responses such as anxiety reactions. The limbic system's association with the brainstem aids in sustaining emotional steadiness and alertness as well as activating the LC to release NE. The cell bodies of the noradrenergic system lie primarily in the LC in the rostral pons and whose projections extend to various brain regions, such as the cerebral cortex, limbic system, brainstem, and spinal cord. The LC-NE-sympathetic nervous system plays a vital role in the body's response to alarm and threat (Alexander, Hillier, Smith, Tivarus, & Beversdorf, 2007). Refer to Table 11–3 for a compilation of biological theories of anxiety.

Typically, stimulation of the adrenergic system involves physiological experiences of NE hyperactivity, palpitations, tachycardia, diaphoresis, sighing, dry mouth, difficulty swallowing, and headache. These manifestations appear to arise from noradrenergic beta-1 postsynaptic receptors. Dysfunction of adrenergic systems seems to reflect dysregulation of inhibitory alpha-2 adrenergic receptors. Stimulation of this brain region also generates feelings of doom and fear and is the potential site of maladaptive anxiety disorders (Simeon et al., 2007; Yehuda, 2006).

In addition, the raphe nuclei, the brain region most responsible for the release of 5-HT, as described in Chapter 9, modulates mood and motivation. 5-HT is integrally involved in the mediation of anxiety via neural pathways originating in the raphe nucleus and innervating various brain regions, including the limbic system, hypothalamus, and thalamus (Ganong, 2005). Overactivity of the 5-HT system may be the basis of many anxiety disorders. Activation of the presynaptic 5-HT_{1A} receptors reduces the release of 5-HT, ultimately producing an increase in 5-HT neurotransmission. The improved response of persons with the type of anxiety disorder characterized by obsessive-compulsive activity and panic disorder to selective serotonin reuptake inhibitors (SSRIs), such as clomipramine, fluvoxamine, and fluoxetine, respectively, suggests that these disorders stem from abnormal 5-HT function. In fact, some of the most compelling data for dysregulation of 5-HT function in anxiety disorders, such as panic disorder (PD), is that agents that inhibit presynaptic 5-HT reuptake, such as SSRIs, are highly effective in the management of these disorders. In addition to the use of SSRIs, serotonin norepinephrine reuptake inhibitors (SNRIs) such as venlafaxine and duloxetine have proven efficacy in generalized anxiety disorder, PTSD, and other disorders (Pae, Lim, Ajwani, Lee, & Patkar, 2007; Sadock, Sadock, & Sussman, 2006; Thase, 2006).

Compelling data implicate the role of genetic vulnerability, personality traits, and psychosocial stressors in the pathogenesis of anxiety disorders and other psychiatric disorders

CRITICAL THINKING

An important biological theory about the cause of anxiety disorders is dysregulation and subsequent activation of NE or the HPA axis. Which set of biological symptoms are clients experiencing anxiety disorders most likely to exhibit when dysregulation or activation of this system occurs?

a. Decreased heart rate, dry skin, muscle tension, and dilated pupils

b. Palpitations, increased respirations, diaphoresis, and paresthesias

c. Normal heart rate and respirations, muscle tension, and "goose bumps"

d. Increased heart rate and respirations, constricted pupils, and dry skin

TABLE 11–3
Compilation of Research Data of Common Biological Theories of Major Anxiety Disorders

Anxiety Disorder	Neuro-Transmitter(s) Involved	Neuroendocrine System	Neuroanatomical Structures	Biological Response	Behavioral Manifestations
Panic disorder	NE or adrenergic system hyperactivity--> stimulates the limbic system and HPA axis	Activation of the HPA and HPS axes--> increase release of CRF, ACTH, GH	Cortical atrophy in the right temporal lobe and decreased volume in the hippocampus (brain region involved in learning and memory)	Tachycardia Tachypnea Palpitations Diaphoresis Sighing	Feelings of doom and fear Avoidant behaviors Hypervigilance Deficits in visual integration, reasoning, memory, and motor coordination performance
	Dysregulation or decrease of 5-HT	Activation of the LC		Dry mouth	
	Decreased GABA levels	(Activation of the ANS)	Abnormalities in glucose metabolism in the frontal, prefrontal, and basal ganglia	Difficulty swallowing Headache	
	Overactivity of serotonin				
Post-traumatic stress disorder	NE hyperactivity	Activation of the HPA and HPS axes--> increase release of CRF, ACTH, GH	Decreased blood flow to the middle temporal lobe, prefrontal cortex (PFC), which plays a role in the interpretation and extinction of fear through inhibition of amygdala function	Tachycardia Tachypnea Palpitations Diaphoresis Sighing	Feelings of doom and fear Avoidant behaviors Hypervigilance
		Activation of the LC		Dry mouth Difficulty swallowing Headache	
Obsessive-compulsive disorder			Abnormalities in the basal ganglia, thalamus, and ventral prefrontal cortex		Deficits in visual integration, reasoning, memory, and motor coordination performance
			Abnormalities in glucose metabolism in the frontal, prefrontal, and basal ganglia		

(continues)

TABLE 11-3
Compilation of Research Data of Common Biological Theories of Major Anxiety Disorders (continued)

Anxiety Disorder	Neuro-Transmitter(s) Involved	Neuroendocrine System	Neuroanatomical Structures	Biological Response	Behavioral Manifestations
GAD	Same as other disorders Widespread activation of cholinergic and noradrenergic centers in the brain stem -N-methyl-dMDA (glutamate receptors appear to play a role in anxiety and fear responses)	Same as other disorders Activation of the amygdala generates worry and fear response Hypothalamus activates stress hormones ("flight/fight" hormones) and brainstem	Total superior temporal gyrus (STG), volume increased with right and left asymmetry Right hemispheric involvement and abnormalities in amygdala and STG increase risk of GAD	Uncontrollable and distressful worrying increases heart rate, muscle tension, sleep disturbances, apprehension, uneasiness, restlessness, agitation, and anticipatory anxiety	Restlessness Unable to "shut mind down" due to worrying Impaired interpersonal relationships and occupational function Avoidance of situations that trigger worrying, reassurance seeking, and checking are used to prevent activation of worrying

Neurotransmitters: GABA, gamma-aminobutyric acid (inhibitory neurotransmitter); NE, norepinephrine (activating neurotransmitter); 5-HT, serotonin (activating neurotransmitter).
Neuroendocrine system: ACTH, adrenocorticotropic hormone; ANS, autonomic nervous system; CRF, corticotropin-releasing factor; GH, growth hormone; HPA, hypothalamic-pituitary-adrenal axis; HPS, hypothalamic-pituitary-somatropin axis; LC, locus ceruleus (specialized neurons that contain the largest number of NE receptors in the ANS).
STG: A structure involved in receptive and nonverbal auditory and language processing.

Note. Adapted from McClure, E. B., Monk, C. S., Nelson, E. E., Parrish, J. M., Adler, A., Blair, R. J., et al. (2007). Abnormal attention modulation of fear circuit function in pediatric generalized anxiety disorder. *Archives of General Psychiatry, 64,* 97–106. Miller, L. A., Taber, K. H., Gabbard, G. O., & Hurley, R. A. (2005). Neural underpinnings of fear and its modulation: Implications for anxiety disorders. *Journal of Neuropsychiatry and Clinical Neuroscience, 17,* 1–6. Richardson, R., Ledgerwood, L., & Cranney, J. (2004). Facilitation of fear extinction by D-cycloserine: Theoretical and clinical implications. *Learning and Memory, 11,* 510–516. Simeon, D., Knutelska, M., Yehuda, R., Putnam, F., Schmeidler, J., & Smith L. M. (2007). Hypothalamic-pituitary-adrenal axis function in dissociative disorders, post-traumatic stress disorder and healthy volunteers. *Biological Psychiatry, 61,* 966–973. Yehuda, R. (2006). Advances in understanding neuroendocrine alterations in PTSD and their implications. *Annals of the New York Academy of Sciences, 1071,* 137–166.

(Zvolensky, Kotov, Antipova, & Schmidt, 2005). Supposedly, the anxiety or arousal modulating system is genetically sensitive or vulnerable to stressful events that contribute to neurotransmitter release and function during intense anxiety states. Anxiety for persons with these characteristics becomes a maladaptive response; heightened anxiety or chronic anxiety generates intense cognitive, biological, and emotional activation (Cloninger, 2006). This chronic anxiety state related to anticipated threat serves to reinforce avoidance behaviors as well as to potentially limit pleasant or new positive experiences (Cloninger, 2006).

The primary theory of anxiety disorders involves dysregulation of benzodiazepine receptors in the central nervous system (CNS). Benzodiazepine receptors have primary binding sites with GABA receptors, which sensitize them to GABA, an inhibitory neurotransmitter. GABA is the principal inhibitory neurotransmitter in the CNS and appears to play a role in modulation and reduction of NE. Presumably, the primary anxiolytic or anxiety-reducing effects of benzodiazepines result from regulating GABA receptors. The inhibitory action of GABA receptors decreases the cells' electrical excitability, hence an anxiolytic effect. Most anxiety symptoms respond positively to both short-acting and long-acting benzodiazepine medications, which activate GABA receptors, such as lorazepam (Ativan) and diazepam (Valium), respectively (Sadock et al., 2006).

Anxiety disorders appear to arise from dysregulation of GABAergic and other neurotransmitter systems. This premise suggests that low levels of GABA or fewer GABA receptors are physiologically incapable of overriding the effects of excessive NE secretion. Lack of regulation or modulation of NE contributes to clinical manifestations of anxiety disorders. Researchers submit that glutamate plays a role in the genesis of anxiety disorders such as GAD, OCD, and social anxiety disorder and major depression. Dysregulation of glutamatergic neurotransmission in the anterior cingulate may be associated with the pathogenesis of OCD and MDD (Phan et al., 2005). Glutamate is posited to have an inverse response with GABA. Low levels of GABA (inhibitory neurotransmitter) increase glutamate (stimulatory neurotransmitter) levels. Based on this premise, low levels of GABA and high levels of glutamate contribute to intense anxiety states. Glutamate antagonists normalize GABA neurotransmission and mitigate symptoms of anxiety disorders. Although these agents have not been approved for psychiatric disorders, preclinical and clinical data (open-label studies) indicate alterations in glutamate modulation in anxiety disorders and the anxiolytic promise for glutamate antagonists (Mathew et al., 2005). Dysregulation of neurotransmitters is one posit of anxiety disorders. Additional biological theories are worthy of discussion.

Neuroanatomical Theories

Neuroanatomical theories, like previous biological theories, support the premise that complex factors contribute to the clinical manifestations of various anxiety disorders. Neuroanatomical studies using positron emission tomography

(PET) and computed tomography reveal abnormalities in glucose metabolism in the frontal and prefrontal cortex and the basal ganglia of the brain in clients with major anxiety disorders, such as PD and obsessive-compulsive disorder (OCD). Researchers also submit that right frontal hemisphere activation seems to represent activation of an avoidance-withdrawal system that gives rise to negative emotions. These data demonstrate asymmetries in the frontal hemisphere resulting in a greater activation of the right frontal-avoidance-withdrawal systems in the client with panic disorder (McClure et al., 2007). The significance of these data is its relationship to anxiety disorders, such as PD, phobias, and PTSD, in which avoidance and withdrawal behaviors are common. Even more important, these data provide a greater understanding of complex alterations in various regions of the brain that give rise to anxiety disorders.

Additional data from other neuroimaging studies suggest that the abnormalities in the basal ganglia and ventral prefrontal cortex are most frequently found in OCD. Based on this premise, adult clients are likely to exhibit decrements on neuropsychological testing, specifically on visual integration, reasoning, memory, and motor coordination performance (de Geus, Denys, Sitskoorn, & Westenberg, 2007).

A consistent PET finding in PTSD clients exposed to combat slides and sounds is a decrease in blood flow (regional cerebral blood flow [rCBF]) in the anterior temporal Broca region (Nemeroff, Bremner, Foa, Mayberg, North, & Stein, 2006). This region plays a major role in the extinction of fear through inhibition of amygdala function. In addition, magnetic resonance imaging (MRI) tests exhibit cortical atrophy in the right temporal lobe of clients experiencing PD and diminished volume of the hippocampus, a brain region involved in learning and memory (Bremner, 2004).

Other neuroanatomical studies suggest that individuals with PD are vulnerable to precipitation of acute anxiety symptoms or physiological arousal by intravenous lactate infusion. Findings from a study conducted in 2007 that tested the physiologic and behavioral effects of naloxone and sodium lactate implicate the role of the endogenous opioid system in modulating biologic underpinnings of PD, particularly shortness of breath or suffocation sensitivity (Sinha, Goetz, & Klein, 2007).

Neurobiological studies implicate alterations in neuroanatomical regions in individuals with various anxiety disorders. Neuroimaging studies involving fractional anisotropy (FA) values revealed that participants with panic disorder exhibited significantly higher FA values in left anterior and right posterior cingulated neural pathways compared to controls. Alterations in cingulated white connectivity in these two regions was positively correlated with severity of symptoms (Abe et al., 2006).

Preliminary findings involving clients with OCD also revealed alterations in the anterior cingulate white matter. Findings from these data parallel neurobiological models, implicating a defect in connectivity in the anterior cingulate basal ganglia-thalamocortical neurocircuitry (Szeszjo et al., 2005).

These data support the premise regarding metabolic dysregulation in individuals with PDs. These researchers, like other scientists, hail these findings as another biological marker of anxiety disorders, specifically PD. Although these findings are not definitive, they support the premise that panic attacks and other anxiety disorders arise from specific brain regions and structures. Figure 11–1 shows specific regions of the brain with a relationship to anxiety disorders.

Genetic Factors

Genetic studies provide strong evidence of familial patterns of anxiety disorders, such as generalized anxiety disorder, OCD, and phobias (Hettema, Prescott, Myers, Neale, & Kendler, 2005; Shih, Belmonte, & Zandi, 2004; Stewart et al., 2007). Perhaps Torgersen (1983) conducted one of the most exhaustive studies linking genetics to familial transmission of PD. Evidence in these data showed that monozygotic (identical) twins were five times more likely to develop a PD than dizygotic (fraternal) twins.

Findings from a 1999 twin study conducted by Stein, Jang, and Livesley (1999) support earlier findings about the heritability of anxiety disorders. In their study of 179 monozygotic twins and 158 dizygotic twins, they identified one psychological risk factor for the development of PD, specifically *anxiety sensitivity*, cognitive risk factor, and a heritable component. This cognitive risk factor arises from the family environment and perception of anxiety symptoms as frightening and that over time this perception becomes part of the individual's personality.

Anxiety sensitivity refers to the fear of anxiety-related physiological sensations (i.e., palpitations, diaphoresis), which clients believe are life threatening. Taylor (1995), an anxiety sensitivity theorist, stated that some people are more vulnerable to this condition than others and they are likely to perceive these symptoms as dangerous and life threatening. Researchers believe that anxiety sensitivity is a risk factor for the development of PD and predict the onset of panic attacks (Schmidt, Zvolensky, & Maner, 2006). They also believe that these findings are consistent with social learning theories that suggest a link between information-processing abnormalities in anxiety disorders and their role in anxiety disorders and sensitivity (Zvolensky & Schmidt, 2007). Findings from this study along with other twin studies suggest a stronger genetic risk or vulnerability to anxiety disorders in identical twins than fraternal twins.

Moreover, these data provide a persuasive argument for collaborating with the client and family to lessen and prevent anxiety sensitivity, particularly in vulnerable populations. Interventions must focus on health teaching symptom management, effective communication, and adaptive coping skills.

The complexity of anxiety disorders makes them difficult to explain from just one theory. A contemporary model for anxiety disorders integrates psychodynamic, existential, cognitive-behavioral, developmental, biological, and genetic theories. These theories are the bases of anxiety across the life span and provide a plausible understanding of diverse treatment approaches across the life span.

ANXIETY ACROSS THE LIFE SPAN

The complexity of anxiety disorders requires a discussion of anxiety on a continuum beginning from infancy to older adulthood. The value of a life span perspective is its holistic model, which integrates psychosocial, developmental, and biological factors and their contributions to anxiety disorders. This model suggests that childhood anxiety is a risk factor or prodromal condition that becomes full circle as adult anxiety disorders.

Presently, there is a paucity of research regarding childhood anxiety disorders. However, over the past decade there has been a compilation of data that indicates childhood and adolescent anxiety disorders as part of a continuum the full expression of which occurs as adult conditions. The significance of these data includes early identification, prevention, education, and reduction in chronicity of anxiety disorders across the life span. It also involves discerning normal childhood and adolescent anxiety from anxiety disorders.

CHILDHOOD AND ADOLESCENT ANXIETY DISORDERS

Anxiety and fear are common childhood experiences that emerge during various aspects of growth and development. For example, during infancy, fear induces the startle reflex in response to sudden movements or loud noises. Similarly, strangers elicit a fear response during the latter part of the first year of life. Jean Piaget's (1954, 1958) research on human growth and development has shown that children's level of logical and cognitive function differs from that of adults, and that they have trouble understanding that although primary caregivers may be out of sight, they still exist. The child's immature logic is the basis of this fear and anxiety when the primary caregivers leave the room. Normally, as the child's cognitive processes mature, he is able to recognize and escape danger and ultimately manages fears or anxiety effectively. Separation anxiety is a normal response to estrangement from primary caregivers and adaptive coping in the child. As the cognitive processes mature and the child masters various developmental tasks, separation anxiety abates.

As their cognitive abilities mature, children's imaginations become vivid, fearing monsters and other imaginary characters. The evolving ego and cognitive function enable children to think about the past and anticipate the future, consequently transforming their responses to fear (Graziano, DeGiorani, & Garcia, 1979).

During late childhood and early adolescence, cognitive and ego function continue to mature, enabling the youth to deal

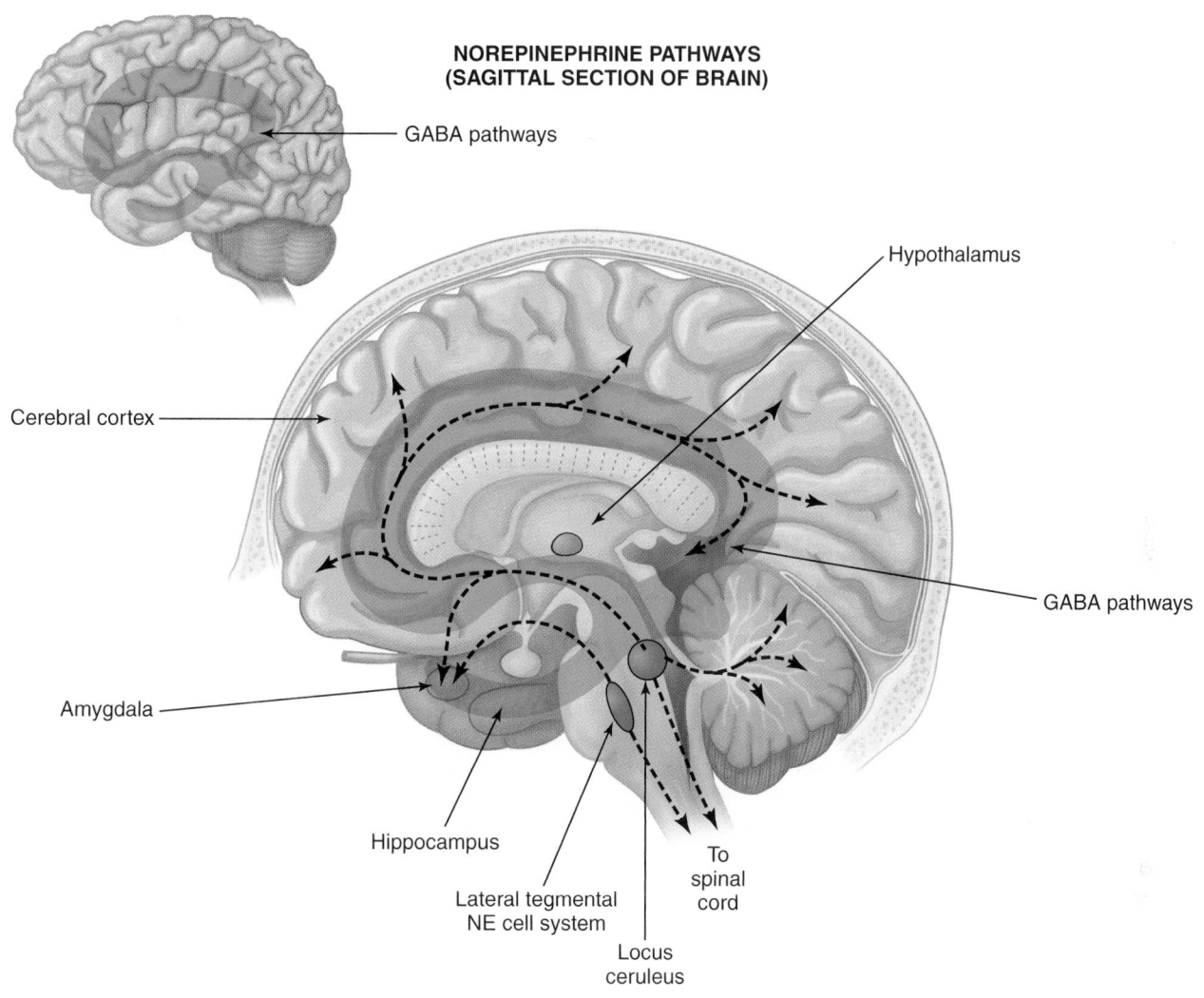

**NOREPINEPHRINE PATHWAYS
(SAGITTAL SECTION OF BRAIN)**

GABA pathways

Hypothalamus

Cerebral cortex

GABA pathways

Amygdala

Hippocampus

Lateral tegmental
NE cell system

To
spinal
cord

Locus
ceruleus

Excessive secretion of the neurotransmitter nor-epinephrine may be a factor in anxiety disorders. Neurons in the locus ceruleus and the lateral tegmental norepinephrine (NE) cell system receive stimuli of sensory pain or potential danger. In re-sponse, they secrete NE in excessive amounts to the cerebral cortex, limbic system (primarily the right temporal lobe), brain stem, and spinal cord to pre-pare for defense or escape. It has not been deter-mined whether the extreme stress felt by a person with an anxiety disorder is caused by overstimulation of a normal NE system or by physiological differences in that person's NE system. Abnormal serotonin func-tioning and glucose metabolism are also believed to play a role in anxiety disorders.

Figure 11–1 Neuroanatomy illustration of specific brain regions associated with anxiety disorders. *(Ilustration concept: Gail Kongable, MSN, CNRN, CCNR, Department of Neurosurgery, University of Virginia Health Sciences Center.)* *(continues)*

GABA PATHWAYS
(CORONAL SECTION)

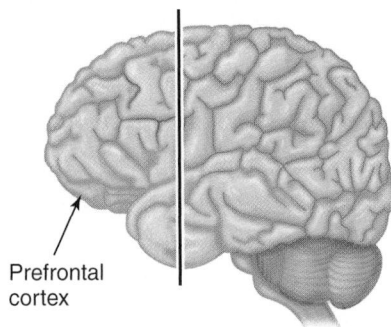

Prefrontal cortex

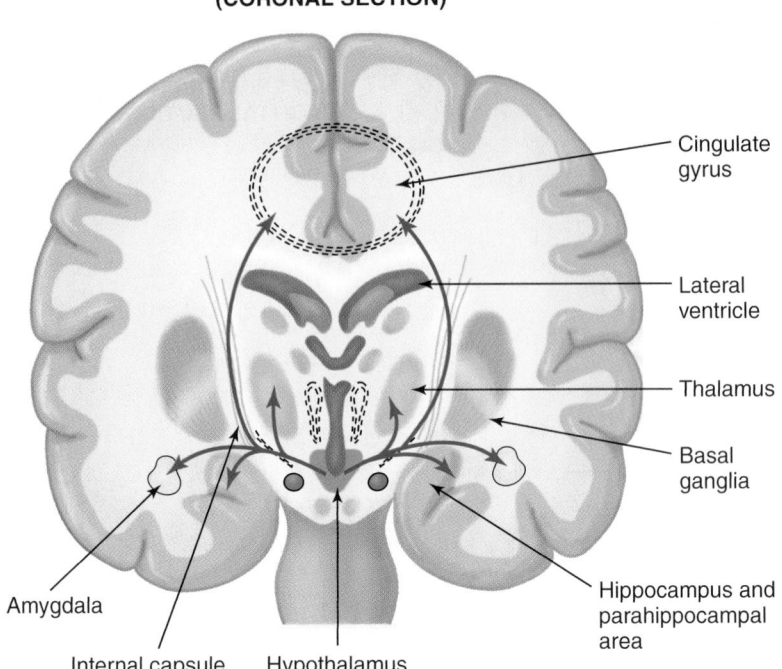

Cingulate gyrus

Lateral ventricle

Thalamus

Basal ganglia

Hippocampus and parahippocampal area

Amygdala

Internal capsule

Hypothalamus

Gamma-aminobutyric acid (GABA), an amino acid that serves as the brain's modulator, is an important inhibitory neurotransmitter. Without adequate GABA biosynthesis, release, and activity, the brain would react to the continuous bombardment of even the smallest external and internal stimuli. GABA receptors throughout the brain counteract the effects of the excitatory neurotransmitters norepinephrine and dopamine, preventing disorganized and frenzied responses to continual stimuli and dampening emotional arousal. A person with low levels of GABA or fewer GABA receptors is theoretically more susceptible to anxiety disorders.

HOW DRUGS WORK IN ANXIETY DISORDERS

Uncontrolled anxiety results from unsuccessful defense against anxiety-provoking stimuli. Sometimes anxiety may be related to chronic depression; in such cases treatment with tricyclic antidepressants or monoamine oxidase inhibitors can cause the anxiety to resolve. Drugs that enhance the action of GABA can also be effective in treating anxiety. *(See Figure 2–4 for an explanation of synaptic structures.)*

1. Norepinephrine (NE) is synthesized from a dopamine and tyrosine hydroxylase reaction. GABA is synthesized from glutamate, a common amino acid.
2. NE and GABA are stored in synaptic vesicles. *Some antihypertensive drugs interfere with the uptake and storage of NE and deplete NE stores. Although they are prescribed for other reasons these drugs may have the side effect of alleviating anxiety.*
3. Vesicles migrate to the presynaptic membrane and release NE and GABA into the synaptic cleft. *Because amphetamines stimulate the release of NE and block its reuptake, they can contribute to anxiety.*
4. Stimulation of GABA receptor sites makes the target neuron less sensitive to stimulation by NE and other neurotransmitters. *Benzodi-*

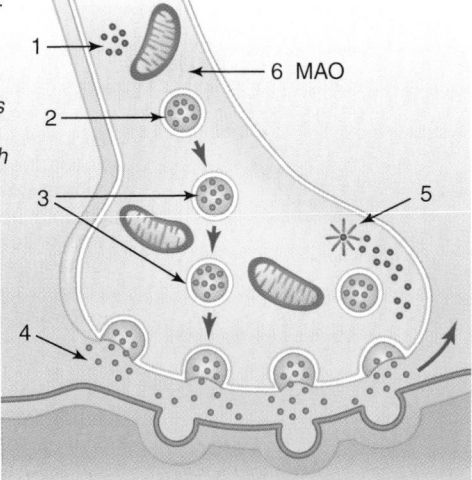

1

6 MAO

2

3

5

4

azepines such as chlordiazepoxide (Librium) and diazepam (Valium) are effective in treating anxiety because they enhance the binding of GABA to its receptor sites.
5. The action of NE is stopped by its resorption into the presynaptic terminal. *The tricyclic drug desipramine (Norpramin), used to treat post-traumatic stress disorder, inhibits the resorption of NE, resulting in larger available amounts that may cause increased anxiety.*
6. NE present in the free state within the presynaptic terminal can be broken down by the enzyme monoamine oxidase (MAO). *MAO inhibitors (MAOIs), sometimes used to treat anxiety disorders caused by underlying depression, prevent the breakdown of NE in the presynaptic terminal.*

Figure 11–1 *(continued)*

more realistically with fear and anxiety. Anxiety tends to vary with age, and fears of strangers and separation decline with age. Origins of normal adolescent anxiety include consolidation of identity, sexuality, performance and achievement, acceptance by peers, formation of meaningful relationships, and independence. Puberty increases vulnerability to various anxiety disorders, particularly PD, agoraphobia, and social phobia. More interestingly, concerns about one's appearance, acceptance, interactions with peers, and self-confidence tend to replace early childhood fears (Bernstein et al., 1996).

Anxiety disorders in childhood and adolescence are more common than previously thought. The APA (2000) lists separation anxiety under childhood and adolescent anxiety disorders in the *DSM-IV-TR*. Other anxiety disorders, such as PTSD, OCD, overanxious disorder, and social phobia are found in this age group.

Separation Anxiety Disorder

Separation anxiety disorder is associated with psychosocial, learning, and genetic factors. It is one of the most common diagnoses in children, affecting girls more than boys. Children with separation anxiety experience panic or excessive worrying about losing their primary caregiver. They are reluctant to go to school or depart from the caregiver because of the fear of separation. These symptoms exist for at least 4 weeks and produce significant or subjective distress (APA, 2000). A number of children may even ruminate or have morbid fears about losing their parents, getting lost, or having accidents. The child's history often reveals significant separations in his life (i.e., hospitalization). Professional help is often sought when the child is unable to adapt socially and cope with the environment. Other behavioral responses include the fear of being harmed, frequent crying when primary caregivers leave the room, and refusal to attend school. These children are often reluctant or refuse to go to sleep, fear the dark, and experience nightmares. Some children may even complain of somatic problems such as nausea, palpitations, faintness, headaches, stomach pain (butterflies in stomach), fretfulness, and whining (APA, 2000).

Diagnosing separation anxiety disorder involves gathering a history of events preceding the separation, response to parents' or primary caretakers' departure, and resulting behaviors. Differential diagnoses of other anxiety disorders, such as PD, overanxious disorder, social phobia, substance-induced anxiety disorder (caffeinism or prescription or nonprescription drugs), mood disorder, medical conditions that produce anxiety, and level of family function, provide the bases of diagnosing separation anxiety disorder. Differential diagnosis of medical conditions that generate anxiety involves a complete physical examination and biopsychosocial assessment.

Considerations for the Caregiver: The Child with Separation Anxiety

Parents or caregivers of a preschool or school-age child often find it frustrating and distressful when the child cries and refuses to go to school. These children often experience intense anxiety and fears. Separation anxiety disorder refers to excessive anxiety concerning separation from home or parents. These children often express fears of something happening to their parents and complain of physical symptoms, such as headaches and stomachaches. It is the most common prepubertal anxiety disorder. Typical anxiety-producing situations include:

- When they are walking out of the house to attend school
- Riding the bus
- When parents walk out of the door or drop the child off at school

The premise behind parental interventions is that environmental "reinforcers" maintain the child's symptoms. Reinforcement include missing school and staying home, attention from the parents, or "goodies" and toys when the child cries or complains about going to school. The following nursing interventions can help parents or caregivers understand their role in reducing their child's symptoms of separation anxiety.

- Assess the parents' understanding about separation anxiety.
- Encourage parents to express their feelings about the child's symptoms.

- Provide health education about separation anxiety and teach cognitive-behavioral approaches to their child's care.
- Make referrals to various community support groups for parents of children with anxiety disorders.

The following interventions are useful in reducing the child's anxiety:

- Recognize that attending school all day is overwhelming to the child.
- Avoid colluding with the child—the child must attend school.
- Consider working with the school and setting up a behavioral approach that involves exposure-based or graded contact (gradual exposure enables the child to gradually adjust and master fears).
- Avoid focusing a lot of attention on the child's behaviors because doing so may reinforce them.
- Set firm and consistent limits—this will help the child develop some internal controls over the environment, subsequently reducing anxiety.
- Consider medications that reduce biological symptoms of separation anxiety when indicated.
- Provide a supportive and caring environment.

Treatment must consist of a multimodal approach that integrates individual psychotherapy, family psychoeducation and therapy, and psychopharmacologic interventions. The basis of treatment emanates from the premise that varied environmental reinforcement maintains symptoms and governs biological responses to anxiety-provoking situations. Primary environmental reinforcers include missing school and staying at home and gaining attention from parents. Positive treatment outcomes must focus on altering current circumstances that sustain these behaviors. Cognitive-behavioral interventions that involve exposure-based or desensitization approaches show promise in the treatment of separation anxiety disorder. This approach uses stepwise exposure that assists the child in confronting fearful situations and focusing on the maladaptiveness of cognitive distortions. Family psychoeducation must focus on teaching parents how to support the child and maintain parent-child boundaries without reinforcing maladaptive behaviors. A comprehensive approach usually involves the child, the parents, and the school, who play key roles in helping the child return and maintain regular school attendance. Initially the parent may be present in school for several weeks or longer; then the parent gradually leaves the child's presence. Deep muscle relaxation techniques enable the child to gain control over biological responses to anxiety-provoking situations (Stein, Jaycox, Kataoka, & Wong et al., 2003; Thurber, Walton, & American Academy of Pediatrics Council on School Health, 2007).

Mainstay treatment for separation anxiety disorder is cognitive behavioral therapy, family and individual therapy, and psychoeducation. Although open-label studies using SSRI antidepressants have been used to treat separation anxiety, few randomized controlled studies have been conducted to determine the long-term effects. Medications must be used with caution, particularly antidepressants, due to the risk of suicide. It is imperative for nurses and other providers to discuss the risk and benefits of using these agents (Clark et al., 2005). See "Considerations for the Caregiver: The Child with Separation Anxiety."

Social Phobia

Social phobia, also known as social anxiety disorder, refers to a fear of performance situations and subsequent avoidance behaviors, particularly when the child fears humiliation or embarrassment when under the scrutiny of others. Social phobia in children and adolescents involves distress in a broad range of interpersonal encounters such as formal speaking, eating in front of others, using public restrooms, and speaking to authority figures (Hirshfeld-Becker et al., 2007).

Avoidant behaviors in children and adolescents are manifested as persistent or extremely constricted social interaction with unfamiliar people to the point of intense social impairment of interaction with peers. These behaviors may occur as early as 2½ years of age and endure for at least 6 months for diagnosis. Behaviors of children tend to be

associated with a desire to be involved with others. If this disorder continues into adulthood, it is linked with avoidant personality disorder (APA, 2000). Factors that increase the risk of social phobia in children and adolescents include modeling of shy, aloof behaviors by the primary caregivers, child abuse, early traumatic childhood losses, chronic medical problems, and impaired social skills.

A multimodal approach that consists of psychosocial and family interventions provides the most effective treatment outcomes for the child with social phobia. Treatment consists of cognitive-behavioral interventions that involve gradual exposure, cognitive reconstructing, coping skills, assertiveness training for shyness, and anxiety self-monitoring. The focus of cognitive reconstructing is modifying maladaptive negative self-statements that interfere with problem-solving behaviors (Cartwright-Hatton, Roberts, Chitsabesan, Fothergill, & Harrington, 2004). Presently, there is lack of clinical data that indicate the effectiveness of pharmacologic agents in the treatment of social phobia in children and adolescents.

Overanxious Disorder

The essential features of overanxious disorder are unwarranted distress over the future of the appropriateness of past behavior, somatic or hyperarousal complaints, and the inability to relax or settle down, all occurring for at least a 6-month period (APA, 2000). Children suffering from this disorder are extremely sensitive, and their overanxious behavior is exaggerated during stressful periods; they need enormous consolation during times of stress. These children tend to be overly concerned about their social performance and competency and possibly exhibit behavioral avoidance.

The treatment of overanxious disorder, like social phobia, primarily involves individual psychotherapy, psychoeducation, family therapy, and cognitive-behavioral interventions that emphasize identification and recognition of anxiety and clarification of anxiety-provoking cognitions. These approaches provide the child and parents with a coping plan that helps evaluate performance and promotes self-approval. It also helps the child to restructure negative self-talk during anxiety-provoking circumstances.

Post-traumatic Stress Disorder

The experience of childhood trauma, like other anxiety disorders, appears to evolve over time and has the potential to produce variable and enduring effects that generate an array of adulthood psychiatric symptoms. This continuum of childhood to adulthood PTSD is more evident in studies of childhood sexual abuse. Clinical findings from contemporary studies also indicate that a failure to provide adequate treatment to children suffering from traumatic experiences, depending on their vulnerability and severity of symptoms, will ultimately evolve into adult PTSD symptoms (Clark,

Rodgers, Caldwell, Power, & Stansfeld, 2007; Copeland, Keeler, Angold, & Costello, 2007).

The relationship between grief and traumatic occurrences in children is a matter that has long been overlooked. Pynoos, Steinberg, and Goenjian (1996) believed that this lack of attention to these issues often impedes the clinicians' ability to assess children's grief and trauma because of their immature ego and cognitive functioning. Immature ego development and cognitive functioning interfere with the child's ability to process trauma and grief issues without experiencing profound emotional pain. The effects of childhood trauma are influenced by several factors, such as the nature of the stressor (e.g., sudden versus foreseen death of a loved one, sexual or physical abuse), available support systems, and the child's ability to work through his pain (Widom, Dutton, Czaja, & Dumont, 2005).

Children are more likely to have difficulty coping with the devastation of physical and emotional trauma than adults, presumably because of their inadequate coping skills. Interestingly enough, the intensity and duration of symptoms parallel several factors, including individual coping style, the degree of self-blame, parental emotional climate and the reactions after disclosure. The last variable, especially if negative reactions occur after disclosure, is most likely to produce negative consequences in later life and is a primary predictor of maladaptation and severe PTSD symptoms over the life span. Presumably, the child who fails to resolve a traumatic experience is likely to cope with it by internalizing depression and anxiety (Goenjian et al., 2005).

The best predictors of psychological well-being after childhood exposure to trauma are adequate emotional support and nurturing families, less exposure to abuse, and absence of family turmoil and self-blaming. Children from healthy families are more resilient and adaptable and are more likely to express feelings about the trauma than those from chaotic, blaming, and nonsupportive families. Furthermore, there is growing evidence that parents of anxious children may also have an anxiety or other mental disorder that interferes with

keeping the child in treatment and providing positive reinforcement (Goenjian et al., 2005; Pynoos et al., 1996).

Interventions must focus on strengthening the youth's individual and family repertoire of coping skills. Adaptive responses to trauma are likely to occur when interventions provide an atmosphere of acceptance and empathy. This process involves fostering enduring adaptation of the child's resilience and facilitating healthy resolution of the traumatic incident. Similarly, it involves facilitating grief resolution in both the child and parents. Finally, treatment must center on preventing the traumatic event to interfere with normal growth and development and minimizing maladaptive responses in the child and family (Pynoos et al., 1996).

The following are suggestions for helping the child experiencing severe trauma to express feelings:

◆ Establish a trusting relationship by assessing the child alone, speaking in a nonthreatening voice tone, affording proper space between the child and the nurse. This process also involves introducing and explaining the purpose of the visit, providing positive experiences to increase confidence, ensuring safety, and considering the child's individual attributes and developmental stage. (See Chapter 6, Therapeutic Communication.)

◆ Engage the child by asking him to draw a picture, or invite the child to play with puppets and other toys.

◆ Tell a story using metaphors that are similar to the youth's traumatic experience, pointing out the character's possible reactions to the incident.

◆ Depending upon the nature of the trauma, developmental stage, and family involvement, facilitate a healthy review and process of the traumatic event while assessing the emotional meaning of the experience, or personal impact. The nurse must be prepared to hear the entire experience, including the horrific details, sadness, and crying that may emerge during this process. This process is enhanced through play therapy, drawing, puppets and other toys, as well as telling a story. More importantly, play and toys afford a safe medium that secures the child's fantasy and play into his expression of the experience (Pynoos et al., 1996). (This depends on the age and the nurse's clinical experience and training.)

In addition, these approaches link intrusive thoughts of the trauma to grief issues that can be explored through assessment of the child's overt and covert behavior and expression. There is no standardized test to assess trauma in children and adolescents, because each one experiences trauma differently (Widom et al., 2005).

Major manifestations of PTSD in the child or adolescent include the following (Copeland et al., 2007; Turner, Finkelhor, & Ormrod, 2006):

◆ Rejection of closeness
◆ Child's sense of a loss of the vigor and magic of youth

CRITICAL THINKING

Ricardo, a first grader, is brought to the school nurse practitioner's office complaining of "stomach pain" and fears of his mother being in an automobile accident. After performing a physical examination and talking to his mother, the school nurse finds no physical basis for the child's stomachaches or fears. Which of the following anxiety disorders is Ricardo more than likely experiencing?

a. Social phobia
b. Specific phobia
c. Separation anxiety
d. Overanxious disorder

- Cognitive impairment or forgetfulness
- Sleep disturbances (e.g., nightmares) that persist more than several days
- Dependency behaviors, such as clinging, separation anxiety, and reluctance to attend school
- Extreme fear of distress associated with events that remind the child of the trauma
- Behavioral or emotional changes
- Dissociation (an unconscious defense mechanism used to detach from painful memories and emotions that arise from a traumatic event)
- Intrusive reexperiencing of the event
- Persistent avoidance of related stimuli
- Regression to previous developmental stage
- Questions about self-worth and expression of need for solitude
- In profound cases, personality development arrest

Often, intrusive thoughts that arise from memories of the violent event interfere with various developmental tasks, increasing the risk of poor school or work performance. Traumatic childhood events include the death of a parent or sibling; child abuse; witnessing violent acts such as murder; and natural disasters such as tornadoes, floods, or earthquakes. See Table 11–4 for the symptoms of childhood PTSD.

The treatment of childhood PTSD, like other childhood anxiety disorders, is multimodal and includes cognitive-behavioral approaches, individual and family therapy, psychoeducation, and pharmacologic interventions. Ideally, treatment occurs during the acute phase or within the first 3 months after the trauma. The cognitive-behavioral model comprises a rapid exposure approach. Currently, there is a lack of empirical data regarding the use of pharmacologic agents in childhood PTSD.

Obsessive-Compulsive Disorder

Obsessive-compulsive disorder (OCD) affects children and adolescents along with adults. One third to one half of adults with OCD report a childhood or adolescent onset, again suggesting the continuum of anxiety disorders across the life span (Stewart et al., 2007). Childhood-onset OCD was once thought to be rare until recent studies of children and adolescents revealed a lifetime prevalence of 2–3 percent of this disorder (Piacentini & Bergman, 2000). Childhood OCD appears to be similar to adult OCD although its pattern regarding specific symptoms and age varies. This childhood anxiety disorder is highly refractory, often presenting with a chronic and episodic course (Ivarsson & Valderhaug, 2005). The emergence of OCD symptoms during childhood generally presents as repetitive, ritualistic behaviors and thoughts. Epidemiological studies of children with OCD show a pattern of the following symptoms:

- Obsessive thoughts with common themes of fears of contamination, sexual, or religious

CRITICAL THINKING

Camellia, a 15-year-old, and her father were recently involved in an auto accident which left her father unconscious for several hours. Camellia was uninjured, but she is experiencing intense guilt and sleep disturbances and has become increasingly more reclusive. She is also feeling guilty about the accident because before leaving home she and her father had had an argument about her dance classes. Camellia has been diagnosed with PTSD. Major predictors of positive outcomes in children with PTSD are all *except* which of the following?

a. The family's response to the child's reactions or disclosure

b. Preventive use of antidepressants shortly after the incident

c. The child's developmental stage and cognitive competency

d. The family's level of conflict and repertoire of coping skills

TABLE 11–4
Symptoms of Post-traumatic Stress Disorder across the Life Span

Childhood/Adolescent

Short-Term Effects

- Sleep disturbances
- Persistent thoughts of trauma
- Fear that another traumatic event will occur
- Hyperalertness
- Regression in young children (i.e., thumb-sucking, bedwetting, and dependent behaviors)

Long-Term Effects

- Antisocial behaviors
- Vandalism
- Psychosomatic illness (i.e., peptic ulcer disease)
- Truancy and conduct disorders
- Mood disorders
- Substance-related disorders
- Eating disorders

Adulthood

- Persistent, recurrent, and intrusive thoughts or dreams of the trauma
- Avoidance behaviors
- Depersonalization
- Biological responses, such as emotional numbing, hypervigilance, and persistent arousal of the sympathetic nervous system

- Rituals, such as washing, checking, arranging, and cognitive rituals
- Repeatedly rewriting a letter or number until it was perfect

A seminal comprehensive study of childhood-onset OCD and tic disorder in 50 children (Swedo et al., 1998) (see Research Abstract) adds another dimension to the biological basis of this complex anxiety disorder. Data from this study show that some disorders may reflect a pediatric autoimmune neuropsychiatric disorder arising from group A beta-hemolytic streptococcal [GABHS] infections (PANDAS). Clinical implications from this study suggest that there is a subgroup of children whose symptom exacerbations are precipitated by GABHS infections. Clearly, these findings also indicate the need for novel pharmacologic interventions, including antimicrobials, immunization, and preventive strategies (see Research Abstract).

Neuropsychological findings implicating the alterations in frontal function in children with OCD, like other anxiety disorders, that evolve over time is well established. These data also implicate that children, unlike adults, may not have clinical symptoms of OCD that interfere with cognitive function during the early course of this illness.

Major treatment modalities for the child with OCD are consistent with adult treatment and include cognitive therapy and psychopharmacology. The developmental stage, severity of symptoms, and parental involvement determine interventions. Cognitive-behavioral therapy is useful for stopping ruminating thoughts. This approach attempts to modify negative perceptions of self and improves the child's self-observation concerning obsessions. It also fosters independence and adaptive behavioral change.

One such approach consists of a 16-session cognitive-behavioral therapy incorporating exposure response prevention (ERP) in conjunction with anxiety management training (AMT). AMT encompasses relaxation, coping skills, breathing exercises, OCD symptom mapping, and coping statements (March, Mulle, & Herbel, 1994). Desensitization, or exposure to biological cues, helps the child and parents recognize fear or anxiety-evoking incidents. The basis of this approach lies in its gradual exposure to these anxiety-evoking situations from the lowest to the highest anxiety levels. This approach, like other CBT techniques, increases confidence and reduces anxiety and stress. Parents also play active roles in the child's treatment program during various stages. Psychoeducation provides a forum for family support and reinforcement techniques that reduce compulsive rituals. Similarly, family therapy is vital to decreasing the family's involvement in the child's rituals and dealing with dysfunctional family dynamics. Group therapy is effective in reducing anxiety, improving social skills, and assessing the meaning of symptoms or behaviors.

RESEARCH ABSTRACT

Pediatric Autoimmune Neuropsychiatric Disorders Associated with Streptococcal Infections: Clinical Description of the First 50 Cases

Swedo, S. E., Leonard, H. L., Garvey, M., Mittleman, B., Allen, A. J., Perlmutter, S., et al. (1998). *American Journal of Psychiatry, 155,* 264–271.

Study Problem/Purpose
To describe the clinical characteristics of a novel group of clients with OCD and tic disorders, designated as pediatric autoimmune neuropsychiatric disorders associated with streptococcal group A beta-hemolytic streptococcal (GABHS) infections (PANDAS).

Methods
The investigators conducted a systematic clinical workup of 50 children who met all of the following diagnostic criteria: presence of OCD or tic disorder, prepubertal onset, episodic symptoms, association with GABHS infections, and neurological deficits. Children with an acute onset or severe exacerbations of OCD or tics were sought through mailings to various child psychiatrists, physicians, pediatric neurologists, and the Tourette's Syndrome Association's national newsletter. More than 270 telephone interviews were conducted, of whom 109 were invited to the NIMH for a face-to-face screening evaluation. Depending on the seriousness of the symptoms, the children were placed in one or two protocols—a placebo-controlled study of penicillin prophylaxis or a randomized-control study of various immunotherapies. Several instruments were used to assess the children's mood, intelligence, and cognitive deficits. Data were gathered from both children and their parents.

Findings
Clinical findings showed that many of these subjects' symptoms had an acute onset and early onset (n = 6.3 years for tics and 7.4 years for OCD) typically triggered by GABHS infections. The clinical course of these episodes were relapsing and remitting with dramatic comorbidity with other mental disorders, such as separation anxiety, nightmares and fears, emotional lability, cognitive deficits, and oppositional behaviors.

These data clearly indicate a homogenous client group whose symptom exacerbations are precipitated by GABHS exposure.

Implications for Psychiatric Nurses
These findings suggest the early influence and course of OCD and other anxiety states in young children exposed to GABHS infections. Nurses need to assess young children presenting with these symptoms for infections to facilitate early identification and reduce the potential risk of serious physical and mental consequences of untreated infections. This also reinforces the need to assess each client's current and past health status to assess a pattern of symptoms that implicates a more serious medical condition.

Psychopharmacologic interventions have been used successfully to treat OCD in children. Major psychotropics, such as those used in adults (SSRIs and tricyclic agents, such as clomipramine) have been among these agents (American Academy of Child and Adolescent Psychiatry, 1998). Despite diverse treatment and the advent of SSRIs and other antiobsessional agents, OCD symptoms persist and have a chronic course for a significant number of clients.

Co-occurring Issues

A major problem associated with childhood and adolescent anxiety disorders is the co-occurrence of anxiety disorders with other psychiatric disorders such as depression, substance misuse, and personality disorders. Coexisting disorders tend to impede the assessment process in children presenting with anxiety reactions. Several diagnostic tools may be used to make a differential diagnosis such as the Revised Children's Manifest Anxiety Scale (Reynolds & Richmond, 1978), the Yale-Brown Obsessive Compulsive Scale (Goodman et al., 1989), and the Child Assessment Schedule (Hodge, McKnew, & Burbach, 1987), which diagnose developmental anxiety. These assessment tools have corresponding forms that parents need to complete regarding their children's behaviors, enabling mental health professionals to assess their children's maladaptive coping patterns. Maladaptive coping patterns include suicide risk and need for continuous monitoring of the client's level of dangerousness toward self and others throughout treatment.

Summary of Childhood and Adolescent Disorders

Overall, childhood and adolescent anxiety disorders tend to become adult anxiety disorders such as agoraphobia, generalized anxiety disorder, and PD. Furthermore, family retrospective and studies support the notion that anxiety disorders form a continuum that evolves from childhood through adulthood (Copeland et al., 2007; Widom et al., 2005)

Like adults with anxiety disorders, children with anxiety disorders may experience feelings of powerlessness, increased dependency, low self-esteem, and have impaired social skills. These problems compromise the youth's ability to cope, consequently increasing the risk of chronicity and persistent avoidance behaviors that impede growth and development. Psychoeducation is a critical aspect of treatment and involves teaching healthy parenting skills in terms of providing positive reinforcement and celebrating small accomplishments, while minimizing feelings of guilt, helplessness, and inadequacy in the parent dealing with the child's illness. Optimally, treatment is multimodal and consists of individual and family therapy, psychoeducation, cognitive-behavioral approaches, and, when appropriate, psychopharmacologic interventions. Table 11–5 lists primary treatment goals for youth experiencing anxiety disorders.

TABLE 11–5
Primary Treatment Goals for Youth Experiencing Anxiety Disorders

- Overcome fear of the threat
- Differentiate among various feelings or responses
- Become familiar with feelings
- Understand the links between feelings, thoughts, biological responses, and behaviors
- Understand that arousal is a symptom of fear
- Enhance problem-solving skills
- Gain a sense of mastery
- Develop adaptive coping behaviors

Note. Data from "Behavioral Assessment and Treatment of Childhood Phobias," by T. H. Ollendick and G. Francis, 1988, *Behavior Modification, 12,* pp. 165–203. Reprinted with permission.

ADULTHOOD DISORDERS

Anxiety is a striking feature of most mental disorders and continues to be one of the most common mental disorders, with an estimated 15 percent of the population experiencing it at some time during their lifetime (Kessler et al., 2005; Regier et al., 1990). More than 25 years ago, anxiety disorders were classified as anxiety neurosis and delineated into panic and generalized anxiety disorders. The *DSM-IV-TR* (APA, 2000) defines a number of anxiety disorders, including generalized anxiety disorder (GAD); PD; phobias such as agoraphobia, social phobia, specific phobia; OCD; acute stress disorder; and PTSD. (See Table 11–1 for a list of specific anxiety disorders.)

The complexity of anxiety disorders and their potential disabling impact across the life span requires accurate identification, accurate diagnoses, and treatment. Before treatment the client must receive appropriate assessment for medical conditions that mimic anxiety disorders. Medical conditions that produce panic-like symptoms include myocardial infarction, mitral valve prolapse, endocrine disorders such as hypoglycemia, respiratory distress, and substance-related disorders. Substance-related disorders such as central nervous system stimulants, anticholinergic intoxication, or alcohol withdrawal pose a challenge to nurses assessing clients with anxiety disorders. Medical examinations are imperative and involve a complete physical examination and other diagnostic tests such as an electrocardiogram (ECG), toxicology screens, and laboratory studies such as electrolytes and cardiac enzymes. The psychobiological assessment provides pertinent information about current prescribed and over-the-counter medications, herbal preparations, past and present medical and psychiatric treatment, nutritional status, and substance-related disorders. Because of the high coexistence with depressive illness, the nurse must also assess the client's risk of dangerousness toward self and others throughout treatment. This also involves assessing the client's past and present coping skills. The client's dietary habits must be a part of this assessment and include caffeine intake; beverages such as coffee, tea, soft drinks; chocolates, and over-the-counter preparations. The nurse must also ask the client and family about alternative or complementary therapies that may also contribute to anxiety such as diet preparations or other stimulants. This holistic database is critical to appropriate diagnosis and treatment of these complex disorders.

Generalized Anxiety Disorder

Historically, the DSM description of GAD referred to chronic anxiety or "free-floating anxiety" or "anxiety neuroses" (APA, 1968). Presently, there is a paucity of research that conceptualizes this anxiety disorder, hence, a distinct definition remains obscure. A lack of clarity also makes it difficult to distinguish from *normal worrying or apprehension*. The *DSM-IV-TR* (APA, 2000) describes the cardinal feature of GAD as apprehensive worrying. It further describes it as a pervasive, frequently *uncontrollable* worrying that extends to concerns about daily living and minor life stressors.

Primary symptoms of GAD include nervousness, irritability, apprehension, agitation, tension, tachycardia, diaphoresis, shortness of breath, difficulty falling and staying asleep, and edginess (APA, 2000). Symptoms of GAD tend to overlap those of panic and depressive disorders. GAD differs from PD in that it rarely remits and its onset occurs during earlier developmental stages, with an absence of autonomic nervous system arousal. The course of GAD is likely to begin during the second decade of life and has chronic episodic course (Connor & Davidson, 1998). Depression is estimated to accompany at least 50 percent of cases of GAD at some time during the course of the illness (Moffitt et al., 2007). Table 11–6 presents the prevalence and primary symptoms of anxiety disorders. See Chapter 9 for an in-depth discussion of depression. Table 11–7 lists anxiety-reducing techniques and interventions and Table 11–8 lists major psychopharmacologic anxiolytic agents for major anxiety disorders.

In brief, the treatment of major anxiety disorders is multimodal and consists of psychopharmacologic and various psychosocial interventions such as cognitive-behavioral-approaches, individual and family therapy, and psychoeducation about the cause, course, and treatment of these disorders and suicide risk. In addition, because of the high comorbidity of depressive disorders, clients presenting with anxiety disorders must be assessed for suicide risk throughout treatment (Sareen, Cox, Afifi, de Graaf, Asmundson et al., 2005).

Panic Disorder

The term *panic* originates from the Greek work *panikos*, meaning "fear." Clinical features of PD vary, and symptoms persist for at least 1 month. Panic attacks have a sudden onset of unanticipated intense anxiety generated by arousal of the sympathetic nervous system such as tachycardia, lightheadedness, diaphoresis, paresthesias, and a sense of doom. Profound fear or sense of imminent danger and an urge to escape may also accompany PD and underlie symptoms of agoraphobia. Normally, panic attacks peak within 10 minutes (APA, 2000). They also vary in their occurrence and intensity, ranging from experiencing multiple episodes for several months at a time to daily attacks for a brief period, with months separating the next episode (Campbell-Sills & Stein, 2006).

PD is rarely found before the peripubertal period; however, retrospective studies of adults show that this disorder probably begins by adolescence or young adulthood. These studies also support a continuum of various anxiety disorders across the life span. Approximately 20 to 40 percent of clients with PD experience their initial panic attack before age 20. Women are two to three times more likely to suffer from a PD than men (Weissman et al., 1997).

In a large replication epidemiological 2006 study from the National Comorbidity Survey (*n* = 9,282), Kessler, Chiu, Jin, Ruscio, Shear, and Walters (2006) found that lifetime prevalence estimates of 3.7 percent for panic disorder without agoraphobia and 1.1 percent for panic disorder with agoraphobia. Severe symptoms were more likely to occur with concomitant PD and agoraphobia (86.3 percent moderate to severe symptoms) along with substantial social impairment and coexisting psychiatric conditions. Women and previously married people consistently demonstrated higher risk for panic, whereas older adults demonstrated a lower incidence of panic. Concomitant anxiety and mood disorders were also found in subjects with PD (Kessler et al., 2006).

Panic attacks result in serious emotional and psychosocial impairment, particularly when they accompany agoraphobia. A number of clients also suffer marital discord and depression, and the suicide rate among persons with PD is high (Friedman, Smith, & Fogel, 1999; Vickers & McNally, 2004).

Sheehan (1986) delineated the possible progression of panic attacks as follows:

Stage 1: Insignificant symptoms

Stage 2: Panic attacks

Stage 3: Hypochrondriasis

Stage 4: Minimal avoidance phobic behavior

Stage 5: Severe avoidance behavior

Stage 6: Secondary depression

Because of the intensity of panic attacks, management of *acute symptoms* of PD involves the use of benzodiazepines such as clonazepam (Klonopin). Long-acting agents are less addictive than shorter-acting, high-potency agents

TABLE 11–6
Symptoms and Prevalence of Primary Anxiety Disorders

	DSM-IV-TR Criteria	Prevalence
Panic Disorder (with or without agoraphobia)	• Shortness of breath • Dizziness • Diaphoresis • Palpitations • Depersonalization • Chest pain • Feelings of doom • Concern of having another attack • Avoidance behaviors • Fear of being in open places	• Isolated recurrent attacks: 10% of adult population • Full criteria for panic attacks: 3.6% of adult population • Full-blown attack: 1.6% of population • Thirty percent to 50% of population with panic attacks have agorophobia (APA, 2000)
Specific Phobia (formerly called Simple Phobia)	• Arousal of anxiety in and avoidance of specific circumstances; natural, environmental type (e.g., snake or spider phobia) or situational (e.g., fear of heights or flying)	• Lifetime prevalence: 10–11.3% (APA, 2000)
Social Phobia	• Persistent fear and avoidance of circumstances that expose one to embarrassment or humiliation (e.g., public speaking or eating in restaurants)	• Lifetime prevalence in men: 1.7% • Lifetime prevalence in women: 2.8% (APA, 2000)
Obsessive-Compulsive Disorder	• Thoughts or images of excessive worries regarding life situations (obsessions) • Ritualistic behaviors such as handwashing, counting, or hoarding (compulsions)	• Lifetime prevalence in U.S.: 1.2–2.4% (APA, 2000)
Post-traumatic Stress Disorder	• Recurrent nightmares • Hypervigilant behavior • Intrusive thoughts of traumatic event • Autonomic arousal generated by nightmares, thoughts, or images • Acute or delayed symptoms • Avoidance behaviors	• Lifetime prevalence in men: 0.5% • Lifetime prevalence in women: 1.2% (APA, 2000)
Generalized Anxiety Disorder	• Restlessness • Tension • Arousal of autonomic nervous system • Agitation/irritability • Free-floating anxiety	• Lifetime prevalence of general population: 5%

Note. Data from *Diagnostic and Statistical Manual of Mental Disorders* (4th edition Revision) (*DSM-IV-TR*), by American Psychiatric Association, 2000, Washington, DC: Author. Adapted with permission.

TABLE 11–7
Anxiety-Reducing Techniques and Interventions

Cognitive-Behavioral Techniques

Cognitive Therapy

Therapy is based on principle of internal dialogue or self-talk and its impact on thoughts and feelings or emotions and behaviors. Major goals are to

- Assess the client's belief systems and cognitive distortions
- Challenge and alter the client's distorted/negative thoughts and self-defeating behaviors
- Strengthen the client's coping skills

Use homework assignments to test cognitions (e.g., stimulus → thoughts → feelings). Various behavioral techniques can be used.

Behavioral Role Rehearsal

The client role-plays anticipated stressful situations. The therapist assesses the client's reactions and provides feedback to the client as a teaching modality. The client can use modeling to shape behavior.

Systematic Desensitization

The client is taught to maintain relaxation while imaging various stages of ranked anxiety-evoking situations. For example, for a client with agoraphobia, situations that evoke an anxiety reaction are ranked from least to most:

1. Going outside
2. Being alone
3. Driving
4. Going to a shopping mall

The client neutralizes anxiety by using deep-muscle relaxation techniques and visual imagery, while the nurse assesses the client's subjective response.

Progressive Relaxation

Visual imagery is the basis of this technique. Directions to the client are as follows:

- Choose a dark, quiet area.
- Close your eyes.
- Focus on all muscle groups from scalp to tips of toes.
- Tense each group of muscles and maintain tension for 4 to 8 seconds.
- Tell yourself to relax and immediately release tension.
- Progress until you have tensed and relaxed all muscles.

Progressive relaxation can also be done using deep-breathing exercises: The client lies on his or her back and inhales through the nose and exhales through the mouth.

Note. Data from *Anxiety Disorders and Phobias: A Cognitive Perspective,* by A. T. Beck, G. Emery, and R. Greenberg, 1985, New York: Basic Books; and *The Practice of Behavioral Therapy,* by J. Wolpe, 1973, New York: Pergamon Press. Adapted with permission.

such as alprazolam (Xanax). Major benefits of clonazepam include its rapid effectiveness and that it is well tolerated. Its long-acting property makes it highly effective in the acute management of PD. These agents should not be used in clients with a history of a substance-related disorder owing to their addictive properties and risk for relapse. In the event of a substance-related disorder or history of substance use, clients can benefit from nonpharmacologic interventions such as deep breathing and relaxation exercises. Maintenance treatment for PD often consists of antidepressant agents such as SSRIs. Antidepressant agents are especially useful in the treatment of PD and co-occurring depressive illnesses.

Historically, the treatment focus of PD was to stop or reduce the frequency of panic attacks. Contemporary treatment extends beyond this approach and centers on treating anticipatory anxiety, phobic avoidance, concomitant depression, and level of functioning. Medications from various classes have proven efficacy in managing major symptoms of panic disorder. These classes comprise SSRIs and tricyclic

TABLE 11–8
Major Psychopharmacological Anxiolytic (Anti-Anxiety) Agents

Selective Serotonin Reuptake Inhibitors (SSRIs) (Antidepressants)

- Broad spectrum anxiolytic efficacy and suitable for first-line treatment of anxiety disorders and co-occurring anxiety-depression.

Escitalopram (Lexapri), paroxetine (Paxil), and sertraline (Zoloft) are most commonly prescribed for anxiety disorders although SSRIs such as fluoxetine (Prozac), fluvoxamine (Luvox), and citalopram (Celexa) also may be prescribed.

Serotonin-Norepinephrine Reuptake Inhibitors (SNRIs) (Antidepressants)

Venlafaxine (Effexor) and duloxetine (Cymbalta) are examples of these agents.

- General anxiety disorder
- Post-traumatic stress disorder
- Social phobia

Tricyclic Antidepressants, such as Clomipramine (Anafranil), Imipramine (Tofranil), and Desipramine (Norpramin)

- Panic disorder
- Post-traumatic stress disorder
- Phobic disorders
- Seasonal affective disorder
- Greater burden of distressful side effects than SSRIs or SNRIs

Monamine Oxidase Inhibitors (Phenelzine [Nardil])

- Panic disorder
- Post-traumatic stress disorder
- Phobic disorders

Beta Blockers (Propranolol [Inderal])

- Panic disorder
- Post-traumatic stress disorder
- Generalized anxiety disorder

Benzodiazepines

- Panic disorder
- Generalized anxiety disorder
- Social phobia
- Effective in the treatment of many anxiety disorders, but should be short-term for specific conditions

Non-benzodiazepines (Serotonin [5-HT$_{IA}$] Partial Agonists [Buspirone, Buspar])

- Generalized anxiety disorder

Note. Data from: "Evidence-based guidelines for the pharmacological treatment of anxiety disorders: Recommendations from the British association for psychopharmacology," by D. S. Baldwin, I. M. Anderson, D. J. Nutt, B. Bandelow, A. Bond, et al., 2005, *Journal of Psychopharmacology, 19,* 567–597; Nutt, D. J. (2005). Overview of diagnosis and drug treatments of anxiety disorders. *CNS Spectrums, 10,* 49–56; and *Journal of Clinical Psychiatry, 60,* Supplement 22, 18–22. "Current concepts in pharmacotherapy for post-traumatic stress disorder," by F. B. Schoenfeld, C. R. Marmar, & T. C. Neylan, 2004, *Psychiatric Services, 55,* 519–531.

antidepressants (Sadock et al., 2006). Other agents include monamine oxidase inhibitors, and calcium channel blockers. (See Chapter 29 for an in-depth discussion of various antipanic agents.) Nonpharmacologic interventions such as behavioral and cognitive therapies have also been reported to enhance antipanic agents. Progressive relaxation, guided imagery, and deep muscle relaxation are examples of these therapies (Barlow, 1997; Beck, Skodol, Clark, Berchick, & Wright, 1992; Loerch et al., 1999). Progressive relaxation is a form of relaxation training that involves visualization and progressive relaxation of specific muscle groups. The goal of this technique is tension and stress reduction. In addition, the client with PD must be continuously assessed for suicide risk and other maladaptive coping behaviors.

Agoraphobia

Most cases of this anxiety disorder arise from PD. Perhaps this premise stems from the notion that over time the treatment of PD also reduces agoraphobia. Clients suffering from

---

My Experience with Panic Disorder (The Client Speaks)

Sometimes when I am driving alone or in the car with my husband, I get this real warm "rush all over my body" and begin sweating. I feel like I have run a mile, because my heart seems to be racing really fast. I become short winded, dizzy and lightheaded, and a little confused. I can hardly talk and feel like I am going to "pass out."

I try not to disturb my husband when he is driving and usually do not complain. Sometimes he looks over at me because I am quiet and asks, "What is wrong?" Many times I tell him that I am all right even though I can hardly talk or breathe. I feel very scared during these periods, and sometimes feel like I am "going to die," but I know that this lasts only a little while.

When I feel like this, I begin to breathe very slowly and check my pulse. Within a short period, which seems like forever, my breath slowly returns and I feel calmer—my heart slows down and I cool off.

These attacks are very frightening because I do not know when they will occur. Fortunately, I am not afraid to go outside or drive. These attacks usually occur when I am extremely tired or have not rested well for several days. These attacks are also frightening to my husband, who is usually driving and feels he needs to stop and do something. I reassure him that I will be okay in a few minutes. I feel guilty about lying because he looks so helpless. When I am alone in the car, I have to take deep breaths because I am afraid to stop on the side of the road.

I do not take medications for these attacks and honestly do not believe I need them because I can take deep breaths and calm myself down.

---

agoraphobia with or without panic attacks generally experience global incapacitation stemming from their avoidant behaviors, which impair their emotional and psychosocial functioning and sense of well-being. The disabling quality of agoraphobia increases the likelihood of maladaptive behaviors such as substance abuse or ineffective coping patterns. Moreover, clients with agoraphobia often find it difficult to seek help despite feeling like they are "going crazy." Symptoms of panic attacks and agoraphobia are often extremely frightening, and clients really feel like they are dying and may often present in emergency departments with symptoms of hyperventilation, chest pains, and flushing.

Social Anxiety Disorder and Specific Phobia

Phobias are common psychiatric disorders. The term *phobia* stems from the Greek word *phobos*, which means *fear* and *flight*. A phobia is an irrational or inexplicable fear that produces intense anxiety and avoidance behaviors. Major classifications of phobias include agoraphobia, social phobia, and specific phobia. Contemporary epidemiological studies show that phobias are one of the most prevalent anxiety disorders with potentially disabling, chronic, and recurrent patterns (Grant et al., 2005). Common phobic disorders are social phobia and specific phobias.

Social Anxiety Disorder

Social anxiety disorder (SAD), similar to other anxiety disorders, is a potentially disabling and chronic course that threatens the client's social, interpersonal, and occupational functioning and overall quality of life. Obviously, these factors underscore the need for early identification, accurate diagnosis, and appropriate interventions of social anxiety disorder. Adult symptoms of social anxiety disorder are comparable to the childhood type and include a fear of performance situations such as public speaking, eating in front of others, or writing in public, ensuing avoidance behaviors. Most people recognize common symptoms of social anxiety disorder; however, few actually recognize and appreciate its potential to generate intense suffering and social impairment. The following case examples illustrate two extremes of social anxiety disorder.

The first case represents the most common form of social anxiety disorder and involves a student who has to do a case presentation in a postclinical conference. Because of the student's fears of ridicule, scrutiny, and humiliation by the instructor and his peers, intense fear and anxiety emerge, producing blushing, increased heart rate and respirations, muscle tension, and, most importantly, a need to "run away from" or avoid doing the presentation all together. This is not only typical of students, but it also occurs at all levels in the organization. Sometimes these fears are so intense that the individual calls in sick a day or two before to avoid anxiety-provoking situations.

Some clinicians refer to this form of social anxiety disorder as generalized social phobia, a more serious and often underdiagnosed condition that carries the profound burden of disability. Social impairment and disability from this pervasive form usually parallels intense fear and avoidance behaviors such as dating, forming and maintaining meaningful relationships, conversing with strangers, and talking to authority figures (Stein & Kean, 2000). Predictably, a lack of meaningful and productive social functioning generates a sense of helplessness, powerlessness, and loss of control over one's life. Over time these negative experiences increase the risk of other maladaptive responses that contribute to depression, suicide risk, and substance-related disorders, particularly alcohol-use disorders.

In contrast to the first case, the second case is more pervasive and presents a greater challenge to the nurse. This is the case of a 39-year-old woman who finds it necessary to seek employment since the recent death of her spouse. She notices that even the thought of seeking employment is overwhelming because of her intense anxiety and fears of scrutiny and humiliation in prospective job interviews. She also notices that even when she goes to the market, she has problems speaking to strangers or greeting neighbors. Before the death of her spouse, she spent most of her time gardening and doing things alone, except when sharing meals with her husband. Her husband, who was also shy, took care of the shopping and other chores because of her difficulty meeting people. Recently her family became involved because of the woman's physical and mental deterioration.

The diverse clinical symptoms of clients experiencing social anxiety disorder are perplexing and require accurate assessment, differential diagnoses, and interventions that reduce its debilitating form and restore quality of life. Interventions for this disorder are similar to other anxiety disorders and include both pharmacologic and nonpharmacologic approaches. Pharmacologic approaches include a broad spectrum of antidepressants, such as SSRIs (Sadock et al., 2006) and SNRIs (Pae et al., 2007). Other researchers are exploring the efficacy of novel anticonvulsants, such as pregabalin (Lyrica), a GABA analog, and tigababine (Gabitril) in the treatment of social anxiety disorder (Dunlop et al., 2007; Schwartz et al., 2005; Tassone, Boyce, Guyer, & Nuzum, 2007). Preliminary findings from these studies indicate these agents may become pharmacological options for social anxiety disorder and other anxiety and mood disorders. Beta-blockers and long-acting benzodiazepines may be used to treat social anxiety disorder. Regardless of pharmacologic agent, clients must be appropriately diagnosed and receive individualized care to manage this chronic and potentially debilitating anxiety disorder.

Nonpharmacologic interventions include various psychotherapies such as individual, cognitive-behavioral therapy, intensive group cognitive treatment, desensitization, rehearsal, an array of homework assignments, progressive muscle relaxation, and abdominal deep breathing exercises (Beck et al., 1985; Mörtberg, Clark, Sundin, & Aberg Wistedt, 2007; Wolpe, 1961, 1973). Frequently, clients with social anxiety disorder gain tremendous relief and hope from holistic approaches that integrate pharmacologic and nonpharmacologic interventions.

Specific Phobia

This phobia, like social anxiety disorder, is a common anxiety disorder and tends to parallel exposure to an anxiety-provoking situation or stimulus. The most common objects that generate intense fears are animals, storms, heights, illness, injury, and death (APA, 2000). These fears appear to arise from anxiety-provoking situations that generate intense emotions, fear, and panic. There are several theories about specific phobia and they are consistent with those of other anxiety disorders, including social or learning behavioral-cognitive, biologic, and genetic risk factors.

One of the most obvious examples of a learning or social influence is modeling. For instance, if a parent sees a snake and begins screaming or running because of his fears and anxiety, the child learns that snakes are dangerous and scary. The next time the child sees a snake or other object, there is some risk of modeling the parent's behavior and developing a fear of snakes—either actual or expected exposure.

The treatment of specific phobias is consistent with that of other phobic disorders. Clients with this disorder can gain relief from pharmacologic and nonpharmacologic treatment approaches that reduce their cognitive, biological, and behavioral responses to anxiety-provoking objects or situations.

Obsessive-Compulsive Disorder

The term *obsession* stems from the Latin *obseus*, meaning to "besiege," and *compulsion* from *compulsus*, meaning "to compel." Obsessions are intrusive, recurrent, and persistent thoughts, impulses, or images. Common patterns of obsessive themes are contamination, washing, need for symmetry or order, pathological doubt, stealing, harming others, sexual, cleanliness or fears of contamination, and somatic concerns (APA, 2000). Compulsions are behaviors that seem purposeful but are enacted in a stereotypical and repetitive manner. Examples of compulsions are repetitive hand washing, counting, checking, touching, cleaning, or hoarding. The client with OCD often attempts to alleviate the anxiety that arises from his obsessions by performing various rituals, or compulsions.

The complexity of OCD challenges nurses to make differential diagnoses, including those with similar clinical presentations, such as obsessive-compulsive personality disorder (OCPD). The primary difference between OCD and OCPD is that the former produces more global functional impairment than the latter. Specifically, because of intrusive thoughts (obsessions) that generate intense anxiety and subsequent rituals (compulsions) or behaviors, OCD is likely to have a greater impact on the client's level of functioning.

Conversely, clinical features of OCPD disorder involve "perfectionism" and emotional constriction, orderliness, rigidity, and indecisiveness. The most obvious impact of these features involves social functioning. Many of these clients have impaired social skills, seem "serious" most of the time, and are inflexible and rigid about their ideas. Moreover,

CRITICAL THINKING

Maria is being seen in the university health center complaining of fears of being contaminated by her college roommate. She admits that since entering college several months ago, she has been bathing at least six times a day because of these fears and anxiety. She also admits knowing that her behavior "does not make sense," but she feels so anxious until she bathes. She also reveals that her skin is very irritated. Her father insisted on her seeing a dermatologist, who, in turn, referred her to the mental health clinic in the university health service. Which of the following most accurately describes Maria's condition?

a. She is delusional and exhibiting characteristic symptoms of a psychotic disorder.

b. She has typical symptoms of obsessive-compulsive disorder.

c. Her behavior is normal and commonly found in college students with roommates.

d. Her fears are irrational and she needs to be hospitalized immediately.

their indecisiveness stems from their need to be perfect and obsessions about routines and orderliness. Despite the potential to affect the client's level of functioning, most respond well to structured, orderly, and stable environments. (See Chapter 15, The Client with a Personality Disorder, for an in-depth discussion of OCPD.)

Because of the disabling character of this anxiety disorder and subsequent feelings of helplessness and powerlessness, these clients often have other co-occurring disorders, such as major depressive disorder, alcohol disorders, eating disorders, and other anxiety disorders (Kessler et al., 2005; Levander et al., 2007).

Major pharmacologic interventions for OCD include SSRIs such as fluvoxamine (Luvox), paroxetine (Paxil), and sertraline, and clomipramine (Anafranil)—a tricyclic with serotonergic properties. Of all of the tricyclic agents, clomipramine is the most selective for serotonin reuptake versus norepinephrine reuptake, which exceeds the efficacy of sertraline and paroxetine. Moreover, this drug was the first drug approved for the treatment of OCD (Clomipramine Collaborative Study Group, 1991). Nonpharmacologic interventions for OCD include cognitive-behavioral therapies (Beck, Emery, & Greenberg, 1985). See Tables 11–7 and 11–8 for the pharmacologic and nonpharmacologic interventions used to treat anxiety disorders.

Acute Stress Disorder

The diagnosis of acute stress disorder was introduced in the *DSM-IV*. Similar to PTSD, this anxiety disorder results from exposure to a traumatic and overwhelming event involving actual or threatened death, physical injury, or other threats to one's or another's integrity. A *stressor* or event (criterion A) represents the client's response and has to comprise intense fear, a sense of helplessness, or horror. Whereas PTSD represents disturbance that endures for more than 1 month, acute stress disorder must last a minimum of 2 days, and a diagnosis can only be made up to 1 month after exposure to the stressor (APA, 2000).

Another clinical difference between acute stress disorder and PTSD is the presence of a dissociative response to the trauma in the former. Hence, the diagnosis of acute stress disorder requires at least three dissociative symptoms (criterion B), such as "being in a daze," derealization, and depersonalization, but only one symptom from each of the reexperiencing or intrusive thoughts (cognitive) (criterion C), avoidance (criterion D), and arousal (biological) (criterion E) categories. Derealization describes a subjective sense that the environment is unreal or strange. Impairment (criterion F) is also necessary to make this diagnosis (APA, 2000). Until now, there was a paucity of empirical studies that explored specific assumptions from this *DSM-IV-TR* diagnostic category. Examples of events that produce acute stress disorder include rape, witnessing a murder or other violent event, violent attacks, combat and other war experience, and surviving natural and man-made disasters.

Because of the potential deleterious and long-term effects (i.e., PTSD) of acute stress disorder, early identification is crucial. Psychiatric nurses must identify high-risk groups and initiate early interventions to promote adaptive resolution of traumatic and stressful events. The constellation and intensity of symptoms direct treatment planning. Crisis Intervention Stress Debriefing (CISD) is a crisis model developed by Mitchell (Mitchell & Dyregov, 1993; Robinson & Mitchell, 1993) for disaster workers exposed to traumatic events who are experiencing acute and chronic symptoms of intense anxiety. The basis of this intervention is the provision of immediate emotional support to individuals suffering from abnormal situations. It offers them a supportive environment that encourages and validates their experience and provides education about current and potential behavioral, psychological, biological, and cognitive responses. As clients express feelings, thoughts, and current reactions to a traumatic stressor, other group members relate to each other and continue to normalize their reactions. Despite the support and advocacy of the CISD model by major organizations, such as the American Red Cross, empirical research fails to support the efficacy of this model in the prevention of PTSD or trauma-related responses (Sijbrandij et al., 2007). The debate concerning the efficacy and prevention of PTSD continues (Jacobs, Horne-Moyer, & Jones, 2004).

Although some clients may benefit from this intervention, others may require professional help, such as psychotherapy or pharmacologic intervention, to manage acute and chronic symptoms such as frightening nightmares, depression, intense and enduring arousal or activation of previous traumatic memories, and PTSD symptoms.

Overall, successful resolution of acute stress disorder requires immediate and supportive interventions and other treatment options to deal with acute and persistent symptoms such as PTSD, depression, and other anxiety disorders.

Post-traumatic Stress Disorder

In the past century, PTSD has appeared in the literature under several names: hysteria, war neurosis, shell shock, and battle fatigue. Regardless of the terminology used, this disorder comprises a complex constellation of symptoms that evolve in survivors of traumatic or overwhelming stressful events. Symptoms usually parallel a traumatic event or circumstance that is beyond the breadth of normal human experience and would be considered stressful to anyone. Exposure to an overpowering event, "resulting in helplessness in the face of intolerable danger, anxiety, and instinctual arousal" (Eth & Pynoos, 1984, p. 173) precipitates and describes psychic traumatic events such as natural disasters, rape, incest, physical or mental torture, combat experiences, and catastrophic accidents and are likely to generate symptoms of PTSD.

The emergence of PTSD symptoms may occur immediately after the event or later. Acute PTSD symptoms may occur within 6 months; after this time, symptoms are referred to as delayed. A preexisting emotional problem or mental illness tends to increase the risk of maladaptive responses to traumatic experiences. The major symptoms of PTSD in adults fall into three major groups:

1. Persistent recurrent and intrusive thoughts; flashbacks (a sense of reliving the event); dreams of the trauma; intense psychological distress at exposure to internal or external cues such as smells, sounds, or visual event)

2. Avoidance behaviors or depersonalization; inability to recall certain aspects of trauma; lack of interest in things that were formerly pleasurable, feeling of detachment, or isolation; restriction in range of feelings (unable to feel happy)

Common Myths about Post-traumatic Stress Disorder (PTSD)

MYTH	FACT
1. PTSD is an adult psychiatric disorder.	1. Although adults may most likely seek treatment for PTSD, this serious anxiety disorder can occur at any age, including childhood and adolescence. The experience of significant childhood trauma often produces enduring effects and contributes to clinical symptoms in adulthood. An increasing number of literature implicates childhood victimization or maltreatment, especially physical and sexual abuse, in the etiology of PTSD (Widom et al., 2005).
2. Exposure to trauma or a disaster always predicts PTSD.	2. PTSD is not an inevitable consequence of exposure to a traumatic event or disaster. Several factors contribute to development of PTSD. First are the nature and intensity of the stressor or event. PTSD is likely to result from trauma or disaster if there are no available resources to assist in debriefing, and if there is a premorbid history of psychiatric problems. It is less likely to occur in the event of immediate emotional support and interventions that promote expression of feelings, thoughts, and responses arising from the event. Premorbid adaptive coping skills along with debriefing also promote emotional healing and resolution of the stressor. (Bremner et al., 2005).
3. PTSD is diagnosed easily.	3. Because of co-occurring disorders that often accompany PTSD, making a differential diagnosis is critical to safe and appropriate treatment. PTSD is commonly misdiagnosed. The nurse and other health care providers must consider PTSD in clients with chronic pain disorder, substance abuse, other anxiety disorders, mood disorders, malingering, and factitious disorder (APA, 2000; Sadock & Sadock, 2005).

3. Biological responses such as emotional numbing, hypervigilance, and autonomic nervous system arousal (APA, 2000). PTSD, like other anxiety disorders, is likely to have other comorbid conditions such as depression, other anxiety disorders, and substance-related disorders.

Treating the client experiencing PTSD requires an understanding of the global impact of traumatic experiences and offering the client and family members a supportive and empathetic environment. Similarly to other anxiety disorders, clients with PTSD often benefit from a holistic treatment approach that integrates pharmacologic and nonpharmacologic interventions such as cognitive-behavioral therapy, desensitization, and progressive relaxation exercises. This program must tailor the client's ability to tolerate intense feelings and biological arousal and motivation for treatment.

A relatively new method of treating PTSD is eye-movement desensitization and reprocessing (EMDR). Shapiro coined this technique in 1989 when she observed that her own disturbing memories and negative self-talk permanently lost their capacity to elicit anxiety when coupled with rapid eye movements. She later used this treatment with her own clients who experienced PTSD and gained a similar positive response. EMDR involves asking the client to imagine an anxiety-provoking or traumatic memory. The primary goal of this technique is to move information and facilitate processing a traumatic experience in a nonthreatening manner when the client's nature processes are blocked (Barron, Curtis, & Grainger, 1998; Rothbaum et al., 2005; Shapiro, 1995). Special training is necessary to perform EMDR.

Because of the high risk of other psychiatric disorders, particularly depression, PD, and substance-related disorder, the nurse must assess clients for these conditions. These conditions increase the risk of suicide and other maladaptive behaviors and require continuous assessment and documentation of client response and level of dangerousness. Health education is an integral part of the client's treatment planning and must include signs and symptoms of PTSD, current treatment options, and the role of family members as a team member.

Summary of Adulthood Disorders

Anxiety disorders in adults, like child and adolescent anxiety disorders, evolve over a continuum. Because of the severity and prevalence of anxiety disorders, early detection and client-centered interventions are necessary to facilitate optimal treatment outcomes. The complexity of anxiety disorders require integrated approaches that reduce recurrence and severity of symptoms across the life span.

Holistic or integrated treatment approaches comprise pharmacologic and psychosocial interventions such as cognitive-behavioral therapies. These interventions reduce the severity and onset of symptoms, restore and enhance adaptive coping behaviors and level of functioning, and reduce the potential acute and chronic debilitating effects of anxiety disorders.

OLDER ADULTHOOD DISORDERS

Anxiety disorders are the most common psychiatric conditions in older adults (Flint, 2005). Despite this high prevalence, there is a paucity of empirical studies that focus on the course and treatment of anxiety disorders in older adults. Of particular interest is the course of PTSD symptoms in older adults. Longitudinal and retrospective data support the PTSD symptom course of acute onset and gradual decline, followed by worsening PTSD symptom among older adult survivors exposed to war-related or remote trauma (Ruzich, Looi, & Robertson, 2005). Because of the chronic and unremitting course of anxiety disorders, it is reasonable for them to persist into older adulthood (Le Roux, Gatz, & Wetherell, 2005). This premise suggests that major anxiety disorders occurring in younger and middle-aged adults also occur in this age group. Major differences in late-onset anxiety disorders, such as PD, include fewer panic symptoms, less avoidance, and lower levels of somatization in older adults when comparing them to earlier-onset illness. Other age-related differences include higher rates of psychiatric and medical problems in older adults presenting with specific phobia (Kessler et al., 2006) and less reexperiencing of traumatic events from PTSD, but more hyperarousal than in younger age groups.

Although anxiety disorders in older adults are likely to evolve over time, distinguishing medical conditions that mimic anxiety disorders is a priority in this age group. These clients are especially susceptible to delirium, which may arise from systemic infections; drug toxicity; polypharmacy; substance intoxication and withdrawal; endocrine disorder, including diabetes mellitus; and fluid and electrolyte imbalance. Depression is also common in older adults and must be ruled out and treated because of the high risk of completed suicide in this age group. Common presentations in older adults with depression and anxiety disorders include vague physical complaints; sleep, appetite, and cognitive disturbances; and self-care deficits. Before treating these clients for anxiety disorders, the treatment team must make a differential diagnosis. Differential diagnoses are contingent on complete physical and psychiatric examinations.

A complete medical and psychiatric workup focuses on differential diagnoses of medical, polypharmacy, substance use, current and past coping skills, and current and past illnesses. Because polypharmacy is a major concern when caring for these clients, the nurse must ascertain information from both the client and family members regarding over-the-counter medications, herbs or other alternative therapies, treatment compliance, suicide risk, and preference. The client's nutritional status, mental status, and functional status are integral aspects of the assessment and treatment planning. Treatment efficacy of anxiety disorders in older adults is comparable with other age groups, specifically cognitive-behavioral and pharmacologic interventions.

Specific Age-Related Issues

Major treatment considerations involve age-related physiological factors that affect prescribing and administering these agents to older adults. Before initiating treatment, the nurse must also assess the quality of the client's support system. This is particularly significant if the client lives alone or has sensory or cognitive deficits. Because of the high rate of drug interactions, polypharmacy, and adverse drug reaction in this age group, the nurse must develop a plan of care that reflects age-specific issues. These clients often require lower and slower increases in drug doses to reduce the risk of cognitive deficits, falls, and promote medication compliance. In addition, because of the high risk of suicide in this age group, they must be assessed throughout treatment for suicide risk and comorbid depressive illness.

Summary of Older Adulthood Disorders

Similar to other age groups, anxiety disorders in older adulthood appear to evolve over time and have developmental origins. Although similarities exist, these clients are vulnerable to medical conditions that mimic anxiety disorder. Before treating anxiety disorders in the older adult, differential diagnoses must be made to rule out various medical and psychiatric illnesses. Similar to other age groups, older adults often present with comorbid depressive illnesses and must be continuously assessed for depression and suicide risk.

Likewise, these clients can benefit from an array of treatment approaches that involve pharmacologic and nonpharmacologic interventions. Age-specific issues such as dosing and observation for drug toxicity or adverse drug reactions are key treatment issues. Health teaching and family involvement are also an integral part of these clients' care. Refer to Table 11–1 for a summary of the *DSM-IV-TR* criteria for specific anxiety disorders.

TREATMENT CONSIDERATIONS FOR THE CLIENT IN COMMUNITY AND HOME SETTINGS

The client with an anxiety disorder is more likely to receive care in the home or community than in an inpatient psychiatric unit. The impact of anxiety disorders on the client and family system is profound, suggesting the need to develop community and home-based treatment approaches. Shifting mental health care from hospital to community and home care may produce intense family tension and overtax their coping skills, thus increasing the risk of treatment failure. Over time, these factors may produce disabling effects on the family or reduce and impair the client's global level of functioning.

Even more disturbing is the growing incidence of concomitant conditions such as depression and substance-related and other psychiatric disorders. These conditions increase the risk of poor treatment outcomes and jeopardize the client's quality of life. Helping the client and family cope

with these disorders remains a treatment priority. Successful treatment outcomes are contingent on collaboration between the nurse, other health care providers, the client and the family. Treatment planning begins by establishing rapport with the client, and family and is based on data from a comprehensive physical and mental assessment that identifies reasons for treatment, current stressors, health status, past and present psychiatric and medical conditions, and a review of the family system. An often overlooked area is assessment of the family, identification of the client strengths and coping skills, and their treatment expectations. The nurse must continuously assess the family's ability to cope with the client's illness, the client's response to treatment, mental and physical status, and potential of violence toward self and others. This holistic approach is basic to community and home-based mental health care.

Mental health care must be family centered, age specific, and focused on assessing client and family needs, cultural and spiritual wishes, health practices, and expectations, health teaching about the course and treatment of anxiety disorders, and strengthening coping skills that facilitate symptom management. The basis of intervention is restoration to a previous or higher level of functioning.

Special treatment considerations must be given to age-specific issues, assessing the developmental stage and educational and cognitive functioning of the client, and family resources. Other treatment considerations include community and family resources. Clients with supportive families and adequate resources are more likely to have more positive treatment outcomes than those who do not. Likewise, the client who is homeless is at a greater risk of nonadherence to treatment and relapse than other populations. These special populations and conditions are challenging to the mental health professional and clearly threaten the client's well-being and return to the highest level of functioning.

Major treatment of anxiety disorders requires a client-centered approach that integrates pharmacologic and non-pharmacologic interventions such as cognitive behavioral therapy. An in-depth discussion of pharmacologic interventions emphasizes the importance of these agents in managing acute and chronic symptoms and their benefits when combined with nonpharmacologic approaches. (See Chapter 29 for an indepth discussion of these agents.)

Major nursing responsibilities for pharmacologic interventions in the home and community include prescribing, administering, and ordering medications; health teaching about desired and adverse effects of various medications; and informing the client about drug interactions between anxiolytic agents and other prescribed and over-the-counter medications. Because of the comorbidity of substance use and depression in clients with anxiety disorders, health education about illicit drugs and alcohol and recognition of suicide risk must be an integral part of treatment. The nurse must also continuously assess for depression, level of dangerousness toward self and others, and substance misuse. Educating the family members about signs and symptoms of these conditions is also essential. Documentation of clinical findings, such as mental status, current stressors, and response to treatment, must occur during each encounter.

Practice implications for nonpharmacologic interventions such as cognitive-behavioral techniques are (Beck et al., 1985):

◆ Psychoeducation. This involves teaching the client and family about anxiety disorders. Initially, this process begins with a didactic approach that helps clients and family members understand the etiology of anxiety disorders, current treatment, and the purpose of *cognitive-behavioral therapy*. Teachings must also include learning about exercises that evoke symptoms and the role of internal cues, including exaggerated fears and their impact on symptoms.

◆ Continuous symptoms monitoring. Clients are actually taught how to log their symptoms using either a diary or other method of record keeping. This strategy helps the client and family in assessing the frequency and intensity of anxiety symptoms and collecting information regarding internal (interoceptive cues, i.e., hot flushes, numbness, tingling, tachycardia, or dizziness) and external cues (i.e., smells, sights) or triggers.

◆ Breathing retraining. This involves teaching the client how abdominal breathing exercises can control physiological responses. This technique reduces anxiogenic responses to symptoms and involves muscle relaxation and diaphragmatic and slow breathing techniques.

◆ Cognitive restructuring. Involves teaching the client to challenge exaggerated fears or worries and attaching realistic meaning of cognitive distortions.

◆ Exposure to trigger or anxiety-provoking events or situations. Involves a gradual exposure on a 0 to 10 basis of the anxiety-provoking or fearful event.

Cognitive-behavioral therapy carries few risks. However, during initial treatment, the client is likely to experience tremendous anxiety. The nurse can reduce these symptoms by informing the client that this may occur. This type of treatment usually lasts from 4 to 16 weeks and is contingent on adjunct treatment. Adjunct treatment may include progressive and deep muscle relaxation techniques, guided imagery, and pharmacology.

Other treatment options for clients experiencing anxiety disorders include individual psychotherapy, group therapy, and marital and family therapy. Nurses often overlook interventions that are basic to all clients, which include sleep manipulation, nutritional counseling, and regular exercise programs. These interventions complement other treatments, offering clients an array of health-promoting activities that foster an optimal level of functioning. Obviously, the choice of therapy is individual and depends on the client and families' needs, nature of symptoms, level of disability,

preferences, and past treatment responses. Providing the client and family members with diverse treatment options affords opportunities to strengthen family support systems, increase confidence and trust in the nurse and treatment team, reduce the incidence of relapse and hospitalization, and promote a high level of functioning. See Chapter 33, Home- and Community-Based Care, for a discussion of the client in the home and community settings.

THE ROLE OF THE NURSE

Caring for the client with an anxiety disorder requires an understanding of complex processes, biological, genetic, and environmental factors and psychosocial stressors that contribute to normal and abnormal anxiety. Moreover, the role of the nurse varies with individual educational preparation, clinical experiences, interest, and clinical setting. Nursing roles and responsibilities vary, from administering to prescribing to offering nonpharmacologic interventions. Responsibilities parallel specific nursing roles that include both the generalist and advanced-practice nurse. Regardless of the nurse's role, interventions focus on helping clients manage their anxiety effectively and facilitating an optimal level of functioning.

THE GENERALIST NURSE

Understanding the underpinnings of anxiety disorders and specific interventions to treat them enables the generalist psychiatric-mental health nurse to identify the mental health needs of the client experiencing anxiety. This approach provides the basis for interventions that reduce the frequency and severity of symptoms of anxiety. Major nursing interventions include establishing rapport, enhancing present coping skills, assessing maladaptive responses, minimizing the deleterious effects of anxiety, and promoting health maintenance. Case management, home health care, and psychoeducation provide diverse opportunities to (American Nurses Association [ANA], 2000):

◆ Enhance coping skills and self-care: teach stress management, assertive communication, and cognitive-behavioral techniques that enable the client to self-regulate anxiety. This may also include administering anxiolytic agents (see Table 11–8), which reduce biological aspects of anxiety such as palpitations and increased heart rate and respirations.

◆ Identify physical and cognitive symptoms that suggest an impending panic attack. Administer medications that minimize the severity and frequency of attacks.

◆ Monitor the client's responses to medication and other treatment modality.

◆ Educate the client and family about the etiology, course, and treatment of anxiety disorders with and without agoraphobia and co-occurring conditions, such as major depressive episode.

- ◆ Teach progressive relaxation, cognitive techniques, self-monitoring, and other anxiety-reducing measures. (See Table 11–7 for specific anxiety-reducing techniques.)
- ◆ Coordinate and mobilize various resources.
- ◆ Provide crisis intervention.
- ◆ Participate in comprehensive care planning.

THE ADVANCED-PRACTICE PSYCHIATRIC REGISTERED NURSE

The advanced-practice psychiatric-mental health nurse incorporates the role of the generalist and autonomously applies advanced clinical skills, knowledge, and experience to complex client needs (ANA, 2000). The role of the advanced-practice psychiatric nurses continues to evolve and responsibilities parallel client needs.

Differential diagnosis is vital to safe and quality care and involves determining the client's current and past health status, course of current symptoms, family and childhood history, and ordering diagnostic studies and interpreting their values. Differential diagnosis also involves collaborating with appropriate health care providers to develop holistic treatment planning and make appropriate referrals.

As the advanced-practice nurse assumes more responsibilities and manages more complex populations, determining differential diagnosis is a major treatment concern. For instance, performing a psychiatric evaluation also entails a review of systems. A review of systems and ordering diagnostic tests, such as ECG, laboratory studies, and drug levels, enable the nurse to gather data about the client's physical and health status and rule out conditions that have a potentially deleterious impact on certain treatment. For instance, the client who seeks treatment for a PD and major depressive episode and also has a diagnosis of Wolff-Parkinson-Wilson syndrome is taking digoxin. Pertinent information about the client's mental and physical status, including diagnostic tests, particularly chemistries and digoxin level, ECG, and bio-pschosocial assessment, determines which antidepressant the nurse will prescribe. In this case, SSRIs, particularly paroxetine (Paxil), are not first choice drugs. These agents act as inducers or drugs that activate liver enzyme systems that reduce digoxin levels and increase the risk of dangerous ventricular tachycardia. This example explains the complexity of the advanced-practice psychiatric nurse's role and inherent responsibilities in providing holistic care. Once the nurse makes the diagnosis, a plan of client-centered treatment planning can be formulated that integrates health education, treatment alternatives, and appropriate referrals.

Psychotherapy, prescription of medications, case management, and evaluation of outcome measures are major treatment foci of the advanced-practice nurse. Psychotherapy enables the nurse to assess the impact of underlying psychodynamic issues such as early childhood traumas and abuse on current symptoms and behaviors. Various theories guide the advanced-practice psychiatric mental health nurse in the decision to provide psychotherapy. Many use an eclectic brief or short-term psychotherapy approach that offers the client didactic and experiential experiences that facilitate adaptive coping skills, self-care activities, emotional support, and reinforcement of adaptive behavioral changes. During the course of treatment the nurse continuously assesses the client's educational needs; risk of dangerousness to self and others; response to treatment, both nonpharmacologic and pharmacologic; and makes appropriate referrals for physical problems.

Understanding pharmacokinetics and pharmacodynamics and the complexity of anxiety disorders is essential to the nurse who prescribes psychotropic medications. Prescribing entails more than writing an order and includes ordering appropriate diagnostic and laboratory studies; making a differential diagnosis of medical and psychiatric conditions; monitoring the client's response to treatment; making decisions to continue the medication, taper the dose, or add another medication such as a mood stabilizer; and providing education about the drug's desired and adverse reactions. Managing medications also involves ordering diagnostic tests, monitoring drug levels, and collaborating with other health care providers, especially those managing the client's medical conditions. This responsibility also involves performing or administering standardized tests to monitor for symptoms reduction and early side effects such as tardive dyskinesias. These tests offer opportunities to evaluate the efficacy of nursing interventions and other treatments and provide invaluable data regarding the efficacy of nursing interventions. Overall, the advanced-practice nurse can offer psychotropic agents and psychotherapy to clients experiencing anxiety disorders in order to reduce their potential chronic and debilitating course. Besides psychotherapy and medication management, the advanced-practice nurse can use case management and research findings to formulate a multidisciplinary holistic plan of care.

THE NURSING PROCESS

Anxiety disorders represent a continuum of symptoms that evolve throughout the life span and affect psychosocial, biological, and occupational well-being. Their comorbidity with other medical and psychiatric disorders, such as endocrine disorders and major depressive episodes, understandably underscore the need for health care professionals to discern the complexity of the human response to internal and external demands and develop effective interventions. Effective interventions require a cultural and age-specific biopsychosocial assessment that integrate data about the client's physical and mental status.

ASSESSMENT

This process begins with a complete medical examination that rules out underlying physical and substance-related conditions. It also entails getting a list of current medications, both prescription and over-the-counter. An often overlooked health assessment area is the client's eating habits. This is particularly important in anxiety disorders because various foods, such as those containing caffeine (e.g., tea, coffee, chocolates) may contribute to exacerbation or interfere with symptom management. Ruling out medical, substance-related, and other mental conditions is critical to holistic treatment of the client with an anxiety disorder.

Determining the client's current physical health status helps the psychiatric nurse to continue the holistic nursing process. Major components of this process include continuous data gathering or assessment of current symptoms and their impact on the client's current level of functioning. In addition, assessing the client presenting with an anxiety disorder requires patience and understanding of these disorders. Likewise, because of the client's intense level of anxiety, the nurse must approach the client in a calm, reassuring, and empathetic manner. Assessing the client also requires assessing the family system to discern current stressors, level of support, academic performance, family stability, coping patterns, level of dangerousness, culture, knowledge about anxiety disorders, and available resources. Performing a mental status examination is part of the assessment process and provides vital information about the client's current mental health, judgment, insight, and strengths. The nurse must assess the client's symptoms and their chronological patterns and other assessment data in order to make accurate diagnoses according to *DSM-IV-TR* and nursing diagnoses.

The mental status examination of these clients often reveals common themes that reflect the severity of symptoms and the client's level of functioning. Common themes of clients seeking treatment for anxiety disorders are fears and feelings of "losing control," fears of a parent dying or not returning, and a sense of helplessness over one's life. Clients with OCD often present with varying thought content such as contamination, need for order, and compulsions to wash, check, count, hoard, or confess. Common behavioral manifestations of various anxiety disorders include avoidant behaviors; staying home from school; ritualistic hand washing or showering; repeating rituals; checking the door, locks, or coffee makers; ordering and arranging; and hoarding. Similarly, clients with anxiety disorders also complain of the biological or physiological distress of their illness.

Biological responses of anxiety disorders arise primarily from autonomic nervous system arousal (i.e., palpitations, shortness of breath, lightheadedness). Because of the intense fears, cognitive distortions, and biological responses, many of these clients suffer significant decline in their previous level of functioning. This decline is likely to increase the risk of various mental and substance-related disorders, particularly major depressive episodes or alcohol abuse. Assessing the distressful nature of these symptoms and their impact on the client's level of functioning is crucial to quality and appropriate treatment planning and resulting in positive outcomes. Appropriate treatment planning involves making accurate diagnoses.

NURSING DIAGNOSES

The assessment component of the nursing process provides the basis of nursing diagnoses. The following nursing diagnoses are common in the client with an anxiety disorder:

◆ Ineffective coping related to . . . as evidenced by a perceived loss of control over self and environment
◆ Risk for self-directed injury as evidenced by risk factors include . . . and evidenced by anxiety, fear, and ineffective coping
◆ Anxiety related to . . . as evidenced by a perception of powerlessness and autonomic nervous system arousal
◆ Disturbed sleep pattern as evidenced by biological disturbances arising from anxiety
◆ Disturbed thought processes as evidenced by negative, irrational, and self-defeating thoughts
◆ Self-esteem disturbance as evidenced by impaired personal and professional role performance
◆ Deficient knowledge as evidenced by a lack of understanding of panic disorder, etiology, course, and treatment
◆ Post-trauma response as evidenced by cognitive and biological disturbances arising from anxiety
◆ Interrupted family processes as evidenced by ineffective family coping responses

Nursing diagnoses guide the nurse in establishing a client-centered treatment plan. This process refers to outcome identification.

OUTCOME IDENTIFICATION

Outcome identification involves identifying individualized outcome measures. These measures are part of the treatment and evaluation process that guide and provide evidence regarding the effectiveness of various interventions. Common outcome measures for the client presenting with anxiety disorders are consistent with nursing diagnoses and include:

◆ Effective individual coping
◆ Symptom management
◆ No self-harm or injury
◆ Return to normal sleeping patterns
◆ Understanding and insight into the anxiety disorder
◆ Healthy family interactions and coping

PLANNING

Successful client outcomes result from holistic treatment planning that involves collaboration among the nurse, client, family members, other health care providers, and community resources. More importantly, treatment planning involves accurate assessment, problem and outcome identification, viable treatment options or interventions, evaluation, and continuous quality improvement.

IMPLEMENTATION

Establishing a therapeutic relationship with the client and significant other is essential (see Chapter 6, Therapeutic Communication). A sound health teaching program begins with education about etiology, course, and treatment of an anxiety disorder. This process begins by teaching the client that symptoms of anxiety disorders arise from internal and external stimuli, which trigger an arousal of the autonomic nervous system to protect the body. Coping with anxiety is a two-part endeavor that consists of the client assessing his perception of the threat and using specific coping behaviors to reduce or eliminate distorted cognitions. For instance, a student with social phobia who has to present a paper before peers is experiencing intense fears of "looking and sounding stupid." These thoughts (cognitive distortions regarding peers' perceptions and scrutiny of the student presenting the paper) trigger intense biological responses, including palpitations, sweaty palms, poor concentration, sleep disturbances, diaphoresis, and shortness of breath, resulting in avoidance behavior. Skipping class or calling in sick are examples of avoidance behavior.

Cognitive-behavioral techniques that the student must use are deep breathing exercises and challenging distorted cognitions. Initially, the student must gain control over biological responses to distorted fears. This process begins with deep breathing exercises that reduce the biological response to these thoughts. By taking 10 slow, deep breaths, the student can gain control over exaggerated biological responses. This may reduce feelings of powerlessness and helplessness and improve thinking processes, which facilitate asking the following questions:

"Where are these fears coming from?"

"Are my fears practical?"

If the student answers "no" to these questions, then he is ready to challenge the fears and explore ways to prepare for the presentation such as using role rehearsal. (See Table 9–2, Cognitive Distortions and Nursing Interventions.) This two-tier process promotes a greater understanding of the student's fears and improves coping responses to future presentations.

Facilitating adaptive coping behaviors through client education is critical to reducing cognitive distortions and empowering the client and family. Teaching strategies must focus on progressive relaxation or deep breathing techniques, which enable the client to control some aspects of anxiety attacks by aborting or reducing emotional and physiological responses to them.

The usefulness of cognitive-behavioral therapy to treat anxiety disorders is the notion that anxiety increases with thoughts and images of social or physical danger. The effectiveness of cognitive-behavioral approaches depends on the completion of structured activities (e.g., homework assignments), which teach clients to recognize or self-monitor and target irrational thoughts or cognitions and replace them with realistic or positive self-talk. Cognitive-behavioral techniques enable the client to recognize adaptive and maladaptive responses and include interruption of self-defeating or negative self-talk and deep breathing and relaxation techniques. Maladaptive responses include substance abuse and avoidance behaviors. (Table 11–7 lists diverse anxiety-reducing techniques that the nurse can recommend or teach the client.)

The client may find cognitive-behavioral strategies, such as meditation and visual imagery, useful ways to reduce anxiety or enhance cognitive techniques (Beck, Emery, & Greenberg, 1985; Ellis, 1962). Furthermore, active participation of significant others in helping the client maintain adaptive coping behaviors is vital to the success of cognitive-behavioral techniques (Lazarus, 1971). Psychotherapy and psychotropics are also vital aspects of treatment planning and, like other strategies, enhance cognitive-behavioral approaches. See Chapters 9 and 26 for discussions of various cognitive-behavioral techniques and psychotherapy.

The overall treatment outcomes for anxiety disorders depend on the client's ability to:

◆ Establish a therapeutic relationship

◆ Acknowledge awareness of anxiety and verbalize related feelings and thoughts

◆ Develop adaptive skills, such as relaxation, deep breathing techniques, and positive self-talk

◆ Avoid maladaptive responses

◆ Reduce the emotional and biological discomforts of anxiety by using anxiety-reducing techniques, including thought blocking and positive self-talk, and having the insight to take prescribed antianxiety agents when indicated

◆ Improve self-esteem and personal control over feelings, thoughts, and behaviors

◆ Perform at an optimal level of functioning

◆ Mobilize support systems and other resources

Psychopharmacology

Nursing implications in the treatment of anxiety disorders include assessing the effectiveness of psychotropics. Prescribing and administering these agents is contingent on the cause and course of specific anxiety disorders, severity of symptoms, the client's preference, the presence of comorbid conditions such as major depressive episode and

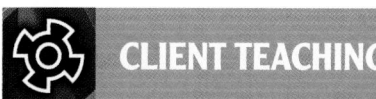

Anxiolytic Agent for the Client with an Anxiety Disorder (Sertraline [Zoloft] a Selective Serotonin Reuptake Inhibitor (SSRI))

- Take the medication during the morning or afternoon to reduce insomnia and restlessness (bedtime only if it produces sedation during the day).
- Administer or take the medication as prescribed. For instance, if you miss a morning dose, take it as soon as you remember (preferably during the morning or afternoon, because taking it at bedtime may interfere with your sleep).
- Avoid taking other antidepressants, or other medications, including over-the-counter medications without discussing it with your health care provider.
- Avoid performing activities that require mental and physical alertness such as driving or operating heavy machinery.
- You will not become addicted to this medication because it is not addictive.
- Avoid taking alcohol or other central nervous system depressants while on this medication.

- You may experience dry mouth: drink plenty of water or use sugarless candy. Constipation may occur, but do not rely on laxatives: increase dietary roughage or discuss taking a stool softener with your health care provider.
- Major side effects of this medication include: insomnia, diarrhea, nervousness, and nausea. This medication may also cause sexual dysfunction and decrease libido.
- If any of the following occur, report them immediately to your provider:
  - suicidal or homicidal ideations or aggressiveness
  - heart palpitations
  - seizures
  - persistent poor appetite, nausea or diarrhea, and excessive weight loss
  - confusion
- Take the medication with food to reduce nausea and diarrhea.

substance-related disorders, previous treatment response, and the client's motivation for treatment. (See Table 11–8 for a list of antianxiety or anxiolytic agents.)

Other nursing implications of psychopharmacologic interventions include client education regarding desired and side effect profile or anxiolytic agents; monitoring and documentation of the client's responses to these agents; and assessment of psychological and physiological dependence, specifically benzodiazepines. Clients experiencing anxiety disorders are at risk for substance abuse and other comorbid conditions such as major depression and other mental illnesses and require continuous assessment for maladaptive responses to minimize relapse and development of chronic ineffective coping patterns. Because of the concomitance of depression and other anxiety disorders, part of the client's assessment and treatment planning must include risk of dangerousness toward self and others. Medications are usually given as an adjunct to cognitive-behavioral therapy to maximize the efficacy of nonpharmacologic interventions. See Client Teaching: Anxiolytic Agent for the Client with an Anxiety Disorder.

Complementary Treatment of Anxiety Disorders

Traditional treatment of anxiety disorders involves prescribing pharmacologic agents, such as anxiolytic and nonanxiolytic agents, and nonpharmacologic interventions, such as cognitive-behavioral therapies. In today's world, one is likely to find other treatments, including complementary therapies. Presumably, more than 60 million Americans are

using daily treatments in the form of herbs. These include a bright yellow flower called St. John's wort; dietary supplements; chamomile tea; and kava and aloe for depression, sleep, and their vitalizing or calming effects. A newer drink that contains St. John's wort and gota kola supposedly "sharpens the mind" and reduces "stress" or helps one "chill out naturally." This blossoming industry offers numerous alternatives to traditional treatment to clients experiencing anxiety and other psychiatric disorders. Nurses must be familiar with these agents and provide health education about their desired and adverse reactions to clients inquiring about or using them.

Clients presenting with anxiety disorders can benefit from several complementary therapies that extend beyond over-the-counter herbs, minerals, and vitamins. Major alternative or complementary therapies include aromatherapy, meditation, massage therapy, exercise, and yoga. Aromatherapy is an ancient treatment that involves the use of plant oils that are absorbed through massage and supposedly reduce stress and anxiety. Olfactory use of these oils may also elicit an array of emotions. Meditation, another ancient treatment, involves entering a calm trance and focusing on a word or sound (or mantra) or stimulus, which produces a sense of calmness. Massage therapy improves circulation and muscle tone and resultant relaxation. Yoga, like alternative therapies, reduces anxiety, stress, and blood pressure.

Other alternative and complementary therapies may already be a part of the nurse's repertoire to reduce stress and

TABLE 11-9
Complementary Therapies for Anxiety Disorders

Mind-Body Interventions	Homeopathic	Herbal Preparations*
Biofeedback	Acupuncture (increases endorphins, serotonin, and other neurotransmitters)	**St. John's Wort** (mixed anxiety and depressive states)
Visualization/Imagery		*Adverse effects:* MAO inhibitor properties--> increase risk of convulsions, death and hypertensive crisis when mixed with cold preparations, antihistamines and tyramine containing foods; unclear effects on P450 liver enzyme system (drug interactions—MAO Inhibitors, serotonin reuptake inhibitors, birth control pills), allergic reactions, fatigue, HA, dry mouth (see Chapter 28)
Stress Management		
T'ai chi		
Meditation		
Yoga		**Kava-kava** (anxiety and sleep disorders)
Exercise		*Adverse effects:* GI disturbances, increased liver enzymes, decreased albumin and protein, increased cholesterol and ataxia and confusion when mixed with a benzodiazepine
Hypnosis		
Progressive Relaxation		**Valerian** (sedative and hypnotic properties)
Centering		*Adverse effects:* GI disturbances, fatigue, chest discomfort, tremors, cardiac disturbances

Caution: Alternative or complementary treatments carry risk profiles and have potentially life threatening consequences, particularly the herbal preparation. This table is not an endorsement of these interventions, but provides a list of alternative therapies that can assist the nurse when clients inquire about them. Herbal preparations are unregulated and there is a lack of standardization regarding doses. This information is also important when discussing them with clients and families.

Note. Data from "Over-the-Counter Psychotropics: A Review of Melatonin, St. John's Wort, Valerian, and Kava-Kava," by E. Heiligenstein and G. Guenther, 1998, *Journal of the American College of Health, 46,* pp. 271-276; and "Kava-Kava Extract WS 1490 versus Placebo in Anxiety Disorders: A Randomized Placebo-Controlled 25-Week Outpatient Trial," by H. P. Volz and M. Kieser, 1997, *Pharmacopsychiatry, 30,* 1–5.

anxiety and promote health restoration. These interventions include therapeutic touch and pet therapy, a regular exercise program, sleep manipulation, and a balanced diet. Soft music and a warm bubble bath also produce calming and therapeutic effects and sleep. Refer to Table 11–9 for alternative and complementary therapies for the client experiencing an anxiety disorder.

Overall, nonherbal complementary therapies enhance other therapies such as visual imagery or other cognitive-behavioral techniques. More importantly, they afford the client experiencing diverse anxiety disorders with an array of traditional and alternative therapies that reduce stress and anxiety.

EVALUATION

Evaluating the effectiveness of nursing interventions is an integral part of the nursing process that begins during the initial assessment phase and continues throughout treatment. It provides invaluable data regarding the client's response to treatment, formation of adaptive coping skills, and potential risk of recurrence of symptoms. Criteria for effectiveness parallel outcome identification, the client and family member's feedback, and observations by the nurse and other mental health professionals regarding the client's response to diverse interventions.

See Nursing Care Plan 11–1, The Client Experiencing Panic Disorder (Ms. Inoh).

Other interventions include prescribing and administering various antipanic/antidepressant agents, such as SSRIs and SNRIs, to manage biological aspects of her illness.

This scenario demonstrates the complexity of an anxiety disorder and multimodal approach that involves client and family education, cognitive-behavioral techniques, and pharmacologic interventions. It also demonstrates the effectiveness of symptom management and self-modulation techniques that promote a sense of control over a potentially controlling anxiety disorder.

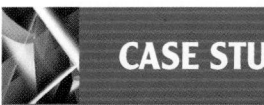

CASE STUDY

The Client Experiencing Panic Disorder (Ms. Inoh)

Ms. Inoh is a 32-year-old woman who presents in the emergency department complaining of chest pains, palpitations, shortness of breath, diaphoresis, lightheadedness, and fears of dying. Her husband reports that she has had these symptoms episodically over the past 4 to 6 months and reports bringing her in today because of his fears of her having a heart attack.

The emergency department physician orders an electrocardiogram and diagnostic studies, including cardiac enzymes, chemistry profile, complete blood count, and a toxicology screen. Her physical examination and diagnostic studies are negative. The physician informs Ms. Inoh and her husband that she does not have a medical problem and tells her that it sounds like she is having panic attacks. She refers Ms. Inoh for a psychiatric consultation with the advanced-practice psychiatric nurse. The couple expresses anger, stating that her symptoms are real and that she is not crazy.

Critical Thinking Questions

1. *What is the most important consideration in the care of this client?*

   The most important consideration for this client is establishing a therapeutic relationship and allaying her fears and anxiety. A therapeutic relationship and rapport are the basis of trust, an essential aspect of this client's care. Clients with panic disorder often feel like they are "losing control" or "going crazy." Establishing rapport and allaying these fears help the client gain some control and validate her feelings, thoughts, and physiological responses arising from panic disorder. Because of the high co-occurrence of depression, suicide, and other mental disorder in clients experiencing panic disorder, the nurse needs to assess for symptoms and continuously monitor her level of dangerousness.

2. *What types of interventions should the nurse provide for this client?*

   Major interventions for this client include psychoeducation about the cause, course, and treatment of panic disorder. Symptoms management and relapse prevention are also crucial aspects of her care. Relapse prevention involves helping the client identify triggers, external (anxiety-provoking situations) and internal (inadequate rest, nutrition, and stress). Symptom management involves using cognitive-behavioral techniques, deep breathing and relaxation exercises, and psychopharmacologic interventions. The basis of these interventions is challenging cognitive distortions (psychological) regarding the fear of having a panic attack and reducing autonomic nervous system arousal (biological). Consequently, the goal is to improve her level of functioning (social, occupational) in both her personal and professional life.

NURSING CARE PLAN 11–1

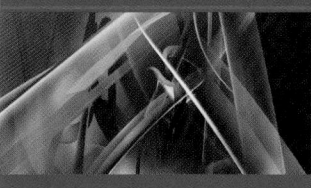

The Client Experiencing Panic Disorder (Ms. Inoh)

Nursing Diagnosis: Ineffective Coping
as evidenced by inadequate level of perception of control

Outcome Identification	Nursing Actions	Rationales	Evaluation
1. By [date], Ms. Inoh will develop adaptive coping behaviors.	1a. Provide a safe, caring environment.	1a. Providing a safe, caring environment promotes expression of feelings and thoughts.	*Goal met:* Ms. Inoh reports that she has had only one panic episode in a 3-month period. She also reports that she feels confident in controlling her attacks and no longer feels helpless and out of control. She is no longer afraid to leave the house and is able to perform household and professional responsibilities.
	1b. Assess Ms. Inoh's present and past coping patterns.	1b. Enables the nurse to discern maladaptive coping patterns.	
	1c. Discuss coping alternatives.	1c. Identifies viable coping options.	

(continues)

Nursing Care Plan 11–1 *(continued)*

Outcome Identification	Nursing Actions	Rationales	Evaluation
2. By [date], Ms. Inoh will be able to identify feelings and thoughts that precede an anxiety attack.	2a. Encourage Ms. Inoh to identify anxiety-provoking situations and her thoughts that arise from them. 2b. Teach Ms. Inoh anxiety-reducing techniques and provide feedback.	2a. Promotes understanding of the meaning of cognitive distortions or erroneous belief systems and gain self-awareness. 2b. Use of anxiety-reducing techniques reduces the intensity and number of anxiety attacks and gives the client a sense of control over situations.	

Nursing Diagnosis: Anxiety

as related to and evidenced by a perception of powerlessness and autonomic nervous system arousal (i.e., increased heart rate and respirations, lightheadedness)

Outcome Identification	Nursing Actions	Rationales	Evaluation
1. By [date], Ms. Inoh will develop a realistic perception of her fears and control her physiological responses to anxiety.	1a. Help Ms. Inoh recognize the relationship between her thoughts, feelings, and biological responses. 1b. Teach Ms. Inoh deep breathing exercises and relaxation techniques.	1a. Recognizing the relationship between thoughts, feelings, and biological responses promotes understanding of the disease process and aspects the client can control. 1b. Deep breathing, relaxation techniques, and anxiolytic agents reduce the intensity of biological and emotional distress of anxiety attacks.	*Goal met:* Ms. Inoh attempts to control the intensity and number of panic attacks she experiences.

Nursing Diagnosis: Disturbed Thought Processes

as evidenced by negative, irrational and self-defeating self-talk

Outcome Identification	Nursing Actions	Rationales	Evaluation
1. By [date], Ms. Inoh will perceive her fears realistically and have fewer cognitive distortions.	1a. Point out Ms. Inoh's self-defeating and negative self-talk. 1b. Explore the basis of Ms. Inoh's negative thinking. 1c. Teach Ms. Inoh cognitive-behavioral techniques (e.g., positive self-talk to challenge irrational beliefs)	1a-c. Challenging self-defeating and negative self-talk facilitates alterations of impaired cognitions, helps the client assess fears realistically, and reduces anxiety.	*Goal met:* Ms. Inoh practices positive self-talk and perceives her fears realistically. Her anxiety attacks decrease in frequency and intensity over time.

(continues)

Nursing Care Plan 11–1 (continued)

Nursing Diagnosis: Situational Low Self-Esteem
as evidenced by self-negating verbalizations

Outcome Identification	Nursing Actions	Rationales	Evaluation
1. By [date], Ms. Inoh will verbalize several positive self-attributes and strengths.	1. Provide successful experiencing paralleling Ms. Inoh's level of functioning.	1. Successful experiences enhance and increase self-esteem.	*Goal met:* Ms. Inoh identifies her strengths and positive attributes.
2. By [date], Ms. Inoh will demonstrate interest in self-care.	2. Provide positive feedback on accomplishments.	2. Positive feedback validates positive attributes and strengths.	Ms. Inoh begins to function at precrisis level.
3. By [date], Ms. Inoh will complete tasks.	3. Explore with Ms. Inoh her current strengths.	3. Successful completion of tasks enhances self-confidence and self-image.	Ms. Inoh directs self-care.

SUMMARY

◆ Anxiety is an integral and innate aspect of the human experience. It arises from arousal, the body's activation of complex biological and neuroendocrine processes.

◆ Clients tend to seek treatment when their anxiety reaches overwhelming proportions and interferes with their psychosocial and biological functioning.

◆ Anxiety symptoms range from mild to severe forms of distress.

◆ Psychiatric nurses must rise to the challenge of assessing clients' adaptive and maladaptive responses and provide clients with quality and safe treatment.

◆ The nursing process is an effective mechanism that identifies disabling symptoms and effective interventions that promote adaptive processes.

◆ Education of the client and his significant others regarding anxiety and their active participation in treatment are critical to successful treatment outcomes.

SUGGESTIONS FOR CLINICAL CONFERENCES

1. Present case histories of clients experiencing anxiety disorders. For each case, identify the (a) psychosocial issues, (b) biological and genetic factors, (c) diverse treatment modalities, (d) life span and developmental issues, and (e) client/family teaching needs.

2. Discuss several treatment modalities for clients experiencing anxiety disorders such as progressive relaxation, visual imagery, and psychopharmacologic interventions.

STUDY QUESTIONS

1. M. B. is a 21-year-old woman who presents in the emergency department crying and distraught, complaining that her date had raped her. After a complete physical examination and laboratory studies, she is referred to the nurse for further assessment. The nurse can most effectively help this client by:
   a. reassuring her that the man will be prosecuted
   b. referring her to a rape crisis center
   c. putting her at ease using active listening techniques
   d. providing her with a tranquilizer to decrease her anxiety

2. M. B. begins screaming and stating she feels so ashamed and that maybe the rape was her fault. What is an appropriate nursing response?
   a. "I can see this is very upsetting to you."
   b. "Please lower your voice because you are disturbing other sick clients."
   c. Remain silent, and allow her to ventilate feelings and thoughts.
   d. Offer her a tranquilizer because she is out of control.

3. J. F., a 15-year-old girl, is admitted to the hospital with numerous somatic complaints, including pain and nausea. Her mother reports that she has had these symptoms for several weeks. J. F. agrees with her and states that she is sick of school and has refused to attend for several days. What information is most pertinent to the treatment team in assisting them in making a definitive diagnosis?
   a. History of substance abuse
   b. Social relationships
   c. History of these symptoms in the past
   d. Present stressors

4. H. M. is seen in his home complaining of fears of going outdoors and grocery shopping. Additionally, he is complaining of intense anxiety manifested by tachycardia, shortness of breath, and lightheadedness. What should the nurse do in this situation?
   a. Inquire about his last dose of alprazolam (Xanax).
   b. Call an ambulance or emergency backup.
   c. Check his vital signs.
   d. Encourage him to express his feelings.

5. Manifestations of childhood anxiety disorders include all of the following *except:*
   a. inability to form trusting relationships
   b. crying and following in infancy
   c. overconcern for the safety of primary caregivers
   d. excessive hand washing and counting

6. In assessing a client for generalized anxiety disorder (GAD), which symptoms would the nurse identify as key in the client's impairment due to this anxiety disorder?
   a. Co-occurrence with major depression
   b. Excessive worrying and free-floating anxiety
   c. Increased sleep and daytime fatigue
   d. Decreased appetite and stable concentration patterns

7. Which of the following would best indicate to the nurse that a child with separation anxiety is improving?
   a. Able to attend school without clinging to mother
   b. Sleeps well through the night
   c. Performs homework with minimal help from mother
   d. Plays with friends in the backyard

8. When teaching relaxation and deep breathing exercises to the client with panic attacks, the nurse knows the client *lacks* understanding when he says which of the following?
   a. "I was able to take a short trip to Canada without feeling short of breath."
   b. "I was able to do a presentation this morning without my heart pounding in my ears."
   c. "I was so nervous today while talking to my boss about a raise."
   d. "I was able to rest last night after completing my homework."

9. In assessing a client for signs of panic disorder, which of the following findings reported to the nurse would indicate a priority for further assessment?
   a. "I get so nervous when I drive my car."
   b. "Sometimes I feel like I am going crazy or dying."
   c. "Sometimes I feel like I am having a heart attack because my chest hurts."
   d. "I feel so down sometimes I don't know if I can live like this."

10. In assessing for post-traumatic stress disorder, which symptoms would the nurse perceive as key in the client's response to trauma?
    a. Emotional numbing and detachment followed by irritability, anxiety, aggressiveness, and hyperalertless
    b. Depression and social withdrawal

c. Intrusive, hyperactive behavior and use of alcohol to soothe symptoms
d. Drug-seeking behavior and hypersexuality as a means to cope

RESOURCES

Please note that because Internet resources are of a time-sensitive nature and URL addresses may change or be deleted, searches should also be conducted by association or topic.

Information regarding the latest research on anxiety disorders is available from the National Institute of Mental Health (NIMH) and other government agencies:

- upcoming programs
- current research
- call for abstract
- nursing research opportunities

Educational materials (handouts for clients) are available regarding the following:

- alternative/complementary therapies
- current medications for various anxiety disorders
- latest information on various anxiety disorders
- support groups for clients experiencing anxiety disorders
- current research on various anxiety and other psychiatric disorders

Professional nursing and mental health professional organizations offer information regarding anxiety disorders such as:

Journal Watch Psychiatry
   E-mail: jwpsych@world.std.com

Internet Resources

http://www.nimh.nih.gov/publicat/NIMHanxiety.pdf
   Anxiety Disorders (2006). National Institute of Health (NIMH) Publication
http://www.nimh.nih.gov/studies/studies_ct.cfm?id=1
   NIMH Clinical Trials: Anxiety Disorders
http://www.psych.org/psych_pract/treatg/pg/ASD_PTSD_05-15-06.pdf   American Psychiatric Practice Guidelines for the Treatment of Patients with Acute Stress Disorder and Post-traumatic Stress Disorder (2004)

Other Resources

National Alliance for the Mentally Ill (NAMI)
   Advocate
   200 N. Glebe Rd., Suite 1015
   Arlington, VA 22203-3754
   (703) 524-7600
   Help line: (800) 950-NAMI
   http://www.nami.org

National Institute of Mental Health
   6001 Executive Blvd., Rm. 8184, MSC 9663
   Bethesda, MD 20892-9663
   (301) 443-4513
   Reliving Trauma
   Post-Traumatic Stress Disorder
   http://www.nimh.nih.gov/publicat/reliving.cfm
   (Retrieved 8/17/2002)
American Psychiatric Nurses Association
   1200 19th St. NW, Suite 300
   Washington, DC 20036-2422
   (202) 857-1133
   http://www.apna.org

REFERENCES

Abe, O., Yamasue, H., Kasai, K., Yamada, H., Aoki, S., & Iwanami, A. (2006). Voxel-based diffusion tensor analysis reveals aberrant anterior cinguluam integrity in posttraumatic stress disorder due to terrorism. *Psychiatry Research, 146,* 231–242.

Abelson, J. L., Curtis, G. C., & Uhde, T. W. (2005). Twenty-four-hour growth hormone secretion in patients with panic disorder. *Psychoneuroendocrinology, 30,* 72–79.

Adams, R. E., & Boscarino, J. A. (2005). Differences in mental health outcomes among Whites, African Americans, and Hispanics following a community disaster. *Psychiatry, 68,* 250–265.

Ainsworth, M. D. S. (1985). Attachment across the life span. *Bulletin of the New York Academy of Medicine, 61,* 792–812.

Ainsworth, M. D. S. (1990). Some considerations regarding theory and assessment relevant to attachments beyond infancy. In M. T Greenberg, D. Cicchetti, & E. M. Cummings (Eds.), *Attachment in the preschool years* (pp. 463–488). Chicago: University of Chicago Press.

Alegria, M., Canino, G., Stinson, F. S., & Grant, B. F. (2006). Nativity and *DSM-IV* psychiatric disorders among Puerto Ricans, Cuban Americans, and non-Latino whites in the United States: Results from the National Epidemiologic Survey on Alcohol and Related Conditions. *Journal of Clinical Psychiatry, 67,* 56–65.

Alexander, J. K., Hillier, A., Smith, R. M., Tivarus, M. E., & Beversdorf, D. Q. (2007). Beta-adrenergic modulation of cognitive flexibility during stress. *Journal of Cognitive Neuroscience, 19,* 468–478.

American Academy of Child and Adolescent Psychiatry. (1998). Practice parameters for the assessment and treatment of children and adolescents with obsessive-compulsive disorder. *Journal of the American Academy of Child and Adolescent Psychiatry, 37,* 1110–1116.

American Nurses Association. (2000). *Scope and standards of psychiatric-mental health nursing practice.* Washington, DC: American Nurses Publishers.

American Psychiatric Association. (1968). *Diagnostic and statistical manual of mental disorders* (2nd ed.). Washington, DC: Author.

American Psychiatric Association. (2000). *Diagnostic and statistical manual of mental disorders* (4th edition, Text Revision) *(DSM-IV-TR).* Washington, DC: Author.

Andrews, G., & Crino, R. (1991). Behavioral therapy of anxiety disorders. *Psychiatric Annals, 21,* 358–367.

Antai-Otong, D. (2001). Critical incident stress debriefing: A health promotion model for workplace violence. *Perspectives in Psychiatric Care, 37,* 125–132.

Barlow, D. H. (1997). Cognitive-behavioral therapy for panic disorder: Current status. *Journal of Clinical Psychiatry, 58*(Suppl. 2), 32–36.

Barron, J., Curtis, M. A., & Grainger, R. D. (1998). Eye movement desensitization and reprocessing. *Journal of the American Psychiatric Nurses Association, 4,* 140–144.

Beck, A. T., Emery, G., & Greenberg, R. (1985). *Anxiety disorders and phobias: A cognitive perspective.* New York: Basic Books.

Beck, A. T., Skodol, L., Clark, D. A., Berchick, R., & Wright, F. (1992). A crossover study of focused cognitive therapy for panic disorders. *American Journal of Psychiatry, 149,* 778–783.

Bernstein, G. A., Borchardt, C. M., & Perwien, A. R. (1996). Anxiety disorders in children and adolescents: A review of the past 10 years. *Journal of American Academy of Child and Adolescent Psychiatry, 35,* 1110–1119.

Bowlby, J. (1969). *Attachment and loss* (Vol. I). New York: Basic Books.

Bremner, J. D. (2004). Brain imaging in anxiety disorders. *Expert Review of Neurotherapeutics, 4,* 275–284.

Bremner, J. D., Vermetten, E., Schmahl, C., Vaccarino, V., Vythilingam, M., Afzal, N., et al. (2005). Positron emission tomographic imaging of neural correlates of a fear acquisition and extinction paradigm in women with childhood sexual-abuse-related posttraumatic stress disorder. *Psychological Medicine, 35,* 791–806.

Breuer, J., & Freud, S. (1957). *Studies in hysteria* (J. Strachey, Trans.). New York: Basic Books. (Original work published 1895)

Briere, J. & Elliott, D. M. (2003). Prevalence and psychological sequelae of self-reported childhood physical and sexual abuse in a general population sample of men and women. *Child Abuse and Neglect, 27,* 1205–1222.

Campbell-Sills, L., & Stein, M. B. (2006). Guideline watch: Practice guideline for the treatment of patients with panic disorder. Available at http://www.psych.org/psych_pract/treatg/pg/Panic.watch.pdf

Cannon, W. B. (1914). The emergency functions of the adrenal medulla in pain and the major emotions. *American Journal of Physiology, 33,* 356–372.

Cartwright-Hatton, S., Roberts, C., Chitsabesan, P., Fothergill, C., & Harrington, R. (2004). Systematic review of the efficacy of cognitive behaviour therapies for childhood and adolescent anxiety disorders. *British Journal of Clinical Psychology, 43,* (Pt 4), 421–436.

Clark, D. B., Birmaher, B., Axelson, D., Monk, K., Kalas, C., Ehmann, M., et al. (2005). Fluoxetine for the treatment of childhood anxiety disorders: Open-label, long-term extension to a controlled trial. *Journal of the American Child and Adolescent Psychiatry, 44,* 1263–1270.

Clark, C., Rodgers, B., Caldwell, T., Power, C., & Stansfeld, S. (2007). Childhood and adulthood psychological ill health as predictors of midlife and anxiety disorders. *Archives of General Psychiatry, 64,* 668–678.

Clomipramine Collaborative Study Group. (1991). Efficacy of clomipramine in OCD: Results of a multicenter double-blind trial. *Archives of General Psychiatry, 48,* 730–738.

Cloninger, C. R. (2006). The science of well-being: An integrated approach to mental health and its disorders. *World Psychiatry, 5,* 71–76.

Connor, K. M., & Davidson, J. R. T. (1998). Generalized anxiety disorder: Neurobiological and pharmacotherapeutic perspectives. *Society of Biological Psychiatry, 44,* 1286–1294.

Copeland, W. E., Keeler, G., Angold, A., & Costello, E. J. (2007). Traumatic events and posttraumatic stress in childhood. *Archives of General Psychiatry, 64,* 577–584.

Craske, M. G., Rowe, M., Lewin, M., & Noriega-Dimitri, R. (1997). Interoceptive exposure versus breathing within cognitive-behavioural therapy for panic disorder with agoraphobia. *British Journal of Clinical Psychology, 36* (Part I), 85–99.

de Geus, F., Denys, D. A., Sitskoorn, M. M., & Westenberg, H. G. (2007). Attention and cognition in patients with obsessive-compulsive disorder. *Psychiatry and Clinical Neuroscience, 61,* 45–63.

Dunlop, B. W., Papp, L., Garlow, S. J., Weiss, P. S., Knight, B. T., & Ninan, P. T. (2007). Tiagabine for social anxiety disorder. *Human Psychopharmacology, 22,* 241–244.

Ellis, A. (1962). *Reason and emotion in psychotherapy.* New York: Lyle Stuart.

Eth, S., & Pynoos, R. (1984). *Post-traumatic stress disorder in children.* Washington, DC: American Psychiatric Press.

Eysenck, H. J. (1981). *A model for personality.* New York: Springer-Verlag.

Eysenck, M. W. (1990). Anxiety and cognitive functioning. In G. D. Burrows, M. Roth, & R. Noyes (Eds.), *Handbook of anxiety: Vol. 2. The neurobiology of anxiety* (pp. 419–435). New York: Elsevier.

Feldman, R. (2007). Parent-infant synchrony and the construction of shared timing; physiological precursors, developmental outcomes, and risk conditions. *Journal of Child Psychology and Psychiatry, 48,* 329–354.

Flint, A. J. (2005). Anxiety and its disorders in late life: Moving the field forward. *American Journal Geriatric Psychiatry, 13,* 7–14.

Flint, A. J. (2005). Generalised anxiety disorder in elderly patients: Epidemiology, diagnosis and treatment options. *Drugs and Aging, 22,* 101–114.

Freud, A. (1936). *The ego and the mechanisms of defense.* New York: International University Press.

Freud, S. (1936). *The problem of anxiety* (H. A. Bunker, Trans.). New York: Psychoanalytic Quarterly Press. (Original work published 1926)

Friedman, S., Smith, L., & Fogel, A. (1999). Suicidality in panic disorder: A comparison with schizophrenic, depressed and other anxiety disorder outpatients. *Anxiety Disorders, 13,* 447–461.

Ganong, W. F. (2005). *Review of medical physiology* (22nd ed.). New York: The McGraw-Hill Companies.

Goenjian, A. K., Walling, D., Steinberg, A. M., Karayan, I., Najarian, L. M., & Pynoos, R. (2005). A prospective study of posttraumatic stress and depressive reactions among treated and untreated adolescents after a catastrophic disaster. *American Journal of Psychiatry, 162,* 2302–2308.

Goodman, W. K., Price, L. H., Rasmussen, S. A., Mazure, C., Delgado, P., Heninger, G. R., & Charney, D. S. (1989). The Yale-Brown obsessive-compulsive scale. II. Validity. *Archives of General Psychiatry, 46,* 1012–1016.

Grant, B. F., Hasin, D. S., Blanco, C., Stinson, F. S., Chou, S. P., Goldstein, R. B., et al. (2005). The epidemiology of social anxiety disorder in the United States: Results from the National Epidemiologic Survey on Alcohol and Related Conditions. *Journal of Clinical Psychiatry, 66,* 1351–1361.

Graziano, A. M., DeGiorani, I., & Garcia, K. (1979). Behavioral treatment of child's fear. *Psychological Bulletin, 56,* 804–830.

Griffin, M. G., Resick, P. A., & Yehuda, R. (2005). Enhanced cortisol suppression following dexamethasone administration in domestic violence survivors. *American Journal of Psychiatry, 162,* 1192–1199.

Grover, R. L., Ginsburg, G. S., & Ialongo, N. (2005). Childhood predictors of anxiety symptoms: A longitudinal study. *Child Psychiatry and Human Development, 36,* 133–153.

Hanna, G. L., Piacentini, J., Cantwell, D. P., Fischer, D. J., Himle, J. A., & Van Ettan, M. (2002). Obsessive-compulsive disorder with and without tics in a clinical sample of children and adolescents. *Depression and Anxiety, 16,* 59–63.

Hettema, J. M., Prescott, C. A., Myers, J. M., Neale, M. C., & Kendler, K. S. (2005). The structure of genetic and environmental risk factors for anxiety disorders in men and women. *Archives of General Psychiatry, 62,* 182–189.

Hirshfeld-Becker, D. R., Biederman, J., Henin, A., Faraone, S. V., Davis, S., Harrington, K., et al. (2007). Behavioral inhibition in preschool children at risk is a specific predictor of middle childhood social anxiety: A five-year follow-up. *Journal of Developmental and Behavioral Pediatrics, 28,* 225–233.

Hodge, K. K., McKnew, D., & Burbach, D. J. (1987). Diagnostic concordance between two structured child interviews, using lay examiners: The child assessment schedule and the Kiddie-SADS. *Journal of the Academy of Child and Adolescent Psychiatry, 26,* 654–661.

Ivarsson, T., & Valderhaug, R. (2005). Symptom patterns in children and adolescents with obsessive-compulsive disorder (OCD). *Behavioural Research and Therapy, 44,* 1105–1116.

Jacobs, J., Horne-Moyer, H. L., & Jones, R. (2004).The effectiveness of critical incident stress debriefing with primary and secondary trauma victims. *International Journal of Emergency Mental Health, 6,* 5–14.

Johnson M. R., Hartzema, A. G., Mills, T. L., De Leon, J. M., Yang, M., Frueh, C., et al. (2007). Ethnic differences in the reliability and validity of a Panic Disorder Screen. *Ethnicity & Health, 12,* 283–296.

Kessler, R. C., Chiu, W. T., Demier, O., Merikangas, K. R., & Walters, E. E. (2005). Prevalence, severity, and comorbidity of 12-month DSM-IV disorders in the National Comorbidity Survey replication. *Archives of General Psychiatry, 62,* 617–627.

Kessler, R. C., Chiu, W. T., Jin, R., Ruscio, A. M., Shear, K., & Walters, E. E. (2006). The epidemiology of panic attacks, panic disorder, and agoraphobia in the National Comorbidity Survey Replication. *Archives of General Psychiatry, 63,* 415–424.

Lazarus, A. A. (1971). *Behavior therapy and beyond.* New York: McGraw-Hill.

Leon, C. A., & Leon, A. (1990). Panic disorder and parental bonding. *Psychiatric Annals, 20,* 503–508.

Le Roux, H., Gatz, M., & Wetherell, J. L. (2005). Age onset of generalized anxiety disorder in older adults. *American Journal of Psychiatry, 13,* 23–30.

Levander, E., Frye, M. A., McElroy, S., Suppes, T., Grunze, H., Nolen, W. A., et al. (2007). Alcoholism and anxiety in bipolar illness: Differential lifetime anxiety comorbidity in bipolar I women with and without alcoholism. *Journal of Affective Disorders, 101,* 211–217.

Loerch, B., Graf-Morgenstern, M., Hautzinger, M., Schlegel, S., Hain, C., Sandmann, J., et al. (1999). Randomised placebo-controlled trial of moclobemide, cognitive-behavioral therapy and their combination in panic disorder with agoraphobia. *British Journal of Psychiatry, 174,* 205–212.

Magee, W. J., Eaton, W. W., Wittchen, H-U, McGonagle, K. A., & Kessler, R. C. (1996). Agoraphobia, simple phobia, and social phobia in the National Cormobidity Survey. *Archives of General Psychiatry, 53,* 159–168.

March, J. S., Mulle, K., & Herbel, B. (1994). Behavioral psychotherapy for children and adolescents with obsessive-compulsive disorder: An open trial of a new protocol-driven treatment package. *Journal of the Academy of Child Adolescent Psychiatry, 33,* 333–341.

Mathew, S. J., Amiel, J. M., Coplan, J. D., Fitterling, H. A., Sackeim, H. A., & Gorman, J. M. (2005). Open-label trial of riluzole in generalized anxiety disorder. *American Journal of Psychiatry, 162,* 2379–2381.

May, R. (1977). *The meaning of anxiety* (2nd ed.). New York: W.W. Norton.

McClure, E. B., Monk, C. S., Nelson, E. E., Parrish, J. M., Adler, A., Blair, R. J., et al. (2007). Abnormal attention modulation of fear circuit function in pediatric generalized anxiety disorder. *Archives of General Psychiatry, 64,* 97–106.

Mitchell, J. T., & Dyregov, A. (1993). Traumatic stress in disaster workers and emergency personnel: Prevention and intervention. In J. P. Wilson & B. Raphael (Eds). *International handbook of traumatic stress syndromes* (pp. 905–914). New York: Plenum.

Moffitt, T. E., Harrington, H., Caspi, A., Kim-Cohen, J., Goldberg, D., Gregory, A. M., et al. (2007). Depression and generalized anxiety disorder: Cumulative and sequential comorbidity in a birth cohort followed prospectively to age 32 years. *Archives of General Psychiatry, 64,* 651–660.

Monk, C. S., Pine, D. S., Charney, D. S. (2002). A developmental and neurobiological approach to trauma research. *Seminars in Clinical Neuropsychiatry, 7,* 137–146.

Mörtberg, E., Clark, D. M., Sundin, O., & Aberg Wistedt, A. (2007). Intensive group cognitive treatment and individual cognitive therapy vs. treatment as usual in social phobia: A randomized controlled trial. *Acta Psychiatrica Scandinavica, 115,* 142–154.

Nemeroff, C. B., Bremner, J. D., Foa, E. B., Mayberg, H. S., North, C. S., & Stein, M. B. (2006). Posttraumatic stress disorder: A state-of-the science review. *Journal of Psychiatric Research, 40,* 1–21.

Nutt, D. J. (2005). Overview of diagnosis and drug treatments of anxiety disorders. *CNS Spectrums, 10,* 49–56.

Ollendick, T. H., & Francis, G. (1998). Behavioral assessment and treatment of childhood phobias. *Behavior Modification, 12,* 165–203.

Pae, C. U., Lim, H. K., Ajwani, N., Lee, C., & Patkar, A. A. (2007). Extended-release formulation of venlafaxine in the treatment of post-traumatic stress disorder. *Expert Review of Neurotherapeutics, 7,* 603–615.

Palapattu, A. G., Kingery, J. N., & Ginsburg, G. S. (2006). Gender role orientation and anxiety symptoms among African American adolescents. *Journal of Abnormal Child Psychology, 34,* 441–449.

Pavlov, I. P. (1927). Conditioned reflexes: An investigation of the physiological activity of the cerebral cortex (G. C. Andrep, Trans. and Ed.). London: Oxford University Press.

Phan, K. L., Fitzgerald, D. A., Cortese, B. M., Seraji-Bozorgzad, N., Tancer, M. E., & Moore, G. J. (2005). Anterior cingulate neurochemistry in social anxiety disorder: 1H-MRS at 4 Tesla. *Neuroport, 16,* 183–186.

Piacentini, J., & Bergman, R. L. (2000). Obsessive compulsive disorder in children. *Psychiatric Clinics of North America, 23,* 519–533.

Piaget, J. (1954). *The construction of reality in the child.* New York: Basic Books.

Piaget, J. (1958). *The growth of logical thinking from childhood to adolescence.* New York: Basic Books.

Pynoos, R. S., Steinberg, A. M., & Goenjian, A. C. (1996). Traumatic stress in childhood and adolescence: Recent developments and current controversies. In B. A. Vander Kolk & A. C. McFarlane (Eds.), *Traumatic stress : The effects of overwhelming experience on mind, body, and society,* (pp. 331–358). NY: Guilford Press.

Regier, D. A., Burke, J. D., & Burke, K. C. (1990). Comorbidity of affective and anxiety disorders in the NIMH Epidemiological Catchment Area Program. In J. D. Maser & C. R. Cloninger (Eds.), *Comorbidity of mood and anxiety disorders* (pp. 112–122). Washington, DC: American Psychiatric Press.

Regier, D. A., Farmer, M. E., Rae, R. S., Locke, B. Z., Keith, S. J., Judd, L. L., et al. (1990). Comorbidity of mental disorders with alcohol and other drug abuse: Results from the Epidemiological Catchment Area (ECA) Study. *Journal of the American Medical Association, 264,* 2511–2518.

Reynolds, C. R., & Richmond, B. D. (1978). What I think and feel: A revised measure of children's manifest anxiety. *Journal of Abnormal Psychology, 6,* 271–280.

Robinson, R. C., & Mitchell, J. T. (1993). Evaluation of psychological debriefings. *Journal of Traumatic Stress, 6,* 367–382.

Rosenbaum, J. F. (1990). A psychopharmacologist's perspectives on panic disorder. *Bulletin of the Menninger Clinic, 54,* 184–196.

Rothbaum, B. O., Astin, M. C., & Marsteller, F. (2005). Prolonged exposure versus eye movement desensitization and reprocessing (EMDR) for PTSD rape victims. *Journal of Traumatic Stress, 18,* 607–616.

Ruzich, M. J., Looi, J. C., & Robertson, M. D. (2005). Delayed onset of posttraumatic stress disorder among male combat veterans: A case series. *American Journal of Geriatric Psychiatry, 13,* 424–427.

Sadock, B. J. & Sadock, V. A. (2005). *Kaplan & Sadock's Pocket Handbook of Clinical Psychiatry,* (4th ed). Philadelphia: Lippincott Williams & Wilkins.

Sadock, J., Sadock, V. A., & Sussman, N. (2006). *Kaplan & Sadock pocket handbook of psychiatric drug treatment* (4th ed.). Philadelphia: Lippincott Williams & Wilkins.

Sareen, J., Cox, B. J., Afifi, T. O., de Graaf, R., Asmundson, G. J., Ten Have, M., & Stein, M. B. (2005). Anxiety disorders and risk for suicidal ideation and suicide attempts: A population-based longitudinal study of adults. *Archives of General Psychiatry, 62,* 1249–1257.

Schmidt, N. B., Zvolensky, M. J., & Maner, J. K. (2006). Anxiety sensitivity: Prospective prediction of panic attacks and Axis I pathology. *Journal of Psychiatric Research, 40,* 691–699.

Schneier, F. R., Goetz, D., Campeas, R., Fallon, B., Marshall, R., & Liebowitz, M. R. (1998). Placebo-controlled trial of moclobemide in social phobia. *British Journal of Psychiatry, 172,* 70–77.

Schwartz, T. L., Azhar, N., Husain, J., Nihalani, N., Simonescu, M., Coovert, D., et al. (2005). An open-label study of tiagabine as augmentation therapy for anxiety. *Annals of Clinical Psychiatry, 17,* 167–172.

Shapiro, F. (1995). *Eye movement desensitization and reprocessing: Basic principles, protocols, and procedures.* New York: Guilford Press.

Sheehan, D. V. (1986). *The anxiety disease* (2nd ed.). New York: Bantam Books.

Shih, R. A., Belmonte, P. L., & Zandi, P. P. (2004). A review of the evidence from family, twin, and adoption studies for a genetic contribution to adult psychiatric disorders. *International Review of Psychiatry, 16,* 260–283.

Sijbrandij, M., Olff, M., Reitsma, J. B., Carlier, I. V., de Vries, M. H., & Gersons, B. P. (2007). Treatment of acute posttraumatic stress disorder with brief cognitive behavioral therapy: A randomized controlled trial. *American Journal of Psychiatry, 164,* 82–90.

Simeon, D., Knutelska, M., Yehuda, R., Putnam, F., Schmeidler, J., & Smith, L. M. (2007). Hypothalamic-pituitary-adrenal axis function in dissociative disorders, post-traumatic stress disorder and healthy volunteers. *Biological Psychiatry, 61,* 966–973.

Sinha, S. S., Goetz, R. R., & Klein, D. F. (2007). Physiological and behavioral effects of naloxone and lactate in normal volunteers with relevance to the pathophysiology of panic disorder. *Psychiatry Research, 149,* 309–314.

Stein, B. D., Jaycox, L. H., Kataoka, S. H., Wong, M., Tu, W., Elliott, M. N., & Fink, A. (2003). A mental health intervention for schoolchildren exposed to violence: A randomized controlled trial. *Journal of the American Medical Association, 290,* 603–611.

Stein, M. B., Fyer, A. J., Davidson, J. R. T., Pollack, M. H., & Wiita, B. (1999). Fluvoxamine treatment of social phobia (social anxiety disorder): A double-blind, placebo-controlled study. *American Journal of Psychiatry, 156,* 756–760.

Stein, M. B., Jang, K. L., & Livesley, W. J. (1999). Heritability of anxiety sensitivity: A twin study. *American Journal of Psychiatry, 156,* 246–251.

Stein, M. B., & Kean, Y. M. (2000). Disability and quality of life in social phobia: Epidemiologic findings. *American Journal of Psychiatry, 157,* 1606–1613.

Stein, M. B., Liebowitz, M. R., Lydiard, R. B., Pitts, C. D., Bushnell, W., & Gergel, I. (1998). Paroxetine treatment of generalized social phobia (social anxiety disorder): A randomized controlled trial. *Journal of the American Medical Association, 280,* 708–713.

Stein, M. B., Torgrud, L. J., & Walker, J. R. (2000). Social phobia symptoms, subtypes, and severity. *Archives of General Psychiatry, 57,* 1046–1052.

Stewart, S. E., Platko, J., Fagerness, J., Birns, J., Jenike, E., Smoller, J. W., et al. (2007). A genetic family-based association study of OLIG2 in obsessive-compulsive disorder. *Archives of General Psychiatry, 64,* 209–214.

Stewart, S. E., Rosario, M. C., Brown, T. A., Carter, A. S., Leckman, J. F., Sukhodolsky, D., et al. (2007). Principal components analysis of obsessive-compulsive disorder symptoms in children and adolescents. *Biological Psychiatry, 61,* 285–291.

Swedo, S. E., Leonard, H. L., Garvey, M., Mittleman, B., Allen, A. J., Perlmutter, S., et al. (1998). Pediatric autoimmune neuropsychiatric disorders associated with streptococcal infections: Clinical description of the first 50 cases. *American Journal of Psychiatry, 155,* 264–271.

Szeszko, P. R., Ardekani, B. A., Ashtari, M., Malhotra, A. K., Robinson, D. G., Bilder, R. M., et al. (2005). White matter abnormalities in obsessive-compulsive disorder: A diffusion tensor imaging study. *Archives of General Psychiatry, 62,* 782–790.

Tassone, D. M., Boyce, E., Guyer, J., & Nuzum, D. (2007). Pregabalin: A novel gamma-aminobutyric acid analogue in the treatment of neuropathic pain, partial-onset seizures, and anxiety disorders. *Journal of Clinical Therapeutics, 29,* 26–48.

Taylor, S. (1995). Anxiety sensitivity: Theoretical perspectives and recent findings. *Behavioral Research Therapy, 33,* 243–258.

Thase, M. E. (2006). Treatment of anxiety disorders with venlafaxine XR. *Expert Reviews of Neurotherapeutics, 6,* 269–282.

Thurber, C. A., Walton, E., & American Academy of Pediatrics Council on School Health. (2007). Preventing and treating homesickness. *Pediatrics, 119,* 192–201.

Torgersen, S. (1983). Genetic factors in anxiety disorders. *Archives of General Psychiatry, 40,* 1085–1089.

Turner, H. A., Finkelhor, D., & Ormrod, R. (2006). The effect of lifetime victimization on the mental health of children and adolescents. *Social Science Medicine, 62,* 13–27.

Vickers, K. & McNally, R. J. (2004). Panic disorder and suicide attempt in the National Comorbidity survey. *Journal of Abnormal Psychology, 113,* 582–591.

Weissman, M. M., Bland, R. C., Canino, G. J., Faravelli, C., Greenwald, S., Hwu, H. G., et al. (1997). The cross-national epidemiology of panic disorder. *Archives of General Psychiatry, 54,* 305–309.

Widom, C. S. (1998). Childhood victimization: Early adversity and subsequent psychopathology. In B. P. Dohrenwend (Ed.), *Adversity, stress, and psychopathology* (pp. 81–95). New York: Oxford University Press.

Widom, C. S., Dutton, M. A., Czaja, S. J., & DuMont, K. A. (2005). Development and validation of a new instrument to assess lifetime trauma and victimization history. *Journal of Traumatic Stress, 18,* 519–531.

Wolpe, J. (1961). The systematic desensitization treatment of neurosis. *Journal of Nervous and Mental Disease, 132,* 189–203.

Wolpe, J. (1973). *The practice of behavioral therapy.* New York: Pergamon Press.

Wolpe, J., & Lazarus, A. (1966). *Behavior therapy techniques: A guide to the treatment of neuroses.* London: Pergamon Press.

Yehuda, R. (2006). Advances in understanding neuroendocrine alterations in PTSD and their implications. *Annals of the New York Academy of Sciences, 1071,* 137–166.

Zohar, A. H. (1999). The epidemiology of obsessive-compulsive disorder in children and adolescents. *Child and Adolescent Psychiatric Clinics of North America, 8,* 445–460.

Zvolensky, M. J., Kotov, R., Antipova, A. V., & Schmidt, N. B. (2005). Diathesis stress model for panic-related distress: A test in a Russian epidemiological sample. *Behaviour Research and Therapy, 43,* 521–532.

Zvolensky, M. J., & Schmidt, N. B. (2007). Introduction to anxiety sensitivity: Recent findings and new directions. *Behavioral Modification, 31,* 139–144.

SUGGESTED READINGS

Bass, E., & Davis, L. (1988). *The courage to heal: A guide for women of child sexual abuse.* New York: Harper Collins.

Beck, A. T. (1976). *Cognitive therapy and the emotional disorders.* New York: International Universities Press.

Boscolo, L., Cecchin, G., Hoffman, L., & Penn, P. (1987). *Milan systematic family therapy.* New York: Basic Books.

Brackbill, R. M., Thorpe, L. E., DiGrande, L., Perrin, M., Sapp, J. H. II, et al. (2006). Surveillance for World Trade Center disaster health effects among survivors of collapsed and damaged buildings. *Surveillance Summaries.* April 7, 2006. 55 (SS02), 1–18 MMWR. Surveillance summaries: Morbidity and mortality weekly report. Surveillance summaries/CDC. http://www.cdc.gov/mmwr/preview/mmwrhtml/ss5502a1.htm

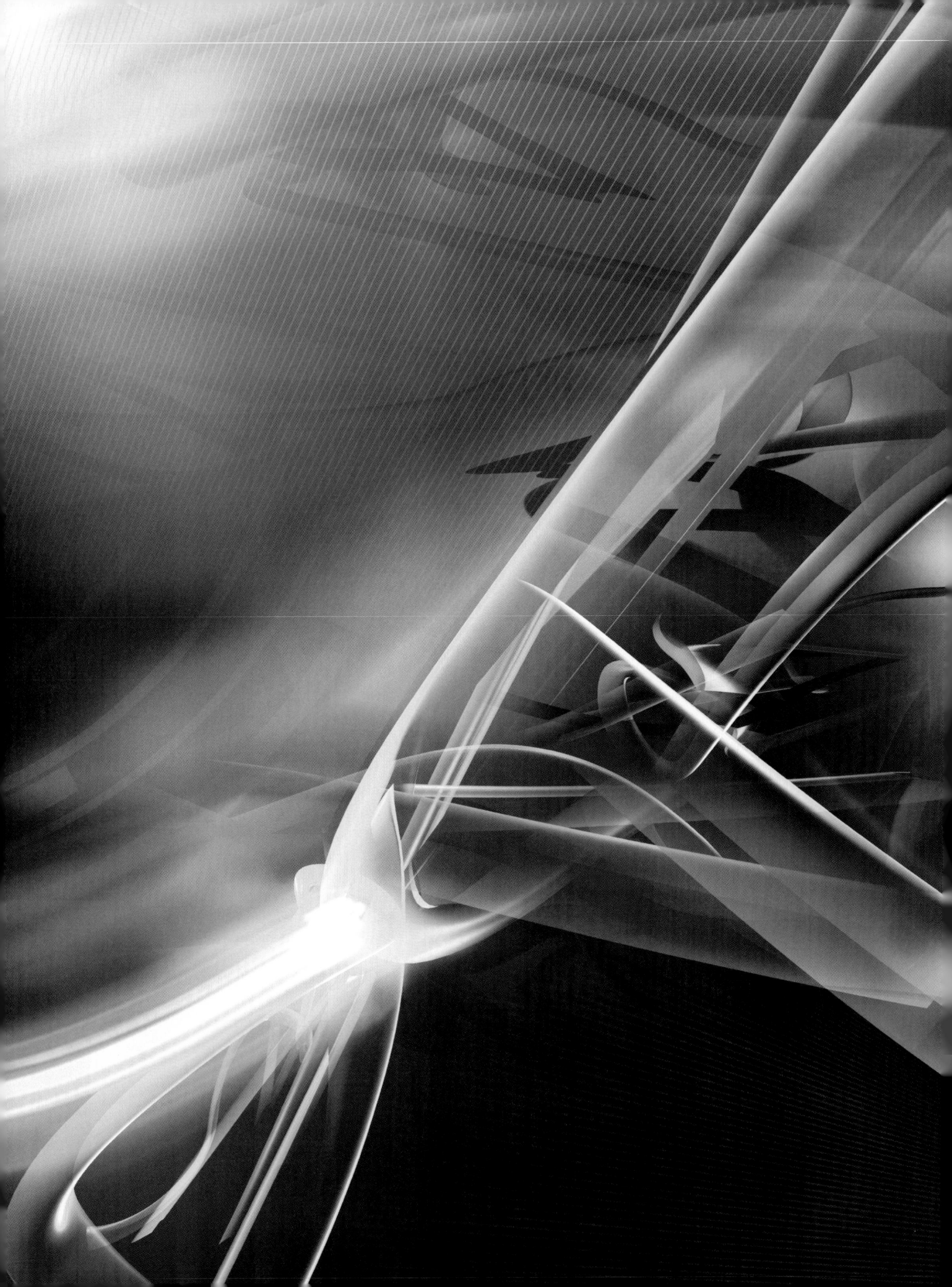

CHAPTER 12

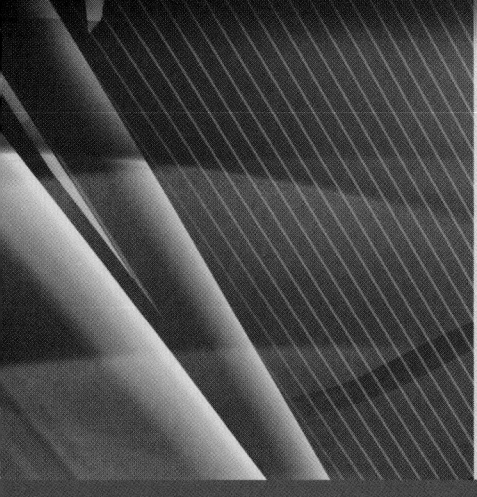

The Client with a Somatization Disorder

Deborah Antai-Otong, MS, APRN, BC, FAAN
Randy Goodwin, RN, MNSc, CS

KEY TERMS

Body Dysmorphic Disorder: A chronic and debilitating mental health condition characterized by a preoccupation with imagined defect in appearance (e.g., a "large" nose, "thinning" hair, or facial "scarring").

Chronic Fatigue Syndrome: A chronic and debilitating disorder characterized by chronic fatigue, flulike symptoms, muscle pain, headaches, and malaise lasting more than 24 hours.

Conversion Disorders: Refer to unexplained physical manifestations or deficits affecting voluntary motor or sensory function that suggest a neurological or other underlying medical condition.

Fibromyalgia Syndrome: A nonspecific condition whose primary symptoms include diffuse musculoskeletal pain, fatigue, distress, and sleep disturbances.

Hypochondriasis: Refers to persistent preoccupation with fears of having, or the idea that one has, a serious disease based on the person's misinterpretation or exaggeration of bodily functions.

Pain Disorder: Disorder whose major symptom is pain in one or more anatomical sites. It is the predominant focus of the clinical presentation and is of sufficient severity that necessitates clinical attention. It also produces significant distress that results in impaired occupational, interpersonal, and social performance.

Somatization Disorder: Refers to a disorder whose primary symptoms are progressive, recurrent, and somatic complaints of pain, sexual, gastrointestinal (GI), and pseudoneurological manifestations. These symptoms produce significant distress and global disability.

Somatoform: Refers to a group of psychiatric disorders whose symptoms are severe enough to cause global impairment or functioning. Typically, these clients present with recurring, multiple, clinically significant somatic complaints. In addition, these complaints are colorful and exaggerated, but lack specific factual information to support the diagnosis.

COMPETENCIES

Upon completion of this chapter, the learner should be able to:

1. Discuss major theories of various somatoform disorders.
2. Differentiate symptoms of somatoform disorders.
3. Analyze causative factors of somatoform disorders.
4. Describe the role of culture on somatoform disorders.
5. Analyze life span issues affecting clients experiencing a somatoform disorder.
6. Delineate major treatment approaches for clients with somatoform disorders.

CHAPTER OUTLINE

Somatoform Disorders

Epidemiology

Causative Factors: Theories and Perspectives

Psychodynamic Theories

Psychosocial and Stress Factors

Attachment Theory

Cognitive-Behavioral Theories

SOMATOFORM DISORDERS

According to the *Diagnostic and Statistical Manual of Mental Disorders* (4th edition, Text Revision) (*DSM-IV-TR*) (APA, 2000), somatoform refers to a group of psychiatric disorders whose symptoms are severe enough to cause global impairment or functioning. Typically, these clients present with recurring, multiple, clinically significant somatic complaints. In addition, these complaints are colorful and exaggerated but lack specific factual information to support the diagnosis. Specific somatoform disorders include somatization disorder, conversion disorder, hypochondriasis, body dysmorphic disorder, and pain disorder.

Despite its apparent significance and the extensive research that has been conducted over the past 20 years, somatoform remains a perplexing concept. Some researchers describe somatoform as two distinct phenomena, specifically, physical symptoms suggesting that a medical condition exists, and, second, the symptoms are not readily defined by a medical condition (American Psychiatric Association [APA], 2000; Leiknes, Finset, Moum, & Sandanger, 2007). Others submit that because of the high co-occurrence with psychiatric and medical conditions, these disorders may be part of a continuum of complex systems (Brown & Jason, 2007; Henningsen, Jakobsen, Schiltenwolf, & Weiss, 2005; Phillips, Didie, & Menard, 2007). Despite different perspectives concerning the complexity of this disorder, most concede that the primary physical symptoms are difficult to explain by underlying medical conditions.

Research indicates that these manifestations have a high prevalence in the general population and all practice settings, including primary care (Fink, Hansen, & Oxhøj, 2004; Kroenke & Rosmalen, 2006). Of particular interest in somatoform disorders is the burden it places on health care resources. The chronic and recurrent patterns of these disorders result in increased use of health care resources, increased disability, and use of days from work (Barsky, Orav, & Bates, 2005; Fink et al., 2004; Kroenke & Rosmalen, 2006). Nurses in vast practice settings are likely to care for a client with a somatoform disorder. In addition, they need to recognize symptoms of these disorders and work with other health care professionals to initiate client-centered interventions that reduce distress and chronicity and facilitate an optimal level of functioning and quality of life.

This chapter focuses on the various somatoform disorders along with major symptoms and treatment modalities. Other disorders that are not classified as somatoform disorders, but are similar in symptomatology, chronicity, and comorbid mental disorders are chronic fatigue syndrome and fibromyalgia, which will also be reviewed. It also explains the role of the nurse in assessing the onset, severity, and duration of symptoms and linking them to physiological influences. Because of the potential disabling course of these disorders, nurses need to recognize the emotional and psychological burden these clients face and work with them and other health care providers to develop client-centered interventions that facilitate adaptive coping behaviors.

EPIDEMIOLOGY

Somatization is a common phenomenon whose definition varies. The two most frequently used diagnoses, somatization disorder and abridged somatization disorder, stem from lifetime unexplained symptoms. Another term that references unexplained symptoms is multisomatoform disorder. Regardless of definition this group of psychiatric conditions are chronic and fluctuate, but rarely remit. Refractory and onset of symptoms may be related to the level of psychopathology and cultural and health beliefs (Gureje, Olley, Olusola, & Kola, 2006).

Typically, criteria occurs before age 25, although initial symptoms may occur during adolescence, such as dysmenorrhea in women. Although the prevalence of somatization disorders vary, most research demonstrates a lifetime prevalence ranging from 0.2 to 2 percent in women and less than 0.2 percent in men (APA, 2000; Rost, Dickinson, Dickinson, & Smith, 2006).

CAUSATIVE FACTORS: THEORIES AND PERSPECTIVES

The precise cause of somatoform disorders remains obscure, but many studies indicate various factors such as genetic, personality style, biological, neuroanatomical, culture, and psychosocial stressors. Many of these disorders coexist with other mental disorders, namely, anxiety and depressive disorders, and challenge nurses to address both their physical and mental conditions.

PSYCHODYNAMIC THEORIES

Evidence of somatoform disorders dates back to ancient Egyptian papyri (Shorter, 1992). Ehlers (1999) describes the *chameleonic* nature of this illness, which is difficult to determine owing to its changing expression or simply taking on characteristics of one's surroundings. It appears that throughout the history of humankind, people have had the capacity to develop symptoms or expressions almost identical to real diseases of the time (Ehlers, 1999). The psychoanalytic theory suggests that symptoms represent a substitution for repressed instinctual impulses and are best depicted by the concept of *hysteria*.

Paul Briquet (1859) first recognized the syndrome characterized by multiple dramatic medical complaints in the absence of a physiological basis. Because of his noted observations, this condition was called *Briquet's syndrome* at one time. Later this syndrome would be referred to as somatization disorder. In comparison, Freud (Breuer & Freud, 1893–1895/1955) foc-used most of his work on the concept of hysteria and postulated that the mechanism of the ego defense mechanism of conversion represented hysteria. That is, this mechanism was conceptualized as converting "psychic energy" into physical manifestations. Briquet's hysteria concept was further refined by adding a quantitative perspective by Purtell, Robins, and Cohen (1951) and further defined by Perley and Guze (1962). Eventually, major symptoms of hysteria involving varied somatic complaints were comorbid with anxiety and depressive symptoms. This particular concept was the precursor of somatization disorder in the *DSM-III* (APA, 1980). Freud and other psychoanalytic theorists used this term throughout their lives and linked it with other concepts, such as *conversion*.

Conversion stems from the premise that the person's physical manifestations depict a symbolic resolution of an unconscious psychological conflict, reducing anxiety and serving to hide the conflict from awareness. This manifestation is referred to as a primary gain. In contrast, secondary gain stems from the conversion symptom or external manifestation, and benefits involve evading negative responsibilities (APA, 2000).

Similar to other psychoanalytic theories and concepts, pain is linked to unmet childhood issues. The psychoanalytic meaning of *pain* involves fulfilling an unconscious need for guilt or masochism (Engel, 1959). Similar to other psychodynamic theories, this concept has been redefined by the *DSM* classification from hysterical conversion disorder to persistent pain disorder.

PSYCHOSOCIAL AND STRESS FACTORS

There is prevailing evidence that somatization is associated with substantial emotional distress expressing underlying anxiety, depression, and stress-related disorders (e.g., adjustment disorders). The Epidemiologic Catchment Area study, a population-based survey of more than 18,000 participants of five communities in the United States demonstrated that present psychological symptoms were found in almost 65 percent of subjects who reported five or more physical complaints, compared to 7 percent of those who denied physical complaints (Barsky, Orav, & Bates, 2005).

The literature consistently reveals that females are more likely to report ill health than males despite some controversy about the true excess prevalence or by female-specific patterns of health care utilization. The incidence of reporting physical symptoms seems even higher in women in low socioeconomic class and high emotional distress (Hiller, Rief, & Brähler, 2006; Kroenke & Rosmalen, 2006; Ladwig et al., 2001). The sick role is often accepted, validated, and reinforced within various social contexts as a coping response. Acceptance of the sick role suggests that they are more likely to frame their bodily changes as ill health. Consequently, women tend to respond more emotionally when their physical function is perceived to be or actually is impaired (Hiller et al., 2006; Kroenke & Rosmalen, 2006; Ladwig et al., 2001). Although women seem to be at a greater risk of developing these disorders, some data also indicate that social class and high emotional stress increase the risk in men (Hiller et al., 2006; Kroenke & Rosmalen, 2006; Ladwig et al., 2001).

Clearly, high emotional stress and psychosocial factors play substantial roles in other somatoform disorders. Although the findings are inconsistent, some researchers have found an increased prevalence of childhood abuse in some cases of these disorders. Co-occurring conditions associated with somatoform disorders include other somatoform disorders, depression, anxiety, and borderline personality disorders (Brown & Jason, 2007; Kroenke & Rosmalen, 2006; Phillips et al., 2005).

These findings have significant treatment implications for psychiatric nurses caring for clients with a somatization disorder. Conducting an extensive health assessment that includes identifying the client's support system, strengths, history of abuse, and duration and severity of distress caused by the disorders, enables the nurse to identify the meaning of the client's symptoms and provide interventions that reduce stress, promote self-efficacy, and improve coping skills.

ATTACHMENT THEORY

A review of the literature concerning somatization disorders indicates that these behaviors may result from complex childhood experiences of illness and the responses of the person's social system to the adult behavior (Stuart & Noyes, 2006). These researchers also submit that early life experiences serve as diatheses, governing illness behavior and resulting in maladaptive coping or personality traits. Likewise, interpersonal stressors occurring during adulthood are likely to generate somatizing behavior in high-risk groups. Based on this premise, health-seeking behavior is synonymous with attachment behavior and assists in procuring or retaining "closeness" to another person for the purpose of receiving care. Unfortunately, this adult attachment behavior (Bowlby, 1973, 1977, 1988) is reinforced each time the client receives attention and "care" for somatization symptoms, thereby gratifying their attachment needs. Maladaptive attachment behaviors tend to be fixed and rigid, often resulting in the client being more sensitive to perceived or actual threats and persistently seeking help from others (Stuart & Noyes, 2006).

When working with clients with somatization disorders it is imperative for the nurse to understand the meaning of their symptoms. Notably, physical symptoms that cannot be explained by an underlying medical condition need to be interpreted as a coping mechanism that enables the client to respond to stressors, similarly to the way anxiety and depression reflect distress. Implications for nursing care include assessing the client's needs, setting firm and consistent limits, and balancing empathy with structure. It is crucial that nurses recognize manipulative behavioral patterns and avoid reinforcing dependency. Clients with somatoform disorders tend to be tenacious and use persistent complaints of pain and physical illness to elicit care from the nurse. Because of the self-defeating nature of these behaviors, nurses may reject clients further reinforcing their somatic symptoms. Formulating nursing interventions that promote self-reliance, confidence, problem solving, and independence are crucial aspects of treatment planning. Psychotherapy and other forms of cognitive therapy and pharmacologic interventions are indicated when the nurse assesses these maladaptive coping patterns.

COGNITIVE-BEHAVIORAL THEORIES

Through complex processes the brain sorts, magnifies, or minimizes afferent and efferent stimuli throughout the body (e.g., pain and perceptual pathways, motor apparatus, and blood vessels) and from the central nervous system. Because of the intimate relationship between the brain and complex physiological processes, it is conceivable that there is dysregulation in perceptions of an event and subsequent physiological responses. Exaggerated appraisal of risk, danger, and vulnerability to disease or illness may play key roles in the cognitive distortion of somatoform disorders (e.g., hypochondriasis). Treatment implications of these cognitive distortions confirm the potential efficacy of cognitive and behavioral therapies to help clients understand and accurately appraise these risks.

NEUROBIOLOGICAL THEORIES

Studies show an array of theories concerning the neurobiological causes of somatoform disorders, ranging from genetics to neurotransmitter dysregulation in pain disorders. According to the *DSM-IV-TR* (APA, 2000), many somatoform disorders have familial patterns and show that male relatives of women with these disorders are predisposed to the risk of personality disorders and other psychiatric conditions (APA, 2000). In addition, recent functional and brain imaging studies reveal that alterations in neuroanatomical structures and decreased activity in frontal and subcortical circuits associated with motor function may accompany some disorders (Vuillemier, 2005).

Another biological theory concerns the gate theory and pain. The *gate* theory may explain the role of the dorsal horn of the spinal cord that modulates afferent pain signals. The dorsal horn represents a "gate" through which pain impulses travel from the periphery to the central nervous system. Activation of this gate results in transmission and the experience of pain. This gate is affected by impulses in the descending tracts of the brain. These collaterals may modify input into other cutaneous sensory systems, including the pain system. Neurotransmitters such as serotonin also play roles in opening and closing the gate of painful sensations. A *closed* gate decreases stimulation of trigger cells, decreases transmission impulses, and thus decreases pain perception, whereas, an *open* gate increases stimulation and transmission and intensifies pain perception. Understandably, cognitive functioning is likely to play a role in modulation of pain perception (Ganong, 2005).

During the data collection process, the psychiatric nurse needs to conduct a thorough family history of symptoms, treatment, and comorbid conditions. Assessment information is relative to understanding family coping patterns, motivation for treatment, and prior treatment outcomes.

CULTURAL CONSIDERATIONS

There is a plethora of strong empirical data concerning the substantial role of cross-culture transition and psychological distress in somatization. In addition, factors such as duration of immigration, self-reported health problems, and help-seeking behaviors appear to contribute to these disorders (Aragona et al., 2005).

Studies consistently show that immigrants worldwide experience significantly more stressful life experiences than those of the native populations and are at a higher risk of somatization (Aragona et al., 2005). These data provide a strong argument for the role of stress, social, cross-cultural, and ethnic factors in symptoms of somatization. A large international study that used 15 primary care centers in 14 countries found that the overall rate of International Classification of Diseases (ICD-10) somatization disorders was almost 3 percent, and that the overall rate, as measured by the Somatic Symptom Index (SSI), was almost 20 percent (Gureje, Simon, Ustun, & Goldberg, 1997).

Prior studies also link other factors such as gender, age, marital status, low educational and socioeconomic status, and minority ethnicity (Interian, Guarnaccia, Vega, Gara, Like, et al., 2005). There are inconsistent data concerning gender issues (Hiller, Rief, & Brähler, 2006; Phillips, Menard, & Fay, 2006).

Despite the explosion of ethnocultural studies, nurses and other health care professionals may find it difficult to accurately interpret the meaning of a client's culture-bound syndromes. For instance, some cultures, such as Southeast Asia, may consider somatic symptoms rather than depressive feelings as a legitimate basis for seeking treatment (Parker, Chan, & Eisenbruch, 2005; Parker, Chan, & Tully, 2006). Understanding the meaning of the client's somatic symptoms and identifying underlying distress enable the nurse to distinguish culture-bound symptoms from somatization. This process requires asking questions that facilitate understanding of symptoms within a social and cultural context (see Chapter 7). Recognizing the high level of distress among immigrants and the need to strengthen their social networks and coping skills and understand the meaning of their symptoms from a cultural perspective are crucial to their care. In addition, psychiatric nurses need to understand the impact of their own culture and its effect on the analysis of the client's experience. These assessment data guide the assessment process, help make an accurate diagnosis, facilitate culturally sensitive nursing interventions, and promote positive outcomes.

Although the complexity of culture-bound symptoms may be an expression of distress, there is a greater need for further research. It is necessary to strengthen the integration of culture and clinical knowledge into client-centered interventions, and embrace the universality of symptoms and culturally sensitive care. See Chapter 7 and Table 12–1, Cultural Expression of Somatization.

Unquestionably, the precise causes of somatoform disorders remain obscure. However, most data suggest an association between underlying psychological distress, neurobiological processes, and symptomatology. These considerations strengthen the argument that these disorders are an integral part of anxiety and depressive disorders continuum. Most studies suggest that treating these disorders is challenging and requires a diverse treatment approach that involves the following principles once the diagnosis is confirmed:

1. Establish a firm and therapeutic relationship with the client and family.
2. Differentiate manipulative and other maladaptive behaviors from cultural factors.
3. Provide health education concerning major symptoms (e.g., inform clients that they are not going "crazy," prognosis, treatment outcomes).
4. Be firm and consistent and provide reassurance.
5. When indicated, treat anxiety and depressive symptoms.

SPECIFIC SOMATOFORM DISORDERS

An overview of specific somatoform disorders ranging from somatization disorder to chronic fatigue provides a broad perspective of these complex disorders. In addition, each disorder delineates various treatment options and the role of psychiatric nurses in facilitating the highest level of function and quality of life.

SOMATIZATION DISORDER

Somatization disorder often perplexes nurses and clients seeking help for unexplainable symptoms. The enigma of this disorder continues to challenge psychiatric nurses to assess core symptoms and initiate holistic treatment that promotes mental and physical health.

Prevalence

Somatization disorder, previously referred to as *Briquet's syndrome* or *hysteria*, is a multiple symptomatic disorder that occurs before age 30 and progresses over the years. Primary symptoms of this disorder are progressive, recurrent, and somatic complaints of pain, sexual, gastrointestinal (GI), and pseudoneurological manifestations (APA, 2000). Somatization rarely remits completely. Earlier onset often occurs during adolescence and may initially manifest as menstrual difficulties. The prevalence of this disorder ranges from 0.2 to 2.0 percent among women and 0.2 percent in men. These clients often grow up in families who are inconsistent, unreliable, and provide little or no emotional support. Recent studies of primary care clients show that the prevalence may be as high as 30 to 60 percent of symptoms

TABLE 12–1
Cultural Expression of Somatization

Culture	Symptoms
West African	*koro*. A culture-bound syndrome, also found in Southeast Asian settings, involving fears of genital retraction as a response to the presence of emotional distress.
Japan	*Work stress*. Has developed over the past decade due to the perceived loss of support from management in Japan's work environment. It is commonly seen in young Japanese employees and is manifested by symptoms of general malaise, nausea, constipation, diarrhea, headache, stiff shoulder, and dizziness.
Cambodia/U.S.	*koucharang*. A culture-bound syndrome found among Cambodian (Khmer) refugees now living in the United States who experienced both physical and emotional trauma secondary to the Khmer Rouge holocaust. It is described as "thinking too much" which is characterized by behavioral changes and somatic complaints. It can become a very disabling condition among this population if not addressed and treated.
India	*Sinking heart*. A syndrome of heart distress found by a sect of Indians from Punjab State. It is an illness in which physical sensations in the heart or chest are experienced and thought to be caused by excessive heat, exhaustion, worry, and/or social failure.

Sources. Dzoko V. A., Adams, G. (2005). Understanding genital-shrinking epidemics in West Africa: Koro, juju, or mass psychogenic illness? *Journal of Cultural Medicine Psychiatry,* Mar;29(1):53–78; Frye, B. A., D'Avanzo, C. (1994). Themes in managing culturally defined illness in the Cambodian refugee family. *Journal of Community Health Nursing,* 11(2):89–98; Krause, I. B. (1989). Sinking heart: A Punjabi communication of distress. *Journal of Social Science Medicine,* 29(4):563–575; Shimla, S., Satoh, E. (2006). Somatoform disorders in the workplace in Japan. *International Review Psychiatry,* Feb;18(1):35–40.

that have no medical basis. Because of the high incidence of co-occurring with other psychiatric disorders, such as anxiety, depression, and personality disorders, some researchers believe that somatization disorders may manifest personality pathology with traits of histrionic, borderline, and antisocial personality disorders (Stuart & Noyes, 2006).

Core Symptoms

Typically, these clients are vague historians, but their presentations are often dramatic and they report detailed and complicated medical problems. They are tenacious in seeking medical attention and are likely to be seeing more than one health provider at a time. Their histories also reveal chaos, impulsiveness, manipulative behaviors, suicidal threats or attempts, unstable occupational and social functioning, and turbulent interpersonal relationships (Stuart & Noyes, 2006). Predictably, these clients are difficult to manage in most practice settings and many clinicians find them difficult to engage in a therapeutic relationship. A major challenge for psychiatric nurses involves patience, empathy, and firm limit setting. Setting limits offers structure and facilitates a supportive environment that fosters a therapeutic nurse-client relationship. See Chapter 15 and Table 12–2, Diagnostic Criteria for Somatization Disorder.

Treatment Modalities

The nurse-client relationship is the cornerstone of managing the care of the client with a somatization disorder. It is very important to understand that the client with this disorder may actually suffer emotionally because of their unyielding belief that they will not be cared for (Stuart & Noyes, 2006). Although there is no physical basis for these concerns, the thoughts of being ill and needing help often result in debilitating depression or anxiety, which need to be treated accordingly (e.g., antidepressants, psychotherapy). Working with the client with somatization disorder challenges the nurse to conduct thorough physical and mental status examinations that assist in making a differential diagnosis of a medical condition or comorbid mental disorder or factitious disorder. Primary symptoms of a *factitious disorder* involve feigning or deliberately injecting a disease on oneself, and the client usually has a severe personality disorder (APA, 2000). Major components of the assessment include history, severity and duration of symptoms; level of functioning; present stressors; coping patterns. The nurse needs to avoid confrontations, and provided instructions must be clear, direct, and respond to crises empathetically. Keep visits for medical complaints brief and assist the client in understanding the symptoms as emotional communication rather than an underlying medical condition. This process generally involves an interdisciplinary approach that facilitates a holistic and client-centered treatment plan.

An important part of the assessment process is the client's illness perception. Danish researchers Fink, Rosendal, and Toft (2002) developed a comprehensive treatment and assessment

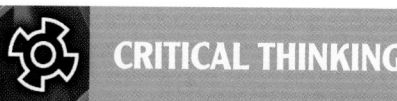

CRITICAL THINKING

Somatization Disorder

Ms. K is a 34-year-old mother of 2 children ages 2 and 4. During her visit to the primary care clinic, she reports vague physical complaints involving her back, headaches, and fatigue. During the nursing assessment she reveals that she works part time as a registered nurse and spends most of her days off taking care of her children and sleeping a lot. She also admits that she is a poor housekeeper and rarely prepares meals until late in the evening despite being home all day. Based on your assessment, what is the most appropriate nursing intervention?

1. Ask if she has a history of psychiatric treatment.

2. Express concerns that she needs to take care of her kids and husband.

3. Ask how her symptoms are interfering with her daily activities.

4. Refer her to a mental health professional.

Answers

1. *Incorrect.* This statement infers that her symptoms are not real and must be "in her head."

2. *Incorrect.* This is a value-laden or judgmental response that will probably engender and anger the client.

3. *Correct.* This question helps the client link her symptoms to everyday life.

4. *Incorrect.* Similar to #1 this implies that she has a psychiatric problem and there is little evidence that supports this assumption.

TABLE 12–2
Diagnostic Criteria for Somatization Disorder

A. A history of many physical complaints beginning before age 30 years that occur over a period of several years and result in treatment being sought or significant impairment in social, occupational, or other important areas of functioning.

B. Each of the following criteria must have been met, with individual symptoms occurring at any time during the course of the disturbance:

- Four pain symptoms: a history of pain related to at least four different sites or functions (e.g., head, abdomen, back, joints, extremities, chest, rectum, during menstruation, during sexual intercourse, or during urination)

- Two gastrointestinal symptoms: a history of at least two gastrointestinal symptoms other than pain (e.g., nausea, bloating, vomiting other than during pregnancy, diarrhea, or intolerance of several foods)

- One sexual symptom: a history of at least one sexual or reproductive symptom other than pain (e.g., sexual indifference, erectile or ejaculatory dysfunction, irregular menses, excessive menstrual bleeding, vomiting through pregnancy)

- One pseudoneurological symptom: a history of at least one symptom or deficit suggesting a neurological condition not limited to pain (conversion symptoms such as impaired coordination or balance, paralysis or localized weakness, difficulty swallowing or lump in the throat, aphonia, urinary retention, hallucinations, loss of touch or pain sensation, double vision, blindness, deafness, seizures, dissociative symptoms such as amnesia, or loss of consciousness other than fainting)

Either (1) or (2):

1. after appropriate investigation, each of the symptoms in Criterion B cannot be fully explained by a known general medical condition or the direct effects of a substance (e.g., a drug of abuse, a medication)

2. when there is a related general medical condition, the physical complaints or resulting social or occupational impairment are in excess of what would be expected from the history, physical examination, or laboratory findings

The symptoms are not intentionally feigned or produced (as in factitious disorder or malingering).

Note. From *Diagnostic and Statistical Manual of Mental Disorders* (4th edition, Text Revision) *(DSM-IV-TR)*, by the American Psychiatric Association, 2000, Washington, DC: Author. Adapted with permission.

approach of functional (somatic) disorders and suggested the following questions for understanding the client's illness perception:

- ◆ Identify the illness: What does the client think is wrong?
- ◆ Cause: What does the client believe is the basis of her symptoms—physical or psychosocial?
- ◆ Duration: How long does the client believe present symptoms will last—acute or chronic?
- ◆ Consequences: What effects will the symptoms have on the client's ability to function?
- ◆ Recovery and self-efficacy: What are the client's prospects of recovering and what types of treatment are available? What kind of control does the client have over the illness, or how much control does the client have over present symptoms?

Assessing the client's illness perception offers crucial data that nurses can use to direct treatment and individual health teaching.

Major mental health treatment needs to focus on a supportive clinical environment and measures that facilitate adaptive coping behaviors. Research demonstrates that several approaches using the cognitive-behavioral model, including dialectical therapy, are showing promising results in the treatment of somatization disorders (Stulemeijer, de Jong, Fiselier, Hoogveld, & Bleijenberg 2005). Group therapy is also helpful in assisting the client in developing adaptive coping skills. This is a cost-effective approach that offers support and opportunity to form healthier interpersonal skills. See Chapters 26 and 28.

CONVERSION DISORDER

Conversion disorder, like other somatoform disorders, challenges psychiatric nurses to understand the underpinnings of this disorder and develop treatment strategies that promote an optimal level of health. In addition, clients with this disorder require nursing interventions that reflect empathy, understanding, and a nonjudgmental approach that enables them to develop adaptive coping behaviors that facilitate a good quality of life.

Prevalence

Conversion disorders refer to unexplained physical manifestations or deficits affecting voluntary motor or sensory function that suggest a neurological or other underlying medical condition. Psychological factors govern symptoms and deficits. Most researchers assert that these disorders also involve a secondary gain or take on a "sick role" (APA, 2000). These disorders are the most frequently occurring of the somatoform disorders. Affected persons can range in age from early childhood into old age. Reported rates of conversion disorder range from 11 in 100,000 to 500 in 100,000 in general population samples and up to 3 percent of outpatient referrals to mental health services (APA, 2000). Like other somataform disorders, conversion

---

TABLE 12–3
Diagnostic Criteria for Conversion Disorders

A. One or more symptoms or deficits affect voluntary motor sensory function that suggest a neurological or other underlying medical condition.

B. Psychological factors are deemed to be associated with the symptom or deficit because the initiation or exacerbation of the symptom or deficit is preceded by conflicts or other stressors.

C. The symptom or deficit is not intentionally produced or feigned (as in factitious disorder or malingering).

D. The symptom or deficit cannot, after appropriate investigation, be fully explained by an underlying general medical condition, or by direct effects of a substance, or as a culturally sanctioned behavior or experience.

E. The symptom or deficit causes clinically significant distress or impairment in social, occupational, or other important areas of functioning or warrants medical evaluation.

F. The symptom or deficit is not limited to pain or sexual function, does not occur exclusively during the course of somatization disorder, and is not better accounted for by another mental disorder.

Specify type or deficit:

   With motor symptom or deficit

   With sensory symptom or deficit

   With seizures or convulsions

   With mixed presentation

Note. From *Diagnostic and Statistical Manual of Mental Disorders* (4th edition, Text Revision) *(DSM-IV-TR)*, by the American Psychiatric Association, 2000, Washington, DC: Author. Adapted with permission.

---

disorders tend to exist with other concomitant medical and mental conditions such as anxiety, depressive, personality, and other somatoform disorders.

Core Symptoms

According to the *DSM-IV-TR* (APA, 2000), the criteria shown in Table 12–3 are necessary for a diagnosis of conversion disorders.

Treatment Modalities

Most conversion symptoms abate spontaneously or respond to cognitive-behavioral and supportive therapy. Major treatment must avoid reinforcing maladaptive behaviors and focus on helping the client develop effective stress management and coping behaviors. If co-occurring conditions, such as anxiety or depression, exist, they need to be treated accordingly with pharmacologic or nonpharmacologic approaches.

PAIN DISORDER

Pain has become the fifth vital sign and offers clients with a pain disorder opportunities for their holistic needs to be assessed by the psychiatric nurse. Efforts to understand the meaning of pain disorder are crucial to the client's mental and physical well-being.

Prevalence

The hallmark of pain disorder is pain of sufficient severity that warrants clinical attention. The association between depression and medically unexplained pain is well documented (Dickens, Jayson, & Creed, 2002; Gupta et al., 2007; Robinson et al., 2005). These data demonstrate that the prevalence of depression ranges from 18 to 31 percent in sample populations. Dickens and colleagues' (2002) findings were inconsistent with other data, namely, concerning excessive pain behavior, which did not indicate underlying anxiety or depression. Regardless of co-occurrence with depression or anxiety, pain produces significant distress and disability in functioning. Annual estimates in the United States show that 10 to 15 percent of adults experience some form of occupational disability owing to back pain.

Core Symptoms

According to the *DSM-IV-TR* (APA, 2000), pain disorder is divided into acute and chronic categories. Table 12–4 lists major criteria of pain disorder.

FIBROMYALGIA SYNDROME

Until recently, fibromyalgia was poorly understood and inappropriately treated. The plethora of research demonstrates the complexity of this disorder and the need for psychiatric nurses to understand the effects it has on the client's functional status and quality of life.

Prevalence

Although fibromyalgia syndrome (FMS) is not considered a somatoform disorder, it is a common and complex musculoskeletal pain disorder whose features are similar to various somatoform disorders, including coexisting and depressive

TABLE 12–4
Diagnostic Criteria for Pain Disorder

A. Pain in one or more anatomical sites is the predominant focus of the clinical presentation and is of sufficient severity that necessitates clinical attention.

B. The pain causes clinically substantial distress or impairment in social, occupational, or important areas of interest.

C. Psychological factors are judged to play an important role in the onset, severity, exacerbation, or maintenance of the pain.

D. The symptom or deficit is not intentionally produced or feigned (as in factitious disorder or malingering).

E. The pain is not better accounted for by a mood, anxiety, or psychotic disorder and does not meet the criteria for dyspareunia.

Specify as:

    Acute: duration of less than 6 months

    Chronic: duration of 6 months or longer

Note. From *Diagnostic and Statistical Manual of Mental Disorders* (4th edition, Text Revision) *(DSM-IV-TR),* by the American Psychiatric Association, 2000, Washington, DC: Author. Adapted with permission.

features. Women are affected more than men, but this syndrome can occur in individuals across the life span. Estimates reveal a prevalence of 2 percent of the general population, but higher incidence has been reported (APA, 2000). These numbers equate to between 3 million and 6 million people in the United States, mainly women in early to middle adulthood.

Depressed states are considered universal among these clients. The exact cause of this pain disorder is unknown; however, the literature indicates that biological, psychosocial, and social factors may predispose, precipitate, and maintain symptoms (Goldstein, et al., 2004). Some clients with fibromyalgia report histories of varied forms of abuse, further strengthening the argument concerning the role of psychosocial factors and stress in this disorder (Ciccone, Elliott, Chandler, Nayak, & Raphael, 2005). Major symptoms include widespread pain and muscle tenderness usually accompanied by sleep disturbances, depression, and fatigue. The lifetime prevalence of fibromyalgia is about 2 percent in community samples, and it occurs twice as often as rheumatoid arthritis, constituting a major health problem.

Core Symptoms

Hallmark symptoms of fibromyalgia include diffuse chronic pain, muscle stiffness and tenderness, sleep disturbances, and profound fatigue. Clients often complain of "aching all over," but common sites involve the neck, shoulders, back, hips, arms, and legs.

Treatment Modalities

In 2007 the FDA approved Lyrica (pregabalin), a GABA agonist—a drug previously used to treat partial seizures and pain syndromes. This is the first FDA-approved drug to treat fibromyalgia. This medication reduces pain, improves sleep, reduces fatigue, and promotes functional status. Like other somatoform disorders, treatment planning should focus on an interdisciplinary and holistic approach. Pharmacologic interventions using tricyclic agents and other antidepressants (e.g., fluoxetine [Prozac], doxepin [Sinequan], nortriptyline [Pamelor]) (Arnold et al., 2004; Antai-Otong, 2005) offer some relief from widespread pain and depression. Other nursing interventions include stress management, meditation and yoga, and sleep manipulation. Assessing the client's risk of danger to self and others is also an integral part of treatment. See Chapter 20.

HYPOCHONDRIASIS

Probably one of the most perplexing somatoform disorders is hypochondriasis. Psychiatric nurses must be able to work with other health providers and discern medical conditions from hypochondriasis and offer an accepting environment that enables the client and family to understand this disorder and formulate a treatment plan that fosters adaptive coping behaviors.

 CRITICAL THINKING

Mr. M is a 40-year-old client who presents in the primary care clinic seeking help with chronic skin problems. While in the waiting area you notice that he gets up a lot and frequently looks in the mirror and frowns. His skin lesions indicate excessive picking. He reports marital discord and problems holding a job the past few years due to concerns about his appearance, specifically he feels his nose is crooked and his hair is too thin. As you are taking his vital signs he asks, "I look awful, don't I?" What is the most appropriate response?

1. "We are concerned about you and have made a referral to the mental health clinic."

2. "This is your third visit to the office in as many weeks. What is going on?"

3. "You sound pretty upset. How have you dealt with your concerns in the past?"

4. "Why are you making negative remarks about yourself?"

Answers

1. *Incorrect.* The nurse must avoid inferring that the client's feelings and thoughts about himself are "all in his head." Clients with somatoform disorders truly do suffer and feel distressed.

2. *Incorrect.* Although the nurse displays empathy toward the client's distress along with some limit-setting, there is also inference that there is something wrong with him due to frequent visits.

3. *Correct.* This response depicts empathy and concern along with a willingness to understand and assess his distress. The inquiry about how he has "dealt" with these concerns in the past helps the nurse assess his current and past coping skills. Furthermore this data enables the nurse and treatment team to improve coping and function rather than eradicate the symptom.

4. *Incorrect.* This response, similar to #1 and #2 minimizes the client's symptoms and conveys a lack of empathy.

Prevalence

The prevalence of hypochondriasis in the general population is 1 to 5 percent. Among primary care populations, the estimates may range from 2 to 7 percent. Like other somatoform disorders, the onset of this disorder could begin at any age, but it is more likely to occur during early adulthood. It is chronic and has a waxing and waning course.

Core Symptoms

Clients with hypochondriasis often focus on their fears of having, or the notion that they have a serious disease owing to an exaggerated appraisal of risk or vulnerability to disease. Oftentimes, these clients sense imminent peril and vulnerability to disease. This sense of heightened physical risk is focused and limited to having a disease or disease-related fears. In addition, the client's history reveals a

TABLE 12–5
Diagnostic Criteria for Hypochondriasis

A. Preoccupation with fears of having, or the idea that one has, a serious disease based on the person's misinterpretation or exaggeration of bodily functions.

B. The preoccupation persists despite appropriate medical evaluation and reassurance.

C. The belief in Criterion A is not of a delusional nature (as in delusional disorder, somatic type) and is not restricted to a circumscribed concern about appearance (as in body dysmorphic disorder).

D. The preoccupation causes clinically significant distress or impairment in social, occupational, or other important areas of functioning.

E. The duration of the disturbance is at least 6 months.

F. Generalized anxiety disorder, obsessive-compulsive disorder, does not better account for the preoccupation disorder, panic disorder, a major depressive episode, separation anxiety, or another somatoform disorder.

Specify if:

With Poor Insight

Note. From *Diagnostic and Statistical Manual of Mental Disorders* (4th edition, Text Revision) *(DSM-IV-TR),* by the American Psychiatric Association, 2000, Washington, DC: Author. Adapted with permission.

CLIENT TEACHING

Hypochondriasis

Hypochondriasis is a psychiatric disorder that affects the lives of millions of people. A major symptom of hypochondriasis involves believing that one has a serious disease and experiencing varying levels of fear and anxiety.

Major symptoms include:

- Misinterpretation of physical sensations as though they represent serious illness

- These symptoms and associated anxiety are real to the client who is not faking

- Sensations often focus on physical sensations and intense anxiety

What should you do?

- Believe the client's experience (e.g., sweating, racing heart, stomach distress, and dizziness)

- Provide reassurance that these symptoms do not indicate a serious illness

- Understand that their condition does not warrant or normally respond to medical interventions

- Recognize that if these symptoms persist they often result in chronic physical disabilities

Treatment of hypochondriasis often involves:

- Working with the primary care provider to discern indications for medical interventions

- Mental health treatment is helpful in dealing with the client's continuous focus on serious medical conditions. A specific approach involves helping the client understand the basis of feelings/fears and related anxiety

- If the client has other psychiatric disorders, such as major depression or anxiety disorders, treatment may involve medications to eliminate symptoms and/or psychotherapy to improve coping skills and behaviors

---

misinterpretation of benign bodily sensations that are mistakenly associated with a suspected and dreaded illness, health hazard, and physical preoccupation. See Table 12–5 for the *DSM-IV-TR* (APA, 2000) diagnostic criteria for hypochondriasis. (See Client and Family Health Teaching.)

Treatment Modalities

Mental health professionals can help clients with hypochondriasis if they are encouraged to seek help. Various psychotherapies, such as cognitive-behavioral therapy can be useful. This treatment approach helps the client understand distorted or problematic thought patterns, beliefs about self and illness, and related emotional distress. When working with these clients the nurse needs to understand the chronicity of this disorder and its potentially disabling course. It is crucial for the nurse and other health care providers to conduct comprehensive mental and physical status examinations to rule out true physical illnesses. Because of their use of health care resources with little resolution, clients with hypochondriasis are likely to express frustration and discouragement about their symptoms. Nurses need to approach these clients with an accepting and nonjudgmental attitude, but should avoid reinforcing preoccupation with bodily functions and illness.

BODY DYSMORPHIC DISORDER

Body dysmorphic disorder, similar to other somatoform disorders, is gaining more attention and better treatment. Because of the high coexistence with other psychiatric disorders, psychiatric nurses must identify core symptoms associated with this disorder and collaborate with the client, family, and mental health team to develop holistic interventions.

Prevalence

Body dysmorphic disorder (BDD) is a chronic and debilitating mental health condition characterized by a preoccupation with imagined defect in appearance (e.g., a "large" nose, "thinning" hair, or facial "scarring") (APA, 2000; Phillips, 2006; Rief, Buhlmann, Wilhelm, Borkenhagen, & Brähler, 2006). It often results in social isolation, unnecessary medical procedures, and occupational and interpersonal impairments. The precise prevalence of BDD in the community remains obscure. In clinical settings, comorbid anxiety and depression occur in 5 to 40 percent of clients with BDD. Normally, this somatoform disorder emerges during adolescence but some believe it can occur during childhood (APA, 2000). A population-based study of BDD showed that it is significantly associated with co-occurring major depression and anxiety disorder. The highest co-occurring anxiety disorders include social phobia and obsessive-compulsive disorder (OCD). These data also demonstrate its overall prevalence of about 0.7 percent in women (Otto, Wilhelm, Cohen, & Harlow, 2001). Phillips and colleagues found a 13.8 percent lifetime history of BDD highest in clients with OCD (Phillips, 2006; Rief et al., 2006). Because of the high co-occurrence with OCD, this disorder has been added to the OCD spectrum. Findings from these studies demonstrate a high co-occurring of anxiety disorders in clients with BDD. A note of interest when dealing with clients with BDD is that a small percentage of them has a history of corrective surgeries ranging from plastic to dermatology (Phillips, 2006; Rief et al., 2006).

Core Symptoms

Chief symptoms of BDD have been previously discussed. Recent studies also show that people with BDD have some cognitive and memory deficits demonstrated by poor performance on neuropsychological tests (Phillips, 2006). Specific deficits seem to indicate poor performance on executive tasks such as learning, long- and short-term memory recall, and organization of verbal and nonverbal memory. These findings are similar to those in individuals with OCD and indicate a neurobiological basis for both disorders (Phillips, 2006). Clinical symptoms that reflect these deficits may include preoccupations that result in

obsessional thinking and compulsive behaviors and avoidance of various tasks, including work, school, and social interactions. See Table 12–6 for the *DSM-IV-TR* criteria for body dysmorphic disorder (APA, 2000).

Treatment Modalities

Currently, there is no mainstay treatment or best practice model for BDD. However, there are promising results from pharmacologic interventions such as the serotonin selective reuptake inhibitors (SSRIs). Clients with BDD seem to require higher doses that are useful in the treatment of BDD with comorbid OCD and depressive symptoms. A partial response of these agents with adjunct buspirone (BuSpar) offer improved treatment. Other studies indicate the efficacy of clomipramine (Anafranil), a tricyclic with potent serotonin properties. Clomipramine is also indicated in the treatment of OCD. A combination of an SSRI medication and cognitive-behavioral therapy, to reframe negative thoughts and maladaptive behaviors, have also demonstrated symptom reduction (Phillips, Pagano, & Menard, 2006).

Although the client with BDD presents a challenging clinical picture, psychiatric nurses need to use an empathic and sensitive approach and assess their preoccupations with personal appearance and resulting emotional distress. Areas of particular interest during the assessment and treatment planning include determining the level of global impairment owing to their preoccupations and excessive time spent worrying about their appearance.

CHRONIC FATIGUE SYNDROME

The complexity of chronic fatigue syndrome and similarities to somatoform disorders explains its relevance to this chapter. There is growing evidence that many clients presenting with this disorder require unique interventions that enable them to manage their fatigue and enhance their functional status.

TABLE 12–6
Diagnostic Criteria for Body Dysmorphic Disorder

A. Preoccupation with an imagined defect in appearance. If a slight anomaly is present, the person's concerns are even greater.

B. The preoccupation causes marked significant distress or impairment in social, occupational, or other important areas of functioning.

C. The preoccupation is not better accounted for by another mental disorder such as dissatisfaction with body shape and size as in anorexia nervosa.

Note. From *Diagnostic and Statistical Manual of Mental Disorders* (4th edition, Text Revision) (*DSM-IV-TR*), by the American Psychiatric Association, 2000, Washington, DC: Author. Adapted with permission.

Prevalence

Although chronic fatigue syndrome (CFS) is not listed as a somatoform disorder, its clinical symptoms are similar to these disorders. The prevalence of CFS remains obscure because of the continued controversy concerning whether it is a mental disorder or a somatic one with psychological components.

Chronic fatigue syndrome (CFS), like fibromyalgia, makes up a number of poorly understood symptoms that challenge nurses and other health clinicians. CFS can affect practically every major system in the body (Sadock & Sadock, 2005). Recent studies indicate hypocapnia as a biological marker for orthostatic intolerance in some clients with chronic fatigue disorder (Natelson, Intriligator, Cherniack, Chandler, & Stewart, 2007). Most clients are not cured, and the majority experience progressive decrease in exercise tolerance. Some symptoms are exacerbated by stress. Studies show that only 10 percent of these clients return to a previous level of functioning and about 10 to 20 percent have actually worsened (Brown & Jason, 2007). Researchers submit that the vagueness of these symptoms may be variants of other somatoform disorders although they do not necessarily share the same maladaptive processes (Brown & Jason, 2007; Henningsen et al., 2005; Phillips et al., 2007).

Causative factors of chronic fatigue disorder stem from the initial premise that it was a form of chronic Epstein-Barr virus (EBV) infections. This theory was dismissed after researchers found high EBV titers in healthy people. To date, there is a lack of strong evidence that links CFS with an infectious process (Natelson, Weaver, Tseng, Ottenweller, 2005). Several researchers surmise that acute infection may activate dysregulation in the immune system, whereas others suggest dysregulation in neuroendocrine processes (Robertson et al., 2005). In addition to a biological basis to this mysterious illness, some assert that CFS is a form of somatization disorder caused by multiple complaints of emotional and physical distress. A link between psychosocial stress and cognitive disturbances has also been suggested (Brown & Jason, 2007). Regardless of the cause of CFS, major symptoms include chronic fatigue, flulike symptoms, muscle pain, headaches, and malaise lasting more than 24 hours.

The 2006 Centers for Disease Control and Prevention (CDC) criteria for CFS include:

A. Severe unexplained fatigue for more than 6 months that is:

- a new onset or definite onset
- not due to postexertion
- not resolved by rest
- functionally impairing

B. The presence of four or more of the following new symptoms:

- sore throat
- impaired memory or concentration
- tender lymph nodes
- muscle pain
- pain in several joints
- new onset of headaches
- unrestful sleep
- postexertional malaise lasting more than 24 hours

Diagnosis of CFS can only be made after medical and psychiatric conditions that cause chronic fatigues have been ruled out (CDC, 2006).

Core Symptoms

Clinical symptoms of BDD include subjective feelings of ugliness or preoccupation with physical flaws or imperfection. Skin is the most common area of concern. Common psychiatric conditions that occur with BDD include avoidant or obsessive-compulsive behaviors and disorders and depression. Suicidal behaviors are common in these clients (Phillips, 2006; Sadock & Sadock, 2005).

Treatment Modalities

The prognosis of CFS is discouraging because most clients have chronic and debilitating symptoms over time. However, owing to the complexity of CFS and poor prognosis, an interdisciplinary approach is necessary to address the clients' holistic physical, emotional, and psychosocial needs. Nurses play key roles in assessing the level of emotional distress, occupational and interpersonal impairment, and quality of life. Providing opportunities to succeed and encouraging clients to participate in stress management and relaxation activities foster a sense of control and promote comfort. Because these clients often have coexisting mental conditions, they need to be assessed for anxiety and depressive symptoms throughout treatment. The clients' occupational or academic performance and social interactions are likely to be further affected by depression and anxiety disorders and require a thorough assessment. Cognitive-behavioral therapies and pharmacologic interventions may provide some relief to some clients, but not necessarily relieve pain. These approaches reduce cognitive distortions arising from unfounded fears and concerns and comorbid mental conditions (Phillips, 2006; Rief et al., 2006).

SOMATOFORM DISORDERS ACROSS THE LIFE SPAN

Understanding the evolution of somatoform disorders over the life span is intriguing. Psychiatric nurses are in pivotal positions to identify high risk groups in childhood and adolescence and work with clients, families, and health care providers to formulate and implement holistic treatment planning.

CHILDHOOD

Impaired family dynamics contribute to childhood somatoform disorders, primarily somatization and conversion disorders.

Common family dynamics include overresponsiveness, limited autonomy, rigidity, overprotectiveness, and rejection. Some of these parents have somatoform disorders themselves and other mental disorders, including depression, anxiety, and self-destructive behaviors (Steinhausen & Winkler-Metzke, 2007). Children presenting with high levels of medical complaints that are difficult to explain should alert the nurse to assess for depressive and anxiety symptoms. Researchers assert that medically unexplainable symptoms appear to be related to prior experience of illness in the family and previously unexplained symptoms during childhood. This may depict a learned behavior during childhood in which the "sick role" or illness experience results in symptom or bodily sensation monitoring. Childhood somatization disorders reflect a family problem and may coexist with a mood or anxiety disorder. It is imperative for the nurse to assess the role of the child's symptoms in the family and cultural factors. The complexity of childhood- and family-related issues concerning somatization require family and other psychotherapies to address these issues. Health education is also an integral part of working with children and their families, and focusing on communication patterns and dysfunctional interactions may reduce tension and family stress. See Chapter 28.

ADOLESCENCE

Some somatization disorders, such as pain and conversion disorder, may occur at any age. However, BDD usually emerges during adolescence, although it can also begin earlier. Despite the onset during childhood or adolescence, symptoms are not readily observed during this developmental stage (APA, 2000). The high prevalence of co-occurring anxiety and depressive disorders requires nurses to assess for these symptoms and formulate interventions that manage specific symptoms. See Research Abstract.

ADULTHOOD

Adulthood somatoform behaviors have been discussed previously in this chapter. Important nursing implications associated with this age group are the same as other groups, including assessing the clients' holistic needs and working with an interdisciplinary team to address their mental and physical conditions.

OLDER ADULTHOOD

The chronic and often unremitting course of somatization disorder is likely to affect the adult and older adult throughout their life span. Treatment considerations include client-centered and age-specific interventions. Many problems relating to somatoform disorders have their bases for development during childhood. The client's level of functioning and quality of life are bound to be impaired after years of these debilitating disorders. Efforts to assess the client's needs and preference and encouraging an optimal level of functioning are major treatment foci for the older adult.

RESEARCH ABSTRACT

Continuity of Functional-Somatic Symptoms from Late Childhood to Young Adulthood in a Community Sample

Steinhausen, H. C., & Winkler-Metzke, C. (2007). *Journal of Child Psychology and Psychiatry, 48,* 508–513.

Study Problem/Purpose

The purpose of this study was to determine the longitudinal course of function-somatic symptoms across the life span from childhood to young adulthood and associations of these symptoms with young adulthood maladaptation.

Methods

Researchers collected data from a large community sample during three data points (1994, 1997, and 2001). The Youth Self-Report (YSR) or Young Adult Self-Report (YASR) was used to evaluate functional-somatic symptoms across this time period.

Findings

Definite functional-somatic symptoms across time were between 1.0 and 2.6 percent for dizziness, 3.0 and 6.7 percent for overtiredness, 1.0 and 2.9 percent for aches and pains, 5.6 and 8.3 percent for headaches, 1.2 and 1.9 percent for nausea, 2.5 and 3.0 percent for stomachache, and 0.2 and 0.8 percent for vomiting. Overall, females were more symptomatic at various times with a greater risk of persistent functional-somatic symptoms across time. Functional-somatic symptoms in childhood and adolescents can be easily assessed in the community. Individuals with high scores were more likely to have persistent behaviors across the life span.

Implications for Psychiatric Nurses

Psychiatric nurses are in key positions to identify children at risk for adulthood somatization disorders. Health education is a critical aspect of primary prevention for children who exhibit early signs of somatization disorders and their parents.

THE ROLE OF THE NURSE

The role of the psychiatric nurse in caring for the client with a somatoform disorder is challenging and requires patience, understanding, and reassurance. It also involves exploring and initiating holistic and culturally sensitive interventions that empower the client and family and promote a sense of well being and health.

THE GENERALIST NURSE

Clients with somatization disorders are found in various practice settings, ranging from inpatient medical units to primary and mental health care settings. The generalist needs to approach the client in a caring, nonjudgmental and firm manner that reduces manipulation or other maladaptive behaviors. Psychosocial stressors appear to exacerbate physical symptoms and emotional distress and must be assessed. Because of the high prevalence of mood and anxiety disorders, the nurse needs to assess the client's level of functioning, reasons for seeking treatment, and risk of dangerousness. Working with the interdisciplinary team enables the generalist nurse to provide structure and firm and consistent limit setting that enable the client to reach an optimal level of functioning and reduce preoccupations with health-seeking behaviors. The assessment process is ongoing and it is key to crisis resolution, symptom management, and appropriate illness perception. Cultural factors must also be assessed to determine their role in symptom manifestation. Stress management techniques, client and family health education, medication administration, and monitoring are important nursing interventions for the client and family presenting with a somatization disorder.

THE ADVANCED-PRACTICE PSYCHIATRIC REGISTERED NURSE

The advanced-practice psychiatric-mental health nurse is likely to collaborate with other health care providers and develop a holistic plan of care that includes pharmacologic and nonpharmacologic interventions. Pharmacologic interventions may include prescriptive authority and medication management. Oftentimes, the advanced-practice nurse collaborates with the medical team or acts as a psychiatric liaison consultant in various inpatient and primary care settings to address the client's physical and mental health concerns. Nonpharmacologic interventions include various psychotherapies, such as individual, family, and group, to improve or reduce cognitive distortions that perpetuate somatization.

THE NURSING PROCESS

Caring for clients with somatoform disorders requires in-depth and comprehensive physical and mental status examinations. The following case study depicts a client presenting with a somatoform disorder.

ASSESSMENT

The nursing assessment for this client needs to focus on gathering data about:

- ◆ Reason for seeking treatment
- ◆ Demographic data
- ◆ Family history, dynamics
- ◆ Cultural and gender-specific factors
- ◆ Perception of health problem
- ◆ Mental and physical status examinations
- ◆ Social interactions and support systems

(See Table 12-7.)

NURSING DIAGNOSES

Major nursing diagnoses for the child presenting with BDD include:

- ◆ Disturbed body image
- ◆ Ineffective coping
- ◆ Self-esteem, low

TABLE 12–7
Strategies for Reducing Somatization Symptoms

- Convey empathetic understanding
- Focus on coping and functioning rather than complete symptoms extinction
- Employ appropriate limit-setting
- Evaluate the client's level of distress and suffering associated with symptoms
- Respond to somatic complaints just as nonsomatic complaints
- Avoid challenging or negating symptoms
- Carefully provide reassurance
- Assess impact of symptoms on daily life and function
- Relate symptoms to quality of interpersonal relationships
- Avoid making inferences or remarks to the client "that it's all in your mind"
- Identify strengths
- Strengthen coping and level of functioning
- Assess for depression and suicide risk

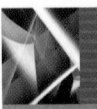

CASE STUDY

The Client with Body Dysmorphic Disorder (Johnny)

Johnny, a 21-year-old man, was recently diagnosed with BDD. As an adolescent, he was very shy and self-conscious about his body. Although he was of slender build, he always perceived himself as being "very skinny" and thus weak. To compensate for his perception of himself, he spent hours working out at a local gym and had gained several pounds. Despite his efforts, he continued to perceive himself negatively. He was also overly self-conscious about his ears, which he thought were too large. He became very obsessed about his ears and sought treatment from a plastic surgeon who told him that he saw no reason to perform surgery. After months of coercion, he finally sought treatment from an advanced-practice psychiatric nurse who diagnosed him with BDD.

OUTCOME IDENTIFICATION AND PLANNING

Outcome identification and planning must be client centered and culturally sensitive. Input from the nurse and interdisciplinary team members are essential and enhance holistic and evidence-based treatment planning.

IMPLEMENTATION

The treatment plan needs to include nursing interventions that reduce mental and physical distress, facilitate adaptive coping skills, and improve the client's functional status. Major nursing interventions need to focus on nursing diagnoses and include those that challenge his negative self-talk and perception of self, enhance his self-esteem, and facilitate adaptive coping behaviors.

EVALUATION

Evaluating the client's responses to interventions is continuous and based on outcome identification. Improved functional status is evidenced by improved physical, emotional, occupational or academic performance, and interpersonal relationships. Evaluation will be based on the nurse and team member's observations of the client's functional status and client and family feedback. Refer to Nursing Care Plan 12–1.

CRITICAL THINKING

1. Mary is a 21-year-old young woman who has been seen in the primary care clinic several times over the past month. Her chief complaints center on vague complaints of pain and all of her laboratory and physical examinations are negative. She asks you to help her get another appointment with her primary care provider. What is the most appropriate response to this client?

   a. Mary, this is your second visit over the past few weeks.

   b. Mary, your next appointment is in 3 months and you cannot see your provider today!

   c. Let me check your vital signs and weigh you.

   d. Mary, I have to see my real "sick" clients today.

2. Martie was seen in the college health center today complaining about a mark on her face that she cannot remove. She appeared upset and reported that her dermatologist told her that the spot was a birthmark. Martie admitted that she has had the mark since childhood, but it really looks "ugly" and she cannot concentrate because of it. As her nurse, which of the following statements reflect your understanding of this student's behavior?

   a. She has a right to be upset if the mark makes her feel bad.

   b. She is a little overly sensitive and is just having a "bad day."

   c. She probably has similar concerns about her body.

   d. She is stressed out about her finals and it is reflected in the way she feels about her body.

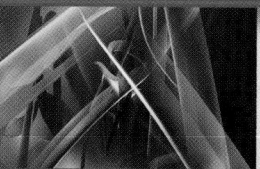

NURSING CARE PLAN 12–1

The Client with a Body Dysmorphic Disorder (Johnny)

Nursing Diagnosis: Disturbed Body Image

Outcome Identification	Nursing Actions	Rationales	Evaluation
1. By [date], client will verbalize realistic perception of self and change in body image.	1a. Establish rapport. Encourage expression of feelings.	1a. Establishes therapeutic interaction. Conveys empathy, caring, and interest.	*Goal met:* Nurse forms therapeutic relationship. Client expresses feelings and acknowledges change in body image.
	1b. Assist in identifying strengths, resources, and coping skills.	1b. Places focus on positive attributes and increased self-esteem.	

Nursing Diagnosis: Ineffective Coping

Outcome Identification	Nursing Actions	Rationales	Evaluation
1. By [date], client will develop realistic perception of present stressor(s).	1a. Explore meaning of recent stessors.	1a. Helps the client understand self and present responses.	*Goal met:* Client develops adaptive coping skills. Client's self-esteem increases.
2. By [date], client will develop enduring adaptive coping skills.	1b. Understand meaning of present stressors.	1b. Validates understanding of meaning of present symptoms.	

Nursing Diagnosis: Self-esteem, low

Outcome Identification	Nursing Actions	Rationales	Evaluation
1. By [date], client will verbalize 2–3 positive attributes and will have increased self-esteem.	1a. Provide successful experiences. 1b. Convey acceptance and empathy. 1c. Encourage active participation in treatment.	1a–c. Positive experiences increase confidence and self-esteem.	*Goal met:* Client's self-esteem increases. Client is able to explore options to deal with present stressors.

SUMMARY

- The complexity of somatoform disorders makes them very difficult to manage.

- Most studies show a correlation between somatoform disorders and co-occurring conditions such as depression and anxiety.

- Working with the client with a somatoform disorder requires patience, empathy, and firm limit setting.

- Causative factors associated with these disorders include psychosocial stress and biological factors.

- Many of the clients have cognitive disturbances manifested by an exaggerated perception of illness and fears of rejection.

- Assessment of the client's illness perception offers invaluable health education data.

SUGGESTIONS FOR CLINICAL CONFERENCES

1. Invite an advanced-practice psychiatric-mental health nurse to present a case conference on somatization disorder.

2. Encourage students to discuss possible cultural issues that may interfere with an accurate diagnosis of somatoform disorders.

3. Encourage students to identify one client case study and discuss various nursing interventions and personal feelings (e.g., fibromyalgia, hypochondriasis).

STUDY QUESTIONS

1. Mercy is a 30-year-old housewife who has made several visits to the emergency department over the past 6 months. Which of the following suggests that she may have a somatoform disorder?
   a. She is doing well in college and optimistic about her future.
   b. She is tearful and stressed and reports having difficulty doing housework.
   c. She is shy and has difficulty describing her symptoms.
   d. Her medical complaints are confirmed by diagnostic laboratory studies.

2. Mrs. Jones is in the primary care clinic for the second time over the past month reporting that she was recently diagnosed with fibromyalgia. Which of the following reflects her condition?
   a. "I am so depressed."
   b. "I believe that the man in the chair next to me can read my mind."
   c. "I need a referral for counseling."
   d. "I need a refill on my medication."

3. Working with the client with a somatoform disorder is challenging for the nurse. What is the most appropriate response to the client with a somatization disorder who continues to come into the college health clinic unscheduled with vague complaints?
   a. "Judy, let's discuss what your provider told you during the last visit."
   b. "Judy, I know that you are hurting and I will do everything for you."
   c. "Judy, this is the second time I have told you to sit down."
   d. "Judy, I do not agree with what your provider said during your last visit."

4. Jerry is a 33-year-old who comes in complaining of numbness and tingling in his legs and that he can hardly stand. He has been informed that there is no physical basis for his symptoms. Which of the following depicts his present complaints?

   a. Hypochondriasis
   b. Conversion disorder
   c. Extrapyramidal side effects
   d. Restless leg syndrome

5. Although classified as a somatoform disorder, body dysmorphic disorder has been hypothesized to be related to which other psychiatric disorder?
   a. Schizotypal personality disorder
   b. Bipolar I disorder
   c. Borderline personality disorder
   d. Obsessive-compulsive disorder

6. Which of the medications listed below has been shown to be the most effective in the treatment of BDD?
   a. Risperidone (Risperdal)
   b. Ziprasidone (Geodon)
   c. Diazepam (Valium)
   d. Clomipramine (Anafranil)

7. The nurse is caring for a client with somatization disorder. Which of the following symptoms will the client be least likely to exhibit?
   a. Clear description of symptoms
   b. Impaired occupational functioning
   c. History of frequent visits to health care facilities
   d. Chaotic, impulsive, and manipulative behaviors

8. Which of the following assessments made by the nurse would be essential in understanding behavior of a client with a conversion disorder?
   a. Physical symptoms are not under voluntary control.
   b. Physical symptoms are experienced as a means to manipulate others to meet self-centeredness.
   c. Physical symptoms are produced through purposeful means to reduce anxiety and maintain dependency.
   d. Physical symptoms are under voluntary control but without intent to reduce secondary gain.

9. When assessing the client with hypochondriasis, the nurse should expect to find all but which of the following?
   a. A pervasive fear of having a serious disease
   b. Misinterpretation of physical sensations as though they depict serious illness
   c. The sensations are not real to the client.
   d. Sensations often center on physical sensations and intense anxiety.

10. The nurse is helping the client with body dysmorphic disorder. The nurse can expect that the client may have which of the following?
    a. Rare co-occurrence with other psychiatric disorders
    b. Memory and cognitive function intact as evidenced by neuropsychological tests
    c. Acute and short-term course
    d. Preoccupation with imagined defect in appearance

11. The nurse is assessing a 12-year-old child. The nurse can expect that the youth may have which of the following?
    a. Few medical complaints easily explained
    b. High co-occurring anxiety and mood disorders
    c. Stable family environment that focuses on health
    d. Family environment that encourages autonomy, flexibility, and empathy

RESOURCES

Please note that because Internet resources are of a time-sensitive nature and URL addresses may change or be deleted, searches should also be conducted by association or topic.

Internet Resources

http://www.medscape.com   Medscape Psychiatry & Mental Health provides an excellent resource for all types of information on mental disorders, pharmacology, and diagnostic testing

http://www.fda.gov/consumer/updates/ fibromyalgia062107.pdf   FDA Consumer Health Information (2007). Living with Fibromyalgia

1. Locate two other sites not listed above that focus on mental illness.
2. Find two articles on Medline that relate to somatoform disorders.
3. Find a site that allows you to view PET scan images of clients with mental disorders.

Other Resources

American Academy of Pain Medicine
    4700 W. Lake Avenue
    Glenview, IL
    (847) 375-4731
    Fax (847) 375-6331
    http://www.painmed.org

American Pain Society
    4700 W. Lake Avenue
    Glenview, IL
    (847) 375-4715
    Fax (847) 375-6315
    http://www.info@ampainsoc.org

REFERENCES

American Psychiatric Association. (1980). *Diagnostic and statistical manual of mental disorders* (3rd ed.). Washington, DC: Author.

American Psychiatric Association. (2000). *Diagnostic and statistical manual of mental disorders* (4th edition, Text Revision) (*DSM-IV-TR*). Washington DC: Author.

Antai-Otong, D. (2005). The art of prescribing. Depression and fibromyalgia syndrome (FMS): Pharmacologic considerations. *Perspectives in Psychiatric Care, 41,* 146–148.

Aragona, M., Tarsitani, L., Colosimo, F., Martinelli, B., Raad, H., Maisano, B., & Geraci, S. (2005). Somatization in primary care: A comparative survey of immigrants from various ethnic groups in Rome, Italy. *International Journal of Psychiatry Medicine, 35,* 241–248.

Arnold, L. M., Lu, Y., Crofford, L. J., Wohlreich, M., Detke, M. J., Iyengar, S., et al. (2004). A double-blind, multicenter trial comparing duloxetine with placebo in the treatment of fibromyalgia patients with or without major depressive disorder. *Arthritis Rheumatology, 50,* 2974–2984.

Barsky, A. J., Orav, E. J., Bates, D. W. (2005). Somatization increases medical utilization and costs independent of psychiatric and medical comorbidity. *Archives of General Psychiatry, 62,* 903–910.

Bowlby, J. (1973). *Attachment and loss: Volume 2. Separation.* New York: Basic Books.

Bowlby, J. (1977). The making and breaking of affectional bonds: Etiology and psychopathology in the light of attachment theory. *British Journal of Psychiatry, 130,* 201–210.

Bowlby, J. (1988). Developmental psychiatry comes of age. *American Journal of Psychiatry, 145,* 1–10.

Breuer, J., & Freud, S. (1893–1895). Studies in hysteria. In J. Strachey (Ed. & Trans.), *The standard edition of the complete psychological works of Sigmund Freud* (Vol. 2, pp. 1–311). London: Hogarth Press. (Original work published 1955.)

Briquet, P. (1859). *Traite clinique et therapeutique y l'hysterie.* Paris: J.B. Balliere & Fils.

Brown, M. M., & Jason, L. A. (2007). Functioning in individuals with chronic fatigue syndrome: Increased impairment with co-occurring multiple chemical sensitivity and fibromyalgia. *Dynamic Medicine, 6,* 6, doi: 10.1186/1476-5918-6-6

Centers for Disease Control and Prevention. *Chronic Fatigue Syndrome: Healthcare Professionals.* http://www.cdc.gov/cfs/healthprofessionals.htm (Accessed Sept. 27, 2006).

Ciccone, D. S., Elliott, D. K., Chandler, H. K., Nayak, S., & Raphael, K. G. (2005). Sexual and physical abuse in women with fibromyalgia syndrome: A test of the trauma hypothesis. *The Clinical Journal of Pain, 21,* 378–386.

Dickens, C., Jayson, M., & Creed, F. (2002). Psychological correlates of pain behavior in patients with low back pain. *Psychosomatics, 43,* 42–48.

Ehlers, L. (1999). Pain and new cultural diseases. *Endodontic Dental Traumatology, 15*(5), 193–197.

Engel, G. L. (1959). Psychogenic pain and the pain-prone patient. *American Journal of Medicine, 26,* 899–918.

Fink, P., Hansen, M. S., & Oxhøj, M. L. (2004). The prevalence of somatoform disorders among internal medical inpatients. *Journal of Psychosomatic Research, 56,* 413–418.

Fink, P., Rosendal, M., & Toft, T. (2002). Assessment and treatment of functional disorders in general practice: The extended reattribution and management mode—an advanced educational program for nonpsychiatric doctors. *Psychosomatics, 43,* 93–131.

Ganong, W. F. (2005). *Review of medical physiology* (22nd ed.). New York: The McGraw-Hill Companies.

Goldstein, D. J., Lu, Y., Detke, M. J., Hudson, J., Iyengar, S., & Demitrack, M. A. (2004). Effects of duloxetine on painful physical symptoms associated with depression. *Psychosomatics, 45,* 17–28.

Gupta, A., Silman, A. J., Ray, D., Morriss, R., Dickens, C., MacFarlane G. J., et al. (2007). The role of psychosocial factors in predicting the onset of chronic widespread pain: results from a prospective population-based study. *Rheumatology (Oxford), 46,* 666–671.

Gureje, O., Olley, B. O., Olusola, E. O., Kola, L. (2006). Do beliefs about causation influence attitudes to mental illness? *World Psychiatry, 5,* 104–107.

Gureje, O., Simon, G. E., Ustun, T. B., & Goldberg, D. P. (1997). Somatization in cross-cultural perspective: A World Health Organization study in primary care. *American Journal of Psychiatry, 154,* 989–995.

Henningsen, P., Jakobsen, T., Schiltenwolf, M., & Weiss, M. G. (2005). Somatization revisited: Diagnosis and perceived causes of common mental disorders. *Journal of Nervous and Mental Disorders, 193,* 85–92.

Hiller, W., Rief, W., & Brähler, E. (2006). Somatization in the population from mild bodily misperceptions to disabling symptoms. *Social Psychiatry and Psychiatric Epidemiology, 41,* 704–712.

Hotopf, M., Mayou, R., Wadsworth, M., & Wessely, S. (1999). Psychosocial development antecedents of chest pain in young adults. *Psychosomatic Medicine, 61,* 861–867.

Interian, A., Guarnaccia, P. J., Vega, W. A., Gara, M. A., Like, R. C., Escobar, J. I., & Diaz-Martinez, A. M. (2005). The relationship between ataque de nervios and unexplained neurological symptoms: A preliminary analysis. *Journal of Nervous Mental Disorders, 193,* 32–39.

Kroenke, K., & Rosmalen, J. G. (2006). Symptoms, syndromes, and the value of psychiatric diagnostics in patients who have functional somatic disorders. *Medical Clinics of North America, 90,* 603–626.

Ladwig, K.-H., Marten-Mittag, B., Erazo, N., & Gundel, H. (2001). Identifying somatization disorder in a population-based health examination survey: Psychosocial burden and gender differences. *Psychosomatics, 42,* 511–518.

Leiknes, K. A., Finset, A., Moum, T., & Sandanger, I. (2007). Course and predictors of medically unexplained pain symptoms in the general population. *Journal of Psychosomatic Research, 62,* 119–128.

Natelson, B. H., Intriligator, R., Cherniack, N. S., Chandler, H. K., & Stewart, J. M. (2007). Hypocapnia is a biological marker for orthostatic intolerance in some patients with chronic fatigue syndrome. *Dynamic Medicine, 6,* 2, doi: 10.1186/1476-5918-6-2

Natelson, B. H., Weaver, S. A., Tseng, C. L., & Ottenweller, J. E. (2005). Spinal fluid abnormalities in patients with chronic fatigue syndrome. *Clinical and Diagnostic Laboratory Immunology, 12,* 52–55.

Otto, M. W., Wilhelm, S., Cohen, L. S., & Harlow, B. L. (2001). Prevalence of body dysmorphic disorder in a community sample of women. *American Journal of Psychiatry, 158,* 2061–2063.

Parker, G., Chan, B., Tully, L., & Eisenbruch, M. (2005). Depression in the Chinese: The impact of acculturation. *Psychological Medicine, 35,* 1475–1483.

Parker, G., Chan, B., & Tully, L. (2006). Recognition of depressive symptoms by Chinese subjects: The influence of acculturation and depressive experience. *Journal of Affective Disorders, 93,* 141–147.

Perley, M., & Guze, S. B. (1962). Hysteria: The stability and usefulness of clinical criteria: A quantitative study based upon a 6–8 year follow-up of 39 patients. *New England Journal of Medicine, 266,* 421–426.

Phillips, K. A. (2006). The presentation of body dysmorphic disorder in medical settings. *Primary Psychiatry, 13,* 51–57.

Phillips, K. A., Coles, M. E., Menard, W., Yen, S., Fay, C., & Weisberg, R. B. (2005). Suicidal ideation and suicide attempts in body dysmorphic disorder. *Journal of Clinical Psychiatry, 66,* 717–725.

Phillips, K. A., Didie, E. R., & Menard, W. (2007). Clinical features and correlates of major depressive disorder in individuals with body dysmorphic disorder. *Journal of Affective Disorders, 97,* 129–135.

Phillips, K. A., Menard, W., & Fay, C. (2006). Gender similarities and differences in 200 individuals with body dysmorphic disorder. *Comprehensive Psychiatry, 47,* 77–87.

Phillips, K. A., Pagano, M. E., & Menard, W. (2006). Pharmacotherapy for body dysmorphic disorder: Treatment received and illness severity. *Annals of Clinical Psychiatry, 18,* 251–257.

Piccinelli, M., & Simon, G. (1997). Gender and cross-cultural differences in somatic symptoms associated with emotional distress: An international study in primary care. *Psychological Medicine, 27,* 433–444.

Purtell, J. J., Robins, E., & Cohen, M. E. (1951). Observations on clinical aspects of hysteria. *Journal of the American Medical Association, 146,* 902–909.

Rief, W., Buhlmann, U., Wilhelm, S., Borkenhagen, A., & Brähler, E. (2006). The prevalence of body dysmorphic disorder: A population-based survey. *Psychological Medicine, 36,* 877–885.

Robertson, M. J., Schacterle, R. S., Mackin, G. A., Wilson, S. N., Bloomingdale, K. L., Ritz, J., et al. (2005). Lymphocyte subset differences in patients with chronic fatigue syndrome, multiple sclerosis and major depression. *Clinical and Experimental Immunology, 14,* 326–332.

Robinson, M. E., Dannecker, E. A., George, S. Z., Otis, J., Atchison, J. W., & Fillingim, R. B. (2005). Sex differences in the associations among psychological factors and pain report: A novel psychophysical study of patients with chronic low back pain. *Pain, 6,* 463–470.

Rost, K. M., Dickinson, W. P., Dickinson, L. M., & Smith, R. C. (2006). Multisomatoform disorder: Agreement between patient and physician report of criterion symptoms explanation. *CNS Spectrum, 11,* 383–388.

Sadock, B. J., & Sadock, V. A. (2005). *Kaplan & Sadock's pocket handbook of clinical psychiatry* (4th ed.). Philadelphia, PA: Lippincott Williams & Wilkins.

Shorter, F. (1992). *A history of psychosomatic illness in the modern era.* New York: Macmillan.

Steinhausen, H. C., & Winkler-Metzke, C. (2007). Continuity of functional-somatic symptoms from late childhood to young adulthood in a community sample. *Journal of Child Psychology and Psychiatry, 48,* 508–513.

Stuart, S., & Noyes, R. (2006). Interpersonal psychotherapy for somatizing patients. *Psychotherapy and Psychosomatics, 75,* 209–219.

Stulemeijer, M., de Jong, L. W., Fiselier, T. J., Hoogveld, S. W., & Bleijenberg, G. (2005). Cognitive behaviour therapy for adolescents with chronic fatigue syndrome: Randomised controlled trial. *British Medical Journal, 330,* doi:10.1136/bmj.38301.587.63

Vuillemier, P. (2005). Hysterical conversion and brain function. *Progress in Brain Research, 150,* 309–329.

SUGGESTED READINGS

CDC website:

Understanding Fatigue Syndrome: A Guide for Patients
http://www.cdc.gov/cfs/pdf/UnderstandingCFS.pdf

Toolkit: Fact Sheets for Healthcare Professionals
http://www.cdc.gov/cfs/toolkit.htm

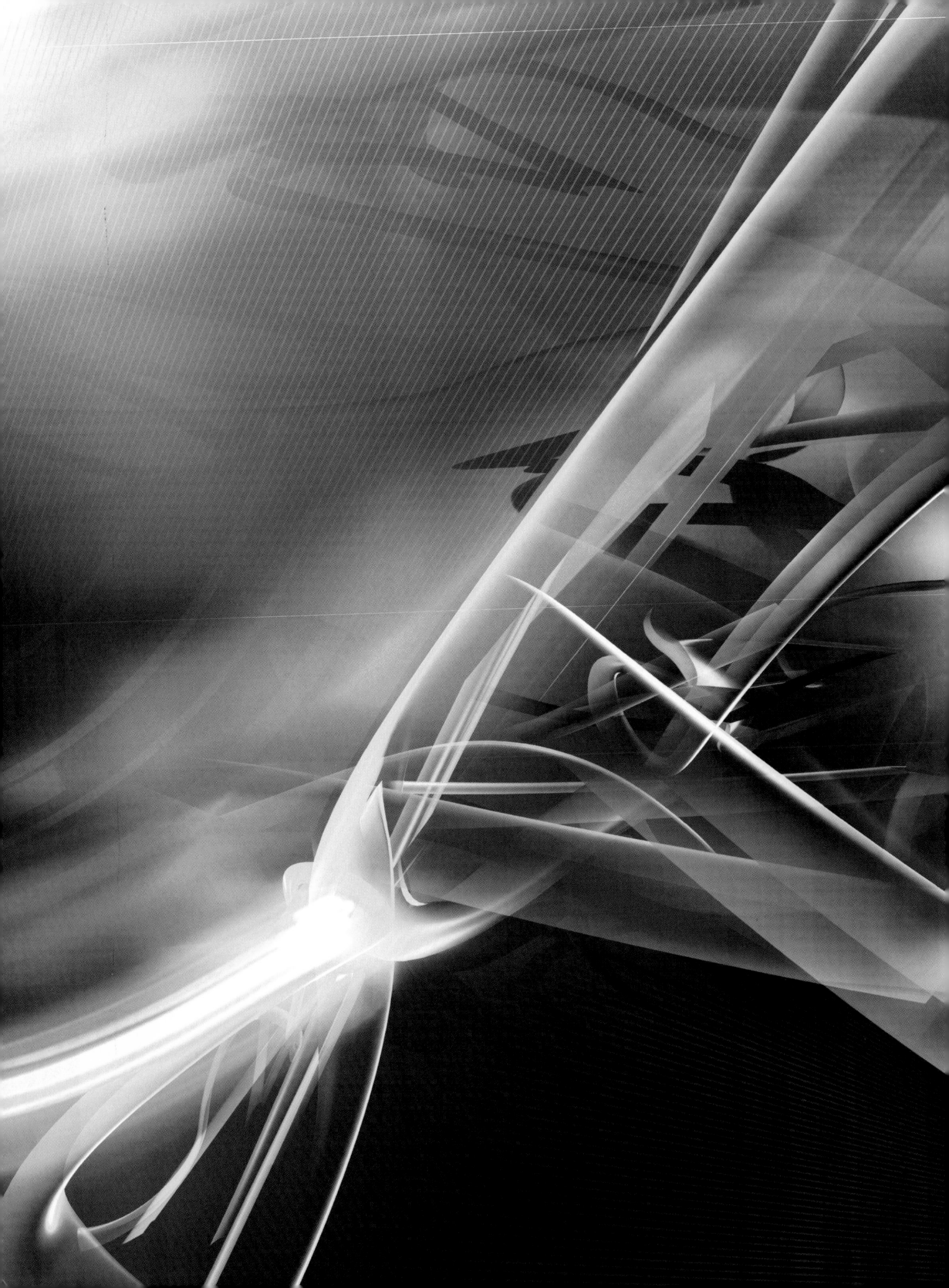

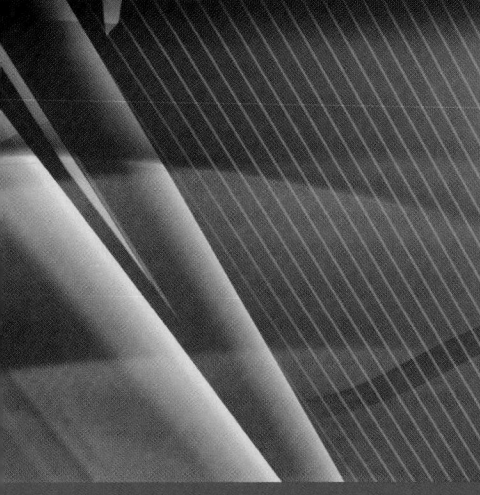

CHAPTER 13

The Client with a Stress-Related Disorder

Lisa A. Jensen, MS, APRN, CS
Deborah Antai-Otong, MS, APRN, BC, FAAN

KEY TERMS

Adaptation: Sustaining homeostasis; the ability to mobilize resources and adjust to demands of internal and external environments.

Catecholamine: Any of the sympathomimetic amines such as epinephrine, dopamine, and norepinephrine. These biochemicals play critical roles in the stress response.

Hardiness: Refers to a personality trait that enables people to maintain health and cope with stressful events.

Psychophysiological Disorder: Denotes emotional states producing or exacerbating physical problems.

Resilience: Successful adaptation to stressful and adverse events. Stressful events may include neurobiological dysregulation, cultural, and environmental challenges.

Sick Role: Dependent, helpless, and ill behavior often associated with control and maintenance of maladaptive relationships.

Stress: A stimulus or demand that has the potential to generate disruption in homeostasis or produce a reaction.

T-cells: Viral- and tumor-fighting lymphocytes (all called natural killer cells) of the immune system. They are referred to as "T" cells because they are processed by the thymus gland.

Type A Personality: A constellation of personality traits, such as highly driven, time-conscious, and competitive behavior, associated with high risk for coronary artery disease.

Type B Personality: A constellation of personality traits opposite from Type A and manifested by "easy-going, laid-back, and reposed" behavior.

COMPETENCIES

Upon completion of this chapter, the learner should be able to:

1. Analyze the role of stress in mental and physical disorders.
2. Discuss psychosocial and biological responses to stress.
3. Formulate a plan of care for clients experiencing psychobiological disorders.
4. Recognize the impact of psychophysiological disorders on the client and family members.

CHAPTER OUTLINE

Definitions

Epidemiology

Causative Factors: Theories and Perspectives

Psychodynamic Theories

Neurobiological Theories

Cognitive and Behavioral Factors: Personality (Coping) Styles

Cultural Considerations

Specific Psychobiological Disorders and Treatment Modalities

Cardiovascular Disorders

    Coronary Heart Disease

    Hypertension

    Treatment Modalities

Pulmonary or Respiratory Disorders

    Asthma

The interrelationship between body and mind is well documented. Emotions and physiological responses are linked with internal and external environments. Franz Alexander (1950) believed that this body-mind relationship arose from intense or prolonged emotions that triggered physiological responses. For example, he hypothesized that underlying anger or rage contributes to heart disease and that helplessness produces gastrointestinal disease. Alexander's premise suggests that humans respond to stressful situations using both neurobiological and psychological resources to maintain and restore homeostasis. Humans are holistic beings, and when stress affects one system, all other systems are influenced. Circumstances that threaten homeostasis activate complex neurobiological, psychosocial, and behavioral coping processes that arise from the autonomic nervous system.

Anger is an example of an intense emotion that triggers the sympathetic nervous system, which in turn stimulates adrenaline production and the flight or fight response. Neurobiological responses usually return to normal levels when anger abates. When people internalize anger or fail to manage it effectively, their bodies keep producing biological responses to stress. The sustained stimulation of the autonomic nervous system in these people results in continual production of catecholamines, which are potent vasopressors. Major catecholamines are norepinephrine and epinephrine. These substances affect all body systems, including the cardiovascular, gastrointestinal, and immunological systems, and chronic levels can produce tissue damage regardless of their origin (Alexander, 1939).

A holistic approach to client care is a major goal of nursing, and it requires assessing complex client needs that relate to emotional and biological responses to stress. Medicine has been dominated by the biomedical model, which proposes that physical problems have a clear-cut scientific explanation. This model does not take into account the influence of stress, social support, resilience, and adaptation to illness. Resilience refers to the ability to adapt to stressful or adverse circumstances. Nurses teach clients strategies that enhance coping skills and reduce stress, and they educate clients and their families about the long-term effects of stress, nonadherence, and ineffective coping patterns.

This chapter focuses on the behavioral and psychological factors that affect nonpsychiatric medical conditions. Nonpsychiatric medical conditions that are caused by behavioral or psychological factors are called psychophysiological disorders. The role of the psychiatric-mental health nurse in identifying clients' high-risk behaviors, reducing stress, and facilitating clients' adaptive coping skills is discussed.

DEFINITIONS

Historically, the term *psychosomatic* was used to describe a physical problem that was caused by an emotional state. The fourth edition of the *Diagnostic and Statistical Manual of Mental Disorders, Text Revision (DSM-IV-TR)* (American Psychiatric Association [APA], 2000) uses the term *psychological factors affecting medical conditions*. To be considered psychophysiological, a disorder must present with a medical condition on Axis III (e.g., hypertension). Other criteria include one of the following:

1. The course of the general medical condition is worsened or triggered by psychological factors (e.g., intense stress).

2. Psychological factors or emotional states unfavorably affect the course or outcome of treatment (e.g., client forgets to take hypertension medication or misses follow-up appointments).

3. Psychological factors or emotional states place the client at greater risk for health problems (e.g., increased risk of stroke or renal failure).

4. Psychological factors hasten stress-related physiological processes that worsen the general medical condition (e.g., hypertension persists in spite of adherence to medication regimen and later the client suffers a stroke or renal failure).

Before the *DSM-IV*, psychophysiological disorders were referred to as "psychological factors affecting physical conditions" (*DSM-III, DSM-III-R*) and "psychosomatic disorders" (*DSM-I, DSM-II*).

EPIDEMIOLOGY

Psychosocial epidemiology as it pertains to the influence of the person's behavior, and to the interrelation of physical and psychiatric illness, is controversial and difficult to discern. It may be that psychological distress represents underlying chronic illness that influences cardiovascular disease and immunological, respiratory, GI, and dermatological disorders. The relevance of neuroscience, neuroendocrinology, and cultural factors to understand the means in which psychosocial exposures affect mental and physical processes is well documented. There is a plethora of evidence that links stress with medical and psychiatric disorders. This chapter provides an in-depth discussion of various stress-related disorders and the role of the psychiatric nurse in caring for clients presenting with specific conditions.

CAUSATIVE FACTORS: THEORIES AND PERSPECTIVES

Human responses to stress involve psychosocial and neurobiological processes. In stressful situations, the body switches on its autonomic nervous system and neurobiological processes in an attempt to maintain homeostasis. Psychosocial adaptive processes are mob1ilized and sustained by temperament and personality traits that help the person cope with stressful situations.

The complexity of psychobiological disorders requires an understanding of the intrinsic relationship between emotions and physiological processes. Physiological processes activated by emotions are both innate and necessary for human survival and adaptation. However, a failure to mobilize resources and manage emotions and physiological processes threaten individual health and integrity. Acute stress responses activate a cascade of intricate survival processes that generate the "fight or flight" response. Prolonged activation of the stress response has potentially deleterious impact on mental and physical health. Implications for the psychiatric nurse include identifying high-risk groups and behaviors, reducing stress, and strengthening the client's repertoire of coping skills. Nurses can work more effectively with the client who presents with a psychophysiological disorder by understanding causative factors such as psychodynamic, neurobiological, culture, and cognitive.

PSYCHODYNAMIC THEORIES

Alexander (1939), a prominent pioneer of psychosomatic medicine and research, described "organ neurosis" or "functional disturbance" as a biological response to psychological stressors. He suggested that every emotional reaction corresponds with biological changes hastened by sympathetic adrenal arousal. Acute stress reactions were perceived as normal everyday responses that generally produced few injurious effects, in comparison with persistent sympathetic

nervous system activation, which produced anatomical changes or physiological disorders.

Later, Alexander (1950) delineated seven psychosomatic disorders: essential hypertension, skin disorders, rheumatoid arthritis, hyperthyroidism, ulcerative colitis, peptic ulcer diseases, and asthma. He believed that visceral or organ dysfunction arose from primarily unconscious personality traits or inadequate coping behaviors that interfered with reduction of intense emotions, such as anger, or repressed, sustained fears, anxiety, and aggression.

Freud (1958) hypothesized that unreleased psychological tension was converted into symptoms such as paralysis or blindness. He termed this reaction *conversion hysteria* and suggested that it stemmed from the inability to express feelings.

A contemporary term for conversion hysteria is *conversion disorder*. The *DSM-IV-TR* (APA, 2000) categorizes these disorders as somatoform disorders and lists several criteria:

◆ The loss or change in physical function is initially associated with a physical cause.

◆ Later, psychological components, such as intense stress and anxiety, are linked to the physical symptoms.

◆ The phenomenon is unintentional and unconscious.

◆ The symptom is not part of cultural mores, general medical condition, or substance misuse.

◆ The symptom is not associated with pain or disturbance in sexual performance.

◆ The symptom interferes with the client's optimal level of function.

See Chapter 12.

NEUROBIOLOGICAL THEORIES

Stress is an integral part of living, and it denotes a stimulus or demand that has the potential to disrupt homeostasis or

---

Myths to Overcome: Psychobiological Disorders

- It is often thought that so-called psychosomatic illnesses are imaginary, or "all in their head." For example, a person complaining of headaches may be thought by others not to be experiencing any pain. In reality, these are physical disorders in which both emotions and thinking play a role. In addition, persons with the disorder are unable to deal effectively with stress in their life.

- Some people believe that having negative or "bad thoughts" can lead to disorders such as cancer. Another popular belief is that having a positive attitude will allow a person to overcome a chronic illness. In reality, although there is a close relationship between the body and the mind, and having a negative attitude may increase one's stress level, people are not able to completely control physical symptoms through their thought processes.

produce a stimulus. Highly complex neurobiological and psychosocial processes are activated by stress, and they determine how internal and external demands are handled. Prolonged stimulation of the autonomic nervous system produces neurobiological changes and affects brain activity. Hans Selye introduced the concept that a person's inability to manage stress effectively increases their vulnerability to illness (Selye, 1976).

The premise of Selye's theory, referred to as General Adaptation Syndrome, is that there is a relationship between stress and neurobiological changes that arise from stimulation of the hypothalamic-pituitary-adrenal axis (Figure 13–1). Effective mastery of stress restores homeostasis and allows adaptation. Adaptation refers to sustaining homeostasis, the ability to mobilize resources and adjust to demands of internal and external environments. See Chapter 4 for an in-depth discussion of adaptation and coping processes.

Stress can alter various immunological processes. The immune system mediates intricate neurobiological processes and behavior to maintain homeostasis. Several studies suggest a relationship between stress and a reduction in natural killer (NK) activity. NK cells are involved in immune responses against certain viruses, bacteria, and parasites (Morikawa et al., 2005; Young & Ortaldo, 2006). Other stress-related alterations include decreased white blood cell, gamma interferon, and T-cell production. Transitory stress-induced change in the immune system is generally considered adaptive, but chronic stress has been associated with an impaired immune system (Akamoto et al., 2007).

Neuroendocrine processes are surmised to parallel dysregulation of the immune system. Prolonged stress is also associated with increased cortisol levels and epinephrine and norepinephrine production, which may alter the immune system (Besedovsky & Rey, 2007; Slack et al., 2007).

More recent studies link immunological suppression with depression, maladaptive coping behaviors, social interactions, substance abuse, cancer, and other physical disorders (Akamoto et al., 2007; Kuloğlu et al., 2007). Inappropriate and chronic release of stress hormones (adrenocorticotropic hormone and cortisol) eventually damages the normal neural and physiological mechanisms that maintain physical and mental adaptation. Long exposure to cortisol has been shown to contribute to systems diseases such as hypertension, atherosclerosis, and myocardial infarction. Perpetual stress has also been shown to destroy brain regions that normally shut down the stress response (i.e., gamma-aminobutyric acid [GABA] pathways), allowing the response to continue unchecked to the point of exhaustion.

The additional biological factor that is influenced by stress and adaptation is *temperament*. Temperament embodies inherited behavioral and genetic factors that make some people vulnerable to allergic reactions and hay fever. The basis of this relationship is that emotional responses affect the sympathetic nervous system, which in turn causes nasal epithelium to react (Kurukulasratchy, Matthews, & Ashad, 2006).

COGNITIVE AND BEHAVIORAL FACTORS: PERSONALITY (COPING) STYLES

Cognitive and behavioral factors that derive from personality styles also affect responses to stress. There is a relationship between personality or coping style and predisposition to certain illnesses. Friedman and Rosenman (1974) introduced the Type A personality and Type B personality more than 20 years ago; these researchers suggested a positive relationship between Type A personality and heart diseases. Type A was delineated by the following behaviors:

- ◆ Rapid speech
- ◆ Rapid walking
- ◆ Irritability
- ◆ Time consciousness
- ◆ Difficulty relaxing
- ◆ Persistent need to stay busy
- ◆ Attempts to do more than one thing at a time

According to the classic work on personality styles (Friedman & Rosenman, 1974), type A people are extremely competitive and aggressively strive for success and achievement. They frequently have high-pressure jobs and are referred to as workaholics, perfectionists, and overachievers. Underlying deficits in self-worth, self-esteem, and self-acceptance and excessive dependence on the approval of others are pervasive characteristics in these people. They are driven, constantly on the run, and tend to internalize their feelings. Psychological and biological needs are frequently ignored, further increasing the risk of stress-related illnesses (Friedman & Rosenman, 1974). Smith (1997) outlines traits with which successful coping are associated. These include general beliefs about the world and responsibility for life problems. These traits include an internal locus of control, a sense of coherence or a person's ability to manage his tensions and have a sense of belongingness, and hardiness, which is comprised of control, commitment, and challenge. Hardiness refers to a personality trait that enables people to maintain health and cope with stressful events. Other coping traits or characteristics are self-efficacy, optimism, hope, constructive thinking, and problem-solving skills. In contrast, traits associated with illness include negative affectivity, neuroticism or a negative view of the world, emotional instability, hostility, introversion, and Type A behaviors. Table 13–1 compares successful coping traits with illness traits. There is controversy regarding Type A personality traits and the risk of coronary disease (see "The More You Know").

People with Type B personalities are less driven than those with Type A and generally are more easy going, laid back, and reposed. Their lifestyles are relaxed and goal directed (Friedman & Rosenman, 1974).

Research suggests that some people are more vulnerable to stress than others. Risk factors include personality traits, genetics, diet, and environmental stressors. A lifestyle of chronic negative emotions, such as hostility, seems to produce neurobiological changes that increase a person's vulnerability

THE STRESS RESPONSE

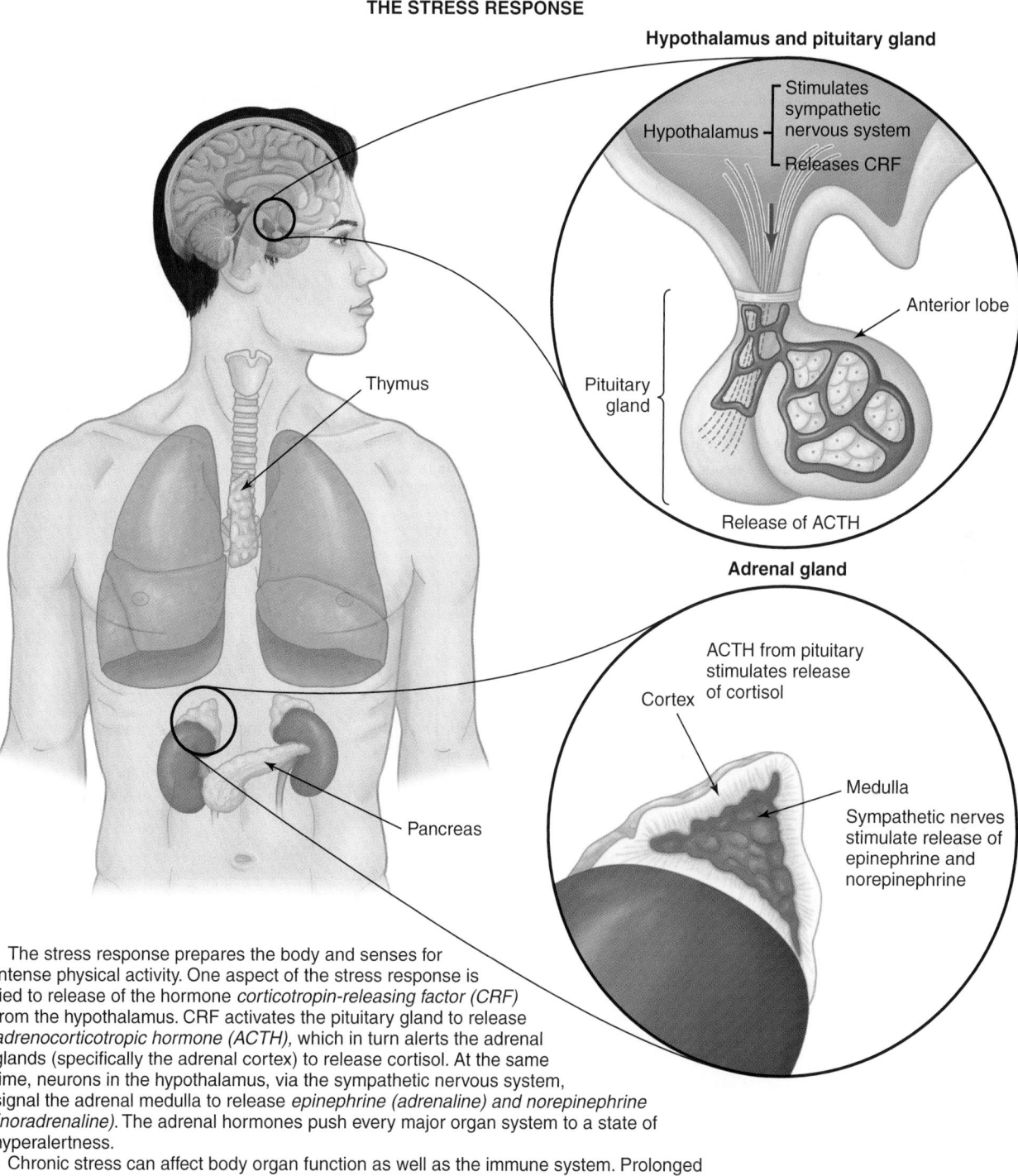

Hypothalamus and pituitary gland

Hypothalamus
- Stimulates sympathetic nervous system
- Releases CRF

Anterior lobe

Pituitary gland

Release of ACTH

Thymus

Pancreas

Adrenal gland

ACTH from pituitary stimulates release of cortisol

Cortex

Medulla

Sympathetic nerves stimulate release of epinephrine and norepinephrine

The stress response prepares the body and senses for intense physical activity. One aspect of the stress response is tied to release of the hormone *corticotropin-releasing factor (CRF)* from the hypothalamus. CRF activates the pituitary gland to release *adrenocorticotropic hormone (ACTH),* which in turn alerts the adrenal glands (specifically the adrenal cortex) to release cortisol. At the same time, neurons in the hypothalamus, via the sympathetic nervous system, signal the adrenal medulla to release *epinephrine (adrenaline) and norepinephrine (noradrenaline).* The adrenal hormones push every major organ system to a state of hyperalertness.

Chronic stress can affect body organ function as well as the immune system. Prolonged and chronic release of cortisol, epinephrine, and norepinephrine eventually exhausts normal mechanisms for maintaining homeostasis, and destroys brain regions (GABA pathways) that normally shut down the stress response. Benzodiazepines (Valium, Librium) are sometimes prescribed for persons vulnerable to chronic stress reactions; these tranquilizers enhance GABA production and uptake, and dampen emotional response.

Figure 13–1 The stress response: the role of hormones and the physical and emotional effects of chronic stress. *(continues)*

PHYSICAL AND EMOTIONAL EFFECTS OF STRESS

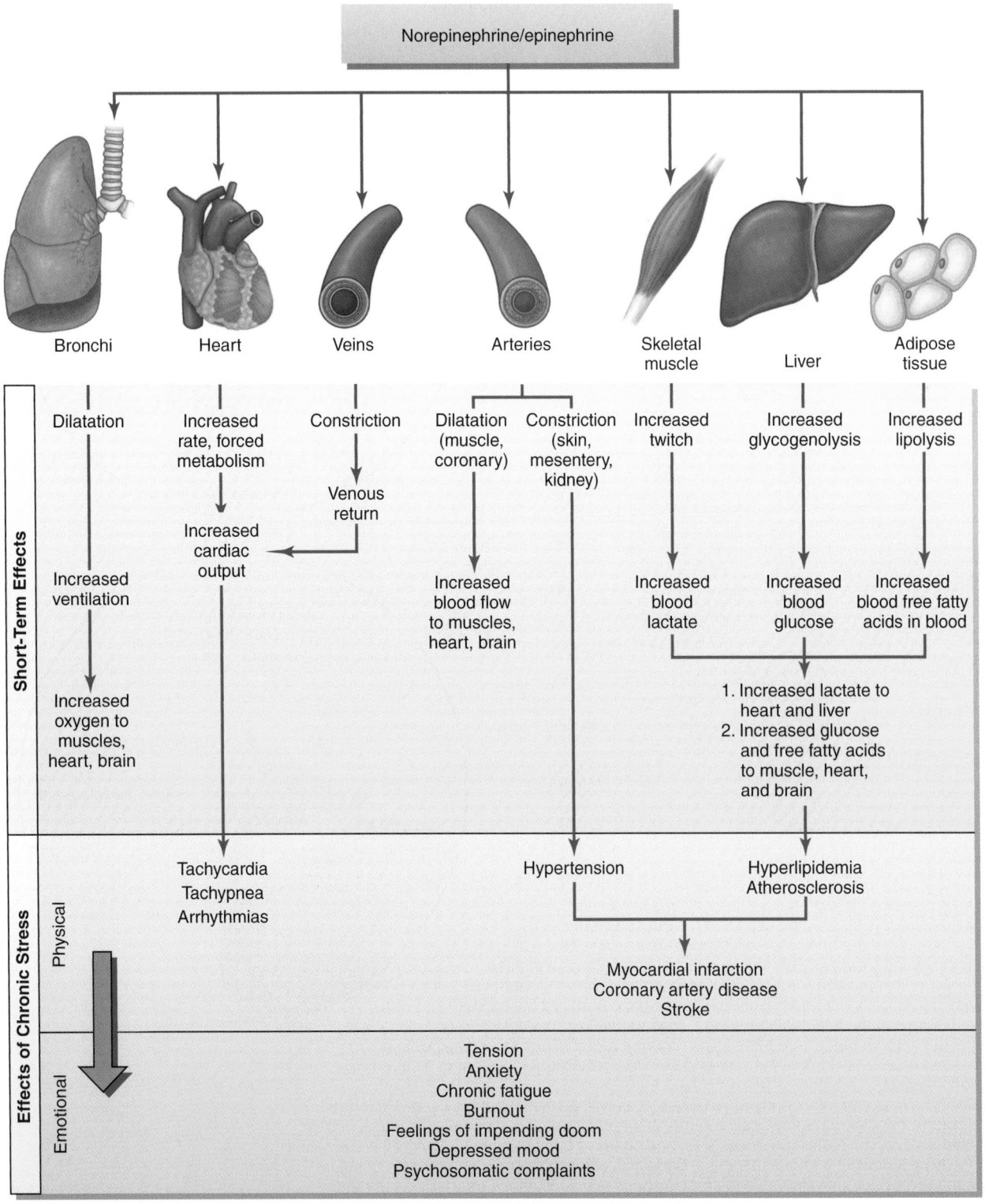

Figure 13–1 *(continued)*

TABLE 13–1
Comparison of Successful Coping Traits and Illness Traits

Successful Coping Traits	Illness Traits
Internal locus of control	Negative affectivity
Hardiness	Anxiety
Self-efficacy	Hostility
Hope	Introversion
Optimism	Type A behaviors
Problem-solving skills	
Constructive thinking	

Note. Data from *Understanding Stress and Coping,* by J. C. Smith, 1997, New York: Macmillan. Adapted with permission.

to stress. People who chronically experience these negative emotions tend to repress their feelings and are likely to abuse substances that further compromise their well-being. The inability to express their feelings is manifested by closed body language, such as folded arms and poor eye contact, an overly appeasing attitude, and an anxious mood. Inability or unwillingness to express feelings has been associated with sustained arousal of the sympathetic nervous system.

Prolonged stress has deleterious effects on neurobiological processes that are understood as the bases of psychophysiological disorders. Responses to stress vary across the life span and depend on mobilization of internal and external resources, which are the bases of adaptation. Nursing implications include identifying high-risk behaviors and formulating interventions that strengthen coping skills and reduce the deleterious effects of stress reactions.

CULTURAL CONSIDERATIONS

An often overlooked area concerning psychophysiological disorders is the role of culture and its impact on the client, family, and communities. Because of the dramatic demographic changes in this country and globally, assessing the role of culture, religion, and spirituality is critical to understanding the client's experiences and symptoms. Implications for nursing practice include self-awareness of one's own culture and its potential impact of perception of the client's experiences. See Chapter 7 for a discussion on culture issues.

SPECIFIC PSYCHOBIOLOGICAL DISORDERS AND TREATMENT MODALITIES

Psychophysiological disorders are divided into several categories: cardiovascular, pulmonary or respiratory, immunological, gastrointestinal (GI), dermatological, and chronic pain.

CARDIOVASCULAR DISORDERS

The cardiovascular system is composed of the heart and blood vessels, which circulate blood and use oxygen, various nutrients, and intricate neurobiological processes to supply cells and deport waste and impurities. Cardiovascular disorders refer to impairment of the heart and blood vessels.

Coronary Heart Disease

Coronary heart disease continues to be the leading cause of death in the United States. It results from blockage of coronary arteries, which interferes with perfusion of blood to the heart and general circulation. The lack of adequate oxygen perfusion and removal of waste products creates hypoxia and angina pectoris (chest pain). Coronary heart disease is linked with a number of high-risk behaviors, including personality traits (e.g., Type A behaviors), elevated cholesterol levels, smoking, lack of regular exercise, and uncontrolled high blood pressure.

It has been hypothesized that Type A behavior is associated with a higher risk of coronary heart disease. Recent

THE MORE YOU KNOW

Is the Type A Personality a Predictor of Coronary Artery Disease?

Despite numerous studies linking Type A personality traits with increased risk of coronary artery disease, controversy prevails. Littman (1998) points out that before 1981, several research studies found Type A behavior (TAB) to be associated with coronary artery disease. He goes on to point out that since 1981, several studies have shown no effect of TAB in patients with coronary disease. Friedman (1996) states that the confusion concerning TAB is caused by the failure of investigators to recognize TAB as a medical disorder, which cannot be diagnosed by a self-report obtained through a questionnaire. He believes that TAB can only be detected by a physical examination.

From Friedman, M. (1996). *Type A behavior: Its diagnosis and treatment* (pp. 31–51). New York: Plenum Press; Littman, A. B. (1998). A review of psychosomatic aspects of cardiovascular disease. In G. A. Fava & H. Freyberger (Eds.), *Handbook of psychosomatic medicine* (pp. 261–293). Madison, CT: International Universities Press.

research conducted since 1981 has had mixed results on this issue (Smith, Glazer, Ruiz, & Gallo, 2004) with the finding that hostility and anger are the specific components of the Type A personality that may be responsible for increasing the risk of heart disease. Vale (2005), in a review of the literature, points to the recognition of the role of negative emotions, personality, and socioeconomic status on coronary heart disease. Although the precise relationship of personality traits to heart disease continues to be studied, growing evidence indicates a positive correlation between anxiety, tension, and hostility (Eaker, Sullivan, Kelly-Hayes, Agostino, & Benjamin, 2005). Gallacher et al. (2003) found Type A personality can be a strong predictor of when, rather than if, coronary heart disease occurs.

Hypertension

Hypertension is another major cardiovascular disease linked with stress. Stress activates the autonomic nervous system, which activates the release of catecholamines (epinephrine and norepinephrine). These biochemicals produce profound changes in the cardiovascular system by raising the blood pressure and heart rate, and causing other physiological changes that produce the flight or fight response. Persistent sympathetic stimulation produces vasoconstriction, increasing the risk of hypertension.

Who is at risk for hypertension? Individuals at risk for this disorder include those with family histories of heart disease, genetics, obesity, hyperlipidemia, smoking, diabetes, and maladaptive personality or coping styles. Psychosocial stressors, such as impoverished living conditions, high-pressured jobs, and strained interpersonal relationships also play key roles in development of hypertension. See "My Experience with Heart Disease."

Treatment Modalities

Prevention is critical to the treatment of hypertension and other cardiovascular disorders. By assessing the client's present stressors and coping styles and developing individualized teaching plans, the nurse can help the client recognize and understand the maladaptive nature and consequences of disease-prone behaviors and explore adaptive ways to manage stress. An interdisciplinary approach is critical to the success of health education and restoration. Major interventions include smoking cessation, weight loss, administration of cardiovascular agents, and adherence to medication regimen, diet restrictions and healthy eating habits, and stress management. Stress management, regular exercise, smoking cessation, psychoeducation, cognitive-behavioral, and various forms of psychotherapy can help clients express feelings and develop effective coping skills. Client education is important in that compliance with antihypertensive treatment may depend on the client's perceptions of the treatment's effectiveness (Paré, Jaana, & Sicotte, 2007). See the Research Abstract. Progressive relaxation exercises teach clients how to relax (see Chapter 26, Individual Psychotherapy, for specific techniques). See Table 13–2 for a description of stress-reducing techniques.

My Experience with Heart Disease

I was diagnosed with heart disease 5 years ago. I was working in sales, a high-stress occupation. I felt pressured to sell more and produce more all the time. I worked many hours, often putting in 60 to 70 hours a week. After my heart attack, I had to make a number of changes in my life. My family and I reassessed our goals in life. I discovered that some of the things I thought were important to me didn't matter at all.

I had to change jobs, finding a position that was much less stressful. My eating and exercise habits have also changed dramatically. Fried foods are pretty much taboo from my diet, as are rich, high-fat desserts. I also have limited my alcohol intake significantly. I exercise every day now. All this has led to quite a weight loss for me. I no longer keep my feelings bottled up inside. When I'm upset with my wife, she and I sit down and talk about it calmly. I write in a journal nearly every day, writing about my feelings and my experiences. I spend more time with my family, just doing fun things like playing with the kids in the park, going for walks, and playing board games at home.

I still worry about my heart, but I know I'm doing the things I need to do to take care of myself. Overall, I feel much better about my life, my future, and myself than I ever have in the past.

PULMONARY OR RESPIRATORY DISORDERS

Breathing patterns reveal emotions. Rapid breathing or hyperventilation is a common sign of anxiety attacks or intense fears. In contrast, shallow breathing or sighs may indicate distress. The parasympathetic (vagal) and sympathetic nervous systems innervate lung tissues. Stimulation of the parasympathetic nervous system, which may be precipitated by dust, cold air, or emotions, causes vasoconstriction.

Asthma

Asthma is a Greek term that means panting, or labored breathing. It is a common respiratory disorder that has numerous causes and is associated with bronchoconstriction, which is the pervasive narrowing of air passages that results from vagal stimulation caused by stress, allergic reactions, cold, dust, or infections. Major manifestations of asthma include coughing, wheezing, shortness of breath, and intense anxiety and fear. Although there is no evidence that stress causes asthma, there is considerable evidence that stress can exacerbate symptoms (Wright, 2005).

Treatment Modalities

Asthma attacks are very distressful, and regardless of the cause, require immediate medical attention. Other interventions include approaching the client in a nonjudgmental manner; identifying the precipitants of the attacks, such as stress, infections, or allergies; developing teaching plans that incorporate stress reduction; and strengthening coping skills. Stress management is indicated because stress causes a change in the immune balance that may increase asthma activity in susceptible individuals (Homnick & DeJong, 2007).

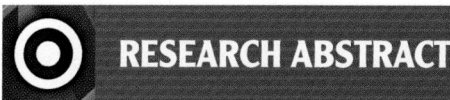

RESEARCH ABSTRACT

Long-term Effects of Two Psychological Interventions on Physical Exercise and Self-regulation Following Coronary Rehabilitation

Sniehotta, F. F., Scholz, U., Schwarzer, R., Fuhrman, B., Kiwus, U., & Voller, H. (2005). *International Journal of Behavioral Medicine, 12*(4), 244–255.

Study Problem/Purpose

To study the role that psychological interventions may play in encouraging clients to engage in regular physical exercise.

Methods

A group of 240 clients were randomly assigned into either of two treatment groups. There was also a standard-care control group. Clients in the two treatment groups produced detailed action plans for regular physical exercise and developed barrier-focused mental strategies. One of the groups kept a weekly diary for six weeks to increase a sense of action control.

Findings

Interventions targeting self-regulatory skills can enable post-cardiac rehabilitation clients to reduce behavioral risk factors and facilitate intended lifestyle changes.

Implications for Psychiatric Nurses

Psychiatric nurses can assist clients in recognizing barriers to carrying out intended behaviors, i.e., regular physical exercise. The nurse can then help the client to make action plans to address these potential barriers. Thus the client will be more successful in their post-cardiac rehabilitation program.

TABLE 13–2
Therapeutic Measures for Stress-Related Illness

Biofeedback

Biofeedback is an electronic indication of a person's stress level that is provided by instrumentation that registers the person's psychophysiological responses. A tone or signal provides the client with immediate feedback. The goal is to keep the tone below a certain threshold for 15 seconds on four occasions. The client learns to observe and control subtle internal body responses (blood pressure, temperature, and muscle tension). This intervention enables clients to modulate physiological responses to stress to play an active role in the promotion of their own health.

Indications: Migraine headaches, hypertension, Raynaud's disease, chronic pain, gastrointestinal disorders.

Deep Muscle Relaxation

The client is taught how to achieve deep muscle relaxation, which is basic to all behavioral stress reduction techniques. The following instructions are given to the client:

- Find a quiet area away from distraction.
- If desired, use a relaxation tape.
- Get into a comfortable position, such as lying on your back.
- Close your eyes and inhale deeply through your nose, allowing your lungs to fill with air and feeling your chest expand. Then slowly exhale.
- Repeat.

The success of deep relaxation depends on daily practice. The goal is to decrease respirations, reduce blood pressure, and reduce peripheral vasodilation.

Indications: Tension headaches, muscle tension, hypertension.

Visual Imagery

Deep muscle relaxation is imperative during visual imagery. A pleasant, quiet, peaceful place is visualized to reduce stress or pain and to enhance relaxation. As with deep muscle relaxation, ongoing practice is necessary for successful use of this technique.

(continues)

TABLE 13–2
Therapeutic Measures for Stress-Related Illness *(continued)*

Indications: Childbirth, gastrointestinal disorders, chronic pain, cancer.

Self-Talk

In this form of cognitive therapy, clients provide themselves with evaluative statements and suggestions to reduce stress and promote relaxation.

Indications: To reduce anxiety, stress, and faulty cognitions.

Note. Definitions are from *The Relaxation Response*, by H. Benson, 1975, New York: William Morrow; and from *Biofeedback: Methods and Procedures in Clinical Practice*, by G. D. Fuller, 1977, San Francisco: Biofeedback Press. Adapted with permission.

IMMUNOLOGICAL DISORDERS

Stress alters people's immunological processes and resistance to illness. Inadequate cellular immune response or alteration in tumor and viral fighting T-cells compromises the immune system, increasing vulnerability to illnesses such as acquired immunodeficiency syndrome; cancer; and the common cold, flu, herpes simplex Type I, and Epstein-Barr viruses (Akamoto et al., 2007; Young & Ortaldo, 2006).

GASTROINTESTINAL DISORDERS

Gastrointestinal (GI) disorders have long been associated with emotions. The GI tract is innervated by the autonomic nervous system and, like other major organs, is affected by stress and tension. Stress and other emotional reactions create tension in the gut and can produce nausea, vomiting, or diarrhea. Emotional factors influence the function of the GI tract (Yates, 2004).

The relationship between emotions and the GI tract can be traced back to the works of Hippocrates and Alexander, who related illness to prolonged stress. The GI tract has been referred to as the "little brain" and associated with expressions such as "gut reactions" or "gut feelings" (Wingate, 1985). In addition, anxiety and other mood disorders have been found in clients experiencing GI disorders. Mood disorders and activation of the GI system are both surmised to result from activation of the autonomic nervous system, particularly the locus ceruleus, which plays a major role in mediating intense feelings and arousal states (Rajkowski, Majczynski, Clayton, & Aston-Jones, 2004).

Major GI disorders include gastroesophageal reflux disease (GERD), irritable bowel syndrome, peptic ulcer disease, ulcerative colitis, and Crohn's disease. The following discussion of irritable bowel syndrome is an example of a psychophysiological GI disorder. (See the Case Study regarding a client with irritable bowel syndrome [Mr. Ekpe] later in this chapter.)

Irritable Bowel Syndrome

According to Locke et al. (2004), higher levels of psychological distress are found in clients with irritable bowel syndrome and should be assessed as a contributing factor. These clients need to be approached in a calm, caring manner so that their concerns and fears are reduced. Identification of their present stressors, coping styles, support systems, and patterns of physical and emotional response is a major aspect of the assessment process. Saito et al. (2004) found a multidisciplinary class for irritable bowel syndrome clients was associated with improvement in symptoms and promotion of healthy lifestyle behaviors. The long-term effects of irritable bowel syndrome are potentially life threatening and debilitating and affect numerous body systems. In addition to adhering to strict medical regimens, the clients and their family have enormous emotional needs and intense psychosocial stress, which stem from feelings of helplessness and a lack of control over their body and life. See Nursing Care Plan 13–1.

Treatment Modalities

Irritable bowel syndrome has been aligned with several mood disorders, including panic, agoraphobia, and depression. People with this syndrome tend to be tense, anxious, depressed, and irritable, and they also tend to internalize feelings (Whitehead et al., 2004). Major interventions for irritable bowel syndrome are relaxation techniques, stress reduction, assertiveness training, and biofeedback. Psychotherapy and psychopharmacology (e.g., anxiolytics or antidepressants) may be indicated for some clients. Major treatment goals focus on strengthening and improving coping behavior and communication skills and reducing psychological and biological stress.

DERMATOLOGICAL DISORDERS

The skin, like other major systems, responds to the environment and is responsive to various emotions such as anger, embarrassment, and terror. The condition of skin often reflects health status. Clammy, cool skin may indicate a serious medical problem or intense fear and anxiety. A generalized rash suggests an allergic reaction or an intense emotional response. Regardless of the cause, skin disorders need to be evaluated and treated immediately to ensure psychological and physiological well-being.

Treatment Modalities

Dermatological or skin disorders considered to be psychophysiological conditions include alopecia, pruritus (itching), psoriasis, and urticaria (hives). Picardi et al. (2005) found a high frequency of psychosocial problems in clients with skin diseases. Psychosocial stress tends to aggravate skin disorders. Nursing implications include identifying stressors and developing interventions that reduce the intensity of stressors and strengthen and develop effective coping skills. In addition, stress reduction interventions, such as cognitive-behavioral techniques and desensitization, provide relief for some clients suffering from stress-induced illnesses (Kim et al., 2006). The chronic nature of some skin disorders creates intense emotional stress arising from feelings of helplessness and decreased self-esteem. See "My Experience with a Skin Condition."

CHRONIC PAIN DISORDERS

The psychophysiological basis of pain is complex. Perman (1954) described pain as a friend because of its lifesaving value. Pain signals both psychological and physiological pain. Emotions generated by pain include rage, fear, and humiliation, and they serve as a force to resolve the situation (Levenson, McDaniel, Moran, & Stoudemire, 1999). Chronic recurrent pain can be emotionally and physically incapacitating and create feelings of guilt, low self-esteem, and discour-

agement (Menninger, 1963). Chronic pain may lead to anxiety, depression, and feelings of hopelessness which in turn may increase the perception of pain (Fluermond & Sharpe 2005).

Treatment Modalities

Major nursing interventions for chronic pain begin with approaching the client in a caring and nonjudgmental manner. This approach is critical to allaying fears of the pain being all in the client's head. Major therapeutic measures include hydrotherapy, massages, physiotherapy, and analgesics. Additional major interventions include behavioral-cognitive techniques, relaxation, distraction, biofeedback, and group psychotherapy (Moore et al., 2007; North, Hong, & Alpers, 2007). See Chapter 26, Individual Psychotherapy, for an in-depth discussion of these techniques. Table 13–2 describes some of the therapeutic measures recommended for clients with stress-related illnesses.

PSYCHOBIOLOGICAL DISORDERS ACROSS THE LIFE SPAN

Psychobiological disorders, like other psychiatric disorders, often expand across the life span. Psychiatric nurses caring for the client with these disorders must explore the role of stress, environmental factors, biological, and genetic factors that contribute to stress-related illnesses and initiate holistic treatment planning that enhances functional status and health promotion across the life span.

CHILDHOOD

Childhood psychophysiological disorders have been linked with the need for protection and attachment to primary caregivers. Separation anxiety plays a key role in formation and exacerbation of physical symptoms. Immature cognitive function and inability to express feelings often compel the child to communicate anxiety and stress through physical symptoms (Garralda & Rangel, 2005). Other childhood stressors include disabling disorders, abuse, family chaos, and unstable living conditions.

Family dynamics play a major role in formation of childhood psychophysiological disorders. Common family dynamics include overresponsiveness, limited autonomy, rigidity, overprotectiveness, and rejection. Many parents of children with psychophysiological disorders are difficult to work with because they lack insight into their role in the child's illness (Liebman, Minuchin, & Baker, 1974).

A case history of a child with a psychophysiological disorder is Baby Judy who was an unplanned birth. Her mother was in the process of a divorce when she discovered her pregnancy. Since her birth, Judy's mother has spent little time with her. Months later, Judy developed symptoms of respiratory distress and was diagnosed with asthma. Because of this illness, her mother is *forced* to spend time

My Experience with a Skin Condition

Over the past few weeks, I have been very stressed. I noticed that I was breaking out in wheals. Before their eruption, I felt burning sensations, similar to an insect bite. At first, I just thought I had been bitten by something, but realized that they erupted when I got off from work, especially after having a stressful day. I thought maybe some Benadryl would help, but opted not to because I was too busy to deal with its sedative effects.

Unfortunately, the wheals would not go away so I decided to go to my physician because I thought something was wrong with me. During the visit, he asked me about the recent events in my life. I told him that my 3-year-old had been pretty sick and the demands at work were "tearing me apart" because I could not be with my child. I also told him that although she was doing better, I wasn't. He told me that my wheals were caused by my stress and that I needed to take a few days off from work and relax. I was so relieved to know that my skin condition was not serious, yet it bothered me that someone else had to point out how "stressed out" I was.

with her. Judy, when ignored or left alone for long intervals, experiences respiratory distress.

Research has shown a positive correlation between childhood asthma symptoms and intense separation anxiety, suggesting that childhood emotional distress affects complex neurobiological responses. This is especially true in children with chronic, severe, and frequent asthma attacks that occur in spite of comprehensive medical management (Marsac, Funk, & Nelson, 2007; Rath et al., 2007).

What role does the child's symptoms play in family dynamics? Minuchin and colleagues' classic work on family dynamics (1975) suggests that childhood psychophysiological symptoms serve as "homeostatic mechanism regulating-family interactions" (p. 1032). This premise suggests that the child's symptoms maintain family "stability." They identified three factors that play major roles in the formation of the child's symptoms:

1. Vulnerability (neurobiological predisposition)
2. Specific family dynamics: enmeshment, overprotective-ness, rigidity, and ineffective conflict resolution (Minuchin, 1974)
3. The usefulness of the sick role in sustaining homeostasis, which serves to reinforce illness

Dysfunctional family interactions tend to create an environment of control and tension. See Chapter 28, Familial Systems and Family Therapy, for an in-depth discussion of family dynamics and interventions.

ADOLESCENCE

The psychological and neurobiological maturation of the adolescent is very perplexing. Adolescence represents a period of intense biological and psychosocial turmoil as the youth searches for a sense of identity and strives to separate from primary caregivers. Other psychosocial stressors are tremendous academic demands and interpersonal relationships, which emerge as important developmental tasks preparing the youth for adulthood.

Healthy family interactions serve as a buffer for the youth, providing emotional support and validating the youth's struggle and need for self-identity and independence. Peer support can also act as a buffer for adolescents, as well as the ability to cognitively appraise stressors. Bodily reactions affected by adolescents in response to stressful situations include recurrent abdominal pain, headaches, chest pain, musculoskeletal pain, chronic fatigue, and nonspecific symptoms such as dizziness or tiredness (Colman, Wadsworth, Croudace, & Jones, 2007).

ADULTHOOD AND OLDER ADULTHOOD

The long-term effects of biological response to chronic stress have been well documented. Certain people seem to be at risk for developing psychophysiological disorders, or they are disease prone. Disease-prone behaviors include certain

TABLE 13–3
Specific Psychophysiological Disorders

System	Disorders/Symptoms
Cardiovascular	• Hypertension • Mitral valve prolapse • Myocardial infarction • Coronary heart disease • Migraine headaches
Pulmonary	• Hyperventilation • Asthma • Allergies
Immunological	• Certain cancers • Autoimmune disease, such as lupus • Herpes zoster • Herpes simplex • Rheumatoid arthritis • AIDS
Gastrointestinal	• Peptic ulcer disease • Crohn's disease • Ulcerative colitis • Irritable bowel syndrome • Gastroesophageal reflux disease (GERD)
Dermatological	• Rashes • Urticaria • Psoriasis • Alopecia • Warts
Endocrine	• Diabetes • Thyroid disorders

personality traits, chronic tension, and internalized emotions. Table 13–3 lists psychophysiological disorders that may be experienced in adulthood.

THE ROLE OF THE NURSE

Nursing care of clients with stress-related disorders requires a holistic perspective that integrates psychosocial, cultural, and medical interventions. Stress-related disorders have the potential to produce significant disabilities and must be treated in a caring and empathetic environment that promotes understanding of the role of stress and coping skills. Nurses across the health care continuum are likely to collaborate with an array of health care providers that address the needs of clients presenting with stress-related disorders.

THE GENERALIST NURSE

The primary roles of the psychiatric-mental health nurse are to assess clients' current and past coping behaviors, help clients resolve crisis situations, minimize exacerbation of symptoms, and strengthen and promote adaptive coping behaviors. Hospitalized clients experiencing acute exacerbation of symptoms require close monitoring so that homeostasis is maintained. Interventions such as adequate dietary intake, hydration, and control of pain involve assessing client response and promotion of self-care. Psychoeducation, crisis intervention, and stress-reducing activities are major nursing interventions for clients experiencing psychophysiological disorders (Table 13–4). It has been found that changing clients' beliefs about their symptoms may improve outcomes, including symptoms, disability, distress, and health care resource use (Price, 2000). As members of the health care team, generalist nurses play a major role in helping clients and their families reduce the deleterious effects of stress in various community settings.

THE ADVANCED-PRACTICE PSYCHIATRIC REGISTERED NURSE

Nurses in advanced-practice also work with clients and families to minimize exacerbation of symptoms and promote self-care and adaptive coping skills. In addition, the advanced-practice nurse identifies complex problems and collaborates with clients to modify behavior and coping patterns. Major interventions include various psychotherapies such as cognitive-behavioral and psychodynamic approaches. Furthermore, prescriptive authority enables the advanced-practice nurse to prescribe various psychotropics that enhance other treatment modalities. Assessing client responses and participating in comprehensive planning in inpatient, community, or home health care settings are critical roles of the advanced-practice nurse.

THE NURSING PROCESS

The following case study is an example of the impact of stress on the GI tract, and it illustrates the nursing care of a client with a psychophysiological disorder.

ASSESSMENT

In treating clients with a psychophysiological disorder, such as Mr. Ekpe, the nurse is challenged to integrate biological concepts to assess client symptoms, identify nursing outcomes, develop effective interventions, and evaluate responses. This process first requires establishing rapport by approaching the client in a caring and nonjudgmental manner; encouraging client and family participation in treatment; and gathering data on current stressors, substance misuse, psychiatric and medical history, present and past symptoms, and coping behaviors. Many clients presenting with psychophysiological disorders have experienced rejection of and skepticism toward their symptoms. In addition, being referred to psychiatry often makes clients feel as though their symptoms are "all in their head." This premise needs to be dispelled quickly to get beyond suspiciousness and anger and focus on building adaptive coping skills.

Inquiring about reasons for seeking treatment and about past treatments and whether they were helpful can reduce these feelings. When past treatment has been unsuccessful, the client's perception of reasons for the lack of success needs to be assessed. Clients with chronic pain disorders are often sensitive to criticism of their illness and may become defensive or argumentative when questioned about pain medication.

TABLE 13–4
Health Teaching for the Angry and Tense Client with a Psychophysiologic Disorder

The next time you find yourself feeling tense and angry, consider using the following techniques:

1. Recognize your anger. Normally, anger and tension manifest as:
   - Increased heart rate and breathing
   - Increased blood pressure
   - Sweating
   - Muscle tension
   - Clenched jaw
   - Need to move around

2. Once you recognize your anger, do the following:
   - Take a time out (get out of the area and away from the stress).
   - Take 10 deep breaths using your abdominal muscles in the following way: Take a deep and slow breath through your nose—as your chest rises, slowly push your abdomen out (this may feel awkward initially, but it is the normal breathing pattern when you are completely relaxed); next exhale slowly through your mouth or nose and gently pull in your abdomen (you should feel relaxed with each breath).
   - Once your body is under control (decreased heart and breathing rate and blood pressure)—your mind and thoughts are clear and focused: ask yourself, "What am I angry about?" If your anger is legitimate, follow up with the person or situation assertively. If it is not legitimate (maybe the feedback was correct and you are overreacting), LET IT GO!

Complete physical and mental status examinations are critical components of the assessment process. Age-appropriate tools can elicit information of life span factors. Children and adolescents must be assessed both individually and in the context of family to determine the significance of the sick role and its impact on homeostasis. Family organization may be tied to the development and maintenance of the child's illness. Assessment of the family's developmental stage and interaction, especially those associated with overprotectiveness, rigidity, and poor problem-solving skills, indicates the family's level of function. Data on the history of symptoms; precipitating stressors, both biological and psychosocial; and symptom maintenance can help the nurse surmise the child's role within the family function (Minuchin et al., 1975).

NURSING DIAGNOSES

♦ Imbalanced Nutrition: Less Than Body Requirements

♦ Ineffective Coping

♦ Deficit Knowledge regarding the role of stress and irritable bowel syndrome

OUTCOME IDENTIFICATION AND PLANNING

Nursing Care Plan 13–1 identifies the desired outcomes for the nursing diagnoses listed above, the nursing actions needed to achieve these outcomes, and the rationales for these actions. In general, major outcomes for clients with stress-related disorders include the following:

1. Development of adaptive coping behaviors

2. Crisis resolution

3. Strengthening and mobilization of support systems

4. Minimization of exacerbation of symptoms

5. Promotion of self-esteem

IMPLEMENTATION

Major nursing interventions have been identified in this chapter in the discussions of specific disorders. Interventions are based on the client's presenting symptoms, developmen-

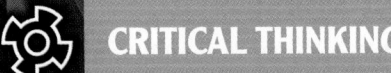

CRITICAL THINKING

An adolescent has lived in the same neighborhood for the past 10 years and has been attending the same high school for the past 2 years. He has made a number of friends at school and has been involved in extracurricular activities. He is, however, somewhat shy and introverted. His parents are divorcing, and he and his mother are moving to another part of the city. This will result in a school change for the teenager.

1. This teen has been physically healthy. Would it be unusual for him to develop physical symptoms at this time?

2. What sort of physical symptoms might one expect to see?

3. What can be done to help this young man adjust to his new situation?

Solutions: Symptoms he could develop might include GI symptoms, anxiety symptoms, or depressive symptoms.

Making him feel comfortable in the new school setting would be important. Encouraging him to maintain contact with his friends from his old school, as well as becoming involved in activities at his new school, would also be helpful in his adjustment.

tal stage, motivation to modify behavior and coping patterns, and access to internal and external resources. Major treatment goals include the development of adaptive stress reduction methods that affect biological processes. Role-playing, various psychotherapies, and psychoeducation regarding the effect of emotions and ineffective coping behaviors on biological processes can enhance clients' coping skills.

Psychophysiological disorders place tremendous demands on clients and families. Family involvement is crucial to the success of interventions. Family members may feel helpless or angry about the client's immense emotional and physical needs, which affect the quality of life. Family life tends to be centered on the client's symptoms, interfering with intimacy and healthy family interactions. Involving the family in the client's treatment decreases feelings of inadequacy, helplessness, and promotes a sense of control and well-being.

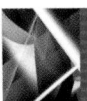

CASE STUDY

The Client with Irritable Bowel Syndrome (Mr. Ekpe)

A 33-year-old man, Mr. Ekpe, is referred to psychiatric triage for evaluation of a recent exacerbation of irritable bowel syndrome. His presenting symptoms—a sudden onset of fear and anxiety, abdominal pain, diarrhea, and nausea—began a week before his visit. His current treatment regimen consists of dietary modifications (e.g., fiber and bulk use) and education about the nature of irritable bowel syndrome.

Mr. Ekpe recently moved to the United States and has experienced great demands from his job and family in the past 18 months. He has recently made several visits to the emergency department complaining of abdominal cramps and diarrhea.

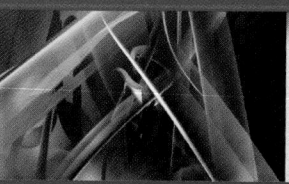

The Client with Irritable Bowel Syndrome (Mr. Ekpe)

Nursing Diagnosis: Imbalanced Nutrition: Less than Body Requirements

Outcome Identification	Nursing Actions	Rationales	Evaluation
1. By [date], client will maintain adequate caloric intake.	1a. Assess nutritional status. 1b. Decrease environmental stress. 1c. Provide diet instructions. 1d. Administer ordered medications.	1a. Determines baseline data. 1b. Stress increases GI motility. 1c. Allows client to gain control over some aspect of care (diet). 1d. Reduces physical stress and promotes comfort.	*Goal met:* Client and family are cooperative in providing baseline data. Client's physical symptoms respond to medication. Client reports decreased stress.

Nursing Diagnosis: Ineffective Coping

Outcome Identification	Nursing Actions	Rationales	Evaluation
1. By [date], client will develop realistic perception of present stressor(s). 2. By [date], client will develop enduring adaptive coping skills.	1a. Explore the meaning of recent present stressors and coping skills. 1b. Encourage ventilation of feelings. 2. Assist in identifying strengths, resources, and coping skills.	1a. Helps the client understand self and present responses. 1b. Validates understanding of meaning of present symptom and disease process. 2. Places focus on positive attributes and increases self-esteem.	*Goal met:* Client returns to prehospitalization level of functioning. Client develops adaptive coping skills. Client's self-esteem increases.

Nursing Diagnosis: Deficit Knowledge
related to the role of stress and irritable bowel syndrome

Outcome Identification	Nursing Actions	Rationales	Evaluation
1. By [date], client will understand the relationship between stress and physical symptoms..	1a. Assess teaching needs (client and family). 1b. Discuss the role of stress and biological responses. 1c. Teach stress management skills. 1d. Inform client and family of symptoms to report.	1a. Helps nurse develop an individualized teaching plan. 1b–d. Increases understanding of disease process and importance of stress management to reduce biological symptoms. Helps client and family gain a greater control over their emotional and physical responses to stress.	*Goal met:* Client and family express understanding the teaching plan and the relationship between stress and physical symptoms.

EVALUATION

Evaluating client responses to interventions is a dynamic process based on outcome identification and includes feedback from the client, family, and other members of the health team. Adaptive behaviors must be strengthened throughout treatment. Changing or eliminating maladaptive behaviors requires patience and understanding because clients with stress-related disorders tend to be extremely demanding, perfectionists, hostile, and sensitive to criticism (Kim et al., 1998, Munakata et al., 1999; Steptoe, 2000). Staff support groups can help the nurse in evaluating treatment outcomes.

SUMMARY

◆ The relationship between the body and mind is well documented.

◆ Stress is an integral part of living and one's ability to mobilize internal and resources to adjust to internal and external demands is crucial to adaptation and health.

◆ Stress affects individuals across the life span, from childhood to older adulthood.

◆ The body's immune system is affected by stress in a number of ways, including a reduction in NK cell activity and decreased white blood cell count and T-cell count.

◆ Nurses are in a unique position to assess stress in the lives of their clients and assist them in the development of effective coping skills.

◆ Adaptation to stress is determined by personality style. Type A and Type B personality styles have been identified.

◆ Individuals with Type A personality have been identified to have an increase in anger, hostility, and aggression, which are risk factors for the development of coronary artery disease (CAD).

◆ Certain traits have been identified as successful coping traits, such as hardiness, whereas other traits have been identified to be associated with illness.

◆ Primary medical conditions that are affected by stress include cardiovascular disorders, pulmonary disorders, immunological disorders, gastrointestinal disorders, dermatological disorders, and chronic pain disorders.

◆ Treatment of these disorders requires making an accurate assessment of all areas of the client's life and the ability to cope with stress.

◆ Major techniques for treatment of stress-related illnesses include psychoeducation, relaxation techniques, assertiveness training, and psychotherapy.

STUDY QUESTIONS

1. All of the following statements may be indications of stress-related alterations *except:*
   a. a decrease in the white blood cell count
   b. a reduction in natural killer cell activity
   c. a decrease in red blood cell count
   d. a decrease in T-cell production

2. Type A personality and Type B personality coping styles affect one's health status. Which of the following states best reflects Type A personality style?
   a. "I have all day to complete this job."
   b. "I am unsure if I can do this!"
   c. "Let's finish eating and go walking!"
   d. "I could just lie back and relax all day."

3. Which of the following are considered successful coping traits with regards to illness?
   a. Extroversion
   b. Introversion
   c. Constructive thinking
   d. Hardiness

4. The nurse learns that Jody's grandfather died 3 weeks ago. He was very close to his grandfather. Additionally, he began the first grade two weeks ago. An important nursing intervention at this time is to:
   a. encourage Jody and his parents to talk about the recent event
   b. talk to the parents alone and encourage them to talk to their son when they return home
   c. assess the family dynamics and the role of the child's illness in keeping the family together
   d. refer the family to the psychiatric APN for family therapy

5. Marty, a 45-year-old woman is in the ambulatory care unit for the third time this week complaining of itching and a skin rash that has not responded to a topical cortisone cream. She is noticeably anxious, tense, and demanding. Which of the following questions reflects an understanding of her situation?
   a. "What recent changes have you experienced over the past 6 months?"
   b. "I noticed that you look pretty anxious. What kind of treatment are you receiving for this condition?"
   c. "When was the last time you had a complete physical?"
   d. "You need to try another medication because this one is not helping you."

6. Stress increases the risk of complex physiological disorders. Which of the following does not represent an alteration in the immune system?
   a. Cancer
   b. Gastroenteritis
   c. Herpes
   d. Epstein-Barr virus

7. When assessing a child with a psychophysiological disorder, namely asthma, the nurse should expect to find which of the following?
   a. A tense and controlling family system
   b. Low-keyed and structured family system
   c. Open and healthy communication among family members
   d. Calm demeanor

8. Which of the following is a common finding in children and adults with stress-related physical conditions?
   a. Internalized emotions
   b. Close family ties
   c. Nonspecific physical complaints
   d. Both a and c

9. The nurse is teaching a client about measures to reduce dermatological reactions to stress. Which of the following *would not* be included?
   a. Antianxiety medication, such as lorazepam, to stay calm
   b. Anger management techniques
   c. Deep breathing exercises
   d. Assertive communication skills

10. Which of the following assessments made by the nurse would be essential in understanding behavior of a client with a stress-related physical condition?
    a. Closed body language, tense, overly appeasing, and negative self-talk
    b. Open body language, outwardly confident, but internally insecure
    c. Openly communicative and cooperative
    d. Closed body language, good eye contact, and calm

RESOURCES

Please note that because Internet resources are of a time-sensitive nature and URL addresses may change or be deleted, searches should also be conducted by association or topic.

Internet Resources

1. Locate on the Internet a site with a life stress test. Complete the test and determine your susceptibility to stress.

2. Locate on the Internet a site containing stress management techniques for coping with stress.

http://www.healthfinder.gov   Office of Disease Prevention and Health Promotion, U.S. Department of Health and Human Services

http://www.plainsense.com   Key website for general health information

http://www.stressfree.com   Stress Free Net

http://www.unl.edu/stress/mgmt/

Other Resources

American Institute of Stress
   124 Park Avenue
   Yonkers, NY 10703
   (914) 963-1200
   http://www.stress.org

REFERENCES

Akamoto, S., Okano, K., Sano, T., Yachida, S., Izuishi, K., Usuki, H., et al. (2007). Neutrophil elastase inhibitor (sivelestat) preserves antitumor immunity and reduces the inflammatory mediators associated with major surgery. *Surgery Today, 37,* 359–365.

Alexander, F. (1939). Psychological aspects of medicine. *Psychosomatic Medicine, 1,* 7–18.

Alexander, F. (1950). *Psychosomatic medicine: Its principles and applications.* New York: W. W. Norton.

American Psychiatric Association. (2000). *Diagnostic and Statistical Manual of Mental Disorders* (4th edition, Text Revision) *(DSM-IV-TR).* Washington, DC: Author.

Benson, H. (1975). *The relaxation response.* New York: William Morrow.

Besedovsky, H. O., & Rey, A. D. (2007). Physiology of psychoneuroimmunology: A personal view. *Brain, Behavior and Immunity, 21,* 34–44.

Colman, I., Wadsworth, M. E., Croudace, T. J., & Jones, P. B. (2007). Forty-year psychiatric outcomes following assessment for internalizing disorder in adolescence. *American Journal of Psychiatry, 164,* 126–133.

Eaker, E. D., Sullivan, L. M., Kelly-Hayes, M., D'Agostino, R. B., & Benjamin, E. J. (2005). Tension and anxiety and the prediction of the 10-year incidence of coronary heart disease, atrial fibrillation, and total mortality: The Framingham Offspring Study. *Psychosomatic Medicine, 67,* 692–696.

Fluermond, J. & Sharpe, I. (2005). Is it all in the head? The psychological effects of chronic pain and the effectiveness of modern therapies. *Ethnicity and Disease, 15*(3 Suppl 4), S4–47–48.

Freud, S. (1958). On psycho-analysis. In J. Strackney (Ed. and Trans.), *The standard edition of the complete psychological works of Sigmund Freud* (Vol. 12, pp. 207–211). London: Hogarth Press. (Original work published 1911)

Friedman, M. (1996). *Type A behavior: Its diagnosis and treatment* (pp. 31–51). New York: Plenam Press.

Friedman, M., & Rosenman, R. H. (1974). Type A behavior and your heart. New York: Knopf.

Fuller, G. D. (1977). *Biofeedback: Methods and procedures in clinical practice.* San Francisco: Biofeedback Press.

Gallacher J. F., Sweetnam, P. M., Yarnell, J. W., Elwood, P. C., & Stansfeld, S. A. (2003). Is type A behavior really a trigger for coronary heart disease events? *Psychosomatic Medicine, 65*(3), 339–346.

Garralda, M. E., & Rangel, L. (2005). Chronic fatigue syndrome of childhood. Comparative study with emotional disorders. *European Child and Adolescent Psychiatry, 14,* 424–430.

Homnick, D. N., & DeJong, S. R. (2007). Parent-reported physician diagnosis is an important factor in asthma management: An elementary school survey. *Clinical Pediatrics (Philadelphia), 46,* 431–436.

Kim, J. S., Yoon, S. S., Lee, S. I., Yoo, H. J., Kim, C. Y., Choi-Kwon, S., et al. (1998). Type A behavior and stroke: High tenseness dimension may be a risk factor for cerebral infarction. *European Neurology, 39*(3), 168–173.

Kim, T. S., Pae, C. U., Jeong, J. T., Kim, S. D., Chung, K. I., & Lee, C. (2006). Temperament and character dimensions in patients with atopic dermatitis. *Journal of Dermatology, 33,* 10–15.

Kuloğlu, M., Atmaca, M., Onal, S., Geçici, O., Bulut, V., & Tezcan, E. (2007). Neopterin levels and dexamethasone suppression test in obsessive-compulsive disorder. *Psychiatry Research, 151,* 265–270.

Kurukulasratchy, R. J., Matthews, S., & Ashad, S. H. (2006). Relationship between childhood atopy and wheeze: What mediates wheezing in atopic phenotypes? *Annals of Allergies, Asthma and Immunology, 97,* 84–91.

Levenson, J. L., McDaniel, J. S., Moran, M. G., & Stoudemire, A. (1999). Psychological factors affecting medical conditions. In R. E. Hales, S. C. Yudofsky, & J. A. Talbott (Eds.), *The American Psychiatric Press textbook of psychiatry* (3rd ed., pp. 635–661). Washington, DC: American Press.

Liebman, R., Minuchin. S., & Baker, L. (1974). The use of structural family therapy in treatment of intractable asthma. *American Journal of Psychiatry, 131,* 535–540.

Locke, G. R., 3rd, Weaver, A. L., Melton, L. J., 3rd, & Talley, N. J. (2004). Psychosocial factors are linked to functional gastrointestinal disorders: A population based nested case-control study, *American Journal of Gastroenterology, 99,* 350–357.

Marsac, M. L., Funk, J. B., & Nelson, L. (2007). Coping styles, psychological functioning and quality of life in children with asthma. *Child: Care and Health Development, 33,* 360–367.

Menninger, K. (1963). *The vital balance.* New York: Viking Press.

Minuchin, S. (1974). *Families and family therapy: A structural approach.* Cambridge, MA: Harvard University Press.

Minuchin, S., Baker, L., Rosman, B. L., Liebman, R., Milman, L., & Todd, T. C. (1975). A conceptual model of psychosomatic illness in children. *Archives of General Psychiatry, 32,* 1031–1038.

Moore, R. K., Groves, D. G., Bridson, J. D., Grayson, A. D., Wong, H., Leach, A., et al. (2007). A brief cognitive-behavioral intervention reduces hospital admissions in refractory angina patients. *Journal of Pain Symptom Management, 33,* 310–316.

Morikawa, Y., Kitaoka-Higashischiguchi, K., Tanimoto, C., Hayashi, M., Oketani, R., Miura, K., Nishijo, M., & Nakagawa, H. (2005). A cross-sectional study of the relationship of job stress with natural killer cell activity and natural killer cell subsets among health nurses. *Journal of Occupational Health, 47,* 378–383.

Munakala, M., Hiraizumi, T., Nunokawa, T., Ito, N. Taguchi, F., Yamauchi, Y., et al. (1999). Type A behavior is associated with an increased risk of left ventricular hypertrophy in male patients with essential hypertension. *Journal of Hypertension, 17*(1), 115–120.

North, C. S., Hong, B. A., & Alpers, D. H. (2007). Relationship of functional gastrointestinal disorders and psychiatric disorders: Implications for treatment. *World Journal of Gastroenterology, 14,* 2020–2027.

Paré, G., Jaana, M., & Sicotte, C. (2007). Systematic review of home telemonitoring for chronic diseases: The evidence base. *Journal of American Medical Informatics Association, 14,* 269–277.

Perman, J. (1954). Pain as an old friend. *Lancet, 1,* 633–635.

Picardi, A., Pasquini, P., Abeni, D., Fassone, G., Mazzotti, E., & Fava, G. A. (2005). Psychosomatic assessment of skin diseases in clinical practice. *Psychotherapy and Psychosomatics, 74*(5), 315–322.

Price, J. R. (2000). Managing physical symptoms: The clinical assessment as treatment. *Journal of Psychosomatic Research, 48*(1), 1–10.

Rajkowski, J., Majczynski, H., Clayton, E., & Aston-Jones, G. (2004). Activation of monkey locus coeruleus neurons varies with difficulty and performance in a target detection task. *Journal of Neurophysiology, 92,* 361–371.

Rath, B., Donato, J., Duggan, A., Perrin, K., Bronfin, D. R., Ratard, R., et al. (2007). Adverse health outcomes after Hurricane Katrina among children and adolescents with chronic conditions. *Journal of Health Care for the Poor and Underserved, 18,* 405–417

Saito, Y. A., Prather, C. M., Van Dyke, C. T., Fett, S., Zinsmeister, A. R., & Locke, G. R. (2004). Effects of multidisciplinary education on outcomes in patients with irritable bowel syndrome. *Clinical Gastroenterolgy and Hepatology 2*(7), 576–584.

Selye, H. (1976). *Stress in health and disease.* New York: McGraw-Hill.

Slack, L. K., Muthana, M., Hopkinson, K., Survana, S. K., Espigares, E., Mirza, S., et al. (2007). Administration of the stress protein gp96 prolongs rat cardiac allograft survival, modifies rejection-associated inflammatory events, and induces a state of peripheral T-cell hyporesponsiveness. *Cell Stress and Chaperones, 12,* 71–82.

Smith, J. C. (1997). *Understanding stress and coping.* New York: Macmillan.

Smith, T. W., Glazer, K., Ruiz, J. M., & Gallo, L. C. (2004). Hostility, anger, aggressiveness and coronary disease: An interpersonal perspective on personality, emotion and health. *Journal of Personality, 72,* 1217–1270.

Steptoe, A. (2000). Psychosocial factors in the development of hypertension. *Annotated Medicine, 32*(5), 371–375.

Vale, S. (2005). Psychosocial stress and cardiovascular disease. *Postgraduate Medical Journal, 81,* 429–435.

Whitehead, W. E., Levy, R. L., VonKorff, M., Feld, A. D., Palsson, O. S., Turner, M., & Drossman, D. A. (2004). The usual medical care of irritable bowel syndrome. *Alimentary Pharmacology & Therapeutics, 20*(11–12), 1305–1315.

Wingate, D. L. (1985). The brain-gut link. *Viewpoints of Digestive Disease, 17,* 17–20.

Wright, R. J. (2005). Stress and atopic disorders. *Journal of Allergy & Clinical Immunology, 116*(6), 1301–1306.

Yates, W. R. (2004). Gastrointestinal Disorders. In Sadock, B. J. & Sadock, V. A. (Eds.), *Kaplan & Sadock's Comprhensive Textbook of Psychiatry Volume II,* (pp. 2112–2123). Philadelphia: Lippincott Williams & Wilkins.

Young, H. A., & Ortaldo, J. (2006). Cytokines as critical co-stimulatory molecules in modulating the immune response of natural killer cells. *Cell Research, 16,* 20–24.

SUGGESTED READINGS

Opolski, M. & Wilson, I. (2005). Asthma and depression: a pragmatic review of the literature and recommendations for future research. *Clinical Practice and Epidemiology in Mental Health 2005, 1*(18), 1–7.

Padwal, R., Campbell, N., & Touyz, R. M. (2005). Applying the 2005 Canadian hypertension education program recommendations: 3. Lifestyle modifications to prevent and treat hypertension. *Canadian Medical Association Journal, 173*(7), 749–751.

Scalco, A. Z., Scalco, M. Z., Serro Azul, J. B., & Neto, F. L. (2005). Hypertension and depression. *Clinics, 60*(3), 241–250.

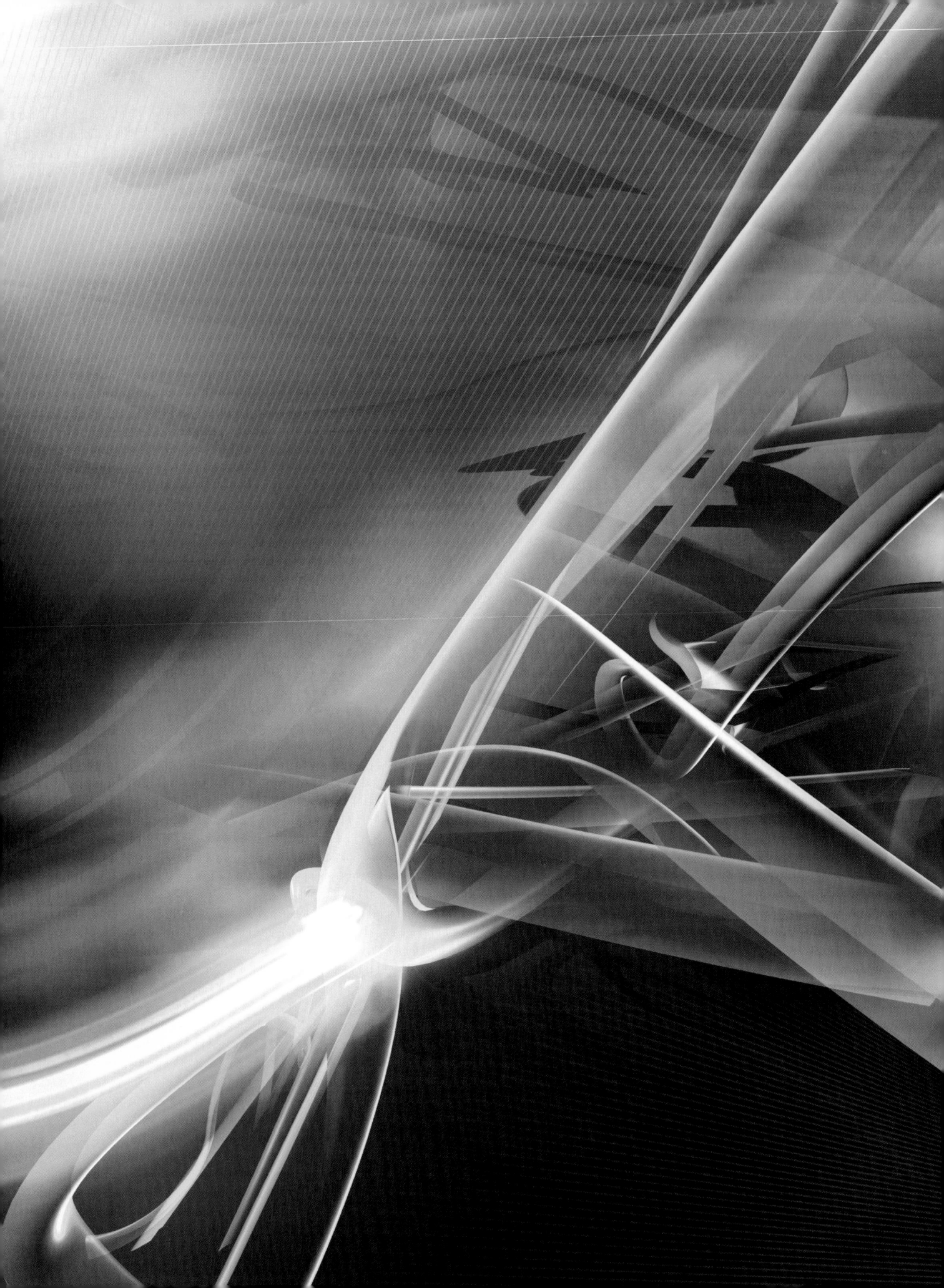

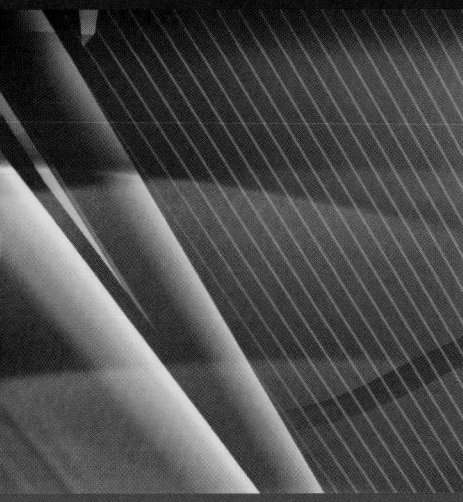

CHAPTER 14

The Client with Schizophrenia and Other Psychotic Disorders

Barbara Jones Warren, PhD, RN, CNS, CS
Deborah Antai-Otong, MS, APRN, BC, FAAN

KEY TERMS

Autism: Denotes the presence of abnormal and impaired development in social and communication skills and severely restricted activity and interests.

Cognitive Enhancement Therapy: A behavioral intervention designed to improve cognition in individuals with schizophrenia who exhibit neurocognitive symptoms.

Cognitive Symptoms: Dissimilar to positive and negative symptoms are discreet and denote poor executive functioning or deficits in attention, working memory, secondary (storage) memory, and semantic memory. Normally, cognitive symptoms are only detected when neuropsychological tests are performed. Cognitive deficits are associated with poor social and occupational functioning in persons with schizophrenia.

Delusion: A fixed false belief unchanged by logic.

Hallucinations: Refer to a false sensory perception occurring in the absence of an external stimulus.

Negative Symptoms: Denote schizophrenic symptoms associated with structural brain abnormalities. Most negative symptoms include blunted affect, inability to experience pleasure, apathy, a lack of feeling, and impaired attention.

Positive Symptoms: Refer to schizophrenic symptoms with good premorbid functioning, acute onset, and positive response to typical and atypical antipsychotics. Common positive symptoms include hallucinations, delusions, disorganized thinking and speech, and gross behavioral disturbances. These symptoms are linked with dysregulation of biochemical processes.

Psychosis: A person's symptom state that refers to the presence of reality misinterpretations, disorganized thinking, and lack of awareness regarding true and false reality.

Reality Testing: The ability to logically and objectively evaluate and judge the world outside self.

Thought Disorder: Often found in individuals with schizophrenia, this term refers to impaired thought processes or disorganized thoughts during which time the client has difficulty organizing thoughts or connecting them logically. Manifestations of disorganized thoughts or thought disorder include incoherent speech, thought blocking, or using unintelligible words (neologisms).

COMPETENCIES

Upon completion of this chapter, the learner should be able to:

1. Describe major symptoms of schizophrenia—positive, negative, and cognitive symptoms

2. Discuss major causative factors of schizophrenia and implications for nursing interventions

3. Explain nursing interventions to manage acute psychotic symptoms

4. Describe pharmacological and psychosocial treatment modalities and implications for nursing practice

5. Discuss nursing interventions for side effects associated with pharmacological agents used to treat schizophrenia

6. Develop a plan of care for a client exhibiting altered sensory perception experience

CHAPTER OUTLINE

DEFINITION AND OVERVIEW

It is generally accepted that the underpinnings of schizophrenia are complex and vast and are associated with genetic influences interacting with environmental insults that result in an array of phenotypes in the schizophrenia spectrum (e.g., schizophrenia, schizoaffective disorder) (Gur et al., 2007). Historically, schizophrenia has been classified as a major psychiatric brain disorder with a chronic, neurodevelopmental, severe, and disabling course. Approximately 1 percent of United States adults or 2.4 million people have schizophrenia. According to the World Health Organization (2005) about 24 million people worldwide suffer from schizophrenia. Schizophrenia is a treatable disorder, in which treatment is more effective in its initial or first episode. The term psychosis refers to a retreat from reality testing that stems from sensory perceptual disturbances, including hallucinations or delusions. Typically, persons with schizophrenia hear voices or see things that others do not hear or see. In addition, they often believe others can read their thoughts or their thoughts are broadcast for others to hear, such as over the television, which results in fearfulness, agitation, isolation, or pacing. Major symptoms of schizophrenia fall into three categories: positive, negative, and cognitive. Together these symptoms lead to deterioration in the level of social, interpersonal, occupational, and academic functioning and impair quality of life. Positive symptoms include hallucinations, delusions, thought disorder, and disorders of movement. Negative symptoms include amotivation or decrease in ability to initiate and sustain planned activity, apathy, and difficulty finding pleasure in daily living. Cognitive symptoms, which may be referred to as cognitive deficits, often interfere with one's ability to plan and organize due to poor executive functioning, attentional deficits, and impaired working memory (the ability to keep recently learned information in mind and use it right away, such as getting someone's telephone number and being able to remember and call). Predominant negative and cognitive symptoms have been associated with poor treatment response, particularly with conventional or typical antipsychotic agents, such as haloperidol (Haldol). The advent of atypical antipsychotic agents has demonstrated promise in reducing negative symptoms and cognitive deficits.

Cognitive deficits can cause significant emotional distress by interfering with the client's ability to attain an optimal level of functioning and be able to lead a normal life. Collectively, positive, negative, and cognitive symptoms can lead to long-term disability. (See Table 14–1, Major Types of Adult Schizophrenia.) Major subtypes of schizophrenia are: paranoid, disorganized, catatonic, undifferentiated, and residual. Specifiers for each subtype are listed in Table 14–1. Symptoms of schizophrenia evolve through two phases: prodromal and active (Table 14–2). The *prodromal phase* of schizophrenia may evolve acutely or have a slower onset. Symptoms within this phase include drastic alteration in the normal behavior patterns, unusual preoccupation concerning other persons, social isolation, and occupational and academic impairment (American Psychiatric Association [APA], 2000). Clinical symptoms of the *acute phase* are hallmark symptoms of schizophrenia that include positive, negative, and cognitive symptoms (APA, 2000).

Current research indicates that the global burden of mental illness is second only to cardiovascular disease worldwide (Lopez, Mathers, Ezzati, Jamison, & Murray, 2006). In the United States, one out of five Americans incurs a mental disorder throughout any year (DHHS, 1999). Statistics for children ages 9 to 17 years are even higher, with 25 percent of them receiving mental health treatment within a year's time (Lopez

et al., 2006). Schizophrenia is a prevalent psychiatric disorder that affects people globally. More than 50 percent of individuals with schizophrenia lack access to mental health services. These numbers are even greater in developing countries (WHO, 2005). Persons from diverse racial and ethnic background have demonstrated poorer treatment outcomes due to limited access to treatment, stigma associated with mental illness, and distrust of the health care system. Despite the advent of atypical antipsychotic agents and a move toward community-based care, schizophrenia remains a high-cost illness because of the enormous health care needs associated with the disorder (Mangalore & Knapp, 2007). Care of individuals with schizophrenia normally occurs in home and community-based settings and by limiting inpatient services to acute symptoms. Active participation by clients and families is critical to treating individuals with schizophrenia. The purpose of this chapter is to describe the multifaceted cause of this brain disorder, treatment considerations, and life span issues. The role of the psychiatric-mental health nurse and implications for nursing practice are also incorporated throughout this chapter.

EPIDEMIOLOGY AND PREVALENCE

As previously discussed, schizophrenia is a prevalent psychiatric disorder worldwide and spans across all cultural groups (Mangalore & Knapp, 2007; WHO, 2005). It is estimated that schizophrenia accounts for approximately 2.5 percent of all health care expenditures. The impact of schizophrenia can be monumental to those individuals diagnosed with it when appropriate treatment is not accessed or is delayed. Schizophrenia generally emerges during adolescence or in one's 20s or 30s. However, it may occur in later adulthood. Among middle-aged and older adults with schizophrenia, about 80 percent have early onset schizophrenia, with the remaining 20 percent with onset after age 40 and very-late onset schizophrenia-like symptoms in the sixth decade of life (Mazak,

---

TABLE 14–1
Major Types of Adult Schizophrenia

Catatonic—marked by a catatonic state or stupor in which the client is unresponsive to his or her surroundings and displays a lack of spontaneous psychomotor activity (rigid posture or bizarre) or mutism

Disorganized—major symptoms include confusion or loose association, disorganized thoughts, and blunt or inappropriate affect

Paranoid—marked by one or more systematic persecutory delusions, auditory hallucinations with a single theme

Undifferentiated—manifested by pronounced delusions, hallucinations, and disorganized thought processes and behavior

Residual—generally there is an absence of pronounced delusions, hallucinations, confusion, or disorganized thoughts or behaviors

Note. Data from *Diagnostic and Statistical Manual of Mental Disorders* (4th ed.), by the American Psychiatric Association, 2000, Washington, DC: Author. Adapted with permission.

RESEARCH ABSTRACT

Self-Care Symptom Management Strategies for Auditory Hallucinations among Inpatients with Schizophrenia at Veterans' Hospital in Taiwan

Tsai, Y.-F., & Ku, Y.-C. (2005). *Archives of Psychiatric Nursing, 19*(4), 194–199.

Study Problem/Purpose

To examine self-care management strategies for auditory hallucinations among persons with schizophrenia on an inpatient unit.

Methods

The researchers used an exploratory descriptive design to understand the severity, degree of interference, and self-care management approaches for auditory hallucinations. Self-report and semistructured questionnaires were employed to identify 36 self-management strategies of 200 clients with schizophrenia on an inpatient unit at a veterans' hospital in Taiwan.

Findings

Data from this study indicated that the most commonly used strategies to manage auditory hallucinations were to ignore them, cover the ears, and watch television. Covering the ears was found to be an ineffective strategy to cope with auditory hallucinations and was considered a passive method in Western cultures. Researchers also found that watching television was the most common approach in Western cultures, whereas clients with schizophrenia in Chinese cultures were more likely to use a more passive method, such as ignoring auditory hallucinations, as a first choice.

Implications for Psychiatric Nursing

Although these findings cannot be generalized due to a convenience sampling and small sample size, they can be used to recognize the importance of client-centered nursing interventions. They also provide interventions that promote self-care management and self-efficacy in clients with schizophrenia.

TABLE 14–2
Schizophrenia: Course of the Illness

Acute (Active) Phase	Prodromal and Residual Phases
Definition Active Phase: presence of psychotic symptoms—at least one from the list of positive symptoms (*DSM-IV* Option A1)	**Definitions** Prodromal phase—clear deterioration in functioning occurring prior to active phase involving minimum of two symptoms listed below. Residual phase—persistence of minimum of two symptoms following active phase.
Symptoms Positive symptoms • Delusion • Hallucination • Disorganized speech • Bizarre or disorganized behavior **Negative symptoms** • Flat affect • Avolition • Alogia • Anhedonia • Attention impairment **Impairment in functioning (one or more major areas)** • Work • Interpersonal relations • Self-care • Failure to achieve expected levels of interpersonal, academic, or occupational development	**Symptoms** • Marked social isolation and withdrawal • Marked impairment in role functioning as wage earner, student, or homemaker • Markedly peculiar behavior • Marked disturbance in speech Circumstantial Poverty of speech and content Vague Overelaborate • Odd beliefs • Unusual perceptual experiences • Marked lack of initiative, interests, energy **Minimum Duration** Continuous signs persisting a minimum of 6 months Must include active-phase period lasting 1 week to 1 month
Minimum Duration 1 month	

Note. Data from *DSM-IV-TR* by the American Psychiatric Association (2000).

Zemishlani, Aizenberg, & Barak, 2005). Regardless of age of onset, data from longitudinal studies implicate that most first-episode clients have had substantial cognitive decline at the time of their initial hospitalization and that it remains fairly stable through at least 10 years of illness (Hoff, et al., 2005; Siegel, et al., 2006). Women generally experience an earlier onset than men do (APA, 2000). The onset of childhood schizophrenia is rare, with only a few cases being documented before age 10. Persons experiencing earlier onset of schizophrenia usually experience more problems with disordered movement from adolescence into adulthood and development of appropriate social relationships and interactions. Emerging epidemiological data suggest that schizophrenia is a neurodevelopment disorder and point to insult to prenatal brain development in the etiology of schizophrenia and implicate environmental influences, such as stress hormones which may predispose individuals to schizophrenia (Rapoport, Addington, Frangou, & Psych, 2005).

Persons with schizophrenia and other psychiatric disorders are overrepresented in jails and prisons. They also represent one-fourth to one-third of the U.S. homeless population (Folsom & Jeste, 2002). Law enforcement, legal, and mental health professionals are concerned that the criminal justice system has become a principal disposition for many difficult-to-manage clients with schizophrenia and other severe mental disorders. The U.S. Department of Justice Bureau of Justice Statistics Report, edited by James and Glaze (2006), reports that about a quarter of both state prisoners and jail inmates had a mental health problem compared to a fifth of those who did not; had served three or more prior incarcerations; and female inmates had higher prevalence of mental health problems than their male counterparts. Of these numbers only 1 in 3 state prisoners, 1 in 4 federal prisoners, and 1 in 6 jail prisoners diagnosed with a psychiatric problem actually received mental health care since their admission (James & Glaze, 2006).

Communities are beginning to address this issue by diversion programs created by local mental health courts and police departments. Preliminary findings indicate success in reducing the number of incarcerations, increasing coordination between police officers and mental health services, and linking clients to appropriate mental health community services and resources. Nurses must be prepared to meet the medical and mental health needs of persons with psychiatric and substance-related disorders by working with staff to establish treatment goals, create a liaison between the treatment team and justice system, provide appropriate and consistent structure, and ensure a safe work situation. Health education with the client and family must be an integral aspect of the treatment plan.

CO-OCCURRING MEDICAL AND PSYCHIATRIC DISORDERS

There is also a higher rate of medical and psychiatric mortality when compared to the general population. Prevalent co-occurring medical conditions include cardiovascular disease, respiratory disease, diabetes, substance use disorders, sexually transmitted diseases, and other infectious diseases (e.g., hepatitis C and HIV) (Buckley & Brown, 2006; Folsom et al., 2005). Suicide is the primary cause of death in persons with schizophrenia. A high percentage of persons with schizophrenia have substance related disorders and depressive symptoms. Co-occuring psychiatric disorders, such as substance-related disorders and depression, are common in persons with schizophrenia and predictably worsen the course of illness. The lifetime co-occurrence of schizophrenia and substance use disorder has increased 20 to 30 percent resulting in about 70 to 80 percent of clients with schizophrenia with a lifetime substance use disorder (Lambert, et al., 2005; Westmeyer, 2006). Male gender, younger age group, and socioeconomic problems appear to be risk factors associated with substance use disorders. There exists a number of negative consequences of substance use among persons with schizophrenia that include nonadherence to treatment, persistent psychosis, relapse, and hospitalization. Addressing this problem is paramount to symptom management and recovery (Wilk et al., 2006). Psychiatric nurses are poised to understand the relationship between substance use disorders and psychosis and to implement primary prevention interventions to identify individuals at risk and provide early treatment of substance use disorders. In comparison, depressive symptoms are common in all phases of schizophrenia (Limosin, Loze, Philippe, Casadebaig, & Rouillon, 2007). The prevalence of depressive symptoms in persons with schizophrenia varies from 7 to 75 percent and may occur during the prodromal phase (Hafner et al., 2005; Siris, 2000). Depressive symptoms are most common during a psychotic episode at a prevalence of about 50 percent (Van der Heiden, Konnecke, Maurer, et al., 2005).

CULTURAL FACTORS

Persons from different cultural and ethnic groups may have health practices unique to their culture that might mimic altered sensory perceptions. When caring for the client who present with symptoms of schizophrenia, it is imperative that the psychiatric-mental health nurse carefully assess the client's preferences, wishes, and perspectives in order to make an accurate differential diagnosis between the client's normal health practices and the presence of hallucinations, illusions, and delusions associated with underlying with psychiatric condition. Behaviors or symptom expressions may be misunderstood. Historically some cultures and ethnic groups who present with psychotic symptoms have been diagnosed with schizophrenia rather than a mood disorder. Psychiatric mental health nurses must take the time to assess and interpret the client's experience and symptoms based on objective and subjective data to ensure that the client receives an accurate diagnosis and mental health care that is congruent with the client's cultural expectations (Brekke, Nakagami, Kee, & Green, 2005). See Chapter 7 for further discussion of cultural factors and mental health.

The precise etiology or pathogenesis of schizophrenia remains unclear, but compelling evidence implicates genetic and environmental interface and alterations; psychodynamic issues; and dysregulation in vast neurobiological processes and alterations in neuroanatomical structures, brain development, and substance abuse (Riley & Kendler, 2006; Westmeyer, 2006).

GENETIC THEORY

The link between genetic susceptibility to schizophrenia is well documented although the question of schizophrenia running in families continues to be explored. Riley & Kendler (2005) submit that data from early family studies involving role of families in the transmission of schizophrenia was inconclusive. Most of the early family studies had three key limitations: no control groups; diagnoses were made unblind (researchers knew the subjects); and there was a lack of structured interviews and clearly defined diagnostic criteria (Riley & Kendler, 2005). Major findings from recent family studies indicate:

◆ The risk of schizophrenia in families varied widely across studies from 1.4 to 16.2 percent.

◆ The risk for schizophrenia in the relatives of non-psychiatric control subjects was consistent across studies—0.2 to 1.1 percent.

◆ The risk of schizophrenia was higher in the relatives of schizophrenia probands than in relatives of control probands (Riley & Kendler, 2005).

Based on these data there is significant evidence to further strengthen the premise that genetics is only one part of the pathogenesis of schizophrenia. Scientists continue to search for a clearer explanation of the interface between genetic susceptibility and specific DNA variants, protein alterations, or neurobiological processes (Riley & Kendler, 2006). Cannon and colleagues (2006) submit there is a critical urgency to translate the complex nature of genotype-phenotype relationships within the vast dimensions of brain structure and function that are compromised in psychiatric conditions such as schizophrenia.

PSYCHODYNAMIC THEORY

The *psychodynamic theory* evolved from the work of Bleuler (1950) and Freud (1959). Their works indicate that schizophrenia developed because of the psychic alterations that occurred within a person. In addition, these alterations are contingent on the poor caregiving that is provided within the child's environment. However, both of these scholars believed that the psychic alterations are somehow tied to the genetic or physiological changes that develop within the growing child's environment.

NEUROBIOLOGICAL THEORY

The neurobiological theory involves the changes that occur within the brains of persons diagnosed with schizophrenia. These changes occur within five system areas: three anatomic systems—prefrontal, limbic, and basal ganglia—and two functional systems—language and memory. In addition, the neurochemical system coordinates the communication between the anatomic and functional systems.

Neuroanatomical Structures

The pathogenesis of schizophrenia is manifold. The most prominent and consistent finding in schizophrenia is an enlarged ventricular system with a subsequent decreased brain volume, with reduced regional hippocampus, thalamus, and frontal lobes (Antonova, Sharma, Morris, & Kumari, 2004). Glutamate is the key excitatory neurotransmitter in the brain and plays a primary role in prefrontal cortical function and vital behavioral activities, including memory and learning. Mounting evidence implicates dysregulation glutamate neurotransmission in the pathogenesis of schizophrenia and prefrontal cortical functioning (Sur & Kinney, 2007).

Overall, normal anatomic brain tissue and capacity are reduced in persons who have schizophrenia. For example, scans of these persons' brains illustrate an enlarged third ventricle, decreased tangles, and less electrical activity. The cortex of the brain is the last section of the human brain to develop. It is responsible for the coordination of information into the rest of the brain, controls arousal and emotions, focuses attention, and assists in the formation of abstract thinking (Hall, 2006). For example, a person with schizophrenia often has trouble concentrating and thinking abstractly. In addition she is often impulsive and may exhibit inappropriate behavior and actions.

The seat of emotions of the limbic system is located under the cortex. It is comprised of the hippocampus, amygdala, and fornix. The limbic system regulates an individual's emotions and memory. Someone with the diagnosis of schizophrenia has a structural change within the limbic system that often creates impulsivity, aggression, and sexually inappropriate behavior. In addition, these individuals often have problems with learning new information owing to the damage within the hippocampus area (Hall, 2006). Figure 14–1 illustrates the degeneration of the coronal section of the limbic system.

The basal ganglia is responsible for the initiation and control of muscle activity and movements as well as postural changes. A person diagnosed with schizophrenia may have problems with her ability to determine where her body is in relationship to others. Thus, she may accidentally run into others as she walks and moves.

Functional Systems Symptomatology

The functional system is comprised of the language and memory systems located within the amygdala and the hippocampus regions (e.g., Broca and Wernicke's areas, respectively) of the brain. The functional system is responsible for the integration of learning and memory within a person's brain. It is postulated that structural changes within these areas may lead to the development of altered sensory perception problems such as hallucinations and delusions. In addition, persons with schizophrenia may have problems understanding language as well as communicating with other persons (Koeda et al., 2006).

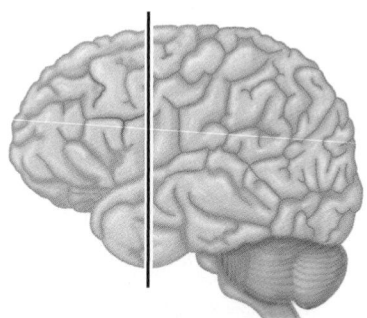

LIMBIC SYSTEM DEGENERATION
(CORONAL SECTION)

Cingulate gyrus*

*These areas show degeneration in schizophrenia

Thalamus

Basal ganglia*

Hippocampus*

Parahippocampal gyrus

Substantia nigra

Hypothalamus

Brain stem

Amygdala*

Medial temporal lobe*

Much is still unknown about the cause of schizophrenia. Biological, genetic, and psychosocial factors combine to make certain people—about 1 in 100—more vulnerable to this disorder. One proposed biological explanation for schizophrenia is that an event during prenatal development of the brain destroyed a significant amount of the neurons of the limbic system. There is radiographic evidence of degeneration in the medial temporal lobe, the cingulate gyrus, the amygdala, the hippocampus, and the basal ganglia that supports the hypothesis of abnormal neurotransmitter activity and response. *(Arrows in drawing indicate dopamine pathways.)*

Figure 14–1 Limbic system degeneration (coronal section).

Neurochemical System

Dysregulation of several neurotransmitters, such as dopaminergic, primarily D_4 and glutamatergic systems in the prefrontal cortex, make this region a target for pharmacotherapy (Mehler-Wex, Riederer, & Gerlach, 2007). Research indicates that D_4 receptor is vital in prefrontal cortex functioning and pathogenesis of schizophrenia and otherneuropsychiatric disorders. Deficits in this brain region also account for neurocognitive deficits associated with schizophrenia, including working memory tasks. Apart from aberrations in D_4 receptor, hypofunction in NMDA receptors has also been implicated in the neurobiology of schizophrenia (Tsai & Coyle, 2002). The interface between NMDA and D_4 receptor in prefrontal pyramidal neuronal regions may play a key role in cognitive and emotional processes in prefrontal neural pathways, making them target sites for antipsychotic medications.

Groupings of neurons are involved in the release of the neurotransmitters of dopamine (DA) (Figure 14–2), norepinephrine (NE), serotonin (5-HT), acetylcholine (M), and gamma-aminobutyric acid (GABA) within the cell body. There is a compatibility with a neurotransmitter (e.g., the key) and receptor (e.g., lock) that causes the activation mechanism of the process. It is postulated that persons with schizophrenia may have too much or too little of the neurotransmitters available. This imbalance creates the development of the positive and negative symptoms that are associated with the disorder (Stahl & Buckley, 2007). Figure 14–3 shows the dopamine pathways of the sagittal section of the brain.

Neurodevelopmental Model of Schizophrenia

Epidemiological studies implicate prenatal maternal infection neurodevelopmental defects and pathological consequences in brain and behavior to cytokine-related inflammatory processes (Meyer et al., 2006). Disturbance to early brain development contributes to brain damage and a heightened risk of neuropsychiatric disorders such as schizophrenia.

The neurodevelopmental assumption of schizophrenia posits that an early event disrupts normal brain development resulting in manifestations of clinical symptoms of puberty or young adult onset (Rapoport, Addington, Frangou, & Psych, 2005). Studies indicate variance among neurodevelopmental models in regard to specificity and timing of genetic and environmental influences, but most implicate insults to prenatal brain development, and these factors collectively interact in the etiology of psychosis. Alterations in brain function and structure in schizophrenia are posited to be genetically mediated, but may also occur in clients with unaffected first degree relatives, while other alterations are present in individuals who exhibit symptom phenotype, but not in relatives at genetic risk (Kirkbride et al., 2006).

SUBSTANCE ABUSE THEORY

The substance abuse theory proposes that persons' use or abuse of alcohol and other v substances create physical and psychological changes that predispose the development of schizophrenia. Although there seems to be a number of

HOW DRUGS AFFECT THE DOPAMINERGIC SYNAPSES

Most of the medications used to treat symptoms of schizophrenia act by blocking dopamine receptor sites. Other medications work by blocking dopamine synthesis or by preventing the breakdown of dopamine. Hallucinogens, amphetamines, and certain prescribed drugs can initiate or exacerbate psychotic episodes by increasing the amount of available dopamine. (See Fig. 2–4 for an explanation of synaptic structures.)

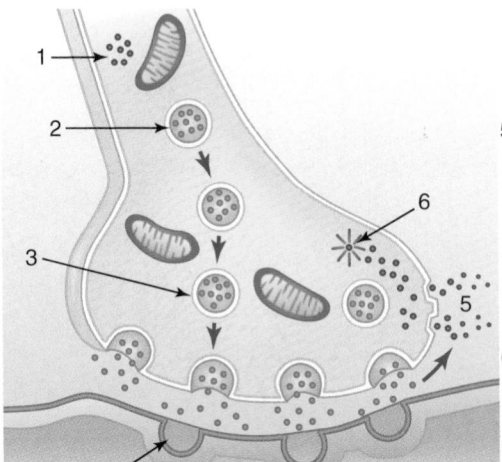

1. Dopamine is synthesized from tyrosine, a basic amino acid.
2. Dopamine is stored in synaptic vesicles.
3. Vesicles migrate to the presynaptic membrane and release dopamine into the synaptic cleft. *Because amphetamines and some antihypertensive drugs stimulate release of dopamine and effectively block reuptake at the presynaptic membrane, they can exacerbate symptoms of schizophrenia and related psychosis.*
4. Receptor stimulation of the postsynaptic membrane initiates an impulse in the dendrite of the next neuron. *Antipsychotic drugs such as perphenazine (Trilafon) and halo-*

peridol (Haldol) block receptor sites to prevent stimulation, alleviating symptoms of schizophrenia.
5. Dopamine activity stops when dopamine is resorbed into the presynaptic membrane. *Benztropine (Cogentin), used to treat the extrapyramidal side effects of antipsychotics, inhibits this reuptake mechanism. In larger doses, Cogentin can precipitate psychosis.*
6. Dopamine is broken down by monoamine oxidase (MAO). *MAO inhibitors prevent the breakdown of dopamine and are used to treat extrapyramidal effects.*

Figure 14–2 How drugs affect the dopaminergic synapses.

reported cases fitting this profile, there has not been adequate research on the subject. Consequently, this theory has less support than the aforementioned theories.

DIATHESIS STRESS THEORY

One of the most popular theories regarding development of schizophrenia is the diathesis stress or combination theory. According to this theory, individuals develop schizophrenia based on the interaction of a number of factors. These factors include genetics, environmental (e.g., both physical and psychological), anatomic and functional systems, and the contribution of stressors (e.g., neurological dysfunction, psychobiological and environmental factors, use of alcohol and other substances, and interpersonal relationships) (Philips et al., 2006). The predisposition to develop schizophrenia is created by changes within a person's physical, psychological, spiritual, or cultural environments in conjunction with the presence of stressors. This combination approach to development of schizophrenia is supported by research regarding the interaction variables. In addition, schizophrenia is likely to evoke from a combination of factors, and the diathesis stress theory is a more holistic examination of the development of the disorder.

ALTERED SENSORY PERCEPTION AND ISSUES OF CARE

The development of schizophrenia in persons is contingent on changes that occur in the anatomic, functional, and neurochemical systems of the brain. This is what makes the disorder

of schizophrenia difficult to diagnose and complicated to treat appropriately. See the *DSM-IV-TR* (APA, 2000) diagnostic criteria for schizophrenia. Anatomic or structural alterations may lead to functional changes in language and memory sections of the brain. In addition, alterations in the neurotransmitter system, at the release, receptor, activation, or reuptake locations, may alter the anatomic or functional systems. The consequences of these changes lead to the basis of schizophrenia positive, negative, and cognitive symptoms (Salgado-Pineda et al., 2007).

ALTERED PERCEPTION PSYCHOSIS AND ISSUES OF CARE

Psychosis refers to a mental state in which the client retreats from reality due to hallucinatory perceptions, including auditory (hearing voices) and visual delusions, such as paranoia, grandiose or persecutory types, disorganized thought processes, and cognitive deficits (APA, 2000). Reality testing is the ability to appraise and judge external and internal stimuli. Psychosis results from impaired reality testing. Consistent findings from postmortem and genetic studies, implicate cognitive impairment, brain functional abnormalities, and environmental factors as the bases of schizophrenia (Addington et al., 2007). Psychosis may occur owing to the presence of medical, neurological, or other psychiatric conditions or substance misuse disorders and pharmacologic agents. Distinguishing underlying factors associated with psychosis requires a differential diagnosis based on a careful and comprehensive examination of the individual's physical and psychological state. During the initial assessment and

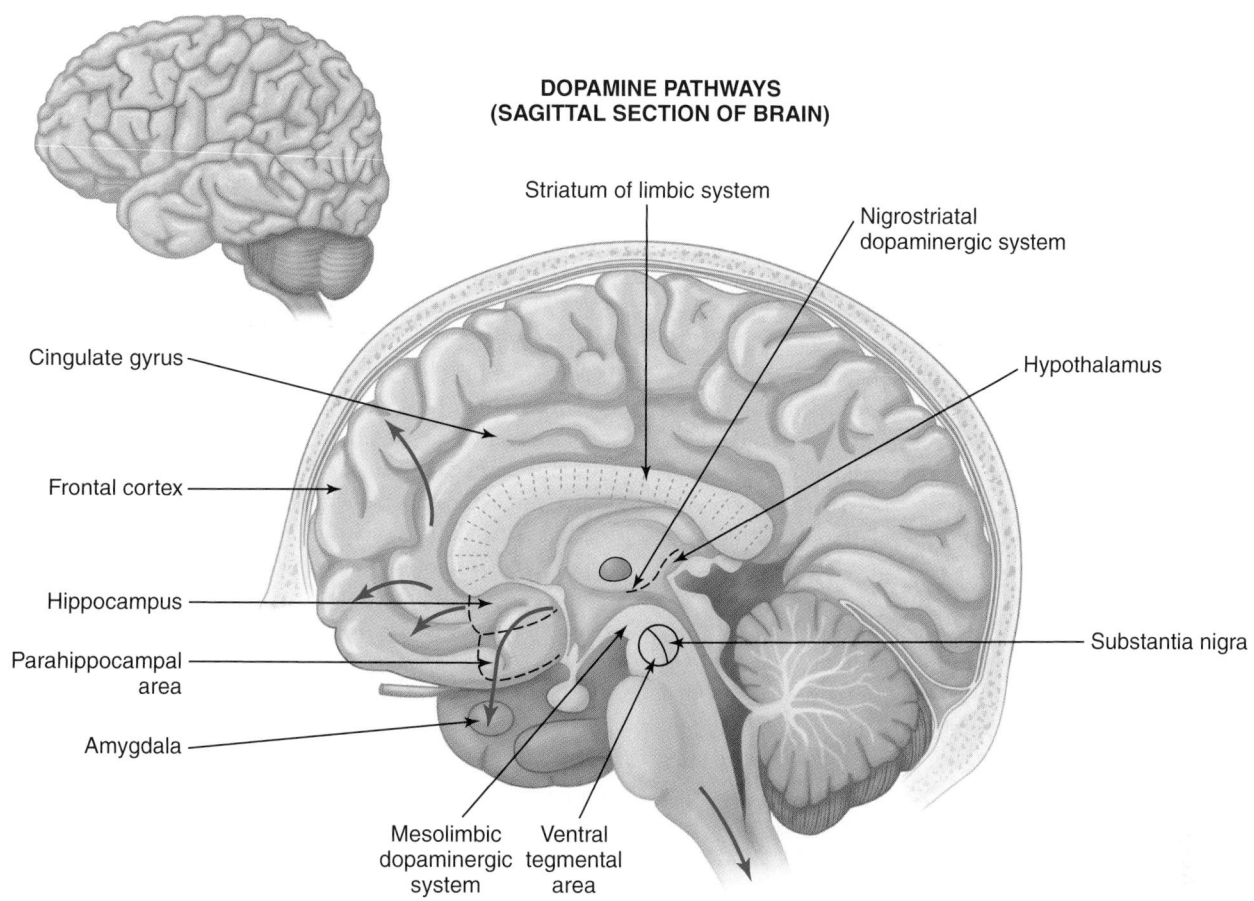

**DOPAMINE PATHWAYS
(SAGITTAL SECTION OF BRAIN)**

Striatum of limbic system

Nigrostriatal
dopaminergic system

Cingulate gyrus

Hypothalamus

Frontal cortex

Hippocampus

Substantia nigra

Parahippocampal
area

Amygdala

Mesolimbic
dopaminergic
system

Ventral
tegmental
area

The major neurotransmitter hypothesis for schizo-phrenia is based on evidence of hyperactivity of the dopaminergic (DA) systems. Excessive dopamine produced in the DA neurons of the substantia nigra stimulates the nigrostriatal tracts. The mesolimbic DA tracts receive a supply of dopamine from the ventral tegmental area and influence processes of the limbic system, amygdaloid body, parahippocampal area, and frontal lobe. This wide distribution of excess dopamine helps explain the variety of symptoms displayed in schizophrenia.

Norepinephrine activity may also be increased in schizophrenia and may lend a paranoid component to the clinical picture *(see text).*

Figure 14–3 Dopamine pathways (sagittal section of the brain).

follow-up, positive and negative symptoms can be assessed with the 30-item Positive and Negative Symptom Scale (PANSS) (Kay, Fiszbein, & Opler, 1987) and the 18-item Brief Psychiatric Rating Scale (BPRS) (Overall & Gorham, 1962). These instruments are used extensively in clinical drug trials and research to monitor symptom management and treatment response. (See Table 14–3 for a list of medical and psychiatric conditions that may cause psychosis.)

This chapter focuses primarily on the person with schizophrenia and this section provides guiding principles for caring for individuals with this serious, chronic, and disabling psychiatric condition. Nursing care of clients with schizophrenia

requires an understanding of psychiatric symptoms unique to these disorders. The symptoms of schizophrenia fall into three broad domains: positive symptoms, negative symptoms, and cognitive symptoms.

Positive symptoms manifest primarily as alterations in thoughts or perceptions and include hallucinations, delusions, thought disorder, and disorders of movement. Typically the client reports auditory or visual hallucinations—"hearing voices" that others do not hear or "seeing things" that others do not see. **Hallucinations** are distorted perceptions of reality and evolve from alterations in complex internal processes. Hallucinations arise from alterations in cognitive processes and are associated with self-generated inner speech that is distorted as externally generated speech. Presumably, during hallucinations activation in cortical regions that mediate the production of inner speech may precede the perception of auditory verbal perception (Picard, Amado, Mouchet-Mages, Olie, & Krebs, 2007; Shergill et al., 2004). (See Figure 14–4.)

Delusions are false beliefs, stemming from inaccurate external inference and do not reflect the individual's culture intelligence; and cannot be corrected by reasoning or logic. For instance, the client who believes that his wife is unfaithful and each time she returns home he accuses her of being with another man or questions her about not being at her desk when he called. Despite explanations about reasons for coming home late or being at lunch when he called, the spouse holds on to his belief or delusion that his wife is unfaithful. This type of delusion is referred to as "delusional jealousy." The nature of most delusions is bizarre, persecutory, paranoid, somatic (e.g., legs are turning into spaghetti) or nihilistic (e.g., fear the world is coming to an end). In addition to having auditory or visual hallucinations, the client usually presents with delusions. For example, the client who feels the FBI has "bugged" his phone or people can read his thoughts or his thoughts are being broadcast on TV may also hear voices that tell her that she needs to hide or turn the TV off and she therefore becomes more fearful, agitated, irritable, and anxious. Others may present with more bizarre delusions, such as aliens landing in his or her backyard and being spied on through birds or squirrels, or thinking someone is "controlling my thoughts." It is imperative to assess the nature of both hallucinations and delusions to determine the level of danger to self and others. Delusions of grandeur refer to an exaggeration of one's importance, wealth, or power.

Thought disorder refers to a disturbance in the form of thought rather than content of thought. Persons with schizophrenia frequently have *disturbed thought processes*. Examples of disturbed thought processes include neologisms (new words created by client), loose associations, and disorganized thinking that causes the client to experience difficulty organizing or having a logical flow of thought. Speech often reflects disturbed thought processes, for instance, with disorganized or incoherent thoughts. Speech is also likely to be disorganized, hard to understand, and incoherent. Clients with schizophrenia may also report "thought blocking" at which time they may say the "thought just disappeared from my head." The following case studies provide opportunities to test critical thinking skills and nursing interventions that promote therapeutic interactions with clients presenting with acute psychosis.

Assessing the client's unique experiences associated with acute psychosis requires therapeutic interventions to allay anxiety, reduce positive symptoms, and ensure personal safety. Pharmacological interventions must be promptly initiated to manage psychosis, anxiety, and agitation. Typically, a conventional or typical agent such as haloperidol and a benzodiazepine such as lorazepam are administered IM to reduce anxiety. If there is a history of a serious adverse side effect to a typical antipsychotic (e.g., neuroleptic malignant syndrome), an IM atypical agent may be administered. Intramuscular administration is necessary to ensure quick action and absorption. It is important to remember that when medications are given against the client's will, this is very traumatic.(See Chapter 29 for an in-depth discussion of typical and atypical antipsychotic medications.) Explain all procedures and let the client know that you are there to help relieve his or her distress.

During the acute period, close observation and documentation of signs and symptoms are equally important. Careful monitoring of symptom management, the client's level of danger to self, and side effects are important nursing interventions during the acute phase and exacerbation of psychosis. Family members are particularly in need of health education about the client's illness and treatment options. Because of the high risk of depression in persons with schizophrenia, nursing care must also include suicide assessment and self-deprecating comments concerning the client's illness, societal stigma, and symptom management. The care of persons with schizophrenia also includes monitoring and treating substance-related disorders. Ideally, treatment planning must be based on a comprehensive integrated model to reduce danger to self and others, abstinence, relapse prevention, and psychosocial rehabilitation.

Negative symptoms manifest as a loss or a decrease in the ability to initiate plans, speak, express feelings, and experience pleasure in activities of daily living. Researchers often link global psychosocial, occupational, and academic functioning and quality interpersonal relationships with negative symptoms and attention (Siegel et al., 2006). Negative symptoms

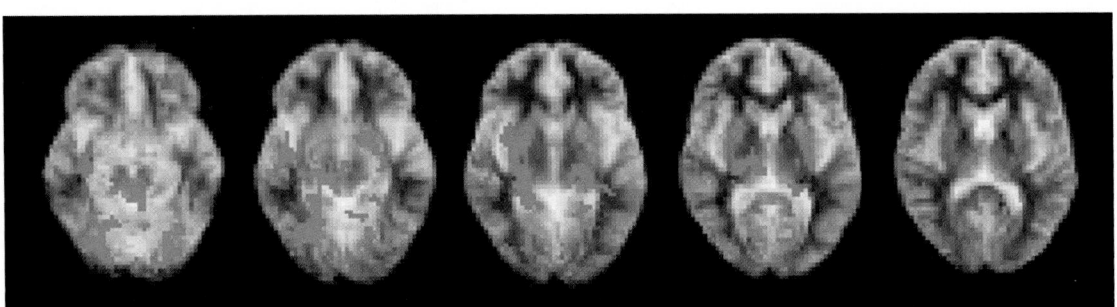

Figure 14–4 Brain regions activated by auditory hallucinations. (*From Shergill, S. S., Bullmore, E., Simmons, A., Murray, R. M., & McGuire, P. [2000]. Functional anatomy of auditory verbal imagery in schizophrenic patients with auditory hallucinations.* American Journal of Psychiatry, 157, *1691–1693. Used with permission.*)

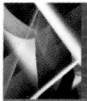

CASE STUDY

Mr. M is a 34-year-old client who was diagnosed with schizophrenia about 10 years ago. For the most part he has had strong family support, able to hold a low-stress job, and taken his medication as ordered. His family reports that he stopped taking his medication several weeks ago and has become more reclusive, irritable, and has lost his job. During the interview, Mr. M appears to be responding to "voices" and is quite fearful and agitated. What is the most appropriate intervention for this client?

1. Ensure personal safety prior to talking to the client.

2. "I understand you were brought in against your will; I am here to help you."

3. "Tell me about your reasons for being here today."

4. All of the above

Answers

1. *Correct.* This client is at high risk of danger to self and others based on his demeanor and behavior and he may respond to "voices" that tell him to protect himself from perceived danger. It is imperative for the nurse to ensure personal safety prior to talking to this client.

2. *Correct.* Establishing a therapeutic relationship with the client requires empathy and understanding of the client's experience. It is important to acknowledge some understanding about reasons for the visit and display empathy and concern. This approach reduces anxiety and promotes trust.

3. *Correct.* Asking the client to provide his side of the story again conveys respect and concern.

4. *Correct.* All of these approaches are correct. Questions are simple and direct and offer opportunities for the client to discuss his situation.

CASE STUDY

Mary is a 24-year-old who has been recently admitted to an acute inpatient unit with a diagnosis of first-episode schizophrenia. During your morning rounds she asks you to come into her room and she asks, "Don't you hear my cousin talking in the corner?" What is the most appropriate response to Mary?

1. "Yes, I do."

2. "Mary, obviously you hear her, but I don't."

3. "Did you take your medication last night?"

4. "No I don't hear your cousin and neither do you!"

Answers

1. *Incorrect.* It is critical to provide reality to clients exhibiting psychotic symptoms and acknowledging that you hear her cousin talking reinforces her retreat from reality.

2. *Correct.* It is imperative for the nurse to acknowledge that the client obviously hears voices, while also reinforcing reality by stating she doesn't hear her cousin's voice. This enables the nurse to provide reality without challenging the client's beliefs and increasing anxiety and agitation.

3. *Incorrect.* Inquiring about taking medication last night prevents the nurse from dealing with the client's present experience of auditory hallucinations.

4. *Incorrect.* The client's hallucinations are "real" to her. By challenging the client's retreat from reality by stating she does not hear voices, the nurse demeans her experience with hallucinations which can result in increased anxiety, agitation, and suspiciousness.

manifest as flat affect, social isolation, aloofness, and diminished ability to plan or manage activities of daily living, including personal hygiene, grooming, and nutritional needs. Psychiatric-mental health nurses must develop a plan of care and nursing interventions to assess the client's needs to ensure that emotional, physical, nutritional, and mental health needs are addressed. Involving the client in his or her care promotes competency and self-esteem.

COGNITIVE SYMPTOMS OR NEUROCOGNITIVE DEFICITS

Persons with schizophrenia consistently exhibit profound neurocognitive deficits in various cognitive domains (Donohoe et al., 2006; Rund et al., 2006). Neurocognitive deficits—disturbances in working memory (keeping information focused), executive function, semantic memory

My Experiences with Psychosis

A person who has struggled with hallucinations and delusions shares some thoughts about her experiences.

I have sought treatment for the last 25 years for a condition now diagnosed as schizoaffective disorder; that is, I have suffered from mood swings and schizophrenic symptoms, such as hearing voices and having delusions.

I began to hear voices when I was 16 years old. These auditory hallucinations were not only very friendly and humorous but they also caused me to feel quite euphoric. They convinced me to stop taking my medication. They also informed me that I was not psychotic, that everyone else hears them, and that I was to keep this psychic phenomenon to myself. The big secret.

I was given an antipsychotic medication and my hallucinations stopped. However, soon thereafter, I began smoking marijuana regularly again, and the voices returned. (My withdrawal from reality was characterized by my thinking that I was telepathic or that I was a very famous person.) I worked and went to school between frequent hospitalizations, as I was constantly up and down and hallucinating. Even though I stopped using street drugs, the hallucinations persisted and became very negative and hateful. This led to the delusion that even loved friends and family hated me. Hence, I became alienated and isolative.

Three years ago I entered a long-term inpatient unit on the East Coast and was taken off all my medication so I could see how I was affected by Clozaril. Since taking the new medication, the hallucinations have been reduced substantially. In addition to the very new medication, therapy and daily activities have really helped me reenter reality.

I have been afflicted by what my treaters and I call "the connective symptom." The messages I get from this "connection" are often misleading, seemingly attempting to make me feel suicidally disappointed, or at least testing my patience and temper. Most often, these messages (what I call "plants"—short for "implanted thoughts"—) are from a boy I dated and was very fond of who died 20 years ago. My treaters explain this experience as my subconscious manifesting my loneliness and grief by creating the imaginary company of a boy I cared about. I read the messages by paying attention to my own and other people's involuntary motions and what they seem to say.

I've been on Clozaril for about 28 months now. While I've had to deal with depression over the lack of my imaginary company in the form of auditory hallucinations, I have been outside the hospital during that time. I have stopped feeling suicidal, I know my friends and family love me, and I'm working on maintaining and developing real relationships. I have improved my concentration and retention regarding what I perceive to an incredible degree.

My coordination has also been impressively improved. I have no craving for street drugs. I have cut down on my consumption of caffeine and nicotine. I have been exercising regularly and eating better and have lost 50 to 60 pounds. All this improvement has led to much better self-esteem and basic relationships with myself and others. Also, I've been getting much more rest and am, in my opinion and according to the observations of treaters, much more consistent and level in my moods.

In closing, I will just say that I feel my treatment and Clozaril have improved the quality of my life, and my life is just getting better and better.

(verbal fluency), visual memory, and verbal memory—are considered core features of schizophrenia. When compared to individuals with depression, persons with schizophrenia tend to score lower in higher-order neurocognitive tests in working memory, executive function, visual memory, and verbal memory. Whereas when compared to normal controls, subjects with nonpsychotic depression scored significantly lower in working memory and reaction time. These data indicate that persons with schizophrenia have pervasive neurocognitive deficits and clients with nonpsychotic depression have milder and restricted cognitive deficits (Rund et al., 2006).

Negative and cognitive symptoms of schizophrenia are associated with retrieval and encoding dysregulation and low levels of dopamine and acetylcholine in the medial prefrontal cortex. Cognitive deficits in persons with schizophrenia are believed to stem from retrieval and encoding dysregulation and low levels of dopamine and acetylcholine in the medial prefrontal cortex. Various genes have been discovered that encode proteins implicated in neurobiological mechanism, including synaptic plasticity, neurotransmission, and neurodevelopment, all of which are dysregulated in schizophrenia (Harrison & Weinberger, 2005). Similar deficits are found in clients who are depressed. The prevalence of depression in clients with schizophrenia must be evaluated and treated. Siblings and offspring of persons with schizophrenia are at risk for the illness and exhibit attentional and memory impairments (Seidman, Giuliano, Smith, Stone, et al., 2006). The goal of pharmacological interventions for cognitive deficits is to increase dopamine metabolism in the mesocortical pathways. Most atypical antipsychotic agents have proven efficacy in improving verbal fluency, attention, and secondary (storage) memory (Lindenmayer, Khan, Iskander, Abad, & Parker, 2007).

Emerging findings from psychiatric research challenge Kraepelin's dichotomy of schizoaffective disorders as being separate from schizophrenia. Issues that fuel this argument include a lack of a clear definition of this psychiatric disorder during the past 70 years and that current diagnostic criteria are unreliable or invalid because they depict a quantitative variance in the etiology and neurobiology of schizophrenia and mood disorders (Craddock, O'Donovan, & Owen, 2005) (see Figure 14–5). Hopefully, the next few years of research of genetic susceptibility will yield a greater understanding of neurobiological underpinnings and psychosis-susceptibility genes are identified and characterized over the generate changes in

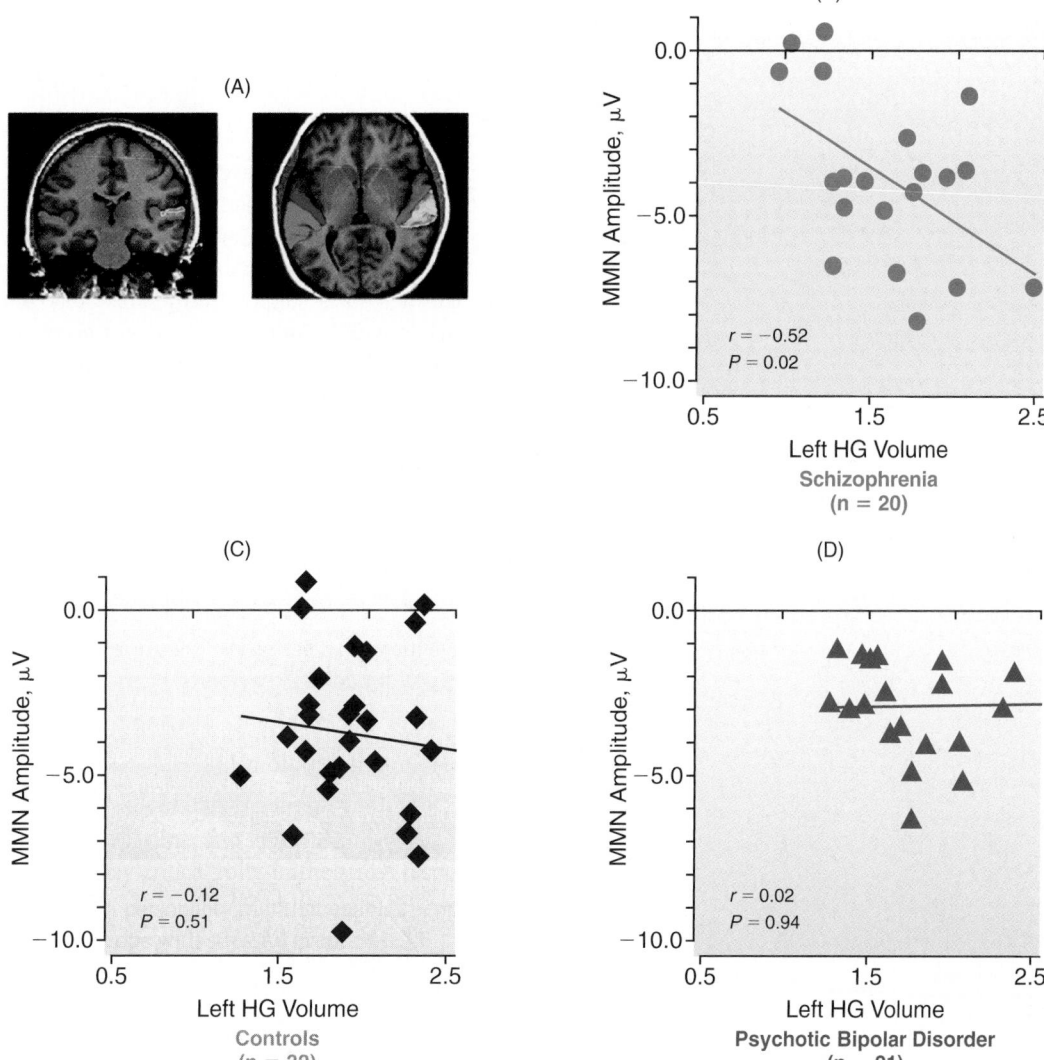

Figure 14–5 Magnetic resonance imaging demarks regions of correlation with mismatched negativity (MMN) at first hospitalization or initial illness. Three-dimensional magnetic resonance imaging constructions of major subdivisions of the superior temporal plane are depicted in **A** and **B**. Heschl gyri (dark blue and dark green) mainly contain the primary auditory cortex. The planum temporale (light blue and yellow-green) contains secondary and tertiary auditory association cortices. The left side of the figure is the left hemisphere, which is has a larger left hemisphere planum temporale. Alterations between MMN and underlying left hemisphere primary auditory cortex volumes during the first hospitalization in individuals with schizophrenia are depicted in **C**. Longitudinally, the interrelated progressive reduction of functional and structural measures implicates progressive pathological processes early in schizophrenia. *(From Salisbury, D. F., Kuroki, N., Kasai, K., Shenton, M. E., & McCarley, R. W. [2007]. Progressive and interrelated functional and structural evidence of post-onset brain reduction in schizophrenia. Archives of General Psychiatry, 64, 521–529.)*

the nosology and the clinical practice of psychiatric mental health care (Craddock, O'Donovan, & Owen, 2006).

Similar to positive and negative symptoms, cognitive deficits interfere with the client's ability to plan and manage activities of daily living. Poor clinical outcomes are associated with persistent negative and cognitive symptoms. Treatment consists of antipsychotic medications to manage symptoms and im-prove the client's level of functioning. Due to the prevalence of depression in clients with schizophrenia, monitoring for de-pressive symptoms and suicide risk are important nursing interventions. Atypical antipsychotic medications have demonstrated efficacy in treating positive symptoms, depression, and much improvement in mitigating negative and cognitive symptoms.

DIFFERENTIAL DIAGNOSIS FOR MEDICAL AND PSYCHIATRIC ALTERED SENSORY BRAIN DISORDERS

Differential diagnosis between medical conditions and psychiatric altered sensory perception disorders is accomplished after a comprehensive physical, psychological, and mental status examination of a person. A diagnostic workup that includes a complete blood count with differential, serum chemistries that include renal and liver panels, thyroid tests (e.g., thyroid stimulating hormone [TSH], T3, T4), and glucose, triglyceride, cholesterol level; urinalysis, drug/toxicology screen, B12, thiamine, and folate, and pregnancy tests help rule out medical conditions that may mimic psychotic symptoms (APA, 2004).

TABLE 14–3
General Medical and Psychiatric Disorders Associated with Psychosis

Medical and Neurological Diseases

- Temporal lobe epilepsy, parkinsonism
- Tumor, stroke, brain trauma
- Endocrine/metabolic disorders
  Porphyria
  Cushing's disease
  Thyroid disorder
- Vitamin deficiency (e.g., B_{12})
- Infectious (e.g., herpes encephalitis, neurosyphilis, acquired immunodeficiency syndrome)
- Autoimmune (e.g., systemic lupus erythematosus)
- Toxic (e.g., heavy metal poisoning—mercury, arsenic)
- Alzheimer's, Huntington's, and Wilson's disease
- Drug induced
  Stimulants—amphetamine, cocaine
  Hallucinogens—phencyclidine
  Withdrawal from alcohol, barbiturates, and anticholinergics

Psychiatric Conditions

Mood Disorder

- Major depressive with psychotic features
- Bipolar disorder, manic, or depressive episode
- Schizoaffective disorder

Delusional Disorders
Personality Disorders

- Paranoid
- Schizotypal
- Borderline

Note. Data from Kirkpatrick, B. & Tek, C. (2005). Schizophrenia: Clinical features and psychopathology concepts. In B. J. Sadock & V. A. Sadock (eds). *Kaplan & Sadock's Comprehensive Textbook of Psychiatry*, (Vol. 1., 8th ed.), (pp. 1416–1436). Philadelphia: Lippincott Williams & Wilkins.

A partial listing of medical and neurological diseases is found in Table 14–3. It is important to use *DSM-IV-TR* (APA, 2000) criteria for schizophrenia and other psychotic disorders as other resources regarding differential diagnosis.

SCHIZOPHRENIA AND OTHER PSYCHOTIC DISORDERS ACROSS THE LIFE SPAN

Life span issues are dependent on the age, maturity, and initial appearance and extent of the disorder. Schizophrenia and other mental disorders are almost always treatable through the use of pharmacologic agents, psychosocial rehabilitation, and psychotherapy.

CHILDHOOD

Schizophrenia is a neurodevelopmental disorder. Childhood-onset schizophrenia, similar to adolescent and adulthood, is manifested by marked neuropsychological deficits in areas of attention, working memory, and executive functions. Findings from recent studies support the premise that schizophrenia is associated with brain damage in that it occurs on a continuum or neurodevelopment course with greater severity associated with childhood-onset schizophrenia (Biswas, Malhotra, Malhotra, & Gupta, 2006).

Psychiatric assessment of children is similar to that for adults. However, differential diagnosis for children is challenging because of the varied developmental stages that they undergo. The following guidelines have been suggested regarding psychiatric diagnosis in children:

- ◆ Delineation between the normal and abnormal developmental behaviors
- ◆ Length and occurrence of symptomatology
- ◆ Presenting symptomatology
- ◆ Social interaction and adaptation
- ◆ Length of abnormal or inappropriate behaviors

Children's normal development is manifested by age-appropriate communication patterns, normal interactions with others, and adaptive play behaviors and patterns (APA, 2000). Misdiagnosis of child psychiatric disorders is generally the result of incorrect assessment of the developmental, psychological, and social stages that a child is experiencing (McClellan & Werry, 2000). Children's psychiatric illness may be precipitated or intensified owing to the presence of trauma, physical illness, mental retardation, environmental factors, learning disabilities, or parental or guardian illness (McClellan & Werry, 2000). As with adults, a complete workup needs to be accomplished. See Table 14–4 for the diagnostic tests.

Interventions for children need to be implemented within the home, school, and social settings. Psychiatric-mental health nurses can be instrumental in the development of these interventions, which need to involve play therapy, age-appropriate counseling and psychotherapy, and psychoeducation. *Psychoeducation* involves assisting parents, children, and others involved with the child to understand the cause of the psychiatric illness. In addition, it is important to help persons with the development and implementation of appropriate interventions and use of resources that maximize recovery within affected persons. In addition, the PMH nurse can be the liaison between children, parents, guardians, teachers, and other professionals. The psychiatric-mental health nurse may use a tool, such as the Child Behavior Checklist or criteria within the *DSM-IV*, in order to rate a child's behavior (APA, 2000; McClellan & Werry, 2000).

TABLE 14-4
Diagnostic Tests: Children and Adolescents with a Suspected Psychotic Disorder

	Tests and Examinations	Rationale
Physical	Configuration and size of head	To assess for microcephaly, hydrocephalus, Down syndrome
	Circumference of head	
	Facial signs; e.g., nose, mouth, brows	
	Handprinting or dermatoglyphics	
Neurological	Skull radiographs	Disturbances in motor areas; e.g., spasticity or hypotonia
	CT scan, MRI	
	Electroencephalogram	Sensory impairments; e.g., hearing, visual cranial defects, central nervous system abnormalities, and seizure disorders, to assess for Down syndrome
Laboratory	Urinalysis and serum	Metabolic disorders
	Hearing and speech evaluations	Enzymatic abnormalities (chromosomal disorders, such as Down syndrome)
		Hearing and speech development, to assess for mental retardation
Psychological	Screening tests such as Gesell, Catell, Bayley (for infants), Stanford-Binet, Wechsler Intelligence Scale for Children—Revised (WISC-R), Bender-Gestalt, Benton Visual Retention tests	Developmental assessment
		Detection of brain damage

CT, computed tomography; MRI, magnetic resonance imaging.

The diagnosis of schizophrenia is rarely made in children. However, there is some evidence indicating that some children who are diagnosed with autism may be diagnosed with schizophrenia once they become adults. Autism is manifested by the presence of abnormal and impaired development in social and communication skills and severely restricted activity and interests. Children with autism may be emotionally aloof and cold, socially isolated, and verbally uncommunicative. In addition, they may exhibit repetitive movements. For example, the child may continually rock back and forth or flush toilets repeatedly. The cause of autism is generally associated with neurobiological damage and stress during pregnancy (i.e., rubella, incompatibility between the mother and fetus) (Vitiello & Wagner, 2007).

Major differences between schizophrenia and autism include the following:

◆ Children with autism are generally diagnosed before 3 years of age and have global dysfunctional patterns.

◆ Onset of schizophrenia occurs in adolescence or adulthood, not in early childhood.

◆ Children with autism have an increased risk of having mental retardation.

Other rare disorders that require differential diagnosis in children include Rett's, childhood disintegrative, and Asperger's disorders. Parents and guardians of children with autism and other psychiatric disorders need respite and support, because the stress is extremely high. Psychiatric nurses can be instrumental in providing respite and support resources for parents.

ADOLESCENCE

Adolescence is a time for rapid and cyclic change and development. This normal aspect of adolescent development makes psychiatric diagnosis even more of a challenge because many of the symptoms of mental disorders mimic those normal patterns within adolescent development. Symptoms of schizophrenia often emerge during adolescence. However, these symptoms are more pronounced than the normal adolescent behavior. Maladaptive behaviors and symptoms may include the ones discussed in the earlier discussion in this chapter as well as the *DSM-IV-TR* (APA, 2000) criteria in Table 14–5 (e.g., extreme social withdrawal and communication problems; presence of hallucinations, delusions, and illusions; bizarre thinking; and behavior patterns).

Parents and guardians need assistance like that for children diagnosed with schizophrenia. In addition, the adolescent also needs support in understanding how to deal with all the normal changes and challenges of adolescence.

TABLE 14–5
DSM-IV-TR Diagnostic Criteria for Schizophrenia

A. *Characteristic symptoms:* Two (or more) of the following, each present for a significant portion of time during a 1-month period (or less if successfully treated):

   (1) delusions

   (2) hallucinations

   (3) disorganized speech (e.g., frequent derailment or incoherence)

   (4) grossly disorganized or catatonic behavior

   (5) negative symptoms, i.e., affective flattening, alogia, or avolition

   Note: Only one Criterion A symptom is required if delusions are bizarre or hallucinations consist of a voice keeping up a running commentary on the person's behavior or thoughts, or two or more voices conversing with each other.

B. *Social/occupational dysfunction:* For a significant portion of the time since the onset of the disturbance, one or more major areas of functioning such as work, interpersonal relations, or self-care are markedly below the level achieved prior to the onset (or when the onset is in childhood or adolescence, failure to achieve expected level of interpersonal, academic, or occupational achievement).

C. *Duration:* Continuous signs of the disturbance persist for at least 6 months. This 6-month period must include at least 1 month of symptoms (or less if successfully treated) that meet Criterion A (i.e., active-phase symptoms) and may include periods of prodomal or residual symptoms. During these prodromal or residual periods, the signs of the disturbance may be manifested by only negative symptoms or two or more symptoms listed in Criterion A present in an attenuated form (e.g., odd beliefs, unusual perceptual experiences).

D. *Schizoaffective and mood disorder exclusion:* Schizoaffective Disorder and Mood Disorder With Psychotic features have been ruled out because either (1) no Major Depressive, Manic, or Mixed episodes have occurred concurrently with the active-phase symptoms; or (2) if mood episodes have occurred during active-phase symptoms, their total duration has been brief relative to the duration of the active and residual periods.

E. *Substance/general medical condition exclusion:* The disturbance is not due to the direct physiological effects of a substance (e.g., a drug of abuse, a medication) or a general medical condition.

F. *Relationship to a pervasive developmental disorder:* If there is a history of Autistic Disorder or another Pervasive Developmental Disorder, the additional diagnosis of Schizophrenia is made only if prominent delusions or hallucinations are also present for at least a month (or less is successfully treated).

Note. From *Diagnostic and Statistical Manual of Mental Disorders* (4th edition Revision) (*DSM-IV-TR*), by the American Psychiatric Association, 2000, Washington, DC: Author. Adapted with permission.

ADULTHOOD

In the past, it was thought that persons with schizophrenia became progressively more debilitated. However, the advent of the concept of recovery, new psychotropic medications, and use of psychotherapy and counseling have been instrumental in facilitating the recovery processes of persons in a different manner. Community-based services and support systems are making a difference in the lives of persons with schizophrenia. They have better access to those services that maximize their recovery and movement through adulthood.

In addition, those persons with schizophrenia may incur physical problems and disorders that will require treatment. Exacerbation of symptoms may occur during times of stress. Therefore, it is important for the nurse to assist clients with knowledge about the symptoms of their disorder and the treatment options for it. In addition, the use of *advance directives* has been beneficial for clients. Advance directives are similar to those for persons with physical illnesses. Clients may make decisions regarding their level of care and use of interventions and pharmacologic treatments while they are at a maximum level of psychological health and wellness. In addition, clients will choose an agent or someone who is responsible for carrying out their wishes when they decompensate or are at a higher level of symptomatology that may require hospitalization and additional treatment.

OLDER ADULTHOOD

Older adults who have physical health problems will need the same assistance and resource development as those without the diagnosis of schizophrenia. This may include attention to management of hypertension, other cardiovascular problems, peri and menopausal care, and oncology issues.

TREATMENT MODALITIES

Treatment issues may involve the use of pharmacologic agents as well as pychosocial rehabilitation and psychotherapy. Of course, each one of these approaches needs to be appropriate for the person's age, cultural reference, and level of symptomatology.

PSYCHOPHARMACOLOGICAL INTERVENTIONS

Traditional or typical and atypical antipsychotic medications are the ones used for treatment of schizophrenia. All of these medications in some way affect the anatomic and functional systems of the brains. Hence, they assist with ending or minimizing the presence of hallucinations, delusions, and illusions that interfere with a person's ability to recover and function appropriately on a daily basis (see Chapters 29 and 32).

Traditional medications were developed during the 1950s. Among these medications are haloperidol, chlorpromazine, and thiothixene. These medications are associated with higher adverse symptoms such as tardive dyskinesia and extrapyramidal side effects (EPS). However, in the 1990s, came the advent of the atypical or newer antipsychotics. These medications are more receptor specific and produce fewer adverse side effects than do the traditional medications. Clozapine (Clozaril) was the first atypical medication. However, additional medications have been developed, including risperidone (Risperdal), olanzapine (Zyprexa), quetiapine (Seroquel), ziprasidone (Geodon), and aripiprazole (Abilify). See Chapter 29, Psychopharmacology Therapy.

Levels and dosages of the antipsychotics need to be adjusted also depending on the age and weight of the client. The use of atypical antipsychotic agents continues to be researched in children. Age-related changes and co-occurring medical conditions must be considered when ordering these agents for older adults.

The use of medications may facilitate the recovery process for persons. However, medications cannot help persons learn about the management of their symptoms, interact with others, and develop a productive life.

PSYCHOSOCIAL INTERVENTIONS AND PSYCHOTHERAPY

In addition to pharmacologic interventions, psychotherapeutics are necessary components of holistic treatment planning. The efficacy of psychoeducation and psychotherapy that focus on schizophrenia, family involvement, coping skills, and psychosocial rehabilitation are well documented. Psychiatric nurses play pivotal roles in the implementation of various psychotherapeutic interventions and monitoring the client's responses throughout treatment planning. See Chapters 31 and 32 for a discussion of community-based care and psychosocial rehabilitation.

Counseling and Psychotherapy

Counseling and psychotherapy are extremely important adjuncts to the use of pharmacologic agents because persons with schizophrenia need a clear understanding of their disorder as well as how to interact with others and manage their symptoms. As previously mentioned, *psychoeducation* provides clients with an understanding of schizophrenia, its management, and resource development to facilitate their recovery process (Roder, Mueller, Mueser, & Brenner, 2006). One of the premier psychoeducational programs is using guidelines from the National Association of the Mentally Ill (NAMI). Their educational programs are geared for persons affected by schizophrenia as well as their families, friends, and significant others.

Social Skills Education

Social skills development and stress and crisis management are other important interventions for clients to develop. The symptoms of schizophrenia may interfere with the developmental process that clients move through. Hence, their ability to know how to interact with others may be altered by the presence of their altered sensory perceptions. The use of medications may eliminate this latter occurrence. However, clients may still need assistance in appropriate social skill use. In addition, as individuals recover, they move toward needing assistance with vocational and career education needs and counseling (see Chapters 32 and 33).

Neurocognitive Enhancement Therapy

Cognitive enhancement therapy, or neurocognitive enhancement therapy (NET), is a recovery-phase approach for stable schizophrenia with social and cognitive impairments (Bell, Bryson, Greig, et al., 2005; Hogarty, Flesher, Ulrich, Carter, et al., 2004). The NET format involves computerized cognitive training and other methods and has been shown to improve working memory and executive function in schizophrenia (Bell et al., 2005; McGurk, Mueser, & Pascaris, 2005).

Stress and Crisis Management Education

Finally, *stress and crisis management* is another important skill for persons to learn in order to establish and maintain their recovery process. As with any chronic illness, exacerbation of symptoms may occur. Persons need to be able to manage the stress that is associated with this occurrence. In addition, stress and crisis situations are often part of everyday existence. Clients' development of knowledge about these techniques also contributes to their recovery progression.

THE ROLE OF THE NURSE

The role of the nurse has been discussed in general terms throughout this chapter. However, there are some specific issues for the generalists and advanced-practice nurses as they provide psychiatric nursing treatment for their clients. Collaboration is the primary role for both the generalist and

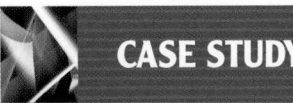

CASE STUDY

The Client with Schizophrenia (Johnny)

Johnny is an 18-year-old admitted to an acute psychiatric unit with a diagnosis of schizophrenia, acute, paranoid type. His parents reported that his grades have dropped from As to Cs, and he has been getting failing grades in school the past 12 months. He has also become increasingly withdrawn, agitated, and irritable during this period. He has been overheard talking and arguing in his room during the day and night. Initially, his parents thought that he was taking drugs and they sought medical treatment. His physical examination and drug screening results were negative. During the past 2 weeks, Johnny has refused to eat and has expressed fears that his mother has been trying to poison him. Additionally, he has refused to attend school or to come out of his room. His parents became concerned about his deteriorating mental and physical condition and brought him to the emergency department. His appearance was disheveled—his hair was uncombed and his clothes were wrinkled. Johnny was pacing, and his mood was irritable and agitated. His eye contact was poor and his thoughts were irrelevant, incoherent, and illogical. He was thinly built, 6 feet tall, and weighed about 137 pounds. He was easily distracted, and his responses were inappropriate. His parents were the chief informants.

advanced-practice PMH nurse. In addition, advocacy for client rights is another important role for both practice roles. Finally, it is important for both practice roles of nurses to provide care in a holistic manner that addresses the cultural mind, body, spirit issues for clients.

THE GENERALIST NURSE

The generalist nurse is involved in the initial development of the nursing treatment plan for the client. The generalist nurse implements and monitors the plan and the client's response to pharmacologic agents. The generalist nurse may be involved in psychoeducation, social skills, and good health habits classes. The nurse may also participate in the collection of data associated with research projects that clients may be involved in. Finally, the generalist nurse needs to be involved in the use of best practices within mental health care as it pertains to direct nursing care.

THE ADVANCED-PRACTICE PSYCHIATRIC REGISTERED NURSE

The advanced-practice psychiatric registered nurse is often the coordinator of care for clients and extends the depth of the nursing process. She may be involved as a case manager and coordinator of care within community settings. In addition, she provides counseling and psychotherapy. The AP PMH nurse may develop and conduct research and evaluation on various aspects of mental health, wellness, and illness. She may practice community settings and use prescriptive authority privileges. The development and use of best mental health nursing practices is another responsibility of the advanced-practice psychiatric registered nurse.

THE NURSING PROCESS

The following nursing care plan provides a useful framework for examining the nusing process in the acute care setting.

ASSESSMENT

Johnny is thinly built (disproportionate weight for height), with a weight loss of 25 to 35 pounds over several months. He demonstrates a disorganized thought process (i.e., disturbances in sensory and perceptual functioning) as well as moderate agitation and irritability.

NURSING DIAGNOSES

- ◆ Imbalanced Nutrition, Less Than Body Requirements
- ◆ Risk for Self-Directed Violence, High Risk for Self-Mutilation
- ◆ Disturbed Thought Processes
- ◆ Self-Care Deficit
- ◆ Disturbed Sensory Perception (Auditory)
- ◆ Anxiety
- ◆ Deficient Knowledge related to lack of information about the illness

PLANNING AND IMPLEMENTATION

Nursing Care Plan 14–1 identifies the desired outcomes for the nursing diagnoses listed and delineates the nursing actions needed to achieve these outcomes, along with the rationales for these actions.

EVALUATION

Evaluation is based on identification of outcomes and feedback from the client, the family, and other mental health professionals. In the case history, Johnny was hospitalized for several weeks and responded rapidly to psychotropics. He was discharged to a partial hospital setting, and his parents continued to play active roles in psychoeducation and provide emotional and psychosocial support during this stressful ordeal.

RESEARCH ABSTRACT

Current Trends in Schizophrenia Research

Conley, R. R. (2006). The CATIE outcome findings are relevant to clinical practice (CON). *Journal of Psychotic Disorders: Reviews & Commentaries, 9,* 3–16.

There exists a plethora of data concerning the etiology and treatment of schizophrenia and other major psychotic disorders, the main emphasis of current and future research. Examples of current trends in research include, but are not limited to:

- Brain imaging and mapping

- Autoimmunity immune system and dysregulation model

- Ethical and legal considerations in high-risk studies of schizophrenia

- Research that extends beyond symptoms management and includes recovery and quality-of-life issues

- Early recognition of early or first-episode psychosis and the longitudinal medications and impact on brain and cognitive function

- Family-centered evaluation of treatment outcomes

- The role of nurses and interdisciplinary teams in developing treatment to address multidimensions of schizophrenia

- Pharmacogenetics and tailored drug treatment

- Follow-up is necessary on the National Institute of Health (NIMH) Clinical Antipsychotic Trials of Intervention Effectiveness (CATIE) project due to its controversial findings. Most critics and researchers cite numerous uncontrolled factors (e.g., provided only pharmacological interventions, no washout period) that flawed the data. Major limitations found include a high dropout rate (e.g., 74%) indicating limitations in the efficacy of study drugs (Conley, 2006).

NURSING CARE PLAN 14–1

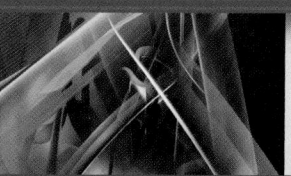

The Client with Schizophrenia (Johnny)

Nursing Diagnosis: Risk for Self-Directed Violence; High Risk for Self-Mutilation

Outcome Identification	Nursing Actions	Rationales	Evaluation
1. Johnny will refrain from harming himself or others during the treatment process.	1a. Assess level of dangerousness (previous attempts, means, and thoughts).	1a. Provides baseline information.	*Goal met:* Johnny does not harm himself or others. Johnny experiences less agitation and fewer hallucinations and delusions after administration of medication. Only medication side effect is sedation.
	1b. Remove dangerous items from the environment.	1b. Removal of dangerous items decreases risk of harm to self or others.	
	1c. Assess for changes in mood, affect, and thoughts (e.g., pacing agitation).	1c. Changes in these areas may indicate imminent danger.	
	1d. Administer antipsychotics/ antianxiety agents.	1d. Medication promotes reality testing and decreases agitation and level of dangerousness.	
	1e. Encourage Johnny to express feelings rather than acting on thoughts.	1e. Expression of feelings enables nurse to assess response to medication.	

(continues)

Nursing Diagnosis: Disturbed Thought Processes (and Disturbed Sensory Perception [Auditory])

Outcome Identification	Nursing Actions	Rationales	Evaluation
1. By [date], Johnny experiences improved reality testing (decreased or alleviated psychotic symptoms).	1a. Administer antipsychotics or antianxiety agents, and assess desired and adverse responses. 1b. Reduce environmental stimuli. 1c. Assess and support reality. 1d. Introduce self to Johnny, and state intentions in simple, short sentences. 1e. Assess nature of Johnny's hallucinations, delusions (verbal and nonverbal cues). 1f. Avoid laughing or whispering in front of Johnny. 1g. Provide information on community-based activities that enhance social, academic, and problem-solving skills. 1h. Counsel Johnny to avoid substance abuse. 1i. Educate Johnny about stress-reducing activities.	1a. Administration of medication promotes reality testing and decreases agitation and level of dangerousness. 1b. Promotes reality testing and reduces agitation. 1c. Enables nurse to assess mental status and response to interventions. 1d. Promotes reality testing. 1e. Important to know what voices are saying to client and the effectiveness of interventions. 1f. These behaviors increase suspiciousness and distrust. 1g. Increases independence and self-esteem. 1h. Increased awareness is associated with prevention. 1i. Enhances coping skills and reduces tension/anxiety.	*Goal met:* Johnny's hallucinations and delusions are gradually reduced. Johnny demonstrates a calm mood and increased trust of the nurse.

Nursing Diagnosis: Imbalanced Nutrition: Less Than Body Requirements

Outcome Identification	Nursing Actions	Rationales	Evaluation
1. By [date], Johnny will maintain adequate nutritional status to meet body requirements.	1a. Assess nutritional status. 1b. Decrease environmental stimuli. 1c. Provide adequate nutrition.	1a. To determine baseline information. 1b. Decreased stimuli minimize anxiety/stress. 1c. Helps ensure adequate intake.	*Goal met:* With parental encouragement, Johnny begins to take in adequate nutrition and demonstrates gradual weight gain.

SUMMARY

◆ Schizophrenia and other psychotic disorders have a biopsychosocial etiology.

◆ These disorders have a profound effect on the lives of persons affected by them as well as the persons who care about and for them.

◆ Physical and structural alterations are affected by the presence and intensity of stressors.

◆ This combination effect may lead to the development of schizophrenia and other psychotic disorders within persons' lives.

◆ The onset of schizophrenia generally occurs within adolescence or early 20s. However, older adults may also incur the disorder.

◆ Treatment issues involve a holistic and interdisciplinary approach that involve the use of pharmacologic and psychotherapeutic interventions.

◆ Emerging data from imaging and genetic studies indicate the complexity of schizophrenia and other psychotic disorders.

◆ Recovery is an important concept in the lives of persons diagnosed with schizophrenia. The presence of recovery promotes a productive and meaningful life for clients even in the presence of their mental illness.

◆ PMH nurses can be instrumental in collaborating with clients throughout all levels and cycles of their recovery processes.

STUDY QUESTIONS

1. The etiology of schizophrenia involves which combination of the following systems?
   a. Sympathetic and autonomic
   b. Central nervous and sympathetic
   c. Anatomic and functional
   d. Sympathetic and anatomic

2. Mrs. J. often hesitates and turns her head to the side when the nurse is speaking with her. This behavior may be indicative of:
   a. inner ear infection
   b. introverted personality behavior
   c. presence of auditory hallucinations
   d. presence of a delusion

3. The atypical antipsychotics are more effective in decreasing or eliminating the negative symptoms of schizophrenia than are the typical antipsychotics.
   a. True
   b. False

4. A person diagnosed with schizophrenia has which of the following brain changes?
   a. Increased brain blood flow
   b. Decreased third ventricle size
   c. Altered sensorium
   d. Decreased brain tissue

5. The nurse is assessing the client admitted to the acute psychiatric inpatient unit with a diagnosis of acute exacerbation of schizophrenia. The nurse can expect the client to exhibit all but which of the following behaviors?
   a. Auditory and/or visual hallucinations
   b. Fears that someone has bugged his phone
   c. Irritable and agitated mood
   d. Intrusiveness, talkativeness, and pressured speech

6. Prior to administering antipsychotic agents to the client with acute psychotic symptoms, it is imperative for the nurse to do which of the following?
   a. Give it as quickly as possible.
   b. Introduce self and explain all procedures.
   c. Make sure the client agrees to take the medication.
   d. Avoid explanations because he is too confused to understand.

7. A client with a diagnosis of schizophrenia is brought to the emergency room with complaints of fever, severe muscle rigidity, confusion, and labile blood pressure. A diagnostic workup reveals neuroleptic malignant syndrome (NMS). When eliciting a history from the client's family, one of the signs of NMS that the nurse should be particularly observant for is which of the following?
   a. Reddish-brown urine
   b. Constricted pupils
   c. Dilated pupils
   d. Hyperreflexia

8. The nurse is assessing the client admitted with neuroleptic malignant syndrome (NMS). The nurse can expect to observe which of the following findings on the mental status examination?
   a. Alert and oriented to person and place
   b. Cooperative and responsive to questions
   c. Waxing and waning level of consciousness
   d. Incoherent speech

9. Which of the following statements is an example of a delusion?
   a. "Every time I call my wife at work her line is busy. She is cheating on me."
   b. "I think my boss is reading my e-mails."
   c. "My best friend has her own publishing company and she has asked me to write a book."
   d. "My boss is harassing me. I can't do anything right."

10. You are assessing a client with acute psychotic symptoms. During the interview the client yells and asks "Can't you hear my father talking to you?" What is the most appropriate response?
    a. "I understand that you hear your father's talking, but I don't."
    b. "Yes, I hear him talking, but I don't understand what he is saying."
    c. "I don't hear him talking and neither do you!"
    d. "I need to give you an injection to make the voice go away."

11. In assessing a client with predominantly negative symptoms of schizophrenia, which symptoms would the nurse perceive as key in the client's response to an atypical antipsychotic medication?
    a. Improved mood, attention, and motivation
    b. Reduced hallucinations and paranoia
    c. Coherent speech and thoughts
    d. Organized thoughts

12. When a client with schizophrenia and a history of non-adherence to medication regimen was first admitted to the hospital, she refused medication and argued with the nurse about her need for it. Which observation by the nurse is the best indication that her goal of adherence with the medication routine has been achieved?
    a. The client requests her medication at scheduled times.
    b. The client verbalizes her need for medication while in the hospital.
    c. The client takes her medication when offered by the nurse.
    d. The client describes reasons that adherence is important.

13. In evaluating side effects in a client who is taking an atypical antipsychotic agent, which of the following is the most important part of the physical assessment?
    a. Weighing the client each visit
    b. Taking the client's blood pressure and temperature
    c. Inquiring about sleeping patterns
    d. Checking the client's pupils for symmetry

14. A 4 year-old-boy is brought into the child psychiatric clinic. He was recently diagnosed with Asperger's disorder. Which of the following behaviors is the nurse least likely to observe in the child?
    a. Impaired social skills
    b. Emotional relatedness, easily engaged
    c. A lack of interest or apathy
    d. Repetitive and stereotypical psychomotor activities

15. A client confides to the nurse that he is being pursued by the Federal Bureau of Investigation because he has access to information that will prevent a dirty bomb. This behavior most likely represents which of the following?
    a. Ideas of reference
    b. Delusions
    c. Hallucinations
    d. Dissociation

RESOURCES

Please note that because Internet resources are of a time-sensitive nature and URL addresses may change or be deleted, searches should also be conducted by association or topic.

Internet Resources

http://www.mentalhealth.com/book/p40-sc01.html
Schizophrenia Handbook for Families

Other Resources

National Institute of Mental Health
    NIMH Genetic Study of Schizophrenia
    (888) 674-6464
http://nimh.nih.gov/sibstudy/
National Institute of Schizophrenia and other
    Allied Disease
    384 Victoria Street
    Darlinghurst NSW 2010
    Australia
    61 2 9295 8407
    Fax: 61 2 9295 8415
    E-mail: nisad@nisad.org.au
http://nisad.org.au/researchDatabase/header.html

REFERENCES

Addington, A. M., Gornick, M. C., Shaw, P., Seal, J., Gogtay, N., Greenstein, D., et al. (2007). Neuregulin (NRG1, 8p12) and childhood onset schizophrenia: Susceptibility haplotypes for diagnosis and brain developmental trajectories. *Molecular Psychiatry, 12,* 195–205.

American Psychiatric Association (APA). (2000). *Diagnostic and statistical manual of mental disorders* (4th edition, Text Revision) (*DSM-IV-TR*). Washington, DC: Author.

American Psychiatric Association. (2004). *Practice guidelines for the treatment of psychiatric disorders*. Washington, DC: American Psychiatic Association.

Antonova, E., Sharma, T., Morris, R., & Kumari, V. (2004).The relationship between brain structure and neurocognition in schizophrenia: A selective review. *Schizophrenia Bulletin, 70,* 457–467.

Bell, M. D., Bryson, G. J., Greig, T. C., Fiszdon, J. M., & Wexler, B. E. (2005). Neurocognitive enhancement therapy with work therapy: Productivity outcomes at 6- and 12-month follow-ups. *Journal of Rehabilitation Research Development, 42,* 829–838.

Biswas, P., Malhotra, S., Malhotra, A., & Gupta, N. (2006). Comparative study of neuropsychological correlates in schizophrenia with onset in childhood, adolescence and adulthood. *European Child and Adolescent Psychiatry, 15,* 360–366.

Bleuler, E. (1950). *Dementia praecox or the group schizophrenias*. New York: International Universities Press.

Brekke, J. S., Nakagami, E., Kee, K. S., & Green, M. F. (2005). Cross-ethnic differences in perception of emotion in schizophrenia. *Schizophrenia Research, 77,* 289–298.

Buckley, P. F., & Brown, E. S. (2006). Prevalence and consequences of dual diagnosis. *Journal of Clinical Psychiatry, 67,* eo1.

Cannon, T. D., Thompson, P. M., van Erp, T. G., Huttunen, M., Lonnqvist, J., Kaprio, J., & Toga, A. W. (2006). Mapping heritability and molecular genetic associations with cortical features using probabilistic brain atlases: Methods and applications to schizophrenia. *Neuroinformatics, 4,* 5–19.

Craddock, N., O'Donovan, M. C., & Owen, M. J. (2005). The beginning of the end for the Kraepelinian dichotomy. *British Journal of Psychiatry, 186,* 364–366.

Craddock, N., O'Donovan, M. C., & Owen, M. J. (2006). Genes for schizophrenia and bipolar disorder? Implications for psychiatric nosology. *Schizophrenia Bulletin, 32,* 9–16.

Donohoe, G., Clarke, S., Morris, D., Nangle, J. M., Schwaiger, S., Gill, M., Corvin, A., & Robertson, I. H. (2006). Are deficits in executive sub-processes simply reflecting more general cognitive decline in schizophrenia? *Schizophrenia Research, 85,* 168–173.

Folsom, D. P., Hawthorne, W., Lindamer, L., Gilmer, T., Bailey, A., Golshan, S., et al. (2005). Prevalence and risk factors for homelessness and utilization of mental health services among 10,340 patients with serious mental illness in a large public mental health system. *American Journal of Psychiatry, 162,* 370–376.

Folsom D., & Jeste D. V. (2002). Schizophrenia in homeless persons: A systematic review of the literature. *Acta Psychiatrica Scandinavica, 104,* 1–10.

Freud, S. (1959). Inhibitions, symptoms, and anxiety. In J. Strachey (Trans. & Ed.), *The standard edition of the complete psychological works of Sigmund Freud* (Vol. 18, pp. 1–64). London: Hogarth Press.

Gur, R. E., Nimgaonkar, V. L., Almasy, L., Calkins, M. E., Ragland, J. D., Pogue-Geile, M. F., et al. (2007). Neurocognitive endophenotypes in a multiplex multigenerational family study of schizophrenia. *American Journal of Psychiatry, 164,* 705–707.

Hafner, H., Mauer, K., Trendler, G., van der Heiden, W., Schmidt, K., Konnecke, R., & Harrow, M. (2005). Schizophrenia and depression: Challenging the paradigm of two separate diseases: A controlled study of schizophrenia, depression and healthy controls. *Schizophrenia Research, 77,* 11–24.

Hall, J. E. (2006). Guyton and Hall. *Physiology Review,* 11th ed. Philadelphia: Elsevier.

Harrison, P. J., & Weinberger, D. R. (2005). Schizophrenia genes, gene expression, and neuropathology: On the matter of their convergence. *Molecular Psychiatry, 10,* 40–68.

Hoff, A. L., Svetina, C., Shields, G., Stewart, J., & DeLisi, L. E. (2005). Ten-year longitudinal study of neuropsychological functioning subsequent to a first episode of schizophrenia. *Schizophrenia Research, 78,* 27–34.

Hogarty, G. E., Flesher, S., Ulrich, R., Carter, M., Greenwald, D., Pogue-Geile, M., Kechavan, M., et al. (2004). Cognitive enhancement therapy for schizophrenia: Effects of a 2-year randomized trial on cognition and behavior. *Archives of General Psychiatry, 61,* 866–876.

James, D. J., & Glaze, L. E. (2006) *Bureau of Justice Statistics Special Reports: Mental health problems of prison and jail inmates.* NCJ 213600 http://www.ojp.usdoj.gov/bjs/pub/pdf/mhppji.pdf

Kay, S. R., Fiszbein, A., & Opler, L. A. (1987). The positive and negative syndrome scale (PANSS) for schizophrenia. *Schizophrenia Bulletin, 13,* 261–276.

Kirkbride, J. B., Fearon, P., Morgan, C., Dazzan, P., Morgan, K., Tarrant, J., Lloyd, T., et al. (2006). Heterogeneity in incidence rates of schizophrenia and other psychotic syndromes: Findings from the 3-Center ÆSOP Study. *Archives of General Psychiatry, 63,* 250–258.

Koeda, M., Takahashi, H., Yahata, N., Matsuura, M., Asai, K., Okubo, Y., et al. (2006). Language processing and human voice perception in schizophrenia: A functional magnetic resonance imaging study. *Biological Psychiatry, 59,* 948–957.

Lambert, M., Conus, P., Lubman, D. I., Wade, D., Yuen, H., Moritz, S., Naber, D., et al. (2005). The impact of substance-use disorders on clinical outcome in 643 patients with first-episode psychosis. *Acta Psychiatrica Scandinavica, 112,* 141–148.

Limosin, F., Loze, J. Y., Philippe, A., Casadebaig, F., & Rouillon, F. (2007). Ten-year prospective follow-up study of the mortality by suicide in schizophrenic patients. *Schizophrenia Research, 94,* 23–28. [Epub ahead of print]

Lindenmayer, J. P., Khan, A., Iskander, A., Abad, M. T., & Parker, B. (2007). A randomized controlled trial of olanzapine versus haloperidol in the treatment of primary negative symptoms and neurocognitive deficits in schizophrenia. *Journal of Clinical Psychiatry, 68,* 368–379.

Lopez, A. D., Mathers, C. D., Ezzati, M., Jamison, D. T., & Murray, C. J. L. (2006). Global and regional burden of disease and risk factors, 2001: Systematic analysis of population health data. *The Lancet, 367,* 1747–1757. Available online at http://www.globalhealth.harvard.edu/documents/LopezADLancet2006.pdf

Managalore, R., & Knapp, M. (2007). Cost of schizophrenia in England. *Journal of Mental Health Policy and Economics, 10,* 23–41.

Mazak, D., Zemishlani, C., Aizenberg, D., & Barak, Y. (2005). Patients with very-late-onset schizophrenia-like psychosis: A follow-up study. *American Journal of Geriatric Psychiatry, 13,* 417–419.

McClellan, J. M., & Werry, J. S. (2000). Introduction-research psychiatric diagnostic interviews for children and adolescents. *Journal of the American Academy of Child and Adolescent Psychiatry, 39,* 19–27.

McGurk, S. R., Mueser, K. T., & Pascaris, A. (2005). Cognitive training and supported employment for persons with severe mental illness: One-year results from a randomized controlled trial. *Schizophrenia Bulletin, 31,* 898–909.

Mehler-Wex, C., Riederer, P., & Gerlach, M. (2007). Dopaminergic dysbalance in distinct basal ganglia neuro-circuits: Implications for the pathophysiology of Parkinson's disease, schizophrenia and attention deficit hyperactivity disorder. *Neurotoxicity Research, 10,* 167–179.

Meyer, U., Nyffeler, M., Engler, A., Uryler, A., Schedlowski, M., Knuesel, I., Yee, B. K., & Feldon, J. (2006). The time of prenatal immune challenge determines the specificity of inflammation-mediated brain and behavioral pathology. *The Journal of Neuroscience, 26,* 4752–4762.

Overall, J. E., & Gorham, D. R. (1962). The brief psychiatric rating scale. *Psychological Report, 10,* 799–812.

Philips, L. J., McGorry, P. D., Garner, B., Thompson, K. N., Pantelis, C., Wood, S. J., et al. (2006). Stress, the hippocampus and the hypothalamic-pituitary-adrenal axis: Implications for the development of psychotic disorders. *Australia and New Zealand Journal of Psychiatry, 40,* 725–741.

Picard, H., Amado, I., Mouchet-Mages, S., Olie, J. P., & Krebs, M. O. (2007). The role of the cerebellum in schizophrenia: An update of clinical, cognitive, and functional evidences. *Schizophrenia Bulletin, June 11,* sbm049v1. Available online at http://schizophreniabulletin. oxfordjournals.org/cgi/reprint/sbm049v1

Rapoport, J. L., Addington, A. M., Frangou, S., & Psych, M.R. (2005). The neurodevelopmental model of schizophrenia: Update 2005. *Molecular Psychiatry, 10,* 434–449.

Riley, B., & Kendler, K. S. (2006). Molecular genetic studies of schizophrenia. *European Journal of Human Genetics, 14,* 669–680.

Riley, B. P., & Kendler, K. S. (2005). Schizophrenia: Genetics. In B. J. Sadock & V. A. Sadock (eds). *Kaplan & Sadock's Comprehensive Textbook of Psychiatry,* 8th ed., Vol. 1 (pp.1354–1371). Philadelphia: Lippincott Williams & Wilkins.

Roder, V., Mueller, D. R., Mueser, K. T., & Brenner, H. D. (2006). Integrated psychological therapy (IPT) for schizophrenia: Is it effective? *Schizophrenia Bulletin, 32* (Suppl. 1), S81–S93.

Rund, B. R., Sundet, K., Asbjørnsen, A., Egeland, J., Landro, N. I., Lund, A., et al. (2006). Neuropsychological test profiles in schizophrenia and non-psychotic depression. *Acta Psychiatrica Scandinavica, 113,* 350–359.

Salgado-Pineda, P., Cadin, A., Baeza, I., Junque, C., Bernardo, M., Blin, O., & Folupt, P. (2007). Schizophrenia and frontal cortex: Where does it fail? *Schizophrenia Research* (e-pub: in print).

Seidman, L. J., Giuliano, A. J., Smith, C. W., Stone, W. S., Glatt, S. J., Meyer, E., Faraone, S. V., Tsuang, M. T., & Cornblatt, B. (2006). Neuropsychological functioning in adolescents and young adults at genetic risk for schizophrenia and affective psychoses: Results from the harvard

and hillside adolescent high risk studies. *Schizophrenia Bulletin, 32,* 507–525.

Shergill, S. S., Brammer, M. J., Amaro, E., Williams, S. C. R., Murray, R. M., & McGuire, P. K. (2004). Temporal course of auditory hallucinations. *The British Journal of Psychiatry, 185,* 516–517.

Siegel, S. J., Irani, F., Brensinger, C. M., Kohler, C. G., Bilker, W. B., Ragland, J. D., Kanes, S. J., Gur, R. C., & Gur, R. E. (2006). Prognostic variables at intake and long-term level of function in schizophrenia. *American Journal of Psychiatry, 163,* 433–441.

Siris, S. G. (2000). Depression in schizophrenia: Perspective in the era of "atypical" antipsychotic agents. *American Journal of Psychiatry, 157,* 1379–1389.

Stahl, S. M., & Buckley, P. F. (2007). Negative symptoms of schizophrenia: A problem that will not go away. *Acta Psychiatrica Scandinavia, 115,* 4–11.

Sur, C., & Kinney, G. G. (2007). Glycine transporter 1 inhibitors and modulation of NMDA receptor-mediated excitatory neurotransmission. *Current Drug Targets, 8,* 643–649.

Tsai, G., & Coyle, I. T. (2002). Glutamergic mechanisms in schizophrenia. *Annual Review of Pharmacology Toxicology, 42,* 165–179.

U.S. Public Health Service, Department of Health and Human Services (DHHS). (1999). *Mental health: A report of the surgeon general.* Retrieved May 12, 2006, from http://www. surgeongeneral.gov/library/mentalhealth.html

Van der Heiden, W., Konnecke, R., Maurer, K., Ropeter, D., & Hafner, H. (2005). Depression in the long-term course of schizophrenia. *European Archives of Psychiatry and Clinical Neuroscience, 255,* 174–184.

Vitiello, B., & Wagner, A. (2007). The rapidly expanding field of autism research. *Biological Psychiatry, 61,* 427–428.

Westmeyer, J. (2006). Comorbid schizophrenia and substance abuse: A review of epidemiology and course. *American Journal of Addictions, 15,* 345–355.

Wilk, J., Marcus, S. C., West, J., Countis, L., Hall, R., Regier, D. A., & Olfson, M. (2006). Substance abuse and the management of medication nonadherence in schizophrenia. *Journal of Nervous and Mental Disorders, 194,* 454–457.

World Health Organization. (2005). *Developing country-specific strategies for reduction of treatment gap in common neuropsychiatric conditions: Report of intercountry workshop, New Delhi, India, 18-20 November 2004.* WHO Project: ICP MN01. Geneva, Switzerland: Author. Available online at http://www.searo.who.int/LinkFiles/ Meeting_reports_18-20Nov-04_Ment-140.pdf

SUGGESTED READINGS

http://www.soros.org/initiatives/justice/articles_publica-tions/publications/cj_mh_consensus_20020601/Consensus%20Project%20Report.pdf Criminal Justice/Mental Health Consensus Project, Council of State Governments 2002. (Accessed September 24, 2006)

http://schizophrenia.com/ Information, support and educa-tion about schizophrenia. (Accessed June 1, 2006)

http://www.shadowvoices.com/resources/default.asp Shadow Voices: Finding Hope in Mental Illness (Accessed June 1, 2006)

Evans, D. L., Foa, E. B., Gur, R. E., Hendin, H., O'Brien, C. P., & Seligman, M. E. P. (2005). *Treating and preventing adolescent mental health disorders*. New York: Oxford University Press.

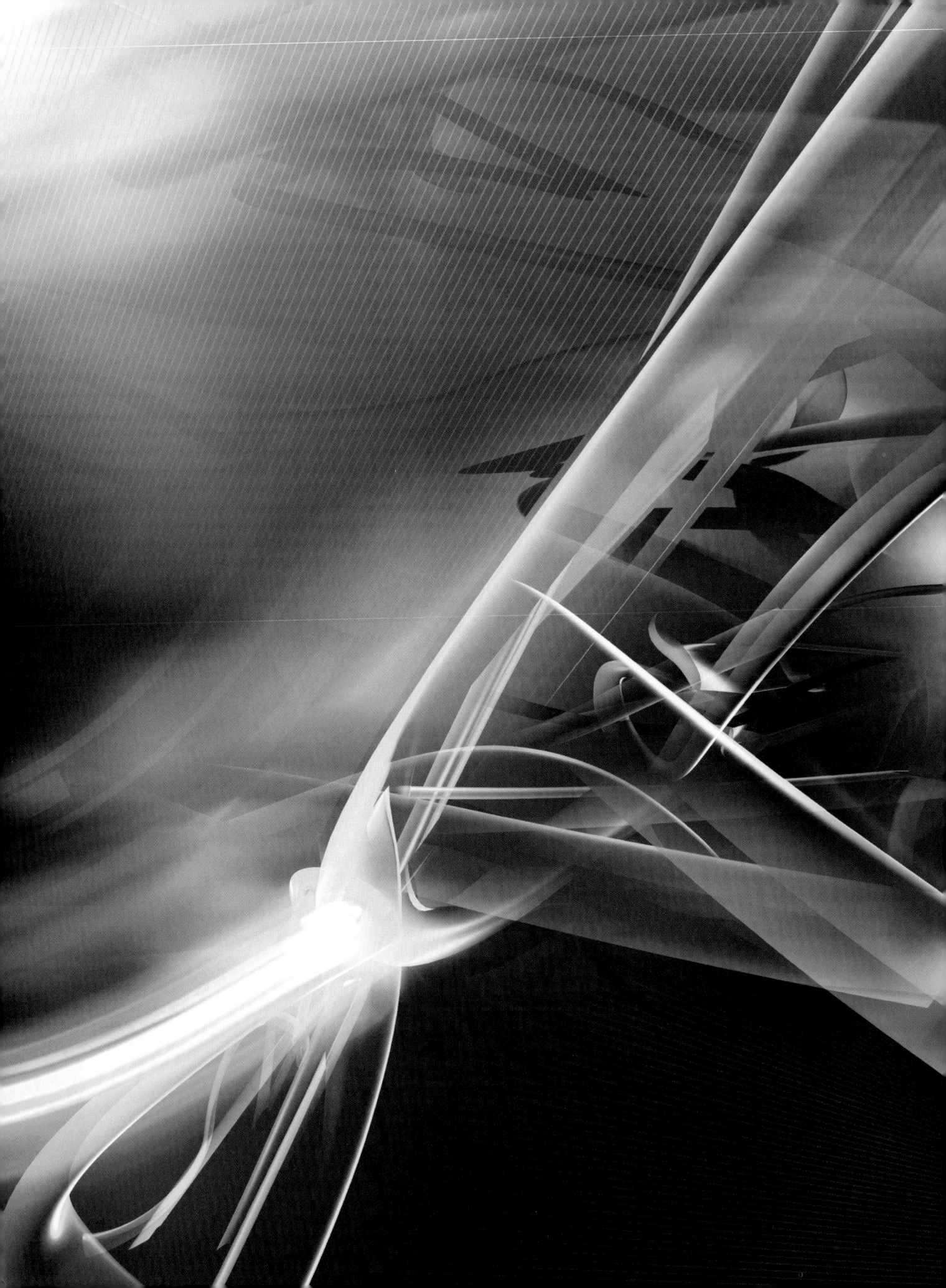

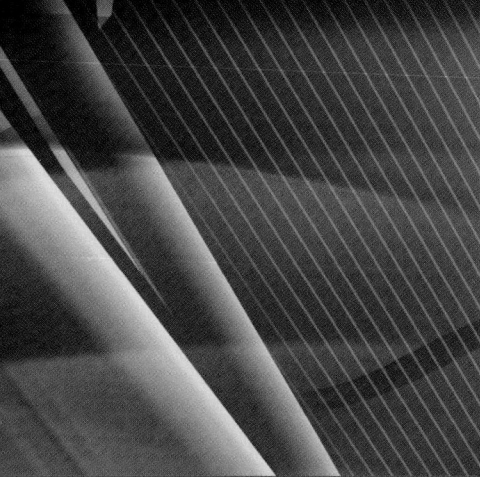

CHAPTER 15

The Client with a Personality Disorder

Sylvia A. Whiting, PhD, APRN, BC

KEY TERMS

Acting Out: Living out unresolved developmental issues or fantasies impulsively in out-of-control behavior.

Attachment Theory: Theory based on the classic works of Bowlby and Ainsworth that define attachment or bonding as an evolutionary and biological process of eliciting and maintianing physical closeness between a child and a parent or primary caregiver. This theory also infers that the infant's relationships with early caregivers are responsible for influencing future interactions and relationships.

Boundary: Refers to rules defining who and how members participate in a subsystem or a relationship. The clearer the boundary, the healthier the relationship.

Character: Learned personality traits that influence behavioral patterns.

Dysphoria: Marked feelings of sadness.

Ego Dystonic: Discomfort in the presence of a disordered mental state.

Ego Syntonic: Personal comfort with symptoms that create discomfort in others.

Evoked Potential: A short train of large slow waves recorded from the scalp to reflect dendritic activity and influenced by many variables—a useful indicator of brain activity in the processing of information.

Internalized Relationships: Those relationships that are maintained as supportive or destructive to the psyche and which continue to affect the individual long after the experience.

Libidinal Object Constancy: The maintenance of the image of the primary caretaker in the growing infant's memory so that the figure remains in the mind even when the object is not immediately present and interactive.

Object Relations: Internalized relationships recollected from early primary caregivers.

Patterns: A person's typical behavioral organization that resists change.

Personality: Characteristic traits that are generally predictable in their influence on cognitive, affective, and behavioral patterns.

Psyche Organizers: Repetitive developmental experiences that guide the person's experience and expectations resulting in the style of reaction that is typical of that person.

Reality Principle: A perception of the environment that fairly matches what others perceive and which fosters adaptive responses toward productivity, enjoyment of life, and maintenance of homeostasis.

Splitting: The internal mechanism wherein the person is unable to evaluate, synthesize, and accept imperfections in others so that a significant other is viewed as all good or all bad, and causing the phenomenon of setting persons up against each other.

Traits: Personality structure that typifies a person's responses in various situations.

COMPETENCIES

Upon completion of this chapter, the learner should be able to:

1. Identify an inclusive list of the personality disorders.

2. Place the personality disorders within their respective clusters.

3. Discuss theories relative to possible or probable causes underlying the development of personality disorders.

4. Describe probable causes and symptom manifestations of various personality disorders across the life span.

5. Discuss epidemiological information regarding various personality disorders.

6. Describe the most appropriate interventions in the treatment of individuals with personality disorders.

7. Acknowledge and discuss the need for nursing research in the field of personality disorders.

Personality is reflected by a person's capacity and skill for managing activities of daily living. Individual responses and interactions to internal and external environmental demands (pressures) are influenced by the constant interplay of genetic, neurobiological, and psychological factors.

Personality is defined as the characteristic traits that are generally predictable in their influence on cognitive, affective, and behavioral patterns of human beings. These patterns develop and evolve over time, are conscious or unconscious, and affect adaptation and response to the environment (American Psychiatric Association [APA],2000). Adaptation is a central core of all personality theories and may include healthy responding (adaptation) or unhealthy responding (maladaptation). Character is generated by early life experience and is represented by learned personality traits that influence behavioral patterns (Hirschfield, 1986).

Hartmann (1958) considered the mastering of reality to be the basis of adaptation, and he related adaptation to productivity, enjoyment of life, and maintenance of homeostasis. Stress is an integral aspect of living; one's capacity to handle it effectively begins at birth and evolves throughout life. Hartmann asserted that the reality principle and its relationship to adaptive responses was integral to life and that the struggle to adjust to environmental disruption was an effort to maintain stability. He concluded that "every stimulus disrupts equilibrium, but not every stimulus causes conflict" (Hartmann, 1958, p. 38).

Adaptive personality traits function to maintain homeostasis through healthy interactions. Everyone is capable of adapting to stress, but the level of adaptation is influenced by one's personality structure or traits. Maladaptive responses influence and often hamper a person's interpersonal relationships and increase the level of internal stress or the various crises that are thus experienced or actually created by their response behaviors. Flexibility is needed in dealing with environmental pressures, and narrow or rigid responses influence the type of coping mechanisms demonstrated by the person.

Maladaptive behavioral patterns are the hallmark of personality disorders and are manifested by the degree of rigidity or inflexibility that exists in attitudes and behaviors within one's coping style. One sees a behavioral pattern in which there is marked deviation from that expected in the individual's culture, and the pattern is seen in two or more of the following areas:

1. cognition (perception and interpretation of self, others, and events)
2. affectivity (the range, intensity, lability, and appropriateness of emotional responses)
3. interpersonal functioning
4. impulse control (APA, 2000)

Howard (2000) provides information about the work of Millon and others in which there are five factors that best account for variability in personalities. These are known as (1) emotional stability; (2) extraversion; (3) culture; (4) agreeableness; and (5) conscientiousness. These may ultimately form the basis for diagnosis of personality disorders in the *DSM-V*. Once a personality trait is established, it is extremely resistant but not impossible to change.

Numerous assumptions have been made regarding personality development. Debate continues as to whether personality traits are genetically (nature) or environmentally (nurture) determined. Both are considered influential in the way that a flower (gene) and fertilizer, soil, and water (environment) are essential to each other. The evolution of personality is a complex issue. It challenges nurses working with clients at various stages of life and requires understanding of adaptive and maladaptive responses that clients use to minimize distress and emotional upheaval.

PERSONALITY DISORDERS

The prevalence of personality disorders challenges psychiatric nurses in various practice settings to recognize symptoms and their impact on treatment outcomes. Personality disorders often complicate the care of clients with co-occurring psychiatric disorders because of their high utilization of mental health resources and emotional demands on psychiatric nurses and other care providers. Although people with personality disorders generally are not considered to be ill and often are not benefited by medications, they do suffer from a life that is not positive, proactive, or fulfilling. Their lives are full of suffering, rejection, and defeat. These never-ending experiences often lead to anxiety, depression, or other Axis I disorders that may require medication and various forms of therapy.

TAXONOMIC CHARACTERISTICS OF PERSONALITY DISORDERS (AXIS II)

The *Diagnostic and Statistical Manual of Mental Disorders* (4th edition Revision) *(DSM-IV-TR)* (APA, 2000) was published after extensive interdisciplinary research and discussion regarding the various conditions constituting the entire domain of psychiatric concern. A total of 10 specific disorders were identified as "Personality Disorders" with an eleventh category entitled "Personality Disorders Not Otherwise Specified" to cover certain conditions not clearly identified by particular symptoms. Conditions classified as personality disorders are placed in a separate category (Axis II) apart from other psychiatric disorders (Axis I) because the underlying causes and presenting behaviors are different and require different treatment approaches. Axis III consists of medical conditions that may coincide, contribute to, or exacerbate Axis I or II conditions. Widiger (2003) differentiates the diagnosis of Axis I from Axis II disorders by time and characteristics of behaviors. Axis I disorders have a rather acute onset during some period of adult life and are readily distinguished from everyday functioning. Axis II disorders have an early onset with chronic features that characterize everyday functioning. In 1999, Widiger reported that response to Millon's three polarity dimensions of active-passive, pleasure-pain, and self-other formed the conditions from which personality disorders derived. Haslam, Reichert, and Fiske (2002), state that because persons diagnosed with an Axis II disorder are socially interactive, attention is drawn to their deviance leading to difficulty in getting along with others.

DEFINITION OF PERSONALITY DISORDERS

Kernberg (1984) defined personality disorders as a spectrum of maladaptive traits that produce or influence considerable psychological and emotional disturbance and impair relationships. The *DSM-IV-TR* (APA, 2000) delineates clinical features of personality disorders as an enduring pattern of feeling (emotions), thinking (cognitive distortions), and behaving (maladaptive in nature) that become rigid and stable over time. Features of personality disorders appear to emerge during adolescence or early adulthood. However, others are less obvious or remit over time, mainly borderline and antisocial personality disorders, whereas this is less accurate for obsessive-compulsive and schizotypal personality disorders (APA, 2000). Behavioral features of personality disorders tend to be rigid and inflexible, resulting in distress or maladaptive coping skills. Such maladaptive responses often lead to personal problems that induce extreme anxiety, distress, and depression in clients, and the ability to perform at optimal levels is constantly compromised. Some clients experience lifelong difficulty adapting to change, tolerating frustration and crises, and forming healthy relationships.

Clients often deny their existing problems and usually lack insight into the maladaptive behaviors that create even more problems for them. These behaviors are symptoms that are described as **ego syntonic** (i.e., comfortable for the individual but usually uncomfortable for others) and thus acceptable to them because they represent aspects of the clients' personality that have become typical and gratifying for them. Clients with personality disorders differ from other clients experiencing anxiety, depression, or other emotional disorders because the latter experience an uncomfortable and unacceptable **ego dystonic** state that forces them to seek psychotherapeutic assistance. Because clients with personality disorders are usually comfortable with themselves and their behaviors, they do not recognize or accept the need for a change in the way they behave, and they tend to use displacement or projection to aid their coping. These clients usually tax the mental and physical resources of the health care team. They often display an uncanny ability to create crisis and uproar. Nurses and other professionals are challenged in developing innovative treatment strategies that meet the needs and demands of these clients without succumbing to manipulation of one kind or another.

TYPES OF PERSONALITY DISORDERS

A large number of clients are admitted for treatment with a single Axis II disorder or for more complex diagnoses consisting of one or more axes. Clients with personality disorders may not seek treatment for their Axis II diagnosis, but there may be many reasons why they present themselves for inpatient or outpatient treatment. They tend to engage in risky behaviors and may attempt suicide, abuse substances, participate in dangerous activities, or have cognitive-perceptual impairments.

The 10 personality disorders are listed as follows: paranoid, schizoid, schizotypal, antisocial, borderline, histrionic, narcis-

sistic, avoidant, dependent, and obsessive-compulsive. The three clusters under which various personality disorders are placed are depicted in Table 15–1. A category for behavioral patterns not falling within the 10 disorders but having characteristics of a personality disorder are found in the *DSM-IV* under *Personality Disorder NOS*. Two of them, *Passive-Aggressive Personality* (having a pattern of negative attitudes) and *Self-Defeating Personality Disorder* (behaving in ways that undermine pleasure and goals) were not included in *DSM-IV* since it was not clear that they constituted separate disorders. The new *DSM-V* may contain very different categories for identifying persons with these problems (http://www.corante.com/brainwaves/archives/2005/05/25the_future_of_psychiatric_diagno).

RECOGNITION OF SPECIAL NEEDS IN CLIENTS WITH PERSONALITY DISORDERS

Clients with personality disorders such as borderline and antisocial types exhibit a wide variety of maladaptive behaviors such as substance abuse, suicidal gestures, and other self-destructive behaviors. Nursing implications for working with these types require attention to the following:

- Understanding factors associated with personality development
- Recognizing the impact of early childhood traumas on coping styles
- Dealing with intense reactions that occur when working with these clients

TABLE 15–1
Personality Disorders Organized By Cluster

	Type of Disorder	Description
Cluster A	Paranoid Schizoid Schizotypal	Clients are withdrawn and engage in odd, eccentric behavior.
Cluster B	Antisocial Borderline Histrionic Narcissistic	Clients seek attention and engage in erratic behavior.
Cluster C	Avoidant Dependent Obsessive-compulsive	Clients seek to avoid or minimize the experience of anxiety or fear.
Personality Disorders NOS	Passive-aggressive Masochistic	Clients are covertly aggressive against others or themselves.

NOS, not otherwise specified.

- Collaborating with other mental health professionals to develop consistency and prevent splitting of staff

- Recognition of the need to maintain boundaries that are extremely clear. Boundary means rules defining who and how members participate in a subsystem or a relationship. For example, it is important for the nurse to maintain a professional boundary between self and the client.

Assessing personality development entails examining the life span and factors such as early relationships with primary caregivers, the impact of these relationships on ego development, and adaptation and coping styles. Clients with personality disorders are often labeled as difficult because of their need for immediate gratification, their lack of empathy, and the intense affect they use in their frequent hostile outbursts and attacks, either verbal or physical. Persons with borderline personality disorder are noted for splitting—a behavior that involves setting up conflicts between others, almost as though saying, "Let's you and he/she fight." It is not uncommon for these clients to create splitting situations among staff members such that the staff become engaged in serious conflict concerning the appropriate management of the client. Such behaviors arouse intense feelings and negative reactions (countertransference) in nurses and other caregivers. Clear boundaries in these settings are essential.

Understanding the origins of these behaviors can play a key role in minimizing negative reactions toward these clients, who are experts in evoking tension in nurses and other professionals. Working with these clients needs to be perceived as a challenge rather than a burden because nurses are challenged to sharpen their skills in patience, self-awareness, creativity, and nonjudgmental approach. Above all, the staff must develop treatment plans that do not allow for splitting of staff; to accomplish this, they must confer frequently.

Most personality theories, regardless of their differences, emphasize the significance of primary caregivers in child growth and development. The child must master the initial demands for socialization within the family, where the foundation is laid for the future emergence of interpersonal relations with all others. These early interactions mediate the infant's perception of the world (Goldstein et al., 2006). Understanding key concepts in personality formation such as ego development and organization is crucial for nurses who must assess the meaning of their own, as well as of clients' maladaptive behaviors, facilitation of adaptive coping behaviors and evaluation of client responses to interventions.

PREVALENCE OF PERSONALITY DISORDERS

Historically, controversy about the precise prevalence of personality disorders has challenged researchers. Gunderson (1988) asserted that the difficulty lies in inconsistent and outdated diagnostic systems.

Today's researchers reiterate these concerns. The distinction between personality diagnoses is often difficult to discern owing to the frequent comorbidity of other diagnoses. Among the most common co-occurring diagnoses are mood disorders, substance-related disorders, anxiety disorders, and attention-deficit hyperactive disorders (ADHD) (Zimmerman, Rothschild, & Chelminski, 2005). Results from the National Comorbidity Survey Replication conducted by Lenzenweger and colleagues (2007) ($n = 5692$) demonstrated the estimates of prevalence of personality disorders (see Table 15–2): Cluster A, 1.5 percent; Cluster B, 6 percent; and Cluster C, 9 percent. These data also implicated that all three clusters were associated with co-occurring Axis I disorders that were subsequently linked to high morbidity (functional impairment)

TABLE 15–2
Available Prevalence Data for Personality Disorders*

Type of Personality Disorder	Prevalence	Rationale for Data
Paranoid	2.4%. More common in males than in females.	These persons are guarded and reluctant to seek treatment.
Schizotypal	0.6%. No gender differentiation provided.	Inferred from familial studies. Use of the diagnosis is highly variable.
Schizoid	1.7%. Found more in males than in females.	Seek treatment only when instigated by family members. Infrequently seen in outpatient settings.
Antisocial	0.7% and 4 to 7% times more frequent in males than in females. Peak prevalence is in the 22- to 44-year age group and drops abruptly after age 45. More prevalent in urban than in rural areas.	Appears by early adolescence. Behaviors are flagrant and easily identified or diagnosed.

(continues)

Type of Personality Disorder	Prevalence	Rationale for Data
Borderline	0.7% and three times more frequent in females than in males. Common in late adolescence and young adulthood, tapering off during the 30s and later.	Most common personality disorder found in outpatient and inpatient populations, occurring in 15 to 25% of all patients.
Histrionic	2.0%. Far more common in females than in males.	Symptoms have feminine connotations in western societies.
Narcissistic	0.8%. No gender differentiation given but diagnosis is generally made after adolescence.	Seen frequently in outpatient settings.
Avoidant	5.0%. Common in outpatient settings.	Not generally used as a primary diagnosis.
Dependent	1%–5%. Very common as a trait across a broad range of psychiatric conditions. More common in females than in males. Dependent behaviors observed at ages 6–10 are likely to continue into adulthood.	More apt to be used as a primary diagnosis in outpatient settings rather than inpatient settings.
Obsessive-compulsive	2.0% of the general population has identifiable traits and about 75% of these are sufficiently dysfunctional to be diagnosed with the disorder. Somewhat more common in females than in males.	Common in outpatient populations.
Personality Disorders NOS Passive-aggressive	1.7%. Passive-aggressive behaviors, however, are highly common, especially when there is a hierarchy of authority and power.	Rare as a primary diagnosis in outpatient populations. It appears likely that accompanying symptoms may lead to Axis II diagnosis.
Self-defeating	0.8%.	Associated with widely masochistic variable of dysfunction in both outpatients and inpatients.

NOS, not otherwise specified.

*Note. Adapted from *Diagnostic and Statistical Manual of Mental Disorders* (4th edition, Text Revision) (*DSM-IV-TR*), by the American Psychiatric Association, 2000, Washington, DC: Author. Adapted with permission.

Note. Data from Lenzenweger, M. F., Lane M. C., Loranger, A.W., & Kessler, R. C. (2007). *DSM-IV* personality disorders in the National Comorbidity Survey Replication. *Biological Psychiatry*. [Epub ahead of print]

(Lenzenweger, Lane, Loranger, & Kessler, 2007). Implications from these findings suggest that psychiatric nurses and other clinicians are challenged to evaluate common Axis I disorders, such as depression, anxiety disorders, and substance-use disorders, and provide appropriate interventions to reduce functional impairment.

CAUSATIVE FACTORS: THEORIES AND PERSPECTIVES

As with other psychiatric disorders, there are no clear-cut single causes for personality disorders. There seem to be a multiplicity of etiological bases for the conditions, with a genetic predis-

position for some (e.g., schizotypal, paranoid, and obsessive-compulsive), environmental causes more likely in others (e.g., narcissism, borderline, dependent, passive-aggressive types), and with mixed causes for still others (e.g., antisocial). Temperament seems to play a significant role in the etiology of some of the conditions. Millon (2000) cited extroversion, introversion, and other Meyers Briggs test components (MBTI) (Myers & McCaulley, 1985) as significant characteristics.

PSYCHODYNAMIC THEORIES

Until the 1970s, Sigmund Freud was the most noted psychoanalytical theorist. Many of his contemporary followers defected in later years and were also responsible for contributing new theories regarding personality development. Freud (1961) proposed that the personality developed by orderly progression through psychosexual stages known as oral, anal, and genital (or oedipal).

Other theorists suggested that these progressions were psychological in nature—that is, they were driven by forces other than libidinal drives proposed by Freud. Harry Stack Sullivan, for instance, suggested that the nature of the relationship between mother and child was the crucial factor in a healthy progression from infancy to childhood. Erik Erikson (1963) proposed a bridge between developmental stages and social functioning or adaptation. He contended that adaptive responses influenced developmental progression.

Theorists who made significant contributions to developmental theory during the era before the 1970s included Klein, Mahler, Kernberg, and Bowlby. More recently, an increasing amount of attention has been given to such areas as ego psychology, self-psychology, temperament, and genetics.

Melanie Klein

An English psychiatrist, Klein (1977) contributed to the evolution of the object relations concept. Her early work focused on the study of personality development as a transformation of primitive object relations. Object relations, defined in simple terms, are internalized relationships recollected from early primary caregivers. This relationship is considered the core of the person's existence, "all other human behavior and experiences . . . are relational derivatives" (Greenberg & Mitchell, 1983, p. 404). Early relationships with caregivers are postulated to be the most significant determinants of the person's ability to adapt and reach optimal growth and health. They also are associated with "emotional gratification [and/or deprivation] . . . and are believed to form the template for all subsequent relationships" (Cashdan, 1988, p. 23).

Margaret Mahler

Mahler's contribution to psychoanalytical theory also centers around her extensive research and study of object relations. Her work with emotionally ill children allowed her to assess growth and development that centered on the faulty object relations between mother and child during early infancy. She proposed that bonding and early childhood separation (separation-individuation) laid the foundation for growth, adaptation, and subsequent relationships. Mahler (1952, 1965a, 1965b) delineated the following three major developmental stages:

1. Autistic (birth to several weeks, when the infant is unaware of others)

2. Symbiotic (when the infant is concerned primarily with meeting basic needs but aware of the primary caregiver)

3. Separation-individuation (includes several phases centering around autonomy)

Mahler postulated that successful resolution of the final stage facilitates internalization of the primary caregiver and allows the child to maintain an image of the caregiver when absent. She named this process libidinal object constancy, a process that allows the child to introject positive and negative

images that influence future perceptions of experience and resulting attitudes.

Successful accomplishment of this task serves as the foundation for the child's ability to function independently of primary caregivers and form subsequent healthy interpersonal relationships. In contrast, unsuccessful or incomplete resolution of the task of integrating the primary caregiver as a model image places the child at risk for developing adult maladaptive behavioral patterns such as responding in an overly dependent or independent manner. Klein, a contemporary of Mahler's termed the inability to achieve resolution as *faulty early object relations* and noted that people with this problem eventually develop psychopathology. Early childhood interactions influence the person's capacity to cope with emotional distress, experience pleasure, and care for others.

Otto Kernberg

Kernberg's (1976, 1984) contribution to object relations theory has been noted in numerous publications and papers. He concurred with other object relations' theorists and noted that the basis of severe personality disorders was related to inadequate or impaired object relations that are ingrained in the personality. He also emphasized that the basis for understanding psychological adaptability and integrity stems from the child's relationship with primary caregivers.

John Bowlby

Bowlby's (1969, 1981) attachment theory also presented the belief that the infant's relationship with early caregivers influences later interactions. He contended that the function of attachment behavior is a process for the protection and development of early ego function. He further stated that by the end of the first year of life the child has internalized cognitive models of himself and others. Early experiences play crucial roles in children's inferences about their value and acceptability. Additionally, Bowlby (1951) surmised that early experiences with primary caregivers provide the basis for appraisals of all future social interactions and situations throughout the life span.

Bowlby viewed attachment behavior as a natural response in periods when certain needs exist. For example, he considered it natural for people to seek closeness during times of illness, and he did not consider these behaviors to be regressive or maladaptive as other psychoanalysts had proposed. On the other hand, Bowlby proposed that infants who have healthy interactions with primary caregivers are enabled to form enduring, mutually satisfying, and close interpersonal relationships with others in adulthood. Those who have unhealthy interactions with primary caregivers are expected to have difficulty in forming relationships and in maintaining closeness that is comfortable; they often experience distrust, fears, intense anxiety, or symbiotic relationships. See Chapter 11.

UNDERSTANDING EGO DEVELOPMENT

Understanding ego development or organization is fundamental to the capacity for aiding effective adaptation to internal and

TABLE 15–3
Comparison of Healthy and Unhealthy Ego Functions

	Healthy Ego Functions (Mature)	Unhealthy Ego Functions (Primitive)
Defense Mechanisms (conflict resolution)	Repression Sublimation Rationalization Displacement Reaction formation Undoing	Denial Projection Splitting Dissociation Isolation Regression Avoidance Conversion reaction
Modulation of Affect (impulsivity)	Postpones gratification needs Tolerates frustration and stress Maintains gratification through sublimation	Low frustration and stress tolerance Poor impulse control Need for immediate gratification
Self-Esteem (competence)	Mastery of environment Sense of worth and confidence	Poor self-esteem Fluctuation in self-worth
Relationship to Others (depth of relationships)	Capacity for object relations Empathic Stable, lasting relationships Capacity to mourn and move on to form new relationships	Places own needs before others Lack of empathy Chaotic relationships Inability to relate to others
Reality Testing	Accurate perceptions and appraisal of inner mental state (insight) Intact ego boundaries Sense of reality	Distorted perceptions Depersonalization Lack of insight into present Fluid ego boundaries Derealization
Cognitive Processes (thinking, learning, judgment)	Tolerates stress Capacity to integrate new experiences Tolerates inconsistency and incongruency in others	Poor tolerance to stress Low capacity to integrate new experiences Rigid, inflexible thinking

external stressors. Evaluating ego function is a major aspect of the nursing process because it provides data that assist in making accurate diagnoses, planning psychotherapeutic interventions, and bringing about therapeutic outcomes. Table 15–3 provides a framework for assessing ego function. This assessment considers the components of interpersonal relationships, affective capabilities, motivation for treatment, capacity for introspection, insight, defensive behavior, and reality testing.

Developmental Stages

Personality is now believed to have its origins in the prenatal period. Early childhood experience and interactions further lay the foundation for the ability to adapt to stress and change and engage in healthy interpersonal relationships. Erikson (1963) stated that the basic component in developing a healthy personality is trust because it serves as the basis for expecting that one's needs will be met, that safety will be provided, and that primary caregivers are reliable. His developmental theory describes trust during the first year of life as the foundation for adaptive responses throughout the life span. See Chapter 2.

Freud's oral stage parallels Erikson's stage of trust. During the oral stage, the infant is totally dependent on the primary caregiver for survival. It is during this period that the primary caregiver's capacity to nurture and modulate the infant's early

TABLE 15–4
Manifested Maladaptive Coping Behaviors Arising from Early Developmental Periods and Continuing across the Life Span

	Maladaptive Behavior	Possible Cause
Infancy	Withdrawal, refusal to enter relationships	Absence of nurturing caregiver
Childhood	Projection, ambivalence, regression, splitting, acting out, denial	Faulty ego development
Adolescence	Boredom, frustration, difficulty dealing with intense feelings, distorted cognitions (impaired reality testing), low self-esteem, acting out, expressing extreme hostility toward authority figures, impaired ability to solve problems, impulsivity, risky tension-reducing activities (e.g., substance abuse, sexual promiscuity, self-destructive and suicidal behaviors)	Impairments in ego and superego development, role confusion
Early and Middle Adulthood	Feelings of emptiness, loneliness, and distress; extremely demanding of relationships; low self-esteem; intense but unacknowledged emotional pain; substance abuse; suicide attempts; destructive relationships and behaviors	Lack of healthy ego functions
Older Adulthood	Intensification of earlier behaviors, suicide, feelings of despair, hopelessness, and helplessness	Nondevelopment of new ego operations; exaggeration of existing defense mechanisms to cope with increased stress associated with loss, retirement, or illness

emotional, psychological, and neurobiological needs is so important to the infant's survival and emotional development. See Chapter 2.

If the child perceives the world as loving, accepting, and safe, a healthy ego is likely to evolve. The process is complex and entails the child's learning how to deal with frustration as well as gratification. Early childhood traumas include conditions such as deprivation, abandonment, abuse, emotional extremes in the primary caregiver and family members, and overindulgence, which hamper the child in developing a healthy ego structure. Table 15–4 provides a list of unhealthy ego functions and their probable causes. Features of personality disorders seem to emerge during adolescence or early adulthood.

NEUROBIOLOGICAL THEORIES

The exact cause of personality disorders is complex. Most data point to an array of factors stemming from environmental factors, such as early childhood trauma to neurobiological modifications in complex biochemistry and neuroanatomical structures, to genetic predisposition. See the Research Abstract.

Recent studies also indicate that when compared to control subjects, clients with schizotypal personality disorders have reduced neocortical gray matter and enlarged sulcal cerebral spinal fluid volumes. Implications these data suggest are that women with schizotypal personality are part of the schizophrenia spectrum and share a genetic susceptibility with schizophrenia which demonstrates similar brain abnormalities (Koo et al., 2006).

Neurotransmitters such as serotonin and dopamine have been implicated in impulsivity, aggression, and suicidal gestures manifested in disordered personalities, especially borderline and antisocial types (Keilp et al., 2006). Several studies have demonstrated that low serotonin levels correlated with impulsive and aggressive behaviors. Sommer and colleagues (2006) and van Goozen and Fairchild (2006) suggested that antisocial behavior and personality result from genetic serotonin dysfunction. In addition, clients with borderline and antisocial personality disorders have been found to have low platelet levels of monoamine oxidase (the metabolizer of dopamine), resulting in higher than normal levels of dopamine, an arousal neurotransmitter. Abnormal testosterone circulation is considered influential in the production of antisocial aggressive behavior that may be impulsive and violent (Sommer et al., 2006; van Goozen & Fairchild, 2006). Brain imaging studies have implicated brain anomalies in persons with antisocial personality (ASP) disorder. Another biological theory implies that antisocial personality disorder has deficits in various brain regions including the amygdala and facial affect recognition. Neuroimaging data implicate corpus callosum deficits or thickness in the lack of attention, arousal, and emotions in individuals with antisocial personality disorder. This brain structure modulates areas of the brain that regulate attention, arousal, and emotion. Because of these deficits, individuals with antisocial personality disorder have deficits in recognition of negative reactions of cues in others—which may account for a lack of emotional responsiveness to others (Baker, Jacobson, Raine, Lozano, & Bezdjian, 2007; Dolan & Fullam, 2006).

The genetic association of schizotypal personality and concordance with those of clients with schizophrenia is well established (Koo et al., 2006). Additional biologic similarities exist between clients with schizophrenia and schizotypal personality disorder such as impaired information processing and abnormal eye movement (Lenzenweger & O'Driscoll, 2006).

Neuroendocrine studies using the dexamethasome suppression test and the thyrotropin-stimulating hormone test used to diagnose depression have recently been applied to clients with personality disorders and have shown abnormalities that suggest a relationship between disordered personality and depressed mood (Benazzi, 2006). Additional neurobiological evidence includes a higher incidence of abnormal electroencephalographic waveforms in the temporal and frontal lobe regions in clients with borderline personality disorder when compared with control subjects. Other studies have shown that some clients with antisocial and borderline personality disorders have abnormal evoked potentials

(Ruchsow et al., 2006). In summary, emerging data from studies of behavioral and cognitive changes associated personality disorders illustrate alterations in multiple brain neurocircuitry and biochemistry. Alterations in serotonergic function in the hippocampus may underlie emotional, mood, and behavioral symptoms in BPD. Specific brain regions implicated in impulsivity and other maladaptive behaviors include the prefrontal cortex, amygdala, anterior and posterior cingulate, and limbic systems (Berlin, Rolls, & Iversen, 2005). Psychiatric nurses are poised to understand these complex underpinnings in working with clients with personality disorders and initiating an interdisciplinary plan of care.

GENETICS

The literature suggests that there are genetic links for certain personality traits such as criminality and other antisocial behavior. Adoption and twin studies suggest a genetic base for antisocial personality (Tuvblad, Eley, Lichtenstein, 2005). Some twin studies have demonstrated higher incidences of personality disorders among monozygotic twins than dizygotic twins, suggesting a genetic basis for personality disorders (Reichborn-Kjennerud, 2007). Other factors are also attributed to criminality such as alcoholism, family violence, and socioeconomic factors.

Controversy concerning the exact role of genetics and personality disorders extrapolated from adoption and twin studies continue to challenge researchers to discern the effects of environmental or parental roles and genetics in twin studies. In this regard, Gunderson (1988) stated that "twin and adoptive studies have pointed to a genetic predisposition to this disorder but have also indicated that its development can be modified by good parental care" (p. 347).

 RESEARCH ABSTRACT

Emotion Process in Borderline Personality Disorders

Bland, A. R., Williams, C. A., Scharer, K., & Manning, S. (2004). *Issues in Mental Health Nursing, 25,* 655–672.

Study Problem/Purpose

The purpose of this descriptive-correlational study was to determine the relationship between the ability to recognize facial affect and affective intensity in women with a diagnosis of borderline personality disorder.

Method

A convenience sample was used to compare women hospitalized with borderline personality disorder and women in the community without a psychiatric disorder. Researchers used several measures: Pictures of facial affect (PFA) and affect intensity measure (AIM).

Findings

Data analysis revealed that women who were hospitalized with borderline personality disorder were significantly less accurate than women in the community in their ability to recognize facial emotion as depicted in the PFA. These women also had significantly higher levels of affect intensity than their counterparts. Researchers found a negative correlation between emotional intensity on the total AIM scale.

Implications for Psychiatric Nurses

When working with individuals with borderline personality disorder, it is imperative to be as objective as possible and recognize the emotional ability often displayed in the client with borderline personality disorder. Learning your own nonverbal cues and their potential impact on the client's perception requires mindfulness, patience, and empathy.

TEMPERAMENT

Temperament refers to innate, genetically based aspects of personality that is thought to influence personality development (Fuertes, Santos, Beeghly, & Tronick, 2006; Kim, Kim, Kim, & Lee, 2006). The impact of temperament as a basis for behavioral disorders and appears to underlie general medical conditions in children who manifest personality disorders or behavioral problems. Specific behaviors include hyperactivity, or distractibility.

Data from genetic studies also associate temperament with a variance between the child and the environment (Duman & Margolin, 2007). For instance, an anxious child who has an anxious mother is more vulnerable to developing a personality disorder. This has been attributed to ineffective parenting styles of parents who are immature and inconsistent. Inadequacy in early caregiver roles often results in chaotic and inconsistent family systems. Children from these families often experience intense outbursts of anger, abuse, and abandonment. Data consistently demonstrated the role of temperament, character, and attachment patterns in borderline personality disorder (Fossati et al., 2007). Although certain conditions may be classified as genetically derived, it is clear that genetic characteristics in combination with environmental forces are most likely the contributing factors in most, if not all, of the personality disorders.

THE ROLE OF CHILD ABUSE

A number of studies have found a high prevalence of child abuse in the histories of clients with maladaptive behaviors. Clients with borderline personality disorders have a high rate of early childhood traumas. Several studies have demonstrated a significant prevalence of sexual abuse among female clients diagnosed with borderline personality disorders. Studies of children and adolescents diagnosed with borderline personality provide strong support for the detrimental impact of early childhood traumas on development. Studies of children and adolescents diagnosed with borderline personality disorder provide strong support for the detrimental impact of early childhood traumas on development. Early traumas identified from these studies included situations of chaotic families, abuse in all forms for extended periods, rejection, and attachment issues (Watson, Chilton, Fairchild, & Whewell, 2006). Childhood histories of adults who exhibit violent behaviors reveal sexual abuse in their childhood to a large degree.

PERSONALITY DISORDER ISSUES ACROSS THE LIFE SPAN

The evolution of personality development and its impact on ego development that underlies life-long coping responses and interpersonal relationships is well documented. The next section overviews the impact of early childhood developmental stages and their role in personality formation.

Psychiatric nurses have numerous opportunities to promote mental health across the life span by recognizing maladaptive behaviors and initiating preventive measures during the formative years. In addition, they can facilitate adaptive handling of difficult situations that may cause behavioral changes by initiating interventions that promote healthy crisis resolution.

INFANCY

Metcalf (1979) described the concept of **psyche organizers** (an idea originally described by Spitz in 1951), which is concerned with the critical biopsychosocial periods of development. In these circumstances a biopsychosocial process takes place throughout early development. Electroencephalographic (EEG) measurements of these developmental changes are possible. Researchers have determined that it is possible to draw a parallel between EEG development (i.e., brain development) and emotional and psychological development. Research was conducted to obtain EEG data from 80 children who were followed from birth through midadolescence. These researchers observed that it is common to find various aberrations in EEGs of normal infants and children and that these variations disappear during early adolescence (Metcalf, 1979). Metcalf stated that "all experience subsequent to the operation of a new psychic organizer is differently organized than prior to that time in development; it is as if the very reality with which the individual deals is now altered" (p. 64). The particular criterion that must be met to serve as psychic organizer is that of a specific affective behavior. The occurrence of a specific affective behavior (e.g., smiling or, later, stranger anxiety) indicates that a new psychic organizer is present, which permits the developmental process to move forward, leading to a new stage of development or "psychological organization." The presence of such an affective signal is required to indicate that an intrapsychic change is occurring, and development can proceed to the next level (Metcalf, 1979).

Emde and Robinson (1979) summarized infant research completed in the 1970s by stating that infants are more active than passive and have a preformed organization, rhythmically organized behaviors, and internal states associated with the organization. These authors note a qualitative difference before and after 2 months of age such that classic conditioning is difficult in the early period and not difficult at all after 2 months of age. Consider, for instance, the erratic sleep patterns of 1-month-old newborns in comparison with those of many 2-month-old infants who may be sleeping all night as well as demonstrating other pattern regularities.

During the second 6 months of life, the infant definitely prefers and attaches to the primary caregiver (Provence, 1979). The infant's awareness and discrimination intensify as an indication of cognitive development and the strengthened maturation of aggressive and libidinal drives. Although self-concept is difficult to measure in infants, there seems to be strong evidence of happy expectation and of satisfaction with self and others in the infant who has been well nurtured.

Also, there is evidence of an increasing variety and number of emotional states such as joy, sadness, anxiety, distaste, perplexity, anger, and reproach (Provence, 1979).

When the nurturing caregiver is absent, the child withdraws and may refuse to enter into any relationship. Allnut (1979) stated that in the absence of an appropriate substitute mother, there is withdrawal of the infant or child and "progressive ego deficits ensue" (p. 376). Thus, the opportunity for trust development is either seriously compromised or diminished altogether.

Developmental studies' concerns about social functions in the adult cortex continue to be debated. As previously mentioned, Metcalf (1979) and others implicate the role of early biopsychosocial interactions with early caregivers as the basis of intrapsychic development that prevails across the life span.

Emerging studies have explored the process in which the adult human brain processes and adapts within social contexts. Interestingly, until lately there was a dearth of data that explained the underpinnings of early social function across the life span. In one study, researchers explored electroencephalography/event-related potential methods, using precursors of human social brain neurocircuitry during infancy in several areas, specifically face and eye gaze processing, perception of emotions, decoding biological motion, and perceiving human behavior (Grossmann & Johnson, 2007; Webb, Long, & Nelson, 2005). Results from these studies are consistent with other studies that implicate the human brain is basically adapted to evolve within a social context as demonstrated in the adult cortex (Hayden, Bhatt, Reed, Corbly, & Joseph, 2007; Webb et al., 2005).

CHILDHOOD

As the child becomes mobile and realizes that he is distinct from the primary caregiver, a sense of separateness evolves. The child still needs to be reassured by a caregiver's encouragement and applause for steps taken by the child toward independence. Healthy families provide this approval and allow the child to wander off in the room—and ultimately to other rooms or places—with the knowledge that he can return at any time for emotional refueling. Dysfunctional families, on the other hand, may be threatened by this newfound sense of freedom and punish the child either by emotional abandonment or other forms of abuse, including continued infantilization.

The second year is also the period of language acquisition. Miller (1979) stated that it is "the prime example of a rule-directed organization of the ego" (p. 127). Miller referred to other theorists who propose that ego is a vocal-auditory apparatus, and that it would be difficult to argue that speech and hearing do not strongly influence the way in which one perceives the environment. One concludes that in the first year, the various speech transactions (sound, tone, pronunciation, accents, and grammatical phrases) are firmly encoded to form the beginning speech patterns of the growing child.

By the time a child reaches ages 2½ to 3, these patterns are already quite fixed and further strengthened in the next year or so. Furthermore, the thinking aspect of the person is strongly influenced by language. Miller stated that the "concept-matching scheme" and "concept formation" both are parts of a process whereby ego is enhanced.

Children with early faulty development frequently maintain primitive defense mechanisms such as projection, ambivalence, regression, splitting, acting out, and denial. These mechanisms often represent the child's survival tools, and they often persist throughout the life span. These early defense mechanisms are used to ward off bad feelings, depression, anxiety, rage, and intense emotional pain.

Kernberg (1984) has attested that clients continue to use these defense mechanisms to protect the ego from intrapsychic (mental) conflicts by rejecting advice from the unconscious ego. Using primitive defense mechanisms decreases the optimal functioning of the ego structure and further compromises the ability to use adaptive coping behaviors such as crying, talking things out, acknowledging one's own failures or weaknesses, changing the weaknesses or the situation if needed, negotiating, laughing at oneself, and asking forgiveness. The primitive defense mechanisms most often resorted to by clients with borderline personality disorder are splitting, displacement, and blaming; clients with paranoid personality disorder often resort to projection; and antisocial personalities use repression and denial to a great extent.

Children with faulty ego structures or maladaptive coping patterns often present with behavioral symptoms or conduct disorder. Their histories are frequently dominated by chaotic or dysfunctional family systems. Some psychodynamic theorists suggest a parallel between early childhood traumas and early object losses as common factors in the histories of clients with personality disorders (Freud, 1957; Kernberg, 1984; Masterson, 2000). Many of these losses are attributed to mental illness, substance abuse, and indifference in primary caregivers (Levy et al., 2006).

It is appropriate to add the problem of ignorance as another factor in considering causes associated with loss. One of the most important tasks of a lifetime is raising healthy children, and yet less attention is given to training in parenting than in any other work endeavor. Presently in the United States, the parental role is often only given lip service. Most caregivers are females who are underpaid and undervalued, a situation which causes concern that inadequate childcare may persist if societal values do not change.

Children reared in these circumstances usually have poor self-esteem, are distrustful, and have poor social skills. Psychodynamic theorists agree that children with faulty ego function have a developmental arrest that begins in early childhood. The role of psychiatric nurses includes assessing areas of impairment, and the process begins by approaching clients and their significant others in a caring nonjudgmental manner. This approach facilitates trust building and enhances the potential success of treatment plan outcomes. Many of these children have disruptive behavior disorders that set the stage for future problems as well. The *DSM-IV-TR* lists the following diagnoses in this category:

◆ Conduct disorder: Childhood-onset type and adolescent-onset type

◆ Disruptive behavior disorder not otherwise specified

Conduct Disorders

The *DSM-IV-TR* (APA, 2000) identifies the essential feature of a conduct disorder as a repetitive and persistent pattern of behavior that violates the basic rights of others or major age-appropriate norms or rules. Certain specific behaviors (at least three) such as lying, truancy, staying out after dark without permission, stealing, vandalism, forced sex, physical cruelty, and use of weapons must have been present during the previous 12 months with at least one criterion present in the past 6 months. The behaviors are grouped according to severity levels of mild, moderate, and severe. These behaviors are also manifestations of antisocial personality disorder in those 18 years of age or older.

Conduct disorder is the most prevalent diagnosis of children and adolescents in both outpatient and hospital settings. In 2006, the National Comorbidity Survey Replication demonstrated the estimated lifetime prevalence of conduct disorder as about 9.5 percent, with 12 percent in boys and 7.1 percent in girls and with a median onset age of 11.6 years (Nock, Kazdin, Hiripi, & Kessler, 2006). The economic and social implications of severe behavioral problems in childhood and across the life span are significant. The underpinnings of conduct disorders are multifaceted and include psychosocial, neurobiological, genetic, and environmental factors. The pathogenesis conduct disorder involves mediation between genetic, familial, and psychosocial factors. Researchers submit that children and adolescents who have conduct disorder may inherit hypothalamic-pituitary-adrenal axis activity, that requires greater stimulation to achieve optimal arousal and may account for their need to engage in sensation-seeking activity associated with conduct disorder. Alterations in neurotransmitters, such as norepinephrine and serotonin are strongly implicated (van Goozen & Fairchild, 2006). Substance-use disorders, psychiatric disorders, family chaos, child abuse, and exposure to antisocial behavior in primary caregivers are significant risk factors for this disorder.

Behavioral problems in preschool-age children who meet diagnostic criteria for conduct disorder require immediate attention and interventions. Early recognition, prevention, and early treatment have the potential to mitigate burden in adulthood. Effective parenting is an important determinant in child behavior. Children have fewer behavioral problems when parents provide consistent limit setting and expect appropriate behaviors. Psychosocial interventions, such as parenting skills programs, demonstrate improved behaviors in children with conduct disorders. (Edwards, Céilleachair, Bywater, Hughes, & Hutchings, 2007).

Table 15–5 depicts the causes and characteristics of conduct disorders.

Interventions and Outcomes

The prognosis of conduct disorders is just as complex as its causes. Diagnosis is critical along with evaluating family dynamics and psychosocial factors that increase the risk of conduct disorder. Initially, it is critical for psychiatric nurses to educate parents by demonstrating clear, direct, and specific communication skills to use with children with behavioral problems. The advent of pharmacological agents to manage severe aggressive behaviors and co-occurring psychiatric conditions, such ADHD, depression, and oppositional defiant disorder, offers hope to some youngsters and their families. A holistic approach that integrates family therapy, pharmacological agents, and behavioral modifications facilitates improved outcomes for the child with conduct disorder. A new approach that involves a Fast Track inpatient intervention, a multiyear, multicomponent intervention designed to decrease violence among children and adolescents, demonstrates promising findings. Results from this study implicate a cost-effective approach to help high-risk youth with conduct disorders (Foster, Jones, & Conduct Problems Prevention Research Group, 2006).

Psychiatric nurses and other clinicians are challenged to work with children and adolescents with conduct disorders. The following section describes major challenges and nursing interventions that facilitate rapport and positive clinical outcomes.

Youth with conduct disorders are difficult to work with, and they frequently tax the emotional resources of caregivers. They often lack empathy, concern, and anxiety or remorse regarding their behavior. Their lack of trust and an inability to engage with healthy peers and adults present nurses with many challenges for devising ways to interact with them (Mishne, 1986). The following are desired outcomes:

◆ Establishing rapport

◆ Completing a comprehensive diagnostic workup (neurobiological, psychological, sociological)

◆ Understanding the meaning of behaviors and associated thoughts and feelings

◆ Maintaining a safe, supportive environment

◆ Improving ego function

Establishing rapport and trust is extremely difficult, but it is crucial if work with these youngsters is to progress. Nurses must form an alliance with such children and the parents (if possible), even though the parent-child relationship is often tenuous. Dysfunctional family dynamics play a crucial role in maladaptive behaviors of children and adolescents (Mishne, 1986), and failure to intervene with parents often results in revictimization of the child. Family therapy may be the major treatment modality, or it may be an adjunct to individual therapy with the child.

Adolescents and children may test nurses and other staff by pressing them to break the rules or by calling them derogatory

TABLE 15–5
Causes and Characteristics of Conduct Disorders

Causes

Psychological

    Chaotic family dynamics

    Lack of parental empathy/affection

    Faulty ego structure (superego)

    Learned behavior

Neurobiological

    Genetics

    Temperament

    Neurological dysfunction, including neurochemical

Sociological

    Low socioeconomic status

    Media environmental violence

    Substance abuse

    Disturbed parent-child relationship (rejection, chaotic interactions, inconsistency)

Characteristics

- Stealing
- Lying
- Running away from home (history of several instances)
- Truancy
- Disrespect for others
- Fire setting
- Cruelty or violence to others and/or animals
- Early experimentation with substances
- Early sexual experimentation

names in their refusal to comply with demands. Nurses must remain steadfast in rule enforcement and limit setting, and they must maintain their composure in the presence of the child. They must be committed to understanding the meaning of the behaviors and their underlying motivations. Impaired impulse control underlies acting-out behaviors. Children often tend to act rather than to think things out or to allow themselves to feel.

Nurses need to be actively involved in the assessment process to determine factors that contribute to the maladaptive behaviors of these children. This process helps in identifying treatment possibilities and determining the possible presence of conditions such as depression, seizure disorder, suicidal attempts, acting-out behaviors, bullying and violence, and school problems. The child may already have experienced run-ins with law officials and other authority figures and may express contempt toward authority; thus it requires a balancing act on the part of the nurse to present as a compassionate, concerned individual with a mandate to protect the child while promoting adherence to the rules required for the protection and safe care of the child. An accepting nonjudgmental attitude during interactions will help to enhance the child's sense of safety in the new environment, which does not hold all the negative influence from which the child is running. Helping these children and their families appreciate the meaning of maladaptive behavior, feelings, and thoughts is crucial to facilitating more adaptive responses from these youngsters. Such children may gain insight in a safe environment where they can say what is on their minds without censure, derision, and punishment. A therapeutic milieu will allow a place for testing and growth as the process of introspection and discussion are fostered and modeled. Group psychotherapy is a helpful intervention modality because it provides opportunities for peer exchanges and for nurses to model healthier attitudes and behaviors.

Self-esteem is influenced by the experiences that have helped to mold the ego. Children who can adapt to changes in their internal and external environments usually feel more secure and can be helped best because their self-esteem is high. Children with low self-esteem tend to perceive their environments as negative and threatening and are more likely to demonstrate depression and faulty super-ego functioning. Building self-esteem is a continuous process that begins with initial contacts in the treatment setting and continues throughout treatment. Acceptance, patience, perseverance, and honest sharing of one's self (as appropriate) are key ingredients for establishing trust and assisting in the process of improvement in the area of developing self-esteem in children with disruptive behaviors.

The single most crucial need is a complete diagnostic evaluation that includes neurobiological, psychological, and sociological aspects of the child's history and present circumstances. Research to determine the long-term effects of previous interventions and intensive multimodal care should be studied and also completed. Juvenile violence remains the major predictor of adult violence, so steps should be taken to assist the child in learning ways to solve problems without resorting to violence (Edwards et al., 2007; Goldstein et al., 2006; Nock et al., 2006).

Oppositional Defiant Disorder

The primary manifestations of oppositional defiant disorder (APA, 2000) are negative, hostile, and stubborn behaviors such as:

- Difficulty in controlling temper
- Frequent arguments with adults, including parents and teachers
- Frequent refusal to follow rules or to do chores or homework
- Frequently being purposely annoying to others

- Being easily agitated or upset by others
- Frequent use of profanity

Causes

Similar to other psychiatric disorders in children and adults, oppositional defiant disorder is highly concomitant with other psychiatric conditions, including ADHD and conduct disorders. Likewise, the cause of oppositional defiant disorder is multifaceted and includes neurobiological, genetic, psychosocial, and environmental influences.

Contemporary research indicates that children with oppositional defiant disorder develop a passive-aggressive response pattern in which there is chronic rebellion against rules and regulations. The contrast between oppositional defiant disorder and conduct disorder is a lack of self-centered manipulative behaviors in the former (Dolan & Fullam, 2006). Recent data indicate that oppositional defiant disorder is more a family characteristic than a child disorder. Several theories about this disorder concerning family dynamic and psychosocial issues are emerging (Steiner et al., 2007):

- Parental discord (too harsh or lacking)
- Overidentification by the child with the parent who has an impulsivity disorder
- A lack of attachment owing to the parent or guardian's lack of emotional and physical warmth

Although psychosocial and family dynamics play key roles in oppositional defiant disorder, neurobiological and temperamental factors may also contribute to this disorder.

As with other psychological conditions of childhood, medical and neurological examinations are suggested to rule out neurological disorders or other illnesses that may contribute to the behaviors. Psychosocial assessment should attend to the type and quality of parent-child interactions, parental skills in disciplining and rewarding, attachment behaviors, and the child's self-perception.

Because of their passive-aggression and poor school performance, these children are often alienated from their peers. Their alienation, coupled with poor self-esteem places these children at risk for depression and self-destructive behaviors such as substance abuse, bullying and violence, cult involvement, promiscuity, and suicide. They must be assessed for symptoms of depression and the level of risk directed at themselves or others throughout treatment.

Interventions and Outcomes

Nursing interventions need to focus on establishing rapport with the child and parents, teaching parental skills in child management, and promoting self-esteem in both child and parents. These children are often searching for reasonable structure or for someone to help them self-regulate their behavior (Marohn, 1992)—a structure that promotes a sense of safety and concern. Realistic limits need to be set and consequences explained in an empathic manner. Therapeutic goals should be established as follows:

- Establishing trust through a therapeutic relationship
- Assisting parents to avoid the use of negative reinforcing behaviors toward the child
- Helping the child to understand the meaning of self-destructive behaviors and obtaining a "no suicide" pact
- Finding ways to build or restore self-esteem
- Building adaptive coping behaviors in children and their parents. See Chapter 19.

Interventions are most effective when they are begun early to prevent the strengthening of dysfunctional behaviors. The high prevalence rate of child abuse is a major concern to mental health caregivers not only because of its effect on the growing child but also because of the long-term effects on adult behaviors. Possibly just as damaging is the current tendency of parents to favor freedom over control, and although children need to be allowed to make choices, their greater need is for nonpunitive structure. Nursing interventions include prevention of abuse, assessment of clients for symptoms of abuse, assistance for the child in learning new coping skills, and provision of safety for children in distress.

ADOLESCENCE

Adolescence, in general, is characterized as a turbulent period in which there are fluctuations of mood, behavior, and ideals. Psychiatric nurses are challenged to differentiate between age-appropriate and non-age-appropriate behavioral fluctuations. Adolescents demonstrate oppositional defiant and conduct disorders as children do, but now the symptoms may intensify. Other aspects of treatment include assessing attitudes and the level of danger in acting-out behaviors. An interdisciplinary team is important in the process of making a differential diagnosis.

Major stressors for adolescents include authority and control (separation-individuation issues). The younger adolescent is shifting from parents to peers in preference, and the older adolescent may be dealing with intimacy and sexual issues. Positive self-esteem is the core struggle in concert with the search for identity (Antai-Otong, 2004). Erikson (1963) identified the primary task of adolescence as identity and found that firm establishment of identity is dependent on successful resolution of previous developmental tasks.

Impairments in ego and superego development are considered to be the major cause of maladaptive behavior. Erikson (1963) contended that if the adolescent were unable to attain a healthy identity, the result would be role confusion that then leads easily into problem behavior. These youngsters are frequently bored and frustrated, and they often experience difficulty dealing with intense feelings such as anxiety, fears, and intimacy (Mishne, 1986). They also have distorted cognitions (impaired reality testing) and low self-esteem. Other maladaptive behaviors include using primitive defense mechanisms such as acting out and expressing extreme hostility or aggression toward authority figures. Their ability to solve problems and control immediate gratification needs (impulsivity) is impaired. Adolescents with personality disorders experience bouts of depression and anxiety and turn to risky tension-reducing activities, including substance abuse, sexual promiscuity, bullying, violence, suicidal behaviors and attempts, and various other antisocial acts to help in coping with their distress (van Lier, Wanner, & Vitaro, 2007).

Assessing the adolescent's level of dangerousness is the same as for adults. Suicidal adolescents present clinicians with a serious emergency situation. Assessing current stressors, the suicide plan, the available means for carrying out the act and previous personal or family history of suicide and gestures can assist the health care team in determining appropriate interventions. The risk of suicide is high and the third leading cause of death in this age group, and the seriousness of the problem is heightened by the impulsiveness of youth as well as by their inability to see past their immediate situation. Although some youngsters provide signals that are quite clear, many give none; therefore, if an adolescent is acting differently than is usual for him or has escalated acting-out behaviors, it may be a signal that he is in serious emotional trouble. If the family has established open communications, it may not be difficult to talk with the adolescent about what is occurring. On the other hand, if communication of the adolescent and family are generally closed and they share little together, or if the parents are too busy, a professional may be the only one who can succeed in making contact. Similarly, for adults who are suicidal, it is important to determine (1) lethality; (2) intent; (3) maladaptation or emotional instability; (4) association of feelings or behaviors with depression or impulsivity; (5) substance abuse; and (6) presence of depression or psychosis (Antai-Otong, 2004; Groholt, Ekeberg, & Haldorsen, 2006).

Clinical features of a personality disorder usually emerge during adolescence or early adulthood (APA, 2000). Adolescents with personality disorders can be demanding and disruptive in clinical settings, and many of their behaviors reflect their unconscious need to re-create their own dysfunctional family systems. Their insatiable need to verbally or behaviorally avoid and minimize intense feelings of anxiety or other emotional pain gives rise to great challenges for psychiatric nurses and other professionals in developing a workable treatment plan for adolescents and their families. Unless these challenges are met, there is a proneness toward failure in the life of the adolescent with school dropout being a major choice leading to disruption of normal progression.

Hospitalization of adolescents for specific personality disorders is indicated when they exhibit destructive behavior toward themselves, toward others, or toward property. These may be suicidal acts or threats to self, eating disorders, substance abuse, homicidal acts and threats to others, or destructiveness to property. Failure to respond to treatment, severe depression, psychosis, or severe family dysfunction may require inpatient care.

Long-term inpatient care may involve a treatment center other than a hospital because there are limited reimbursement mechanisms now available for inpatient treatment, and psychotherapeutic interventions require considerable time and involvement. Therefore, the adolescent may be admitted to a hospital for diagnostic purposes and referred elsewhere for ongoing intervention. This may be to a residential treatment program or a group home, depending on the seriousness of the condition. Short-term treatment focuses on crisis resolution, and long-term care focuses on the facilitation of attitudinal and behavioral change in the adolescent and his family. The overall aim of care is to minimize acting-out behaviors and to increase ego strength. Egan (1986) stated that the following purposes are served when the adolescent's ego is strengthened:

- ◆ Increased impulse control
- ◆ Delayed need gratification
- ◆ Improved self-esteem
- ◆ Decreased dysphoric feelings (sadness) and anxiety
- ◆ Increased problem-solving skills

Building ego capacity in adolescents and other age groups can be facilitated in therapy. An array of therapeutic modalities are available to treat clients with personality disorders and include psychotherapies, group, and milieu; activity and educational therapies; behavior modification; and pharmacology.

Although the most useful treatment modality was once the therapeutic milieu, treatment has now shifted to outpatient settings where there is less opportunity for long-term exposure. Now, the major modality is physiological with the prescription of medication and one-to-one treatment in private settings. The impact of staff nurses must generally occur during a 3- to 5-day hospital stay, in outpatient individual or group therapy or in home/school visits; and these are definitely not as available as one would like. Group therapy can be very helpful; however, there is the problem of association with other troubled youngsters who may increase the tendency of a youngster to act out in order to gain peer approval. Family therapy and multifamily therapy groups are helpful ways to provide therapeutic help.

Pharmacologic Interventions

Pharmacologic treatment depends on the adolescent's symptoms. For instance, if the youth presents with symptoms of depression, such as dysphoric mood and sleep and appetite disturbances, antidepressants may be prescribed. Because of the risk of suicide associated with taking antidepressants, the youth must be closely monitored for suicide risk along with psychoeducation to both client and family about symptoms to report, such as suicidal ideations or thoughts of dying. Symptoms such as aggressive or impulsive acting out may respond to carbamazepine (Tegretol); lithium; divalproex sodium (Depakote); atypical antipsychotic agents, such as risperidone (Risperdal), to modulate mood and agitation; atomoxetine (Strattera) to manage co-occurring ADHD; and mood stabilizers, such as lithium (Eskalith), to manage aggressive-hostile behaviors because of fewer side effects (Biederman et al., 2007; Turgay, 2005). However, some of the newer drugs seem to offer promise of hope even though there is ongoing controversy about the prescription of these medications to children and adolescents. Psychopharmacologic agents are used as an adjunct to behavioral and psychosocial interventions to maximize the treatment.

Working with adolescents can be an exhausting experience. Their endless demands and limit-testing tax the patience and fortitude of nurses and the health care team. Staff nurses and their staff members are probably the most vulnerable of the health care team because they are required to staff inpatient units for 24 hours every day of the week instead of just 1 or 2 hours at a time. Strategies that help to maximize resources when working with demanding clients include the following:

◆ Examining personal reactions to these clients

◆ Determining the meaning of client behaviors

◆ Participating in professional and peer supervision activities to sort out feelings and reactions

◆ Having sufficient time and opportunity to take care of professional needs

◆ Developing realistic client outcomes

ADULTHOOD

As previously mentioned, healthy adult behavior depends on mastering early childhood and adolescent tasks and the development of an ego capable of mastering reality issues and relationships successfully. Capacity for maturation, optimal level of functioning, and adaptability to life are at their apex (Erikson, 1963). See Chapters 2 and 19. The characteristics associated with interdependence as opposed to dependence and dysfunctional independence were identified (Whiting, 1997) as typical for healthy adults.

Resolving crises and dealing with changes are integral aspects of adulthood. One's ability to use adaptive coping behaviors is influenced by the person's emotional repertoire, the experience and perception of stressors, and available support systems. Adaptive coping methods allow people to reduce, modify, or eliminate their stress. Adults can usually be expected to demonstrate resilience in the face of crisis if internal and external resources are available.

Clients with personality disorders often perceive crises or change as overwhelming. Their lack of internal and external resources compromises their ability to use adaptive coping methods to reduce or eliminate intense feelings. A lack of healthy ego functions interferes with a person's ability to perceive stress accurately or realistically, to minimize his anxiety effectively, and to establish and maintain healthy relationships. The capacity for intimacy is lacking. Erikson (1963) described self-absorption as the antithesis of intimacy. These persons often experience feeings of emptiness and loneliness in spite of their numerous efforts to form

relationships in some cases. This also may be extremely demanding of the relationships that they do have, and this is representative of the unmanageable anxiety that they may have but fail to acknowledge because many or most tend to remain in an ego-syntonic state. Distress usually results from the inability to cope and deal with emptiness, low self-esteem, and intense but often unacknowledged emotional pain. Clients experiencing these feelings are at risk for using other maladaptive behaviors such as substance abuse, suicide attempts, and destructive relationships and behaviors. The more florid acting-out and socially disturbing behavior of earlier years tend to drop off or abate as the person grows older (Gunderson, 1988).

OLDER ADULTHOOD

Personality disorders are postulated to endure throughout the life span with only minor changes dependent on the variety of learning experiences and models to which one may be exposed. Long-term follow-up studies of personality disorders indicate the course is variable across the life span. Over time, older adults reach greater stability in social and occupational function (Stone, 1990). Clients with these disorders generally tend to be influenced by internal and external stimuli. Older adults are challenged to use their previous life experience to cope with biological and neurological changes associated with the aging process. Erikson (1963) described the eighth stage of development as old age, with the primary developmental task being ego integrity. In some instances, however, despair rather than integrity is the outcome because the person does not perceive himself to have had any or many positive experiences for which to be proud; in effect, the task of generativity was not accomplished and probably neither were other earlier tasks. See Chapter 19.

As mentioned earlier, the antisocial behaviors that may have been present in earlier years have generally become less of a problem as time passes; however, some of the disorders may intensify (e.g., the suspiciousness of the paranoid personality or the seclusiveness of the schizoid personality) because there often are accentuations of personalities in older persons. This occurs because new ego operations do not develop, and the person exaggerates defense mechanisms already present to cope with increased stress in association with loss, retirement, illness, and other circumstances of later life (Berezin, Liptzin, & Salzman, 1988).

Older adults who have never developed healthy ego functions, as well as those with physical and mental problems, are at risk for experiencing despair (Erikson, 1963). Lacking accomplishment, the person may face what is left of life with hopelessness and helplessness. He may believe that any chance to make anything out of life is gone and that there is no reason to be cheerful or ambitious about anything. Because of the numerous losses in this period, there is a vulnerability to depression, and the rate of suicide among men is high (Berezin et al., 1988). Relative to losses, one older adult remarked, "All my friends have either gone to Florida or to Heaven."

Cultural and age-appropriate behaviors must be assessed in addition to all the physical problems likely to be present. Individualized care plans must be established. This is emphasized because there is a tendency for young people to perceive older adults as all alike, and this is far from the truth. There are very wide variations in behavior and personality just as there is in physical status of older adults.

There is need for research to determine age-specific needs of clients with personality disorders. These efforts may be useful in minimizing feelings of hopelessness and helplessness in older adults and also in the nurses who work with them as appropriate interventions are established.

SPECIFIC PERSONALITY DISORDERS AND TREATMENT MODALITIES

Phillips and Gunderson (1999) describe people with personality disorders presenting with problems that are complex and demanding. Some clients have intense dependency needs to form a relationship, while others fear rejection and avoid relationships. Still others devalue relationships and have self-concept concerns and feel they do not exist. Because these characteristics describe a spectrum of personality disorders and who clients really are, nurses are challenged to recognize disorders in their clients and the level of distress they experience. Because of their core personality traits, most clients exhibit maladaptive behaviors and coping patterns.

Blashfield and Intoccia (2000) report that their search of the literature revealed limited growth of literature relating to personality disorders, contrary to expectations, and that only three personality disorders have slightly growing literatures. These disorders receiving some attention since the publication of the *DSM-IV-TR* are antisocial personality disorder (ASPD), found in Cluster B; borderline personality disorder (BPD), found in Cluster B; and schizotypal personality disorder, found in Cluster A. Table 15–1 summarizes the three clusters of personality disorders as defined by Gunderson (1988).

Researchers continue to evaluate the scope of potential answers to difficulties with the current *DSM-IV* diagnostic criteria and have made recommendations for revisions of diagnostic criteria to reduce limitations inherent in the current system. To address these concerns, these researchers proposed a prototype matching approach to personality disorder diagnosis. Issues involving diagnostic categories for personality continue to be debated (Shedler & Westen, 2004; Westen, Shedler, & Bradley, 20016).

CLUSTER A

The first cluster of personality disorders comprises those in which clients are considered withdrawn, odd, or eccentric. These disorders include paranoid, schizoid, and schizotypal types.

Paranoid Personality Disorder

Kraeplin first coined the term "paranoia" and described it as systemized delusions devoid of global deterioration. People with pervasive distrust and suspiciousness of others such that their motives are interpreted as malevolent are more likely to develop this disorder, and it is the basis for *DSM-IV-TR* criteria for paranoid personality disorder. The following characteristics are defined in the *DSM-IV-TR* (APA, 2000).

- ◆ Suspects, without sufficient basis, that others are exploiting, harming, or deceiving him
- ◆ Is preoccupied with unjustified doubts about the loyalty or trustworthiness of friends or associates
- ◆ Is reluctant to confide in others because of unwarranted fear that the information will be used maliciously against him
- ◆ Reads hidden demeaning or threatening meanings into benign remarks or events
- ◆ Persistently bears grudges, that is, is unforgiving of insults, injuries, or slights
- ◆ Perceives attacks on his character or reputation that are not apparent to others and is quick to react angrily or to counterattack
- ◆ Has recurrent suspicions, without justification, regarding fidelity of spouse or sexual partner

Interventions

Interventions are planned to draw the client into a nurse-client relationship in which a measure of trust can be established. See the key interventions. However, all personality disorders are ingrained, fixed patterns of behavior that are extremely resistant to change. Nurses must be scrupulously attentive to keeping their word in all situations because the client will look for chinks in the armor of any professional who attempts to become involved in a therapeutic relationship. The pattern of suspiciousness was established a long time before the professional relationship; and because the client has not felt sufficiently able to trust others previously, there is no guarantee that it will happen in these instances either.

These clients rarely seek treatment because of these personality traits. They are distant and guarded, and it is difficult to establish rapport with them because they consistently perceive people as untrustworthy. They are hypersensitive to criticism, and they have impaired interpersonal and work relationships. They have generally not been successful in establishing intimacy.

Clients with paranoid personality disorder often feel the need to be on guard all the time in an effort to deal with perceived threats or attacks from others. (This characteristic is known as hypervigilance.) Their moods are irritable and agitated, and they are distant. Such behaviors make it difficult for nurses to establish a nurse-client relationship. Interventions that are helpful in these situations include approaching the client in a calm, empathic manner, avoiding overzealousness. These suspicious clients may interpret all behavior as threatening and react in an aggressive manner. Nurses need to assess verbal and nonverbal behaviors for signs that suggest increased agitation and aggression. Signs of impending aggression include pacing, speaking loudly, glaring, and clenching the fist and jaw. These clients are not good candidates for intensive or intrusive therapy, especially group therapy, because these approaches may intensify suspiciousness and increase the risk of escalating thoughts and behaviors. Some of these clients show a slight response to low-dose antipsychotics, benzodiazepines, and antidepressants for symptoms of agitation, anxiety, and aggression.

The key nursing interventions for the client with paranoid personality disorder are:

◆ Establish rapport
◆ Minimize potential for aggressive behavior
◆ Support adaptive behaviors

Schizoid Personality Disorder

Individuals with this disorder demonstrate a pervasive pattern of detachment from social relationships and manifest a restricted range of emotional expression with others. The pattern is apparent by early adulthood in a variety of contexts (APA, 2000). These loners choose solitary activities that do not require much participation with others. They may be very adept at computer or mathematical games. There is little interest in sexual activity with another person, and there is minimal pleasure sought from sensory, bodily, or interpersonal experience. There are generally no close friends except possibly a first-degree relative. There is no seeking out of approval from others and they seem oblivious to what others think of them. Affect is constricted and they appear cold and aloof even to the point of showing no anger when provoked by others. There seems to be no direction to their lives and responses are passive to negative experiences. Under extreme stress, these individuals may experience very brief psychotic episodes and the condition may be a premorbid antecedent condition to schizophrenia or delusional disorder. These persons may do well in work conditions where they are socially isolated and may perform well when left alone. Persons with schizoid personality disorder are not likely to seek therapy even though the characteristics may have been present since childhood in which there were limited relationships and they were underachievers in school.

Schizotypal Personality Disorder

Individuals with this disorder demonstrate a pervasive pattern of social and interpersonal deficits accompanied by marked discomfort with and limited capacity for close relationships along with cognitive and perceptual distortions and behavioral eccentricities (APA, 2000). They are poor candidates for treatment and are at risk for developing schizophrenia. Clients with this disorder usually have positive neurobiological and genetic markers similar to those found in schizophrenia. Gunderson (1988) stated that there may be greater differences between schizoid and schizotypal disorders than previously supposed. Isolation, limited peer relationships, social anxiety, school underachievement, hypersensitivity, peculiarities in thought and language, and bizarre fantasies are all characteristics often found in schizotypal personalities as early as childhood and adolescence (APA, 2000). Gunderson (1988) suggested that there may be a need for further delineation between these types if their similarities are borne out.

Clients with schizoid or schizotypal disorders may have positive family backgrounds of schizophrenia (Koo et al., 2006). Some of these children are at risk for developing schizophrenia in adolescence or later life, but there is dispute about how many actually do. Gunderson (1988) stated that the schizotypal individuals rarely need institutional care, and schizoid personalities rarely seek treatment because of their interpersonal detachment. Clients with these disorders are more likely to be located as inpatients for medical or surgical intervention or in home health care situations, and the psychiatric nurse may be called on as a consultant rather than as primary caregiver. A study by Mittal, Dhruv, Tessner, Walder, and Walker (2007) revealed that adolescents with schizotypal disorders in a comparative study with other personality disorders and those with no disorders were found to have more minor physical abnormalities and dermatological abnormalities than the normal comparison group and higher cortisol levels than the other two groups. Table 15–6 compares the symptoms as identified in the past for schizoid and schizotypal disorders (APA, 2000); it remains to be seen whether new studies will bring about revisions in the diagnostic criteria.

One can readily see that there are similarities in the descriptions of the schizoid and schizotypal disorders described in Table 15–6. Basically, the differences seem to be in degree more than in substance, with the client with schizotypal-type

CLINICAL EXAMPLE

The Client with Paranoid Personality Disorder

Mr. Jones came into the psychiatric triage unit with his wife of 6 months. He stated that he is seeking help because his wife is threatening to leave him. He says she complains of his intense jealousy and constant accusations of infidelity. Mrs. Jones reported that her husband calls her at work constantly trying to find out whom she is talking to in her workplace. Her boss has threatened to terminate her employment if he calls again. Mr. Jones denied having a basis for his accusations, but he admitted that when someone calls their home and has the wrong number, he believes it is some man trying to reach his wife. Two weeks ago, he lost his fourth job within a 10-month period and admitted, also, that his jealousy had increased during this period. When questioned about the basis of his jealousy, he became argumentative and defensive, stating he doesn't know why his wife feels there is something wrong with him: "After all, if a man loves his wife he is going to guard her and protect her from someone else, isn't he?"

personality disorder more likely to be disabled, more likely to have a genetic predisposition, and demonstrating more ongoing disability than does the schizoid type (Gunderson, 1988). Further differentiation seems to be in the fact that while the client with schizotypal disorder fears social interaction, the schizoid client is basically disinterested in them.

Interventions and Outcomes

Working with clients with schizotypal and schizoid disorders requires that nurses understand the need for establishing rapport and that the clients are difficult to engage and establish positive affective interactions. Feedback will be limited, but in addition to rapport, the nurse will need to work at establishing a reality base and developing adaptive behaviors. Specific interventions to achieve these outcomes for the client with schizoid or schizotypal disorder are listed in the key nursing interventions that follow:

◆ Approach the client in a calm manner

◆ Maintain a comfortable distance based on the client's verbal and nonverbal communication

◆ Administer psychotropics (e.g., risperidone [Risperdal], olanzapine [Zyprexa], and quetiapine [Seroquel]) and observe the client's responses—both desired and adverse

◆ Engage supportive groups to provide feedback on the client's behaviors

◆ Provide for structured social interactions

CLUSTER B

The second cluster of personality disorders consists of those in which clients seek attention and engage in erratic behaviors. These disorders include antisocial, borderline, histrionic, and narcissistic personalities.

Antisocial Personality Disorder

The oldest known personality disorder is that termed antisocial (Blashfield & McElroy, 1987). Throughout history it has been given several names, including moral insanity by Prichard in 1830, constitutional psychopathic insanity by Koch in the nineteenth century, and sociopathy in the twentieth century. Cleckley (1964) considered it a disorder to be distinguished from other psychiatric or behavioral abnormalities. Regardless of the label, antisocial personality has typically referred to socially deviant persons who were societal outcasts because they refused to conform to societal norms. Gunderson (1988) stated that although these people appear to be enviably free from worry, the essential "flatness and barrenness" from within becomes

---

TABLE 15–6
Comparison of Symptoms: Schizoid and Schizotypal Disorders

Schizoid Disorder	Schizotypal Disorder
• Neither desires nor enjoys close relationships, including being part of a family	• Ideas of reference (excluding delusions of reference)
• Almost always chooses solitary activities	• Odd beliefs or magical thinking that influences behavior and is inconsistent with subcultural norms (e.g., superstitious belief in clairvoyance, telepathy, or "sixth sense"; in children and adolescents, bizarre fantasies or preoccupations
• Has little, if any, interest in having sexual experiences with another person	• Unusual perceptual experiences, including bodily illusions
• Takes pleasure in few, if any, activities	• Odd thinking and speech (e.g., vague, circumstantial, metaphorical, overelaborate, or stereotyped)
• Lacks close friends or confidants other than first-degree relatives	• Suspiciousness or paranoid ideation
• Appears indifferent to the praise or criticism of others	• Inappropriate or constricted affect
• Shows emotional coldness, detachment, or flattened affectivity	• Behavior or appearance that is odd, eccentric, or peculiar
	• Lack of close friends or confidants other than first-degree relatives
	• Excessive social anxiety that does not diminish with familiarity and tends to be associated with paranoid fears rather than negative judgments about self

Note. Adapted from *Diagnostic and Statistical Manual of Mental Disorders* (4th edition, Text Revision) *(DSM-IV-TR)*, by American Psychiatric Association, 2000, Washington, DC: Author. Adapted with permission.

apparent when their activities fail to provide the desired long-term satisfactions. Typical characteristics include the following (APA, 2000):

◆ Failure to learn from experience

◆ Regular engagement in impulsive and risky behavior

◆ Lack of guilt demonstrated toward repetitive misbehavior

◆ Exploitation of others

◆ Chronic disregard for the rights of others

◆ Lack of fidelity, loyalty, and honesty

Onset should be documented by antisocial behaviors before the age of 15 and by failure to demonstrate a positive work role after the age of 18 (APA, 2000). Specific interventions aimed at achieving positive outcomes are noted as in the key interventions for antisocial disorders. Most twin and adoption studies of conduct disorder and antisocial personality disorder demonstrate modest genetic vulnerability and substantial contributions of environmental factors (Goldstein et al., 2006). Findings from a study conducted by Kim-Cohen and colleagues (2006) concerning the role of genotype in the cycle of violence in maltreated children indicate that genotypes also play a role in modulating the children's sensitivity to environmental insults. These data confirm previous findings that implicate the role of genetic and environmental factors in the development of conduct problems and antisocial behaviors. Implications from these data suggest the importance of recognizing high-risk children and family systems and early interventions, such as parenting classes, to reduce perpetuation of maltreatment and resulting conduct disorders and antisocial behaviors during childhood.

Clients with antisocial personality disorders tend to participate in high-risk behaviors involving substance abuse. These clients present several treatment problems in that treatment successes are low and risk is increased so that workups are needed to assess behavioral style and resulting illnesses. Other necessary preventive measures include education regarding high-risk behavior and the facilitation of more adaptive coping skills. A study conducted by Dolan and Fullam (2006) supports previous findings that demonstrated a structural brain deficit in persons with antisocial personality disorder. The deficit is a prefrontal structural one that underlies characteristic features of low arousal, poor fear conditioning, lack of conscience, and decision-making deficits.

Other treatment concerns center on the clients' ability to charm and manipulate because these usually quite intelligent people possess excellent verbal and nonverbal skills. An inexperienced nurse may unwittingly fall into a trap that involves flattery and favors. The nurse, lacking sophistication in this treatment arena, may be swayed by the seemingly rational arguments so skillfully presented by these clients. When a nurse fails to respond with firm and consistent limits to maladaptive behavior, the behavior is reinforced, boundary limits breached, and greater problems ensue.

Mental health professionals are often hesitant, resistant, and pessimistic about treating antisocial clients for a number of reasons because their characteristics include the following (APA, 2000):

◆ A lack of conformity to social norms and lawful activity by repetitive illegal activity

◆ A lack of honesty as evidenced in lying, adoption of aliases, and conning others as personal gain

◆ A lack of planning as seen in impulsive behavior

◆ A history of fights and assaults manifesting irritability and aggression

◆ A disregard for the safety of self and others

◆ A failure to be consistent in work or financial obligations

◆ A lack of remorse evidenced by indifference and rationalization of mistreatment of others

Although these clients have long been considered to be poor candidates for treatment, some studies have given some hope for success in developing insight. The studies have demonstrated that structure in confined settings, along with peer pressure and confrontations, are essential aspects of treatment (Bender, 2005). Professional nurses must learn to approach these clients in a sensitive and nonjudgmental manner to facilitate trust and rapport because they fear and mistrust intimacy and closeness. Their self-destructive and criminal behaviors allow them to maintain distance in relationships. It must also be recognized that, contrary to earlier thought, persons with this disorder may demonstrate a considerable degree of anxiety reflected by jitteriness, panic attacks, obsessions and compulsions, and some of the specific anxiety disorders. Neither do some escape anxiety and suicidal behavior, which are, in fact, more prevalent in this group than in the general population (Black, 1999). However, an attempt has been made to base diagnosis of ASP on objective rather than subjective criteria such as arrests, use of aliases, and angry outbursts rather than perceived motives and thought patterns (Black, 1999). Additionally, according to Black, ASP is much more prevalent in males, occurring two to eight times more often in men than in women (p. 28); although the disorder may be diagnosed less frequently in females because of a different way of manifesting symptoms. The condition is linked with poverty and homelessness, most likely propelled by a disinterest in employment and the adherence to rules that employers require. In spite of the fact that poverty and homelessness are common, there is no evidence that ethnicity predominates in the disorder. As to etiology, there is no well-defined understanding of this in ASP, and Black (1999) states, "If science ever manages to locate . . . a gene, the search will not end there. The next step will be to determine what the gene products are and how they function at the cellular level to create a vulnerability to antisocial personality disorder" (p. 108).

Borderline Personality Disorder

The next area within Cluster B, and one frequently encountered inside and outside of inpatient units, is BPD. Gunderson (1988) stated that of all the personality disorders, this one is the most varied and unstable. Once thought to be associated with schizophrenia, the condition is now more closely aligned with affective disturbances. In many ways it shares commonalties with several other personality disorders. One study (Becker, Grilo, Anez, Paris, & McGlashan, 2005) considered the variants of hostility between those with APD and those with BPD. Those with APD had an extroverted manifestation of hostility while those with BPD manifested an introverted type.

Causal Confusion

Borderline personality has been consistently associated with other illnesses. Deutsch (1942) described the "as if" character. Grinker, Werber, and Drye (1968) called it borderline schizophrenia; and Kernberg (1975) described it as a continuum of pathology associated with severity of symptoms at corresponding levels of development.

Neurobiological studies of clients have demonstrated abnormal EEGs, and pharmacologic trials have demonstrated positive results using anticonvulsants and antidepressants for target symptoms of impulsivity or dyscontrol and dysphoria. Results from a study conducted by New, Hazlett, Buchsbaum, Goodman, Mitelman, Newmark, and others (2007) were consistent with other findings that implicate abnormalities in the amygdala-prefrontal cortex in persons with borderline personality. Abnormalities in these neurocircuitry pathways account for impulsivity, dysphoria, and suicide risk in this population. Early childhood trauma and other adverse experiences are believed to modulate alterations in these neural pathways. In some instances, these become active rather late in development and are then limited in coordinating disparate elements in the central nervous system. Certain symptom clusters may be investigated using psychometric and brain imaging techniques. Also, because the symptoms are related to experience, they are considered reversible, at least partially, through therapy.

A wide spectrum of behaviors or symptoms is associated with this disorder, ranging from intense anxiety to psychosis. Numerous factors have been associated with the development of borderline personality such as attachment problems, early childhood traumas or abuse (emotional, physical, or sexual), genetic predisposition, and various neurobiological causes.

Typical Characteristics

Borderline disorder refers to people who have poorly integrated and fragile ego structures. Their dysfunction manifests itself in the lack of a sense of self-identity, the use of primitive defense mechanisms, and impairment in reality testing. They tend to regress during stressful times and often resort to splitting, denial, and projection. Gunderson (1988) stated that the essential feature of the disorder is fear of and intolerance for aloneness, and clients frequently report intense and excessive feelings of loneliness, emptiness, and rage. Their rage is often translated into self-abusive behaviors such as hitting walls; head-banging; skin scratching and tearing; and suicide attempts, gestures, or threats. Relationships are often unstable and are manifested by devaluation, manipulation, dependency, and self-denial. They may, at times, have psychotic-like perceptual distortions, become dissociative, or experience paranoid episodes (Gunderson, 1988). The *DSM-IV-TR* (APA, 2000) lists the following behaviors:

- Attempts to avoid abandonment, either real or imagined, that are frantic
- Alternating extremes of idealization and devaluation leading to relationship instability
- Poor and unstable self-image and sense of self
- Self-damaging impulsivity in at least two areas such as spending, sexual behavior, substance abuse, reckless drinking, or binge eating
- Gestures, threats, self-mutilation, or actual suicidal behavior that is recurrent
- Marked mood reactivity, lasting a few hours to days
- Chronic feelings of emptiness
- Anger that is inappropriately intense, uncontrolled, and frequent
- Stress-related paranoid thinking or severe dissociative symptoms that are transient

Management Issues

As with some of the other personality disorders, clients with borderline disorders are particularly difficult to work with and may tax the emotional and physical resources of even the most experienced nurse. This occurs because of the intense demands of dependency or neediness (immense emotional demands), poor insight into their behaviors, and extreme fears of abandonment. These behaviors often trigger countertransference responses in nurses and other health care professionals. No other group of clients has a greater ability to create chaos and stress within a system than these.

Because of their dependency needs, these clients often seek therapeutic assistance in their frequently occurring crises. Stressors tend to precipitate a crisis (there may be a new and different crisis every day, and strangely, the one from the previous day may not even be mentioned in the latest encounter). These clients are prone to telephone abuse by calling for help at any time, especially at night; and this may be in response to loneliness and the sense or fear of abandonment. One pattern in clients with BPD is that of omitting important details in their communication exchanges, and these distortions seem to be related to the common phenomenon of family invalidation (Allen & Whitson, 2004). Abandonment or separation issues, particularly those that arise in close relationships, most often precipitate crises.

Nursing interventions must center on assessing the meaning of crises, identifying current stressors and coping behaviors, and minimizing self-destructive behaviors. A preferable

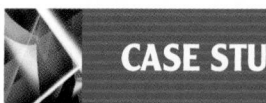

CASE STUDY

The Client with Borderline Personality Disorder (Louise)

Louise is a 30-year-old school teacher who has three older brothers. She has a history of broken relationships, having been engaged twice previously, and now with another broken relationship after 5 months of serious dating and consideration of marriage. Louise has never been married but says she is looking for the perfect man, "like my Grand dad." She relates the breakup to her boyfriend's complaints that she was smothering him and that he could not handle her need to control his every move. Furthermore, she had told him that she would never be willing to move away from her hometown "because I need to be close to people I know." She admits that these problems were the bases of her previous relationship problems. Her history also shows that she drinks three to four cans of beer each night and that she consumes more during periods of stress. She says that she does not drink to get drunk, but "just to feel relaxed." She also admits to binging and purging after drinking too many beers, and she has a history of several suicidal gestures. She had expressed suicidal thoughts just before this hospitalization, which was what prompted her eldest brother to take her to the emergency department. She had told her brother, "I might as well just check out since John doesn't want me anymore." Her family has never taken her suicide attempts very seriously because none of her threats or attempts were serious enough to cause permanent injury, and she was never hospitalized in the past. She had been seen through crisis intervention services on several occasions. Louise does not appear to be significantly depressed; however, she seems to want to latch on to one or two nurses who have become her favorite, and she shows a good bit of disdain toward the others whom she sees as not catering sufficiently to her needs. When asked about her family relationships, she replies, "None of them ever wanted me; I was an afterthought."

Inpatient treatment typically focuses on crisis stabilization. The challenges in working with these clients has already been described, but it must be stressed that the ego development of these clients is insecure and a great deal of structure, gentle confrontation, and limit setting similar to that used with the antisocial client is needed. See Nursing Care Plan 15–1.

method of intervention is related to a careful consideration of the client's developmental level and experience. The need for psychopharmacologic intervention must also be considered as treatment for the affective components that frequently accompany this condition. The client is assisted to identify the reasons for the present hospital or outpatient experience; the coping methods used in the present situation and the alternative behaviors that might work better; and past coping methods and their outcomes. Because these clients are likely to resort to the use of substances and to attempt suicide, it is important to assess and discuss these issues as unproductive coping methods during therapeutic encounters. *Dialectical Behavior Therapy* (Linehan, 1987, 1993) has been described as the most successful and effective psychotherapeutic approach (Swenson, Torrey, & Koerner, 2002). This method teaches the client how to learn to better control their lives, emotions, and themselves using a self-knowledge, regulation of emotions, and cognitive restructuring.

Kernberg (1984) defined splitting as the dichotomous manner in which clients perceive the world, that is, all good or all bad. These clients have difficulty seeing both positive and negative qualities in one situation or person at a given time. This defect may be the result of early developmental arrests associated with a lack of opportunity or ability to have integrated these qualities from positive or helpful parenting experiences.

An example of splitting can be seen when the client perceives the nurses as either good or bad, and this depends on some arbitrary or unrealistic perception retained by the client at a given time. Good nurses are seen as those who allow the client to break the treatment rules or those who

rescue (overprotect) the client. Bad nurses are seen as those who insist on limit setting or who provide negative responses to the client. When "good" and "bad" nurses argue over what the client needs, intense feelings toward the client emerge along with chaos on the unit. The scenario represents a re-creation of the client's family of origin. Splitting is unconscious and needs to be assessed as a coping behavior requiring consistent interventions. Key nursing interventions for these clients are:

◆ Form a nurse-client alliance based on clearly stated, realistic expectations

◆ Assist in reduction of self-destructive behavior and intent

◆ Acknowledge problem behaviors

◆ Assist the client to develop adaptive coping patterns

◆ Encourage verbalization of feelings about self

Johnson and Silver (1988) stressed that the treatment of persons with borderline personality disorder is a stressful experience potentially full of conflict between clients and staff. They suggest that these clients probably evoke more intense staff reactions than other clients do. Some methods for minimizing conflict and promoting growth in clients are suggested as follows:

◆ Identify and state the treatment, although not necessarily the goals, from the outset

◆ Use staff development meetings to discuss conflicts and problem-solving methods

◆ Seek and use professional staff supervision

- Help create an environment for the honest expression of feelings regarding unit conflicts
- Maintain open communication between staff and members of the interdisciplinary team

Clients with borderline personality disorder have particular difficulty with boundaries, and they may become intrusive into the life and activities of others if permitted to get past appropriate limits. Gutheil and Gabbard (1993) defined boundaries as "parameters of a relationship." The nurse must remain firm from the outset if there is to be some later assurance that there will be no intrusions on the part of the client. Furthermore, the client needs help in understanding the nature of the problem, the expectations of the nurse (and others in the client's life), and responsibilities for changing old behavioral patterns surrounding this issue. These boundary problems exist because of the client's lack of ego integration, and his frail self-identity (or fluid ego boundaries) contributes to difficulty in recognizing where his boundaries end and others' begin.

Another area of difficulty for clients is placing the blame for their own behavior and its outcomes on others and to avoid any consideration of their own role in continuing the problems in their lives. It is important for them to learn to take responsibility and to recognize that it is not bad to fail. Clients with borderline disorder often believe that they are bad because they often have received the message that they are throughout their lifetime. In addition, they have often been sexually abused and generally have a great sense of guilt, believing that they were responsible for what occurred to them. They also may have been held responsible either by the victimizer or even by their mother.

Because of the circumstances of their entire life, clients with borderline disorder often believe they are bad, worthless, hopeless, and helpless, even though they generally have an amazing amount of ingenuity and ability to maneuver through many difficult circumstances. Their negative self-beliefs lead to dysphoria and sometimes the desire to die. Also, because they feel so alone and often abandoned, they come to believe they are of no consequence with no place or belonging in the world. They may feel the need to test these beliefs by threatening suicide in order to find out if there really is anyone who cares enough to rescue them. Therefore, the nurse or others involved in their care may feel caught in a bind because there is a need to rescue on the one hand and a need not to be manipulated on the other. When a trust relationship has been formed, the nurse can reassure the client that he will be there (although not necessarily always physically present) and that there is confidence that the client will begin to make wise decisions. The nurse needs to promise to check in later at a specified time to assure the client that he is valued and to discuss the issue with problem-solving in mind when there is no immediate crisis. When the nurse and client talk the next time, the client will most likely have moved on to something else and will seem already to have put the issue in the past. It is almost as if a crisis lasts until the client has been told in some way that he is significant and then works

through it alone so that by the next contact, the issues are changed and the client presents a new set of concerns. There actually seems to be an incredible amount of personal strength that the client never acknowledges and this most likely occurs because of the number and extent of past crises and difficult periods he has lived through. This particular behavior is reminiscent of la belle indifference, a behavior related to secondary gain in conversion reactions except that, in this instance, it is related to emotional upheaval rather than to physical symptoms.

Self-Destructive Behaviors

As stated earlier, these clients often manifest poor impulse control; it is seen most often in suicidal behavior or self-mutilation. Self-mutilation or injurious behaviors is distinct from suicidal behavior in intent, bodily injury, frequency, and technique (Favazza & Rosenthal, 1993). In addition, borderline personality is often present (Favazza & Rosenthal, 1993). Studies also link self-injurious behaviors with traumatic experiences, particularly sexual and physical abuse, and co-morbid dissociative symptoms (Foote, Smolin, Kaplan, Legatt, & Lipschitz, 2006). (See Chapter 19.) These acts may be carried out as spur-of-the-moment impulses; however, as noted earlier, it also is not unusual for the client to make telephone calls to see if someone will respond. The nurse can make more accurate predictions and determine interventions if there is an accurate assessment of past behaviors already recorded and at hand. If the client is in denial or is ashamed about these past events, there may be unwillingness to share the information. The nurse needs to check the skin of the hands, arms, face, and neck to observe for any old or new scars and record the client's report about the occurrence of self-mutilation. Freeman and Gunderson (1989) suggested that these destructive behaviors are germane to maladaptive responses in borderline clients.

Favazza and Rosenthal (1993) defined self-mutilation as a "deliberate alteration or destruction of body tissue" (p. 134), without the intent of killing oneself. Self-mutilation is associated with a myriad of conditions encompassing psychosocial, neurobiological and cultural components (Krysinska, Heller, & De Leo, 2006). Acts considered to be self-mutilating include plucking eyebrows completely; eye enucleation; castration; head banging; and skin burning, cutting, or carving. Vincent van Gogh provided an example of this behavior in cutting off his ear during an episode of mental derangement.

Favazza and Rosenthal (1990) categorized self-mutilation as three types: major, stereotypical, and superficial or moderate. Major mutilation can appear in a wide variety of disorders encompassing psychosis, substance abuse (acute intoxication), and schizoid personality disorder in addition to BPD. Clients at risk include those who are religiously or sexually preoccupied. Some of these acts may be responses to command hallucinations. Clients who self-mutilate tend to be calm after the act, suggesting that the act temporarily relieves unconscious emotional pain or conflict. Stereotypical mutilation is the most common type. The highest rates are found in autistic children and clients who are mentally retarded. Other clients who may exhibit these behaviors include those with schizophrenia, drug-induced psychosis, brief reactive psychosis, obsessive-compulsive disorder, and eating disorders.

Effective Therapeutic Intervention

Linehan (1993) and Koerner and Linehan (2000) stressed the role of the therapist in helping clients gain insight into the meaning of their behaviors, teaching them adaptive coping skills and continually assessing their level of dangerousness. Linehan's use of Dialectical Behavior Therapy is defined by determining specific treatment targets, treatment strategies, and therapist attitudes. In this type of therapy the client is taught that all of life exists on a continuum and that the extreme viewpoints are limiting to one's appreciation and enjoyment of life. The model assumes that individuals and environments are continuously interactive, interdependent, and reciprocal, with constant adaptation and influencing taking place. Consistent limit setting allows nurses to provide external controls for these clients until they are able to do so for themselves. See Chapters 2 and 27.

Nurses need to take advantage of any hospital experience that these clients may have because it might be the only access that a professional has to a continuous opportunity for interacting and intervening into maladaptive behavior as it occurs. It can be a time when the client makes tremendous strides if optimal use is made of the time and experience. Hospital stays are generally not extended stays, and good use needs to be made of the contacts that are now quite limited.

The focus of specific therapies includes targeting the maladaptive behaviors and the feelings and perceptions associated with interpersonal relationships (Gunderson et al., 2006). These interventions can teach clients how to modulate their feelings and rage episodes and minimize their feelings of helplessness and sensitivity to criticism. Supportive and group therapies can facilitate development of adaptive social skills associated with learning about how one's behavior affects others. See the Research Abstract included for BPD.

Psychopharmacologic Therapy

There has been limited success in the use of psychotropic medications in clients with borderline personality disorder. Mood stabilizers, such as divalproex (Depakote) and lithium (Eskalith), antipsychotics, and serotonin reuptake inhibitors have provided some relief for dyscontrol, impulsivity, self-injurious behaviors, and depression. Results from most studies implicate limited efficacy in those clients with severe childhood trauma and co-occurring psychiatric and substance use disorders. Most studies consistently demonstrate that the treatment of personality disorders requires an integrated psychobiologic approach that includes pharmacologic and psychotherapeutic interventions. Other clients have responded favorably to antidepressants (e.g., tricyclics and the newer agents such as sertraline [Zoloft] and paroxetine [Paxil]). A number of studies have demonstrated increased effectiveness of combined psychotherapy and pharmacologic treatment (Livesley, 2000; Soloff, 1998, 2000). However, Clarkin, Marziali, and Munroe-Blum (1992) suggested that multiple causal pathways exist in the client with BPD; thus, it may be that the same holds true for the affective component of the condition because mood oscillation is one of the symptoms identified for the disorder.

Histrionic Personality Disorder

Early psychoanalytic literature coined the term "hysteria," now known as histrionic personality disorder. Manifestations of this disorder included exaggerated labile emotions, sexualization of relationships, and dramatic emotional states. The behaviors ranged from higher ego function (attention seeking and sociability) behaviors to lower ego function (promiscuity, impulsivity, and psychosis) (Reich, 1949).

Symptoms of histrionic personality tend to be manifested by attention-seeking behaviors in which clients exhibit the following behaviors (APA, 2000):

◆ Discomfort in situations where he is not the center of attention
◆ Inappropriate sexually seductive behavior with others
◆ Rapidly shifting and shallow emotional expressions
◆ Excessively impressionistic style of speech that lacks detail
◆ Self-dramatization, theatrics, or exaggerated emotional expressions
◆ Suggestibility
◆ Attitude that relationships are more intimate than they are

This disorder is most often diagnosed in women. Their interpersonal relationships are superficial, flighty, and their melodramatic expressions are flamboyant, apparently designed to gratify early unmet dependency needs; they anticipate these will be met through their therapists. Their ego functioning is disorganized, and they tend to fantasize and idealize their relationships with the therapists; that is, they secretly love them and consider themselves special to the therapists (Freeman & Gunderson, 1989). Their major defense mechanisms include repression and dissociation. Other maladaptive behaviors may include temper tantrums, manipulation, and endless demands. They also tend to evoke intense emotional reactions in nurses such as anger and a sense of inadequacy. Treatment is similar to that of some other personality disorders and focuses on consistency, understanding, managing countertransference issues, and providing an environment that minimizes maladaptive coping patterns.

In addition to the trust and rapport-building activities and identifying the client's particular maladaptive behaviors, it also is necessary to gain understanding about infantile fantasies (feelings). As these tasks are accomplished, the client can be helped to develop more adaptive coping skills by finding alternatives to previous destructive behaviors. Encouragement and assistance in developing and recognizing how new behaviors will lead to increased self-worth will be needed. The nurse who is skillful in helping the client accomplish these outcomes also needs to recognize how extremely sensitive to rejection and depressive moods and episodes these clients tend to be. A detailed discussion of treatment strategies are similar to that found in the section on BPD.

Psychopharmacologic approaches center on depression, anxiety, and psychosis that may occur in these clients.

Narcissistic Personality Disorder

The term *narcissism* is associated with self-love and self-absorption as depicted in Greek mythology when young Narcissus fell in love with the image of himself, which he saw reflected in a pool. Psychoanalytical theory proposes that narcissism is a necessary part of the early developmental stages. Freud described these personality types as having no tension between ego and superego and with no preponderance of erotic needs because the main interest was self-preservation. Narcissistic individuals are independent, not easily intimidated, and quite aggressive. They prefer loving to being loved and enjoy serving as champions to others (Freud, 1957). Freud described three types of narcissism, namely, erotic obsessional (superego restriction of libidinal life), erotic narcissistic (unity of opposites so that there is considerable amount of aggressiveness and activity), and narcissistic obsessional (capacity for vigorous action and strengthening of the ego over against the superego). Rothstein (1991) summarized earlier theoretical works of Kernberg and Kohut, stating that some narcissistic personalities adapt well vocationally but generally seek help for problems relating to difficulties in intimate relations with others; others suffer in their object relations and seek treatment because they experience neurotic symptoms, sexual difficulties, and chronic feelings of emptiness. The third group functions on a borderline level with nonspecific symptoms of ego weakness.

Children whose parents are aloof, aggressive, rejecting, and emotionally cold are at risk for developmental arrest at the early narcissistic stage because the person is prevented from achieving a sense of self-worth and value. They tend to seek approval and recognition throughout life and experience emptiness, low self-esteem, self-absorption, and somatic symptoms (Kohut, 1971, 1977). Shengold (1999) referred to the narcissistic effect of parents as "Soul Murder."

The *DSM-IV-TR* (APA, 2000) states that five or more of the following characteristics must be present to diagnose this disorder:

- Has a grandiose sense of self-importance (e.g., exaggerates achievements and talents, expects to be recognized as superior without commensurate achievements)
- Is preoccupied with fantasies of unlimited success, power, brilliance, beauty, or ideal love
- Believes that he is "special" and unique and can only be understood by, or should associate with, other special or high-status people (or institutions)

- Requires excessive admiration
- Has a sense of entitlement, that is, unreasonable expectations of especially favorable treatment or automatic compliance with his expectations
- Is interpersonally exploitive, that is, takes advantage of others to achieve his own ends
- Lacks empathy; is unwilling to recognize or identify with the feelings and needs of others
- Is often envious of others or believes that others are envious of him
- Shows arrogant, haughty behaviors or attitudes

Because of their self-centeredness, inability to be empathic, greediness, parasitism, and coldness, clients with this disorder experience relationship problems. However, this grandiose facade covers feelings of low self-esteem, insecurity, and inadequacy. These adults are referred to by Miller (1981) as "Prisoners of Childhood."

As with other personality disorders, nursing interventions first require that the nurse be aware of his own reactions around clients who evoke a great deal of tension in their demands for attention. Kohut (1971) contended that the establishment of therapeutic alliances is important for increasing self-esteem. The nature of narcissism is such that these clients are preoccupied with themselves and need assistance in understanding and valuing events that occur outside their internal environments. To do this, they must first begin to view themselves from a different perspective, and this demands therapeutic intervention requiring much time and effort. Other nursing interventions are the same as those listed in the section on BPD.

Inpatient hospitalization is usually precipitated by depression, suicidal behaviors, and mood swings that often follow failure or rejection. The primary focus of hospitalization is treatment of these target symptoms; attention to the underlying cause may be neglected because of the longer time needed to provide such treatment. Clients may avoid group therapy because it would require their balancing the desire for a special client-therapist relationship and because they fear confrontation by group members (Freeman & Gunderson, 1989). It may be necessary to provide a period of individual psychotherapy either before or concomitant with a lengthier period of group therapy to achieve the greatest benefit. Individual psychotherapy is often the treatment of choice and allows clients an opportunity to introject or incorporate the adaptive aspects of the therapist (Meissner, 1988) and to avoid the regressive use of primitive defenses such as rage, splitting, and projection.

CLUSTER C

The third cluster of personality disorders comprises conditions in which the prominent symptoms are anxiety and fear. Major symptoms include avoiding or minimizing the experience of anxiety by avoiding relationships. Disorders in this cluster include avoidant, dependent, and obsessive-compulsive.

Avoidant Personality Disorder

Major manifestations of avoidant personality disorder are avoidance of activity based on fears of criticism, disapproval, or rejection; unwillingness to be involved without guarantees of acceptance; restraint within intimate relationships because of insecurity; preoccupation with criticism and rejection; interpersonal inhibition based on a sense of inadequacy; a view of self as unappealing, inept, and inferior; and a reluctance to engage in new activity because of a potential risk of embarrassment (APA, 2000). Seclusiveness differs from that seen in schizoid personality disorder by the capacity and desire to form meaningful relationships. Fears of rejection coupled with self-doubt interfere with the ability to risk entry into a relationship; these clients are constantly assessing their interactions for signs of devaluation and deception. Even positive social events are avoided so that clients often have no one to whom they relate. They tend to "make mountains out of molehills" and often attend to negative responses in their environments. They are easily hurt by criticism.

These conditions of distrust make it imperative that nursing interventions create an environment that engenders trust through the formation of reliable and dependable nurse-client alliances. This helps to minimize anxiety sufficiently to permit the exploration of old behaviors and to consider ways to change and feel better. Specific attention needs to be given to relaxing, because mistrust causes hypervigilance, and to developing other relationships in which trust can be expected. The inpatient unit is an ideal place for helping this process, and the nurse is urged to take advantage of every opportunity to promote trust because hospital stays are so brief, if indeed one would be hospitalized at all. It is important to recognize the need for therapy as an outpatient; appropriate referrals are needed to continue what was begun in an inpatient or other therapeutic setting.

Dependent Personality Disorder

The hallmark of dependent personality disorder is the pervasive pattern of dependency and submissiveness. These clients rely on others exclusively for their support. They rarely make their own decisions, and they place tremendous demands on others for reassurance and advice. They attach and cling tenaciously to anyone who will take care of them, tell them what to do, or make their decisions for them. They are fearful of many things and become the willing shadow of anyone who will take care of them. Their behavior is often childlike in their hesitation to stand on their own as responsible adults.

Dependency is a normal process in nurse-client interactions but must always be redirected as long as the client has the ability to do for self. The need for constant redirection is needed because they ask for advice or assistance in doing things they are able to do. For instance, the client may ask the nurse to make a telephone call and request information that he is perfectly capable of obtaining, or there may be requests for advice that most others would not ask for or for which answers have already been previously given. The following is an example of an intervention that may occur with a dependent client:

In this example, the nurse has not given advice but has offered some ways to begin the process of helping the client to begin thinking independently and taking some action. The nurse has provided support and a broad suggestion about

Client: "Oh, I'm so upset about getting a job. I have to go to work and I don't know where to go."

Nurse: "You don't know where to go?"

Client: "No. What do you think I should do?"

Nurse: "What kinds of things have you thought about doing?"

Client: "I can't think of anything. I need help with this."

Nurse: "What kind of help do you need with this?"

Client: "Someone to pick out places for me."

Nurse: "What things have you already considered?"

Client: "I haven't considered anything. I'm waiting for someone to help me."

Nurse: "You haven't looked into any possible solutions?"

Client: "No. This is just too hard for me. I need help."

Nurse: "Perhaps you might get the phone book and look up some job placement centers in the newspaper. We can get back together again this afternoon, and you can tell me what you've discovered. Then we can talk about some of the options you've considered. I'd be interested in hearing about that."

possible job sources along with the offer to listen to problem-solving activities later in the day. Thus, the nurse supports and empowers the client in the beginning steps of a decision-making process. Later, it will become possible to promote even more responsibility on the client's part so that there would not even be a need to suggest use of the telephone book or the newspaper. In this instance, the nurse might say instead, "Tell me what you think are some of the places where you can find job opportunities."

Nurses who need to sustain dependent interactions with clients fail to promote autonomy and growth in their clients. In this situation the nurse must examine the meaning of their own dependent needs. Nurses may also err by responding to dependent needs by becoming hostile and negative in their responses to the client. These countertransference responses suggest the need for supervision in which the nurse is given opportunity to explore and evaluate his behavior.

In all therapeutic endeavors, the most apparent need is the reduction of anxiety, and in nearly all instances, a concomitant need for increasing self-esteem. This is no less true for

dependency. A skillful balancing act is needed to provide enough but not too much in the process of helping clients grow into a more adaptive lifestyle. The nurse-client relationship may be the only place in which this is given an opportunity to begin. Nurses are urged to consider the dependent-independent-interdependent need construct of themselves and their clients (Whiting, 1994).

Psychotherapeutic intervention may take place through individual therapy that fosters the development of insight and individual change. The techniques may be interpersonal, behavioral, analytical, or cognitive. Other appropriate modalities include group therapy, family therapy, and psychoeducation to provide decision-making models and assertiveness training.

Obsessive-Compulsive Personality Disorder

Obsessive-compulsive disorder (OCD) is characterized by a pervasive rigidity and preoccupation with control and power and an exaggerated fear of losing control. Most clients with OCD personality disorder recognize the irrational and maladaptive nature of their behavior but have difficulty controlling it. Researchers are exploring the underpinning and nosological description of OCPD as it relates to OCD to determine if it is part of the OCD spectrum or a true personality disorder (Eisen et al., 2006; Fineberg, Sharma, Sivakumaran, Sahakian, & Chamberlain, 2007). Their emotional expression is extremely constricted and they give little of anything, either emotionally or materially. They may be described as perfectionists, and these behaviors interfere with relationships. These tendencies also interfere with task completion because their overly strict standards cannot be met. Preoccupation with detail causes them to lose sight of the goal (APA, 2000). See Chapter 11.

Treatment Issues for the Client with Obsessive-Compulsive Personality Disorder

The same needs exist for anxiety reduction and increased self-esteem as with other disorders previously described. Understanding and decreasing maladaptive behaviors are the goals, and they depend on specific manifestations of the disorder. In addition to the nurse-client relationships, psychoanalytical, behavioral, or cognitive therapy may be helpful. An expert panel of 69 clinicians (an 87 percent response rate) participated in a study conducted by March, Frances, Carpenter, and Kahn (1997) relative to the most appropriate treatment strategies. Most of the experts favored combined treatment. The cognitive behavior therapy (CBT) method is generally considered by these researchers to be more effective than thought stopping and distraction or contingency management. Sessions are generally held weekly for a total of 13 to 20 sessions, but intensive therapy may be conducted in severe cases on a daily basis for 3 weeks. Homework may be assigned and the format may include individual, family, or group therapy.

March et al. (1997) recommend first-line treatment with selective serotonin reuptake inhibitors (SSRIs) that include fluvoxamine ([Luvox] 100–300 mg; average dose 200 mg); fluox-etine ([Prozac] 20–80 mg; average dose 50 mg); clomipramine (Anafranil), a tricyclic antidepressant (100–300 mg; average dose 200 mg); sertraline ([Zoloft] 75–225 mg; average dose 150 mg); or paroxetine ([Paxil] 20–60 mg; average dose 50 mg). The expert panel considered 8 to 13 weeks as an adequate medication trial before changing medication or augmenting with another agent, 4 to 6 weeks if there is no response at a maximum dose, and a 2- to 4-week interval between increases. If the SSRIs are not ultimately effective, the clinician may consider using venlafaxine (Effexor), monoamine oxidase inhibitors (MAOIs), and clonazepam (Klonopin) as a third line of treatment.

In the event that the regimen described above does not become effective, the addition of other approaches such as using a new and different CBT technique (i.e., satiation, stopping, habit reversal, relaxation), making the CBT more intensive, changing the setting or therapist, or changing the modality (e.g., group instead of family or individual and so on). Other medication augmentation strategies may include conventional antipsychotics, buspirone (BuSpar), risperidone (Risperdal), or a second SSRI added to the first. These are especially important considerations in the event of a co-occurring condition. Maintenance will require a gradual reduction in visits, and a continuation of medication for 1 to 2 years, with gradual elimination of them. Longer-term medication use may be needed if there are relapses of various kinds. This has been shown to effectively reduce symptoms commonly seen in these clients and has offered hope in treatment. Side effects that are usually dose and time dependent must be considered. Tolerance often develops over 6 to 8 weeks.

THE ROLE OF THE NURSE

Clients presenting with personality disorders often challenge the patience of psychiatric nurses more than those with other psychiatric disorders. For these reasons, psychiatric nurses must initiate interventions that address the needs of clients exhibiting maladaptive coping skills and facilitate adaptive behavioral changes. Frequently, the psychiatric nurse overlooks the bases of disorders that stem from early childhood trauma and neglect resulting in comorbid conditions, such as depression, anxiety, and substance-related disorders. The role of the psychiatric nurses must involve collaboration with the client, family members, and other health care providers can facilitate adaptive behavioral changes and an optimal level of functioning.

THE GENERALIST NURSE

The generalist nurse will most likely encounter the majority of clients with personality disorders in the acute inpatient or community settings. These may occur in medical-surgical situations as well as in mental health situations. These clients, especially those with borderline, dependent, or antisocial personality disorders, often look for ways to penetrate the nurse's boundaries. They seem to possess an uncanny ability to sense where the nurse is most vulnerable. It is helpful for the nurse to examine personal responses with the following questions:

◆ What feelings do I have about the client?

◆ How often do I find myself in conflict with other team members regarding this client?

◆ What are the behaviors that trigger the most emotion in me?

◆ What emotional response do I have when I find myself assigned to this client?

The generalist nurse may need to role play responses in a supervisory setting or talk about the feelings engendered by such clients. He needs to recognize when there is a need for a nurse with advanced skills and make the proper referral as

well as to seek supervision from an advanced-practice registered nurse (APRN). The client with a personality disorder is particularly difficult to manage and needs the services of a nurse therapist to assist in changing pathological and destructive behavioral patterns. The generalist can provide support for change that occurs in therapy.

The care of clients with a personality disorder is difficult and often frustrating because they demonstrate behaviors that challenge even the experts. Interventions must be specific to the behaviors, which can vary widely from time to time and from client to client. Overall, however, some of the behaviors of clients with a personality disorder can be categorized using the *DSM-IV-TR* (APA, 2000) personality disorders' section. Table 15–7 outlines the diagnoses and some of the typical behaviors that have prevented these clients from establishing

---

TABLE 15–7
Typical Behaviors of Clients with Personality Disorders According to *DSM-IV-TR* Diagnostic Groupings and Suggested Interventions

Diagnoses	Typical Behaviors	Suggested Interventions
Avoidant Obsessive-compulsive disorder Paranoid Passive-aggressive Schizoid Schizotypal	Anger Dysfunctional independence Isolation Mistrust and suspicion Withdrawal	1. Offer self on a regular basis without intrusion 2. Acknowledge observed behaviors with the client 3. Be particularly attentive to trust building 4. Work at drawing the client into one-on-one interactions that promote enjoyment of a relationship 5. Involve the client in establishing at least one relationship and in working to increase the number of social involvements
Borderline Dependent Histrionic Narcissistic (sometimes)	Attention-seeking Dependence Neediness	1. Assess the type and frequency of demands for attention 2. Establish a trusting relationship that allows confrontation of behaviors, and assist in acknowledging the behavior 3. Set specific goals and methods for achieving greater independence 4. Provide reinforcement of independent functioning
Antisocial Narcissistic (dishonest at times)	Aggression Entitlement Manipulation Risk-taking	1. Provide and maintain a team-developed set of rules that are reasonable and strictly followed 2. Remind the client of expectations before the temptation sets in to deviate 3. Develop an atmosphere of trust in which sincere confrontation is possible 4. Provide pleasurable activities that serve as a substitute for the previous deviant activities no longer permitted 5. Recognize that many of these clients have operated for a long time and have a pattern of behavior that is difficult, if not impossible, to change

Note. Adapted from *Diagnostic and Statistical Manual of Mental Disorders* (4th edition, Text Revision) (*DSM-IV-TR*), by the American Psychiatric Association, 2000, Washington, DC: Author. Adapted with permission.

or maintaining meaningful relationships throughout their lifetime. The nurse must take every opportunity to use the short periods when these clients are available to provide honest confrontation and limit setting within a milieu that is open and trusting; this is not a simple assignment and requires diligence and knowledge about the various personality disorders.

THE ADVANCED-PRACTICE PSYCHIATRIC REGISTERED NURSE

In addition to treating clients with a personality disorder in acute care or community mental health settings, the APRN may encounter these clients in a variety of other clinical settings (e.g., in the liaison nurse role). Many opportunities exist for providing care either directly or indirectly in liaison roles, independent practice roles, and through supervision and consultation.

Because the predominant etiologic theory for BPD is that of separation-individuation, a developmental framework is useful and necessary for understanding, guiding, and treatment. It also is a helpful framework for working with all other types of personality disorders, especially those who are stuck at the level of "I want what I want when I want it." The advanced-practice nurse will encounter many clients with self-centered, dramatic, seductive, ambivalent, hostile, isolated, dependent, or independent behaviors that challenge the ability to respond without losing control and demeanor.

There are many risks involved in the direct care of clients who use treatment as a relationship they may never have had or to replace relationships they have damaged by their attitude or behavior. Many clients seek a relationship that is nurturing and expect undivided attention from the therapist they claim as their own. For example, the dependent client may want a "mother"; the seductive client, a lover; and the narcissistic client, an admirer. In contrast, the paranoid client may be so mistrusting as to push the nurse away; the avoidant client, afraid; and the obsessive-compulsive client, too controlling. The therapist needs to be extremely careful in responding to these demands. Each of the behaviors challenges the nurse's ingenuity for trust building and countering certain behaviors that prevent the formation of trust between individuals.

The advanced-practice nurse is warned to be alert to the skillful maneuvers of seduction and neediness by maintaining constant and clear boundaries. The client feels safe and will honor the boundaries that aid him in maintaining self-control. Also, there is the need to recognize that many of these clients are not suited to brief encounters or therapy, so the advanced-practice nurse must be willing to commit to long periods and a process for building new behavioral patterns—a process that is tedious and requires great patience, commitment, and strength.

THE NURSING PROCESS

The nursing process enables the nurse to assess patterns of maladaptive and adaptive coping behaviors while collaborating with the client to identify individual needs. In addition, treatment planning and nursing intervention must focus on adaptive coping behaviors that promote safety, facilitate effective coping, and enhance meaningful interpersonal relationships.

ASSESSMENT

Evaluating the client coping skills (often tied to ego functioning) is a major aspect of the nursing process because it provides data necessary for making accurate diagnoses, planning therapeutic interventions, and bringing about therapeutic outcomes. The assessment considers the components of interpersonal relationships that have not worked on the client's behalf; affective capabilities and problems, motivation for treatment, capacity for introspection, insight, defensiveness, memory, judgment, and reality testing.

Assessing personality development entails examining the life span and factors such as early relationships with primary caregivers, their impact on ego development, their adaptation, and coping style. Understanding key concepts in personality formation such as ego development and organization is crucial in assessing the meaning of maladaptive behaviors, facilitating adaptive coping behaviors, and evaluating client responses to interventions.

The role of the psychiatric nurse includes assessing areas of impairment that begins with approaching clients and their significant others in a caring and nonjudgmental manner. The approach facilitates trust building and enhances the potential success of treatment plan outcomes. Interventions are planned to encourage the client into a nurse-client relationship, in which a measure of trust can be established early in the process. However, it must be remembered that all personality disorders are ingrained, fixed patterns of behavior that are extremely resistant to change; and the nurse must not be discouraged when only small initial gains are made. Indeed, the overall outcome may produce negligible results, but this will not be the fault of the professional who uses appropriate interventions and maintains an attitude of acceptance.

NURSING DIAGNOSES

Once the assessment is completed, the nurse analyzes the data to arrive at the nursing diagnoses. Clients with a personality disorder are difficult to treat, so to determine what is preventing the client from making adequate adjustment and engaging successfully in relationships, it is necessary to identify the specific behaviors that hamper success. It is typical to find, in all clients with a personality disorder, a pattern of immaturity, narcissism, inflexibility, and hostility that may be either overt or covert. Examples of nursing diagnoses include the following:

◆ High risk for self-directed violence

◆ Chronic Low Self-Esteem

◆ Disturbed thought process

◆ Impaired social interaction

◆ Risk for Self-Mutilation

◆ Powerlessness

◆ Ineffective coping

◆ Defensive coping

OUTCOME IDENTIFICATION AND PLANNING

Goal setting and outcome criteria enable the nurse to schedule activities that are helpful to the client and to evaluate outcomes. Goals (long term) and outcome criteria (short term) are measurable. Examples of three goals and outcome criteria as related to the diagnoses listed previously are as follows:

Goal I. Client will report at least one satisfying relationship in three weeks.

Outcome criteria:

1. Client will list at least five positive personal characteristics by the next interaction on (date).
2. Client will describe the type of person with whom he or she would like to be friends within the next several meetings.
3. Client will identify the things in self that he believes are hindering development of relationships within the next three meetings.
4. Client will identify within the next week at least three behaviors that interest him.
5. Client will demonstrate definite effort toward establishing contact with the person who was identified as a desirable friend within 3 weeks.

Goal II. Client will demonstrate more appropriate cognitive functioning by the time of discharge (or the end of the contract with the nurse).

Outcome criteria:

1. Client will listen to alternative ideas and beliefs as offered by group members (or nurse).
2. Client will accept confrontation by group members (or nurse) within 1 week.
3. Client will verbalize alternatives for faulty thoughts or ideas when challenged by group members (or nurse) within 2 weeks.
4. Client will begin to challenge faulty thinking of self and other group members within 3 weeks.

Goal III. Client will demonstrate improved interactions with peers.

Outcome criteria:

1. Client will become acquainted with peers through attendance at group meetings for the next 4 weeks.
2. Client will acknowledge behaviors in self that group members identify as detrimental to relationships within 2 weeks.
3. Client will respond to in-group critiques by acknowledging what he needs to work on within 2½ weeks.
4. Client will verbalize the behaviors in self that create interpersonal problems within 3 weeks.
5. Client will demonstrate less interest in self and more interest in others within 4 weeks.

Refer to Nursing Care Plans for borderline personality and antisocial personality disorders.

INTERVENTIONS

Interventions are planned and carried out in accordance with the steps identified in the section on outcome criteria. All formal and informal interactions are considerate of the goals and outcome criteria. The nurse is most helpful by remaining cognizant of the specific needs of the client throughout every contact. This means that each contact is goal and client centered and aimed at taking advantage of every available (and costly) moment. This is especially important in these times when treatment contact is short and every contact is significant. Interventions for the above goals may include interactions such as the following:

Nurse:	"Hi, Louise. I see that you have spent only 10 minutes applying your makeup today."
Client:	"Yes, I remembered what the group said last time, and I didn't want them to jump on me again today."
Nurse:	"You didn't want them to 'jump' on you again today?"
Client:	"No way."
Nurse:	"Louise, I'm aware that you used to spend 2 hours plus numerous remakes on your makeup each day. What changed?"
Client:	"I think I'm beginning to see that I was spending too much time on that and keeping others away from me by my self-centeredness."

The nurse-client interaction indicates the effectiveness of group intervention coupled with nurse interventions. These occur both internally and externally as the client begins to think and then to act out the new behaviors. Nehls (1992) decried the lack of information in the literature about group approaches for BPD (see the Research Abstract display).

EVALUATION

When nursing diagnoses are directly related to goals and outcome criteria that in turn are directly related to the interventions, there is greater likelihood that the client will make obvious progress toward a goal. Clients with a personality disorder are, however, likely to regress and need frequent, sometimes constant, reinforcement. It may take years to fully accomplish the original goals, but the client will be able to hear and respond to criticism or confrontation when it is skillfully applied within the context of treatment and given with sincere care. Clients with a personality disorder are capable of identifying the nurse's weak spots and often appear to be working to defeat the nurse's attempts to help. Unless the nurse is extremely secure, there may be a tendency to give up in despair. The nurse must be willing to persevere even when success seems elusive.

Evaluations are completed at the times designated in the goals and outcome criteria. The nurse and client meet together and discuss the evaluation so that they are able to experience satisfaction over completion. This fosters a sense of partnership when the client can verbally acknowledge feeling better or having success in one of the areas where there was great struggle in the beginning. It may be the first

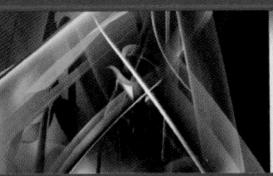

The Client with a Borderline Personality Disorder (Louise)

Nursing Diagnosis: High Risk for Self-Directed Violence related to suicidal gesture as evidenced by history of suicide attempts

Outcome Identification	Nursing Actions	Rationales	Evaluation
1. By [date], client will verbalize the absence of suicidal ideations or plan.	1a. Assess level of dangerousness.	1a. Using a suicide risk assessment tool assists in determining the kind of action toward the client that maintains safety.	*Goal met:* Client denies suicidal ideations. Client agrees not to harm self and identifies other options of coping. Client exhibits gradual mood changes and superficial expression of feelings.
	1b. Provide safe environment, e.g., remove potential or actual dangerous objects from environment.	1b. Clients are often impulsive and may use suicidal behavior to gain the attention they need. Safety is a major concern in a psychiatric setting.	
	1c. Discuss "no suicide" verbal contract.	1c. No-suicide contracts have proved to be effective in eliciting client's cooperation and in assuring the client that someone else is concerned enough to provide boundaries such as contracts. Many clients do not really want to die but see no other way to get their needs met or to control their environment. Contracts help place control in the client's hands.	
2. By [date], client will discuss options to deal with present stressors.	2a. Encourage examination of available options to cope with present stressors.	2a. An inpatient experience is an excellent place and opportunity for testing, evaluation, and learning more effective alternative behaviors.	
	2b. Observe for sudden changes in mood.	2b. Mood changes *may* reflect a decision to carry out a suicidal threat if underlying depression is present. The nurse can also use the mood shift to determine behavioral patterns in clients.	

(continues)

Outcome Identification	Nursing Actions	Rationales	Evaluation
	2c. Encourage expression of feelings.	2c. The expression of feelings is important for helping clients to get in touch with themselves, something that they are not typically accustomed to doing.	

Nursing Diagnosis: Ineffective Coping
as evidenced by fear of abandonment

Outcome Identification	Nursing Actions	Rationales	Evaluation
1. By [date], client will develop an awareness of the meaning of present behaviors.	1a. Facilitate understanding of client's behaviors.	1a. Cognitive information aids clarify about behaviors that interfere with productive relationships.	*Goal met:* Client returns to previous, or new, level of function. Client develops adequate coping skills. Client displays decreased anxiety.
	1b. Assist in problem solving.	1b. Assisted problem solving helps promote greater future independence.	
	1c. Confront maladaptive behaviors.	1c. Fair and consistent confrontation by a trusted model assists in the establishment of needed boundaries.	

Nursing Diagnosis: Self Esteem, Low

Outcome Identification	Nursing Actions	Rationales	Evaluation
1. By [date], client verbalizes feelings of self worth.	1a. Encourage identification of 1 or 2 positive attributes.	1a. This activity promotes cognitive functioning that serves as a foundation for promotion of improved self-esteem based on factual information.	*Goal met:* Client verbalizes at least one positive quality. Client presents self in positive manner (e.g., groomed).
	1b. Provide positive age-appropriate realistic experiences.	1b. This activity provides here-and-now experience that promotes future healthy behavior.	
	1c. Provide constructive feedback regarding accomplishments.	1c. Praise and honest feedback from a trusted model enhance formation of a healthier self-concept.	
2. By [date], client interacts with others assertively.	2. Reinforce adaptive behaviors.	2. Reinforcement in the form of praise and acknowledgment help enhance positive self-esteem.	

(continues)

Nursing Diagnosis: Impaired Social Interaction
related to personal inadequacy as evidenced by behaviors that cause anger in others, low self-esteem, or poor social skills

Outcome Identification	Nursing Actions	Rationales	Evaluation
1. Form nurse-client relationship	1a. Approach client in accepting manner.	1a. A nonjudgmental approach is a necessary prerequisite for relationship development. It paves the way for the client to lay aside hesitancy to be open in sharing thoughts and feelings.	*Goal met:* Client is able to interact appropriately with others. Acting-out behaviors decrease. Client receptive to limit setting and is less demanding. Client actively participates.
	1b. Use active listening.	1b. Active listening demonstrates to the client that she is being heard because the nurse repeats the client's statements or pays very close attention.	
2. By [date], client will recognize that this behavior impacts relationships.	2. Develop and maintain realistic/consistent limit setting.	2. Clients who are needy, dependent, testy, or manipulative have weak or poorly-defined boundaries and benefit best in a therapeutic setting that maintains clear and understandable boundaries.	
3. By [date], client will be able to control impulses to meet immediate gratification needs.	3a. Confront maladaptive responses.	3a. Gentle confrontation offers the client an opportunity to clarify appropriate expectation and establish a stronger sense of boundaries.	
	3b. Actively involve client in treatment.	3b. Clients who are involved in their treatment program are assisted in establishing greater independence of thought and decision making that will ultimately help them become more independent in their overall functioning.	

(continues)

Nursing Care Plan 15–1 *(continued)*

Nursing Diagnosis: Impaired Social Interactions
related to anxiety as evidenced by dependent behaviors

Outcome Identification	Nursing Actions	Rationales	Evaluation
1. By [date], client will verbalize needs directly.	1. Develop environment that fosters trust.	1. Trust is best established when others are honest, consistent, reliable, and dependable.	*Goal met:* Client asks for assistance. Client adheres to treatment goals. Client is able to make simple decisions.
2. By [date], client will assume responsibility for problem solving.	2a. Maintain consistent limit setting.	2a. Limit setting is essential for clients whose anxiety prevents them from setting their own limits and establishing their own appropriate boundaries.	
	2b. Offer alternatives/ options to present stressors.	2b. Alternatives and options allow clients to decide and choose what makes them comfortable thus promoting growth toward a more independent level of functioning.	
	2c. Encourage client to assess behaviors.	2c. Personal assessment of own behaviors by clients aids them in the cognitive activity required for looking at self and changing.	

time the client has experienced any success or partnership in any endeavor, and it needs to be recognized as an accomplishment for the client.

SUMMARY

◆ Personality development is a complex process involving innate neurobiological, genetic, psychological, and sociological factors. Numerous theories abound about the influence of early caregivers on the developing personality.

◆ Maladaptation appears in many forms, and it is imperative that all nurses have an understanding about adaptive and maladaptive relationship styles, both in themselves and in others. Therapeutic nurse-client relationships can be effective in developing trust and providing an opportunity for intervening in maladaptive behavioral patterns.

◆ Personality disorders represent a continuum of maladaptive coping patterns and are currently organized into three clusters centering on certain pattern types.

◆ Overall, the personality disorders are characterized by inflexible, compulsive responses that are specific to the conditions involved. Within these behavioral clusters are generalized distress, rejection issues, restricted expression, insecure attachment, conduct problems, intimacy problems, social impairment, and cognitive distortion.

◆ Nurses are challenged to use the nursing process to assess client experience of chronic distress, fragmented ego functioning, and impaired social skills. Clients with a personality disorder often experience an overlay of other psychiatric problems and may present with a complexity of problems.

◆ These clients present a challenge to the nurses because they may take a significant amount of powerful and potentially toxic medications and place themselves in situations taut with frustration, tension, manipulation, rejection, and disparagement.

◆ Nurses need to maintain their sense of adequacy and self-esteem by recognizing that these behaviors are representative of client illness and not aimed at personal destruction of the nurse. When the nurse is able to grasp this concept, it becomes easier to be nonjudgmental and caring enough to minimize the overwhelming distress these clients experience. Mastery of feeling and response in the nurse can set the stage for the modeling of adaptive behavior that reflects clear boundaries and health-promoting activities between nurse and client.

SUGGESTIONS FOR CLINICAL CONFERENCES

1. Role-play countertransference reactions such as malice, hate, and anger, and examine the feelings engendered by the exercise.

2. Discuss adaptive and maladaptive behaviors using the nursing process.

3. Analyze developmental issues associated with a client's present behaviors.

4. Compare major concepts of personality theories and apply them to several case histories.

5. Role-play a situation where boundaries between nurse and client are not maintained, and demonstrate the correct way to manage the same event.

Conference I

For an individual or group assignment:

1. Identify one of the clients on the assigned unit in whom there are obvious clinical signs of a personality disorder.

2. Describe the classical symptoms observed and cite rationale for determining this as opposed to selecting an alternative personality disorder. Discuss the preferred plan of care, specific areas in which caution is necessary, and rationale for the decisions made.

Conference II

1. Select a client with obvious signs of obsessive-compulsive disorder and describe the symptoms.

2. Discuss the etiology for this condition and describe the treatment plan, including all aspects of nursing management. Discuss the potential outcomes for the client.

Conference III

1. Discuss the characteristics of a client with antisocial disorder. Consider the various etiological theories that might apply to the selected client's situation. List strengths and weaknesses.

2. Consider ultimate potential outcomes for the client and state rationale for the beliefs presented.

Conference IV

1. Select one of the suggested readings at the end of the chapter and present opinions relative to the most likely personality disorder presented in the book. Discuss etiology of the condition based on history of the individual about whom the book is written.

STUDY QUESTIONS

1. John Bowlby is a theorist concerned with attachment behavior. Attachment theory refers to the:
   a. type of love relationship that occurs between two adults
   b. attachment that exists between mother and infant immediately after birth
   c. ability to engage in relationships throughout life based on early life experiences
   d. ability of toddlers to ambulate early in the presence of caregivers

2. You are a nurse working in the residential treatment center where most of the clients are youngsters who have experienced poor home conditions, and many of the female clients are diagnosed as borderline. You realize that you will encounter the characteristic of "splitting." This means that:
   a. a person cannot leave or exist apart from the primary object
   b. one idealizes another and tends to see them as "all good" or "all bad"
   c. a person loves another so much that he or she refuses to let others participate with the beloved person
   d. a person expects persons with authority to make decisions for him

3. You are requested to do a clinical presentation on Cluster B personality disorders. You know that the characteristics found in Cluster B are:
   a. withdrawal and odd and eccentric behavior
   b. attention-seeking and erratic behavior
   c. fear and anxiety
   d. a combination of features that imply ambivalence

4. As a registered nurse working on a psychiatric-mental health unit, you realize that the outstanding features of personality disorder are:
   a. related to thinking problems and inability to function well at intellectual pursuits
   b. highlighted by failure to maintain mood stability
   c. dysfunctional in their failure to relate to others
   d. behavioral patterns that are maladaptive

5. You are a nurse assigned to a unit where the majority of clients have a personality disorder. You would expect that treatment of personality disorders is:
   a. likely to be successful because of the responsiveness to psychotropic medications
   b. likely to be resistant because of the inflexibility of behavioral patterns
   c. highly responsive because of the desire to relate to others and therefore respond to psychotherapy
   d. successful about 75 percent of the time because most personality disorders have a clear-cut etiological basis

6. The eleventh *DSM-IV-TR* category, personality disorder NOS, refers to conditions such as:
   a. schizophreniform and paranoid personality disorders
   b. hypochondriacal and multiple personality disorders
   c. affective and thinking disorders
   d. passive-aggressive and masochistic disorders

7. Libidinal object constancy refers to:
   a. maintaining the memory of the primary caregiver when that individual is not present
   b. maintaining the memory of the beloved object only when that person is present
   c. idealizing the primary object and refusing to move past the stage when it peaks
   d. desiring to remain with the primary object long after the time when it is appropriate to separate

8. A client is described as ego syntonic. This means that he is:
   a. comfortable with symptoms that cause discomfort in others
   b. uncomfortable with symptoms that make others uncomfortable, almost as if the two were one person
   c. uncomfortable all the time
   d. uncomfortable with one's own mental state

9. Christine demonstrates a behavior common to borderline clients, and there tends to be a great deal of discussion about her in staff conferences with much disagreement concerning her. The staff seem to take sides for or against her requests because she shows favoritism to certain staff and strong dislike for others. The behavior that creates this condition is known as:
   a. conditioning
   b. selective manipulation
   c. splitting
   d. reality testing

10. The nurse is caring for a client with borderline personality disorder. The client asks the nurse to allow her to participate in an activity that will interfere with her current treatment plan. When the nurse says no to this request, the client responds by saying, "You are not like the other nurses because they let me do what I want. Why are you so mean to me?" What is the most appropriate response?
    a. "I don't care what the other nurses let you do. You understand the rules."
    b. "I recognize you are unhappy about my decision to ask you to follow the treatment plan."
    c. "Every time you agree to participate in treatment you want to break the rules. This is not helpful to you."
    d. "I am really a nice person, but I can't change your treatment plan because you agreed to follow it."

11. The nurse is caring for a client with a personality disorder. The client complains that the nurse never tells personal things about herself, yet she is always asking the client personal questions. She states that she would really like to get to know the nurse better because she is so easy to talk to. What is the least appropriate response to this client?
    a. "I like you too and also feel we have a special relationship, but it is limited to me working with you in the clinic."
    b. "I am glad to know it's easy to talk to me, but it is important for us to focus on helping you get through this crisis."
    c. "Once you get through the crisis and you are no longer in the clinic maybe we can be friends."
    d. "Let's focus on you. What does this have to do with me?"

12. The nurse is planning care for a client with schizotypal personality disorder. Which one of the following is the nurse *least* likely to observe?
    a. Appropriate affect and calm demeanor
    b. Odd and eccentric behavior
    c. Socially aloof and withdrawn
    d. Suspiciousness and distrust

13. A 9-year-old child is brought to the pediatric psychiatric clinic with his mother. During the assessment the nurse observes the youth being easily upset, refusing to follow instructions, and his mother has difficulty getting him to obey directions. His mother also reports he has few friends and is doing poorly in school. What is the best explanation for his behavior?
    a. The mother has poor parenting skills
    b. The child has a conduct disorder
    c. The child has oppositional defiant disorder
    d. The child is just acting like a normal 9-year-old

14. A client with antisocial personality uses manipulation to gain access to a vending area close to the entrance of the hospital, where he attempts to leave the hospital grounds. Which is the best nursing intervention for manipulative behavior?
    a. Place client in restraints for illegal behaviors
    b. Help the client identify patterns of manipulative behavior and the consequences as determined by the treatment team
    c. Deal with each incident of client manipulation on an individualized basis, dependent on the context of the situation and the nurse involved
    d. Restrict the client from all unit activities, to provide time for reflection on social behavior

15. Which statement would be least expected when the nurse assesses a client with borderline personality disorder?
    a. "I was totally wrong and am willing to take full responsibility for my actions."
    b. "John is responsible for what I did. I trusted him and he let me down."
    c. "If you hadn't rushed me I would have been able to make the right decision."
    d. "Why does everyone always blame me for things out of my control?"

16. Key interventions for a client with antisocial personality disorder include all but which one of the following?
    a. Assisting him to identify and clarify his feelings
    b. Changing staff assigned to a client at his request
    c. Making expectations about his behavior clear as well as consequences for same
    d. Setting firm limits with clear consequences

17. The nurse would formulate which of the following outcome criteria for a client with borderline personality disorder? The client
    a. displays anger frequently
    b. acts out her neediness
    c. experiences troubling thoughts without using self-injurious behaviors
    d. idolizes her nurse

RESOURCES

Please note that because Internet resources are of a time-sensitive nature and URL addresses may change or be deleted, searches should also be conducted by association or topic.

Internet Resources

Contact various Internet sources devoted to mental health to gain the latest information regarding research in the area of personality disorders. Use these Internet sites to strengthen clinical conference discussions and papers that are required.

http://www.intelihea...m/IH/ihtIH/WSIHW)))/8271/8885.html

http://www.toad.net/~arcturus/dd/schtypal.htm

http://web4.infotrac.galegroup.com/itw/i...89&dyn=7!xrn_1_0_A54823489?sw_aep=miller

http://www.ncbi.nlm.nih.gov/entrez/query.fcgi?CMD=Display&DB=PubMed

http://www.mentalhealth.com/dis1/p21-pe03.html

http://www.iop.kcl.ac.uk/main/ResRep/Antisoc.htm

http://www.mhsanctuary.com/BPDr/index.htm

http://mentalhelp.net/guide/person.htm

http://mentalhelp.net/disorders/sx13t.htm

http://www.suite101.com/welcome.cfm/npd

http://www.healthgate.com/cgi-bin/q-format.cgi

Other Resources

American Psychiatric Nurses Association
    1200 19th St. NW, Suite 300
    Washington, DC 20036-2422
    (202) 857-1133
International Society for Psychiatric-Mental
        Health Nurses (ISPN)
    1211 Locust Street
    Philadelphia, PA 19107

(215) 545-2843
Fax (215) 545-8107
E-mail: ispn@nursecominc.com

REFERENCES

Allen, D. M., & Whitson, S., (2004). Avoiding patient distortions in psychotherapy with borderline personality disorder patients. *Journal of Contemporary Psychotherapy, 34*(3), 211–229.

Allnutt, B. L. (1979). The motherless child. In J. D. Noshpitz (Ed.), *Basic handbook of child psychiatry* (pp. 373–378). New York: Basic Books.

American Psychiatric Association (APA). (2000). *Diagnostic and statistical manual of mental disorders* (4th edition, Text Revision) (*DSM-IV-TR*). Washington, DC: Author.

Antai-Otong, D. (2004). *Psychiatric emergencies: How to accurately assess and manage the patient in crisis.* Eau Claire, WI: Professional Educational Systems, Inc.

Baker, L. A., Jacobson, K. C., Raine, A., Lozano, D. I., & Bezdjian, S. (2007). Genetic and environmental bases of childhood antisocial behavior: A multi-informant twin study. *Journal of Abnormal Psychology, 116,* 219–235.

Becker, D. F., Grilo, C. M., Anez, L. M., Paris, M., & McGlashan, T. H. (2005). Discriminant efficiency of antisocial and borderline personality disorder criteria in Hispanic men with substance use disorders. *Comprehensive Psychiatry, 46,* 140–146.

Benazzi, B. (2006). Borderline personality-bipolar spectrum relationship. *Progress in Neuropsychopharmacology Biological Psychiatry, 30,* 68–74.

Bender, D. S. (2005). The therapeutic alliance in the treatment of personality disorders. *Journal of Psychiatric Practice, 11,* 73–87.

Berezin, M. A., Liptzin, B., & Salzman, C. (1988). The elderly person. In A. Nicholi (Ed.), *The new Harvard guide to psychiatry* (pp. 665–680). Cambridge, MA: Belknap Press.

Berlin, H. A., Rolls, E. T., & Iversen, S. D. (2005). Borderline personality disorder, impulsivity, and the orbitofrontal cortex. *American Journal of Psychiatry, 162,* 2360–2370.

Biederman, J., Spencer, T. J., Newcorn, J. H., Gao, H., Milton, D. R., Feldman, P. D., et al. (2007). Effect of comorbid symptoms of oppositional defiant disorder on responses to atomoxetine in children with ADHD: A meta-analysis of controlled clinical trial data. *Psychopharmacology (Berlin), 190,* 31–41.

Black, D. W., Jr., (with Larson, C. L.). (1999). *Bad boys, bad men: Confronting antisocial personality disorder.* New York: Oxford University Press.

Blashfield, R. C., & McElroy, R. A. (1987). The 1985 journal literature on the personality disorders (review). *Comprehensive Psychiatry, 28*(6), 536–546.

Blashfield, R. K., & Intoccia, V. (2000). Growth of the literature on the topic of personality disorders. *American Journal of Psychiatry, 157*(3), 472–473.

Bowlby, J. (1951). *Maternal care and maternal health.* (Monograph Series, No. 2). Geneva, Switzerland: World Health Organization.

Bowlby, J. (1969). *Attachment and loss. Volume I: Attachment.* New York: Basic Books.

Bowlby, J. (1981). *Attachment and loss. Vol. 3: Loss, sadness and depression.* Hammondsworth, England: Penguin.

Cashdan, S. (1988). *Object relations therapy.* New York: W. W. Norton.

Clarkin, J. F., Marziali, E., & Munroe-Blum, H. (1992). *Borderline personality disorder: Clinical and empirical perspectives.* New York: The Guilford Press.

Cleckley, H. (1964). *The mask of insanity* (4th ed.). St. Louis: C. V. Mosby.

Deutsch, H. (1942). Some forms of emotional disturbances and their relationship to schizophrenia. *Psychoanalysis, 11,* 301–321.

Dolan, M., & Fullam, R. (2006). Face affect recognition deficits in personality-disordered offenders: Association with psychopathy. *Psychological Medicine, 36,* 1563–1569.

Duman, S., & Margolin, G. (2007). Parents' aggressive influences and children's aggressive problem solutions with peers. *Journal of Clinical Child and Adolescent Psychology, 36,* 42–55.

Edwards, R. T., Céilleachair, A., Bywater, T., Hughes, D. A., & Hutchings, J. (2007). Parenting programme for parents of children at risk of developing conduct disorder: Cost effectiveness analysis. *British Medical Journal, 334,* 682. Available online at http://www.bmj.com/cgi/reprint/334/7595/682

Egan, J. (1986). Etiology and treatment of borderline personality disorder in adolescents. *Hospital and Community Psychiatry, 37*(6), 613–618.

Eisen, J. L., Coles, M. E., Shea, M. T., Pagano, M. E., Stout, R. L., Yen, S., et al. (2006). Clarifying the convergence between obsessive-compulsive personality disorder criteria and obsessive compulsive disorder. *Journal of Personality Disorders, 20,* 294–305.

Emde, R. N., & Robinson, J. (1979). The first two months: Recent research in developmental psychobiology and the changing view of the newborn. In J. D. Noshpitz (Ed.), *Basic handbook of child psychiatry* (pp. 72–125). New York: Basic Books.

Erikson, E. (1963). *Childhood and society* (2nd ed.). New York: W. W. Norton.

Favazza, A., & Rosenthal, R. J. (1990). Varieties of pathological self-mutilation. *Behavioral Neurology, 3,* 77–85.

Favazza, A., & Rosenthal, R. J. (1993). Diagnostic issues in self-mutilation. *Hospital and Community Psychiatry, 44*(2), 134–140.

Fineberg, N. A., Sharma, P., Sivakumaran, T., Sahakian, B., & Chamberlain, S. (2007). Does obsessive-compulsive personality disorder belong within the obsessive-compulsive spectrum? *CNS Spectrum, 12,* 467–482.

Foote, B., Smolin, Y., Kaplan, M., Legatt, M. E., & Lipschitz, D. (2006). Prevalence of dissociative disorders in psychiatric outpatients. American *Journal of Psychiatry, 163,* 623–629.

Fossati, A., Barrat, E. S., Borroni, S., Villa, D., Grazioli, F., & Maffei, C. (2007). Impulsivity, aggressiveness, and DSM-IV personality disorders. *Psychiatry Research, 149,* 157–167.

Foster, E. M., Jones, D., & Conduct Problems Prevention Research Group. (2006). Can a costly intervention be cost-effective? An analysis of violence prevention. *Archives of General Psychiatry, 63,* 1284–1291.

Freeman, P. S., & Gunderson, J. G. (1989). Treatment of personality disorders. *Psychiatric Annals, 19*(3), 147–153.

Freud, S. (1957). On narcissism: An introduction. In J. Strachey (Ed. and Trans.), *The standard edition of the complete psychological works of Sigmund Freud* (Vol. 19, pp. 69–102). London: Hogarth Press. (Original work published 1923)

Freud, S. (1961). *Beyond the pleasure principle.* New York: Norton.

Fuertes, M., Santos, P. L., Beeghly, M., & Tronick, E. (2006). More than maternal sensitivity shapes attachment: Infant coping and temperament. *Annals of the New York Academy of Sciences, 1094,* 292–296.

Goldstein, R. B., Grant, B. F., Huang, B., Smith, S. M., Stinson, F. S., Dawson, D. A., et al. (2006). Lack of remorse in antisocial personality disorder: Sociodemographic correlates, symptomatic presentation, and comorbidity with Axis I and Axis II disorders in the National Epidemiologic Survey on Alcohol and Related Conditions. *Comprehensive Psychiatry, 47,* 289–297.

Greenberg, J. R., & Mitchell, S. A. (1983). *Object relations in psychoanalytic theory.* New York: Basic Books.

Grinker, R., Werber, B., & Drye, R. (1968). *The borderline syndrome.* New York: Basic Books.

Groholt, B., Ekeberg, O., & Haldorsen, T. (2006). Adolescent suicide attempters: What predicts future suicidal acts? *Suicide and Life Threatening Behavior, 36,* 638–650.

Grossmann, T., & Johnson, M. H. (2007). The development of the social brain in human infancy. European *Journal of Neuroscience, 25,* 909–919.

Gunderson, J. G. (1988). Personality disorders. In A. M. Nicholi (Ed.), *The new Harvard Press guide to psychiatry* (pp. 337–357). Cambridge, MA: Harvard Press.

Gunderson, J. G., Daversa, M. T., Grilo, C. M., McGlashan, T. H., Zanarini, M. C., Shea, M. T., et al. (2006). Predictors of 2-year outcome for patients with borderline personality disorder. *American Journal of Psychiatry, 163,* 822–826.

Gutheil, T. G., & Gabbard, G. O. (1993). The concept of boundaries in clinical practice: Theoretical and risk-management dimensions. *American Journal of Psychiatry, 15*(2), 188–196.

Hartmann, H. (1958). *Ego psychology and problem of adaptation* (D. Rapaport, Trans.). New York: International Universities Press.

Haslam, N., Reichert, T., & Fiske, A. P., (2002). Aberrant social relations in the personality disorders. *Psychology and Psychotherapy: Theory, Research and Practice, 75*(1), 19–31.

Hayden, A., Bhatt, R. S., Reed, A., Corbly, C. R., & Joseph, J. E. (2007). The development of expert face processing: Are infants sensitive to normal differences in second-order relational information? *Journal of Experimental Child Psychology, 97,* 85–98.

Hirschfield, R. M. A. (1986). Personality disorders. In A. J. Franced & R. D. Hales (Eds.), *American Psychiatric Association annual review* (Vol. 5, pp. 233–239), Washington, DC: American Psychiatric Press.

Howard, P. J. (2000). *The owner's manual for the brain: Everyday applications from mind-brain research,* (2nd ed.). Austin: Bard Press.

Johnson, M., & Silver, S. (1988). Conflicts in the inpatient treatment of the borderline patient. *Archives of Psychiatric Nursing, 2*(5), 312–318.

Keilp, J. G., Gorlyn, M., Oquendo, M. A., Brodsky, B., Ellis, S. P., Stanley, B., et al. (2006). Aggressiveness, not impulsiveness or hostility, distinguishes suicide attempters with major depression. *Psychological Medicine, 36,* 1779–1788.

Kernberg, O. (1975). *Borderline conditions and pathological narcissism.* New York: Jason Aronson.

Kernberg, O. (1976). *Object relations theory and clinical psychoanalysis.* New York: Jacob Aronson.

Kernberg, O. (1984). *Severe personality disorders.* New Haven, CT: Yale University Press.

Kim, S. J., Kim, Y. S., Kim, C. H., & Lee, H. S. (2006). Lack of association between polymorphisms of the dopamine receptor D4 and dopamine transporter genes and personality traits in a Korean population. *Yonsei Medical Journal, 47,* 787–792.

Kim-Cohen, J., Caspi, A., Taylor, A., Williams, B., Newcombe, R., Craig, I. W., et al. (2006). MAOA, maltreatment, and gene-environment interaction predicting children's mental health: New evidence and a meta-analysis. *Molecular Psychiatry, 11,* 903–913.

Klein, M. (1977). Some theoretical considerations regarding the emotional life of the infant. In M. Klein (Ed.), *Envy and gratitude and other works: 1946–1963* (Vol. 4). New York: Delacorte Press.

Koerner, K., & Linehan, M. M. (2000). Research on dialectical behavior therapy for patients with borderline personality disorder. *Psychiatric Clinics of North America, 23,* 151–167.

Kohut, H. (1971). *The analysis of self.* New York: International Universities Press.

Kohut, H. (1977). *The restoration of self.* New York: International Universities Press.

Koo, M. S., Levitt, J. J., McCarley, K. W., Seidman, L. J., Dickey, C. C., Niznikiewicz, M. A., et al. (2006). Reduction of caudate nucleus volumes in neuroleptic-naïve female subjects with schizotypal personality disorder. *Biological Psychiatry, 60,* 40–48.

Krysinska, K., Heller, T. S., & De Leo, D. (2006). Suicide and deliberate self-harm in personality disorders. *Current Opinion in Psychiatry, 19,* 95–101.

Lenzenweger, M. F., Lane, M. C., Loranger, A. W., & Kessler, R. C. (2007). DSM-IV Personality Disorders in the National Comorbidity Survey Replication. *Biological Psychiatry.* [Epub ahead of print]

Lenzenweger, M. F., & O'Driscoll, G. A. (2006). Smooth pursuit eye movement and schizotypy in the community. *Abnormal Psychology, 115,* 779–786.

Levy, K. N., Meehan, K. B., Kelly, K. M., Reynoso, J. S., Weber, M., Clarkin, J. F., et al. (2006). Change in attachment patterns and reflective function in a randomized control trial of transference-focused psychotherapy for borderline personality disorder. *Journal of Consulting and Clinical Psychology, 74,* 1027–1940.

Linehan, M. M. (1987). Dialectical behavioral therapy: A cognitive approach to parasuicide. *Journal of Personality Disorders, 1,* 328–333.

Linehan, M. M. (1993). *Cognitive-behavioral therapy of borderline personality disorder.* New York: Guilford.

Livesley, W. J. (2000). A practical approach to the treatment of patients with borderline personality disorder. *Psychiatric Clinics of North America, 23,* 211–232.

Mahler, M. (1952). On child psychosis and schizophrenia: Autistic and symbiotic psychosis. *Psychoanalytic Study of the Child, 7,* 206–305.

Mahler, M. (1965a). On early infantile psychosis: The symbiotic and autistic syndromes. *Journal of the Academy of Child Psychiatry, 4,* 554–568.

Mahler, M. (1965b). On the significance of the normal separation-individuation phase: With reference to research in symbiotic child psychosis. In M. Shur (Ed.), *Drives, affects, behaviors* (Vol. 2, pp. 161–169). New York: International Universities Press.

March, J. S., Frances, A., Carpenter, D., & Kahn, D. A. (1997). The expert consensus guideline series: Treatment of obsessive-compulsive disorder. *Journal of Clinical Psychiatry, 58*(Suppl. 4), 1–72.

Marohn, R. C., (1992). Management of the assaultive adolescent. *Hospital and Community Psychiatry, 43*(6), 622–624.

Masterson, J. F. (2000). *Psychotherapy disorders: A new look at the developmental self and object relations approach.* Phoenix, AZ: Tucker.

Meissner, W. W. (1988). The psychotherapies: Individual, family and group. In A. Nicholi (Ed.), *The new Harvard guide to psychiatry* (pp. 449–480). Cambridge, MA: Belknap Press.

Metcalf, D. R. (1979). Organizers of the psyche and EEG development: Birth through adolescence. In J. D. Noshpitz (Ed.), *Basic handbook of child psychiatry* (pp. 63–71). New York: Basic Books.

Miller, A. (1981). *Prisoners of childhood: How narcissistic parents form and deform the emotional lives of their gifted children.* New York: Basic Books, Inc.

Miller, R. (1979). Development from one to two years: Language acquisition. In J. D. Nospitz (Ed.), *Basic handbook of child psychiatry* (pp. 127–144). New York: Basic Books.

Millon, T. (2000). *Personality disorders in modern life.* New York: John Wiley & Sons.

Mishne, J. M. (1986). *Clinical work with adolescents.* New York: Free Press.

Mittal, V. A., Dhruv, S., Tessner, K. D., Walder, D. J., & Walker, E. F. (2007). The relations among putative biorisk markers in schizotypal adolescents: Minor physical anomalies, movement abnormalities, and salivary cortisol. *Biological Psychiatry, 61,* 1179–1186.

Myers, I., & McCaulley, M. (1985). *Manual: A guide to the development and use of the Myers-Briggs Type Indicator.* Palo Alto, CA: Consulting Psychologists Press.

Nehls, N. (1992). Group therapy for people with borderline personality disorder: Interventions associated with positive outcomes. *Issues in Mental Health Nursing, 13*(3), 255–269.

New, A. S., Hazlett, E. A., Buchsbaum, M. S., Goodman, M., Mitelman, S. A., Newmark, R., et al. (2007). Amygdala-prefrontal disconnection in borderline personality disorder. *Neuropsychopharmacology, 32,* 1629–1640.

Nock, M. K., Kazdin, A. E., Hiripi, E., & Kessler, R. C. (2006). Prevalence, subtypes, and correlates of DSM-IV conduct disorder in the National Comorbidity Survey Replication. *Psychological Medicine, 36,* 699–710.

Phillips, K. A., & Gunderson, J. G. (1999). Personality disorders. In R. E. Hales, S. C. Yodofsky, & J. A. Talbott (Eds.), *Textbook of psychiatry* (3rd ed., pp. 795–823). Washington, DC: American Psychiatric Press.

Provence, S. (1979). Development from six to twelve months. In J. D. Noshpitz (Ed.), *Basic handbook of child psychiatry* (pp. 113–117). New York: Basic Books.

Reich, W. (1949). *Character analysis.* New York: Noonday Press.

Reichborn-Kjennerud, T., Czajkowski, N., Neale, M. C., Ørstavik, R. E., Torgersen, A., Tambs, K., et al. (2007). Genetic and environmental influences on dimensional representations of *DSM-IV* cluster C personality disorders: A population-based multivariate twin study. *Psychological Medicine, 37,* 645–653.

Rothstein, A. (1991). An exploration of the diagnostic term *narcissistic person.* In M. R. F. Kets de Vries & S. Perzow (Eds.), *Handbook of character studies: Psychosocial explorations* (pp. 303–318). Madison, CT: International Universities Press.

Rubinstein, M., Yeager, C. A., Goodstein, C., & Lewis, D. O. (1993). Sexually assaultive male juveniles: A follow-up study. *American Journal of Psychiatry, 150*(2), 262–265.

Ruchsow, M., Walter, H., Buchheim, A., Martius, P., Spitzer, H., Kachele, H., et al. (2006). Electrophysiological correlates of error processing in borderline personality disorder. *Biological Psychiatry, 72,* 133–140.

Shedler, J., & Westen, D. (2004). Refining personality disorder diagnosis: Integrating science and practice. *American Journal of Psychiatry, 161,* 1350–1365.

Shengold, L. (1999). *Soul murder revisited.* New Haven: Yale University Press.

Soloff, P. H. (1998). Algorithms for pharmacological treatment of personality dimensions: Symptom specific treatments for cognitive-perceptual, affective, and impulsive-behavioral dysregulation. *Bulletin of Menniger Clinic, 62*(2), 195–214.

Soloff, P. H. (2000). Psychopharmacology of borderline personality disorder. *Psychiatric Clinics of North America, 23,* 169–192.

Sommer, M., Hajak, G., Döhnel, K., Schwerdtner, J., Meinhardt, J., & Müller, J. L. (2006). Integration of emotion and cognition in patients with psychopathy. *Progress in Brain Research, 156,* 457–466.

Steiner, H., Remsing, L., & Workgroup on Quality Issues. (2007). Practice parameter for the assessment and treatment of children and adolescents with oppositional defiant disorder. *Journal of the American Academy of Child and Adolescent Psychiatry, 46,* 126–141.

Stone, M. H. (1990). *Long-term follow-up of borderline patients: The fate of borderlines.* New York: Guilford.

Swenson, C. R., Torrey, W. C., & Koerner, K. (2002). Implementing dialectical behavior therapy. *Psychiatric Services, 53,* 171–178.

Turgay, A. (2005). Treatment of comorbidity in conduct disorder with attention-deficit hyperactivity disorder (ADHD). *Essential Psychopharmacology, 6,* 277–290.

Tuvblad, C., Eley, T. C., & Lichtenstein, P. (2005). The development of antisocial behaviour from childhood to adolescence. A longitudinal twin study. *European Child and Adolescent Psychiatry, 14,* 216–225.

van Goozen, S. H., & Fairchild, G. (2006). Neuroendocrine and neurotransmitter correlates in children with antisocial behavior. *Hormones and Behavior, 50,* 647–654.

van Lier, P. A., Wanner, B., & Vitaro, F. (2007). Onset of antisocial behavior, affiliation with deviant friends, and childhood maladjustment: A test of the childhood- and adolescent-onset models. *Developmental Psychology, 19,* 167–185.

Watson, S., Chilton, R., Fairchild, H., & Whewell, P. (2006). Association between childhood trauma and dissociation among patients with borderline personality disorder. *Australia and New Zealand Journal of Psychiatry, 40,* 478–481.

Webb, S. J., Long, J. D., & Nelson, C. A. (2005). A longitudinal investigation of visual event-related potentials in the first year of life. *Developmental Science,* 8, 605–616.

Westen, D., Shedler, J., & Bradley, R. (2006). A prototype approach to personality disorder diagnosis. *American Journal of Psychiatry, 163,* 846–856.

Whiting, S. A. (1994). A delphi study of the defining characteristics of interdependence and dysfunctional independence. *Issues in Mental Health Nursing, 13*(1), 37–47.

Whiting, S. A., (1997). Development of the person. In B. S. Johnson (ed.). *Psychiatric-mental health nursing: Adaptation and growth.* (4th ed.), 357–373. Philadelphia: Lippincott.

Widiger, T. A. (1999). Millon's dimensional polarities. *Journal of Personality Assessment, 72*(3), 365–389.

Widiger, T. A. (2003). Personality disorder and axis I psychopathology: The problematic boundary of axis I and axis II. *Journal of Personality Disorders, 17*(2), 90–108.

Zimmerman, M., Rothschild, L., Chelminski, I. (2005). The prevalence of *DSM-IV* personality disorders in psychiatric outpatients. *American Journal of Psychiatry, 162,* 1911–1918.

SUGGESTED READINGS

Evans, D. L., Foa, E. B., Gur, R. E., Hendin, H., O'Brien, C. P., & Seligman, M. E. P. (2005). *Treating and preventing adolescent mental health disorders.* New York: Oxford University Press.

McCourt, F. (1999). *'Tis: A memoir.* New York: Scribner.

Morton, A. (1999). *Monica's story.* New York: St. Martin's Press.

Peck, M. S. (1983). *People of the lie: The hope for healing human evil.* New York: Simon & Schuster.

Redl, F., & Wineman, D. (1951). *Children who hate.* Glencoe, IL: Free Press.

Stone, M. (1993). *Abnormalities of personality: Within and beyond the realm of treatment.* New York: W. W. Norton.

Stowers, C. (1995). *Sins of the son.* New York: St. Martin's Press.

Toobin, J. (1996). *The run of his life: The people v. O. J. Simpson.* New York: Random House.

Wallace, M. (1986). *The silent twins.* New York: Prentice Hall Press.

Webster-Stratton, C., & Hancock, L. (1998). Training for parents of young children with conduct problems: Content, methods, and therapeutic processes. In C. E. Schaefer & J. M. Briesmeister (Eds.), *Handbook of parent training.* New York: John Wiley.

Weinstein, D. D., Diforio, D., Schiffman, J., Walker, E., & Bonstall, R. (1999). Minor physical anomalies, dermatoglyphic asymmetries, and cortisol levels in adolescents with schizotypal personality disorder. *American Journal of Psychiatry, 156,* 617–623.

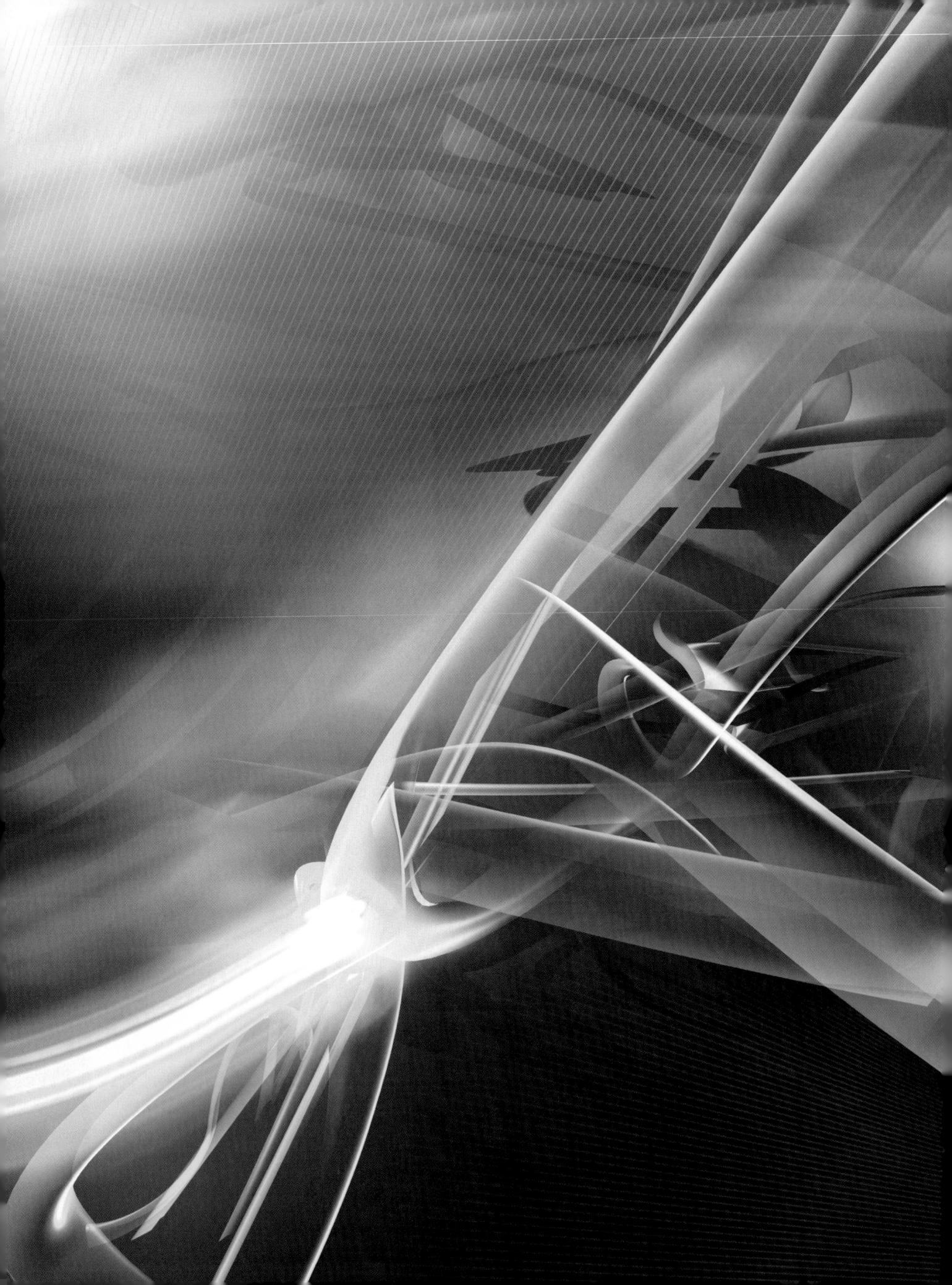

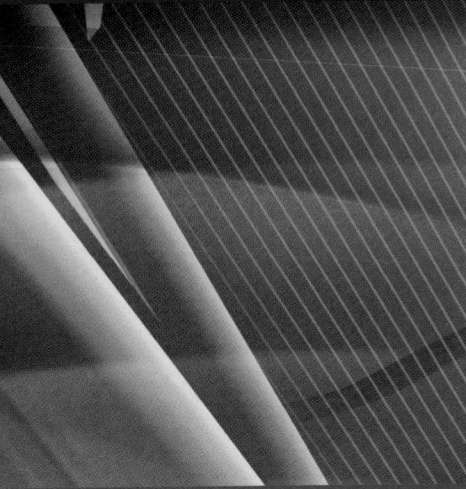

CHAPTER 16

The Client with Delirium, Dementia, Amnestic, and Other Cognitive Disorders

Jacqueline M. Stolley, PhD, RN, CS
Tracy Poelvoorde, MS, RN

KEY TERMS

Acute Confusion: Refers to the cognitive phenomenon of delirium (rapid onset of a disturbance in consciousness and cognition) before the actual diagnosis is made.

Alzheimer's Disease (AD): A condition characterized by progressive loss of memory, intellect, language, judgment, and impulse control. Neurofibrillary tangle and neuritic plaques are found in the cerebral cortex, particularly the hippocampus.

Anomia: Inability to recall or recognize names of objects.

Aphasia: Loss of power of expression by speech, writing, or signs of loss of comprehension of spoken or written language owing to brain injury or pathology.

Apraxia: Loss of ability to carry out familiar, purposeful movements in the absence of paralysis or other motor or sensory impairments, especially the inability to make proper use of an object.

Asimultanagnosia: Inability to visually integrate the components of an ordinarily complex scene into a coherent whole.

Brain Lesion: A condition in which an abnormality is noted in the brain such as a tumor or hematoma. A potentially reversible dementia.

Chorea: The ceaseless occurrence of a wide variety of rapid, jerky but well-coordinated movements performed involuntarily.

Choreiform: Resembling chorea.

Cognitive Disorders: Those conditions in which "the predominant disturbance is a clinically significant deficit in cognition or memory that represents a significant change from a previous level of functioning" (APA, 2000).

Creutzfeldt-Jakob Disease (CJD): A syndrome of motor, sensory, and mental disturbances. There is widespread degeneration and atrophy of the cerebral cortex, basal ganglia, and thalamus. Course of disease months to years.

Decerebrate: A sign characterized by adduction and extension of the arms, pronated wrists, and flexed fingers. The legs are stiffly extended, with plantar flexion of the feet. This sign indicates upper brain stem damage and usually heralds neurological deterioration.

Decorticate: A sign characterized by adduction and flexion of the arms, with wrists and fingers flexed on the chest. The legs are extended and internally rotated with plantar flexion of the feet. Most often, it results from cerebrovascular accident or head injury. It is a sign of corticospinal damage and carries a more favorable prognosis than decerebrate posture.

Delirium: A medical syndrome characterized by acute onset and impairment in cognition, perception, and behavior. Also known as acute confusion.

Dementia: A condition manifested in the insidious development of memory and intellectual deficits, disorientation, and decreased cognitive functioning.

Dysarthria: Imperfect articulation of speech caused by muscular weakness resulting from damage to the central or peripheral nervous system.

Executive Function: Ability to set a goal, make decisions, and implement appropriate activities toward meeting that goal.

Fetal Alcohol Syndrome (FAS): A pattern of birth defects, learning, and behavioral disabilities associated with exposure to alcohol during pregnancy.

Focal Neurological Signs: Specific signs of neurological impairment such as blurred vision, aphasia, and the like.

Korsakoff's Disease (KD): A psychosis that is usually based on chronic alcoholism, and which is accompanied by disturbance of orientation, susceptibility to external stimulation and suggestion, falsification of memory, and hallucinations.

Lewy Body: Proteinaceous structures composed of a central core with radiating filaments, located in the substantia nigra in Parkinson's disease and in the cortex in diffuse Lewy body disease.

Life Expectancy: Refers to the age at which an individual born into a particular cohort is expected to die.

Life Span: The maximum age that could be attained if an individual were able to avoid or be successfully treated for all illnesses and accidents.

Multi-infarct Dementia (MID): A probable irreversible dementia caused by many small strokes, or a large stroke.

Myoclonus: Shocklike contractions of a portion of a muscle, an entire muscle, or a group of muscles, restricted to one area of the body or appearing synchronously or asynchronously in several areas.

Neuritic Plaques: A patch or flat area of neurons.

Neurofibrillary Tangles: Tangles of the neurofibril, the delicate threads running in every direction through the cytoplasm of the body of a nerve and extending into the axon and the dendrites of the cell.

Normal Pressure Hydrocephalus (NPH): A condition in which the cerebral spinal fluid pressure reading is normal or high normal, but excessive fluid exists in the ventricles of the brain.

Parkinson's Disease: The chronic condition marked by rigidity, tremor with intention. Pathology in the substantia nigra.

Pick's Disease (PD): A rare, fatal degenerative disease of the nervous system, occurring mostly in middle-aged women. Characterized by signs of severe frontal or temporal lobe dysfunction. Overall symptomatology is very similar to Alzheimer's disease.

Potentially Reversible Dementia: A condition characterized by an acute onset, causing neurological symptoms and changes in level of consciousness. If treated in time, the condition may be reversed. See delirium.

Probable Irreversible Dementia: Progressive loss of intellectual functioning caused by permanent brain damage.

Visual Memory: Ability to remember what is seen.

COMPETENCIES

Upon completion of this chapter, the learner should be able to:

1. Identify causes and symptoms of the most prevalent cognitive disorders across the life span.

2. Differentiate between reversible and irreversible cognitive disorders.

3. List signs and symptoms for major cognitive disorders.

4. Develop a plan of care for the client with a reversible or irreversible dementia.

5. Recognize appropriate tests used to diagnose cognitive disorders.

6. Understand the appropriateness of medications to treat the symptoms of cognitive disorders.

CHAPTER OUTLINE

Cognitive Disorders across the Life Span

Development of the Brain

Child and Adolescent Development

Adult Development

Physiological Changes

Psychosocial Changes

Potentially Reversible Dementias

Delirium

Treatable Brain Lesions

Normal Pressure Hydrocephalus

Probable Irreversible Dementias

Mental Retardation

Fetal Alcohol Syndrome

The Epilepsies

Mild Cognitive Impairment

Alzheimer's Disease

Vascular Dementia

Cortical Degenerative Syndromes

Huntington's Disease

Creutzfeldt-Jacob Disease

Acquired Immune Deficiency Syndrome

Korsakoff's Disease or Alcohol Amnestic Disorder

Other Cognitive Disorders

Cognitive disorders are those conditions in which "the predominant disturbance is a clinically significant deficit in cognition or memory that represents a significant change from a previous level of functioning" (American Psychiatric Association [APA], 2000, p. 135). In the third revised edition of the *Diagnostic and Statistical Manual of Mental Disorders (DSM-III-R)*, the term "organic" was applied to many cognitive disorders in which psychological and behavioral abnormalities are "associated with transient or permanent dysfunction of the brain" (APA, 1987, p. 98). Organic mental disorders and syndromes are heterogeneous; therefore, no single description can characterize all of them. The different clinical presentations of organic mental disorders reflected differences in the localization, mode of onset, progression, duration, and nature of the underlying pathophysiological process. Because the term "organic mental disorder" implies that "nonorganic" mental disorders do not have a biological basis, the term was not used in *DSM-IV-TR* (APA, 2000). The subtitle of Organic Mental Disorders versus "inorganic" mental disease in the *DSM-III-R* suggests a mind-body dualism. Therefore, in the *DSM-IV-TR*, disorders known to be caused physically are listed under the category that best describes the psychiatric features, so that a mood disorder induced by substance abuse is listed as a mood disorder. Delirium, dementia, and amnestic disorders are categorized as "cognitive disorders." In this way, organic disorders refer to a condition caused by something outside a mental disorder, but the mind-body dualism is softened.

Included among cognitive disorders discussed in this chapter are those that affect younger persons, such as fetal alcohol syndrome and mental retardation, and those that generally affect older persons, such as dementia and delirium. These syndromes are highly variable; they will be different from person to person and over time in the same individual. More than one disorder may be present in a person simultaneously (e.g., Delirium superimposed upon Dementia), and one syndrome may succeed another (e.g., thiamine-deficiency Delirium or Wernicke's encephalopathy followed by Alcohol Amnestic Disorder Korsakoff's disease).

The *DSM-IV-TR* classifies cognitive disorders according to etiology, so that the appropriate treatment may be initiated. The psychiatric nurse who is devoted to biological, psychological, social, and spiritual care of clients must also search for contributing factors related to cognitive disorders in an effort to identify the full array of potential nursing interventions.

COGNITIVE DISORDERS ACROSS THE LIFE SPAN

It is not the purpose of this chapter to review in detail all prevailing theories of growth and development as they relate to cognitive disorders. However, discussion will address general concepts and principles that are germane to understanding the relationship between brain and behavior in child and adolescent psychiatric and mental health nursing. Additionally, certain general issues must be remembered.

First, child and adolescent psychiatric and mental health nursing is concerned with *developing* brain, behavior, and biology. Although growth and change are a continuous process throughout the life span, they will never progress at this rapid rate again. Second, there is still a wide gap between theory and practice. There is also disagreement about application of some theories. This often leads to polarized approaches to the same problem behavior. Finally, it is not difficult to see that in some areas, etiological breakthroughs that will affect clinical practice are imminent and demand that psychiatric nurses stay abreast of developing theories and research in these areas.

DEVELOPMENT OF THE BRAIN

Life begins as a single cell; however, by the time of birth, billions of neurons are created, differentiated, and in place. Initially, the biological focus is on formation, but in later fetal life, there is a shift to differentiating and fine-tuning. After birth, the most significant development in the brain is the development and proliferation of efficient nerve conduction. The brain continues to grow through early childhood. Although approximately 75 percent of brain growth (as shown by weight) occurs by the age of 2 years, and 90 percent by the age of 4 years the process of differentiation continues at a decelerating rate until adulthood, and axonal and dendritic growth continues until final senescence (Goetz, 1999; Hockenberry et al., 2003). During intrauterine life the developing brain is exquisitely sensitive to changes in the biochemical environment and the supply of essential nutrients, especially glucose and oxygen. If disrupted this can result in temporary or permanent impairment. Additionally, injury and localized brain disease can result in the direct loss of nervous tissue (Figure 16–1 and see Figure 16–2). Obviously, if these disruptions or assaults occur early in fetal life, they can and often do have catastrophic results. Examples include congenital malformations and severe mental retardation. The birth process itself can be a difficult transition when the most dangerous occurrence is anoxia, which is worsened when combined with prematurity.

Changes occur in the brain throughout life. Genetics, environment, and general health affect the timing, development, and magnitude of damage. After age 50 brain cells die at the rate of 1 percent per year, and brain weight decreases 6 to 11 percent by age 80 (Crigger & Forbes, 1997). Even though these losses may result in slow impulse transmission, they do not have a measurable effect on cognition. With age, there is an impairment in neurotransmission, especially with the serotonin, cholinergic, and dopamine systems (Strong, 1998). These changes may predispose the older person to signs of cognitive and affective disorders. Pronounced deficits may be related to severe cognitive disorders in older adults.

CHILD AND ADOLESCENT DEVELOPMENT

An understanding of normal growth and development provides a framework for assessing the child or adolescent with a psychiatric or medical condition. Although theoretic concepts differ, theorists agree that development proceeds in a sequential manner along a prescribed continuum. Stages defined in each model are characterized by certain tasks or goals that must be mastered before a child can successfully progress to the next level. Although growth and development proceeds in a sequential manner, the pace of this development can exhibit tremendous variation within specific developmental stages.

As assessment and treatment proceed, it is important for the psychiatric nurse to remember that when using a developmental framework there is a wide variation within "normal" development. Growth and development occur fairly rapidly from birth to 3 years but is less dramatic through the latency period. During puberty and adolescence the rate of growth increases sharply and behavior is more labile again.

ADULT DEVELOPMENT

Contrary to popular opinion, intellectual decline is not a normal part of aging. There are changes in reaction time, recall, slight changes in short-term memory, and an increased cautiousness that lead one to believe that the older adult is unsure. However, there is an increase in intelligence in the normal older adult that is related to life experience and wisdom that is not found in younger persons.

Physiological Changes

Many physiological changes occur in the older adult that can affect memory function. There are changes in fat-to-lean body mass ratios and water balance that make medication prescription and electrolyte balances challenging. Liver and kidney dysfunction may occur and can also affect these areas. This must be kept in mind when prescribing medication or diagnosing an older adult who presents with "confusion."

Psychosocial Changes

Sociologists have theorized several reasons for aging. These include the disengagement, activity, and continuity theories. Thus far no theory of aging, whether biological or sociological, has been supported definitively.

Psychosocial changes seem to occur with aging that affect coping and general health. Losses occurring with aging include aspects of all five physical senses and changes in body functioning that affect psychosocial activity. In addition, elders frequently experience the loss of a spouse, friend, sibling, occupation, home, income, and possibly a child. These losses can present extraordinary burdens on the older person and must be kept in mind when caring for a geriatric patient. Textbooks on geriatrics or gerontology can provide the reader with in-depth information regarding these theories, which is beyond the scope of this chapter. Developmental changes associated with age are summarized in Table 16–1.

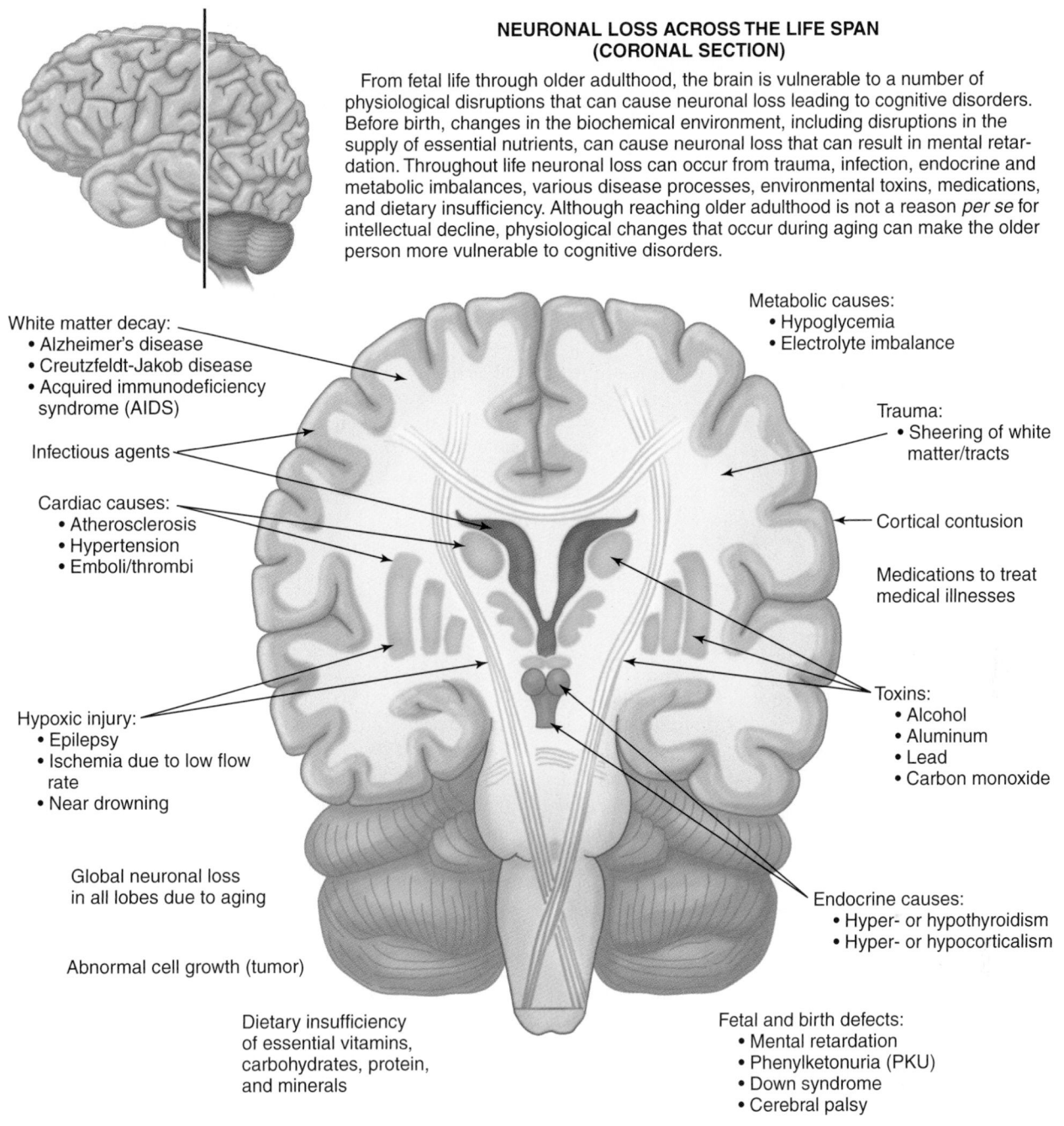

**NEURONAL LOSS ACROSS THE LIFE SPAN
(CORONAL SECTION)**

From fetal life through older adulthood, the brain is vulnerable to a number of physiological disruptions that can cause neuronal loss leading to cognitive disorders. Before birth, changes in the biochemical environment, including disruptions in the supply of essential nutrients, can cause neuronal loss that can result in mental retardation. Throughout life neuronal loss can occur from trauma, infection, endocrine and metabolic imbalances, various disease processes, environmental toxins, medications, and dietary insufficiency. Although reaching older adulthood is not a reason *per se* for intellectual decline, physiological changes that occur during aging can make the older person more vulnerable to cognitive disorders.

White matter decay:
• Alzheimer's disease
• Creutzfeldt-Jakob disease
• Acquired immunodeficiency syndrome (AIDS)

Infectious agents

Cardiac causes:
• Atherosclerosis
• Hypertension
• Emboli/thrombi

Hypoxic injury:
• Epilepsy
• Ischemia due to low flow rate
• Near drowning

Global neuronal loss in all lobes due to aging

Abnormal cell growth (tumor)

Dietary insufficiency of essential vitamins, carbohydrates, protein, and minerals

Metabolic causes:
• Hypoglycemia
• Electrolyte imbalance

Trauma:
• Sheering of white matter/tracts

Cortical contusion

Medications to treat medical illnesses

Toxins:
• Alcohol
• Aluminum
• Lead
• Carbon monoxide

Endocrine causes:
• Hyper- or hypothyroidism
• Hyper- or hypocorticalism

Fetal and birth defects:
• Mental retardation
• Phenylketonuria (PKU)
• Down syndrome
• Cerebral palsy

Figure 16–1 Neuronal loss across the life span.

POTENTIALLY REVERSIBLE DEMENTIAS

It is important to differentially diagnose clients with dementias so that the appropriate treatment can be instituted. Similarly, the psychiatric nurse must remember that a potentially reversible dementia can be superimposed on a probable irreversible dementia, causing excess disability. Excess disability can be defined as "a reversible deficit that is more disabling than the primary disability, existing when the magnitude of the disturbance in functioning is greater than might be accounted for by basic physical illness or cerebral pathology" (Dawson, Kline, Wiancko, & Wells, 1986, p. 299). When stressors causing excess disability are removed, cognitive and physical functioning may improve. If not, the client becomes stressed, resulting in further disability and possibly death. The most common potentially irreversible medical syndrome is delirium.

TABLE 16–1
Developmental Changes with Age

Stage	Age (yr.)	Task
Young adulthood	20–28	Development of life dream; separation from nuclear family. Erikson: Intimacy vs. isolation
Adulthood	29–39	Changing commitments; childbearing and childrearing; self-identity. Erikson: Generativity vs. stagnation
Middle adulthood	40–65 or 70	Reintegration of self-identity; launching family; accepting physical aging; redefined attitudes about money, religion, and death. Erikson: Generativity vs. stagnation
Late adulthood	65–70	Capacity to feel whole in spite of diminishing health; adjusting to decreased physical strength, health; to retirement; reduced income; death of spouse. Feeling of enduring significance; adjusting and adopting social roles; maintaining maximum independence. Erikson: Ego integrity vs. despair

Note. From *Childhood and Society*, by E. Erikson, 1963, New York: W.W. Norton.

Delirium

The words *delirium, acute confusional state* (ACS), and acute confusion (AC) are used by health care professionals to describe a particular type of cognitive impairment. Delirium is a diagnosis described in the *DSM-IV-TR* as a condition in which the individual experiences a rapid onset of a disturbance in consciousness and cognition (APA, 2000; Bhat & Rockwood, 2007). ACS and AC are broad descriptive terms that refer to the cognitive phenomenon before the actual diagnosis of delirium is made. No matter how this phenomenon is defined, it is vital to differentiate acute confusion/delirium (acute, reversible) from dementia (chronic, irreversible), as well as from depression, another common condition that may impair cognition. Delirium is a condition distinguished by an acute, fluctuating change in mental status. Clients with delirium show signs of diminished attentiveness to their surroundings, fluctuating consciousness, and a varying capacity to focus, sustain, or change attention (Bhat & Rockwood, 2007).

Delirium is the most common psychiatric disorder encountered by health care personnel. Five to eighty percent of all persons admitted to acute hospitals experience acute confusion delirium (Foreman, Wakefield, Culp, & Milisen, 2001). Unfortunately, only 3 of 10 cases are recognized by physicians or nursing staff because of incomplete assessment or preconceived notions of aging. Delirium superimposed on dementia is even less likely to be recognized.

A pioneer in the study of delirium, Lipowski (1990) described delirium as the most common and important form of psychopathology in later life. More than 20 terms have been used to describe delirium (i.e., organic brain syndrome, acute confusional state, acute brain failure, etc.). From a clinical standpoint it is crucial that delirium be recognized and an etiologic factor determined promptly. In older adults, delirium is often the first sign of an underlying medical problem (such as an acute infection, fecal impaction, or myocardial infarction) and if it is not diagnosed and properly treated, it may result in an extended hospital stay, functional decline and institutionalization, or death.

The essential features of delirium are reduced ability to maintain attention to external stimuli and to appropriately shift attention to new external stimuli, and disorganized thinking, as manifested by rambling, irrelevant, or incoherent speech. The disorder also presents with altered or clouded consciousness with sensory misperceptions (hallucinations, delusions, or illusions); disturbances in the sleep-wake cycle and level of psychomotor activity (agitation to stupor); disorientation to person, place, or time; and memory impairment. The onset is rapid and the course typically fluctuates throughout the day and night. The duration is typically brief and death ensues if underlying medical conditions are not resolved (Cook, 2004).

Associated features of delirium include anxiety, fear, depression, irritability, anger, euphoria, and apathy. Emotional disturbances are very common and quite variable with delirium. Some persons experience rapid and unpredictable changes from one emotional state to another. Fear is commonly experienced as a response to threatening hallucinations or delusions (Cook, 2004). These responses can result in the individual's attempts to escape the environment and subsequent falls; removal of medical equipment such as catheters and intravenous lines; disturbing vocalizations such as yelling and screaming; and a predilection to attack others (Bhat & Rockwood, 2005; Cook, 2004). Delirium can occur at any age, but it is especially common in children and those over the age of 60.

Persons at risk for delirium may have co-occurrences such as dementia, chronic obstructive pulmonary disease (COPD), hypertension, polypharmacy, and cerebral vascular accident (CVA) (Hanley, 2004). Other conditions that contribute to the incidence of delirium are infection, hypoxia, metabolic disturbance, fractures, pain, nutritional deficiencies, and acute illness. Additionally, medications can contribute to the development of delirium (Cook, 2004). Some of these contributing factors are highlighted in Table 16–2.

Delirium can be categorized into three types: hyperactive, hypoactive, and mixed (Cook, 2004). Recognition of hyperactive delirium is most common, but hypoactive is often unrecognized and untreated (Hanley, 2004). Recognition of the type of delirium may be helpful in determining appropriate treatment.

Prodromal signs and symptoms of delirium are insomnia, distractibility, excessive sensitivity to light and sound, drowsiness, anxiety, vivid dreams or nightmares, complaints of difficulty remembering, disproportionate fatigue, and a short attention span (Stanley, Blair, & Beare, 2005). Autonomic signs (tachycardia, sweating, flushed face, dilated pupils, and elevated blood pressure) commonly occur. Chronic conditions experienced by so many older adults can contribute to confusion. These include cardiac and respiratory problems, myocardial infarctions, arrhythmias, and respiratory problems, all of which can affect the central nervous system. Other factors that may lead to delirium are infections such as pneumonia, urinary tract infections, dehydration, and drugs, even those prescribed to treat an acute or chronic condition (Bhat & Rockwood, 2007; Cook, 2004). Refer to Table 16–3 for drugs most likely to be linked with the incidence of delirium. Because of physiological changes that occur with normal aging, the psychiatric nurse must be aware of the dictum "start low and go slow," which means that the dose of medication should be the lowest possible therapeutic dose, and increases in dose must be made slowly, after assessing for effects. Older adults are also likely to take many medications for multiple chronic conditions, which may be prescribed by multiple practitioners (Cole, 2004). Withdrawal syndromes may contribute to episodes of delirium. When a person suddenly discontinues use of sedative-hypnotics or alcohol, a withdrawal delirium can result.

Nursing Implications

Interventions can be classified into those targeted to physiological etiologies and supportive interventions (Stanley et al., 2005). Initial physiological interventions include detecting early signs, aggressively searching for the cause, and treating any underlying medical conditions. Drug reactions or interactions and infection should be ruled out first (Cook, 2004). Often, delirium can be attributed to new drugs and urinary tract and respiratory infections. Changing the medication regimen and treating infections can produce reversal of the disorder. Correction of underlying medical conditions must be initiated slowly, with frequent monitoring (Stanley et al., 2005). These may include correction of blood glucose levels, treating metabolic disturbances, hydration, replacing electrolytes, and balancing the acid-base systems. Delirium is prevalent after surgery and during major physical crises, such as burns, and must be treated proactively. The older adult and the very young are very susceptible to the development of delirium. If they do develop delirium, it is a grave prognostic sign, perhaps resulting in coma and death. Thus, recognition and prompt treatment are imperative.

DSM-IV-TR Diagnostic Criteria for Delirium Due to . . .

(Indicate the general medical condition.)

A. Disturbance of consciousness (i.e., reduced clarity of awareness of the environment) with reduced ability to focus, sustain, or shift attention.

B. A change in cognition (such as memory deficit, disorientation, language disturbance) or the development of a perceptual disturbance that is not better accounted for by a preexisting, established, or evolving dementia.

C. The disturbance develops over a short period of time (usually hours to days) and tends to fluctuate during the course of the day.

D. There is evidence from the history, physical examination, or laboratory findings that the disturbance is caused by the direct physiological consequences of a general medical condition.

Coding Note: If delirium is superimposed on a preexisting Dementia of the Alzheimer's Type or Vascular Dementia, indicate the delirium by coding the appropriate subtype of the dementia, e.g., 294.1 Dementia of the Alzheimer's Type, With Late Onset, With Delirium.

TABLE 16–2
Factors Associated with the Development of Delirium

Category	Factor	Category	Factor
Body fluids and kidney function	Fluid/electrolyte disturbances		Limited social contact (suggested, nonsignificant relationship)
	Dehydration/volume depletion		Admission from an institution
	Hypocalcemia	Infection and trauma	Symptomatic infection
	Hypokalemia		Urinary tract infection
	Abnormal sodium level		Respiratory infection
	Low serum albumin		Elevated white blood cell count at admission
	High blood urea nitrogen (BUN)		
	Elevated creatinine		Emergency admission
	Azotemia		Fracture
	Proteinuria		Falls
	Chronic renal disease		Orthopedic surgery
Sensory and neurological function	Sensory disturbances		Physical illnesses (usually two or more in conjunction)
	Pain (unmanaged or poorly managed)		Severity of illness
	Neurological disease	Effects of pharmaceuticals	Multiple medications (usually greater than four)
	Cognitive impairment/brain damage/dementia (one of the most commonly identified risk factors, especially in older adults)		Drugs with anticholinergic or central nervous system (CNS) effects
Circulation and oxygenation	Low blood pressures		Drug toxicity
	Cardiovascular disease		Psychoactive drug use
	Congestive heart disease		Narcotic use
	Aortic aneurysm surgery		Drug or alcohol abuse
	Elevated prothrombin time (PT)		Drug withdrawal
	Low hematocrit	Impaired physical or functional ability	Activity of daily living (ADL) impairment
	Abnormal arterial blood gases		Urinary problems/incontinence
	Respiratory insufficiency		
	Noncardiac thoracic surgery		
Metabolism and body temperature	Metabolic disturbances		
	Nutritional deficiencies		
	Abnormal blood glucose		
	Elevated aspartate aminotransferase (AST)/serum glutamic oxaloacetic transaminase (SGOT)		
	Abnormal body temperature		
Age, gender, and living arrangement	Age 65 and older (higher incidence at age 80 or older)		
	Male gender (suggested, nonsignificant relationship)		

Note. From Bhat & Rockwood, 2007; Cook, 2004.

TABLE 16–3
Commonly Used Drugs Causing Delirium

Group	Examples
Analgesics	Opiates, salicylates
Antiarrhythmics	Lidocaine, procainamide
Antibiotics	Cephalexin, gentamicin, penicillin
Anticonvulsants	Phenytoin
Antihypertensives	Methyldopa
Anti-inflammatory	Indomethacin, steroids
Antineoplastic	5-fluorouracil, methotrexate
Antiparkinsonian	Levodopa, bromocriptine
Gastrointestinal	Cimetidine
Psychotropics	Antidepressants, barbiturates, benzodiazepines, lithium, antipsychotics
Antihistamines	Diphenyldramine (Benadryl)
Sympathomimetics	Amphetamines, phenylephrine
Miscellaneous	Drug withdrawal (alcohol, barbiturates, benzodiazepines)
	Bromides
	Disulfiram
	Timolol eyedrops
	Theophylline

Supportive interventions have shown promise in decreasing the degree of confusion and prompt restoration of cognitive function (Stanley et al., 2005). These include environmental interventions controlling noise and external stimuli, providing adequate lighting, and maintaining an uncluttered environment. Other interventions include reassuring and calming communication, gentle reality orientation, validation of feelings, and the involvement of family and significant others. Reality orientation is best used by integrating information such as the date, time, place, and reason for hospitalization into a more casual conversation. Restraint-free approaches are strongly encouraged.

The *DSM-IV-TR* describes delirium according to etiology. Several etiologies are presented in the text and include delirium caused by a general medical condition, substance-induced delirium, substance withdrawal delirium, and delirium caused by multiple etiologies (APA, 2000). These disorders and associated criteria are further described later in this chapter.

Treatable Brain Lesions

Most **brain lesions** can be detected with computerized tomography (CT) scan or magnetic resonance imaging (MRI). Vascular occlusion, cerebral infarction, subarachnoid hemorrhage, and cerebral hemorrhage are acute lesions. Primary or metastatic brain tumors, subdural hematomas, or brain abscesses can also lead to delirium or confusional states but develop over a longer period of time. Timely and accurate differentiation is imperative because the therapeutic approaches to each of these can differ.

The varied clinical picture is prominent, and rapid changes are often seen. The most prominent manifestation is any change in level of consciousness, with an attendant disorientation to time, place, or person. The syndrome is more common in older adults, particularly those with baseline cognitive impairment, but it can appear at any age. Primary brain tumors are less common in the very old than earlier in life, except for meningiomas. Brain tumors in the adult are most often a metastatic process from a site outside of the cranium. Frontal lobe tumors may present a dementia-like picture. Personality and affect changes occur frequently, with symptoms of giddiness, irritability, inappropriate behavior, fearfulness, excessive energy, and possibly psychotic features such as hallucinations or paranoia. Contradictory emotions are often displayed in the same individual within a short time span. Disordered speech with prominent slurring is often observed, along with rapidity, neologisms, aphasic errors, or chaotic patterns.

Confusion regarding day-to-day events and daily routine, as well as individual roles, is common. Normal patterns of sleeping and eating are usually grossly distorted. Physical restlessness is often seen in the form of pacing, but apathy can also be a manifestation of acute processes. In fact, the

CRITICAL THINKING

Mr. K is a 75-year-old retired engineer seen in the emergency room with his wife of 50 years who reports that her husband is confused, agitated, and has been seeing and hearing things that were not there. A major nursing intervention in caring for Mr. K must include which of the following?

a. Assess duration of symptoms

b. Inquire about his current and over-the-counter medications, including if new medications have been added recently

c. Inquire about substance abuse/dependence history

d. All of the above

Answers

Answers a, b, and c are all correct, but the *correct answer is d* because depending upon duration of symptoms, recent changes in medications and data about substance use are critical assessment data that help the nurse and staff distinguish between dementia and delirium. As a rule, delirium has a rapid onset and transitory course, whereas dementia has a slower, chronic, and insidious course.

RESEARCH ABSTRACT

Antipsychotic Drug Use and Mortality in Older Adults with Dementia

Gill, S. S., Bronskill, S. E., Normand, S. L., Anderson, G. M., Sykora, K., Lam, K., et al. (2007). *Annals of Internal Medicine, 146,* 775–786.

Study Problem/Purpose

The purpose of this study was to determine the association between treatment with conventional and atypical antipsychotics and all-cause mortality in older adults with dementia.

Methods

Researchers used a population-based, retrospective cohort study of older adults (*n* = 27,259) living in community or long-term care who were treated between April 1997 and March 2003. The risk of death was evaluated at 30, 60, 120, and 180 days after antipsychotic agents were initiated. Two pair-wise comparisons were made: atypical versus no antipsychotic use and conventional versus atypical antipsychotic use. Groups were stratified by place of residence.

Findings

Scientists found that the use of atypical antipsychotics were associated with a statistically significant increase in the risk for death at 30 days compared with nonuse in both the community-dwelling cohort (adjusted hazard ratio,

1.31 [95 percent CI, 1.02 to 1.70]; absolute risk difference, 0.2 percentage point) and the long-term care cohort (adjusted hazard ratio, 1.55 [CI, 1.15 to 2.07]; absolute risk difference, 1.2 percentage points). Increased risk of death appeared to persist to 180 days. The results may have been linked to unequal rates of censoring over time. In reference to atypical antipsychotic use, conventional antipsychotic use was associated with a higher risk for death at all data points. Researchers concluded that atypical antipsychotic use was associated with a greater risk of death compared with nonuse among older adults with dementia, whereas the risk for death seemed greater with conventional antipsychotic agents than with atypical antipsychotic agents. The cause of death was not revealed in this study.

Implications for Psychiatric Nursing

Antipsychotic medications are often used to manage dementia-related behaviors. Psychiatric nurses must be strong advocates for appropriate medications for older adults with dementia. They should monitor clients for adverse side effects and collaborate with interdisciplinary teams to ensure clients receive the lowest effective medication.

severity and progression of each of these symptoms may vary widely among clients and time periods. Family members and friends may report that the recent changes in behavior are alarming and "out of character" for the patient. The time course for these changes is rarely more than hours or days, and they almost always precipitate a medical emergency.

Confusional states, which are milder cases of this cascade of symptoms, develop more slowly and persist for weeks or even months before being detected. The symptoms of confusional states may resemble those of delirium but may be less obvious and less likely to require an emergency consultation. Rapid evaluation of persons with confusional states is imperative because the underlying condition often changes acutely and is sometimes reversible. In the absence of a known cause, a thorough evaluation should include a detailed history (including information from as many relatives or caregivers as possible), physical examination, and mental status examination. If the lesion is resectable, a neurosurgeon will perform a craniotomy to remove the lesion, or create bur-holes to relieve pressure. Return of function may be slow or rapid, depending on the location and size of the lesion.

Older adults are particularly susceptible to hematomas because the danger of falling increases with age (Stolley, Lewis, Moore, & Harvey, 2001). Because the normal older adult experiences some cerebral atrophy, the brain can "bounce around" inside the skull more readily, causing subarachnoid or subdural hematomas. Subarachnoid hematomas develop relatively quickly, but subdural hematomas may develop over a period as long as 3 months. The neurologist or neurosurgeon may elect to observe the client with a subdural hematoma, which may be resorbed by the body.

Normal Pressure Hydrocephalus

Chronic communicating hydrocephalus with "normal" pressure can cause an insidiously developing dementia, which occurs in mid to late middle age. It is rare but potentially correctable, and it affects men more than women (Geldmacher, 2004). Therefore, it must always be considered when dementia is suspected. Such persons are slow and slovenly, in contrast to the more alert behavior characterizing Alzheimer's disease (AD). Unsteady, slow, and shuffling gait, and episodes of urinary incontinence are common. Gait changes include difficulty initiating the gait and reduced step height. This results in a type of shuffling in which the feet appear to be "stuck to the floor." It is important to remember that the triad of shuffling gait, mental impairment, and incontinence are hallmarks of this disease, but gait impairments may be unaccompanied by bladder symptoms or mental changes. Pathogenesis is based on an impeded cerebral spinal fluid (CSF) circulation and absorption. There may have been a previous attack of meningitis, encephalitis, or head injury, and a few persons have tumors, particularly of the midbrain (Geldmacher, 2004). CT scans show large, dilated ventricles with little or no cortical atrophy. The CSF pressure is normal or high normal. Some improvement may follow the introduction of ventriculoatrial shunt, especially when gait disorders precede or outweigh mental decline. Thus, this disorder is considered potentially reversible, but it may become irreversible if untreated.

PROBABLE IRREVERSIBLE DEMENTIAS

Dementia is a global impairment of cognitive functioning, memory, and personality that occurs without a disturbance in consciousness or level of alertness. Dementias are acquired, unlike mental retardation, which is usually congenital. Although dementia is found predominantly in older adults, some neuropsychiatric disorders (epilepsy, brain tumors, traumatic head injury, or AIDS) may cause dementia in childhood and adolescence. It is important for the psychiatric nurse to remember that the onset, course, and clinical management of dementia in children, adolescents, and adults depend heavily on the underlying etiology.

The most common probable irreversible disorders seen in children are mental retardation (MR) and epilepsy, although epilepsy can occur throughout the life span. Alzheimer's disease (AD) is the most prevalent form of dementia in adults followed by vascular dementia (VaD) and dementia with Lewy bodies (DLB), or a mixed type of dementia (AD with VaD). Because MD, epilepsy, and AD are the most commonly seen probable irreversible organic diseases, the main focus on this section is on these diseases.

Mental Retardation

Significantly subaverage intellectual functioning that originates during the developmental period and accompanied by deficits in adaptive functioning is defined as mental retardation (APA, 2000). The subaverage intellectual functioning is accompanied by significant limitations in adaptive functioning in two of the following skills: communication, self-care, home living, social or interpersonal skills, use of community resources, self-direction, functional academic skills, work, leisure, health, and safety. The etiology of mental retardation is often unknown, but causes of mental retardation can be grouped into two main factors: heredity and acquired. Table 16–4 summarizes these factors.

Standardized tests to measure intelligence quotient (IQ) are used in the determination of mental retardation. A variety of tests are available to evaluate infant through adult IQ. The person whose performance on these tests is similar to others of the same age is considered to have average intelligence (a score of 100). The IQ score expresses the relationship of "mental age" to "chronological age." The basic formula is:

$$\frac{\text{Mental Age}}{\text{Chronological Age}} \times 100 = IQ$$

The specific IQ cutoff point used to define mental retardation is 70. Mental retardation is divided into four broad categories: mild (IQ = 50–70), moderate (IQ = 35–50), severe (IQ = 20–35), and profound (IQ = below 20). The person with mild retardation is educable and can function at a mental age of 8 to 12 years. A moderately mentally retarded individual can achieve a mental age of 3 to 7 years, and severely and profoundly mentally retarded individuals can attain the mental age of a toddler and infant, respectively (APA, 2000).

TABLE 16–4
Causes of Mental Retardation

Genetic	Acquired
Down syndrome	Rubella and prenatal Viruses
Klinefelter's syndrome	Toxins
Phenylketonuria (PKU)	Placental insufficiency
Hypothyroidism	Blood type incompatibility
Tay-Sachs disease	Anoxia
Fragile X syndrome	Birth injury
Autism	Prematurity
	Infection—meningitis, encephalitis
	Poisons—lead, medicine, chemicals (FAS)
	Poor nutrition
	CNS insult
	Sociocultural factors
	Hydrocephalus

THE MORE YOU KNOW

Cellular Discoveries: Genetic and Biological Advances Help Unlock Mysteries of Mental Retardation

New research is uncovering the biological dysregulation at the base of mental retardation. Recently scientists have found numerous abnormal genes that deter brain cells from working correctly. For instance, some of the genetic abnormalities that result in mental retardation affect tiny knobs referred to as dendrite spines nerve cells in the brain. Mutations in dendrite spines appear to interfere with the ability of the dendrite spines' necks to expand. Because these spines link billions of nerve cells in the brain, scientists believe this expansion of the neck is crucial to conveying messages throughout the brain.

New research is offering a greater understanding of the many causes of mental retardation. For example, in the brains of clients with Down syndrome, cells that are responsible for producing nerve cells make too few. In people with Fragile X syndrome, the most prevalent cause of mental retardation, nerve cell connections may be too immature.

From Ambrose, S. G. (2002). *Texas Living,* (p. 12C). Dallas, TX: Dallas Morning News.

The long-term outcome of mental retardation is variable. Those with severe and profound forms often experience progressive deterioration and premature death, as early as the teens or early 20s. Many individuals with moderate retardation also experience a somewhat reduced life expectancy. Diagnosis of mental retardation may be made at birth relative to a specific genetic syndrome or disorder. However, some cases of MR may not be diagnosed until suspicion is raised because the child has failed to meet developmental milestones. In some cases, a child enters the school system and exhibits subaverage progress, thus raising suspicion. In all cases, developmental screening and standardized testing is implemented to identify MR.

Fetal Alcohol Syndrome

Fetal alcohol syndrome (FAS) is characterized by a specific pattern of malformation seen in the offspring of women who consume alcohol during pregnancy. In the United States it has been suggested that FAS is the most commonly recognized cause of mental retardation, with an estimated incidence of 1 to 3 per 1,000 live births with alcohol-related neurodevelopmental disorder (ARND) occurring at a rate 10 times that of FAS (Caley, Kramer, & Robinson, 2005). However, when infants with more mild manifestations of the syndrome were included, a rate of 1 in 300 was estimated. Since its initial description in 1973 (Jones, Smith, Ulleland, & Streissguth, 1973), it has become clear that the most severe manifestations of FAS represent only the tip of the iceberg. Perhaps most tragic is the recognition that this form of mental retardation is entirely preventable if the mother consumes no alcohol during pregnancy.

The principal features of FAS are outlined in Table 16–5. These abnormalities are produced through the teratogenic effect of alcohol acting directly on the developing fetus or indirectly by changing maternal or placental physiology. The exact mechanisms by which teratogens cause birth defects is not completely understood. However, three basic mechanisms have been established. Agents like alcohol affect normal fetal development by killing cells, disturbing cell differentiation or migration, or causing the cells to malfunction in response to normal stimuli. There is no indication that there is a minimum or safe dosage of alcohol that may be consumed without potential harm to the fetus. The fetus is placed at risk for the effects of alcohol when the amount consumed exceeds the liver's ability to detoxify the substance.

The structure most sensitive to the prenatal effects of alcohol is the developing brain. These effects are apparent in the presentation of neurological manifestations (see Table 16–5). Although the average IQ score of individuals with FAS is 63, a wide range of developmental outcomes have been documented, from children with profound mental retardation to children with normal intelligence who display learning disorders and behavioral abnormalities that lead to significant difficulties in adaptation. Developmental and behavioral problems occur in the vast majority of affected children.

TABLE 16–5 Fetal Alcohol Syndrome: Patterns of Malformation	
Affected Area	**Patterns of Malformation**
Growth	Microcephaly
	Postnatal growth deficiency
	Prenatal growth deficiency
Neurological	Developmental delay & motor retardation
	Hyperactivity
	Poor attention span
	Irritability
	Poor school performance
	Mental retardation
	Hearing disorder
Facial features	Short palpebral fissures
	Smooth philtrum
	Thinned upper lip
	Micrognathia or prognathia in adolescence
	Ptosis
	Strabismus
	Myopia
	Hypoplastic maxilla
Skeletal	Joint dysfunction, including congenital hip dislocation
	Abnormal palmar crease pattern
	Thoracic cage abnormalities
Cardiac	Ventral septal defect
	Atrial septal defect
Other	Cleft lip/palate
	Low set posteriorly rotated ears
	Strawberry hemangioma
	Maldeveloped teeth

The differential diagnosis of mental retardation is important, though complex, owing to the frequent comorbidity of other childhood disorders. Differential diagnosis includes such things as ADHD, academic skills disorder, autism, and childhood psychosis. The psychiatric nurse must also remember that seizure disorders are common in children with mental retardation.

The Epilepsies

Epilepsy is a condition characterized by sudden, recurrent, and transient disturbances of mental functioning or body movements that result from excessive discharging of groups of brain cells (Goetz, 1999). Based on this definition, the psychiatric nurse will recognize that epilepsy is not a specific disease but is comprised of a group of symptoms that have different causes in different individuals.

Grand mal seizures are a tonic-clonic attack with a loss of consciousness. These are the most common form of generalized seizures. Many clients experiencing grand mal seizures will report vague warning symptoms of discomfort, anxiety, mood changes, or physical discomfort such as headache, upset stomach, sweating, or changes in body temperature. An aura often immediately precedes a full-blown seizure. Dizziness, fainting, and sensory phenomena (lights, dots, sounds, odors, and tastes) are the more frequent kinds of auras.

The tonic phase is a dramatic stiffening of the muscles throughout the body. The head and neck are thrown back, the back is arched, and the extremities are in maximum extension. Respiration is halted, sometimes for as long as a minute and the individual may appear cyanotic. Often the force of the seizure and the rigid body position places the patient at risk for injury. The tonic phase ends when repetitive jerking of all body muscles begins. This signals the clonic phase of the seizure. The client may bite the tongue or lose bladder and bowel control. The clonic phase ends with the person appearing to be in a deep coma, eyes turned upward, and pupils dilated and nonreactive to light.

A postictal phase follows. Clients awaken from the seizure dazed and sometimes confused. Amnesia for the seizure, headache, and sleepiness are common occurrences, which diminish over the following 1 to 4 hours. Safety is of great concern during the postictal phase.

Petit mal seizures are a common seizure type often beginning in childhood. They may consist of one of three types. The first is a brief lapse of consciousness for 15 to 30 seconds, with very little twitching, a blank stare, and amnesia for the seizure. The second type consists of a similar lapse of consciousness with some twitches, and the third type is an episode of a rather sudden loss of muscle tone and consciousness.

The term *psychomotor epilepsy* is often used to refer to epileptic disturbances of the temporal lobe. The term is used very broadly and includes increased tonicity of the muscles and movements of the head, neck, and gulping or swallowing movements. There may be automatic behavior (automatisms) of various degrees of complexity. Buttoning, unbuttoning movements; complicated "wandering" fugue states; or speech automatisms may be present.

Psychic seizures, as the name implies, consist of perceptual or affective symptoms. The diagnosis is confirmed with clinical data and electroencephalogram results.

Focal discharge seizures are classified according to the location of the seizure discharged. These seizures may begin with twitching of a muscle, then spread to the extremities. If skin sensation is involved, these seizures are called sensory seizures.

The diagnosis of epilepsy involves two processes: determining the type of seizure experienced and attempting to ascertain the cause of the epileptic event. A history of the seizure activity along with a complete physical and neurological examination are conducted. Laboratory studies are utilized to rule out metabolic, infective, renal, hepatic, or metastatic etiologies. The EEG is a valuable diagnostic tool, giving information relative to type and possible cause of the seizure.

Mild Cognitive Impairment

Mild cognitive impairment (MCI) has been the subject of recent research and is considered to be an early stage of dementia, particularly AD (Panza et al., 2005; Solfrizzi et al., 2004). MCI is characterized by mild memory or cognitive loss that cannot be accounted for by a specific medical or psychiatric condition. This predementia syndrome may be a prodromal phase of AD or VaD, with the majority of persons progressing to AD. Since its initial definition in 1991, MCI has been the subject of intense research to determine the pathology and potential to progress to full-blown dementia. Memory impairments are mild and disability is minimal, so it is difficult to differentiate MCI from forgetfulness that is normally experienced in old age, benign senescent forgetfulness (BSF). However, BSF tends to be stable, and MCI, although mild, progresses to dementia. Ongoing research will further define, describe, and test interventions for MCI (Panza et al., 2005; Solfrizzi et al., 2004).

Alzheimer's Disease

Alois Alzheimer first described AD neuropathology in 1907, describing neurofibrillary tangle and neuritic plaque in the brain of a 55-year-old woman. This neurological disorder occurs primarily in middle or late life, but it may occur earlier, depending on the cause. Several causes have been postulated, but except for a genetic component of some types of AD, no definitive cause has been found. The disease is characterized by progressive loss of memory, especially short term; language impairments; poor impulse control; and poor judgment. The course of the disease is anywhere from 2 to 20 years, with 10 years being the average. Experts stage the disease in three stages, four stages (Hall & Buckwalter, 1987; Smith, Gerdner, Hall, & Buckwalter, 2004), and seven stages (Reisburg, Ferris, De Leon, & Crook, 1982). For purposes of this chapter, the four-stage measurement is used. The four stages of AD and associated symptoms are listed in Table 16–6.

Causative Factors

Four genes have been located that are associated with AD. Autosomal dominant genes on chromosomes 1, 14, and 21 are associated with earlier onset AD, and a gene on chromosome 19 carries a risk factor that is connected with later onset AD; 92. The early-onset (ages 30–50) familial AD is associated with the 14th chromosome discovered in 1992 (Mullan et al., 1992; Schellenberg et al., 1992; Van Broeckhoven et al., 1992). The genes on chromosomes 1 and 21 are associated with AD that has an onset from age 49 to 65 (Levy-Lahad et al., 1995; St. George-Hyslop et al., 1992). It is interesting to note that the genetic anomaly associated with Down syndrome is located on the 21st chromosome, and persons with Down syndrome who survive to age 40 almost always in older age develop symptoms of AD. Late-onset AD is associated with chromosome 19 (Pericak-Vance et al., 1991).

The etiology of AD cannot totally be explained by genetics. Persons with AD who have at least one other relative affected are categorized as familial, which could include genetics or some environmental trigger. Persons with AD with no known family history are classified as sporadic.

A clear biochemical abnormality associated with AD was discovered in 1976. This chemical, choline acetyltransferase (CAT) was reduced by 90 percent in the hippocampus and cerebral cortex of AD patients. CAT is a catalyst for the neurotransmitter, acetylcholine, which is responsible for functioning of the hippocampus, paramount in the formation of memory (Figure 16–2). Other neurotransmitters such as norepinephrine, serotonin, and somatostatin have been found to be deficient in the brains of persons with AD and may contribute to behavioral impairments manifested by persons with AD (Caselli, Beach, Yaari, & Reiman, 2006). Cholinesterase inhibitors (CEIs) have been used and seem to slow the progression of the disease (Warner, Butler, & Arya, 2005). The earliest of these was tacrine (THA or Cognex), but side effects of the drug, including gastrointestinal (GI) and liver abnormalities, have reduced its popularity. The CEI Aricept (donepezil) has been used with fewer reported side effects. In April 2000, another CEI, Exelon (rivastigmine tartrate), was approved by the U.S. Food and Drug Administration (Alzheimer's Association, 2000). Exelon therapy has been effective in improving global functioning and cognition. Nausea and vomiting are most common but are decreased with slow titration and continued use. In late 2003, the drug memantine was approved by the U.S. FDA for treatment of moderate to severe AD. Research has shown that memantine may improve cognitive and global functioning and result in reduced care dependence in people with severe AD and VaD (Warner et al., 2005). Other therapies under investigation are estrogen for postmenopausal women, anti-inflammatory agents, and antioxidants. Persons with AD and other dementias who demonstrate agitation, aggression, or psychotic features may need to be treated with psychoactive agents such as non-benzodiazepines and low-dose a typical antipsychotics. See Chapter 28 for information about medications.

Symptoms of AD

Although symptoms are usually categorized by stages, the course of AD is insidious, with one stage running into another. The progression of the disease is gradual, and staging is done for the benefit for professionals caring for or researching persons with AD (see Table 16–6).

Losses are associated with AD in the form of cognitive or intellectual, affective or personality, and conative or planning. By reviewing the behaviors associated with each state, the psychiatric nurse can clearly determine the progression of the disease. In addition to these three clusters of loss, Hall has postulated a fourth cluster of losses, the progressive inability to handle stress (Hall & Buckwalter, 1987; Smith et al., 2004). As a result of her theoretical framework and research, Hall has developed a conceptual model for caring for persons with AD and related dementias, including those discussed in the following pages, termed the Progressively Lowered Stress Threshold (PLST) Model of Care. This model of care is incorporated in the interventions section of this chapter and can usually be used for irreversible dementias of all types, excluding Pick's disease and Korsakoff's disease.

Hall postulates that persons with AD have three possible behavioral responses: baseline, anxious, and dysfunctional (Hall, 1991, 1997; Hall & Buckwalter, 1987; Smith et al., 2004). Baseline behaviors include a basic awareness of the environment and ability to interact and function, limited

TABLE 16–6
Stages of Alzheimer's Disease

Stage	Manifestations
1. Forgetfulness	Short-term memory losses: Misplace, forget, lose things
	Compensate with memory aides: Lists, routine, organization
	Express awareness of problem: Concern about abilities
	May become depressed: Complicates symptoms and makes worse
	Not diagnosable at this stage
2. Confusion	Progressive memory decline: interferes with all abilities; short term most impaired, long term follows later
	Disorientation: Time, place, person, thing
	Instrumental activities of daily living (IADLs): Money management, legal affairs, transportation difficulties, housekeeping, cooking
	Denial is common but give clues that fear "losing their mind"
	Depression is more common; aware of deficits and frightened
	Confabulation and stereotyped word usage: Covering up for memory losses
	More problems when: Stressed, fatigued, out of own environment, ill
	Day care and in-home assistance is commonly needed
3. Ambulatory dementia	Functional losses in ADLs (in approximate order of loss): willingness and ability to bathe, grooming, choosing among clothing, dressing, gait and mobility, toileting, communication, reading, and writing skills
	Loss of ability to reason, to plan for safety, and communicate verbally
	Frustration is common
	Becomes more withdrawn and self-absorbed
	Depression resolves as the person's awareness of her memory loss and disability decreases
	Becomes less "accessible" to others—unable to retain information or use past experiences to guide her behavior
	Communication becomes more and more difficult with loss of language
	Behavioral evidence of reduced stress threshold: up at night, wandering, pacing, confused, agitated, belligerent, combative, withdrawn
	Institutional care is usually needed
4. Endstage	Does not recognize family members, or even her own image in a mirror
	No longer walks; little purposeful activity
	Is often mute and may yell or scream spontaneously
	Forgets how to eat, swallow, and chew; weight loss is common and may become emaciated
	Develops problems associated with immobility: Pneumonia, pressure ulcers, urinary tract infections, and contractures
	Incontinence is common; may have seizures
	Most certainly institutionalized at this point

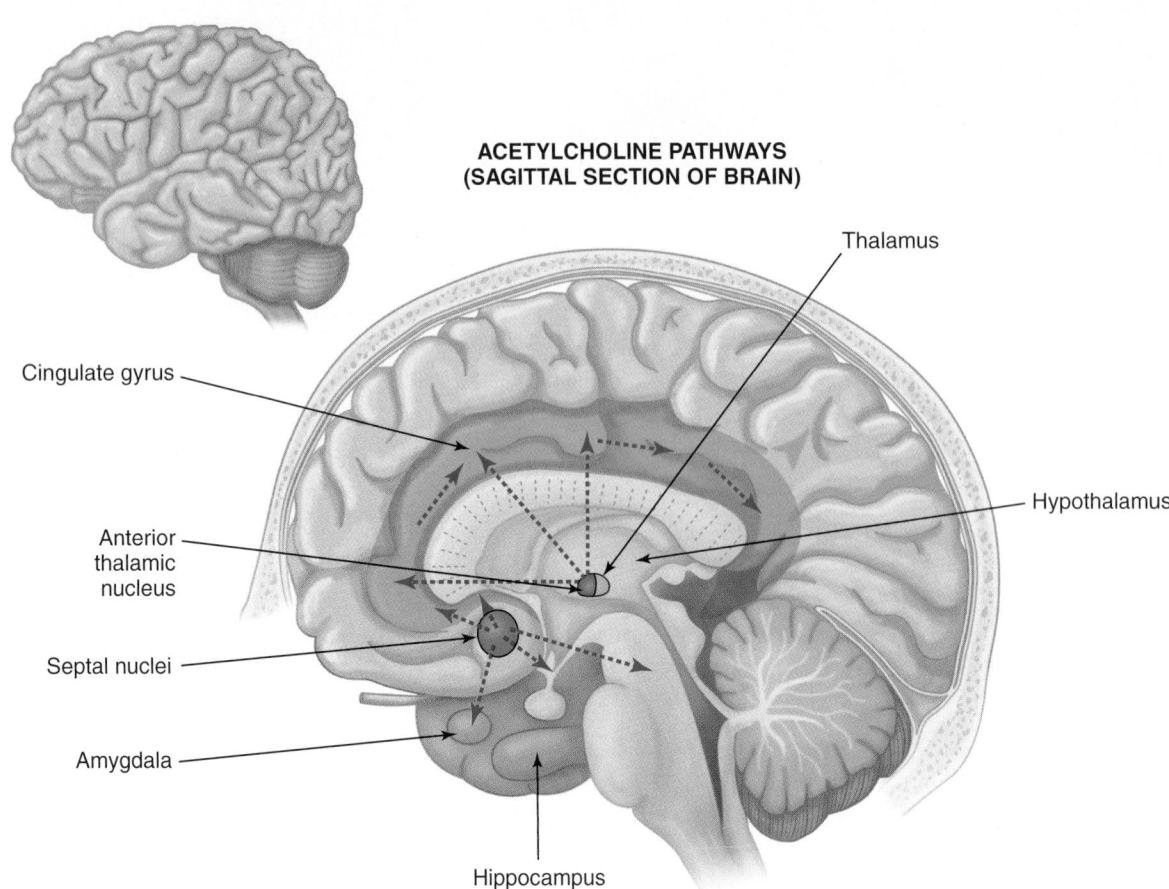

ACETYLCHOLINE PATHWAYS
(SAGITTAL SECTION OF BRAIN)

Thalamus

Cingulate gyrus

Hypothalamus

Anterior thalamic nucleus

Septal nuclei

Amygdala

Hippocampus

The neurotransmitter acetylcholine stimulates the higher brain functions of learning and memory. In the normal brain, acetylcholine is synthesized mainly in two clusters of nerve cells (cholinergic neurons): the *septal nuclei* in the anterior forebrain and the *anterior thalamic nucleus*. Acetylcholine travels from these neuronal bodies to the hippocampus, the cerebral cortex, the limbic system, the hypothalamus, and the thalamus. In people with Alzheimer's disease, there is a pattern of neuronal loss, mostly in the frontal, anterior temporal, and parietal lobes. Profound neuronal loss in the septal nuclei leads to a 60 percent to 90 percent loss of choline acetyltransferase, the enzyme that catalyzes the synthesis of acetylcholine.

Figure 16–2 The role of neuronal loss in cognitive disorders.

only by the amount of neurological deficits. The client becomes functionally impaired if stress levels continue or increase. When the client becomes anxious, he is beginning to feel stress. The client may complain of feeling uneasy. Eye contact is poor or absent and increase in psychomotor activity may appear in response to noxious stimuli. However, the client remains intact.

The client becomes dysfunctional if stress levels continue or increase. As a result, the client becomes catastrophic and cognitively and socially inaccessible. Communication is impaired and the client is unable to interpret the environment appropriately. The individual may actively avoid the noxious stimuli and become fearful and panic

stricken. The result is increased confusion, purposeful wandering, night awakening, "sundowner's syndrome," agitation, fearfulness, panic, combativeness, and sudden withdrawal. The person may experience these symptoms early in the disease at times, but with disease progression, they increase in frequency and intensity.

Six factors can contribute to anxious and dysfunctional behavior. The purpose of the intervention is to control these factors and provide a safe environment. These factors are:

1. Fatigue
2. Change in routine, caregiver, or environment
3. Multiple competing stimuli

4. Demands to achieve beyond capabilities

5. Affective responses to losses

6. Physiologic causes such as elimination problems (urinary retention or constipation), pain, infection, medication, and electrolyte imbalances (see previous discussion on delirium)

Assumptions underlying the PLST model were derived using psychological theories of coping and adaptation. In addition, concepts of rhythmicity and self-esteem were incorporated. These assumptions are basic principles of nursing care for all clients and should be used in caring for all persons with dementia (Hall & Buckwalter, 1987):

1. All humans require some control over their person and their environment and need some degree of unconditional positive regard.

2. All behavior is rooted and has meaning; therefore, all catastrophic and stress-related behaviors have a cause.

3. The confused or agitated client is not comfortable and should be regarded as frightened. All clients have the right to be comfortable.

4. The client exists in a 24-hour continuum. Care cannot be planned or evaluated on an 8-hour shift basis. If the client has a problem during the night, some changes need to be implemented during the day.

Brief descriptions of other probable irreversible dementias are now described. Many of the symptoms are similar to those of AD, with variations as delineated. It is important to remember that persons who suffer from dementia are individuals and that the disease presentation is as heterogeneous as the population it affects.

Vascular Dementia

Vascular dementias (VaD) are associated with ischemic cerebral injury. The most common vascular dementia is multi-infarct dementia (MID) which results from vascular diseases that cause multiple small or large cerebral infarcts. These infarcts can produce dementia as a dominant symptom. The onset is generally acute, and unlike AD, the stages are clear cut or stepwise, with clear decline associated with each infarct. The client may have a history of transient ischemic attacks (TIAs), hypertension, strokes, diabetes mellitus, vasculitis, and cardiac arrhythmias. Family history of stroke or cardiovascular disease are common (Gorelick, 2004; Roman, 2003). Several subtypes of vascular dementia have been identified by APA. They are vascular dementia with delirium, with delusions, with depressed mood, or uncomplicated (APA, 2000).

The person with VaD may have more language difficulties than the person with AD, as well as focal neurological signs and symptoms. Emotional lability, depression, and crying spells are frequently observed. Other deficits may include dysarthria, hemi-neglect, movement disorders, or a subtle paresis. The course of the disease is fluctuating and intermittent. Delirium may occur with each infarct, clearing with time, with no return to baseline cognitive functioning. Some persons with VaD may benefit from anticoagulation therapy and treatment of underlying disease, especially hypertension, which is the most important risk factor.

Cortical Degenerative Syndromes

This section describes characteristics of several common atypical syndromes of cortical degeneration and suggests how those presentations might be accommodated in care provision.

Identifying atypical presentations, whether histologically linked to AD or not, can only help practitioners and caregivers to understand observed behaviors, distinguish between primary and secondary symptoms, and plan care accordingly. Several categories of atypical cortical dementias are discussed next, including progressive aphasias, perceptual-motor syndromes, frontal degenerative syndromes, and bitemporal syndromes. Because of its initial presentation with symptoms of cortical decline, diffuse Lewy body syndrome is often mistakenly diagnosed as AD. Therefore, this syndrome is also addressed.

Progressive Frontal Lobe Syndromes (FLS)

Persons suffering from Pick's disease and other FLS often provide some of the greatest caregiving challenges encountered. In the very early stages of the disease, people developing FLS often appear quite normal and rational, yet caregivers note changes in behavior patterns and judgment. This produces conflict and crises among family members (Kumar-Singh & Van Broeckhoven, 2007; Lantz & Buchalter, 2005).

Although some medical literature describes persons with FLS in passive terms, in a care setting such as the home, day care center, or nursing home, they often have little insight into their limitations, make poor choices, and can be disruptive, posing risks to themselves and others. Many are disinhibited and act on impulse seemingly without reason. Clients with damage to prefrontal areas may verbalize risks and alternatives, yet consistently make poor decisions. The greatest concern with FLS is maintaining safety for clients and those around them.

The person with FLS may refuse to stop driving, make unusually large purchases, use power tools inappropriately, have social outbursts, or eat nonfood items such as glass ornaments. Their lack of insight and disinhibition may produce inconsistent behavior despite making verbally appropriate statements, constantly catching caregivers off guard.

A structured environment whereby the daily schedule, the level of noise, extraneous stimuli, and potential hazards can be controlled is one way to decrease the need for one-to-one supervision for persons with FLS. Yet, the FLS client may not benefit from the structured program in the same way as the person with dementia of an Alzheimer's type, meaning outcomes of appearing calm, interacting with others appropriately, sleeping through the night, or participating in activities will not be reached. A structured environment will, however, decrease the need for client judgment, eliminate many potential safety hazards, and enhance the likelihood of bathing

DSM-IV-TR Diagnostic Criteria for Dementia of the Alzheimer's Type

A. The development of multiple cognitive deficits manifested by both memory impairment (impaired ability to learn new information or to recall previously learned information)

1. One (or more) of the following cognitive disturbances:

   a. **aphasia** (language disturbance)

   b. **apraxia** (impaired ability to carry out motor activities despite intact motor function)

   c. agnosia (failure to recognize or identify objects despite intact sensory function)

   d. disturbance in **executive functioning** (i.e., planning, organizing, sequencing, abstracting)

B. The cognitive deficits in criteria A1 and A2 each cause significant impairment in social or occupational functioning and represent a significant decline from a previous level of functioning.

C. The course is characterized by gradual onset and continuing cognitive decline.

D. The cognitive deficits in Criteria A1 and A2 are not due to any of the following:

1. Other central nervous system conditions that cause progressive deficits in memory and cognition (e.g., cerebrovascular disease, Parkinson's disease, Huntington's disease, subdural hematoma, normal-pressure hydrocephalus, brain tumor)

2. Systemic conditions that are known to cause dementia (e.g., hypothyroidism, vitamin B_{12} or folic acid deficiency, niacin deficiency, hypercalcemia, neurosyphilis, HIV infection)

3. Substance-induced conditions

E. The deficits do not occur exclusively during the course of delirium.

F. The disturbance is not better accounted for by another Axis I disorder (e.g., Major Depressive Disorder, Schizophrenia).

Code based on type of onset and predominant features:

Without Behavioral Disturbance: if the cognitive disturbance is not accompanied by any clinically significant behavioral disturbance.

With Behavioral Disturbance: if the cognitive disturbance is accompanied by a clinically significant behavioral disturbance (e.g., wandering, agitation).

Specify Subtype:

With Early Onset: if onset is at age 65 years or below

With Late Onset: if onset is after age 65 years

and meeting basic needs. Moreover, structured settings often offer specialized training to employees about FLS, whereby the individual will receive unconditional positive regard.

Progressive Aphasia

Five types of progressive aphasia have been identified: nonfluent, fluent, anomic, mixed, and aphasia associated with motor neuron disease (Weder, Aziz, Wilkins, & Tampi, 2007). Each type differs in the following areas: client understanding, type of language deficit, ability to comprehend written materials, write, and name things. Careful assessments by a neurologist and ongoing speech pathology consultations can assist caregivers with defining exact losses and identifying appropriate compensatory interventions.

Nonfluent aphasia is characterized by halting, effortful, labored speech production, whether expressing original ideas or repeating. The client may still be able to read, and visual memory is generally preserved. Persons with nonfluent aphasia, therefore, may be safe to live alone. They may be able to use language boards, lists, and written materials, and they can generally respond to pictures and signs.

The person with fluent aphasia can produce language, but it is flawed. Comprehension may be impaired and the client often makes paraphasic errors (e.g., calling a couch a "frouch"). The person is unable to recognize and describe things, but she can repeat what is said to her. Persons with fluent aphasia generally have severe language deficits with preserved cognition for about 2 years of an 8-year disease course (Grossman & Ash, 2004; Weder et al., 2007).

Anomia is a pure localized inability to name. Probably the two most troubling progressive aphasias are the mixed type, in which the client demonstrates impairments in all aspects of language, and the aphasia associated with motor neuron disease.

DSM-IV-TR Diagnostic Criteria for Vascular Dementia

A. The development of multiple cognitive deficits manifested by both

1. memory impairment (impaired ability to learn new information or to recall previously learned information)

2. one (or more) of the following cognitive disturbances:

   a. aphasia (language disturbance)

   b. apraxia (impaired ability to carry out motor activities despite intact motor function)

   c. agnosia (failure to recognize or identify objects despite intact sensory function)

   d. disturbance in executive functioning (i.e., planning, organizing, sequencing, abstracting)

B. The cognitive deficits in Criteria A1 and A2 each cause significant impairment in social or occupational functioning and represent a significant decline from a previous level of functioning.

C. Focal neurological signs and symptoms (e.g., exaggeration of deep tendon reflexes, extensor plantar response, pseudobulbar palsy, gait abnormalities, weakness of an extremity), or laboratory evidence indicative of cerebrovascular disease (e.g., multiple infarctions involving cortex and underlying white matter) that are judged to be etiologically related to the disturbance.

D. The deficits do not occur exclusively during the course of a delirium.

Code based on predominant features:

With Delirium: if delirium is superimposed on the dementia

With Delusions: if delusions are the predominant feature

With Depressed Mood: if depressed mood (including presentations that meet full symptom criteria for a Major Depressive Episode) is the predominant feature. A separate diagnosis of Mood Disorder due to a general medical condition is not given.

Uncomplicated: if none of the above dominates in the current clinical presentation

Specify if:

With Behavioral Disturbance

DSM-IV-TR Diagnosis Criteria for Dementia Due to Other General Medical Conditions

A. The development of multiple cognitive deficits manifested by both

1. memory impairment (impaired ability to learn new information or to recall previously learned information)

2. one (or more) of the following cognitive disturbances:

   a. aphasia (language disturbance)

   b. apraxia (impaired ability to carry out motor activities despite intact motor function)

   c. agnosia (failure to recognize or identify objects despite intact sensory function)

   d. disturbance in executive functioning (i.e., planning, organizing, sequencing, abstracting)

B. The cognitive deficits in Criteria A1 and A2 each cause significant impairment in social or occupational functioning and represent a significant decline from a previous level of functioning.

C. There is evidence from the history, physical examination, or laboratory findings that the disturbance is the direct physiological consequence of one of the general medical conditions listed below.

D. The deficits do not occur exclusively during the course of a delirium.

Code based on presence or absence of a clinically significant behavioral disturbance:

Without Behavioral Disturbance: if the cognitive disturbance is not accompanied by any clinically significant behavioral disturbance

With Behavioral Disturbance: if the cognitive disturbance is accompanied by a clinicaly significant behavioral disturbance (e.g., wandering, agitation)

Motor neuronal disease usually advances rapidly and is associated with dysarthria and dysphagia. If diagnosed early the client may be trained in use of alternative communication devices such as a light writer. Swallowing function and management of secretions must be closely monitored with the increasing danger of aspiration. The individual and family need to be counseled regarding advance directives for alternatives to oral feeding.

Persons with progressive aphasias generally may be able to maintain daily function longer than people with global cognitive decline, although they will need assistance with emergency planning and communication aids to live independently. Moreover, because their level of comprehension may be high, persons with progressive aphasia should be evaluated for depression and treated, if present, in order to prevent excess disability and maintain optimum function.

Perceptual-Motor Syndromes

Three perceptual-motor syndromes have been described (Weder et al., 2007). The first two are visual syndromes. Asimultanagnosia limits the client's ability to perceive a common scene as a whole. Although able to understand bits and pieces of their environment, these individuals are unable to comprehend "the big picture." The second, visual agnosia, is a failure to recognize objects and, more commonly, people. The visual perceptual deficits have been well documented by Sacks (1985), who described a case of a music professor who mistook his wife's hand for a hat.

When working with persons with asimultanagnosia, the caregiver must provide continuous verbal input, describing actions and the environment. Clients often learn to rely heavily on other sensory modalities, including hearing, touch, and smell, to function in their environment. Caregivers would want to provide distinct identifying odors and tactile textures to areas of the environment to enable recognition. However, extraneous environmental stimuli, such as large crowds and high noise levels, could potentially add to the person's disability by taxing remaining senses. Sacks (1985) suggests having caregivers wear a single identifying object, such as a brightly colored hat or flower, to assist the client with caregiver recognition.

Persons with visual agnosia do not recognize day-to-day objects. They must be supervised and assisted when using objects, such as feeding utensils, inappropriately. It is not uncommon to see people with visual agnosia put ketchup on their cereal instead of milk or request help to find something while appearing to gaze directly at the object.

The two visual syndromes may confuse direct care providers because although the client is able to "see," vision is often not functionally useful. Having the client describe what she is seeing helps train direct caregivers. For example, a farmer explained that he saw tractors and trees piled atop of one another. Although he recognized the information he was receiving was impaired, he was unable to develop compensatory strategies to enhance function. Ongoing work with occupational therapists and neuropsychological testing can help care providers to modify the environment to meet the client's needs. Services for people who are visually impaired may be helpful for these families. Caregivers must also remain alert for signs and symptoms of auditory and additional sensory deficits that may accompany this syndrome.

The third group of perceptual-motor syndromes is progressive motor syndromes. Clients develop inexorably progressive hemiparesis, hemispasticity, and disabling apraxias. One of the more "common" of these syndromes is corticobasal ganglionic degeneration (CBGD). Over time people with CBGD become increasingly disabled with spasticity and loss of motor planning for purposeful movement. They can develop cramping and contractures. Visual loss may result from impaired eye movement. Speech and swallowing difficulties are common problems. Persons with CBGD have impairments in performance on neuropsychological testing; however, insight into their condition remains and may produce depression or acute anxiety.

With severe apraxias and hemiparesis, occupational and physical therapies can be used to maintain function. Occupational therapists assist by assessing levels of function using task analyses and training caregivers to assist clients with tasks by breaking them into progressively simpler components that clients should be able to perform. Physical therapists assist families by demonstrating passive and active range of motion exercises, positioning, and measures to manage spasticity and maximize function in affected extremities. Clients also report increased comfort with massage therapy.

CRITICAL THINKING

Mr. C has recently been admitted to the geriatric and extended stay unit and during your assessment you ask questions to evaluate his orientation. Which of the following responses may indicate that he is depressed?

a. "I don't know what day of the week it is and I don't care."

b. "Why are you asking me all these dumb questions?"

c. "I believe it's the beginning of the week."

d. a and b.

Answers

a. Correct response (incorrect answer) because this is a common response from depressed older adults.

b. Correct response (incorrect answer) (same as #a)

c. *Incorrect.* This response indicates disorientation about the day of the week and is more indicative of dementia than depression.

d. Correct because a and b are common responses to orientation questions in depressed older adults.

Scrupulous skin care is required to maintain skin integrity and prevent breakdown over bony prominences, in contracted extremities, and in areas exposed to secretions or excreta. Botox injections have been used to release contracted hands, allowing for hygiene when there is danger of skin breakdown.

Accommodations for loss of coordinated eye movements can be accomplished by providing care and activities slowly and simplifying the environment. The slowed purposeful movement accompanied by verbal description can help clients gather more "perceptual information" as they try to focus on activities. Caregivers should try to stand directly in front of clients and place items within the field of vision. Consistent, calm caregiving provides reassurance and continuity when clients are aware of continuing loss of control over their environment. In the final stages of motor syndromes, clients may become immobile and mute. Difficulties with swallowing, coughing, and excretory functions occur in the late stages of the disease. As with any degenerative condition, it is important to determine client care preferences using an advance directive before the onset of aphasia. Clients must be observed for aspiration pneumonia, constipation, urinary retention, and skin breakdown. Bowel and bladder regimens, feeding techniques, range of motion exercises, skin care, and care for immobility must be taught to caregivers.

At the end of the disease, clients become unable to chew or swallow. Rapid weight loss ensues. Providing high-calorie, protein-rich, vitamin-enriched soft foods such as custards can help to maintain weight and nutritional status. A multiple vitamin syrup may also be given. Swallowing studies can determine optimal food consistencies to prevent aspiration. Use of an enteral feeding system may be selected to minimize the danger of aspiration pneumonia. Hospice care is an excellent alternative for care during terminal stages because personnel are trained to manage pain, secretions, fear, and help with family support.

Bitemporal Syndromes

Bitemporal degeneration is characterized by severe progressive amnesia (Short, Broderick, Patton, Arvanitakis, & Graff-Radford, 2005). Clients differ from those with AD in that they lack other areas of cognitive impairment. In a case described by Sacks (1985), a man who appeared to converse and reason in a perfectly normal manner totally forgot the encounter after the neurologist left the room. Sacks describes the man as doomed to repeat the same encounter over and over. Moreover, because the amnesia was so complete, it was impossible to convince the individual of his deficit. The client did not comprehend the passage of time, so he remained "frozen" at age 23. He could not believe that ages of family members increased, thereby arguing over their claims to be his relatives. Because of the severity of the amnestic syndrome, the man could never live independently.

Nursing care of people with amnestic syndrome includes making sure they wear identification because they appear and sound normal. In early stages of the disease, clients may benefit from concrete memory aids such as calendars (marked off by others), schedules, and clocks. Later, careful supervision is required because clients may become lost in all but the most overlearned environments. Direction and supervision would be required for completion of basic daily activities because clients would not know if tasks had not been completed. Moreover, the clients' lack of insight into deficits challenges caregivers to evaluate all statements made by clients—especially answers to questions requiring any memory at all such as "Did you have lunch?"

An environment offering 24-hour supervision would be required to ensure safety and provide the necessary structure. Family and caregiving staff would require extensive ongoing training because clients appear and sound perfectly lucid. Moreover, clients might be vulnerable to dependent adult abuse because caregivers might perceive their actions to be purposeful.

Dementia of the Lewy Body Type (DLB)

Although its relationship to AD is the subject of debate, DLB is thought to be the second most common dementia. Often misdiagnosed, DLB is mistaken for AD with parkinsonian features, AD with psychosis, or Parkinson's disease with AD (Olichney et al., 2005). The early course of the disease closely resembles AD, but with progression the character of the symptoms change to include parkinsonian features, which can include bradykinesia, rigidity, or tremor. Psychotic symptoms appear in about half of cases. The early psychotic symptoms may include paranoid delusions, visual and auditory hallucinations, and illusions accompanied by dementia. These may escalate until the client becomes quite violent or may lose touch with reality altogether. Studies of DLB are small and behavioral findings are often conflicting, but there have been no differences between AD and DLB reported for severity of cognitive decline or duration of illness.

Using medications to control parkinsonian features or to manage psychotic features is difficult owing to competing side effects and increased potential for sensitivity to adverse effects of antipsychotics. Anti-Parkinson's medications are strongly anticholinergic, producing increased confusion and potentiating psychosis, whereas many antipsychotics produce dopamine blockade, worsening symptoms of Parkinson's disease. Moreover, increased susceptibility to neuroleptic malignant syndrome has been noted in people with DLB. For the person with DLB, medications should be used as a last resort. When seeking medications, primary consideration must be given to maintaining safety of both clients and those around them. This may mean focusing and providing dopamine only to clients who are immobile or antipsychotics only to those who are violent owing to psychotic features. There are some studies of the use of acetylcholinesterase inhibitors (donepezil) in persons with DLB, suggesting improved movement and cognition with no increase in psychotic symptoms (Ballard et al., 2007).

Nursing care of the persons with DLB consists of encouraging families to seek appropriate neurological diagnosis and follow-up. Additionally, persons with DLB may be followed by a psychiatrist. These clients require a multidisciplinary approach and, often, several medical subspecialties working in concert.

Much of the care focuses on helping the family to understand the disease process, providing for basic physical care, and safety. Persons with DLB often behave far differently than those with AD or vascular dementias. Families are often in conflict about behavioral presentations because the caregiver may become quite fearful of the client. Moreover, relatives living long distances from the client may express disbelief at caregiver reports of psychotic or aggressive behaviors.

People with DLB are at high risk for falls and injury to themselves from decreased mobility during simple tasks, including eating and drinking. Exercise and range of motion activities may help maintain mobility. A quiet, structured environment with few misleading stimuli may help to minimize hallucinations and combative behaviors. Avoidance of fatigue and caffeine can assist with stability of mood. Yet, despite the best intentions, these clients may become psychotic.

Management of early disease includes careful assessment of psychotic behaviors including descriptions of presenting symptoms; numbers, duration, and timing of episodes; antecedents (triggers) to episodes; and measures that provide relief. Safety hazards must be removed and documented. Even though the client may be a resident of a long-term care setting, careful documentation must be achieved for this client both to plan care and measure outcomes. A primary care approach to staffing using psychiatric consultation, ongoing consultation from psychiatric consultation-liasion nurse (PCLN) (see Chapter 35), and supervision by professional nurses is desirable. Supervisory personnel must evaluate direct caregiving staff for fatigue and burnout that might potentiate employee injury or client abuse. If the person with DLB becomes unmanageably violent, placement in a long-term psychiatric institution where staff are specially trained in management of assault may be required.

Huntington's Disease

Huntington's disease (HD) results in an FLS presentation characterized by intellectual deterioration, and advanced HD results in impairment of memory, intelligence, and verbal fluency. Early stages elicit deficits in learning ability, but verbal fluency is only mildly impaired. Intelligence is within normal ranges. However, memory is more impaired in recognition than are recall tasks. Impairment in long-term memory is present as well as an inability to learn skills. Language functioning is usually intact. Impairments are also seen in visuospatial capacity, along with personal orientation in space. The classic presentation is general chorea, with intensity correlating with the severity of the cognitive

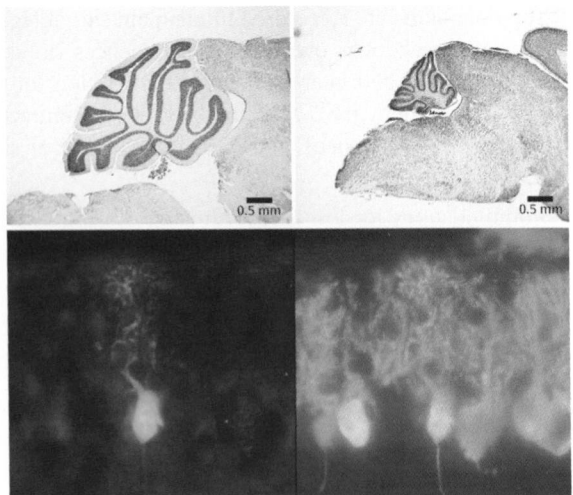

Figure 16–3 Cellular Death. *(From Vogel, M. V. [2005]. Cell death.* American Journal of Psychiatry, 162, *1503. Used with permission.)*

deficits. Mild choreiform movements are present in the earlier stages, but these increase in severity as the disease progresses. The absence of rapid eye movements is the most striking of oculomotor disturbances. See Figure 16–3, Cellular Death, as underpinning of dementia.

Creutzfeldt-Jakob Disease

Creutzfeldt-Jakob disease (CJD) is another form of presenile dementia. It is a progressive, fatal disease of the CNS that usually begins in late life, after age 50. The disease has been observed in younger persons, however. CJD evolves rapidly, with death occurring within 2 years, although its course may be longer. The disease is characterized by loss of neurons in all lobes and the cerebellum, along with a proliferation of hypertrophied astrocytes. The brain takes on a sponge-like appearance, which is termed status spongiosus.

Mental deterioration begins early in CJD, and presents as memory loss, behavioral abnormalities, and higher cortical dysfunction (aphasia, apraxia, agnosia). Myoclonus, early or late in the course of the disease, is characteristic of CJD. Sensory stimuli such as loud noises, flashing lights, movement, or touch can produce myoclonus. Visual disturbances, headache, vertigo, and dizziness are common.

Several types of CJD have been identified. Iatrogenic CJD is a disorder caused by medical treatment with contaminated injections, hormones, and tissue. A second form is thought to be inherited as a result of a mutated prion protein gene which makes the disease more likely. A third type, sporadic CJD, involves cases of the disease that occur randomly throughout the world and have no relationship to familial tendencies or iatrogenesis. A fourth type of CJD has been more recently described. This type is called variant CJD (vCJD) and is linked to bovine spongiform encephalopathy (BSE) (Akhvlediani, Gochitashvili, & Tsertsvadze, 2007). BSE is more popularly known as "mad cow disease" and is transmitted by the consumption of infected animals.

The disease progresses rapidly, and changes can be noted on a daily basis. With progression of the illness, the person becomes bedridden, mute, and unable to move voluntarily. Decerebrate, decorticate posturing and rigidity are common in the later states, and the person eventually lapses into a coma.

The disease is thought to be caused by a specific virus that is highly resistant to destruction. The source of infection and pathogens are considered to be blood, cerebrospinal fluid, and CNS tissue. Universal precautions should be used when caring for a person with CJD to prevent exposure to blood, cerebral fluid, tissues, or urine. A familial history of CJD has been observed in about 10 percent of the cases, consistent with an autosomal dominant mode of inheritance.

Acquired Immune Deficiency Syndrome

Acquired immune deficiency syndrome (AIDS) is one of the most serious health problems confronting our society today. The virus causing the disease, human immunity deficiency virus (HIV), is the infecting organism. An estimated 39.4 million adults and children are living with HIV/AIDS throughout the world (UNAIDS, 2005). Of this number, 94.4 percent are adults, 44.7 percent are women, and 5.6 percent are children less than 15 years of age.

AIDS cases are caused by HIV-infected blood through homosexual or heterosexual contact, transfusions, or mother to child transmission. Most children with AIDS will exhibit central nervous system abnormalities. Deficits in behavioral, motor, and communication abilities are not uncommon. With language skills, expressive language is affected more commonly and profoundly than receptive language skills. AIDS dementia complex (ADC) is frequently misdiagnosed as AD. ADC is a subcortical dementia in which the HIV virus begins to infect the CNS without overt signs of dementia observed. Before clinical symptoms occur, cerebral atrophy may be seen on the CT scan. Early symptoms include gradual cognitive impairment, forgetfulness, problems with concentration, flat affect, poor insight, and indifference. These symptoms may lead to functional disabilities. Balance problems and leg weakness may occur. Behavioral changes vary and are unresponsive to antidepressant medications. There may be verbal and motor slowing, as well as gait ataxia and hyperreflexia. Later, ADC symptoms frequently include a spontaneous tremor or myoclonus, paraparesis, urinary and fecal incontinence, and mutism.

It is estimated that 40 to 70 percent of people with AIDS will develop a discernible neurological syndrome during the course of the illness. In about 10 percent of all HIV-positive persons, the presenting symptom is neurological impairment (Scaravilli, Bazille, & Gray, 2007). Because the disease is spread through body fluids, psychiatric nurses caring for people with an HIV infection must use universal precautions to prevent transmission to themselves.

Korsakoff's Disease or Alcohol Amnestic Disorder

Dementia caused by chronic alcoholism is called Korsakoff's disease (KD). In KD, recent memory is impaired, and these clients fail to learn and remember new information despite the fact that they can effectively retrieve and use previously acquired knowledge. Clients are frequently able to learn and perform complex skills and procedures but are unable to recall the context in which these procedures were learned. There is dissociation between knowing how to do something and recalling what was learned. People with KD frequently lack motivation or initiative and appear apathetic. CNS functions other than memory are usually normal.

OTHER COGNITIVE DISORDERS

The prevalence of various cognitive disorders challenges the psychiatric nurse to recognize patterns and duration of symptoms that assist in making an accurate diagnosis. Even more significant is initiating an appropriate treatment plan that facilitates holistic treatment planning.

Amnestic Disorder Caused by a General Medical Condition

The main features of amnestic syndrome are inability to remember recent events and its relatively uncommon occurrence in children (APA, 2000). It may be found in childhood and adulthood, however, if the individual has experienced head trauma, hypoxia, lead or carbon monoxide poisoning, or herpes simplex encephalitis. It may also be related to alcohol withdrawal, sedative hypnotic, or anxiolytic intoxication in adults. The *DSM-IV-TR* classifies amnestic disorders as those caused by a general medical condition such as physical trauma or vitamin deficiency; Substance Induced Persisting Amnestic Disorder, which includes medications that are prescribed for the client; and Amnestic Disorder Not Otherwise Specified. The primary feature of amnestic disorders is the loss of short-term memory that is directly caused by a physical disorder or a substance such as a medication, alcohol, or a toxin (APA, 2000).

Personality Change Caused by a General Medical Condition

This syndrome is characterized by a persistent personality disturbance, either a lifelong disturbance or a disturbance that represents a change or exaggeration of a previously characteristic trait, caused by a specific organic factor (APA, 2000). Clinical features include emotional instability, aggressive outbursts, impaired social judgment, apathy and, sometimes, suspiciousness and paranoid ideation. Common causes include tumors, head trauma, and cerebrovascular disease.

THE ROLE OF THE NURSE

It is imperative that the nurse understand the normal or common physiological and psychosocial changes that are part of the developmental and aging process. In this way, the nurse can deliver holistic care that empowers the client and family and allows for maximum physical and psychosocial functioning.

THE GENERALIST NURSE

The nurse must recognize the importance of family, the support of significant others, the school, and the community, and include these persons in all stages of the nursing process. Not all older adults are isolated and without family involvement. However, there exists a stereotype, termed "ageism," coined by Butler in 1982, which asserts that all old persons are senile, decrepit, isolated, lonely, and useless. Nothing could be further from the truth. The psychiatric nurse must recognize the valuable resources available to society in the form of our older population.

As we age, individuals are more susceptible to chronic diseases. It is estimated that all persons over age 65 suffer from at least one chronic disease, and those persons in middle age may be beginning to develop chronic disease conditions. Many persons suffer from more than one chronic condition, most commonly, perceptual deficits, especially vision and hearing losses; arthritis, hypertension, and heart disease. It is obvious that as we age, the incidence and frequency of chronic illness increase. As a result, interactions occur between and among the illnesses and drug therapy and may result in psychosocial repercussions. Therefore, it is important for the nurse to be cognizant of concomitant illnesses and their symptoms, as well as the psychosocial effect of these illnesses.

Similarly, the nurse must have knowledge of normal growth and development of younger persons when caring for those with cognitive deficits. Even though the child or adolescent is developmentally challenged because of mental retardation, she is an individual and must be assessed and treated at the appropriate developmental level. By recognizing and intervening, the nurse can take measures to educate and enhance the understanding of developmental and physical changes these clients will experience.

Persons with seizure disorders may or may not have cognitive deficits, and it is important for the nurse to recognize both disabilities and abilities. Providing counseling to those clients and their families is essential in helping the client lead life as normally as possible. A delicate balance may exist between preventing further disability and promoting a healthy emotional life.

When caring for a client with a cognitive disorder, some general guidelines can be followed:

◆ Perform a thorough assessment to ascertain the client's physical, emotional, and mental health status, focusing on strengths and weaknesses. This assessment includes results of diagnostic tests, use of medications, and the course of the disorder.

◆ Explore the client's previous environment and consult with caregivers to develop a care plan that is individu-

alized and will enhance quality of life. Initiate the services of the interdisciplinary team and incorporate recommendations into a total plan of care.

◆ Modify the environment to promote optimal functioning. Most clients with cognitive disorders need structure and modified stimulation, and it is important to identify the client's likes and dislikes to help her feel secure.

◆ Monitor medications and diagnostic tests and be alert for signs and symptoms of delirium, especially in the very young and very old. Monitor the effects of medication and report any untoward effects. If delirium is suspected, implement interventions immediately.

◆ Include the family or primary caregivers in the plan of care. Often these primary caregivers are forgotten when the professional "takes over." Persons who have been caring for these clients can feel "left out" and frustrated if their valuable knowledge and experience is not sought after or used. Educate the family or primary caregiver on the course of the disorder, appropriate medications, signs of illness, and the need to take care of their own health.

◆ Initiate the services of the case manager or social worker to help coordinate continuity of care and obtain the necessary support services across the continuum of health care and home settings.

◆ If the client is in the school system, involve teachers, the school nurse, school counselors, and parents in the plan of care. Individualized Education Plans (IEP) foster input from all involved individuals and promote optimal development in the client with a cognitive disorder.

THE ADVANCED-PRACTICE PSYCHIATRIC REGISTERED NURSE

In addition to guidelines for the generalist nurse, the advanced-practice psychiatric registered nurse (APRN) performs according to her licensure or role in an agency. An APN can be either a nurse practitioner or a clinical nurse specialist. In general, the advanced-practice psychiatric nurse practitioner and clinical nurse specialist function independently in mental health and primary care settings. However, the roles and functions of APRNs may vary from region to region depending on state boards of nursing.

The APN can evaluate clients with mental retardation, seizure disorders, and FAS. In doing so, the APN can make recommendations for interventions that can minimize disability. This may include activities such as ordering and assessing diagnostic tests and prescribing appropriate medications. Working with pregnant women and teaching about the importance of abstaining from alcohol can be a large role of the APN, along with counseling and psychotherapy that target problematic behaviors of the expectant mother. Additionally, the psychiatric APN can develop treatment plans for persons with cognitive disorders, working with families, staff, and the community to educate and enhance quality of life. The APN may function as a case manager, educator, researcher, or primary care mental health provider.

For the older adult client, the psychiatric APN or gerontologic APN can be involved in caring for older adults with cognitive disorders. The APN makes differential diagnoses, orders diagnostic laboratory studies, and collaborates with primary care providers to rule out medical and psychiatric disorders. An astute APN can elicit causes of delirious states through careful evaluation of diagnostic tests, medications, and physical state. She can prescribe appropriate medications for the disorder, such as CEIs for clients with AD, or medications to treat dysfunctional behaviors and psychotic symptoms. Of course, medications targeted at controlling behaviors must only be prescribed after careful assessment of contributing factors has been done. Most likely, the environment can be modified and use of unnecessary drugs can be avoided. Regardless of where the client enters the health care continuum, the APN is part of an interdisciplinary team that develops an integrated plan of care for the client with Alzheimer's disease and other cognitive disorders.

For clients of all ages, the APN can track the client's progress using psychometrically sound instruments such as the mini mental state exam or a depression rating scale. Depression left unrecognized and untreated can result in excess disability and diminished functioning. Family or caregiver counseling and teaching can take place on an individual basis or in a group setting. APNs can conduct or facilitate support groups for the family or caregivers of clients with a cognitive disorder, and even the client herself.

An important function of the APN is to use research that results in the best practices in caring for persons with cognitive disorders. The APN can be a change agent in transforming an environment from one of chaos and confusion to one of structure and security using models such as the PLST model of care. Many models of care and nursing interventions can be implemented in the institutional or home setting, and the APN can guide caregivers in this implementation and facilitate changes that may need to be made.

Finally, the APRN functions in a leadership capacity by role modeling, teaching, and providing resources for caregivers of persons with cognitive disorders. Through advanced education and experience, the APN is in a position to institute change and support others through the stages of making changes. Leadership abilities enhance credibility and respect for the APRN, and the nursing profession.

COLLABORATION

The interdisciplinary team is important in designing comprehensive, holistic care for the person who is ill. This team consists of nurses, physicians, social workers, teachers and, possibly, special therapists such as physical and occupational therapists. The interdisciplinary team can develop a plan of inpatient and outpatient care that is appropriate for the person who is ill and her family on both inpatient and outpatient bases. Community resources such as partial hospitalization, special education, case management, day programs, assisted living, visiting nurses, and respite are examples. In caring for the cognitively impaired child or adult, it is necessary for the psychiatric nurse to recognize the importance of caring for the caregiver as well. With a healthy caregiver, positive outcomes are possible. If a caregiver becomes physically or psychologically ill because of the burdens of caregiving, dire consequences can result. It is not uncommon for the caregiver of a cognitively impaired person to develop physical illness or even die because of the physical and psychological demands of caregiving. Therefore, it is important to follow through with comprehensive community support through work with the interdisciplinary team.

MEDICAL DIAGNOSIS AND MANAGEMENT

Cognitive disorders are complex and often result from underlying general medical conditions. It is imperative for the psychiatric nurse to collaborate with various health care providers and discern underlying causes. This process involves a comprehensive physical examination, psychosocial assessment, mental status examination, and developmental screening as appropriate.

SPECIFIC DISEASE STATES

Cognitive disorders may be classified as potentially reversible or probable irreversible conditions. Potentially reversible conditions are common and frequently unrecognized by health care professionals. If a potentially reversible condition is not recognized, the condition may develop into an irreversible condition, and may even result in death.

DATA COLLECTION

For any cognitive disorder, the emphasis of data collection is on the underlying general medical or psychiatric condition. A thorough history, mental status assessment, medical examination, behavioral observations, neurological evaluation, neuropsychological testing, and selected laboratory tests are all essential components of the diagnosis and treatment of the organic mental disorders and syndromes.

SYMPTOMATOLOGY

There are a limited number of cognitive disorders, but there are innumerable conditions that give rise to them. The psychological condition can result in several different clinical syndromes, and thus the psychiatric manifestations of a depends more on the disease process itself than on etiology. For example, the psychiatric symptoms associated with a brain tumor depend not only on the cellular morphology but also on the location, size, and extent of tissue involvement and speed with which the tumor is growing. The clinical expression of symptoms may also be affected by the person's genetic makeup, intelligence, premorbid personality, support network, coping mechanisms, environment, and past experiences.

HISTORY

The history probably provides the most important clues to the etiology of the cognitive disorder. The history indicates whether the psychiatric symptoms are acute or chronic, whether they change throughout the day and night, whether there are any recent psychosocial stressors, whether the client's medication or health status has changed recently, and so on. The review of systems, medical history, social history, school history, past psychiatric history, family psychiatric history, and description of the current symptoms are essential for making an accurate diagnosis of underlying etiology for the psychiatric symptoms.

DIAGNOSTIC TESTS

In the medical examination, the physician and other health care providers look for any underlying medical disorders that might cause the symptoms associated with cognitive disorders. The neurological evaluation is not usually helpful when the psychiatric symptoms are caused by a medical condition. The neurological examination is usually normal and remains so until the disorder or disease is far advanced.

Neuropsychological Testing

Neuropsychological testing is only a quantitative assessment of several specific behaviors. Cognitive impairment found through neuropsychological testing is no more certain evidence of treatable disorders than is cognitive impairment demonstrated by a mental status assessment. The neuropsychological test may be helpful when a cognitive disorder is suspected, but it cannot be substantiated on the basis of other diagnostic measures (i.e., history, physical examination, mental status assessment, and laboratory tests). It may reveal subtle but undeniable losses that point toward the underlying medical condition. Neuropsychological testing is also very useful in measuring changes in function over time. The nurse can continue to monitor the disease by administering psychometrically sound instruments such as the mini mental state exam (MMSE), cognitive capacity screening tool (CCST), and others.

Laboratory and Radiologic Testing

Laboratory testing includes a blood chemistry profile (urine and blood cultures if sepsis is suspected), a complete blood count with differential, a venereal disease research laboratory (VDRL) test, a urinalysis, B_{12}, folate, an electrocardiogram, thyroid function tests, and a toxicology screen. A test for Lyme disease may be ordered, because a form of dementia can result from this infection. Further evaluation with a chest x-ray, CT scan of the brain, MRI, and a CSF examination is indicated if the cause has not yet been determined. An EEG is used for new onset and recurring seizure activity.

Ancillary Diagnostic Procedures

Ancillary diagnostic procedures are essential to the search for the etiology of cognitive disorders. These include neurodiagnostic procedures, such as electroencephalography, average evoked responses, as well as an array of biochemical measures of bodily function. Additional diagnostic tests used in the diagnosis of cognitive disorders include computed tomography (CT) of the brain, positron emission tomography (PET) imaging of the brain, and magnetic resonance imaging (MRI).

Differential Diagnosis

Differential diagnosis of cognitive disorders from other psychiatric diagnoses rests primarily on evidence gathered from the history, physical examination, or laboratory tests of a specific factor judged to be etiologically related to the disorder. There are three types of diagnostic errors related to cognitive disorders. The first error is when there is failure to determine the etiology for psychiatric symptoms; the second diagnostic error is made when the disorder is diagnosed and there is none; and the third error is made when a diagnosis of only one disorder is made when, in fact, more than one are present.

Medical Diagnosis

Diagnosis is based on symptoms, results of physical examination and history, and *DSM III-R-TR (IV)* criteria. Diagnostic criteria for delirium, dementia, and ADHD are presented in the *DSM-IV-TR* boxes in this chapter.

The methods described for collecting data to diagnose and treat general medical disorders and syndromes are very complex and often do not yield definitive results. The progression from history and psychiatric interview to medical examination, observation of behavioral changes, and ancillary diagnostic procedures may or may not lead to an etiologic explanation for the psychiatric symptoms. The nurse who cares for persons with mental disorders must learn to function comfortably within a complex framework in which diagnostic uncertainty often prevails.

THE NURSING PROCESS

Throughout this chapter, emphasis is on the role of psychiatric nurses in caring for the client with a cognitive disorder. Nurses play essential roles in identification of symptoms, collaborating with various health care providers to initiate holistic treatment planning, and monitoring the client's response to individualized interventions. In addition, because of the emotional and physical demands placed on caregivers, their needs and participation must also be an integral part of treatment planning.

ASSESSMENT

The psychiatric interview must contain a description of the client's mental status with a thorough description of behavior, flow of thought and speech, affect, thought processes and mental content, sensorium and intellectual resources, cognitive status, insight, and judgment. Serial assessment of psychiatric status is necessary for determining fluctuating course and acute changes in mental status. Interviews with family members should be included and can be crucial in the treatment of infants and young children with cognitive disorders. In interviews with children and adolescents, it is essential to include developmental screening.

NURSING DIAGNOSES

Nursing diagnoses for persons with organic mental syndromes or disorders include:

- Disturbed thought processes
- Acute confusion
- Chronic confusion
- Impaired verbal communication
- Risk for injury
- Risk for other-directed violence
- Disturbed sensory perception
- Impaired memory
- Delayed growth and development
- Risk for interrupted family processes
- Risk for altered bonding and attachment

Other nursing diagnoses that may be seen with cognitive disorders are: Noncompliance; Situational low self-esteem; Disturbed sleep pattern; and Impaired social interaction.

Etiology of the nursing diagnosis depends on the medical diagnosis. For example, if the person has chronic confusion related to AD, the etiology could be MID, Korsakoff's psychosis, AD, or CVA. If a person has acute confusion related to delirium, the etiology could be age over 60 years, alcohol abuse, delirium, dementia, and drug abuse.

Defining characteristics target behaviors that need attention. Defining characteristics of chronic confusion related to probable irreversible brain damage could be any or all of the following: altered interpretation/response to stimuli, clinical evidence of physical and mental impairment, progressive/longstanding cognitive impairment, altered personality, impaired memory (short- and long-term); impaired socialization, or no change in level of consciousness.

With Hall's model, defining characteristics could include the following losses as described previously: cognitive, affective, conative, and progressively lowered stress threshold.

Defining characteristics of altered growth and development may include any or all of the following: delay or difficulty in performing skills (motor, social, expressive) typical of age group, inability to perform self-care or self-control activities appropriate for age, flat affect, listlessness, and decreased responses.

PLANNING

Treatment outcomes for cognitive disorders that are potentially treatable differ from disorders that are probably untreatable. In addition, outcome measures that are developmentally appropriate should be used. The psychiatric nurse individualizes care and sets realistic goals.

OUTCOME IDENTIFICATION FOR ACUTE CONFUSION

It is expected that the client with a potentially reversible dementia will be determined by the individual's premorbid personality. Possible outcomes are:

- Full recovery
- Progression to an irreversible organic brain syndrome
- Progression to a functional psychosis
- Death

Although full recovery is common, it is not always swift. Despite effective treatment, delirium may be prolonged, especially in the older adult. Full recovery is most difficult with the client who manifests a variety of emotional sequelae. Progression to an irreversible cognitive disorder sometimes occurs, especially in those cases in which the etiology cannot be treated effectively. Progression to functional psychosis has been documented, but the incidence is low. Finally, death does occur in some people with a delirium, but it is presumed that for the most part, death is due to the diseases that caused the delirium and is not a result of the delirium itself.

OUTCOME IDENTIFICATION FOR CHRONIC CONFUSION

Because this condition will probably not improve, it is essential to measure outcomes against cerebral pathology. In order to evaluate the plan of care, the psychiatric nurse must objectively evaluate client comfort and safety using the following measures (Hall, 1991, 1997; Smith et al., 2004):

- The number of hours the client sleeps at night should increase, and episodes of confused night wakening should decrease.
- The client's weight should stabilize or increase without special supplements. Food intake at mealtimes should increase, and caloric expenditure will decrease as pacing and agitation disappear.
- Episodes of combative behavior will be eliminated. Agitated episodes will diminish or be eliminated.
- The client's degree of socialization, including voluntary participation in small-group activities, should increase.
- Functional level may improve briefly as excess disability disappears.

- The need for sedatives and tranquilizers should decrease.
- Once family members understand the care program, their satisfaction with the care plan and empathy with the staff should increase.

IMPLEMENTATION

Nursing interventions must be individualized according to the client's needs. When addressing client needs, the developmental level as well as cognitive ability must be considered. Family members should be involved to the fullest extent possible.

Delirium Management

Delirium management is the provision of a safe and therapeutic environment for the individual who is experiencing an acute confusional state.

Activities include: identify etiological factors causing delirium; initiate therapies to reduce or eliminate factors causing the delirium; provide unconditional positive regard; provide the client with information about what is happening and what can be expected to occur in the future; avoid demands for abstract thinking, if the client can think only in concrete terms; limit the need for decision making, if frustrating/confusing to the client; respond to the theme/feeling or tone, rather than the content, of the hallucination or delusion; remove stimuli, when possible, that create misperception in a particular client (e.g., pictures on the wall or television); maintain a well-lit environment that reduces sharp contrasts and shadows; inform client of person, place, and time, as needed; provide a consistent physical environment and daily routine; provide caregivers who are familiar to the client; use environmental cues (e.g., signs, pictures, clocks, calendars, and color coding of environment) to stimulate memory, reorient, and promote appropriate behavior; provide a low-stimulation environment for client in whom disorientation is increased by overstimulation.

Dementia Management

Dementia management is the provision of a modified environment for the person who is experiencing a chronic confusional state.

Activities include: include family members in planning, providing, and evaluating care, to the extent desired; identify usual patterns of behavior for such activities as sleep, medication use, elimination, food intake, and self-care; determine physical, social, and psychological history of the client, usual habits, and routines; determine type and extent of cognitive deficit(s) using standardized assessment tool; monitor cognitive functioning using a standardized assessment tool; provide a low-stimulation environment (e.g., quiet, soothing music; nonvivid and simple, familiar patterns in décor; performance expectations that do not exceed cognitive processing ability; and dining in small groups); provide a consistent physical environment and daily routine; give one simple direction at a time; speak in a clear, low, warm, respectful tone of voice; use distraction, rather than confrontation, to manage behavior; provide unconditional positive regard; provide caregivers who are familiar to the client (e.g., avoid frequent rotations of staff assignments); avoid unfamiliar situations, when possible (e.g., room changes and appointments without familiar people); provide rest periods to prevent fatigue and reduce stress; monitor nutrition and weight; avoid frustrating the client by quizzing with orientation questions that cannot be answered; provide cues—such as current events, seasons, location, and names—to assist orientation; select television or radio activities based on cognitive processing abilities and limit the number of choices the client has to make, so as not to cause anxiety; avoid use of physical restraints; monitor carefully for physiological causes of increased confusion that may be acute and reversible.

Limit Setting

Limit setting is establishing the parameters of desirable and acceptable client behavior. Activities include: discuss concerns with client about behavior; establish reasonable expectations for client behavior, based on the situation and the client; establish consequences (with client input, when appropriate) for occurrence/nonoccurrence of desired behaviors; communicate the established behavioral expectations and consequences to the client in language that is easily understood and nonpunitive; communicate established behavioral expectations and consequences with other staff who are caring for the client; modify behavioral expectations and consequences, as needed, to accommodate reasonable changes in the client's situation; initiate the established consequences for the occurrence/nonoccurrence of the desired behaviors; decrease limit setting, as individual behavior approximates the desired behaviors.

Medication Management

At times, clients with delirium may be so agitated, assaultive, or paranoid that immediate symptomatic control is required, either to prevent these clients from harming themselves and others or to quiet them sufficiently for medical evaluation and treatment to be accomplished. Sometimes clients must be treated symptomatically even before a definite diagnosis can be made. The antipsychotics and nonbenzodiazepines are the drugs most often used to help control patients in these out-of-control situations. There is little evidence that one group is more effective than another in managing delirium. Each class of medication has certain advantages and disadvantages. The choice is often made on the basis of the specific effect desired or the specific side effect to be avoided. Many of the same medications are used to manage the behaviors of the person with a probable irreversible dementia.

It is imperative that behaviors be monitored before the medication is implemented to determine possible external causes of the behavior such as stimuli, time of day, or a certain caregiver. It is then important to monitor behaviors after beginning medication management to determine the effect of the medication. In addition, the client should be monitored for possible side effects on a continual basis, particularly because the client is likely unable to voice concerns. The following is an overview of medications used for delirium and dementia. For a more in-depth discussion of these medications, refer to Chapter 29, Psychopharmacologic Therapy.

Of the antipsychotic medications, recent studies indicate the atypical agents have fewer extrapyramidal side effects than the older agents. Examples of atypical antipsychotic medications include quetiapine (Seroquel) and risperidone (Risperdal). Although these agents have a more positive side effect profile than typical antipsychotics, major side effects include weight gain, diabetes, and metabolic disturbances. Similar to the administration of all psychotropic agents, the client's vital signs and mental status must be closely monitored and documented. Psychoeducation must be an integral part of nursing interventions that include both the client and family members.

Because the incidence of extrapyramidal side effects (especially acute dystonic reactions) is high with antipsychotic agents, particularly with adolescents and young adults, it may be necessary to give benztropine mesylate (Cogentin) with the antipsychotic agent. In older adults, it may not be advisable to add a medication such as Cogentin for two reasons. First, older adults do not demonstrate the dystonic reactions as frequently as young persons do. Secondly, it may be desirable to avoid the use of potent anticholinergic agents

unless they are essential. With chronic use of antipsychotics, the client must be monitored with the Abnormal Involuntary Movement Scale (AIMS). Older adults are at higher risk for tardive dyskinesia (see Chapter 29).

The benzodiazepines must be used sparingly in the client with cognitive disturbances to reduce sedation, cognitive disturbances, and risk of falls and fractures. This is particularly significant when treating delirium. Long-acting agents should be avoided in older clients due to their long half-lives and potential to worsen cognitive states and produce ataxia.

Not all clients with delirium or dementia require psychopharmacologic agents for relief or control of their symptoms. On the contrary, because these conditions are manifestations of altered cerebral metabolism and because psychopharmacologic agents further alter cerebral metabolism, the possibility that these agents will cause further damage is very real.

Pharmacologic treatment of the symptoms of delirium and dementia is necessary when:

◆ The symptoms interfere seriously with medical evaluation or treatment.

◆ The individual's behavior is dangerous to self or others.

◆ The symptoms cause the client intense personal distress.

Specific symptoms targeted for treatment include: intense anxiety, fearfulness, paranoid delusion, insomnia, hallucinations, irritability, intense anger, restlessness, incessant

CASE STUDY

The Client with Alzheimer's Disease (Mrs. Miller)

Mrs. Miller is a 77-year-old female who was admitted to the SCU (special care unit) of a local nursing facility 2 years ago with a diagnosis of Alzheimer's disease, diagnosed 5 years previously. She is in the third stage of AD, moving quickly to the fourth. She had been living in her home with live-in help until her admission, but her mental condition had deteriorated so much that it was unwise to keep her at home. She became increasingly dependent in her activities of daily living (ADLs), began wandering, and experiences night wakening. Her caretaker was unable to cope. It was felt that Mrs. Miller should be placed near her younger son in a nursing facility. Mrs. Miller also has another daughter and son who live in another state. Mrs. Miller's only other diagnosis is emphysema with no presenting symptoms and for which she is not treated. Mrs. Miller takes only a multiple vitamin daily, and prn medication for constipation.

Mrs. Miller is dependent in all ADLs. Her son visits infrequently, because Mrs. Miller no longer recognizes him and it is distressing for him to see her with such cognitive decline. Most of the day, Mrs. Miller wanders around her room, chattering and tearing the bedsheets off the beds. She does respond to her name and seems to recognize her frequent caregivers, whom she wants to touch and hug.

Mrs. Miller's speech is jargon, with many words meaningless to others. When focused by staff, she will follow simple directions, will dance with staff, and even hum along to old-time songs when staff are singing to her. Mrs. Miller hates to be left alone and will eat only if she can sit on someone's lap or at least very near the person. She will not nap unless someone lies in bed with her to get her to sleep.

Mrs. Miller's communication is limited. At times her speech is spontaneous—"Leave me alone," when someone is doing something she doesn't like, such as combing her hair, and profanity comes easily, illustrating the lowered inhibitions frequently observed in persons with AD. Sometimes she will cry for no apparent reason but accepts the comfort offered by the staff. Mrs. Miller detests bathing or showering, and this is one of the most difficult aspects of her care. Staff is very affectionate with Mrs. Miller and she seems appreciative of this acceptance.

Mrs. Miller responds well to touch, which is her main form of communication. Her attention is focused only on certain cues, which include touch, imitation of her chattering, and singing. She listens briefly when her name is called and, when in distress, Mrs. Miller is able to make appropriate sounds. Her language

(continues)

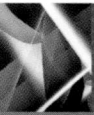

and reality base have been altered because of her cognitive deficits, but she is able to interpret affection and caring with an applicable response. According to her family, Mrs. Miller has never wanted to be alone, and this social response remains intact. She frequently reaches out for caregivers as they pass her by. Her attention span is poor, but hugging, dancing, or singing will maintain her focus for several minutes at a time. She is unable to participate actively in communication unless directed by staff. Her major strength is her love of human contact and the warm manner in which she responds to touch.

When developing interventions for Mrs. Miller, her primary mode of communication must be considered. Touch and affection are used to get her attention and to comfort her when she is distressed. The staff of the nursing facility were able to use several of the interventions that flow from the PLST model and incorporated in *NIC:*

1. Always call Mrs. Miller by name whenever communicating with her. Identify yourself. In this way, Mrs. Miller's attention can be focused, even if for only moments, and her social role can be preserved.

   Rationales:

   a. Calling by name attracts the client's attention; using surname preserves dignity and social role.

   b. Short-term memory loss inhibits a client with AD from remembering. Identifying self helps the client "save face" and may orient the client to the nurse's position.

2. Use touch and hugs whenever possible except when Mrs. Miller is not receptive (when she is angry). Mrs. Miller is particularly dependent on nonverbal language, and is able to actively participate in physical touch and communication.

   Rationales:

   a. Client may not be receptive to touch if angry.

   b. Dependence on nonverbal language necessitates using touch or exaggerated facial expressions.

3. Use exaggerated facial expressions and gestures when communicating. This will enhance verbal communication with nonverbal cues.

   Rationales:

   a. Exaggerated facial expressions help to convey verbal information.

   b. Clients with AD tend to lose the ability to understand verbal communication.

4. Mimic Mrs. Miller's jargon to get her attention, then proceed with the task at hand.

   Rationales:

   a. This intervention will serve to catch the client's attention.

   b. Clients with AD may not be able to understand more than one step at a time.

5. Sing with Mrs. Miller, perhaps dance with her too.

   Rationales:

   a. In order to have an effective quiet time together, engage clients with AD in activities they enjoy.

   b. A sense of security and congruity with the environment and caregivers can be achieved by keying into the symbolic meaning of the client's attempts at communication.

6. Make sure Mrs. Miller is an active participant in communication and other interactions. Do not talk about Mrs. Miller or others in her presence.

   Rationales:

   a. Active participation in an interaction will serve to facilitate the client's communication and enhance a sense of security.

   b. To preserve the client's social functioning and dignity, do not exclude her from conversations when she is present.

7. Redirect inappropriate behavior: if angry or hostile, leave and return in 5 minutes or have another caregiver take over.

   Rationales:

   a. Because of impairments in communication, it is fruitless for staff to explain or reason with her.

   b. Use whatever communication abilities the client possesses at the time, and do not expect more than that of which she is capable.

(continues)

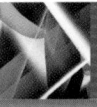

CASE STUDY *(continued)*

8. Provide for assistance in activities of daily living. Bathe, dress, and groom Mrs. Miller in privacy, taking one step at a time.

   Rationales:

   a. The psychiatric nurse acts as a "prosthetic memory" for clients with AD.

   b. Privacy is essential for all clients with AD during hygiene procedures.

   c. Clients with AD may be unable to understand more than one step at a time because of conative losses.

9. Provide for adequate nutrition. Because of Mrs. Miller's wandering and fear of being alone, it is necessary to have her sit on the caregiver's lap to be spoon fed.

   Rationales:

   a. Clients with AD are frequently unable to attend to task at hand.

   b. Nutritional considerations are important for clients with AD because of changes in glucose metabolism, frequent nonstop activity, and forgetting to eat.

10. Provide for rest periods. It is frequently necessary for a caregiver to lie in bed with Mrs. Miller in order to get her to rest.

    Rationales:

    a. Rest periods are important in preventing fatigue and subsequent anxiety and dysfunctional behavior.

    b. Some clients require unusual interventions to facilitate rest.

11. Provide for safety. Keep all toxic materials such as cleaning fluids, perfumes, and even some plants out of reach. Assess her walking ability and provide for rest if she seems unsteady. Because of diminished perceptions and interpretation of the environment, keep furniture arranged in a way that maximizes safe ambulation. Keep all areas well lit and avoid glare.

    Rationales:

    a. Clients with AD have poor judgment and may consume toxic substances.

    b. Because of age-associated changes in vision and gait, the client is at risk for falling.

---

hyperactivity, assaultiveness, and self-injurious actions. Older adults or debilitated clients should receive one third to one half of the initial recommended dosage of antipsychotic or anxiolytic medication, and then adjustments made upward or downward, depending on the response of the client. When treating symptoms of delirium, the problem is most often the appropriate amount rather than the drug of choice. Too little will be ineffective; too much may be toxic and may actually worsen the delirium. The client's condition must be assessed repeatedly and interventions initiated to keep implications, but when used in the right child for the right reasons, it seems highly effective in ameliorating target behaviors and providing impetus for change in other areas.

EVALUATION

Evaluation of the medical and nursing diagnoses relies greatly on etiologic factors and defining characteristics and should be an ongoing process during intervention. Outcomes for cognitive disorders that are potentially reversible will be different from those that are probably irreversible, and measures that are developmentally appropriate should

be used. It is important for the psychiatric nurse to individualize care and set realistic outcomes or goals. The *NOC* outcome labels and indicators can be used to set goals and determine the extent to which an indicator is achieved.

SUMMARY

◆ Cognitive disorders can affect people across the life span and have many causes.

◆ Psychiatric nurses are in pivotal positions to identify high risk behaviors and offer health education to minimize risk factors.

◆ Researchers are on the cusp of making new discoveries that explain biological and genetic underpinnings of various disorders, such as, mental retardation and the role of environmental factors.

◆ By understanding these complex causative factors psychiatric nurses become more adept at developing comprehensive and holistic treatment planning when caring for the client with a cognitive disorder.

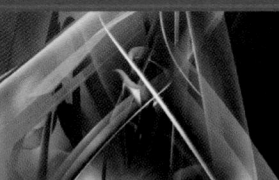

The Client with Alzheimer's Disease (Mrs. Miller)

Nursing Diagnosis: Chronic Confusion
related to progressive and long-standing cognitive impairment

Outcome Identification	Nursing Actions	Rationales	Evaluation
1. By [date], the number of hours Mrs. Miller sleeps at night will increase, and episodes of confused night wakening will decrease.	1a. Identify Mrs. Miller's usual sleep patterns.	1a. Familiar habits are easy to implement and comforting to client.	*Goal met:* Mrs. Miller is able to sleep 6 hours throughout night without waking. Documentation:
	1b. Provide structured rest periods.	1b. Periodic rest prevents accumulation of stress and facilitates relaxation.	Document number of hours slept and night wakenings.
	1c. Provide low-stimulation environment.	1c. Low or modified stimulation prevents anxiety and promotes relaxation.	
2. By [date], Mrs. Miller's weight will stabilize or increase without special supplements.	2a. Identify Mrs. Miller's usual eating patterns.	2a. Familiarity with foods and rituals optimizes clients' eating abilities.	*Goal met:* Client will maintain or gain weight. Documentation:
	2b. Seat Mrs. Miller at small table in group of three to five or seat her alone at a table.	2b. Because of clients' inability to process multiple stimuli, eating in small groups or alone reduces stimuli.	Document weight and possibly caloric intake if client is undernourished.
	2c. Provide finger foods.	2c. Client may be unable to sit to eat but will eat finger foods while moving, thus taking in adequate nutrition.	
	2d. Decrease noise levels while Mrs. Miller is eating.	2d. Noise distracts clients from eating.	
3. By [date], episodes of combative or agitated behavior will be eliminated or diminished.	3a. Determine Mrs. Miller's physical, social, and psychological histories to find familiar interventions.	3a. Clients find comfort in the familiar and are likely to be more cooperative.	*Goal met:* Episodes of agitation and combative behavior decrease.

(continues)

Nursing Care Plan 16–1 (continued)

Outcome Identification	Nursing Actions	Rationales	Evaluation
	3b. Determine appropriate behavioral expectations for Mrs. Miller.	3b. Depending on orientation level, behaviors may or may not be alterable. It is important to set realistic goals.	Documentation: Document episodes of confusion/agitation/combative behavior on log; who, what, when, how, why.
	3c. Identify potential changes in Mrs. Miller's environment.	3c. Because of poor judgment, clients may misinterpret the environment, causing harm or injury.	
	3d. Provide consistent routine and environment.	3d. Consistency provides predictability and security for memory-impaired clients.	
	3e. Use touch and unconditional positive regard when interacting with Mrs. Miller.	3e. Communication, especially nonverbal, determines the tone of interactions.	
	3f. Avoid situations that are unfamiliar to Mrs. Miller.	3f. The unfamiliar is frightening to memory-impaired clients and can cause catastrophic behaviors.	
	3g. Provide structured rest periods.	3g. Rest periods allow clients' stress level to return to baseline.	
	3h. Decrease noise levels and stimulation.	3h. Overstimulation leads to increased confusion and agitation.	
	3i. Monitor causes of increased confusion in Mrs. Miller.	3i. Agitation and confusion may be caused by fatigue, changes, stimuli, demands, and physiological disorders.	
4. By [date], Mrs. Miller's socialization will increase.	4a. Determine Mrs. Miller's previous history of socialization.	4a. Clients are more likely to participate in familiar activities.	*Goal met:* Mrs. Miller's socializing increases.
	4b. Select activities (using TV or radio carefully) for Mrs. Miller based on her interests.	4b. Client may not be able to tolerate the stimulation of the TV or radio.	Documentation: Document participation in activities and episodes of socialization.
	4c. Select one-to-one activities as appropriate.	4c. Because of clients' diminished ability to tolerate stimuli, one-to-one and small-group activities are best.	

(continues)

Nursing Care Plan 16–1 (*continued*)

Outcome Identification	Nursing Actions	Rationales	Evaluation
	4d. Label familiar pictures and objects.	4d. This practice assists caregivers and visitors in identifying important items, events, and people in client's life, and provides opportunity for socialization through reminiscence.	
5. By [date], Mrs. Miller's functional level may improve briefly as excess disability disappears.	5a. Determine Mrs. Miller's functional history prior to confusion.	5a. It is unrealistic to expect clients to function differently from previous optimal level.	*Goal met:* Mrs. Miller's functional ability improves.
	5b. Provide consistency in all daily activities.	5b. Consistency reduces feeling of insecurity and fear, and enables clients to concentrate on task at hand.	Documentation: Observe ability to perform self-care and document actions that facilitate functioning.
	5c. Decrease multiple competing stimuli in Mrs. Miller's environment.	5c. Competing stimuli precipitate frustration and inability to accomplish tasks.	
	5d. Limit the number of choices Mrs. Miller has to make.	5d. Clients can concentrate on only one or two choices at a time. Breaking down tasks into steps helps simplify and promote self-care.	
	5e. Provide positive feedback.	5e. Provides encouragement to clients.	
	5f. Instruct family and staff that it may be impossible for Mrs. Miller to learn new tasks.	5f. Because of loss of cerebral cortex function, new material cannot be learned, and it is frustrating to all for clients to try.	
	5g. Refrain from using physical restraints.	5g. Physical restraints inhibit movement and self-care and cause frustration and agitation.	

SUGGESTIONS FOR CLINICAL CONFERENCE

1. List the suggestions a nurse could give the parents of a 9-year-old mildly mentally retarded boy regarding limit setting in the home.

2. List the nursing interventions for a 20-year-old client recently admitted to the hospital for evaluation of grand mal seizures.

3. Discuss the differences and similarities between dementia and delirium in the older adult, and specify assessment and intervention strategies for dementia and delirium.

4. Discuss why it is important to distinguish between reversible and irreversible disorders. What nursing implications are different?

5. Identify the topics that need to be reviewed in the education of the parents of a 7-year-old child who has grand mal seizures.

STUDY QUESTIONS

1. Ms. Johnson is 2 months pregnant and seeking crisis intervention to deal with a recent separation from spouse of 2 years. During the assessment process, she acknowledges drinking several times a week. Which of the following is the most important nursing intervention during the assessment?
   a. Provide health education about the effects of alcohol and fetal alcohol syndrome (FAS).
   b. Make appropriate referrals for prenatal care.
   c. Instruct her to calm down because of the potential effects of stress.
   d. Encourage her to attend parenting classes.

2. Mr. Jones has recently been discharged after being diagnosed with vascular dementia. His family brings him in today for an evaluation because he is having problems with his memory. What is the most nursing appropriate response?
   a. "Tell me what you understand about your loved one's condition."
   b. "You must take him back to the emergency room immediately."
   c. "You really do not need to worry, his memory will clear up."
   d. "With plenty of therapy, his memory will improve."

3. Mr. Murphy has been admitted to the Alzheimer's Unit to provide respite care for his wife. Based on your understanding of Alzheimer's disease, what is a major implication for the psychiatric nurse?
   a. Mr. Jones is likely to have fluctuation in his sensorium.
   b. Mr. Jones will benefit from explaining and teaching concerning the unit.
   c. Mr. Jones will benefit from having the same caregiver for a week.
   d. Mr. Jones may have periods when he is forgetful, but he will benefit from frequent orientation.

4. Miss Miller is an 86-year-old retired physician who is seen in the psychiatric emergency room. Her son reports that over the past few days she has been very confused and combative. The most important question to ask her son is?
   a. "Does mental illness run in your family?"
   b. "Has she been started on any new medications recently?"
   c. "How often do you visit your mother?"
   d. "When was the last time you saw her like this?"

5. Mr. Ekpa, an 88-year-old retired engineer, is brought to the emergency room with his daughter who reports that over the past 6 months her father has become progressively more confused and she is concerned about him living alone. She also reports that he has begun refusing to eat. An important question to ask Mr. Ekpa and his daughter is?
   a. "Has he had any major changes in his life over this period?"
   b. "Why have you waited so long to bring him in?"
   c. "Does he have a history of drinking?"
   d. "Have you thought about putting him in a nursing home for safety reasons?"

6. A client is admitted to a medical unit with symptoms of "seeing spiders," high anxiety, and agitated and irritable mood. His sensorium waxes and wanes between alertness and confusion. In planning for his care, the nurse's highest priority is to do which of the following?
   a. Administer medications to reduce hallucinations and agitation
   b. Maintain safety and closely monitor physical and mental status
   c. Offer fluids to prevent dehydration
   d. Leave client alone to promote sleep

7. A client with suspected prodromal signs of delirium is seen in the emergency room for evaluation and treatment. Which of the following is the nurse *least* likely to observe?
   a. Increased sensitivity to light and noises
   b. History of insomnia or sleep disturbances
   c. Memory difficulties
   d. Increased fluid consumption

8. A 78-year-old client is seen in the primary care clinic complaining of shuffling gait, episodic urinary incontinence, and memory disturbances. The most likely explanation for his symptoms is which of the following?
   a. Parkinson's disease
   b. Side effects from an antipsychotic medication
   c. Normal pressure hydrocephalus
   d. Pick's disease

9. A client with Alzheimer's disease has a self-care deficit related to his cognitive impairment. He has difficulty

dressing himself. The best action for the nurse to take is which of the following?

   a. Have the client wear hospital gowns

   b. Explain to the client why he should dress himself

   c. Give the client step-by-step instructions for dressing himself

   d. Allow enough time for the client to dress himself

10. The family of a client with Alzheimer's disease indicates to the nurse an understanding of the prognosis when they say,

   a. "Does another hospital have a better treatment?"

   b. "Will change in diet help his memory?"

   c. "Won't his medication cure him?"

   d. "What supports are available for the long haul?"

11. A client with severe Alzheimer's disease has violent outbursts, wanders, and is incontinent. He can no longer identify familiar people or objects. In developing a nursing care plan, the nurse would give highest priority to which nursing diagnosis?

   a. High risk for injury

   b. Impaired verbal communication

   c. Self-care deficits

   d. Altered pattern of urinary elimination: incontinence

12. A 72-year-old was recently admitted to a nursing home due to confusion, disorientation, and negativistic behavior. Which activity would you engage the client in at the nursing home?

   a. Reminiscence groups

   b. Sign-alongs

   c. Discussion groups

   d. Exercise class

13. Which of the following would be an appropriate nursing intervention in reorienting a confused client to where his room is?

   a. Place pictures of his family on the bedside

   b. Put his name in large letters on his clothes

   c. Remind the client where he is

   d. Let the other clients know where the client's room is

RESOURCES

Please note that because Internet resources are of a time-sensitive nature and URL addresses may change or be deleted, searches should also be conducted by association or topic.

Internet Activities

1. Locate Alzheimer's support group meetings in your area by searching for Alzheimer's Association on the Internet. Are there support group meetings in your area? How do you access them?

2. Locate the virtual hospital on the Internet (http://vh.org/). Search the site for information on cognitive disorders. What kind of information is provided? Is it adequate for nurses? For family? For the community?

Internet Resources

http://www.thearc.org   Arc of the United States (formerly the Association for Retarded Persons in the United States)

Joint United Nations Programme on HIV/AIDS (UNAIDS) http://www.unaids.org/en/   Accessed March, 5, 2007

GeroNurse.Org (Information on competencies in gerontological nursing) http://www.GeroNurseOnline.org Accessed March, 5, 2007

The Alzheimer's Disease Education and Referral (ADEAR) Center (comprehensive Alzheimer's disease [AD] information and resources from the National Institute on Aging [NIA]. http://www.nia.nih.gov/alzheimers Accessed March, 5, 2007

Alzheimer's Publication: Understanding Memory Loss http://www.nia.nih.gov/Alzheimers/Publications/ UnderstandingMemoryLoss/   Accessed March, 5, 2007

Alzheimer's Association http://www.alz.org/index.asp Accessed March, 5, 2007

http://unaids.org   Uniting the World Against AIDS (UNAIDS), the Joint United Nations Programme on HIV/AIDS (a joint initiative between ten United Nations system organizations to the global AIDS response)

http://GeroNurseOnline.org   (information on competencies in gerontological nursing)

http://www.nursing.uiowa.edu/centers/gnirc/protocols.htm (provides evidence-based protocols for geriatric nursing, including AD, and acute confusion)

Other Resources

Alzheimer's Association

   919 North Michigan Avenue, Suite 1000

   Chicago, IL 60611-1676

   (312) 335-8700 or (800) 272-3900

   http://www.alz.org

Alzheimer's Disease Education and Referral Center (ADEAR)

   P.O. Box 8250

   Silver Spring, MD 20902-8250

   (800) 438-4380

   http://www.alzheimers.org/adear

REFERENCES

Akhvlediani, T., Gochitashvili, N., & Tsertsvadze, T. (2007). Prion diseases—mysterious persistent infections. *Georgian Medical News, 146,* 38–42.

Alzheimer's Association, Mississippi Valley Chapter. (2000). New drug approved for Alzheimer's treatment. *Alzheimer's Association, Mississippi Valley Chapter Newsletter, 4*(3), 5.

American Psychiatric Association. (1987). *Diagnostic and statistical manual of mental disorders* (3rd ed.—Revised). Washington, DC: Author.

American Psychiatric Association. (2000). *Diagnostic and statistical manual of mental disorders* (4th edition, Text Revision) *(DSM-IV-TR)*. Washington, DC: Author.

Ballard, C. G., Chalmers, K. A., Todd, C., McKeith, I. G., O'Brien, J. T., Wilxcock, G., et al. (2007). Cholinesterase inhibitors reduce cortical Abeta in dementia with Lewy bodies. *Neurology, 68*, 1726–1729.

Bhat, R., & Rockwood, K. (2007). Delirium as a disorder of consciousness. *Journal of Neurology and Neurosurgery Psychiatry, 8.* [Epub ahead of print]

Butler, R. (1982). *Aging and mental health* (3rd ed.). St. Louis: Mosby.

Caley, L. M., Kramer C., & Robinson, L. K. (2005). Fetal alcohol spectrum disorder. *Journal of School Nursing, 21*, 139–146.

Caselli, R. J., Beach, T. G., Yaari, R., & Reiman, E. M. (2006). Alzheimer's disease a century later. *Journal of Clinical Psychiatry, 67*, 1784–1800.

Cole, M. (2004). Delirium in elderly patients. *American Journal of Geriatric Psychiatry, 12*(1), 7–12.

Cook, I. A. (2004). *Guideline watch: Practice guideline for the treatment of patients with delirium.* Arlington, VA: American Psychiatric Association. Available online at http://www.psych.org/psych_pract/treatg/pg/Delirium.watch.pdf

Crigger, N., & Forbes, W. (1997). Assessing neurologic function in older patients. *American Journal of Nursing, 97*(3), 37–40.

Dawson, P., Kline, K., Wiancko, D., & Wells, D. (1986). Preventing excess disability in patients with Alzheimer's disease. *Geriatric Nursing, 1*(6), 298–330.

Foreman, M., Wakefield, B., Culp, K., & Milisen, K. (2001). Delirium in elderly patients: An overview of the state of the science. *Journal of Gerontological Nursing, 28*(4), 12–20.

Geldmacher, D. S. (2004). Differential diagnosis of dementia syndromes. *Clinics in Geriatric Medicine, 20*, 27–43.

Goetz, G. C. (1999). *Textbook of clinical neurology.* New York: W.B. Saunders.

Gorelick, P. B. (2004). Risk factors for vascular dementia and Alzheimer disease. *Stroke, 35*(suppl 1), 2620–2622.

Grossman, M., & Ash, S. (2004). Primary progressive aphasia: A review. *Neurocase, 10*(1), 3–18.

Hall, G. R. (1991). Altered thought processes: SDAT. In M. Maas and K. Buckwalter (Eds.), *Nursing diagnoses and interventions in the elderly.* Menlo Park, CA: Addison-Wesley.

Hall, G. R. (1997). Alzheimer's disease and chronic dementing illnesses In M. Titler (Series Ed.). Iowa City: The University of Iowa Gerontological Nursing Interventions Research Center.

Hall, G. R., & Buckwalter, K. C. (1987). Progressively lowered stress threshold: A conceptual model for care of

adults with Alzheimer's disease. *Archives of Psychiatric Nursing, 1*(6), 399–406.

Hanley, C. (2004). Delirium in the acute care setting. *MEDSURG Nursing, 13*(4), 217–225.

Hockenberry, M. J., Wilson, D., Winkelstein, M. L., & Kline, N. E. (2003). *Wong's Nursing Care of Infants and Children.* St. Louis: Mosby

Jones, K. L., Smith, D. W., Ulleland, C. N., & Streissguth, P. (1973). Pattern of malformation in offspring of chronic alcoholic mothers. *Lancet, 1*, 1267–1271.

Kumar-Singh, S., & Van Broeckhoven, C. (2007). Frontotemporal lobar degeneration: Current concepts in the light of recent advances. *Brain Pathology, 17*, 104–114.

Lantz, M. S., & Buchalter, E. N. (2005). Pick's disease. *Clinical Geriatrics, 13*(6), 14–17.

Levy-Lahad, E., Wasco, W., Pookaj, P., Ramano, D. M., Oshima, J., Pettingell, W. H., et al. (1995). Candidate gene for the chromosome 1 familial Alzheimer's disease locus. *Science, 269*, 973–977.

Lipowski, Z. J. (1990). *Delirium: Acute confusional states.* New York: Oxford University Press.

McCloskey, J. C., & Bulechek, G. M. (2000). *Nursing interventions classification (NIC)* (3rd ed.). St. Louis: Mosby.

Mullan, M., Houlden, H., Windelspecht, M., Fidani, L., Lombardi, C., Diaz, P., et al. (1992). A locus for familial early-onset Alzheimer's disease on the long arm of chromosome 14, proximal to the alpha 1-antichymotrypsin gene. *Natural Genetics, 2*(4), 340–342.

Olichney, J. M., Murphy, C., Hofstetter, C. R., Foster, K., Hansen, L. A., Thal, L. J., et al. (2005). Anosmia is very common in the Lewy body variant of Alzheimer's disease. *Journal of Neurology and Neurosurgery Psychiatry, 76*, 1342–1347.

Panza, F., D'Introno, A., Calacicco, A. M., Capurso, C., DelParigi, A., Caselli, R. J., et al. (2005). Current epidemiology of mild cognitive impairment and other predementia syndromes. *American Journal of Geriatric Psychiatry, 13*(8), 633–644.

Pericak-Vance, M. A., Bebout, J. L., Gaskell, P. C., Yamaoka, L. H., Hung, W. Y., Alberts, M. J., et al. (1991). Linkage studies in familial Alzheimer disease: Evidence for chromosome 19 linkage. *American Journal of Human Genetics, 48*(6), 1034–1050.

Reisburg, B., Ferris, S. H., DeLeon, M. J., & Crook, T. (1982). The global deterioration scale (GDS): An instrument for the assessment of primary degenerative dementia. *American Journal of Psychiatry, 139*(9), 1136–1139.

Roman, G .C. (2003). Vascular dementia: Distinguishing characteristics, treatment and prevention. *Journal of the American Society of Genriatrics, 51*, S296–S304.

Sacks, O. (1985). *The man who mistook his wife for a hat and other clinical tales.* New York: Harper Perennial.

Scaravilli, F., Bazille, C., & Gray, F. (2007). Neuropathologic contributions to understanding AIDS and the central nervous system. *Brain Pathology, 17,* 197–208.

Schellenberg, G. D., Bird, T. D., Wijsman, E. M., Orr, H. T., Anderson, L., Nemens, E., et al. (1992). Genetic linkage evidence for a familial Alzheimer's disease locus on chromosome 14. *Science, 258*(5082), 668–671.

Schutte, D. L. (2004). The evolving role of genomics in shaping care for persons with dementia. *Nursing Clinics of North America, 39,* 581–592.

Short, R. A., Broderick, D. F., Patton, A., Arvanitakis, Z., & Graff-Radford, N. R. (2005). Different patterns of magnetic resonance imaging atrophy for frontotemporal lobar degeneration syndromes. *Archives of Neurology, 62,* 1106–1110.

Smith, M., Gerdner, L. A., Hall G. R., & Buckwalter, K. C. (2004). History, development, and future of the progressively lowered stress threshold: A conceptual model for dementia care. *Journal of the American Society of Geriatrics, 52,* 1755–1760.

Solfrizzi, V., Colacicco, A. M., D'Introno, A., Capurso, C., Torres, F., Grigoletto, F., Maggi, S., Del Paragi, A., Reiman, E. M., Caselli, R. J., Scafato, E., Farchi, G., Capurso, A. (2004). Vascular risk factors, incidence of MCI, and rates of progression to dementia. *Neurology, 63*(10), 1882–1891.

Stanley, M., Blair, K. A., & Beare, P. G. (2005). *Gerontological nursing: Promoting successful aging with older adults,* (3rd ed., pp. 347–354). Philadelphia: F. A. Davis.

St. George-Hyslop, P., Haines, J., Rogaev, E., Mortilla, M., Vaula, G., Pericak-Vance, M., et al. (1992). Genetic evidence for a novel familial Alzheimer's disease locus on chromosome 14. *Natural Genetics, 2*(4), 330–334.

Stolley, J. M., Lewis, A., Moore, L., & Harvey, P. (2001). Risk for injury: Falls. In M. L. Mas, K. C. Buckwalter, M. D. Hardy, T. Tripp-Reimer, M. G. Titler, & J. P. Specht (Eds.), *Nursing care of older adults. Diagnoses, outcomes, & interventions* (pp. 23–33). St.Louis, Mosby.

Strong, R. (1998). Neurochemical changes in the aging human brain: Implications for behavioral impairment and neurodegenerative disease. *Geriatrics, 53*(Suppl. 1), S9–S12.

UNAIDS. (2005). *Joint United Nations programme on HIV/AIDS*. Available at http://www.unaids.org

Van Broeckhoven, C., Backhovens, H., Cruts, M., DeWinter, G., Bruyland, M., Crass, P. L., et al. (1992). Mapping of a gene predisposing to early-onset Alzheimer's disease to chromosome 14q24.3. *Natural Genetics, 2*(4), 335–339.

Warner, J. P., Butler, R., & Arya, P. (2005). Dementia. In Fiona Godlee (Ed.). *Clinical Evidence*. London: BMJ Publishing Group.

Weder, N. D., Aziz, R., Wilkins, K., & Tampi, R. R. (2007). Frontotemporal dementias: A review. *Annals of General Psychiatry, 6,* 15. [Epub ahead of print] Available online at http://www.annals-general-psychiatry.com/content/6/1/15

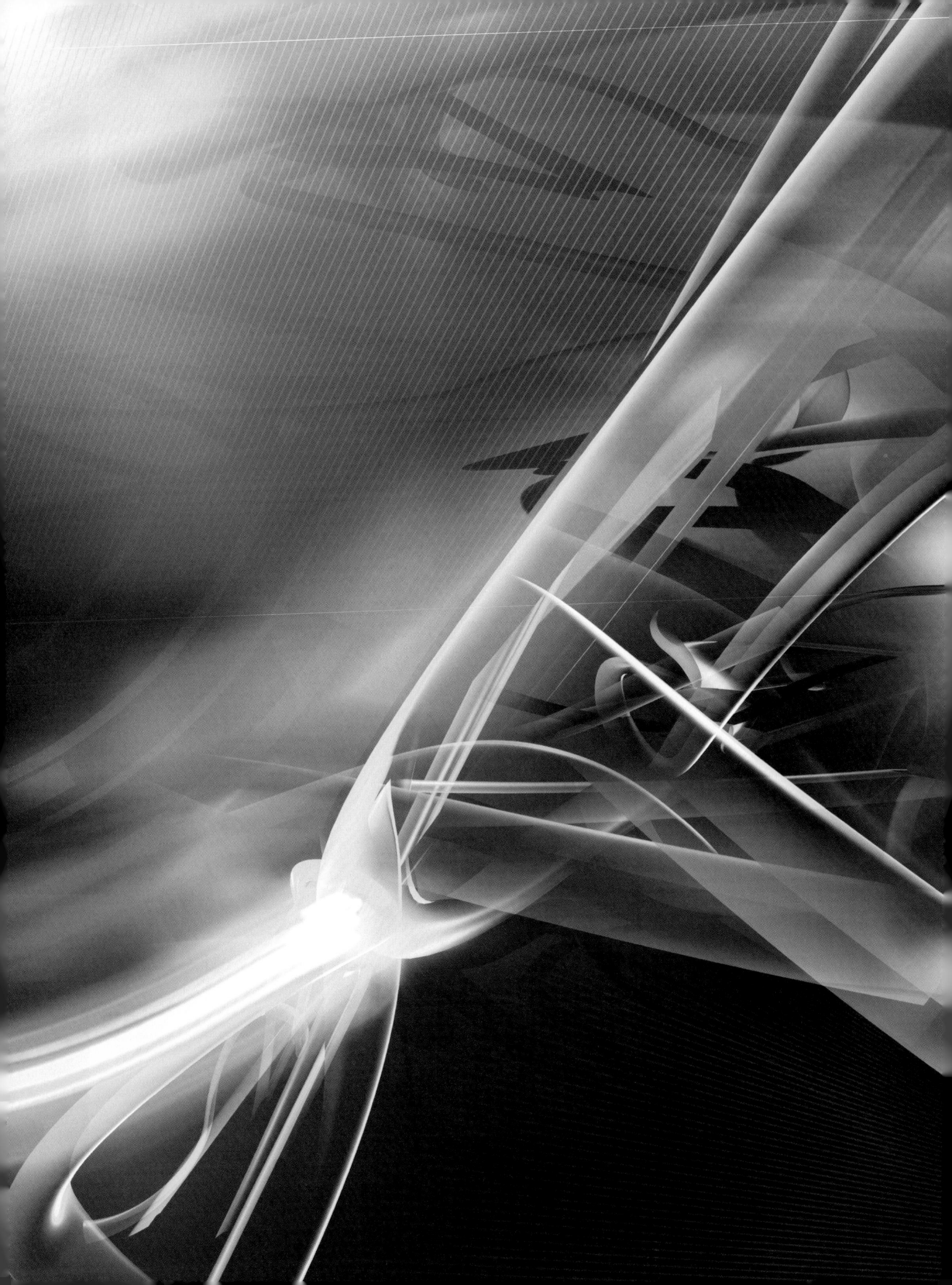

CHAPTER 17

The Client with Attention-Deficit Disorder

Cindy Parsons, DNP, APRN, BC

KEY TERMS

Aggressive: Physical or verbal behavior that is forceful, hostile, or enacted to intimidate others.

Behavior Management Plans: A plan designed to reinforce positive and reduce negative behaviors through the use of visual cues, charts, communication tools, and reward systems.

Cognitive: The mental process involved in obtaining knowledge, including the aspects of perceiving, thinking, reasoning, and remembering.

Co-occurrence: Psychiatric or physical disorder that occurs with a primary psychiatric disorder.

Conflict: The opposition of mutually exclusive impulses, desires, or tendencies; controversy or disagreement.

Cues: Internal and external response signals that, if noticed, predict when, where, and what response will occur.

Disruptive: To throw into disorder or confusion; to disturb a balance.

Distractibility: The inability to maintain attention, shifting from one area or topic to another with minimal provocation, or attention being drawn too frequently to unimportant or irrelevant external stimuli.

Emotional Lability: An affective disturbance characterized by excessive and inappropriate emotional response.

Gratification: To be satisfied; receive pleasure from.

Hyperactivity: Extra active; having too much energy to handle. An activity level that is out of proportion for the situation, setting, and person's developmental level.

Impulsivity: A tendency to act suddenly and without thought. An inability to delay gratification, which reflects a lack of personal control and inability to manage feelings and emotions.

Inattention: A failure to focus attention on those elements of the environment that are most relevant to the task at hand.

Learning Disability: A condition that makes it difficult for a person to learn information in a usual manner.

Neurotransmitters: Biochemicals found in the central nervous system involved in the transmission of impulses across the synapses between neurons.

Overarousal: To be excessively excited or stimulated.

Personal Boundaries: A mental idea of how one experiences and maintains a line of separation between oneself and the world.

Psychostimulants: A class of medications that temporarily increases the functioning activity of the brain.

COMPETENCIES

Upon completion of this chapter, the learner should be able to:

1. Discuss the history of the diagnosis and recent advances in understanding attention-deficit hyperactivity disorder (ADHD) as a neurobiological disorder.

2. Identify the *DSM-IV-TR* criteria for the diagnosis of ADHD and describe the various subtypes.

3. Recognize and describe the symptoms of ADHD throughout the life span.

4. Discuss the impact of the three major ADHD subtypes on a person's ability to function in a variety of settings.

5. Identify the various components of a comprehensive assessment to achieve the diagnosis of ADHD.

6. Develop a comprehensive plan of care for the client with ADHD, including managing at home, in school, and in community settings.

7. Discuss the role of pharmacotherapy in treating the client with ADHD, including the various types of medications, indications for use, efficacy, dosing guidelines, and potential side effects.

8. Discuss the role of behavioral interventions in the treatment of the client with ADHD.

Attention-deficit hyperactivity disorder (ADHD) is the most common neurobehavioral disorder among school-age children. The main characteristics of the disorder are inattention, impulsivity, and hyperactivity. Its estimated prevalence is between 3 and 8 percent, which makes it one of the most frequently encountered chronic health disorders in mental health clinics that treat children (Barkley, 1996). The brain possesses limited capacity for processing simultaneous information. It relies on a complex process to narrow the scope and focus of information to be processed and assimilated. ADHD is characterized by attention skills that are developmentally inappropriate for the clients' age and may include the symptoms of hyperactivity and impulsivity.

In 2006, results of the National Comorbidity Survey Replication revealed that the estimated prevalence of adult ADHD was 4.4 percent and had significant correlates with adults of male gender, previously married, unemployed, and non-Hispanic white. Consistent with other data concerning ADHD, this disorder was highly concomitant with other psychiatric disorders and is associated with considerable morbidity and disability (Kessler et al., 2006). Overall, ADHD is a neurobehavioral disorder, with multiple etiologies including genetic, environmental, and biological factors. This disorder persists into adolescence and adulthood across the life cycle, and coexisting psychiatric and medical disorders are distinct clinical features of both childhood and adult ADHD (Spencer, Biederman, & Mick, 2007).

The child with attention difficulties, impulsive behaviors, and increased motor activity presents a challenge to parents, teachers, peers, and health care providers. These symptoms create problems for the child and family in many settings, with the demands of the setting influencing the severity of the symptoms. At some point in the child's life the impact of these symptoms on his academic, social, or leisure functioning causes the child to be brought to the attention of mental health providers.

The goal of this chapter is to discuss ADHD and its etiology, diagnosis, and the role of the nurse in developing and implementing an integrated biopsychosocial treatment plan.

EPIDEMIOLOGY

It is estimated that 3 to 5 percent of all school-age children have ADHD. This translates into a probability of 1 to 2 students in a typical classroom. Estimations of the number of affected adults vary widely, from 30 to 70 percent of those diagnosed in childhood experiencing ongoing symptoms. The incidence of occurrence in males exceeds females by a 4 to 1 ratio.

Symptoms of ADHD are usually first noticed in early childhood. The symptoms of excess motor activity are frequently detected when the child is a toddler, although children this age are normally active and curious. The child with ADHD, however, will be more active and impulsive than his peers. Symptoms of inattention in toddlers or preschool age children are not easily observable because young children rarely experience demands for sustained attention. As children mature the symptoms become more conspicuous. By late childhood or early adolescence, the symptoms of excess motor activity are less common and have been replaced by restlessness or fidgeting (APA, 2000). In most individuals, symptoms attenuate during late adolescence and adulthood, although a minority will experience the full complement of symptoms into adulthood.

Co-occurrence is common with ADHD. Coexisting disorders often include learning disabilities, bipolar disorder, oppositional defiant disorder, conduct disorder, depression, and anxiety disorders (Wilens et al., 2002). Recognition of coexisting disorders is important because these conditions may influence the outcomes of medical and treatment interventions.

In response to public and professional concern regarding the possible over diagnosis of ADHD and possible over prescription of stimulant medications used to treat the illness, the American Medical Association commissioned a study to review relevant evidence. The study concluded, "ADHD is one of the best researched disorders in medicine and the overall data on its validity are far more compelling than for

most mental disorders and even for many medical conditions (Goldman et al., 1998).

CAUSATIVE FACTORS: PERSPECTIVES AND THEORIES

Although the exact cause of ADHD is unknown, recent studies indicate an array of factors that play key roles in the cause of this complex disorder. Causative factors of ADHD include environmental factors associated with pregnancy and delivery complications, alterations in biochemical processes, genetics, and other biological influences.

BRAIN INJURY

In the early 1900s, the symptom cluster that now represents ADHD was hypothesized to evolve from brain injury (Still, 1902). This theory gained wide acceptance supported by evidence of cognitive and behavioral symptoms in children and adults who had suffered from encephalitis. Most children with these symptoms, however, had no evidence of definitive brain injury (Bond & Partridge, 1926). The concept of minimal brain damage then emerged and was to children who had symptoms but no observable neurological signs of injury. This was based on the assumption that a lesser degree of injury could cause behavioral symptoms without other signs of brain injury (Knobloc & Pasaminick, 1959).

Most families with children manifesting symptoms of ADHD could identify difficulties during pregnancy or with labor or delivery occurring. The theory of minimal brain damage resulting from pre- or perinatal injury persisted through the 1950s. Major studies done during the 1960s and 1970s, however, did not validate the hypothesis. Routh (1978) reported that there was little evidence to support the theory that brain damage was the underlying cause of ADHD.

DIETARY INTAKE

During the 1970s, food and food additives became popular suspects as causal factors. Feingold (1974) developed a hypothesis, based on anecdotal observations, that certain foods and food additives caused behavioral deterioration. He postulated that a group of food constituents called natural salicylates yielded a toxic effect, thereby contributing to behavioral disturbances. Furthermore, he proposed that elimination of these substances from the diet would produce substantial improvement in the child's behavior. Feingold again supported this hypothesis with anecdotal observations. There are no studies that provide data to support this.

Conners and Taylor (1980) also performed studies on the effects of artificial colors and food additives. He placed children on an additive-free diet and evaluated their behavior using the Conners' Parent Rating Scale to determine severity of symptoms. He then reintroduced the additives in a double-blind manner. The findings demonstrated that, initially, when children were placed on an additive-free diet, there was improvement in their behavior. However, with the addition of additives there was no clear deterioration of behavior that could be correlated. To date there are no definitive studies demonstrating a clear causal relationship between food additives and behavioral problems in children.

ENVIRONMENTAL TOXINS

The developing brain is very susceptible to toxins and other chemicals during the prenatal period. The neurotoxic effects of alcohol, drugs and lead often result in brain damage, attention deficits, and behavioral problems.

Fetal Exposure to Alcohol and Drugs

Alcohol and other drugs ingested by the mother are transferred through the placenta to the fetus. Steinhaus, Williams, & Spohr (1993) studied children suffering from fetal alcohol syndrome. They found attention deficits and behavioral problems similar to those of ADHD children; however, they also found that the children who were affected by alcohol were more impaired intellectually. These findings were further supported by studies conducted (Kodituwakku, Coriale, Fiorentino, et al., 2006).

In Holland, a long-term longitudinal study looked at children exposed prenatally to amphetamines, cocaine, and heroin. These children showed impairment in cognitive functioning. The children exposed to amphetamines also exhibited more **aggressive** behavior. However, they did not find evidence of an increase in ADHD symptoms in the children exposed to these substances. Studies to date validate behavioral and cognitive problems related to fetal exposure to drugs or alcohol. There is no clear evidence that this exposure represents a significant risk factor for the development of ADHD.

Lead

Lead is a trace element that has no known use in human bodies. Ingestion of lead from paint, contaminated soil, or other sources can poison the brain. This poisoning produces a swelling of the brain, causing a decrease in general brain function. It also could lead to convulsions, if it is not detected and treated. Studies of children with significant lead ingestion demonstrate deficits in global IQ function, visual and fine motor coordination, and in behavior. School failure resulting from learning and behavior problems was also more frequent in the group exposed to lead.

These findings suggest that there may be a group of children with ADHD symptoms that are at least in part a result of lead exposure. The studies provided no evidence that treatment for lead poisoning would improve the cognitive or behavioral functioning of these children (Braun, Kahn, Froehlich, Auinger, & Lanphear, 2006.

GENETICS

The majority of children with ADHD are found to have a positive family history of ADHD. For many, it is a close family member such as a parent. Studies of parental psychopathology demonstrate that attention-deficit symptoms are more common in the fathers and uncles of ADHD children than in the relatives of non-ADHD children (Smith, Daly et al., 2003). Biederman and colleagues (1986) found that hyperactivity is present four times more often in parents of hyperactive children than those of a control sample.

Studies of identical twins demonstrated a strong element of heredity. Findings showed that identical twins are more likely to demonstrate hyperactive behaviors than do fraternal twins (Willerman, 1973). Subsequent studies have produced similar findings. Heredity appears to represent the most common identifiable factor in children who develop ADHD.

NEUROBIOLOGICAL BASIS

The attention system consists of a brainstem center composed of dopamine, serotonin, and noradrenaline neurons that project to many areas of the brain, basal ganglia, and frontal lobes. Limbic, frontal, and right hemispheric cells also are part of this system. This network, which projects to all areas of the brain, is important for a regulating system whose purpose is to modulate whole brain activity (Goldstein, 2006). Dopamine and norepinephrine are **neurotransmitters** that help transmit information from one brain cell to another. The dopamine neurons have cell bodies that originate in the brainstem. The noradrenaline neuron cell bodies originate and lie within the locus ceruleus, whereas the serotonin neuron cell bodies lie in the midline raphe of the medulla. Within the cerebral hemispheres, information from the senses is converted into electrical impulses that are sent to specific areas of the cerebral cortex. Certain areas of the cerebral hemispheres are involved in translating sensory input to prepare a response. Several areas of the brain responsible for this task have been identified to function differently in children with ADHD.

One area identified is the frontal lobes. The frontal lobes are the area of the brain responsible for the executive functions. These functions consist of initiating and sustaining activities, prioritizing, strategizing, and inhibiting impulses until the brain can weigh the possible consequences of the activity rationally. The basal ganglia are also an affected area. The basal ganglia assist the frontal lobes by helping to prioritize input and by organizing and executing actions decided on by the frontal lobes. The third area is the cerebellum. The cerebellum was once thought to be involved primarily in muscular coordination, balance, and movement. It is now recognized to play a role in emotion and higher level cognitive functions. These areas of the brain work together to take in information, process it, and act on it. Being able to sustain attention and process information before acting on it is an important component of this interrelationship.

The attention system may regulate the processing of information and concentration through coordination of several groups of nerve cells, primarily serotonin, dopamine, and norepinephrine. This system adjusts the sensitivity of the brain to stimuli and regulates the degree of activity, attention, concentration, as well as impulsivity. For example, the attention system regulates a person's ability to concentrate on reading and the cerebral cortical centers determine comprehension.

Attention and concentration are not an all-or-nothing phenomenon. There are times when it is appropriate to be inattentive to certain stimuli. For example, when driving, the driver's attention is focused primarily in front of the vehicle, and although a loud noise or commotion may momentarily distract him, the driver is able to filter out stimuli and attend to the task of safe driving. Most people are able to adjust their attention and concentration abilities so that they can be less inhibited in certain situations yet remain focused in others. The disorder known as ADHD can be viewed as a dysfunction of the attention system.

A breakdown in any one of the parts of the system would produce dysfunction in the system. Children with ADHD likely have varying degrees of differences within this system. They are unable to change their degree of attention appropriately as required by tasks or situations. The high degree of variability of ADHD symptoms could be seen as variability in effectiveness of the attention system.

Studies at the Child Psychiatry Branch of the National Institute of Mental Health involving neuroimaging through positron emission tomography (PET) and functional magnetic resonance imaging (FMRIs) provide findings of structural and functional differences in three areas of the brain: the frontal lobes, the basal ganglia, and the cerebellum (Spencer, Biederman, Madras, et al., 2007). These findings support the hypothesis that ADHD has a brain-based cause and provide the basis for future research.

DIFFERENTIAL DIAGNOSIS

Major symptoms of ADHD mimic those of various medical and psychiatric conditions. It is imperative to rule out these conditions to ensure an accurate diagnosis and appropriate nursing interventions and treatment. The most common misdiagnosis of ADHD is bipolar disorder. Making a differential diagnosis of mania opposed to ADHD is difficult. Elevated mood, flight of ideas, racing thoughts, and decreased need for sleep and delusions of grandeur are the most distinguishing symptoms between bipolar disorder and ADHD. Furthermore, symptoms of bipolar disorder are episodic in comparison to ADHD symptoms, which are relatively stable or chronic. An additional challenge of distinguishing these two disorders is the high rate of co-occurrence of ADHD among childhood and adolescent onset bipolar disorder and from the overlap of specific *DSM-IV* criteria for mania and ADHD, such as hyperactivity, attention difficulties, accelerated speech, and impulsive behavior (Masi et al., 2006; Nierenberg et al., 2005). Psychiatric-mental health nurses must work with other staff to make accurate decisions regarding treatment by gathering data from the youth and family members to grasp the longitudinal patterns of ADHD. Relevant diagnostic studies including serum chemistries, thyroid panel, renal and liver function tests, and toxicology screens are indicated to rule out medical conditions. There is a growing number of adults who are being diagnosed later in life and a comprehensive history of symptoms, treatment, maladaptive coping patterns, and substance misuse offer vital information necessary to make a differential diagnosis.

HISTORICAL PERSPECTIVES

Historical perspectives associated with attention-deficit disorders have evolved over the past century and were linked to moral and neurological factors. The moral deficit theory most likely paralleled social norms concerning mental illness. Attempts to link biological factors to these disorders were first associated with some form of brain injury. Over the past decade there has been growing evidence that indicates that the cause of these disorders are far more complex than ever imagined and they are linked by neurobiological, neurocognitive, genetic, and environmental factors.

MORAL DEFECT

Over the past century, the childhood cognitive and behavioral disorders categorized as disorders of attention, impulsivity, and hyperactivity have presented a challenge for psychiatric clinicians. In 1902, George F. Still first defined the disorder as a problem resulting from a defect in moral control. He defined moral control as "the control of action and conformity with the idea of the good of all" (p. 1008). He noted that this problem prevented these children from internalizing rules and limits; he also identified a pattern of restless, inattentive, and overaroused behavior in these children. Still based his observations and research on the prevailing theories of the 1890s, which stated that this pattern of behavior occurred in individuals with brain injury. He suggested that children with these symptoms had experienced brain injury, which had caused some type of brain damage or dysfunction, and associated the defect in moral control with impairment in intellect. Still did note that this pattern of behavior could have resulted not only from injury, but also from heredity or environmental experience. He further hypothesized that the aim of these behaviors was self-gratification and could not be treated; therefore, these children should be institutionalized at an early age.

BRAIN INJURY

In 1917 and 1918, following a worldwide outbreak of encephalitis, health professionals observed groups of children who had recovered from encephalitis who presented a pattern of restless, inattentive, impulsive, easily aroused, and hyperactive behavior not exhibited before the encephalitis (Ng, Lim, Yeoh, & Lee, 2004). It was thought that this pattern of behavior resulted from some type of brain injury caused by the disease process and was described as postencephalitic disorder (Bender, 1942).

MINIMAL BRAIN DAMAGE

From 1930 through the 1940s, behavior disorders with overactivity as a primary symptom continued to be associated with the hypothesis of brain damage or injury. Gradually, these symptoms or patterns of behavior were recognized even in children without identifiable brain damage. The hypothesis then shifted to a suspicion that these children had suffered some type of prenatal neurological insult or trauma during labor and delivery, which left the children with a slight injury or minimal brain damage.

The first studies using psychostimulants to treat these behaviors were performed at the Emma Pendleton Bradley Home in Providence, Rhode Island. Charles Bradley and his colleagues used dextroamphetamine to treat children with syndromes of cerebral dysfunction or organic brain syndrome (Bradley, 1937). Bradley documented improvements in a variety of tasks in 60 to 75 percent of these children regardless of specific diagnosis or level of intellectual functioning. (Bradley, 1937, 1950; Bradley & Bowen, 1941). These studies continued over the course of the next 40 years. At about the same time, Molitch and Eccles (1937) investigated the effects of Benzedrine on intelligence scores in children. Although noting no improvement on intelligence scores, they observed an improvement in general behavior, compliance, and attending skills.

HYPERKINETIC REACTION OF CHILDHOOD

In 1957, Laufer and Denhoff, working at the same facility as Bradley, were credited with the first behavioral description of the hyperactivity syndrome. Short attention span, poor concentration, variability of behavior, behavioral impulsiveness, and the inability to delay gratification were considered characteristics of this syndrome. These authors suggested that these behaviors could be observed in infancy or childhood and that it was observed more frequently in males.

The 1950s saw a growth in the use of psychotropic medications, including renewed interest in the use of medications for children, specifically use of stimulants. Laufer and Denhoff's (1957) tripartite set of hyperactive, impulsive, and inattentive symptoms was an early target of medication trials. In the second edition of the *Diagnostic and Statistical Manual of Mental Disorders*, the disorder is categorized as Hyperkinetic Reaction of Childhood (APA, 1968).

ATTENTION-DEFICIT DISORDER

By the 1970s, research strongly suggested that the core problem was not excessive activity, but inattention (Douglas & Peters, 1979), leading to a major shift in the focus of research, diagnosis, and treatment. Through the 1980s, the

idea that the symptoms of impulsiveness and hyperactivity, but primarily inattention, were biologically based and caused multiple developmental and later life problems became popular (Goldstein, 2006). Research in the field grew at a rapid pace, and so did the rate of diagnosis of the disorder. Through the 1980s and 1990s, research had shifted to the concept of ADHD as a lifelong disorder that can affect all areas of an individual's functioning. It is now accepted that inattentiveness can yield lifelong problems.

The third edition of the *Diagnostic and Statistical Manual of Mental Disorders* (APA, 1980) greatly expanded the definition of the disorder and retitled it Attention-Deficit Disorder with and without Hyperactivity. It included attention disorders with or without hyperactivity as well as a category for those who do not present with symptoms but whose history clearly demonstrates a period when the full disorder was exhibited. The two sets of core symptoms, inattention and hyperactivity, were arranged in three distinct areas, with hyperactivity and impulsivity separated. The third, revised edition of the *DSM* grouped these symptoms together, despite strong research supporting the distinction between children with an attention disorder with and without hyperactivity (Lahey, Schaughency, Hynd, Carlson, & Nieves, 1987).

ATTENTION-DEFICIT DISORDER WITH OR WITHOUT HYPERACTIVITY

Despite criticism, the *DSM-III-R* (APA, 1987) criteria represented an attempt to improve the operational definition of ADHD. These criteria required that symptoms present before children reached age 7; symptoms be experienced for 6 months or more; and could not be better accounted for from pervasive developmental disorder, mental retardation, schizophrenia, or severe emotional or behavioral problems. There, however, could be a coexisting diagnosis of ADHD for those populations, if the ADHD symptoms were excessive even in light of these disorders.

Although the *DSM-III-R* provided a thorough description of behavioral problems present with ADHD, it did not eliminate the need for the clinician to understand the impact of growth and development and social, environmental, and life experiences on a child's behavior. The categorical model of the *DSM-III-R* is generalized and may have yielded over-inclusion of children meeting the criteria for ADHD. Symptoms of ADHD are a good start to differential diagnosing, but it is important to gather data from a number of sources; otherwise, children with a wide variety of behavioral, emotional, and developmental problems may be diagnosed inappropriately with ADHD.

DSM-IV AND *DSM-IV-TR*— ATTENTION-DEFICIT HYPERACTIVITY DISORDER (ADHD)

The *DSM-IV* criteria resulted from more comprehensive and better-structured field studies and represent an attempt to categorize ADHD as more than a unipolar disorder. The

DSM-IV-TR defines ADHD as a persistent pattern of inattention or hyperactivity-impulsivity, or both, that is more frequent and severe than is typically observed in individuals at a comparable level of development (APA, 2000). Some hyperactive-impulsive or inattentive symptoms that cause impairment must have been present before age 7 years. Age of onset before age 7 had not been established by empirical data but it has become a mainstay of the diagnostic criteria (Applegate et al., 1997). A clinical study of 380 children ages 4 to 17 received a diagnosis of ADHD. Out of the children receiving a diagnosis of inattentive type, 50 percent did not meet the criteria for age of onset. Some impairment from the symptoms must be present in at least two settings (e.g., home and school or work). There must be clear evidence of interference with developmentally appropriate social, academic, or occupational functioning. Lastly, the symptoms do not occur exclusively during the course of another disorder, such as Pervasive Developmental Disorder, a psychotic disorder, mood, or other mental disorder. The *DSM-IV-TR* criteria are displayed in Table 17–1.

The *DSM-IV-TR* criteria are further broken down into symptoms of inattention and hyperactivity-impulsivity. These symptoms are behavioral and can be measured through direct observation of the client in the home, school, or work environment. A variety of observation rating scales have been developed that help identify and measure the severity of the core symptoms of inattention, impulsivity, and hyperactivity. Many of these include ratings of social relationships. Some of the more well-known scales are the Conners' Parent-Teacher Rating Scale, the Vanderbilt Rating Scale, and the Achenbach Child Behavior checklist. These scales are well established and have high degrees of interrater reliability. See the sample Behavior Rating Scale and instructions for use.

Field trial studies for the criteria resulted in some interesting findings. Of 276 children diagnosed with ADHD, 55 percent had the combined type, 27 percent had the inattentive type, and 18 percent had the hyperactive-inattentive type. Females accounted for 20 percent of the hyperactive-impulsive type, 12 percent of the combined type, and 27 percent of the inattentive type. This validates clinician perceptions that males are affected more often than females and that females more often demonstrate the inattentive type (Silverthorn, Frick, Kupper, & Ott, 1996).

The current *DSM-IV-TR* criteria are well defined and comprehensive. Before establishing a diagnosis it is important to collect data, history, and observations from a variety of sources to determine that the child meets symptom criteria in more than one setting. Children with language, socialization, cognitive, and other behavioral difficulties that are the result of life experiences because of abnormal development or illness also exhibit attention-related problems (Goldstein, 2006).

In 1998, Goldstein and Goldstein proposed a practical definition of ADHD to provide a logical framework from which to understand the patterns of behavior that constitute ADHD. They are outlined as follows:

1. Impulsivity: Children with ADHD have difficulty thinking before they act. They know what to do but they do not do what they know. Their difficulty following rule-governed behavior (APA, 2000) appears to result directly from their inability to separate experience from response, thought from emotion, and action from reaction. They are impetuous and unthinking in their behavior. They require more parental or teacher supervision. They frustrate their parents and teachers with their inability to learn from experience. Frequently, parents and teachers label this behavior as purposeful, noncaring, or oppositional, which is not accurate and often leads to punitive and ineffective interactions between the adult and the child.

2. Inattention: Children with ADHD have difficulty remaining on-task and focusing attention compared with children without ADHD (APA, 2000). Normally as children get older they become more efficient in their ability to sustain attention. By the first grade or age 6 we expect children to sustain attention and work at a task for at least one-half hour at a time. Children with ADHD have an inability to invest and sustain attention to task, especially repetitive, effortful, uninteresting, or unchosen tasks.

3. Hyperactivity and overarousal: Children with ADHD tend to be restless, overactive, and easily overaroused emotionally. They have difficulty controlling bodily movements in situations where they are required to sit still or stay in place for an extended period of time. They are quicker to become overaroused. Whether happy or sad, the speed and intensity of the emotion is much greater than that of a peer of the same age. This problem reflects their impulsive inability to separate thought from emotion.

4. Difficulties with gratification: As a result of impulsivity children with ADHD require immediate, frequent, predictable, and meaningful rewards. They experience greater difficulty working toward a long-term goal. They do not appear to respond to rewards in a manner similar to other children without ADHD (Haenlin & Caul, 1987). Because of this problem, children with ADHD often require more time to master a task. It is therefore important to provide a sufficient number of structured, supervised, and reinforced experiences for the children to learn. This includes simple tasks, such as making a bed, to more complex tasks, such as playing a team sport.

It also appears that children with ADHD tend to receive more negative reinforcement and feedback than children without ADHD. Because of the child's impulsivity and inconsistency, adults may place great pressure on them or the child perceives it this way. The child responds to this by completing tasks to the best of their ability but to gain relief from the adults' negative attention. It is important when establishing a plan of care to remember that children with ADHD respond positively to rewards and not to punishment.

5. Emotions and locus of control: Children with ADHD are often on a roller coaster of emotions owing to their impulsiveness and emotional overarousal. When they

A. Either (1) or (2)

    (1) Six (or more) of the following symptoms of inattention have persisted for at least 6 months to a degree that is maladaptive and inconsistent with developmental level:

        (a) often fails to give close attention to details or makes careless mistakes in schoolwork, work, or other activities

        (b) often has difficulty sustaining attention in tasks or play activities

        (c) often does not seem to listen when spoken to directly

        (d) often does not follow through on instruction and fails to finish schoolwork, chores, or duties in the workplace (not due to oppositional behavior or failure to understand instructions)

        (e) often has difficulty organizing tasks and activities

        (f) often avoids, dislikes, or is reluctant to engage in tasks that require sustained mental effort (such as schoolwork or homework)

        (g) often loses things necessary for tasks or activities (e.g., toys, school assignments, pencils, books, or tools)

        (h) is often easily distracted by extraneous stimuli

        (i) is often forgetful in daily activities

    (2) Six (or more) of the following symptoms of hyperactivity-impulsivity have persisted for at least 6 months to a degree that is maladaptive and inconsistent with developmental level:

    Hyperactivity

        (a) often fidgets with hands or feet or squirms in seat

        (b) often leaves seat in classroom or in other situations in which remaining seated is expected

        (c) often runs about or climbs excessively in situations in which it is inappropriate (in adolescents or adults, may be limited to subjective feelings of restlessness)

        (d) often has difficulty playing or engaging in leisure activities quietly

        (e) if often "on the go" or often acts as if "driven by a motor"

        (f) often talks excessively

    Impulsivity

        (a) often blurts out answers before questions have been completed

        (b) often has difficulty awaiting turn

        (c) often interrupts or intrudes on others (e.g., butts into conversations or games)

B. Some hyperactive-impulsive or inattentive symptoms that caused impairment were present before age 7 years.

C. Some impairment from the symptoms is present in two or more settings (e.g., at school [or work] and at home).

D. There must be clear evidence of clinically significant impairment in social, academic, or occupational functioning.

E. The symptoms do not occur exclusively during the course of a Pervasive Developmental Disorder, Schizophrenia, or other Psychotic Disorder and are not better accounted for by another mental disorder (e.g., Mood Disorder, Anxiety Disorder, Dissociative Disorder, or Personality Disorder).

Code based on type:

314.01 ADHD, Combined Type:
        Both Criteria A1 and A2 are met for the past 6 months

(continues)

314.00	ADHD, Predominantly Inattentive Type:
	Criterion A1 is met, but Criterion A2 is not met for the past 6 months

314.01	ADHD, Predominantly Hyperactive-Impulsive Type:
	Criterion A2 is met but Criterion A1 is not met for the past 6 months

Coding note:

For individuals (especially adolescents and adults) who currently have symptoms that no longer meet full criteria, "In Partial Remission" should be specified

314.9	ADHD, Not Otherwise Specified:
	There are prominent symptoms of inattention or hyperactivity-impulsivity that do not meet criteria for ADHD

Note. From *Diagnostic and Statistical Manual of Mental Disorders* (4th edition, Text Revision) *(DSM-IV-TR)*, by the American Psychiatric Association, 2000, Washington, DC: Author. Reprinted with permission.

Quick Guide to Using the Abbreviated ADHD Symptom Checklist

The Abbreviated ADHD Symptom Checklist-4 (ADHD-SC4) is a behavior rating scale whose items are based on the 18 behavioral symptoms of attention-deficit hyperactivity disorder (ADHD) as defined by the American Psychiatric Association's *Diagnostic and Statistical Manual of Mental Disorders* (*DSM-IV*). Individual items are worded to be easily understood by caregivers. Physicians can use the Abbreviated ADHD-SC4 as a brief screening device with parents and teachers who are concerned about child behavior at home and in school. The findings from a number of studies indicate that the Abbreviated ADHD-SC4 is a reliable and valid screening instrument for ADHD in children 3 to 18 years old, and it is a reliable and valid measure for assessing response to treatment. The checklist can be completed in less than 2 minutes, and it is quick and easy to score.

Scoring procedures. There are two different ways to score the Abbreviated ADHD-SC4: Symptom Count scores and Symptom Severity scores. The weights assigned to the response choices are as follows:

SYMPTOM COUNT: Never = 0, Sometimes = 0, Often = 1, Very Often = 1

SYMPTON SEVERITY: Never = 0, Sometimes = 1, Often = 2, Very Often = 3

Symptom Count scores are used to screen for specific disorders. The *DSM-IV* identifies three types of ADHD: the predominantly inattentive type (Items 1–9), the predominantly hyperactive-impulsive type (Items 10–18), and the combined types (Items 1–18). The *DSM-IV* also specifies the number of symptoms necessary for a diagnosis. The minimum number of symptoms for each of the three types of ADHD is as follows: the predominantly inattentive type (six symptoms), the predominantly hyperactive-impulsive type (six symptoms), and the combined type (six symptoms of each the inattentive and hyperactive-impulsive types). Items that are checked as "Often" and "Very Often" are considered to be clinically significant.

Symptom Severity scores are used to assess the overall severity of child symptoms after a diagnosis has been established. This method of scoring is most useful when evaluating response to treatment.

Parent and teacher ratings. The accuracy of the Abbreviated ADHD-SC4 is enhanced when information is obtained from both parents and teacher(s). However, parent and teacher ratings do not always agree. Discrepancies between parent and teacher scores may indicate that either the child's behavior is different in the two settings or one of these care providers is a more accurate informant about certain child behaviors. Because this is a screening instrument, parent or teacher indications of ADHD behavior should be investigated further when the child's behavior is considered to be a serious problem by either informant.

Interpreting Symptom Count scores. The Abbreviated ADHD-SC4 does not provide diagnoses; it is simply a screening instrument. Furthermore, Symptom Count scores cannot be interpreted as verifying the presence or absence of specific disorders. If a child's Symptom Count score meets the minimum number of symptoms required for a diagnosis of ADHD, then a comprehensive clinical evaluation is necessary to determine if (a) the child really had ADHD, (b) some other variable (e.g., environmental stressor) can explain the symptom, or (c) another disorder can account for the ADHD symptoms. In addition to the behavioral symptoms, a diagnosis of ADHD requires information about the age of onset and duration of symptoms, extent of impairment in functioning, and the exclusionary conditions and disorders. According to the *DSM-IV,* onset must be by age 7 years, symptoms must have been

(continues)

Quick Guide to Using the Abbreviated ADHD Symptom Checklist *(continued)*

present for a minimum of 6 months, symptoms must cause difficulties in at least two settings, symptoms must cause clinically significant distress or impairment in functioning, and symptoms are not caused by other disorders (e.g., pervasive developmental disorder, schizophrenia, mood and anxiety disorders).

User qualifications. Users of the Abbreviated ADHD-SC4 should have an understanding of the basic principles and limitations of psychological and psychiatric screening and diagnostic procedures. Only qualified professionals can render diagnoses after a thorough evaluation.

TABLE 17–2
Historical Evolution of the Diagnosis of Attention-Deficit Hyperactivity Disorder

1900–1920s	Brain Injury
1930–1950s	Minimal Brain Damage
1960s	Minimal Brain Dysfunction
1968–1970s	Hyperkinetic Reaction of Childhood, *DSM-II*
1980	Attention-Deficit Disorder with or without Hyperactivity, *DSM-III*
1987–1993	Attention-Deficit Hyperactivity Disorder, *DSM-III-R*
1994	Attention-Deficit Hyperactivity Disorder, *DSM-IV*
2000	Attention-Deficit Hyperactivity Disorder, *DSM-IV-TR*

CRITICAL THINKING

Attention-deficit hyperactivity disorder (ADHD) is a neurobiological disorder characterized by:

a. a high degree of consistency in the frequency of symptoms among patients with ADHD

b. developmentally inappropriate levels of inattention

c. a predictable and consistent pattern of functional impairment associated with the symptoms of ADHD

d. inappropriately high levels of attention

are happy they are so excited and exuberant that people tell them to calm down. When they are angry or upset they are so volatile and intense that people tell them to calm down. They learn emotions are not to be valued, instead that they may lead to trouble or to being reprimanded.

The combination of these qualities—feedback received for emotional lability, lack of ability to develop the skills necessary to control emotions, and the disruption in relationships—exerts a significant impact on the child's emerging sense of self, locus of control, and likely subsequent personality. Refer to Table 17–2 for a historical time line of the diagnosis.

ADHD SYMPTOMS ACROSS THE LIFE SPAN

Historically, attention-deficit disorders were thought to be limited to childhood and adolescence. Longitudinal studies indicate that core symptoms of attention-deficit disorders persist over time (Connors & Jett, 1999). Psychiatric nurses are in unique positions to recognize the potentially disabling and adverse outcomes of these disorders across the

life span and work with the client, caregivers, and other mental health professionals, and develop holistic treatment planning to facilitate an optimal level of functioning and quality of life.

CHILDHOOD

The symptoms of ADHD appear to arise on average between the ages of 3 to 7. This is true primarily for the symptoms of hyperactivity and impulsivity. Hyperactivity is often seen as restlessness, excessive running, inability to sit still for an age-appropriate length of time, fidgeting, or excessive talking. Impulsivity is exhibited as acting before thinking, not being able to take turns, poor personal boundaries, intrusive behavior, and frequently interrupting others. Many of these symptoms are behaviors often seen in young children who have not learned the skills of delayed gratification or impulse control. Refer to Table 17–3 for symptoms of ADHD across the life span.

Children with hyperactivity and impulsivity in infancy are often described as difficult or temperamental. They are frequently very active, easily overstimulated, become very upset with changes in routine, and sleep poorly. They nap infrequently, fall asleep late, and wake early. As toddlers their exuberance is out of proportion to their peers'. They are overactive, respond poorly to direction or requests, exhibit an intensity of emotional response, have frequent temper tantrums, and increased accidental injury.

Inattentiveness is a more discreet symptom and may not be identified until the child is in a structured situation requiring

Abbreviated ADHD Symptom Checklist–4

Child's Name _____ Date _____

Name of Person Completing Form _____ Relationship to Child _____

Directions: Indicate the degree to which each item below is a problem. Please respond to all items. Consider the child's behavior on the following days: _____

	Never	Sometimes	Often	Very Often
1. Doesn't pay attention to details; makes careless mistakes	0	1	2	3
2. Difficulty paying attention	0	1	2	3
3. Does not seem to listen	0	1	2	3
4. Difficulty following instructions; does not finish things	0	1	2	3
5. Difficulty getting organized	0	1	2	3
6. Avoids doing things that require a lot of mental effort	0	1	2	3
7. Loses things	0	1	2	3
8. Easily distracted	0	1	2	3
9. Forgetful	0	1	2	3
10. Fidgets with hands or feet; squirms in seat	0	1	2	3
11. Difficulty remaining seated	0	1	2	3
12. Runs about or climbs on things	0	1	2	3
13. Difficulty playing quietly	0	1	2	3
14. "On the go"; acts as if "driven by a motor"	0	1	2	3
15. Talks excessively	0	1	2	3
16. Blurts out answers to questions	0	1	2	3
17. Difficulty awaiting turn	0	1	2	3
18. Interrupts others or butts into their activities	0	1	2	3

Note. Data from *ADHD Symptom Checklist-4 Manual,* by K. D. Gadow & J. Spafkin, 1997, Stony Brook, NY: Checkmate Plus. Adapted with permission; and from *Child Symptom Inventory-4 Norms Manual,* by K. D. Gadow & J. Spafkin, 1997, Stony Brook, NY: Checkmate Plus. Reprinted with permission.

sustained attention to tasks, such as school. Inattentiveness is often seen as distractibility, inability to complete tasks or assignments, forgetfulness, poor listening skills, or disorganization. Children with the inattentive subtype tend to miss essential details with schoolwork and often lose the tools or materials required for class work or play. Because they have difficulty sustaining attention they will avoid activities that

require concentration and mental effort. They also have more difficulty staying on topic or following the rules of a game once it has started.

In addition to the core symptoms discussed, children with ADHD may experience low self-esteem and difficulties with interpersonal relationships. They may exhibit mood swings, low frustration tolerance, temper tantrums, negativism, oppositional

TABLE 17–3
Symptoms across the Life Span

Preschool (3–5 Years Old)	School Age (6–12 Years Old)	Adolescent (13–18 Years Old)	Adult
• Increased motor activity	• Easily distracted	• Decreased/poor self-esteem	• Disorganized, poor planning skills
• Aggressive to others	• Homework poorly organized, frequent errors, careless mistakes, not complete	• School work is disorganized	• Forgetful, frequently loses things
• High curiosity level	• Blurts out answers before question is completed	• Difficulty completing long-term assignments	• Difficulty in initiation and completion of tasks, projects, assignments
• Spills, breaks things		• Fails to work independently	
• Rough play (often breaks, damages toys, frequent accidental injuries)	• Frequently interrupts, disrupts class	• High-risk-taking behaviors	• Poor time management skills—misjudges available time
• Demanding, argumentative	• Fails to wait turn in games	• Poor peer relations	
• Noisy, frequently interrupts others	• Often out of seat	• Difficulty with rules, laws, and authority figures	• Frequent job changes
• Excessive temper tantrums (severe and frequent)	• Perceived as being immature by adults		• Marital difficulties
• Low level of compliance with adult's requests	• Unwilling or unable to complete chores at home		• Continued inattention/concentration problems
	• Often interrupts or intrudes on peers		• Poor frustration tolerance
	• Poor peer relations/few friends		
	• Difficulty playing games, unable to follow directions		

Note. Adapted from *Attention Deficit Disorder (In Adults and Children): The Latest Assessment and Treatment Strategies*, by C. K. Conners & J. L. Jett, 1999, Kansas City, MO: Compact Clinicals.

---

behavior, bossiness, and poor response to authority. School problems are common and they frequently are described as lazy, stubborn, or unmotivated. **Conflicts** within the family are common owing to the child's impulsivity, disorganization, difficulty with obeying rules, and academic problems.

ADOLESCENCE

It is estimated that 50 to 80 percent of children with ADHD will continue to experience symptoms in adolescence. Adolescents with ADHD of the hyperactive-impulsive subtype will exhibit increasing difficulty with authority and an increase in high-risk-taking behaviors. They continue to have academic difficulties primarily in the area of assignment completion and organization of schoolwork. If the children have been able to channel their energy into sports, they may exhibit difficulty showing up on time for practices or following the coach's instruction. Refer to Table 17–3.

Adolescents with ADHD are often seen as underachievers academically. Symptoms that persist and contribute to poor performance are inability to organize work, even having the proper tools, failing to follow directions, or forgetting to turn in assignments. By their teens many children with ADHD have experienced some academic failure either course or complete grade failure.

Adolescents with ADHD continue to experience age-inappropriate levels of emotions. They are described as silly, overly sensitive to teasing by peers, or they are seen to excessively "fool around." They continue to be restless or fidgety, frequently interrupt others, and have poor frustration tolerance. The high levels of overactivity and excessive talking have diminished but are still present at levels above that of same-age peers.

Taylor, Chadwick, Heptinstall, and Dancharets (1996) completed a follow-up study of a large community survey of children with severe hyperactivity or conduct problems identified at age 6 to 7 by parent and teacher ratings. The follow-up study was done when the children were ages 16 to 18. The authors concluded that children with hyperactivity demonstrated a much higher risk for development of other psychiatric disorders, including persistent hyperactivity, antisocial behaviors, and problems with peers. Achenbach and McConaughy (1996) tested the long-term effects of inattention on the development of conduct problems. After controlling for initial conduct problems, the authors concluded that initial problems with attention made little contribution to the development of later conduct problems. Adolescents with untreated ADHD of the hyperactive-impulsive subtype appear to be at higher risk for development of conduct problems, antisocial behaviors, academic failures, and substance abuse problems.

ADULTHOOD

Historically, ADHD was considered to be a disorder of childhood. There has been limited research done into the persistence of symptoms of ADHD into adulthood. Estimates are that from 40 to 60 percent of clients with ADHD eventually outgrow the symptoms or develop the skills to effectively manage the symptoms. Prospective studies that followed children diagnosed with ADHD through age 25 years demonstrated that over 50 percent continued to exhibit symptoms of the disorder into adulthood. They exhibit continued problems in the ability to sustain attention and inhibit impulsivity (Barkley, Fisher, Edelbrook, & Smallish, 1990; Searight, Rottnek, & Abby, 2001). Their findings further demonstrated that 23 percent of these adults had dropped out of high school. They also found that nearly 25 percent had progressed into conduct disorder and developed a pattern of antisocial behavior, including interpersonal difficulties, occupational instability and substance abuse. Refer to Table 17–3.

In 1995, Achenbach, Howell, McConaughy, and Stanger followed a sample of youngsters with ADHD into young adulthood. They found a common syndrome among young adults who had previously been diagnosed with ADHD inattentive type in adolescence: they exhibited a pattern of irresponsible behavior. The attention problems continued to affect significantly more females than males. The researchers suggested that when clinicians evaluate adults for ADHD, they should assess for problems related to irresponsibility. Common problems that would be exhibited are frequent firings from jobs, problems making decisions, and low self-confidence. The authors further concluded that the symptoms of overactivity and overimpulsivity might not be evident in the adult syndrome.

Deficits in sustained attention and concentration are likely to remain and become more apparent or problematic as responsibilities increase. Impulsivity can take the form of socially inappropriate behavior such as blurting out thoughts,

interrupting others, or being rude. Although many of these symptoms are reported by significant others, adults with ADHD often present with complaints of an inability to be organized. They may also experience difficulties in prioritizing, giving simple tasks inordinate time and attention while procrastinating or not completing important ones (Vollmer, 1998).

Diagnosis of ADHD in adults, not previously identified in childhood, requires that the individual meet the diagnostic criteria as identified in the *DSM-IV TR* (4th ed.). Clinicians should obtain diagnostic information from significant persons involved with the adult, such as spouses/partners, colleagues, supervisors, and parents. If available, clinicians should review data from various phases of the client's life (report cards/transcripts, school evaluations, reports of legal violations if they exist, and any previous medical evaluations). It is estimated that nearly 75 percent of adults with ADHD have a comorbid condition (i.e., anxiety disorder, bipolar II disorder, or personality disorder) (Bailey & Weiss, 2003). Adults with ADHD are at considerable risk for substance abuse problems (alcohol, marijuana), smoking, antisocial behaviors (stealing, violence, and vandalism), however, the risk is diminished with appropriate treatment of ADHD (Elliott, 2002).

Results from the 2006 National Comorbidity Survey Replication of adults with ADHD are consistent with these findings in which concomitant psychiatric disorders are highly prevalent across the life span (Kessler et al., 2006).

Adults with ADHD often are attracted to occupations that can be characterized as exciting, risky, or active (such as stock broking, sales, or involving traveling). Many adults with ADHD report frequent occupational problems such as difficulties planning, disorganization, failing to complete projects/tasks, and frequent changes in jobs. Interpersonally, they may experience problems with unstable relationships, social isolation, managing their personal schedule, and organizing their homes. Their choice of leisure activities are ones that are higher risk or very stimulating such as downhill skiing, high-contact sports, or surfing the Internet.

Other symptoms noted in adults can include:

◆ Being argumentative
◆ Becoming bored easily
◆ Chronic tiredness and fatigue
◆ Poor frustration tolerance
◆ Narcissism
◆ Poor short-term memory
◆ Impaired spatial perception
◆ Increased incidence of spousal or child abuse
◆ Low degree of motivation

Adults with ADHD are not the only ones affected by their symptoms. Relatives, spouses, employers, coworkers, and teachers also experience the disruptive impact of their symptoms. Disruptive refers to throwing into disorder or confusion. Appointments, social commitments, and deadlines may frequently be forgotten. These symptoms often lead to difficulties in sustaining employment, friendships, or even marriages. Adults with ADHD are often labeled as poor performers, lazy, unmotivated, self-centered, or slow learners. Over the course of their lives a minority of those with ADHD are at significant risk for development of comorbid disorders of oppositional defiant disorder, conduct disorder, antisocial behaviors, learning disabilities, depression, or bipolar disorder (Biederman, Petty, et al., 2007).

TREATMENT CONSIDERATIONS FOR THE CLIENT IN THE HOME AND COMMUNITY SETTINGS

Clients with ADHD will receive the majority of their care in the home and community. Impact of the symptoms of ADHD on the client, family, and social systems can be profound. Symptoms can range from mild to severe and extremely disruptive. Symptoms occur across a variety of settings, making it important to have a holistic treatment approach that incorporates home- and community-based interventions. Children with ADHD can present a challenge, and response to treatment interventions is individualized and unpredictable.

ADHD is often complicated by the existence of comorbid conditions such as oppositional defiant disorder, conduct disorder, anxiety, or affective disorders (Biederman, Spencer, 2007; Turgay, 2005). These conditions have an impact on and may complicate treatment outcomes. The nurse must be familiar with a wide range of disorders and symptoms that can overlap or mimic ADHD, such as the overactive behaviors that can occur with bipolar disorder. The goal of treatment should be to identify and reduce disruptive symptoms and to promote improvement in family, peer, and social relationships. Successful treatment outcomes rely heavily on involving family and significant adults (teachers, mentors, coaches, clergy). The nurse needs to collaborate closely with all individuals involved with the client to identify symptoms and implement treatment strategies that best meet the client's individual needs.

To identify appropriate and effective interventions, the nurse should first perform an in-depth biopsychosocial assessment. The assessment should include identification of significant symptoms by both client and the adults involved with the client, physical health status (including nutrition, vision, and hearing), past and present academic performance, presence of comorbid conditions, and identification of the components of the family system. Because family members are often the most affected and are the primary providers of behavioral interventions, the assessment should include clinical interviews with the client and family and it must be comprehensive. It should assess family structure, communication patterns, strengths, weaknesses, styles of discipline, and social support network.

RESEARCH ABSTRACT

Does Methylphenidate Cause a Cytogenetic Effect in Children with Attention Deficit Hyperactivity Disorder?

Walitza, S., Werner, B., Romanos, M., Warnke, A., Gerlach, M., & Stopper, H. (2007). *Environmental Health Perspectives, 115*, 936–940.

Study Problem/Purpose
Researchers explored the possible correlation between methylphenidate (MPH) and risk of developing cancer later in life after long-term use of MPH therapy.

Method
A prospective study was used to analyze genetic damage in children with ADHD (n = 38 children [initial]) before and 1 (30 children), 3 (21 children), and 6 (8 children) months after the start of MPH therapy. The researchers also examined a group of 9 children receiving long-term MPH therapy. Subjects were recruited within the researchers' inpatient and outpatient Clinical Research Group on ADHD in the Department of Child and Adolescent Psychiatry and Psychotherapy. Genomic damage was measured by frequency of micronuclei in serum lymphocytes samples.

Findings
Researchers concluded that concerns raised by El-Zein and colleagues (2005) could not be replicated and concerns about the risk of developing cancer later in life after long-term MPH treatment was not supported.

Implications for Psychiatric Nurses
More research is needed to determine the precise long-term effects of medications on children and adults across the life span. Medications used to treat children must be carefully monitored and based on the absolute need for treatment with specific medications, such as MPH. Informed consent with the youth and family are an integral part of any treatment. Short- and long-term adverse risks must be discussed and monitored throughout treatment across the life span.

Another very important aspect of the nursing assessment is client and family educational needs. The nurse will serve an important role in educating the client, family, and significant adults about ADHD, its signs and symptoms, treatment options and prognosis. Because ADHD occurs across the life span, mental health care needs to be age specific and individualized to the client. Educational materials and teaching strategies must be appropriate for the client and family's cognitive level and include verbal information and visual and written materials.

Treatment considerations need to include family and community resources. Clients with supportive families and strong social support are more likely to have positive treatment outcomes (Murphy, 2005; Weiss, Hechtman, & The Adult ADHD Research Group, 2006). Financial resources are another consideration; lack of insurance or limited finances are likely reasons that access to required care will be impeded, because medical visits and pharmacologic agents can be costly. Assessing for potential barriers and incorporating these into the treatment plan can improve compliance.

Nursing responsibilities for management of the client's plan of care may include administering medications. Health teaching about the indications for use, effects, and potential side effects of medication is a major nursing responsibility. Clients and families will require education and nutritional counseling because many of the pharmacologic agents can affect the appetite.

Nonpharmacologic strategies should include the client, family, and other involved adults' education as well as behavioral management skills. These skills begin with parent training and follow a progression. Parents and teachers first need to be educated about ADHD—its causes, symptoms, presentation across the life span, and various treatments. A goal of education should be to help these adults to recognize ADHD as a chronic condition with symptoms, which vary in response to surroundings but which respond to interventions, much like diabetes. Family members need to be helped to modify their expectations of the child with ADHD because his performance in tasks may differ from his peers. They should be encouraged to assume the role of advocate for their child and work with school, sports, or group leaders to provide the support and structure that will help enhance the child's performance.

Interventions in the classroom and at school will require the support of the child's teacher. A teacher who is knowledgeable about ADHD can help to effectively implement behavioral interventions, modify classroom setting, and provide valuable feedback on treatment efficacy. Behavioral interventions in the classroom may include moving the desk to a less-distracting location, daily report cards, visual cues, token or reward systems, and rules for time-out (Barkley & Murphy, 1998). It may also include workload or assignment modifications, peer tutoring, or individualized education plans.

When first implementing treatment it is important to decrease the impact of the symptoms of inattentiveness, distractibility, disruptive behavior, and overactivity. These symptoms are the most disturbing to the child and the adults who live or work with him on a daily basis. An initial goal of treatment should be to increase individual productivity (completing assignments correctly) rather than total workload. This will help the child experience successes and internalize new skills.

Younger children benefit from token or reward systems that are used consistently across multiple settings such as the home, school, and day care. The system should be used in similar fashion but address areas of functioning specific to the setting. Home areas may focus on chores, family relationships, and general behavior. School areas may focus on assignment completion, following class rules, and peer relationships. The behaviors need to be defined in a clear, concise manner, and the token or reward should be given frequently and immediately in response to desired behaviors. Figure 17–1 provides a sample behavior and reward contract.

For teenagers, classroom strategies will need to be modified. Teens should be allowed greater responsibility and involvement in developing a behavior management plan. By adolescence, many teens are very aware of their specific symptoms and which strategies are most effective. Home rules will begin addressing areas such as curfews, dating, and even driving. Rewards can be modified to be immediate and long term, such as earning points for an evening or weekend outing. School strategies should include the use of organizers and calendars, scheduling harder classes in the mornings, and use of adult mentors.

Other nonpharmacologic interventions may include the use of psychoeducational groups such as social skills or anger management. Individual or family therapy may be added to address issues related to communication, relationships, or symptoms from other co-occurring conditions. The type of therapy should be individualized and specific to the needs of the client and family, severity of symptoms, personal preference, and past response to treatment.

THE ROLE OF THE NURSE

Providing care for the client with ADHD requires an understanding of the complexity of the disorder, symptom variations, and the influence of social, environmental, and biological factors. The role of the nurse will vary according to educational preparation, use of nursing theoretical frameworks, clinical experience, personal interest, and the clinical care setting. Nursing roles and responsibilities vary, from administering medications to developing and implementing holistic treatment plans. Responsibilities will be commensurate with educational preparation and legal parameters. State practice acts define and regulate the nurse's scope of practice at each level of nursing. Regardless of the level of practice, the nurse's role is to assess, diagnose, plan, implement, and evaluate the client's response to interventions. Interventions should be designed so as to minimize symptoms, improve relationships, and enhance client functioning.

THE GENERALIST NURSE

The nurse in a generalist role may work with clients with ADHD in a variety of settings. Nurses working in mental health clinics, pediatricians' offices, and schools have the most contact with these clients. Understanding the disorder, its etiology, symptoms, and types of treatment enables the nurse to work with the client and family and identify their specific mental health needs. The nurse may choose a specific theoretical framework to guide his practice, or he may follow clinical guidelines developed at the work setting. The initial goal of the nurse is to identify problems and establish a plan of intervention to reduce the frequency and severity of symptoms. Interventions include establishing the nurse-client relationship, enhancing the coping skills of the client and family, identifying maladaptive responses, and decreasing the negative impact of the symptoms of hyperactivity, impulsivity, and inattention. Another important nursing intervention is medication administration, patient education, and monitoring patient response.

The nurse will establish outcome criteria to measure client response. Improved relationships within the home and school environment, improved academic performance, improved sleep pattern, and ability to delay gratification can serve as outcome measures. Treatment modalities can include case management, group therapy, and psychoeducation.

Psychoeducation can be effective in:

◆ Fostering age-appropriate behaviors, improving interactions with peers, dealing with aggressive impulses, and improving social skills (e.g., taking turns, following rules, and not interrupting others).

◆ Setting and helping the child respond to and adhere to limits through the use of time-outs, behavior charts, or earning and losing privileges.

◆ Assisting the parents in developing systems to improve self-esteem by providing tasks or activities in which the child can succeed.

◆ Helping the family, child, and teachers understand the disorder, client-specific symptoms, and interventions, which will help decrease the symptoms. These may be pharmacologic or behavioral, or both.

Behavioral Contract

I, _____, agree to do the following:
(name of child)

1. _____
2. _____
3. _____
4. _____
5. _____

Each period of _____ that I will do these will earn me one of the following rewards:

1. _____
2. _____
3. _____
4. _____
5. _____

I understand that if I do not complete these responsibilities, I will not earn the rewards on this contract.

I agree to try to fulfill this contract to the best of my abilities.

Signed,   Date

child: _____   _____

parent: _____   _____

teacher: _____   _____

Figure 17–1 Behavioral contract.

The nurse in the generalist role may encounter the client with ADHD in a variety of settings. He may work in a clinic as part of the direct treatment team or be an external partner located in the child's school. It is essential for the nurse to work as part of the team in order to deliver consistent care and provide reinforcement in the use of new skills by the child or parent. The nurse also plays an important role in assessing the efficacy of treatment interventions and he can serve as a liaison between the child and family and the other members of the treatment team, including the child's teachers.

THE ADVANCED-PRACTICE PSYCHIATRIC REGISTERED NURSE

The advanced-practice nurse (APN) is a nurse with a master's degree, who has the ability to apply knowledge, skills, and experience autonomously to complex mental health problems (ANA, 2000). The APN may function in the role of clinical specialist, psychotherapist, or nurse practitioner. The APN can perform all the role functions of the generalist nurse but additionally may use psychobiological interventions to diagnose and treat mental health disorders. These interventions can include ordering diagnostic tests, evaluating symptoms and making differential diagnoses, prescribing pharmacologic agents, or providing psychotherapy.

Establishing a diagnosis involves gathering information on the client's current health status, family system, functional capacity, growth and development, course of symptoms, and ordering diagnostic tests. Data collection can involve communication and collaboration with other health care providers. Assessment data will include a review of body systems, mental status evaluation, psychosocial history, and interpretation of diagnostic information. Analysis of these data allows the APN to rule out certain conditions and establish a diagnosis.

Comprehensive physical and psychiatric assessments converge and form the basis for pharmacologic intervention. Before prescribing a medication, the APN should perform a psychopharmacologic assessment, including (ANA, 2000):

- Target symptoms and selection of treatment methods
- Side effect profile of selected agents
- Client response to previous medication(s)
- Concomitant medication usage
- Drug allergies
- Client and family treatment preferences
- Therapeutic response of first-degree family members to medications prescribed for similar problems

After collecting, analyzing assessment data, and establishing a diagnosis, the APN will collaborate with other health care providers, the client, and family to establish a treatment plan. The plan of care may include a variety of interventions such as use of behavioral charts, reward systems, pharmacotherapy, and psychotherapy.

APNs in psychiatric-mental health are educated to perform independently in a primary therapist role. Their knowledge and skills as a therapist will depend on the types of modalities they were trained in, their clinical experience, and the clients' diagnoses. Psychotherapy enables the APN to assess the impact of symptoms on the clients' self-esteem, the influence of social and environmental factors on symptom severity, and client communication patterns with family, peers, and adults. The choice of therapeutic modality is influenced by many factors, including client needs, care setting, cost, and research validating positive response of similar diagnoses to treatment. Research has not validated a positive response of ADHD clients to individual psychotherapy (MTA Cooperative Group, 1999). Use of cognitive-behavioral interventions (coaching, skills training) initially offers the client and family experiences to promote adaptive coping skills, improve communication, resolve conflict, and reinforce positive behavioral changes (Murphy, 2005; Safren et al., 2005; Weiss et al., 2006).

Through advanced training and education, the APN is qualified to initiate and monitor pharmacotherapy. An understanding of the pharmacokinetics, pharmacodynamics, and the biological basis of ADHD guides the APN in prescribing psychotropic medications. Before initiating any pharmacologic agent, the APN must obtain the informed consent of the client and parents or guardians. Informed consent involves providing information about the medication, its intended effects, and potential side effects, and discussing alternative medications or treatment options. Medication prescription includes the ordering of medication, monitoring effect and symptom response, titration of dosage as warranted by symptoms, and client and family education. Over the course of treatment the APN continuously assesses the client's response to interventions, educational needs, and makes appropriate referrals for identified health care needs.

The APN, through the use of advanced knowledge, skills, and experience, offers a comprehensive approach to the care of clients with ADHD, combining a variety of interventions, pharmacologic and behavioral, to meet the client's individual needs.

THE NURSING PROCESS

ADHD is composed of a range of symptoms that evolve and change throughout the client's life span. The incidence of comorbidity of other psychiatric disorders (anxiety, major depression, conduct, and oppositional defiant disorders) reinforces the need for nurses to understand the complexity of human responses to actual or potential mental health problems. This understanding provides the basis for development of effective interventions. The nursing process provides a guide for nurses to address these problems systematically. Development of a comprehensive plan of care requires an age-specific biopsychosocial assessment integrating data about the client's physical and mental status.

ASSESSMENT

The assessment process begins with ruling out other potential illnesses or factors yielding symptoms that mimic ADHD. A complete medical examination, including hearing and vision evaluations, is the initial step. Data collection should also include a review of currently used prescribed and over-the-counter medications, dietary habits, and an assessment of the client's living environment. Dietary habits are important to assess because many food additives can exacerbate symptoms. Data about the client's living environ-ment should be carefully gathered to identify potential contributing factors such as exposure to lead, inadequate living or sleeping space, or exposure to community violence.

Eliminating other diagnoses and medical conditions then allows the nursing assessment to focus on identification of symptoms and their impact on client functioning. Assessing the client with ADHD requires an understanding of normal growth and development because this disorder most often first manifests itself in early childhood.

The establishment of the nurse-client relationship and development of trust and rapport begin during the assessment phase. It requires skill and patience in interviewing, because the client may be very overactive, impulsive, and distractible. The clinical interview may need to be broken into shorter visits, or the setting may need to be modified to minimize distractions and promote client participation.

The mental status examination is an important component of the assessment process, providing data about the client's current mental health, judgment, cognitive functioning, thought processes, impulse control, insight, and strengths. Data collected can be used to classify ADHD into its various subtypes: inattentive, hyperactive, or combined type. The mental status examination will provide data regarding the symptoms, severity, and impairment in functioning as well as allow the nurse to identify possible comorbid conditions.

The family system is another important area of assessment. The nurse will need to focus the interview and data collection process to identify current stressors, communication patterns, social support systems, parenting and discipline styles, parents' knowledge about ADHD, and available resources. Family systems are often disrupted by the client with ADHD. Parents are frustrated with their inability to help their child, sibling relationships are impaired owing to the client's poor skills in relating to others, and support systems are often diminished because of the impact of the client's symptoms.

Common behavioral manifestations of ADHD comprise difficulties with task completion, impaired peer relationships, frequent accidental injuries, and a high level of family conflict and tension. Clients with the inattentive type of ADHD often do not exhibit the disruptive behaviors and are often not identified until their school years, where they have difficulty with task completion, focusing, and concentration. Their academic performance suffers and they are frequently identified because of school failure.

Symptoms of ADHD are evident across a variety of settings, and the frequency and severity are determined by the demands placed on the client in the particular environment. For instance, a child may exhibit only mild symptoms in the home and social situations but symptoms greatly exacerbate within the school setting because of the structure and performance demands. Assessing the frequency, areas of occurrence, and impact on the client's level of functioning is essential to accurate diagnosis and treatment planning.

NURSING DIAGNOSES

Nursing diagnoses should be based on an analysis of assessment data. The nurse working with the client with ADHD should consider the following diagnoses in developing the plan of care (NANDA, 2007):

◆ Risk for Injury: Related to Impulsivity

◆ Imbalanced Nutrition: Less than Body Requirements Related to Excessive Motor Activity

◆ Disturbed Sleep Pattern: Related to Medication Side Effects

◆ Impaired Social Interaction: Related to Ineffective Social Skills

◆ Chronic or Situational Low Self-Esteem: Possibly related to rejection by Family, Peers, and Adults

◆ Deficient Knowledge: Related to a Lack of Understanding of ADHD, etiology, Course and Treatment

◆ Impaired Parenting: Related to Knowledge Deficit about ADHD

Nursing diagnoses guide the nurse in developing an individualized, client-centered treatment plan. It identifies patterns of human response to actual or potential health problems. Nursing care is holistic in nature and focuses not only on the client but also on the family or others affected by the client's symptoms. The goal of treatment is to return the client to optimum level of functioning and restore equilibrium within the family system and other affected environments. The effectiveness of treatment is measured by establishing outcomes and continuously evaluating patient progress against these targets.

OUTCOME IDENTIFICATION

Outcome identification involves establishing individualized outcome measures. These measures are incorporated into the treatment plan. Outcome measures logically flow from the nursing diagnosis and planned interventions. They provide evidence regarding the effectiveness of planned interventions and they are measurable and objective. Common outcome measures for clients with ADHD include:

◆ Adequate management of symptoms

◆ Adequate nutrition

- Normal sleep and rest patterns
- Understanding and insight about the nature of ADHD, its symptoms, causes, and treatments
- Effective individual coping
- Healthy family, peer, and adult interactions

PLANNING

Achieving successful outcomes are the result of effective treatment planning, which should be holistic and collaborative. Collaboration needs to occur between the nurse, client, family, teachers, other health care providers, and community resources.

Treatment planning involves accurate assessment, problem identification, development of easily implemented interventions, and achievable outcome measures. Interventions should be designed to target specific symptoms and reduce or eliminate their impact on the client and others. Treatment plans are dynamic and fluid, requiring continuous evaluation and revisions in accordance with changes in the client and family.

IMPLEMENTATION

During the assessment phase the nurse has established a therapeutic relationship with the client, family, and others involved in the client's treatment. From this relationship trust evolves along with the rapport needed to successfully implement treatment. Client and family education are a fundamental component of treatment of the client with ADHD.

Parents require education about causal factors, hereditability, and chronicity in order to modify their expectations of their child. Clients with ADHD will need time, patience, understanding, and ongoing treatment to achieve their full potential. Parents need assistance to develop advocacy skills so that they can assist in identifying environmental, academic, or systems problems that affect the child and facilitate change. Education about the variety and range of symptoms, effective interventions, and correcting misinformation is a primary goal of treatment. Clients and families should be educated as to the role of pharmacotherapy, the symptoms most likely to respond to medication, and potential side effects or problems that may result from the use of medication.

Individual and family therapies have not been demonstrated to be effective in the treatment of ADHD (MTA Cooperative Group, 1999). However, psychoeducation groups that focus on skill improvement, such as social skills or anger management, do serve to enhance client strengths. Social skills training can be effective in promoting listening skills, developing conflict resolution skills, and enhancing peer relations. Social skills training is more effective when taught in a group setting such as summer camp, after-school programs, or school-based groups (Sheridan, Dee, Morgan, McCormick, & Walker, 1996).

Psychosocial interventions will need to be taught to parents and teachers. The focus of parent training includes establishing a consistent, supportive, and structured environment for the client. Establishing household rules; giving commands that are specific, clear, and positive; ignoring mild inappropriate behavior, and praising positive behaviors are interventions designed to reduce the severity of disruptive symptoms and enhance self-esteem. Use of behavioral contracting, chart systems, and daily report cards serve to identify target behaviors and improve home-school communication while providing the client with consistent expectations. Figure 17–2 provides an example of a daily report card.

Behavioral interventions focus on positive learning experiences that reduce symptom impact, enhance coping skills, and provide opportunities for success for the client with ADHD. Active participation of family and teachers in helping the client adapt and develop coping skills is vital to the success of treatment. The overall treatment outcomes for the family and client with ADHD are:

- Identify and implement interventions to reduce target symptoms.
- Develop an understanding of triggers that exacerbate symptoms.
- Develop adaptive skills that enhance relationships and personal functioning in school or work and the community.
- Avoid maladaptive responses.
- Use community resources and support systems effectively.

Treatment must consider a combination of pharmacologic and behavioral interventions. Simultaneous use of this combination of interventions provides superior outcomes rather than the use of either intervention alone.

EVALUATION

Evaluation of the effectiveness of the established behavioral management plan should be ongoing. The nurse, family, and child should meet on a regularly established timetable to review agreed-upon outcomes, academic and social progress, and whether or not problematic behaviors have improved. To achieve objectivity and consistency, the nurse may use a rating scale administered by teachers and parents, report cards, and reports from leaders of community-based activities. To accurately measure the child's progress and improvement, it is important to use the same rating scale throughout the course of treatment. As the child ages and matures, it will be necessary to modify the plan of care to meet the needs of the child, family, and other adults involved in his life.

PSYCHOPHARMACOLOGY

Pharmacologic treatment of ADHD is the most studied and best understood of all pyschopharmacologic treatments in children and adolescents. Nursing implications in the treatment of

SUBJECTS	1	2	3	4	5	6
Participates in class						
Follows class rules						
Gets along with peers						
Performs assignments in allotted time						
Homework is complete						
Teacher's initials and comments						
Parent's initials and comments						

TONIGHT'S HOMEWORK: _____

_____

LONG-TERM PROJECTS: _____

Figure 17–2 Daily report card.

ADHD vary with the nursing role but at either level includes assessing efficacy of psychotropics and patient and family education.

The APN will be involved in prescribing or recommending medications to treat the symptoms of the disorder. In order to effectively prescribe pharmacologic agents, maximize efficacy, and minimize risk, the APN must have an understanding of basic and clinical sciences. These include biochemistry, pharmacology, anatomy, physiology, cardiology, endocrinology, and neurology.

Diagnosis and symptom identification are key in determining the choice of pharmacologic agent. The core symptoms of ADHD—inattention, impulsivity, distractibility, and hyperactivity—have been shown to respond favorably to pharmacotherapy. Psychostimulant medication has clearly been demonstrated to be the treatment of choice in those clients who are able to tolerate them.

Before prescribing a medication, the APN will need to identify any existing comorbid conditions. ADHD often presents with concomitant conditions of depression, anxiety, conduct disorder, oppositional defiant disorder, tic disorder, or Tourette's syndrome. Clients with ADHD and either conduct or oppositional defiant disorder often do fine with psychostimulant medication (Preen, Calver, Sanfilippo, Bulsara, & Holman, 2007). Clients with ADHD and the concomitant conditions of depression, anxiety, bipolar disorder, Tourette's syndrome, or schizophrenia are less likely to respond favorably to these medications and will require further assessment.

STIMULANTS

Psychostimulants are the most widely prescribed and best-researched medication used to treat ADHD. They increase the availability of certain neurotransmitters and have been found to improve focus and concentration. Common psychostimulant medications used in the treatment of ADHD include methylphenidate (Ritalin), mixed salts of a single-entity amphetamine product (Adderall), and dextroamphetamine (Dexedrine). Pemoline (Cylert) was once used first line, but because of the risk of development of serious side effects (liver failure), it is no longer recommended. The majority of these medications are short acting, with effect lasting from 4 to 6 hours. There are a few psychostimulants with longer duration of action such as dextroamphetamine spansules, methylphenidate SR (a single dose of which can last for up to 8 hours), Metadate CD, and Adderall XR. Currently, both Adderall and methylphenidate have been produced with a different delivery system providing efficacy up to 12 hours.

The specific dose of medicine must be determined for each individual. There are ranges based on dose per unit of body weight that are recommended and that provide guidelines for initiation of treatment. However, there are no consistent relationships among the height, weight, and age of the child and response to medication. A medication trial is often used to determine the most beneficial dosage. Medication is started at a low dose and gradually increased in frequency of administration and dosage until optimal effect is achieved. This also provides the opportunity for identification of side effects early in treatment.

Psychostimulants have been used successfully for over 50 years to treat ADHD. Although they have been found to be safe and effective, side effects may occur. The most common side effects are reduced appetite, headache, and difficulty sleeping. A relatively uncommon side effect may be the unmasking of latent tics such as eye blinking, shrugging, and clearing of the throat. Psychostimulant medications can facilitate the emergence of a tic disorder but are not a direct cause. Often the tic(s) will stop once the medication is discontinued. Some children experience a rebound effect as the medication wears off. They demonstrate a negative mood, increased irritability, or increased hyperactivity. Side effects are usually managed by an adjustment in dosage and scheduling of the medication. (See Chapter 29, Psychopharmacologic Therapy.)

ALTERNATIVE MEDICATIONS

Although psychostimulants are first-line agents in the treatment of ADHD, there are individuals who are not responsive to or cannot tolerate these medications. However, there are a variety of nonstimulating agents that have demonstrated efficacy. Strattera (atomoxetine) is the first FDA-approved treatment for ADHD that is not a stimulant. It is a novel agent that enhances nonadrenergic function through highly selective blockade of the presynaptic norepinephrine transporter (Adesman, 2002). Table 17–4 provides an overview of medications used to treat ADHD and their mechanism of action. Tricyclic antidepressants and bupropion act on the neurotransmitters norepinephrine and dopamine. These medications have demonstrated a positive response in symptom reduction. Clonidine, originally an antihypertensive medication, has shown some positive response, primarily, in reduction of the symptoms of hyperactivity, impulsive behaviors, intrusiveness, and sleep disturbance. The selective serotonin reuptake inhibitors have not demonstrated efficacy in treatment of the core symptoms of ADHD. They have been effective in treatment of concomitant disorders such as depression and anxiety. These medications have been less studied and are not approved by the FDA for treatment of ADHD. However, they are frequently used off-label in the treatment of individuals with ADHD (Turgay, 2005).

Medication Assessment

Baseline assessment data to be collected before initiation of medication include:

1. Complete blood count (CBC) with differential.
2. Height, weight, heart rate, and blood pressure.
3. Behavioral rating scales from a variety of adults who observe the child in different settings such as parents,

extended family members, teachers, coaches, or adult mentors. Some common rating scales are Conners' Parent-Teacher Rating Scale, ADHD Rating Scale, or the Vanderbilt ADHD Rating Scale. Refer to the ADHD checklist for an example of a behavior rating scale and instructions for use.

4. A complete physical examination, including hearing and vision evaluation and electrocardiogram if TCAs are used.

The choice of medication will be contingent on assessment data, patient symptoms, previous response to medications, patient or family preference, and social or environmental factors. Table 17–5 lists guidelines for diagnosis.

Other nursing implications of pharmacotherapy include client and family education about desired effects, potential side effects, timing of administration, monitoring, and documenting response to medication. Psychostimulants often require two-to-three-times-a-day dosing owing to their short-acting nature (Kutcher, 1997). This may necessitate administration of medication during school hours. It is important to work with the parents and the school to time dose administration to be effective and as least disruptive as possible. Trying to ensure medication administration during a child's lunch or recess time will decrease drawing attention to the child and avoid disruption of class time. It is also important to time administration after meals to minimize appetite disturbance. The nurse's role in medication administration will be two fold: assessing the effects of medication and assessing the child's response to the process. Table 17–6 provides medication education guidelines for the client on a stimulant medication.

Treatment of ADHD is usually long term. ADHD does not just disappear nor do children "grow out of it." There is no evidence to support that clients develop a tolerance to or develop dependence on stimulant medications. Periodic evaluations of the continued efficacy of medication should be incorporated into the treatment plan. For children and adults with ADHD, medication is an integral part of treatment. Pharmacologic treatment of ADHD has been shown to be the most effective treatment in reduction and long term management of symptoms (Turgay, 2005).

TABLE 17–4
Medications Used in the Treatment of ADHD

Name	Type	How it Works	Target Symptoms
Tofranil (imipramine) Pamelor (nortryptiline)	Tricyclic antidepressants (TCAs)	Inhibits the reuptake of norepinephrine and serotonin	Helps with impulsivity and hyperactivity and sleep disturbance; not effective with inattention
Ritalin, Concerta, Metadate CD or ER (methylphenidate) Dexedrine, Spansule or Dextrostat Adderall, Adderall XR	Stimulants	Acts as a mild cortical stimulant with CNS action	Helps with focusing, concentration, and overactivity
Catapres (clonidine) Tenex (guanfacine)	Antihypertensives	Stimulates alpha-adrenergic receptors to inhibit sympathetic nervous system	Helps with tic disorders, aggressive behaviors, and impulsivity. Does not help with inattention
Wellbutrin (bupropion)	Antidepressant	Inhibits the reuptake of dopamine and norepinephrine	Improves mood and possibly inattention; some decrease in overactivity noted in adolescents and adults
Remeron (mirtazapine)	Antidepressant	Inhibits reuptake of norepinephrine and dopamine	Helps improve mood and sleep disturbance in children with concomitant mood and sleep disorders
Strattera (atomoxetine)	Nonstimulant	Inhibits reuptake of norepinephrine	Helps improve symptoms of inattention

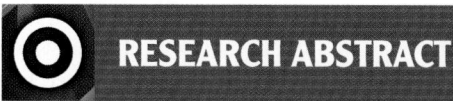

RESEARCH ABSTRACT

Efficacy and Safety of Mixed Amphetamine Salts Extended Release (Adderall XR) in the Management of Attention-Deficit/Hyperactivity Disorder in Adolescent Patients: A 4-Week, Randomized, Double Blind, Placebo-Controlled, Parallel-Group Study

Spencer, T. J., Wilens, T. E., Biederman, J., Weisler, R. H., Read, S. C., & Pratt, R. (2006). *Clinical Therapeutics, 28*, 266–279.

Study Problem/Purpose

The chief goal of the study was to examine the efficacy and safety of combination treatment of mixed amphetamine salts extended release (MAS XR) in the treatment of adolescents with ADHD.

Method

A 4-week randomized, multicenter, double blind, placebo-controlled, parallel-group, forced-dose-titration study that comprised adolescents ages 13 to 17 years old with ADHD. Adolescents were randomized to 1 to 4 active treatments of MAS XR 10, 20, 30, or 40 mg/day. The principle efficacy measure was change from baseline to end point in ADHD Rating Scale-IV score. The secondary efficacy measure was the score on the Clinical Global Impressions-Improvement (CGI-I) scale for ADHD. Safety was ensured and monitored, recording adverse events, vital signs, and weight during all study visits and 30 days after drug discontinuation.

Findings

Of the 287 randomized subjects, 258 completed the study. Most adolescents were male (65.5 percent) and white (73.7 percent). Adolescents with ADHD treated with 10 to 40 mg/day MAS XR up to 4 weeks demonstrated substantial improvements in ADHD symptoms compared to those who received placebo, and once-a-day dosing with MAS XR up to 40 mg was efficacious and well tolerated by adolescents with ADHD.

Implications for Psychiatric Nurses

Psychiatric nurses must understand major treatment for clients with ADHD. Psychoeducation is critical to helping clients and families understand the illness and available medications and potential side effects. As with all medications, particularly stimulants, it is imperative to monitor the client's physical and mental health status throughout treatment.

TABLE 17–5
The American Academy of Pediatrics Guidelines for Diagnosis

1. Initiate an evaluation for ADHD in a child aged 6 to 12 years who presents with inattention, hyperactivity, impulsivity, academic underachievement, or behavior problems.

2. A diagnosis of ADHD requires that a child meet criteria set forth in the *Diagnostic and Statistical Manual of Mental Disorder,* 4th edition Revision (*DSM-IV-TR*).

3. A diagnosis of ADHD requires evidence from parents or caregivers concerning the core symptoms of Attention-Deficit Hyperactivity Disorder in various settings, the age of onset, duration of symptoms, and the degree of functional impairment.

4. A diagnosis of ADHD requires evidence from the child's classroom teacher or other school professional concerning the core symptoms of ADHD, the duration of symptoms, the degree of functional impairment, and coexisting conditions.

5. Include an assessment for coexisting conditions in the evaluation of the child with ADHD.

6. No other diagnostic tests are routinely indicated to establish a diagnosis of ADHD.

TABLE 17–6
Patient Education Guide for the Client on a Stimulant Medication

- Take the medication as prescribed. If you miss a dose, do not "make it up." Just resume the medication at the next scheduled time.

- Avoid taking other medications, including over-the-counter medications, without discussing it with your health care provider or checking with your pharmacist to be sure there are no drug interactions.

- Take the medication after eating to avoid appetite problems or stomach upset.

- Avoid taking the medication late in the evening because it may disturb sleep.

- Some common side effects of this medication are:

  1. Stomach upset, appetite loss, vomiting

  2. Insomnia

  3. Rapid heartbeat, chest pain

  4. Headache

  5. Irritability, nervousness, or confusion

- Keep all regularly scheduled appointments with your health care provider so that medication effects can be monitored. This may include laboratory tests, blood pressure or pulse checks, height and weight checks, or other tests like ECGs.

BEHAVIORAL INTERVENTIONS

Treatment modalities associated with attention-deficit disorders must be holistic and include pharmacologic, behavioral, psychotherapy, and psychoeducation. Psychiatric nurses play key roles in implementing mutimodal interventions that involve symptom management, improve self-esteem, facilitate adaptive coping behaviors, and a higher level of functioning in the client, caregivers, and family systems.

TIME-OUT

Time-out procedures are quite effective in the management of the child with ADHD and should be incorporated into an overall behavior management plan. Time-out can be as simple as having the child sit in an isolated portion of the room, placing his head down on his desk, or sitting quietly for a few minutes. Time-out should be used to target unwanted behaviors that have previously been identified to the child, noncompliance, or to decelerate behavior.

BEHAVIOR MANAGEMENT PLANS

Behavior management plans are very effective in decreasing unwanted behaviors and promoting desired behaviors. The plan should be developed by the adults involved with the children and incorporate behaviors across different environments such as the home, the school, public places (stores, restaurants), day care, and church. The behaviors should be clearly and simply stated and written to provide the child with visual cues. Barkley (1997) identified a number of principles to use to enhance the efficacy of a behavior management plan:

◆ Be positive. It is important to tell the child with ADHD what you want to happen rather than what is not desired.

◆ Provide the child with simple, clear directions. The child with ADHD has difficulty complying with multiple or complex instructions. This information should be shared with the child's teacher. Because teachers frequently must give multiple or complex instructions to a group of students, they can be encouraged to check with the child with ADHD and have him repeat the instructions to ensure his understanding.

◆ State rules. Rules and desired behaviors need to be stated simply and clearly. They must also be reviewed and repeated frequently.

◆ Provide cues. The client with ADHD responds positively to visual and auditory cues. Cues such as audiotapes or cards taped to the desk that provide reminders to keep working have been shown to decrease off-task behavior.

◆ Use reinforcers. Provide reinforcement of positive by use of multiple and frequent reinforcers. The reinforcers do not need to be fancy or expensive and can be as simple as stickers or tokens.

◆ Provide a consistent routine but keep things changing. A child with ADHD functions better in a consistent, predictable setting. Frequent changes in daily activity schedule may confuse the child or increase his disorganization.

◆ Within this consistent routine, however, the child with ADHD will function better with multiple shortened work periods, opportunities for choice among work tasks, and reinforcers that are enjoyable.

SOCIAL SKILLS TRAINING

The social problems of ADHD are pervasive and varied; children with the hyperactive subtype tend to be overactive, impulsive, and aggressive, whereas the inattentive subtype have difficulty focusing, are socially inattentive, and can be withdrawn. These tendencies can directly or indirectly interfere with social interactions and the formation of peer relationships or friendships over time. It has been suggested that over 50 percent of children with ADHD have problems with interactions with peers (Barkley, 1996). Treatment of this deficit in social skills is an important part of the overall treatment of the client with ADHD.

According to social learning theory, social behaviors are acquired through observation and reinforcement (Bandura, 1977). The most common form of social skills intervention using social learning principles is modeling. Modeling is typically carried out in three steps. First is skill instruction involving the use of videotapes, audiotapes, or live demonstration showing the skill to be acquired. Social skills' training entails identification of skill components, discussion about the particular social skill, and information about skill performance.

The second step is skill demonstration. A skill trainer, teacher, peer, or video demonstration models the behavior. The child is instructed to observe the behavior and identify the components previously discussed. The third and final step is skill performance. The child is required to demonstrate the skill after completion of the first two steps. This is usually done through role playing. Active and constructive feedback is provided to the child for attempts at skill performance. Skill performance demonstration will continue until the desired behavior is accurately displayed.

Social skills training can be done one-on-one or in a group context. Several curricula are available that focus on social skills training with children and adolescents. Most programs are based on skill or use a problem-solving approach. Programs that focus on preventing aggression and violence have been developed recently and implemented with youth at risk.

PARENT TRAINING AND EDUCATION

Training parents to more effectively manage the behavior of children with ADHD is one component of parent training.

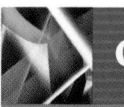

CASE STUDY

The Client with Attention-Deficit Hyperactivity Disorder (Joe C.)

Joe C. is an 8-year-old male referred by his pediatrician for evaluation of academic and behavioral problems of at least 1-year duration. His parents accompany him. He has two siblings, both girls, ages 10 and 6. His parents are married and there has been no history of marital discord. The parents are concerned about Joe's grades, his behavior at home, school, and with his soccer team. They comment that "he seems a lot more immature than the other boys his age."

Joe is currently in the second grade after failing reading and language arts (writing skills) last year. Currently he is continuing to perform very poorly in these areas. He is currently in a class of 24 children. Joe has few friends and his classmates identify him as one of the least-liked children in the class. His teacher notes the following problem areas:

- Is frequently out of his seat
- Appears to be daydreaming when he is supposed to be working on an assignment
- Has difficulty getting along with peers during recess or free time
- Has trouble following the rules of games
- Becomes easily angered and can be aggressive with other children
- Is intrusive with others (adults and children)
- Wants to switch from activity to activity, becomes bored easily

His parents are frustrated with his behavior and feel overwhelmed by complaints from school, soccer, and parents of other children. Their concerns about his behavior are:

- He rarely completes his chores, even the simple ones (make bed, put toys away, and help take out the trash once a week).
- He frequently fights with his siblings.
- He cannot sit still through a meal.
- He requires constant supervision to complete his homework.
- Even though he is in bed by 8:30 P.M., he is rarely asleep before midnight.
- He has had more accidental injuries (scrapes, bruises, cuts) than his siblings.

While practicing and playing with his soccer team, Joe's parents have observed the following behaviors:

- He has difficulty following the coach's instruction; he appears to forget what he's been told.
- He is aggressive with teammates.
- During games he is easily distracted by the crowd noise.

The pediatrician has provided a copy of Joe's latest physical examination, including current laboratory results, immunization record, and vision and hearing assessments.

The parents are anxious, frustrated, and want Joe fixed.

Scenario Questions

1. *What is the most important nursing consideration in the care of this client and his family?*

   The most important consideration is establishing a therapeutic relationship with the family and the client. Establishing trust and rapport are the basis of the nursing relationship and essential to the care of the client. Parents of children with ADHD often seek treatment when they have reached the peak of their frustration. Establishing trust and rapport can allow the nurse to work with the parents to decrease their frustration, gain an understanding of the nonvoluntary nature of the behavior, and develop a sense of hope. Once the anxiety and tension are decreased the family can be engaged in the assessment phase of treatment.

   The nurse's relationship with the client is extremely important, because children with ADHD have frequently received negative feedback about themselves in relation to their impulsive and overactive behavior. Their self-esteem and a feeling of mastery over their environment are usually quite low.

2. *What important assessment data should the nurse collect as the next step in treatment?*

   - Information regarding the mother's course of pregnancy, including labor and delivery, any history of maternal substance use during pregnancy, any family history of attention or excess motor activity, any history of head injury
   - Information about the child as an infant, toddler, and preschooler, including activity level, developmental milestones, sleep pattern, any significant illnesses or hospitalizations, relationships with siblings and peers, any history of lead ingestion, and use of medications

(continues)

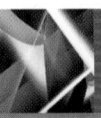
- Child's school behavior, including information from the teacher and parents and child, ability to perform academically, quality of work, need for frequent reminders, child's report of boredom, and ability to get along with others

- Any history of sleeping, eating, or self-care problems

- Child's response to limit setting, ability to follow rules, parent and teacher's perception of child's activity level, attention span, and response to authority

- Parent and teacher behavior rating scales

3. *The child is started on a psychostimulant. What interventions should the nurse provide for the client and family?*

   The primary focus is psychoeducation of the family, client, and teacher related to the disorder, etiology, symptoms, and treatment options. Education about physical self-care (nutrition, exercise, and sleep and rest pattern). Behavioral strategies need to be developed and implemented as an integrated plan of care.

   Reduction of symptoms and ongoing management involve pharmacologic and nonpharmacologic interventions. Outcome criteria should address stability of symptoms, medication administration and monitoring, acceptable and unacceptable behaviors, improvement in relationships with family and peers, and improved academic performance.

This case study demonstrates the variety and range of symptoms, the complexity of the disorder, and its impact across multiple environments. It outlines an approach based on client and family involvement, psychoeducation, and behavioral and pharmacologic interventions. It also demonstrates the effectiveness of involving the client and family in treatment planning.

NURSING CARE PLAN 17-1

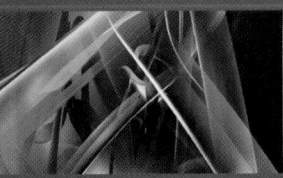

The Client with Attention-Deficit Hyperactivity Disorder (Joe C. [Age 8])

Nursing Diagnosis: Impaired Social Interaction

Outcome Identification	Nursing Actions	Rationales	Evaluation
1. By [date], Joe C. will complete assignments in class in allotted time.	1. With Joe's teacher, identify distracters in the classroom and modify the environment to decrease stimulation (e.g., move desk close to teacher, do not place desk near doors or windows).	1. By decreasing stimuli the child with ADHD can more easily focus on tasks, assignments, or projects and become distracted less easily or frequently.	*Goals met:* By the end of the first month, Joe, his parents, and teachers report a marked improvement in task completion.
2. By [date], Joe C. will remain in his seat for 20 minutes consecutively.	2. With Joe, his parents', and teacher's input, develop a daily report card outlining expected behaviors. Develop a reward system to recognize immediately and reward positive behaviors.	2. Children respond positively to structure and rules. Children with ADHD require frequent visual reminders, rewards, and recognition to reinforce behaviors. Communication between home and school is essential to identify any new or recurrent problems.	Daily report cards contain more positive behavior checks and comments.

(continues)

Nursing Care Plan 17–1 *(continued)*

Nursing Diagnosis: Impaired Social Interaction (cont'd)

Outcome Identification	Nursing Actions	Rationales	Evaluation
3. By [date], Joe C. will not interrupt the teacher or disrupt class for 30 minutes.	3. Monitor and assess response to medication, recommending scheduling changes, observed side effects, or poor response.	3. Each child will respond to medication and dosage individually. During the early phase of treatment, monitoring of response, effect, side effects, and modification of regime is often required to achieve optimal response.	*Goals met:* Joe C. graduates from Social Skills group at the end of 10 sessions. Joe's medication dose and schedule was adjusted, achieving maximum effect and no side effects are reported.
4. By [date], Joe will graduate from Social Skills group.	4. Joe is assigned to a twice-a-week Social Skills group that meets after school.	4. Social skills are often impaired in children with ADHD. Small group work that focuses on clearly defined skills and behaviors provide a safe environment for the child to learn new behaviors.	Joe C. graduates from Social Skills group at the end of 10 sessions.
5. By [date], Joe will have had three play dates with no episodes of fighting.	5a. With Joe's parents, identify two classmates Joe enjoys playing with. Educate Joe's parents to supervise play without being critical or intervening often. Role play a scenario where Joe becomes angry over a game not going his way and demonstrate interventions to help calm Joe down and redirect him.	5a. Supervising play and structuring activities ensures the child with ADHD receives clearly defined expectations and early interventions when problems arise. Parents often need the opportunity to practice their newly acquired intervention and redirection skills before using them in real-life activities.	He has had two classmates over on three separate occasions, and his parents supervised the play dates. The visits were kept to 1½ hours with two activities planned along with a small juice and snack break. The parents report the visits went well with no arguments or temper tantrums from Joe.
	5b. Educate Joe's parents about the types of groups and activities that support his development of positive social skills.	5b. Children with ADHD often have difficulty in group activities. Activities that are geared to use of large muscle with minimal directions provide the child opportunity to burn energy and be part of a team. The parents should discuss the child's diagnosis with coaches or leaders to help them be aware of the child's symptoms.	

(continues)

Nursing Care Plan 17–1 (continued)

Nursing Diagnosis: Impaired Social Interaction (cont'd)

Outcome Identification	Nursing Actions	Rationales	Evaluation
		Group and peer interaction is important for all children. Groups with clearly defined rules allow children with ADHD to practice new skills in a safe and supervised environment. Enlisting the help of the group leader can provide the child opportunity to receive feedback for rule violations.	

Nursing Diagnosis: Chronic Low Self-Esteem
related to rejection by peers, negative feedback from parents and teachers, and classroom failures

Outcome Identification	Nursing Actions	Rationales	Evaluation
1. Joe's parents will demonstrate by verbal report an understanding of behavior management plans, including the use of charts, daily report cards, and rewards.	1. Educate Joe's parents about the use of daily behavior charts and token systems for positive reinforcement.	It often seems that children with ADHD are getting into trouble. Despite frequent reminders, their behavior does not change. Visual cues, clearly defined rules, and reward systems provide the type of stimulation and reinforcement that promote change in these children. Requests to do chores should be phrased as follows: "Your room will be neat with the bed made and toys put away" rather than "Clean your room." This helps the child to understand the request and follow rules. Children with ADHD require frequent and immediate feedback (rewards), or they forget what had occurred.	*Goal met:* Joe's parents and teacher are able to identify the five most difficult school behaviors he exhibits. They develop and implement a home behavior chart, a school daily report card, and a reward system. The parents and Joe establish five household rules and chores and design posters outlining these. The posters are hung in Joe's room and in the kitchen.
2. By [date], Joe's parents will have identified four major negative behaviors and established a behavior management plan to target these behaviors for change.	2. Work with the parents to identify both positive and negative behaviors, help to develop a plan that will cover behaviors in at least two environments (home and school) and will include communication tools for use at home and school. The plan will include the use of rewards for positive behaviors. Input/feedback from the teacher.		

(continues)

522 **UNIT 2** Response to Stressors across the Life Span

Nursing Care Plan 17–1 *(continued)*

Nursing Diagnosis: Chronic Low Self-Esteem (cont'd)

Outcome Identification	Nursing Actions	Rationales	Evaluation
3. By [date], Joe's parents will have successfully used a behavior management plan at home and school for 3 weeks.	3. At home the parents will develop posters with behaviors and tasks outlined. This will include targets for task completion. Posters will be posted in Joe's room and in the kitchen to provide visual cues for him. Task completion by expected date and following rules will be rewarded.	When the child misbehaves, time-out is a useful intervention; it removes the child from the situation and provides time for calming down. Reward systems of tokens or marks provide the child with visual feedback about his behavior. Together these components form an effective behavior management plan.	

Parents must also be taught to identify and modify causative or aggravating factors in the environment and advocate for their children within the educational and social environments. Nurses can be instrumental in implementing and facilitating parent education classes. It is important to help parents understand that parenting classes offer a means to obtain new skills, develop problem-solving strategies, enhance communication, and develop conflict resolution skills. General parenting education classes may not be effective for the parents of children with ADHD.

Barkley (1997) suggests incorporation of eight principles within the parent training classes and recommends emphasis of the following:

1. The use of immediate consequences.
2. The use of consequences at a greater frequency.
3. The use of meaningful consequences.
4. Use of incentives before punishment.
5. Focus on consistency.
6. Plan ahead for problem situations.
7. Keep a disability perspective. This requires parents to recognize the need for consistent behavior management over a long period of time.
8. Practice acceptance and forgiveness.

Barkley's program targets nonadherence. Parents are first taught the typical causes of child misbehavior. They are then taught how to attend to and interact with the child appropriately, how to use time-out to decrease noncompliance, and how to generalize procedures learned at home to other environments. Assisting the parents to develop the awareness of causes of behavior and develop effective skills to manage the behavior promotes positive outcomes for both the child and family.

SUMMARY

◆ Attention-deficit hyperactivity disorder (ADHD) is a psychiatric illness characterized by attention skills that are developmentally inappropriate and, in some cases, impulsivity and hyperactivity.

◆ ADHD is a neurobiological disability that affects between 3 and 8 percent of all children in the United States.

◆ ADHD can have long-term serious consequences without diagnosis and appropriate treatment. These can include school failure, low self-esteem, and dropout, conduct disorder or antisocial behaviors, failed relationships, and even substance abuse.

◆ ADHD symptoms are often first detected in early childhood and are chronic, lasting at least 6 months, with onset before age 7.

◆ ADHD symptoms that may be exhibited are overactivity, academic difficulties (distractible, does not complete assignments, out of seat frequently), impaired family and social relationships, and frequent accidental injury.

◆ Before the late 1990s it was believed that most children outgrew ADHD in adolescence. It is now known that many symptoms of ADHD continue through adolescence and into adulthood.

◆ Adults with ADHD may experience difficulties at work and in relationships. Many adults with ADHD are restless, easily distracted, have difficulty sustaining attention, are impulsive or impatient, have poor frustration tolerance, and are disorganized or poor planners. They may also develop the co-occurring disorders of depression, anxiety, or antisocial behaviors.

◆ Psychiatric nurses play an integral role in the diagnosis and treatment of ADHD.

- Nursing roles and responsiblities include assessment, planning, and implementation of interventions and on-going evaluation of progress. Assessment data from a variety of sources are useful in clarifying symptoms and subtype classification.

- Treatment of ADHD is a multidisciplinary process that relies heavily on patient and family education regarding the etiology, symptoms, and pharmacologic and behavioral interventions.

- Psychostimulants are the most widely used medication for the treatment of ADHD, with between 70 and 80 percent of children with ADHD responding positively. The nurse plays an important role in working with the client and family to monitor efficacy and symptom response.

- The nurse also plays an important role in helping the client and family to develop new and more effective coping skills through social skills and parent training classes, and psychoeducation.

SUGGESTIONS FOR CLINICAL CONFERENCES

1. Present several case histories of clients with attention-deficit hyperactivity disorder (ADHD); the cases should be representative of clients across the life span. For each case, identify (a) biological, environmental, and hereditary factors, (b) life span and developmental issues, (c) psychosocial issues, (d) diverse treatment modalities, (e) client and family education needs.

2. Discuss several treatment modalities for the treatment of clients with ADHD, such as pharmacologic options, social skills training, classroom modifications, and behavioral management plans.

STUDY QUESTIONS

1. ADHD is a disorder that often coexists with other psychiatric disorders. Which of the following is not a commonly identified co-occurring disorder?
   a. Major depression
   b. Learning disabilities
   c. Tourette's syndrome
   d. Social phobia

2. ADHD has been categorized as a psychiatric disorder for many years. In the early 1900s ADHD was thought to be a disorder deriving from:
   a. deficiencies in parenting
   b. brain injury or damage
   c. poor nutrition
   d. fetal exposure to drugs or alcohol

3. The *DSM-IV-TR* criteria for ADHD require that the onset of symptoms occur:
   a. before the age of 7
   b. after the age of 7

c. before adolescence
d. before the age of 5

4. ADHD screening tools include all of the following except:
   a. Conners' Parent-Teacher Rating Scale
   b. Achenbach Child Behavior Checklist
   c. Vanderbilt Rating Scale
   d. Young Mania Rating Scale

5. Which of the following medications used to treat the symptoms of ADHD is *not* classified as a psychostimulant?
   a. Ritalin
   b. Dexedrine
   c. Wellbutrin SR
   d. Adderall

6. Adolescents with untreated ADHD (hyperactive-impulsive type) are at high risk for development of:
   a. conduct disorders
   b. depression
   c. aggressive behaviors
   d. anxiety disorders

7. Adults with ADHD (inattentive type) continue to exhibit problems in the area of:
   a. overactivity
   b. high-risk-taking behaviors
   c. organization skills
   d. emotional lability

8. In conducting the nursing assessment of a child with symptoms of ADHD, the nurse may do the following to minimize distractions:
   a. include all family members in the first session
   b. observe the child in the classroom setting before the interview
   c. establish a small number of shortened interview sessions
   d. talk with the child without the parents or other family members

9. The most effective treatment plan for the client with ADHD includes:
   a. family therapy and pharmacotherapy
   b. behavior management plan and pharmacotherapy
   c. individual therapy and pharmacotherapy
   d. behavior management plan and parent education

10. A common side effect of psychostimulant medications is:
    a. lethargy
    b. decreased blood pressure
    c. increase in activity level
    d. decreased appetite

11. The parents of a 10-year-old with ADHD indicates to the nurse an understanding of the child's illness when they say which of the following?
    a. "How will we know if our son is addicted to his medication?"
    b. "Will a change in his sugar intake help his behavior?"
    c. "Will allowing him to do what he wants help him?"
    d. "Does another psychiatrist have a better treatment?"

12. In teaching a youth and his family about a psychostimulant medication, methylphenidate (Ritalin), the nurse should include which of the following?
    a. Caution the client and family to avoid foods high in sugar.
    b. Instruct the client to take the medication at bedtime.
    c. Instruct the client that treatment is usually short term.
    d. Take the medication after eating to avoid GI disturbances.

13. When caring for the client with ADHD it is important for the nurse to include which of the following in the medical assessment?
    a. Height, weight, and blood pressure
    b. Eye examination
    c. Drug screen
    d. Thyroid function tests

RESOURCES

Please note that because Internet resources are of a time-sensitive nature and URL addresses may change or be deleted, searches should also be conducted by association or topic.

Internet Resources

The latest information on attention-deficit hyperactivity disorders and treatment recommendations can be accessed at:

http://www.health-center.com

http://www.chadd.org

http://www.add.org

Many of these sites provide chat rooms, bulletin boards, or answers to frequently asked questions (FAQs).

Information regarding the latest research on attention-deficit hyperactivity disorders is available from the National Institute of Mental Health (NIMH) and other government agencies:

- ◆ Current research
- ◆ Guidelines for diagnosing
- ◆ Nursing research opportunities
- ◆ Call for abstracts

Professional Nursing and Mental Health Professional Organizations:

http://www.apna.org   American Psychiatric Nurses Association

http://www.psychnurse.org   Alliance for Psychosocial Nursing

http://www.nami.org   National Alliance for the Mentally Ill (NAMI)

Other Resources

Children and Adults with Attention Deficit Disorder (CHADD)
8181 Professional Place, Suite 201
Landover, MD 20785
http://www.chadd.org/

Learning Disabilities Association of America
4156 Library Road
Pitsburgh, PA 15234
http://www.ldanatl.org/

The National Attention Deficit Disorder Association (ADDA)
PO Box 972
Mentor, OH 44061
http://www.add.org/

National Institute of Mental Health
Office of Communications and Public Liaison
6001 Executive Blvd.,
Rm 8184, MSC 9663
Bethesda, MD 20892-9663
http://www.nimh.nih.gov/publicat/adhdmenu.cfm

Reading Resources for Families

Parents

Barkley, R. A. (2005). *ADHD and the nature of self-control.* New York: Guilford Press.

Barkley, R. A. (2005). *Attention-deficit hyperactivity disorder: A handbook for diagnosis and treatment* (3rd ed.). New York: Guilford Press.

Barkley, R. A. (2000). *Taking charge of ADHD.* New York: The Guilford Press.

Barkley, R. & Benton, C. M. (1998). *Your defiant child: 8 steps to better behavior.* New York: Guilford Press.

Bender, P. S. (1997). *How to keep your kids from driving you crazy: A proven program in improving your child's behavior and regaining control of your family.* New York: Wiley.

Brown, T. E. (2005). *Attention deficit disorder: The unfocused mind in children and adults.* New Haven, CT: Yale University Press.

Horacek, H. J. (1998). *Brainstorms: Understanding and treating the emotional storms of attention deficit hyperactivity disorders from childhood through adulthood.* Northvale, NJ: J. Aronson.

Wachtel, A. & Boyette, M. (1998). *The attention deficit answer book: The best medications and parenting strategies for your child.* New York: Plume.

Wender, P. H. (2002). *ADHD: Attention-deficit hyperactivity disorder in children and adults.* New York: Oxford University Press.

Children

Corman, C. L. & Trevino, E. (1995). *Eukee the jumpy elephant.* Plantation, FL: Specialty Press.

Janover, C. (1997). *Zipper the kid with ADHD.* Bethesda, MD: Woodbine House.

Moss, D. M. (1989). *Shelley: The hyperactive turtle.* kensington, MD: Woodbine House.

Quinn, P. O. & Stern, J. M. (1991). *Putting on the brakes: young people's guide to understanding attention deficit hyperactivity disorder (ADHD).* New York: Magination Press.

Shapiro, L. (1993). *Sometimes I drive my mom crazy, but I know she's crazy about me.* King of Prussia, PA: Center for Applied Psychology.

REFERENCES

Achenbach, T. M., Howell, C. T., McConaughy, S. H., & Stanger, C. (1995). Six-year predictors of problems in a national sample of children and youth: II. Signs of disturbance. *Journal of the American Academy of Child and Adolescent Psychiatry, 34,* 488–498.

Achenbach, T. M., & McConaughy, S. H. (1996). *Empirically based assessment of child and adolescent psychopathology: Practical applications* (2nd ed.). Thousand Oaks, CA: Sage.

Adesman, A. R. (2002). New medications for the treatment of children with attention deficit hyperactivity disorder: Review and commentary. *Pediatric Annals, 31,* 514–522.

American Academy of Pediatrics. (2000). Clinical practice guidelines: Diagnosis and evaluation of the child with attention deficit hyperactivity disorder. *Pediatrics, (105),* 1158–1168.

American Nurses Association. (2000). *Scope and standards of psychiatric-mental health nursing practice.* Washington, DC: Author.

American Psychiatric Association. (1968). *Diagnostic and statistical manual of mental disorders* (2nd ed.).Washington, DC: Author.

American Psychiatric Association. (1980). *Diagnostic and statistical manual of mental disorders* (3rd ed.). Washington, DC: Author.

American Psychiatric Association. (1987). *Diagnostic and statistical manual of mental disorders* (3rd ed., Rev.). Washington, DC: Author.

American Psychiatric Association. (2000). *Diagnostic and statistical manual of mental disorders* (4th edition, Text Revision) *(DSM-IV-TR)* Washington, DC: Author.

Applegate, B., Lahey, B. B., Hart, E. L., Biederman, J., Hynd, G. W., Barkley, R. A., et al. (1997). Validity of the age of onset criterion for ADHD. A report from the *DSM-IV* field trials. *Journal of the American Academy of Child and Adolescent Psychiatry, 36,* 1211–1221.

Bailey, R. & Weiss, M. (2003). Advances in the treatment of adult ADHD: Landmark findings in nonstimulant therapy. *Medscape.* Retrieved December 15, 2005 from http://www.medscape.com/viewprogram/2530.

Bandura, A. (1977). *Social learning theory.* Englewood Cliffs, NJ: Prentice Hall.

Barkley, R. A. (1996). Attention-deficit hyperactivity disorder. In E. J. Mash & R. A. Barkley (Eds.), *Child Psychopathology,.* (pp. 63–112). New York: Guilford Press.

Barkley, R. A. (1997). *Attention deficit hyperactivity disorder and the nature of self-control.* New York: Guilford Press.

Barkley, R. A., Fisher, M., Edelbrook, C. S., & Smallish, L. (1990). The adolescent outcome of hyperactive children diagnosed by research criteria: I. An eight-year prospective follow-up study. *Journal of the American Academy of Child and Adolescent Psychiatry, 29,* 546–557.

Barkley, R. A., & Murphy, K. R. (1998). *Attention deficit hyperactivity disorder: A clinical workbook.* New York. Guilford Press.

Bender, L. (1942). Post-encephalitic behavior disorders in children. In J. B. Neal (Ed.), *Encephalitis: A clinical study.* New York: Grune & Stratton.

Biederman, J., Munir, K., Knee, D., Habelow, W., Armentano, M., Autor, S., et al. (1986). A family study of patients with attention deficit disorder and normal controls. *Journal of Psychiatric Research, 20,* 263–274.

Biederman, J., Petty, C. R., Fried, R., Fontanella, J., Doyle, A. E., Siedman, L. J., et al. (2007). Can self-reported behavioral scales assess executive function deficits? A controlled study of adults with ADHD. *Journal of Nervous and Mental Disorders, 195,* 240–246.

Biederman, J., Spencer, T. J., Newcorn, J. H., Gao, H., Milton, D. R., Feldman, P. D., et al. (2007). Effect of comorbid symptoms of oppositional defiant disorder on responses to atomoxetine in children with ADHD: A meta-analysis of controlled clinical trial data. *Psychopharmacology (Berlin), 190,* 31–41.

Bond, E. P., & Partridge, C. E. (1926). Post encephalitic behavior disorders in boys and their management in the hospital. *American Journal of Psychiatry, 6,* 103.

Bradley, C. (1937). The behavior of children receiving Benzedrine. *American Journal of Psychiatry, 94,* 577–585.

Bradley, C. (1950). Benzedrine and Dexedrine in the treatment of children's behavior disorders. *Pediatrics, 5,* 24–36.

Bradley, C., & Bowen, M. (1941). Amphetamine (Benzedrine) therapy of children's behavior disorders. *American Journal of Orthopsychiatry, 11,* 92–103.

Braun, J. M., Kahn, R. S., Froehlich, T., Auinger, P., & Lanphear, B. P. (2006). Exposures to environmental toxicants and attention deficit hyperactivity disorder in U.S. children. *Environmental Health Perspectives, 114,* 1904–1909.

Conners, C. K., & Jett, J. L. (1999). *Attention deficit disorder (in adults and children): The latest assessment and treatment strategies.* Kansas City, MO: Compact Clinicals.

Conners, C. K., & Taylor, E. (1980). Pemoline, methylphenidate and placebo in children with brain dysfunction. *Archives of General Psychiatry, 37,* 922–930.

Douglas, V. I., & Peters, K. G. (1979). Toward a clearer definition of the attentional deficit of hyperactive children. In G. A. Hale & M. Lewis (Eds.), *Attention and the development of cognitive skills.* New York. Plenum Press.

Elliott, H. (2002). ADHD in adults: A guide for the primary care physician. *Southern Medical Journal, 95*(7), 736–742.

Feingold, B. F. (1974). *Why your child is hyperactive.* New York: Random House.

Gadow, K. D., & Spafkin, J. (1997). *ADHD symptom checklist-4 manual.* Stony Brook, NY: Checkmate Plus.

Gadow, K. D., & Spafkin, J. (1997). *Child symptom inventory-4 norms manual.* Stony Brook, NY: Checkmate Plus.

Goldman, L. S., Genel, M., Bezman, R., et al. (1998). Diagnosis and treatment of Attention Deficit Hyperactivity Disorder in children and adolescents. *Journal of the American Medical Association,* (279), 1100–1107.

Goldstein, L. B. (2006). Neurotransmitters and motor activity: Effects on functional recovery after brain injury *NeuroRX, 3,* 451–457.

Haenlin, M., & Caul, W. F. (1987). Attention deficit disorder with hyperactivity: A specific hypothesis of reward dysfunction. *Journal of the American Academy of Child and Adolescent Psychiatry, 26,* 356–362.

Kessler, R. C., Adler, L., Barkley, R., Biederman, J., Conners, C. K., Demler, O., et al. (2006). The prevalence and correlates of adult ADHD in the United States: Results from the National Comorbidity Survey Replication. *American Journal of Psychiatry, 163,* 716–723.

Knobloc, H., & Pasaminick, B. (1959). The syndrome of minimal cerebral damage in infancy. *Journal of the American Medical Association, 70,* 1384–1386.

Kodituwakku, P., Coriale, G., Fiorentino, D., Aragon, A. S., Kalberg, W. O., Buckley, D., Gossage, J. P., Ceccanti M. & May, P. A. (2006). Neurobehavioral characteristics of children with alcohol spectrum disorders in communities from Italy: Preliminary results. *Alcohol and Clinical Experimental Research, 30,* 1551–1561.

Kutcher, S. P. (1997). *Child and adolescent psychopharmacology.* Philadelphia: W.B. Saunders.

Lahey, B. B., Schaughency, E. A., Hynd, G. W., Carlson, C. L., & Nieves, N. (1987). Attention deficit disorder with and without hyperactivity. *Journal of the American Academy of Child and Adolescent Psychiatry, 26,* 718–723.

Laufer, M. W., & Denhoff, E. (1957). Hyperkinetic behavior syndrome in children. *Journal of Pediatrics, 50,* 463–474.

Masi, G., Perugi, G., Toni, C., MIllepiedi, S., Mucci, M., Bertini, N., & Pfanner, C. (2006). Attention-deficit hyperactivity disorder-bipolar comorbidity in children and adolescents. *Bipolar Disorder, 8,* 373–378.

Molitch, M., & Eccles, A. K. (1937). Effects of Benzedrine sulphate on intelligence scores of children. *American Journal of Psychiatry, 94,* 587–590.

MTA Cooperative Group. (1999). Fourteen-month randomized clinical trial of treatment strategies for attention deficit hyperactivity disorder. *Archives of General Psychiatry, 56,* 1073–1086.

Murphy, K. (2005). Psychosocial treatments for ADHD in teens and adults: A practice-friendly review. *Journal of Clinical Psychology, 61,* 607–619.

NANDA International. (2007). *Nursing diagnoses: Definitions and classification, 2007–2008* (7th ed.). Philadelphia: Author.

Ng, B. Y., Lim, C. C., Yeoh, A., & Lee, W. L. (2004). Neuropsychiatric sequelae of Nipah virus encephalitis. *Journal of Neuropsychiatry and Clinical Neuroscience, 16,* 500–504.

Nierenberg, A. A., Miyahara, S., Spencer, T., Wisniewski, S. R., Otto, M.W., Simon, N., Pollack, M. H. et al. (2005). Clinical and diagnostic implications of lifetime attention-deficit/hyperactivity disorder comorbidity in adults with bipolar disorder: Data from the first 1000 STEP-BD patients. *Biological Psychiatric, 57,* 1467–1473.

Preen, D. B., Calver, J., Sanfilippo, F. M., Bulsara, M., & Holman, C. D. (2007). Patterns of psychostimulant prescribing to children with ADHD in Western Australia: Variations in age, gender, medication type and dose prescribed. *Australia and New Zealand Journal of Public Health, 31,* 120–126.

Routh, D. K. (1978). Hyperactivity. In P. R. Magrab (Ed.), *Psychological management of brain damaged patients* (Vol. 2). Baltimore: University Press.

Safren, S. A., Otto, M. W., Sprich, S., Winett, C. L., Wilens, T. E., & Biederman, J. (2005). Cognitive-behavioral therapy for ADHD in medication-treated adults with continued symptoms. *Behaviour Research and Therapy, 43,* 831–842.

Searight, H. R., Rottnek, F., & Abby, S. L. (2001). Conduct disorder: Diagnosis and treatment in primary care. *American Family Physician, 63*(8), 1579–1588.

Sheridan, S. M., Dee, C. C., Morgan, J., McCormick, M., & Walker, D. (1996). A multi-method intervention for social skills deficit in children with attention deficit hyperactivity disorder and their parents. *School Psychology Review, 25,* 57–76.

Silverthorn, P., Frick, P. J., Kupper, K., & Ott, J. (1996). Attention deficit hyperactivity and sex: A test of two etiological models to explain male predominance. *Journal of Clinical Child Psychology, 25,* 52–59.

Smith, K. M., Daly, M., Fischer, M., Yiannoutsos, C.T., Bauer, L., Barkley, R., et al. (2003). Association of the dopamine beta hydroxylase gene with attention deficit hyperactivity disorder: Genetic analysis of the Milwaukee longitudinal study. *American Journal of Medical Genetics B and Neuropsychiatry Genetics, 119,* 77–85.

Spencer, T. J., Biederman, J., Madras, B. K., Dougherty, D. D., Bonab, A. A., Livni, E., et al. (2007). Further evidence of dopamine transporter dysregulation in ADHD: A controlled PET imaging study using altropane. *Biological Psychiatry,* May 16. [Epub ahead of print]

Spencer, T. J., Biederman, J., & Mick, E. (2007). Attention-deficit/hyperactivity disorser: Diagnosis, lifespan, comorbidities, and neurobiolgy. *Journal of Pediatric Psychology, 32,* 631–642.

Steinhaus, H. C., Williams, J., & Spohr, H. L. (1993). Long term psychopathological and cognitive outcomes of children with fetal alcohol syndrome. *Journal of the*

American Academy of Child and Adolescent Psychiatry, 32, 990–994.

Still, G. F. (1902). The Coulstonian lectures on some abnormal physical conditions in children. *Lancet, 1,* 1008–1012.

Taylor, E., Chadwick, O., Heptinstall, E., & Dancharets, M. (1996). Hyperactivity and conduct disorders as risk factors for adolescent development, *Journal of the American Academy of Child and Adolescent Psychiatry, 35,* 1213–1226.

Turgay, A. (2005). Treatment of comorbidity in conduct disorder with attention-deficit hyperactivity disorder (ADHD). *Essential Psychopharmacology, 6,* 277–290.

Vollmer, S. (1998). ADHD: It's not just in children. *Family Practice Recertification, 20,* 45–46.

Weiss, M., Hechtman, L., & The Adult ADHD Research Group. (2006). A randomized double-blind trial of paroxetine and/or dextroamphetamine and problem-focused therapy for attention-deficit/hyperactivity disorder in adults. *Journal of Clinical Psychiatry, 67,* 611–619.

Wilens, T. E., Biederman, J., Brown, S., Tanguay, S., Monuteaux, M. C., Blake, C., & Spencer, T. J. (2002). Psychiatric comorbidity and functioning in clinically referred preschool children and school-aged youths with ADHD. *Journal of the American Academy of Child and Adolescent Psychiatry, 41,* 262–268.

Willerman, L. (1973). Activity level and hyperactivity in twins. *Child Development, 44,* 288–293.

SUGGESTED READINGS

Barkley, R. A. (1995). *Taking charge of ADHD: The complete authoritative guide for parents.* New York: Guilford Press.

Barkley, R. A. (1998). *Attention deficit hyperactivity disorder, a handbook for diagnosis and treatment* (2nd ed.). New York: Guilford Press.

Barkley, R. A. (2000). *Taking charge of ADHD.* New York: The Guilford Press.

Barkley, R. A. (2005). *Attention-deficit hyperactivity disorder: A handbook for diagnosis and treatment* (3rd ed.). New York: Guilford Press.

Barkley, R. A. (2005). *ADHD and the nature of self-control.* New York: Guilford Press.

DuPaul G. J., & Stoner, G. D. (1998). *ADHD in the schools: Assessment and intervention strategies associated with attention deficit hyperactivity disorder in children* (2nd ed.). New York: John Wiley & Sons.

Goldstein, S., & Goldstein, M. (1998). *Managing ADHD in children, a guide for practitioners* (2nd ed.). New York: John Wiley & Sons.

Greene, R. (1998). *The explosive child.* New York: HarperCollins.

Parker, H. (1999). *Put yourself in their shoes.* New York: Specialty Press.

Weiss, L. (1996). *Give your ADD teen a chance: A guide for parents of teenagers with attention deficit disorder.* Colorado Springs, CO: Pinon Press.

Wilens, T. (1999). *Straight talk about psychiatric medicine for kids.* New York: Guilford Press.

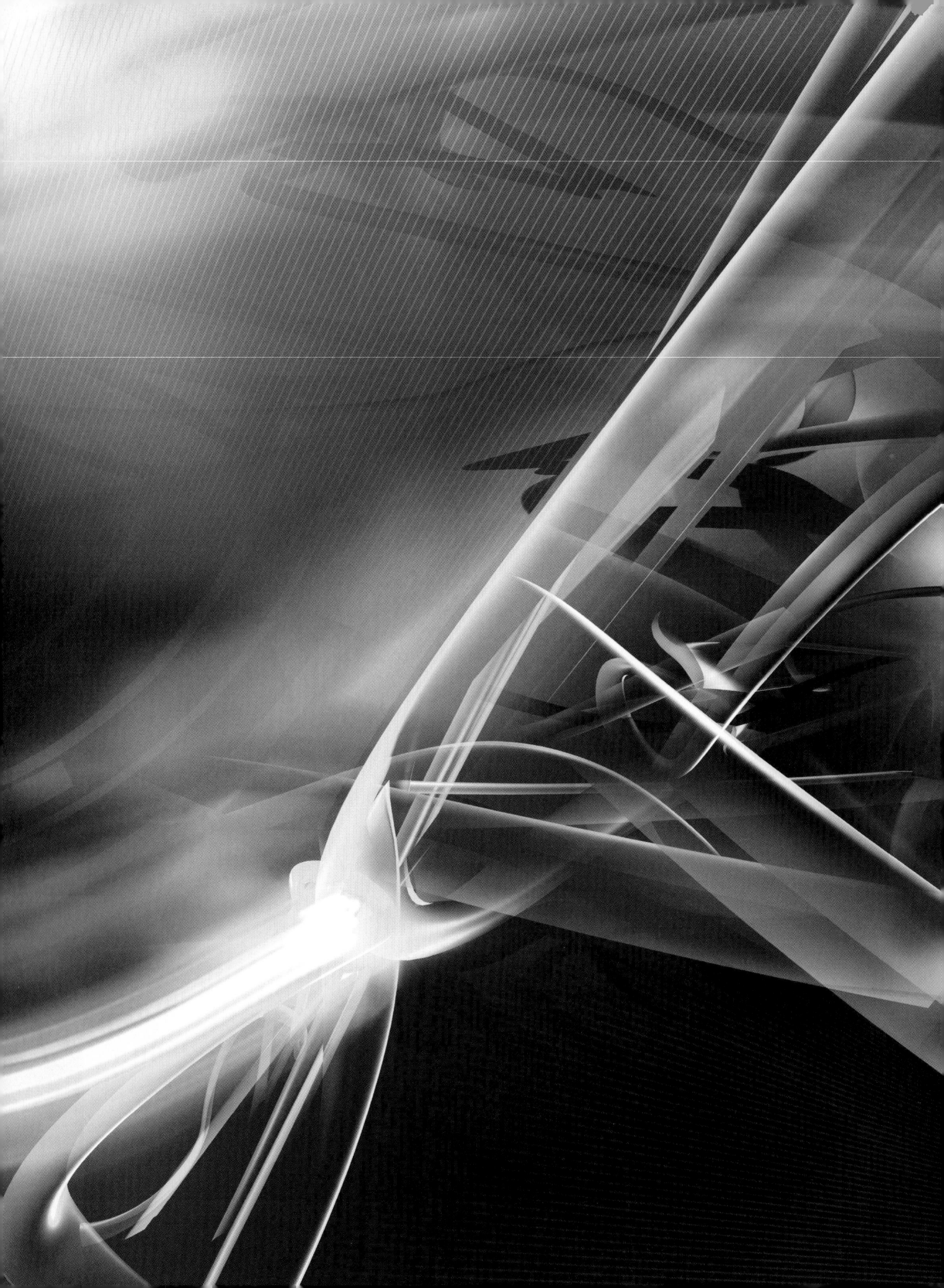

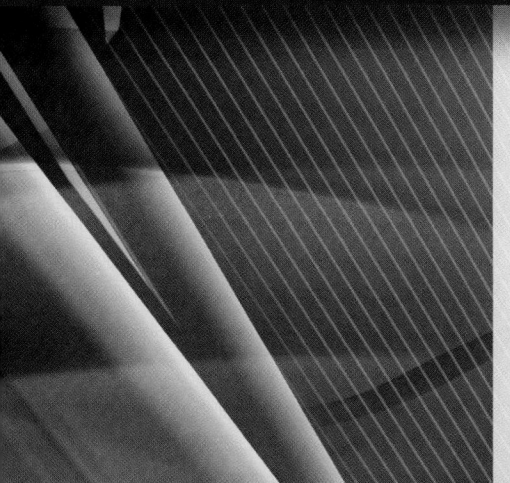

CHAPTER 18

The Client with a Dissociative Disorder

Lisa A. Jensen, MS, APRN, CS
Catherine Pawlicki, MSN, RN, CS

KEY TERMS

Alters: A distinct identity with its own enduring pattern of perceiving, relating to, and thinking about the world and the self.

Dissociation: The separation of thoughts, feelings, or experiences from the normal stream of consciousness and memory.

Dissociative Disorders: A continuum of disorders experienced by individuals exposed to trauma, including depersonalization disorder, dissociative amnesia, dissociative fugue, and dissociative identity disorder. These disorders involve a disturbance in the organization of identity, memory, perception, or consciousness.

Personality: Enduring patterns of perceiving, relating to, and thinking about the world and oneself.

Secondary Gain: Attempting to earn the sympathy of others, receiving financial gain, or obtaining other benefits by suffering from a disorder.

Switching: The process in which one alter is changed into another.

Trauma: An event that results in long-standing distress to the individual experiencing that event.

COMPETENCIES

Upon completion of this chapter, the learner should be able to:

1. Analyze major components of dissociation.

2. Discuss the influence of the nature of the stressor on the identified dissociative disorder.

3. Assess a client for the presence of dissociation.

4. Analyze life span issues that influence the development of dissociative disorders.

5. Intervene with a dissociating client to promote continuity of the self.

6. Formulate a plan of care for the client with a dissociative disorder.

CHAPTER OUTLINE

Epidemiology

Causative Factors: Perspectives and Theories

Interpersonal Theory and Personality Development
    Good-Me Aspect
    Bad-Me Aspect
    Not-Me Aspect

Biological Factors
    Neurocircuitry System

The Role of Family Dynamics

Cultural Considerations

Dissociative Disorders across the Life Span

Childhood

For centuries, people have been exposed to trauma through natural disasters such as earthquakes, tornadoes, floods, tidal waves, forest fires, and hurricanes. Trauma is also experienced through man-made disasters, including motor vehicle accidents, house fires, combat, and physical and sexual assaults. Most people witnessing or experiencing such traumas and atrocities are able to recover fully. A number of people, however, will suffer from long-term emotional symptoms. These symptoms make up a spectrum of disorders known as dissociative disorders. According to Spiegel and Maldonado (1999, p. 453), "the dissociative disorders involve a disturbance in the integrated organization of identity, memory, perception, or consciousness. Events normally experienced on a smooth continuum are isolated from the other mental processes with which they would ordinarily be associated." Bernstein and Putnam (1986) define dissociation as the separation of thoughts, feelings, or experiences from the normal stream of consciousness and memory. In the late nineteenth century, Pierre Janet, a French psychiatrist, studied in depth the effects of traumatic events on psychopathology (Bob, 2003; Nemiah, 1999). He postulated that traumatic events are stored in the memory differently than normal events. Today all aspects of the concept of dissociation continue to be researched.

This chapter discusses dissociative disorders as sequelae of the experience of trauma. Causative factors are reviewed looking at biological factors as well as family dynamics. Developmental influences across the life span explain the impact of these issues in the formation of dissociative disorders. Specific dissociative disorders identified in the Diagnostic and Statistical Manual of Mental Disorders (4th edition, Text Revision) (DSM-IV-TR) (APA, 2000) are reviewed, along with the role of both the generalist nurse and the advanced-practice nurse in working with clients with these disorders.

According to Sullivan, dissociation is an anxiety-reducing mechanism that functions by restricting awareness. If circumstances require a child to adapt by using dissociation excessively, the child becomes limited in her ability to make meaningful connections between an event and her thoughts and feelings about the event (Sullivan, 1953). Using Sullivan's theory, Peplau (1952) operationally defined dissociation, which is presented in Table 18–1.

Continual exposure to overwhelming experiences in the absence of an external comforter can lead to life events being managed by varying degrees of dissociation. Dissociative phenomena exist along a continuum, from mild and common to pathological forms (Steinberg, Barry, Sholomskas, & Hall, 2005). Minor forms of dissociation can be inconspicuous everyday occurrences of "spacing out," for example, while driving a car or sitting in class. Midpoint on the continuum would be reported out-of-body, near-death experiences, wherein the clients have an experience of viewing their body from a vantage point above or to the side of their body. Individuals who have near-death experiences describe the occurrence of dissociative phenomena during their experience (French, 2005). The more pathological forms of dissociation are amnesia, fugue, and identity disorder. They are related to traumatic, intense anxiety antecedents (Figure 18–1).

TABLE 18–1
Operational Definition of Dissociation

1. In early life, certain thoughts, feelings, and/or actions of the client are disapproved by significant other persons.

2. Significant people's standards are incorporated as the client's own.

3. Later in life, the client experiences one of the disapproved thoughts, feelings, or actions.

4. Anxiety increases to a severe level.

5. The feelings are barred from awareness.

6. Anxiety decreases.

7. Dissociated content continues to appear in disguised form in the client's thoughts, feelings, and actions.

Note. Adapted from *Interpersonal Relations in Nursing*, by H. Peplau, 1952. New York: G. F. Putnam.

The core conflict in the person experiencing trauma is the wish to deny the horrible experience, while simultaneously wishing to proclaim it to everybody (Herman, 1991). The traumatic experience is usually prolonged and engenders in the victim a deep sense of being helpless to control her own survival. The repertoire of coping mechanisms available depends on the age of the victim during the traumatic event and determines the extent to which dissociation serves as the primary or persistent defense mechanism. Research has demonstrated a significant relationship between early childhood traumas, especially sexual abuse, and chronic dissociation (Diseth, 2005; Karadag et al., 2005).

In the normal or minor process of dissociation, the sense of self or of the affect and thought belonging to the self is never lost. In pathological dissociation, the sense of self is disconnected from the experience. Affect or thought is disowned (psychogenic fugue and amnesia) or attributed to another self, or "not me" (dissociative identity disorder). When the intensity of the trauma increases, there is a greater loss of the sense of self as well as an increasing notion of personal estrangement (Meares, 1999). Repeated application of dissociation leads to its indiscriminate use in response to a variety of stressors.

Dissociation does help a person survive and escape an overwhelming reality such as child abuse. It provides relief and time for the person to gather resources to cope with the trauma. When trauma persists, as is usually the case in child abuse, the use of dissociation persists and greatly influences personality development. Estimates of the incidence of child abuse have increased dramatically in the last decade. Extensive review of research in this area (Diseth, 2005) indicates that child abuse is almost always part of the history of individuals with dissociative identity disorder. Until further quantitative research becomes available that links dissociative disorder to the major public health problem of child abuse, the psychiatric nurse will be the frontline case finder of these clients. Therefore, the psychiatric nurse needs to have a firm grasp of dissociative disorders.

EPIDEMIOLOGY

Dissociative disorders are prevalent around the world and often occur with other psychiatric disorders such as depression, post-traumatic stress disorder, substance use disorders, and borderline personality. Elmore (2000) notes studies in North America find a lifetime prevalence of dissociative disorders of about 10 percent. Empirical data support the relation between trauma and dissociation, particularly adult and childhood trauma stemming from sexual and physical abuse (Foote, Smolin, Kaplan, Legatt, & Lipschitz, 2006; Pearlman & Courtois, 2005; Sar, Akyüz, & Dogan, 2007). Sexual abuse, its severity, and combination with physical abuse and neglect have been found to be strongly linked to adult dissociation as well as problems with affect regulation, memory and attention, and self-perception (van der Kolk et al., 2005).

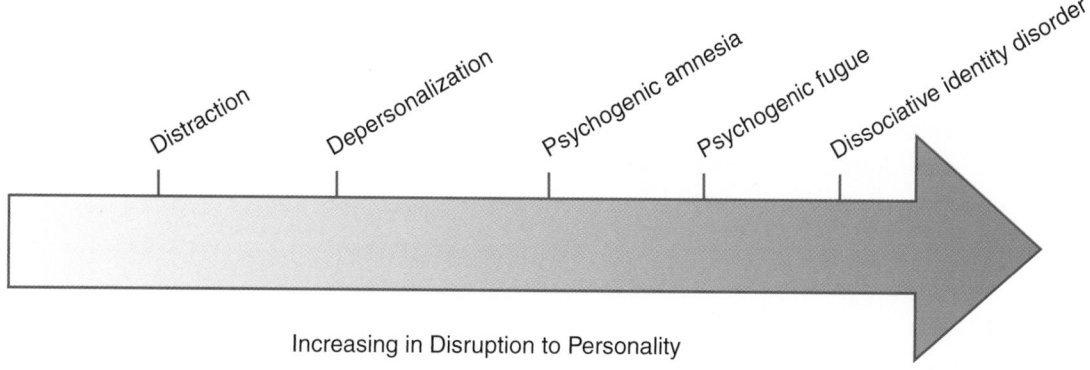

Distraction Depersonalization Psychogenic amnesia Psychogenic fugue Dissociative identity disorder

Increasing in Disruption to Personality

Figure 18–1 Dissociative disorder continuum.

Overall, the dissociative disorders continue to stir controversy among clinicians. They represent a complex component of mental illness (Steinberg et al., 2005). Normally, these disorders are treatable, with psychotherapy as the primary treatment modality.

CAUSATIVE FACTORS: PERSPECTIVES AND THEORIES

Theories and causative factors associated with dissociative disorders remain an enigma, although theories and causative factors associated with these disorders continue to emerge. Research in brain imaging, neurobiological and psychosocial studies indicate the exact causes of dissociative disorders are multifaceted, but indicated a link between emotional trauma and intensity of clinical symptoms.

INTERPERSONAL THEORY AND PERSONALITY DEVELOPMENT

A significant part of personality development is the lifelong process of assimilating experiences (thoughts, feelings, and actions) and using the assimilated product (understanding) to observe the self and make judgments of present-day interpersonal interactions.

In Sullivan's theory of personality development, Interpersonal Theory, the personality is conceptualized as a self-system that consists of three mutually interacting aspects: *good me, bad me,* and *not me.* The development of each aspect is based on significant interpersonal experiences and the intensity of anxiety caused by each experience. According to Sullivan (1953), the self-system, or personality, develops around attempts to modulate anxiety internally in the context of an interaction with a significant other.

Good-Me Aspect

This good-me aspect of the self-system consists of experiences from infancy on that are soothing and indicative of approval and acceptance by a significant other. Good me is the part of self that is available to conscious awareness and comfortably revealed to others throughout life. The following example illustrates the good-me dynamic: A toddler is playing and runs away from her mother into the next room. A little later, the toddler reappears and races and puts her head into her mother's lap. Laughing, the mother picks up her daughter and hugs her. The daughter smiles, and when she is put down, runs away again.

In this interaction, the toddler is experimenting with separation. The crucial issue is the degree of control over separation that she and her mother can tolerate without either one becoming overwhelmingly anxious.

Bad-Me Aspect

Experiences that elicit disapproval from significant others and result in a high degree of anxiety for a person constitute that part of the self-system known as bad me. This aspect of the personality is available to a person's conscious awareness, but defense mechanisms (e.g., splitting or sublimation) are used in an effort to control the internal anxiety experience. The following is an example of the bad-me dynamic: A 5-year-old girl wants the toy her 3-year-old brother is playing with. The brother does not give it to her, so the 5-year-old slaps the toy out of his hand. The little boy cries loudly, and their mother comes over, picks her son up, and tries to comfort him. The mother asks the little girl why she did that, and the little girl states that she wanted the toy. The mother sternly tells the daughter "That was not nice," and says she should not do it again.

In this incident, the girl tried to meet her need through aggression directed toward her brother. As the mother comforted her brother, the little girl became more anxious, because not only did she not get her need met, she also did not receive comfort. As she assimilates this experience, her bad me will come to involve the notion that attempting to get her needs met through aggression will cause her more anxiety.

Not-Me Aspect

Experiences that are intensely overwhelming and elicit little or no soothing from a significant other are relegated to the not-me aspect. This aspect of the self is kept in the unconscious; that is, it is dissociated. Even though this part of the self-system is dissociated, it continues to exert powerful influences on the rest of the person's development, interpersonal world, and behavior. Maturation involves discovering and bringing to conscious awareness this aspect of the self and assimilating it with other known experiences of the self. The mature person experiences the self as whole and continuous. The not-me dynamic is demonstrated in the following example: Her father repeatedly sexually abuses a little girl. Each time he is done abusing her, he tells her he did it for her own good, but that she must never tell because her mother may die. The little girl never tells and believes she is now responsible for keeping her mother alive. Somehow, she must learn to live with the overwhelming experience of being abused without seeking comfort from a significant other.

This little girl will dissociate the abuse experience as well as her feelings and needs associated with it in order to survive the ordeal psychologically and physically. As an adult, she will be vulnerable to self-mutilation and dissociation any time she becomes angry. Her personality development will be seriously compromised because her experiences and feelings are so overwhelming that she cannot assimilate them or make emotional and conceptual connections about her self. She will adapt through dissociation, disowning this aspect of her self-system but continuously being affected by it.

BIOLOGICAL FACTORS

There is growing evidence of the role of trauma on intricate neurobiological and neuroanatomical structures in dissociative disorders. Early childhood trauma, witnessing or exposure to traumatic or violent incidents, apparently has the potential to produce enduring alterations on brain chemistry, neuro-endocrine processes, and memory. Psychiatric nurses are likely to encounter clients exposed to trauma in various practice settings and must be able to understand the basis of symptoms and use them to guide treatment modalities and prevent acute and chronic traumatic responses.

Neurocircuitry System

An impressive body of research has charted the neuro-circuitry underpinnings of stress reactions and fear (Farinelli, Deschaux, Hugues, Thevenet, & Garcia, 2000; Quirk, Garcia, Gonzalez-Lima, 2006; Rauch, Shin, & Phelps, 2006; Simeon et al., 2007). The amygdala, hippocampus, and prefrontal cortex play crucial roles in modulating fear responses. There is strong clinical evidence that indicates that the amygdala is a central structure in the brain neurocircuitry and plays a pivotal role in conditioned or (learned) fear responding (Farinelli et al., 2006; Quirk et al., 2006). The hippocampus and prefrontal cortex have modulatory roles in fear conditioning by processing information about the environmental context (unconditioned stimulus). Dysregulation of the amygdala or the hippocampus, or both, results in poor contextual stimulus discrimination (misinterpretation) and leads to overgeneralization of fear responding cues (Davis, 2000; Farinelli et al., 2006; Quirk et al., 2006; Weike et al., 2005). When overgeneralization of an environmental cue occurs, the prefrontal cortex loses the capacity to extinguish fear and anxiety or discriminate between threatening situations and innocuous situations (or repeated stimuli). Alterations in these complex brain regions contribute to maladaptive stress and trauma responses.

Many years of research with nonhuman primates have indicated that early and prolonged detachment from the significant caretaker directly affects the development of the limbic system (van der Kolk & Saporta, 1991). Because the limbic system is where memories are processed, early trauma experiences will remain unassimilated to the degree the stress of detachment affected the limbic system. This could account for the hyperarousal caused by stimuli similar to the original trauma that then precipitate dissociation.

Significant early traumatic experiences and the lack of attachment have also been demonstrated to have long-term effects on neurotransmitters, specifically serotonin, which has been identified as a primary neurotransmitter involved in the regulation of affect (Casper, 1998). Kraemer (1997) has determined through research with nonhuman primates that the usual regulation of the neurotransmitters norepinephrine, serotonin, and dopamine is dependent on early interactions with a maternal caregiver. There is reason to expect that research will demonstrate a positive relationship between dissociation and serotonin levels.

Clients with a dissociative disorder often present with a multitude of somatic complaints. Thus the nurse must thoroughly assess the client's physical status as the first intervention. Simultaneously, the nurse will want to keep in mind that if the client has a history of very early trauma, the somatic complaint may be representative of a memory laid down along primitive neurological pathways that is being stimulated by something in the current environment (van der Kolk & Saporta, 1991). The client often experiences the nurse's attention to her physical complaints and the nurse's education about "body memories" to be helpful and soothing.

Any sudden onset of symptoms of dissociative disorder should first be evaluated for a possible medical etiology (Table 18–2). Prolonged sleep deprivation, fever, and hyperventilation can present with symptoms of amnesia, depersonalization, or identity disturbance (Cochen et al., 2005; Löf, Berggren, & Ahlström, 2006). Clients with head injuries, seizure disorders, or brain lesions can present with symptoms of dissociation. Clients arriving in the emergency room after overdosing on street drugs may present with dissociative symptoms.

In the nineteenth century, Charcot and others attributed dissociative processes to various forms of epilepsy involving the temporal lobe. Research that continues in this area today presents supporting evidence of temporal lobe involvement in dissociation.

Research on stress and trauma has also demonstrated altered limbic system function in response to chronic stress, with concurrent suppression of hypothalamic activity and dysregulation of the neurocircuitry systems. It is possible that the stress hormones released (cortisol and adrenaline) precipitate dissociative episodes directly or through influence on the amygdala, hippocampus, and prefrontal cortex. Dissociation may be precipitated by physiological or emotional changes, and the nurse must thoroughly assess the client in all domains to gain understanding of contributing factors.

THE ROLE OF FAMILY DYNAMICS

The role of family dynamics in the dissociative process is highly potent for the child experiencing trauma such as physical or sexual abuse.

Personality development in the child is fostered by the family and is initially concentrated in the mother-child interaction. Healthy interactions between the mother and child protect and soothe the child when she is confronted by anxiety-provoking experiences. Healthy caretaking by the whole family facilitates the child's developing into an adult family member who is able to protect and soothe the self. This ability is manifested in appropriate affect regulation and a continuous experience of the self.

Behaviors such as sucking, crying, clinging, and smiling are evolutionarily adapted to elicit caretaking from the mother (Bowlby, 1969). When the mother responds calmly and reciprocally to the infant, attachment behavior is facilitated. Once young children learn that behavior can elicit comfort and security from the mother figure, they can start to develop a whole range of behaviors that enable them to attach to others and comfort themselves.

The perception of a secure base in the mother generalizes to the family as a whole. The members of a healthy, dynamic family protect and soothe each other through the maintenance of permeable but stable boundaries, defined and

TABLE 18–2
Medical and Other Psychiatric Diagnoses with Symptoms Similar to Those of Dissociative Disorders

Dissociative Disorder	Signs and Symptoms	Medical or Other Psychiatric Diagnosis	Signs and Symptoms
Depersonalization disorder	Parts of body feel unreal Client has sensation of body change Client is aware of perceptual distortions	Accompanies numerous other psychiatric disorders: electrolyte disturbance, seizure disorder Ganser's syndrome (seen in men with severe personality disorder) Factitious disorder: client fabricates symptoms Toxic disorders Neoplasms	Hard to differentiate Has factitious quality—symptoms are worse when client is aware of being observed Blood chemistry is abnormal Magnetic resonance imaging, computed tomography, and positron emission tomography are abnormal
Dissociative amnesia	Begins abruptly Client is aware of memory loss and is alert before and after Depression is usually associated Physical assessment is normal	Transient global amnesia Postconcussion amnesia	Client is upset about amnesia Memory loss is generalized Amnesia *gradually* subsides Central nervous system examination is abnormal
Dissociative fugue	Client travels away from home and takes on a new identity May be associated with alcohol ingestion Evidence of secondary gain is clear	Cognitive disorder	Temporal lobe epilepsy Wandering does not result in socially adaptive behavior
Dissociative identity disorder	Changes in behavior are dramatic or sudden Client experiences either co-consciousness of or amnesia for alters Physical assessment is usually normal	Cognitive disorder	Central nervous system examination is abnormal Intoxication Street drugs are used

fulfilled roles and functions for each family member, resilience in the face of danger, and the ability to communicate across generations and family roles.

In an incestuous family, little, if any, protection or soothing occurs. The members of the family experiencing incest are usually closed, not only to each other, but also to the outside world. Often the father is a controlling figure who dominates through physical force. He may present himself as a quiet family man, a good provider, and a churchgoer, but often he is actually quite introverted and preoccupied with sex. His relationship with the wife is conflicted. She is often weak or absent (detached) and physically or emotionally disabled. The child exposed to early trauma will often form a negative view of self (van der Kolk et al., 2005). She is living an experience that is violent and overwhelming. The experience and fear drive the child to a desperate search for attachments. When there is no protective figure to attach to, the need is so great that she will attach to the abuser. This attachment manifests itself in a phenomenon known as "internalization of the abuser." The child searches a means to "join" a significant other on an unconscious level. In order to join or to be attached to the other, part of the child's self will mirror and eventually even mold to the abuser's self. This "attachment" is a survival defense for the child's internal self. In dissociative identity disorder, one **alter**, or personality fragment, is usually rageful, sadistic, and potentially homicidal.

A child may react to her incestuous family by defensively detaching the abandoning parent. The defensive detachment is usually manifested in a dissociative disorder. Dissociative symptoms help a child maintain a sense of reality during exposure to trauma. In a healthy family, the child is able to develop a wide range of soothing behaviors because of effective and protective family response, whereas in an abusive family, the only soothing the child is able to take into adulthood is a well-developed dissociative disorder. Any relationship that signals danger will elicit attachment behavior that is alternated with behavior that maintains distance (e.g., self-mutilation or dissociation).

Incestuous families often deny they have problems. Excessive use of denial by a family is fertile ground for physical and sexual abuse. There usually is a rationale for abusive behavior, such as claims that it is "deserved," "unintentional," or "forgivable." A child attempting to cope through dissociation and surrounded by a family in denial struggles in treatment with the issue of what is real and what is not real. She may go through life excessively seeking validation or engaging in retraumatizing behavior in an effort to make the trauma real and develop some mastery over it.

Family dynamics around the abused child leave her with a rigid perception of interpersonal roles. That is, the child perceives all people to fall into one of the following roles: abuser, victim, rescuer, or neglectful or powerless bystander (Herman, 1991) (see Chapters 24 and 27).

The nurse who is interacting with the dissociating client will be placed in one of these roles as the client re-creates the family experience. The nurse needs to observe the developing role pattern and assist the client in describing her perception of their interactions. Nursing interventions such as limit setting or confrontation will cause the client to perceive the nurse as an abuser. The client's threats or acts of self-destructive behavior can initiate the dynamic, whereby the nurse perceives and experiences herself as a target of violence or powerless bystander.

As each of these re-created family patterns is enacted, the nurse assists the client to identify her present need and to think about how to get it met. The goal is to foster a secure base for the client in the various treatment relationships so that security will eventually be internalized.

CULTURAL CONSIDERATIONS

The phenomena of dissociation are pervasive in most cultures, particularly in Third World countries. Because of their prevalence, most researchers are reluctant to label them as mental disorders. The *DSM-IV-TR* (APA, 2000) highlights culture-bound syndromes and idioms of distress as a means of offering nurses and clinicians a list of terms and their meanings unique to some cultures. These symptoms are

CLINICAL EXAMPLE

The Client with a Dissociative Disorder

Lucy, a 30-year-old client experiencing episodes of dissociation, visits with the psychiatric nurse at the mental health clinic every 2 weeks. Her father and a neighbor sexually and physically abused Lucy severely until she was 18 years old and left home. Since that time, she has been experiencing severe alcohol and drug abuse, self-mutilation, and dissociation. Lucy reports that whenever she was upset at home, her mother would tell her to "put on a happy face."

Lucy has been meeting with the nurse for 3 months, having stated that she wanted to "feel better." Early in treatment, Lucy would start a session stating everything was going "pretty good." However, she would come in the following session with scratches on her arms and say she didn't remember what she had said in the preceding session. After seeing this pattern develop, the nurse pointed out to Lucy that she would come in and say that everything was okay but end up mutilating herself a short time later. Lucy and the nurse worked on what the pattern might mean. Eventually, Lucy was able to tell the nurse that she came in determined to talk about her anger but started worrying that the nurse could not handle hearing about it. Her wish for the nurse to know her anger and her simultaneous fear of the consequences if that should happen resulted in dissociation and self-mutilation. Lucy was afraid of being angry in front of the nurse and believed the nurse "couldn't handle it"—the powerless bystander role. Lucy used the "happy face" her mother had wanted and engaged in dissociation, to detach and manage the internal conflict, and in self-mutilation, to punish and soothe herself.

culturally shaped and prescribe ways of depicting distress. Most researchers submit that the most common clinical features of these disorders vary, but include trance states of amnesia, emotional lability, and loss of identity. These states are likely to occur as an idiom of distress, but they are not necessarily perceived as normal within the sociocultural context. They are generally accepted as part of the sociocultural context and religious practice (APA, 2000; Escobar & Vega, 2006; Tseng, 2006; Van Duijl et al., 2005). (See Chapter 7 for a discussion of culture-bound syndromes.)

Psychiatric nurses need to familiarize themselves with behaviors that are unique to various cultures and assess the significance of the clients' symptoms to ensure an accurate diagnosis. The nursing assessment needs to include a thorough spiritual and religious assessment along with other aspects of the mental status and physical examination to make an accurate description of the clients' symptoms. (See Research Abstract.)

DISSOCIATIVE DISORDERS ACROSS THE LIFE SPAN

Exposure to traumatic or overwhelming stressful situations occurs across the life span requiring psychiatric nurses to assess various clinical symptoms of dissociative disorders.

Infants as well as older adults require nursing interventions that assist in modulating the overwhelming impact of stressful situations and preventing their negative sequel. The following section entails dissociative disorders and their impact across the life span.

CHILDHOOD

Dissociation is an early primitive defense mechanism available to children until they mature and gain greater psychological capacity to accommodate ambiguity and tolerate conflict. Putnam (1997) labeled this a "normative dissociation." It is normally manifested in fantasy play and other imaginary activities. It is common for children to have elaborate, imaginary companions, and the phenomenon should not be considered pathological unless it is carried into adolescence. Normative dissociation usually peaks at 10 years of age if the child has not experienced a traumatic event and has had supportive and empathetic parenting.

Empathetic parenting allows the child to develop the cognitive and emotional schemata with which to understand ambiguous and conflicting thoughts and feelings. The child is provided comfort and protection while experimenting in the world and can verbalize her experience to the parent with a sense of safety.

A child with a dissociative disorder is most likely to have a history of early sexual or physical abuse and has not been able to develop attachment because of the absence of empathetic parenting.

Children with a dissociative disorder are often difficult to differentiate from children with attention-deficit disorder. Clients with dissociative disorders can manifest mild-to-moderate inattention and sustained concentration deficits on psychological testing (Cromer, Stevens, DePrince, & Pears, 2006). The abrupt changes in behavior and short attention and memory spans seen in hyperactive children are similar to episodes of dissociation. Sadly, children with pathological dissociation will be labeled as liars when they accurately state that they cannot remember homework, behavior, and so on. Often, these children suffer self-hatred and appear anxious and depressed. Silberg (1998) identified the following behavioral features common in children with dissociative disorder diagnoses:

◆ Amnesia, or forgetting test responses
◆ Staring, indicative of trance states
◆ Unusual or odd motor behaviors
◆ Fearful and angry reactions to stimuli
◆ Expressions of internal conflict

ADOLESCENCE

At its best, adolescence is a turbulent time for the individual. Affect and behavior become more erratic than they were in childhood, and the search for identity necessitates some fantasy thinking. Fantasy provides the healthy adolescent an opportunity to redefine her power and role in relation to significant others (Putnam, 1997). It can be normal for adolescents who are under temporary, severe stress to regress and cope through depersonalization.

Symptoms of pathological dissociation in adolescence can be consistent with the diagnosis of conduct disorder. More defense mechanisms are available to the adolescent, and the dissociative process—the struggle to keep the not-me out of awareness—will be confused with the adolescent's search for identity and intimacy. The adolescent with dissociative identity disorder is likely to be the more vunerable to the pressures of peer groups and use alters to respond to each demand. In a study looking at a spectrum of traumatic events and the development of dissociative symptoms in adolescents, Reigstad, Jørgensen, and Wichstrøm (2006) found that even less severe forms of abuse and neglect may have a significant impact on the development of dissociative symptoms in adolescents (see the research abstract).

In an effort to counteract a not-me personification of powerlessness, the adolescent may become more aggressive and act out sexually. Denial, along with dissociation, will present in an adolescent who not only does not recall trauma but also rejects any suggestion that she is the least bit troubled.

Having never experienced parental soothing and attachment, the adolescent who is dissociative will attempt to provide soothing for herself through drug abuse and sexual promiscuity and to meet attachment needs through gang membership. Management of affect, especially sadness, is accomplished by self-mutilation in the form of excessive tattoos or ear piercing.

The Role of the Nurse Working with Children and Adolescents

When working with the child or adolescent with a dissociative disorder, the nurse's first goal is to ensure the client's safety. The protection and soothing that were unavailable in the client's early development must be present in the nurse-client relationship and therapeutic environment. The nurse should accept the experiences of alters in children and adolescents with dissociative identity disorder. Excessive switching between alters is usually the result of an environmental or interpersonal trigger similar to past trauma. A therapeutic intervention occurs when the nurse, who is in the here-and-now, reassures the client. Structure in the nurse-client relationship and physical milieu helps the client experience her self in a continuous manner. In addition the continuity of the client's self may be facilitated by the use of clearly defined limits and consequences for inappropriate behavior. Emphasis should be on talking or writing about feelings, rather than on acting on them. Children can be encouraged to keep art journals.

The nurse in advanced practice may have success in using a group therapy process for adolescents. An expressive group process will help the adolescent normalize some feelings as well as provide a consistent and healthy peer group experience.

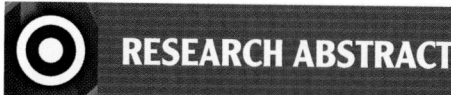

RESEARCH ABSTRACT

Cultural Issues and Psychiatric Diagnosis: Providing a General Background for Considering Substance Use Diagnoses

Escobar, J. I., & Vega, W. A. (2006). *Addiction, 101*(Suppl 1), 40–47.

Study Problem/Purpose

To construct a general perspective on the concept of cross-cultural diagnosis and provide guidance concerning application to substance use disorders.

Methods

Researchers performed a comprehensive analysis of the literature on psychiatric diagnosis and cross-cultural and ethnic issues and formulated a context to make recommendations for substance-use diagnoses.

Findings

Data analysis reveals inconsistencies in the broad use of cross-cultural and ethnic issues in the diagnosis of psychiatric disorders. Researchers also submit that the current *Diagnostic and Statistical Manual for Mental Disorders (DSM)* criteria are difficult to apply to unique populations.

Implications for Psychiatric Nurses

The growing diversity of society requires a greater understanding of the unique needs of all clients seeking psychiatric treatment. Psychiatric nurses are poised to explore the nature of client symptoms and experience to accurately diagnose and treat individuals with psychiatric disorders.

Promotion of the client's self-soothing is a major goal for the psychiatric nurse. The child client will need concrete direction in this area. Does she have a soothing stuffed toy or a favorite story or something or someone to turn to when frightened? The adolescent can be assisted to use sports or imagery that involves relaxation as a means of soothing.

ADULTHOOD

The healthy adult continues the development of the three aspects of her self-system that originated in childhood, with the not-me aspect continually being uncovered and brought into conscious awareness. However, even in healthy adults, the experience of a traumatic event, such as a flood, earthquake, or car crash, may result in dissociation. Dissociation allows the individual to distance oneself from the trauma (Morgan et al., 2004). Dissociation of the experience is adaptive in the sense that it gives the person time to gather her defense mechanism resources. This gathering of resources will help the person assimilate the experience without being psychologically overwhelmed. The dissociative process paces the assimilation of the experience into consciousness and modulates the anxiety. For example, after a natural disaster, such as a hurricane or earthquake, it is not uncommon for people not to remember the event or to be found wandering, unsure of where they live. It is quite common after a car crash not to remember what happened during hours immediately after the crash.

As with any other age group, it is important to differentiate between a general medical condition and a psychological etiology for a dissociative process in an adult. In amnesia with an underlying medical condition, such as severe electrolyte imbalance or head injury, general information is lost before personal information. Thus, elderly clients may wander away from home and, when found, be able to state their name but not have a sense of their general location or how long they have been wandering. Clients with psychological amnesia, on the other hand, have no sense of who they are, who their family members are, or what their occupation is.

The psychiatric nurse can make major contributions to the diagnostic process. The nurse observes patterns of apparent dissociation in terms of particular time of day and the presence or absence of possible environmental factors. The nurse correlates these observations with the objective physiological data. The advanced-practice nurse in the community will use her extensive knowledge of physiology as well as interviewing skills to identify trauma in the assessment of a client presenting with "lost time" or a sense of "not being myself."

The adult with a dissociative disorder frequently goes undiagnosed or is misdiagnosed (Foote, Smolin, Kaplan, Legatt, & Lipschitz, 2006). Several factors account for this unfortunate phenomenon. First, the person, having grown up in a chaotic family, may not know that losing time is an abnormal experience. Unless the behavior becomes disruptive, she may go through life with a dissociative disorder. Second, some adults may be in the mental health system for years being treated for depression, and the dissociation becomes evident only after a triggering event such as puberty or pregnancy. Adults with dissociative identity disorder have usually developed skill at keeping secret all the alters and their activities. Often, the dissociative disorders of adult survivors of incest will come to the fore when one of their children reaches the age that they were victimized. Adult men with undiagnosed dissociative disorders end up incarcerated in prison because of aggressive behaviors such as assaults on men or women, serial killing, or drug-related activities. The problem for these men is poor affect regulation, which results in episodes of rage or attempts at intimacy that only recreate the abuse they experienced as children.

SPECIFIC DISSOCIATIVE DISORDERS

The diagnosis and clinical features of various dissociative disorders requires recognition of the continuum of symptoms and appropriate diagnoses. Psychiatric nurses must also be able to implement individualized treatment planning that reduces the intensity of dissociative symptoms and facilitates healthy resolution when possible.

DEPERSONALIZATION DISORDER

Depersonalization disorder is a rapid-onset, persistent dissociative process in which the client's experience of the self or perception of the reality of the self or environment is changed. The client is able to observe the process as it occurs and verbalize discomfort (APA, 2000).

Etiology

The client is overwhelmed by feelings during a current event that is similar to a traumatic event in the past (APA, 2000).

DISSOCIATIVE AMNESIA

Dissociative amnesia is a dissociative process that results in a sudden identity disturbance owing to the client's inability to recall significant personal information. Underlying general medical conditions, brain injury, and substance abuse have been ruled out as possible causes (APA, 2000). Dissociative amnesia is the most common of the dissociative disorders. A person may experience secondary gain, or psychogenic amnesia could be a means of gaining media attention or escaping from financial responsibility.

Etiology

Dissociative amnesia is usually a defense mechanism that occurs in response to an emotional conflict or an external stressor, for example, the sudden loss of a significant other.

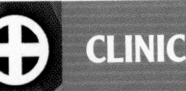

CLINICAL EXAMPLE

The Client with a Depersonalization Disorder

Ed, a 20-year-old hospitalized male, has just had a visit from his family, with whom he has not lived for 5 years. His mother, a recovering drug abuser, would violently beat Ted and then tell him to "forget everything" before he went to school. His greatest concern before the family visit was that he would "just hold it together." After his family left, Ted was observed sitting rigidly in a chair. He reported feeling like the floor was sinking and the walls were falling out. The episode lasted 2 to 3 minutes.

CLINICAL EXAMPLE

The Client with Dissociative Amnesia

Louise was admitted to the psychiatric unit after her daughter found her sitting on her porch. Louise did not recognize her daughter or know her own name or the name of the town in which she lived. Louise was given a thorough medical evaluation, and no general medical cause was found for her amnesia. Louise had no history of psychiatric treatment. Louise's daughter told the nurse that her mother had discovered her husband having an affair and had been planning to divorce him, but he was killed in a car wreck 10 days ago. Louise had told her daughter the day before the accident that she was so angry with her husband that she wished he was dead.

DISSOCIATIVE FUGUE

Dissociative fugue is a dissociative process that results in an identity and memory disturbance manifested by sudden travel away from the home or work environment along with confusion about personal identity or, rarely, the assumption of a new identity. The travel may be brief or extensive. These patients appear normal, not attracting the attention of others.

Myths to Overcome

- People with dissociative identity disorder are often portrayed in the media as nonfunctional, out-of-control individuals, who can appear to others as frightening and bizarre. In reality, there are many people with this disorder who function effectively in relationships, raise children, and are gainfully employed in jobs that require high skills and training.

- Dissociative disorders often result from abuse experienced during childhood. The media have reported that therapists may have suggested memories of this abuse when adult clients are in hypnotic states. In reality, children are at times subjected to horrific abuses. It is often difficult to corroborate this abuse

because of the time that has elapsed, and because family members are hesitant to admit to their own involvement in the abuse.

- Many people who have been victims of traumas, such as childhood abuse, loss of significant others, or natural disasters, are encouraged by others to "just get over" these traumas. In reality, these memories have a significant impact on a person's emotions, cognition, and body, even many years after the incident occurred.

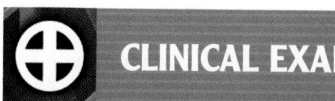

CLINICAL EXAMPLE

The Client with Dissociative Fugue

Bob was a 54-year-old insurance salesman with a wife and three teenage children. One day he did not come home from work, and all efforts to locate him proved unsuccessful. Before his disappearance, Bob had sought a promotion but was passed over for a much younger employee. Bob had always worked 7 days a week. He had been proud of the fact that his wife had never had to work outside the home. After hearing that he had been rejected for the promotion, Bob got in his car to drive home, but he ended up going to the Northwest coast, where he lived alone, worked as a bartender, and gambled on the side. He called himself Rex and felt vague about his past, but he calmed himself by saying "life is for having fun and spending money."

Etiology

The origin of dissociative fugue is usually the desire to withdraw from emotionally painful experiences (Coons, 2000).

DISSOCIATIVE IDENTITY DISORDER

Dissociative identity disorder was previously known as multiple personality disorder. It is considered the most serious of the dissociative disorders. Clients have two or more distinct personalities, each with its own behavior and attitudes (APA, 2000).

The following are the signs and symptoms of dissociative identity disorder:

- Unremembered behaviors
- The discovery of items in the client's possession for which she cannot account
- Loss of time
- Behavior characteristics that represent distinctly different ages
- Changes in appearance and dress
- Use of different voices

Etiology

Dissociative identity disorder is most likely caused by a severe childhood trauma. The trauma is usually severe sexual abuse that overwhelms the child's nondissociative defenses. Subsequently, the abuse experience is dissociated and aspects of the experience (memory of it and affect related to it) later appear in the form of various personalities.

TREATMENT MODALITIES

Presently, there is little empirical evidence that indicates a particular pharmacologic intervention for dissociative disorders. However, with the high concomitance of psychiatric disorders, including major depression, somatization disorder,

borderline personality disorder, and psychosis, antidepressants and other medications may be indicated (Sar et al., 2007). Currently, there is a dearth of randomized controlled trials that demonstrate the efficacy of antidepressants or other pharmacologic interventions for clients with dissociative disorders. Yet, data indicate the efficacy of various psychotherapeutic interventions that enable the client to manage the distress arising from some of these disorders.

PHARMACOLOGIC INTERVENTIONS

There is no particular drug or combination of drugs that is specific to the treatment of a client with a dissociative disorder. Pharmacologic interventions may be most useful in treating the target symptoms that often accompany dissociative identity disorder, as well as intrusive and hyperarousal symptoms (Loewenstein & Putnam, 2004). See Chapter 29 for more specific information on psychopharmacology.

Depression is also a common presenting symptom of clients with dissociative disorder and may be what first brings them into the mental health system. No particular class of antidepressant is more effective than another; each needs to be evaluated on an individual basis.

Anger and severe internal disequilibrium accompany dissociation in varying degrees. Antipsychotics can be a useful adjunct to treatment to assist the client in periods of dyscontrol or rapid dissociation. Atypical antipsychotics can be effective. It should be noted that the alters of the client with dissociative identity disorder may have varying degrees of responsiveness to neuroleptics. This is not manipulation, but a basic difference in psychological responsiveness.

The nurse's role in pharmacotherapy is to educate the client about the medication, including the purpose of the medication, the dose schedule, and possible side effects. The nurse must assess the client for medication adherence, which can be disrupted by dissociative episodes. An emphasis on client responsibility, especially persons with dissociative identity disorders, is paramount for medication adherence and safety.

PSYCHOSOCIAL INTERVENTIONS

General principles that can guide the nurse in caring for clients with dissociative disorders involve interventions that help the client modulate and cope with constant anxiety and high arousal states, such as relaxation techniques, deep breathing exercises, and meditation. Thought-blocking techniques and cognitive behavioral therapy help reduce preoccupations and obsessive thoughts. Grounding techniques help the client manage the immediacy of the current experience and acute emotional states.

Intensive psychotherapy is probably the most effective treatment for the dissociative disorders, particularly dissociative identity disorder. The psychotherapy will be long term in nature. Hypnosis is also a technique that has been found to be useful in treating these disorders. The advanced-practice nurse may be involved in these treatment modalities.

Additional psychosocial interventions include assessing and monitoring the client's risk of danger to self and others, assisting in developing adaptive coping skills, and providing opportunities to succeed in activities that increase self-esteem.

CLIENT GROUNDING TECHNIQUES

Grounding, as a concept, is meant to convey the notion of "not going away," that is, dissociating. The following techniques help clients concentrate on the here and now and move toward verbalizing what is occurring in their internal world. The nurse should teach clients these techniques.

Safe Place

Finding a safe place is a concept very familiar to survivors of abuse. The dissociative person should be encouraged to find a reasonable place in the environment where she can go and guarantee the nurse and herself safety and freedom from destructive impulses. A typical place could be a particular chair or room.

Ice in Hands

Ice helps the client focus on a physical sensation that is not harmful. When the warning signs of dissociation are present, the nurse may encourage the client to hold an ice cube securely in each hand until she can report feeling calmer.

Counting Forward or Backward

Counting forward or backward is a technique used mostly by clients with dissociative identity disorder. Counting is a form of hypnosis that can be used to let an alter that is overwhelmed go in and another come forward with behavior appropriate to the situation.

CLIENT EDUCATION

Providing clients with skills to cope with their dissociative disorder is an important function of the psychiatric nurse. Essential skills are relapse prevention and journaling.

Relapse Prevention

Relapse prevention is an important skill drawn from working with chemically dependent persons. The client is taught to recognize contributing factors (triggers) to dissociation. The client and nurse then develop a concrete plan to interrupt the stimulation of a dissociative episode. The plan could include activities such as listening to music, staying with people, or engaging in a task. Then the plan is shared with the family and other health care professionals involved in the client's treatment to enlist support in implementing it whenever it is needed.

Journaling

Writing in a journal helps the client achieve several outcomes: feelings are put into words, a sense of continuity of the self is developed in the journal, and the impact of triggers is diminished.

If the client has not had journals before, she should start with a 5-minute daily exercise. The client should be encouraged to pick an event that occurred during the day and write down her thoughts and feelings about it. The client needs to share the journal with the nurse on a regular basis. Journal work should be an essential part of each client's day. The structure can vary according to the client's threshold of dissociation and phase of treatment. Children and adolescents can be encouraged to keep an art journal, rather than a written one.

THE ROLE OF THE NURSE

Because of the complexity of dissociative disorders, psychiatric nurses must assess the client's coping skills, risk of self-injury, and provide a safe and empathetic environment that promotes symptom management. Educational and clinical preparation will determine the role of the psychiatric nurse working with the client with a dissociative disorder.

THE GENERALIST NURSE

The psychiatric nurse is pivotal in the care of the client vulnerable to or diagnosed with dissociative disorder. The

---

My Experience with Dissociative Identity Disorder

My wife suffers from dissociative identity disorder (DID). For years, we did not know what was wrong with her. I have always known that she grew up in a very abusive home, and that she had had a difficult childhood and adolescence. When we first met, she told me that she had had psychiatric treatment, and that she had been called "crazy" by various people, even labeled as schizophrenic at one time. I also knew that she had attempted suicide on more than one occasion before we were married.

A few years after we married, she began experiencing memories of her childhood, as well as flashbacks of abuse she had experienced. These flashbacks were frightening for both of us.

Her different "personalities" or alters began coming out. At times she was like a very small child, at other times like a mean, nasty teenage boy. Most of the time, she was still my loving wife. Our lives became very chaotic during this period. We both knew she needed help, but did not know where to turn.

Eventually, my wife found a therapist she could trust and began opening up to that therapist. She was given a diagnosis of DID. We both have been involved in the therapy at times. Our lives are much more intact now, but she continues to struggle with processing the memories of her childhood and learning to live with those memories.

generalist nurse will be on the front line of identifying the undiagnosed dissociative disorder. The nurse's other important role is to help the client develop adaptive coping skills and achieve basic symptom management, including appropriate use of medications. The nurse needs to continually assess the client's level of danger to self and others throughout treatment.

THE ADVANCED-PRACTICE PSYCHIATRIC REGISTERED NURSE

The advanced-practice nurse may often encourage the client in a psychotherapy or case management process. Psychotherapy is the arena in which the client may retrieve memories in a controlled manner to consider their impact on her life. Advanced-practice nurses require specialized training to work with clients with dissociative disorders, particularly when working with alters. The nurse needs to assess client safety continually, using short hospital stays if necessary, to help clients retrieve their capacity to feel safe.

THE NURSING PROCESS

Caring for the client with dissociative disorder involves a comprehensive and holistic approach. The nursing process enables the nurse to participate in the data collection process of potential causes and high risk factors and client needs. Analyzing the data also helps ensure an accurate diagnosis and appropriate plan of care for clients with dissociative disorders.

ASSESSMENT

Early case finding is an important function of the nurse working with children. Recognition that a child is being abused or is experiencing early school failure can help interrupt progression toward a much more problematic dissociative disorder in adulthood.

Psychological assessment involves collecting both subjective and objective data. The client may not always be able to report sexual or emotional trauma because the event is dissociated. The nurse should watch for signs of abuse: startle reaction, erratic sleep, and fear of objects or other people. Because some clients are not aware they dissociate, the nurse should also observe for a pattern of not remembering events and a pattern of unexplained behaviors. van der Kolk (1996) explains that clients who chronically engage in self-destructive behavior or who repeatedly seek medical help for problems with no organic basis may be dealing with issues of trauma.

More than any other psychiatric disorder, dissociation is assessed basically through observation and a period of repeated interaction with the client. Because dissociation is episodic and not continual, many clients learn to adjust to their dissociation experience. Psychological tests do not always reveal dissociation.

NURSING DIAGNOSES

Possible nursing diagnoses include:

- Risk for self-directed violence
- Disturbed personal identity
- Ineffective Coping: escape through dissociation
- Anxiety severe related to acute stressor

OUTCOME IDENTIFICATION AND PLANNING

The process of working to identify desired outcomes is empowering. Outcomes need to be very short term in nature, so that clients are able to appreciate their progress. Planning, whether in a community or hospital setting, should be reviewed frequently.

The client and psychiatric nurse should mutually identify the desired outcomes of their working together. The outcome that is most likely to be achieved is the one the client values. In most cases, clients with dissociative disorders need environmental and interpersonal safety to be established first. A core part of trauma is the sense of helplessness and loss of control of one's body.

IMPLEMENTATION AND EVALUATION

As the client works with the nurse to implement a plan of care, the client should experience a form of support that has been missing in her life. Regardless of setting, intervention should be flexible but emphasize consistency and predictability. The nurse who is working with the client with

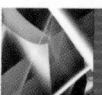

CASE STUDY

The Client with Dissociative Identity Disorder (Penny)

Penny is a 35-year-old woman who suffered sadistic sexual abuse by both of her parents and their friends from infancy through 15 years of age. She is admitted to the hospital in a dissociated state, claiming that she is Mary and does not understand how she got to the unit, except that Penny must have tried to commit suicide again. A nursing assessment elicits a description of five alter personalities ranging in age from 6 months (the children) to 35 (Mary). Each of the personalities is described as manifesting a particular affect. The "host" personality is Mary. Lily is 5 years old and looking for a "mommy and daddy." Sue is 16 years old and the protector; she wishes to kill people when they do not do as she says. Penny is 12 and feels all the pain. Mary states she tries to keep Penny from hearing things that are "going on outside."

Nursing Care Plan 18–1 identifies the desired outcomes for this case study, the nursing actions needed to achieve these outcomes, and the rationales for these actions.

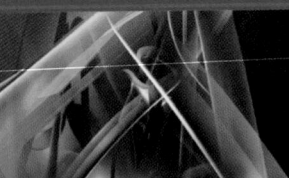

The Client with Dissociative Identity Disorder (Penny)

Nursing Diagnosis: Risk for Self-Direct Violence

Outcome Identification	Nursing Actions	Rationales	Evaluation
1. By [date], Penny will verbalize the absence of suicidal thoughts or plans.	1a. Assess the level of danger.	1a. This enables the nurse to identify interventions to reduce suicidal risk.	*Goal met:* Penny • denies suicidal ideations.
	1b. Provide a safe environment. Remove potential or actual dangerous objects from the environment.	1b. Removing objects reduces access to lethal or harmful objects and lessens the risk of self harm and suicide.	• does not harm herself. • is able to identify options. • demonstrates gradual mood changes and is able to express superficial feelings.
	1c. Discuss a "no suicide" verbal contract.	1c. Encouraging the client to agree to a "no suicide contract" helps her understand the seriousness of the situation and verbalize feelings concerning suicide or self harm.	

Nursing Diagnosis: Disturbed Personal Identity as evidenced by dissociative phenomena

Outcome Identification	Nursing Actions	Rationales	Evaluation
1. By [date], Penny will identify at least two warning signs of impending dissociation.	1a. Teach Penny to write in journal every day, especially after a dissociative episode.	1a. Keeping a journal is a method of documenting events and feelings that are otherwise difficult to retrieve because of dissociation.	*Goal met:* Penny discovers that her handwriting changes dramatically around 11:00 each evening.
	1b. Review Penny's journal with her.	1b. Working with the client on the journal enhances the value of the journal.	Penny has started to list six warning signs by reviewing the past 48 hours of her journal.
	1c. Have Penny make a list of possible warning signs of dissociation.	1c. The first step in mastering dissociation is achieving conscious awareness of warning signs.	

Nursing Diagnosis: Risk for Self-Directed Violence: Directed at Others as evidenced by presence of alter (Sue) with homicidal rage

Outcome Identification	Nursing Actions	Rationales	Evaluation
1. By [date], Penny will identify one strategy for managing the feeling of abandonment.	1a. Emphasize to Penny that she is responsible for all parts of herself.	1a. Teaches client that the "personalities" are all part of her and under her control (Putnam, 1997).	*Goal met:* Penny makes an effort to communicate verbally with staff about Sue's rage.

(continues)

Nursing Care Plan 18–1 *(continued)*

Outcome Identification	Nursing Actions	Rationales	Evaluation
	1b. Empathize with the original purpose of the rage—to provide protection from sadistic abuse.	1b. All defense mechanisms serve a purpose. Behavior cannot be changed without understanding the original motivation for it.	Chart requested restraints because "didn't want to hurt innocent people" when feeling angry.

Nursing Diagnosis: Risk for Impaired Parent/Child/Attachment as evidenced by continued wish for idealized parents and lack of integrated sense of self

Outcome Identification	Nursing Actions	Rationales	Evaluation
1. By [date], Penny will identify one strategy for managing the feeling of abandonment.	1a. Help Penny identify the dysfunctional coping strategy she presently uses when she is feeling abandoned.	1a. Expectations of others and behaviors when needs are not met must be brought to client's awareness before they can be changed.	*Goal met:* Penny makes plans to offer "Lily" (the 5-year-old alter) extra time in her room near shift change.
	1b. Encourage Penny to develop a coping plan for potential times of feeling abandoned.	1b. Anticipation of an event promotes observance of behavior and sense of control over impact of the event.	

dissociative identity disorder needs to set appropriate and consistent boundaries in treatment, i.e., acceptable behavior and firm limits (Loewenstein & Putnam, 2004).

The client should be encouraged to write in her journal about the effectiveness of the care plan as often as possible.

Evaluation should be a mutual affair and based on as much behavioral data as possible.

The following case study illustrates the application of the nursing process to the client with a dissociative disorder.

Standard of Care for the Client with a Dissociative Disorder

Nursing Diagnosis: Disturbed Personal Identity

Client Outcome: By (date), client will demonstrate or verbalize increased continuity in one or all parameters of the self: identity, memory, experience.

Defining Characteristics:

Nursing Domain	Client Outcome	Nursing Interventions
Psychotherapeutic interventions	1. Client states what personality is interacting with nursing staff.	1a. Collaborate with client in mapping out the alters and the purpose and function of each.
		1b. Instruct client that she is responsible for letting staff know which alter is out.
		1c. Identify with client which alters are caretakers (internal self-helpers) and can be elicited in stressful situations.
		1d. Before the client goes off the unit, have her contract to have only an appropriate alter out when off the unit.
		1e. Emphasize that all alters are responsible for care and behavior of body.
		1f. Respond to client as a whole person.
		1g. Encourage host personality to engage all alters in writing in a journal.

(continues)

Standard of Care for the Client with a Dissociative Disorder *(continued)*

Nursing Domain	Client Outcome	Nursing Interventions
	2. Client relates memories of self-system to present peer relationship patterns.	2a. Educate client about dysfunctional attachment/trust patterns from past abuse. 2b. Initiate *brief* contact frequently with client during first 72 hours of hospitalization. 2c. Problem-solve with client regarding how she may feel safe in the presence of another client or nurse who reminds client of trauma.
	3. Client maintains progressively longer experience of here-and-now reality.	3a. Teach client basic structure of journal: Work 5 to 10 minutes daily. Choose one event of day. Write about thoughts and feelings related to the event. 3b. Review journal work with client on a regular basis. 3c. Review nursing care plan and sleep patterns with client on a regular basis. 3d. Assess client for what, if any, grounding techniques she currently uses. 3e. Support client in use of following client-appropriate grounding techniques: Going to safe place Holding ice in hands Placing feet on the floor and grasping a chair Staying out of the room Blowing her nose Listening to tapes that provide pleasant memories Washing face Counting forward or backward Requesting quiet room Requesting p.r.n. medicines Requesting restraints Deep breathing exercises Relaxation techniques, meditation
Therapeutic milieu	1. Client identifies triggers in environment that lead to dissociation.	1a. Educate client about concept of trigger. 1b. If client switches rapidly, start flow sheet to identify pattern of triggers. 1c. Provide client with feedback about when dissociation was observed.
	2. Client participates in promotion of safe milieu.	2a. Explore with client how the need to feel safe is met. 2b. Educate client about the need to not allow own behavior to become alarming to other clients (abuse is unacceptable). 2c. Develop plan with client to contain violent or self-destructive alters when and if they come out. 2d. Encourage client to have child alters come out only in privacy of her room. 2e. Support client in stating when another client's behavior seems similar to past abuse.

(continues)

Standard of Care for the Client with a Dissociative Disorder *(continued)*

Nursing Domain	Client Outcome	Nursing Interventions
Activities of daily living	1. Client maintains a structured day.	1a. Assess client's ability to make up a daily schedule.
		1b. Support client in keeping appointments by providing positive feedback.
		1c. Provide client with unit-restricted schedule if she is being kept on the unit.
		1d. Actively support client in adhering to schedule.
		1e. Document any dissatisfaction client expresses with schedule.
		1f. Assist client in structuring time for alters to come out.
	2. Client participates in development of safe nighttime environment.	2a. Help client identify her patterns of sleep and wakefulness.
		2b. Problem-solve periods of wakefulness.
		2c. Encourage identification and use of specific self-soothing techniques as a part of bedtime preparation.
Health teaching	1. Client verbalizes purpose, side effects, and dose of medication.	1a. Provide client with appropriate information about medications.
		1b. Explain the value of consistent medication dosage.
		1c. Encourage client to identify which alters, if any, are resistant to medication.
		1d. Problem-solve resistance to use of medication.
	2. Client verbalizes understanding of nursing care plan development and implementation.	2a. Explore understanding of nursing care plan in development of care plan.
		2b. Identify with the client the value of participating in development of care plan.
		2c. With client, practice identifying problem goal and intervention.
	3. Client demonstrates use of journal as tool to facilitate continuity of experience.	3a. Assess client's experience with journal writing: how often:_____ technique:_____ tools:_____
		3b. Teach client journal structure and value of using journal consistency.
		3c. Review client's journal writing with her.
		3d. Encourage journal writing as a substitute for acting out and as method to self-soothe.
	4. Client demonstrates use of safe place.	4a. Assess client's history of using safe place: where:_____ when:_____ how long:_____
		4b. Teach client value of still using safe place as an adult.
		4c. Encourage client to identify safe place on the unit.
		4d. When client appears overstimulated, remind her of safe place.
		4e. If client harms self or others in safe place, repeat b and c.
		4f. Encourage client to use safe place for alters via imagery.

(continues)

Standard of Care for the Client with a Dissociative Disorder *(continued)*

Nursing Domain	Client Outcome	Nursing Interventions
Somatic therapies	1. Client adheres to prescribed medication regimen.	1a. Encourage client's input regarding most effective time structure of doses.
		1b. Assist client in encouraging resistant alters to help take care of the body.
		1c. Teach client to use p.r.n. medication as a preventive basis using warning signs.
	2. Client uses self-soothing techniques for grounding.	2a. Assess client's repertoire of self-soothing techniques.
		2b. Encourage attendance at group activities promoting body awareness.
		2c. Assist client in use of grounding techniques listed under Psychotherapeutic interventions.
Discharge planning	1. Client develops relapse prevention plan for triggers that lead to dissociation.	1a. Review relapse prevention plan with client.
		1b. Practice prevention plan with client.
		1c. Help client identify people with whom she will share plan after discharge.

STANDARD OF CARE

The accompanying Standard of Care for clients with a dissociative disorder provides the nurse with a menu of client outcomes and nursing interventions within the six domains of nursing: psychotherapeutic intervention, therapeutic milieu, health teaching, activities of daily living, somatic therapies, and discharge planning.

SUMMARY

◆ Dissociative disorders are usually the result of trauma.

◆ Clients with underlying general medical conditions can present with symptoms of dissociative disorder, and a general medical condition should be ruled out in a thorough evaluation.

◆ The severity of the dissociative disorder is determined by the severity and nature of the trauma, the age at which the trauma was experienced, the neurobiological predisposition of the victim, and the presence or absence of a soothing caretaker.

◆ Dissociative disorders are treated with psychopharmacology, psychotherapy, and psychoeducation.

◆ The nurse's role in the care of the client with a dissociative disorder is that of a case finder, consultant, and coach in affect regulation.

◆ The nurse helps the client observe the pattern of dissociation and develop coping strategies to interrupt or minimize the process.

SUGGESTIONS FOR CLINICAL CONFERENCES

1. Briefly describe trauma a client has experienced and identify one factor that has been helpful.

2. Discuss myths you have heard about people with dissociative disorders.

STUDY QUESTIONS

1. Symptoms of dissociative identity disorder include all of the following *except:*
   a. loss of time
   b. changes in appearance and dress
   c. unexplained extensive travel away from home
   d. use of different voices

2. Which of the following is the most effective treatment for dissociative disorders?
   a. Antidepressant medications
   b. Psychotherapy
   c. Behavioral therapy
   d. Client grounding techniques

3. In Sullivan's theory of personality development, all of the following make up the mutually interacting aspects *except:*
   a. okay me
   b. not me
   c. good me
   d. bad me

4. All of the following statements regarding the role of family dynamics in dissociative disorders are true *except*:
   a. Dissociative symptoms help a child maintain her sanity during exposure to trauma.
   b. In an incestuous family, the father usually appears to outsiders as a violent man, absent from the family.
   c. The child in an abusive family may join or mold to the abuser's self.
   d. The members of a healthy family have stable, but permeable, boundaries.

5. The following describes which dissociative disorder? A dissociative process that results in a sudden identity disturbance owing to the inability to recall significant personal information is:
   a. dissociative amnesia
   b. dissociative fugue
   c. dissociative identity disorder
   d. depersonalization disorder

6. Sharon is a 20-year-old college junior whose friends saw her wandering the streets. Her friends brought her to the college health clinic where you practice. The friends say that when they asked Sharon what she was doing, she did not recognize them. Sharon has just finished her final exams for the academic year. One of the following factors you want to assess is:
   a. how much coffee and sleep she has had over the past few weeks
   b. whether Sharon has a history of sexual trauma
   c. whether Sharon has a history of a head injury
   d. what could be the secondary gain from acting "weird"

7. A major goal for the nurse working with a child or adolescent with a dissociative disorder is:
   a. encouraging the client to express her feelings appropriately
   b. promotion of client self-soothing practices
   c. explaining to the client what defense mechanisms she is using
   d. reminding the child to "come back to reality" when she engages in fantasy play

8. W. T. is admitted to the psychiatric department with a diagnosis of depersonalization. One of the nursing interventions is to teach W. T. how to use a journal. The expected outcome of this nursing intervention is:
   a. W. T. will develop better writing skills.
   b. W. T. will have a record of his week to show his psychotherapist.
   c. W. T. will not experience depersonalization.
   d. W. T. will develop a greater and continuous sense of himself.

9. Ms. Melvin brings 8-year-old Terri to the clinic for a checkup. Terri is in Ms. Melvin's care as a foster child, having been removed from her parents because of profound neglect and abuse. As part of a psychosocial assessment to rule out any chronic dissociative pattern of coping on Ms. Melvin's part, the nurse would ask about:

   a. the presence of other siblings in the home
   b. play patterns with other children
   c. odd, contradictory displays of behavior
   d. 24-hour nutritional intake

10. A young woman is found wandering on campus after a fraternity party. She is disheveled and does not know who she is. She has no recollection of the evening. At the student health service she is diagnosed with dissociated amnesia subsequent to a rape. The most appropriate nursing diagnosis for the nurse to formulate is which of the following?
    a. Ineffective individual coping
    b. Personal identity disturbance
    c. Anxiety related to alteration in memory
    d. Risk of violence, self-directed

11. The nurse would formulate which of the following outcome criteria for a client with a dissociative disorder. The client
    a. identifies triggers in the environment that lead to dissociation
    b. uses deep breathing exercises to control dissociative states
    c. controls dissociative states using antidepressants
    d. avoids people, places, and things associated with traumatic event

12. Which of the following indicates to the nurse that a client with a dissociative disorder is improving? The client
    a. has improved sleep
    b. uses self-soothing techniques for grounding
    c. discusses her feelings with minimal anxiety
    d. maintains progressively shorter experience of here-and-now reality

RESOURCES

Please note that because Internet resources are of a time-sensitive nature and URL addresses may change or be deleted, searches should also be conducted by association or topic.

Internet Resources

1. Locate organizations that provide support for individuals with dissociative identity disorder.

2. Locate an Internet site addressing trauma and its effects, and find definitions for the following terms:
   ◆ Amnesia
   ◆ Attachment
   ◆ Derealization
   ◆ Hypermnesia
   ◆ Ego States
   ◆ Losing Time
   ◆ Trance
   ◆ Unification

http://www.healinghopes.com Support forum for abuse/trauma survivors

http://www.issd.org International Society for the Study of Dissociation

Other Resources

Traumatic Stress Foundation
200 E. Joppa Road, Suite 207
Towson, MD 21286
(410) 825-8888
http://www.sidran.org

National Alliance for the Mentally Ill
Colonial Place Three
2107 Wilson Blvd., Suite 300
Arlington, VA 22201-3042
(800) 950-NAMI (6264)
http://www.nami.org

New England Society for the Treatment of Trauma and Dissociation
P.O. Box 506
Malden, MA 02148-7837
(617) 489-1504
http://www.nesttd.org

REFERENCES

American Psychiatric Association. (2000). *Diagnostic and statistical manual of mental disorders* (4th edition, Text Revision) *(DSM-IV-TR)*. Washington, DC: Author.

Bernstein, E. M., & Putnam, F. W. (1986). Development, reliability, and validity of a dissociation scale. *Journal of Nervous and Mental Disease, 174*(12), 727–735.

Bob, P. (2003). Dissociation and neuroscience: History and new perspectives. *International Journal of Neuroscience, 113*(7), 903–914.

Bowlby, J. (1969). *Attachment and loss: Vol. 1. Attachment.* New York: Basic Books.

Casper, R. C. (1998). Serotonin, a major player in the regulation of feeding and affect [editorial]. *Biological Psychiatry, 44*(9), 795–797.

Cochen, V., Arnulf, I., Demeret, S., Neulat, M. L., Gourlet, V., Drouot, X., et al. (2005). Vivid dreams, hallucinations, psychosis and REM sleep in Guillain-Barre syndrome, *Brain, 128,* 2535–2545.

Coons, P. M. (2000). Dissociative fugue. In B. J. Sadock & V. A. Sadock (Eds.), *Comprehensive textbook of psychiatry* (Vol. I, pp. 1549–1552). Philadelphia: Lippincott Williams & Wilkins.

Cromer, L. D., Stevens, C., DePrince, A. P., & Pears, K. (2006). The relationship between executive attention and dissociation in children. *Journal of Trauma & Dissociation, 7,* 135–153.

Davis, M. (2000). The role of the amygdala in conditioned and unconditioned fear and anxiety. In Aggleton, J. P. (Ed.), *The Amygdala,* (Vol. 2, pp. 213–287). Oxford: Oxford UP.

Diseth, T. H. (2005). Dissociation in children and adolescents as reaction to trauma—An overview of conceptual issues and neurobiological factors. *Nordic Journal of Psychiatry, 59*(2), 79–91.

Elmore, J. L. (2000). Dissociatve spectrum disorders in the primary care setting. *Primary Care Companion to The Journal of Clinical Psychiatry, 2*(2), 37–41.

Escobar, J. I., & Vega, W. A. (2006). Cultural issues and psychiatric diagnosis: Providing a general background for considering substance use diagnoses. *Addiction, 101*(Suppl 1), 40–47.

Farinelli, M., Deschaux, O., Hugues, S., Thevenet, A., & Garcia, R. (2006). Hippocampal brain stimulation modulates recall of fear extinction independently of prefrontal cortex synaptic plasticity and lesions. *Learning & Memory, 13,* 329–334.

Foote, B., Smolin, Y., Kaplan, M., Legatt, M. E., & Lipschitz, D. (2006). Prevalence of dissociative disorders in psychiatric outpatients. *American Journal of Psychiatry, 163,* 566–568.

Foote, B., Smolin, Y., Kaplan, M., Legatt, M. E., & Lipschitz, D. (2006). Prevalence of dissociative disorders in psychiatric outpatients. *American Journal of Psychiatry, 163,* 623–629.

French, C. C. (2005). Near-death experiences in cardiac arrest survivors. *Progress in Brain Research, 150,* 351–367.

Herman, J. (1991). *Trauma and recovery.* New York: Basic Books.

Karadag, F., Sar, V., Tamar-Gurol, D., Evren, C., Karagoz, M., & Ekiran, M. (2005). Dissociative disorders among inpatients with drug or alcohol dependency. *Journal of Clinical Psychiatry, 66*(10), 1247–1253.

Kraemer, G. W. (1997). Psychobiology of early social attachment in rhesus monkeys. Clinical implications. *Annals of the New York Academy of Sciences, 807,* 401–418.

Loewenstein, R. J., & Putnam, F. W. (2004). Dissociative disorders. In Sadock, B. J. & Sadock, V. A. (Eds.), *Kaplan & Sadock's comprehensive textbook of psychiatry, Volume 1* (8th ed., pp. 1844–1901). Philadelphia, PA: Lippincott Williams & Wilkins.

Löf, L., Berggren, L., & Ahlström, G. (2006). Severely ill ICU patients' recall of factual events and unreal experiences of hospital admission and ICU stay—3 and 12 months after discharge. *Intensive and Critical Care Nursing, 22,* 154–166.

Meares, R. (1999). The contribution of Hughlings Jackson to an understanding of dissociation. *American Journal of Psychiatry, 156*(12), 1850–1855.

Morgan, C. A., III, Southwick, S., Hazlett, G., Rasmusson, A., Hoyt, G., Zimolo, Z., et al. (2004). Relationships among plasma dehydroepiandrosterone sulfate and cortisol levels, symptoms of dissociation, and objective performance in humans exposed to acute stress. *Archives of General Psychiatry, 61,* 819–825.

Nemiah, J. (1999). The psychodynamic basis of psychopathology. In A. Nicholi (Ed.), *The Harvard guide to* psychiatry (3rd ed., pp. 203–219). Cambridge, MA: Belknap Press of Harvard University Press.

Pearlman, L. A., & Courtois, C. A. (2005). Clinical applications of the attachment framework: Relational treatment of complex trauma. *Journal of Traumatic Stress, 18*(5), 449–459.

Peplau, H. (1952). *Interpersonal relations in nursing.* New York: G.F. Putnam & Sons.

Putnam, F. W. (1997). *Dissociation in children and adolescents. A developmental perspective.* New York: Guilford Press.

Quirk, G. J., Garcia, R., & González-Lima, F. (2006). Prefrontal mechanisms in extinction of conditioned fear. *Biological Psychiatry, 60,* 337–343.

Rauch, S. L., Shin, L. M., & Phelps, E. A. (2006). Neurocircuitry models of posttraumatic stress disorder and extinction: Human neuroimaging research—past, present, and future. *Biological Psychiatry, 60,* 376–382.

Reigstad, B., Jørgensen, K., & Wichstrøm, L. (2006). Diagnosed and self-reported childhood abuse in national and regional samples of child and adolescent psychiatric patients: Prevalences and correlates. *Nordic Journal of Psychiatry, 60,* 58–66.

Sar, V., Akyüz, G., & Doğan, O. (2007). Prevalence of dissociative disorders among women in the general population. *Psychiatry Research, 149,* 169–176.

Sar, V., Koyuncu, A., Ozturk, E., Yargic, L. I., Kundakci, T., Yazici, A., et al. (2007). Dissociative disorders in the psychiatric emergency ward. *General Hospital Psychiatry, 29,* 45–50.

Silberg, J. L. (1998). Dissociative symptomatology in children and adolescents as displayed on psychological testing. *Journal of Personality Assessment, 71*(3), 421–439.

Simeon, D., Knutelska, M., Yehuda, R., Putnam, F., Schmeidler, J., & Smith, L. M. (2007). Hypothalamic-pituitary-adrenal axis function in dissociative disorders, post-traumatic stress disorder, and healthy volunteers. *Biological Psychiatry, 61,* 966–973.

Spiegel, D., & Maldonado, J. R. (1999). Dissociative disorders. In R. E. Hales & S. C. Yudofsy (Eds.), *Essentials of clinical psychiatry* (3rd ed., pp. 453–469). Washington, DC: American Psychiatric Press.

Steinberg, M., Barry, D. T., Sholomskas, D., & Hall, P. (2005). SCL-90 symptom patterns: Indicators of dissociative disorders. *Bulletin of the Menninger Clinic, 69,* 237–249.

Sullivan, H. (1953). *The interpersonal theory of psychiatry.* New York: G. F. Putnam & Sons.

Tseng, W-S. (2006). From peculiar psychiatric disorders through culture-bound syndromes to culture-related specific syndromes. *Transcultural Psychiatry, 43,* 554–576.

van der Kolk, B. A. (1996). The complexity of adaptation to trauma. Self-regulation, stimulus discrimination, and characterlogical development. In B. A. van der Kolk, A. C. McFarlane, & L. Weisaeth (Eds.), *Traumatic stress: The effects of overwhelming experience on mind, body, and society* (pp. 182–213). New York: Guilford Press.

van der Kolk, B. A., Roth, S., Pelcovitz, D., Sunday, S., & Spinazzola, J. (2005). Disorder of extreme stress: The empirical foundation of a complex adaptation to trauma. *Journal of Traumatic Stress, 18*(5), 389–399.

van der Kolk, B., & Saporta, J. (1991). The biological response to psychic trauma: Mechanisms and treatment of intrusion and numbing. *Anxiety Research, 4,* 199–212.

Van Duijl, M., Cardena, E., & De Jong, J. T. (2005). The validity of DSM-IV dissociative disorders categories in south-west Uganda. *Transcultural Psychiatry, 42*(2) 219–241.

Weike, A. I., Hamm, A. O., Schupp, H. T., Runge, U., Schroeder, H. W. S., & Kessler, C. (2005). Fear conditioning following unilateral temporal lobectomy: Dissociation of conditioned startle potentiation and autonomic learning. *The Journal of Neurosceince, 25*(48), 11117–11124.

SUGGESTED READINGS

Anonymous. (1994). Living and working with MPD. *Journal of Psychosocial Nursing, 32*(8), 17–22.

Benishek, D., & Wichowski, H. C. (2003). Dissociation in adults with a diagnosis of substance abuse. *Nursing Times, 99*(20), 34–36.

Brimmer, J. (1998). Treating multiple personality patients. *Nursing Spectrum, 8*(7), 4.

Holden, M. A., Van Hassel, D. J., & Holden, M. S. (1997). Care of the dissociative identity disordered patient on a medical-surgical unit: Nursing implications. *Medsurg Nursing, 6*(1), 47–51.

Kaplow, J. B., Dodge, K. A., Amaya-Jackson, L., & Saxe, G. N. (2005). Pathways to PTSD, part II: Sexually abused children. *American Journal of Psychiatry, 162*(7), 1305–1310.

Pope, H. G., Barry, S., Bodkin, A., & Hudson, J. I. (2006). Tracking scientific interest in the dissociative disorders: A study of scientific publication output 1984–2003. *Psychotherapy and Psychosomatics, 75*(1), 19–24.

Riggs, S. R., & Bright, M. A. (1997). Dissociative identity disorder: A feminist approach to inpatient treatment using Jean Baker Miller's Relational Model. *Archives of Psychiatric Nursing, 11*(4), 218–224.

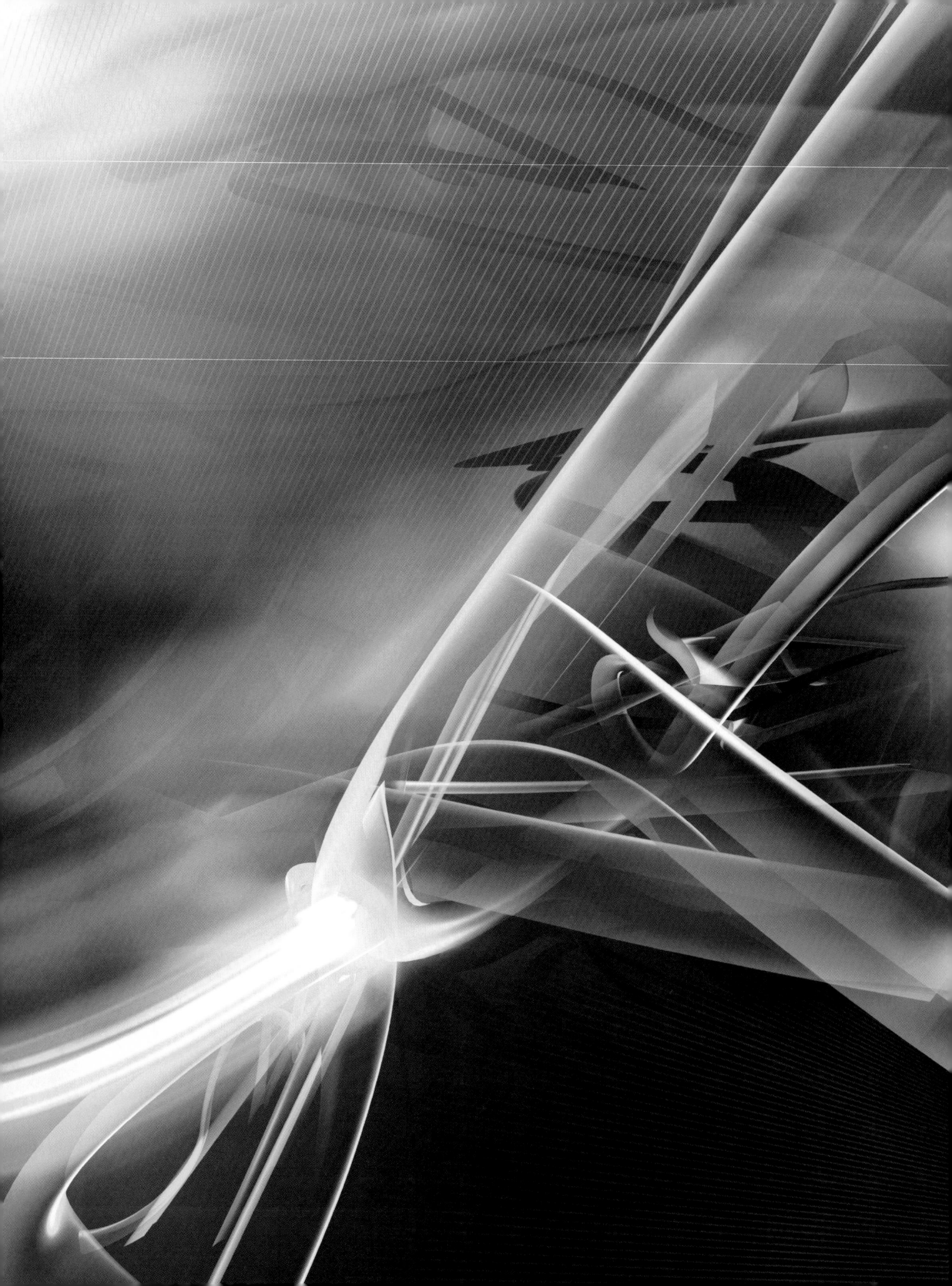

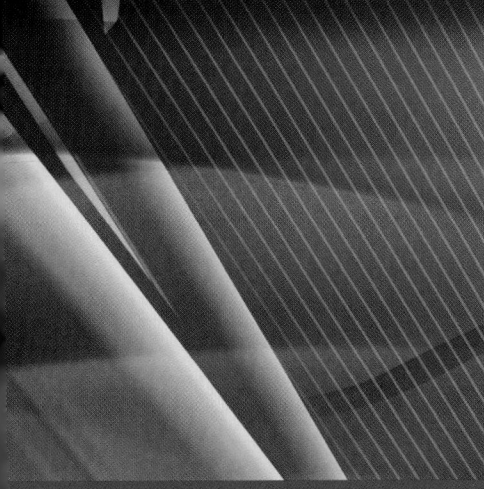

CHAPTER 19

The Client at Risk of Suicidal and Self-Destructive Behaviors

Deborah Antai-Otong, MS, APRN, BC, FAAN

KEY TERMS

Hopelessness: A state of despondency and absolute loss of hope.

Impulsivity: The act of spontaneous actions without thinking about consequences.

Lethality: Level of dangerousness or injury.

Psychological Autopsy: A standard procedure following a suicide that involves team members presenting and discussing the case with other staff with the intent of evaluating issues of quality of care and learning from the experience. It also offers an opportunity for staff to process their feelings and thoughts about the tragedy.

Self-Destructive: Behavior that has the potential to harm or destroy self.

Self-Mutilation: The act of self-induced pain or tissue destruction void of the intent to kill oneself.

Suicidal Ideation: A thought or idea of suicide.

Suicidal Intent: Refers to the degree to which the person intends to act on his suicidal ideations.

Suicidal Threat: Verbalization of imminent self-destructive action, which, if carried out, has a high probability of leading to death.

Suicide: The act of killing oneself.

COMPETENCIES

Upon completion of this chapter, the learner should be able to:

1. Discuss cultural factors that increase the risk of suicidal behavior.
2. Describe sociological theories of suicide.
3. Identify clients at risk across the life span.
4. Describe the various levels of suicidal lethality.
5. Develop a nursing care plan for the suicidal child and adolescent.
6. Differentiate self-mutilating and suicidal behaviors.
7. Analyze key aspects of the psychological autopsy.
8. Explain personal reactions to the suicidal client.

CHAPTER OUTLINE

Epidemiology

Definitions

Suicide

Self-Destructive and Self-Injurious Behaviors

Causative Factors

Psychodynamic Theories

Sociological Theories

Cultural Considerations

Neurobiological Theories

Psychosocial Factors

Harm associated with suicide is a major health care concern worldwide. The need for preventive measures that target high-risk groups is great. Because mental illness is a powerful risk factor for suicide, psychiatric nurses must play key roles in its prevention. Preventive measures must include recognizing risk factors across the life span cycle, understanding causative factors, assessing self-destructive behavioral patterns, and implementing a client-centered plan of care.

EPIDEMIOLOGY

The prevalence of suicide in the United States is approximately 12 per 100,000 persons annually. The frequency of suicide in the United States has remained constant since 1950 (Centers for Disease Control and Prevention [CDC], National Center for Injury Prevention and Control, 2004). Over 30,000 people per year commit suicide in the United States, making it a significant public health problem. Suicide is the eighth leading cause of death in this country and the third leading cause of death in 15- to 24-year-old persons (Anderson & Smith, 2003; CDC, 2004). The incidence rates among this age group have nearly tripled, from 4.5 percent in 1950 to 13 percent in 1992 (CDC, 2004; Indian Health Service, 1996). These data are conservative because not all suicides are recorded. A large percentage of clients who commit suicide have experienced profound psychological and emotional disturbances. Tragically, suicide also creates profound distress in surviving family and friends.

Variances in gender, age, race, and geographic areas prevail among those who commit suicide. Men commit suicide more often than women; however, women are more likely to attempt suicide than men. European American males commit suicide more frequently than African Americans. The peak age of suicide among African American men is 25 to 34 years, compared with that of European Americans, which is older than 65 years in the United States (Patel, Webb, & White, 2006). In addition, a disproportionate number of young Native American males between the ages of 15 and 24 accounted for about 64 percent of this group from 1979 to 1992 (Wallace, Calhoun, Powell, O'Neil, & James, 1996). Suicide rates tend to be above the national average in the western states and lower in the eastern and midwestern states (CDC, 1997).

Findings from a large population-based longitudinal study demonstrated that a preexisting anxiety disorder is an independent risk factor for suicidal ideation and attempt (Sareen et al., 2005). Psychiatric nurses and other mental health providers must use these data as a guide to assess coexisting anxiety and other psychiatric disorders in clients and initiate treatment that mitigates suicide in high-risk groups.

Suicide crosses all boundaries, affecting the rich and poor, people of all ages, and all socioeconomic and religious groups. Illnesses such as depression, bipolar disorder, alcoholism, personality disorders, and schizophrenia increase the risk of suicide (Dumais et al., 2005; Grunebaum et al., 2006; Sher, 2006; Shields, Hunsaker, & Hunsaker, 2007). Fifteen percent of clients with major depression eventually kill themselves. These data are based primarily on inpatient studies. Most outpatient studies indicate that the range of individuals who are depressed who eventually commit suicide is 2 to 10 percent (Dumais et al., 2005; Nierenberg, Gray, & Grandin, 2001). Concomitant conditions with mood and anxiety disorders also increase the risk of suicide across the lifespan. Other risk factors include male gender, previous attempts, accessibility to firearms, sexual orientation, psychotic disorders, European American ethnicity, genetic or familial influences, panic disorder, social isolation, and aging. Suicide and suicide attempts are highly concomitant with psychiatric disorders, including mood disorders, alcoholism, and schizophrenia (Baldessarini, Pompili, & Tondo, 2006; Dumais et al., 2005; Palmer, Pankratz, & Bostwick, 2005; Sher, 2006). Developmental and biological factors also place individuals at risk for suicide. See Table 19–1, Clinical Factors of High Suicide Risk.

The incidence of adolescent and older adult suicides are on the rise, presenting mental health professionals with challenges to develop innovative strategies to identify persons at risk. Advances in neuroscience have identified biological markers such as platelet serotonin receptors and a deficit in brain serotonin (5-HT) transmission in depressed clients, which place those clients at risk for suicide and other self-destructive behaviors (Samuelsson, Jokinen, Nordström, & Nordström 2006).

It is a common fallacy that people who threaten to kill themselves are not likely to commit suicide. The opposite is

Myths about Suicide

Myth: People who talk about suicide do not commit suicide.

Fact: The majority of people who kill themselves express thoughts of suicidal intention. All suicidal threats, behaviors, or gestures must be taken seriously.

Myth: Asking about suicide puts ideas into the client's head.

Fact: Asking the client about suicide is legally and ethically necessary. In fact, it is an integral part of the nursing process or evaluation of clients seeking psychiatric treatment and particularly those who are experiencing a crisis. This process enables the nurse to explore the client's thoughts, assess adaptive coping behaviors, and determine treatment planning.

Myth: Suicide usually happens without warning.

Fact: Most suicidal clients give cues of their intent. Nurses must be aware of these cues and intervene to prevent suicidal behavior.

Myth: Suicidal clients are likely to act on their thoughts when they are tired and have little energy.

Fact: Suicidal clients tend to act on their thoughts when their energy level increases, and it is during these times that nurses must assess the clients' level of danger to self and others.

TABLE 19–1
Clinical Factors of High Suicide Risk

Psychological

Hopelessness

Helplessness

Depression

Cognitive Impairment

Panic attacks, anxiety

Current suicidal ideations, intent, plan

Behavioral

History of suicide attempts

Poor impulse control

Alcoholism

Substance abuse

Sociocultural

Family history of suicide or attempts

Previous attempts

Recent significant loss

Poor support systems

Chaotic or disorganized family systems

Poverty status

Living alone

Psychosocial crisis

Neurobiological

Neurochemical dysregulation

Genetic

Hormonal imbalances (e.g., as detected by dexamethasone suppression and thyroid-stimulating hormone tests)

Major Demographic

Unmarried (separated, divorced, widowed)

Male older than 65 years of age

White (European American)

Protestant

Mental illness (e.g., depression, schizophrenia)

Bipolar disorder

Alcoholism or substance abuse

Medical Conditions

HIV, AIDS

Terminal and debilitating illnesses

Coronary Artery Disease

Chronic Obstructive Pulmonary Disease (COPD)

(continues)

TABLE 19–1
Clinical Factors of High Suicide Risk *(continued)*

Chronic pain

Certain neurological conditions, including brain tumors and multiple sclerosis

HIV, human immunodeficiency virus.

1. The child who states "I want to kill myself" (ideation)
2. The adolescent who says "I am going to hang myself" (threat)
3. The older person who says "I have a plan and a gun and want to kill myself" (intent and means)

Suicidal ideations or threats must always be taken seriously, especially when they are expressed by children. In fact, a child or adolescent who expresses suicidal ideations is just as serious as an adult who commits suicide.

true: an estimated 20 to 30 percent of clients who commit suicide have made previous threats or attempts to do so (Wingate, Joiner, Walker et al., 2004). The mistaken premise that suicidal threats or gestures are mere manipulative behaviors often generates negative reactions toward suicidal clients and impedes objective decision making. Increased awareness and knowledge about suicide are crucial to evaluating clients at risk for self-destructive behaviors such as suicide. There is no absolute predictor of suicide and it remains an enigma.

The focus of this chapter is to analyze salient biological and psychosocial concepts that increase the risk of suicide or other self-destructive behaviors. Psychiatric nurses play a crucial role in assessing, preventing, and evaluating self-destructive behaviors in clients using maladaptive coping patterns.

DEFINITIONS

The following section is a discussion of various concepts associated with suicide and self-destructive behaviors. Understanding these concepts enable psychiatric nurses to implement interventions that promote safety in clients exhibiting these behaviors.

SUICIDE

The term suicide stems from the Latin word *sui*, of oneself, and *cidus* from *caedre*, "to kill." Shneidman (1985) described suicide as "the conscious act of self-induced annihilation" (p. 203), and he emphasized the importance of psychosocial stressors and the inability to resolve intolerable pain by stopping "consciousness" (p. 203). Suicidal ideations are thoughts of injury or demise of self but not necessarily a plan, intent, or means. Suicidal intent refers to the degree to which the person intends to act on his suicidal ideations. Suicide intent is the most significant determinant of parasuicides or repeated attempts and eventual suicide. This is particularly true of single men with a psychiatric condition (Kumar, Mohan, Ranjith, & Chadrasekaran, 2006). A suicidal threat is verbalization of an imminent self-destructive action, which, if carried out, has a high probability of leading to death (Shneidman, 1985). The following is an example of these terms:

SELF-DESTRUCTIVE AND SELF-INJURIOUS BEHAVIORS

Roy (1985) classified self-destructive behaviors as direct or indirect. *Direct patterns of self-destruction* refer to those behaviors that directly affect the client's physical and mental well-being such as suicide, anorexia, alcohol and substance abuse, and self-mutilation. *Indirect patterns of self-destruction* include high-risk behaviors that may cause harm such as promiscuity, unsafe sexual practices, prostitution, abusive relationships, dangerous sports, and compulsive gambling.

Self-destructive behaviors occur on a continuum and present a challenge to psychiatric nurses. The most severe is suicide. These behaviors may appear as bizarre, distressful, and unexplainable. Other actions include other self-mutilation behaviors such as hair pulling, nail biting, burning, picking at wounds, and hacking or cutting. Winchel and Stanley (1992) defined self-mutilation behaviors as those that cause deliberate harm to one's body without the conscious intent of suicide. Injuries sustained by these behaviors frequently cause tissue damage, such as cutting (usually superficial) one's skin, especially the wrists and forearms. Self-injurious behaviors also include destruction of nails, cuticles, injurious masturbation, trichotillomania (hair pulling), head banging, or rocking. High-risk groups for self-mutilating are clients with mental retardation, those with pervasive developmental disorders such as autistim, those with psychosis, those who have a history of childhood abuse, or those with borderline personality disorders. Clients who self-mutilate are likely to be highly distressed and afraid, and they are distrustful of the nurse who wants to help.

Self-mutilation is frequently described as experiences of depersonalization or dissociative states. These acts of self-induced pain stimulate the opiate system in the brain, producing endorphins. Many clients state that they do not *feel* pain when they injure themselves (Bohus et al., 2000). (See the section on borderline personality disorder in Chapter 15, The Client with a Personality Disorder, and Chapter 18, The Client with a Dissociative Disorder, for more information about self-mutilation.)

Self-mutilating behaviors in adolescents is a growing public health concern. Researchers suggest that the increase in these behaviors parallel the prevalence of depression, hostility, and anxiety in American youth. Self-mutilation may be a coping behavior in adolescents who are using it to cope with despair, hopelessness, distress, low self-esteem, and intense emotional states. Principal means of self-injurious behaviors in this age group include using razors, scissors, knives or other sharp objects, or burning to mitigate intense anxiety, tension, and emotional distress. Coupled with trends in music and media that emphasize self-injurious behaviors and violence adolescents may lose sight of the seriousness of their behavior. Multimodal approaches that integrate antidepressant therapy, psychotherapy for the youth and family provide hope in the treatment of self-mutilation (Derouin & Bravender, 2004). (See Chapter 18, The Client with a Dissociative Disorder, for an in-depth discussion of self-mutilation when it occurs.)

CAUSATIVE FACTORS

Early perceptions of suicide still affect current beliefs, assumptions, and practices. Most mental health professionals do not consider suicide a rational act. The perception of suicide is generally based on religious, cultural, and social factors that have prevailed for centuries. Suicide is considered a taboo by many societies and religions, and it is frequently labeled a sin.

PSYCHODYNAMIC THEORIES

Early psychodynamic theorists described suicide as an escape from intolerable life stressors—an act of valor, insanity, and seductiveness. The act symbolized aggression directed at a loved one or society. Freud's (1961) classic psychoanalytical theory of suicide described suicidal clients as ambivalent, integrating concepts of love and hate in the decision to kill themselves. He surmised that guilt generated by self-destructive impulses toward object relations (early caregivers) motivated clients to suicide. Suicide was perceived as a kind of self-murder and accepted as internalized aggression.

Karl Menninger's (1938, 1947) contribution to the understanding of suicide was based on Freud's earlier concepts. He postulated that suicide is anger turned inward, and in his classic contributions, *Man against Himself* and *The Human Mind*, Menninger (1947) linked depression and suicide and described them as an "ever-present spectra" (p. 122). Depressed clients are always at risk for suicide. Moreover, he delineated three components of hostility in suicide:

1. The wish to kill
2. The wish to be killed
3. The wish to die

In other words, he perceived suicide as an integration of anger, malice, remorse, retaliation, and despair that were too great to be resolved realistically and that the act is a "flight from reality" or "submission to punishment." This premise proposes that suicide is a symptom of mental illness and the murder of self by self (Menninger, 1947).

SOCIOLOGICAL THEORIES

Emile Durkheim's (1951) classic work, *Suicide*, focused on the sociological aspects of suicide. His writings centered on deaths by suicide, and he analyzed patterns of death from health statistics. He contended that several sociological theories involving the integration and regulation of society contributed to suicide. He defined four types of suicides as follows:

1. *Egoistic suicide:* The person no longer finds acceptance or is insufficiently integrated into a social group and lacks close meaningful relationships (higher rates of suicides among single, socially isolated).
2. *Altruistic suicide:* The individual is too integrated into society, or the suicidal behavior is a response to cultural expectation (i.e., cult members may be willing to kill as group suicide or hara-kiri).
3. *Anomic suicide:* Society is insufficiently regulated; social instability (i.e., lack of norms or values).
4. *Fatalistic suicide:* Society is too regulated (i.e., group suicide regulated by rigidity and control or suicide pact).

CULTURAL CONSIDERATIONS

Cultural factors play pivotal roles in the prevalence of suicide across the life span. The plethora of research data that reflects this ominous societal trend offers the psychiatric nurse opportunities to identify high-risk factors, mobilize resources, and develop culturally appropriate interventions that nurture resilience and adaptation in high-risk groups.

Although culture often serves as a protection from suicide, research indicates children and adolescents share common risk factors across all cultures. In a community study of participants from a community population of African American children and adolescents, first recruited at age 6 and followed up over time through ages 19 to 20, the researchers found that depressed mood was the best predictor of adolescents and young adults who attempted suicide. Findings from the study indicated that African American children's self-reported depressed mood as early as the fourth grade may be invaluable in predicting suicide risk in later adolescence and young adulthood. Implications for the psychiatric nurse include early identification of suicide in this age group and making timely referrals for further evaluation and treatment to decrease suicide risk during adolescence and young adults.

Hendlin's notable 1987 study of youth suicide examined a broad spectrum of cultural and psychosocial aspects of suicide. The subjects of his study were youths from Scandinavian countries, Harlem, the white middle class, and colleges. He explored the relationship of completed suicides and social influences. His findings demonstrated that for the first 70 years in the twentieth century, the suicide rates among New York urban African Americans aged 15 to 30 were consistently higher than the rates among European American whites of the

In 2006, the United States and its territories and Canada hosted a Collaborative Agenda: Indigenous Suicide Prevention and Research and Programs conference. Attendees included service organizations, diverse tribes and villages, and government agencies. Major themes identified included the high incidence of suicide among youth.

◆ Suicide is the second leading cause of death for American Indian and Alaska Native youth, ages 14 to 24, and is 2.5 times higher than the national average.

◆ Suicide rates for aboriginal youth are 5 to 7 times that of non-aboriginal youth.

◆ Suicide rates for Inuit youth are among the highest in the world, at 11 times the national average in Canada (Langlois & Morrison, 2002). Suicide rates have been steadily on the rise in Micronesia and Guam, with suicide being the leading cause of death among young men in Micronesia.

◆ Suicide for Native Hawaiians ages 15 to 24 years old is about 5 times the national rate and over 7 times the national average rate for ages 25 to 44 years old.

Centers for Disease Control and Prevention, National Center for Injury Prevention and Control (Producer). (2004). *Web-based injury statistics query and reporting system* (WISQARS) [Online]. Available online at http://www.cdc.gov/ncipc/wisqars/default.htm. Langlois, S., & Morrison, P. (2002). Suicide deaths and suicide attempts. *Health reports, 13,* 9–22.

National Institute of Mental Health. (2006). *Indigenous suicide prevention research and programs in Canada and the United States: Setting a collaborative agenda.* Held in Albuquerque, NM, February 7–9, 2006. Summary available online at http://www.nimh.nih.gov/scientificmeetings/2006/indigenous-suicides.cfm

same age group. These findings were consistent with other metropolitan areas across the country (Castle, Duberstein et al., 2004). High suicide rates among African American youths were related to marked histories of childhood violence and rage. Overt cultural rejection among young African Americans often reinforced feelings of rage, worthlessness, and powerlessness, which their families cultivated, resulting in distorted self-images. Self-image—personal meaning of life and death—for youths is determined by cultural and subcultural social structures. (Hendlin, 1987). Contemporary studies indicate that African American adolescents who commit suicide are more likely to come from families with a higher socioeconomic status compared with those from the general population of African American youth. Researchers from this study also concluded that there has been a dramatic rise in the rate of suicides among African Americans since 1987 (Garlow, Purselle, & Heninger, 2005). Others surmised that educational and employment opportunities resulted in closer identification with European American whites, and loss of some protective African American traditional values contributed to this increase (Joe, Baser, Breeden, Neighbors, & Jackson, 2006; Oquendo et al., 2001).

Obviously, cultural norms affect the rate of suicide throughout the life span, and particularly among older adults. For instance, societies or cultures that value their older adults tend to foster integrity, positive self-regard, and importance. Subsequently, these societies regard older adults as role models for future generations for their wisdom and family contributions. In comparison, societies or cultures that devalue older adults and discount their importance are likely to engender feelings of alienation and hopelessness, impair their sense of integrity, and view suicide as a coping option. Of course, other factors contribute to suicide in older adults, such as significant losses.

Socioeconomic, ethnic, and cultural factors influence suicide rates. Some cultures seem to be relatively protected or buffered against suicidal behavior (Garlow, Purselle, & Heninger, 2005; Oquendo et al., 2005). While the precise cause for these differences among cultures and ethnicities is unknown, principal influences include:

◆ Negative perceptions of suicide

◆ Strong social support systems

◆ Networking generated by families who experience discrimination or extreme stress. Conversely, cultures that condone substance abuse, neglect, social isolation, and violence increase the risk of suicide (Gibbs, 1988).

◆ Strong religious beliefs

◆ Family cohesion

◆ Self identification with culture

Current studies indicate an alarming and growing rise in suicides among Native American and Alaska Native tribes. Suicide is a paramount concern of Native American tribes. Of all the ethnic groups and cultures in the United States, Native Americans and Alaska Natives have the highest suicide rates (Harrop, Brant, Ghalia, & Macathur, 2007; Langlois & Morrison, 2002). It is the second leading cause of death among Native American and Alaska Native youth ages 15 to 24. Suicide rates among this population have increased drastically over the past 10 years. For example, the rates of suicide among the Navajo reflect the national average, approximately 12 per 100,000. In contrast, the Apache tribes have suicide rates as high as 43 per 100,000 (Berlin, 1987). Suicide rates vary among tribes and are related to decreased ties with traditional Native American practices. Tribes that practice traditional rituals are usually more stable and promote a sense of belonging and support among members. In contrast, tribes in turmoil and those that do not support their members have higher rates of substance abuse, feelings of alienation, neglect, alcoholism, and emotional and physical abuse. These factors increase the risk of suicide among adolescents and young adults in Native Americans and other populations (CDC, 2004).

A study conducted by the University of Minnesota (Borowsky, Resnick, Ireland, & Blum, 1999) analyzed survey responses from one of the most comprehensive databases available on rural, reservation-based Native American and

Alaska Native youth. Moreover, data from this study reflected previous studies that indicate high-risk groups and appropriate culturally sensitive interventions. Researchers found that 22 percent of girls and 12 percent of boys surveyed reported previous suicide attempts. Previous suicides were the most correlate for youth suicide and indicated that for every 13 suicide attempts, 1 results in a completed suicide in the Native American population (May, 1987). Data from this study also indicated that additional risk factors among this population included having a friend or family member commit suicide and physical or somatic symptoms, such as headaches, stomach disturbances, a history of sexual or physical abuse, and alcohol or marijuana use. Being a male, gang member, and having a history of emotional problems also increased suicide attempts among Native American and Alaska Native youths. During 1989–1998, suicide rates among Native American and Alaskan children remained stable and were especially high in the Alaska, Aberdeen, and Tucson regions. In comparison, the rate has declined in New Mexico due partly to the Community Suicide-Prevention Center and Network with a community-based approach involving school-based youth, mental health professionals, and outreach to families (CDC, 2004). Interestingly enough, girls who had access to guns and had been in special education classes were at high risk for suicide. Protective factors identified by these data include being able to express feelings with friends and family members, having good emotional health, and having a sense of connectedness with family. (See The More You Know box.)

Findings from the CDC (2004) also demonstrate a growing trend among Hispanic females. This report indicates a 21 percent prevalence of suicide attempts in this population, whereas African American and non-Hispanic white females have rates of 10.8 percent and 10.4 percent, respectively (CDC, 2004). Several researchers of Hispanic females submit that this population is ethnically and racially diverse and includes Puerto Rican, Dominican Republic, Mexican, and Nicaraguan adolescents (Evans, Hawton, Rodham, & Deeks, 2005; Guiao & Thompson, 2004). Zayas, Lester, Cabassa, and Fortuna (2005) integrated salient factors that contributed to a pattern of sociocultural, familial, developmental, and psychological circumstances of suicide attempts. See Table 19–2, Cultural Factors Increasing the Risk of Suicide among Hispanic Females.

There are inconsistent research findings about the role of social and cultural influences on the prevalence of suicide or suicide attempts. Some of these studies have been criticized for biased sampling because they showed a significant number of suicides among the poor. However, recent studies indicate an alarming rate of suicides among diverse cultures, thus providing a stronger argument for the provision of culturally sensitive psychiatric nursing care.

NEUROBIOLOGICAL THEORIES

Recent advances in neuroscience and neurobiology suggest a relationship between suicide and altered neurological factors such as genetics, neuroendocrine, and neurochemical

TABLE 19–2
Cultural Factors Increasing the Risk of Suicide among Hispanic Females

Family domain	Low family unity
	Familial and marital chaos and discord
	Family violence
	Minimal parental empathy and support
	Traditionalism (patriarchal and male dominance)
	Absence of father
	Mother-daughter conflict
Developmental factors	Mother-daughter conflict
	Lack of self-validation
	Pressures to conform to traditionalism
	Parental adjustment to new culture
	Autonomy-separation issues
Sociocultural domain	Acculturation
	Rituals and traditions
	Generational gaps
	Hispanic cultural factors
Psychological domain	Depression
	Low self-esteem
	Lack of confidence
	Ineffective coping and problem-solving skills
	Difficulty coping with stressful events
	Inability or permission to express anger effectively

Note. Data from "Understanding Suicide Attempts by Adolescent Hispanic Females," by L. H. Zayas, C. Kaplan, S. Turner, K. Romano, and G. Gonzalez-Ramos, 2000, *Social Work, 45*, pp. 53–63.

functioning in the brain. For example, there may be an association between major depression and dysregulation of the hypothalamic-pituitary-adrenal axis. Studies have been done using dexamethasone suppression test (DST), which is performed to determine the body's response to additional steroid administration. In normal health, the dexamethasone would suppress adrenocortical production of cortisol; however, in major depression, the neuroendocrine challenge shows high production of urinary-free cortisol and nonsuppression of plasma cortisol. This has been found in suicidal clients, suggesting that cortisol secretion is poorly regulated by the hypothalamic-pituitary-adrenal process (Pfennig et al., 2005).

Perhaps, most significantly, the serotonergic system is believed to play a pivotal role in suicide risk, because serotonin modulates mood and modifies feelings of fearfulness, despondency, and depression (Vogt, 1982). Major depression is represented by a constellation of core *neurovegetative* behaviors such as altered mood, abnormal sleeping patterns, diminished libido, abnormal eating patterns, and impaired cognitive function. Abnormalities in the production and metabolism in serotonin and other neurotransmitters, such as dopamine and norepinephrine, directly affect these same behaviors (see Chapter 9, The Client with a Depressive Disorder). Abnormally low levels and activity of 5-hydroxyindoleacetic acid (5-HIAA, a major metabolite of serotonin) have been found in the spinal fluid of depressed suicidal clients (Boldrini, Underwood, Mann, & Arango, 2007; Mann & Currier, 2007), indicating low brain serotonin production. (See Figure 19–1.) Finally, because of substantial evidence linking low serotonergic activity to suicidal behavior, aggression, and alcoholism, perhaps low serotonergic activity underlies all three conditions and may mediate genetic, developmental effects of these behaviors (Boldrini, Underwood, Mann, & Arango, 2007; Mann & Currier, 2007).

Aggression and self-injurious behaviors also have been linked to decreased serotonergic levels in clients diagnosed with borderline personality disorder. Recent studies link aggression, impulsivity, and borderline personality with genetic and early life experiences such as physical and sexual abuse (Coccaro, 2006). High free testosterone levels in the cerebrospinal fluid are also associated with aggressive and thrill-seeking behaviors in violent alcoholic criminals. Some studies have found that high levels of testosterone and low levels of serotonin produce a synergistic process that enhance the risk of aggressive behaviors (Coccaro, 2006). Serotonin reuptake inhibitors have consequently been effective in the treatment of self-injurious behaviors, and depression suggests a biological component to these disorders. Self-injurious behaviors, such as nail-biting and hair-pulling symptoms, have been relieved by fluoxetine (Prozac) and clomipramine (van Minnen et al., 2003).

Genetic factors have also been linked to the prevalence of major depression and suicidal behavior. Twin and adoption studies suggest that genetic traits play a significant role in the cause of depression and vulnerability to maladaptive coping patterns (Brezo, Paris, & Turecki, 2006). Despite these findings, the exact role of genetic influences remains controversial. Other environmental factors such as psychosocial stressors, parent-child conflict, culture, and modeling contribute to depression and suicidal behaviors.

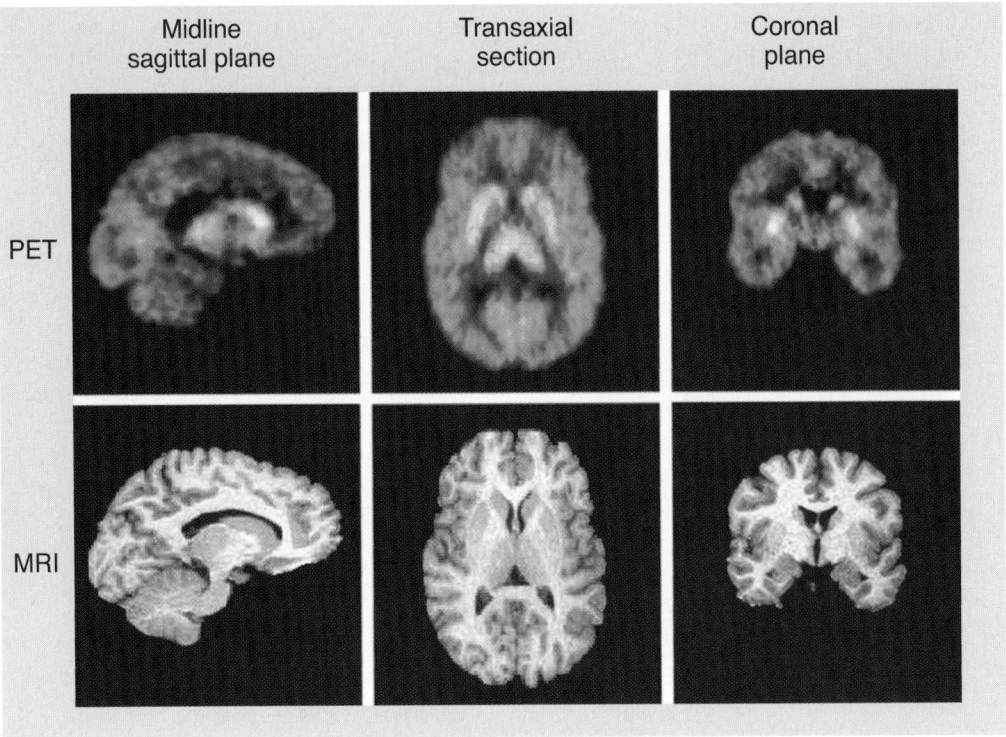

	Midline sagittal plane	Transaxial section	Coronal plane
PET			
MRI			

Figure 19–1 Alterations in brain serotonin circuitry in individuals with impulsive aggression. (*From Frankle, W. G., Lombardo, I., New, A. S., Goodman, M., Talbot, P. S., et al. [2005]. Brain serotonin transporter distribution in subjects with impulsive aggresssivity: A positron emission study with [¹¹C] McN 5652. American Journal of Psychiatry, 162, 915–923. Used with permission.*)

PSYCHOSOCIAL FACTORS

Suicide is a response to a crisis, and it is an effort to cope with intolerable psychosocial and neurobiological stressors generated by life experiences. Significant adverse life situations, such as financial and legal turmoil, bereavement, and intense relationship problems, also heighten the risk of suicide. Developmental crisis generates enormous stress for the person who is challenged to master the next life phase. People with close family ties are less likely to commit suicide than are those with distant ties. Meaningful interpersonal relationships can buffer people from experiencing stress as intolerable and decrease the deleterious effects of crisis.

The two developmental stages in which suicide peaks are adolescence and older adulthood. Social problems such as chaotic family systems, child-parent conflict, divorce, violence, access to firearms, or child abuse increase the likelihood of adolescent suicide. Furthermore, family conflict manifested by rejection, a lack of warmth, abuse, and ineffective communication patterns are common among adolescents who commit suicide (Renaud, Berlim, McGirr, Tousignant, & Turecki, 2007).

Older adult clients who suffer significant losses, such as personal and spousal health problems, social and emotional isolation, depression, impaired cognitive function, alcoholism, or financial security, experience enormous psychological and physical stress. The rise in the suicide rate of older European American white men ages 65 and older over the past two decades are well documented. In fact, this group has the highest rate of completed suicide in the United States (Conwell, Duberstein, & Caine, 2002). In an epidemiological study that examined trends in suicide by firearms among older white and black men over a 13-year period (1979–1991), researchers concluded that the highest risk were white men ages 75 and older and black men between the ages of 75 and 84 (Adamek & Kaplan, 1996).

Data from this study also revealed that firearm suicides increased substantially over time among white males in all three groups. Findings from the 1993 National Mortality Followback Survey conducted by Joe and colleagues (2007) are inconsistent with these findings. Analyses of data from the survey of variables associated with firearms used in suicides in men 15 and older, mental illness, and other variables demonstrated that African American men were twice more likely to use firearms in completed suicides than Caucasians (Joe, Marcus, & Kaplan, 2007). Despite inconsistency concerning the use of firearms and completed suicide, it is imperative for psychiatric nurses to perform a firearm assessment with all clients, regardless of age, who are depressed or suicidal.

Older adults also make fewer attempts per completed suicide and often report a history of seeing a health care provider shortly before their demise (CDC, 2004). Clinical implications from these data suggest that nurses must use proactive approaches to reduce the risk of suicide, which constitutes assessing every older adult for depression, suicide risk, quality of social systems, and firearm availability. Protective factors that reduce the incidence of suicide among older adults include having stable and close interpersonal relationships to help this age group cope more effectively.

STRESS FACTORS

Living can be thought of as a continuum of stress and adaptation. Perceptions of stress are influenced by the frequency of stressful life events and their severity, and the individual's ability to mobilize internal and external resources to handle them. Stress plays a major role in adaptation, and an inability to resolve stress results in crisis. Crisis often generates disorganization and feelings of helplessness and hopelessness. Reorganization and crisis resolution are determined by ego integrity or a function of the individual's ability to mobilize psychosocial and biological resources (Caplan, 1961). Suicide becomes a viable option in the face of poor ego function and a lack of resources to cope with stress (see Chapter 31, Crisis Intervention Management: The Role of Adaptation).

OTHER RISK FACTORS

Other risk factors associated with suicide are mood disorders, such as major depression and bipolar disorders, hopelessness, borderline personality disorder, schizophrenia, previous attempts, lack of psychosocial support, alcoholism and substance abuse or dependence, major health problems (psychiatric or physical), and a family history of suicide.

Recognizing the risk factors for suicide provides a basis for understanding nursing interventions and prevention. Predicting suicide remains a mystery, but certain behaviors and circumstances increase its risk. The nursing assessment is a vital part of identifying populations at risk for suicide. The client needs a comprehensive physical and psychosocial assessment to determine reasons for seeking treatment, level of dangerousness to self and others, present and past coping patterns, and the quality of current support systems.

CLINICAL EXAMPLE

The Client at Risk for Suicide

Mr. Jones is a 46-year-old man who recently had a massive heart attack. His business is failing and his wife of 20 years has decided that she does not want to be married to an "invalid." He has few social supports. He is referred to a mental health professional on a psychiatric consultation. His mood is sad and depressed and he is expressing feelings of hopelessness about his situation and thoughts of dying. He reports a poor appetite, concentration difficulties, loss of interest in things that were once pleasurable (anhedonia), and extreme fatigue since the heart attack.

What places Mr. Jones at risk for suicide? He is depressed and has feelings of hopelessness, a major physical health problem, an impending divorce, and he is preoccupied with dying.

Depression

Mood Disorders: Depression and Bipolar Disorders

Mood disorders have a significant impact on suicide risk and completed suicide. Persons with depression or bipolar disorder have a 3 to 12 times greater risk for suicide than other populations. Clients who commit suicide usually have major depression, but not all depressed clients commit suicide. Clients with depression often feel hopeless, worthless, inadequate, and guilty. These clients have already given up and feel they do not deserve happiness. Suicide may be an act of desperation for clients or a way out of immense psychological pain. Preoccupation with suicide reflects the client's perception that current conditions are hopeless.

Hopelessness

Hopelessness is a fundamental suicide predictor. People who feel hopeless are more likely to kill themselves because they believe that suicide is the only viable option to managing "insoluble problems" (Beck et al., 1990). Psychotic depression increases the risk of suicide. Symptoms of this disorder include delusions, excessive worrying, guilt, shame, and hallucinations.

Borderline Personality Disorder

Estimates of the lifetime risk of death by suicide among clients with borderline personality disorder range from 8 to 10 percent, which is similar to the prevalence among those diagnosed with major depression (Gunderson, 2001). A review of published studies by Duberstein and Conwell (1997) estimated that 30 to 40 percent of clients who commit suicide have an Axis II diagnosis, of which the most frequent was borderline personality disorder. Personality traits such as impulsivity may constitute a temperamental vulnerability to suicide especially in the presence of maladaptive coping behaviors arising from mood disorders, substance abuse, and anxiety disorders on Axis I. Additional risk factors include a history of childhood trauma, previous suicide attempts, concurrent psychiatric disorders, and affective instability.

Schizophrenia

An estimated 10 to 13 percent of clients with schizophrenia will commit suicide. These data parallel suicide in clients who experience depression and alcoholism. Young men recently diagnosed with schizophrenia have the highest suicide rates, especially during the first four years (Shields et al., 2007). In addition to being a young male, other risk factors in persons with schizophrenia include having multiple previous episodes or previous suicide attempts (Limosin, Loze, Philippe, Casadebaig, & Rouillon, 2007). Psychosis is often manifested by command auditory hallucinations, that is, voices telling the client to commit suicide. The nature of psychosis increases impulsivity or aggressive behaviors and impairs judgment and cognitive function. Impulsivity is the act of spontaneous actions without considering the consequences and, when coupled with other symptoms of schizophrenia, increase the likelihood of suicide.

Previous Attempts

A previous suicide attempt is often the best predictor of death by suicide (Suominen, Isometsä, Ostamo, & Lönnqvist, 2004). Suicide attempts usually occur 8 to 10 times more

---

RESEARCH ABSTRACT

Risk Factors for Suicide Completion in Borderline Personality Disorder: A Case-Control Study of Cluster B Comorbidity and Impulsive Aggression

McGirr, A., Paris, J., Lesage, A., Renaud, J., & Turecki, G. (2007). *Journal of Clinical Psychiatry, 68,* 721–729.

Study Problem/Purpose

Researchers employed a case-control design and investigated clinical and behavioral risk factors for suicide completion in borderline personality disorder.

Methods

Researchers used 120 subjects meeting *DSM-IV* criteria for borderline personality disorder and used structured diagnostic instruments and personality trait assessments to conduct proxy-based interviews of 50 controls and 70 who died by suicide between 2001 and 2005.

Findings

Persons with borderline personality disorder suicides had fewer psychiatric hospitalizations and suicide attempts than the controls with borderline personality disorder. Individuals with borderline personal-ity disorder suicides often met criteria for current and lifetime substance use disorders and concomitant Axis I diagnoses and Cluster B diagnoses. The lethality of borderline personality disorder suicide attempts increases with coexisting impulsivity and violent-aggressive features and cluster B comorbidity. Data from this study confirm the high risk of completed suicide with concomitant Axis I and Axis II disorders.

Implications for Psychiatric Nursing

Identifying risk factors associated with completed suicide and suicide attempts provides an infrastructure for psychiatric nurses to collaborate with clients, interdisciplinary mental health teams, and primary care providers to use a comprehensive assessment process to discern these conditions and implement a holistic plan of care to reduce suicide in clients with borderline personality disorder.

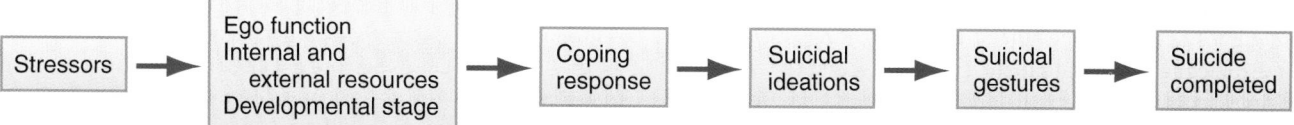

Stressors → Ego function / Internal and external resources / Developmental stage → Coping response → Suicidal ideations → Suicidal gestures → Suicide completed

Figure 19–2 Suicide continuum.

often than completed suicides. Most people who commit suicide have made previous attempts. The severity of suicide attempts is a continuum, and the severity of attempts evolves over time until they end with a completed suicide (Garland & Zigler, 1993). Figure 19–2 shows a suicide continuum.

Past suicide attempts must be explored along with reasons for their failure and whether the client was under the influence of alcohol or other intoxicants. This information is invaluable because it helps the nurse understand about the client's impulsivity, seriousness of intent, and coping behaviors. Nurses can explore the meaning of past suicide attempts by asking clients the following questions:

◆ How many suicide attempts have you made?

◆ How have you tried to kill yourself (actual behavior)? Did you want to die? When was the last time?

CRITICAL THINKING

You are working the evening shift on a medical unit and one of your clients states, "I just can't deal with this pain anymore. I wish I were dead!" Based on your understanding of this situation, what is the most appropriate response?

1. Do nothing because most people who kill themselves don't give a warning.

2. Ask, "What do you mean you wish you were dead?"

3. Go immediately to the charge nurse and report that he is going to kill himself.

4. Ask him about his religious beliefs.

Answers

1. *Incorrect.* This is a myth; most people who kill themselves do give verbal and nonverbal warnings, such as giving away cherished personal items.

2. *Correct.* It is imperative to further assess the client's statement to understand the meaning of his comments and distress.

3. *Incorrect.* Reporting his comments to the charge nurse or physician is important, but since there is no evidence of his imminent danger to self or others, it is imperative to evaluate his comments first and then act on them appropriately.

4. *Incorrect.* Asking religious questions reflects the nurse's personal beliefs and values and interferes with exploring the meaning of the client's experience.

◆ What are your feelings about the uncompleted attempt(s) (clues about the client's attitude regarding the attempt)?

◆ What were the circumstances of each (i.e., What types of stressors [changes] were you experiencing at the time?)?

◆ What happened before the attempt that made you believe killing yourself was an option?

◆ Did you plan the attempt or did you do it on the spur of the moment (impulsivity)?

◆ Were you drinking or abusing substances at the time or shortly before the attempt?

◆ What type of treatment did you receive after the attempt(s)?

Questions about past suicide attempts serve as the basis for developing nursing interventions to prevent or reduce the incidence of present or future suicides. Assessing the meaning of present and past coping patterns needs to include verbal and nonverbal cues. An example is the client who admits making attempts in the past and his facial expression or voice tone reflects remorse about the impact it has had on family members. Another client shows no affective response when discussing past attempts. The client who exhibits remorse or feelings is more likely to be concerned about the impact of future attempts that will affect the family's well-being. Conversely, the client who displays little affect or emotion is less likely to consider the effect of suicide on others. Each client provides information about coping patterns, substance abuse, and interpersonal relationships. Clients with histories of poor impulse control, such as those with personality disorders, psychosis, and alcoholism, are at risk for suicide.

Lack of Psychosocial Support

Psychological support is crucial to crisis resolution. Recently divorced, widowed, or socially isolated clients are at far greater risk for suicide than those who have strong family ties or interpersonal relationships. Support systems provide emotional renewal and validation of self-worth. Depressed clients may willfully distort their experiences and isolate themselves from loved ones to resolve their perception of being a burden or to be remorseful of their present illness.

Suicide generally occurs within chaotic and stressful environments or relationships (Oquendo et al., 2005). Suicidal threats and attempts are forms of communication with families and may represent expressing feelings of stress or despair that the client has difficulty verbalizing. Incidences such as the adolescent who overdoses after failing a class or the man who drives his car off a bridge the day his divorce is final are examples of communicating stress and feelings of helplessness. Clients who commit suicide often generate feelings of helplessness, negative reactions, and anxiety in the nurse. These feelings often stem from the belief that nurses are supposed to save lives, and when clients commit suicide, the inability to save them triggers anger and guilt.

General Considerations

Approaching the client in a calm, nonjudgmental manner is the basis of a therapeutic alliance. The primary intervention of working with the suicidal client is prevention. Effective communication is fundamental to helping the client understand his behavior. Assessing suicide risk involves recognizing risk factors and understanding the effect of psychosocial stressors on biological processes and cognitive functioning. Several considerations can assist in evaluating suicide risk. They include:

◆ Determining whether the client has a suicidal plan. The client may express thoughts of dying, such as "I want to kill myself" or "I wish I could go to sleep and not wake up." Most clients who have killed themselves have planned their demise. Suicidal plans need to be taken seriously because they indicate that thorough planning and working through have already taken place. A suicide note suggests that the client is resolved to kill himself, and the ambivalence of wanting to live or die has been worked through. Assessing for suicidal plans includes asking "Are you having thoughts of killing yourself?" There is a myth that asking clients about suicide "plants" ideas. Contrary to this belief, clients often welcome the opportunity to discuss their feelings about suicide. Nurses need to make sure that they are speaking the same language as the client, because he may not know what the word *suicide* means. An example is the client who is asked, "Are you having thoughts of hurting yourself?" He may respond "no," but actually, he is not having thoughts of hurting himself, but killing himself. Consequently, the client should be asked if he is having thoughts of killing himself.

◆ Determining the dangerousness of the suicide attempt. It is essential to assess the level of lethality. The term lethality refers to the potential degree of injury caused by suicidal gestures or attempts. Direct questions need to be asked about the suicide to assess the suicidal potential. Degrees of lethality range from high risk (e.g., shooting, hanging, stabbing, or using carbon monoxide) to lower risk (e.g., overdosing on 5 acetaminophen [regular-strength] tablets). The client's perception of the incident determines the seriousness of the attempt, except in cases when the attempt is minimized.

When the client is assessed to have a definite suicidal plan, the next question involves assessing lethality. Shneidman (1985) defined lethality as the probability of the person killing self in the immediate future. He ranked lethality into four levels: (1) high; (2) medium; (3) low; and (4) absent. The second concern is providing safety and preventing suicide. This is generally done by offering the client referral for evaluation for acute inpatient psychiatric or other means of treatment, such as the crisis mobile team or day hospital, to provide crisis intervention and further evaluation of suicidality and the treatment of underlying mental illness.

Preoccupation with suicide or dying is a symptom of distress and ineffective coping reactions. Suicidal thoughts and plans must be thoroughly assessed to determine their duration and how they have been responded to in the past. It is also important to assess the client's reasons for not acting on the thoughts. An acute suicidal ideation is more likely to generate greater concern than chronic ideations or threats. This does not mean that chronic suicidal thoughts are less serious than acute ones. The client who admits having thoughts of dying for 10 years and has not acted on it for whatever reason is indicating some degree of impulse control. This information needs to be documented, and the client needs to be assessed for level of dangerousness to self and others at the present time. The client also needs to be asked about specific circumstances that would make him act on the thoughts.

Most suicidal clients tend to be ambivalent about dying. That is, a part of them usually wants to die and another part wants to live. The part that wants to live usually communicates despair and pain though verbal and nonverbal cues. These cues must be taken seriously and their meaning must be thoroughly assessed. The client who has a specific plan, means, and intent is at serious risk for suicide. Questions such as, "What has stopped you from acting on these thoughts or plans in the past?" elicit information about the imminence of suicide. Some clients may respond with "I don't want to hurt my family" or "I know this is a silly idea." Inquiring about ways they have handled similar thoughts is useful in assessing impulse control and coping patterns.

Alcoholism and Substance Abuse or Dependence

The risk of suicide increases when alcohol or substance misuse occurs during a crisis, stressful life events, or major losses, and it is likely to occur within 6 weeks of these events. Major losses account for about a third of suicides among alcoholic clients. Intoxication impairs cognitive function and lowers inhibitions that impair cognitive ability, judgment, reasoning, decision making, and reality testing. People who are actively drinking are particularly vulnerable to suicide when they have concomitant depression or bipolar disorder and have experienced a recent loss. Chronic alcoholism tends to impair meaningful interpersonal relationships and increase isolation and alienation from support systems. Contemporary studies add neurobiological factors as additional risk factors to alcoholism and suicide. Researchers implicate 5-HT dysregulation in alcoholism and this population. Low levels of 5-HT and its metabolite 5-HIAA have been found in the blood and cerebrospinal fluid of alcohol-dependent people who attempted suicide (Sher, 2006).

Moreover, the prevalence of alcoholism among clients with schizophrenia increases the risk of suicide. Besides, alcoholism accounts for 15 percent of suicides (Sher, 2006). A noteworthy observation is the growing trend of a dramatic increase in the number of adolescents who kill themselves under the influence of alcohol and drugs. Adolescents using violent means tend to kill themselves when intoxicated. Nursing implications from these findings indicate the need to assess the clients' present and past substance abuse history, particularly when comorbid psychiatric and physical conditions exist.

Major Health Problems

Major health problems have the propensity to generate feelings of hopelessness, helplessness, and despair. These factors interfere with the clients' internal and external sense of control, and subsequent depression results. Chronic illnesses such as renal failure, chronic pain, chronic lung disease, HIV/AIDS, and terminal and debilitating illnesses interfere with the clients' livelihood and quality of life. Clients with chronic and debilitating illnesses need to be assessed for depression and suicide potential (see Chapter 34, Psychosocial Care in Medical-Surgical Settings).

SUICIDE RISK ACROSS THE LIFE SPAN

Suicide crosses all boundaries of the life span. Understanding coping patterns throughout the life span helps the nurse recognize the significance of prevention and health promotion.

Table 19–3 summarizes the prevalence and causative factors of suicide across the life span.

CHILDHOOD

Children and adolescent suicide has perplexed poets, composers, artists, and authors for years (e.g., Shakespeare's *Romeo and Juliet*). Early descriptions of suicidal children were noted in several nineteenth century foreign journals. The authors postulated that the risk of suicide increased with age and that suicide was more likely to occur in urban than rural communities. Other commonalties among suicidal children included: the death of a significant family member, parent-child strife, and the school's role in discipline. Freud (1961) asserted that parent-child turmoil and incest influenced childhood suicides.

Family factors have generally played a major role in childhood suicide. Accordingly, two of the most salient characteristics of suicidal children are parental behavior and depression. Modeling suicidal behavior from parents increases the risk for suicide. Family discord is also a risk factor for childhood suicide (Enns et al., 2006). Children and adolescents who commit suicide typically live in homes of family chaos owing to substance misuse with fears of abandonment and inconsistent discipline styles.

TABLE 19–3
Prevalence and Causative Factors of Suicide across the Life Span

	Prevalence	Causative Factors
Childhood	Unknown (some accidents may be suicide); predicted to increase 13% for ages 10–14 years by 2000	Affective disorder (depression), family and developmental factors Death of parent
Adolescence	6–13% have attempted suicide	Affective disorders, conduct and antisocial disorders, substance abuse, family disorganization, social withdrawal, hopelessness, sexual abuse
Early and Middle Adulthood	15% of those with major depression commit suicide; 15% of those with schizophrenia commit suicide; 80% of those who commit suicide have made previous attempts; 15% of alcoholics commit suicide	Depression, schizophrenia, previous attempts, lack of psychosocial resources, alcoholism and substance abuse, major psychiatric and physical health problems
Older Adulthood	17% have attempted suicide	Loss, feelings of isolation, poor physical health status
Total Population	12% have attempted suicide	Mental illness, alcoholism

Note. Center for Disease Control & Prevention, (2004).

Negative parent-child relationships generate low self-esteem, which arises from anger and rejection. Low self-esteem has been observed in abused, depressed, and suicidal children. These children tend to blame themselves and feel responsible for family problems (Barbe, Williamson, Bridge, Birmaher, Dahl et al., 2005; Shneidman, 1975).

Major predictors of childhood emotional distress and suicide (Shaffii, Carrigan, Whittinghill, & Derrick, 1985) include:

◆ Affective disorder (depression or bipolar disorder)
◆ Family factors (chaos, abuse, divorce, or death; lack of nurturing and empathy)
◆ Developmental factors, including early major losses
◆ Hopelessness
◆ Aggression
◆ Death of a parent

Researchers consistently submit that the most notable psychosocial risk factors for child and adolescent suicide include school problems, a family history of suicidal behavior, poor parent-child communication, and stressful life events (Enns et al., 2006). Children as young as 2 or 3 years of age have been found to have suicidal behaviors, such as attempting to jump from high places, verbalizing wishes to kill oneself, and attempting to hang oneself or ingest poison (CDC, 2004).

Suicidal behavior is the most common psychiatric emergency in children and adolescents. It is the third leading cause of death in this age group. Demographic findings show that girls contemplate suicide three times as often as boys, but boys kill themselves four times more frequently than girls (CDC, 2004).

Suicidal ideation is far more serious when expressed by children than when expressed by adults because of children's immature ego and cognitive development. Ego function is affected by relationships with primary caregivers, previous life experiences, present stressors, and affect modulation. Immature ego function interferes with the capacity to cope with stress, modulate feelings, feel good about oneself and relate to others. Depression affects cognitive function and interferes with the way the child thinks of himself and situations. Depression has been positively correlated with suicide as a major risk factor (Ialongo, Koenig-McNaught, Wagner, Pearson et al., 2004; Pfeffer, 2002). When adaptive mechanisms fail to allay the child's emotional pain and distress, the risk of acting on suicidal ideations heightens. Children have a distorted and inadequate sense of time and death. Their limited capacity for abstract thinking interferes with believing the finality and absoluteness of death. The concept of death is beyond their comprehension (Pfeffer, 1986).

Furthermore, children do not command a realistic comprehension of death to suicide. Similarly, they have a difficult time expressing emotional pain and problems, and suicide is often perceived as the solution to immense distress.

Although some children report feelings of sadness and hopelessness, others have difficulty verbalizing thoughts, feelings, and ideas, and they may act on them. Unlike their adult counterparts who have a depressed or sad mood, depressed children are more likely to have an irritable or agitated mood (APA, 2000). Children are capable of planning and carrying out suicide, and their behavior provides invaluable cues about their intent. Predominant behaviors among suicidal children include aggression, preoccupation with death, social isolation, depression, and antisocial symptoms (Pfeffer, 2002; Shaffer & Pfeffer, 2001). Pfeffer (1986) also identifies three common behaviors of a suicidal child. First, the play, activities, and interests are inappropriate for the child's developmental stage. Second, the child's play is repetitive, dangerous, and reckless, usually involving use of his body as a play object. Finally, a suicidal child's play involves acting out fantasies of death or aggression. Nurses are challenged to determine if these behaviors are suicidal because they are also seen in children who are not suicidal. In today's world of technological advances and exposure to violence on the internet, iPods, television, and other media, children are likely to mimic what they watch, including violent or aggressive behavior (Brady & Matthews, 2006).

Many childhood accidents may have been suicides. Pfeffer (1986) asserted two reasons that children do commit suicide accidentally: (1) they misjudge the impact of the suicide act (e.g., placement of gun or the number of pills); and (2) they miscalculate the time for others to save them. They often use deadly methods such as shooting, hanging, and ingesting poisons. It is difficult to determine if a child's death is accidental or intentional because of social embarrassment, remorse, and cultural and socioeconomic reasons (Pfeffer, 1986).

The Nursing Process

Children exhibiting suicidal behaviors are experiencing serious distress and emotional pain. Early detection and prevention of childhood suicide are crucial to helping depressed or mentally disturbed children and families. The following case study provides a useful framework in which to examine the nursing process.

Assessment

Childhood suicidal behaviors often represent a family problem. Ideally, assessing the children should take place in an emotionally and physically safe environment. For older children, a quiet room is adequate. Younger children require a room with ample space for toys and art materials. Assessing the child's role within the family context is important to evaluating the meaning of suicidal behavior (Antai-Otong, 2004). Children's understanding about death is crucial in determining the lethality of any ideation. Asking about previous experiences with death, such as the death of a pet or family member, provides some understanding about the child's grasp of death. When children are preoccupied with death and exhibit little fear or dislike of death, their risk of suicide is high (Barbe et al., 2005; CDC, 2004). Factors such as motivation and current stressors play key roles in the children's

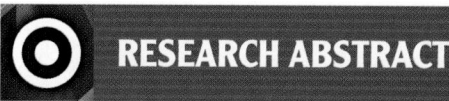

RESEARCH ABSTRACT

Current Psychiatric Morbidity, Aggression/Impulsivity, and Personality Dimensions in Child and Adolescent Suicide: A Case-Control Study

Renaud, J., Berlim, M.T., McGirr, A., Tousignant, M., & Turecki, G. (2007). *Journal of Affective Disorders.* [Epub ahead of print]

Study Problem/Purpose

The researchers sought to evaluate psychiatric risk factors for child and adolescent suicide and discern the association between impulsivity and aggression and additional personality traits and completed suicides in these subjects.

Methods

Researchers used psychiatric diagnoses, impulsive-aggressive and other personality traits, and employed semistructured proxy-based interviews; and questionnaires were assessed in 55 children and adolescents who committed suicide and 55 community controls.

Findings

The major psychiatric risk factors linked to child and adolescent suicides were depressive disorders, substance/alcohol abuse disorder, and dis-ruptive disorders. Moreover, youths who killed themselves demonstrated higher scores on lifetime aggression/impulsivity and harm avoidance. However, after logistic regression, the sole independent striking predictors of suicide in this age group were the incidences of depressive disorders.

Implications for Psychiatric Nursing

Whilst the sample size was relatively small and researchers used a cross-sectional design, researchers confirm depression, substance-use disorders, and disruptive disorders as risk factors for individuals across the life span, including children and adolescents. It is imperative for psychiatric nurses to understand risk factors associated with suicide, identify persons at risk and implement nursing intervention to treat various psychiatric disorders, and mitigate the risk of suicide in all age groups.

CASE STUDY

Ms. M is a 34-year-old client who was recently admitted to the ER with renal complications associated with lupus. She is alert and oriented, but appears fatigued.

NURSE: Good evening Ms. M. My name is Linda and I am your nurse. What's brought you in today?

CLIENT: My husband wanted me to come to the hospital because I am having kidney problems.

NURSE: Kidney problems?

CLIENT: Yes. I may have to go on dialysis. I would rather die than be put on dialysis.

NURSE: What do you mean you would rather die than be put on dialysis?

CLIENT: My mother died after they put her on one of those machines.

NURSE: I understand your concerns and am sorry to hear about your mother, but how long ago did she die?

CLIENT: She died 20 years ago when I was very young.

NURSE: I understand your concerns about dialysis, but many advances have occurred since your mother died. Besides, we really don't know if you need to be dialyzed yet.

CLIENT: I know, but it seems like the past year has been so hard because of chronic pain and now my kidneys.

NURSE: Have you had these feelings or thoughts in the past?

CLIENT: Yes.

NURSE: How did you resolve them?

CLIENT: I thought about my children and my husband. I would never hurt myself or anyone else.

NURSE: I am glad to hear this. It sounds like lots of folks love you.

CLIENT: I know. They do. I guess everyone has days when life seems so hard.

NURSE: You are right.

CLIENT: Thanks for listening.

NURSE: I believe your husband is asking to see you. I will get him and check on you later. Please let me know if you need to talk again.

(continues)

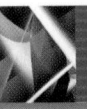
In this case study the nurse used empathy and open-ended questions to evaluate the client's reasons for not acting on her suicidal ideations. Through patience and genuine concern she underscored the client's importance to her loved one and reasons to live. Clients with suicidal ideations tend to feel hopeless and often alone. The nurse was able to help the client focus on the positive aspects of her life rather than the negative. Negative thinking and feelings often co-exist with depression. Strategies to move to positive thinking are important nursing interventions when working with the client at risk for suicide.

ability to cope. Motivations of childhood suicidal threats include manipulation, revenge, escape from distress, desire to join a dead friend, or response to auditory hallucinations. Table 19–4 presents guidelines for assessing the suicidal child.

In the case study, Lillie was depressed about the death of her friend. Additionally, her mother reported a recent separation from Lillie's father and a current custody dispute. Shortly after her father moved out of the home, Lillie's grades began to drop, her appetite decreased, and she spent more time with her best friend until her death. The nurse interviewed the child and mother separately and together to assess the parent-child interaction. It is crucial to assess the child in this manner because the nurse can obtain data that the parent may not be aware of, including sleep disturbances, irritable or sad mood, and suicidal ideations. Questions that often elicit information about the child's suicide potential include "Do things ever get so bad that you think about hurting yourself?" or "Have you ever wished or tried to kill yourself?" (Pfeffer, 1986, p. 178). Pfeffer (1986) also advocates that a

child with suicidal ideations must be asked about the specific method, plan for the attempt, and absence of barriers. The parent-nurse interview enables the nurse to gather salient data such as home and academic performance. It also affords the nurse an opportunity to assess the parent's mental status, the ability to provide safety for the child, and the response to the child's suicidal ideations (i.e., empathy and concern). In this case study, the major family stressors identified involved several losses, mainly the death of a close friend and Lillie's father moving away from home, and, consequently, the family disorganization generated by an impending divorce. Other fears included losing her parents.

Pfeffer (1986) asserted that suicidal children often have fantasies and wishes to be cared for by kind and devoted people, and these fantasies can be fulfilled during the initial family-child assessment. The child becomes the center of attention, acquires a sense of hopefulness, and renews the wish to live and work out problems rather than to commit suicide.

Nursing Diagnoses

- ◆ High Risk for Self-Directed Violence
- ◆ Ineffective Coping
- ◆ Bereavement

Planning

Nursing Care Plan 19–1 identifies the desired outcomes for the nursing diagnoses listed earlier and delineates the nursing actions necessary to achieve these outcomes, along with the rationales for these actions.

TABLE 19–4
Assessing the Suicidal Child: Major Concepts

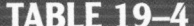

Understand developmental factors and suicidal behaviors in children

Examine feelings regarding death and suicide

Explore meaning of ideations, thoughts, and attempts

Assess imminence of suicide risk (lethality)

Obtain "no suicide" contract from the child

Actively involve the family

Encourage the child to talk about suicidal feelings and thoughts

---

Note. From "Basic Principles of Assessing Childhood Suicidal Risk." In *The Suicidal Child* (p. 178), by C. R. Pfeffer, 1986, New York: Guilford Press.

CASE STUDY

The Child at Risk for Suicide (Lillie)

Lillie is a 10-year-old girl who was brought to the emergency department by her mother, who reported that she expressed feelings of wanting to die and join her best friend. Lillie has become increasingly despondent over the past 2 weeks since the death of her best friend, who died from complications of cystic fibrosis.

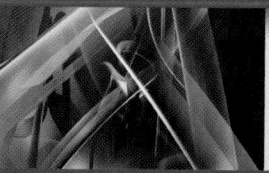

The Child at Risk for Suicide (Lillie)

Nursing Diagnosis: Risk for Self-Directed Violence

Outcome Identification	Nursing Actions	Rationales	Evaluation
1. By [date], Lillie will verbalize the absence of suicidal ideations or plans.	1a. Assess the level of danger.	1a. All suicidal threats, plans, or ideations must be explored to determine if the child is at risk of harming or killing herself.	*Goal met:* Lillie • denies suicidal ideations. • does not harm self. • is able to identify options. • shows gradual mood changes. • is able to express superficial feelings.
	1b. Provide a safe environment. Remove potential or actual dangerous objects from the environment.	1b. A safe environment provides structure and the controls needed to reduce impulses to harm or kill oneself.	
	1c. Establish an agreement with the child to inform the staff/nurse of suicidal ideations or aggressive behavior.	1c. This agreement provides an agreement and understanding between the child and the nurse and stresses the seriousness of the child's suicidal ideations.	
2. By [date], client will discuss options to deal with present stressors.	2a. Encourage examination of available options to cope with present stressors.	2a. Exploring options and resources enhances coping skills.	
	2b. Observe for sudden changes in mood.	2b. Sudden mood changes, especially decreased depression, may signal the increased energy needed to act on suicidal ideations or plans.	
	2c. Encourage expression of feelings.	2c. Expression of feelings decreases internalization of emotional distress and mechanism to process meaning of present stressors/crisis.	
	2d. Encourage participation in therapeutic grief group activities with peers.	2d. Enhances social interactions and facilitates the grief process.	
	2e. Teach the child to identify symptoms of sadness, preoccupation with death, and suicide.	2e. Encourages expression and understanding of feelings.	

(continues)

Nursing Care Plan 19–1 (continued)

Nursing Diagnosis: Ineffective Coping

Outcome Identification	Nursing Actions	Rationales	Evaluation
1. By [date], Lillie will develop an awareness of the meaning of present behaviors.	1a. Facilitate an understanding of Lillie's present behaviors.	1a. Understanding the meaning of maladaptive behaviors enhances adaptive coping responses and provides an opportunity for growth and mobilization of adaptive coping behaviors.	*Goal met:* Lillie • returns to previous level of functioning. • develops adequate coping skills. • displays less anxiety. • resolves grief effectively.
	1b. Assist in problem solving.	1b. Crisis situations often overtax coping and problem-solving skills. This action affords an opportunity to enhance coping and problem solving.	
	1c. Confront maladaptive behaviors.	1c. Confronting maladaptive behaviors allows the client to understand the meaning of them and develop adaptive coping responses.	
2. By [date], Lillie's family will understand and use available community resources.	2. Provide the family with information about local resource groups for suicide prevention.	2. Group participation can provide an environment that enables the client to express feelings and thoughts.	

Families should never be blamed for the client's suicidal behavior. Nurses need to provide emotional support to families coping with crisis, and form therapeutic relationships to protect the child. Crisis intervention is a useful strategy to teach parents and the child to identify and enhance their strengths, teach effective coping skills, reinforce family cohesiveness, and increase the family's ability to handle stress (Langley & Kaplan, 1968). Each situation must be assessed to determine interventions that ensure the child's safety and effective resolution of crisis situations.

Implementation

Major nursing interventions include:

◆ Establishing rapport with the child and parents

◆ Ensuring the child's safety

◆ Assessing the parent's mental status and response to the child's behavior

◆ Assessing the parent-child relationship

◆ Assessing the family system

◆ Informing the family about legal rights regarding treatment

Crisis intervention with the child and parent helps reestablish effective communication and expression of feelings and thoughts of the family crisis. It also helps the nurse identify family stressors, strengths, resources, and vulnerability. Involving the family in the initial assessment infers the seriousness of the situation and understanding that the child's behavior reveals family problems. Additionally, the nurse is able to assess the family's understanding and willingness to make rapid changes to ensure the child's safety.

Encouraging the child to talk about suicidal behavior during the initial assessment emphasizes the significance of this behavior. Verbalization of feelings may be difficult for some children, and other means of communication, such as play or art therapy, can be useful in assessing the child's behavior.

Evaluation

In the case study, Lillie stated that she wanted to live and that she would not kill herself. Her mother was genuinely concerned and reassured her that she would not leave her and that she loved and wanted her. They were given bi-weekly parent-child (family therapy) follow-up appointments and Lillie was discharged from the emergency department. Her mother was encouraged to observe the child for behavioral changes that suggested despondency, worsening irritability, suicidal ideations, and social isolation. She was also given a list of community referrals, including the emergency department, assessment, and treatment resources for children, and she was instructed to call the nurse or family therapist or community 24-hour hotline in case of emergency. The child agreed to report any recurrent suicidal ideations to her mother or other family members or school nurse. Refer to Nursing Care Plan 19–1.

ADOLESCENCE

There is growing concern about the increased suicidal rates in adolescents. The suicide rate in this age group increased more than 200 percent, compared to an increase of 17 percent in the general population from 1968 to 1991. The greatest risk for suicide among youths is among young white males; yet the most rapid increase the past decade has been among American Indians and Alaskan Natives (Bernard, Paulozzi, & Wallace, 2007; Harrop et al., 2007). Recent studies also indicate that suicide continues to occur less often among black youths compared with white youths (Bernard et al., 2007). Adolescent males tend to use more violent means (e.g., shooting, hanging) than females. Most adolescents who attempt suicide do not seek or receive psychiatric treatment. Suicidal ideations are prevalent among adolescents, but only 10 percent have specific plans (CDC, 2004).

Risk Factors

Adolescence is a time of intense emotional and biological changes. Puberty increases vulnerability to stress and impaired self-concept as youths search for identity within society. The turbulent adolescence also contributes to ineffective coping patterns, low self-esteem, inadequate support systems, and increase the risk of maladaptive responses to stress. Suicidal behavior is a symptom of maladaptive or ineffective coping. Adolescent suicidal behavior in any form such as ideation, threat, gesture, or attempt increases the risk of lethality (Enns et al., 2006). As with adults, most studies indicate that the most robust predictor of suicide in adolescents is a prior attempt.

Accordingly, youth suicidal behavior may be associated with other precipitants similar to childhood factors such as mental illness (in the youths and family members), positive family history of suicide, previous attempts, ineffective coping skills, family disorganization, and substance abuse. Most adolescents who commit suicide have at least one mental disorder. Major mental illnesses include affective (mood) disorder, aggression, attention-deficit disorder or attention-deficit hyperactive disorder, sexual identity issues, impulsive behavior, anxiety disorder, conduct or antisocial disorders, and substance abuse. They tend to perform poorly academically and experience family conflict and legal problems (Reinhertz,

Tanner, Berger, Beardslee, & Fitzmaurice, 2006; Rohde, Lewinsohn, Klein, & Seeley, 2005).

Depressed adolescents, like depressed adults, usually experience impaired cognitive function and coping skills. They also tend to view themselves and the world as negative or hopeless. Ineffective interpersonal and problem-solving skills further compromise their ability to express emotional pain and worries and problem-solve effectively.

Gibbs (1988) stressed the significance of sociocultural factors in assessing depression in adolescents. She noted that African American youths from lower socioeconomic families are more likely to communicate depression and suicidal feelings with verbal abuse, hostility, and acting out in school and with their peers and society. Furthermore, Gibbs associated these experiences with underlying feelings of isolation, pessimism, and discouragement generated by enormous life stressors.

Family disorganization also increases the risk of mental illness and suicide in adolescents. Numerous studies support the notion that family competence affects coping behaviors in its members. Mental illness and substance abuse affect the parent's ability to provide stable nurturing environments. Changing times, a mobile society, and a lack of extended families increase stress in the youth (Gould et al., 2003). Mobilizing family resources and strengths buffers the adolescents' coping skills.

Healthy or functional families provide immediate emotional and physical support for the youth during a turbulent period of rapid biological, emotional, and behavioral changes. They also recognize behaviors in the youth that suggest distress and ineffective coping responses. Healthy families also tend to seek assistance from professionals and community resources when they exhaust their own coping and problem-solving skills. In contrast, dysfunctional families lack the capacity to mobilize adaptive coping skills and support the adolescent during stressful periods. A lack of support coupled with inadequate structure and limit setting increases stress in the adolescent. Poor child-parent interactions heighten the risk of maladaptive behaviors, such as substance abuse and suicidal and other self-destructive acts, to soothe emotional turmoil and pain.

Additionally, peer groups are significant to adolescents. They serve functions similar to families, providing a sense of belonging, validation, acceptance, and camaraderie. Interpersonal communication and sharing serve as psychological buffers and enable youths to effectively cope with crisis situations. Because peer groups provide adolescents with a sense of validation and acceptance, rejection or alienation from one's peers increases the risk of maladaptive coping responses such as suicidal behaviors. A risk factor that contributes to adolescent isolation and alienation from peers is homosexuality. Unfortunately, nurses often overlook or ignore this issue and its impact on the adolescents' mental health.

There is growing evidence that homosexuality is a risk factor for adolescent suicidal behavior. In one study, researchers found that sexual orientation per se was not the cause of suicidal behavior. Instead they submitted that early and middle adolescents were less able to cope with isolation and the stigma of homosexuality identity than older adolescents (Eisenberg & Resnick, 2006). Gay-related suicides are associated with a lack of understanding or support from parents, psychological abuse, negative parental reactions to youth's sexual orientation, and verbal abuse. It is imperative for psychiatric nurses to examine their own perspectives about the youth's sexual orientation to provide support to the youth and to educate his family and significant others. Equally important is the assessment of the family's response to the youth and their level of empathy concerning his sexual orientation.

Treatment Modalities

Treating youths at risk for suicidal behaviors requires an interdisciplinary approach whose aim is to ensure safety, reduce acute suicidal behaviors, decrease risk factors, stabilize biological factors, and reduce vulnerability to future suicidal behavior (Pfeffer, 1986). Assessing the adolescent requires establishing an alliance. Sometimes this process can be lengthy and requires patience. Forming an alliance with an adolescent requires a nonthreatening approach. The nurse can begin the process with inquiries about neutral topics such as school and interests before asking about reasons for seeking treatment or family problems. This process must start as soon as possible and include taking dynamic efforts to assess the client's mental and physical status. These early nurse-client interactions foster trust and provide immediate emotional support to the adolescent and family in crisis.

All suicidal gestures are significant in children and adolescents. The youth with a history of previous attempts must be protected and probably hospitalized to evaluate the risk for harm when presenting behaviors that are dangerous to the youth or others or when outpatient treatment has failed. Outpatient treatment is appropriate when the youth does not pose an imminent danger to self or others and the family is motivated to participate in treatment. Treatment strategies are usually multimodal, consisting of crisis intervention and psychodynamic, psychopharmacologic, cognitive, behavioral, and family therapy. An emphasis on building hope and establishing healthy family interactions is vital to all treatment. This may involve family members monitoring the youth for signs of danger or worsening symptoms 24 hours a day. Assessing family interactions, strengths, manner of discipline, roles, and nurturing patterns provides information that can improve communication between the youth and his parents (Pfeffer, 1986). See Chapter 28, Familial Systems and Family Therapy, for an in-depth discussion of family therapy.

In brief, adolescence is a challenging and turbulent developmental stage. It is also a time for growth and health that allow youths to move into adulthood using adaptive coping skills. The youth who attempts or completes suicide has immense emotional pain and is unable to cope with the turbulence of adolescence. Nurses play a major role in helping troubled adolescents and their families by identifying high-risk behaviors and working with these clients to build adaptive coping behaviors that protect youths and promote health.

ADULTHOOD

Adults, like children and adolescents, face numerous stressful life events. A previous discussion of theories and contributing factors for suicide in adults is found in the initial part of this chapter. Factors that affect one person's ability to mobilize adaptive coping responses and another person's use of maladaptive behaviors challenge the psychiatric nurse to establish rapport and focus on risk factors, individual strengths, and support systems. This process involves crisis intervention and other therapeutic measures that help clients cope with overwhelming and painful internal and external life events. Some of these stressors include significant losses, deteriorating health problems, child rearing, and caring for aging parents. Sometimes these life span stressors exhaust the person's repertoire of coping behaviors and increase the risk of maladaptive behaviors, including suicide.

OLDER ADULTHOOD

As our society ages and people live longer, older adults, like other age groups, confront vast challenges to cope with life's stressors. Suicide in older people is a major national health problem, and reducing its occurrence is a national priority. People 65 years old and older have the highest rate of completed suicides in the United States (19 deaths per 100,000 persons), and these rates are six times higher than the national average (Harwood, Hawton, Hope, Harriss, & Jacoby, 2006). The highest rate of suicide is in the depressed older, widowed or divorced, medically or mentally ill, white male. Approximately 75 percent of these clients have visited their primary care physician within 4 weeks of their suicide, and 39 percent commit suicide within a week of a visit to their physician (Carney, Rich, Burke, & Fowler, 1994; Clark, 1991). Older adults make fewer attempts than younger clients, but they have a higher rate of completed suicides because they tend to use more lethal means.

Risk Factors

As previously discussed in this chapter, several factors such as significant losses, feelings of isolation, and poor physical health, in addition to those shown in Figure 19–3, have been found to be consistent predictors of suicidal behaviors in the older adult.

Loss

The first factor is loss. Older adults face numerous losses, which consist of health, financial, and social status and the death or deteriorating health of a loved one. Inadequate or ineffective coping skills also increase the risk of depression and maladaptive responses to loss. Depression is a major predictor of suicide among the older adult and assessing it is critical to prevention and development of effective treatment.

Ageism or Myths about Aging

Myths and stereotypes about the aging process may interfere with assessing depression in the older adult. Nurses

and ignoring suicidal behaviors in this age group can be deadly. Older adult clients perceive this unresponsiveness as indifference and devaluation, which reinforces their sense of worthlessness and hopelessness.

Feelings of Isolation

The third factor is isolation stemming from a lack of social ties and a sense of belonging. Older adult clients with strong family ties and a sense of integrity are less likely to become depressed or suicidal than those who are socially isolated. Roskow (1967) believed that many older adults feel alienated from society because their social roles are devalued by their families and communities. See "My Experience with Suicidal Ideations and Hopelessness."

Poor Physical Health

The final factor is physical status. Physical illness places tremendous stress on older adults, threatening their quality of life, comfort, and a sense of well-being. These stressors compromise coping mechanisms, self-esteem, and interpersonal relationships, and generate feelings of despair (Cohen & Lazarus, 1979). The client's personality and coping style and whether mental illness and alcoholism are present influence coping with physical illness.

The older adult client with physical illnesses needs to be assessed for depression because he is at risk for suicide. It is imperative for nurses to be aware of life span issues that make an impact on older adults' perception of mental health care. Older adults are often stoic and have difficulty asking

can dispel these misconceptions by working with the mental health team to assess age-related symptoms and those associated with depression. Contrary to popular belief, that dementia is part of the normal aging process, clients who present with cognitive impairment (i.e., memory loss, acute mood changes) require a comprehensive assessment to determine if depression exists. Depression in the older adults is significant because of its relationship to suicidal behavior

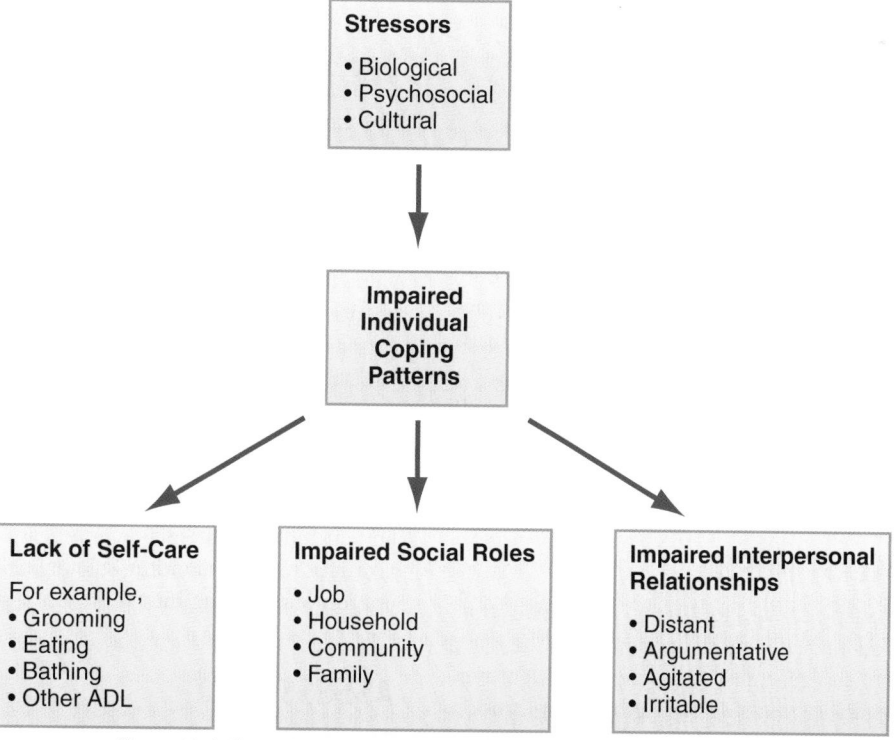

Figure 19–3 Factors that may put the elderly at high risk for suicidal behaviors. *(From "Toward Classification of Aging Behavior," by L. Miller, 1979, Gerontologist, 19, pp. 283–290.)*

for help, particularly mental health issues. Many of them perceive asking for help as a sign of weakness and inadequacy. Involving families or significant others in the client's care is helpful. Major treatment goals include helping clients express their feelings and mobilizing psychosocial resources.

Suicidal behaviors in older adults, as in other age groups, must be assessed early, and measures to prevent it are major nursing goals. Establishing therapeutic relationships are critical to this process because nurses can identify client resources and develop effective interventions that increase self-esteem and adaptive coping skills.

THE ROLE OF THE NURSE

The role of the nurse has been explicated throughout this chapter. Primary responsibilities focus on prevention that involves identifying high-risk groups, assessing age-specific considerations, and implementing nursing interventions that reduce suicide and facilitate adaptive coping behaviors. As societal stress increases and affects the mental health of its people, psychiatric nurses must prepare themselves to meet the challenge of caring for clients at risk of suicide and preventing this tragedy. The next section focuses on the roles of the generalist and advanced-practice nurse in caring for the suicidal client.

THE GENERALIST NURSE

Suicidal clients challenge nurses to develop innovative strategies that facilitate adaptive coping skills and reduce the risk of suicide. The role of the generalist nurse includes identifying clients at risk for suicide, assessing coping behaviors, and intervening to minimize the risk of suicide among all age groups in various clinical settings. Additionally, the generalist nurse collaborates with clients, families, and other mental health

professionals to develop a comprehensive plan of care that reduces the risk factors of suicide. Major strategies include crisis intervention, case management, psychoeducation, administration of psychotropics, and monitoring of client responses.

THE ADVANCED-PRACTICE PSYCHIATRIC REGISTERED NURSE

Nurses in the advanced-practice role must respond to complex needs of clients in distress, and the suicidal client is of particular challenge in this regard. The complexity of suicidal behaviors suggest a need to understand the factors that increase the risk of self-destructive behaviors, such as biochemical aspects of mental illness, developmental issues, and family dynamics. Managing the care of these clients involves making accurate and differential diagnoses. Establishing a differential diagnosis involves a comprehensive mental status examination, physical examination, and ordering and interpreting the results of appropriate diagnostic studies. The advanced-practice nurse also collaborates with appropriate health care providers and develops appropriate evidence-based interventions for the suicidal client. Most interventions include prescriptive authority, case management, consultation-liaison, individual and family psychotherapy, and working with other disciplines to develop a comprehensive plan of care. Psychopharmacologic agents used to treat impulsivity and aggressive behaviors in suicidal clients include antidepressants such as the selective serotonin reuptake inhibitors; mood stabilizers such as lithium; valproic acid; and atypical antipsychotic agents (e.g., olanzapine) (Ernst & Goldberg, 2004; Glick et al., 2004; Hollander, Swann, Coccaro, Jiang, & Smith, 2005).

THE NURSING PROCESS

The care of suicidal clients often generate feelings of uneasiness, anger, and helplessness in the nurse. These feelings usually stem from conflicts or ambivalence associated with personal values and beliefs and ethical and professional considerations. Nursing is a helping profession, and life is valued—suicide is the antithesis of this premise. Suicidal clients challenge nurses to use sensitive, nonjudgmental and caring approaches to manage profound emotional pain and suffering. Regardless of the number of suicide attempts, each one depicts the client's inability to cope effectively. Unfortunately, some nurses may even have difficulty relating to suicidal clients because they perceive their problems as self-imposed. Nurses must explore their own perceptions and attitudes about suicide and death. This personal process is crucial to understanding suicidal behaviors and developing appropriate nursing interventions.

ASSESSMENT

The care of suicidal clients can be effectively managed by an interdisciplinary approach, and nurses are crucial to this process. Initially, there must be an evaluation of the level of suicide risk or danger. Evaluation is a continuous process that requires accurate and prompt documentation of the clients' behavior and response to treatment.

The therapeutic relationship is the basis of the assessment process. Cultural and life span factors must be an integral part of the assessment and data-gathering process. Encouraging clients to discuss suicidal ideations, feelings, and plans allays their anxiety and disputes the notion that asking about suicide "puts thoughts into the client's head." Suicidal clients are frightened about their impulses and wishes to kill themselves. Suicidal thoughts must be assessed in all clients as part of the mental status examination. Questions such as "Are you having thoughts of killing yourself?" or "Have you attempted to kill yourself in the past?" are parts of this assessment. Most suicidal clients feel relieved about the opportunity to discuss these feelings. Most suicidal clients who eventually kill themselves have communicated clues about their intent. Exploring suicidal intent communicates that the cry for help has been assessed and relief is achievable.

Once the client has been assessed to be a suicide risk, the decision to hospitalize is considered. Criteria for hospitalization are based on several factors:

- The nature of the suicide attempt (e.g., gunshot, hanging, carbon monoxide)
- The client's expression of a plan, intent, and means to carry out the plan
- History of previous attempt or impulsivity
- Lack of a quality social support system
- Active substance use or withdrawal
- Male gender, older adulthood (when accompanied by suicidal ideations, plan, and intent)
- Psychosis in the presence of suicidal ideations, plan

Clients presenting with suicidal ideations realize they are in trouble. Hospitalization is a viable option to further protect clients from suicide and evaluate psychosocial and biological stressors. This process can begin with discussing treatment options with the clients and family. If the clients are unwilling to enter the hospital voluntarily and this is clearly indicated, an involuntary admission may be initiated by the psychiatrist. Laws governing this process vary, and nurses must familiarize themselves with statutes for emergency detention and involuntary admissions (see Chapter 8, Legal and Ethical Considerations, for an in-depth discussion of this process). See Table 19–5 for legal considerations regarding the care of the suicidal client.

The first priority when caring for the suicidal client is managing the crisis situation with the least restrictive treatment to ensure safety. This can be accomplished by the following (Antai-Otong, 2004):

- Placing the client in a room free of sharp or dangerous items that can be used to harm self or others such as glass, razors, knives, or metal
- Checking the client's personal belongings and clothing for medication or potential weapons

TABLE 19–5
Legal Considerations Regarding the Suicidal Client

- Careful documentation
- Clear and complete documentation of the decision-making process surrounding the discharge
- Development of a postdischarge and aftercare plan
- Appropriate referral (call and confirm)
- Provide written instructions to the family and patient
- Instruct client and/or family to remove weapons from the home
- Family, friend, and patient need to be able to call on interim basis in case of an emergency
- Documentation of weapons-availability assessment

- Making sure that the client is not left alone
- Placing the client in a hospital gown or pajamas
- Approaching the client in a calm and reassuring manner
- Using active and assertive communication skills

Even when safety measures are instituted by the emergency department of hospitalization, the risk for suicide exists throughout treatment. A small number of clients may commit suicide on psychiatric units, especially during the first week of hospitalization. Preventing suicide begins with recognizing high-risk behaviors, minimizing the risk, and developing effective treatment plans that ensure safety and effective coping behaviors. Times of high risk within the hospital routine include weekends and holidays, visiting hours (if the client has no visitors), change of shifts or mealtime, rotation of staff, or times of unit chaos (Occupational Safety and Health Administration [OSHA], 2004).

When clients are determined to commit suicide, the greatest efforts will not stop them. These clients tend to wait and watch for opportunities when there is chaos or less staff on the unit or even when they leave on pass or elopement (without medical advice or approval). High-risk clients need to be observed continuously and assessed for change in mood, behaviors, or ideations. A sudden change in mood from a depressed to elated or energetic mood increases the risk of suicide because of improved cognitive function, a lack of ambivalence about dying, and ability to carry out a plan. Nurses must document all observations when caring for suicidal clients and report any changes in their mental or physical status.

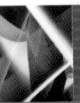

CASE STUDY

The Adult at Risk for Suicide (Mr. Leonard)

Mr. Leonard is a 45-year-old man who had reported having thoughts of killing himself because his 13-year-old son recently died of bone cancer. He was despondent and expressed guilt because he was unable to spare his son from intense pain and suffering. He has a history of chronic back pain and associated this pain to his son's suffering. His mood was depressed, and he cried often during the assessment. He denied having made suicide attempts in the past or actively abusing alcohol or other drugs. He has thoughts of shooting himself. When questioned about reasons for not acting on these thoughts in the past, he replied that his son would not approve of it.

NURSING DIAGNOSES

- ◆ Risk for Self-Directed Violence
- ◆ Ineffective Coping
- ◆ Dysfunctional Grieving
- ◆ Spiritual Distress

Mr. Leonard is in tremendous emotional pain, and his suicidal thoughts and plan place him at high risk for lethality. He is currently on one-to-one suicide precaution, which means that a staff person is constantly with him until his condition improves (i.e., he no longer expresses suicidal ideations or plans). Suicidal clients need to be encouraged to express feelings and thoughts about their problems and suicide. This helps them sort out the reality of their situation and incorporate adaptive coping patterns through crisis intervention. Mr. Leonard openly discussed his pain and despair about losing his son. His sense of helplessness in not being able to save his son mirrored his intense emotional suffering. Conveying care and instilling hope are major aspects of suicide prevention.

PLANNING

The following are desired outcomes identified for Mr. Leonard:

- ◆ Expresses feelings and thoughts of suicide rather than acting on them
- ◆ Identifies reasons for wanting to die
- ◆ Acquires adaptive coping skills
- ◆ Develops hope regarding the future
- ◆ Forms adequate support system
- ◆ Effectively resolves grief

NURSING INTERVENTION

Nursing Care Plan 19–2 delineates the nursing action needed to achieve some of these outcomes and the rationales for each action.

NURSING CARE PLAN 19–2

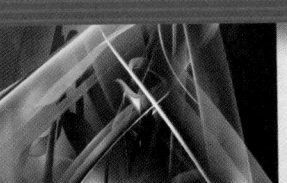

The Adult at Risk for Suicide (Mr. Leonard)

Nursing Diagnosis: Risk for Self-Directed Violence

Outcome Identification	Nursing Actions	Rationales	Evaluation
1. By [date], client will verbalize the absence of suicidal ideations or plans.	1a. Assess the level of danger.	1a. This enables the nurse to identify interventions to reduce suicidal risk.	*Goal met:* Mr. Leonard • denies suicidal ideations. • does not harm self. • is able to identify options. • shows gradual mood changes and is able to express superficial feelings.
	1b. Provide a safe environment. Remove potential or actual dangerous objects from the environment.	1b. Removing objects reduces access to lethal weapons and lessens the risk of suicide.	

(continues)

Outcome Identification	Nursing Actions	Rationales	Evaluation
	1c. Discuss a "no suicide" verbal contract.	1c. Encouraging the client to agree to a "no suicide contract" helps him or her understand the seriousness of the situation and verbalize feelings regarding suicide.	
2. By [date], client will discuss options to deal with present stressors.	2a. Encourage the examination of available options to cope with present stressors.	2a. Increasing the client's options decreases the lone option of suicide; it also enhances the client's coping skills.	
	2b. Observe for sudden changes in mood.	2b. Sudden mood changes (decreased depression) signal increased energy and ability to carry out a suicide plan.	
	2c. Encourage the expression of feelings.	2c. Expression of feelings reduces tension and frustration and is an important aspect of the nurse–client relationship.	

Nursing Diagnosis: Ineffective Coping

Outcome Identification	Nursing Actions	Rationales	Evaluation
1. By [date], client will develop an awareness of the meaning of present behaviors.	1a. Facilitate an understanding of the client's present behaviors.	1a. Understanding the meaning of maladaptive behaviors enhances adaptive coping responses and provides an opportunity for growth and mobilization of adaptive coping behaviors.	*Goal met:* Mr. Leonard • returns to previous level of functioning. • develops adequate coping skills. • displays less anxiety.
	1b. Assist the client in problem solving.	1b. Crisis situations often overtax coping and problem-solving skills. This action affords an opportunity to enhance coping and problem-solving skills.	
	1c. Confront maladaptive behaviors.	1c. Confronting maladaptive behaviors allows the client to understand the meaning of them and develop adaptive coping responses.	

(continues)

Nursing Diagnosis: Dysfunctional Grieving

Outcome Identification	Nursing Actions	Rationales	Evaluation
1. By [date], client will realistically accept loss.	1a. Form a meaningful nurse-client relationship. 1b. Assess the meaning of the loss to the client. 1c. Determine stage of grief.	1a–b. This relationship provides emotional support and enables the nurse to assess the significance of the loss. 1c. This helps the nurse to assess the client's needs and conveys empathy.	*Goal met:* Mr. Leonard • forms a meaningful relationship with the nurse. • expresses feelings regarding the death of his son and how life has been without him.
2. By [date], client will actively participate in the grief process.	2a. Provide a calm, accepting, and empathic environment. 2b. Encourage expression of feelings regarding loss. 2c. Educate the client and family about the grief process.	2a. This alleviates anxiety and promotes trust. 2b. This facilitates understanding the meaning and acceptance of the loss. 2c. This facilitates understanding and participation in the grief process.	• begins working through the grief process and works through his guilt. • reestablishes a relationship with family members.
3. By [date], client will participate in activities that promote social interaction.	3. Encourage participation in social activities.	3. This decreases social isolation and facilitates the establishment of new and meaningful relationships.	

IMPLEMENTATION

The primary intervention of working with the suicidal client is prevention and development of adaptive coping behaviors.

EVALUATION

Mr. Leonard was discharged after a brief hospitalization. He was assessed for suicidal risk and tendencies during hospitalization and on discharge. During his hospitalization he was not suicidal after the first day, and he began to openly express his pain and sadness. He decided that suicide was not the solution to his present stressors. At discharge he was referred to a day hospital program for several weeks. He was able to use group therapy to resolve his grief and develop effective coping skills. No medication was prescribed at the time of discharge to the day hospital program.

This case study demonstrated how crisis intervention can be used to help a suicidal client. All situations do not end this way and the client sometimes completes a suicide. Completed suicides can be devastating to nurses, other mental health professionals, and families. How can these situations be dealt with?

WHEN A CLIENT COMMITS SUICIDE

In spite of heroic efforts to save clients, some of them manage to kill themselves. The suicidal client is not the only victim when this occurs. Family members and friends have to deal with the emotional aftermath of completed suicides. General staff reactions include "What did I miss?" or "I should have been able to prevent this suicide." Feelings of guilt, helplessness, inadequacy, and anger are common staff reactions when a client commits suicide. Similar reactions emerge in the relatives or friend survivors of suicide. Many of them openly attack nurses and other staff, projecting their own sense of guilt, helplessness, and anger about losing a loved one. Nurses can work through these feelings and form an interdisciplinary approach with a psychological autopsy.

Litman, Curphey, Shneidman, Farberow and Tabachnick (1963) defined psychological autopsy as a process for evaluating whether a death was suicidal or accidental. This process involves exploring the circumstances of the suicidal client's life by reconstructing it through interviews with the family and friends. Components of the psychological autopsy include:

◆ Interviewing the family or significant others who were familiar with the client

- Reviewing the client's behavior before death
- Discussing the client's medical and psychiatric history
- Identifying the client's significant family history concerning suicide and mental illness
- Determining the presence or absence of substance or alcohol abuse

This process facilitates interaction between staff and provides opportunities to express feelings and thoughts about the suicide. Team members can work through the crisis of suicide while grasping the reality that it was the client's decision to follow through with the act.

Interviewing significant others provides the staff with pertinent information about familial interactions, lifestyle, personal attributes, and coping patterns. Family may be hesitant to discuss these issues with staff because of guilt and remorse generated by the suicide. Families can be referred to age-appropriate community suicide survivors' support groups.

NURSING RESEARCH

The emergence of evidence-based approaches to understanding the psychosocial and neurobiological aspects of suicidal and other self-destructive behaviors prompts psychiatric-mental health nurses to explore these major concepts. Nurses can examine and identify factors that increase the risk or vulnerability for suicide as part of data collection from clients, families, and records (see the Research Abstract). Collaborating with other disciplines is a critical aspect of research because it integrates the expertise of a team approach to assessing, intervening in, and evaluating self-destructive behaviors across the life span. Other studies involve investigating the effects of psychotropics on behavior. Major nursing roles in drug trials include prescribing, administering research drugs, observing clients for desired and adverse responses, and participating in structured interviews and evidence-based treatment planning.

SUMMARY

- Suicide is a significant health problem that affects approximately 12 out of 100,000 people in the United States.
- Adolescents and older adults are the age groups most likely to commit suicide.
- Additionally, clients with histories of mental illness and alcoholism are likely to commit suicide.
- The complexity of suicide suggests that nurses must identify clients at risk and collaborate with other mental health professionals to develop effective evidence-based interventions to prevent suicide.
- Suicide prevention is crucial, alleviating stress and a sense of crisis.

- When a client commits suicide, families, friends, and staff are affected.
- Nurses can provide immediate emotional support, mobilize resources, and promote a sense of hope in otherwise overwhelming situations through therapeutic relationships.

SUGGESTIONS FOR CLINICAL CONFERENCES

1. Interview a client who is suicidal in the presence of a registered nurse and present the data to peers. Discuss the feelings generated by the interview/assessment
2. Present a case history of a client with self-destructive behaviors
3. Role play as client who is suicidal with a peer and discuss interactions and feelings generated
4. Present a case history of an adolescent and older adult and compare assessment process

STUDY QUESTIONS

1. Mrs. Annie Wilson, a 76-year-old woman, has been brought to the mental health center by her daughter because she has been isolating herself and refusing to eat over the past 2 weeks. Which of the following questions is essential in assessing this client for suicide?
   a. "Annie, what has brought you in today?"
   b. "Mrs. Wilson, how are you doing today?"
   c. "Mrs. Wilson, are you depressed?"
   d. "Mrs. Wilson, tell me how long you have been spending time alone?"

2. Mrs. Wilson reports that she can no longer do the things she used to do since injuring her knee several weeks ago and feels like a burden to her daughter. A critical question to ask a depressed older client is which of the following?
   a. "Mrs. Wilson, why are you spending so much time alone?"
   b. "How hopeful are you about doing the things you used to do?"
   c. "How often does your daughter visit you?"
   d. "Have you thought about going to a local adult day center?"

3. Marty, a 15-year-old boy, is brought into the school nurse's office by a teacher who reports that one of his friends reported that he has been boasting about a teenage suicide pact. Which of the following best describes the *sociological theory* behind his suicidal comments?
   a. Altruistic suicide
   b. Egoistic suicide
   c. Anomic suicide
   d. Fatalistic suicide

4. Alcoholism and schizophrenia increase the risk factors of suicidal behavior. Which of the following *best* describes the basis of these risk factors?
   a. Increased impulsivity or disinhibition
   b. Increased cognitive functioning
   c. Increase the risk of major depressive episode
   d. Increased ability to problem-solve

5. Mary is a 10-year-old girl who expresses thoughts of not wanting to wake up some mornings. Her mother states that sometimes she does not want to get up either. The nurse's most appropriate response to this mother is:
   a. "Your child's comments are serious and require further evaluation."
   b. "Sometimes most of us do not want to wake up."
   c. "Her comments are not serious and they are just part of being a child."
   d. "You are a good mother; do not worry about her comments."

6. Of the following, which is the *best* predictor of suicide?
   a. Family history
   b. Previous attempts
   c. Alcoholism
   d. Recent loss

7. Patience is a 15-year-old adolescent brought into the emergency department by her mother expressing concerns about the cuts on her wrists. Her mother reports noticing this behavior off and on over the past year but never took them seriously until now. She is expressing concerns about her daughter trying to take her life. Patience denies trying to kill herself. Which of the following statements are important for the nurse to make to her mother?
   a. "Her wounds are not life threatening, but we need to further assess her behavior."
   b. "Your daughter really is trying to commit suicide and needs immediate attention."
   c. "This is not a serious act. Just watch her and bring her back if she cuts herself again."
   d. "You need to consider putting her on medication to reduce this behavior."

8. Mr. Sanders, a 35-year-old client who has a history of depression, dies in the emergency department from a self-inflicted gunshot wound. The nurses are angry, sad, and upset. What statement best describes their reactions to the client's suicide?
   a. Judgmental reactions that reflect a lack of empathy
   b. Normal reactions that reflect a sense of helplessness and inability to save the client
   c. Normal reactions that reflect being overworked and tired
   d. Unprofessional reactions because it is normal for clients to die in emergency rooms

9. The nurse caring for a client at risk for violence should always put her safety first. One of your clients is pacing and yelling in the waiting room. What is the most appropriate response to the client?
   a. "Mary, I know you are upset, but it is difficult for me to help when you are yelling."
   b. "Mary, please be quiet, you are disturbing the other clients."
   c. "Mary, if you don't lower your voice we are going to put you in restraints."
   d. "Mary, I have already called security. Sit down!"

10. When caring for a client with major depression she expresses thoughts of hurting herself. Which is the most appropriate response to the client's statement?
    a. "What kind of thoughts are you having about hurting yourself?"
    b. "Have you thought about the effects hurting yourself will have on your family?"
    c. "How long have you been depressed?"
    d. "Does your family know about your thoughts?"

11. The nurse is developing a plan of care for a 15-year-old with major depression who is taking an antidepressant medication. Which of the following is most appropriate to include in the plan of care?
    a. Monitoring mood changes and thoughts of suicide
    b. Encouraging the client to interact more often with family and friends
    c. Warning the client not to smoke
    d. Reporting all side effects from the antidepressant

RESOURCES

Please note that because Internet resources are of a time-sensitive nature and URL addresses may change or be deleted, searches should always be conducted by association or topic.

Internet Resources

http://www.healthfinder.gov   Department of Health and Human Services

http://www.cf.nlm.nih.gov   National Institute of Health

http://www.nimh.nih.gov   National Institute of Mental Health

http://www.nami.org   National Alliance for the Mentally Ill National Web Page

http://www.reidpsychiatry.com   Psychiatry and the Law

http://nursingworld.org/anp/pcatalog.cfm   American Nurses Association's website at Nursesbooks.org (for information about the psychiatric-mental health generalist and advanced-practice nurse's role)

http://www.suicidology.org   American Association of Suicidology

http://www.epo.cdc.gov   CDC Prevention Guidelines Database-aepo-xdv

http://www.cdc.gov/ncipi/dvp/yvt/suicide/htm   Suicide Prevention Fact Sheet http://www.cdc.gov./safeusa/suicide.htm   Preventing Suicide—SAFEusa

http://www.cdc.gov/mmwr/preview/mmwrhtml/0031525.htm   Programs for Prevention of Suicide among Adolescents and Young Adults

http://www.cdc.gov/mmwr/preview/mmwrjtml/00051966.htm   Suicide Prevention Evaluation in a Western Alhabaskan American Indian Tribe

http://www.spanusa.org/home.htm   Suicide Prevention Advocacy Network (SPAN)

http://www.nami.org/Content.NavigationMenu/Inform_Yourself/About_NAMI/About_NAMI.htm   National Alliance on Mental Illness (NAMI)

Family, Child, and Adolescent

http://www.nami.org/Content/ContentGroups/Helpline1/Suicide_in_Youth.htm   (Accessed February 22, 2006)

http://www.aacap.org/publications/factsfam/suicide.htm   American Academy of Child and Adolescent Psychiatry, Facts for Families Teen Suicide (Accessed February 22, 2006)

http://www.aacap.org/publications/factsfam/depressed.htm   The Depressed Child (Accessed February 22, 2006)

http://wonder.cdc.gov/wonder/prevguid/p0000024/p0000024.asp   Youth Suicide Prevention Program—A Resource Guide (Accessed February 22, 2006)

Spanish Resources

References: http://quetzalcoatlhernandez.com/referencias.html   (Accessed February 22, 2006)

Information: http://www.suicidioadolescente.info/suicidologia.html   (Accessed February 22, 2006)

Prevention: http://www.suicidioadolescente.info/prevencion.html   (Accessed February 22, 2006)

REFERENCES

Adamek, M. E., & Kaplan, M. S. (1996). Firearm suicide among older men. *Psychiatric Services, 47,* 304–306.

Adams, K. S. (1985). Attempted suicide. *Psychiatric Clinics of North America, 8,* 183–201.

American Psychiatric Association. (2000). *Diagnostic and statistical manual of mental disorders* (4th edition, Text Revision). Washington, DC: Author.

Anderson, R. N., & Smith, B. L. (2003). Deaths: Leading causes for 2001. *National Vital Statistics Report, 52,* 1–86.

Antai-Otong, D. (2004). *Psychiatric emergencies: How to accurately assess and manage the patient in crisis (revised).* Eau Claire: PESI Healthcare Inc.

Baldessarini, R. J., Pompili, M., & Tondo, L. (2006). Suicide in bipolar disorder: Risks and management. *CNS Spectrums, 11,* 465–471.

Barbe, R. P., Williamson, D. E., Bridge, J. A., Birmaher, B., Dahl, R. E., Axelson, D. A., & Ryan, N. D. (2005). Clinical differences between suicidal and nonsuicidal depressed children and adolescents. *Journal of Clinical Psychiatry, 66,* 492–498.

Beautrais, A. L. (2003). Suicide and serious suicide attempts in youth: A multiple-group comparison study. *American Journal of Psychiatry, 160,* 1093–1099.

Beck, A. T., Brown, G., Berchick, R. J., Stewart, B. L., & Steer, R. A. (1990). Relationship between hopelessness and ultimate suicide: A replication with psychiatric outpatients. *American Journal of Psychiatry, 147,* 190–195.

Berlin, I. N. (1987). Suicide among American Indian adolescents: An overview. *Suicide and Life Threatening Behaviors, 17,* 218–232.

Bernard, S. J., Paulozzi, L. J., & Wallace, L. J. D. (2007). Fatal injuries among children by race and ethnicity—United States, 1999–2002. *Surveillance Summaries: Mortality and Morbidity Weekly Reports (MMWR), 56,* (SS05), 1–16.

Bohus, M., Limberger, M., Ebner, U., Glocker, F. X., Schwarz, B., Wernz, M., & Lieb, K. (2000). Pain perception during self-reported distress and calmness in patients with borderline personality disorder and self-mutilating behavior. *Psychiatric Research, 95,* 251–260.

Boldrini, M., Underwood, M. D., Mann, J. J., & Arango, V. (2007). Serotonin-1A autoreceptor binding in the dorsal raphe nucleus of depressed suicides. *Journal of Psychiatric Research,* June 14. [Epub ahead of print]

Borowsky, I. W., Resnick, M. D., Ireland, M., & Blum, R. W. (1999). Suicide among American Indian and Alaska Native youth: Risk and protective factors. *Archives of Pediatric and Adolescent Medicine, 153,* 573–580.

Brady, S. S., & Matthews, K. A. (2006). Effects of media violence on health-related outcomes among young men. *Archives of Pediatric and Adolescent Medicine, 160,* 341–347.

Brezo, J., Paris, J., Turecki, G. (2006). Personality traits as correlates of suicidal ideations, suicide attempts and suicide completions: A systematic review. *Acta Psychiatrica Scandinavia, 113,* 180–206.

Caplan, G. (1961). *An approach to community mental health.* New York: Grune & Stratton.

Carney, S. S., Rich, C. L., Burke, P. A., & Fowler, R. C. (1994). Suicide over 60: The San Diego study. *Journal of the American Geriatric Society, 42,* 174–180.

Castle, K., Duberstein, P. R., Meldrum, S., Conner, K. R., & Conwell, Y. (2004). Risk factors for suicide in blacks and whites: An analysis of data from the 1993 National Mortality Followback Survey. *American Journal of Psychiatry, 161,* 452–458.

Centers for Disease Control and Prevention, National Center for Injury Prevention and Control. (2004). Web-based injury statistics query and reporting system (WISQARS) [Online]. Available at http://www.cdc.gov/ncipc/wisquars/default.htm

Centers for Disease Control and Prevention. (1999). Suicide surveillance for injuries and violence among older adults. *Morbidity and Mortality Weekly Reports, 48*(SS-8), 27–34.

Centers for Disease Control and Prevention. (1997). *Regional variations in suicide rates—United States, 1990–1994, 46*(34), 789–793.

Clark, D. C. (1991). *Suicide among the elderly*. (Final report to the AARP Andrus Foundation), Washington, DC: American Association of Retired Persons.

Coccaro, E. F. (2006). Association of C-reactive protein elevation with trait aggression and hostility in personality disordered subjects: A pilot study. *Journal of Psychiatric Research, 40*, 460–465.

Cohen, F., & Lazarus, R. (1979). Coping with stresses of illness. In G. Stone, F. Cohen, & N. Adler (Eds.). *Health and psychology: A handbook* (pp. 217–255). San Francisco: Jossey-Bass.

Conwell, Y., Duberstein, P. R., & Caine, E. D. (2002). Risk factors for suicide in later life. *Biological Psychiatry, 52,* 193–204.

Derouin, A., & Bravender, J. (2004). Living on the edge: The current phenomenon of self-multilation in adolescents. *MCN American Journal of Maternal and Child Nursing, 29,* 12–18.

Duberstein, P., & Conwell, Y. (1997). Personality disorders and completed suicide: A methological and conceptual review. *Clinical Psychology: Science and Practice, 4,* 359–376.

Dumais, A., Lesage, A. D., Alda, M., Rouleau, G., Dumont, M., Chawky, N., et al. (2005). Risk factors for suicide completion in major depression: A case-control of impulsive and aggressive behaviors in men. *American Journal of Psychiatry, 162,* 116–124.

Durkheim, E. (1951). *Suicide* (2nd ed.). J. A. Spaulding & G. Simpson (Trans.). New York: Free Press. (Original work published 1897)

Eisenberg, M. E., & Resnick, M. D. (2006). Suicidality among gay, lesbian and bisexual youth: The role of protective factors. *Journal of Adolescent Health, 39,* 662–669.

Enns, M. W., Cox, B. J., Afifi, T. O., De Graaf, R., Ten Have, M., & Sareen, J. (2006). Childhood adversities and risk for suicidal ideation and attempts: A longitudinal population-based study. *Psychological Medicine, 36,* 1769–1778.

Ernst, C. L., & Goldberg, J. F. (2004). Antisuicide properties of psychotropic drugs: A clinical review. *Harvard Review of Psychiatry, 12,* 14–41.

Evans, E., Hawton, K., Rodham, K., & Deeks, J., (2005). The prevalence of suicidal phenomena in adolescents: A systematic review of population-based studies. *Suicide and other Life Threatening Behaviors, 35,* 239–250.

Freud, S. (1961). Economic problems of masochism. In J. Strachey (Ed. and Trans.), *The standard edition of the complete psychological works of Sigmund Freud* (Vol. 19, pp. 159–170). London: Hogarth Press. (Original work published 1923)

Garland, A. F., & Zigler, E. (1993). Adolescent suicide prevention. *American Psychologist, 48,* 169–182.

Garlow, S. J., Purselle, D., & Heninger, M. (2005). Ethnic differences in patterns of suicide across the life span. *American Journal of Psychiatry, 162,* 319–323.

Gibbs, J. T. (1988). Conceptual, methodological, and sociological issues in black youth suicide: Implications for assessment and early intervention. *Suicide and Life-Threatening Behavior, 18,* 73–89.

Glick, I. D., Zaninelli, R., Hsu, C., Young, F. K., Weiss, L., Gunay, I., & Kumar, V. (2004). Patterns of concomitant psychotropic medication use during a 2-year study comparing clozapine and olanzapine for the prevention of suicidal behavior. *Journal of Clinical Psychiatry, 65,* 679–685.

Gould, M. S., Fisher, P., Parides, M., Flory, M., & Shaffer, D. (1996). Psychosocial risk factors of child and adolescent completed suicide. *Archives of General Psychiatry, 53,* 1155–1162.

Gould, M. S., Greenberg, T., Velting, D. M., & Shaffer, D. (2003). Youth suicide risk and preventive interventions. A review of the past 10 years. *Journal of the American Academy of Child and Adolescent Psychiatry, 42,* 386–405.

Grunebaum, M. F., Ramsay, S. R., Galfalvy, H. C., Ellis, S. P., Burke, A. K., Sher, L., et al. (2006). Correlates of suicide attempt history in bipolar disorder: A stress-diathesis perspective. *Bipolar Disorders, 8,* 551–557.

Guiao, I. Z., & Thompson, E. A. (2004). Age and problem behaviors among adolescent multi-ethnic females. *Issues in Mental Health Nursing, 25,* 147–164.

Gunderson, J. G. (2001). *Borderline personality disorder: A clinical guide*. Washington, DC: American Psychiatric Publishing Inc.

Harrop, A. R., Brant, R. F., Ghalia, W. A., & Macathur, C. (2007). Injury mortality rates in Native and non-Native children: A population-based study. *Public Health Reports, 122,* 339–346.

Harwood, D. M., Hawton, K., Hope, T., Harriss, L., & Jacoby, R. (2006). Life problems and physical illness as risk factors for suicide in older people: A descriptive and case-control study. *Psychological Medicine, 36,* 1265–1274.

Hendlin, H. (1987). Youth suicide: A psychosocial perspective. *Suicide and Life-Threatening Behavior, 17,* 151–165. Washington, DC: American Psychiatric Press.

Hollander, E., Swann, A. C., Coccaro, E. F., Jiang, P., & Smith, T. B. (2005). Impact of trait impulsivity and state aggression on divalproex versus placebo response in borderline personality disorder. *American Journal of Psychiatry, 162,* 621–624.

Ialongo, N. S., Koenig-McNaught, A. L., Wagner, B. M., Pearson, J. L., McCreary, B. K., Poduska, J., & Kellam, S. (2004). African American children's reports of depressed mood, hopelessness, and suicidal ideation and later suicide attempts. *Suicide and Life-Threatening Behavior, 34,* 395–407.

Indian Health Service. (1996). *Trends in Indian health*. Rockville, MD: U.S. Department of Health and Human Services.

Joe, S., Baser, R. E., Breeden, G., Neighbors, H. W., & Jackson, J. S. (2006). Prevalence of and risk factors for lifetime suicide attempts among blacks in the United States. *JAMA, 296*, 2112–2123.

Joe, S., Marcus, S. C., & Kaplan, M. S. (2007). Racial differences in the characteristics of firearm suicide decedents in the United States. *American Journal of Orthopsychiatry, 77*, 124–130.

Kumar, C. T., Mohan, R., Ranjith, G., & Chadrasekaran, R. (2006). Characteristics of high intent suicide attempters admitted to a general hospital. *Journal of Affective Disorder 91*, 77–81.

Langley, D., & Kaplan, D. (1968). *Treatment of families in crisis*. New York: Grune & Stratton.

Langlois, S., & Morrison, P. (2002). Suicide deaths and suicide attempts. *Health Reports 13*, 9–22.

Limosin, F., Loze, J. Y., Philippe, A., Casadebaig, F., & Rouillon, F. (2007). Ten-year prospective follow-up study of the mortality by suicide in schizophrenic patients. *Schizophrenia Research*, June 15. [Epub ahead of print]

Litman, R. E., Curphey, T., Shneidman, E. S., Farberow, N. L., & Tabachnick, N. (1963). Investigation of equivocal suicides. *Journal of the American Medical Association, 184*, 924–929.

Mann, J. J., & Currier, D. (2007). A review of prospective studies of biologic predictors of suicidal behavior in mood disorders. *Archives of Suicide Research, 11*, 3–16.

May, P. A. (1987). Suicide among American Indian youth: A look at the issues. *Child Today, 16*, 22–25.

Menninger, K. A. (1938). *Man against himself*. New York: Harcourt, Brace, & World.

Menninger, K. A. (1947). *The human mind*. New York: Alfred A. Knopf.

Miller, L. (1979). Toward classification of aging behavior. *Gerontologist, 19*, 283–290.

Nierenberg, A. A., Gray, S. M., & Grandin, L. D. (2001). Mood disorders and suicide. *Journal of Clinical Psychiatry, 62*, (Suppl 62), 27–30.

Occupational Safety and Health Administration. (2004). *Guidelines for preventing workplace violence for health care & social service workers*. U.S. Department of Labor, OSHA 3148-01R. Available online at http://www.osha.gov/Publications/OSHA3148/osha3148.html

Oquendo, M. A., Ellis, S. P., Greenwald, S., Malone, K. M., Weissman, M. M., Mann, J. J. (2001). Ethnic and sex differences in suicide rates relative to major depression in the United States. *American Journal of Psychiatry, 158*, 1652–1658.

Palmer, B. A., Pankratz, V. S., Bostwick, J. M. (2005). The lifetime risk of suicide in schizophrenia: A reexamination. *Archives of General Psychiatry, 62*, 247–253.

Patel, N., Webb, K., & White, D. (2006). Homicides and suicides—national violent death reporting system, United States, 2003–2004. *MMWR, 55*, 721–724. Available online at http://www.cdc.gov/mmwr/PDF/wk/mm5526.pdf

Pfeffer, C. R. (1986). *The suicidal child*. New York: Guilford Press.

Pfeffer, C. R. (2002). Suicide in mood disordered children and adolescents. *Child and Adolescent Psychiatric Clinics of North America, 11*, 639–647.

Pfennig, A., Kunzel, H. E., Kern, N., Ising, M., Majer, M., Fuchs, B., Ernst, G., Hosboer, F., & Binder, E. B. (2005). Hypothalamus-pituitary-adrenal system regulation and suicidal behavior in depression. *Biological Psychiatry, 57*, 336–342.

Reinhertz, H. Z., Tanner, J. L., Berger, S. R., Beardslee, W. R., & Fitzmaurice, G. M. (2006). Adolescent suicidal ideation as predictive of psychopathology, suicidal behavior, and compromised functioning at age 30. *American Journal of Psychiatry, 163*, 1226–1232.

Renaud, J., Berlim, M. T., McGirr, A., Tousignant, M., & Turecki, G. (2007). Current psychiatric morbidity, aggression/impulsivity, and personality dimensions in child and adolescent suicide: A case-control study. *Journal of Affective Disorders*. [Epub ahead of print]

Rohde, P., Lewinsohn, P. M., Klein, D. N., & Seeley, I. R. (2005). Association of parental depression with psychiatric course from adolescence to young adulthood among formerly depressed individuals. *Journal of Abnormal Psychology, 114*, 409–420.

Roskow, I. (1967). *Social integration of the aged*. New York: Free Press.

Roy, A. (1985). Suicide and psychiatric patients. *Psychiatric Clinics of North America, 8*, 181, 227–241.

Samuelsson, M., Jokinen, J., Nordström, A-L., & Nordström, P. (2006). CSF 5-HIAA, suicide intent and hopelessness in the prediction of early suicide in male high-risk suicide attempters. *Acta Psychiatrica Scandinavia, 113*, 44–47.

Sareen, J., Cox, B. J., Afifi, T. O., de Graaf, R., Asmundson, G. J., ten Have, M., et al. (2005). Anxiety disorders and risk for suicidal ideation and suicide attempts: A population-based longitudinal study of adults. *Archives of General Psychiatry, 62*, 1229–1257.

Shaffer, D., Pfeffer, C. R. (2001). Practice parameters for the assessment and treatment of children and adolescents with suicidal behavior. *Journal of the American Academy of Child and Adolescent Psychiatry, 40*, 24S–51S.

Shaffii, M., Carrigan, S., Whittinghill, J. R., & Derrick, A. (1985). Psychological autopsy of completed suicide in children and adolescents. *American Journal of Psychiatry, 142*, 1061–1064.

Sher, L. (2006). Alcoholism and suicidal behavior: A clinical overview. *Acta Psychiatric Scandinavia, 113*, 13–22.

Shields, L. B., Hunsaker, D. M., & Hunsaker, J. C. (2007). Schizophrenia and suicide: A 10-year review of Kentucky medical examiner cases. *Journal of Forensic Sciences, 52*, 930–937.

Shneidman, E. S. (1975). Psychiatric emergencies: Suicide. In A. M. Freedman, H. Kaplan, & B. J. Sadock, (Eds.). *Comprehensive textbook of psychiatry* (Vol. 2), (pp. 1774–1785). Baltimore: Williams & Wilkins.

Shneidman, E. S. (1985). *Definition of suicide*. New York: Wiley.

Suominen, K., Isometsä, E., Ostamo, A., & Lönnqvist, J. (2004). Level of suicidal intent predicts overall mortality and suicide after attempted suicide: A 12-year follow-up study. *BioMed Central Psychiatry, 4,* 11. Published online 2004 April 20. doi: 10.1186/1471-244X-4-11

van Minnen, A., Hoogduin, K. A. L., Keijsers, G. P. J., Hellenbrand, I., & Hendriks, G-J. (2003). Treatment of trichotillomania with behavioral therapy and fluoxetine. *Archives of General Psychiatry, 60,* 517–522.

Vogt, M. (1982). Some functional aspects of central serotonergic neurons. In N. N. Osbow (Ed.), *Biology of serotonergic neurotransmission* (pp. 299–316). Chichester, England: John Wiley & Sons.

Wallace, J. D., Calhoun, A. D., Powell, K. E., O'Neil, J., & James, S. P. (1996). *Homicide and suicide among Native Americans, 1979–1992. Violence surveillance summary series, no. 2.* Atlanta: CDC, National Injury and Prevention and Control.

Winchel, R. M., & Stanley, M. (1992). Self-injurious behavior: A review of behavior and biology of self-mutilation. *American Journal of Psychiatry, 148,* 306–317.

Wingate, L. R., Joiner, T. E. Jr., Walker, R. L., Rudd, M. D., & Jobes, D. A. (2004). Empirically informed approaches to topics in suicide risk assessment. *Behavioral Science Law, 22,* 651–665.

Zayas, L. H., Lester, R. J., Cabassa, L. J., & Fortuna, L. R. (2005). Why do so many latina teens attempt suicide? A conceptual model for research. *American Journal of Orthopsychiatry, 75,* 275–287.

SUGGESTED READINGS

Ganong, W. F. (1999). *Review of medical physiology* (19th ed.). Stamford, CT: Appleton & Lange.

Spector, R. E. (1996). *Cultural diversity in health & illness* (4th ed.). Stamford, CT: Appleton & Lange.

The Indian Health Services. (2005). The Indian Health Service suicide prevention work plan. *The IHS Primary Care Provider, 30,* 1–20. Available online at http://www.ihs.gov/NonMedicalPrograms/nspn/file/Sept05_Provider.pdf

Waern, M., Runeson, B. S., Allebeck, P., Beskow, J. Rubenowitz, E., Skoog, I., et al. (2002). Mental disorder in elderly suicides: A case-control study. *American Journal of Psychiatry, 159,* 450–455.

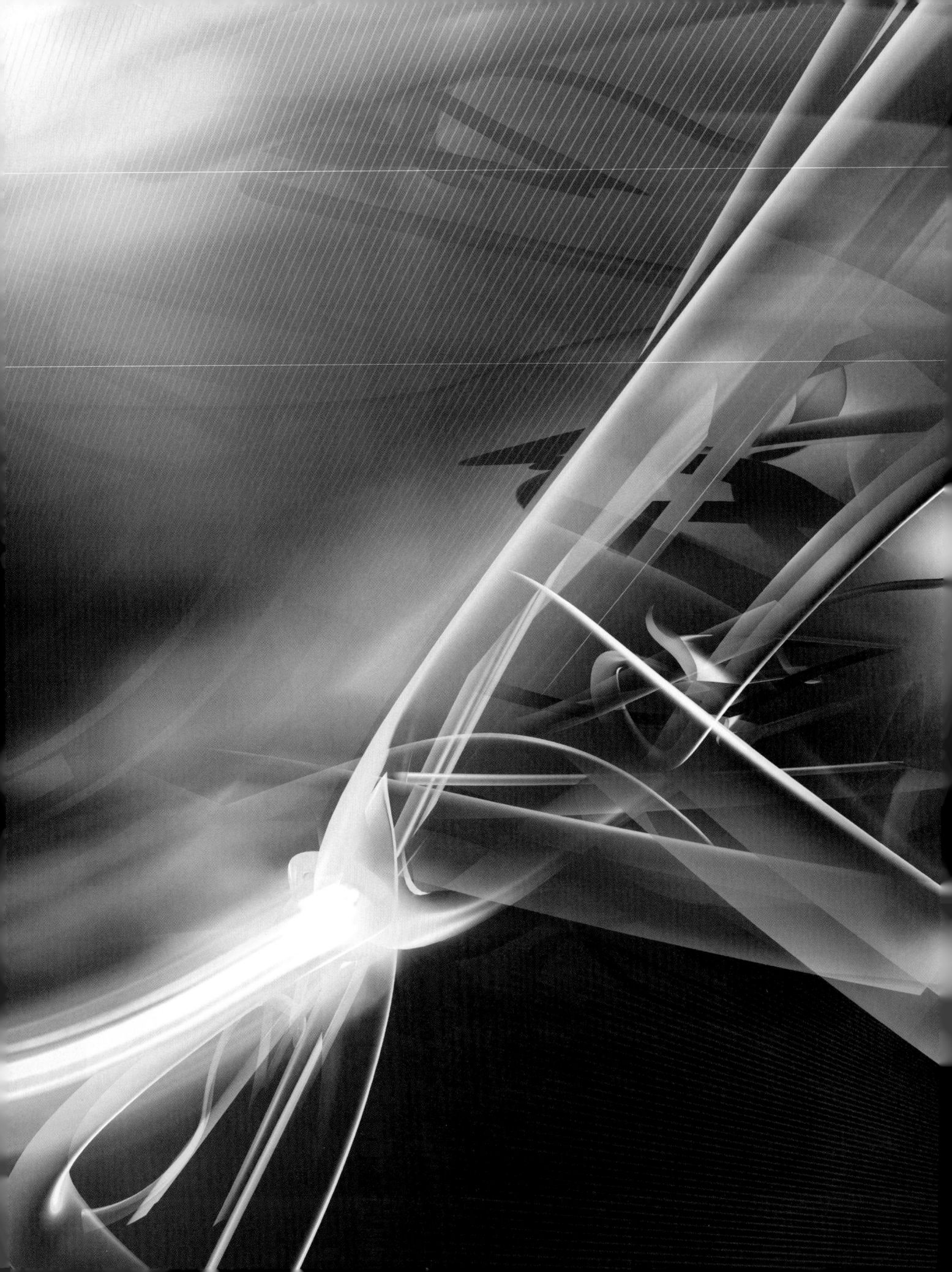

CHAPTER 20

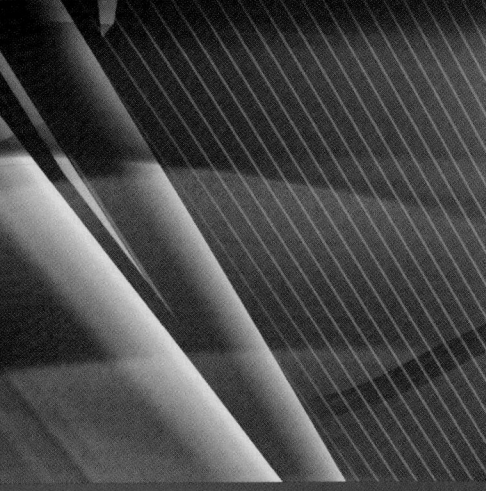

The Client Exhibiting Aggression, Hostility, and Violence

Deborah Antai-Otong, MS, APRN, BC, FAAN

KEY TERMS

Acting Out Refers to living out unresolved developmental issues or fantasies impulsively in behavior.

Aggression: Refers to hostile, injurious, or destructive behavior or outlook, particularly when caused by frustration.

Agitation: To give motion to or disturb. It also refers to a state of increased mental and motor activity.

Assault: A violent physical or verbal attack.

De-escalation: Refers to verbal interventions that aim to defuse potentially and actual volatile situations using empathetic, calm, yet firm limit-setting approaches.

Defuse: To reduce tension and harm in a potentially violent situation.

Frustration: A condition that emerges when a goal is blocked. The stronger the frustration, the greater the potential for aggression. It is the single most potent means of provoking aggression.

Hostility: Refers to overt antagonism, opposition, or resistance in thought or principle.

Impulsivity: Closely related to disinhibition and central to conceptions of attention-deficit/hyperactivity disorder (ADHD) and personality disorders and the aggressive spectrum or disruptive behaviors disorders.

Physical Assault: Attacks ranging from slapping and beating to rape, homicide, and the use of weapons such as knives, firearms, or bombs.

Physical Restraint: Any physical or mechanical device, material, or equipment that is attached to or placed adjacent to the client's body that cannot be removed easily by the client and limits freedom of movement or normal access to one's body.

Restraint: A physical or chemical intervention to deter a client from movement that results in injury.

Seclusion: Placing and keeping a client in a bare room (free of sharp or dangerous objects) for the purpose of containing a clinical situation that may evolve or has evolved into an emergent situation.

Stress Debriefing: A crisis intervention technique that relies on three therapeutic modalities: provide an opportunity to express one's feelings in the context of group support, facilitate normalization of reactions to an abnormal event, and learn about postdisaster reactions.

Time-Out: A behavior modification method that involves restriction of the youth for a period of time to an assigned area from which the child is not physically restricted from leaving for the purpose of providing the child an opportunity to regain self-control.

Violence: Verbal abuse or threatening behavior, damage to property, self-harm, and physical aggression.

COMPETENCIES

Upon completion of this chapter, the learner should be able to:

1. Understand causative factors of aggression, hostility, and violence.
2. Identify high-risk factors for aggressive and violent behavior.
3. Recognize behaviors that preclude aggression.
4. List the steps of defusing and de-escalation.
5. Discuss the role of the nurse in caring for the client who exhibits or is at risk for aggression, hostility, and violence.
6. Identify legal and ethical responsibilities about violence and threats to harm others.
7. Discuss the purpose and major aspects of stress debriefing.

A **36-year-old man** shows up in the emergency department (ED) smelling of alcohol and demanding to be seen. He is pacing, talking loudly, and cursing nursing staff. This scenario occurs often in EDs and psychiatric, geriatric, and primary care settings. Nurses are on the frontline of health care and at great risk of harm unless they are appropriately trained to defuse these situations and recognize that violence in any form must be taken seriously. Results from a 2003–2005 national audit of inpatient and outpatient settings in the United Kingdom found that 36 percent of inpatients, 41 percent of clinical staff, and nearly 80 percent of nursing staff in psychiatric mental health experienced violence or threats of violence

(Healthcare Commission and Royal College of Psychiatrists, 2005). Defuse means to reduce tension and harm in a potentially volatile situation. De-escalate is another term that applies to tense situations. Nurses use de-escalation by employing verbal limit setting or interventions that aim to defuse potentially and actual volatile situations.

The prevalence and nature of client aggression and violence in health care have long been minimized and neglected. Client aggression occurs more often than client violence, with a substantial number of psychiatric nurses generally being threatened. Anecdotal data suggest that psychiatric nurses are less likely to report violent incidents, hence the failure to implement proactive policies for preventing violent events. This premise supports the debate that violence is often seen as part of the job. Fortunately, nowadays, concerns about the severity and frequency of client violence toward nurses and other health care providers are being reported more frequently perhaps because of the resulting serious morbidity for clients and staff (Bowers, Allan, Simpson, Nijman, & Warren, 2007).

Violence in various practice settings, including psychiatric inpatient, geriatrics, ED, and inpatient settings, is well documented and has become a significant health care concern in many facilities (Bowers et al., 2007; Occupational Safety and Health Administration [OSHA], 2004).

According to a survey of health care workers at one ED in Vancouver, respondents in this study reported a 1-year prevalence of 92 percent for physical assault and 97 percent for physical threats, and 66 percent reported verbal abuse at least once per shift. Nurses and male physicians were at a greater risk of assault, and receptionists were at the least risk (Fernandes et al., 1999).

Violence is not limited to the ED although it has become the portal for persons with psychiatric disorders who lack access to health care. Data from several studies exploring the risk of violence in inpatient psychiatric facilities demonstrate that violence is most likely to occur during times of high activity and interactions with clients, such as meal times, bathing hours, and client transportation. Violence is also likely to occur when services are denied, when clients are involuntarily admitted, or when health care providers set limits on eating, drinking, smoking, or consuming other drugs (Badger & Mullan, 2004). One particular study conducted by Crilly, Chaboyer, and Creedy (2004) showed that most nurses (n = 71) in their study of violence in the ED found that clients were often seen during the evening hour, under the influence of alcohol and other drugs, and exhibited behaviors and symptoms of mental illness. Many studies show that assaults usually occur when there is interaction between nurses and clients, for instance, when clients are asked to take medication, and use of duress or limit setting.

The aim of this chapter is to introduce the learner to major assumptions and theories associated with violence and aggression across the life span. It also emphasizes the significance of personal, staff, and client safety; preventive approaches to violence; and legal implications. Finally, it describes the role of the nurse and the implementation of the nursing process when caring for the client at risk for violent and aggressive behaviors.

DEFINITIONS

Agitation originates from the Latin word *agitatus* and means "to give motion to or disturb." It also refers to a state of increased mental and motor activity. Clients exhibiting agitated states are often verbally and physically threatening and can abruptly become violent.

Aggression stems from the Latin word *aggressus*, which means "to attack." It is further defined as a forceful unprovoked act described as hostile, injurious, or destructive, particularly when caused by frustration. Aggressive behaviors involve those that are marked by combativeness readiness, driving forceful energy, or initiative. Perception, intolerance, miscommunication, and a sense of powerlessness or helplessness often fuel aggression.

Assault stems from the French word *assaltus*, which means "a violent or verbal attack and effort to do harm to another."

Hostility, or hostile, is marked by unfriendliness, antagonism, or opposition and stems from the Latin word *hostilis* and "relates to the enemy." Hostile people are distant, distrustful, and antagonistic and are in a mode that prepares them to defend themselves by attacking others. Behaviors associated with hostility include restlessness, defensiveness, argumentativeness, pacing, irritability, and agitation.

Impulsivity has become a key concept in the determinants of violence and aggression. Impulsiveness and impulsive aggression have significant correlation with physical violence. Loss of impulse control is associated with disinhibition and is central to conceptions of borderline, antisocial and other personality disorders, attention-deficit/hyperactivity disorder (ADHD), and medical conditions such as delirium and dementia, and substance-related disorders.

Violence, or violent, refers to the Latin word *violare*, which means "to violate." Violence is linked to hostility and aggression and generates high energy in both the survivor and perpetrator. Examples of violence include kicking, beating, grabbing, spitting, choking, pushing, forcing sex, and using a weapon.

Perhaps the single issue that concerns most nurses is the client at risk for aggression and violence. Clients exhibiting violent and aggressive behaviors evoke fear, anger, a sense of helplessness, and thoughts of retaliation. Despite these challenges nurses can successfully manage personal reactions by making personal safety a priority and by implementing proactive interventions that reduce the risk of violence and promote personal safety.

Knowledge of causative and risk factors associated with aggression and violence can help nurses assess and manage risk. The following section discusses the epidemiology and incidence of violence and reviews major underpinnings associated with aggressive and violent behaviors.

EPIDEMIOLOGY AND INCIDENCE

Growing empirical studies implicate psychiatric disorders as a risk factor for aggressive and violent behaviors across the life span (Fazel & Grann, 2006; Swanson et al., 2006). Higher rates are now firmly established most prominently for persons with diagnoses of substance-related disorders, followed by cluster B personality disorders (e.g., borderline, antisocial) and less frequently in persons with schizophrenia (Corrigan & Watson, 2005). While violence is less likely to occur in persons with schizophrenia, researchers submit that persons with schizophrenia and bipolar mania, particularly with active psychotic symptoms and specifically paranoid delusions and command hallucinations, have been associated with a history of assaults (Beck, 2004). Albeit delusions can precipitate violence in some cases, there is a lack of consensus that show that they increase the overall risk of violence in persons with mental illness discharged from acute inpatient units (Beck, 2004). Despite this debate, nurses must assess for delusions and other psychotic symptoms and base their assessment of the potential for aggression and violence on individual symptoms and risk factors (e.g., coexisting substance-related disorders).

Further research is necessary to determine the degree to which a single factor is predominant in causing assaults committed by individuals over time. Despite controversy, the risk of violence results in serious morbidity in nurses caring for persons with sundry psychiatric disorders. While there is a high prevalence of violence among clients with psychiatric disorder, not all violent people are mentally ill nor are all persons with psychiatric conditions violent. Comprehending the etiology of aggression and violence offers nurses a rational basis for using the nursing process to assess, diagnose, identify outcomes, utilize nursing interventions, and evaluate treatment outcomes involving aggressive and violent behaviors.

CAUSATIVE FACTORS

Aggression results from the interaction of an array of systems and processes. It can be defined as predatory, impulsive, or it can stem from underlying medical conditions. Environmental stress or trauma, dysregulation of multiple biochemical processes including dopamine and serotonin transmission, and alterations in neuroanatomical structures within the context of impulsivity heighten the likelihood of aggressive and disruptive behaviors.

Collectively interactions among systems interfere with the person's ability to reason, control impulses, and employ nonviolent means and effective coping skills and expand the risk of violence. This section reviews various theories that have been proposed to account for aggression and violence.

PSYCHODYNAMIC THEORIES

Sigmund Freud's (1960) psychoanalytic theory views aggression as a basic drive (like thirst). He held that many of our actions are determined by instincts, particularly sexual. When expression of these instincts is frustration, aggressive drives emerge. He believed that from birth to death a person possesses two conflicting instincts: a life instinct (eros) that encourages a person to grow and survive, and a death instinct (thanatos) that drives people to redirect the death instinct or self-destructiveness from self toward others. His theory also proposes that the body constantly generates energy for self-destructiveness and if the individual fails to channel or modulate this energy effectively, it eventually amasses and is released in a maladaptive or aggressive manner. He also submitted that antisocial behavior involves a defective ego that is combined with an immature or ineffective superego, resulting in the individual being unable to control or modulate his or her behavior, but experiencing little guilt due to his or her inability. His theory also proposed that one way to minimize accumulation of noxious energy was to drain it off safely through catharsis (a Greek word for *purification* or *cleansing*) through crying, verbalization, physical activities, or various symbolic means. Freud's theory on aggression has been criticized for its failure to delineate factors that could be used to predict aggression or its specific character.

Konrad Lorenz (1966), an ethologist, endorsed Freud's theory of catharsis, and asserted that people should engage in competitive sports in order to reduce aggression. His theory also emphasized the innateness of aggression based on animal studies. He submitted that people share certain instincts with other organisms and that aggression is spontaneous and crucial for survival. He further submitted that aggression stems from territoriality and an innate drive to gain and defend property. He also postulated that a certain balance exists between inclinations to fight and flight, with the inclination to fight being the strongest in the center of the territory and the inclination to flight being the strongest when it was farthest from the center. Based on his assertions, aggression emerges as a function of the sum of accumulated energy and the presence of aggression-releasing stimuli.

SOCIAL LEARNING THEORIES

Social learning theorists view aggression as a learned response that is based on the assumption that role modeling, identification, and human interactions shape learning and behavior (Dutton, 2000; Trocki & Caetano, 2003). This model stresses the role of transmitting both specific behavior and emotional responses. Aggression can be learned through observation or imitation, and the more often it is reinforced, the more likely it occurs. According to Albert Bandura (1977, 1986), observing violence is likely to lead to violence, particularly during childhood and adolescence. This argument has been strengthened by other studies that implicate exposure to family violence and temperament as a predictor of adult antisocial behaviors (Bartholow, Sestir, & Davis, 2005). Most people have observed children imitating adults in a variety of ways, such as reading the newspaper and yelling at the dog. Another example of observation and imitation is a child who observes a parent hitting the family pet and later mocks the parent by hitting the pet. The relationship between exposure to aggression in the media and children's aggression has been well researched (Bartholow et al., 2005).

In addition, children who experience abuse or severe punishment are likely to be more aggressive than average; the parents role model the learned behavior. A number of children who participated in studies involving exposure to violent video games and subsequent violent and aggressive behavior found that the students rated their peers' aggressive behavior and reported that they perceived the world as scary and mean. Hence, observing violence introduces new ways to be violent and activate cardiovascular arousal, diminishes helping behaviors, and makes violence more sociably acceptable. Data also showed that playing video games could lead to the automatic learning of aggressive self-views (Anderson, 2004; Uhlmann & Swanson, 2004). Most studies indicate that irrespective of age, observing violence with repeated exposure to real life and to entertainment may alter cognitive, affective, and behavioral processes, perhaps resulting in desensitization. Albeit these findings are disturbing, new data indicate that when interventions to reduce television, videotapes, and video games were implemented, aggression in elementary children was decreased. These data support the causal relationship between media and aggression and the potential benefits of reducing media exposure in this age group (Bartholow et al., 2005; Ulhmann & Swanson, 2004). (See Controversy Box.)

While some theorists assert that psychodynamic and social factors may explain some aspects of violent and aggressive behaviors, most believe that they fail to explain the complexity of innate and social and complex biological and genetic influences associated with violence.

BIOLOGICAL THEORIES

Technological advances in neurobiology provide a better explanation of the role of genetics and complex biological processes that mediate stress, environmental, and social factors in the etiology of aggression and violence.

Neurobiological and Neuroanatomical Factors

The advent of brain imaging research makes it possible to directly assess brain functioning. Typically, emotion is regulated in the human brain by a complex circuit comprised of the orbital frontal cortex, amygdala, anterior cingulate cortex, and several interconnected pathways. Genetic and environmental factors mediate the structure and function of this circuitry. Faulty wiring of this neural circuitry pathway or emotional modulation is a possible prelude to impulsive aggressive and violent behaviors (Berlin, Rolls, & Iversen, 2005).

In addition, the hippocampus and amygdala (located within the temporal lobe), which are involved in emotional responsiveness, may be activated by an interpersonal trigger. This process is facilitated by serotonin in the orbitofrontal cortex (OFC) and anterior cingulated gyrus (ACG) regions (Berlin et al., 2005). The ACG region is implicated in the affective-cognitive activity, and the OFC is implicated in the sensory processing and possibly fear-generating stimuli. Dysfunction or decreased activation or damage in the OFC and ACG regions may play a role in the regulation of negative emotion through reduced serotonin-mediated activation of the prefrontal cortex, and heighten the risk of impulsive aggression, hostility, and violence (Berlin et al., 2005).

Several studies also implicate abnormalities in the amygdala and the prefrontal cortex with the hyperarousal-dyscontrol control states observed in clients with intermittent explosive disorder (IED) and antisocial personality disorder (Dolan & Fullam, 2006). Other studies have substantiated these conclusions and found that persons with IED exhibited poor impulse control, explosive aggressive outbursts, and lack of sensitivity in response to interpersonal emotional cues such as perceived rejection or disrespect. These behaviors often occurred within the context of intact cognitive, motor, and sensory function (Berlin et al., 2005).

A host of additional brain regions, such as white mater tracts in impulse-control disorders are associated with violence and aggression (Dyer, Bell, McCann, & Rausch, 2006). Specifically, persons with histories of traumatic brain injury (TBI) and other brain disorders have exhibited poor impulse control and behavioral symptoms due to neurophysiological deficits. Aggressive behaviors associated with post TBI and other neuropsychiatric conditions, especially during the acute period, can prevent clients from receiving necessary care and disrupt their rehabilitation process. These behaviors must be quickly assessed and managed to facilitate positive treatment outcomes.

 CRITICAL THINKING

Do Violent Video Games and Other Media Really Contribute to Violence in Our Youth?
There is growing evidence that link media violence with childhood and adolescent aggression and violence. Some argue that violent video games and other media violence have minimal impact on violence in these age groups and that this controversy is overemphasized. Others disagree with this notion and have strong evidence that strengthens the argument that exposure to media violence and violent video games have a definite negative impression on children and adolescents and increase the risk of aggression and violence. Regardless, nurses must develop proactive approaches and educate parents, teachers, religious organizations, and youth about the potential harmful effects of media violence, including violent video games, on violence and aggression among our youth and society.

Neuroanatomical alterations resulting from TBI may result in deactivation of the lateral and dorsal prefrontal cortices and enhance activation of various limbic structures, including the amygdala (Jorge et al., 2004). Implications from these findings suggest that these clients have difficulty modulating their emotional response and are at high risk for impulsive aggression and violence. Likewise, clients with other compromised frontal lobe and executive function neurophysiological deficits (e.g., Alzheimer's disease, schizophrenia), particularly with psychosis, are also at a greater risk of these behaviors (Dyer et al., 2006; Naudts & Hodgins, 2007). Other studies indicate that hypometabolism or atrophy in the right inferior frontal region and orbital frontal areas correlate with clinical severity of delusions in AD (Dyer et al., 2006; Naudts & Hodgins, 2007).

Neurophysiological Influences

Early scientists suspected that gross brain dysfunction increased the risk of violent behaviors. Studies using electroencephalogram (EEG), and neurological and cognitive tests in clients with partial seizures who exhibited violent behavior repeatedly found the temporal lobe to be the brain region responsible for aggressive behavior. These findings, however, were mainly nonspecific and researchers were unable to replicate them owing to methodological flaws (Raine, Lencz, Bihrle, LaCasse, & Colletti, 2000). Despite these early assertions, the role of the temporal lobe, epilepsy, and violence continues to be debated.

Researchers continue to link various brain regions, including specific areas in the temporal lobe, to aggressive and violent behaviors. In a study of the relationship of EEG abnormalities and violent criminal behavior in 222 defendants referred for psychiatric evaluation, Pillman and his colleagues (1999) discovered left hemispheric focal (temporal lobe) abnormalities in a large number of violent offenders. Most of these cases were comorbid with other brain disorders, including intellectual disabilities, epilepsy, or early brain damage. Findings from this study strengthen the debate that links the propensity for violence in individuals with abnormalities in the temporal lobe brain regions. Contemporary neuroimaging data confirm earlier findings that demonstrate alterations in neuroanatomical regions, namely the prefrontal cortex and amydala, and their role in violent and aggressive behaviors and an increase in white matter volume (Coccaro, McClosky, Fitzgerald, & Phan, 2007; Yang et al., 2007).

Biochemical Theories

There is compelling evidence that links abnormalities in central serotonin activity to impulsive aggression (Frankle et al., 2005; Völlm et al., 2006). Supposedly, reduced central serotonin (5-HT) system function is associated with decreased behavioral constraint and subsequent higher risk of aggressive behaviors. Many behavioral problems and violent impulse control exhibited in persons with ADHD and antisocial personality appear to be mediated by brain serotonergic systems. Most data support the notion that decreased cerebrospinal fluid (CSF) and 5-HT metabolite, 5-hydroxyindoleacetic acid (5-HIAA) may be a biological marker of impulsivity rather than a specific type of violence. Furthermore, these findings indicate that 5-HT plays a role in inhibiting, aggressive behavior in persons with personality disorders and may play a role in suicide and other aggressive behaviors (Frankle et al., 2005; Völlm et al., 2006).

Additional biochemical theories associated with impulsive aggression and violence involve aberrations in dopaminergic and noradrenergic systems that are limbic in nature. Abnormalities in these regions and neural pathways may also contribute to cognitive impairments, as manifested by executive function deficits, reduced moral reasoning, and impaired empathetic ability and the likelihood of adult antisocial behavior and violent impulse-control disorders (Dyer et al., 2006).

Neuroendocrine Theories

Many hormones, including testosterone, progesterone, luteinizing hormone, renin, ß-endorphin, prolactin, and melatonin are involved in the mediation of aggressive behavior. Most studies involving animal and human subjects indicate that aggression is mediated by the hypothalamus-pituitary-adrenal (HPA) axis and that stimulation of various brain regions in this area and activation of cortisol, past experiences, and social influence play critical roles in the neuroendocrinology of aggression. Findings from animal studies demonstrate that mild electrical stimulation of specific brain regions in the hypothalamus produce aggressive and sometimes fatal behavior. In contrast, studies using higher mammals, such as instinctive patterns of aggression, found that aggression was controlled by the cortex and influenced by experience and social influences.

Biological markers involving the neuroendocrine system have been indirectly corroborated by neuroendocrine challenges. Specifically, neuroendocrine challenges using a single dose of fenfluramine increase plasma levels of prolactin. Serotonin mediates this response; hence the prolactin elevation measures central 5-HT activity (Frankle et al., 2005; Oquendo et al., 2006). Prolactin response is reduced in aggressive subjects and is believed to be more sensitive than the CSF 5-HT. As previously discussed the aggressive behaviors are associated with dysregulation of serotonin activity (Frankle et al., 2005; Oquendo et al., 2006).

Studies assessing CSF 5-HIAA concentrations or neuroendocrine responses to challenge doses of 5-HT agonist (fenfluramine) have consistently demonstrated either inverse correlations with indices of aggression and prolactin response (Frankle et al., 2005; Oquendo et al., 2006) or diminished function in some aggressive individuals. Findings from a prospective study that examined the relationship between serotonin function measured in prepubertal children with ADHD and adult antisocial personality disorder demonstrated that decreased serotonergic responsivity evaluated in children predicted the development of antisocial personality disorder (Flory, Newcorn, Miller, Harty, & Halperin, 2007). These data implicate that the differences between adult responses to the neuroendocrine challenge and those found in prepubertal boys may be associated with their age or ADHD (Flory et al., 2007).

Recent studies of low resting cortisol levels and aggression in preadolescents and adolescents have generated considerable interest. This potential biological marker or predictor of dyscontrol behaviors in this age group continues to be debated, while some studies indicate that it may be predictive of personality traits (e.g., antisocial) over time (van Goozen, Fairchild, Snoek, & Harold, 2007). Similar findings have been seen in children with comorbid ADHD and conduct disorders (CD) that demonstrated lower cortisol concentrations at rest and response to stress (van Goozen et al., 2007). Even as the precise mechanism that links low cortisol concentration and persistent aggression is poorly understood, results from some animal studies implicated prenatal and early developmental stress that produced alterations of the HPA axis.

The ability to modulate these complex processes is guided by numerous factors, including biochemical, neuroanatomical, and neurobiological processes that may be compromised in persons already at high risk for impulsive aggression or violence, such as those with major psychiatric disorders and medical conditions. Adaptive physiological arousal and responsiveness to a threatening or fearful event are likely to enable the client to resolve the situation effectively. Failure to mediate adaptive process increases the risk of frustration and aggressive or destructive behavior.

Neuroimaging Studies

Neuroimaging studies consistently demonstrate abnormalities in three brain regions: dorso-lateral prefrontal cortex, regions of the basal ganglia, and the cerebellum. Abnormalities in these regions are found in persons with ADHD when compared to control groups (Makris et al., 2007; Yang et al., 2007). Abnormalities in these structural regions have also been found in adults with antisocial personality disorder and disruptive behaviors associated with ADHD and CD. Hereditary influences, neuroimaging data, and the efficacy of psychopharmacological agents as anti-aggressive agents strengthen the connection between ADHD and aggressive and violent behaviors and biological substrates (see Chapter 17, The Client with Attention-Deficit Disorder).

GENETIC INFLUENCES

There is a preponderance of evidence from family, pedigree, twin, adoption, and molecular genetic studies of the heritability of some psychiatric disorders such as ADHD, disruptive behavior disorder (DBD), oppositional defiant disorder (ODD), and CD. Data from these findings suggest that these and other disorders associated with aggression are highly heritable and are impacted by environmental influences (American Psychiatric Association [APA], 2000; Kutcher et al., 2004; Scourfield, van den Bree, Martin, & McGuffin, 2004). The notion that a child with ADHD is likely to have at least one parent with this disorder also implicates the role of genetic vulnerability.

Several studies directed at elucidating the link between genetic predisposition of violence show variation in physical aggression and heritability estimates as high as 0.58 in adults and 0.32 in adolescents (Baker, Jacobson, Raine, Lozano, & Bezdjian, 2007; Bartels et al., 2007; Rowe, Almeida, & Jacobson, 1999). Regardless of diagnosis, some scientists have attempted to subtype aggression that can be demonstrated in various psychiatric conditions, including ADHD, DBD, borderline personality disorder, ODD, exacerbation of psychotic conditions, and neurodegenerative disorders.

GENDER

People often assume that men are more violent than women with psychiatric disorders because in the general population men are more physically aggressive than women on numerous measures of aggression (Maguire & Pastore, 2003). Findings from some studies indicate the opposite and suggest that psychiatric disorders actually reduce the gender difference and in some cases eliminate them completely (Krakowski & Czobor, 2004). More detailed analysis of violence showed that male clients have a greater prevalence of more serious violence involving weapons and injury in the 4 months preceding hos-pitalization than women, but there were no gender differences when measures of violence that were more inclusive were used. Other data suggest that women were more violent than men during the 3 days post admission (Krakowski & Czobor, 2004). Most researchers assert that there is an overlap in the expression of violence and in the factors that contribute to its emergence in men and women, specifically psychosis and behavioral disturbances and other inclinations that vary according to gender. For example, in women, physical violence may occur with high arousal and excitation associated with acute psychosis, whereas acute symptoms in men may play a lesser role in the emergence of violence, but psychosis may foster more chronic inclinations associated with antisocial behaviors (Krakowski & Czobor, 2004).

In a 2006 national study of violence in persons with schizophrenia, researchers found that younger women with coexisting substance-use disorders were more likely to engage in minor violence than men (Swanson et al., 2006). These findings are consistent with previous studies that indicate that staff often underestimate violence among females and overestimate violence in males. For these reasons, data continue to support the premise that injuries to staff members on inpatient units treating men and women are as likely to be caused by women as by men. Implications from these findings suggest that when a female exhibits signs of escalation, her behavior should not be minimized on the basis of gender.

MOOD DISORDERS

In addition to previously discussed psychiatric disorders, mood disorders, particularly bipolar disorders, increase the risk of violence. Agitated psychotic depression associated with hypomania or mania refers to a mixed state manifested by depressed mood, psychomotor agitation, and flight of ideas. Like other psychiatric disorders, these symptoms increase the risk of violence. Additional symptoms of agitated depression in bipolar I disorder (history of at least one manic episode) include severe agitation, intractable insomnia, suicidal obsessions and impulses, restlessness, racing thoughts, despair, depressed mood, and unendurable sexual excitement. Other psychiatric disorders not mentioned in this chapter, such as post-traumatic stress disorder, are also associated with aggression and assaultive behaviors.

ENVIRONMENTAL AND SOCIOECONOMIC FACTORS

Environmental factors often contribute to aggression and violence such as exposure and learned behavior either prenatally, due to childhood abuse; witnessing violence either through one's family, culture, or the media; or owing to socioeconomic factors such as poverty and family disorganization. Prenatal influences include exposure to toxins, such as alcohol and resultant brain damage that results a high propensity for neurobehavioral anomalies, cognitive deficits, and impaired executive function (Hazen, Connelly, Kelleher, Barth, & Landsverk, 2006).

Home environments play a prominent role in shaping behavior, including violence (Hazen et al., 2006), and are continuously mediated by genetic and other environmental influences. Childhood frustration, violence in the home, oppression, and hostility have been linked to various psychiatric conditions where individuals are at a high risk of aggressive behaviors, such as intermittent explosive disorder (APA, 2000). Accessibility to guns and exposure to violent media, videos, and television are linked to violence among children (Bartholow et al., 2005).

PSYCHOSOCIAL FACTORS

Psychosocial factors associated with aggression and violence include inadequate social skills required to resolve conflicts or violent encounters. This belief suggests that anger is morally and social acceptable or expected. Numerous studies link ineffective anger management with violence, particularly among persons with intellectual disabilities, and psychiatric and medical disorders that involve impaired cognitive and executive functioning (Novaco & Taylor, 2004; Smith, Waterman, & Ward, 2006).

Common causes of anger and aggression also include a sense of powerlessness, loss of self-esteem, or the belief that someone else has been treated unfairly. In addition, ineffective coping skills and an inability to cope with and manage anger effectively, misinterpretations of the intentions of others, low self-esteem, and a sense of hopelessness about the future are key contributors to aggression across the life span.

SAFETY CONSIDERATIONS

A safe environment is everyone's responsibility. There is no single solution to preventing violence or ensuring workplace safety. However, proactive and preventive measures are necessary to ensure workplace safety and afford emotional support during the aftermath of a violent or traumatic incident. The following section focuses on the role of administrators and staff in creating a safe work environment.

ADMINISTRATIVE AND STAFF RESPONSIBILITIES

Personal and staff safety must be a priority for all nurses regardless of their practice setting. Several strategies are required to ensure personal safety. First, administrative staff must create a culture of zero tolerance of violence. Policies must be established that guide staff, consumers, and clients and their families about this expectation. Environmental factors that increase the risk of violence include a lack of administrative support to maintain a safe work environment, including poorly written policies that fail to mandate annual training for all staff. See Box 20-1 for additional environmental factors that reduce workplace safety. Additional administrative responsibilities that foster safer work environments include:

- Allocating and implementing emergency signals, alarms, and monitoring systems
- Installing security devices such as metal detectors, strategically placed cameras, and good lighting in the hallways and parking areas

Box 20–1: Risk Factors for Violence—Environmental

- Working with high-risk groups
- Transporting clients
- Long waits for service
- Working alone
- Poor environmental design
- Inadequate or inappropriately trained security or staff
- Crowdedness
- Loud noises
- Access to firearms and other weapons
- Inappropriate interviewing or treatment arranged room
- Lack of staff training and policies on the prevention and management of disturbed behaviors
- Lack of administrative support for zero tolerance of workplace violence
- Unrestricted movement of the public
- Poorly lit corridors, rooms, parking lots, and other areas

- Providing security escorts to the parking lot at night
- Developing waiting areas to accommodate and assist visitors and clients
- Designing the triage area, emergency rooms, and other public areas to reduce the risk of assault
- Establishing a call system that alerts teams to assist staff involved in potential and actual violent situations

Awareness and Training

One of the most critical components of a facility or agency's violence prevention is training. Training is necessary for nurses and other employees and supervisors who may be involved in responding to violent incidents. Participation in training sessions helps staff recognize and report incidents of violence, intimidation, and threatening and disruptive behaviors. Developing policies and providing staff training on the management of disruptive behaviors enable nurses to advance proactive activities within their organization and create safer workplaces. Ideally, annual training concerning the prevention and management of disturbed behaviors should be provided, and policies that delineate zero tolerance of violence should be implemented. Non-mental health staff may opt for annual training that entails verbal de-escalation and escape techniques. Refer to the dialogue box for an example of how to communicate with an aggressive client.

Secondly, prior to taking a client into a room, particularly alone, it is imperative to inquire about weapons, such as "Mr. Jones, are you carrying a weapon?" Any object can be used as a weapon. Nurses should never see an armed client. Remember, most clients carrying or holding a weapon are just as frightened as the nurse. All weapons must be surrendered to trained security. In the event that a client brings a weapon into the assessment or evaluation area, it important for the nurse to remain calm and use strategies listed in the dialogue box "When a Client Has a Weapon."

Thirdly, if the client is deemed dangerous (e.g., yelling, physically aggressive, threatening) before taking him or her into the office, a decision of whether to actually see the client in the waiting area, a safe place (e.g., security), or an office alone must be made immediately. If the nurse opts to see the client alone in an office, the door must remain open and a third person should stand near or outside the door to ensure safety. It is imperative to afford adequate personal space to reduce anxiety and mitigate the client's symptoms and defuse a potentially volatile situation. A failure to create and maintain a safe work environment places the nurse, staff, and clients at risk of dire consequences, including serious injury and death.

Finally, provisions for safety also involve arranging furniture that allows the nurse to sit between the client and the door without obstructing the space. Easy access to the door affords a safe escape in the event of an escalating or violent episode and/or the need to summon assistance. Chairs should be equal in height and the nurse must avoid towering or standing over the client or vice versa. Remove all dangerous objects, such as scissors and other sharps from the desk.

It is imperative to be familiar with policies and procedures concerning restraints, seclusion, and the use of panic buttons. Uninformed staff may perceive panic buttons or alerts as a false sense of security. Depending on the workstation, staff response to panic alerts varies and is often unreliable.

Certain clients may pose a greater risk of violence than others do. Clients who are overtly confused or delirious, intoxicated or in withdrawal from a substance, or exhibiting high-risk behaviors such as yelling or threatening either verbally or with a weapon are at high risk for violence. Nurses must immediately summon appropriately trained security. Delusions must be assessed for degree of severity, nature, and power to influence the client's action. Never approach an openly hostile client alone. Common sense is a critical part of personal and staff safety regardless of whether you know the client. (See Box 20–2: Individual Characteristics Associated with Violence.)

If you feel uneasy about a clinical situation based on "gut feelings" or assessment of nonverbal cues such as increased agitation, yelling, or restlessness before or during an interview, it is imperative to discontinue the assessment and seek

Nurse-Client Dialogue Box

The client who is yelling and screaming in the waiting area is likely to respond to the nurse who maintains her composure and allows adequate space (e.g., at least a leg's length) to reduce anxiety and speaks in a normal but firm voice.

CLIENT: yells "You make me sick! You remind me of my _____ ex-husband."

NURSE: "Martha, I can see that you are pretty upset. How can I help you?"

CLIENT: yells "You betcha!"

NURSE: "Martha, please lower your voice. It is very difficult for me to help you when you are yelling and cursing."

CLIENT: "That's too damn bad!"

NURSE: "I know that you are upset and I want to help, but if you lower your voice and stop cursing I will do whatever is necessary to help you."

CLIENT: "I am sorry, but I have had a bad day."

NURSE: "I see. Tell me more about your day."

Providing directions such as "lower your voice" or "please sit down" are examples of limit setting. Limit setting provides structure and may decrease anxiety and agitation in clients who already feel anxious, helpless, and out of control. Each situation must be handled based on individual circumstances—there is no such thing as "one size fits all." Depending on the underlying causative factor, medications may be indicated to control psychosis, or a calm approach may reduce her anxiety and assist in de-escalation.

When a Client Has a Weapon

1. Acknowledge that you are afraid, and that it is difficult to help under these circumstances. "Mr. Jones, it is difficult to help you with a gun pointed at me."

2. Assume the client is in control and let him know.

3. Move slowly, cautiously, and deliberately. Avoid startling the client.

4. Maintain a calm, reassuring, and normal voice tone.

5. Maintain eye contact and avoid looking around the room.

6. If the client is willing to surrender the gun, avoid taking it directly, instead ask him to put it on the desk or floor. "Mr. Jones, I want to help you and if you put the weapon on the table or desk, I can."

7. Avoid provoking the client.

8. If the client refuses to surrender the weapon, leave the situation as quickly as possible; push the panic button when escape is impossible.

Box 20–2: Individual Characteristics Associated with Violence

- Loner
- Withdrawn
- Poor interpersonal skills
- Unemployment
- Suspicious of others
- Problems with authority figures
- Mental illness (acute exacerbation of symptoms)
- Frequent mood swings
- History of violence, including domestic violence
- Child abuse history
- Personality disorder (e.g., borderline, antisocial)
- Low frustration tolerance
- Blames others for problems
- Bullied
- History of incarceration
- Juvenile delinquency
- Economic instability
- Lack of concern for others

assistance. In the event of escalating circumstances or overt aggression and violence, personal safety skills listed in Box 20–3 are helpful in de-escalating and defusing a situation. In addition, set firm limits to assist the client in maintaining control by using the following suggestions:

- Be clear, direct, and supportive.
- Exhibit respect for others.
- Offer options if possible (e.g., medication).
- Seek to ensure personal dignity and establish a therapeutic relationship.
- "I understand that you are upset, but it is difficult to assist when you are yelling and threatening."
- "How can I help you?"
- Offer food, beverage or other assistance, or voluntary medication before moving to more intrusive interventions.
- "I will do whatever is necessary to assist you and help you regain control."
- State consequences if necessary.
- Immediately remove yourself from the area and call for assistance if the client continues to escalate or when the violence is imminent.
- Consider restraints when the client is deemed so dangerous to self or others that he or she poses a severe threat that cannot be managed using least restrictive measures. Typically, parenteral medications, such as antipsychotic and benzodiazepine medication, are administered as needed to ensure safety and facilitate the psychiatric assessment. During this period, the client must be closely monitored for side effects, such as emesis or seizures.

- Prevent an involuntary client from eloping before assessment or transfer to a locked facility (sometimes).

Normally, restraints or seclusion are used as a temporary intervention to receive medication, or longer if medication is inappropriate. It is important to explain reasons for using restraints and conditions for them to be removed. Staff training about the application of these procedures and devices is imperative, and every effort must be used to provide the least restrictive measures before putting the client in restraints. Never bargain with a violent client about restraints/seclusion once the decision has been made to use these interventions. For further information about restraints and seclusion refer to:

- Your facility's policies and procedures for the use of restraints and seclusion
- Standards stipulated by the Joint Commission (TJC) (see Internet Resources)
- Legislation stipulated by the Center for Medicaid and Medicare Services (CMS) (see Internet Resources)

Albeit there is no precise measure to predict violence, remember, given the right set of conditions or circumstances, everyone has the potential for violence in order to regain control. Nurses must pay attention to situation-specific cues for the aggressive behaviors in their clients. They must also employ common sense to determine and secure personal

Box 20–3: De-escalation: Personal Safety Skills

- Be concerned about personal safety.
- Use common sense.
- Remain calm and convey being in control.
- Use a normal voice tone.
- Give suggestions, not orders.
- Avoid matching the threats.
- Avoid personalizing comments.
- Approach the client in an unhurried manner.
- Use active listening skills.
- Acknowledge the client's feelings, such as "I know you are angry and upset."
- Afford adequate space—at least a leg's length.
- Avoid using threatening body language (e.g., pointing, hands on hip, yelling, standing over the client, making sudden movements, touching).

safety when assessing, planning, and working with actual and potentially violent clients. It is prudent to ensure personal safety before interviewing a client, particularly before taking a client into a room or area alone. Most clients exhibit warning cues before becoming physically violent. Clients are most likely to exhibit impulsive aggressive or violent behaviors when they are acutely ill and cognitively impaired, such as with withdrawal or delirious states. Using an unhurried and calm approach and using astute observational skills are essential steps in creating a safe work environment. When verbal de-escalation fails to reduce violence, other steps must be taken to ensure staff and client safety, such as restraints and seclusion, as a last resort.

Restraints and Seclusion: Life Span Considerations

Historically, restraints and seclusion were overused to control disruptive and dangerous behaviors, which ultimately resulted in negative treatment outcomes. Excessive reliance on these methods interfered with nurses and other staff creating therapeutic environments and fostering environments that helped clients develop adaptive coping skills to manage stressors in the community. Today, there is a greater public concern and legislation that emphasizes the least restrictive approach to manage aggressive and violent behaviors in adults that involves more behavioral interventions. Most of these changes occurred as a result of heightened media and legislative attention on the use of restraints and seclusion in psychiatric settings, especially among the youth and other populations. As a result of these concerns the Department of Health and Human Services and Health Care Financing Administration (HCFA), now the Centers for Medicare and

Medicaid Services, were created. This legislation was mandated in August 1999, the Interim Financial Rule, for the use of seclusion and restraint in all psychiatric treatment facilities that receive government funding (DHHS, HCFA, 1999). This document was published in the Federal Register on January 22, 2001 (see Box 20–4: Legislative Guidelines on Restraints and Seclusions). Nurses must follow policies and guidelines of their organization for these interventions.

Lastly, seclusion and restraints must never be used to punish the client. Nor should they be applied when the client has a history of previous self-harm or aggressive behavior. Each incident must be individually assessed and based on the current situation and symptoms.

Annual staff training on workplace violence and managing disruptive behaviors is imperative to ensure client and staff safety. Once a decision is made to restrain or seclude, the client must be given ample time to comply. Before placing a client in a gown, he or she must be searched for sharps, belts, or any potentially dangerous object. (See Chapter 8, Legal and Ethical Considerations, for further discussion about legal and ethical issues.)

VIOLENCE AND AGGRESSION ACROSS THE LIFE SPAN

The next section focuses on specific implications for nurses caring for clients exhibiting aggression and violence across the life span.

CHILDHOOD AND ADOLESCENCE

Aggressive and disruptive behaviors in our youth are common and pose serious health care concerns. The precise basis of these behaviors continues to be debated. However, most researchers and clinicians agree that they are multifaceted and stem from psychiatric disorders, neurobiological processes, genetic influences, and social and environmental factors.

Violence in any form during childhood and adolescence has potentially debilitating effects on healthy growth and development in children and adolescents. Its effects have been especially devastating to males and minority youth. Exposure to violence during childhood at home, in school, or in the community is predictably associated with violence and aggression across the life span (Bartels et al., 2007; Hazen et al., 2006). It produces psychological distress, such as depression, poor school and academic performance, and subsequent injury. Most researchers assert that these behaviors also predict poor treatment outcomes and heighten the risk of serious antisocial behaviors in adulthood.

A study conducted by Kosterman, Graham, Hawkins, Catalana, and Herrekenkohl (2001) of violent behaviors in children and young adults between the ages of 13 to 21, identified predictions of violence at age 10. Logistic regression was used to determine the developmental patterns of violence in this group. They found that male gender childhood fighting, early individual characteristics, and early antisocial influences best predicted violence in adolescence. In comparison, these data showed that Asian male gender, prosocial development, female gender, and early school achievement were protective against violence during this period. These results have implications for prevention of violence, particularly during early childhood (Kosterman et al., 2001). Contemporary studies consistently support these findings and implicate adverse childhood events as a predictor of violence across the life span (Herrenkohl et al., 2007; Swaim, Henry, & Kelly, 2006).

Obviously, the transition from childhood to adolescence to adulthood requires adequate adult supervision and guidance, especially including an awareness of the youth's friendship network. Aggression during this period requires immediate attention and interventions, and must be distinguished from normal childhood and adolescent acting out and rebellious behaviors. Acting out refers to living out unresolved developmental issues. Acting out may also be associated with early childhood trauma and conflicting parental attitudes and behaviors and failure to form healthy parental relationships. Observations associated with acting out include "testing limits," "breaking rules," and engaging in high-risk and self-destructive behaviors.

Psychiatric Disorders among Children and Adolescents

Several factors increase the risk of aggressive behaviors in children and adolescents. Of particular interest are childhood psychiatric disorders. Attention-deficit hyperactivity disorder (ADHD) is the most commonly diagnosed psychiatric disorder in 3 to 5 percent of school-age children and adolescents (Swaim et al., 2006). Clinical features of ADHD include persistent impairments in attention or concentration and/or symptoms of hyperactivity and impulsivity. This is a chronic condition, associated with poor treatment outcomes. Comorbid conditions such as conduct disorder, substance abuse, and oppositional defiant disorder (ODD) further heighten the risk of aggressive behaviors during this period. Children with ODD are likely to demonstrate sustained patterns of argumentative, hostile, resentful, and defiant behaviors toward adult authority (Swaim et al., 2006). Children and adolescents with these psychiatric conditions are likely to enter the juvenile justice system, have a history of persistent aggressive and antisocial behaviors, and develop substance-related disorders in adulthood (Swaim et al., 2006).

Substance-related disorders are the strongest predictors of violence in youth. Data from the 2005 National Survey on Drug Use and Health revealed that substance use among

1. Karen is a 30-year-old client seen in the emergency department. During the visit she starts pacing, yelling, and wringing her hands. What is the *most appropriate initial* response to this situation?

    a. Alert the security guard because she is dangerous.

    b. Touch her on the shoulder and provide reassurance.

    c. Approach her cautiously and maintain a safe distance.

    d. Ignore her behavior and let her calm down.

2. Mr. Jones, who has a diagnosis of chronic schizophrenia, walks into the community mental health center and accuses staff of stealing his money. He is agitated, irritable, and intrusive. What is the *most appropriate* response to this patient?

    a. "Mr. Jones, it sounds like you are pretty upset, how can I help you?"

    b. "I am afraid you are mistaken. No one in the clinic would steal your money."

    c. "Mr. Jones, our staff is very honest and we resent your accusations."

    d. "You are right, let me talk to my supervisor about your concerns."

3. An angry family member approaches you and demands information about one of your clients. She is loud, rude, and threatening. What is the most appropriate response?

    a. Tell her you cannot provide information due to confidentiality issues.

    b. Ask her to leave until she gets herself under control.

    c. Acknowledge her anger, but let her know that it is difficult to assist when she is yelling and threatening.

    d. Touch her on the shoulder and let her know that her family member is doing fine.

4. Marty is a 20-year-old client who is brought to your facility by the local police after he is picked up for shouting and threatening his supervisor. He is currently being treated for bipolar disorder, manic episode. What is the most appropriate initial nursing intervention?

    a. Attempt to establish rapport and maintain a safe distance.

    b. Ask the police to leave the room to ensure confidentiality.

    c. Put him in restraints and medicate him as soon as possible.

    d. Let him know that his behavior is inappropriate.

---

youth has declined, but marijuana was the most commonly used illicit drug in 9.9 percent of adolescents ages 12 to 17: 6.8 percent used marijuana; 3.3 percent used prescription drugs for nonmedical purposes; 1.2 percent used inhalants; and 0.6 percent used cocaine (Substance Abuse and Mental Health Services Administration [SAMHSA], 2006).

In a study conducted by Mason and his colleagues (2004) of children ages 10 and 11 years, they found that children who reported higher levels of behavioral problems were almost four times as likely to experience a depressive episode in early adulthood. These data offer implications for the potential value of intervening to reduce childhood conduct problems as a primary prevention approach for not only violence, but also depression (Mason et al., 2004).

Neurobiological Factors

Neurobiological factors associated with violence in children and adolescents are similar to those in adults with the exception of developmental and environmental influences. The relationship between childhood and adolescent psychiatric disorders and aggression and delinquent behaviors is well documented. Implications from these findings show that these disorders have a genetic and neurobiological basis, mainly neuroanatomical dysfunction in the HPA, specifically low activity, which is a correlated with protracted and severe aggression. Delinquent behaviors in boys, particularly those exhibiting physical aggression, demonstrate that they have low resting cortisol levels. Researchers have also discovered these findings in girls with conduct disorder who had no other psychiatric condition. These findings are consistent with early theories and studies that implicate abnormalities in the HPA axis, specifically cortisol secretion, as a risk factor for violence across the life span in male and female adolescents.

Developmental and Environmental Factors

Environmental factors, including perinatal exposure to toxins, child rearing, and parenting influences have been previously discussed. Prenatal and perinatal factors are also associated with genetic vulnerability and mediated by developmental and environmental factors and stress. Individual development is influenced by the quality of social systems in which the family resides or participates. Social structures provide consistency, safety, and a sense of belonging, beginning with families and, later, peers, who are nested in a larger social context. Identifying family strengths can bolster family functioning. Just as significant is identification of high-risk families; developmental, ethno-cultural, and environment factors; and implementing client and family-centered interventions that focus on these issues. These conditions often result in a stressful or unstable home life, combined with ineffective parenting practices and failure to provide adequate supervision, which produce distant and unhealthy child-parent relationships. Children whose parents have substance-related disorders are also more likely to experience difficulty coping and modulating their emotions and often exhibit aggressive behaviors.

Finally, media violence has been overlooked as a contributor to childhood and adolescent aggression. Both video game and movie violence exposure have been associated with stronger providence attitudes. The process of playing video games, the intense emotional and physical engagement, and the propensity to be translated into the fantasy play provide a simplistic explanation for the negative impact. However, the specific impact on the desensitization varies and is based on the youth's individual differences and vulnerabilities to violence (Anderson, 2004; Funk, Baldacci, Pasold, & Baumgardner, 2004; Uhlmann & Swanson, 2004).

Major treatment goals include early identification of high-risk youth, mitigation of symptoms, de-escalation of potentially volatile situations, promotion of healthy family systems, and adherence to treatment.

Assessment

Astute assessment and management of disruptive and aggressive or violent behavior in youths are a challenge for the nurse. Early identification and recognition of imminent violence and a clear understanding of the spectrum of violence are critical to ensure the safety of clients and staff. Initially, the nurse must collaborate with the family and client to establish rapport and trust to elicit important information about the youth's aggressive behavior, current stressors, and level of distress. This collaborative approach also enables the nurse to assess and honor client preferences and facilitate favorable treatment outcomes. It is also essential for the nurse to assess the parents' parenting skills, level of stress, and child-rearing practices. In the event of impending violence, the nurse must remove self from the situation and call for help (e.g., appropriately trained security, staff). Report all violent incidents to your manager and document the incident in a timely manner. If available seek assistance from staff involved in debriefing employees in the aftermath of a violent situation.

A thorough assessment provides crucial data about the child's psychiatric and medical status, which includes vital signs, visual examination "eyeball," medical history, and brief psychiatric assessment. This process requires talking and listening to the client; collaborating with the youth's parents, pediatrician, or provider; and obtaining information about developmental milestones and family psychiatric and mental history. A focused medical assessment must be performed to rule out medical conditions, including endocrine disorders. Drug screens and a Breathalyzer exam should be performed when alcohol intoxication is suspected. If medical conditions are the bases of the client's symptoms, these problems must be addressed and treated as soon as possible.

Assessment data must include a screening mental status examination (MSE). The mental status examination is an integral part of the assessment process and provides general information about the youth's overall appearance, attitude, mood, speech, concentration, thought processes and content, judgment, level of dangerousness to self and others, insight into illness, and motivation for treatment. All threats of violence must be taken seriously. Additional information to obtain from the youth and family include:

- Target symptoms or behaviors (e.g., restlessness, agitation, hitting)—often a reason for seeking treatment
- Severity of symptoms—guides nursing interventions
- Common triggers or precipitating factors—may range from a social situation, such as bullying by another student to exacerbation of a psychiatric condition
- Early signs of escalation
- Successful or effective interventions
- Context of past incidents (e.g., school, home)

Recent changes in the youth's behavior, including isolation from peers, drug or alcohol use, secretiveness, and increased time spent away from the house are red flags that nurses must recognize as the bases for serious psychiatric disorders such as depression. The following information about the family is also crucial to determining the child's level of distress and the parents' ability to provide safety:

- Quality of the couple/parent relationship
- Past and present psychiatric histories
- Past violent or aggressive episodes and methods of resolving
- Coping styles and disciplining practices (consider ethnocultural factors)
- Parent-child relationship (e.g., conflict, abuse, neglect)
- Ethno-cultural factors that impact parental style and approaches and response to violent and aggressive bahaviors
- Substance use
- Level of empathy

(See Chapter 5, The Nursing Process, for a further discussion on data collection.)

In effect, nurses and interdisciplinary team members must quickly differentiate medical conditions from psychiatric disorders and rapidly determine whether they are conditions that warrant specific interventions (e.g., behavioral, pharmacotherapy), or if behaviors depict a misunderstood appropriate developmental incident. An accurate synthesis and interpretation of data is required to make an accurate diagnosis.

Diagnosis

- High risk for other violence
- Ineffective coping
- Anxiety
- Risk for self-directed violence
- Low self-esteem
- Parent-child problem
- Deficit knowledge: parenting skills, psychiatric disorder(s), and treatment considerations

An accurate diagnosis is necessary before appropriate client and family goals are established and appropriate treatment can begin.

Outcome Identification/Planning and Implementation

Major goals during this period are the provision of staff and client safety, maintaining client autonomy, reducing the target symptoms, and establishing a therapeutic relationship and milieu (dosReis, Barnett, Love, Riddle, & the Maryland Youth Practice Improvement Committee, 2003). During this period the nurse and interdisciplinary team must determine the level of intervention required for managing the client's symptoms when there is potential or looming danger.

Major Nursing Interventions

- ◆ Ensure staff and client safety.
- ◆ Establish and maintain a therapeutic relationship.
- ◆ Assess and monitor the youth's mental status and level of peril to self and others.
- ◆ Assess and strengthen the parent-child relationship.
- ◆ Administer or order appropriate pharmacological and nonpharmacological treatment.
- ◆ Provide activities to succeed and generate positive feelings.
- ◆ Assess and provide client-centered psychoeducation.

The level of interventions involves behavioral strategies that foster trust and hope, such as active listening. The primary aim of this goal is to maintain the milieu or limit setting and promote autonomy. Early intervention defuses the situation and should be implemented as soon as mild agitation is assessed.

Pharmacological Interventions

Although there is no consensus on the treatment of disruptive and aggressive behaviors, a number of studies involving children and medications used to treat these conditions show promise. Psychotropic use of chemical restraint in youths is an evolving clinical approach. Normally, this intervention is required for the child's, nurses', and other staff safety and to advance the medical and psychiatric evaluation.

The decision to administer psychotropic agents to children and adolescents exhibiting agitation and violent and psychotic symptoms must be determined by a differential diagnosis. Data from nurses and members of the interdisciplinary team or pediatric and medical consultants are crucial in making this decision.

There are controversies surrounding some of these psychotropic agents because there is paucity of data that have focused on this subject in this population. Once a decision is made to use these agents, nurses and other providers must be aware of available options along with complications associated with their side-effect profile (Sorrentino, 2004; Staller,

2007). Nurses and other providers need to be as conservative as possible concerning safety and to reduce antipsychotic exposure when treating children.

If required, antipsychotic agents should be one of the atypical medications, such as olanzapine, quetiapine, aripiprazole, and risperidone, rather than typical drugs, such as haloperidol, due to their side-effect profile (Sorrentino, 2004; Staller, 2007). Consider oral medications as the first-line treatment for aggression and violence, when appropriate, followed by intramuscular (injectable/parenteral) medication and seclusion; the least acceptable resort is physical restraints. Clients receiving injections perceive this as physically and mentally traumatic, and it may compromise the nurse-client relationship. Whatever measures are initiated, these considerations must go into treatment planning decisions.

Antipsychotic agents may be used to reduce severely disruptive behaviors or aggression, despite limited efficacy and safety data and side-effect profile. Psychostimulants have also been used to treat various disorders, such as CD and ADHD, with a lack of agreement concerning the efficacy of these agents. Lithium is safe and effective for short-term use for aggression in inpatients with CD, although it is also associated with adverse side effects. Its efficacy in treating other childhood disorders and disruptive behaviors remains controversial. Specific pharmacological interventions for psychiatric conditions in children and adolescents (e.g., CD, ADHD) are discussed in Chapter 17, The Client with Attention-Deficit Disorder, and other childhood and adolescent aggressive disorders.

Behavioral Interventions

The last resort for treating the child exhibiting disruptive or unmanageable behaviors is seclusion and restraints. Nurses and team members must use various guidelines previously mentioned to determine the appropriateness of chemical and physical restraints. Other interventions show great promise in reducing the progression of these behaviors and should be considered as first-line interventions, such as time-outs and other behavior interventions, family-centered care, and psychoeducation (Multisite Violence Prevention Project, 2004).

Various approaches are used to manage disruptive and unmanageable behaviors in youths. Time-out is commonly used with children exhibiting aggressive and violent behaviors, including those with psychiatric disorders and learning disabilities. This term means the restriction of the youth for a period of time to an assigned area from which the child is not physically restricted from leaving, for the purpose of providing the child an opportunity to regain self-control. This behavioral intervention reduces the use of restraint and can be used to mold the child's behavior. Children and their parents perceive this intervention as less punitive than seclusion and restraints.

Other behavioral interventions that show promise in controlling these behaviors include therapeutic holding (Berrios & Jacobowitz, 1998). In a study conducted by Sourander,

Ellilia, Valimaki, and Piha (2002) of 504 children and adolescents, the researchers looked at the use of holding, restraints, seclusion, and time-out on an inpatient unit. Time-out was used 28 percent, holding 26 percent, seclusion 8 percent, and mechanical restraints 4 percent. Findings from this study indicated that therapeutic holding was more likely to occur with younger children less than 13 years and with diagnoses of attachment disorder and autism. In contrast children with psychosis, suicidal acts, and older than 13 were more likely to be secluded and be mechanically restrained. The researchers also concluded that the high prevalence of restraint techniques used indicated a need for nurses to receive guidelines on the use of these interventions that should consider the child's need for protection from his impulses, and the legal rights of the youth (Sourander et al., 2002).

Family Interventions

Criticism of or blaming the family is counterproductive. The family is the most immediate and influential social system for children at risk for aggression and violence. The nurse and staff must provide feedback to the family and youth about the situation, and involve them in outcome identification and treatment planning.

During this stressful period, families need emotional support and mutually defined interventions that bolster their resources to facilitate healthy resolution of the present crisis and reduce future occurrences. Family-centered interventions need to focus on the importance of consistent child management at home, opportunities to help the youth in need of control of aggressive and disruptive behaviors. Debriefing and crisis intervention are useful strategies that can teach families about triggers, educate them about de-escalation techniques, reinforce family cohesiveness, and strengthen their ability to cope and handle future stress and crises.

Appropriate referrals for family therapy, medication management, and individual psychotherapy for the child are critical aspects of follow-up and maintenance. Parental involvement and multiple family groups also offer families opportunities to address parental practices surrounding discipline and monitoring, communication, and investment in the youth's academic performance. Understanding parental approaches within the family and youth's social, ethnic, and cultural communities are crucial to working with the family and child during stressful periods (Gorman-Smith, Henry, & Tolan, 2004; Multisite Violence Prevention Project, 2004). Psychoeducation is an integral part of treatment planning and provides opportunities to impart crucial health education that strengthens the client and family's knowledge of psychiatric conditions, the importance of treatment adherence, stress management, and the significance of structure and consistent parenting in mitigating disruptive behaviors and violence.

Evaluation

Ideally, the nurse and appropriate staff defuse and de-escalate the situation by enlisting the client and parents/caretakers in the assessment, outcome identification, and treatment process. During this aspect of treatment it is imperative for the nurse and interdisciplinary team to discuss the situation and use it to improve treatment outcomes. It is also important for staff to discuss the situation and use it to improve health care. Feedback facilitates interactive dialogue with the family, client, and staff and facilitates greater knowledge of the risks and benefits of various interventions. Staff can also reassess the contributing or precipitating factors and determine the level of treatment and violence toward self or others.

Documentation is an integral part of this process. It should include pertinent information about triggers, early warning signs, and efficacy of interventions as evidenced by reduced symptoms or de-escalation and amelioration of symptoms.

ADULTHOOD

Personal and client safety has been previously discussed as a priority in dealing with violence across the life span. Additional factors are associated with violent and aggressive behaviors such as psychiatric disorders, substance-related disorders, medical conditions, and ineffective coping styles. Presumably these factors result in ineffective coping behaviors; inability to manage frustration, anger, and stress; low self-esteem, and emotional pain and distress. Psychiatric disorders, learned behaviors, history of childhood abuse and neglect, and substance-use disorders may increase the risk of aggression and violence during adulthood.

Assessment

The nurse must approach the client confidently and convey caring and empathy. Establishing rapport is critical to the success of resolving potentially violent situations. Clients must be observed for signs and behaviors associated with impending violence throughout the assessment and treatment process (e.g., yelling, threatening gestures, signs of alcohol). Specific interventions were previously discussed in this chapter. Regardless of educational background, psychiatric nurses must perform a thorough biopsychosocial assessment and work with the interdisciplinary team and make a differential diagnosis. Nursing responsibilities may vary but generally include ordering appropriate diagnostic studies, including drug screens, reviewing the results, and sharing them with members of the treatment team.

The case study is an example of the unpredictable nature of aggression and violence. Staff training on the prevention and management of disruptive behavior (PMDB) is crucial. Major goals in this situation included preventing further violence, protecting others from harm, and using the least restrictive interventions to defuse a violent situation. In this case, the client was physically aggressive and responding to hallucinations, which increased his risk of violence and harm. The staff responded appropriately to this violent situation by implementing physical and chemical interventions to contain the violence, reassure the client, and mitigate auditory hallucinations and anxiety. They also attended to the needs of the assaulted client.

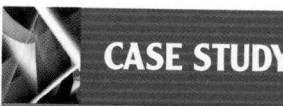

CASE STUDY

During lunch, Melvin, a 33-year-old client with a diagnosis of schizophrenia, yelled that he was hearing voices and he wanted to eat alone. Another client inadvertently sat at his table and was struck in the face. Staff attended the assaulted client, and other staff immediately restrained Melvin from further assault and slowly put him on the floor. Throughout the course of the incident, staff talked calmly and reassured him that he was not going to be hurt. He continued to yell that he was hearing voices. Despite receiving an injection of haloperidol and lorazepam, he continued to fight and attempt to get up. The staff continued to talk calmly to him and reassure him that he was not going to be hurt and that they wanted to make sure he was safe along with other clients and staff. Within 25 to 30 minutes, Melvin calmed down, became cooperative, and was able to complete his meal and return back to the unit. He was debriefed after the incident to assess his feelings about the situation and assessed for further violence. The assaulted client was also debriefed, allowed to eat, and sent back to the unit.

Diagnosis

- Risk for other directed violence
- Acute confusion
- Risk for suicide
- Ineffective coping
- Anxiety
- Powerlessness

Outcome Identification/Planning and Implementation

- Prevent harm to self and others
- Maintain staff and client safety
- Improve coping skills
- Increase self-esteem

Nursing Interventions

Nursing interventions must be tailored to improve the nurse-client relationship, ensure safety, improve clinical skills in de-escalation and defusion, and recognize personal characteristics and interpersonal skills that impact the incidence of aggression and violence. Specific nursing interventions include:

- Establish rapport
- Observe for high-risk behaviors (e.g., restlessness, agitation, pacing)
- Remain calm
- Maintain quality nurse-client interactions
- Avoid power struggles and authoritarian approaches
- Maintain personal space
- Participate in annual training on the PMDB
- Avoid contact with an openly aggressive client alone

Major nursing interventions must focus on establishing rapport, maintaining quality nurse-client interactions, and avoiding authoritarian approaches or power struggles. Depending on the etiology of aggression and violence, interventions include behavioral or pharmacological or both.

(See the Nurse-Client Dialogue Box and Case Study.)

Behavioral Interventions

De-escalation and defusion have been discussed extensively in this chapter (see Box 20–3). The effectiveness of behavioral interventions are influenced by the nurse's attitude and verbal and nonverbal communication. The following self-assessment checklist can be helpful:

- How am I reacting? Nervous, anxious, calm, reassuring
- How's my tone of voice? Loud, demanding, calm, firm
- How's my body language?
- Check personal space
- Am I wearing anything dangerous?
- What are my "gut" feelings?

When a condition involves an imminent danger to the client or others and behavioral interventions fail to de-escalate the situation, other measures, such as restraints and seclusion, are used as the last resort.

The legal tenet that determines the use of seclusion and restraint involves using the least restrictive interventions to manage imminent violence to the client and others. It also involves implementing applications that minimally deprive the client of personal freedom to achieve the purposes of the intervention. When asked about their preferences for the least restrictive, most clients answered medication over physical restraint. Many clients view these interventions as a form of punishment rather than a treatment strategy. Implications from these perceptions include the importance of using these applications appropriately and providing health education surrounding their purpose, and debriefing to reduce stress. Some nurses believe that there will always be a need to contain a severely mentally disturbed client as a means of protection, especially when there are limited alternatives. This notion is an inappropriate reason to restrain or seclude.

Pharmacological Interventions

Pharmacological interventions should be considered when there are clear clinical indications, such as acute psychosis, intense agitation, severe cognitive deficits, and the threat of violence. Interventions for aggressive and violent behaviors in adults are similar to those for children and older adults. Early identification of warning cues include pacing, restlessness, physical arousal, and yelling and threatening body cues. Whether the client is angry and taking out frustration on others, or experiencing psychosis due to nonadherence to treatment, or experiencing hallucinations and delusions caused by illicit or licit drug use, staff and client safety must be a priority.

Typical medications used to treat acute agitation, psychosis, drug intoxication or withdrawal, and aggression include antipsychotic agents and benzodiazepines. For clients presenting with acute schizophrenia and mania, the drugs of choice include traditional antipsychotic agents such as haloperidol 5 mg IM and lorazepam 2 mg IM. These drugs are given in combination to reduce psychosis, agitation, and anxiety. Combined with lorazepam, the haloperidol can be reduced to minimize the potential for extrapyramidal side effects during rapid tranquilization.

Normally, violence decreases within 20 minutes after an injection of haloperidol, and improvement of psychosis occurs within 6 hours. Lorazepam has a rapid onset and produces sedation within one hour. Haloperidol is contraindicated in clients with a history of neuroleptic malignant syndrome (NMS) or tardive dyskinesia (TD).

Atypical agents, such as ziprasidone and risperidone injection or rapid dissolving pill should be considered in clients who report a history of NMS or other serious adverse drug reactions (e.g., TD). Alternatives are oral risperidone and oral lorazepam, which show similar efficacy when compared to IM haloperidol and lorazepam (Allen et al., 2005). It is noteworthy to repeat that most clients perceive IM medication as a form of mental and physical trauma. Every effort to ask the client to take oral medications, when appropriate, should be used to promote rapport and a therapeutic nurse-client relationship.

Benzodiazepines, such as lorazepam and diazepam, are part of the treatment facility's protocol for alcohol withdrawal. Although these drugs have proven efficacy in sedating agitated clients and reducing the risk of seizures, they must be monitored closely and assessed for signs of disinhibition—a behavior that further increases the risk of impulsive aggression and violence.

Haloperidol and other typical antipsychotics should be limited to acute care and should be avoided to minimize serious adverse drug reactions. Other drugs used as maintenance treatment to manage impulsivity, aggression, and disruptive behaviors are the mood stabilizers (e.g., lithium) and anticonvulsants, such as lamotrigine and divalproex. Lithium and valproate acid have also shown promise for reducing aggressive behavior in adults, again with inconsistent results in children and adolescents. Monitoring and documenting the client's response to all interventions are important nursing interventions during and after these agents are given. (See Chapter 29 for a discussion on pharmacologic agents.)

Evaluation

Positive outcomes for managing aggressive and violent behaviors include safety, resolution of violent situation, and implementation of appropriate intervention associated with underlying causative factors. Underlying causative factors may include amelioration of psychosis, correction of a medical condition such as diabetes ketoacidosis, or a severe adverse drug reaction. A positive treatment outcome indicates that the client's condition is stable and there is no evidence of untoward reactions from treatment or interventions.

OLDER ADULTS

Aggression is a common behavioral symptom of dementia, delirium depression, and other psychiatric and medical disorders in the older adult. As previously discussed, aggression in this population and other age groups is associated with frontotemporal dementia, cognitive decline, impulsivity, poor executive functioning, and subsequent behavioral and psychological disturbances. Unfortunately, aggressive and violent behaviors in older adults result in high chemical restraints and caregiver distress and depression. Increased psychotropic use in older adults is likely to result in a greater risk of sensitivity to drugs, side effects, and risk of toxicity due to age-related changes.

Implications for the nurse include recognizing these changes and working with the interdisciplinary team to develop and implement age-specific interventions that reflect the individual's preferences and cultural needs that reduce the risk of adverse treatment outcomes and facilitate a higher level of functioning.

Geriatrics and Extended Care Settings

Persons residing in nursing homes are vulnerable to intentional injury, particularly resident-to-resident violence. Aggressive behavior can lead to institutionalization, overmedication and physical restraint. Efforts to provide care and maintain the client's dignity is a daunting task. It often requires educating the staff about alternative measures to reduce or minimize aggressive behaviors, such as implementing restraint-free environments.

High-risk factors associated with violence among residents include dementia, psychosis, male gender, younger age, pain, and facilities that have a large proportion of residents with dementia (Shinoda-Tagawa et al., 2004). According to findings from the Centers for Medicare and Medicaid Services (CMS), close to 90,000 nursing home residents in the United States have exhibited physical aggressive behavior in the week before their assessment with the Minimum Data Set (MDS). (See Box 20-2: Individual Characteristics Associated with Violence.)

Target symptoms include psychosis (e.g., hallucinations, delusions, agitation) and severe agitation, which are the most common symptoms reported in clients with neurodegenerative disease. Paranoid or persecutory delusions are the most common forms of delusions, especially in those with Alzheimer's disease (Sink, Holden, Yaffe, 2005). The significance of delusions and hallucinations in these clients is their level of distress and high risk of agitation and aggression. Typically, delusions involve a belief that people are stealing things from them, that their home is not theirs, and that their spouse is unfaithful. They are also troublesome and distressful to caregivers, which are often cited as reasons for institutionalization. Violence may also occur if the client acts on his or her delusions or hallucinations. Additional behaviors associated with these disorders include a history of sleep disturbances, apathy, pacing, noisy vocalizations, physical aggression, restlessness, hypersexuality, and confusion.

Assessment

Behavioral disturbances and psychosis are common manifestations of neurogenerative conditions and may be drug induced or linked to an underlying medical condition, or both. Regardless of the cause, safety must be a priority. It is imperative to approach the aggressive older client cautiously and maintain personal and client safety. Collaboration with the client, family, and other appropriate staff is crucial to the data collection process and understanding the client's preferences, previous level of functioning, and quality of life. Additional questions include duration of current mental status changes (e.g., acute confusion, disorientation, agitation), current medications, recent surgeries, and medical conditions.

Considerations for age-related changes must also be taken into account, such as speaking slowly, and addressing the client by his or her preferred name per the client or family. Use an unhurried approach and allow the client and family to respond to queries. Assess and recognize the impact of age-related sensory deficits on the client's behavior and ability to respond to questions. Because of potential cognitive deficits in the older client that may stem from an underlying medical or psychiatric condition, this approach reduces anxiety and frustration even when the client is hostile. It is reassuring to the client and family when the nurse conveys patience and empathy during this difficult situation.

Screening tools, such as the Mini Mental State Exam (MMSE) is also useful in the data collection process. This 10-minute screening tool provides invaluable client data in the following areas:

◆ Orientation
◆ Attention
◆ Concentration
◆ Memory
◆ Language
◆ Visuospatial ability
◆ Calculation

Appropriate laboratory and diagnostic studies, such as a complete blood count with differential, a liver panel, toxicology screens, an oxometry, chemistries, Vitamin B_{12}, folic acid, thiamine, a urinalysis, and an electrocardiogram should be ordered as soon as possible to rule out underlying medical conditions

Several psychiatric and medical conditions are associated with aggression and physical assault in older adults. The most common reasons are psychiatric disorders, acute medical conditions such as endocrine disorders and fluid and electrolyte disturbances, substance use, and neurodegenerative conditions. Neurodegenerative disorders include extrapyramidal disorders (e.g., Parkinson's disease, Alzheimer's disease), mylein disorders such as amyotropic lateral sclerosis (ALS), cortical disease, dementia, and delirium. Once medical conditions are confirmed the client must be transferred to an appropriate provider, or treatment should be initiated immediately.

Diagnosis

◆ Acute confusion
◆ Risk for injury
◆ Risk for other directed injury
◆ Risk for self-directed danger
◆ Anxiety
◆ Disturbed sleep patterns
◆ Caregiver role strain

Outcome Identification, Planning, and Implementation

Treatment planning for Mr. Jones will focus on staff and client safety. An evaluation will be conducted of his symptoms and underlying medical conditions that may have been

---

CASE STUDY

Mr. Jones is an 80-year-old married man who is brought to the emergency room by his 83-year-old wife, who reports that he has been accusing her of taking his things, wandering around at night, and screaming at her and their grandchildren. She reports that she is tired and depressed and needs help in caring for her spouse.

Data from the assessment reveal that Mr. Jones has been recently started on medication for arthritis (2 weeks ago). He has been taking it as ordered, but his wife reports that he has refused to take all of his medication over the past few days. She describes him as a "good-natured" man and explains that she has never seen him like this before. Mr. Jones' mental status examination indicates that he is extremely agitated, restless, uncooperative, confused, and disoriented. The most remarkable history is his new medication for arthritis that he began 2 weeks ago. His wife denies other changes or stress in their lives. He has a negative history of alcohol or other drugs. His medical examination is unremarkable. He is admitted to the hospital to further evaluate his delirious and acute confusional state.

caused by an adverse reaction to his new medication. Outcome identification will focus on:

- Maintaining a safe environment
- Improving his mental status and restoring his baseline level of functioning
- Reducing the risk of danger and injury to self or others
- Improving his sleep patterns
- Lessening his anxiety
- Reducing his caregiver's distress

Interventions

Although dementia is common in older adults, it is imperative to rule out such conditions before making assumptions.

Pharmacological Interventions

There is some evidence that psychotic symptoms improve modestly with antipsychotic medication. Risperidone has been the most often studied of the atypical antipsychotic agents, confirming its efficacy in reducing aggression and psychosis (Katz et al., 2007).

Typically, aggressive and violent behaviors in this age group is treated with a low-dose antipsychotic agent that reduces psychosis, agitation, and anxiety. After coaxing from the staff and his wife, Mr. Jones took a low dose (1 mg) of risperidone liquid by mouth. Several hours later he was calmer and the staff was able to complete his examination.

It is well documented that risperidone and other atypical antipsychotics, such as olanzapine and quetiapine, significantly improve symptoms of psychosis and aggression in persons with severe dementia (Katz et al., 2007; Kryzhanovskay et al., 2006). Major benefits of atypical medications include their favorable side-effect profile in older adults and their efficacy that is at least equal to haloperidol. Due to risk of toxicity, side effects, and drug sensitivity, older adults are usually prescribed one half or one third of adult doses.

Behavioral Interventions

In this case study, staff did not believe that restraints or seclusion were indicated because of the potential for actual adverse outcomes. Historically, restraints were used in various settings, including intensive care units, older age, cognitive deficits, dementia, immobility, and physical dependence. Studies that demonstrated a positive correlation between length of stay (LOS) in facilities and restraint use are well documented. The LOS was at least twice as long for the restrained client as the nonrestrained clients. Clinical findings associated with these interventions have demonstrated negative psychological and physical consequences. These consequences include loss of muscle strength, formation of pressure ulcers, incontinence, strangulation, psychological distress, and death, regardless of whether the appliance was put on appropriately.

Contemporary data have emerged that indicate that facilities have moved from restraints and seclusion to restraint-free or least restrictive environments (Wagner et al., 2007). Music therapy and alarm devices and corrective environmental and equipment changes, including beds without side rails, are showing great promise in reducing aggressive behaviors, particularly in older adults with cognitive deficits and dementia.

Behavioral interventions used with Mr. Jones included reorientation, music therapy, and a restraint-free environment. He was taken off all medications to determine if one of them caused acute mental status changes. The nurse and other staff worked with the client and his wife and created a "safe" environment that allowed her to participate throughout his hospital stay and play a key role in developing client-centered and culturally sensitive health care. She also participated in a psychoeducation group that centered on medications, stress management, and treatment adherence. (See Nursing Care Plan 20–1.)

Evaluation

Outcome identification was used as a parameter for the evaluation process. (See Nursing Care Plan 20–1.)

LEGAL AND ETHICAL ISSUES RELATED TO VIOLENCE

Dealing with a violent or aggressive situation requires balancing the client's right to freedom and autonomy using least restrictive means and the communities' right to protection from violence. Psychiatric nurses must distinguish between various forms of restraints and/or seclusion, including pharmacotherapy for personal protection, and use them to assist the client and society. Normally, restraints and seclusion are the last alternative to manage assaultive and aggressive behaviors after verbal de-escalation or defusing and other behavioral interventions fail as evidenced by continued escalation. Ideally, facilities have policies and codes that are used to guide staff in the event that physical interventions are necessary. It is imperative to explain reasons for verbal and physical interventions and ensuring that steps will be taken to help the client regain control regardless of the client's mental status. This approach conveys concern and respect and reduces anxiety in the already agitated or aggressive client who may feel helpless and frightened. Of particular importance are the following medical and legal issues. See Chapter 8 for an in-depth discussion of legal and ethical issues involving clients exhibiting aggressive and violent behaviors.

WHEN VIOLENCE OCCURS: STRESS DEBRIEFING

Self-care during the aftermath of violence is crucial and helps nurses cope with trauma and fears associated with these incidents. Historically, psychiatric and other nurses

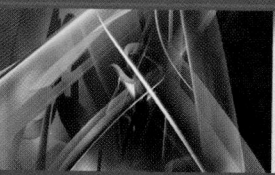

Mr. Jones (Case Study)

Nursing Diagnosis: Acute Confusion and Anxiety

Outcome Identification	Nursing Actions	Rationales	Evaluation
1. By [date], client will be alert and oriented to person, place, and time.	1a. Establish rapport and reassurance that he is safe.	1a. Establishes therapeutic interaction. Conveys empathy, caring, and interest.	*Goal met:* Nurse forms therapeutic relationship. Client is oriented and anxiety is reduced. Client responds to orientation and reassurance and his risk of dangerousness to self and others is achieved.
	1b. Orient the client as needed. Use short and direct sentences.	1b. Present reality, orientation, and reduce anxiety and agitation.	
	1c. Allow spouse to remain with client. Assess level of dangerousness.	1c. Provides safety and orientation to surroundings.	
	1d. Observe for mood changes. Ask wife to notify staff of mood changes.	1d. Change in mood or anxiety level increases risk of dangerousness.	

Nursing Diagnosis: Risk for Injury

Outcome Identification	Nursing Actions	Rationales	Evaluation
1. By [date], client mental status returns to pre-confusional state.	1a. Establish rapport and reassurance that he is safe.	1a. Establishes therapeutic interaction. Conveys empathy, caring, and interest.	*Goal met:* Nurse forms therapeutic relationship. Client is oriented and anxiety is reduced. Client's mental status returns to pre-confusional state. Client responds to orientation and reassurance and his risk of dangerousness to self and other is achieved.
	1b. Orient the client as needed. Use short and direct sentences.	1b. Present reality, orientation, and reduce anxiety and agitation.	
	1c. Allow spouse to remain with client.	1c. Provides safety and orientation to surroundings.	
	1d. Continuously assess the client's mood and anxiety level.	1d. Change in mood or anxiety level increase risk of dangerousness.	

Nursing Diagnosis: Risk for Other-Directed Injury

(same as previous interventions and goals)

Nursing Diagnosis: Risk for Self-Directed Danger

(same as previous interventions and goals)

(continues)

Nursing Care Plan 20–1 (continued)

Nursing Diagnosis: Disturbed Sleep Patterns

Outcome Identification	Nursing Actions	Rationales	Evaluation
1. By [date], client's normal sleeping patterns return to optimal level.	1a. Assess normal sleeping patterns from spouse. 1b. Maintain quiet environment. 1c. Implement sleep hygiene techniques such as avoiding heavy meals and fluids 2–3 hours before sleep.	1a. Helps nurse identify normal sleeping patterns. 1b–c. Promotes rest, sleep	*Goal met:* Client's normal sleeping patterns return and are maintained.

Nursing Diagnosis: Caregiver Role Strain

1. By [date], spouse and other caregiver verbalize present stressors and ways to effectively manage them.	1a. Inquire and assess present stressors. 1b. Reassure that this is a temporary situation and that all is being done to assist spouse. 1c. Convey acceptance and empathy. 1d. Provide health education on various topics including delirium and acute confusion.	1a–c. Gathering this data helps the nurse gain a greater understanding of caregiver's present confusional state and coping pattern. 1d. Health education helps family members understand their loved one's medical condition and reduces undue stress and anxiety.	*Goal met:* Client has a clearer understanding of present stressors. Client's self-esteem increases. Client is able to explore options to deal with present stressors.

were told that violence was part of their job. Violence should never be an acceptable part of nursing regardless of setting. Once it occurs, nurses need to seek support and opportunities to process the event and put it into perspective. Ideally, organizations provide internal services, such as stress debriefing. **Stress debriefing** is a logical process during which clients or staff can discuss what they have experienced, and normalize their reactions by comparing their reactions with those of others (Antai-Otong, 2001). Although there is a lack of consistent empirical data (Boris, Ou, & Singh, 2005; Sijbrandij, Olff, Reitsma, Carlier, & Gersons, 2006) that stress debriefing prevents PTSD, most agree that it offers immediate emotional support and education about normal stress responses.

THE ROLE OF THE NURSE

Regardless of one's role on the interdisciplinary team, violence prevention is everyone's responsibility. Nurses must advocate for their personal safety and participate in proactive endeavors that ensure healthy work environments.

THE GENERALIST/STAFF NURSE

Generalist nurses are likely to spend more time gathering data at the bedside or in groups with individuals at high risk of violence during acute stages of their illness than other staff. Steps that facilitate and promote safe work environments have been aforementioned. The nursing process guides the interviewing process and helps the nurse make appropriate queries about the client's symptoms, including previous history of violence, current medications, and reviewing laboratory studies to help team members determine an accurate diagnosis.

Primary responsibilities of the generalist include assessment, outcome identification, working with the interdisciplinary team, and making an accurate differential diagnosis. Major nursing interventions include medication administration, implementing behavioral interventions, and psychoeducation. Monitoring the results of laboratory and other diagnostic tests are also part of the generalist role. Reporting adverse effects, abnormal laboratory results, and worsening violence is an integral part of this process. Throughout the assessment and treatment process the nurse must monitor and document client responses to pharmacological and behavioral interventions.

THE ADVANCED-PRACTICE PSYCHIATRIC REGISTERED NURSE

Major responsibilities of the advanced-practice psychiatric registered nurse are the same as the generalist nurse's regarding safety issues. The APPRN also performs psychiatric and physical evaluation to rule out psychiatric and medical conditions that contribute to aggression and violence. Ordering diagnostic studies and interpreting these findings and prescribing medications are vital aspects of the APPRN's responsibilities. As a part of the interdisciplinary team the nurse also discusses relevant data to make accurate diagnosis of underlying causes and treatment to reduce these behaviors.

Advanced-practice psychiatric registered nurses must also advocate for staff and client safety by initiating dialogue and working with interdisciplinary teams and facility administrators and developing policies that mandate safe and healthy work environments. This process must also afford nurses, clients, families, and other staff opportunities to cope with immediate emotional reactions during the aftermath of violent incidents (e.g., stress debriefing).

THE NURSING PROCESS

ASSESSMENT

Major principles guiding the nursing process were discussed earlier and focused on life span issues. Strategies that facilitate differential diagnosis and guide the decision-making process in making accurate diagnosis are crucial in establishing outcome identification, treatment planning, and evaluation. (See Chapter 5, The Nursing Process, for information about the nursing process.)

DIAGNOSIS

Various nursing diagnoses involving aggressive and violent behaviors have been previously mentioned. Listed diagnoses include injury to self and others, anxiety, chronic low self-esteem, and powerlessness.

OUTCOME IDENTIFICATION/PLANNING AND IMPLEMENTATION

Prevention is a key element surrounding outcome identification, planning, and implementation. Prevention of violence and mitigation of symptoms must be systemic and involve strategies that control or prevent these behaviors in clients and the workplace.

NURSING INTERVENTIONS

Nursing interventions must focus on prevention and on personal, client, and staff safety. Issues such as life span consid-erations, differential diagnosis, and the importance of inter-disciplinary teams are important components that reduce the causative factors associated with aggressive and disruptive behaviors and positive treatment outcomes.

EVALUATION

Evaluations are based on treatment outcomes and the level of safety facilitated by nursing interventions.

NURSING RESEARCH

The growing incidence of workplace violence in vast practice settings is an area of interest for nursing research. Nursing theorists have explored numerous factors associated with workplace violence, the incidence of violence in specific practice settings, and interventions that reduce its incidence. There is a great need for the psychiatric nurse researcher to develop evidence-based interventions that reduce the incidence of violence across the life span.

There is also a dearth of data on the effectiveness of behavioral interventions that reduce aggressive behaviors in children and adolescents. This specialty needs further research to determine the efficacy of age-specific interventions and opportunities to discover innovative approaches to managing aggressive and assaultive behaviors in this age group.

Other areas of interest include developing models of care for the growing aging populations that exhibit aggression and violence. As our society ages, there is a growing need to develop evidence-based age-specific interventions that embrace the concept of restraint-free interventions and the role of chemical restraints that ensure safety, dignity, and respect of older adults. (See Research Abstract.)

SUMMARY

- ◆ Violence can and does occur everywhere.
- ◆ Aggressive and violent behavior across the life span is a major public health problem.
- ◆ Nurses and other health care providers are at a high risk of violence.
- ◆ Personal safety is a priority in maintaining workplace safety.
- ◆ Proactive measures are key to the prevention of workplace violence.
- ◆ Numerous factors contribute to violent, disruptive, and aggressive behaviors.
- ◆ Nurses must advocate for personal safety and dismiss the notion that workplace violence is part of their job.
- ◆ Psychiatric nurses participate in policy making and other administrative decisions to ensure their personal safety.
- ◆ Nurses must work toward creating restraint-free inpatient units.

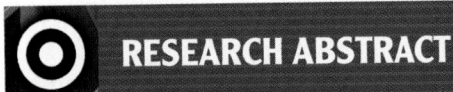

Perilous Work: Nurses' Experiences in Psychiatric Units with High Risks of Assault

Kindy, D., Petersen, S., & Parkhurst, D. (2005). *Archives of Psychiatric Nursing, 19*, 169–175.

Study Problem/Purpose

Provide a venue for psychiatric mental health registered nurses to describe their experiences associated with working in environments with high risk of assault.

Methods

A qualitative descriptive and interpretative phenomenological approach was employed to answer the research question "What is the lived experience of registered nurses working in an environment where assault is a continual threat?" Ten registered nurses participated in the open-ended interviews.

Findings

Analyses of interviews generated four categories (namely, safety fortifications, catalysts for violence, perplexing aftermath, and pervasive invasive sequelae) and 13 subcategories under the principal construct of "perilous work." Overall these data implicate the stressful nature of working in environments of high-risk assault and the emotional aftermath of workplace violence.

Implications for Psychiatric Nursing

Whilst the sample size was relatively small, researchers provided a venue for registered nurses to describe their experiences associated with working in high-risk work environments. Psychiatric nurses are on the frontline of mental health care and are continually exposed to potential and actual environments of high risk for violence. It is imperative to recognize high-risk groups and verbal and nonverbal behaviors associated with violence and to seek emotional support in its aftermath. Findings from this study strengthen the importance of developing policies and training that ensure safe work environments.

◆ Research indicates that behavioral and pharmacologicals interventions are safer than seclusion and restraints in managing violence across the life span.

SUGGESTIONS FOR CLINICAL CONFERENCES

1. Train students in verbal de-escalation and defusing.

2. Invite an advanced-practice registered psychiatric nurse to discuss the role of the nurse in psychiatric triage or in a crisis center. Ask the nurse to focus on verbal and nonverbal cues that indicate active or imminent violence and environmental factors that create a safer workplace.

3. Set up a scenario and ask students to role play an aggressive client and nurse (switch roles) and discuss their feelings about each role, and ask them to critique the interactions.

4. Invite a nurse who has actually had a serious encounter with a violent client to discuss what happened, lessons learned, and what services the nurse used to cope with the situation.

5. Invite the program leader of the facility Critical Incident Team or someone from the American Red Cross Mental Health Disaster Team to share their goals in dealing with the aftermath of a violent incident.

STUDY QUESTIONS

1. Which of the following increases the risk of aggression and violence?
   a. Previous history of violence
   b. An untreated psychiatric disorder
   c. History of domestic violence
   d. All of the above

2. Which of the following statements best describes social learning theories about violence?
   a. Aggression is learned through modeling or observation.
   b. The relationship between exposure to violence in media and children has not been documented.
   c. Repeated exposure to violence has little impact on behavior or emotions.
   d. Frequent exposure to violence does not result in desensitization.

3. Which of the following statements best describes limit setting?
   a. "Ms. Marsh, it is difficult for me to help you when you are screaming."
   b. "Mr. Johnson, I understand that you are upset, but please lower your voice."
   c. "Jonathan, it's time for a time-out."
   d. All of the above

4. One of your colleagues witnessed a violent attack in the emergency room. She is overtly upset and tearful. What is the best explanation for her behavior?
   a. She is overly reacting because she was not physically injured.
   b. Her behavior is a normal reaction to an abnormal event.
   c. She has "personal problems."
   d. Her behavior is abnormal and requires a referral to a mental health professional.

5. All nurses must be cognizant of their personal safety. Which of the following is the *least* proactive approach to workplace safety?
   a. Gather as much information about the client as possible.
   b. Know where staff is at all times.
   c. Remove all sharps from the work environment.
   d. Allow the client to sit between you and the exit.

6. Which of the following clients poses the *least* risk of violence?
   a. The client with acute psychosis
   b. The older client with Alzheimer's disease
   c. The client in alcohol withdrawal
   d. None of the above

7. When working with the aggressive, hostile, and violent client the *highest priority* for the nurse is to do which of the following?
   a. Convey concern for the client's well-being
   b. Secure self-limits and muster help if needed
   c. Maintain personal safety
   d. Use verbal de-escalation to manage the situation

8. An adult was placed in four-point restraints 3 hours ago after he attempted to hit the nurse. Which observation by the nurse is the best indication that the client's restraints could be discontinued?
   a. The client has had one hand and one leg free for the past hour and has made no aggressive moves.
   b. The client apologizes to the nurse and explains that he doesn't want to hurt anyone.
   c. The nurse has explained the importance of not striking out in anger and the client verbalized understanding.
   d. The medication administered to the client has been effective and he is now sleeping.

9. One of your clients is obviously upset and is pacing and raising his voice. What is the *least* appropriate nursing intervention to manage this situation?
   a. Put your hands on the client's shoulders and tell him to calm down.
   b. Set verbal limits and ask the client to lower his voice.
   c. Assess the client's needs.
   d. Offer medications if indicated.

RESOURCES

Please note that because Internet resources are of a time-sensitive nature and URL addresses may change or be deleted, searches should also be conducted by association or topic.

Internet Resources

http ://www. redcross.org   American Red Cross.

http://community.nursingspectrum.com   Antai-Otong, D. (2003). Workplace violence. *Nursing Spectrum.*

http://www.hcfa.gov   Centers for Medicare and Medicaid Services

http://.paproviders.org   Department of Health and Human Services, Health Care Financing Administration: Medicare and Medicaid Programs. (1999). *Conditions of Participation: Patients' Rights. Interim Financial Rule, 42,* CFR 482. Federal Register 64:36069-36089

http://www.jointcommission.org/AccreditationPrograms/Hospitals/Standards/FAQs/Provision+of+Care/Restraint+and+Seclusion/Restraint_Seclusion.htm   The Joint Commission: Behavioral Health Care Restraint and Seclusion

http://grants.nih.gov   NIH Guide: Workplace Violence Prevention Research

http://www.cdc.gov   NIOSH. (2002). Violence: Occupational Hazards in Hospitals.

http://albany.edu   Pastore, A. L., & Maguire, K. (1999). Sourcebook of Criminal Justice Statistics.

http://www.usda.gov   The USDA Handbook on Workplace Violence Prevention and Responses

http://www.wps.org   Workplace Solutions

Other Resources

NIOSH Violence: *Occupational hazards in hospital publication* (public domain)
NIOSH-Publications Dissemination
4676 Columbia Parkway
Cincinnati, OH 45226-1998
E-mail: pubstaft@cdc.gov

REFERENCES

Allen, M. H., Currier, G. W., Carpenter, D., Ross, R. W., Docherty, J. P., & Expert Consensus Panel for Behavioral Emergencies 2005. (2005). The expert consensus guideline series. Treatment of behavioral emergencies. *Journal of Psychiatric Practice, 11,* (Suppl 1), 5–108.

American Psychiatric Association. (2000). *Diagnostic and statistical manual of mental disorders 4th edition text revision.* Washington, DC: American Psychiatric Association.

Anderson, C. A. (2004). An update on the effects of playing violent video games. *Journal of Adolescence, 27,* 113–122.

Antai-Otong, D. (2001). Critical incident stress debriefing: A health promotion model for workplace violence. *Perspectives in Psychiatric Care, 37,* 125–132.

Badger, F., & Mullan, B. (2004). Aggressive and violent incidents: Perceptions of training and support among staff caring for older people and people with head injury. *Journal of Clinical Nursing, 13,* 526–533.

Baker, L. A., Jacobson, K. C., Raine, A., Lozano, D. I., & Bezdjian, S. (2007). Genetic and environmental bases of childhood antisocial behavior: A multi-informant twin study. *Journal of Abnormal Psychology, 116,* 219–235.

Bandura, A. (1977). *Social learning theory*. Englewood Cliffs, NJ: Prentice-Hall.

Bandura, A. (1986). *Social foundations of thought and action: A social cognitive theory*. Englewood Cliffs, NJ: Prentice-Hall.

Bartels, M., van Beijsterveldt, C. E., Derks, E. M., Stroet, T. M., Polderman, T. J., Hudziak, J. J., et al. (2007). Young Netherlands Twin Register (Y-NTR): A longitudinal multiple informant study of problem behavior. *Twin Research and Human Genetics, 10,* 3–11.

Bartholow, B. D., Sestir, M. A., & Davis, E. B. (2005). Correlates and consequences of exposure to video game violence: Hostile personality, empathy, and aggressive behavior. *Personality and Social Psychology Bulletin, 31,* 1573–1586.

Beck, J. C. (2004). Delusions, substance abuse, and serious violence. *Journal of the American Academy of Psychiatry and Law, 32,* 169–172.

Berlin, H. A., Rolls, E. T., & Iversen, S. D. (2005). Borderline personality disorder, impulsivity, and the orbitofrontal cortex. *American Journal of Psychiatry, 162,* 2360–2370.

Berrios, C. D., & Jacobowitz, W. H. (1998). Therapeutic holding. Outcomes of a pilot study. *Journal of Psychosocial Nursing and Mental Health Services, 36,* 14–18.

Boris, N. W., Ou, A. C., & Singh, R. (2005). Preventing post-traumatic stress disorder after mass exposure to violence. *Biosecurity and Bioterrorism, 3,* 154–163.

Bowers, L., Allan, T., Simpson, A., Nijman, H., & Warren, J. (2007). Adverse incidents, patient flow and nursing workforce variables on acute psychiatric wards: The Tompkins Acute Ward Study. *International Journal of Social Psychiatry, 53,* 75–84.

Coccaro, E. F., McClosky, M. S., Fitzgerald, D. A., & Phan, K. L. (2007). Amygdala and orbitofrontal reactivity to social threat in individuals with impulsive aggression. *Biological Psychiatry, 62,* 168–178.

Cornell, D. G., Peterson, C. S., & Richards, H. (1999). Anger as a predictor of aggression among incarcerated adolescents. *Journal of Clinical and Consulting Psychology, 67,* 108–115.

Corrigan, P. W., & Watson, A. C. (2005). Findings from the National Comorbidity Survey on the frequency of violent behavior in individuals with psychiatric disorders. *Psychiatry Research, 136,* 153–162.

Crilly, J., Chaboyer, W., & Creedy, D. (2004). Violence towards emergency department nurses by patients. *Accident and Emergency Nursing, 12,* 67–73.

Department of Health and Human Services, Health Care Financing Administration: Medicare and Medicaid Programs. (1999). *Conditions of participation: Patients' rights. Interim Financial Rule, 42, CFR 482.* Fed. Reg. 64:36069–36089. Retrieved April 27, 2004, from http://paproviders.org.

Dolan, M., Anderson, I. M., & Deakin, J. F. W. (2001). Relationship between 5-HT function and impulsivity and aggression among male offenders with personality disorders. *British Journal of Psychiatry, 178,* 352–359.

Dolan, M., & Fullam, R. (2006). Face affect recognition deficits in personality-disordered offenders: Association with psychopathy. *Psychological Medicine, 36,* 1563–1569.

Dollard, J., Doob, L. W., Miller, N. E., Mowere, O. H., & Sears, R. R. (1939). *Frustration and aggression* (pp. 438–439). New Haven, CT: Yale University Press.

dosReis, S., Barnett, S., Love, R. C., Riddle, M. A., & the Maryland Youth Practice Improvement Committee. (2003). A guide for managing acute aggressive behavior of youth in residential and inpatient treatment facilities. *Psychiatric Services, 54,* 1357–1363.

Dutton, D. G. (2000). Witnessing parental violence as a traumatic experience shaping the abusive personality. *Journal of Aggression, Maltreatment and Trauma, 3,* 59–67.

Dyer, K. F., Bell, R., McCann, J., & Rauch, R. (2006). Aggression after traumatic brain injury: Analysing socially desirable responses and the nature of aggressive traits. *Brain Injury, 20,* 1163–1173.

Fazel, S., & Grann, M. (2006). The population impact of severe mental illness on violent crime. *American Journal of Psychiatry, 163,* 1397–1403.

Fernandes, C. M. B., Bouthillette, F., Raboud, J. M., Bullock, L., Moore, C. F., Christenson, J. M., et al. (1999). Violence in the emergency department: A survey of health care workers. *Canadian Medical Association Journal, 161,* 1245–1248.

Flory, J. D., Newcorn, J. H., Miller, C., Harty, S., & Halperin, J. M. (2007). Serotonergic function in children with attention-deficit hyperactivity disorder: Relationship to later antisocial personality disorder. *British Journal of Psychiatry, 190,* 410–414.

Frankle, W. G., Lombardo, I., New, A. S., Goodman, M., Talbot, P. S., Huang, Y., et al. (2005). Brain serotonin transporter distribution in subjects with impulsive aggressivity: A positron emission study with [11C]McN 5652. *American Journal of Psychiatry, 162,* 915–923.

Freud, S. (1960). Psychopathology of everyday life. In J. Strachey (Ed.), *The standard edition of the complete psychological works of Sigmund Freud.* London: Hogarth Press. (First English edition, 1904).

Funk, J. B., Baldacci, H. B., Pasold, T., & Baumgardner, J. (2004). Violence exposure in real-life, video games, television, movies, and the Internet: Is there desensitization? *Journal of Adolescence, 27,* 23–34.

Gorman-Smith, D., Henry, D. B., & Tolan, P. H. (2004). Exposure to community violence perpetration: The protective effects of family functionality. *Journal of Clinical Child and Adolescent Psychology, 33,* 439–449.

Hazen, A. L., Connelly, C. D., Kelleher, K. J., Barth, R. P., & Landsverk, J. A. (2006). Female caregivers' experiences with intimate partner violence and behavior problems in children investigated as victims of maltreatment. *Pediatrics, 117,* 99–109.

Healthcare Commission and Royal College of Psychiatrists. (2005). *The national audit of violence (2003-2005).*

Available online at http://www.rcpsych.ac.uk/pdf/HC%20Commission-funded%20NAV-2005%20-2006.pdf

Herrenkohl, T. I., McMorris, B. J., Catalano, R. F., Abbott, R. D., Hemphill, S. A., & Toumbourou, J. W. (2007). Risk factors for violence and relational aggression in adolescence. *Journal of Interpersonal Violence, 22,* 386–405.

Jorge, R. E., Robinson, R. G., Moser, D., Tateno, A., Crespo-Facorro, B., & Arndt, S. (2004). Major depression following traumatic brain injury. *Archives of General Psychiatry, 61,* 42–50.

Katz, I., de Deyn, P. P., Mintzer, J., Greenspan, A., Zhu, Y., Brodaty, H., et al. (2007). The efficacy and safety of risperidone in the treatment of psychosis of Alzheimer's disease and mixed dementia: A meta-analysis of 4 placebo-controlled clinical trials. *International Journal of Geriatric Psychiatry, 22,* 475–484.

Kosterman, R., Graham, J. W., Hawkins, J. D., Catalana, R. F., & Herrekenkohl, T. I. (2001). Childhood risk factors for persistence of violence in the transition to adulthood: A social developmental perspective. *Violence and Victims, 16,* 355–361.

Krakowski, M., & Czobor, P. (2004). Gender differences in violent behaviors: Relationship to clinical symptoms and psychosocial factors. *American Journal of Psychiatry, 161,* 459–465.

Kryzhanovskaya, L. A., Jeste, D. V., Young, C. A., Polzer, J. P., Roddy, T. E., Jansen, J. F., et al. (2006). A review of treatment-emergent adverse events during olanzapine clinical trials in elderly patients with dementia. *Journal of Clinical Psychiatry, 67,* 933–945.

Kutcher, S., Aman, M., Brooks, S. J., Buitelaar, J., van Daalen, E., Fegert, J. et al. (2004). International consensus statement on attention-deficit/hyperactivity disorder (ADHD) and disruptive behaviour disorders (DBDs): Clinical implications and treatment practice suggestions. *European Neuropsychopharmacology, 14,* 11–28.

Lorenz, K. (1966). *On aggression.* New York: Harcourt Brace Jovanovich.

Maguire, K., & Pastore, A. L. (Eds.). (2003). Sourcebook of Criminal Justice Statistics [online] http://www.albany.edu/sourcebook Accessed August, 2004.

Makris, N., Biederman, J., Valera, E. M., Bush, G., Kaiser, J., Kennedy, D. N., et al. (2007). Cortical thinning of the attention and executive function networks in adults with attention-deficit/hyperactivity disorder. *Cerebral Cortex, 17,* 1364–1375.

Mason, A. W., Kosterman, R., Hawkins, J. D., Herrenkohl, T. I., Lengua, L. J., & McCauley, E. (2004). Predicting depression, social phobia, and violence in early adulthood from childhood behavior problems. *Child & Adolescent Psychiatry, 43,* 307–315.

Multisite Violence Prevention Project. (2004). The multisite violence prevention project: Background and overview. *American Journal of Preventive Medicine, 26*(1S), 3–11.

Naudts, K., & Hodgins, S. (2006). Neurobiological correlates of violent behavior among persons with schizophrenia. *Schizophrenia Bulletin, 32,* 562–572.

Novaco, R. W., & Taylor, J. L. (2004). Assessment of anger and aggression in male offenders with developmental disabilities. *Psychological Assessment, 16,* 42–50.

Occupational Safety and Health Administration. (2004). *Guidelines for preventing workplace violence for health care & social service workers.* US Department of Labor, OSHA 3148-01R. Available online at http://www.osha.gov/Publications/OSHA3148/osha3148.html

Oquendo, M. A., Krunic, A., Parsey, R. V., Milak, M., Malone, K. M., Anderson, A., et al. (2005). Positron emission tomography of regional brain metabolic responses to a serotonergic challenge in major depressive disorder with and without borderline personality disorder. *Neuropychopharmacology, 30,* 1163–1172.

Pillman, F., Rohde, A., Ullrich, S., Draba, S., Sannemuller, U., & Marneros, A. (1999). Violence, criminal behavior, and the EEG: Significance of left hemispheric focal abnormalities. *Journal of Neuropsychiatry and Clinical Neuroscience, 11,* 454–457.

Raine, A., Lencz, T., Bihrle, S., LaCasse, L., & Colletti, P. (2000). Reduced prefrontal gray matter volume and reduced autonomic activity in antisocial personality disorder. *Archives of General Psychiatry, 57,* 119–127.

Rowe, D., Almeida, D., & Jacobson, K. (1999). School context and genetic influences on aggression in adolescence. *Psychology Science, 10,* 277–280.

Scourfield, J., Van den Bree, M., Martin, N., & McGuffin, P. (2004). Conduct problems in children and adolescents. *Archives of General Psychiatry, 61,* 489–496.

Shinoda-Tagawa, T., Leonard, R., Pontikas, J. McDonough, J. E., Allen, D., & Dreyer, P. I. (2004). Resident-to-resident violent incidents in nursing homes. *Journal of the American Medical Association, 291,* 591–598.

Sijbrandij, M., Olff, M., Reitsma, J. B., Carlier, I. V., & Gersons, B. P. (2006). Emotional or educational debriefing after psychological trauma. Randomised controlled trial. *British Journal of Psychiatry, 189,* 150–155.

Sink K. M., Holden K. F., & Yaffe K. (2005). Pharmacological treatment of neuropsychiatric symptoms of dementia: A review of the evidence. *JAMA, 293,* 596–608.

Smith, P., Waterman, M., & Ward, N. (2006). Driving aggression in forensic and non-forensic populations: Relationships to self-reported levels of aggression, anger and impulsivity. *British Journal of Psychology, 97,* (Pt3), 387–403.

Sorrentino, A. (2004). Chemical restraints for the agitated, violent, or psychotic pediatric patient in the emergency department: Controversies and recommendations. *Current Opinion in Pediatrics, 16,* 201–205.

Sourander, A., Ellilia, H., Valimaki, M., & Piha, J. (2002). Use of holding, restraints, seclusion, and time-out in children and adolescent psychiatric in-patient treatment. *European Child and Adolescent Psychiatry, 11,* 162–167.

Staller, J. A. (2007). Psychopharmacologic treatment of aggressive preschoolers: A chart review. *Progress in Neuropsychopharmacology of Biological Psychiatry, 31,* 131–135.

Substance Abuse and Mental Health Services Administration. (2006). *Results from the 2005 National Survey on Drug Use and Health: National Findings.* Rockville, MD: Office of Applied Studies, NSDUH Series H-30 DHHS Publication No. SMA 06-4194.

Swaim, R. C., Henry, K. L., & Kelly, K. (2006). Predictors of aggressive behaviors among rural middle school youth. *Journal of Primary Prevention, 27,* 229–243.

Swanson, J. W., Swartz, M. S., Van Dorn, R. A., Elbogen, E. B., Wagner, H. R., Rosenbeck, R. A., et al. (2006). A national study of violent behavior in persons with schizophrenia. *Archives of General Psychiatry, 63,* 490–499.

Trocki, K. F., & Caetano, R. (2003). Exposure to family violence and temperament factors as predictors of adult psychopathology and substance use outcomes. *Journal of Addictions Nursing, 14,* 183–192.

Uhlmann, E., & Swanson, J. (2004). Exposure to violent video games increases automatic aggressiveness. *Journal of Adolescence, 27,* 41–52.

van Goozen, S. H., Fairchild, G., Snoek, H., & Harold, G. T. (2007). The evidence for a neurobiological model of childhood antisocial behavior. *Psychological Bulletin, 133,* 149–182.

Völlm, B., Richardson, P., McKie, S., Elliott, R., Deakin, J. F., & Anderson, I. M. (2006). Serotonergic modulation of neuronal responses to behavioural inhibition and reinforcing stimuli: An fMRI study in healthy volunteers. *European Journal of Neuroscience, 23,* 552–560.

Wagner, L. M., Capezuti, E., Brush, B., Boltz, M., Renz, S., & Talerico, K. A. (2007). Description of an advanced practice nursing consultative model to reduce restrictive siderail use in nursing homes. *Research in Nursing & Health, 30,* 131–140.

Yang, Y., Raine, A., Narrm, K. L., Lencz, T., LaCasse, L., Colletti, P., et al. (2007). Localisation of increased prefrontal white matter in pathological liars. *British Journal of Psychiatry, 190,* 174–175.

SUGGESTED READINGS

Antai-Otong, D. (2004). *Psychiatric emergencies.* Eau Claire, WI. Professional Education Institute.

Coccaro, E. F., Beresford, B., Minar, P., Kaskow, J., & Geracioti, T. (2007). CSF testosterone: Relationship to aggression, impulsivity, and venturesomeness in adult males with personality disorder. *Journal of Psychiatric Research, 41,* 488–492.

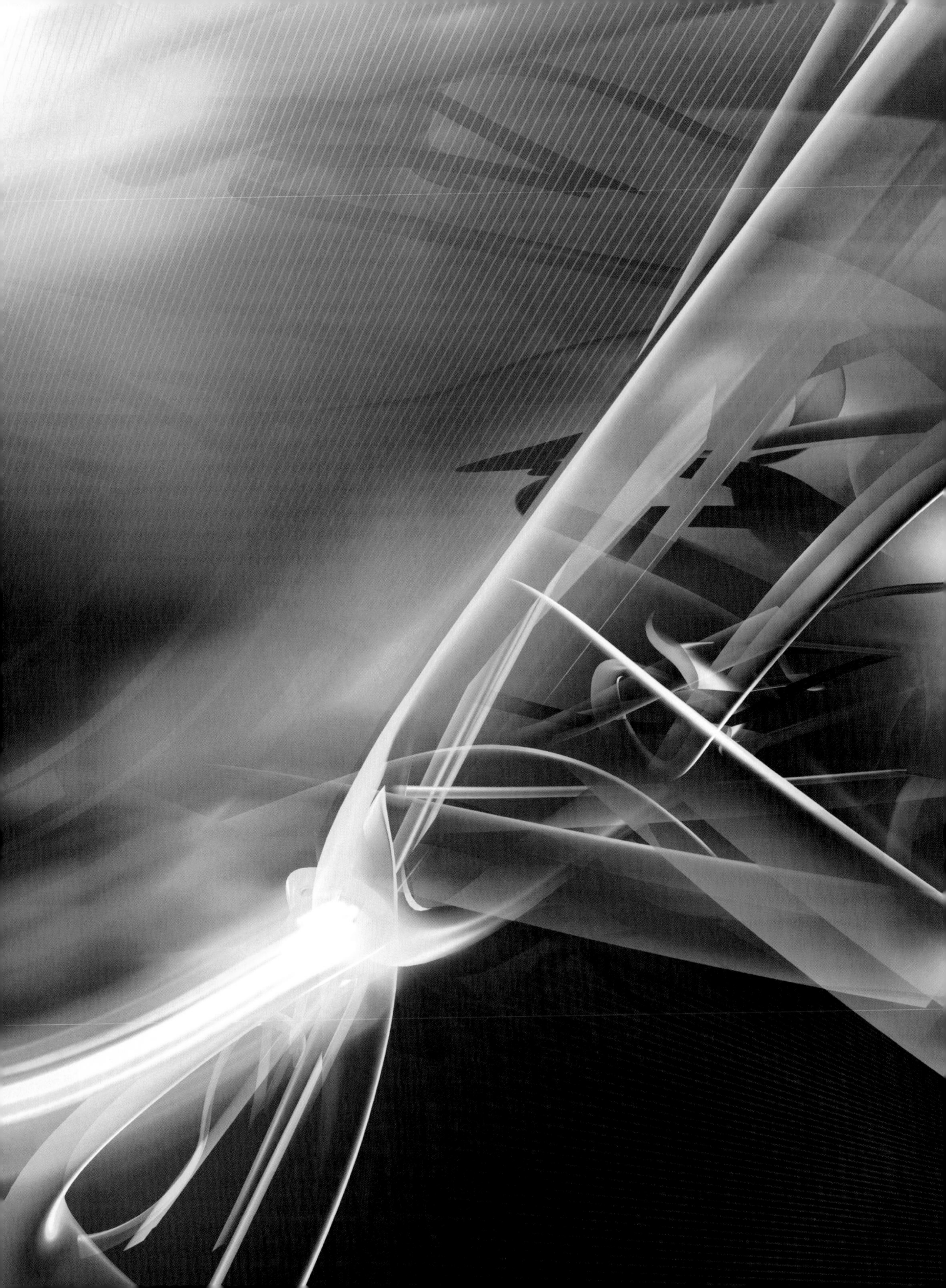

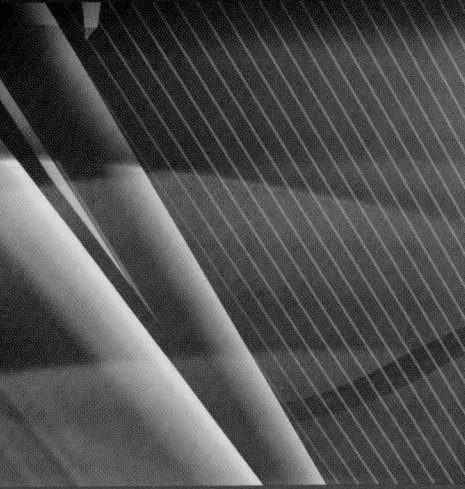

CHAPTER 21

The Client with a Substance-Related Disorder

Susan Beyer, MSN, APRN, BC, LCDC
Deborah Antai-Otong, MS, APRN, BC, FAAN

KEY TERMS

Abstinence: Refers to avoidance of all substances with abuse potential. It denotes cessation of addictive behaviors, such as substance abuse/dependence.

Addiction: A pattern of out-of-control or compulsive use of psychoactive substances in which use continues despite negative consequences; often used interchangeably with the terms *chemical dependency or substance dependence*.

Al-Anon: A self-help group for spouses, parents, or significant others of alcoholics.

Alcoholics Anonymous: An international self-help organization whose purpose is to help alcoholics achieve and maintain sobriety.

Binge Use: Five or more drinks at the same time or within two hours of each other at least once in the past month (SAMHSA, 2004).

Chemical Dependency: A pattern of out-of-control or compulsive use of psychoactive substances in which use continues despite negative consequences; a popular term often used interchangeably with the terms *addiction* or *substance dependence*.

Delirium Tremens (DTs): The most serious form of alcohol withdrawal that can be potentially fatal; characteristic symptoms include profound confusion, disorientation, and autonomic arousal; also known as alcohol withdrawal delirium.

Denial: An assertion that an allegation is false despite evidence to the contrary.

Dual Diagnosis: Refers to the condition of a person who has been diagnosed with a mental disorder and substance use or abuse. The term *dual diagnosis* may also be used to describe a person who has a mental disorder and mental retardation or developmental disability diagnosis. May also be known as a comorbid diagnosis.

Freebase Cocaine: A purer form of cocaine produced by removing the water-soluble base; commonly referred to as "crack" or "rock" cocaine.

Pseudoaddiction: A syndrome of behaviors resembling addiction that develops in chronic pain management; with adequate pain management, drug-seeking behaviors cease.

Recovery: Refers to a state of wellness or function characterized by symptom management and attaining an optimal level of function and quality of life. It is client-centered and based on principles of hope, healing, and optimism. In substance-use treatment, it refers to a state of physical and psychological health in which abstinence from dependency-producing drugs is complete and comfortable.

Relapse: Use of psychoactive substances after a maintained period of abstinence.

Substance Abuse: Repeated intentional use or misuse of a psychoactive substance; use is modified or discontinued with the occurrence of significant adverse consequences.

Substance Dependence: The accepted diagnostic term for a pattern of out-of-control or compulsive use of psychoactive substances in which use continues despite negative consequences; often used interchangeably with the terms *addiction* or *chemical dependency*.

Substance Intoxication: Substance-specific physical, psychological, and cognitive effects produced as a result of ingesting a psychoactive substance.

Tolerance: A pharmacologic property of certain substances in which increased amounts over time are necessary to achieve similar results as in earlier use.

Wernicke-Korsakoff Syndrome: A complication of Wernicke's encephalopathy characterized by profound memory impairment and an inability to learn new material.

Wernicke's Encephalopathy: A reversible delirium seen in alcoholics; it is associated with thiamine deficiency.

Withdrawal Syndrome: Substance-specific signs and symptoms precipitated by the abrupt cessation or reduction of a substance that produces tolerance and dependence after prolonged use.

COMPETENCIES

Upon completion of this chapter, the learner should be able to:

1. Define common terms and concepts related to substance-related disorders.

2. Describe biopsychosocial perspectives for understanding substance use disorders.

3. Identify major substances of abuse and patterns of abuse and dependency.

4. Describe the signs and symptoms of intoxication and withdrawal.

5. Distinguish medical complications commonly associated with abused substances.

6. Assess the impact of substance abuse and dependency on the individual, the family, and the community.

7. Discuss pharmacologic and psychosocial treatment approaches.

8. Apply the nursing process to the care of clients and families experiencing substance use disorders.

9. Recognize attitudes and opinions that enhance or inhibit health promotion and maintenance.

10. Identify referral resources for persons and family members affected by substance use disorders.

Advances in neurobiology are rapidly providing new and expanded knowledge of human behavior, health, and disease. The role of biochemical processes has enhanced our understanding of health maintenance, prevention, and treatment of many illnesses. Addictionology—the diagnosis and treatment of addictive disorders—has greatly benefited from this knowledge explosion. Nevertheless, disagreement exists among health professionals regarding the etiology, progression, and treatment of substance use disorders. Despite technology's advances, the specific causes continue to elude us. Treatment remains multidimensional as well with no one approach rigorously supported by research. Neither psychosocial or biochemical processes fully explain the complexities of substance abuse and dependence nor offer us the best answer to treatment. Though this lack of knowledge can be frustrating, persons with substance use disorders are not uncommon. They will need nursing care at some point in their lives. The professional nurse will provide the highest quality of care prepared with a basic understanding of the biopsychosocial-spiritual concepts related to substance use disorders.

HISTORICAL PERSPECTIVES

References to the use of mind-altering substances can be found from antiquity forward. Substance use and misuse are cited in the Bible, Chaucer's *The Canterbury Tales* (2000) written in the fourteenth century, and in Shakespeare. The excessive use of alcohol became a focus of American medicine between 1780 and 1830 (White, 1998). In the late 1800s, magazines offered unregulated mail-order medicines containing alcohol, opium, and cocaine. The number of individuals exhibiting short- and long-term mental status changes related to alcohol dependence increased. There was also an epidemic of syphilis and its neuropsychiatric complications, and the number of treatment facilities known as asylums multiplied during this era (Shorter, 1997). The syringe appeared on the scene in the Civil War era and some soldiers returned home dependent on morphine. Morphine's efficacy as an analgesic was well known by this time and there was an emerging awareness of its addictive properties. The Sears catalogue offered 50 cent cures for alcohol habits and 75 cent cures for morphine habits (White, 1998). As the new century emerged, the antialcohol temperance movement gained strength. Alcohol was blamed for a variety of individual and societal ills. Unwittingly, it may have promoted the use of opiates. No respectable person of good social standing, particularly women, wanted to be seen drinking. Opiate use was much less public and medicinal use may have preceded subsequent dependency. Concerns began to emerge that doctors were overmedicating their patients, producing opium fiends. The Harrison Narcotic Act of 1914 regulated the manufacture, distribution, and prescribing of opiate substances. Efforts to outlaw alcohol culminated in 1920 with the passage of the 18th amendment to the Constitution prohibiting the sale, manufacture, or transportation of intoxicating liquors. Organized crime was born to satisfy the public's appetite for alcoholic beverages, which continued despite legal prohibitions. Underground saloons and private stills emerged, as did the gangsters who did most of the trafficking in illegal liquor. During World War II tobacco cigarettes were issued as part of standard gear to soldiers fighting for America's freedom. The 1960s, 1970s, and 1980s saw an explosion of the drug culture and the attitude "if it feels good do it." Soldiers serving in Vietnam had access to a ready supply of heroin. Many of America's long trusted institutions and mores were being questioned as the country fought an unpopular war in a faraway, little understood part of the world. Some veterans came back home as drug or alcohol abusers or addicts. As drug use became part of the scene in white middle-class youths, laws at the state and federal levels emerged, further regulating or prohibiting a variety of psychoactive substances. Whereas criminalizing alcohol in the 1920s did little to effectively deter demand, the drug laws of the late 20th century produced an exploding prison population of drug offenders, with mixed impact on supply or demand.

SUBSTANCE ABUSE IN THE TWENTY-FIRST CENTURY

Substance-related disorders in the late twentieth and early twenty-first centuries are viewed as a public health problem. By inclusion in Healthy People 2010 (United States Department of Health and Human Services [U.S. DHHS], 1999), the nation's public health agenda, there is broad recognition of the negative impact on individuals, families, and society. Economic impact is in the billions. Disruption to relationships, marriage, and family; lost productivity in the workforce; criminal justice costs; and health consequences add up to over $1000 for every individual in America when all costs are considered (U.S. DHHS, 1999). Every nurse in every health care setting will encounter individuals and families who have been affected directly or indirectly by what is considered a major public health problem. A basic understanding of the physical, psychological, social, and spiritual dimensions of substance-related disorders is part of a broad-based fund of knowledge the nurse can use in promoting health and preventing disease.

DEFINITIONS AND OVERVIEW

The complexity of substance-related disorders lies in its neurobiological and behavioral underpinnings. The following section provides an overview of major concepts associated with substance-related disorders that include addiction, tolerance, withdrawal, and dependence. Understanding these concepts enables the nurse to integrate biological and behavioral concepts into holistic nursing care and facilitate positive treatment outcomes.

ADDICTION, TOLERANCE, WITHDRAWAL, AND DEPENDENCE

The term addiction is used to describe a dependent pattern of behavior on drugs or alcohol in which the ability to moderate or stop use is repeatedly unsuccessful. There can be a sense of craving in the absence of the substance and an uncontrollable compulsion to use it again despite the knowledge of negative consequences. The loss of control over frequency or amount of use is a key indicator of addiction.

Tolerance is a pharmacologic property of some substances in which chronic use produces changes in the central nervous system so that more of the substance is needed to produce desired effects. With cessation or reduction of use, depending on the pharmacologic properties of the substance, a withdrawal syndrome may occur. Typically, the symptoms of withdrawal are the opposite of the effects of the substance. Addiction can be present even if a withdrawal syndrome does not occur. Tolerance and withdrawal can occur without addiction. Withdrawal syndromes are specific to the individual substance. All classes of substances, with the exception of caffeine and nicotine, may cause delirium and psychosis during intoxication as well as varying degrees of depression or anxiety with

intoxication or after withdrawal. There are abused substances that do not produce tolerance or withdrawal, yet they are highly addictive. Cocaine is highly addictive, yet its withdrawal syndrome is not as intense physiologically and does not require the degree of medical intervention ideally needed to manage opiate or alcohol withdrawal.

Chemical dependency and substance dependence are often used interchangeably with the term *addiction*. Although addiction and chemical dependency are not diagnostic labels in the *Diagnostic and Statistical Manual of Mental Disorders* (4th edition, Text Revision) *(DSM-IV-TR)* (American Psychiatric Association [APA], 2000), they are terms commonly used (and misused) by health care professionals and the general public. Substance abuse and substance dependence are diagnostic terms with standard criteria that describe patterns of misuse and resulting adverse effects of mood-altering substances (Table 21–1).

There is concern by some (Jaffe & Anthony, 2005) in the psychiatric field that continuing to use the terms *addict* or *addiction* promotes a derogatory labeling of the individual with substance dependence. These terms are still widely used by many mental health and addictions professionals and are not intended to promote negative images. Substance-related disorders have neurobiological foundations and should be seen as legitimate medical problems, not moral failings. Others may disagree as to the emphasis on biological explanations and see substance abuse or dependence as a disturbance more rooted in psychosocial or spiritual causes. The evidence is strong, nonetheless, that just about every substance of abuse shares common neurochemical processes and pathways and sets in motion a cascade of biochemical responses. These drive the compulsive use and loss of control that characterize addiction (Kalivas & Volkow, 2005; Liu, Bubar, Lanfranco, Hillman, & Cunningham, 2007). Individual, environmental, and social factors are also important in understanding addictive disorders. The complex interplay of various factors more than likely contributes to the fact that no one particular treatment method is scientifically supported as being significantly superior. It is also important to note that the majority of individuals using drugs or alcohol to excess have substance abuse rather than substance dependence disorders.

INTOXICATION AND WITHDRAWAL

Substance intoxication occurs when an individual is exposed to a specific substance. Features are characteristic to the specific substance and eventually subside. Changes can be produced in alertness, coordination, attention, judgment, and thinking as well as in pulse, respiration, and blood pressure. Different substances can produce similar patterns of intoxication as in cocaine and amphetamine as stimulants, or alcohol and benzodiazepines as central nervous system (CNS) depressants. Medical and nursing interventions must be tailored to the features of the specific substance. As in the management of withdrawal syndromes, knowing the substance that has been used guides the plan of care in both degree and intensity of intervention (Table 21–2).

TABLE 21–1
DSM-IV-TR Diagnostic Criteria for Selected Substance-Related Disorders

Disorder	Criteria
Substance Abuse	A. A maladaptive pattern of substance use leading to clinically significant impairment or distress, as manifested by one (or more) of the following, within a twelve-month period:

A. A maladaptive pattern of substance use leading to clinically significant impairment or distress, as manifested by one (or more) of the following, within a twelve-month period:

1. Recurrent substance use resulting in a failure to fulfill major role obligations at work, school, or home (e.g., repeated absences or poor work performance related to substance use; substance-related absences, suspensions, or expulsions from school; neglect of children or household).

2. Recurrent substance use in situations in which it is physically hazardous (e.g., driving an automobile or operating a machine when impaired by substance use).

3. Recurrent substance-related legal problems (e.g., arrests for substance-related disorderly conduct).

4. Continued substance use despite having persistent or recurrent social or interpersonal problems caused or exacerbated by the effects of the substance (e.g., arguments with spouse about consequences of intoxication, physical fights).

B. The symptoms have never met the criteria for Substance Dependence for this class of substance.

Substance Dependence

A maladaptive pattern of substance use, leading to clinically significant impairment or distress, as manifested by three (or more) of the following, occurring at any time in the same twelve-month period:

1. Tolerance, as defined by either of the following:

   a. A need for markedly increased amounts of the substance to achieve intoxication or desired effect

   b. Markedly diminished effect with continued use of the same amount of the substance

2. Withdrawal, as manifested by either of the following:

   a. The characteristic withdrawal syndrome for the substance

   b. The same (or closely related) substance is taken to relieve or avoid withdrawal symptoms

3. The substance is often taken in larger amounts or over a longer period of time than was intended.

4. There is a persistent desire or unsuccessful efforts to cut down or control substance use.

5. A great deal of time is spent in activities necessary to obtain the substance (e.g., visiting multiple doctors or driving long distances), use the substance (e.g., chain smoking), or recover from its effects.

6. Important social, occupational, or recreational activities are given up or reduced because of substance use.

7. The substance use is continued despite knowledge of having a persistent or recurrent physical or psychological problem that is likely to have been caused or exacerbated by the substance (e.g., current cocaine use despite recognition of cocaine-induced depression, or continued drinking despite recognition that an ulcer was made worse by alcohol consumption).

Substance Intoxication

1. The development of a reversible substance-specific syndrome due to recent ingestion (or exposure to) a substance.

2. Clinically significant maladaptive behavioral or psychological changes that are due to the effect of the substance on the central nervous system (e.g., belligerence, mood lability, cognitive impairment, impaired judgment, impaired social or occupational functioning) and develop during or shortly after use of the substance.

3. The symptoms are not due to a general medical condition and are not better accounted for by another medical disorder.

(continues)

TABLE 21–1

DSM-IV-TR Diagnostic Criteria for Selected Substance-Related Disorders *(continued)*

Disorder	Criteria
Substance Withdrawal	1. The development of a substance-specific syndrome due to the cessation of (or reduction in) substance use that has been heavy and prolonged.
	2. The substance-specific syndrome causes clinically significant distress or impairment in social, occupational, or other important areas of functioning.
	3. The symptoms are not due to a general medical condition and are not better accounted for by another medical disorder.

Note. From *Diagnostic and Statistical Manual of Mental Disorders* (4th edition, Text Revision) *(DSM-IV-TR),* by the American Psychiatric Association, 2000, Washington, DC: Author. Adapted with permission.

The occurrence and potential seriousness of withdrawal or intoxication varies according to the specific substance, amount used, and the unique biology of the individual. A debilitated, older adult with an alcohol problem who has gone through multiple episodes of withdrawal will be at higher risk for a more dangerous medical course than an otherwise healthy younger adult in the first withdrawal episode. It is possible that the first time cocaine is nasally ingested, one individual feels a euphoric high and another suffers a cardiac arrest.

Detoxification refers to the process of systematically and safely managing withdrawal from a substance. Going through "detox" is often the first step of formal drug or

TABLE 21–2

Selected Substances: Peak Time of Withdrawal Onset and Period of Detection

Substance	Peak Time for Onset After Last Use	Detectable in Body
Alcohol	12–24 hours	6–10 hours
Benzodiazepines		1–6 weeks
Short acting	12–24 hours	
Long acting	5–8 days	
Barbiturates		2–10 days
Short acting	12–24 hours	
Long acting	5–8 days	
Nicotine	24 hours	1–2 days
Cocaine	4–6 hours	2–4 days
Crack cocaine	30–60 minutes	2–4 days
Amphetamines	12–24 hours	1–2 days
Heroin	10–12 hours	2–3 days
Methadone	24–96 hours	1 day–1 week
Marijuana		2 days–5 weeks
LSD		8 hours
PCP		2–8 days

LSD, lysergic acid diethylamide; PCP, phencyclidine.

alcohol treatment. Less-informed nurses assume a difficult drug or alcohol withdrawal ("let him go cold turkey") will motivate the individual to stop abusing substances. This is not accurate. The fear or discomfort of withdrawal can play a part in promoting continued compulsive use, particularly if dependence is on alcohol or opiates.

DENIAL AND RELAPSE

Denial is an integral part of addiction and fuels the addictive behaviors. The client minimizes or disconnects from the reality of the negative impact of chemical use. Although it may be painfully clear to others that problems exist, the client with a substance-related disorder may offer little to no acknowledgment. The client may insist there are no problems and any expression of concern or suggestion to get help is viewed as unwelcome meddling. The client with a substance-related disorder may rationalize use of substances as a way to solve problems, fit in with a social group, expand creativity, enhance sexual drive, or cope with boredom, anxiety, or depression. And although some of those things may be true, serious consequences such as loss of job, school failure, disrupted interpersonal relationships, or health problems are routinely minimized, rationalized, or negated in the addict's view of reality. Working with someone in denial is often a source of frustration for the nurse, especially when the client fails to take advantage of treatment resources or returns again and again to substance use. Facilitating a client's move out of denial requires patience, willingness to appropriately confront distorted thinking, and an acceptance that the individual is ultimately in charge of taking any steps toward recovery.

Increasingly, substance dependence is being understood as a chronic, relapsing disorder with similarities to other long-term chronic illnesses such as diabetes or chronic obstructive lung disease. Abstinence, avoiding all substances with abuse potential, is strongly encouraged as part of recovery. For the substance-dependent individual, recovery is the process of experiencing life without the use of substances with abuse potential. Most in the addictions field define successful recovery in broader terms than just abstinence. This view of recovery includes an ongoing process of willingness to live a balanced lifestyle with a wellness focus within the context of healthy spiritual and interpersonal relationships. A relapse for the client implies the return to using substances in the characteristic dependent manner. As in most chronic diseases, relapses are often part of the course of illness. The person with hypertension, diabetes, or hypercholesterolemia is not considered a hopeless failure when health deteriorates due to poor self-care. With the most diligent medical and personal management of chronic illness, relapses or exacerbations occur. In viewing addiction similarly, it is unproductive and possibly life threatening to "give up" on the chemically dependent. It is equally unreasonable to judge treatment as having failed if relapse occurs. Treatment outcomes need to be viewed as effective on the basis of the decrease in substance use and the length of time that the person has been drug or alcohol free (Leshner, 1997). Minimum expectations of the professional

nurse working in any capacity with substance addicted or abusing clients must include a baseline understanding of addiction science. Judgmental attitudes and shaming behaviors can be avoided. Recovery can be promoted.

THE DISEASE CONCEPT

The disease concept of addiction recognizes substance dependence as a complex biogenetic psychosocial disorder that is chronic, progressive, and potentially fatal. Some object to the use of the term "disease" because using a substance the first time is a personal choice. We have yet to fully understand why most individuals stop at experimentation or occasional use, whereas others find it is the first step to a lengthy, if not lifelong, struggle with addiction. Much remains to be discovered about the interplay of genetics, neurobiology, learning, motivation, environment, and social factors. How these factors affect the onset, course, treatment, and resolution of substance use disorders will guide improved prevention and treatment. It is possible to envision a day when we no longer have to speculate about the impact of nature, nurture, and individual choice.

EPIDEMIOLOGY

Substance-related disorders are major health problems in the United States. They challenge psychiatric nurses to differentiate between symptoms of substance-related and psychiatric disorders and recognize they often co-exist. Given the potential for detrimental effects on individuals, families, and communities, it is important to understand the scope of substance use and abuse.

THE NATURE AND EXTENT OF SUBSTANCE USE IN THE UNITED STATES

Substance use and abuse have been monitored routinely since the 1970s by the federal government. Data gathered in interviews with thousands of Americans have revealed patterns and trends used to guide research and intervention efforts. Despite regulation of all psychoactive substances and national, state, and local antidrug efforts, substance misuse remains a major problem with significant economic, social, and interpersonal consequences. The 2004 National Survey on Drug Use and Health (Substance Abuse and Mental Health Services Administration [SAMHSA], 2004) found 19.1 million Americans—almost 8 percent of the total population over age 12—had used an illicit substance in the past month. Marijuana is the most commonly used drug—6.1 percent. This figure is small when compared to the 50.3 percent of Americans who use alcohol. It is important to differentiate among substance ex-perimentation, abuse, and dependence. An estimated 22.5 million—almost 10 percent—were substance dependent on either drugs or alcohol.

Particularly troubling is the fact that drug and alcohol use is very much a part of the youth experience in America. Males and females between ages 12 and 17 have similar rates of substance abuse and dependence at approximately 9 percent.

Substance use can be a gateway to criminal involvement. Almost 40 percent of the criminal justice population demonstrates problematic substance use patterns.

An estimated 23 million people needed treatment for a substance use problem in 2004. Only about 10 percent received it. Cost or insurance barriers were the main reasons desired treatment was not received. Of the 4.6 million with both a mental health and a substance use disorder, less than 6 percent received treatment addressing both health issues (SAMHSA, 2005).

ALCOHOL

Alcohol remains the most used and abused substance in all age groups. Most of those abusing or dependent on alcohol work either full or part time. Approximately 23 percent binge use (five or more drinks on the same occasion in the past month). Heavy drinking (five or more drinks on the same occasion on each of five or more days in the past month) occurs in about 7 percent. Problem alcohol use is highest in the American Indian and Alaskan Native populations at 20.2 percent and lowest in Asians at 4.7 percent. Males misuse alcohol at about twice the rate of females.

Although consumption of alcoholic beverages is illegal for those under age 21 in most states, 10.8 million adolescents between ages 12 and 20 report current alcohol use. Almost 20 percent meet the criteria for binge drinking and 6.3 percent for heavy drinking. Binge patterns in youth are highest in rural areas. Compared to other age groups, those between the ages of 18 and 25 have the highest rates of binge and heavy drinking, peaking at about age 21 (SAMHSA, 2005). In 2004,19 percent of eighth graders, 35 percent of tenth graders, and 48 percent of twelfth graders admitted to drinking alcohol in the month prior to their being surveyed. By the end of high school, 77 percent of students have tried alcohol and 60 percent have been drunk. (Johnston, O'Malley, Bachman, & Schulenberg, 2004). The younger one begins to drink the more likely a pattern of abuse or dependence will develop. Trying alcohol for the first time by age 14 increases the likelihood of problem drinking by adulthood—approximately 17 percent versus 4 percent for those whose first use was after age 18 (SAMHSA, 2005).

TOBACCO, PRESCRIPTION DRUGS, AND ILLICIT SUBSTANCES

With the increase in use of marijuana in the 1960s, illicit substance use increased to a peak of 25 million users in 1979. Illicit substances include marijuana/hashish, stimulants, inhalants, hallucinogens, heroin, and nonmedically used prescription drugs. At the beginning of the twenty-first century, approximately 45 percent had used some type of illicit substance in their lifetime. The figure drops to about 15 percent if marijuana is excluded. In the 2004 Household Survey of Drug Use (SAMHSA, 2005), 19.1 million individuals had used an illicit substance in the prior month, representing 7.9 percent of the population. Marijuana, prescription pain relievers, cocaine, and hallucinogens were the most abused substances. The most common illicit drug combination was alcohol and marijuana.

The stereotype drug user as a down-and-out street person is not supported as 75 percent of those who had used an illicit drug in the prior three months were employed. Employed youths were more likely to have used alcohol or an illicit drug during the past month (SAMHSA, 2005). The prevalence of illicit drug use among persons age 12 to 64 in families receiving some sort of government assistance (9.6 percent) is slightly higher than among persons in families receiving no government assistance (6.8 percent). College graduates used illicit substances at a rate of 5.6 percent versus approximately 8 percent for those with lesser education. About 50 percent of adults who had completed four years of college had tried drugs in their lifetime compared to 37 percent of those who had not completed high school (SAMHSA, 2005).

The highest rate of current use, 13.3 percent, was reported among those characterized by two or more races. The rate for American Indians or Alaskan Natives was 12.3 percent. Rates for the predominant racial groups were similar at 8.1 percent in whites, 7.2 percent in Hispanics, and 8.7 percent in blacks. Asians had the lowest rate at 3.1 percent. In youths, similar trends emerged with the highest rates of current illicit drug use among American Indians and Alaskan Natives. The rates were more than twice that of youths of other races, 26 percent versus 10.6 percent. Youths in families with lower incomes had a slightly higher rate of lifetime illicit drug use than those in families with income above $75,000, 33 percent versus 27 percent (SAMHSA, 2004).

The National Institute on Drug Abuse (NIDA) has collected youth substance use data annually since 1975 (Johnston et al., 2004). The overall rate of use in youths, ages 12 to 17, dropped by half by the late 1970s. This trend began to change by 1992 when rates began to increase. By 2001 the rate had doubled from 5.3 percent in 1992 to 10.8 percent. The earlier drug use begins the greater the risk for dependence in adulthood (SAMHSA, 2000). Cocaine, hallucinogens, prescription drugs, and heroin are used for the first time between ages 17 and 21. Illicit substance use is highest in adolescence peaking between the ages of 18 and 21 (SAMHSA, 2005) (Figure 21–1).

In 2004, results from nearly 50,000 students in over 400 secondary schools revealed older students had an annual rate of illicit drug use holding steady at about 10.6 percent. Eighth graders have shown a gradual decline from a peak of nearly 24 percent in 1996 to approximately 15 percent in 2004. Notable decline in the use of marijuana, LSD, ecstasy (MDMA), steroids, and cigarettes has occurred since 2002. Marijuana was used in the month prior to the survey by 6 percent of eighth graders, 16 percent of tenth graders, and 20 percent of twelfth graders.

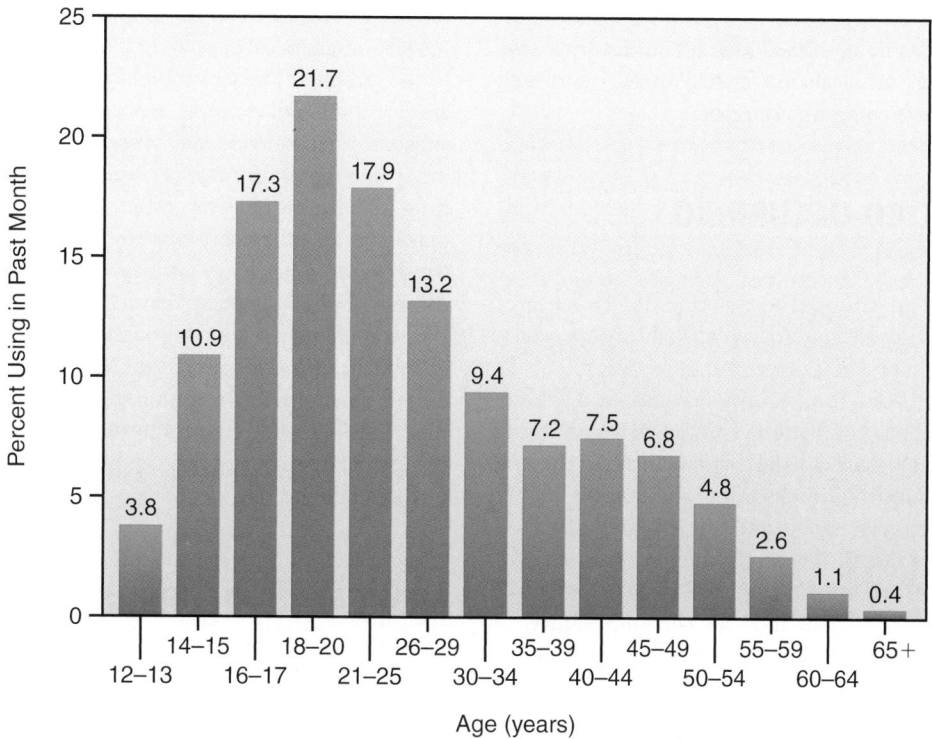

Figure 21–1 Past month illicit drug use among persons aged 12 or older, by age, 2004. (*Overview of Findings from the 2004 National Survey on Drug Use and Health, by the Substance Abuse and Mental Health Services Administration, 2005 Rockville, MD: Author.* http://oas.samhsa.gov/NSDUH/2k4NSDUH/ 2k4Overview/2k4Overview.pdf.)

Over a third of adolescents have used marijuana by the twelfth grade but in 2004 greater numbers of youth expressed disapproval of its use. Heroin use doubled between 1992 and 2000 but has leveled in the past few years. Since its peak in the 1990s, amphetamine use has declined in older students. Diazepam (Valium™) and alprazolam (Xanax™) are the most popular "downers." Hydrocodone and acetaminophen (Vicodin™) and oxycodone (Oxycontin™) were the most frequently abused prescription drugs at 5 and 10 percent, respectively. Given the health dangers, particularly neurological in nature, it is alarming that inhalant use had an upward trend across all grades (SAMHSA, 2005).

Approximately 20 to 30 percent of adults and high school students currently smoke cigarettes. Health risks are well known and rates have dropped significantly. Cigarette smoking is the leading cause of preventable death in the United States. The prevalence of lifetime cigarette use in high school students has declined from approximately 70 percent in 1999 to approximately 58 percent in 2003. The percentage of adult smokers using greater than 25 cigarettes a day has dropped from 19 percent to 12 percent between 1993 and 2003. Current smokers have three to four times the rates of binge and heavy alcohol use compared to nonsmokers. Similar patterns exist for illicit drug and cigarette use. The average age of first use of cigarettes is 15.4 and 16.7 for smokeless tobacco. There are about 4000 new regular smokers daily and more than half are under the age of 18. More disturbing are findings from the National Epidemiologic Survey on nicotine and psychiatric disorders, which indi-

cated that individuals with concomitant psychiatric disorders and nicotine dependency consumed 70 percent of all cigarettes in the United States (Grant, Hasin, Chou, Stinson, & Dawson, 2004).

GENDER DIFFERENCES

Drug use among males is about twice that of females. Factors in the progression toward addiction and its consequences play out differently for men and women. Drug abuse comes later for women and is often woven within the context of intimate relationships. Women become involved with cocaine often to develop or maintain an intimate relationship. Men's cocaine use is associated with friends and in relation to the drug trade. The onset of drug abuse occurs later for females, and a preexisting psychiatric disorder is often present. Histories of childhood sexual abuse and drug- or alcohol-dependent parents are more common for women. Subsequent victimization (homicide, domestic violence) occurs more frequently in women (Harris, Fallot, & Berley, 2005; Morrissey et al., 2005).

Physiologically, women are more susceptible to the effects of alcohol because they absorb more alcohol through the gastrointestinal tract than men. Men have a greater amount of alcohol dehydrogenase in their gastric mucosa. This enzyme metabolizes alcohol and lowers blood alcohol concentration. Greater sensitivity to alcohol may explain why women progress more rapidly from abuse to dependence (Antai-Otong, 2006). Alcohol dependence is more commonly a primary disorder in men, whereas depressive disorders often occur before alcohol dependence in women (Compton, Thomas, Stinson, & Grant, 2007). Men often find their way to treatment because of legal problems. Women often seek treatment in response to health concerns.

PSYCHIATRIC CO-OCCURRING DISORDERS

Dual diagnosis is a term used to describe the presence of substance-related disorders and psychiatric disorders occurring at the same time. The co-occurrence between various mood and anxiety disorders and substance-related disorders is pervasive in the U.S. population. These data also indicate that co-occurring psychiatric disorders may increase the risk of more serious illicit drug use disorders and that the higher the relationship between mood and anxiety and drug use disorders among women suggests a higher incidence of antisocial behaviors in women who use drugs than men. Implications from these data indicate the importance of early identification of high-risk populations, prevention, and appropriate interventions to treat both disorders (Conway, Compton, Stinson, & Grant, 2005). This has prompted more research and treatment providers to reevaluate their programs. The Epidemiologic Catchment Area Study reported that over 70 percent of alcohol-dependent individuals met the criteria for another psychiatric disorder, including drug dependency. In the general population, lifetime prevalence rates for dual disorders were 3 percent or less. Of the affective disorders 16 to 18 percent of those with major depression have a co-occurring alcohol or drug problem. Bipolar disorder was the most common affective disorder to occur with substance use disorders. Schizophrenia and antisocial personality disorder have a particularly high co-occurrence of substance disorders at 50 percent or more (Conway et al., 2005; Kessler et al., 2005).

Diagnosis is often complicated because symptoms of one disorder may mask or mimic those of another. The mechanisms behind dual disorders are as yet not well understood. Possible explanations include the role of genetics and neurobiology. Psychiatric and substance use disorders often have familial patterns and involve the same or similar neurobiological systems. Being vulnerable to one psychiatric illness may increase the risk for developing another. For example, someone experiencing a depressive or anxiety disorder may self-medicate with a stimulant or sedative, seeking symptom relief and laying the foundation for addiction. Diagnostic classifications and criteria change as technology and research reveal new explanations for the etiology, course of a disorder, and more effective treatment. It is possible that some disorders are more alike than different, and current diagnostic classifications have yet to reflect this. For example, some of the behavioral manifestations of addiction share features of personality disorders. Are these two separate entities or, rather, manifestations along a symptom spectrum? Diagnostic classifications and criteria are continually evolving.

As the neurobiology of psychiatric and substance use disorders is better understood, nurses who want to practice in the mental health area can no longer align themselves as solely "psych" or "chemical dependency." Consideration must be given to the potential impact multiple disorders have on treatment and outcome. For example, a client with bipolar disorder and substance dependence may neglect to take mood stabilizers, increasing the risk for mania or severe depression. The risks of drug interactions must be considered. A client taking a benzodiazepine for an anxiety disorder may be at risk for a lethal drug overdose if actively abusing alcohol. Suicide is greater in those with dual disorders, particularly substance use and depression (Cottler, Campbell, Krishna, Cunningham-Williams, & Abdallah, 2005; Sher, 2006; Wines, Saitz, Horton et al., 2004). The nurse in any setting should help clients learn about their illnesses, the opportunity for treatment, and encourage the use of any resources that can help improve functioning and quality of day-to-day life.

MEDICAL CO-OCURRING DISORDERS

Hospitals and health care agencies provide care for premature illness and injury often associated with addiction and substance abuse. Misuse of substances even without a pattern of dependency can produce serious health consequences affecting various body systems. Health promotion and maintenance are not priorities to those in the depths of an addiction. Acute and long-term medical care needs are enormous when considering the types of illness and injury typically associated with substance abuse and dependence. Drug-related HIV/AIDS, hepatitis, tuberculosis, endocarditis, and vascular disease are chronic problems. About 54 to 60 percent of hospitalized clients have a co-existing medical problem in addition to the listed reason for admission. Drug and alcohol abuse are in the top 10 concomitant medical disorders in hospitalized adults aged 18 to 64. In this same age group, excluding pregnancy-related causes, alcohol-related liver disease is one of the top four causes of in-hospital mortality (Merrill & Elixhauser, 2005). Additional costs are associated with those who do not abuse substances but are affected by them such as drug-exposed infants, those exposed by a user to TB, HIV/AIDS, or hepatitis B and C, and victims of drug-related violence or trauma.

ECONOMIC AND HUMAN COSTS

Costs related to drug abuse have risen steadily since the late 1970s with the epidemic of cocaine use in the 1980s, HIV, and enormous expenditures related to crime (Meara & Frank, 2005; Rockette et al., 2005; National Institute on Alcohol Abuse and Alcoholism, 2000). Economic costs are in the billions related to lost productivity from incarceration, crime careers, illness, and premature death. According to findings from SAMHSA's National Survey on Drug Use and Health from 2002 to 2004, approximately 1.2 million adults 18 years of age and older were more likely to be involved in serious violent or property crimes and arrested for murder, rape, robbery, and aggravated assault. Most offenses involved adults who had used illicit drugs in the past year. Those arrested were more likely than those not arrested to have had consumed marijuana, cocaine, crack cocaine, methamphetamines, heroin, and prescription drugs nonmedically (SAMHSA, 2005).

Drug offenses, across all racial groups, are the most common reason for incarceration. About 30 percent of jail inmates were using drugs or alcohol at the time of their offense. About 60 percent of white inmates met criteria for substance abuse or dependence compared to about 45 percent of black or Hispanic inmates. Whites received treatment at double the rate of black or Hispanic inmates (Karberg & James, 2005). Blacks and Hispanics are in jail for drug offenses at rates about 10 percent higher than whites. Whites and Hispanics were four times more likely than blacks to be in jail for driving while intoxicated (James, 2005).

In 2002, two-thirds of all jail inmates met the criteria for either substance abuse or dependence. Marijuana and cocaine were the most frequently abused substances. Inmates were more likely to have been homeless in the year before their incarceration. Over a third had grown up in a home where the parent or guardian abused drugs or alcohol. Sixty-three percent had participated in some form of treatment program in the past with almost half participating while in a correctional system. (Karberg & James, 2005).

The growth of the prison population related to drug offenses, the over-representation of minorities in the criminal justice system, and the lack of community-based treatment programs have prompted discussion concerning the War on Drugs approach of the last 20 years. The majority of dollars has gone to law enforcement at the expense of prevention and treatment. Is prison the best way to make treatment available? The long-term community and societal impact of

incarcerating large numbers of young men, particularly minority men, has yet to be fully realized.

Contemporary data continue to demonstrate a lack of dollars to deter substance use and for diagnosis and treatment (Figure 21–2). Federal, state, and local governments; private insurers; and those directly affected by a drug or alcohol abuser bear the majority of the costs (Rajendram, Lewison, & Preedy, 2006; Rockette et al., 2005). The average American paying federal, state, and local taxes and ever-increasing health insurance premiums, is bearing the cost of failing to adequately address substance use issues.

NATIVE AMERICANS AND THE MYTH OF FIREWATER

With over 500 Native American tribes with differing languages, customs, and ceremonies, problem alcohol use is by no means equally distributed among them. Native Americans, at 1 percent of the American population, however, experience some of the most serious alcohol-related health problems and death rates. Alcohol-related discharge rates for Indian Health Service or tribal-run hospitals were almost 12 percent higher than all other general, short-stay hospitals. Findings from 2002 to 2005 indicated that American Indians and Alaska Natives suffered disproportionately from alcohol-related and other substance use when compared to other ethnic groups (i.e., 10.7 versus 7.6 percent) (Office of Applied Science [OAS], 2006). The firewater myth is one of many factors believed to affect participation and support of prevention and treatment efforts. It holds Native Americans to have a unique genetic predisposition, making them more sensitive to alcohol's effect and thereby more susceptible to problem drinking.

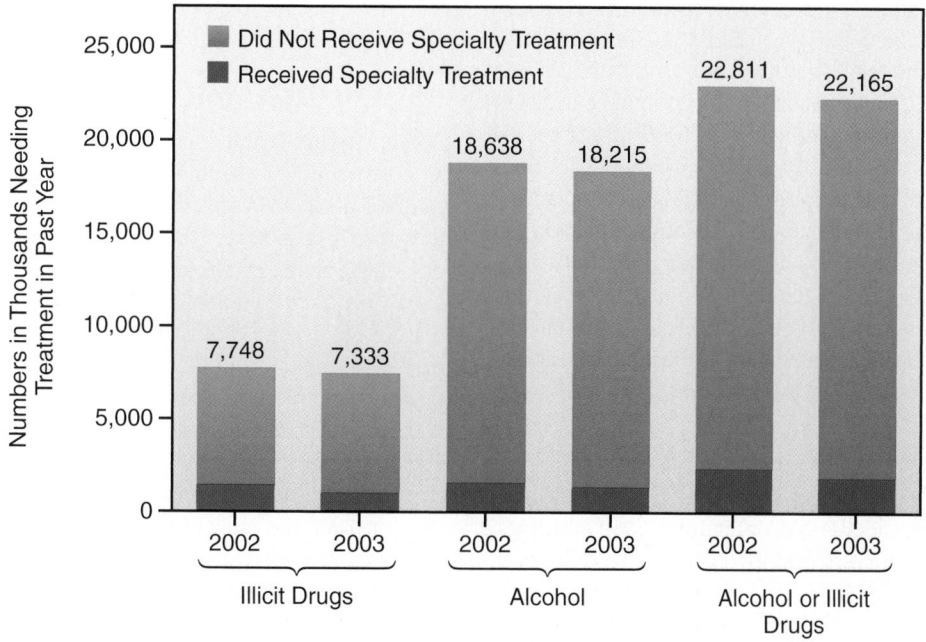

Figure 21–2 Past year need for and receipt of specialty treatment for any illicit drug or alcohol use among persons aged 12 or older, 2002 and 2003 (*From The 2003 National Survey on Drug Use and Health: National Findings, Substance Abuse and Mental Health Services Administration, 2004.* http://oas.samhsa.gov/nhsda/2k3nsduh/2k3Results.htm#toc.)

This myth is not supported by the scientific literature examining objective (biology) and subjective (perception) factors (Ehlers, Wall, Garcia-Andrade et al., 2001). Efforts to understand problem alcohol use and develop prevention and treatment programs should not discount biological factors but examine them within the context of cultural, social, and economic factors as well (Spicer, Bezdek, Manson, & Beals, 2007) Traditional treatment approaches tend to be less successful with the Native American population without the incorporation of culturally relevant concepts and customs.

SUBSTANCE-RELATED DISORDERS: THEORIES AND PERSPECTIVES

Although the exact cause of substance-related disorders remains obscure, there is a plethora of evidence that indicates that they have multifarious underpinnings. Most studies indicate the role of social, biological, and psychosocial factors.

CLASSIC THEORY

If substance use disorders could be definitively explained by one compact theory, effective prevention and treatment efforts would be much easier to develop and implement. Until recently, most research has centered on alcoholism. For over 30 years, the cornerstone theory in addiction science has been E. M. Jellinek's (1960) disease concept of addiction. The most recent definition of alcoholism by the American Society of Addiction Medicine uses many of Jellinek's concepts (Figure 21–3). Although no known cause is apparent, alcoholism is viewed as a chronic, progressive disease that follows a predictable natural history. It progresses in predictable stages, with death as the eventual outcome barring some degree of intervention. In Johnson's classic book *I'll Quit Tomorrow* (1980) alcoholism is referred to as a disease that "swallows up all differences and creates a *universal alcoholic profile*" (p. 5). More recent developments in understanding addiction do not support such a predictable, universal profile. One of the major contributions of the disease model was to move away from viewing addiction as a problem of flawed character. The individual with an addiction is seen, not as a hopeless moral failure, but someone in need of help to overcome a serious problem that involves physical, mental, psychological, and spiritual elements. There is widespread agreement at this time that addiction involves biological, genetic, psychological, and social factors (Figure 21–4).

When individuals have a disease they *are not blamed* for having it; they are, however, held *responsible for participating in the management* of their disease for optimum health outcomes. Disease management in addiction involves a recovery process. Most addiction professionals view recovery as a lifelong process of abstinence, and physical, emotional, and spiritual healing. Some addiction professionals do not consider a spiritual component as necessary to managing addictive behavior. More emphasis is placed on correcting faulty cognitive processes. There

Alcoholism is a primary, chronic disease with genetic, psychosocial, and environmental factors influencing its development and manifestations. The disease is often progressive and fatal. It is characterized by continuous or periodic: impaired control over drinking, preoccupation with the drug alcohol, use of alcohol despite adverse consequences, and distortions in thinking, most notably denial.

Figure 21–3 The American Society of Addiction Medicine definition of alcoholism. *(From The American Society of Addiction Medicine, approved 1990.* www.asam.org*.)*

is little disagreement that for the substance-dependent individual, abstinence is an essential element of the recovery process.

Despite growing understanding of the complex interplay of factors, addiction continues to carry a stigma. Pronouncements that clients with substance-related disorders are weak in character and lack a moral compass are still heard. This outdated moralistic frame of reference fails to take into account the knowledge explosion in the neurobiology of addiction of the last decade. Today, researchers are able to see living images of the brain and map the molecular processes of the nerve cell. The advances gained in neurobiology and genetics over the past decade in no way diminish the interactive nature of social and environmental factors in the genesis and maintenance of addiction. Successful prevention efforts and treatments will follow expanded knowledge of the relationships between the human organism, social systems, and environmental influences. The significance of integrative understanding and implementation of interdisciplinary efforts is to facilitate stronger interface between research and clinical practice. This concept is widely accepted as mainstay treatment of substance-related disorders and highly endorsed by substance abuse and mental health clinicians.

PSYCHODYNAMIC THEORY

Recent psychodynamic thinking emphasizes the role of the ego as a structure of the individual's personality that regulates thinking and controls instinctual drives, most notably drives for pleasure. Ego defenses protect against anger, boredom, emptiness, rage, shame, guilt, and depression. From the psychodynamic perspective, persons with substance-use disorders lack mature ego defenses and thus do not cope well with painful or unpleasant emotion. Impulsive acting out with little ability to postpone gratification is an immature defense. Denying reality and rationalization are narcissistic and neurotic ego defenses. Lacking more effective ego defenses, substance use is an effort to enhance pleasure or self-medicate to soothe emotional distress or pain. The roots of initial substance use lie in this basic unconscious underlying psychopathology. As part of treatment psychotherapy commonly uses psychodynamic principles. The therapist helps the individual or group develop self-awareness, interpersonal growth, and the resolution of current conflicts that may be rooted in the past (Frances, Frances, Franklin, & Borg, 1999).

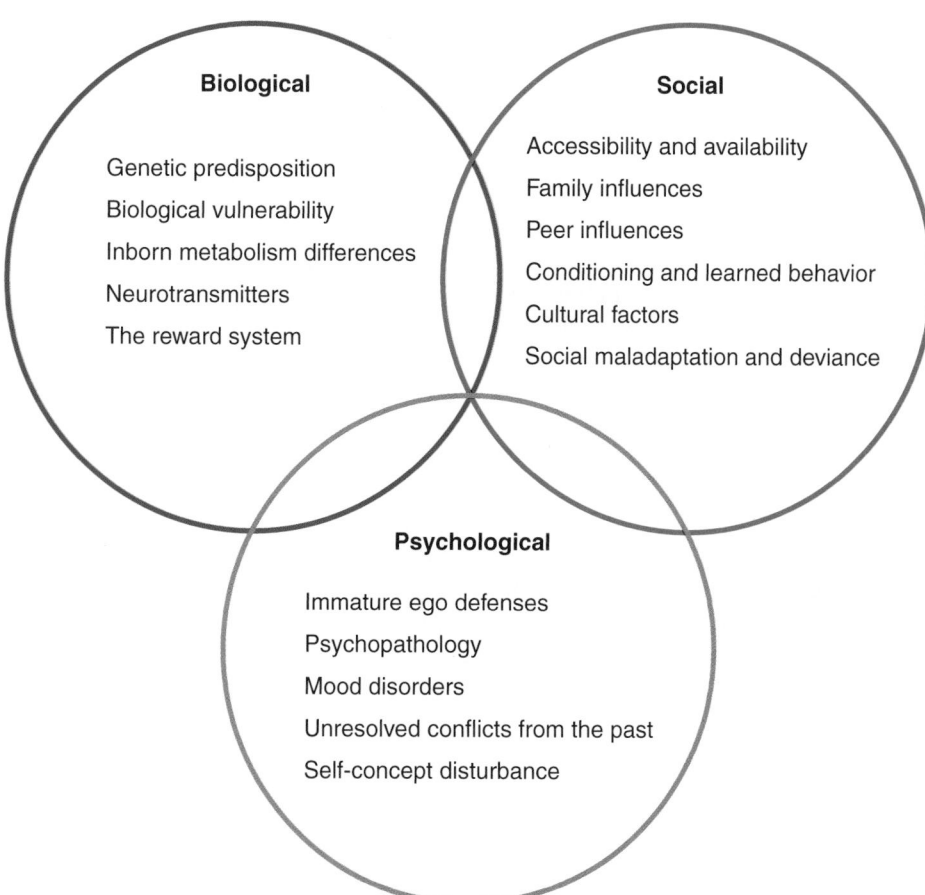

Figure 21–4 Substance use disorders and biopsychosocial influences.

SOCIAL AND ENVIRONMENTAL INFLUENCES

Initial use of drugs or alcohol is influenced by many factors, such as peers and cultures. One's beliefs about the substance and perceptions about its effects and potential dangers may encourage or inhibit experimentation. Availability and cost are important considerations not only for initial but also continued use. Psychopathology and biological vulnerability appear to play a larger role in the development of dependence. The Vietnam era is a good example of the interplay of availability, vulnerability, and environment. Many young soldiers were away from home for the first time in often horrific circumstances with readily available drugs, particularly heroin. Although factors such as prior arrests, school expulsion, and drunkenness predicted drug use, the risk for relapse, and thus dependence, was most associated with being older and white with parents with alcohol-related problems who had been involved in criminal activity (Jaffe & Anthony, 2005).

SOCIAL LEARNING AND CONDITIONING THEORIES

B. F. Skinner's theory of operant conditioning asserts that behavior that produces reward will continue. Rewards reinforce behavior so the likelihood of the behavior continuing can be predicted. Using drugs or alcohol can produce a "rush"—feelings of relaxation, euphoria, elation, and an enhanced sense of well-being. Anxiety, depression, shyness, and social awkwardness are relieved at least temporarily. In some groups social acceptance is gained and maintained by the use of drugs or alcohol. The "drug scene"—meaning the people, places, and things associated with using a substance—promote continued use, because they are associated with the feelings that are produced by drug use. Clients, particularly in early recovery, are urged to avoid their "drug hangouts" and the people with whom they used drugs because these can trigger the craving or the urge to use again.

THE NEUROBIOLOGY OF REWARD AND REINFORCEMENT

"More is known about abused drugs and the brain than is known about almost any other aspect of brain function" (Leshner, 1998, p. 5). Animal studies have provided compelling evidence that virtually all substances of abuse activate the brain's pleasure and reward mechanisms. The reward and pleasure systems reside in what is termed the "old brain," or "primitive brain." The median forebrain bundle is the major site of action of addicting drugs. Neurotransmitters are the chemical message carriers between neurons. They are released from the neuron, travel across the synapse (the space between nerve cells), and exert an effect in the next cell. Dopamine, serotonin, and norepinephrine are the neurotransmitters most understood in the process of addiction. Dopamine is the neurotransmitter most associated with the pleasure and reward system (see Figure 21–5).

The neurochemical processes of this system had to have existed from the origins of human development because they are essential to survival. The brain's release of neurotransmitters ensures repetition of survival behaviors. Not only do these behaviors enhance individual survival but, ultimately, survival of the human species. The fight or flight response to threat, the urge and motivation to eat or drink fluids, and even sexual desire all serve to meet basic survival needs. Satisfying these needs through behavior also produces a sense of well-being, safety, and pleasure. Survival behaviors are thus reinforced time and time again.

Before understanding the neurobiology of reward and reinforcement, compulsive use of a substance was thought to arise from a predisposing internal drive or "addictive personality." Much emphasis was also placed on the role tolerance and withdrawal play as a primary driving force for continued use (Pillolla et al., 2007). Abused substances significantly activate the brain reward system that laboratory animals will continue to self-administer substances even to the point of foregoing food and mating behavior. Using the substance becomes more important than basic survival behaviors. Avoiding the discomfort of withdrawal is no doubt a reinforcement to continued use, but animals (and humans) will compulsively self-administer substances even in the absence of tolerance (Pillolla et al., 2007). Substance-dependent individuals do describe a strong desire to avoid withdrawal symptoms, but if withdrawal avoidance were the key force in maintaining compulsive use, other substances that do not produce significant tolerance and withdrawal syndromes would not be used in a characteristically addictive manner. Although cocaine typically does not produce a withdrawal syndrome with the spectrum of physical symptoms seen in opiates and alcohol, from laboratory animal evidence, it is the most pharmacologically powerful reinforcer of drug-taking behavior (Jaffe & Anthony, 2005).

GENETICS

Although alcohol and alcoholism have been studied most extensively, research is rapidly expanding our understanding of genetic factors associated with other substances of abuse. Studying twins born to parents with alcoholism, but raised in nonalcoholic homes, has provided strong evidence that the tendency to become alcoholic is inherited. Similar studies examining abused drugs also support an increased vulnerability to addiction when a family history is present (Hicks, Krueger, Iacono, McGue, & Patrick, 2004). Family history of addiction does not guarantee the development of alcoholism or drug dependency but it makes an individual at higher risk. Substance disorders are not genetic disorders as of the current state of scientific knowledge. Although no specific genetic link has been identified it is only a matter of time until the role of genetic influence on addictive behavior is better understood.

SUBSTANCE-INDUCED NEUROBIOLOGICAL CHANGES

The way the brain changes after acute and chronic exposure to drugs and alcohol is better understood today than ever before. Tolerance and withdrawal are biochemical processes that occur after repeated use of substances with these pharmacologic properties. Although they are not the only factors associated with addiction, their role cannot be ignored. Postwithdrawal or protracted withdrawal syndromes are thought

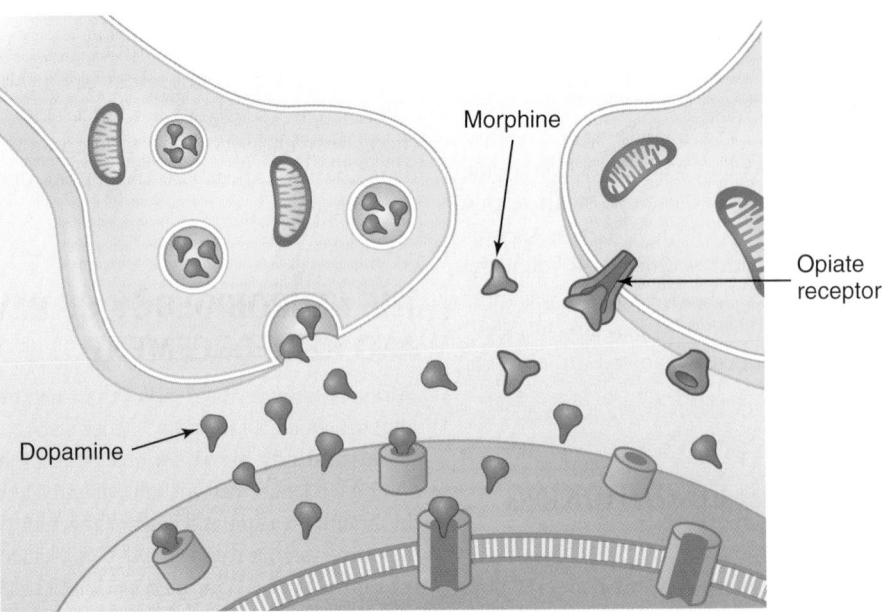

Figure 21–5 Opiates bind to opiate receptors in the nucleus accumbens, resulting in increased dopamine release.

to be associated with relapse risk. Mood abnormalities and anhedonia, particularly in opiate-dependent individuals, may prompt the urge to use again. The syndromes appear to be associated with neurobiological changes resulting from chronic substance exposure and the brain's impaired ability to maintain proper neurochemical balance. Inadequate amounts of gamma-aminobutyric acid (GABA) and dopamine are associated with increased anxiety and depression.

The role of abnormal neuroendocrine response to stressors is becoming better understood in relation to relapse risk, particularly for individuals addicted to opiate and cocaine. Those addicted to opiate and cocaine show a neuroendocrine hypersensitivity to stress exposure. Opiates inhibit the stress system, whereas cocaine activates it. Because cocaine also acts in the pleasure centers of the brain, the "rush" masks the unpleasant feelings produced by the stress response but only as long as the "rush" lasts. Heroin is short acting and individuals addicted to it often experience withdrawal several times a day. Withdrawal produces a rise in stress hormones and related neurotransmitters. The frequent switching on and off of the stress response appears to produce hypersensitivity and the brain produces an outpouring of stress hormones. Compared to nondependent individuals, exposure to mild stress produces an out of proportion stress response (Siegrist et al., 2005). The discomfort and uneasy feelings associated with stress exposure (tension, anxiety, irritability, and anger) are alleviated almost instantly when the drug is used. This quick removal of discomfort and distress may provide the reinforcement for continued use.

Emerging evidence confirms that addiction is a pathological brain disease whose underpinnings include dysregulations in complex neural mechanisms of learning and memory that relate to the quest of rewards and the cues that predict them (Hyman, 2005). Of particular interest are neuroimaging findings such as positron emission tomography (PET) studies which indicate that cue-induced craving is associated with the activation of specific brain regions involved in the reward processes, memory, and attentional mechanisms. Data from these studies expand studies of the neurobiology of addiction (Olbrich, Valerius, Paris, et al., 2006).

Evidence continues to accumulate identifying common as well as specific neurochemical mechanisms of addictive substances (Huang et al., 2007). Despite the ability to demonstrate the brain's consistent neurochemical response to addictive substances, science has yet to determine definitively what makes certain individuals vulnerable to addiction. It is safe to say much remains to be discovered. The role of pharmacologic agents as part of standard substance disorder treatment will grow as more is learned about the brain's function in response to addictive substances.

FAMILY DYNAMICS

The presence of substance abuse or dependence, physical or sexual abuse, emotional abandonment, or any number of family stressors can profoundly affect interpersonal relationships in a family system. Family systems theory maintains that what

affects one family member affects other family members. The system functions to maintain homeostasis even if pathological behavior is necessary to achieve and maintain this balance. An example would be a child starting to use drugs as her parent's marriage begins to disintegrate. The child becomes the "identified patient" in an attempt to draw a unified parental response. The parents' working together to focus on the child's problem accomplishes homeostasis by postponing or thwarting divorce or separation. Families in which addiction is present may deny or rationalize the problem in an effort to maintain homeostasis. This is often referred to as enabling behavior and can become a treatment issue. If the family is to be an effective element in the treatment process, enabling behavior must be identified and addressed. An example of enabling behavior would be the grandmother who takes out a personal loan to cover legal expenses for her grandson who has relapsed again and is arrested on drug charges.

Jaffe and Anthon, (2005) described similarities that have been observed in families with multigenerational substance dependence. These include absence of a parent, particularly from divorce, abandonment, or incarceration; an overprotective, overcontrolling parent; a cold or emotionally distant parent; and the presence of drug-using children who remain overly dependent on the family well into adulthood. The pain of unresolved grief associated with family of origin losses might be a factor in addictive behavior. Although many who are seeking treatment reveal a family history of addiction to various substances, particularly alcohol, there is no universal pattern of pathological family function that fits across the spectrum of abused substances. Difficulties in studying the impact of family function include the variability of self-report when different family members describe similar events in different ways versus the way a researcher or therapist might.

CULTURAL CONSIDERATIONS

Data from the U.S. Census Bureau (2000) indicate that the United States has a growing and more diverse population. In addition, findings from the 2005 National Survey on Drug Use and Health: National findings (NSDUH) (SAMHSA, 2005) indicate that the prevalence of substance-related disorders is higher in large cities (8.4 percent) than in smaller cities (6.9 percent). Beyond the growing diverse population and incidence of substance misuse in high-risk populations, recent studies demonstrate a substantial disparity in availability of health care for minority groups regarding substance-related disorders and mental health care. Substance use patterns vary within social and cultural domains and parallel ethnic group mores and attitudes and extent of acculturation to the larger society. Substance use mores and attitudes are tied to strong predictors of drinking (Bell, Harford, Fuchs, McCarroll, & Schwartz, 2006).

Much of the disparity in mental health care and substance abuse treatment is associated with a lack of culturally sensitive care. Culturally sensitive care requires identifying high-risk groups, reducing barriers to appropriate treatment, and assessing the role of families, communities, spirituality, and religion within the sociocultural context. The sociocultural context shapes the meaning of substances and affects treatment outcomes (Rockett et al., 2005). Self-awareness, accurate diagnosing, and trust and family involvement are critical issues that must be addressed when working with the client with a substance-related disorder.

SUBSTANCES OF ABUSE AND DEPENDENCE

The term *narcotic* can be confusing because it is used to describe a variety of substances. It may be of value to seek clarification as to what specifically is meant when someone uses the term *narcotic*. It comes from the Greek word for stupor and it is used commonly to describe opioid substances. Legally defined in the Controlled Substances Act, narcotic refers to opioids, cocaine, and coca leaves. Cocaine and coca technically are not narcotics. Yet another way the term is used is as a global reference to all substances with abuse potential.

Although the various categories of substances are described individually, it is important to realize that many drug users have a pattern of using multiple substances. Sometimes in the absence of the drug of choice, others will be substituted. Some users intentionally mix substances to produce a particular result, as in combining heroin and cocaine ("speedball"). If no one particular substance is the predominant drug of choice, this pattern is defined as polysubstance dependence (APA, 2000).

CENTRAL NERVOUS SYSTEM (CNS) DEPRESSANTS

CNS depressants induce sedation and drowsiness, and they can produce respiratory depression, coma, and death. Taken in combination they potentiate effects on the CNS. Alcohol, sedative-hypnotics, anxiolytics, and opioids are CNS depressants. They can produce a variety of sensations, including a feeling of relaxation, euphoria, and disinhibition. All have the potential for abuse and dependence.

Alcohol

The most commonly abused drug is alcohol. It is a staple of many social, cultural, and religious rituals and practices. It is used to celebrate good fortune and to drown sorrows. In some societies and cultures, alcoholic beverages with meals are part of every day life and have been for centuries. In others, any form of alcohol for any reason is strictly prohibited. Although research has found that modest drinking is not necessarily dangerous and possibly even beneficial in some ways, for those susceptible to impaired control alcohol use, it can produce devastating physical, emotional, and social effects.

Alcohol is absorbed quickly from the stomach and small intestine, and it is metabolized by the liver at a fixed rate—about one drink (1 ounce) an hour. Alcohol is both fat and water soluble, and it is distributed throughout the body. Its effects are dose dependent (Table 21–3). In its concentrated form alcohol is toxic to nerve cells, whereas in diluted form it is a nerve cell irritant. Thus, long after the drinker eliminates alcohol from the body, a hangover produced by irritated nerve cells may persist. Alcohol stimulates the release of the body's own opioids, endorphins and enkephalins, which turn on the central dopamine reward system.

Frequently, individuals seek medical care for ailments resulting from alcohol use, but alcohol abuse and dependence are underdiagnosed and undertreated in primary care settings. Psychosocial consequences related to legal, occupational, and interpersonal relationship difficulties are frequently part of the history. A history of vehicle crashes, falls, or other traumas should trigger further assessment of alcohol use.

Chronic alcohol use affects all body systems and predisposes a person to a variety of health problems. The classic physical appearance of an alcoholic includes a flushed face, spider angiomas, bulbous nose, abdominal fat accumulation, and a wasted appearance of the extremities. In chronic drinkers, inspection and palpation of the abdomen may reveal an enlarged liver, increased girth related to ascites, and snake-like veins around the umbilicus (caput medusae related to the effects of portal vein obstruction). Bruising and other signs of traumatic injury are common.

Medical complications of chronic alcohol dependence affect all body systems. Commonly seen medical problems are listed in Table 21–4. Alcohol use is also related to increased sexual risk taking such as risk for exposure to HIV infection and other sexually transmitted diseases. When working with older adults, evaluations for dementia must include a history of alcoholism. Chronic, excessive use results in the destruction and shrinkage of neurons, particularly in the frontal cortex of the brain (Liu, Lewohl, Harris, Dodd, & Mayfield, 2007).

Tolerance and dependence occur in heavy alcohol use. Individuals with high tolerance can show little sign of intoxication at blood alcohol levels in which nontolerant individuals would be exhibiting significant impairment. "Anyone who does not show significant levels of impairment at about 150 mg/dL probably has significant pharmacodynamic tolerance" (Schuckit, 2005, p. 961). The misconception exists among many that drinking beer or wine will not cause as many problems as hard liquor. Over time heavy drinking produces tolerance, whether the ethanol is delivered via very expensive bottles of Scotch whiskey or six packs of beer. This is a key point to emphasize when providing health education about alcohol use.

Withdrawal is associated with neuronal excitation in the face of abrupt cessation of the depressant action of alcohol. Its development is related to the amount of alcohol ingested on a daily basis. It is dose dependent in that heavier drinkers are more likely to develop withdrawal—the brain adapts to regular doses and cannot function sufficiently without the presence of alcohol. Withdrawal is mild in the majority of individuals who develop it, and it does not occur in every alcohol-dependent person. Early withdrawal can occur within hours of the last drink or with a decrease in the amount of drinking. The time the last drink was taken is an

TABLE 21–3
Blood Alcohol Level (BAC) and Effects

BAC	Number of Drinks* Male	Female	Effects**
.02	1	½	Relaxed; congenial
.05	2½	1½	Mood changes; loosening inhibitions; ↓ judgment; slight euphoria
.10	5	<2	↓ muscle coordination; ↓ reaction time; impaired vision; driving impaired
.20	10	<5	Staggering; poor emotional control; poor frustration tolerance, poor impulse control; memory loss; passing out
.25	12½	6½	Worsening of above
.30–.40	15–20	7½–10	.30 mental confusion, stupor .40 coma .50+ respiratory depression; death

*One drink (12 g ethanol) = 12 oz beer; 4 oz wine; 1–1½ oz 80 proof liquor.
**Based on the average 150# male and average 120# female.

important assessment question. Tremor, commonly referred to as "the shakes," is the hallmark sign of withdrawal. Some individuals will show no sign of external tremor but complain of an internal sense of shakiness (McIntosh & Chick, 2004). Tremors, particularly mild ones, can be detected best by asking the person to hold the arms outstretched in front.

TABLE 21–4
Medical Consequences of Alcoholism

Brain atrophy	Gastritis
Dementia	Peptic ulcers
Esophagitis	Acute and chronic pancreatitis
Esophageal varices	
Alcoholic cardiomyopathy	Testicular atrophy
	Alcoholic myopathy
Lowered resistance to infection	Coagulation deficits
	Anemia
Alcoholic hepatitis	Thiamine deficiency
Cirrhosis	Elevated lipids
Hypersplenism	Peripheral neuropathy

An "eye opener" refers to the need to have a morning drink to calm the nerves and stop tremors.

Withdrawal is also characterized by hyperarousal in the form of the individual being easily startled, anxious, or irritable. Insomnia, loss of appetite, tachycardia and elevated blood pressure, nausea, vomiting, diarrhea, flushing, or diaphoresis can occur. Hallucinations can occur and take the form of misinterpreting noises as voices, spots on the wall as bugs, or shadows as people not there (McIntosh & Chick, 2004). Typically, symptoms peak at about 4 days after the last drink and gradually subside over a period of days. Symptoms can persist for 1 to 2 weeks. Withdrawal can become a life-threatening medical emergency, particularly in the presence of medical co-occurrences such as cardiovascular or renal disease.

Seizures and alcohol withdrawal delirium (delirium tremens, or DTs) comprise the most serious forms of alcohol withdrawal, and they can occur in a small percentage of individuals. Seizures can indicate the development of DTs. Profound confusion and disorientation are classic symptoms. Hallucinations can be present along with significant autonomic nervous system arousal. This is evidenced by hyperpyrexia, hypertension, significant tachycardia, coarse tremor, and agitation. Early withdrawal signs and symptoms may still be present but at a more intense level of severity. Without medical intervention, ketoacidosis, seizures, hyperthermia, cardiovascular collapse, and death can occur.

Prompt identification of withdrawal risk can be more readily detected through an adequate nursing admission assessment regardless of setting. Repeated episodes of developing tolerance and experiencing withdrawal can increase the risk of seizure in subsequent withdrawal episodes. The client should be asked directly how many times she has gone through withdrawal (or detoxifications) and whether or not DTs or seizures have occurred. Early management of withdrawal is preferable to managing DTs. Although no optimal treatment exists for withdrawal delirium, symptoms can be minimized and managed by appropriate pharmacotherapeutic agents.

Individuals at high risk for withdrawal delirium are frequently encountered in acute care hospital settings. Many treatment or rehabilitation centers are not equipped to provide the aggressive medical support required to optimally manage DTs and will refer the client to a medical setting for detoxification management. Clients admitted to acute care hospital settings for medical or surgical reasons not directly related to alcoholism may not disclose their heavy drinking even when queried on routine nursing admission assessment. The nurse discovers the client's alcoholism a few days after admission when the patient develops DTs. The importance of adequate assessment and early intervention cannot be overemphasized. The nurse may often be the one who discovers substance abuse issues not previously disclosed to the treating physician. Communicating this important piece of information is a nursing responsibility and should be documented in the medical record. Some physicians may not be familiar or comfortable with detoxification management and request assistance from psychiatric consultation liaison resources or physicians who specialize in addiction medicine.

Pharmacotherapy promotes prevention of serious withdrawal but it is not a guarantee. Benzodiazepines are the drugs of choice for managing alcohol withdrawal syndrome according to the American Society of Addiction Medicine's evidence-based practice guidelines (Mayo-Smith et al., 2004). They promote rest and decrease the risk for seizures and severe alcohol withdrawal syndrome (McIntosh & Chick, 2004). They are cross-tolerant with alcohol in that each enhances GABA. GABA produces inhibitory effects in the central nervous system. Chlordiazepoxide (Librium), diazepam (Valium), or lorazepam (Ativan) are typical medications given in progressively tapered doses over the course of several days to facilitate safe alcohol withdrawal. An objective withdrawal assessment scale, such as the Clinical Institute Withdrawal Assessment-Alcohol (CIWA-Ar) Tool (Table 21–5) is recommended to monitor the severity of symptoms and response to treatment. Dosing should be individualized based on severity of the withdrawal and half-life considerations. Benzodiazepine selection and dosing should also be guided by whether the client has a healthy liver, by potential drug interactions, and by the presence of any coexisting conditions that could create additional risks for respiratory depression, which can occur with benzodiazepine administration. When frank hallucinations or delusions occur, especially when severe agitation is present, antipsychotics, such as haloperidol, are indicated. Anticonvulsants are not routinely recommended for use in alcohol withdrawal. Reports are mixed regarding the benefit of adding anticonvulsants to routine benzodiazepine treatment. There are reports in the literature of anticonvulsant use in treating mild alcohol withdrawal. For persons with preexisting seizure disorders, the use of anticonvulsants appropriate to the type of seizure in addition to benzodiazepines is appropriate but routine use of anticonvulsants is not standard practice.

Vitamin therapy with parenteral thiamine 100 mg should also be given as soon as possible, followed by daily doses of 50 to 100 mg. Persons with alcohol dependence are at risk for thiamine deficiency owing to inadequate nutritional intake or poor gastrointestinal absorption. Thiamine administration is administered as treatment of choice to try to prevent Wernicke's encephalopathy, a reversible condition associated with thiamine deficiency. Symptoms include ataxia, delirium, and palsy of the sixth cranial nerve (abducens muscle of the eye). Thiamine administration may not prevent delirium in all clients. Untreated, Wernicke's encephalopathy can progress to Wernicke-Korsakoff syndrome. This syndrome is characterized by profound memory impairment and an inability to learn new material. It can be a permanent condition in over 50 percent of cases. Daily doses of thiamine may help a little, but not all recover (Schuckit, 2005).

Sedative-Hypnotics and Anxiolytics

Sedative-hypnotic and anxiolytic drugs are important pharmacotherapeutic agents. They are commonly used to treat chronic and acute anxiety, as adjunctive therapy in other psychiatric disorders, and for preoperative and conscious sedation. The majority of these medications are taken orally and used for less than 1 month. When used for a short time tolerance, dependence, or withdrawal are usually not of concern. Although the risk for abuse and dependence exists, compared to other substances they are not widely abused. Benzodiazepines with shorter half-lives such as alprazolam have greater abuse potential than longer-acting agents. Benzodiazepines rank behind heroin, cocaine, all other opiates, marijuana, barbiturates, and stimulants in terms of mood-altering affects. Individuals who misuse these drugs typically seek a time-limited effect such as mild euphoria or relaxation. Abuse and dependence patterns usually consist of obtaining prescriptions from multiple physicians. Intravenous abuse usually occurs in young adults (Ciraulo & Sarid-Segal, 2005). One of the difficulties that may be encountered in prescription drug dependence is the difficulty breaking through denial. When the drug has been obtained legally through legitimate health care providers, its use may not be seen as problematic because "my doctor prescribed it for me."

Commonly prescribed anxiolytics from the benzodiazepine group include lorazepam (Ativan), alprazolam (Xanax), clonazepam (Klonopin), and diazepam (Valium). These three agents have been reported to produce the best high when compared with other benzodiazepines (Ciraulo & Sarid-Segal, 2005). Sedative-hypnotic benzodiazepine agents include temazepam (Restoril), flurazepam (Dalmane), and triazolam (Halcion). Since the availability of benzodiazepines, barbiturates are used much less frequently for sedative-hypnotic purposes. Phenobarbital is still used as an anticonvulsant and as a sedative in children. Combination analgesics, such as Fiorinal,

TABLE 21–5
The Clinical Institute Withdrawal Assessment-Alcohol (CIWA-Ar) Tool

Patient:_____ Date: ____/____/____ Time: _____ : _____
                                          y   m   d   (24 hour clock, midnight = 00:00)

Pulse or heart rate, taken for one minute: _____ Blood pressure: _____/_____

NAUSEA AND VOMITING—Ask "Do you feel sick to your stomach? Have you vomited? Observation.

0 no nausea and no vomiting
1 mild nausea with no vomiting
2
3
4 intermittent nausea with dry heaves
5
6
7 constant nausea, frequent dry heaves, and vomiting

TREMOR—Arms extended and fingers spread apart. Observation.

0 no tremor
1 not visible, but can be felt fingertip to fingertip
2
3
4 moderate, with patient's arms extended
5
6
7 severe, even with arms not extended

PAROXYSMAL SWEATS—Observation.

0 no sweat visible
1 barely perceptible sweating, palms moist
2
3
4 beads of sweat obvious on forehead
5
6
7 drenching sweats

ANXIETY—Ask "Do you feel nervous?" Observation.

0 no anxiety, at ease
1 mildly anxious
2
3
4 moderately anxious, or guarded, so anxiety is inferred
5
6
7 equivalent to acute panic states as seen in severe delirium or acute schizophrenic reactions

TACTILE DISTURBANCES—Ask "Have you any itching, pins and needles sensations, any burning, any numbness, or do you feel bugs crawling on or under your skin?" Observation.

0 none
1 mild itching, pins and needles, burning, or numbness
2 mild itching, pins and needles, burning, or numbness
3 moderate itching, pins and needles, burning, or numbness
4 moderately severe hallucinations
5 severe hallucinations
6 extremely severe hallucinations
7 continuous hallucinations

AUDITORY DISTURBANCES—Ask "Are you more aware of sounds around you? Are they harsh? Do they frighten you? Are you hearing anything that is disturbing to you? Are you hearing things you know are not there?" Observation.

0 not present
1 very mild harshness or ability to frighten
2 mild harshness or ability to frighten
3 moderate harshness or ability to frighten
4 moderately severe hallucinations
5 severe hallucinations
6 extremely severe hallucinations
7 continuous hallucinations

VISUAL DISTURBANCES—Ask "Does the light appear to be too bright? Is its color different? Does it hurt your eyes? Are you seeing anything that is disturbing to you? Are you seeing things you know are not there?" Observation.

0 not present
1 very mild sensitivity
2 mild sensitivity
3 moderate sensitivity
4 moderately severe hallucinations
5 severe hallucinations
6 extremely severe hallucinations
7 continuous hallucinations

HEADACHE, FULLNESS IN HEAD—Ask "Does your head feel different? Does it feel like there is a band around your head?" Do not rate for dizziness or lightheadedness. Otherwise, rate severity.

0 not present
1 very mild
2 mild
3 moderate
4 moderately severe
5 severe
6 very severe
7 extremely severe

(continues)

TABLE 21–5
The Clinical Institute Withdrawal Assessment-Alcohol (CIWA-Ar) Tool *(continued)*

AGITATION—Observation.

0 normal activity

1 somewhat more than normal activity

2

3

4 moderately fidgety and restless

5

6

7 paces back and forth during most of the interview, or constantly thrashes about

ORIENTATION AND CLOUDING OF SENSORIUM—Ask "What day is this? Where are you? Who am I?"

0 oriented and can do serial additions

1 cannot do serial additions or is uncertain about date

2 disoriented for date by no more than 2 calendar days

3 disoriented for date by more than 2 calendar days

4 disoriented for place and/or person

Total CIWA-A Score _____

Rater's Initials _____

Maximum Possible Score   67

This scale measures 10 symptoms associated with alcohol withdrawal. The scale can be administered by a nurse in about 5 minutes.

SCORING:

0–10	mild withdrawal
11–20	mild/moderate withdrawal
21–25	moderate withdrawal
>25	severe withdrawal, possible impending delirium tremens (DT)

Scores 11–20   Indicate the use of medication is optional.

Scores 21–25   Require close monitoring either in an inpatient setting or outpatient setting where the patient can be reevaluated every hour until the score is below 20. Medication is required.

Scores >25   Require inpatient detoxification until the patient is stable and the score is below 20. Medication is required.

Note: CIWA does not evaluate blood pressure (BP) or pulse. Neither BP nor pulse correlate with the severity of withdrawal. The indices measured by the CIWA are more reliable indicators of the severity of withdrawal. (Sullivan et al., 1989)

The physician must, however, monitor vital signs as an integral part of detoxification, prescribing medication as necessary to control BP and/or tachycardia.

Elevated body temperature >100°F, though not addressed in the CIWA or in CIWA studies, may signal incipient DT or early infection. The physician is advised to closely monitor any rise in body temperature over 100°F and to consider a hospital admission if DT is a possibility.

often have a barbiturate component. Barbiturates have the highest addiction liability and hold the greatest risk for respiratory depression in intoxication and overdose states. Benzodiazepines have a larger margin of safety, but when benzodiazepines or barbiturates are combined with any other central nervous system depressant there is serious risk for overdose and death.

The time from discontinuation to the appearance of withdrawal symptoms depends on the half-life of the drug. Symptoms can begin to develop within 24 hours and peak around 48 hours in short-acting agents. Alprazolam is particularly associated with immediate and severe withdrawal symptoms. Longer half-life agents (diazepam) may not have peak symptom development until about 2 weeks after discontinuation. Symptoms include anxiety, irritability, insomnia, fatigue, headache, muscle twitching, tremor, dizziness, sweating, tachycardia, agitation, nausea, vomiting, and concentration difficulties. Serious withdrawal symptoms include hallucinations, depression, paranoia, delirium, and seizures. Barbiturates have similar withdrawal symptoms. Discontinuation of these agents should ideally be done by tapering the dosage by a planned amount over time, depending on the total daily dose and length of time on the drug.

Opioids

Opioids are natural or synthetic agents possessing morphine-like properties and are primarily used for analgesia. The seedpods of the poppy plant are the naturally occurring source of opium. Medicinal use of opium dates to the time before Christ. Morphine and codeine were isolated from opium in the first half of the nineteenth century, replacing opium for medical use. Heroin, a semisynthetic form processed from morphine, became available in the late nineteenth century and it is most associated with abuse and addiction. Use of an alcohol and opium concoction called laudanum was used widely in the Victorian era. It helped relieve aches and pains and its abuse crossed all socioeconomic classes.

In the 1940s, meperidine (Demerol) and methadone (Dolophine) became available for medical use and were the first purely synthetic opioids (Jaffe & Strain, 2005). Other synthetic analgesic agents include hydromorphone (Dilaudid), fentanyl (Duragesic), propoxyphene (Darvon), hydrocodone (Vicodin, Lorcet, Lortab), and pentazocine (Talwin). Codeine is used in preparations for cough suppression, and diphenoxylate (Lomotil) is used as an antidiarrheal agent.

Lately there have been growing concerns about the illicit use of fentanyl, an opioid analgesic. Fentanyl is an opioid analog whose chemical compounds are similar to heroin in its effects although it differs slightly in its chemical structure. It is especially perilous because it is 50 times more potent than heroin and can instantly cause apnea and death from overdose. Fentanyl also has a shorter duration of action than heroin and is most frequently used intravenously, but it may also be smoked or snorted. Fentanyl (e.g., Duragesic, Actiq, Sublimaze) has several street names that include *dance fever, TNT,* china *white,* and *goodfella* (National Institute on Drug Abuse [NIDA], 2005). Recent reports from major national papers, including the *New York Times* (May 28, 2006) indicate a deadly trend of heroin and cocaine users overdose deaths due to a combination of fentanyl, cocaine, and/or heroin. Up until now, most of these deaths have been reported in several U.S. cities in the northeast and midwest, including Detroit, Philadelphia, and Chicago. Medical examiners attribute deaths to suppression of the natural impulse to breathe. The Centers for Disease Control (CDC) is currently investigating the deaths and community organizations are rushing to disseminate this information.

The site of action of all opioids is the reward centers of the brain. Acting on various receptors (mu, kappa, delta) of the cell membrane, a cascade of neurochemical processes occurs, altering the perception of pain in the brain and spinal cord. Neuronal excitability is reduced and neurotransmitters (glutamate and substance P) that communicate pain messages are inhibited. Stimulation of opioid receptors not only produces analgesia but the commonly seen effects of respiratory depression, pupillary constriction, decreased gastrointestinal motility (constipation), euphoria, as well as physical dependence. Taken in overdose, respiratory depression can result in coma or death. Naloxone hydrochloride (Narcan) competes for receptor binding sites and reverses the depressant effects.

The potential for opioids to produce tolerance, dependence, and withdrawal has been recognized for centuries. Opioids have a high abuse potential because they produce sedation, euphoria, and, depending on the agent, a sudden pleasurable sensation (a "rush"). Heroin addiction is a serious public health problem with significant adverse effects for the individual and the community. The recent trend of increased heroin use in younger age groups is disturbing. Heroin can be used either intravenously or nasally ("snorting"). Although there are no hard data for the numbers of prescription opioid abusers, law enforcement sources cite hydrocodone as a common drug of choice. Prescription drug abusers obtain drugs by calling in fraudulent prescriptions, altering legitimate prescriptions, producing computer-generated prescriptions, and obtaining prescriptions from multiple doctors and emergency rooms.

The majority of medical users of opioids do not become substance abusers. Despite widespread agreement that opioid analgesics are the treatment of choice for pain relief, physicians

Myths to Overcome: Pain Management in Chemically Dependent Clients

1. Adequately managing pain with narcotic pain medication will not worsen a preexisting drug dependency.

2. The likelihood of causing an individual to become drug dependent ("addicted") during medical hospitalization is practically nonexistent.

3. The goal of effective pain relief should be no different in the client with a substance-related disorder than any other client.

4. An effective pain management plan is a collaborative effort among the client, physician, nurse, and other key members of the client's health care team. When multiple physicians are involved, one should be designated to direct the pain management regimen. That physician should discuss the plan with the client, be the only one to write analgesic orders, evaluate daily, and modify as needed.

5. Current or past alcohol- or opiate-dependent clients may have a physiologically based tolerance to narcotic analgesics, making typical dose ranges ineffective for pain relief.

6. If clinically appropriate, a client-controlled analgesia (PCA) pump should be used. If PCA is not used, scheduled doses are preferable to as-needed dosing.

7. "Drug-seeking behavior" may be an effort to achieve adequate pain relief when ordered doses of pain medication are too low or the period between doses is too long.

8. If a client requests pain medicine for pain relief and it can be given within the parameters of the physician's orders, the medication should be given whether or not the client looks like she is in pain or the nurse thinks the client is trying to be manipulative.

9. Withholding clinically indicated and physician-ordered pain medicine is unethical and may violate state laws regulating nursing practice.

10. Opiate-dependent clients in recovery may choose to avoid narcotic pain medication for fear of triggering relapse. Alternatives should be explored with the client. If non-narcotic methods are not adequate or are clinically inadvisable for managing the client's pain, the client needs to be reassured that the medication is provided within a controlled environment for a limited time. The client may want to contact a support person involved with her recovery.

and nurses often fear they will contribute to the genesis of an addiction. Clients also hold this fear and may forego beneficial treatments. Individuals recovering from addiction are often hesitant to use clinically indicated pain medication. Many suffer needlessly. There are many myths associated with managing pain in substance-dependent individuals. See Myths to Overcome, Pain Management in Chemically Dependent Clients. There is no indication an increase in abuse coincides with the appropriate medical use of opioids for pain management (Simpson, Messina, Xie, & Hale, 2007).

The concept of **pseudoaddiction** describes a syndrome of behaviors that develops as a result of inadequate pain management. Response to pain and pain tolerance are highly individualized. Typically recommended dosing ranges of narcotic pain medication do not uniformly relieve pain across the spectrum of medical disorders and individuals. Not only may clinicians avoid clinically appropriate opioids out of fear of producing dependence, there can also be a fear of law enforcement scrutiny if prescribing patterns appear excessive. If prescribed, the medication or dose may be inadequate. The person in pain begins to repeatedly request, then complain, and eventually become demanding of more pain medication. Pain severity or intensity may be overstated in an effort to secure an effective pain relief regimen. The behaviors begin to appear like those of an addict. A crisis of mistrust develops between the person and the health care team (Lusher, Elander, Bevan, Telfer, & Burton, 2006). When pain is adequately treated, however, so-called drug seeking behavior ceases and function is not impaired.

Few serious complications occur with appropriate medical use of opioids. Taken in overdose or in combination with other CNS depressants, respiratory depression and death are risks. Unhygienic practices associated with the abuse of opioids via the intravenous route are the usual culprits for medical complications. Pulmonary emboli, endocarditis, septicemia, meningitis, and brain abscesses can be life threatening. Infectious disease risks from needle sharing include hepatitis B and C, tetanus, osteomyelitis, and HIV. In the presence of addiction, even medical professionals with access to clean syringes will neglect infection control techniques and share or use dirty needles.

Opiate withdrawal is seldom fatal. Withdrawal symptoms appear about 6 to 8 hours after the last dose of heroin and peak in about 36 to 48 hours. Withdrawal resolves within 7 to 10 days. Because of methadone's longer half-life, withdrawal symptoms are seen in about 2 to 3 days after the last dose and peak several days later. Complete symptom resolution can take up to 2 weeks. Levomethadyl acetate hydrochloride (*L*-alpha-acetyl-methadol, or LAAM) is a long-acting derivative of methadone with a duration of action up to 72 hours. Withdrawal symptoms can be quite prolonged because of its long half-life.

In 2002 the U.S. Food and Drug Administration approved buprenorphine as a schedule III drug for the treatment of opioid dependency. When compared to LAAM and high-dose methadone, buprenorphine appears to be just as effective in the treatment of opioid dependence (Donaher & Welsh, 2006; Gowing, Ali, & White, 2006; Marsch, Stephens, Mudric, Strain, et al., 2005). Major advantages of buprenorphine over other narcotics, such as methadone, are its lower risk of respiratory depression, overdose risk, and less severe withdrawal. The safer profile increases accessibility to opioid treatment, including office-based practice (Jones, 2004; Kosten & Fiellin, 2004). Treatment guidelines for buprenorphine therapy indicate it should be started at the onset of withdrawal symptoms and dosing should be governed by the nature of withdrawal symptoms and cravings.

Severity of symptoms depends on dose, continuous or sporadic use, duration of use, and how quickly the opioid is removed from the cell receptors (Jaffe & Strain, 2005). Although rarely life threatening, individuals with addiction compulsively seek a continued supply of drugs to avoid withdrawal ("getting sick"). A variety of symptoms can occur—restlessness, anxiety, insomnia, craving, body aches, abdominal cramps, nausea, vomiting, rhinorrhea, increased lacrimation, diaphoresis, and dilated pupils. Chills and piloerection ("gooseflesh" or "goose bumps") are the bases for the term "going cold turkey" as a reference to withdrawing suddenly from opioids. More serious symptoms from autonomic arousal can include fever, elevated blood pressure and pulse, tremors, agitation, and muscle spasms. The risk of adverse outcome from withdrawal is greatest in those who have other medical illnesses.

For prescription opioid dependence, a gradual tapering over time can provide an effective and safe withdrawal. Opioids are cross-tolerant, which means drugs in the same class act in similar ways. Cross-tolerance allows methadone to be used for managing heroin withdrawal. Clonidine, though not an opioid, reduces sympathetic nervous system stimulation. Hypotension is the major adverse side effect, therefore, blood pressure must be monitored. Clonidine is not effective for muscle aches, restlessness, insomnia, or craving. Muscle relaxants, anxiolytics, and antiemetics are used to promote comfort and provide relief from cramping, anxiety, nausea, and vomiting. Warm baths can provide soothing relief. Though limited in availability and still being researched, a rapid detoxification process that must occur within a medical setting shortens withdrawal to 2 or 3 days. Medication to rapidly reverse the effects of opioids is provided under anesthesia or heavy sedation.

CENTRAL NERVOUS SYSTEM STIMULANTS

Caffeine, nicotine, cocaine, and amphetamines are the major CNS stimulants. Nicotine and caffeine are much less potent stimulants than cocaine and amphetamine.

Stimulants act primarily through the dopamine system of the brain. Dopamine receptors are prevalent in the limbic system. Rather than a specific lobe or hemisphere, the limbic system consists of structures associated with the very earliest development and survival of the human species. Considered part of the "primitive brain," the limbic system plays a role in basic survival by regulating basic functions such as sexual response, hunger, aggression, expression of emotion, and memory. It is the center of the emotional brain and plays a role in reinforcing behaviors. The limbic system is associated with the "reward pathways" of the brain. There is increasing evidence that drug-induced changes in this area of the brain play a role in the chronic brain changes that are associated with addiction (Hope, 1998). The slang "fried brain" is a rather accurate description of the neurotoxicity associated with stimulant abuse.

Caffeine

There is no diagnosis of caffeine dependence in the *DSM-IV-TR* (APA, 2000), and caffeine use is not an addictive process. Consuming large amounts of caffeine can produce an intoxication syndrome but repeated intoxication is not pursued. Avoidance of the unpleasant symptoms experienced when routine consumption is abruptly stopped is the primary reinforcement for continued use. Caffeine discontinuation syndrome includes headaches, drowsiness, fatigue, nausea, or vomiting. Doses consistent with drinking two or three cups of coffee (approximately 85 mg per cup) produce mild to moderate CNS effects—feeling motivated and energized and less fatigued or drowsy. Dopamine may play a role. At higher doses (300 mg to 800 mg) an unpleasant experience of nervousness, anxiety, and sleep disturbance occurs.

Nicotine

According to the surgeon general (U.S. Public Health Service, 2000, June) tobacco use is most responsible for avoidable illness and death in millions of Americans. Approximately one third of all tobacco-dependent users will die prematurely. Tobacco contains nicotine, a psychoactive substance. Nicotine dependence is considered an addictive disorder. A key criterion for addiction is the continued use of the substance despite substance-related consequences. Nicotine-dependent individuals will continue use despite significant tobacco-related problems, primarily related to health. Nicotine has the pharmacologic properties of tolerance and withdrawal. The first cigarette in the morning provides a boost of nicotine to the brain and is more potent than those smoked later in the day. Inhaled tobacco smoke provides nicotine to the CNS in a matter of seconds and has a half-life of about 2 hours. Dopamine is increased with nicotine use, and serotonin, epinephrine, and norepinephrine may also play a role in the reward and reinforcement processes that sustain dependence. Anger is decreased, mood is stabilized, hunger is decreased, and metabolic rate is increased. Nicotine may enhance performance on long, boring tasks (Hughes, 2005).

Amphetamine and Cocaine

The abuse potential of cocaine and amphetamines is high because they markedly elevate mood and produce euphoria. Cocaine has the highest addiction potential of all abused substances. Cocaine inhibits the uptake of dopamine, serotonin, and norepinephrine in the presynaptic neurons, leaving an abundance of neurotransmitters in the synapse. Dopamine is particularly implicated in the reinforcing effect of cocaine as well as other drugs of abuse (Chocyk, Czyrak, & Wedzony, 2006; Le Foll, Goldberg, & Sokoloff, 2005). Repeated use leads to tolerance and craving for the drug when it is absent. Amphetamines stimulate release of dopamine and norepinephrine. The addicted user seeks the rush again and again. Intense craving is common. There is evidence that chronic stimulant use produces lasting changes in the chemistry and structure of the neurons. Even after years of cocaine abstinence, craving can still persist, and it can be triggered just by watching someone use cocaine.

Stimulant users will exhibit grandiosity, restlessness, pacing, talkativeness, hypervigilance, suspiciousness, anxiety, irritability, paranoia, and hallucinations. Appetite is suppressed sometimes to the point where users appear cachectic. Hyperpyrexia and seizures can occur. Cardiovascular effects include tachycardia, arrhythmias, elevated blood pressure, vasoconstriction, myocardial infarction, heart failure, and spinal cord and brain hemorrhages. Vasoconstriction can produce toxic renal complications. Although sudden death can occur at any time cocaine or amphetamines are used, there is evidence that continued use produces some degree of tolerance to cardiovascular effects. One of the most publicized cocaine-related deaths was that of Len Bias in 1986. He was a healthy, well-conditioned, talented University of Maryland athlete and was bound for a professional basketball future. At age 22 he died in his dormitory room of cocaine-induced sudden cardiac death. He was not known to be a regular drug user and it is speculated that it was the first time he had used cocaine.

Routes of administration include oral, nasal ("snorting" or "sniffing") or buccal absorption via the mucous membranes, intravenous, and inhalation. Intravenous and inhalation routes produce effects almost instantly. Sniffing powdered forms of stimulants can produce nasal mucosa ulceration and septal perforations. Chronic users will often have repeated nosebleeds. Freebase cocaine has been vaporized to remove its water-soluble base to extract a purer form of cocaine. "Crack" is freebase cocaine. Crack (crackles when heated) or "rock" (looks like a small rock or a piece of rock salt) cocaine is placed into pipes and smoked. Its appearance on the drug scene in the 1980s produced a dramatic peak in cocaine use because of its low cost (several doses cost less than $20) and ready availability.

Stimulant withdrawal does not produce the physiologic instability that can occur with alcohol or opiates. Dysphoria, sleep disturbance, anhedonia, and fatigue are symptoms of the withdrawal syndrome. Pharmacotherapy is usually not required (Klein, 1998). Depression, anhedonia, and irritability are common after chronic use. Mood disorders can be triggered or become more serious after withdrawal from cocaine and amphetamines. These pose significant relapse risks. The symptoms are associated with the depletion of dopamine and serotonin in the neurons.

HALLUCINOGENS

Lysergic acid diethylamide (LSD), commonly referred to as "acid," is the substance most commonly associated with hallucinogen use. It has been studied most extensively. Other hallucinogenic substances include psilocybin, methylenedioxyamphetamine (MDA), methylenedioxymethamphetamine (MDMA), also known as ecstasy, and mescaline. The substance is ingested orally from small pieces of paper called blotters or stamps that are soaked with the drug. Less common forms come in sugar cubes or gelatin. Doses are usually no more than $25 and can be as inexpensive as a few dollars. Hallucinogen use more often fits abuse rather than dependence criteria. Its use is most common in adolescents and fits a pattern of experimentation.

The experience produced by taking hallucinogens is referred to as a "trip" and if adverse reactions occur, a "bad trip." The personality of the user strongly influences the overall experience. Sensory perceptions are altered while the individual remains aware of self and surroundings. There can be a sense of altered time and self. Colors and sounds can be vivid and pronounced. Visual illusions and hallucinations are predominant. Hallucinogenic potency is associated with binding to serotonin receptors. Sympathetic nervous system stimulation occurs, and arousal, elevated blood pressure, tachycardia, hyperreflexia, tremor, and pupillary dilation can be present. Dizziness, poor coordination, anxiety, and panic can occur. The impact on mood is affected by the feeling state of the user at the time of ingestion. Effects last between 4 and 12 hours. The hallucinogenic experience has often been compared to the psychotic state of schizophrenia, but advanced technology in brain imaging has shown that this is not accurate. Treating an acute episode can involve supportive presence while the episode plays out on its own over several hours. Administration of 20 mg of diazepam (Valium) to alleviate hallucinogen intoxication is preferable (Jones, 2005). Serious complications are most associated when the hallucinogen has been laced with another substance, or alcohol, cocaine, or other drugs are taken concomitantly. Otherwise healthy individuals do not usually experience a sudden reoccurrence of symptoms, referred to as a "flashback."

CANNABIS

The most widely used illicit substance comes from the cannabis plant that contains the chemical compound tetrahydrocannabinol (THC) responsible for the psychoactive effects. Marijuana refers to the dried leaves, flowers, and stems that are used to make cigarettes ("joints" or "reefers"). Marijuana is also referred to as "Mary Jane," "pot," "weed," and "grass." Hashish is part of the cannabis plant and contains a higher concentration of THC. Route of ingestion is usually inhalation by smoking. The effects of smoking range from very mild to moderate because of the variations in THC concentration. The drug affects several neurotransmitter systems and the chemicals that regulate them. These include dopamine, GABA, acetylcholine, histamine, serotonin, norepinephrine, opioid peptides, and prostaglandins. Cannabinoids have both neurotransmitter uptake inhibition and stimulation properties (Hall & Degenhardt, 2005).

Although acute intoxification effects vary widely among individuals, common effects include an enhanced sense of well-being and euphoria. There can be a sense of time passing slowly, and perceptions can be distorted. Physical effects can include tachycardia, appetite stimulation, conjunctival injection, and dry mouth. Short-term memory is impaired. A sense of relaxation, drowsiness, or lethargy often follow the initial effects. There has been no scientifically rigorous evidence that links chronic marijuana use to an amotivational syndrome characterized by social withdrawal, apathy, and loss in interest in achievement. Withdrawal from chronic high-dose use can include irritability and restlessness, which typically subside in a few days.

INHALANTS

Inhalants are primarily used by adolescents, with most discontinuing use after a few times. Studies indicate that about 30 percent of young persons have experimented with inhalants as early as the eighth grade when most students are only 13 and 14 years old (Johnston et al., 2004). The attraction to youth lies in the low cost and ready availability, often in common household products. They are easy to conceal, and few legal or regulatory obstacles exist. Peer pressure to fit in with the group and apparent rewarding effects can be considered factors that reinforce continued use. Fumes from volatile substances found in fuels, propellants, solvents, thinners, and nitrites are inhaled via breathing in deeply through the nose or mouth ("huffing") or pouring the substance into a plastic bag and inhaling the fumes ("bagging"). Butane (lighter fluid, hair spray, room freshener), acetone (nail polish remover), and mothballs are also examples of commonly used inhalants. Prolonged use of moth balls, which contains the aromatic compound naphthalene, can cause severe hemolytic anemia, liver failure, cardiac arrhythmias, and other organ damage. Inhalant use during pregnancy can also cause fetal anomalies. Though the exact action at the cellular level is not clear, they appear to be CNS depressants. Intoxication effects can include elated mood, slurred speech, slowed reflexes, ataxia, disorientation, hallucinations, anxiety, irritability, concentration difficulties, and lethargy. Differential diagnosis of inhalant abuse is challenging and relies mainly on a comprehensive history of substance use; acute behavioral changes; smell or odor on breath; residue (e.g., oil) on skin or clothing; spots or sores or cracked areas around the mouth and nasal area associated with contact from the inhalant, red eyes, rhinorrhea; stained nails (e.g., paint), or confused state (Crowley & Sakai, 2005). Psychiatric nurses must provide psychoeducation to children and adolescents, parents, caregivers, and professionals about the signs and symptoms and dangers of inhalant abuse. There is evidence of tolerance. Withdrawal is not common but discontinuation after chronic use can include sleep disturbance, irritability, nausea, and shakiness. Inhalant use should be suspected when an individual presents with an odor of solvents or evidence of perioral or nasal residue. Paraphernalia includes paper or plastic bags to contain the substance or soaked rags that are placed over the nose and mouth. Inhalants have serious adverse effects, particularly damaging neurological effects. With long-term exposure there is evidence of brain atrophy and decreased blood flow. Other organ systems also can be affected, including hepatic, renal, cardiac, and pulmonary. Accidents and injury related to driving or engaging in any other task that requires mental sharpness can occur. Death can occur from respiratory depression, cardiac arrhythmia, asphyxiation, or aspiration.

CLUB DRUGS

Club drugs is a term given to a group of substances used primarily by adolescents and young adults in social gatherings at nightclubs, bars, or all-night parties called raves. Use is touted as a way to enhance the experience of the club or party scene. MDMA ("ecstasy") produces hallucinogen and amphetamine effects. Rohypnol ("roofies" or "rophies"), gamma hydroxybutyrate (GHB), and Ketamine ("vitamin K") are CNS depressants that have been associated with "date rape" drugs because of their use in setting up an unsuspecting victim for sexual assault. All of these drugs produce sedation; Rohypnol produces amnesia. They are often used with alcohol or other CNS depressants for enhanced sedative effects. Respiratory depression, seizures, coma, and death can occur.

MISCELLANEOUS SUBSTANCES OF ABUSE

Phencyclidine (PCP), also known as "angel dust," is a substance that produces dependence and withdrawal. Its characteristic behavioral manifestations include hyperactivity, aggressiveness, impulsivity, belligerence, impaired judgment, decreased responsiveness to pain, and psychosis. Behavior can be dangerously unpredictable. Physical effects reflect neuronal hyperexcitability with tachycardia, hypertension, and hyperthermia. Seizures, coma, and death can occur. There is no drug that can reverse the effect of PCP. The symptom picture guides treatment of acute intoxication. Low environmental stimulation is warranted in addition to indicated medical support. Agitation can be managed with either benzodiazepines or antipsychotics. Restraints may be necessary to protect the person as well as the treatment staff. Average half-life for PCP is about 20 hours, and once symptoms clear there is complete symptom resolution barring any medical complications.

Anabolic steroids (Anadrol, Oxandrin, Dianabol, Winstrol, Durabolin) are synthetic substances related to testosterone. In the United States, a prescription is required but they can be obtained through mail order from other countries where prescriptions are not required. The primary medical uses of anabolic steroids are the treatment of delayed puberty, some types of impotence, and wasting syndromes associated with HIV and other diseases. They facilitate the growth of skeletal muscle,

and their use by athletes started in the 1950s. Their misuse and abuse occur primarily among adolescent and young adult males involved in athletics or body building. Although adverse effects are usually reversible, when a child or adolescent takes anabolic steroids, the resulting artificially high sex hormone levels can prematurely halt normal bone growth. Steroids increase low density lipoproteins (LDL) cholesterol and decrease high density lipoproteins (HDL) cholesterol, setting up increased risk for cardiovascular disease. Other effects are acne, baldness, testicular atrophy, gynecomastia, and low sperm count and motility. Withdrawal symptoms include a depressed mood, fatigue, restlessness, decreased libido, insomnia, and anorexia. Although a particular brain mechanism associated with reward has not been identified, compulsive use is reinforced socially by the admiration that is given a muscular appearance, as well as by winning athletic events (Elliott, Cheong, Moe, & Goldberg, 2007). Clinically significant depressive disorders can persist after discontinuing steroid use. Psychotic symptoms are uncommon but they can occur.

SUBSTANCE-RELATED DISORDERS ACROSS THE LIFE SPAN ISSUES

Addiction is a complex family problem that often evolves prenatally and continues through older adulthood. Psychiatric nurses must be able to recognize the actual and potential impact of addiction and its pervasiveness across the life span. In addition, they must collaborate with the client and family and implement interventions that promote health across the life span.

EFFECTS OF ADDICTION ON FAMILY

Addiction is a problem that affects every member of a family. Families adapt in many ways and by no means does growing up in an addicted family necessarily predict an adult life burdened by personal difficulty. Family life with an addict can be stressful and painful, yet many come through the experience more or less emotionally intact. Interpersonal functioning may be compromised nonetheless. Society expects the family unit to provide for the care, growth, and development of children. When a family member becomes addicted, particularly a parent, that parent becomes unable in some capacity to fulfill the responsibilities of the adult role of spouse (or partner) and parent. Other family members may compensate by taking on those roles and responsibilities, even when they do not have the developmental or emotional maturity needed to do so. Because the onset of addiction is often insidious and woven so tightly within the fabric of the family's day-to-day existence, denial and rationalization become major ways to cope. Day-to-day family life can be filled with an undercurrent of tension of not knowing what will happen next. Depending on the severity of the addiction, the individual who is addicted can be loving and kind for a short time and then change, almost Jekyll and Hyde-like. Black (1991) and Bradshaw (1988) discuss the impact of growing up in an addicted family under unwritten but ever so apparent rules of *don't talk, don't trust,* and *don't feel.*

The spouse or significant other of the individual with a substance-related disorder may devote inordinate amounts of time and energy trying to control the addicted person's behavior and forestall or soften a variety of impending disruptions or crises. Energy needed to support the growth and development needs of children is diverted toward efforts to control the addicted person. An external focus on something and someone that cannot be controlled can become an almost obsessive focus to the neglect of other important responsibilities to self and others, particularly the needs of developing children. A term that many still use to describe this type of behavior is *codependency*.

Women with substance-related disorders often experience an array of feelings and beliefs about their disease and its potential impact on their children's well-being. Unresolved feelings of guilt and shame may result in perceptions of failure in the maternal role, and ultimately serve as barriers to positive clinical outcomes and recovery for substance-related disorders (Ehrmin, 2001). The high prevalence of long-term psychosocial, socioeconomic, developmental, physical, and academic consequence of substance-related disorders on families and children necessitates early identification of families and individuals at risk, increased access to appropriate treatment, and interventions that ensure recovery, address the needs of children and family members, and provide long-term supportive services (Eiden, Stevens, Schuetze, & Dombkowski, 2006).

Growing up in a home with addiction or other forms of inadequate functioning can interfere with developing a healthy sense of self. Being totally dependent on caregivers for basic survival, children assume that the environment in which they live is basically adequate even when it is far from any semblance of healthy functioning. They may interpret the family morass as somewhat their responsibility by not having been good enough to prevent problems or at least make things better. An internal sense of shame may result. Shame differs from healthy guilt. Healthy guilt allows one to take proper responsibility when an action is taken that violates the predominant expectations for appropriate behavior. It basically lets an individual admit "I have done wrong," Healthy guilt is illustrated in the Twelve Steps of Alcoholic's Anonymous, a self-help group of individuals who come together to promote recovery from alcoholism (Table 21–6). Steps 8 and 9 (Alcoholics Anonymous World Services, 1997) involve admitting you have done something that harmed another and offering to the extent possible to repair the damage done, but only if doing so will not create more damage to the other person. "I am wrong" is representative of shame. Shame is a sense of internal defectiveness and unworthiness. Children do not have the capacity to fully understand the impact of various forms of parental abuse, neglect, or abandonment. Physical and sexual abuse inflicts significant damage in many ways. Emotional abuse or abandonment that can occur in the addicted family can also compromise the child's ability to develop a healthy sense of self-efficacy, self-confidence, and a clear definition of interpersonal boundaries. Often the lesson learned in the addicted family is there is no safe, predictable, consistent place in the world that allows the authentic self to be expressed and accepted. This flawed fundamental perspective can accompany the child into adulthood, bringing with it a sense of shame and compromised ability to have healthy interpersonal relationships.

MATERNAL-INFANT ISSUES

In general, alcohol and other drugs used during pregnancy present a spectrum of risks to maternal and fetal health. Polysubstance use is not uncommon. Substances can interfere with the normal physiological processes of pregnancy, causing fetal demise, physical abnormalities, prematurity, and obstetrical complications. Acute intoxication can increase risk for injury related to accidents, falls, or other trauma. Lack of prenatal care, nutritional inadequacies, and an overall physical neglect can contribute to a variety of problems. Substances that produce physical dependence can cause

---

TABLE 21–6
The Twelve Steps of Alcoholics Anonymous

1. We admitted we were powerless over alcohol—that our lives had become unmanageable.

2. Came to believe in a Power greater than ourselves could restore us to dignity.

3. Made a decision to turn our will and our lives over to the care of God as we understood Him.

4. Made a searching and fearless moral inventory of ourselves.

5. Admitted to God, to ourselves, and to another human being the exact nature of our wrongs.

6. Were entirely ready to have God remove all these defects of character.

7. Humbly asked Him to remove our shortcomings.

8. Made a list of all persons we had harmed, and became willing to make amends to them all.

9. Made direct amends to such people wherever possible, except when to do so would injure them or others.

10. Continued to take personal inventory and when we were wrong promptly admitted it.

11. Sought through prayer and meditation to improve our conscious contact with God *as we understood Him,* praying only for knowledge of His will for us and the power to carry that out.

12. Having had a spiritual awakening as the result of these steps, we tried to carry this message to alcoholics, and to practice these principles in all our affairs.

Note. From *Twelve Steps and Twelve Traditions,* by Alcoholics Anonymous World Services, 1997, New York: Author.

withdrawal syndromes in the newborn infant as well as in the postpartum mother. Because of impaired interpersonal, occupational, and social functions of the mother and family, an adequate home for newborn care and nurturing may not be available. Maternal-infant bonding may be deficient. State agencies involved in child welfare may have to be called in to provide safe placement for the infant.

Because women with substance-related disorders have a greater propensity toward abusive or neglectful behaviors their infants are vulnerable to impaired bonding, ineffectual parenting skills, abuse, and neglect. The potential deleterious impact of substance use on the psychological and developmental well-being of infants and children requires early interventions that ensure access to treatment for mothers and families. Nurses are poised to play key roles in this process and initiate interventions that prevent prenatal exposure to drugs and alcohol; facilitate maternal-child bonding; and promote overall health in the mother and child and normal childhood development.

The most consistent sequelae from drug and alcohol use during pregnancy are intrauterine growth retardation and smaller than normal head and chest measurements. Exposure to alcohol in utero can produce a spectrum of abnormalities known as fetal alcohol syndrome (FAS). The range of abnormalities appears to be related to the point of fetal development at which exposure occurs. Low birth weight, neurological abnormalities, developmental delays, behavioral dysfunction, intellectual impairment, and skull or brain malformations can occur. The face has a characteristic appearance of shortened eye openings, thin upper lip, and an elongated, flattened face with an enlarged groove in the middle of the upper lip. FAS is one of the leading known causes of mental retardation in the Western world. Problems in learning, attention, memory, and problem solving along with incoordination, impulsiveness, and speech and hearing impairment persist (Warren & Foudin, 2001). Heavy alcohol consumption throughout pregnancy results in a wide variety of effects characteristic of FAS, whereas episodic binge drinking at high levels results in partial expression of the syndrome known as alcohol-related neurodevelopmental disabilities (ARND). The exact time or exact amount capable of causing the most damage is not known. FAS and ARND are completely preventable, and their effects are irreversible and lifelong. No amount of alcohol is considered safe during pregnancy.

Cocaine's effects on pregnancy and fetal development may be related to its vasoconstrictive effects entirely. There is increased risk for placental abruption and spontaneous abortion, preterm labor, maternal seizures, intercranial bleeds, ruptured uterus, and maternal death. The most common fetal effects associated with poor outcomes are prematurity, intrauterine growth retardation, low birth weight, and placental abruption. Resultant risks include intracranial lesions, fetal hypoxia, and cardiac defects. "Pregnancy seems to increase the toxicity of cocaine" (Plessinger & Woods, 1998, p. 103). Unlike the specific physical and behavioral effects of FAS, long-term effects associated with prenatal cocaine exposure are not well defined. An epidemic of impaired children ("crack babies") produced when crack cocaine became prevalent in the 1980s has not materialized.

An array of obstetrical, maternal, and fetal complications are associated with opioid dependence. Most prominent effects are those most often associated with a lack of prenatal care and the medical complications that can occur from intravenous drug abuse. Premature labor, intrauterine growth retardation, and fetal death are risks. Although not without debate, women maintained on methadone have fewer complications than those who remain on heroin. Fetal exposure to opioid withdrawal presents a higher risk for seizures, premature delivery, and death. If withdrawal is to occur during pregnancy, fetal monitoring is necessary (Kuschel, 2007). Newborns do experience an opioid withdrawal syndrome, usually appearing within 72 hours of delivery, that can be treated without any lasting untoward effects.

CHILDHOOD AND ADOLESCENCE

Studies of the impact of substance-related disorders on children have primarily been on children of alcoholics. The long-term effects of fetal exposure to alcohol are well known. There is also good evidence that familial history of alcoholism is a risk factor for development of the disorder. Growing evidence also demonstrates the adverse effects of substance use across the life span including childhood and adolescence. Apart from data that link various substances to life-long developmental, physical, mental, psychological, and academic performance during this vulnerable period, researchers submit the necessity to intervene during the prenatal period to prevent and reduce substance use. Genetic susceptibility to substance use disorders, parental psychopathology, and quality of parenting continues to be examined in relationship to outcomes on children's psychological health and function. It is accurate to say that both nature and nurture play a role in the development of psychopathology and substance use disorders. Multiple studies, including adoption studies, have found a link among familial alcoholism, dysfunctional parenting styles, and personality disorders in the parent to subsequent substance abuse and behavioral problems in children (Button et al., 2007). (See Figure 21–6.)

Initial onset of drug abuse often occurs during adolescence, although younger aged children may also abuse drugs. Adolescence is believed to be a vulnerable period to substance use disorders and is associated with social, genetic predisposition and developmental neurocircuitry associated with motivation and impulsivity. Impulsivity and novelty-seeking are an integral part of transitional trait behavior, which is modulated by developmental changes in frontal cortical and subcortical neurotransmitter systems. Affective dysregulation and neurobehavioral disinhibition coupled with functional immaturity of prefrontal cortices heightens vulnerability to the onset of substance-related disorders, psychiatric illness, and poor judgment during adolescence (Kalivas & Volkow, 2005). (See Research Abstract.)

Adolescents may try drugs or alcohol to experience the pleasurable feelings of getting high, to cope with family or

RESEARCH ABSTRACT

Perceptions of Risk and Resiliency Factors Associated with Rural African American Adolescents' Substance Abuse and HIV Behaviors

Brown, E. J., & Waite, C. D. (2005). *Journal of the American Psychiatric Nurses Association, 11,* 88–100.

Purpose/Aim of Study

The purpose of this study was to select and refine an integrated substance abuse and HIV prevention model for rural African American adolescents based on feedback from adolescents, religious leaders, and school officials.

Methods/Design

This qualitative descriptive study consisted of 21 adolescents and 17 adults (n=38) drawn from 10 rural counties in North Central Florida who participated in four focus groups. The two adolescent groups consisted of 11 adolescents between ages 13 to 15 and 10 adolescents aged 16 to 18. The two adult groups comprised 7 and 8 subjects, respectively. Participants were recruited from churches in the counties, all middle and high school truancy officers, and guidance counselors. Five topics were used to guide discussion and data collection in the focus groups: drug-related risk factors; HIV-related risk factors; drug-related resiliency factors; HIV-related resiliency factors; and acceptable programs, activities, or strategies that parents would permit their teens to participate in and effective intervention models.

Findings

Major themes from this qualitative study related to peer influence for drug risk factors, parental monitoring for drug resiliency factors, early and unprotected sex for HIV risk factors, and recognition of the consequence of engaging in high-risk sexual behaviors and focus on activities of HIV-resiliency factors. Curiosity and boredom were also associated with drug and HIV risk. A lack of recreational activities; the few programs that existed were not culturally sensitive, limited social interactions outside school; and peer pressure to engage in high-risk behaviors were discussed as contributing factors to drug use in adolescent participants.

Implications for Psychiatric Nurses

Psychiatric nurses can play a key role in early identification of youth at risk for substance abuse and HIV risk. Working with adolescents and their parents, school officials, and religious leaders offers numerous opportunities for health education, collaboration with community centers to develop integrated programs unique to individuals, families, and communities to reduce the risk of substance abuse and high-risk sexual behaviors.

social stressors, or to fit in with the peer group and have a good time. Becoming increasingly involved with the regular use of mind-altering substances delays normal developmental maturation and increases risk-taking behavior. Parents may not be alert to the changes in friends, personality, school performance, social activities, eating, and sleeping patterns that can signal substance use. They may attribute these changes to normal adolescent challenges, sometimes with tragic consequences. Suicide risk is higher in adolescents who abuse substances (Esposito-Smythers & Spirito, 2004; Spremo & Loga, 2005). (See Figure 21–6).

Results from the 2004 National Survey on Drug Use and Health (Office of Applied Studies [OAS], 2005) indicate a high prevalence of major depression among adolescents. Data from this study demonstrated approximately 14 percent of adolescents aged 12 to 17 (an estimated 3.5 million adolescents) had experienced at least one major depressive episode (MDE) in their lifetime, and about 9 percent, or approximately 2.2 million adolescents, had at least one MDE in the past year. Adolescents aged 12 to 17 who had an episode of MDE were more likely to use substances than adolescents who did not experience an episode of MDE (see Figure 21–7). Other highlights from this study found that adolescents aged 16 or 17 were more than twice as likely to report past year MDE as those aged 12 or 13 (12.3 versus 5.4 percent) and that females were more likely than males to have a past year MDE (13.1 versus 5.0 percent). These rates were found among all racial/ethnic populations and socioeconomic status (OAS, 2005).

Major implications from these data suggest the necessity to assess adolescents presenting with substance-related disorders for co-occurring major depression and other psychiatric disorders. It is equally imperative to determine if the substance-related disorder is primary or secondary (see Figure 21–7).

Behavioral problems and adolescent substance use go hand in hand (Table 21–7). Treatment for the adolescent ideally involves the entire family in an attempt to return the teen to normal growth and development. The earlier in life drinking behavior begins, the more likely alcohol use disorders will develop. Interventions aimed at postponing drinking until age 15 or 16 can avert substantial harm from drinking later in life (Saha, Chou, & Grant, 2006). The most successful prevention approaches involve parents, schools, and the community, but parents have the greatest influence.

Youth with substance-use disorders challenge psychiatric nurses to carefully assess developmental, psychosocial, and medical needs. A comprehensive biopsychosocial assessment helps determine a differential diagnosis and formulate a holistic plan of care (see Table 21–7).

ADULTHOOD

Evidence of addiction is most likely to appear during adulthood. Most of those who are going to initiate substance use in their lifetime do so by adulthood. Those who start in adolescence begin to experience more consequences of their

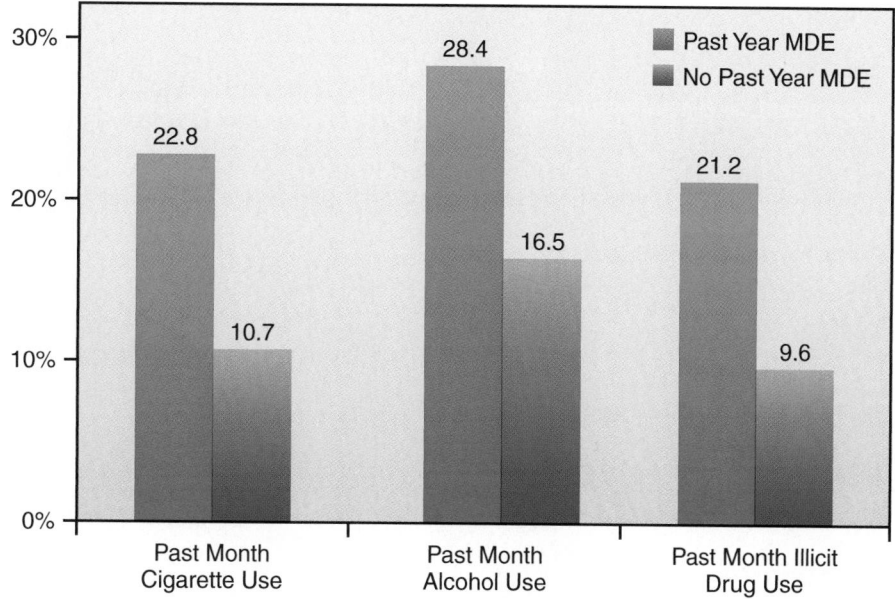

Figure 21–6 Cigarette, alcohol, and illicit drug use among adolescents with a past year of MDE. (*From Office of Applied Studies. National Household Survey on Drug Abuse, by the Substance Abuse and Mental Health Services Administration, 2005. Rockville, MD: Author.* http://oas.samhsa.gov/2k5/youthDepression/youthDepression.htm. *Accessed May 28, 2006.*)

substance use during adulthood. Crossing the line from patterns of abuse to dependence often becomes evident at this time. Some authors have attempted to describe a sequence of phases in the development of addiction. No one generic pattern of progression applies to all who eventually become substance dependent. Alcoholism has been described as progressing through predictable phases (Jellinek, 1960), but not all persons with alcohol-related problems follow this pattern.

To cope with the greater responsibilities of adulthood and associated stressors, substance use may increase. Psychosocial stressors that are often cited as precipitants to chemical use include divorce, death of a spouse or child, and loss of job. The alcohol user may increase drinking to the point where blackouts begin to occur. Blackouts are periods in which the individual is drinking heavily but is awake and later has no memory of that time. They can occur in adolescent drinkers as well. It is important for clinicians to assess for underlying psychiatric illness, which can be a factor in excessive substance use. Assessment for the use of substances should be a routine part of any health assessment. Physical complaints may have their basis in alcohol or drug abuse. The advanced-practice nurse should consider substance use disorders when making differential diagnoses.

Adolescents Aged 12 to 17 Who Experienced an MDE in the Past Year, by Age Group: 2004

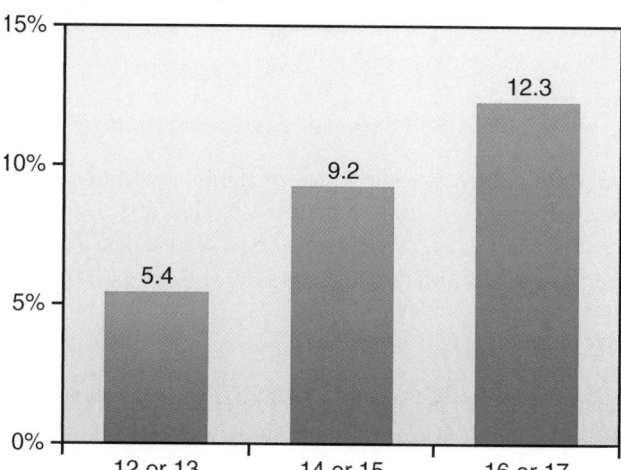

Past Year Treatment for Depression among Adolescents Who Experienced a Past Year MDE, by Age Group: 2004

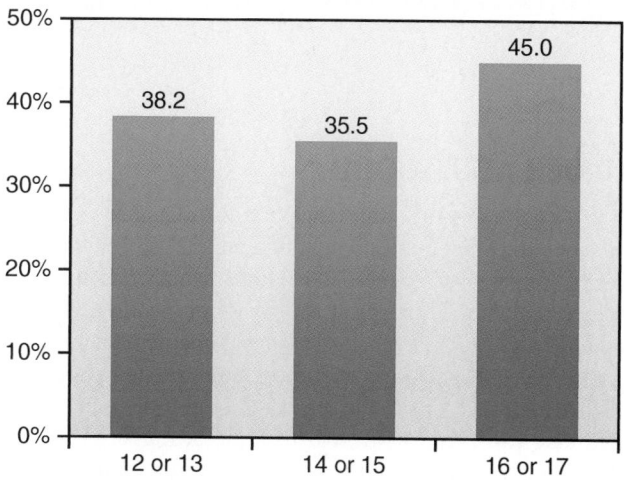

Figure 21–7 Past month substance use among adolescents 12 to 17, past year MDE. (*From Office of Applied Studies, National Household Survey on Drug Abuse, by the Substance Abuse and Mental Health Services Administration, 2005, Rockville, MD: Author.* http://oas.samhsa.gov/2k5/youthDepression/youthDepression.htm. *Accessed May 28, 2006.*)

TABLE 21–7
Assessment Considerations for the Adolescent with a Substance-Related Disorder

Gather information about physical and mental status

- Diagnostic studies, including laboratory tests, toxicology screens
- Determine need for HIV or sexually transmitted disease screening and tests
- Perform mental status examination
- Determine if substance-related disorder is a primary or secondary disorder
- Perform focused physical exam

Interview the adolescent alone

- Discuss confidentiality issues
- Assess suicide and homicide risk
- Previous attempts
- Current stressors
- Assess strengths
- Describe relationship with parents, siblings, and friends
- Positive family history of suicide
- Friend or classmate suicide
- Inform the youth of matters that will not remain confidential (e.g., danger to self or others)
- What substance, how often used, last used, and how long
- Assess the nature and seriousness of substance use and its impact on physical, social, cognitive, and mental status and academic and occupational performance

Interview the parents

- Provide data about the youth's behavior, academic and social performance, legal involvement, and personality changes
- Evaluate marital and family stress, coping styles, and level of empathy
- Assess family strengths and resources
- Describe relationship with youth

Interview the family

- Assess family dynamics and communication patterns
- Assess family stressors and coping styles
- Provide psychoeducation about substance use disorders
- Address their concerns

OLDER ADULTHOOD

It is a myth to assume substance use disorders have no relevance to the older adult population (Table 21–8). A complex set of factors place some older adults at high risk for substance problems. Changes at this phase of life often include major losses and role changes. Late life depression is not a normal part of aging. It is a serious illness and it is associated with a high risk for suicide, particularly in older adult men. Drinking can be a way to self-medicate in the face of overwhelming losses. The older adult is more susceptible to the effects of substances owing to the normal physiologic changes of aging. There is less gastric alcohol dehydrogenase produced, which is responsible for the first step in alcohol metabolism. Body water content is less, and renal and liver clearance is not as efficient, making blood concentrations higher for any substances that are ingested. Older adults are often taking a variety of medications that can produce adverse reactions in the presence of alcohol or other abused substances. A history of multiple falls or evidence of related trauma needs to be evaluated comprehensively, including medical conditions and substance use.

Several patterns of substance abuse may be seen in the older adult. First, there are those who have abused alcohol or drugs for many years and continue to do so. Often by this time in

TABLE 21-8
DSM-IV-TR and the Older Adult with Alcohol Problems

Criteria	Special Considerations for Older Adults
1. Tolerance	May have problems with even low intake due to increased sensitivity to alcohol and higher blood alcohol levels
2. Withdrawal	Many late onset alcoholics do not develop physiological dependence
3. Taking larger amounts or over a longer period than was intended	Increased cognitive impairment can interfere with self-monitoring; drinking can exacerbate cognitive impairment and monitoring
4. Unsuccessful efforts to cut down or control use	Same issues across life span
5. Spending much time to obtain and use alcohol and to recover from effects	Negative effects can occur with relatively low use
6. Giving up activities due to use	May have fewer activities, making detection of problems more difficult
7. Continuing use despite physical or psychological problem caused by use	May not know or understand that problems are related to use, even after medical advice
	May cause serious drug interactions with current medications

Note. From *Treatment Improvement Protocol Series 26 Substance Abuse Among Older Adults* (DHHS Publication No. SMA 98-3179), by the Substance Abuse and Mental Health Services Administration Center for Substance Abuse Treatment, 1998, Rockville, MD: Department of Health and Human Services; and *Diagnostic and Statistical Manual of Mental Disorders* (4th edition, Text Revision) (*DSM-IV-TR*), by the American Psychiatric Association, 2000, Washington, DC: Author.

life, there can be significant health deterioration. Second, there are those who began using drugs or alcohol abusively late in life to cope with grief and loss and the emptiness of finding themselves alone. Third, there are those whose consumption is not much different than it had been over their adult years but because of age-related changes the same amount of substance places them at higher risk for adverse outcomes.

Many family members, nurses, and other health care providers may minimize the seriousness of substance abuse in the older adult. Believing it is too late to try to change these patterns is erroneous. Sadly, a major illness or injury can be the ultimate event that brings about the cessation of substance use. By that time, the consequences may be so severe that a return to a premorbid state physically or socially is no longer possible. Identifying substance use early and aggressively intervening to promote abstinence can greatly affect quality of life. When appropriately confronted, particularly by health professionals, with the reality of the cognitive and physical problems caused by substance abuse, many are willing and able to quit and enjoy a healthier lifestyle. Involving the family is often crucial. Treatment needs to be tailored to the needs and issues of the older adult. Treatment settings with a predominantly young population may not be appropriate. Many older adults are not comfortable with the casual use of profanity by many younger substance abusers. The grief and loss issues at this stage of life are usually different from those in the earlier stages of life.

Coming to terms with being in the last stages of life may need to be a treatment focus.

TREATMENT AND RECOVERY

The complexity of substance-related disorders requires innovative and evidence-based treatment planning that integrates biological and psychosocial concepts. Psychiatric nurses are in key positions to work with the client, family, and other health providers to develop individualized treatment planning that restores health and reduces the serious long-term effects of various substances.

SUBSTANCE DEPENDENCE AS CHRONIC ILLNESS

Treatment for substance use disorders is best understood when viewed from the perspective of how other chronic illnesses are treated. Different levels of care are needed at different times in the course of the disorder. Treatment effectiveness is a function of the severity of the disorder and the motivation of the individual to actively participate in managing it. The accessibility and availability of treatment options and social factors such as quality of social support affect treatment outcome. Unfortunately, there is a prevailing view among many that addiction treatment does not work. The failure to view substance disorders in the same light as other chronic health conditions by the public, insurance companies, and many doctors and nurses has contributed to significant inequities in treatment availability and funding for research. Few public or private health care systems fund addiction treatment anywhere near the level that is provided for other chronic, relapsing illnesses. It is hoped that the day will come when access to treatment will at least be as available as treatment for other chronic illnesses.

Treatment planning requires understanding the nature and general course of the substance use disorder, knowing what modalities are best suited to the substance being abused, and a willingness to individualize to best serve the client. To expect a single episode of treatment to be curative shows a lack of understanding of the nature of chronic illness. For example, diabetes often becomes more difficult to control with coexisting infection, and coronary artery disease will likely worsen if dietary guidelines are not followed. Individuals with diabetes or heart disease are rarely, if ever, stigmatized and stereotyped when they fail to follow recommended care guidelines. Under certain circumstances, such as periods of increased psychosocial stress, substance abusers are at higher risk for a return to previous patterns of excessive use.

In the absence of one scientifically superior method known to cure addiction or effectively prevent its occurrence, research continues for ways to reduce morbidity and mortality, reduce substance use, relieve symptoms of withdrawal, and promote abstinence. Nevertheless, large studies of thousands of drug users confirm reduced drug use as well as decreases in criminal behavior following inpatient, outpatient, and residential treatment for drug addiction. For all drugs, with the exception of crack cocaine, those remaining in treatment the longest were more likely to reduce or eliminate abuse of substances following treatment. Adolescents were the only group who failed to follow this pattern, pointing out the challenge to the research and treatment communities in this area. The cost of incarceration more than doubles the cost of the most expensive treatment intervention, long-term residential care.

THE PROCESS OF CHANGE

It is true that many individuals "just quit" without any form of treatment or attendance at self-help support groups. For others treatment or help in some form is needed to provide the support and encouragement to steadily move along in a recovery process. It is increasingly recognized that a combination of behavioral, pharmacologic, and social service interventions comprise the best approach to treating addiction. Multiple interventions have an additive effect. Because addiction is not strictly biological or psychosocial in nature, it makes sense that a combination of treatment modalities would offer more success.

It is important to assess the client's readiness to change. Treatment modalities ideally should match the needs of the client based on where she is in the change process. The trans-

theoretical model of health behavior change describes five stages of change (Anatchkova, Velicer, & Prochaska, 2005; Prochaska, DiClemente, & Norcross, 1992; Prochaska & Velicer, 1997). At *precontemplation* there is no desire to change behavior in the foreseeable future. Applied to addiction, the individual may not yet have experienced the quantity or severity of adverse outcomes to spur any desire to change behavior. If any action does occur it is only at the insistence of an outside influence. In the absence of an external motivator, return to problem behavior occurs. Resistance is the hallmark of precontemplation. *Contemplation* is when awareness of a problem begins to occur, with thoughts of doing something about it but no readiness to take action. The individual may begin to tire of her family's expressions of concern about chemical use and adverse consequences. Consideration is given to what it will take to tackle the problem. This stage would lend itself to education and awareness-raising activities. Providing educational material would be an appropriate intervention at this stage. *Preparation* is when the individual intends to move forward with change. Reduction in chemical use can occur but abstinence has not yet been achieved. Providing encouragement to talk to a health care or mental health professional would be better accepted at this stage. *Action* is when concerted effort and time are spent changing behavior, experiences, and the environment. Attendance at self-help groups, pursuing or resuming a religious faith, changing friends, avoiding drug- or alcohol-related activities, exploring spirituality, or formal treatment could all be incorporated at this stage. *Maintenance* is when the work of staying clean and sober one day at a time occurs. Relapse prevention strategies are put in place. Retreat to a former stage can occur at any stage and recycling through the stages is not uncommon in addiction. Experiencing emotional distress related to job, spouse or partner relationships, legal problems, finances, or grief and loss can present a risk for relapse. When faced with a significant stressor or multiple stressors, an attitude of "why bother" may be expressed even after a prolonged period of abstinence. For example, after completing a treatment program and remaining abstinent for a year, the spouse still decides to move out and seek a divorce. The recovering person is at risk for relapse as a response to the psychosocial stressor of divorce. The change model helps explain why experiencing consequences or having gone to treatment one time may not cement an addict's resolve to change.

THE TASKS OF TREATMENT

The goals of recovery in substance use disorders are learning to live without chemicals and coping with the realities of everyday life. This begins, but does not end, with abstinence. Most addiction professionals subscribe to the belief that true recovery also means recovering from being a "dry drunk." This term is used to describe an individual who may be abstinent but who has made little to no effort to change distorted thinking and dysfunctional behavior patterns that accompany addiction. Although chemical use may stop, behavioral problems such as poor frustration tolerance, a lack of regard for others, lying, an impaired ability to delay gratification, and an excessive desire for control can continue. The process of developing emotional maturity is impeded when chemicals take the primary focus in life. Learning to cope with the emotional waves associated with living every day life without rushing to chemically blunt, obliterate, or control is crucial. Other more practical matters may need to be addressed as part of cleaning up the debris of addiction. Getting or keeping a job, debt management, or meeting court-ordered activities may require vocational or social services support. If the addiction has become especially severe, the basic things in life that most take for granted may have to be put in place, such as a place to stay and regular meals. Long-neglected family relationships may need to be reestablished. Learning new ways of having fun usually involves giving up relationships, old and new, with substance-abusing friends and acquaintances. A daily routine without chemicals needs to be developed. Boredom and too much idle time are enemies of abstinence, particularly early in recovery. The chances for maintaining abstinence improve if the individual with addiction can find "new playgrounds and new playmates."

The most common models of treatment usually consist of the following components:

1. Withdrawal management as indicated by substance(s) of choice.

2. Client and family education about the disease of alcoholism and drug dependency.

3. Group work that focuses on challenging rationalization, minimization, and denial.

4. Introduction to Alcoholics Anonymous (AA) meetings or its counterpart Narcotics Anonymous (NA) and the 12 Steps. The 12 Steps originated from the experience of the early founders of AA. They are a list of core components they found useful to a program of personal recovery. Individuals are encouraged to find a sponsor, an active AA or NA member who has been clean and sober for at least 1 year. The sponsor serves as an identifiable resource who is available one on one as an additional link in resources to support sobriety. (See Table 21–6).

5. Initiating "Step Work"—readings and activities, often written assignments discussed later with individual staff or in a group, that involve the study and application of the 12 Step principles in day-to-day living. No one is required to adopt the steps but to keep an open mind about the role they can play in a recovery program.

6. Raising awareness and building skills to recognize relapse triggers and adopt strategies to promote abstinence. Cognitive therapy approaches are often useful.

7. Development of a discharge plan to promote an ongoing program of recovery. Many treatment centers incorporate "after-care" programs. These often include the availability of regularly scheduled group meetings for those who have been discharged from the program.

It should be noted that individuals with coexisting psychiatric disorders and substance use disorders often do not respond well to highly confrontational techniques frequently encountered in traditional treatment approaches. Program content and process should take into consideration the impact that severe brain disorders may have on cognitive processes. Group work may not be the best approach for all clients. Some communities offer self-help groups designed as a forum for discussion of psychiatric disabilities, medications, and substance abuse (Naegle, 2000). These may be referred to as dual diagnosis groups.

Inpatient stays at treatment centers are usually reserved for the medical management of withdrawal. Advanced-practice nurses may assess individuals for appropriateness for admission and, with prescribing authority, manage the pharmacologic treatment of withdrawal. The generalist nurse assesses the client's status on admission and throughout detoxification, provides patient and family education, and participates in the discharge planning process. Length of stay is usually short, about 5 days or less, barring any withdrawal complications. Before the changes over the past decade spurred by managed health care, treatment often meant a 30-day inpatient stay. An outpatient setting is now typical. Outpatient treatment programs are usually offered at various times, including day and evening hours. Individuals who managed to keep their jobs despite their addiction can still take advantage of a formal treatment program at hours compatible with their work schedule. Evening programs meet anywhere from one night to several nights over a period of several weeks. Funding for treatment for those without insurance or personal wealth is woefully inadequate, and programs often have extensive waiting lists. Specialized services for the dually diagnosed are even less accessible. Waiting for program admission often bypasses individuals motivated at the time to seek treatment. By the time space is available, the motivation may have passed.

Depending on the focus of the program, a physician and nurse may or may not be part of the treatment staff. Long-term residential settings such as therapeutic communities are highly structured settings with a planned length of stay of about 6 to 12 months. The program focus is broad. Staying chemical free is but one objective. The overall emphasis is on developing the skills and abilities consistent with being a responsible, productive, and chemical-free member of society. The residents, treatment staff, and all activities, even routine chores, are all considered to have therapeutic value.

Successful treatment settings are structured so that strong cohesiveness develops among those in the program. The person can then begin to face life without chemicals with the support of others striving for the same goal and potentially facing similar obstacles. Healthy relationships with people rather than chemicals provide a support system to promote and sustain recovery. Group and family therapy as well as education are major parts of the treatment experience. A committed family involved in the treatment process is associated with better outcomes. Not having an extensive criminal background is also associated with better outcomes.

Cognitive behavioral therapy is often a part of the treatment process helping the addict recognize faulty thinking, substitute more rational thoughts, and in turn decrease emotional distress. Learning ways to decrease emotional distress is a relapse prevention strategy.

A staff member may be assigned to each client for drug counseling or psychotherapy but, traditionally, the majority of structured therapeutic activity occurs in group settings. In some settings nurses with adequate background in addictions serve as counselors and therapists. Generalist nurses often are responsible for psychoeducation and medication groups. Advanced-practice nurses may function in the role of psychotherapist. It is important for staff in both individual and group settings to be willing to appropriately confront the distortions and rationalizations commonly heard from the addicted person. Modeling respectful, yet honest and forthright communication should be a requirement for all treatment team staff. It is inappropriate and nontherapeutic to attack a person's humanity in adversarial confrontations. Treatment staff and loved ones also have to come to terms with the fact that they have no control over the eventual choices the individual might make once she leaves treatment.

RELAPSE ISSUES

Relapses are part of addiction. Most will relapse within the first year after treatment. This does not mean that treatment failed. Patterns of remission and exacerbation are common in most chronic conditions. In chemical dependency, relapse is the exacerbation. Learning to identify the cues that can trigger cravings for the drug of choice is a key part of treatment. Prevention strategies can then be developed and rehearsed. It is important for the recovering person to learn about relapse triggers and the types of situations or events that can begin to chip away at the foundation of recovery. It is essential to recognize the thinking distortions that begin to develop on the road to relapse. Relapse does not occur at the time abstinence ends; it begins with a series of steps leading up to using the drug of choice. Relapse can begin by being in places associated with using drugs or being around people who are using drugs. Old patterns of thinking and reality distortion creep back into consciousness and promote the illusion of being able to control substance use. Thinking

distortions such as, "one drink (or hit) won't hurt" or "I've had a rough day, I deserve a little relief" often occur before actual use. Having access to a support system such as AA can offer a much-needed reality check and a chance at interrupting or shortening the relapse.

PHARMACOLOGIC AND COMPLEMENTARY THERAPIES

Medical treatment options are expected to increase as the knowledge of the biochemical processes of addiction are further discovered. Klein (1998) asserts that the success of any addiction treatment medication must be judged by the achievement of a sustained effect, measured quantifiably. Short-term usage reduction, though beneficial, is of little lasting value. Outcomes must also take into consideration the physical, environmental, and social factors associated with addiction. As in psychosocial treatments, the best pharmacologic approach has yet to be identified. Pharmacologic agents are not a substitute, but often an adjunct, to psychosocial approaches. Unless a preexisting psychiatric disorder is known or diagnosed after detoxification is complete, antidepressants, anxiolytics, mood stabilizers, and antipsychotics are not routinely used in substance use disorders.

An older medication used for treating alcohol disorders is disulfiram (Antabuse). It blocks alcohol metabolism, and if alcohol is ingested the person experiences nausea, vomiting, and a burning sensation in the face and stomach. If drinking resumes, the physical discomfort provides negative reinforcement and extinguishes the desire to drink. Its use is not widely accepted because it produces no effects superior to placebo and it can produce life-threatening complications in those with concomitant medical conditions such as diabetes and cardiovascular disease. Naltrexone (ReVia) is a newer agent, an opiate antagonist (blocks opiate receptors). Alcohol activates the opiate receptors in the brain. Naltrexone blunts the rewarding effects of alcohol by blocking these receptors. When used in combination with psychosocial therapies, it has the potential to decrease the amount consumed and the number of days drinking. It can play a role in preventing craving and relapse. It can be particularly helpful to the client in early recovery. This is a critical time when the alcoholic is learning to restructure her life and adopt psychosocial strategies to sustain sobriety.

Many chronic heroin users are not successful in maintaining abstinence via traditional treatment approaches. Methadone or long-acting methadone (LAAM) maintenance prevents the medical complications and behavioral destabilization associated with heroin use. Methadone typically does not produce euphoria. It can reduce craving and illicit use. Traditional treatment elements such as counseling and relapse prevention are part of a comprehensive rehabilitation program for methadone clients. Because physical dependence and a withdrawal syndrome occur with chronic use of methadone and LAAM, detractors argue that it is merely substituting one addiction for another. Because

---

Myths about Persons with Substance-Use Disorders

Myth: "All addicts are the same."

Reality: Persons with addiction or substance-related problems are individuals. Treatment approaches must be holistic and based on culture, ethnicity, gender, and client wishes, preferences, and health practices.

methadone does not produce the quality "high" and craving, as do other opioids, the abuse potential is much lower. In addition to treating opioid dependence, methadone is used in the treatment of chronic pain. Methadone is not an appropriate agent for acute pain management, because it will not adequately relieve acute pain. Methadone maintenance patients should not have methadone discontinued if at all possible when they receive acute hospital care. Abrupt discontinuation will produce the typical opiate withdrawal syndrome.

Naltrexone is also used in treating opioid addiction because it blocks the effects of heroin. The theory behind its use as a treatment option is that when used regularly, all the effects of self-administered opiates, including euphoria, are completely blocked. With repeated inability to experience the effects, the desire for the drug will gradually cease. Buprenorphine (Buprenex) is a newer pharmacotherapeutic agent. It can be used to medically manage withdrawal and helps maintain long-term abstinence from opiates when it is used as a maintenance medication. Major adverse effects of buprenorphine are similar to other opioids. The most serious side effects include hepatitis and hepatic necrosis. Clients taking this medication must be closely monitored for signs of liver disease, which include increased liver enzymes, jaundice, abdominal pain, malaise, and icteric sclera. It should be used cautiously in clients with liver disease (Herve, Riachi, Noblet, Guillement, et al., 2004). A common problem with pharmacotherapy is the client's failure to take the agent as prescribed. Successful use of any pharmacologic treatment is promoted by an established therapeutic relationship, accompanied by counseling, and monitoring of medication compliance. Those highly motivated to maintain abstinence have the best outcomes.

Methadone maintenance clients do not usually find acceptance in traditional 12 step groups and many traditional treatment centers will not accept them. Methadone Anonymous groups do exist, though in much fewer numbers than AA or NA. The philosophy is consistent with traditional groups in that abstinence from all substances of abuse, including alcohol, is the goal of recovery. The fellowship developed with members of the group seeks to encourage a healthy lifestyle and help others find and maintain recovery. Methadone is viewed as one tool, not the only tool, available to combat opioid addiction.

Contemporary studies continue to demonstrate promise in the treatment of substance-use disorders. Data from a recent study implicated agonist therapy in the treatment of cocaine and other stimulant addiction (Rothman, Blough, & Baumann, 2007). This approach involves prescribing stimulant-like drugs such as dual dopamine/serotonin releasers. Researchers concluded that dual DA/5-HT releasers may be effective adjuncts in the treatment of cocaine and alcohol addiction, mitigating withdrawal syndromes and preventing relapse (Rothman, Blough, & Baumann, 2007). Further randomized controlled studies are justified to find an effective medication for the treatment of stimulant addiction and withdrawal syndromes.

THE ROLE OF THE NURSE

The role of the psychiatric nurse in caring for the client with substance-related disorders is associated with the nurse's educational level and clinical expertise. The clinical setting and area that the client enters the health care system also determine it. If the client enters through the emergency department, efforts to manage mental and physical symptoms are a priority. On the other hand, if the client is admitted to an inpatient psychiatric unit in alcohol withdrawal, the nurse will coordinate holistic treatment planning with other health care providers.

THE GENERALIST NURSE

The role of the generalist nurse is based on basic nursing education that prepares the nurse to do a nursing assessment that includes taking vital signs, monitoring the client's response to treatment, and providing a safe and therapeutic healing environment. The generalist nurse's practice also includes 24-hour monitoring of the client's physical and medical status concerning withdrawal and intoxication from various substances. Assessing the client's safety requires close observation and continuous monitoring of her level of danger to self and others. Other responsibilities include psychoeducation; facilitating self-help groups; administering medications, monitoring the client's response, and reporting adverse reactions; and collaborating with the client, family, and other clinicians to provide holistic care.

THE ADVANCED-PRACTICE PSYCHIATRIC REGISTERED NURSE

The advanced-practice nurse's practice is based on advanced educational and clinical expertise in managing complex client populations. Major responsibilities include collaborating with other clinicians to provide holistic care, prescribing psychotropic agents as allowed by the nurse's state regulation concerning prescriptive authority, and providing psychotherapy and health education. An in-depth discussion of the nurse's role in caring for the client with a substance-related disorder is forthcoming in this section.

THE NURSING PROCESS

Clients presenting with substance-related disorders are likely to present with serious psychiatric and physical signs of withdrawal or intoxication. The nursing process enables the nurse to gather critical data, accurately diagnosis symptoms, determine outcome criteria and nursing interventions, and continuously evaluate the client's responses.

ASSESSMENT

The complexity of substance-related disorders challenges psychiatric nurses to explore their own reactions to the clients who present at various stages of their addiction. Nurses must also educate themselves about the recovery process, addiction, and sobriety in order to assess the client's needs and implement individual health care. Issues involving denial, relapse, and maladaptive behaviors often generate frustration and interfere with establishing a therapeutic nurse-client relationship. The following discussion offers strategies for dealing with these issues.

Attributes of the Nurse

Assessment of the client who is abusing substances is sometimes a difficult process because of the pervasiveness of denial. In addition to a variety of reasons why the client is reluctant to openly disclose substance use, other factors can hinder the process. How well informed the nurse is about addiction science and the nurse's own attitudes can influence the quality of the nurse's contribution to the assessment and treatment process. A nurse who had grown up in a home or had a relationship with the client with a substance-related disorder may be reminded of unresolved anger and pain associated with the experience. This may make developing a therapeutic relationship difficult. It is imperative for nurses to be aware of their attitudes toward those who abuse substances and to accept them as people in need of help managing a serious health problem. The American Nurses Association's (ANA) *Code for Nurses with Interpretive Statements* (1985) clearly defines the goals, values, and ethical expectations that guide the profession of nursing. The 2001 House of Delegates updated the code but there was no change in the basic expectation of the professional nurse to provide care respecting human dignity and unrestricted by the client's personal attributes or type of health problem (ANA, 2001). Having a professional supervision relationship established with another nurse who practices in the addictions area can provide valuable support and guidance. Al Anon, Adult Children of Alcoholics (ACA), and Codependents Anonymous (CoDA) are self-help groups for those who currently or in the past have had a close relationship with the client with a substance-related disorder. The chaos of living with a loved one who has an addiction can produce many conflicting feelings and set in place unhealthy patterns of interpersonal relating. The 12 step philosophy serves as a guide for focusing on living fully in the present and releasing the burdensome distress of the past. The nurse may benefit from the support of self-help groups or psychotherapy.

Nurses are not protected from substance use disorders by their knowledge and experience. Nursing practice can be compromised, sometimes dangerously so, by the nurse in the midst of her own addiction. Impaired nurses will drink or use drugs while on duty. They will divert narcotic analgesics from patient supplies, replacing morphine or meperidine with normal saline, or falsifying narcotic records. Being a nurse, an educated health care professional, is no insurance against addiction. For the addicted nurse, help may be available in the form of peer assistance programs. These programs seek to protect the public from unsafe nursing practice while providing the impaired nurse an opportunity to receive treatment, achieve and maintain sobriety, and preserve her state license. License preservation is dependent on satisfactory completion of treatment and maintenance of sobriety. Some programs assign a peer advocate to serve as a support person to the nurse and also to monitor the individual's compliance with program requirements. Some specialty groups, such as the American Association of Nurse Anesthetists, have extensive resources available to assist their impaired colleagues—their co-workers and managers. Educational aids, policy and procedure recommendations, resource directories, links to Internet sites, and published guidelines for nurse managers are helpful tools. There are specialty 12 step groups for impaired nurses as well as treatment programs tailored to the needs of health care professionals. Treatment staff often includes recovering health care professionals. Having "been there" offers a closer therapeutic alliance as well as intimate understanding of denial and relapse triggers.

Substance Abuse History

Asking for information on current and past use of drugs and alcohol is part of a basic health history. Depending on the setting where health information is being gathered, it may be useful to begin asking about the use of less-threatening substances such as caffeine and nicotine. Clients may underestimate the quantity and frequency of use. To identify problematic use of mind-altering substances, not only do the type, amount, and frequency need to be assessed but also the consequences resulting from patterns of use. Information needed to perform a thorough assessment includes:

- ◆ Types of substances used
- ◆ Amounts typically used
- ◆ Time and amount of last use (critical in assessing for intoxication or withdrawal states)
- ◆ Duration and frequency of use
- ◆ Routes of use for those substances that are administered by various means
- ◆ Past history of any withdrawal states and characteristics of those states
- ◆ Occurrence and degree of adverse consequences
- ◆ Experience with any prior treatment modalities
- ◆ Cultural needs, health practices, and preferences

The client should also be asked about any medical problems, past or current, that are often associated with substance use.

In a setting not specifically focused on addiction treatment, the nurse may feel uncomfortable directly asking about substance use. An explanation of the value this information provides the medical team and an expression of the desire to promote the patient's safety and comfort can go a long way to break down the defensive and guarded demeanor many addicted individuals bring to a medical setting. Many fail to recognize the dangers of untreated alcohol or opioid withdrawal in the presence of medical illness. Assessment of education needs and provision of appropriate information and guidance are responsibilities of the professional nurse. Unfortunately, for many persons with an addiction, past experiences with health care professionals have not been positive.

Screening and Assessment Tools

Numerous screening, assessment, treatment planning, and outcome evaluation tools are available. Selection is often based on the setting in which they are to be used and the intended objective for their use. One of the most commonly used assessment tools is the CAGE questionnaire. It is short (only four questions), it can be administered using informal language, and it is particularly suited to use as part of a general health history. It is used in a variety of settings and holds up to tests of reliability and validity (Soderstrom et al., 1997). Results are more valid if it is administered before questions are asked about quantity and frequency of alcohol use (Steinweg & Worth, 1993). The individual is asked whether or not he has ever felt the need to cut down on drinking, felt *Annoyed* by criticism or complaining by others about alcohol use, felt *Guilty* about drinking, or if an *Eye* opener in the morning has ever been needed to calm nerves or treat a hangover. Two or more affirmative answers indicate a clinically significant alcohol use disorder (Ewing, 1984). Other commonly used tools include the Michigan Alcohol Screening Test, the Alcohol Use Disorders Identification Test (AUDIT), and the Addiction Severity Index (ASI) (NIAAA, 1998).

Physical Assessment

The level of preparation and setting may determine the degree and extent to which the nurse conducts a physical assessment. Basic components include:

1. Baseline vital signs
2. Neurological signs, including pupil size and reaction to light, abnormal movements, and gait

TABLE 21–9
Routes and Effects of Major Classes of Abused Substances

Drug and Routes	Effects	Overdose	Withdrawal Syndrome
Alcohol: Central nervous system depressant Route: Oral	Sedation, decreased inhibitions, relaxation, decreased coordination, impaired judgment; slowed reflexes; slurred speech; nausea; euphoria; depression; sexual dysfunction	Respiratory depression, stupor, circulatory collapse, cardiac arrest, coma, death Effects potentiated by combination with other central nervous system depressants	Tremors; increased temperature, pulse and respiration; psychomotor agitation; impaired attention and memory; illusions (misinterpretation of stimuli); auditory, visual, or tactile hallucinations; delusions; seizure, delirium tremens; circulatory collapse; death
Opiates: Central nervous system depressant Morphine Codeine Diacetylmorphine (heroin) Hydromorphone (Dilaudid) Dolophine (Methadone) Meperidine (Demerol) Hydrocodone (Vicodin) Propoxyphene (Darvon, Darvocet) Oxycodone (OxyContin) Tramadol [Tramdal] (atypical opioid) Fentanyl (Duragesic) Routes: Oral, inhalation, IM, IV, smoking	Analgesia; euphoria, calming sensation, sedation; clouding of consciousness; memory and concentration impairment; psychomotor retardation; constricted pupils; constipation; decreased libido	Respiratory depression, stupor; circulatory collapse; coma; death Effects potentiated by combination with other central nervous system depressants	Yawning; rhinorrhea; lacrimation; abdominal cramps; diaphoresis; irritability; restlessness; anxiety; agitation; sleep disturbance; body aches; muscle cramps; "goose bumps"; sensations of hot and cold; nausea; diarrhea; anorexia; fever; dilated pupils; muscle twitching; increased blood pressure, pulse, respiration; dysphoria; craving

(continues)

Drug and Routes	Effects	Overdose	Withdrawal Syndrome
Sedative-Hypnotics and Anxiolytics: Central nervous system depressants *Barbiturates* Amobarbital (Amytal) Butabarbital (Butisol) Butalbital compound (Esgic, Fioricet) Pentobarbital (Nembutal) Phenobarbital (Luminal) Secobarbital (Seconal) *Barbiturate-like* Chloral hydrate (Noctec) Ethchlorvynol (Placidyl) *Benzodiazepines* Alprazolam (Xanax) Chlordiazepoxide (Librium) Clonazepam (Klonopin) Clorazepate (Tranxene) Diazepam (Valium) Flurazepam (Dalmane) Lorazepam (Ativan) Oxazepam (Serax) Quazepam (Doral) Temazepam (Restoril) Triazolam (Halcion) Rohypnol ("date rape drug") *Other* Meprobamate (Equanil, Miltown) Glutethimide (Doriglute) Routes: Oral, IM, IV	Relief of anxiety, euphoria; sedation; reduced libido; impaired judgment; dizziness; lack of coordination; impaired memory	Somnolence; hypotension; hypotonia; respiratory depression; coma; cardiac arrest; death Effects potentiated by combination with other central nervous system depressants	Tremor; nightmares; diaphoresis; blepharospasm; dilated pupils; agitation; ataxia; increased respiration and blood pressure; vomiting; hallucinations; delusions; apprehension; rebound anxiety or panic; clouded consciousness; muscle twitching; confusion; disorientation; memory impairment; seizures
Stimulants: Central nervous system stimulants Cocaine ("crack," "rock") Dextroamphetamine (Dexedrine) Dextroamphetamine and Amphetamine (Adderall) Methylphenidate (Ritalin) Pemoline (Cylert) Routes: Oral, buccal absorption, inhalation, smoking, IV	Alertness; reduced fatigue; euphoria; initial CNS stimulation then depression when "coming down"; sleep disturbance; irritability; decreased appetite; paranoia; impaired judgment; hypertension; slowing of cardiac conduction; aggression; dilated pupils; tremors; palpitations	Cardiac arrhythmias/arrest; sudden cardiac death; elevated or lowered blood pressure; chest pain; vomiting; seizures; hallucinations; confusion; dyskinesias; dystonias; weakness; lethargy; dysphoria; coma	Fatigue then insomnia; increased appetite; psychomotor retardation then agitation; severe dysphoria, anxiety; cravings; disturbed sleep; suicide

(continues)

Drug and Routes	Effects	Overdose	Withdrawal Syndrome
Cannabis santiva (marijuana, hashish) Routes: Usually inhalation by smoking; can be ingested orally ("Alice B. Toklas brownies")	Euphoria or dysphoria; relaxation; drowsiness; anxiety; panic attack; heightened perception of color, sound; loss of coordination; spatial perception and time distortion; unusual body sensations; dry mouth; conjunctival injection (blood shot eyes); food cravings; learning and memory impairment; increased heart rate	Unlikely	No recognized syndrome
Inhalants *Gases* Household: butane, propane, refrigerant gases, whipping cream aerosol Propellants: aerosols—paint, hair spray, deodorants, air fresheners, fabric protectors, cooking oil spray Medical anesthetics: nitrous oxide, halothane, chloroform, ether *Solvents:* Household: Cleaning agents—spot removers, dry cleaning fluid, degreasers, lighter fluid, acetone, spot removers, gasoline Adhesives: airplane glue, rubber cement *Art/Office Supplies:* Felt tip marker, correction fluid *Nitrites:* amyl, butyl, cyclohexyl Route: Inhalation ("huffing")	Euphoria; giddiness; excitation; disinhibition; loss of consciousness; ataxia; nystagmus; dysarthria	Central nervous system depression; heart failure; coma; seizures; death	Similar to alcohol but milder, with anxiety, tremors, hallucinations, sleep disturbance

(continues)

Drug and Routes	Effects	Overdose	Withdrawal Syndrome
Hallucinogenic Agent Phencyclidine (PCP) "Angel Dust" Routes: Oral, inhalation, smoking	Feelings of strength, power, invulnerability and a numbing effect on the mind; decreased awareness of and detachment from the environment; elevated pulse, respiration, blood pressure; flushing; disphoresis; ataxia; dysarthria; decreased pain perception; paranoid delusions; disordered thinking; catatonia; garbled and sparse speech	Decreased pulse respirations, blood pressure; extreme aggression; suicidality; nausea; vomiting; rapid eye movement; blurred vision; drooling; hallucinations; seizures; coma; death	None—supportive care with benzodiazepines or low dose antipsychotic agent for drug-induced psychosis
Caffeine Route: Oral	Stimulation; increased mental acuity; inexhaustability	Restlessness, nervousness; excitement; insomnia; flushing; GI distress; muscle twitching; rambling flow of thought and speech; tachycardia or cardiac arrhythmia; agitation	Headache; drowsiness; fatigue; craving; impaired psychomotor performance; difficulty concentrating; yawning; nausea
Nicotine Routes: Smoking, chewing	Stimulation; enhanced performance and alertness; appetite suppression	Anxiety	Mood changes; craving; anxiety; poor concentration; sleep disturbance; headaches; GI distress; increased appetite

3. Mental status—level of consciousness, orientation, memory, mood, affect, reality testing, judgment, suicidal or homicidal ideation

4. Presence of any intoxication or withdrawal symptoms

5. Nutritional status

6. Assessment of skin integrity

Having a basic understanding of the expected effects of substances likely to be abused is helpful when assessing a client's behavior (Table 21–9).

NURSING DIAGNOSES

The nurse selects nursing diagnoses based on conclusions supported by assessment data. Diagnoses serve to provide clear direction for focused intervention. The standards of addictions nursing practice (ANA, 1998) group potential responses to health problems associated with addiction under biological, cognitive, psychosocial, and spiritual dimensions.

Examples of common nursing diagnoses in each dimension include the following.

Biological

◆ Disturbed sensory perception (visual, auditory, tactile) related to substance withdrawal/intoxication (specify) evidenced by increasing misperception of environmental stimuli

◆ Risk for infection related to intravenous drug abuse and needle sharing evidenced by open skin lesions and prior history of endocarditis

◆ Acute pain related to opioid withdrawal evidenced by protective positioning and grimacing

Cognitive

◆ Deficient knowledge related to lack of understanding of the relapse process evidenced by continuing relationships with drug abusing acquaintances

- Noncompliance related to craving evidenced by prior against medical advice (AMA) discharges
- Ineffective denial related to inability to cope without alcohol evidenced by second DWI (driving while intoxicated) charge in six months

Psychosocial

- Chronic low self-esteem related to shame evidenced by verbalizing doubt about ability to obtain sobriety
- Compromised family coping, potential for growth related to active participation in family groups and Al Anon evidenced by limit setting on inappropriate behaviors of the addicted family member
- Risk for other directed violence related to altered perceptions and poor impulse control evidenced by poor frustration tolerance and verbal aggression

Spiritual

- Spiritual distress related to multiple personal losses evidenced by isolative behaviors
- Powerlessness related to unwillingness to accept treatment for co-occurring psychiatric illness evidenced by multiple relapses
- Hopelessness related to failing physical health evidenced by non-adherence to medically prescribed health regimen

OUTCOME IDENTIFICATION

Being able to set specific measurable outcomes provides a way to judge the effectiveness of interventions. Some outcomes are directly related to nursing and medical interventions. Others relate more specifically to the client and her recovery. Outcomes or goals should be reasonable, and when appropriate, jointly set with the client. Family involvement may also be indicated. Examples of outcomes include:

- Decrease in pain score to below 5 on a 1 to 10 scale
- Identifies home AA group and has a temporary sponsor by discharge
- Vital signs remain stable throughout the withdrawal process
- Selects nonsubstance outlets for managing feelings of anger, frustration, anxiety, and sadness
- Communication patterns within the family improve, evidenced by decreased conflict
- Expresses realistic, positive appraisal of strengths and limitations
- Scores on the Beck Depression Scale improve from baseline
- Identifies anticipated relapse triggers and avoidance strategies
- Experiences decreased craving
- Sensorium remains clear throughout detoxification

PLANNING

A plan of nursing care is developed after an adequate assessment, identification of nursing diagnoses or problems, and selection of desired outcomes. The plan of care delineates interventions directed at meeting outcomes. In a treatment setting, the nursing care plan is often part of the multidisciplinary plan of care. The collaborative efforts of team members allow the strengths of each discipline to be directed at maximizing outcomes. The involvement of the client and those who can play a positive role in supporting the client's recovery is an important factor in successfully obtaining treatment goals. Treatment resources are often limited, depending on a variety of factors. With this in mind, outcomes should be developed, taking into consideration the resources available in the community, the quality of the client's social support system, and any physical, neurocognitive, or psychiatric factors. It is unreasonable to expect all clients to benefit from 12 step work. The treatment team must remain flexible and creative.

IMPLEMENTATION

Nursing interventions include both independent and dependent actions. They are implemented across a diversity of settings: acute care hospitals, treatment centers, client homes, jails, the street, and the homeless shelters. A genuine desire to help, intuitive interpersonal communication skills, and research-based psychotherapeutic techniques are as valuable as strong technical skills (Figure 21–8). For example, the nurse must be able to take care of the client in alcohol withdrawal by understanding the medications being used and monitoring and responding to vital sign changes. Equally valuable is being able to communicate effectively and help the client decide to stay after announcing a desire to leave against medical advice in the midst of detoxification. Engaging the client and family in a therapeutic relationship, promoting a treatment environment conducive to health and healing, providing education aimed at health promotion and

Research-based nursing practice
Honesty
Ability to confront reality without shaming
Patience
Empathy
Hope
Flexibility
Ability to work in a team
Intellectually curious
Willing to change perspectives in light of new evidence
Ability to listen
Nonjudgmental
Self-awareness of limitations
Willingness to seek help and guidance from others
Ability to expect and tolerate setbacks
Informed optimism
Capacity to tolerate not being in control of outcomes
Healthy boundaries

Figure 21–8 Promoting health and wellness: Caring attributes of nurses working with clients who abuse substances.

maintenance, and providing links to community resources are interventions within the psychosocial scope of nursing practice. In a generalist role, the nurse applies a basic knowledge of nursing theory as it relates to the client with substance use disorders when applying the nursing process. The nurse in an advanced-practice role will use advanced theoretical knowledge and clinical skills, implementing aspects of medical care as well as nursing care. The scope of practice for the advanced-practice nurse often is determined by the setting and structure of the treatment team. Typical roles include consultation liaison (psychiatric-addictions nursing consultation in the medical-surgical setting), consultant to the nursing or multidisciplinary team in chemical dependency settings, psychotherapist, and medication management consistent with statutory provisions regulating prescriptive authority. Regardless of the level of nursing practice, implementation of a plan of care requires effective collaboration with the client and family and other members of the health care team and a respect for the contribution each has to offer.

Interventions

Standards of addictions nursing practice identify six key nursing interventions. These span the health-illness continuum and are directed at helping the client and the family healthily adapt to the problems stemming from substance abuse and addiction (ANA, 1988).

Therapeutic Alliance

The nurse's ability to use effective interpersonal communication skills and model genuine respect and concern for all persons builds relationships based on trust. This is referred to as therapeutic use of self, and it is crucial in working with a population often stigmatized and dismissed by many health care providers. This alliance helps clients develop awareness of the attitudes and behaviors that contribute to poor health and encourages the client to take alternative actions.

Psychoeducation

Clients, families, and the community benefit from gaining knowledge about the process of addiction, acute and chronic effects of substance use, and ways to promote and sustain recovery. Topics often needing to be addressed include the value of discussing concerns with others, developing problem-solving alternatives to chemical use, delaying gratification, using relaxation or other anxiety- or anger-reducing techniques, and interpersonal skills. Many clients have little to no understanding of what constitutes a healthy lifestyle. Nutrition, rest, exercise, recreation (without chemicals), and sexual health topics may all need to be discussed. These topics lend themselves to health teaching across the continuum of health care settings. The nurse does not have to be practicing in an addictions setting to be able to offer useful health information.

The family may have a variety of learning needs. If spousal or partner abuse is suspected, the nurse should explore this and direct the family member to appropriate community resources. Many communities have domestic violence services that also include counseling and other support services. The spouse or partner may choose not to acknowledge abuse or indicate intention of not following up with resources. The nurse must accept the choices adults make for themselves regarding living in abusive situations. The client's cultural needs, preferences, and health practices must be an integral part of the assessment process and treatment plan. Encouraging the individual to make a tentative escape plan can promote empowerment. If child abuse or neglect is suspected there may be statutory reporting requirements. Social service professionals are often helpful colleagues to consult with questions in this area.

The nurse uses a variety of educational tools, including written or audiovisual materials. Readiness to learn and how best the learner learns must be assessed, and education strategies are developed with this in mind. With the explosion of information on addiction, the Internet offers many useful sites aimed at both public and professional learners. There may be other valuable resources in the community. The nurse should assess the client's needs and make appropriate referrals.

Self-Help Groups

The nurse needs to have a working knowledge of the array of self-help groups that are available to those seeking or working a recovery program. Although groups based on the 12 step model—AA, NA, Al Anon—are usually available in most communities, the nurse must assess the appropriateness of the client for this type of involvement. Any group that helps the client learn to alter distorted, self-destructive thinking patterns, supports constructive behavior change to achieve and maintain sobriety, and provides motivation and support benefits clients. AA alternatives include variations of Albert Ellis' Rational Emotive Behavior Therapy (Ellis, 1973). Cognitive distortions in the form of irrational thoughts are seen as critical elements in sustaining addictive patterns and promoting relapse. Recognizing these distortions and replacing them with more accurate representations of reality form the basis for more appropriate behavior choices. Rational Recovery (Trimpey, 1996) asserts that the individual can adopt new thinking and behaving patterns without attending support groups whose focus is mainly spiritual. Secular Sobriety is a self-help group with similarities to AA yet without the emphasis on a higher power. Focus is placed on empowerment and self-reliance (Table 21–10). Some clients may find faith-based support groups and activities such as pastoral counseling very helpful. The nurse can help the client understand the variety of choices available to promote and maintain abstinence.

Pharmacologic Therapies

The nurse may have various responsibilities related to pharmacotherapy. As with any medication administered by the nurse, she must comply with the Five Rights: the right patient or client, the right drug, the right dose, the right route, and the right time. The nurse must understand the

TABLE 21–10
Secular Sobriety: How to Stay Sober

To break the cycle of denial and achieve sobriety, we first acknowledge that we are alcoholics or addicts.

We reaffirm this truth daily and accept without reservation the fact that, as clean and sober individuals, we can not and do not drink or use, no matter what.

Since drinking or using is not an option for us, we take whatever steps are necessary to continue our Sobriety Priority lifelong.

A quality of life—"the good life"—can be achieved. However, life is also filled with uncertainties. Therefore, we do not drink or use regardless of feelings, circumstances, or conflicts.

We share in confidence with each other our thoughts and feelings as sober, clean individuals.

Sobriety is our Priority, and we are each responsible for our lives and our sobriety.

desired effects, the potential side effects, and must monitor the client's response. If in an advanced-practice role the nurse must function under any applicable physician partner protocols, she can only prescribe those medications within her clinical scope of practice. To safely provide nursing care related to pharmacologic treatment, the nurse must equip herself with an understanding of the pharmacologic properties of cross-tolerance, food and drug interactions, and the impact of any coexisting medical disorders. The nurse at both the advanced and generalist levels often assumes the major responsibility for educating clients and their families about medications. She may be the key information resource regarding pharmacologic agents to other multidisciplinary team members. Maintaining current knowledge via continuing education offerings and self-study is an expectation of professional nursing practice.

Therapeutic Environment

Regardless of the setting, the nurse has an important role in establishing an environment that satisfies physical, cultural, gender, and emotional needs, models healthy conflict resolution, and promotes the client's sense of self-worth, self-confidence, and self-efficacy. This is a collaborative process. In those settings where there is a 24-hour nursing presence, the nurse provides the foundation for the therapeutic environment. A safe treatment environment is essential in any setting. Staffing should be at a client or patient-to-staff ratio where basic safety is ensured. Access to appropriate physician or nurse practitioner resources should be present in settings where detoxification is provided. It is important to have a basic knowledge of regulatory requirements regarding environmental safety, client rights and responsibilities, and how to appropriately pursue remedy when unsafe practices are occurring. The nurse assists the client in understanding behavioral expectations and appropriately intervenes to maintain human dignity yet ensure safety and a healing environment. Nursing should take responsibility for implementing or teaching rituals that model healthy self-care and building interpersonal relationships such as morning goal setting or end-of-the day "cool down" activities. The nurse keeps an awareness of the "pulse" of the environment whether in a facility or the client's home. Although the nurse's role is critical in promoting and maintaining a therapeutic environment, the quality of the relationships among team members is crucial. The team must be able to accept and discuss differing clinical viewpoints, assessments, and interventions. Disagreements must be respectfully resolved.

Counseling

Counseling is focused therapeutic communication. The acute intoxication or withdrawal period does not lend itself to the minimum level of cognitive engagement needed for an effective counseling relationship. Counseling provides support and guidance to the client and family as they learn more about the nature of substance use disorders, interpersonal factors that promote or inhibit recovery, and the importance of awareness and accountability for choices. It also allows for exploration of distorted thinking processes and resultant behavior and holds the client accountable for her choices. The family has the opportunity to explore its part in the addiction process and how to support a healthy recovery for all family members.

Counseling occurs within the framework of a helping relationship and focuses on the here and now. Although not rejecting events of the past that may trouble the client, recovery requires a willingness to begin to accept what has been and move on with new thinking and behavior. Patience is needed on the part of the nurse. Entrenched denial does not fade equally nor rapidly for all individuals. Entrenched family denial can be especially frustrating. The nurse in a counseling role will appropriately confront the client (or family member) who projects blame on others, intellectualizes, rationalizes, minimizes, or otherwise excuses or explains away the consequences related to substance use. Continually drawing a connection between substance use and the harmful outcomes the client has experienced erodes the façade of denial. The nurse confronts the client's selective thinking by highlighting any incongruity with reality. An example would be the client who sustains injuries after driving while intoxicated: when questioned about the role of alcohol in the crash, the client denies drinking. Providing a copy and explanation of the blood alcohol level drawn on admission to the emergency department challenges denial and reinforces reality.

It is important that the nurse use a matter-of-fact yet attentive, interested approach. Humor has a role at times. It is never appropriate to humiliate or shame a client.

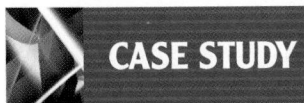

CASE STUDY

The Client with Dual Diagnosis in the Acute Care Setting (Mrs. Richardson)

Mrs. Richardson, a 49-year-old female, was admitted to the trauma surgical floor after having fallen on the stairs at her apartment. She fell 3 days before but did not come to the emergency department (ED) because neither she nor her family believed that she had injured herself other than some soreness, scrapes, and bruises. Her family brought her to the ED when she began to exhibit confusion. They were concerned she had a worse injury than originally thought. She also lived alone. They did not know if in her confusion she had forgotten or taken extra doses of her psychiatric mainte-nance medications. She had told them at the time of the fall that she had not been "knocked out" but had hit her head "pretty hard." There was no indication she had experienced any changes in level of consciousness (LOC) since the fall. She was evaluated in the ED and was admitted to the hospital after x-rays revealed a pelvis and humerus fracture. A computed tomography (CT) scan of the head revealed no acute abnormalities but evidence of an old infarct.

The client's daughter was the informant for the nursing admission assessment. Mrs. Richardson was a regular client at the county mental health clinic. She had a diagnosis of bipolar I disorder and was taking Depakote (divalproex) and Paxil (paroxetine). The daughter had brought her mother's current prescription bottles with her and the doses were verified. Mrs. Richardson had been psychiatrically stable over the past 5 years. The divalproex level drawn in the ED indicated therapeutic blood levels. The drug screen was positive for opioids. She was also a recovering heroin user and was on methadone maintenance. The daughter believed her mother's dose of methadone was 35 mg daily. To the daughter's knowledge, her mother had been compliant with the methadone program and had not used illicit drugs or alcohol "for years." There was nothing in the recent past to indicate any rea-son to suspect her mother had relapsed.

Medical evaluation and monitoring continued over the next 48 hours, and surgery was determined not to be necessary. The physician ordered home medications restarted 24 hours after her admission and began a rapid taper of methadone, thinking that methadone, in addition to the par-enteral morphine being given for pain, would increase risks for respiratory depression. She was also receiving p.r.n. doses of lorazepam (Ativan) for anxiety. Her confusion worsened, she became somnolent, and began to hallucinate and have paranoid delusions. The admitting physician stopped all of her home psychiatric medications, discontinued the methadone and lorazepam, and changed from morphine to oral hydrocodone for pain control. After 24 hours, she was less somnolent but her mental status was not improving. The psychiatric consultation liaison team was consulted. A neuro-logical assessment was performed and a repeat CT of the head was ordered, which showed no change from the prior CT. Hydrocodone was discon-tinued. The consultation liaison psychiatric nurse verified the patient's methadone dose by contacting her methadone clinic. Mrs. Richardson had been on methadone for 13 years and her current dose was 60 mg. Methadone and her psychiatric medications were restarted. Within the next 24 hours her mental status began to clear, and by discharge there was no evidence of confusion, hallucinations, or delusional thinking.

Critical Thinking

1. *What is important to know about a client's medication history?*

   It is very important to obtain accurate information about a client's current medications as soon as possible after admission. This should include prescription medications and any over-the-counter and herbal preparations. Verification of doses and time of last dose are vital pieces of data. Although it is not always possible to obtain complete information, efforts should be made to gather as much information as possible. The psy-chiatric medications were easily verified in this case study but no effort was made to verify the methadone dose. Efforts should have been made to contact the methadone clinic and verify the dose. Methadone clinics usually provide each client with a card listing the clinic name, phone number, and a list of precautions associated with methadone use. In a medical emergency, many psychiatric and methadone providers are allowed by statute to release pertinent information. Most methadone clinics will also provide recommendations that have been developed with the clinic's medical director for managing methadone when medical or surgical care is required.

2. *What factors contributed to Mrs. Richardson's altered mental status?*

   The case study demonstrates the challenge presented by clients with co-occurring medical, psychiatric, and substance-use disorder. Although there is no one clear etiology for Mrs. Richardson's unusual presentation and hospital course, a combination of acute effects of trauma, pain, anxiety, and medication were the culprits in her worsening mental status. CNS depressants potentiate each other. In this case, a combination of parenteral morphine and lorazepam (Ativan) caused oversedation. Because methadone is not an agent useful for acute pain relief, particu-larly in those clients on maintenance, the addition of the morphine and, eventually, hydrocodone, was very appropriate. The sedation cleared when morphine, hydrocodone, and lorazepam were all eventually discontinued. The continued confusion and sensory perceptual changes could be linked to morphine. Many times clients report hallucinations when given morphine. The methadone taper and eventual discontinuation were not effective strategies. Methadone withdrawal typically is not associated with confusion or psychosis but it can occur. Opioid taper can be a time of increased risk of psychosis, particularly in those with preexisting CNS illness (Shreeram, McDonald, & Dennison, 2001). Mrs. Richardson had evidence of an old cerebral event and she had also probably suffered an acute, mild head injury. Detoxification of methadone mainte-nance clients during any period of acute illness is generally not recommended. If this occurs, there must be appropriate documentation of the rationale for this decision, which must also include an angreement between the client, attending physician, and treatment team to initiate methadone detoxification. Methadone should be prescribed at the client's usual dose, and pain should be managed by the addition of appro-priate narcotic or non-narcotic agents at adequate doses. An additional lesson this case provides is that nurses and physicians who do not spe-cialize in the addictions field are more than likely to be unfamiliar with methadone maintenance issues.

Holding a client accountable for her choices is appropriate. The nurse should use open-ended, specific, factual questions that do not lend themselves to evasiveness or vague generalities. Hostile responses can be expected, and the nurse reflects the stated or implied feeling. Reflecting the tone of the feeling that the client expresses promotes engagement in the therapeutic process. Hostility can be a strategy to divert the nurse to less relevant topics as are changing the subject or sidestepping a question. The nurse must tactfully stick to the task and stay focused. The nurse should not attempt to quell expressions of strong or intense emotion. Acknowledging and appropriately responding to the range of feelings being expressed models active listening and acceptance of the client where she is at that particular moment. Limits must be set on abusive, threatening behavior with appropriate consequences pursued. The effects of the nurse's efforts may not be evident initially. Resistance or outright refusal to acknowledge substance-related problems does not mean that the nurse's interventions have failed. The reinforcement that more than likely will come at other times and places will build on the nurse's efforts.

EVALUATION

The purpose of evaluation is to revise diagnoses and interventions as needed. The following are major criteria for evaluation of nursing care:

1. The client safely undergoes detoxification and withdrawal.

2. The client realizes the use of substances is detrimental. This is a major criterion, and the likelihood it will be realized with one treatment episode is unrealistic. If the client has acknowledged even a small increment of awareness, then progress has been made. It is increasingly understood that the progress made in prior treatment episodes or other health-promotion activities builds a stronger foundation for ongoing recovery.

3. The client connects use of substances to problems experienced. An appropriate evaluation criterion would be the client acknowledging that substance use had a role in at least one adverse event.

4. The client and family agree to some form of continued care toward recovery from substance abuse.

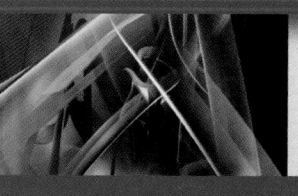

NURSING CARE PLAN 21–1

The Client with Dual Diagnosis in the Acute Care Setting (Mrs. Richardson)

Nursing Diagnosis: Disturbed Sensory Perceptions (visual hallucinations) related to biochemical imbalance evidenced by confusion, visual hallucinations, and paranoia

Outcome Identification	Nursing Actions	Rationales	Evaluation
1. By [date], Mrs. Richardson will be fully oriented and sensory perceptual alterations will be resolved.	1a. With a calm, relaxed approach, orient to person, place, time, and situation at each interaction and do not argue with the client regarding her hallucinations. Acknowledge the patient's experience while clarifying reality—"I know you see your children in the room but I don't see them right now."	1a. Arguing with the client's inaccurate perceptions can provoke increased anxiety and agitation. A sense of safety is promoted when the nurse approaches the client with a calm, relaxed demeanor and remains a consistent link to reality.	*Goal met:* Within 24 hours of discontinuation of narcotic pain medication and benzodiazepines, Mrs. Richardson is awake and alert and the confusion is starting to clear.

(continues)

Nursing Care Plan 21–1 (*continued*)

Outcome Identification	Nursing Actions	Rationales	Evaluation
	1b. Monitor and document response to the addition or discontinuation of pharmacologic agents.	1b. It is important to identify and discontinue as soon as possible any offending agents that may be responsible for acute mental status changes. The physician or advanced practice nurse relies on the nurse's timely and astute observations to help determine needed changes.	Within 24 hours of methadone being restarted at 30 mg a day, hallucinations and paranoia are no longer present. She was able to be discharged home with no special precautions and resume her usual activities.
	1c. Cautiously use touch to gain the client's attention and be alert to a heightened startle response.	1c. Appropriate touch provides a link to reality and can convey care and safety. Caution should be taken because those experiencing perceptual alterations can misperceive touch as a threat or attack, sparking a defensive response such as hitting or biting. It can help to alert the person to the touch by saying "I am going to touch your shoulder, Mrs. Richardson."	
2. By [date], Mrs. Richardson will no longer be guarded or suspicious.	2a. Provide a safe environment, being careful to do nothing that could be interpreted as secretive. Answer questions honestly and avoid excessive sensory stimulation.	2a. Activities perceived as suspicious heighten the sense of fear and anxiety. Excessive external stimulation in the presence of compromised mental status overloads the person's ability to process and respond appropriately. Aggression can occur if the person has perceptual-sensory deficits.	Mrs. Richardson's paranoia did not persist and she was able to complete her hospital stay free of agitation or aggression. Restraints were not required.
	2b. Make frequent, brief contacts identifying yourself each time and not demanding any particular task.	2b. Successful interactions build trust and allow the client to gather internal resources to maintain a sense of self and safety within the environment and those in it.	

(continues)

Nursing Care Plan 21–1 (continued)

Outcome Identification	Nursing Actions	Rationales	Evaluation
	2c. Provide simple explanations and answer questions honestly without excessive detail.	2c. Simple explanations provide less material for distortion and require less effort to process.	
	2d. Avoid restraints.	2d. Unless absolutely required to keep the client or others safe, restraints are to be avoided. They heighten paranoia and will be interpreted as a threat.	
	2e. Monitor oxygen saturation and vital signs.	2e. Acute alterations in mental status may indicate inadequate oxygenation. When multiple central nervous system depressants are administered, they place clients at risk for marked sedation, respiratory depression, aspiration, coma, and death.	

It is the nurse's responsibility to promote client safety and effective outcomes. Whether or not the physician acts within standard expectations for medical management, the nurse may be held legally accountable for pursuing all reasonable measures to prevent poor clinical outcomes. Every nurse should know and pursue available resources to assist with complicated situations. If unsafe or inappropriate medical practice is a concern, the nurse needs to understand how to follow procedures for accessing the chain of command structure in the agency or institution where she practices.

SUMMARY

◆ Substance abuse and dependence disorders are maladaptive patterns of using mood- and mind-altering chemicals to the point where, despite a variety of interpersonal, occupational, psychological, or physical problems, use continues. Addiction is synonymous with substance dependence.

◆ The precise mechanism by which a user progresses from occasional or experimental substance use to patterns of abuse and dependence is not clearly understood. A combination of biopsychosocial factors such as genetic predisposition, learned behavior, environmental influences, neurotransmitter alterations, and stress response are implicated.

◆ Abused substances are classified as CNS depressants, CNS stimulants, hallucinogens, cannabis, inhalants, and club drugs. Of all substances, alcohol, a CNS depressant, is most widely abused. Cannabis is the most widely abused illicit substance.

◆ A substance can produce dependence (addiction) even if it does not produce a withdrawal syndrome. Withdrawal syndromes are marked by effects opposite the effects of the substance when it is used for intoxication. Medical comorbidity can increase the risk for adverse outcomes in alcohol and opioid withdrawal.

◆ A wide array of medical sequelae can occur, ranging from mild and transient to fatal. Serious complications, including death, can occur whether or not the individual has a dependent pattern of substance use.

◆ The economic impact of drug abuse has risen steadily over the past 30 years as a result of increased cocaine use, HIV, and crime. The jail populations have exploded

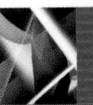

CASE STUDY

Focus on Denial

Mr. M is a 47-year-old client who has been seen in the primary clinic several times a month requesting pain medication. He has a history of a severe back injury several months ago during which time he was started on hydrocodone. The following scenario depicts a nurse-client interaction during the last visit.

NURSE: "Mr. M, I noticed that this is your third visit this month in which you came in requesting pain medications." (Points out current situation)

CLIENT: "I take this medication because I am depressed and in pain."

NURSE: "Mr. M, your pain medication is a depressant and will worsen your depression." (Reminds the client of the reality of how the medication may cause more problems)

CLIENT: "You are bringing this up because you don't care. Just give me my medication!"

NURSE: "Mr. M, I am actually bringing this up because I am concerned and care about your health." (Conveys caring and empathy)

CLIENT: "It's my business. It sounds like you think I am a drug addict. The doctor prescribed this medication because I need it! Who are you to question what I take?"

NURSE: "I know you feel depressed and it sounds like your pain is pretty intense. Let's discuss other ways to manage your pain and cope with your present stressors." (Conveys empathy, caring, and concern)

with drug offenders and are disproportionately represented by black males.

◆ There is no cure for substance-use disorders. Treatment is most successful when a combination of modalities is used. Those with strong family and social support systems have better outcomes.

◆ The nurse has an ethical and moral obligation to provide quality and culturally sensitive nursing care to persons with substance-use disorders.

◆ A variety of resources within the health care system and the community to support a recovery process. Alcoholics Anonymous and similar self-help groups are most widely known but they are not universally beneficial to every individual wanting help to overcome addiction.

◆ Because the effects of substance use show up in a variety of health care settings, the nurse should have a basic understanding of the addictions process and know how to assist clients and families in accessing appropriate resources.

SUGGESTIONS FOR CLINICAL CONFERENCES

1. Invite your local AA and request that a recovering person attend a clinical conference. Inquire about their recovery process and the role of a 12 step program in their life.

2. Discuss your attitudes about persons with substance-related disorders.

3. Attend an open AA, NA, or Alanon meeting. Discuss what happened. What feelings did you experience?

STUDY QUESTIONS

1. A 50-year-old male began drinking a six-pack of beer daily 10 years ago. He now requires 12 to 16 beers a day to achieve the same effect. He is experiencing:
   a. withdrawal
   b. altered mental status
   c. tolerance
   d. ineffective coping

2. A 35-year-old female has chronic pain related to congenital orthopedic malformations and subsequent corrective surgeries. She was recently in a car accident that aggravated her pain. Usual routine of massage, relaxation techniques, and p.r.n. Darvocet-N 100 (propoxylphene napsylate) are no longer effective in providing pain relief. This is the fourth visit to her primary care clinic since the accident. The nurse at the primary care clinic tells the physician she believes the client is addicted to her current medication and exhibits drug-seeking behavior. The doctor gives the client a prescription with two refills for hydrocodone (Vicodin). She has had no further clinic visits and has not called requesting more prescriptions. The client was displaying a pattern of behavior consistent with:
   a. narcotic addiction
   b. withdrawal
   c. personality disorder
   d. pseudoaddiction

3. A 29-year-old female has tried several times to stop drinking in the past 5 years. Each time she has stopped she has either had a driving while intoxicated charge, a job loss, or a breakup with a boyfriend. Within a few months, she returns to excessive drinking. This pattern of impaired control even after experiencing adverse consequences is a hallmark sign of:
   a. alcohol abuse
   b. major depression
   c. alcohol dependence
   d. tolerance

4. What factors are believed to be associated with the development of a substance addiction?
   a. Genetic predisposition
   b. Environmental influences
   c. Chemical changes in the brain
   d. All of the above

5. Pharmacotherapeutic agents commonly used to medically manage alcohol withdrawal are:
   a. haloperidol (Haldol) and calcium channel blockers such as diltiazem (Cardizem)
   b. vitamin therapy in the form of thiamine and benzodiazepines such as chlordiazepoxide (Librium)
   c. antidepressants such as SSRIs and vitamin C
   d. intravenous alcohol drip in decreasing doses

6. A 38-year-old male is in employer-mandated drug treatment after testing positive for cocaine in a random drug test. He has lost a previous job because of drug-related problems. His wife has given him an ultimatum—if he does not stay clean she will divorce him. He tells the nurse the company tricked him, and his wife puts too much pressure on him to make money. His cocaine use helps him have the energy to do what is expected of him. Which of the following statements are accurate?
   a. His wife is making too many demands on him.
   b. He was erroneously tested for drugs even though he signed an acknowledgment form that random drug testing was company policy.
   c. His drug of choice is cocaine and he does not use other substances therefore he cannot be substance dependent.
   d. He is demonstrating rationalization and denial and the nurse should not accept distortions of reality.

7. Which of the following interventions might be helpful to the person who is chemically dependant seeking recovery and abstinence?
   a. Regular attendance at Alcoholics Anonymous or Narcotics Anonymous meetings
   b. Naltrexone or methadone maintenance
   c. Family education and pastoral counseling
   d. All of the above

8. Encephalopathy associated with thiamine deficiency, if left untreated, can progress to a potentially irreversible syndrome of profound memory loss and inability to learn new material known as:
   a. dissociative disorder
   b. Alzheimer's disease
   c. Wernicke-Korsakoff syndrome
   d. Pick's disease

9. A recent nursing graduate is working in a trauma intensive care unit in a large city. He is surprised to find himself wanting to avoid those clients whose injuries are related to substance use, and on two occasions has knowingly delayed administering pain medication with no valid clinical reason. His older brother has an active alcohol and heroin addiction. The nurse resents the fact that his parents went through all their savings, including his college fund, trying to help his brother. What can he do to prevent himself from potentially endangering a client and help him cope with the distress he feels about his family situation?
   a. Seek out a fellow experienced colleague and discuss what he's experiencing.
   b. Attend Al Anon.

   c. Talk to the hospital's psychiatric consultation liaison advanced-practice nurse.
   d. All of the above.

10. You are working in an outpatient substance disorder clinic during which time you find out that one of your clients has been started on buprenorphine. Which of the following requires immediate attention?
    a. Hyperalertness, increased heart rate, and elevated blood pressure
    b. Complaints of malaise, clay-colored stools, and icteric sclera
    c. Dilated pupils, mild sweating, and rhinitis
    d. Complaints of sleep disturbances, agitation, and anxiety

11. A characteristic common to most substance abusers is difficulty in effectively doing which of the following?
    a. Coping with stress and anxiety
    b. Interacting socially
    c. Performing in work-related settings
    d. Setting limits

12. Signs and symptoms that a client is developing impending alcohol withdrawal delirium include diaphoresis, tremors, and which of the following?
    a. bradycardia and hypertension
    b. bradycardia and hypotension
    c. tachycardia and hypertension
    d. tachycardia and hypotension

13. A 14-year-old male client is admitted to the emergency room after ingesting a high dose of PCP and subsequently injuring himself in a fall. An effective action for the nurse to take is which of the following?
    a. An attempt to talk the client down
    b. Withhold fluids
    c. Place the client in a quiet, dimly lit room
    d. Administer a PRN antipsychotic medication

14. The nurse on a medical unit smells alcohol and notices that the relief nurse's words are slurred and she is giggling inappropriately. The best initial action for the nurse to take is which of the following?
    a. Double-assign the nurse's clients
    b. Ask the relief nurse if she has been drinking
    c. Report the nurse to the licensing board
    d. Refer the nurse to an employee assistance program

15. A 16-year-old girl is admitted to a detoxification unit with a history of cocaine abuse. Her pupils are dilated and she complains of nausea and feeling cold. She states that she is not addicted, but uses cocaine occasionally with friends. Which one of the following nursing diagnoses is appropriate for the nurse to make?
    a. Impaired verbal communication related to substance use as evidenced by giving untrue information
    b. Altered growth and development related to substance use as evidenced by the age of onset
    c. Perceptual alteration related to substance use as evidenced by distortion of reality
    d. Ineffective denial related to substance use as evidenced by refusal to admit problem

RESOURCES

Please note that because Internet resources are of a time-sensitive nature and URL addresses may change or be deleted, searches should also be conducted by association or topic.

Internet Resources

http://www.pbs.org/wnet/closetohome/home.html
Journalist Bill Moyers examined addiction and recovery in America with the five-part series *Moyers on Addiction: Close to Home*, which premiered on March 29, 1998, on PBS. The website features original reporting, animated illustrations of the neurochemistry of addictive substances, and personal stories of struggles and triumph. Links to related sites and information are provided.

http://www.streetdrugs.org provides an extensive database of drug information that can be used by the public and the nursing or teaching professional for health education purposes. Pamphlets, posters, audio-video, and CD-ROM training materials are available, some for a fee. Many of the pages have useful content that could be adapted to meet the teaching needs of a variety of client populations. Detailed information on all abused substances is readily accessible as well as related information on gangs, law enforcement, workplace issues, and topics of concern to parents.

http://pubs.niaaa.nih.gov/publications/MakeADiff_HTML/makediff.htm   Make a Difference: Talk to Your Child About Alcohol (Accessed May 22, 2006)

http://pubs.niaaa.nih.gov/publications/Practitioner/CliniciansGuide2005/guide.pdf   Helping Patients who Drink Too Much (Accessed May 22, 2006)

http://www.mentalhealth.samhsa.gov/media/ken/pdf/toolkits/illness/02.IMR_Users.pdf   Illness Management and Recovery (Accessed May 21, 2006)

Other Resources

Alcoholics Anonymous
A.A. World Services, Inc.
P.O. Box 459
New York, NY 10163
(212) 870-3400
http://www.alcoholics-anonymous.org

Adult Children of Alcoholics World Service Organization
P.O. Box 3216
Torrance, CA 90510
(310) 534-1815 (message only)
http://www.adultchildren.org

Al-Anon Family Group Headquarters
Al-Anon and Al-a-Teen
1600 Corporate Landing Parkway
Virginia Beach, VA 23454-5617
(757) 563-1600
http://www.al-anon-alateen.org

American Society of Addiction Medicine
4601 North Park Ave.

Arcade Suite 101
Chevy Chase, MD 20815
(301) 656-3920
http://www.asam.org

Hazelden Foundation
P.O. Box 11 CO3
Center City, MN 55012-0011
(800) 257-7810
http://www.hazelden.org

International Nurses Society on Addictions
P.O. Box 10752
Raleigh, NC 27605
(919) 821-1292
http://www.intnsa.org

Mothers Against Drunk Driving
P.O. Box 541688
Dallas, TX 75354-1688
(800) GET-MADD
http://www.madd.org

Narcotics Anonymous World Service Office
P.O. Box 9999
Van Nuys, CA 91409
(818) 773-9999
http://www.na.org

National Association of Alcoholism & Drug Abuse Counselors
1911 N. Fort Myer Dr.
Suite 900
Arlington, VA 22209
(800) 548-0497
http://www.naadac.org

National Institute on Drug Abuse (NIDA)
6001 Executive Blvd.
Bethesda, MD 20892-9561
(301) 443-1124
http://www.nida.nih.gov

Secular Organizations for Sobriety/Save Ourselves (SOS)
5521 Grosvenor Boulevard
Los Angeles, CA 90066
(310) 821-8430
http://www.secularsobriety.org

SMART Recovery
7537 Mentor Avenue, Suite #306
Mentor, OH 44060
(440) 951-5357
http://www.smartrecovery.org

Substance Abuse and Mental Health Services Administration (SAMHSA)
Room 12-105 Parklawn Building
5600 Fishers Lane
Rockville, MD 20857
(301) 443-4795
http://www.samhsa.gov

REFERENCES

Alcoholics Anonymous World Services. (1997). *Twelve steps and twelve traditions*. New York: Author.

American Nurses Association. (1985). *Code for nurses with interpretive statements*. Washington, DC: Author.

American Nurses Association. (1988). *Standards of addictions nursing practice with selected diagnoses and criteria*. Washington, DC: Author.

American Nurses Association. (2001). *Code of ethics for nursing with interpretive statements*. Washington, DC: American Nurses Publishing.

American Psychiatric Association. (2000). *Diagnostic and statistical manual of mental disorders* (4th edition, Text Revision) *(DSM-IV-TR)*. Washington, DC: Author.

American Society of Addiction Medicine. (1982). *Public policy of ASAM: State of recovery*. Retrieved September, 2002, from http://www.asam.org/asam

Anatchkova, M. D., Velicer, W. F., & Prochaska, J. O. (2005). Replication of subtypes for smoking cessation within the contemplation stage of change. *Addictive Behavior, 30*, 915–927.

Antai-Otong, D. (2006). Women and alcoholism: Gender-related medical complications: Treatment considerations. *Journal of Addictions Nursing, 17*, 33–45.

Bell, N., Harford, T. C., Fuchs, C. H., McCarroll, J. E., & Schwartz, C. E. (2006). Spouse abuse and alcohol problems among white, African American, and Hispanic U.S. Army soldiers. *Alcohol, Clinical and Experimental Research, 30*, 1721–1733.

Black, C. (1991). *It will never happen to me*. New York: Ballantine.

Bradshaw, J. (1988). *Healing the shame that binds you*. Deerfield Beach, FL: Health Communications.

Brent, D. A., Baugher, M., Bridge, J., Chen, T., & Chiappetta, L. (1999). Age and sex related risk factors for adolescent suicide. *Journal of the American Academy of Child and Adolescent Psychiatry, 38*(12), 1497–1505.

Button, T. M., Rhee, S. H., Hewitt, J. K., Young, S. E., Corley, R. P., & Stallings, M. C. (2007). The role of conduct disorder in explaining the comorbidity between alcohol and illicit drug dependence in adolescence. *Drug and Alcohol Dependence, 87*, 46–53.

Chaucer, G. (2000). *The Canterbury tales in modern English*. (N. Coghill, Trans.). New York: Penguin.

Chocyk, A., Czyrak, A., & Wedzony, K. (2006). Acute and repeated cocaine induces alterations in FosB/DeltaFosB expression in the paraventricular nucleus of the hypothalamus. *Brain Research, 1090*, 56–68.

Ciraulo, D. A. & Sarid-Segal, O. (2005). Sedative-, hypnotic-, or anxiolytic-related disorders. In B. J. Sadock & V. A. Sadock (Eds.), *Kaplan & Sadock's Comprehensive Textbook of Psychiatry,* (8th ed., Vol. 1, pp. 1300–1318). Philadelphia: Lippincott Williams & Wilkins.

Compton, W. M., Thomas, Y. F., Stinson, F. S., & Grant, B. F. (2007). Prevalence, correlates, disability, and comorbidity of DSM-IV drug abuse and dependence in the United States: Results from the national epidemiologic survey on alcohol and related conditions. *Archives of General Psychiatry, 64*, 566–576.

Conners, N. A., Bradley, R. H., Mansell, L. W., Liu, J. Y., Roberts, T. J., Burgdorf, K., & Herrell, J. M. (2003). Children of mothers with serious substance abuse problems: An accumulation of risks. *American Journal of Drug and Alcohol Abuse, 29*, 743–758.

Conway, K. P., Compton, W. M., Stinson, F. S., & Grant, B. F. (2005). Lifetime comorbidity of DSM-IV mood and anxiety disorders and specific drug use disorders: Results from the National Epidemiologic Survey on Alcohol and Related Conditions. *Journal of Clinical Psychiatry, 67*, 247–257.

Cottler, L. B., Campbell, W., Krishna, V. A., Cunningham-Williams, R. M., & Abdallah, A. B. (2005). Predictors of high rates of suicidal ideation among drug users. *Journal of Nervous and Mental Disorders, 193*, 431–437.

Crowley, T. J. & Sakai, J. (2005). Inhalant-related disorders. In B. J. Sadock & V. A. Sadock (Eds.), *Kaplan & Sadock's Comprehensive Textbook of Psychiatry,* (8th ed., Vol. 1, pp. 1247–1257). Philadelphia: Lippincott Williams & Wilkins.

DeWit, D. J., Adlaf, E. M., Offord, D. R., & Ogborne, A. C. (2000). Age at first alcoholism: A risk factor for the development of alcohol disorders. *American Journal of Psychiatry, 157*(5), 745–750.

Dodd, P. R., & Lewohl, J. M. (1998). Cell death mediated by amino acid transmitter receptors in human alcoholic brain damage: Conflicts in the evidence. In S. F. Ali (Ed.), *Annals of the New York Academy of Sciences: The neurochemistry of drugs of abuse* (Vol. 844). New York: New York Academy of Sciences.

Donaher, P. A. & Welsh, C. (2006). Managing opioid addiction with buprenorphine. *American Family Physician, 73*, 1573–1578.

Ehlers, C. L., Wall, T. L., Garcia-Andrade, C., & Phillips, E. (2001). Effects of age and parental history of alcoholism on EEG findings in mission Indian children and adolescents. *Alcohol Clinical Experimental Research, 25*, 672–679.

Ehrmin, J. T. (2001). Unresolved feelings of guilt and shame in the maternal role with substance-dependent African American women. *Journal of Nursing Scholarship, 33*, 47–52.

Eiden, R. D., Stevens, A., Schuetze, P., & Dombkowski, L. E. (2006). Conceptual model for maternal behavior among polydrug cocaine-using mothers: The role of postnatal cocaine use and maternal depression. *Psychology of Addictive Behavior, 20*, 1–10.

Elliott, D. L., Cheong, J., Moe, E. L., & Goldberg, L. (2007). Cross-sectional study of female students reporting anabolic steroid use. *Archives of Pediatric and Adolescent Medicine, 161*, 572–577.

Ellis, A. (1973). *Humanistic psychotherapy: The rational-emotional approach*. New York: The Julian Press.

Enoch, M. A., & Goldman, D. (1999). Genetics of alcoholism and substance abuse. *Psychiatric Clinics of North America, 22*(2), viii, 289–299.

Esposito-Smythers, C. & Spirito, A. (2004). Adolescent substance use and suicidal behavior: A review with implications for treatment research. *Alcohol and Clinical Experimental Research, 28,* 5 Suppl, 77S–88S.

Ewing, J. A. (1984). Detecting alcoholism: The CAGE questionnaire. *Journal of the American Medical Association, 252,* 1905–1907.

Frances, R., Frances, J., Franklin, J., & Borg, L. (1999). Psychodynamics. In M. Galanter & H. D. Kleber (Eds.), *Textbook of substance abuse treatment* (2nd ed., pp. 309–322). Washington, DC: American Psychiatric Press.

Gowing, L., Ali, R., & White, J. (2006). Buprenorphine for the management of opioid withdrawal. *Cochrane Database Systematic Review,* CD002025.

Grant, B. F., Hasin, D. S., Chou, S. P., Stinson, F. S., & Dawson, D. A. (2004). Nicotine dependence and psychiatric disorders in the United States: Results from the national epidemiologic survey on alcohol and related conditions. *Archives of General Psychiatry, 61,* 1107–1115.

Hall, W. & Degenhardt, L. (2005). Cannabis-related disorders. In B. J. Sadock & V. A. Sadock (Eds.), *Kaplan & Sadock's Comprehensive Textbook of Psychiatry,* (8th ed., Vol. 1, pp. 1211–1220). Philadelphia: Lippincott Williams & Wilkins.

Harris, M., Fallot, R. D., & Berley, R. W. (2005). Qualitative interviews on substance abuse relapse and prevention among female trauma survivors. *Psychiatric Services, 56,* 1292–1296.

Herve, S., Riachi, G., Noblet, C., Guillement, N., Tanasescu, S., Goria, O., Thuillez, C., Tranvouez, J. L., et al. (2004). Acute hepatitis due to buprenorphine administration. *European Journal of Gastroenterology and Hepatology, 16,* 1033–1037.

Hicks, B. M., Krueger, R. F., Iacono, W. G., McGue, M., & Patrick, C. J. (2004). Family transmission and heritability of externalizing disorders: A twin-family study. *Archives of General Psychiatry, 61,* 922–928.

Hope, B. T. (1998). Cocaine and the AP-1 transcription factor complex. In S. F. Ali (Ed.), *Annals of the New York Academy of Sciences: The neurochemistry of drugs of abuse* (Vol. 844). New York: New York Academy of Sciences.

Huang, S. Y., Lin, W. W., Wan, F. J., Change, A. J., Ko, H. C., Wang, T. J., et al. (2007). Monoamine oxidase-A polymorphisms might modify the association between the dopamine D2 receptor gene and alcohol dependence. *Journal of Psychiatry Neuroscience, 32,* 185-192.

Hughes, J. R. (2005). Nicotine-related disorders. In B. J. Sadock & V. A. Sadock (Eds.), *Kaplan & Sadock's Comprehensive Textbook of Psychiatry,* (8th ed., Vol. 1, pp. 1257–1264). Philadelphia: Lippincott Williams & Wilkins.

Hyman, S. E. (2005). Addiction: A disease of learning and memory. *American Journal of Psychiatry, 162,* 1414–1422.

Jaffe, J. H. & Anthony, J. C. (2005). Substance-related disorders: Introduction and overview. In B. J. Sadock & V. A. Sadock (Eds.), *Kaplan & Sadock's Comprehensive Textbook of Psychiatry,* (8th ed., Vol. 1, pp. 1137–1168). Philadelphia: Lippincott Williams & Wilkins.

Jaffe, J. H. & Strain, E. C. (2005). Opioid-related disorders. In B. J. Sadock & V. A. Sadock (Eds.), *Kaplan & Sadock's Comprehensive Textbook of Psychiatry,* (8th ed., Vol. 1, pp. 1265–1290). Philadelphia: Lippincott Williams & Wilkins.

James, D. J. (2005). *Profile of jailed inmates, 2002.* Washington, DC: Bureau of Justice Statistics, U.S. Department of Justice.

Jellinek, E. M. (1960). *The disease concept of addiction.* New Haven, CT: College & University Press.

Johnson, R. E., Chutuape, M. A., Strain, E. C., Walsh, S. L., Stitzer, M. I., & Bigelow, G. E. (2000). A comparison of levomethadyl acetate, buprenorphine, and methadone for opioid dependence. *New England Journal of Medicine 343,* 1290–1297.

Johnson, V. E. (1980). *I'll quit tomorrow* (Rev. ed.). New York: Harper & Row.

Johnston, L. D., O'Malley, P. M., Bachman, J. G., & Schulenberg, J. E. (2004). *Monitoring the Future National Results on Adolescent Drug Use: Overview of Key Findings, 2005* (NIH Publication No. 06-5882). Bethesda, MD: National Institute on Drug Abuse. Available at: http://monitoringthefuture.org/pubs/monographs/overview2005.pdf

Jones, H. E. (2004). Practical considerations for the clinical use of buprenorphine. www.drugabuse.gov/PDF/Perspectives/vol2no2/02Perspectives-Practical.pdf (Accessed May 27, 2006).

Jones, R. T. (2005). Hallucinogenic-related disorders. In B. J. Sadock & V. A. Sadock (Eds.), *Kaplan & Sadock's Comprehensive Textbook of Psychiatry,* (8th ed., Vol. 1, pp. 1238–1247). Philadelphia: Lippincott Williams & Wilkins.

Kalivas, P. W. & Volkow, N. D. (2005). The neural basis of addiction: A pathology of motivation and choice. *American Journal of Psychiatry, 162,* 1403–1413.

Karberg, J., & James D. J. (2005). *Substance dependence, abuse, and treatment of jail inmates, 2002.* Washington, DC: Bureau of Justice Statistics, U.S. Department of Justice.

Kessler, R. C., Chiu, W. T., Demler, O., Merikangas, K. R., & Walters, E. E. (2005). Prevalence, severity, and comorbidity of 12-month DSM-IV disorders in the National Comorbidity Survey Replication. *Archives of General Psychiatry, 62,* 617–627.

Klein, M. (1998). Research issues related to development of medications for treatment of cocaine addiction. In S. F. Ali (Ed.), *Annals of the New York Academy of Sciences: The neurochemistry of drugs of abuse* (Vol. 844). New York: New York Academy of Sciences.

Kosten, T. R. & Fiellin, D. A. (2004). Buprenorphine for office-based practice: Consensus conference overview. *The American Journal on Addictions, 13,* Suppl 1, S1–S16.

Kuschel, C. (2007). Managing drug withdrawal in the newborn infant. *Seminars in Fetal and Neonatal Medicine, 12,* 127–133.

Le Foll, B., Goldberg, S. R., & Sokoloff, P. (2005). The dopamine D3 receptor and drug dependence: Effects on reward or beyond? *Neuropharmacology, 49,* 525–541.

Leshner, A. I. (1997). Addiction is a brain disease, and it matters. *Science, 278*(3), 45–47.

Leshner, A. I. (1998). Drug addiction research: Moving toward the 21st century. *Drug and Alcohol Dependence, 51,* 5–7.

Liu, S., Bubar, M. J., Lanfranco, M. F., Hillman, G. R., & Cunningham, K. A. (2007). Serotonin (2C) receptor localization in GABA neurons of the rat medial prefrontal cortex: Implications for understanding the neurobiology of addiction. *Neuroscience, 146,* 1677-1688.

Liu, J., Lewohl, J. M., Harris, R. A., Dodd, P. R., & Mayfield, R. D. (2007). Altered gene expression profiles in the frontal cortex of cirrhotic alcoholics. *Alcohol, Clinical and Experimental Research,* July 11. [Epub ahead of print]

Lusher, J., Elander, J., Bevan, D., Telfer, P., & Burton, B. (2006). Analgesic addiction and pseudoaddiction in painful chronic illness. *The Clinical Journal of Pain, 22,* 316–324.

Marsch, L. A., Stephens, M. A., Mudric, T., Strain, E. C., Bigelow, G. E., & Johnson, R. E. (2005). Predictors of outcome in LAAM, buprenorphine, and methadone treatment for opioid dependence. *Experimental and Clinical Psychopharmacology, 13,* 293–302.

Mayo-Smith, M. F, Beecher, L. H., Fischer, T. L., Gorelick, D. A., Guillaume, J. L., Hill, A., Jara, G., Kasser, C., Melbourne, J., & Working Group on the Management of Alcohol Withdrawal Delirium, Practice Guidelines Committee, American Society of Addiction Medicine. (2004). Management of alcohol withdrawal delirium. An evidence-based practice guideline. *Archives of Internal Medicine, 164,* 1405–1412.

Meara, F. & Frank, R. G. (2005). Spending on substance abuse treatment: How much is enough? *Addiction, 100,* 1240–1248.

McIntosh, C., & Chick, J. (2004). Alcohol and the nervous system. *Journal of Neurology, Neurosurgery and Psychiatry, 75,* (Suppl 3), 16–21.

Merrill, C. T., & Elixhauser, A. (2005). *Hospitalization in the United States, 2002.* Rockville, MD: Agency for Healthcare Research and Quality, HCUP Fact Book No. 6 AHRQ Publication No. 05-0056 ISBN 1-58763-217-9. Available online at http://www.ahrq.gov/data/hcup/factbk6/factbk6.pdf

Morrissey, J. P., Jackson, E. W., Ellis, A. R., Amaro, H., Brown, V. B., & Najavits, L. M. (2005). Twelve-month outcomes of trauma-informed interventions for women with co-occurring disorders. *Psychiatric Services, 56,* 1213–1222.

Naegle, M. A. (2000). Mental health and substance-related health care. In M. A. Naegle & C. E. D'Avanzo (Eds.), *Addictions and substance abuse: Strategies for advanced practice nursing.* Upper Saddle River, NJ: Prentice Hall.

National Institute on Alcohol Abuse and Alcoholism (NIAAA). (1998). *Alcoholism assessment and treatment instruments.* Bethesda, MD: Retrieved September, 2002, from http://silk.nih.gov/silk/niaaa1/publication/aa13.htm

National Institute on Alcohol Abuse and Alcoholism. (2000). *Ninth special report to the U.S. Congress on alcohol and health.* Bethesda, MD: Author, NIH Publication 00–1583.

National Institute on Drug Abuse. (2005). Fentanyl http://www.drugabuse.gov/drugpages/fentanyl.html (Accessed March 2, 2007)

Office of Applied Studies. (2005). *Results from the 2004 National Survey on Drug Use and Health: National findings* (DHHS Publication No. SMA 05-4062, NSDUH Series H-28). Rockville, MD: Substance Abuse and Mental Health Services Administration. http://www.oas.samhsa.gov/p0000016.htm#2k4 (Accessed May 28, 2006).

Office of Applied Studies. (2006). *Results from the 2005 National Survey on Drug Use and Health: National findings.* Rockville, MD: Substance Abuse and Mental Health Services Administration, DHHS Publication No. 06-4194 NSDUH Series H-30. Available online at http://oas.samhsa.gov/2k7/AmIndians/AmIndians.pdf

Olbrich, H. M., Valerius, G., Paris, C., Hagenbuch, F., Ebert, D., & Juengling, F. D. (2006). Brain activation during craving for alcohol measured by positron emission tomography. *Australian New Zealand Journal of Psychiatry, 40,* 171–178.

Pillolla, G., Melis, M., Perra, S., Muntoni, A. L., Gessa, G. L., & Pistis, M. (2007). Medial forebrain bundle stimulation evokes endocannabinoid-mediated modulation of ventral tegmental area dopamine neuron firing in vivo. *Psychopharmacology, 191,* 843–853.

Plessinger, M. A., & Woods, J. R. (1998). Cocaine in pregnancy. *Obstetric and Gynecology Clinics of America, 25*(1), 99–118.

Prochaska, J. O., DiClemente, C. C., & Norcross, J. C. (1992). In search of how people change: Applications to addictive behaviors. *American Psychologist, 47*(9), 1102–1113.

Prochaska, J. O., & Velicer, W. F. (1997). The transtheoretical model of health behavior change. *American Journal of Health Promotion, 12*(1), 38–48.

Rajendram, R., Lewison, G., & Preedy, V. R. (2006). Worldwide alcohol-related research and the disease burden. *Alcohol and Alcoholism, 41,* 99–106.

Rockett, I. R., Putnam, S. L., Jia, J., Chang, C. F., & Smith, G. S. (2005). Unmet substance abuse treatment need, health services utilization, and cost: A population-based emergency department study. *Annals of Emergency Medicine, 45,* 118–127.

Rothman, R. B., Blough, B. E., & Baumann, M. H. (2007). Dual dopamine/serotonin releasers as potential medications for stimulant and alcohol addictions. *The American Association of Pharmaceutical Scientists Journal, 9,* E1–10.

Saha, T. D., Chou, S. P., & Grant, B. F. (2006). Toward an alcohol use disorder continuum using item response theory: Results from the National Epidemiologic Survey on Alcohol and Related Conditions. *Psychological Medicine, 36,* 931-941.

Schuckit, M. A. (2005). Alcohol-related disorders. *Comprehensive textbook of psychiatry* (8th ed., Vol. 1, pp. 1169–1188). Philadelphia: Lippincott Williams & Wilkins.

Sher, L. (2006). Alcoholism and suicidal behavior: A clinical overview. *Acta Psychiatrica Scandinavia, 113,* 13–22.

Shorter, E. (1997). *A history of psychiatry: From the era of the asylum to the age of Prozac.* New York: John Wiley & Sons.

Shreeram, S. S., McDonald, T., & Dennison, S. (2001). Psychosis after ultrarapid opiate detoxification. *American Journal of Psychiatry, 158,* 970.

Siegrist, J., Menrath, I., Stocker, T., Klein, M., Kellerman, T., Shah, N. J., et al. (2005). Differential brain activation according to chronic social reward frustration. *Neuroport, 16,* 1899-1903.

Simpson, D. M., Messina, J., Xie, F., & Hale, M. (2007). Fentanyl buccal tablet for the relief of breakthrough pain in opioid-tolerant adult patients with chronic neuropathic pain: A multicenter, randomized, double blind, placebo-controlled study. *Clinical Therapeutics, 29,* 588-601.

Soderstrom, C. A., Smith, G. S., Kufera, J. A., Dischinger, P. C., Hebel, J. R., McDuff, D. R., et al. (1997). The accuracy of the CAGE, the Brief Michigan Alcoholism Screening Test, and the Alcohol Use Disorders Identification Test in screening trauma center patients for alcoholism. *Journal of Trauma, 43*(6), 962–969.

Spicer, P., Bezdek, M., Manson, S. M., & Beals, J. (2007). A program of research on spirituality and American Indian alcohol use. *Southern Medicine Journal, 100,* 430-432.

Spremo, M., & Loga, S. (2005). The relationship between suicidal thoughts and psychoactive substances. *Bosnia Journal of Basic Medical Science, 5,* 35–38.

Steinweg, D. L., & Worth, H. (1993). Alcoholism: The keys to the CAGE. *American Journal of Medicine, 94*(5), 520–523.

Substance Abuse and Mental Health Services Administration Office of Applied Studies. (1998). *Services research outcomes study.* Rockville, MD: Author. Retrieved September, 2002, from http://www.samhsa.gov/oas/sros/httoc.htm

Substance Abuse and Mental Health Services Administration (SAMHSA). (2000). *1999 National household survey on drug abuse.* Rockville, MD: Author. Retrieved September, 2002, from http://www.samhsa.gov/oas/NHSDA/1999/Table%20of%20Contents.htm

Substance Abuse and Mental Health Services Administration Center for Substance Abuse Treatment. (2000). *National treatment improvement evaluation study.* Rockville, MD: Author. Retrieved September, 2002, from http://www.health.org/govstudy/f027/index.htm

Substance Abuse and Mental Health Services Administration (SAMHSA) (2004). Overview of Findings from the 2004 National Survey on Drug Use and Health http://www/oas.samhsa.gov/NSDUH/24kNSDUH/2k4overview/2k4overview.pdf

Substance Abuse and Mental Health Services Administration and Office of Applied Studies (2005). Illicit durg use among persons arrested for serious crimes. The National Survey on Drug Use & Health. *NSDUH Report,* Office of Applied Studies, SAMHSA. Available online at http://www.oas.samhsa.gov/2k5/arrests/arrests.pdf

Sullivan, J. T., Sykora, K., Schneiderman, J., Naranjo, C. A., & Sellers, E. M. (1989). Assessment of alcohol withdrawal: The revised Clinical Institute Withdrawal Assessment for Alcohol scale (CIWA-AR). *British Journal of Addictions, 84,* 1353–1357.

Trimpey, J. (1996). *The small book: A revolutionary approach to overcoming drug and alcohol dependence* (Rev. ed.). New York: Dell. Retrieved September, 2002, from http://www.rational.org/recovery/

U.S. Census Bureau. (2000). *Census 2000 redistricting (Public Law 94–171) summary file, table 1.* Washington, DC: Government Printing Office.

United States Department of Health and Human Services, Office of Disease Prevention and Health Promotion of the Office of Public Health and Science. (1999). *Healthy people 2010, conference edition* (Vols. I and II). Washington, DC: Author.

United States Public Health Service. (2000, June). *Treating tobacco use and dependence.* Retrieved September, 2002, from http://www.surgeongeneral.gov/tobacco/smokesum.htm

Warren, K. R., & Foudin, L. L. (2001). Alcohol-related birth defects, the past, present and future. *Alcohol Research and Health, 25*(3). Retrieved September, 2002, from http://www.niaa.nih.gov/publications/arh25-3/153-158.htm

White, W. L. (1998). *Slaying the dragon: The history of addiction treatment and recovery in America.* Bloomington, IL: Chestnut Health Systems.

Wines, J. D. Jr., Saitz, R., Horton, N. J., Llyod-Travaglini, C., & Samet, J. H. (2004). Suicidal behavior, drug use and depressive symptoms after detoxification: A 2-year prospective study. *Drug and Alcohol Dependence, 76* Suppl, S21–S29.

SUGGESTED READINGS

Alcoholics Anonymous. (1986). *Alcoholics Anonymous: The big book.* New York: Author.

Gorski, T. T. (1997). *Passages through recovery: An action plan for preventing relapse.* Center City, MN: Hazelden Information Education.

Hesley, J. W., & Hesley, J. G. (1998). *Rent two movies and let's talk in the morning: Using popular movies in psychotherapy.* New York: John Wiley and Sons.

Hogdson, B. (2001). *In the arms of Morpheus: The tragic history of laudanum, morphine, and patent medicines.* Toronto, Ontario, Canada: Firefly Books.

Hughes, T. L. (1995). Chief nurse executives' response to chemically dependent nurses. *Nursing Management, 26*(3), 37–40.

Johnson, V. (1989). *Intervention: How to help someone who doesn't want help, a step-by-step guide for families of chemically dependent persons.* Washington, DC: Johnson Institute.

Kuhn, C., Swartzwelder, S., & Wilson, W. (1998). *The straight facts about the most used and abused drugs from alcohol to ecstasy.* New York: W.W. Norton & Company.

McDowell, D. M., & Spitz, H. I. (1999). *Substance abuse from principles to practice.* Philadelphia: Brunner/Mazel.

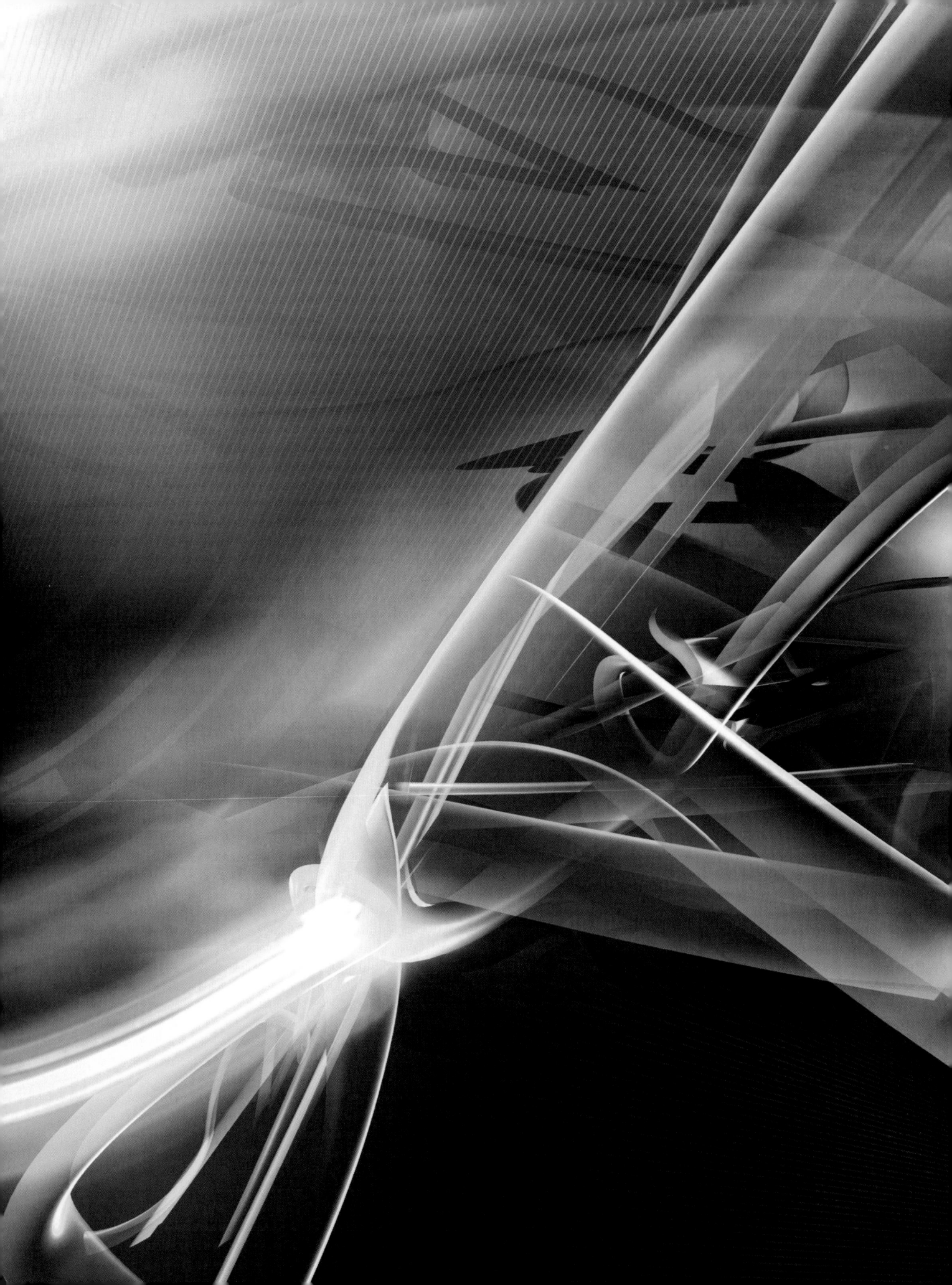

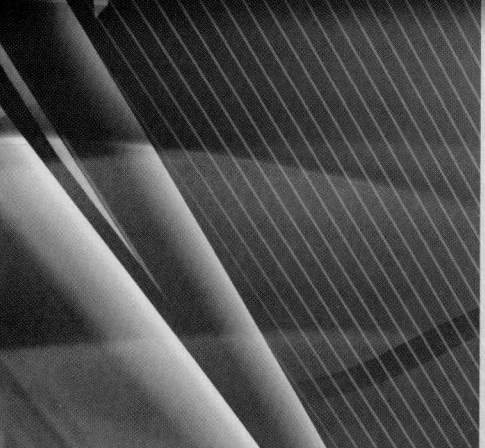

CHAPTER 22

The Client with an Eating Disorder

Michele L. Zimmerman, MA, APRN, BC

KEY TERMS

Alexithymia: Refers to a lack of introceptive awareness, mistrust of self and others, cognitive dysfunction, and starvation-induced depression.

Anorexia Nervosa (AN): Self-induced starvation resulting from fear of fatness; not caused by true loss of appetite.

Binge: A period of uncontrolled eating in which a large amount of food is consumed unrelated to physical hunger.

Body Image Disturbance: Refers to a distortion in the image of the body that is of near or actual delusional proportions; may include strong feelings of self-loathing projected onto the body, body parts, or perceived fat.

Body Mass Index (BMI): Refers to a mathematical formula that is highly correlated with body fat. It is weight in kilograms

divided by height in meters squared (kg/m^2). In the United States and in the United Kingdom, people with BMIs between 25 and 30 kg/m^2 are considered overweight and those with BMIs of 30 kg/m^2 are categorized as obese.

Bulimia Nervosa (BN): Binge eating followed by self-inflicted vomiting, laxative or diuretic abuse, or starvation.

Eating Disorder (ED): A general term for abnormalities in behavior toward food, growing out of fear of fatness and pursuit of excessive thinness.

Purge: Self-induced vomiting or misuse of laxative, diuretics, or enemas.

COMPETENCIES

Upon completion of this chapter, the learner should be able to:

1. Discuss medical and nursing diagnoses for eating disorders.
2. Analyze the etiologies of eating disorders.
3. Recognize risk factors for eating disorders and the nurse's role in prevention.
4. Investigate the neurobiological implications associated with eating disorders.
5. Discuss co-occurring psychiatric and medical conditions associated with eating disorders.
6. Describe medical interventions used in treatment of eating disorders.
7. Implement a plan of care for the client with an eating disorder.
8. Discuss psychopharmacologic interventions used in treating eating disorders.

CHAPTER OUTLINE

Eating disorders (EDs) are a significant health problem among children, adolescents, and young women. The eating disorder, anorexia nervosa, has the highest mortality rate of any mental illness. Western society places an emphasis on physical attractiveness, and, in this century, there is an extreme emphasis on thinness as the epitome of feminine beauty. Cultural values, particularly since the 1970s, have promoted images of willowy, gaunt young women as the ideal female form. Dieting, weight loss, exercise, fitness, and small size are relentlessly promoted in all of the media, and the comment "You look great . . . you've lost weight . . . !" is a high form of praise to both men and women in American society. Thus, the message—that to be attractive, desirable, and successful is to be thin, small, and slender—and losing weight are constantly broadcast to children, adolescents, and young adults in our society. The range of age of onset has been declining and young children are increasingly diagnosed. Simultaneously, there has been an explosion in the number and variety of high-fat, high-calorie fast foods as well as in food advertising, and there is an increase in the number of markedly obese people of all ages, except for the elderly. The rate of obesity among children has doubled in the last decade (U.S. DHHS, Mental Health of the Surgeon General, 1999). Although EDs are increasing all over the world, there is evidence to suggest that Western women are at greater risk for developing them, and the degree of westernization increases the risk (Cummins & Lehman, 2007).

While there is uncertainty about the prevalence of eating disorders, the general consensus among experts is that full blown EDs occur in 1 (anorexia nervosa) to 3 percent (bulimia nervosa) of women at some point. Rates among men are one-tenth of those observed in women (Walsh & Cameron, 2005). Only recently have EDs been recognized as distinct clinical entities, with bulimia nervosa first appearing in the *Diagnostic and Statistical Manual of Mental Disorders* (3rd edition) *(DSM III)* in 1980. High-risk professions for EDs include female gender athletes, dancers, and models (Torstveit, Rosenvinge, & Sundgot-Borgen, 2007). Because preoccupation with appearance and weight is so commonplace, and thinness is culturally sanctioned, with weight loss recognized as a goal to strive for, a youngster's disorder may go unrecognized by her family and loved ones. This complicates prevention, case finding, and treatment.

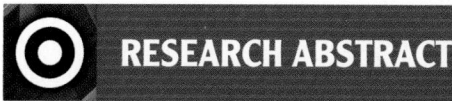

RESEARCH ABSTRACT

A Randomised Controlled Treatment Trial of Two Forms of Family Therapy in Adolescent Anorexia Nervosa: A Five-Year Follow-up

Eisler, I., Simic, M., Russell, G. F., & Dare, C. (2007). *Journal of Child Psychology and Psychiatry, 48*, 552–560.

Study Problem/Purpose

The purpose of this study was to evaluate the long-term impact of two forms of outpatient family intervention, formerly evaluated in a randomized controlled trial in the treatment for adolescent anorexia nervosa.

Methods

A 5-year follow-up was conducted on a cohort of 40 clients who had participated either in conjoint family therapy (CFT) or separated family therapy (SFT). For the 38 subjects who agreed to be re-evaluated, face-to-face interviews were used in 29 cases and telephone interviews were conducted in 3 cases; 6 subjects completed questionnaires and/or agreed for parents and grandparents to be interviewed.

Findings

Results from the study demonstrated insignificant differences between the two therapies at the 5-year follow-up and that more than 75 percent of subjects were free of eating disorder symptoms. There were no mortalities in the subjects and only 8 percent who achieved a normal weight by the end of treatment reported any kind of relapse. Three patients developed bulimic symptoms but only one met diagnostic criteria of bulimia nervosa. The one difference between the treatments was in clients from families with high levels of maternal criticism. This group of clients had a poorer response to treatment at the end of treatment. This study corroborates the efficacy of family therapy for adolescent anorexia nervosa, demonstrating that those who respond well to outpatient family intervention generally have prolonged results.

Implications for Psychiatric Nurses

Findings from this study corroborate the efficacy of family therapy for adolescents with anorexia nervosa. They offer hope to families and adolescents with anorexia nervosa. Psychiatric nurses can also use these findings to identify high-risk populations, particularly ones in which there is high family criticism, to prevent eating and other psychiatric disorders associated with family stress and turmoil.

EDs are common in the United States, affecting from 1 to 4 percent of the population (Hudson, Hiripi, Pope, & Kessler, 2007; Torstveit et al., 2007). Cross-cultural studies have also been reviewed extensively and demonstrated the global prevalence of eating disorders (Chamorro & Flores-Ortiz, 2000; Hudson et al., 2007; Torstveit et al., 2007). About 8 percent of the obese population meet criteria for binge eating disorder (BED). (Hudson et al., 2007). These conditions are characterized by an extreme disturbance in eating-related behaviors. Most people with EDs are greatly ambivalent about seeking treatment because treatment may be associated with weight gain. AN and bulimia are seen in a heterogeneous population and it is important not to generalize or stereotype persons with these disorders. Although AN, bulimia nervosa (BN), and BED are classified as separate disorders by the *Diagnostic and Statistical Manual of Mental Disorders* (4th edition, Text Revision) *(DSM-IV-TR)* (American Psychiatric Association [APA], 2000), they are frequently comorbid conditions, as well as comorbid with other Axis I and Axis II disorders.

A summary of 68 treatment studies published between 1953 and 1989 of 3,104 people, with a length of follow-up of 1 to 33 years, found that 43 percent of people recover completely (range 7 to 86 percent), 36 percent improve (range 1 to 69 percent), 20 percent develop a chronic ED (range 0 to 43 percent), and 5 percent die from AN (range 10 to 21 percent) (Treasure & Schmidt, 2001). Clinicians agree that persons with EDs experience low self-esteem and associated emotional mental problems owing to a variety of reasons associated both with the etiology of these disorders and their sequelae (Signorini et al., 2007).

DEFINITIONS AND CRITERIA

Clients with eating disorders often present with a host of psychiatric and medical conditions that require immediate attention and management. Effective treatment management requires a holistic and interdisciplinary approach stemming from an accurate diagnosis that parallels specific criteria for each disorder. The following section defines specific eating disorders and promotes a greater understanding of these complex and life-threatening psychiatric and medical conditions.

ANOREXIA NERVOSA

Anorexia nervosa (AN) refers to a syndrome manifested by self-induced starvation resulting from fear of fatness rather than from true loss of appetite. Anorexia nervosa normally begins around the onset of puberty. The word *anorexia* is derived from Greek and is translated as "loss of appetite due to nerves," but the term is a misnomer. Persons with AN continue to feel hunger but persist in denying themselves food. The onset is usually in an adolescent female who perceives herself to be overweight. In her classic work, Hilde Bruch (1973) described one of the central features of this disorder as "the relentless pursuit of thinness." Other features include amenorrhea, an intense fear of gaining weight or becoming fat, refusal to maintain a normal body weight (e.g., less than 85 percent of expected weight for age and height, or body mass index [BMI] less than 17.5 kg/m²), failure to gain expected weight during growth (Treasure & Schmidt, 2001),

DSM-IV-TR Diagnostic Criteria for Anorexia Nervosa

A. Refusal to maintain body weight at or above a minimally normal weight for age and height (e.g., weight loss leading to maintenance of body weight less than 85 percent of that expected; or failure to make expected weight gain during period of growth, leading to body weight less than 85% of that expected).

B. Intense fear of gaining weight or becoming fat, even though underweight.

C. Disturbance in the way in which one's body weight or shape is experienced, undue influence of body weight or shape on self-evaluation, or denial of the seriousness of the current low body weight.

D. In postmenarchal females, amenorrhea, i.e., the absence of at least three consecutive menstrual cycles. (A woman is considered to have amenorrhea if her periods occur only following hormone, e.g., estrogen, administration.)

and a distorted body image. Other psychological characteristics include fear of loss of control, alexithymia, lack of introceptive awareness, mistrust of self and others, cognitive dysfunction, and starvation-induced depression. Anorexia nervosa has the highest mortality of all psychiatric disorders.

Although AN has been described in the medical literature for hundreds of years, it was not until the 1960s that the disorder was considered a treatable psychiatric condition. Clients with this disorder usually are not seen in the treatment setting until the weight loss or failure to gain expected weight is marked. The *DSM-IV-TR* (APA, 2000), in considering the client's age and height, uses less than 85 percent of expected weight as the guide (see the display on diagnostic criteria for AN). Physiological findings present as a result of the severe starvation and weight loss (Table 22–1).

The course of AN varies: it most often consists of a single episode with return to normal weight, but it may be episodic or unremitting until it leads to death (Signorini et al., 2007). It is a deadly psychiatric disorder. Mortality rates of this disorder vary due to methodological issues, but most studies have demonstrated a standardized mortality ratio between 4 and 13 for anorexia nervosa. Early diagnosis and intensive treatment may reduce mortality in this population. Favorable factors include early age at onset and short interval between onset of symptoms and the beginning of treatment—the mortality rate is higher for people with lower weight and with older age at presentation (Signorini et al., 2007). Unfavorable factors and increased risk and fatal outcome of AN are chronicity, binging and purging, and comorbid substance-related and mood disorders (Fichter, Quadflieg, & Hedlund, 2006).

BULIMIA NERVOSA

Bulimia nervosa (BN) is more prevalent than AN. This disorder appears to have a later onset than AN. The term *bulimia* is translated as "ravenous appetite" and refers to a syndrome of episodes of binge eating, followed by self-induced vomiting, or purge behavior, accompanied by an excessive preoccupation with weight and body shape. There is a feeling of a lack of control over eating behavior when binging, and the measures to prevent weight gain include use of laxatives, cathartics, enemas, and diuretics; periods of strict dieting or fasting; and strenuous exercise. Weight may be normal but there may be a history of AN or restrictive dieting. Some clients with bulimia discover and abuse syrup of ipecac, a high-risk behavior because of the drug's cardiotoxicity.

Binge refers to "eating in a discrete period of time an amount of food that is definitely larger than most individuals would eat under similar circumstances." See the display on diagnostic criteria for BN. Typical binge food is sweet and high in calories. It is consumed rapidly with little chewing and often in secret. The client with bulimia nervosa (BN) purges by vomiting, laxative and diuretic abuse, and/or excessive exercise after the binge to get rid of the excess calories ingested during the binge (APA, 2000).

Clients with bulimia may have a normal weight, be overweight, or be underweight. Clients with this disorder characteristically have a thin body with swollen cheeks, owing to enlarged salivary glands, and exhibit signs of fluid retention. The skin tends to be dry with cuts and abrasions, particularly over the knuckles, owing to the repeated trauma of putting the fingers down the throat to induce vomiting (Russell's sign). The repeated vomiting causes erosion of the dental enamel, and any of the purging mechanisms may lead to dehydration and electrolyte imbalance, particularly of potassium. The condition is often first discovered by dental examination. Blood-streaked vomitus is not unusual, but frank bleeding may signal a life-threatening gastric or esophageal tear. Serious complications may also include cardiac arrhythmias owing to electrolyte imbalances, which can cause sudden death (Mitchell & Crow, 2006).

BN usually begins in late adolescence or early adulthood, and the disorder can follow a chronic and intermittent course over many years. Parents of clients with this disorder may be obese or markedly underweight, and there is a higher rate of major depression than expected in first-degree relatives. The families may be overly preoccupied with food and appearances. Clients with bulimia themselves commonly have a depressive disorder and may concurrently abuse psychoactive substances, most frequently alcohol, sedatives, or stimulants. They tend to have less superego control than their counterparts with anorexia. Disorders of impulse control such as compulsive shopping and shoplifting have been associated with bulimia. Persons with bulimia also reportedly have increased rates of obesity, parental problems, disturbed family dynamics, histories of sexual and physical abuse, parental weight or shape concern, anxiety disorders, low self-esteem, mood disorders, substance abuse, perfectionism, bipolar

TABLE 22–1
Physiological Findings in Eating Disorders

Physical Symptoms	Cold intolerance, constipation, abdominal discomfort, dizziness, bloating, and hyperactivity
	Lethargy is worrisome because it may indicate cardiovascular compromise
Physical Examination	Appearance is younger than chronological age
	Multiple layers of clothing, cachexia, and breast atrophy
	Dry skin, bradycardia, hypotension, hypokalemia, lanugo, alopecia, edema of the lower extremities, and dental enamel erosion
Medical Complications	Cardiovascular, hematologic, gastrointestinal, renal, neurologic, endocrine, and skeletal
Cardiovascular Complications	ECG abnormalities
	Prolonged QT intervals, and emetine-induced myocardial damage may be life threatening
	Long-standing bradycardia due to regular exercise
Hematologic Changes	Mild anemia 30% of cases
	Leukopenia up to 50% of cases
Gastrointestinal Complications	Decreased gastric motility and delayed gastric emptying
Renal Abnormalities	Dehydration results in increased levels of blood urea nitrogen
	Polyuria due to decrease in renal concentrating capacity and abnormal vasopressin secretion producing partial diabetes insipidus
	Peripheral edema in 20% of cases
Neurologic Abnormalities	Rarely found
Endocrine Complications	Amenorrhea is hallmark of anorexia, due to starvation-induced hypogonadism
Skeletal Complications	Osteopenia; skeletal fractures

ECG, electrocardiogram. RT, portion of the cardiac complex on the electrocardiogram that extends from the beginning of the Q wave to the end of the T wave.

I disorder, and dissociative disorders (Hudson et al., 2007). Positive outcomes involving BN are associated with shorter duration of illness, younger age of onset, and higher socioeconomic status. Negative outcomes, similar to other eating disorders, include co-occurring psychiatric disorders and premorbid and parental obesity.

BINGE EATING DISORDER

Binge eating disorder (BED) is a disorder newly described in the *DSM-IV-TR* (APA, 2000). See the display on research criteria for BED. Clients with BED experience recurrent binge eating but do not regularly engage in the purging behaviors or compulsive exercise that clients with bulimia use to avoid weight gain. Spitzer et al. (1993) studied 2,802 subjects drawn from client and nonclient community samples. More than one half of the total sample (1,785 subjects) were participants in weight control programs, and 20 percent of these met the criteria for BED. In both the weight control and community samples, BED was associated with a lifetime history of fluctuating weight and severe obesity. The female-to-male ratio in the study by Spitzer et al. was 3:2.

Characteristics of the BED population include impairment in work and social functioning; preoccupation with weight and shape; general psychopathology; significant time and energy devoted to dieting; and a history of depression, alcohol, or drug abuse and treatment for emotional problems (Hudson et al., 2007). According to findings from the 2007 National Comorbidity Replication study, the lifetime prevalence estimates of BED are 3.5 percent in women and 2 percent in men (Hudson et al., 2007).

OBESITY

Obesity is recognized as a serious health problem but is not classified by itself as an eating disorder, at least in the *DSM-IV-TR* (APA, 2000). According to the National Heart, Lung, & Blood Institute (1998) *overweight* and *obesity* refer to ranges of weight that are greater than what is generally considered for a

DSM-IV-TR Diagnostic Criteria for Bulimia Nervosa

A. Recurrent episodes of binge eating. An episode of binge eating is characterized by both of the following:

1. Eating, in a discrete period of time (e.g., within any 2-hour period), an amount of food that is definitely larger than most people would eat during a similar period of time and under similar circumstances

2. A sense of lack of control over eating during the episode (e.g., a feeling that one cannot stop eating or control what or how much one is eating)

B. Recurrent inappropriate compensatory behavior in order to prevent weight gain, such as self-induced vomiting; misuse of laxatives, diuretics, enemas, or other medications; fasting; or excessive exercise.

C. The binge eating and inappropriate compensatory behaviors both occur, on average, at least twice a week for 3 months.

D. Self-evaluation is unduly influenced by body shape and weight.

E. The disturbance does not occur exclusively during episodes of Anorexia Nervosa.

DSM-IV-TR Diagnostic Criteria for Binge Eating Disorder

A. Recurrent episodes of binge eating. An episode is characterized by both of the following:

1. Eating, in a discrete period of time (e.g., within any 2-hour period), an amount of food that is definitely larger than most people would eat during a similar period of time under similar circumstances.

2. A sense of lack of control during the episode (e.g., a feeling that one cannot stop eating or control what or how much one is eating).

B. The binge-eating episodes are associated with three (or more) of the following:

1. Eating much more rapidly than normal.

2. Eating until feeling uncomfortably full.

3. Eating large amounts of food when not feeling physically hungry.

4. Eating alone because of being embarrassed by how much one is eating.

5. Feeling disgusted with oneself, depressed, or feeling very guilty after overeating.

C. Marked distress regarding binge eating is present.

D. The binge eating occurs, on average, at least 2 days a week for 6 months.

Note: The method of determining frequency differs from that used for bulimia nervosa; future research should address whether the preferred method of setting a frequency threshold is counting the number of days on which binges occur or counting the number of episodes of binge eating.

E. The binge eating is not associated with the regular use of inappropriate compensatory behaviors (e.g., purging, fasting, excessive exercise) and does not occur exclusively during the course of anorexia nervosa or bulimia nervosa.

---

given height. Weight is also correlated with the risk or likelihood of diseases and associated health problems. For adults this is determined by using weight and height to calculate the BMI. An adult who has a BMI of 25 to 29.9 is considered overweight. In comparison, an adult who has a BMI of 30 or higher is considered obese. Many medical diseases and complications are associated with obesity, including hypertension, gallbladder disease, diabetes, trauma to weight-bearing joints, and increased risk of cardiovascular disease, especially when there is an excess accumulation of fat in the abdominal region. A precise measure of obesity is the amount of fat in the body or the BMI, which is calculated by the following formula:

$$BMI = [body\ weight\ in\ kg] \div [height\ in\ m^2]$$

BMI correlates with morbidity and mortality (Adams, Schatzkin, Harris, et al., 2006). Prevalence statistics indicate that obesity is found more commonly in women than in men and that the condition increases with age up to 60 years, when it begins to decrease. According to findings from a 2007 epidemiologic study (Wang & Beydoun, 2007), the prevalence of obesity in the United States has risen from 13 percent to 32 percent between the 1960s and 2004. The prevalence of obesity and overweight has increased at an average rate of 0.3 to 0.8 percentage points across socioeconomic groups over the past 3 decades. Some minority and lower socioeconomic status populations are disproportionately affected by obesity. Researchers who conducted this study describe the increased rate of obesity as "alarming" and a public health crisis (Wang & Beydoun, 2007). Implications from these findings include the need to identify high-risk groups and provide psychoeducation concerning the consequences of obesity and the importance of healthy eating habits and regular exercise across the life span.

In spite of the widespread popularity of weight loss programs, most studies from the 1970s have shown that significant weight loss is rare and losses that do occur are not well maintained. Evidence is overwhelming that restrictive dieting serves to actually trigger weight gain once normal eating resumes.

Although obesity is not yet considered an ED in the psychiatric nomenclature, it is considered a risk factor for AN and BN. With the new category of BED, people with simple obesity must be differentiated from those with the more complex features of that disorder.

PICA

Pica refers to the persistent eating of a nonnutritive substance. The name is derived from the Latin word for magpie, a bird known to eat a variety of objects. Infants with this disorder may eat hair, cloth, plaster, paint, or string; and older children may eat sand, leaves, insects, pebbles, or animal droppings. Almost all children occasionally ingest such substances, and the behavior is not considered abnormal in children 18 months of age and younger. Pica is common in children as old as 6 years of age, with greater occurrence in severely mentally retarded or children with psychosis (APA, 2000). Pregnant women may also exhibit pica.

Pica is believed to result from iron and zinc deficiencies or related to lack of stimulation and adult supervision. Medical complications include lead poisoning from the ingestion of paint or paint-soaked plaster. *Toxoplasma* or *Toxocara* infections may result from the ingestion of feces or dirt. Hair-ball tumors may cause intestinal obstruction. The *DSM-IV-TR* (APA, 2000) includes only two diagnostic criteria for pica, as listed in the accompanying display.

RUMINATION DISORDER

Rumination disorder is a rare phenomenon, seen equally in male and female infants. It usually appears between 3 months and 1 year of age but may show up later in children who are mentally retarded or in adolescents. This disorder can be serious, with a reported 25 percent mortality rate from malnutrition. Even when children with this disorder survive, the failure to gain expected weight and malnutrition may lead to general developmental delays and severe impairment.

This disorder is marked by repeated regurgitation of food, with resultant weight loss or failure to gain expected weight (see the display on diagnostic criteria for rumination disor-

der of infancy). It develops following a period of normal functioning. There is no accompanying self-disgust, nausea, vomiting, or other associated gastrointestinal disorder. Ruminating infants typically regurgitate milk and partially digested food either spontaneously or after inserting their fingers into their mouth. They may chew and reswallow the regurgitated food, or they may vomit the food. The characteristic posture is described as straining and arching the back with the head held back.

Even though the infant seems to be satisfied, as evidenced by sucking movements and sounds, the parent or caretaker may avoid the infant. This avoidance behavior occurs either because of frustration or discouragement with failure to gain or because of the noxious odor of the regurgitated food. Thus there is a danger of disrupted bonding or understimulation. An additional feature is that the infant is often irritable and hungry between episodes of regurgitation. There are no known predisposing factors.

Rumination disorder must be differentiated from other disorders that cause regurgitation, such as pyloric stenosis and infections of the gastrointestinal system. When the disorder occurs in adolescence, the behavior appears involuntary and may be related to a disturbance of esophageal motility. Some of these affected adolescents have a history of self-induced vomiting and a fear of becoming fat. They are able to achieve vomiting more and more easily over time, and then the disorder resembles rumination of infancy (*DSM-IV-TR*) (APA, 2000).

CO-OCCURRING PSYCHIATRIC AND MEDICAL CONDITIONS

Co-occurring psychiatric and medical conditions are commonly found in clients with eating disorders. Common concomitant psychiatric conditions associated with eating disorders include anxiety disorders, substance-use disorder, and mood and personality disorders. Clinical implications for psychiatric nurses are the high relapse rate, chronic course, and poor response to treatment when co-occurring disorders

TABLE 22–2
Mental Status Examination and Co-occurring Psychiatric Conditions with Eating Disorders

Mental Status Examination	Variable affective range cheerful and hyperactive to hypomanic
	Sad and hypoactive to depressed; generally, affect restricted
	Limited capacity for self-observation, insight, psychological mindedness
	Resistance to treatment and denial of disorder
	Body image disturbance: cognitive distortion that client is fat in spite of emaciation
	All or nothing thinking: "If I am not perfect I am a complete failure"
	Faulty perception of inner sensations: unable to identify inner sensations of hunger with constant thoughts of food
	Sense of personal ineffectiveness
Personality Characteristics	Obsessional traits, insecurity, minimization of emotional expression, perfectionism, excessive conformance, rigid impulses control, highly industrious, competitiveness, enviousness, and responsible
Co-occurring Disorders	Depressive disorders
	Anxiety disorders, including dissociative disorders
	Substance abuse
	Obsessive-compulsive disorder
	Personality disorders: commonly avoidant, schizoid, borderline, narcissistic
	Psychosis
	Trauma history
	Impulse control disorders: shoplifting, compulsive shopping, and spending

Note. From *Practice Guidelines for the Treatment of Patients with Eating Disorders* (2nd ed., Compendium 2000, pp. 627–697), by the American Psychiatric Association, 2000, Washington, DC: Author; and Steiger, H., Gauvin, L., Israel, M., Kin, N. M., et al. (2004). Serotonin function, personality-trait variations, and childhood abuse in women with bulimia. *Journal of Clinical Psychiatry, 65,* 830–837.

exist in the client with an eating disorder. See Table 22–2, Mental Status Examination and Co-occurring Psychiatric Conditions with Eating Disorders.

MAJOR DEPRESSIVE DISORDERS

Several family and twin studies demonstrated the high co-occurring EDs and major depressive disorders. Estimates demon-strate that familial risk factors for depression in clients with eating disorders is highly prevalent (Fernandez-Aranda et al., 2007; Spindler & Milos, 2007). Despite the co-occurrence of eating disorders and major depression, most researchers assert that they are two distinct disorders.

ANXIETY DISORDERS

Research indicates that the prevalence of anxiety disorders in general and OCD in particular was much higher in people with anorexia nervosa and bulimia nervosa than in a nonclinical group of women in the community. Anxiety disorders commonly had their onset in childhood before the onset of an eating disorder, supporting the possibility that they are a vulnerability factor for developing anorexia nervosa or bulimia nervosa (Kaye, Bulik, Thornton, Barbarich, & Masters, 2004; Spindler & Milos 2007).

SUBSTANCE ABUSE

The co-occurrence of substance-use disorders and eating disorders is widely documented and associated with poor treatment response, suicide risk, and chronicity (Conason, Brunstein, Klomek, & Sher, 2006; Conason & Sher, 2006). Brewerton (1995) reviewed the relationship of serotonin (5-HT) in the development of alcoholism and other addictions and looked at a unified theory of 5-HT dysregulation to eating and other disorders. The relationship of problems of impulsive control leads the client with bulimia to experience the uncontrolled eating as more ego dystonic than the client with anorexia and more likely to seek help. See Chapter 21 for a review of substance abuse disorders.

BORDERLINE PERSONALITY DISORDER

The client with a coexisting personality disorder and ED presents unique challenges for nurses and therapists. Clients with personality disorders and EDs can be considered aggressive toward others and toward themselves. They share characteristics of impulsivity, self-mutilation, and disinhibition. They may evidence frequent suicide attempts, drug and alcohol use, and angry behavior, and the health care team may be challenged by the manipulative or immature qualities evidenced in behaviors (Franko & Keel, 2006). This is consistent with a 5-HT deficiency theory. See Chapter 15 for an in-depth discussion of personality disorders.

CHILDHOOD TRAUMA

Much has been written about trauma, and sexual abuse in particular, in the development of eating disorders. Individuals with eating disorders are more likely to have trauma histories than those without. However, among individuals with AN and BN, only a minority have such histories. The occurrence of childhood trauma increases one's chances of developing many emotional and behavioral problems. Such trauma is more properly viewed as a nonspecific risk factor for a range of problems later in life (Walsh & Cameron, 2005).

CAUSES OF EATING DISORDERS: THEORIES AND PERSPECTIVES

The complexity of EDs challenges psychiatric nurses to have some basic understanding of causative factors. There are three distinct theories about the cause of EDs. They are derived from biological, psychodynamic, and psychosocial perspectives.

BIOLOGICAL FACTORS

The most common ED is bulimia nervosa in women who maintain normal weight. These women exhibit symptoms usually found in women with AN, such as disturbed appetite, abnormal body image, depression, and neuroendocrine changes that precipitate menstrual irregularities. However, because these women are of normal weight, the changes cannot be attributed to weight loss.

Brewerton's extensive research (1995) postulates a unified theory of 5-HT dysregulation in clients with eating and related disorders. Clients with ED exhibit several clinical features and biologic findings indicative of 5-HT dysregulation as well as a failure of neurotransmitter regulation, rather than a simple increase or decrease in activity. These include feeding disturbances, depression and suicidal behavior, impulsivity and violence, anxiety and harm avoidance, obsessive-compulsive features, substance abuse, seasonal variation of symptoms,

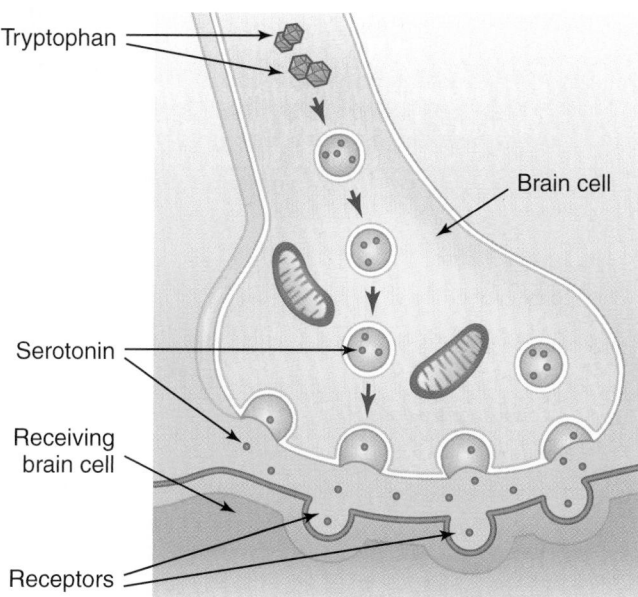

Figure 22–1 Serotonin dysregulation in eating disorders.

disturbances in neuroendocrine and vascular tissues, and neurochemical systems linked to 5-HT such as temperature. Research review supports a 5-HT dysregulation hypothesis and that a variety of psychobiological stressors, such as dieting, binge eating, purging, drug abuse, photoperiodic changes, as well as psychosocial-interpersonal stress, perturb a vulnerable 5-HT system (see Figure 22–1). The interaction with a variety of psychobiological stressors perturbs the vulnerable 5-HT system, leading to further dysregulation. Review Chapter 3 to help understand the Behavioral-Biological Interface to give further understanding for Brewerton's theory of 5-HT dysregulation hypotheses. See Table 22–3 for the interaction of stressors with vulnerable 5-HT system. Twin studies implicate the heritability of eating disorders. Several studies indicate that biological and psychosocial changes during adolescence heighten the risk of eating disorders in vulnerable youth (Klump, Perkins, Alexandra Burt, McGue, & Iacono, 2007). Psychiatric nurses are poised to identify risks associated with eating disorders and work with clients, families, and interdisciplinary teams to develop holistic treatment plans.

PSYCHODYNAMIC FACTORS

Body image disturbance is an essential characteristic of AN. Although it is related to a more generalized misperception of internal states, such as hunger and emotions, it specifically involves the inability of the client with anorexia to identify her appearance as abnormal. This misperception can be extremely dangerous because it can become almost delusional as the client with anorexia defends an emaciated body shape.

In the psychoanalytical framework, EDs are viewed as a form of neurosis representing a regression to the oral stages of development. Just as Freud connected oral drives and sexual drives, Bruch (1973) expounded on his connection when she addressed the abhorrence of the client with anorexia to her own sexuality.

TABLE 22–3
5-HT Dysregulation Hypotheses of Eating Disorders: Interaction of Stressors with Vulnerable 5-HT System

- Dieting; fasting
- Binge eating
- Purging; dehydration
- Compulsive exercising
- Alcohol and drug use
- Photoperiodic changes
- ED clients exhibit disturbances in other neurochemical systems linked to 5-HT, including:
  - Hypothalmic-Pituitary Adrenal (HPA) axis
  - Noradrenergic system
  - Dopaminergic
  - Isatin, an endogenous MAO-like compound
  - Neuropeptides, e.g., ß-endorphin, dynorphin, cholecystokinin, neuropeptide Y and YY, galanine, arginine, vasopressin
  - Leptin

5-HT, serotonin. MAO, monoamine oxidase.

Note. From *Serotonin Dysregulation in the Eating Disorder Adolescent*, by T. D. Brewerton, 1997, paper presented at Eating Disorders at AACAP, Toronto, Ontario, Canada.

PSYCHOSOCIAL FACTORS

Psychosocial factors associated with eating disorders often mediate various biological and genetic factors. Because of the high co-existence with other psychiatric disorders, it is highly likely that various psychosocial factors, such as chaotic or dysfunctional family dynamics, culture, deprivation, and trauma play are linked to eating disorders.

Familial Factors

The genesis of EDs may be viewed from a family systems theory framework. Ideally, the family is to provide a child with the nurturance and opportunities needed to develop as an individual. This is done through parental guidance and promotion of the autonomy needed in adult life. Family systems theorists view the family interactions of the family system in which there is a member with anorexia or bulimia as discouraging the development of independence and autonomy. This results in a self-perception of powerlessness and helplessness on the part of the child. This theory views a pattern of unconscious collusion where the family "agrees" to divert the conflict onto the symptomatic family member (Minuchin, Rosman, & Baker, 1978).

In the 1950s, with the emphasis on psychoanalytic theory, it was believed that particular patterns of family interaction, especially early in life, were causative factors in the development of eating disorders. Investigators today are more cautious about ascribing the risk of EDs to the family environment. There is often dysfunction in the family when a child has anorexia nervosa or bulimia nervosa. It is difficult to know whether such problems have any role in the development of the disorder or whether they are manifestations of distress about an ill child in an otherwise normally functioning family (Walsh & Cameron, 2005).

SOCIOCULTURAL FACTORS

Obviously, we live in a diet-conscious society in which thinness is viewed as attractive and healthy. Images and messages, both blatant and subtle, bombard young girls and women, promoting thinness, dieting, and weight loss as attractive and associated with sex appeal and achievement. The phenomenon of EDs has been described mainly in Western culture, where there is an extreme idealization of thinness.

It has been thought in the past that certain sociocultural groups, specifically white females, were at highest risk for these disorders; however, current clinical practice indicates that the most assimilated minority cultures are at as great risk as white females. This incorrect perception, that EDs are mainly a disease of white females, has led to a general lack of awareness among clinicians and subsequent failure to diagnose disturbed eating behaviors in minority clients. African American women report laxative and diuretic abuses as well as fasting behaviors to avoid weight gain. Research indicates that younger, more educated, and perfection-seeking African American women were most at risk for succumbing to these disorders. There are similarities as well as important differences between Caucasian and African American women with BED. Among Latinos, EDs are also directly related to acculturation (Alegria et al., 2007). Models, actresses, and others in the entertainment industry have a high frequency of EDs. Gymnasts and ballet dancers are at extremely high risk. These assumptions about the incidence of EDs across cultures are supported by cross-cultural studies. Data from repeated cross-cultural studies show that EDs are prevalent worldwide (Alegria et al., 2007; Jackson & Chen, 2007).

In addition, there is tremendous pressure on women today to achieve in separate arenas simultaneously. They must be successful, independent, and competitive professionally while competently maintaining their traditional role as wife, mother, and homemaker. The stressors inherent in this situation may be overwhelming to those women who may be predisposed to EDs.

Although numerous theories about EDs exist, none can explain the current increase in their incidence.

PERSONALITY FACTORS

Clients with AN are described by clinicians as having specific personality characteristics, as shown in Table 22–4.

TABLE 22–4
Personality Factors

Anorexia Nervosa (AN)

- Resistance to acknowledging they have a problem
- Obsessional thoughts about doing things right
- Hyper-rigid behaviors
- Difficulty learning from experience
- Greater risk avoidance (compared to controls)
- Emotionally restrained
- Conformity to authority
- Trait obsessionality
- Inflexible thinking
- Social introversion
- Limited social spontaneity

Bulimia Nervosa (BN)

- Problems identifying internal states contributing to feelings of helplessness (self-regulation)
- Variable moods: fatigue and depression to agitation, which contribute to impulse control difficulties
- Sense of loss of control related to bodily experience (probably related to early experiences with abuse/trauma); children of alcoholic parents
- Low self-esteem, personal efficacy, leading to self-doubt and uncertainty
- Highly self-critical and punitive in self-evaluation
- Self-conscious, sensitive to rejection from others

INTIMACY AND MARITAL ISSUES

Issues of disturbance in sexuality and intimacy have been associated with EDs. The early experiences of sexual and physical abuse may affect the libido, and the association with mood disorders may decrease the libido. Persons who restrict food intake appear to have decreased libido and be less interested in sex, whereas those who binge or binge and purge seem to have more frequent sexual activity and interest. The latter is sometimes interpreted as part of the larger issue of impulse control, but it may also be caused by age differences. Anorexia has been interpreted psychologically as a fear of sexuality or an attempt to delay or prevent sexual development and menses. The person with ED with obesity also experiences a fear of intimacy and may use food as a substitute. Food is more dependable and does not evoke issues of trust and vulnerability that emerge in relationships, including marriage. Most clients with ED experience shame and disgust with their bodies, whether they are obese, of normal weight, or very thin. These feelings obviously interfere with any enjoyment or pleasure in physical touching or joining.

Additional intimacy issues include hiding or not showing their bodies to partners or spouses and projecting feelings of disgust when looked at or touched. Some obese women have reported much anxiety when dieting in the context of becoming more attractive and thus sexually appealing. It would appear that the ED syndrome might provide comfort, safety, and anxiety reduction when the client is presented with the fears and conflicts of intimacy.

POPULATIONS AT RISK

Persons in occupations that stress appearance and weight management as a mark of achievement, such as models, ballet dancers, and gymnasts, are at high risk. Although women are at highest risk, subgroups of men include athletes (runners, wrestlers) and homosexuals (Baum, 2006; Feldman & Meyer, 2007). Risk factors include behavioral and attitudinal factors connected to developmental issues such as excessive weight concerns and dieting. Peer pressure, including teasing and low self-confidence, is a risk factor, as well as worry about size, and family history of eating or affective disorders (which may support the biological determinants of the disorder as well as the familial determinants), in conjunction with social and peer factors. Recognition of the patterns and risk factors of ED is crucial for early identification and school and parental education about these serious comorbid disorders. Nurses are in pivotal positions to provide health education and primary prevention in vast practice settings.

EATING DISORDERS ACROSS THE LIFE SPAN

Because of the unique biological and life-threatening challenges presented by the client with an ED, special circumstances must be considered in the treatment plan based on the development needs of the client. The pediatric specialist, child and adolescent psychiatrist, and child and adolescent advanced-practice registered nurse must be consulted in developing treatment strategies for this population.

See Table 22–5 for an overview of when specific EDs occur in relation to the life stage.

EARLY CHILDHOOD

The young child with an ED is one who is in a prepubertal stage of development and is considered to be preadolescent—classic *DSM* criteria may not be applicable. However, *DSM-IV-TR* now addresses feeding disorders that occur in childhood before the age of 6 years (see the box on diagnostic criteria for feeding disorder of infancy or early childhood). For instance, a child does not have to lose the percentage of weight appropriate for an adult with an ED. Prepubertal children have a lower percentage of body fat. A child who is thin at the start of the weight loss process may reach an unhealthy state quickly. In addition, children tend to eliminate fluids, including water,

TABLE 22–5
Occurrence of Eating Disorders Throughout the Life Span

	Anorexia	Bulimia	Obesity	Rumination Disorder	Pica	Binge Eating Disorder
Infant (Birth–1 yr)				X		
Toddler (2–5 yr)			X		X	
Early School Age (6–9 yr)			X			
Late School Age (10–12 yr)	X		X			
Adolescence (13–18 yr)	X	X	X			X
Adulthood (18 yr +)	X	X	X			X

as well as food. It is helpful to continually plot out the child's progression on the growth chart, accounting for both height and weight. This important tool quickly demonstrates developmentally inappropriate positions on the chart that need specific attention. In addition, both boys and girls present with infantile or childhood anorexia, whereas bulimia is extremely unusual. Symptoms of depression are also usually present and need to be addressed.

Within the psychotherapeutic process, developmental theory continues to be of great importance. Infants or younger children are still very involved in the family and may react strongly to changes within the household and stressful family events. The infant who refuses food or fails to thrive is a medical and life-threatening emergency. Failure to successfully deal with this issue may be caused by a genuine medical problem, such as esophageal atresia, or maternal retardation, depression, or lack of information. Immediate and accurate assessment must be done quickly before permanent damage occurs. A major component of treatment should be family education and individual treatment for the caregiver as well as family therapy. A child protective services referral, with a service plan instituted for the family, may need to be instituted. Individual therapy for the child, depending on age, may also prove helpful. Issues in attachment problems usually refer to loss and unresolved grief with the caregiver's own family of origin, for example, the mother who could not respond to the needs of her infant had not recieved appropriate nurturing herself. Mothers with substance-use disorders have been unable to respond emotionally to their infants' needs, and these babies are at risk for the development of attachment problems and failure to thrive.

DSM-IV-TR Diagnostic Criteria for Feeding Disorder of Infancy or Early Childhood

A. Feeding disturbance as manifested by persistent failure to eat adequately with significant failure to gain weight or significant loss of weight over at least 1 month.

B. The disturbance is not due to an associated gastrointestinal or other general medical condition (e.g., esophageal reflux).

C. The disturbance is not better accounted for by another mental disorder (e.g., Rumination Disorder) or by lack of available food.

D. The onset is before age 6 years.

ADOLESCENCE

The clinical picture presented by the adolescent also needs to be considered within a developmental framework. Central to the ED are those issues relative to puberty, such as increased independence from the family and increased autonomy in problem solving; family and peer pressures, including sexuality; and initiation in the process of major life choices.

The issue of sexuality is noteworthy because clients with anorexia tend to have difficulty with interpersonal intimacy and closeness. Both groups of clients with anorexia and bulimia may reveal a history of childhood sexual trauma, which would have implications for future sexual relationships. The adolescent with an ED will benefit from a variety of therapies, including individual, family, and group work (see Chapters 27 and 28 regarding adolescent, group, and family therapy).

ADULTHOOD: SPECIAL POPULATIONS

Most studies demonstrate that college women have higher rates of eating disorders than other age groups and gender. Despite this evidence, there are special populations with eating disorders, including young men.

The Adult Male

EDs typically present in the male with the same core psychopathological features as in the female; however, there are some unique features. Eating disorders in men appear to be more prevalent in the community than had previously been thought (Goldfield, Blouin, & Woodside, 2006; Hudson et al., 2007). According to contemporary researchers, men and women share similar motivation to engage in eating disorders, but men have fewer psychosocial issues. They tend to focus less on perfectionism and self-destructive behaviors than women and have fewer co-occurring psychiatric conditions than women. Woodside and colleagues (2004) also noted that 10 percent of men with eating disorders report a history of sexual abuse. Males usually share a history of involvement with sports such as wrestling before developing the ED. In addition, males tend to exhibit more sexual anxiety related to issues of homosexuality and bisexuality. A variation of extreme body awareness seems to be occurring among young men who do not meet the "idealized" masculine image of hypermuscularity promoted by the media.

The Client with Diabetes

The prevalence of EDs among the population with diabetes is unknown, yet the lethality possible in this combination cannot be overemphasized. Food is an integral component of the diabetic regimen. Researchers believe that diabetes may predispose one to the development of an ED, because a person can attempt to control weight by manipulating an insulin dosage (Colton, Olmsted, Daneman, Rydall, & Rodin, 2007). Recent research on diabetic women indicates that for those who meet criteria for eating disorders, overall outcome was poor; serious microvascular complications were common and mortality was high. There were significant relationships between disordered eating habits, insulin misuse, and microvascular complications (Peveler et al., 2005). Many women with diabetes equate insulin usage with weight gain and therefore reduce their insulin dosage to decrease their weight. This method results in glycosuria and the life-threatening consequence of diabetic ketoacidosis (DKA). An ED should be suspected in a female with diabetes who presents with a history of multiple incidents of DKA and unexplainable difficulties in the regulation of blood glucose levels. This situation becomes even more complex in an adolescent who is confronting developmental issues in addition to those related to the chronic nature of diabetes. The registered nurse may plan to monitor the results of the glyco-

sylated hemoglobin tests. This blood test monitors the glucose levels of the client with diabetes over the past 3 months. The normal values for this test range from 4 to 8 percent, so a result between 12 and 20 percent would indicate uncontrolled blood glucose levels. In other words, if a client with diabetes claims to have had normal blood glucose levels at home, a glycosylated hemoglobin test will validate or invalidate this claim. Most important, appropriate control of the diabetes must be the first goal of treatment.

TREATMENT MODALITIES FOR EATING DISORDERS

The complexities of eating disorders and their life threatening potential require an interdisciplinary, comprehensive, and holistic treatment plan. The role of the psychiatric nurse is crucial to identifying high-risk groups along with other health care providers who work to facilitate healthy nutrition and physical stability. The following section focuses on the importance of the interdisciplinary team approach in working with clients with eating disorders.

THE INTERDISCIPLINARY APPROACH

The care of the person with an ED is complex and multifaceted. The optimal form of treatment is via the team approach. This method helps diffuse the heavy burden of dealing with these clients and their families. The ability to share the responsibilities with others helps each professional maintain perspective because working with these clients is quite challenging. Essential members of the team include a family physician or pediatrician, a psychotherapist from one of the designated mental health professions, a dietician, a consulting psychologist to administer standardized tests, and a consulting psychiatrist to assess the need for psychotropic medication. During inpatient hospitalization, the nursing staff plays an integral role in the care also. See the section on the nurse's role later in this chapter.

Clients receiving treatment for an ED can be extremely manipulative and may try to "split" the professionals on the team. It is essential that team members communicate and firmly abide by the boundaries of their particular role; otherwise, the goals of treatment may be sabotaged. A major function of the team is to provide support, clarification, and feedback to the mental health professional acting in the role of primary therapist. Team conferences may be held frequently and regularly to optimally aid the client and family being treated. Changes in reimbursement for inpatient treatment have resulted in the development of intensive outpatient programs (IOPs) for ED treatment.

PSYCHOTHERAPY

The use of psychotherapy in treatment may take more than one form—many clients benefit from a combination. For instance, a 15-year-old client with AN may find both individual and family work necessary for recovery. A 30-year-old client with BN may need both individual and marital therapy. Many clients with EDs, especially bulimia, seem to benefit from group work. It is essential that the group therapist have advanced preparation in group leadership skills as well as in ED treatment because of the issues mentioned previously. The primary goal of any therapeutic relationship is the establishment of trust (see Chapters 6 and 26). The issue of confidentiality should be addressed early in therapy. However, any indication of an issue involving self-harm (or maltreatment in the case of a child) needs to be addressed with family members. This should be explicitly shared with the identified client, and the family, if appropriate.

Individual Psychotherapy

In today's cost-conscious mental health environment, newer forms of treatment have emerged, which aim at decreasing symptoms while enhancing personal efficacy and responsibility for self in conjunction with using medication evaluation and management. Solution-focused approaches have shown a degree of success over older, traditional forms of psychotherapy. Cognitive behavioral treatment emphasizes changing old patterns that maintain the illness. Emphasizing change instead of illness is especially important with clients with ED for two reasons:

1. Because the client with ED experiences low self-esteem, which is a factor in developing and maintaining the disorder
2. The tendency for the client with ED to engage in all-or-nothing thinking in which they view themselves as all good or all bad, and discount any progress that is not absolutely perfect

Another behavioral approach to EDs, particularly when they are comorbid with borderline personality disorder, is dialectical behavior therapy (DBT) (Linehan et al., 2006). Studies show that DBT reduced relapse in clients with BN and other EDs. Major behavioral changes and benefits involved enhanced coping skills, modulation of distress and emotions, and a decrease in binge-purge behaviors.

Solution-focused approaches emphasize progress and look at small changes as evidence of even greater possibilities in the future. The emphasis in solution-focused approaches is on increasing the client's perceptions of personal capabilities and resources. Instead of focusing on past mistakes, the emphasis is on future possibilities and empowering the client by strengthening resources and skill building to achieve the goals mutually set.

Halmi (1997) developed an outpatient treatment protocol using cognitive-behavioral therapies and psychopharmacologic treatments. The core assumptions about anorexia used by the treatment team is that AN is essentially a food phobia and that AN serves a positive function in providing escape from aversive developmental issues and distressing life events. Thus, the prospect of relinquishing the disorder is highly frightening to the client. This approach involves a treatment plan that identifies problems and client-generated solutions. The client identifies and selects coping strategies, defines steps for coping, carries out the strategy, and evaluates the process. The goal is to overcome the food phobia, restore weight, and restructure the cognitive operations. This takes place for approximately 37 sessions over a 12-month period with more intensity initially, then tapered in an intensive outpatient format. See Chapter 26 for an in-depth discussion of individual psychotherapy. Cognitive-behavior therapy has been found more effective than nutritional counseling after 1 year posthospitalization in relapse prevention of AN (Pike et al., 2003).

Family Therapy

All the issues discussed earlier also need to be addressed within family therapy if the client lives with her parents and is under age 18. However, the family usually defines the problem in the context of eating behaviors and weight (Dare & Eisler, 1997). They believe that if the client gives up these behaviors, then any remaining problems would be solved. This misconception will need further clarification because the family will need insight into the working of the family as a system. They need to see how the person with ED has contributed to the functioning of the family system. Some family members become extremely angry and upset when the therapist suggests that everyone needs to work on changes, not just the person with ED. Conflicts and disagreements need to be openly acknowledged and compromises need to be worked out. This open acknowledgment of conflict and problems can be threatening to these families, because the image of perfection may be extremely important to them. Transgenerational family therapy moves beyond present issues to exceed symptomatic relief and emphasizes restoring familial resources for growth and strength to cope with future stress. The family of origin consultation may be used to elicit multiple perspectives on the problem. Transgenerational issues involve using a genogram to create a "map" of the structure and interrelationships over generations, while providing an analysis of the family structure, life cycle, and multigenerational patterns over at least three generations (Dare & Eisler, 1997; Roberto 1986, 1992). Family therapy may be used to educate members about the disorder, support the family as they deal with guilt and stigma about having a member with the disorder, and focus on fostering open, healthy interaction patterns (Eisler, Simie, Russell, & Dare, 2007). Family therapy issues are covered in Chapter 28.

Marital Therapy

Sometimes within the context of individual therapy, the need for marital therapy will be uncovered. This may occur with an adult client attempting to deal with relationship issues in her own marriage. Leadership, power, autonomy, and decision-making issues may need further exploration within the privacy of marital sessions. A transgenerational focus may also be used in assisting each member of the marital dyad to recognize how each brings unresolved issues from their parents' marriages to their marriage. Marital therapy may focus on the messages or pressure that the spouse may be projecting onto the ED partner to maintain a certain weight and appearance, while at the same time denying the existence of a life-threatening ED. From a transgenerational perspective, it can be said that marital therapists really are dealing with multiple couples in the therapy room: the presenting couple, each one of the couples' parental marriages (and their grandparents), the therapist's marriage, as well as the therapist's family of origin (see Chapter 28).

Group Therapy

Group work can be an effective tool in the treatment of clients with an ED. Clients with bulimia especially seem to benefit from the support of a group. Clients with anorexia may have difficulty with the group setting because it may be too threatening to speak so openly about relevant issues. The client with anorexia is usually less skilled socially than the client with bulimia and may fear the intimacy created by the group situation. The group leaders must be aware of the potential for competition in the group. For instance, the members with anorexia may begin to compete with each other in weight loss to see who can be the thinnest. The groups need the supervision of highly skilled professionals who are knowledgeable about group dynamics. The advanced-practice nurse can be an effective member of the team in providing care for this population. Chapter 27 provides a comprehensive discussion of group therapy principle.

PHARMACOTHERAPY

Assessment of the need for medication includes:

1. establishing differential diagnosis
2. implementing a complete medical and psychological evaluation
3. systematically reviewing weight, dieting, purging and nonpurging compensatory behaviors
4. assessing comorbid psychiatric illness
5. screening for suicide risk
6. prior and current response to psychotherapy
7. capacity to be compliant with medication management.

Pharmacolgic treatment is highly individualized and specific to co-occurring disorders and stage of illness. It is offered in the context of psychotherapy and medical monitoring. Data is limited on medication for EDs in children and adolescents.

Anorexia Nervosa

No specific medication has been shown to be generally clinically useful for the primary symptoms of AN, although other agents (antidepressants, anxiolytics) may be helpful in treating comorbidities. Becker (2005) reports possible benefits with risperidone and olanzapine in promoting weight gain as well as improvement in insight and pre-meal compliance. Citalopram may be useful in improving associated depression and obsessional thinking. Transdermal testosterone improved depression and spatial cognition in depressed patients with AN and testosterone deficiency (Miller et al., 2005).

Fluoxetine (Prozac) has been shown to reduce the obsessive-compulsive behavior, anxiety, and depression seen in classic anorexia symptoms, carbohydrate craving, and other pathologic eating behaviors. Mirtazapine, an atypical antidepressant, because of its well-known tendency to quickly add weight, shows promise as a medicine that may be helpful for anorectics whose health status is severely compromised. However, any weight-promoting medication should be used judiciously and with full informed consent of the patient. Patients with AN should have calcium supplementation of 1000 to 1500 mg daily and a multivitamin containing 400 to 800 IU of vitamin D daily.

Bulimia Nervosa

Numerous studies have demonstrated short-term moderate efficacy of multiple agents in symptom reduction, however remission rates are low and relapse high. The best established medication is fluoxetine (60 mg/d). It is the only agent to have received FDA approval for bulimia treatment. Medications with unacceptable risk include bupropion due to seizure risk and is **not** recommended for bulimic patients. Monoamine oxidase inhibitors (MAOIs) pose a greater risk of hypertensive reactions among bulimic patients due to dietary indiscretion and diet pill use. There have been no studies on medication efficacy for EDNOS or children with eating disorders (Becker, 2005). Stahl (2000) in discussing the antibulimic profile of SSRIs generally states, "The usual starting dose is higher than for other indications, the onset of response may be faster than for other indications, it may not be as effective as for other indications in maintaining acute effects chronically, fluoxetine has the best efficacy data to date and also serotonin 2C ($5\text{-}HT_{2C}$) properties and the target symptoms do not worsen on initiation of treatment" (p. 233). Psychopharmacology is reviewed in Chapter 29.

MEDICAL CONSIDERATIONS

Ideally, an outpatient regimen is the method of choice when treating a person with an ED. After the initial evaluations with the EDs team, the client may carry on with usual daily activities. Concurrently, she meets regularly with the therapist, dietician, family physician, and psychiatrist as needed. In this way, progress is monitored closely, and any indication of need for hospitalization will be noted quickly and acted on accordingly. Seriously ill or emaciated clients may need to be hospitalized when seen for the first assessment on an outpatient basis. Involuntary commitment, to stave off further deterioration or possible death, may be initiated; however, the establishment of trust following the decision to ask for detention may be counterproductive. The financial considerations of a managed care climate must also be determined. Clients with anorexia are especially upset at the need for hospitalization because they may be in a state of profound denial. Most clients with bulimia acknowledge the maladaptive aspects of their eating behaviors but may still resist an inpatient stay. See Table 22–6, Physiological Assessment in Eating Disorders.

Medical Management

The medical management of the client with an ED is critically important. Along with the history, laboratory examination should augment the physical examination. Laboratory tests include determination of the following:

- Complete blood count with differential
- Renal function
- Thyroid function
- Electrolytes
- Blood glucose
- Trace minerals
- Cholesterol and triglycerides
- Hepatic profile
- Muscle enzymes
- Urinalysis may be used to detect the use of stimulants, laxatives, or diuretics. An electrocardiogram (ECG) may also be helpful.
- Drug/toxicology screen

The main goal of a medical admission is emergent medical stabilization. Correction of the body weight of the client with anorexia is of supreme importance. Liquid supplements or tube feedings may be employed along with intravenous fluids. Extreme care is needed to prevent fluid overload that may possibly result in congestive heart failure.

TABLE 22–6
Physiological Assessment in Eating Disorders

Anorexia

Clients with anorexia will present themselves as "fine," although that is a far cry from reality. There is often a history of lethargy or frenetic energy, or both.	*Gastrointestinal* symptoms, including gastric emptying, constipation, bloating, and abdominal pain are frequent.
	Cardiovascular symptoms such as bradycardia, orthostatic hypotension, mitral valve prolapse, and electrocardiographic (ECG) abnormalities.
	Endocrine abnormalities include amenorrhea, osteoporosis, hypothermia, elevated growth hormone levels, and changes in thyroid function. During fluid restriction there may be changes such as an increased blood urea nitrogen (BUN) level, decreased glomerular filtration rate, renal calculi, and edema.
	Dermatological abnormalities include hair loss, dry skin, and development of lanugo hair. Metabolic changes include trace mineral deficiencies (e.g., zinc), osteopenia, and increased plasma cholesterol and triglyceride levels. The client with anorexia may show signs of anemia, leukopenia, and thrombocytopenia.

Bulimia

Clients with bulimia also present a complex clinical picture.	*Gastrointestinal* symptoms include constipation, bloating, abdominal pain, and nausea owing to delayed gastric emptying. Chronic laxative abuse can result in the loss of normal peristalsis, and recurrent vomiting of stomach acid can result in esophagitis. Forceful vomiting can cause tears in the esophagus (Mallory-Weiss syndrome) and possible gastrointestinal bleeding—esophageal rupture is a life-threatening situation. Chronic vomiting causes salivary and parotid gland enlargement.
	Cardiovascular symptoms include dehydration, orthostatic hypotension, arrhythmias owing to electrolyte imbalance (e.g., potassium), bradycardia, myocardial changes related to ipecac poisoning, and possible congestive heart failure.
	Endocrine changes include irregular menses.
	Pulmonary complications usually take the form of aspiration pneumonia secondary to vomiting. Fluid and electrolyte imbalance is extremely serious and results in dehydration, hypokalemia, hypochloremia, metabolic acidosis and alkalosis, hypophosphatemia, hyponatremia, and hypocalcemia. Vomiting induced with the use of a finger produces calluses and abrasions on the fingers and knuckles. The teeth are eroded by stomach acid, and there may be increased dental caries.
	Renal symptoms such as an elevated BUN level is usually noted owing to fluid restriction and loss. Another renal symptom includes a reduced glomerular filtration rate. There may be polydipsia and polyuria.

In the client with bulimia, the focus may be on the interruption of the binge-purge cycle and the associated abuse of laxatives, diuretics, and ipecac. The abrupt cessation of laxatives results in constipation, whereas the discontinuation of diuretics may result in reflex edema. The constipation may be handled through the use of roughage intake, exercise, and hydration. The normalization of fluid imbalance will usually occur spontaneously.

Nutritional Management

During hospitalization, the dietician plays a major role in the rehabilitation process. Using a nonjudgmental approach enables the dietician to provide support and establish rapport. The dietician supplies nutritional education, helps the client explore extreme misperceptions and use of food, and recommends realistic goals to the client and the treatment team. The dietician attempts to reestablish regular eating patterns with the client. Dieticians use the BMI as a measure of nutritional status (Table 22–7).

Inpatient Management

Overall, weight restoration is a central goal during the hospitalization of the client with anorexia. A behavioral management program may be employed using both positive and negative reinforcements, and this may influence the rate at which the client with anorexia progresses. Lenient behavioral plans may be as effective as the strict programs because they enlist the client's cooperation and increase the sense of control and autonomy. A drawback of the strict behavioral regimen is that conflict may develop between the client and the staff over "control" of the client. This may be a reproduction of the power struggle already occurring at home for the

adolescent client who is rebelling against his parents. The behavioral plan must be carefully delineated by the involved professionals and clearly understood by everyone involved. Even then, misunderstandings between the client and the staff occur over the parameters of the plan. Clear limits need to be established with the client.

The following are nursing interventions that are used during the hospitalization of a client with anorexia or bulimia.

1. Implement behavioral protocol for gradual weight gain.
2. Supervise meals to ensure adequate intake of nutrients.
3. In collaboration with the dietician, determine the number of calories required to provide adequate nutrition and weight gain.
4. Remain with the client during mealtime for support and to observe amount ingested.
5. Strictly document intake and output.
6. Weigh client daily on arising.
7. Once the nutritional status is stable, explore with client feelings associated with fears.
8. Observe weighing activity to ensure that the client is not secreting weights to falsify data.

The length of hospital stay may vary, depending on factors such as physical acuity, resolution of emotional crises, and financial status. Some clients may require multiple hospitalizations for their ED, because this illness can take a course of chronicity. Recidivism after hospitalization is high, and hospitalization should be seen only as part of a lengthy course of treatment.

THE ROLE OF THE NURSE

Nursing care of clients with eating disorders requires an integration of physical and psychotherapeutic measures, which focus initially on proper nutrition and hydration and later on exploring the basis of these life-threatening disorders. Depending on the nurse's educational level and clinical expertise, major responsibilities may range from monitoring intake and output and food intake to psychotherapy that facilitates adaptive coping skills as well as medication management by those APRNs with prescriptive authority. Regardless of the role, major responsibilities include health maintenance, safety, and an optimal level of functioning.

THE GENERALIST NURSE

The treatment of a person with an ED is challenging for all involved, and considerable knowledge, skill, and energy are required. The ED team meets with the nursing staff to review treatment and facilitate clear communication among the members of the team. The primary nurse assumes responsibility for the care plan.

Generalist nurses have an important role to play because they enforce the therapeutic milieu of the unit. They must be

---

TABLE 22–7
How to Calculate Ideal Weight Using the Body Mass Index

Body mass index (BMI) is a measure of relative body weight, in which the weight in kilograms (2.2 pounds) is divided by the square of the height in meters (39.37 inches). For example,

$$\frac{\text{Weight (kg)}}{\text{Height (m)}^2} = \frac{35 \text{ kg}}{(1.54 \text{ m})^2} = \frac{35 \text{ kg}}{2.37 \text{ m}} = 14.76 \text{ BMI}$$

This is an example of a woman with anorexia who is approximately 5'1½" tall and weighs 77 lbs. A desirable BMI is in the range of 19 to 23. As can be seen, her BMI is far lower than would be expected for a healthy woman

Note. "Definition, Measurement and Classification of the Syndromes of Obesity," by G. A. Bray, 1978, *International Journal of Obesity, 2*, pp. 99–112.

empathic and supportive but clearly able to define boundaries and set appropriate limits with these clients. It is essential that the nursing staff is well versed in nutritional and physiological information relative to EDs in addition to having a solid background in medical nursing. There is commonly manipulation and "splitting" done by the client with an ED, and nurses must be aware of these dynamics even before they occur. Most generalist nurses are invaluable in their ability to establish trust within the therapeutic relationship. In order for the nurse-client relationship to be effective it must be empathic with unconditional positive regard and acceptance; the nurse must be warm and committed as well as nonjudgmental. Nurses need ongoing support and preparation in order to deal effectively with this population. Their conversations and exchanges with the client with ED may serve to strengthen and augment the relationship between the client and the primary psychotherapist.

In addition, it is essential that the nurse explore feelings about clients with EDs. These include the following: sharing society's obsession with thinness, revulsion at the binge-purge behavior, and envy of the client (especially one who is "model thin"). The nurse with eating or weight problems must be prepared to deal with his own issues relative to weight through supervision or therapy when working on an ED unit in order to be able to deal with these issues in a nondefensive way. The slender nurse may have to deal with the ED client's anger or hostility. The generalist nurse also provides client teaching to the client with ED regarding medication actions, side effects, and encourages family support of medicine, as well as clears up misconceptions about medicine. The nurse provides physical assessment and implements the weight management program, while stressing to the client with ED that the primary concern is regaining health through better nutrition. Milieu issues are covered in Chapter 32. See the Family Health Education display that follows.

THE ADVANCED-PRACTICE PSYCHIATRIC REGISTERED NURSE

The advanced-practice registered nurse (APRN) may participate in a variety of roles. The APRN with prescriptive authority may provide medication management in an outpatient setting, either while providing psychotherapy or in conjunction with another psychotherapist. The advanced-practice nurse may participate as part of the specialized ED team as a primary psychotherapist. The APRN is also responsible for individual, family, marital, or group therapy. Additional responsibilities may include being the program director of an ED team, which involves coordination of services and consultation to facilitate restoration of health and an optimal level of functioning for clients with EDs. The APRN in private practice may see the client with an ED in short-term or long-term outpatient therapy. Outpatient mental health care also involves collaborative work with other members of the treatment team owing to the multisystem impairment and potentially life-threatening nature of this illness. Finally, the APRN may be a member of the research team studying EDs and their treatment. In general, the role of the nurse in the treatment of clients with EDs is governed by the practitioner's level of education and clinical expertise with the treatment of this special population. Assuming management of the treatment of clients with EDs requires advanced-practice clinical expertise, as well as those acquired through institutes, supervision, and continuing education.

THE NURSING PROCESS

Clients with EDs often present with complex psychopathology, physical symptoms, and maladaptive eating and coping behaviors. The nursing process is used to develop an individualized, holistic, comprehensive, continuous plan of care.

The following case study provides a useful framework in which the nursing process can be examined.

Psychosocial assessment begins with establishing a trusting relationship with the client and family members. Major components of the psychosocial assessment include identifying the client's reasons for seeking treatment, present and past history of impaired eating and coping patterns, family involvement, and the impact of family members on the client's well-being. A complete family assessment is a critical part of assessing clients with EDs. Assessing family interactions, communication

---

Family Health Education: Living with Someone with an Eating Disorder

The strain of stress of living with someone with an eating disorder generates tension for the family. Common feelings include:

- Confusion about the eating disorder and recovery process
- What caused it?
- How should I deal with it or approach my family member?
- Grief and anger
- Guilt or fear

The best way to approach the family member is:

- Express your concerns honestly and tactfully
- Be positive and open
- Let the person know that you are talking to her out of concern rather than criticism
- Offer health education (e.g., services, resources)
- Select a time when both are at ease to talk
- Anticipate the family member's intense emotional reaction (e.g., anger, denial, or relief)
- Encourage professional help
- Encourage the family member to see the positive aspects of life without an ED

patterns, conflict resolution, family developmental issues, personal boundaries, coping patterns, and management of stress are major aspects of this process. See Chapter 28 for a comprehensive review of family dynamic and therapy.

ASSESSMENT

Assessing the client with an ED is a multifaceted process that must include a review of the medical assessment and biological history of the client, review of the psychological evaluation, and a comprehensive psychosocial history of both the client and the family.

The client's medical condition must be assessed to determine the extent of nutritional deprivation and potential complications. A complete physical examination includes laboratory tests and cardiac evaluation.

Other aspects of the assessment process include the following:

◆ Mental status examination

◆ Substance abuse history

◆ Family and social history, including employment history

◆ Academic achievement and performance

◆ Present and past psychiatric and medical treatment

◆ Current and past medications; drug and other allergies

◆ Quality of support system and other resources

◆ Level of danger to self or others

◆ Individual and family strengths

◆ Current stressors

◆ Cultural and gender needs

NURSING DIAGNOSES

Major nursing diagnoses for clients with EDs include:

◆ Imbalanced Nutrition: Less than Body Requirements related to dysfunctional eating patterns

◆ Disturbed Body Image related to fear of weight gain

◆ Powerlessness related to lack of control over food avoidance

◆ Anxiety related to fear of weight gain as evidenced by rituals associated with food intake

◆ Constipation related to erratic eating patterns

◆ Decreased Cardiac Output related to inadequate caloric and fluid intake

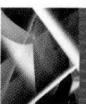

CASE STUDY

The Client with an Eating Disorder (Tiffany)

Tiffany Dale, a 15-year-old girl, was seen with her mother for an initial family interview in an eating disorders program for children and adolescents. This first meeting was conducted on an outpatient basis. Mrs. Dale expressed concern about her daughter's physical status. Tiffany is 5'4" tall and weighs 80 lb. She has lost 40 lb from her original weight of 120 lb over the last 8 months and she has experienced amenorrhea for the last 4 months.

Tiffany admitted to eating very little food, consisting mostly of raw green vegetables. She drinks only water and diet soda on a restricted basis. She admitted to using vomiting only when her mother forces her to eat. She denied any use of diuretics, laxatives, or ipecac, although she did complain of constipation. Tiffany has exercised every day for 2 hours but can no longer do this because she is too exhausted. Lanugo hair was evident on both her forearms, and her lips were dry and cracked. Tiffany wore layers of clothing and complained of constantly being cold. She kept her coat on throughout the interview. Her affect was flat, and she said little. She maintained minimal eye contact on interview. She was tearful at times. Answers given by Tiffany were slow and laborious in coming.

Family history revealed that Mr. and Mrs. Dale had divorced when Tiffany was 3 years old. She has two older sisters. Mrs. Dale stated that Mr. Dale had been physically abusive of her and their girls. She also questioned the possibility of sexual abuse of Tiffany by her father. Tiffany has always denied this. The family history was positive for depressive disorder and alcoholism on the paternal side. Tiffany admitted to long-standing insomnia, decreased concentration, and suicidal ideation. Tiffany continues to attend high school, where she maintains a 4.0 grade point average. Tiffany used to be active in school clubs, cheerleading, and dance. However, she has withdrawn from all extracurricular activities and stays home isolated in her room. She rarely spends time with friends.

Because of the findings revealed by the interview, Tiffany was hospitalized immediately in children's hospital on an adolescent medical unit. Her primary care physician was a pediatrician who consulted the eating disorders team, including the team's child psychiatrist. A complete physical examination was done and appropriate laboratory tests were ordered. These showed severe metabolic acidosis, hypophosphatemia, elevated cholesterol and low serum zinc levels, and anemia. There was bradycardia in the range of 45 to 49 beats per minute. An ECG was done, and Tiffany was placed on strict bed rest with a cardiorespiratory monitor. She was started on intravenous fluids, and a nasogastric tube was placed for feedings, which she resisted. The team dietician met with Tiffany and began to work on food-related issues. The APRN on the team was designated as primary therapist. The team psychiatrist recommended a trial dose of fluoxetine. A behavioral plan was instituted. The team psychologist later conducted a full psychological profile. The primary nurse worked closely with the eating disorders team and constructed a plan of care for Tiffany. See Nursing Care Plan 22–1.

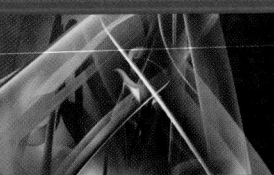

NURSING CARE PLAN 22–1

The Client with an Eating Disorder (Tiffany)

Nursing Diagnosis: Imbalanced Nutrition: Less than Body Requirements related to self-starvation

Outcome Identification	Nursing Actions	Rationales	Evaluation
1. By [date], Tiffany will verbalize increased understanding of appropriate nutritional needs.	1. Discuss fundamentals of health nutrition; i.e., basic four food groups and/or food pyramid.	1. Increased understanding of basic nutritional requirements may encourage more appropriate food intake.	Goal met: Tiffany expresses understanding of the need to eat more and increase food intake. Tiffany has fewer complaints of bloating and gas, and there is no sign of cardiac overload. Improvement is noted in phosphorus and carbon dioxide levels.
2. By [date], Tiffany will increase oral intake.	2a. Provide small frequent feedings.	2a. Small, frequent feedings limit stress on the gastrointestinal and cardiac systems.	
	2b. Monitor intake and output.	2b. Appropriate intake and output will ensure meeting of caloric requirements.	Tiffany's weight has increased.
3. By [date], Tiffany will show appropriate weight gain as specified by the team dietician.	3a. Monitor weight gain.	3a. Weight gain will validate appropriately met metabolic needs.	
	3b. Monitor the results of laboratory studies.	3b. Laboratory studies will indicate improvement in metabolism and fluid and electrolyte balance.	
4. By [date], Tiffany will cooperate with tube feeding regimen.	4. Educate the client and family concerning the rationale for tube feedings.	4. Client may be unable to meet caloric needs by oral intake. Tube feedings provide a caloric supplement.	

Nursing Diagnosis: Constipation related to erratic eating patterns

Outcome Identification	Nursing Actions	Rationales	Evaluation
1. By [date], Tiffany will have more frequent bowel movements.	1a. Provide small, frequent feedings.	1a. Small, frequent feedings will improve intake and limit stress on the gastrointestinal system.	*Goal met:* Tiffany exhibits more normal bowel habits.
	1b. Monitor bowel function.	1b. Regular assessment will indicate whether or not there is improvement in bowel function.	

(continues)

Nursing Diagnosis: Decreased Cardiac Output
related to inadequate caloric and fluid intake

Outcome Identification	Nursing Actions	Rationales	Evaluation
1. By [date], Tiffany will experience alleviation of bradycardia and increased normalization of pulse.	1a. Provide small, frequent feedings.	1a. Small, frequent feedings limit stress on the cardiovascular system.	*Goal met:* Tiffany shows improvement in cardiac status and increased metabolism. Laboratory results are improved. No sign of respiratory or cardiac distress.
	1b. Monitor vital signs. 1c. Use cardiorespiratory monitor.	1b. and c. Regular vital sign readings and use of monitor will help with assessment of pulse and cardiac status.	
2. By [date], Tiffany will avoid congestive heart failure during the refeeding process.	2a. Monitor serum electrolytes, urine specific gravity, and blood urea nitrogen.	2a. Regular assessment of laboratory studies will indicate improvement in cardiovascular system.	
	2b. Offer small amounts of fluid.	2b. Small amounts of fluid will prevent cardiac overload.	
	2c. Measure intake and output.	2c. Appropriate intake and output will ensure meeting of caloric requirements.	

Nursing Diagnosis: Ineffective Coping
related to feelings of lack of control, fears of growing up, and symptomatic response to family stress

Outcome Identification	Nursing Actions	Rationales	Evaluation
1. By [date], Tiffany will explore and identify feelings associated with perception of self.	1a. Encourage expression of feelings. 1b. Explore misperceptions between perceived and actual self.	1. These actions will contribute to increased self-awareness and realization of low self-esteem.	*Goal met:* Tiffany: Begins to express feelings, both positive and negative.
2. By [date], Tiffany will use viable options for coping with negative feelings and self-perceptions.	2a. Explore use of assertiveness techniques.	2a. Use of assertiveness technique enables client to express herself.	Begins to use assertiveness techniques in discussions with her mother.
	2b. Encourage realistic expectations of self.	2b. Encourages examination of perfectionism.	Expresses awareness of her own unrealistic expectations of self.
3. By [date], Tiffany will actively participate in social activities.	3. Encourage participation in unit activities.	3. Clients with anorexia tend to be socially isolated and have limited interpersonal skills.	Begins to go to the activity room on her own accord.
4. By [date], Tiffany will verbalize a more positive perception of self.	4. Encourage positive verbalization about self.	4. Clients with anorexia tend to have extremely low self-esteem.	Is able to verbally share her positive traits.

(continues)

Nursing Diagnosis: Compromised Family Coping
related to impaired interactions and ineffective management of stress

Outcome Identification	Nursing Actions	Rationales	Evaluation
1. By [date], Tiffany will improve patterns of family communication as family increases knowledge of underlying dynamics in anorexia nervosa.	1a. Develop a trusting relationship with family.	1a. Trust is the basis for therapeutic relationships.	*Goal met:* Tiffany and her family: Freely voice worries and concerns.
	1b. Assess patterns of family communication.	1b. Lack of family communication about health contributes to anorexia.	Begin to express perceptions and needs more clearly.
	1c. Assist family in the identification of inherent patterns of communication.	1c. Family may not be aware of ineffective patterns of communication; i.e., may need to learn more appropriate methods of conflict resolution.	Begin to implement more effective methods of conflict resolution. Begin to examine with therapist what changes in communication patterns need to occur.
	1d. Encourage expression of thoughts and feelings.	1d. Family may not encourage expression of conflicts or differences.	Agree to long-term plan of care.
	1e. Share information on the process of anorexia nervosa with the family.	1e. Increased knowledge will increase awareness of need to examine family communication patterns.	
2. By [date], Tiffany's family will be in agreement with extended therapeutic plan of care.	2. Assist family in the development of a long-term plan of care.	2. Family will need to continue treatment on an outpatient basis, as treatment is long term.	

◆ Ineffective Coping related to feelings of lack of control, fears of growing up, denial of the severity of the ED and symptomatic response to family stress

◆ Compromised Family Coping: Disabling related to impaired interactions, poor conflict resolution and ineffective management of stress

OUTCOME IDENTIFICATION

Expected outcomes include an increase in oral intake without binging or purging, appropriate weight gained and maintained (85 percent of expected body weight), and alleviation of the physical manifestations of food deprivation. Vital signs, blood pressure, and laboratory serum studies are within normal limits and the client verbalizes the importance of adequate nutrition. Expected psychosocial outcomes include an increase in the client's identification and expression of feelings, and recognition by the client of unrealistic self-expectations. Additional outcomes include the use of viable coping behaviors

to deal with negative self-perceptions, increased use of social support mechanisms, and improved communication patterns within the family.

PLANNING

Planning for and implementing a plan of care for clients with EDs is a detailed process that requires a multidisciplinary, comprehensive, and continuous approach. The health care team often includes an internist or pediatrician, the nursing staff, a dietician, a child psychiatrist, and an APRN.

Treatment planning and milieu interventions for clients with EDs require an interdisciplinary approach that integrates biological and psychotherapeutic interventions.

Milieu interventions for AN include:

◆ Weighing the client at specific intervals

◆ Providing for safety and physical needs

- Sitting with and observing during and 1 hour following meals
- Encouraging the client to share feelings with the staff
- Teaching relaxation techniques
- Discussing factors interfering with client's inability to eat
- Educating the client about the negative effects of dietary restriction and low weight and the rationale for maintaining a normal weight
- Monitoring and documenting intake and output
- Instructing the client on how to increase caloric intake and developing strategies for coping with anxiety associated with such eating behaviors
- Validating the client's fear of relinquishing anorexia and the challenges associated with behavioral changes

Milieu interventions for BN include:

- Behavioral diaries
- Encouraging the expression of feelings
- Reinforcing healthy coping
- Teaching recognition of cues for hunger and satiation
- Education about physical consequences of binging, self-induced vomiting, and laxative or stimulant abuse
- Limiting exercising
- Limiting food records, frequent weighing, obsessive calorie counting, cooking for others, reading recipes
- Providing nutritional consultation to the client
- Monitoring fluid and electrolyte status
- Teaching the client to reduce caloric anxiety with staff support and coaching
- Using reality-based statements and providing positive affirmations

Medical interventions depend on the extent of nutritional alterations. Major interventions focus on restoring fluid and caloric intake while monitoring for medical complications such as cardiac arrhythmia. Furthermore, close monitoring of laboratory studies, cardiac status, intake and output, and vital signs enables the health care team to assess responses to treatment.

Psychosocial interventions include solution-focused approaches, cognitive-behavioral interventions, assertiveness techniques and family therapy, as well as psychoeducational approaches. Cognitive-behavioral techniques increase self-awareness, including realization of low self-esteem and maladaptive coping patterns. Relapse prevention should include coping strategies, identifying triggers, developing support systems, distracting activities, contacting friends, and anticipating problem situations in advance. Assertiveness techniques encourage self-expression, improve interpersonal skills, and increase self-esteem. Family psychoeducational techniques facilitate improved communication patterns and increase knowledge of underlying family dynamics in AN and BN.

EVALUATION

The evaluation of client and family response to treatment is continuous and based on outcome identification. Outcomes for AN include stabilizing body weight without loss and being able to ingest food intake, whereas for BN the client will abstain from purging and will decrease time spent calculating calories and obsessing about appearance.

DIRECTIONS FOR FURTHER RESEARCH

The care of clients with EDs is extremely complex. More formal research is needed because the study of disturbed eating patterns is relatively recent. Collaboration of researchers from different disciplines is essential. The following are required:

- Continued development of sophisticated measurement tools
- Replication of previous studies using these newer tools
- Family studies
- Comparison of different psychotherapy techniques
- Longitudinal study of the long-term effects of EDs on health status
- Continued study of at-risk populations and identification of causative factors as well as focus on prevention
- Cross-cultural studies, which include Asian subgroups and Native Americans
- Psychopharmacologic intervention studies
- Continued study in the neurobiological area and other physiological implications of an ED

SUGGESTIONS FOR CLINICAL CONFERENCES

1. Discuss similarities between various eating disorders.
2. Discuss how nursing care of the client with AN differs from a client with BN.
3. Explore the possibility that cultural expectations support the continuation of ED.
4. Present case study of client with eating disorders and discuss your feelings and thoughts.

SUMMARY

- The client with an ED presents with complex symptoms and clinical findings.
- There are some similarities and symptom overlaps, which may make diagnosis confusing.
- There are distinct clinical differences that determine modifications in treatment approaches.
- Theories concerning possible causality encompass the neurobiological, psychological, family, and psychosocial perspectives.

An interdisciplinary team whose members focus on the medical, nursing, psychological, and nutritional needs of the client best manages treatment of the client with an ED.

A research agenda is essential, particularly in the area of prevention and treatment.

STUDY QUESTIONS

JP, a 15-year-old girl, has been admitted to a medical unit owing to complications from her out-of-control bulimia. She is 5 ft. 3 inches tall and weighs 122 pounds. She has a number of binge episodes each week and purges three times per day. When the nurse asks, JP admits to irregular "heartbeats" at times and menstrual periods. JP is tearful throughout the interview and admits to sporadic suicidal thoughts and chronic insomnia. She denies any history of suicidal gesture. The nurse is assessing JP's current physical status.

1. Which of the following would most likely be seen in a client with bulimia nervosa?
   a. Lanugo hair, amenorrhea
   b. Swollen parotid glands, callused knuckles
   c. Hepatomegaly
   d. Hair loss

2. Restoration of fluid and electrolyte balance is important to the care of the client with bulimia. Disturbances of which electrolyte is most responsible for the client's irregular pulse?
   a. Zinc
   b. Potassium
   c. Magnesium
   d. Chloride

3. In planning JP's comprehensive nursing care while she is in the hospital, which nursing diagnosis would assume initial priority?
   a. Chronic low self-esteem
   b. Nutrition imbalanced: Less than Body Requirements
   c. Deficit Fluid Volume
   d. Impaired Social Interaction

4. JP continues to say that she feels "bloated and fat." Which response by the nurse would be most appropriate?
   a. "You look just fine."
   b. "You're too thin."
   c. "You may perceive yourself as fat, but you are at a healthy weight for your height."
   d. "Why would you feel that way?"

5. Family therapy has been ordered while JP is in the hospital, with the hope that it will continue once she is discharged. The parents are "not sure" that they need to participate. What would be the most helpful response by the nurse in reference to the parents' ambivalence?
   a. "As parents, you need to understand how you helped to cause this."
   b. "You can't expect JP to handle this by herself."
   c. "You need to go because your physician has ordered the therapy."

d. "Participation in family sessions may help everyone understand how family relationships make an impact on JP's eating disorder."

6. A 16-year-old is hospitalized for treatment of anorexia nervosa. While admitting the client, the nurse discovers a bottle of pills that the client calls antacids. She takes them because her stomach hurts. The nurse's best initial response is which of the following?
   a. "Tell me more about your stomach pain."
   b. "These do not look like antacids. I need to get an order for you to have them."
   c. "Tell me more about your drug use."
   d. "Some girls take pills to help them lose weight."

7. All but which of the following are important nursing interventions for the client with an eating disorder?
   a. Monitoring vital signs
   b. Weighing the client 3 times per week at alternate times
   c. Checking to be sure the client has not water loaded or hidden heavy objects before being weighed
   d. Measuring intake and output

8. Which of the following behaviors may be indicative of an eating disorder?
   a. The client routinely goes to the bathroom shortly after eating.
   b. The client takes a nap shortly after a meal.
   c. The client exercises prior to a meal.
   d. The client complains of being overweight.

9. Mary is a 21-year-old administrative assistant who has recently been hospitalized due to excessive weight loss and electrolyte imbalance. During your assessment you notice she is preoccupied with being thin. Which of the following statements best describes additional features of anorexia nervosa?
   a. "I have always avoided sports."
   b. "I am cold all the time. Do you have an extra blanket?"
   c. "I know I am too thin."
   d. "I have always been last in my class."

10. A 21-year-old is admitted with a diagnosis of anorexia nervosa. Which of the following should the nurse include in her plan of care?
    a. Allow her as much time as she needs for each meal.
    b. Explain the importance of an adequate diet.
    c. Observe her during and one hour after each meal.
    d. Use a random pattern for surprise weights.

RESOURCES

Please note that because Internet resources are of a time-sensitive nature and URL addresses may change or be deleted, searches should also be conducted by association or topic.

Internet Resources

http://eating.ucdavis.edu   University of California, Davis website

http://overeatersanonymous.org   Overeaters Anonymous

http://www.healthyplace.com/communities/
Eating_Disorders   Healthy Place Web Tour: Eating
Disorders

http://www.nationaleatingdisorders.org   The National
Eating Disorders Association

www.something_fishy.org   Online chat for families and
patients

www.nimh.nih.gov/publicat/eatingdisorders.cfm
National Institute of Mental Health

Other Resources

The following organizations are good resources for eating
disorders:

Academy for Eating Disorders
60 Revere Drive, Suite 500
Northbrook, IL 60062-1577
(847) 498–4274
www.aedweb.org

Alliance for Eating Disorders Awareness
Box 13155
North Palm Beach, FL 33408–3155
info@eatingdisorderinfo.org

Anorexia Nervosa and Related Eating Disorders, Inc.
603 Stewart Street
Seattle, WA 98101
(800) 931–2237
www.anred.com

Center for the Study of Anorexia and Bulimia
A Division of the Contemporary Institute for
Psychotherapy
1841 Broadway, 4th floor
New York, NY 10023
(212) 333–3444
www.csabnyc.org

Eating Disorders Anonymous
www.eatingdisordersanonymous.org

National Association of Anorexia Nervosa and Associated
Disorders (ANAD)
P.O. Box 7
Highland Park, IL 60035
(847) 831–3438
http://www.anad.org

Overeaters Anonymous, Inc.
World Service Office (WSO)
6075 Zenith CT, NE
Rio Rancho, NM 87124
(505) 891–2664
http://www.overeatersanonymous.org

The Academy for Eating Disorders
6728 Old McLean Village Drive
McLean, VA 22101
(703) 556–9222
Fax (703) 556-8729
http://www.aedweb.org

http://www.cdc.gov/nccdphp/dnpa/bmi/children_BMI/
about_childrens_BMI.htm#How%20is%20BMI%
20used%20with%20children%20and%20teens
CDC: How to Calculate BMI in Children and Teens
(Accessed September 25, 2006)

Additional resources can be found through local libraries,
your health care provider, and the Yellow pages under "Social
Service Organizations."

REFERENCES

Adams, K. E., Schatzkin, A., Harris, T. B., Kipnis, V., Mouw,
T., Ballard-Barbash, R., Hollenbeck, A., & Leitzman, M. F.
(2006). Overweight, obesity and mortality in a large
prospective cohort of persons 50 to 71 years old.
New England Journal of Medicine, 355, 763–778.

Alegria, M., Woo, M., Cao, Z., Torres, M., Meng, X. L., &
Striegel-Moore, R. (2007). Prevalence and correlates of
eating disorders in Latinos in the United States. *International Journal of Eating Disorders.*

American Psychiatric Association. (2000). *Diagnostic and statistical manual of mental disorders,* (4th edition, Text
Revision). Washington, DC: Author.

Baum, A. (2006). Eating disorders in the male athlete. *Sports
Medicine, 36,* 1–6.

Becker, A. E. (2005). Eating disorders: Integrating medication into management. Harvard Institute of Psychopharmacology. Boston, Massachusetts.

Bray, G. A. (1978). Definition, measurement, and classification of the syndromes of obesity. *International Journal of
Obesity, 2,* 99–112.

Brewerton, T. D. (1995). Toward a unified theory of serotonin dysregulation in eating and related disorders.
Psychoendocrinology, 2016, 561–590.

Brewerton, T. D. (1997, October). *Serotonin dysregulation in
the eating disorder adolescent.* Paper presented at the meeting of eating disorders at American Academy of Child and
Adolescent Psychiatry (AACAP): Toronto, Ontario,
Canada.

Bruch, H. (1973). *Eating Disorders: Obesity, anorexia and the
person within.* New York: Basic Books.

Chamorro, R., & Flores-Ortiz, Y. (2000). Acculturation and
disordered eating patterns among Mexican American
women. *International Journal of Eating Disorders, 28,*
125–129.

Colton, P. A., Olmsted, M. P., Daneman, D., Rydall, A. C., &
Rodin, G. M. (2007). Natural history and predictors of
disturbed eating behaviour in girls with Type 1 diabetes.
Diabetic Medicine, 24, 424–429.

Conason, A. H., Brunstein Klomek, A., & Sher, L. (2006).
Recognizing alcohol and drug abuse in patients with eating disorders. *Quarterly Journal of Medicine, 99,* 335–339.

Conason, A. H., & Sher, L. (2006). Alcohol use in adolescents with eating disorders. International *Journal of Adolescent Medicine and Health, 18,* 31–36.

Cummins, L. H., & Lehman, J. (2007). Eating disorders and body image concerns in Asian American women: Assessment and treatment from a multicultural and feminist perspective. *Eating Disorders, 15,* 217–230.

Dare, C., & Eisler, I. (1997). Family therapy for anorexia nervosa. In D. M. Carner & P. E. Garfinkel (Eds.), *Handbook of Treatment of Eating Disorders* (pp. 307–324). New York: Guilford Press.

Eisler, I., Simic, M., Russell, G. F., & Dare, C. (2007). A randomised controlled treatment trial of two forms of family therapy in adolescent anorexia nervosa: A five-year follow-up. *Journal of Child Psychology and Psychiatry, 48,* 552–560.

Feldman, M. B., & Meyer, I. H. (2007). Eating disorders in diverse lesbian, gay, and bisexual populations. *International Journal of Eating Disorders, 40,* 218–226.

Fernandez-Aranda, F., Pinheiro, A. P., Tozzi, F., Thornton, L. M., Fichter, M. M., Halmi, K. A., et al. (2007). Symptom profile of major depressive disorder in women with eating disorders. *Australia and New Zealand Journal of Psychiatry, 41,* 24–31.

Fichter, M. M., Quadflieg, N., & Hedlund, S. (2006). Twelve-year course and outcome predictors of anorexia nervosa. *International Journal of Eating Disorders, 39,* 87–100.

Franko, D. L., & Keel, P. K. (2006). Suicidality in eating disorders: Occurrence, correlates, and clinical implications. *Clinical Psychology Review, 26,* 769–782.

Goldfield, F. S., Blouin, A. G., & Woodside, D. B. (2006). Body image, binge eating, and bulimia nervosa in male bodybuilders. *Canadian Journal of Psychiatry, 51,* 160–168.

Halmi, K. A. (1997, October). *Outpatient treatment of anorexia nervosa: Cognitive-behavioral and pharmacological therapies. Institute VI Adolescent Eating Disorders: A panorama.* Academy of Child & Adolescent Psychiatry Institute and Conference, Toronto, Ontario, Canada.

Hudson, J. I., Hiripi, E., Pope, H. G., & Kessler, R. C. (2007). The prevalence and correlates of eating disorders in the National Comorbidity Survey Replication. *Biological Psychiatry, 61,* 348–358.

Jackson, T., & Chen, H. (2007). Identifying the eating disorder symptomatic in China: The role of sociocultural factors and culturally defined appearance concerns. *Journal of Psychosomatic Research, 62,* 241–249.

Kaye, W., Bulik, C. M., Thornton, L., Barbarich, N., & Masters, K. (2004). Cormorbidity of anxiety disorders with anorexia and bulimia nervosa. *American Journal of Psychiatry, 161,* 2215–2221.

Klump, K. L., Perkins, P. S., Alexandra Burt, S., McGue, M., & Iacono, W. G. (2007). Puberty moderates genetic influences on disordered eating. *Psychological Medicine, 37,* 627–634.

Linehan, M. M., Comtois, K. A., Murray, A. M., Brown, M. Z., Gallop, R. J., Heard, H. L., et al. (2006). Two-year randomized controlled trial and follow-up of dialectical behavior therapy vs therapy by experts for suicidal behaviors and borderline personality disorder. *Archives of General Psychiatry, 63,* 757–766.

Miller, K. K., Grieco, K. A., & Klibanski, A. (2005). Testosterone administration in women with anorexia nervosa. *Journal of Clinical Endocrinology and Metabolism, 90,* 1428–1433.

Minuchin, S., Rosman, B., & Baker, L. (1978). *Psychosomatic families: Anorexia nervosa in context.* Cambridge, MA: Harvard University Press.

Mitchell, J. E., & Crow, S. (2006). Medical complications of anorexia nervosa and bulimia nervosa. *Current Opinions in Psychiatry, 19,* 438–443.

National Heart, Lung, & Blood Institute. (1998). *Clinical guidelines on the identification, evaluation, and treatment of overweight and obesity in adults.* National Institute of Health publication No. 98-4083. http//www.nhlbi.nih.gov/guidelines/obesity/ob_gdlns.pdf

Peveler, R. C., Bryden, K. S., Neil, H. A., Fairburn, C. G., Mayou, R. A., Dunger, D. B., & Turner, H. M. (2005). The relationship of disordered eating habits and attitudes to clinical outcomes in young adult females with type I diabetes. *Diabetes Care, 28,* 84–88.

Pike, K. M., Walsh, B. T., Vitousek, K., Wilson, G. T., Bauer, J. (2003). Cognitive behavior therapy in the posthospitalization treatment of anorexia nervosa. *American Journal of Psychiatry, 160,* 2046–2049.

Roberto, L. G. (1986). Bulimia: The transgenerational view. *Journal of Marital and Family Therapy, 12,* 231–240.

Roberto, L. G. (1992). *Transgenerational family therapies.* New York: Guilford Press.

Signorini, A., De Filippo, E., Panico, S., De Caprio, C., Pasanisi, F., & Contaldo, F. (2007). Long-term mortality in anorexia nervosa: A report after an 8-year follow-up and a review of the most recent literature. *European Journal of Clinical Nutrition, 61,* 119–122.

Spindler, A., & Milos, G. (2007). Links between eating disorder symptom severity and psychiatric comorbidity. *Eating Behaviors, 8,* 364–373.

Spitzer, R. L., Yanoski, S., Wadden, T., Wing, R., Marcus, M. D., Stunkard, A., et al. (1993). Binge eating disorder: Its further validation in a multisite study. *International Journal of Eating Disorders, 13,* 137–153.

Stahl, S. M. (2000). *Essential psychopharmacology neuroscientific basis and practical applications* (2nd ed.). New York: Cambridge University Press.

Torstveit, M. K., Rosenvinge, J. H., & Sundgot-Borgen, J. (2007). Prevalence of eating disorders and the predictive power of risk models in female elite athletes: A controlled study. *Scandinavian Journal of Medicine & Science Sports.*

Treasure, J., & Schmidt, U. (2001). *Anorexia nervosa in clinical evidence, 6,* 705–714. London, UK: British Medical Journal Publishing Group.

U.S. Department of Health and Human Services. (1999). *Mental Health: A Report of the Surgeon General—Executive Summary.* Rockville, MD: U.S. Department of Health and

Human Services, Substance Abuse and Mental Health Services Administration, Center for Mental Health Services, National Institutes of Health, National Institute of Mental Health.

Walsh, B. T. & Cameron, V. L. (2005). If Your Adolescent Has an Eating Disorder. New York: Oxford University Press.

Wang, Y., & Beydoun, M. A. (2007). The obesity epidemic in the United States—gender, age, socioeconomic, racial/ethnic, and geographic characteristics: A systematic review and meta-regression analysis. *Epidemiological Reviews, 29,* 6–28.

Woodside, D. B., Bulik, C. M., Thornton, L., Klump, K. L., Tozzi, F., Fichter, M. M., et al. (2004). Personality in men with eating disorders. *Journal of Psychosomatic Research, 57,* 273–278.

SUGGESTED READINGS

Costin, C. (1996). *Your dieting daughter.* New York: Brunner Mazel.

Costin, C. (1997). *The eating disorder sourcebook.* Los Angeles: Lowell House.

Fairburn, C. (1995). *Overcoming binge eating.* New York: Guilford Press.

Hornbacher, M. (1998). *Wasted: A memoir of anorexia and bulimia.* New York: Harper Collins.

Siegel, M., Brisman, J., & Weinshel, M. (1988). *Surviving an eating disorder: Strategies for family and friends.* New York: Harper & Row.

Smith, G. P. (1998). *Satiation from the gut to the brain.* New York: Oxford University Press.

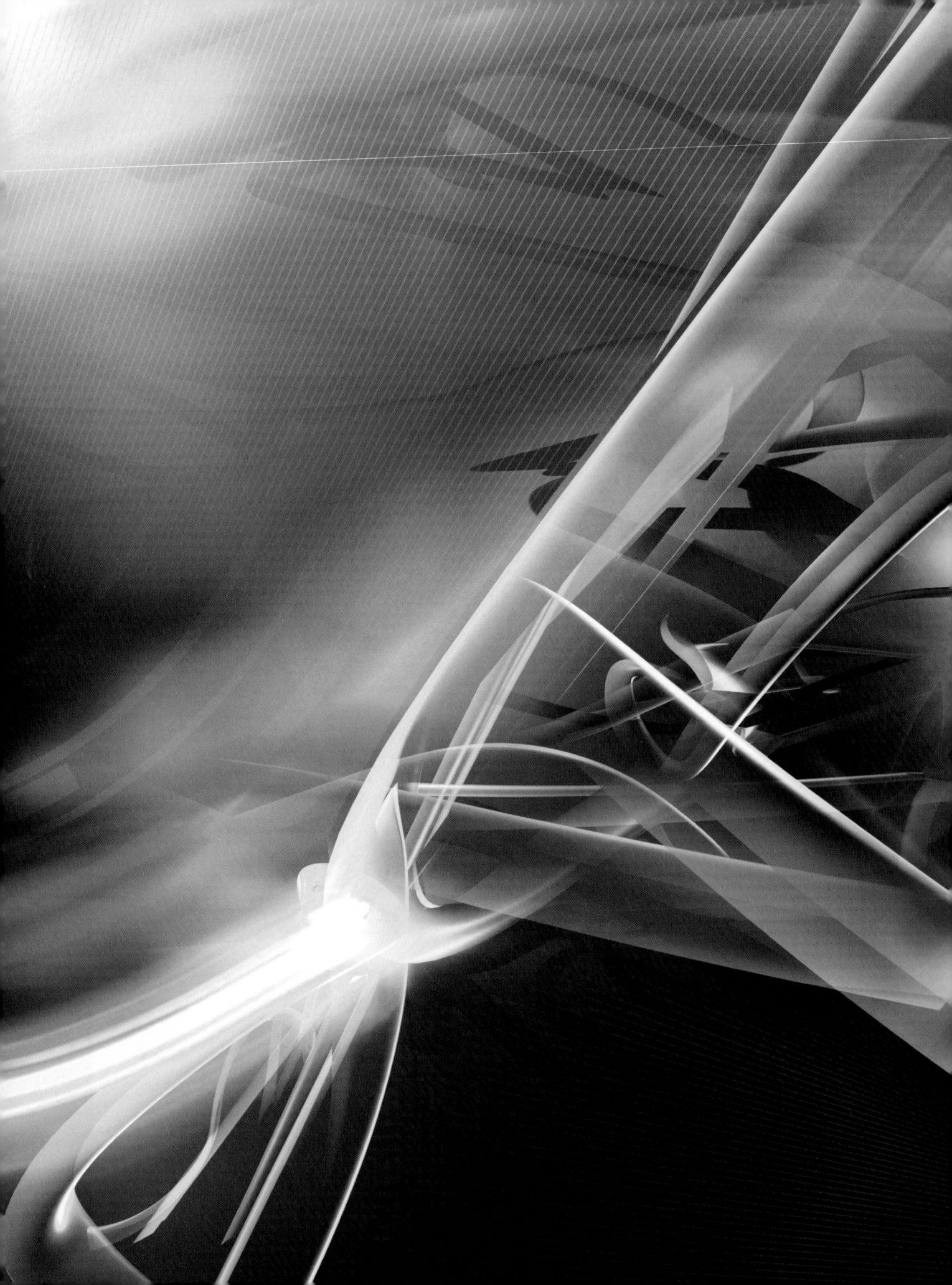

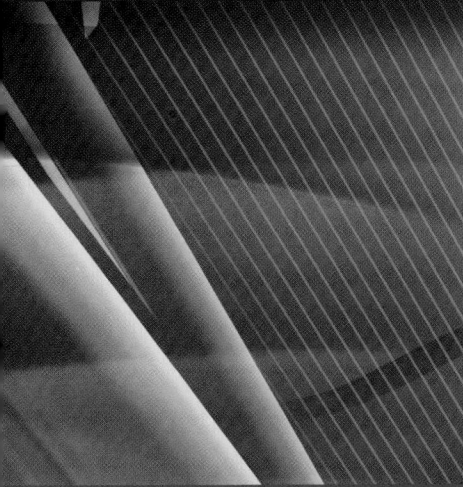

CHAPTER 23

The Client with a Sleep Disorder

Sheryl A. Innerarity, RN, PhD, FNP, CS

KEY TERMS

Advanced Sleep Phase Syndrome (ASPS): A circadian rhythm disorder common in the older adult, with early bedtime and related early rising time, inability to remain asleep during the night, and the perception of being "out of sync" with the rest of the population. Associated with napping, which worsens the problem.

Cataplexy: Sudden loss of motor control while awake, usually occurring with strong emotions, associated with narcolepsy.

Chronic Insomnia: Refers to insomnia that lasts more than one month and occurs most often in women, older adults, and clients with medical and psychiatric conditions.

Circadian Rhythm: Biological cycles occurring over an approximate 24-hour period and influencing biochemical, biological, and behavioral processes.

Delayed Sleep Phase Syndrome (DSPS): A circadian rhythm disorder, common in adolescence, with late sleep onset, and resultant desire to oversleep.

Enuresis: Bedwetting after having been toilet trained; generally resolves by school age.

Hypersomnia: Excessive daytime sleepiness, associated with disordered, non-restorative sleep.

Insomnia: The perception of not sleeping well, including difficulty in falling asleep, early awakening, and disrupted sleep; includes a perception of inadequate sleep quantity as well as quality.

Narcolepsy: A rare disorder of chronic daytime sleepiness, cataplexy, and sleep paralysis. No amount of normal sleep ameliorates the disorder; individuals have disturbed nocturnal sleep, including vivid dreams, nightmares or night terrors, or both.

Non-rapid Eye Movement (NREM) Sleep: Four stages of sleep occur: Stage I is light sleep; Stage II, eye movements are minimal or absent; Stages III and IV, slow EEG wave activity, with difficulty in arousal.

Non-Restorative Sleep: Associated with fatigue, difficulty awakening, poor concentration, and low productivity.

Parasomnias: Also called arousal disorders; include nightmares or night terrors, sleepwalking, and confusion with arousal.

Psychophysiologic Insomnia (PI): Refers to complaints of difficulty attaining or maintaining sleep during a normal sleep period.

Rapid Eye Movement (REM) Sleep: Associated with relative paralysis of skeletal muscles, rapid eye movement, penile erection, and dreaming.

Restless Leg Syndrome (RLS)/Periodic Limb Movement Disorder (PLMD): Motor movement during sleep characterized during the day by akathesia, which is the inability to sit still, and a "deep uneasy" feeling in the legs, as well as aching, and "crazy legs," which is uncommon in the daytime, with an onset in the evening or at bedtime; associated with renal failure and iron deficiency anemia.

Restorative Sleep: Refers to sleep that restores normal brain activity and equilibrium in the central nervous system and bodily processes.

Shift Work Sleep Disorder (SWSD): Develops in shift workers and is characterized by insomnia or excessive sleepiness unrelieved by sleep.

Sleep Apnea: Various disorders arising from respiratory obstruction to cessation; associated with decreased oxygenation, fragmented sleep, and increased risk for injury, particularly with coexisting medical disorders such as chronic obstructive pulmonary disease (COPD), congestive heart failure (CHF), coronary artery disease (CAD), and myocardial infarction (MI). Characterized by snoring, gasping, or absence of breathing.

Sleep Cycles: Composed of cycles of REM and NREM sleep, with REM sleep occurring every 1 to 2 hours in normal situations.

Sleep Deprivation: Chronic lack of sleep, but may occur acutely, inability to get the needed 8.3 hours of sleep nightly.

Sleep Paralysis: Associated with narcolepsy, inability to move or speak just after or before awakening; breathing is not affected.

COMPETENCIES

Upon completion of this chapter, the learner should be able to:

1. Differentiate types of sleep disorders.
2. Analyze relevant client history data associated with sleep disorders.
3. Compare physical and behavioral characteristics that are associated with sleep disorders.
4. Describe relevant components of the nursing assessment and physical examination associated with sleep disorders.
5. Acquire an understanding of various approaches that facilitate restorative sleep.
6. Contrast common medical, surgical, and psychiatric factors that contribute to sleep disorders.
7. Develop a nursing care plan for clients presenting with sleep disorders.

CHAPTER OUTLINE

Biology and Physiology of Normal Sleep

Epidemiology of Sleep Disorders

Causative Factors: Theories and Perspectives

Biological Factors

Psychiatric Disorders

Medical Conditions

Cognitive and Behavioral Factors

Psychosocial Factors

Dietary, Pharmacologic, and Other Preparations

Environmental Factors

Specific Sleep Disorders

Developmental Perspectives

Infancy and Childhood

Adolescence

Adulthood

Older Adulthood

Diagnostic Strategies

Treatment Modalities

Pharmacologic and Other Biological Interventions

Complementary Therapies

Psychosocial Interventions

The Role of the Nurse

The Generalist Nurse

The Advanced-Practice Psychiatric Registered Nurse

The Nursing Process

Assessment

Nursing Diagnoses

Outcome Identification

Planning

Implementation

Evaluation

Implications for Research

Healthy individuals generally sleep well and wake up feeling refreshed. Normally, restorative sleep is controlled by homeostatic sleep processes, circadian rhythm, and sleeping environment. Generally, the circadian rhythm opposes the homeostatic sleep drive for about 16 hours daily, facilitating the wakeful state (Russo, 2005). Human behavior has a major impact on the normal sleep process and can disrupt sleep even when homeostasis, circadian rhythm, and environments are normal. In addition, normal circadian temperature curve governs sleep because during this period, the body temperature is at its lowest setting then rises on awakening (Russo, 2005). The relevance of body temperature and sleep is the time that most nurses measure the clients' temperature. Nurses tend to measure temperature at one of the lowest points of the day, rather than between 4:00 P.M. and 8:00 P.M., when it is at its highest normal. In addition, nurses need to be concerned about elevated temperatures that occur during the normally low period, from bedtime to wakening.

Individuals with health problems, either psychological or physiological, often have disturbed or non-restorative sleep. Sleep patterns are often linked to disease and those who have sleep problems often eventually become ill, or existing chronic illness can become more severe. Because of the profound impact that sleep has on mental and physical functioning, nurses need to develop assessment skills that enable them to reduce sleep disturbances and develop a plan of care that restores health. A review of basic sleep physiology is helpful in understanding the significance of restorative sleep and the potential health risks associated with non-restorative sleep.

BIOLOGY AND PHYSIOLOGY OF NORMAL SLEEP

Although the exact purpose of sleep is unknown, most researchers agree that it has restorative powers that promote health. Considering that most people spend about a third of their lives sleeping, it is important to know the role of sleep in health promotion.

Regardless of the purpose of sleep, most researchers submit that this physiological process is mediated by neurochemical, neuroendocrine, and neuroanatomical structures. Serotonin is believed to play a role in sleep and other brain function along with other neurotransmitters (e.g., norepinephrine). Synthesis and release of serotonin by its receptors are mediated by the availability of L-tryptophan, an amino acid precursor of this neurotransmitter. Clients who inject large amounts of L-tryptophan have reduced latency sleep, whereas low levels of this chemical reduce rapid eye movement (REM) sleep. Norepinephrine and dopamine also play a role in the regulation of sleep. Drugs, such as stimulants, that mimic the actions of norepinephrine produce marked reduction in REM sleep, whereas dopamine-blocking agents increase sleep time (Kalia, 2006).

Sleep is a perplexing multistage and predictable process. During sleep many biological, biochemical, and neuroendocrine restorations occur. In addition it restores and maintains cardiovascular function, muscle tone, and thermoregulation and plays a crucial role in restoring the brain and complex physiological processes, such as protein and ribonucleic acid synthesis (Kalia, 2006).

The brain consumes an equal amount of energy during sleep and wakefulness. There is a plethora of research that indicates a predictable pattern of brain activity during sleep. Sleep physiology or energy is captured by polysomnography (PSG), an electroencephalogram (EEG), and an electroculogram to measure parameters of sleep. These physiological tests provide information about the onset of sleep (amount of time necessary to fall asleep), latency to the first REM sleep, total of sleep cycles, and number of awakenings and time of sleep. Sleep cycles are marked by cycles of REM and non-rapid eye movement (NREM) sleep.

Normally, there are two physiological states of sleep: non-rapid eye movement (NREM) sleep and rapid eye movement (REM) sleep. During NREM, four additional distinct electrophysiologic sleep stages occur: Stages I through IV (see Figure 23–1).

Stage I: light sleep (falling asleep), alpha waves interspersed with low-frequency theta waves; slow eye movement

Stage II: high K-complexes, sleep spindles, and slow eye movements

Stage III: slow sleep or "delta sleep"; slow waves on EEG; low-frequency delta waves with occasional sleep spindles and slow eye movements

Stage IV: delta waves. See Table 23–1, Non-rapid Eye Movement Sleep Stages.

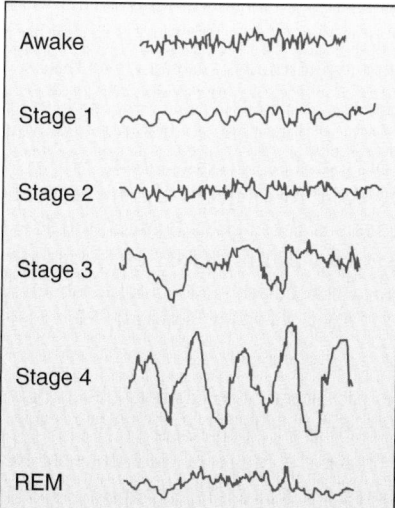

Figure 23–1 Brain activity during sleep stages. (*From National Institute of Brain Disorders and Strokes. Brain basics: Understanding sleep.* http://www.ninds.nih.gov/disorders/brain_basics/understanding_sleep.htm#dynamic_activity. *[Accessed December 4, 2006]. Brain Resources and Information Network.*)

TABLE 23–1
Non-rapid Eye Movement (NREM) Sleep Stages

Stage	Physiological Process
Stage I: light sleep (falling asleep); (alpha waves interspersed with low-frequency theta waves; slow eye movement (transitional stage between wakefulness and sleep)	• Inhibition of the reticular formation (arousal mechanism) in the cerebral cortex occurs. • Basal metabolic decreases. • Cerebral blood flow to brainstem and cerebellum decreases. • Heart rate, respirations, temperature, and muscle tone decrease. • Pupils constrict.
Stage II: high K-complexes, sleep spindles, and slow eye movements (light voltage sleep)	• Cerebral blood flow to brainstem and cerebellum decreases.
Stage III: (slow sleep or "delta sleep"); slow waves on EEG; low-frequency delta waves with occasional sleep spindles and slow eye movements (restorative sleep)	• Blood flow to cortex decreases.
Stage IV: delta waves (restorative sleep)	• Blood flow to cortex decreases. • Growth hormone is released and corticosteroid and catecholamines decrease.

EEG, electroencephalogram.

Note. Data from "Sleep disorders," by T. C. Neylan, C. F. Reynolds, D. F. Kupfer, 2003, in *Textbook of Clinical Psychiatry* (4th ed., pp. 975–1000), by R. E. Hales, S. C. Yudofsky (Eds.), Washington, DC: American Psychiatric Press. Adapted with permission.

REM sleep is characterized by a high volume of brain activity and physiological activity levels similar to those of wakefulness. Active dreaming occurs during this stage of sleep, along with decreased muscle tone, cardiovascular, and respiratory function. During REM sleep there is also an increase of 20 percent in metabolism, and EEG changes are consistent with wakefulness (Neylan, Reynolds, & Kupfer, 2003). EEG patterns during REM sleep are characterized by low-voltage, fast activity that occurs every 90 minutes after 1 to 2 hours of NREM sleep. Alternating periods of REM and NREM sleep, occur throughout the night, with the REM becoming longer as the night advances and less NREM toward the morning. During REM sleep, vast physiological and biochemical processes occur including an increase in cerebral blood flow to both hemispheres (Neylan et al., 2003).

In essence, the sleep cycle consists of a progression from wakefulness to Stages I, II, III, and IV sleep, then it continues back to Stage III, Stage II, and the first REM period. Initially, REM sleep lasts 5 to 7 minutes, but because the sleep cycle recurs four to six times during the night, the REM becomes longer as the night advances. Older adults spend less time in delta sleep and REM sleep and have less total sleep time than younger age groups. They also tend to awaken more often during the night and nap during the day (Foley et al., 2007).

Sleep patterns vary across the life span. Newborns sleep up to 20 hours a day, whereas older adults require less sleep but have more difficulty falling asleep. REM and NREM sleep are not fully differentiated until 3 to 6 months of age (Russo, 2005). In addition, older adults are less likely to tolerate sleep deprivation than younger age groups (Foley et al., 2007).

Regardless of sleep stage, disruption often results in negative physiological results such as various psychiatric and medical disorders. Because of the profound impact that sleep has on mental and physical functioning, nurses need to understand its relevance when caring for the client who presents with psychiatric and medical conditions. In addition, nurses must recognize intricate factors that prevent normal or restorative sleep and develop a plan of care that restores it.

EPIDEMIOLOGY OF SLEEP DISORDERS

Estimates of sleep problems vary, from 40 to 50 percent of people who occasionally or intermittently have sleep problems to 10 to 15 percent who report that they have chronic sleep problems. In worldwide studies, sleep disorders were reported by 13 to 49 percent of subjects, and insomnia by 3 to 19.4 percent of participants (Roth, 2005; Stewart et al., 2006). Likewise, 10 percent of clients seen in primary care reported current insomnia; 25 percent had symptoms of restless leg syndrome and 13 to 33 percent reported symptoms of obstructive sleep apnea (Alattar, Harrington, Mitchell, & Sloane, 2007). The incidence of insomnia increases with age and people 65 years and older tend to complain about it 1.5 times more than younger age groups. Approximately 12 percent of adolescents and adults report significant sleep disturbances (Foley et al., 2007). Surprisingly, less than 15 percent of people with insomnia receive treatment.

Although the term insomnia is often used to describe sleep problems, there is general lack of its meaning among clinicians. Generally, this term refers to a subjective description of inadequate sleep. Most complaints of inadequate sleep range from difficulty falling asleep, staying asleep, early morning wakening, and resultant daytime sleeping caused by insomnia. In older adults, these estimates increase to 15 to 25 percent of people with chronic insomnia (Foley et al., 2007). Many times people have various complaints concerning insomnia, ranging from acute to chronic complaints that parallel the duration of symptoms. Chronic insomnia refers to sleep disturbances lasting more than 3 weeks. These estimates fail to capture the significant number of people who do not have access to health care and who are never asked about their sleep or report difficulties with sleep. Self-imposed sleep deprivation is a malady of the stress-filled lifestyle of many people who do not know that they are sleep deprived. "I can function just fine" is a common refrain of the typical worker.

Sleep deprivation is a chronic lack of sleep but may vary according to the person's normal sleep requirements. Sleep deprivation is pervasive and often goes unrecognized. Common consequences of sleep deprivation include decreased job performance stemming from concentration and memory difficulties, increased health care costs, and poorer general health (Sigurdson & Ayas, 2007). Unfortunately, the consequences of falling asleep while driving a vehicle or operating machinery are often fatal. General health problems include functional impairment and disability and higher use of health care services.

In addition, there are forms of impaired sleep such as obstructive sleep apnea (OSA) that generate subsets of the populations with sleep disorders. Sleep apnea comprises a variety of disorders, ranging from respiratory obstruction to cessation. These disorders often result in decreased oxygen saturation, fragmented sleep, and potential risk of injury. OSA affects up to 30 percent of the population intermittently—men (4 percent) twice as often as women (2 percent) (Alattar et al., 2007). Upper airway resistance syndrome (UARS) affects about 11 percent of individuals with sleep disorders. Uncommon forms of sleep disorders, such as

narcolepsy, affect .02 to .05 percent of the population, which has a genetic linkage.

Shift work sleep disorder (SWSD) develops in approximately 10 percent of shift workers. More than 6 million Americans work the night shift on a regular basis (Schwartz & Roth, 2006) and sleep studies indicate an estimated 5 to 10 percent of night-shift workers suffer the sleep–wake disturbance which is severe enough to meet criteria for shift-work sleep disorder (APA, 2000; Drake, Roehrs, Richardson, Walsh, & Roth, 2004). Even those hours fail to relieve excessive sleep. Shift work sleep disorder results in significant sleep disturbances, fatigue, impaired insight and judgment, reduced productivity, mood swing, irritability, and decreased motivation and subsequently increased work-related accidents and sick leave use (Drake et al., 2004).

The prevalence of sleep disorders is phenomenal because of the potential health, quality of life, societal, and economic consequences. Indirect and direct costs of sleep disorders are estimated to be in the tens of billions of dollars per year (NIH, 2005). Because of potential and actual adverse consequences of sleep disorders, psychiatric nurses need to understand their complexity and collaborate with clients to develop evidence-based treatment strategies that promote sleep, restore health, and improve overall quality of life.

CAUSATIVE FACTORS: THEORIES AND PERSPECTIVES

Psychiatric and medical conditions are likely to occur as a consequence of comorbidity with sleep disorders. Because many illnesses are associated with disruption of sleep, one must determine if sleep disruption contributed to the development of the illness, or whether it resulted from the illness. Understanding the etiology of insomnia has clinical implications for the psychiatric nurse. It helps the nurse recognize the importance of asking about sleeping patterns and sleep aids, assess symptoms that suggest sleep disturbances, and promote quality of life.

BIOLOGICAL FACTORS

Biochemical process involving various neurotransmitters such as serotonin and norepinephrine play roles in sleep regulation. Drugs and medical or psychiatric conditions that alter brain chemistry contribute to sleep disorders. (Saper, 2006).

Neuroanatomical studies also link sleep disorders to dysregulation in the hypothalamic-pituitary-adrenal (HPA) axis, which plays a role in cortisol release (Otte et al., 2007). These data consistently indicate that low cortisol levels are found in post-trauma clients, whereas depressed clients are likely to have high cortisol levels (Otte et al., 2007). Sleep deprivation is associated with increased slow wave sleep, resulting in

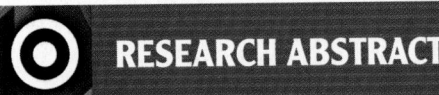
Sleep Patterns in Battered Women Living in Transitional Housing

Humphreys, J., & Lee, K. (2005) *Issues in Mental Health Nursing, 26,* 771–780.

Study Problem/Purpose

To illustrate objective and subjective sleep in a convenience sample of 29 battered women living in specialized transitional housing programs compared to 30 women living in their own homes.

Methods

Objective sleep was determined by an actigraph worn by each participant that recorded continuous activity using a battery-operated micropressor that detected motion with an electric beam and movement in all three axes. Activity was recorded in 30-second intervals and used to determine sleeping patterns (e.g., sleep onset latency, number of wake episodes). Subjective sleep was captured in a daily sleep diary based on when the participants fell asleep at night and how many times they woke during the night.

Findings

Compared to healthy controls, battered women living in transitional housing had a higher incidence of longer sleep onset latency based on subjective and objective measures and higher percentage of time awake during the night by objective measure. Data indicate that battered women in transitional housing programs may improve daytime alertness and benefit from interventions that center on reducing sleep onset latency and increasing total sleep time.

Implications for Psychiatric Nurses

Women in transitional housing experience sleep disturbances. Psychiatric nurses can use these data to guide the assessment process of women living in transitional housing to improve sleeping patterns, encourage dialogue and identify personal stressors, and offer emotional support during a stressful transitional period in the life of women dwelling in these situations.

significant reduction in cortisol and growth hormone (GH) secretion the following day. Some researchers suggest that reduced cortisol levels arising from sleep deprivation may provide a temporary relief from depression. These data also strongly suggest that deep sleep has an inhibitory effect on the HPA axis, whereas it enhances the activity of the GH axis. These findings are consistent with data concerning idiopathic hypersomnia and HPA axis and activation of chronic insomnia. (See Research Abstract).

Additional research indicates that when compared to controls, clients with insomnia demonstrate elevated global cerebral glucose metabolism on positron-emission tomography when awake and asleep (Perlis, Smith, & Pigeon, 2005). Data also indicate a familial incidence of insomnia. Clients with sleep disorders often report a positive history of sleep disturbances, particularly in women (Hamet & Tremblay, 2006). A genetic locus on chromosomes 8q, 12q, 13q, and 22q11 is also linked to the etiology of enuresis (Bayoumi et al., 2006). Likewise, narcolepsy has a genetic etiology, and, recently, researchers from UCLA and Stanford discovered that individuals with narcolepsy have missing critical cells in the hypothalamus. These cells secrete a hormone called hypocretin, previously known as orexin, which is involved in the regulation of sleep. The researchers feel that the cells have been destroyed, most likely because of some autoimmune process. Narcolepsy is a rare sleep disorder. Its primary symptoms include chronic daytime sleepiness or "sleep attacks," abnormal REM sleep manifestations, including *hypnagogic hallucinations*, cataplexy, and sleep paralysis (APA, 2000). Sleep paralysis is associated with narcolepsy and an inability to move or speak just before and after awakening. Hypnagogic hallucinations refer to a misinterpretation of sensory perception occurring while falling asleep and are normally not associated with a mental disorder.

A thorough nursing assessment or evaluation is crucial to making an accurate diagnosis of a sleep disorder. By asking questions, such as the client's current sleeping patterns, family history, substance abuse history, caffeine consumption, current medications, both prescribed and over-the-counter (OTC), the nurse can make an accurate diagnosis. Oftentimes, sleep disorders are directly associated with alterations in brain chemistry precipitated by these risk factors.

PSYCHIATRIC DISORDERS

Mood, anxiety, and substance-related disorders often result from insomnia. In addition, dementia is highly associated with disrupted sleep and, in fact, is a hallmark of Alzheimer's dementia (Moran et al., 2005). Other mental illnesses that affect, and are affected by, sleep include schizophrenia and other psychotic disorders. Clients in a manic episode tend to have sleep disturbances manifested by severe insomnia and a reduced need for sleep (APA, 2000). In addition, clients with mood disorders, such as bipolar I and major depressive episodes and anxiety disorders, have difficulty achieving REM sleep (Theorell-Haglow, Lindbery, & Janson, 2006). See Chapters 9 and 10 for a discussion of mood disorders.

Sleep disturbances are often prodromal to relapse in psychiatric disorders (Sierra, Livianos, Argues, Castelló, & Rojo, 2007). Common prodromal symptoms include psychomotor agitation, mood changes, and increased anxiety. Clients with psychiatric disorders are able to recognize prodromal symptoms of relapse. Psychiatric nurses implement interventions that facilitate early identification of clients at risk, provide psychoeducation of early symptoms of relapse, and enhance coping skills to help the client manage and reduce stress and anxiety.

Seasonal affective disorder (SAD) (APA, 2000) is another psychiatric disorder that is associated with prolonged days without sunlight. It can result in hypersomnia, depression, and a cycle of worsening sleep until sunlight returns. Hypersomnia is excessive daytime somnolence, associated with non-restorative sleep (APA, 2000). Seasonal changes and sleep disturbances tend to occur in global regions where there is prolonged darkness and days of light. These factors have a biological effect on sleep quality. Assessing the client's sleeping patterns need to be an integral part of treatment planning beginning with an initial assessment and throughout

treatment. The nurse must collaborate with the client and family and identify effective measures to restore and maintain restorative sleep. See Table 23–2, Common Medical Disorders, Psychiatric Disorders, and Medications That Cause Insomnia.

MEDICAL CONDITIONS

Somatic illnesses, once thought to be purely psychiatric disorders, include chronic fatigue syndrome and fibromyalgia, which are both strongly associated with sleep disorders. In fact, lack of Stage IV non-REM sleep is used to help make the diagnosis of fibromyalgia as well as symptoms of fatigue and reduced physical endurance (Antai-Otong, 2005).

Psychophysiologic factors, such as anxiety about not sleeping, may result when there is a temporary cause of insomnia. Poor sleep patterns may continue long after the

---

TABLE 23–2
Common Medical Disorders, Psychiatric Disorders, and Medications That Cause Insomnia

Medical Conditions	Psychiatric Disorders	Medications
Cardiovascular diseases	Major depressive episode	Diuretics
Chronic obstructive pulmonary disease	Bipolar I and II disorders	Alcohol
Endocrine disorders, such as diabetes and thyroid disease	Seasonal affective disorder	CNS stimulants
Dementia	Post-traumatic stress disorder	Diphenhydramine (Benadryl)
Menopause	Obsessive-compulsive disorder and other anxiety disorders	Caffeine
Pain	Schizophrenia and other psychotic disorders	Theophylline
Nocturia	Substance-related disorders	Selective serotonin reuptake inhibitors (e.g., fluoxetine [Prozac])
Periodic limb movement disorder	Somatoform disorders	Antipsychotic agents
Restless leg syndrome	Personality disorders	Cortisone
Fluid and electrolyte imbalance	Attention-Deficit/Hyperactivity Disorder (ADHD)	Thyroid replacement hormone
Delirium	Night terrors	
Allergies—rhinitis, sinusitis	Sleep walking	
Bronchitis	Generalized anxiety disorder	
Gastroesophageal reflux disease (GERD)	Anxiety disorders	
Peptic ulcer disease		
Malignant tumors		
Fibromyalgia		
Benign prostatic hypertrophy (BPH)		
Congestive Heart Failure (CHF)		
Parkinson's disease		
Sleep apnea		
Snoring		

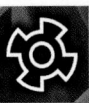
betics in poor control, have frequently interrupted sleep. Men with benign prostatic hypertrophy often have nocturia as a classic symptom, with multiple awakenings to void. The seriousness of these problems is related to the individual's ability to return to deep sleep within a reasonable period of time. However, clients who are awakening three or four times a night are more likely to have non-restorative sleep. See Table 23–2 for the major medical conditions associated with sleep disorders.

COGNITIVE AND BEHAVIORAL FACTORS

Cognitive factors associated with sleep disorders often parallel other psychiatric disorders such as anxiety and mood disorders. Frequently, the inability to sleep stems from worrying about staying awake or faulty distortions, such as "I need to get 8 hours of sleep every night." An important part of the nursing assessment is identifying the cause of the client's distress. Questions concerning the meaning of sleep and excessive worrying can provide invaluable information about the client's coping skills. Health education about exercise, diet, and maladaptive behaviors reduces stress and restores normal sleeping patterns.

There are many behavioral factors associated with sleep disorders. Most commonly, it is associated with self-induced sleep deprivation because of stress and hectic irregular schedules. Women who work outside of the home and who are also responsible for the care of the home and the children of adult parents are commonly sleep deprived. Many feel that this is a state to be expected and never seek help for their poor sleep or their exhaustion. Choices may be made that interfere with getting adequate restorative sleep. Even if more hours of sleep are achieved, the quality of the sleep is often impaired owing to stress and worry or other behavioral choices.

PSYCHOSOCIAL FACTORS

Individuals who worry excessively and have difficulty "shutting down" to sleep, may tend to have sleep disturbances. Any major stressor can disrupt sleep; for example, starting college, moving, marrying, a new job, a new baby, or the loss of a loved one. Other stressors include significant losses, pain, illness, development of health problems, or need for surgery, all of which have the potential to disrupt sleep.

DIETARY, PHARMACOLOGIC, AND OTHER PREPARATIONS

Oftentimes clients resort to using various sleep aids, such as OTC medications that contain diphenhydramine (Benadryl), or have an alcoholic beverage. Alcohol relaxes the individual, increasing drowsiness and the ability to fall asleep. However, with more than two drinks, and especially if they are ingested within a couple of hours of bedtime, alcohol interferes with normal sleep architecture so that the quality of sleep is impaired. In addition, OTC sleep preparations containing

original cause of the insomnia has disappeared. This is called **psychophysiologic insomnia**. Poor sleep hygiene is a major factor in this situation. In this type, the cause of the sleep disorder is the client's behaviors (Espie, Broomfield, MacMahon, Macphee, & Taylor, 2006).

Many medical disorders affect sleep. Some of the most common are thyroid disorders, hypothyroidism (excessive sleep) and hyperthyroidism (sleep deficit), and any pain syndrome. Chronic obstructive pulmonary disease (COPD) and coronary artery disease (CAD) are both associated with sleep apnea. The sleep apnea increases the risk of a major cardiovascular event occurring in this population. Restless leg syndrome (RLS), and periodic limb movement disorder (PLMD) interfere with the quality of sleep, and further affect daytime quality of life through continued limb symptoms. These include a classic "creepy-crawly" feeling, deep-aching, inability to sit still, and a deep powerful aching in the legs (Alattar et al., 2007).

Another major medical condition that impairs sleep is nocturia or urinary frequency (Petit, Touchette, Tremblay, Boivin, & Montplaisir, 2007). Nocturia can occur in the form of enuresis in children and occasionally continues into young adulthood, but nighttime awakening to void is more common in the middle-aged and older adult. Individuals who are taking diuretics or who have osmotic diuresis, such as dia-

diphenhydramine (Benadryl) may also produce paradoxical side effects that disturb sleep.

Caffeinated drinks are known causes of sleep disruption. Various dietary and nutritional preparations contain caffeine, including chocolates and certain teas. Women taking female hormones also clear caffeine much more slowly, so they may have to limit caffeine much earlier in the day to achieve sleep after initiating hormone therapy. Many people who "sleep fine" after caffeine are really not achieving the deep sleep needed for normal physiological processes. Also, use of any headache medicines that contain caffeine interfere with the sleep, which may help relieve the headache. Sometimes questions concerning OTC medications, dietary preparations, and beverages are overlooked during the nursing process. Because these agents interfere with normal sleeping patterns, nurses need to ask about them and provide appropriate health teaching to address these concerns.

ENVIRONMENTAL FACTORS

Environmental factors that contribute to sleep disorders include noise in the sleep setting, inability to achieve a dark room, and season of the year. Likewise, admission to a health care facility interferes with sleep through many of the mechanisms mentioned previously, especially environmental changes, including having a roommate and having strangers and nurses entering the sleep environment, sometimes without warning. Administration of medications, treatments, and taking of vital signs and blood all interfere with sleep. The more disruptive and frequent the intrusion, the more difficult to return to a state of sleep that is restorative.

In most health care facilities, ambient temperature, noise, and physical comfort are out of the individual's control, increasing stress and negatively affecting sleep. Repeated interruptions create difficulty with maintaining deep sleep, which then worsens the physiologic response, creating a vicious cycle. Generally, admission to a hospital or long-term care facility indicates serious or chronic illness, which obviously have the potential to disrupt sleep and result in sleep deprivation. Obviously, hospital environments increase tension and stress and reduce the quality of sleep in various clinical settings.

Sleep disturbances in acute care are common (Weinhouse & Schwab, 2006). Environmental factors in these settings often result in sleep deprivation or non-restorative sleep. Polysomnographic studies indicate that sleep and fragmentation are common in acutely ill clients. These data also show that the predominance of Stage I sleep with a reduction of time spent in other sleep stages, including REM and slow wave sleep, increased awakening and more daytime sleep. Of particular interest are clients with acute MI and neurological and respiratory conditions. Common complaints from these clients include "not feeling rested" or complaints of poor quality sleep and increased requests for sleeping aids. Because sleep deprivation produces significant stress during acute illness, nurses must identify these high-risk groups, modify environmental factors, and promote rest and sleep. Nurses need to initiate interventions such as active listening, music, back rubs, and therapeutic touch that reduce pain and anxiety and promote a relaxation response.

Other environmental factors that contribute to sleep disturbances arise from alterations in the circadian rhythm. Circadian rhythm is the variation in sleep tendency over a period slightly greater than 24 hours. The core body temperature, neurotransmitter and hormonal secretion, and light and dark exposure modulate circadian rhythms. Circadian rhythm sleep disorders arise from various causes, including *delayed sleep phase type, jet lag type,* and *shift work type.* Delayed sleep phase type is marked by sleep and wake times that are considerably later than desired, with a resultant difficulty in falling asleep and awakening at a desired time. Jet lag type normally occurs when people cross various time zones that are different from their normal zone time. This sleep disorder usually spontaneously corrects itself after several days. (See My Experience with Jet Lag.) Shift work type occurs in people who repeatedly and rapidly change work schedules. The effects of these disorders vary among individuals and reflect alterations in one's normal sleep-wake cycle. See Chapter 30 for an in-depth discussion of circadian rhythms and their treatment.

SPECIFIC SLEEP DISORDERS

The *Diagnostic and Statistical Manual of Mental Disorders* (4th edition, Text Revision) (*DSM-IV-TR*) (APA, 2000) for sleep disorders include the following:

◆ Primary sleep disorders—includes dyssomnias and parasomnias
◆ Sleep disorders related to another mental condition
◆ Other sleep disorders
◆ Sleep disorders due to a general medication condition
◆ Substance-induced sleep disorders

Primary insomnia is diagnosed when other causes of insomnia are eliminated. The *DSM-IV-TR* diagnosis of primary insomnia requires that a client has difficulty falling or maintaining asleep or has non-restorative sleep, and experiences marked distress or social, occupational, or other area disturbances (APA, 2000). Moreover, this sleep disturbance is not related to other psychiatric or medical conditions previously listed under these criteria (APA, 2000).

In addition to insomnia, the most common include restless leg disorder, periodic limb movement disorder, obstructive sleep apnea, and upper airway resistance syndrome. **Restless leg syndrome (RLS)** and **periodic limb movement disorder (PLMD)** are motor movements that occur during sleep and are characterized during the day by akathesia or inability to sit still. These limb disorders are associated with renal failure and iron deficiency anemia. Other disorders include the **parasomnias**, which include narcolepsy, sleepwalking, and sleep terrors. A thorough family history is useful in these cases, because narcolepsy, particularly, has a strong genetic component (APA, 2000). The parasomnias are more rare conditions, as is narcolepsy. Signs and symptoms of narcolepsy present during adolescence and are often misdiagnosed.

Active dreaming occurs during REM sleep, as well as decreased muscle tone, irregular heart and respiratory rates, and the individual is difficult to arouse during this period, even though people normally awaken during a period of REM sleep. In addition the brain is extremely active in REM sleep, with an increase in metabolism of 20 percent, and EEG changes are consistent with those during wakefulness (Kalia, 2006).

Regardless of the stage of sleep, disruption results in negative physiologic outcomes, and restorative sleep contributes to health and a perception of well-being. Of further interest to nurses, sleep deprivation is associated with depression of the immune system, including decreased neutrophils and natural killer T-cells (Ranjbaran, Keefer, Stephanski, Farhadi, & Keshavarzian, 2007). Nurses, in particular, should be aware of the processes associated with sleep, because in institutionalized clients, they have a great deal of control over enhancing or disrupting restorative sleep.

DEVELOPMENTAL PERSPECTIVES

This section discusses how sleep disorders vary among people in different stages of life.

INFANCY AND CHILDHOOD

According to the 2003 National Survey of Children's Health, approximately 15 million U.S. children are affected by inadequate sleep. Parents of children with sleep problems are more likely to report decreased academic performance and poor health (Smaldone, Honig, & Byrne, 2007). Sleep varies significantly with age, with newborns sleeping two thirds of the day, and the older adult sleeping less than a third of a day.

GH is secreted during sleep, which results in growth and healing in the young, and inability to replace and repair cells in the aging individual. In terms of psychiatric illness, children more commonly have a disorder within the parasomnias, such as nightmares, sleep terrors, talking in their sleep, and sleepwalking (Mahendran, Subramaniam, Cai, & Chan, 2006).

Unfortunately, instead of exhibiting excessive daytime sleepiness, they often appear to be hyperactive, or irritable, preventing correct diagnosis. Children also suffer more from **enuresis** (refers to bedwetting after being toilet trained), with concurrent psychological stresses associated with parental sleep deficit and disapproval and fear of peer knowledge of the disorder. These children may develop social isolation when they do not interact with other children, attend or host sleepovers, or have school-associated problems owing to the stress and sleep issues. Stressors of this type tend to worsen the sleep issues and may be associated with development of anxiety, depression, and other mental illnesses.

ADOLESCENCE

Sleep disturbances and insomnia appear to be chronic and common in adolescents with a median onset of age 11. The lifetime prevalence of insomnia in this age group is almost 11 percent of which about 53 percent have a comorbid psychiatric disorder. Developmental factors include menarche and pubertal development. Onset of menses is associated with 2.75-fold increased risk of insomnia. In comparison, the risk of insomnia in males was not associated with the onset of maturational development (Johnson, Roth, Schultz, & Breslau, 2006). Parents of adolescents with sleep problems are likely to report they have frequent headaches and skin rashes.

Adolescence and early adulthood are often times in which sleep is either a priority, like Saturday and Sunday mornings, or not necessary, like Friday and Saturday nights. Teenagers are particularly prone to **delayed sleep phase syndrome (DSPS)**, with difficulty or delay of falling asleep, and thus difficulty waking. Individuals with narcolepsy often present with signs and symptoms during this period, but are often not diagnosed because teenagers often doze off at unexpected times, owing to their tendency to stay up late, and then arise early to attend school. Typically, narcolepsy is not diagnosed until the 30s or 40s, by which time serious life consequences may already have occurred (APA, 2000).

Growth and development are major physiologic issues during this time, and disruption of normal sleep patterns can result in negative physiologic effects, which spill over into school and work. In adolescents, major physiological and hormonal changes are occurring, including major growth spurts, voice changes, and secondary sexual characteristic development.

In and of themselves, these changes are stressful; however, in the face of sleep deficit, these processes are impaired, and sleep deprivation at this time increases the stress, and thus a vicious cycle ensues. In addition, repeated nights of impaired sleep are linked to psychosis and other mental illnesses.

ADULTHOOD

As individuals take on the tasks of adulthood, sleep, or lack of it, may have a serious impact on the activities of daily living. Marriage and learning to live and sleep with another individual may be a challenge that has negative consequences if coping skills are lacking. Managing to attend work in a timely fashion, staying employed, and dealing with shift work, all become tasks adults must strive to complete successfully.

Once adults begin to deal with the challenges of adding children to the family, sleep deficit can become a serious issue, especially for the primary caregiver(s). Sleep deprivation is associated with the raising of small children, and young adults are often dealing with more than one child at a time. Adults who do not plan for necessary sleep to be achieved begin to suffer the effects of sleep deficit, which drift into all aspects of their lives.

Work and financial stressors also contribute to sleep problems. These worries are common in adulthood, as individuals are striving to manage the tasks of achieving a successful career, maintaining financial stability, and planning for the future. Whenever these tasks are difficult to achieve, sleep becomes an early casualty. Individuals in this age group often have the most difficulty with sleep hygiene issues.

OLDER ADULTHOOD

In the older adult, almost 40 percent have some type of sleep disorder, with complaints of early morning awakenings, disturbed sleep, daytime sleepiness, decreased total nocturnal sleep time, increased delayed onset of sleep, and fragmented sleep with frequent arousal (Wolkove, Elkholy, Baltzan, & Palayew, 2007). The sleep pattern in the older adult commonly results in a decrease in deep sleep cycles, with an increase in wakefulness. Recall that deep sleep results in GH secretion, so the less deep sleep, the more problems that may occur with healing and cell growth and repair.

Older adults tend to go to sleep earlier and arise earlier. If an individual plans to sleep at 8 P.M., then it would be reasonable to arise at 4 A.M. This tends to be perceived as abnormal by many clients. If the individual then goes to sleep later, but continues to awaken at 4, sleep deficit will result. These changes are called advanced sleep phase syndrome (ASPS) and are common in the older adult. Daytime napping may worsen the problem, with delayed onset of nighttime sleep, further decreasing restorative deep sleep.

In addition, older adults are more prone to the sleep disorders such as restless leg syndrome, sleep apnea, or snoring. If the older adult has a partner with any of these problems, then both partners will need to be treated to resolve the issues. Disorders of mental health can cause or exacerbate sleep, and the neurodegenerative disorders such as Alzheimer's disease commonly result in disordered sleep (Wolkove et al., 2007).

Older adults are particularly prone to be receiving medications that alter normal sleeping patterns. Common suspects should include the selective serotonin reuptake inhibitors (SSRIs), decongestants, bronchodilators, diuretics, antianxiety agents, and many OTC "sleep aids." Diphenhydramine (Benadryl) is a common active ingredient in many OTC sleep products, and although it does create drowsiness, it also contributes to falls from the sedation. It also has drying effects that may cause further problems in this age group. In addition, diphenhydramine does not support normal sleep architecture, so it is a poor choice if there is an ongoing sleep disorder, especially in older adults.

All of these result in daytime problems such as decreased concentration, poor memory, difficulty driving, or difficulty performing other physical activities, which may be perceived as the beginnings of dementia, when, in fact, they are a result of sleep deprivation or depression, or both. These problems increase the risk of falls and fractures, which may be terminal events in this age group.

Not all older adults have sleep disturbance. Studies indicate that healthy older adults who exercise early in the day, and who have bright light exposure, have less sleep fragmentation and a perception of better sleep quality (Wolkove et al., 2007). The authors also note that there were indications that a structured daily routine gave cues that were important for sleep and rest, and that a short routine afternoon nap might not be detrimental.

CRITICAL THINKING

Mary is a 34-year-old executive secretary who is seen in the primary care clinic with complaints of daytime sleepiness, irritable mood, and concentration difficulties. During your assessment she reports that she drinks 1 to 2 glasses of wine at night. Based on your understanding of her reasons for seeking treatment at this time, which of the following might she also report?

a. "I can usually fall asleep when I drink, but I wake up several times during the night."

b. "I have a very restful sleep after drinking wine."

c. "I feel irritable and agitated when I wake up after having a glass of wine."

d. "Wine does not affect my sleep at all."

Answers

a. *Correct.* Drinking wine or alcohol prior to sleep results in fragmented sleep.

b. *Incorrect.* Alcohol results in fragmented and decreased restorative/restful sleep.

c. *Incorrect.* Although alcohol may interfere with restful sleep, irritability and agitation are not common in clients who use alcohol to sleep.

d. *Incorrect.* Alcohol does impair sleep and it is unlikely that it will not affect the quailty of sleep.

Regardless of age, restorative processes are associated with restorative sleep, such as GH, which peaks in slow wave sleep. Inadequate REM sleep has been associated with interference with learning and memory, decreased daytime functioning, and risk of health problems (Zammit, 2007).

DIAGNOSTIC STRATEGIES

In clients with chronic sleep disorders, polysomographic (PSG) testing should be considered when a sleep-related breathing disorder, such as obstructive sleep apnea (OSA), is suspected. Clients with daytime sleepiness, snoring, observed periods of apnea, and body mass index (BMI) above 35 have a 70 percent risk of having sleep apnea. Other candidates for PSG include those with narcolepsy, sleepwalking, and individuals who are pilots or truck drivers (Pack et al., 2006).

TREATMENT MODALITIES

Effective treatment modalities for sleep disorders vary, but are likely to parallel underlying causative factors. For instance, if a client complains of sleep disorders, it is important for the nurse to inquire about dietary habits, such as tea or coffee or other stimulants before going to bed. More than likely, the client with a sleep disorder will benefit from a holistic treatment plan that includes pharmacotherapy agents and psychotherapeutic interventions, such as sleep hygiene.

PHARMACOLOGIC AND OTHER BIOLOGICAL INTERVENTIONS

Making a diagnosis of insomnia requires a complete physical and psychiatric evaluation to rule out medical and psychiatric conditions. Psychiatric nurses play key roles in the data collection process and must ask questions that elicit relevant data concerning the client's sleeping pattern, current medication, substance abuse, and family history of sleep disorders. The assessment process helps the nurse and other clinicians undercover causative factors and initiate appropriate treatment planning. For example, if sleep disturbances arise from an underlying mood or anxiety disorder, antidepressant agents are usually prescribed. If the client has an underlying medical condition, such as sleep apnea or drug-induced insomnia, once these conditions are corrected, normal sleeping patterns often return with nonpharmacologic interventions, such as sleep hygiene.

Pharmacologic interventions are the most common treatment strategy for primary insomnia (Perlis, McCall, Krystal, & Walsh, 2004; Roth, Soubrane, Titeux, Walsh, Zoladult Study Group, 2006). Symptoms of primary insomnia may respond to various medications, such as hypnotics. Hypnotics are the mainstay treatment for acute insomnia and play a limited role in chronic insomnia. Examples of common hypnotics include benzodiazepines (e.g., temazepam [Restoril]) and nonbenzodiazepines (zolpidem [Ambien], zaleplon [Sonata]).

Historically, prescription drugs used to treat insomnia were mainly benzodiazepines. The advent of benzodiazepine receptor agonists, such as zaleplon (Sonata), zolpidem (Ambien), and eszopiclone (Lunesta) and the melatonin-receptor agonist, Ramelteon (Rozerem), offers additional pharmacological agents to manage insomnia. Regardless of drug class, optimal use of these agents is short term. Data from randomized studies indicate the efficacy of zolpidem and zaleplon for short-term insomnia, which is defined as lasting one to four weeks, while eszopiclone has demonstrated efficacy in the treatment of chronic insomnia (Roth et al., 2006). Ramelteon is primarily for sleep-onset insomnia. It targets MT1 and MT2 receptors in the brain's suprachiasmatic nucleus (SCN). The SCN modulates circadian rhythms and the sleep-wake cycle. Major side effects associated with Ramelteon include somnolence, dizziness, decreased testosterone levels, and increased prolactin levels (Karim, Tolbert, & Cao, 2006). Due to its effects on hormonal levels, menses, sex drive, or fertility, health education about these and other side effects associated with hypnotics must be an integral part of treatment along with monitoring and documenting signs and symptoms. An in-depth discussion of hypnotic agents is discussed in Chapter 29.

Off-label pharmacologic agents used to manage insomnia but are not FDA approved for insomnia include trazodone (Desyrel). Precaution must be used when these agents are prescribed for older adults, owing to potential side effects (Antai-Otong, 2006; Lieberman, 2007). See Table 23–3 Pharmacologic Agents Used to Treat Insomnia and Specific Medical Conditions. See Chapter 29 for further discussion of pharmacologic agents.

Specific treatment should be initiated for disorders that are associated with sleep, such as RLS and PLMD, Parkinson's disease, and other dementias. Parkinson's disease, RLS, and PLMD generally respond to dopaminergically active medications such as pergolide (Permax), bromocriptine (Parlodel), and carbidopa/levodopa (Sinemet). Gabapentin (Neurontin) is another option for insomnia (Arnold et al., 2007), and duloxetine has demonstrated efficacy in treating sleep problems in depressed clients with chronic pain problems (Gupta, Nihalani, & Masand, 2007).

Regardless of the pharmacologic agent, psychiatric nurses must assess their clients for desired and adverse side effects associated with these medications. Pharmacologic considerations for older adults taking sleep agents include monitoring their blood pressure and asking them to rise slowly from lying and sitting positions to reduce orthostatic hypotension. Encouraging hydration and oral hygiene reduces dry mouth and oral care. Cautioning clients to avoid operating vehicles and machinery is crucial to reduce fatal or dangerous accidents. Because of the risk of suicide among clients with chronic medical and psychiatric conditions, nurses need to assess the client's risk of danger to self and others throughout treatment planning. Certain diagnostic studies are necessary before and during some treatments, specifically when tricyclic antidepressants are used.

TABLE 23–3
Pharmacologic Agents Used to Treat Insomnia and Specific Medical Conditions

Medication	Side Effects	Nursing Implications
Benzodiazepines flurazepam (Dalmane) temazepam (Restoril)	Psychological and physiological dependence CNS sedation Rebound insomnia	• Provide health education about sleep disorders • Educate about sleep hygiene • Monitor for signs of dependence or abuse (increase dose to achieve same effects) • Encourage to use nonpharmacologic (adjunct) interventions, including relaxation techniques • Assess level of danger to self and others • Encourage to keep sleep diary
Nonbenzodiazepines/Benzodiazepine receptor agonists (short-term use with various psychiatric disorders; sleep latency problems) zolpidem (Ambien) zaleplon (Sonata) eszopiclone (Lunesta) ramelteon (Rozerem)	Contraindicated in clients with substance-related disorders and pregnancy Nausea Drowsiness/daytime sedation Sleepwalking Delirium Headache Potential for abuse/dependence	• Same as above—particularly for signs of abuse and psychological dependence • Encourage to use nonpharmacologic (adjunct) interventions, including relaxation techniques
Antidepressants (tricyclic) doxepin (Sinequan), useful in the treatment of chronic pain syndromes imipramine (Tofranil), helpful in the treatment of enuresis	Anticholinergic: dry mouth, blurred vision, constipation, urinary retention Cardiotoxic (lethal in overdosing) Sedation Orthostasis Weight gain Delirium* Cognitive deficits*	• Health education, same as above • Assess for suicide throughout treatment • Provide health education that reduces anticholinergic side effects (e.g., high roughage diet and fluids [if not contraindicated]) • Encourage a regular exercise program (as medically safe) • Order baseline ECG prior to beginning tricyclics, including children • Instruct to rise slowly to reduce dizziness and falls—risks associated with orthostasis • Due to the high lethality associated with overdose of TCAs it is imperative to perform a thorough suicide assessment both initially and throughout treatment.
Antidepressants trazodone (Desyrel), increases Stages III and IV	Anticholinergic properties Priapism Sexual dysfunction	• Same as above, except encourage men to report erectile or sexual difficulties (women the latter)

(continues)

TABLE 23–3
Pharmacologic Agents Used to Treat Insomnia and Specific Medical Conditions *(continued)*

Medication	Side Effects	Nursing Implications
Anticonvulsants (restless leg syndome and pain syndromes) gabapentin (Neurontin)	Neurotoxic Sedation Ataxia Confusion Weight gain	• Same usted on previous page except for erectile problems and liver enzymes

ECG, electrocardiogram.

*Higher risk in older adults.

Note. Data compiled from "Gabapentin in the treatment of fibromyalgia: A randomized, double-blind, placebo-controlled, multicenter trial," by L. M. Arnold, D. L. Goldenberg, S. B. Stanford, J. K. Lalonde, H. S. Sandhu, P. E. Keck, et al., 2007, *Arthritis and Rheumatism, 56,* pp. 1336–1344; "Effects of psychiatric medications on sleep and sleep disorders," by N. A. DeMartinis and A. Winokur, 2007, *CNS and Neurological Disorders—Drug Targets, 6,* pp. 17–29; "Treatment of sleep dysfunction and psychiatric disorders," by P. M. Becker, 2006, *Current Treatment Options in Neurology, 8,* pp. 367–375.

COMPLEMENTARY THERAPIES

The explosion of complementary or alternative therapies offers clients with various sleep disorders an array of preparations. Most of the agents are derived from the dietary supplement melatonin and plants and include valerian and kava kava (Bressler, 2005). Likewise, foods such as turkey and potatoes and, of course, warm milk, have tryptophan, which may promote rest and sleep.

Valerian comes from the root of the *Valeriana officinalis* and has been used for more than 1,000 years. Its action is thought to increase gamma-aminobutyric acid (GABA), an inhibitory neurotransmitter, whose properties are similar to benzodiazepines; however, its exact action remains unknown (Bressler, 2005). Major adverse side effects of valerian are headache, gastrointestinal complaints, and daytime sedation. Rare side effects include dystonias (movement disorders) and liver toxicity. Safety in pregnancy has not been determined (Mischoulon, 2007).

Melatonin is a neurohormone secreted by the pineal gland and plays a role in modulating the circadian rhythms. Like other herbal or alternative therapies, there are inconsistent data concerning its efficacy in managing sleep problems such as jet lag (Arendt & Skene 2005). Major side effects of melatonin include sedation, drowsiness, fatigue, hypothermia, and increased risk of seizures in children .

Kava kava is extracted from the *Piper methysticum root.* Its usefulness lies in its calming, relaxing effects without lasting sedation. Although side effects from kava kava are rare, they include gastrointestinal distress, headaches, allergic skin reactions, and liver toxicity (Mischoulon, 2007).

Although alternative therapies such as herbal and melatonin facilitate sleep, their precise actions remain obscure and their efficacy has yet to be supported by research. Of particular concern is that because the Federal Drug Administration (FDA) does not regulate manufacture of these drugs, it is conceivable that some preparations may have minimal amounts of active ingredients. Also of concern in the case of a preparation like tryptophan is that it may have contaminants that cause undesirable effects; for example, lead has been found in some Chinese herbal preparations, resulting in lead poisoning.

PSYCHOSOCIAL INTERVENTIONS

Regardless of the treatment approach, psychiatric nurses play key roles in providing pharmacologic and nonpharmacologic interventions. Nonpharmacologic nursing interventions include psychosocial approaches such as deep breathing exercises, sleep hygiene stress management, relaxation, and cognitive-behavioral therapies. Deep abdominal breathing exercises and stress management techniques help the client gain control of physiological manifestations of anxiety and stress. Brisk walks, regular exercise, and a balanced diet also promote health and promote rest. Stressing the importance and role of sleep in health promotion through health education using sleep hygiene and a sleep diary provides the client with a sense of control. Ultimately, health teaching and other psychosocial interventions return the client's normal sleeping patterns and improve quality of life. See Table 23–4, Behavioral Rules for Good Sleep Hygiene.

Cognitive-behavioral therapy is another psychosocial and behavioral intervention that is limited to the advanced-practice psychiatric nurse practitioner who is educationally prepared

TABLE 23–4
Behavioral Rules for Good Sleep Hygiene

1. Avoid using bed for activities other than sleep and sex.
2. If sleep does not occur after lying awake for 15 minutes (whether initially or on early awakening), get out of bed and do something that facilitates sleep, such as reading a boring book, until sleepiness occurs.
3. Avoid caffeine after 6 P.M. (some say noon, or no caffeine at all).
4. Use relaxation techniques.
5. Go to bed and arise at planned times on a daily basis.
6. Avoid worrying or trying to resolve issues before bedtime.
7. Avoid alcohol before bedtime.
8. Avoid napping during the day.
9. Eliminate pre-sleep activities that create arousal, such as exercise, watching violent television, work, or socializing.
10. Remove the clock from the bedroom, or face the numbers away from the bed.
11. Create a quiet, dark sleep environment.
12. Avoid nicotine.
13. Avoid large meals close to bedtime, but do not go to bed hungry.
14. If using diuretics, take them early in the day, and empty the bladder before going to bed.
15. If using a hypnotic or other medications for sleep, avoid using them on a daily basis.
16. Maintain a cool room temperature because it facilitates sleep if the individual has adequate covering; a room that is too hot or too cold will interfere with sleep.

Myths to Overcome about Sleep Disorders

1. "Alcohol helps individuals to sleep." Alcohol may facilitate getting to sleep, but then about 4 hours later, the individual wakes and has difficulty getting back to sleep. Alcohol interferes with normal sleep architecture.
2. "Reading in bed until you are tired helps to fall asleep." Bed should be reserved for sleep and intimate activities with one's significant other. Using the bedroom as a living area interferes with the perception of bed as a place to fall asleep. Insomniacs who awaken and cannot get back to sleep should get up and read in another room until they feel sleepy again.
3. "If sleep deprivation occurs, afternoon naps are a good idea." Actually, napping worsens sleep by advancing the sleep phase so that the individual goes to bed later but then has to awaken at the set time.
4. "If I exercise about 15 minutes before going to bed I will sleep better." Exercise shortly before bedtime is actually stimulating and has the opposite effect. However, exercise or aerobic fitness promotes sleep if done earlier in the day.

and nationally certified. Major goals of cognitive-behavioral therapy include reducing cognitive and biological arousal and helping the client challenge distorted cognitions, such as "all or none" thinking that generate distress. Clients presenting with various pain syndromes, anxiety, and mood disorders can benefit from cognitive-behavioral therapy.

Disorders such as post-traumatic stress syndrome, of which insomnia is a major manifestation, should benefit from ongoing therapy as well as a variety of medications that may be helpful, such as antidepressants and antianxiety agents. Clients with panic and anxiety disorders often benefit more from combination therapy, counseling, and medications than from medications alone, because triggering the episodes may

be linked to specific stimuli that the client needs help to work through.

THE ROLE OF THE NURSE

Health promotion is an integral part of nursing practice. Facilitating the clients' return to normal or restorative sleep is a major concern for psychiatric nurses. Health promotion begins by establishing a trusting relationship with the clients, families, and significant others.

THE GENERALIST NURSE

The generalist nurse offers an array of health-promoting activities. This process begins by assessing the client's holistic needs and stressing the importance of health-promoting activities that restore normal sleeping patterns. A thorough nursing assessment needs to include the client's normal sleeping patterns, duration of sleep disturbances, psychiatric and medical histories, level of danger to self and others, and cultural and personal preferences. The generalist nurse also collects data concerning the client's physical health, including vital signs, neurological status, and relevant aspects of the mental status examination. In addition, the generalist nurse reviews client data and synthesizes data that assist the mental health team in making a differential diagnosis. Once the diagnosis is confirmed, the nurse provides appropriate interventions such as crisis intervention, stress management, and relaxation techniques. Health education is an integral part of health-promoting activities. It involves the application of knowledge concerning causative factors associated with various sleep disorders and the importance of sleep and health promotion.

THE ADVANCED-PRACTICE PSYCHIATRIC REGISTERED NURSE

The role of the advanced-practice psychiatric nurse, like the generalist nurse, needs to focus on health promotions that facilitate restorative sleep. Additional responsibilities of the advanced-practice nurse include assessing the appropriateness of pharmacologic and nonpharmacologic interventions, such as prescribing medications and cognitive behavioral therapy (CBT) to treat co-occurring psychiatric conditions and sleep disorders, and assessing the client's health educational needs, preferences, and motivation to participate in psychotherapy. Initially, the advanced-practice nurse performs a comprehensive mental status and physical examination and orders appropriate diagnostic studies to rule out medical and psychiatric disorders. Once a differential diagnosis is made, the advanced-practice nurse will develop an individualized treatment plan.

THE NURSING PROCESS

The nursing process involving sleep disorders requires a thorough assessment of the client's symptoms and a basic understanding of causative factors. Issues, such as recent stressors, physical or mental conditions, and client preferences must be considered throughout, using the nursing process to facilitate an accurate diagnosis, appropriate interventions, and treatment outcomes.

ASSESSMENT

Characteristics associated with sleep disorders are easily assessed through interviewing the client and her significant other(s). It assesses the likeliness of dozing in a variety of situations, such as while reading, sitting, and talking to someone, and at the extreme, in a car while stopped in traffic. The individual can simply be asked if she sleeps well, for about 8 hours, and if she wakes up feeling refreshed, all of which are necessary components of restorative sleep. Use of a scale in a clinical setting is very helpful, because it may help diagnose a problem initially (and provides documentation), and it can be reused to follow and document the course and treatment of a problem.

Other questions should address any difficulties falling asleep; early awakenings; sleep interruptions; the perception of not sleeping; falling asleep when not stimulated (as in a boring meeting); fatigue or lack of energy, difficulties with concentration, memory, and psychiatric symptoms such as anxiety and changes of mood. Asking the client and significant other to complete a sleep diary also offers important data that assists in making an accurate diagnosis.

Apart from asking the client questions to determine quality and nature of sleep disturbances, it is equally important to discuss and gather data from the bed partner, parent, or caregiver (Lee & Ward, 2005). Lifestyle habits also should be assessed and include sleep schedule during the week and weekends; alcohol and caffeine consumption; bedtime routine, such as sleeping with the radio or TV on; and the length of time falling asleep after going to bed. Questioning the client in the following areas provides important data concerning the client's sleeping patterns:

◆ Hours of sleep
◆ Time the client goes to bed and time he/she actually falls asleep
◆ Frequency of awakening and sleep
◆ Sleep position
◆ Type of bed, mattress, pillow
◆ Eating habits prior to sleep
◆ Confusional arousal
◆ Enuresis
◆ Teeth grinding (bruxism)
◆ Disordered breathing (Lee & Ward, 2005; Silber, 2005)

Observing the client is essential, and, typically, the sleepless client presents with apparent fatigue, dark circles under the eyes, yawning, or even dozing while waiting to be seen. Sleepless clients can be irritable and impatient as well. Many of the signs of sleeplessness also are seen with anemia, hypoxia, cognitive deficits, and mental illness. A complete physical examination is always useful to rule out other, or concurrent, disease.

Other diagnostic criteria include sleep studies and monitoring for abnormal laboratory results, which might indicate sleep problems such as an elevated or depressed thyroid-stimulating hormone (TSH), elevated or depressed potassium, calcium, or magnesium levels, which can lead to muscle spasms or somnolence. Other studies include complete blood count to rule out anemia and diagnostic studies to rule out arrhythmias.

The following case study offers an opportunity to use the nursing process when caring for the client with a sleep disorder.

NURSING DIAGNOSES

The following are potential nursing diagnoses that can be considered for the client who presents with a sleep disorder (North American Nursing Diagnosis Association [NANDA], 2007):

◆ Disturbed Sleep Pattern
◆ Ineffective Coping
◆ Risk for Self-Directed Violence
◆ Fatigue
◆ Situational Low Self-Esteem
◆ Anxiety

An accurate nursing diagnosis is crucial for appropriate treatment planning. In the case of Mr. Martin, who reports sleep disturbances since his recent hospitalization, the nurse, client, and his wife need to collaborate and identify measurable

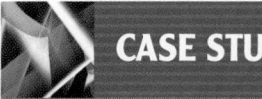

CASE STUDY

The Client with Sleep Disturbance (Mr. Martin)

Mr. Martin, an 80-year-old man, is seen during a mental home health visit shortly after his discharge post myocardial infarction. During his hospitalization he was begun on an antidepressant. He and his wife complain that he is more irritable, and that he has had frequent awakenings since his discharge. His wife also complains of having problems sleeping because of his sleeplessness. Both complain of daytime sleepiness, fatigue, anxiety, and difficulty falling and staying asleep during the night. Mr. Martin reports that he feels so useless but denies suicidal or homicidal ideations. He and his wife report that they understand the teaching instructions regarding his activities and that it takes time to recover from his recent heart attack. The following nursing process reflects this case study.

client outcomes. Outcome measures need to focus on promoting restoration of normal sleeping patterns and facilitating an optimal level of functioning.

OUTCOME IDENTIFICATION

The client's goals for sleep are often much different from the nurses' goals for the client. Client goals that facilitate major client outcomes include:

- The client will be able to express feelings rather than acting on them.
- The client will be able to express feelings appropriately and express that he feels in control of life again.
- Reduce the number of times the client gets up during the night from three to one.
- List two or three positive personal attributes.
- The client will express feeling less fatigue and be able to tolerate performing specific activities of daily living within 2 weeks.

PLANNING

The psychiatric nurse and the client need to collaborate a plan of care that reflects identified nursing diagnoses and outcome measures. Treatment considerations need to be evidence-based and client centered. In addition, nursing interventions need to integrate biological, psychosocial, and cognitive modalities that facilitate sleep restoration and help the client manage medical and psychiatric conditions. Family and significant others must be included in the treatment planning process, which can elicit the client's goals related to his personal needs for sleep and rest.

IMPLEMENTATION

Implementing a plan of care for the client with a sleep disorder requires using an array of interventions that promote

sleep. Depending on the practice settings, nursing interventions may range from structuring the client's environment by reducing noise or light, such as in an extended care unit, to teaching the client cognitive-behavioral techniques to reduce cognitive distortions. Medication administration and prescriptive authority reduce biological aspects of the sleep disorder, whereas psychosocial interventions can strengthen coping skills and increase self-esteem.

In the case study, the nurse needs to establish rapport with the client and his wife and focus on sleep hygiene, stress management, and health education. See Nursing Care Plan 23–1. Refer to the behavioral rules for good sleep hygiene in Table 23–4 for further health teaching ideas.

Clients seen in home health or other community centers can benefit from measures of nursing interventions such as therapeutic touch, which can be used to promote rest and sleep. Therapeutic touching methods, such as a back rub before bedtime, can be very relaxing to stressed clients, and a warm glass of milk can also be helpful. Attempting to reestablish the clients' normal sleeping and waking times can be very helpful. Asking them about their normal sleep routines can be enlightening. Nurses have the opportunity to teach the clients and their families the elements of good sleep hygiene, including methods to decrease worrisome behavior before bedtime and short-term use of antianxiety agents and sedative antidepressants. See Nursing Care Plan 23–1.

EVALUATION

Evaluation focuses on client responses. In this case, major outcome measures and evaluation include the following:

- Develop adaptive coping skills to manage present stressors and restore confidence and self-esteem.
- Return to the prehospitalization sleeping patterns.
- Increase energy (self-report) and be able to perform designated activities (gradually) as medical condition permits.

IMPLICATIONS FOR RESEARCH

The issue of quality sleep and its relationship to mental and physical health continue to be researched. Complaints of sleep disturbances are well documented and common in individuals with psychiatric and medical conditions. One out of three adults is likely to report difficulty falling or staying asleep. Major clinical challenges for nurses and other clinicians are making an accurate diagnosis of insomnia and other sleep problems and initiating client-centered interventions to promote rest and quality sleep. Currently there is a lack of consensus or variance about the concept of insomnia. Sleep disorders associated with schizophrenia are well researched and current data comes from sleep difficulties associated with mood disorders. Of particular interest are sleep disturbances in anxiety disorders, the long-term use and efficacy of hypnotics, and psychotherapeutic interventions.

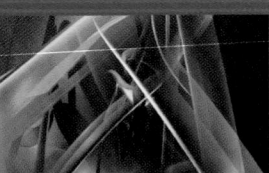

The Client with Sleep Disturbance (Mr. Martin)

Nursing Diagnosis: Risk for Self-Directed Violence

Outcome Identification	Nursing Actions	Rationales	Evaluation
1. By [date], client verbalizes feelings rather than acting on them.	1a. Establish rapport. Encourage expression of feelings.	1a. Establishes therapeutic interaction. Conveys empathy, caring, and interest.	*Goal met:* Nurse forms therapeutic relationship. Client expresses feelings Client does not express suicidal ideations or act on thoughts.
	1b. Maintain a safe environment. Assess level of dangerousness.	1b. Provides safety and control and decreases acting-out behaviors.	
	1c. Observe for mood changes. Ask the client's wife to notify staff if mood changes.	1c. Change in mood or anxiety level increase risk of dangerousness.	

Nursing Diagnosis: Ineffective Coping

Outcome Identification	Nursing Actions	Rationales	Evaluation
1. By [date], client develops realistic perception of present stressor(s).	1a. Explore meaning of recent job loss and other stressors.	1a. Helps the client understand self and present responses.	*Goal met:* Client returns to pre-hospitalization level of functioning. Client develops adaptive coping skills. Client's self-esteem increases.
	1b. Understand meaning of present stressors (recent MI).	1b. Validates understanding of meaning of present symptoms.	
2. By [date], client develops enduring adaptive coping skills.	2. Assist in identifying strengths, resources, and coping skills.	2. Places focus on positive attributes and increase self-esteem.	

Nursing Diagnosis: Disturbed Sleep Pattern

Outcome Identification	Nursing Actions	Rationales	Evaluation
1. By [date], client's normal sleeping patterns return to optimal level.	1a. Assess normal sleeping patterns.	1a. Helps the nurse identify normal sleeping patterns.	*Goal met:* Client's normal sleeping patterns return and are maintained.
	1b. Maintain quiet environment.	1b–d. Promotes rest, sleep.	
	1c. Provide health education about sleep hygiene.		
	1d. Encourage to keep a sleep diary.		

(continues)

Nursing Care Plan 23–1 *(continued)*

Nursing Diagnosis: Situational Low Self-Esteem

Outcome Identification	Nursing Actions	Rationales	Evaluation
1. By [date], client verbalizes two or three positive attributes.	1a. Provide successful experiences. 1b. Convey acceptance and empathy. 1c. Encourage active participation in treatment.	1a–c. Positive experiences increase confidence and self-esteem.	*Goal met:* Client's self-esteem increases. Client is able to explore options to deal with present stressors.

Nursing Diagnosis: Fatigue

Outcome Identification	Nursing Actions	Rationales	Evaluation
1. By [date], client will verbalize feeling less fatigued and able to tolerate performing specific tasks.	1a. Encourage client and wife to list designated tasks (within medical post-MI treatment plan). 1b. Stress importance of recognizing physical tolerances.	1a. Promotes a sense of control and personal importance. 1b. Promotes healing and helps client understand strengths and limitations.	*Goal met:* Client is able to perform activities of daily living as tolerated with increased endurance.

During the past decade, leaders in the field of sleep research continue to explore dimensions of sleep disorders and contribute to the knowledge of these complex conditions (Humphreys & Lee, 2005; McEnany & Lee, 2005). Psychiatric nurses are poised to participate in research studies that address these and other issues that impact the quality of sleep, cognitive and physical functioning, and overall health.

SUMMARY

◆ Most sleep disorders coexist with medical and psychiatric conditions.

◆ Clients who describe difficulty falling asleep, difficulty staying asleep, difficulty returning to sleep after being awakened, and who do not wake up feeling rested and refreshed have a sleep disorder.

◆ Suspect a sleep disorder when a client complains of fatigue, has dark circles under the eyes, is unable to stay awake, and has an irritable mood.

◆ High-risk groups for sleep disorders include individuals with a history of mental illness, particularly depression and anxiety; heart disease; chronic pain syndromes; situational stress; chronic obstructive pulmonary lung disease; or a family history of narcolepsy or enuresis.

◆ Pharmacologic and nonpharmacologic interventions are available to clients experiencing sleep disorders.

Psychiatric nurses must assess reasons for sleep disturbances and initiate holistic interventions that promote rest and restore the client's level of functioning.

◆ Researchers continue to explore and develop ideal sleep medications.

STUDY QUESTIONS

1. Mary, a 22–year-old young woman, has been staying up late for finals. She is seen shortly before taking her exams complaining of difficulty with concentration and fatigue. What is the most appropriate response to this client?
   a. "You probably need a sleep medication."
   b. "Describe your normal sleeping patterns."
   c. "Tell me how long you have been depressed."
   d. "You are just having finals jitters."

2. One of your clients reports having sleep disturbances. He reports that he seems to dream "all night long" and feels exhausted on awakening. What is the best explanation for his statement?
   a. He has increased REM sleep.
   b. He has decreased REM sleep.
   c. He has increased Stages III and IV sleep.
   d. He has decreased Stages I and II sleep

3. Mr. Jones has been recently started on zolpidem (Ambien). He is expressing concerns about becoming

"addicted" to this medication. Which answer reflects your understanding about this medication?

  a. "You have every reason to be concerned because it is highly addictive."

  b. "No problem, because this medication is not addictive."

  c. "I understand your concerns, but you are only going to be on it 2 weeks."

  d. "If I were you, I would not take it."

4. Ms. Mooneyham, an 82-year-old woman, is seen during a home health visit. You notice that she is sleeping during your visit and has difficulty staying awake. Her daughter expresses concerns about her sleepiness over the past week. What is the most appropriate response?

  a. "How long and how often have you been napping during the day?"

  b. "Please stay awake, I need to talk to you for a few minutes."

  c. Express concerns to her daughter about the daytime drowsiness.

  d. Tell the daughter and client that if she is tired, it is okay to nap.

5. Mr. Jones comes into the community mental health clinic complaining of how much he worries about falling and staying asleep and he needs something stronger than his present sleep medication. Which of the following indicates an understanding of Mr. Jones' present situation?

  a. He might benefit from a referral to the APN for cognitive-behavioral therapy.

  b. He needs a stronger medication so he can stop worrying so much.

  c. He needs a complete physical examination.

  d. His medications need to be changed to something more effective.

6. One of your clients complains of difficulty sleeping the past few months and related fatigue and increased agitation. An important question to ask during the nursing assessment when a client presents with sleep disturbance is which of the following?

  a. "Have you had any major life changes the past few months?"

  b. "Tell me more about your sleep routine."

  c. "Describe your past sleeping patterns and how they have recently changed."

  d. "How often do you get up to go to the bathroom during the night?"

7. Mr. K. is a 43-year-old client who has recently been diagnosed with bipolar disorder, manic most recent episode. Which of the following sleep patterns do you expect to see in this client?

  a. Increased and prolonged sleep up to 12 hours a night

  b. Decreased need for sleep associated with about 4 hours each night

  c. Normal sleeping patterns of 6 to 8 hours per night

  d. Early morning wakening with difficulty falling back to sleep

8. A client presents in ambulatory care complaining of increased sleepiness, difficulty concentrating, irritability, and reduced job productivity. He also reports his wife is complaining about his mood swings and lack of motivation to do things with the family since he changed jobs. An important question to ask is which of the following?

  a. "What shift do you work?"

  b. "Tell me about your current medications."

  c. "List your current medical problems."

  d. "How long has your wife been concerned about your behavior?"

9. All but which of the following statements about non-benzodiazepine sleep medications are accurate?

  a. They are generally prescribed for short-term use.

  b. They have a short half-life and may require more than one nightly dose.

  c. They can be used safely in clients with a history of substance-related disorders.

  d. They can be used in conjunction with sleep hygiene measures to improve sleep.

10. Which of the following sleeping patterns is likely to be found in the client with generalized anxiety disorder?

  a. Frequent early morning awakenings

  b. Difficulty falling asleep

  c. Normal sleeping patterns

  d. Both difficulty falling asleep and early morning wakening

RESOURCES

Please note that because Internet resources are of a time-sensitive nature and URL addresses may change or be deleted, searches should also be conducted by association or topic.

Internet Resources

http://www.americansleepassociation.org   American Sleep Association (Accessed May 13, 2006)

http://www.asda.org   American Sleep Disorders Foundation

http://bisleep.medsch.ucla.edu   Sleep Home Pages

http://www.sleeping.org.uk/contents/homefrm.htm British Sleep Society (Accessed May 13, 2006)

http://www.css.to/sleep/brochures.htm   Canadian Sleep Society (brochures on various sleep disorders) (Accessed May 13, 2006)

http://consensus.nih.gov/2005/2005InsomniaSOS026PDF.pdf   NIH state-of-the-science conference statement on manifestations and management of chronic insomnia in adults, 2005 Jun 13–15. *National Institute Consensus State of Science Statements, 22,* 1–30.

http://www.nlm.nih.gov/medlineplus/sleepdisorders.htm National Institute of Health: Medline Plus: Sleep Disorders (Government Resources and Research); Patient education (tutorial available in both English and Spanish) (Accessed May 13, 2006) http://www.nhlbi.nih.gov/health/public/sleep/healthy_sleep.htm "Your Guide to Healthy Sleep," (PDF document, 60 pages) (Accessed May 13, 2006)

http://www.sleepfoundation.org National Sleep Foundation

http://www.aasmnet.org American Academy of Sleep Medicine

http://www.rls.org Restless Leg Syndrome Foundation

REFERENCES

Alattar, M., Harrington, J. J., Mitchell, C. M., & Sloane, P. (2007). Sleep problems in primary care: A North Carolina Family Practice Research Network (NC-FP-RN) Study. *Journal of the American Board of Family Medicine, 20,* 365–374.

American Psychiatric Association. (2000). *Diagnostic and statistical manual of mental disorders* (4th edition, Text Revision) (*DSM-IV-TR*). Washington, DC: Author.

Antai-Otong, D. (2005). The art of prescribing. Depression and fibromyalgia syndrome (FMS): Pharmacologic considerations. *Perspectives in Psychiatric Care, 41,* 146–148.

Antai-Otong, D (2006). The art of prescribing. Risk and benefits of non-benzodiazepine receptor agonists in the treatment of acute primary insomnia in older adults. *Perspective in Psychiatric Care, 42,* 196–200.

Arendt, J., & Skene, D. J. (2005). Melatonin as a chronobiotic. *Sleep Medicine Reviews, 9,* 25–39.

Arnold, L. M., Goldenberg, D. L., Stanford, S. B., Lalonde, J. K., Sandhu, H. S., Keck, P. E., et al. (2007). Gabapentin in the treatment of fibromyalgia: A randomized, double-blind, placebo-controlled, multicenter trial. *Arthritis and Rheumatism, 56,* 1336–1344.

Bayoumi, R. A., Eapen, V., Al-Yahyaee, S., Al Barwani, H. S., Hill, R. S., & Al Gazali, L. (2006). The genetic basis of inherited primary nocturnal enuresis: A UAE study. *Journal of Psychosomatic Research, 61,* 317–320.

Bressler, R. (2005). Herb-drug interactions: Interactions between kava and prescription medications. *Geriatrics, 60,* 24–25.

Drake, C. L., Roehrs, T., Richardson, G., Walsh, J. K., & Roth, T. (2004). Shift work sleep disorder: Prevalence and consequences beyond that of symptomatic day workers. *Sleep, 27,* 1453–1462.

Espie, C. A., Broomfield, N. M., MacMahon, K. M., Macphee, L. M., & Taylor, L. M. (2006). The attention-intention-effort pathway in the development of psychophysiologic insomnia: A theoretical review. *Sleep Medicine Reviews, 10,* 215–245.

Foley, D. J., Vitiello, M. V., Bliwise, D. L., Ancoli-Israel, S., Monjan, A. A., & Walsh, J. K. (2007). Frequent napping is associated with excessive daytime sleepiness, depression, pain, and nocturia in older adults: Findings from the National Sleep Foundation "2003 Sleep in America" Poll. *American Journal of Geriatric Psychiatry, 15,* 344–350.

Gupta, S., Nihalani, N., & Masand, P. (2007). Duloxetine: Review of its pharmacology, and therapeutic use in depression and other psychiatric disorders. *Annals of Clinical Psychiatry, 19,* 125–132.

Hamet, P., & Tremblay, J. (2006). Genetics of the sleep-wake cycle and its disorders. *Metabolism, 55,* (Suppl 2), S7–S12.

Humphreys, J., & Lee, K. (2005). Sleep disturbance in battered women living in transitional housing. *Issues in Mental Health Nursing, 26,* 771–780.

Johnson, E. O., Roth, T., Schultz, L., & Breslau, N. (2006). Epidemiology of DSM-IV insomnia in adolescence: Lifetime prevalence, chronicity, and an emergent gender difference. *Pediatrics, 117,* 247–256.

Kalia, M. (2006). Neurobiology of sleep. *Metabolism, 55,* (Suppl 2), S2–S6.

Karim, A., Tolbert, D., & Cao, C. (2006). Disposition kinetics and tolerance of escalating single doses of ramelteon, a high-affinity MT1 and MT2 melatonin receptor agonist indicated for treatment of insomnia. *Journal of Clinical Pharmacology, 46,* 140–148.

Lee, K. A., & Ward, M. W. (2005). Critical components of a sleep assessment for clinical practice settings. *Issues in Mental Health Nursing, 26,* 739–750.

Lieberman, J. A. (2007). Update on the safety considerations in the management of insomnia with hypnotics: Incorporating modified-release formulations into primary care. *Primary Care Companion Journal of Clinical Psychiatry, 9,* 25–31.

Mahendran, R., Subramaniam, M., Cai, Y., & Chan, Y. H. (2006). Survey of sleep problems amongst Singapore children in a psychiatric setting. *Social Psychiatry & Psychiatric Epidemiology, 8,* 669–673.

McEnany, G. W., & Lee, K. A. (2005). Effects of light therapy on sleep, mood, and temperature in women with nonseasonal major depression. *Issues in Mental Health Nursing, 26,* 781–794.

Mischoulon, D. (2007). Update and critique of natural remedies as antidepressant treatments. *Psychiatric Clinics of North America, 30,* 51–68.

Moran, M., Lynch, C. A., Walsh, C., Coen, R., Coakley, D., & Lawlor, B. A. (2005). Sleep disturbance in mild to moderate Alzheimer's disease. *Sleep Medicine, 6,* 347–352.

Neylan, T. C., Reynolds, C. F., & Kupfer, D. F. (2003). Sleep disorders. In R. E. Hales, S. C. Yudofsky, (Eds.), *Textbook of Clinical Psychiatry,* (4th ed., pp. 975–1000). Washington, DC: American Psychiatric Publishing.

NIH state-of-the-science conference statement on manifestations and management of chronic insomnia in adults, 2005 Jun 13–15. *National Institute Consensus State of Science Statements, 22,* 1–30. Available online at http://consensus.nih.gov/2005/2005InsomniaSOS026PDF.pdf

North American Nursing Diagnoses Association (NANDA). (2007). *Nursing diagnoses: Definitions and classification 2007–2008.* Philadelphia: Author.

Otte, C., Lenoci, M., Metzler, T., Yehuda, R., Marmar, C. R., & Neylan, T. C. (2007). Effects of metyrapone on hypothalamic-pituitary-adrenal axis and sleep in women with post-traumatic stress disorder. *Biological Psychiatry, 61,* 952–956.

Pack, A. I., Maislin, G., Staley, B., Pack, F. M., Rogers, W. C., George, C. F., & Dinges, D. F. (2006). Impaired performance in commercial drivers: Role of sleep apnea and short sleep duration. *American Journal of Respiratory Critical Care Medicine, 174,* 446–454.

Perlis, M. L., McCall, W. V., Krystal, A. D., & Walsh, J. K. (2004). Long-term, non-nightly administration of zolpidem in the treatment of patients with primary insomnia. *Journal of Clinical Psychiatry, 65,* 1128–1137.

Perlis, M. L., Smith, M. T., & Pigeon, W. R. (2005). Etiology and pathology of insomnia. In M. H. Kryger, T. Roth, W. C. Dement (Eds.), *Principles and Practice of Sleep Medicine,* (4th ed., pp. 714–725). Philadelphia: Elsevier/Saunders.

Petit, D., Touchette, E., Tremblay, R. E., Boivin, M., & Montplaisir, J. (2007). Dyssomnias and parasomnias in early childhood. *Pediatrics, 119,* e1016–1025.

Ranjbaran, Z., Keefer, L., Stephanski, E., Farhadi, A., & Keshavarzian, A. (2007). The relevance of sleep abnormalities to chronic inflammatory conditions. *Inflammatory Research, 56,* 51–57.

Roth, T. (2005). Prevalence, associated risks, and treatment patterns of insomnia. *Journal of Clinical Psychiatry, 66,* Suppl 9, 10–13.

Roth, T., Soubrane, C., Titeux, L., Walsh, J. K., Zoladult Study Group. (2006). Efficacy and safety of zolpidem-MR: A double-blind, placebo-controlled study in adults with primary insomnia. *Sleep Medicine, 7,* 397–406.

Russo, M. B. (2005). Normal sleep, sleep physiology, and sleep deprivation: General principles. www.emedicine.com/neuro/topic444.htm

Saper, C. B. (2006). Staying awake for dinner: Hypothalamic integration of sleep, feeding, and circadian rhythms. *Progress in Brain Research, 153,* 243–252.

Schwartz, J. R., & Roth, T. (2006). Shift work sleep disorder: Burden of illness and approaches to management. *Drugs, 66,* 2357–2370.

Sierra, P., Livianos, L., Argues, S., Castello, J., & Rojo, L. (2007). Prodromal symptoms to relapse in bipolar disorder. *Australia and New Zealand Journal of Psychiatry, 41,* 385–391.

Sigurdson, K., & Ayas, N. T. (2007). The public health and safety consequences of sleep disorders. *Canadian Journal of Physiology and Pharmacology, 85,* 179–183.

Silber, M. H. (2005). Chronic insomnia. *New England Journal of Medicine, 353,* 803–810.

Smaldone, A., Honig, J. C., & Byrne, M. W. (2007). Sleepless in America: Inadequate sleep and relationships to health and well-being of our nation's children. *Pediatrics, 119,* (Suppl 1), S29–S37.

Stewart, R., Besset, A., Bebbington, P., Brugha, T., Lindesay, J., Jenkins, R., et al. (2006). Insomnia comorbidity and impact and hypnotic use by age group in a national survey population aged 16 to 74 years. *Sleep, 29,* 1391–1397.

Theorell-Haglow, J., Lindberg, E., & Janson, C. (2006). What are the important risk factors for daytime sleepiness and fatigue in women? *Sleep, 29,* 751–757.

Weinhouse, C. L., & Schwab, R. J. (2006). Sleep in the critically ill patient. *Sleep, 29,* 707–716.

Wolkove, N., Elkholy, O., Baltzan, M., & Palayew, M. (2007). Sleep and aging: 1. Sleep disorders commonly found in older people. *Canadian Medical Association Journal, 176,* 1299–1304.

Zammit, G. K. (2007). The prevalence, morbidities, and treatments of insomnia. *CNS and Neurological Disorders— Drug Targets, 6,* 3–16.

SUGGESTED READINGS

Lichstein, K. L., & Morin, C. M. (2000). *Treatment of late-life insomnia.* Thousand Oaks, CA: Sage Publishers.

Owens, J. BEARS. www.aassmnet.org/MEDSleep/

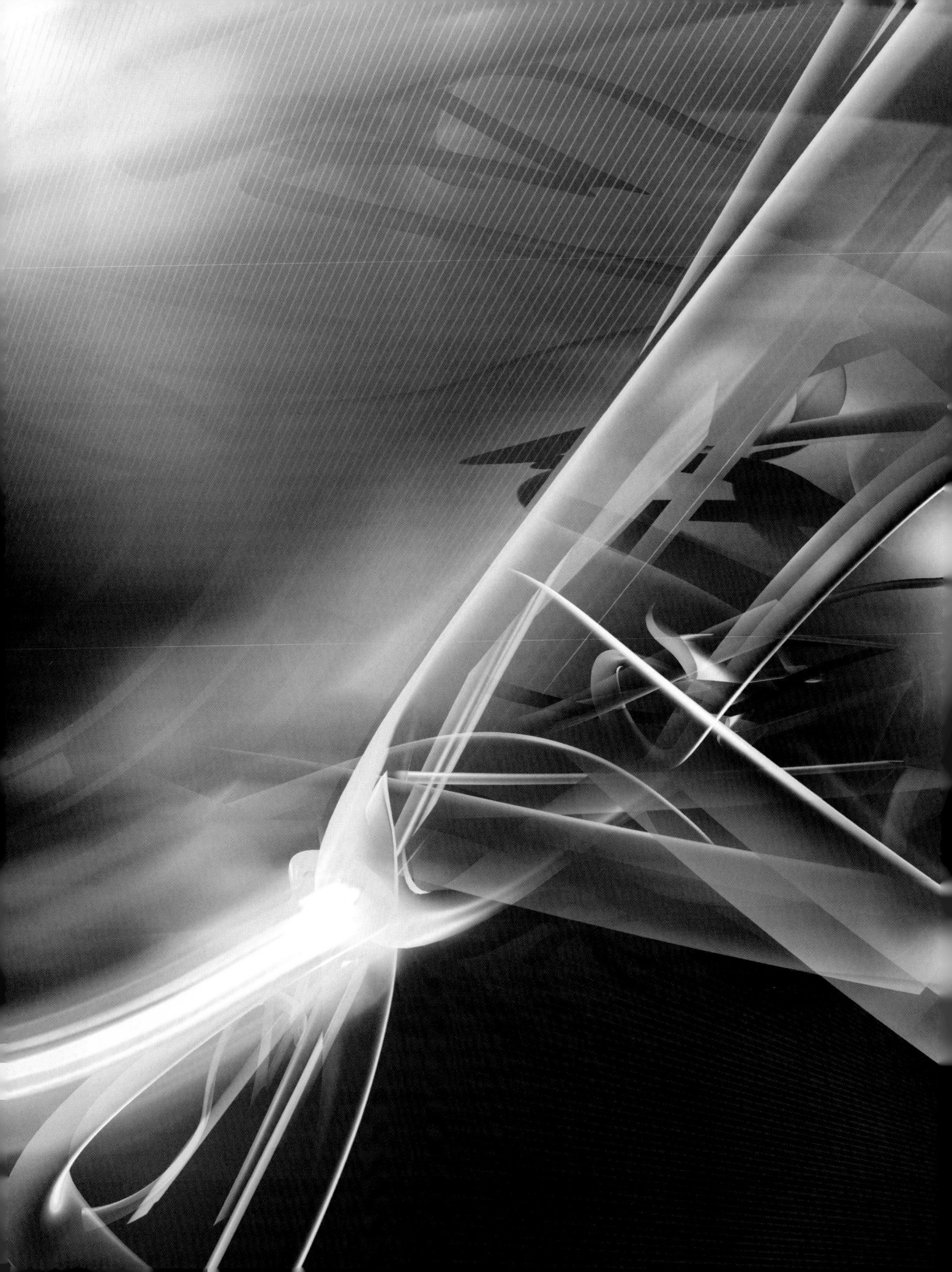

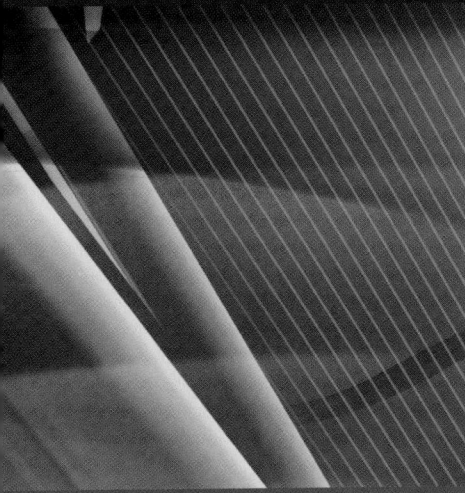

CHAPTER 24

The Client with a Sexual Disorder

Dona H. Caine-Francis, MSN, Psychiatric CNS, PMH-NP
Margaret Brackley, PhD, RN, CS

KEY TERMS

American Association of Sex Educators, Counselors, and Therapists (AASECT): A multidisciplinary national organization of professionals dedicated to the study, education, and role of spokesperson for sexuality.

Declaration of Sexual Rights: A document that identifies 11 human rights stating sexuality is an integral part of the personality of every human being.

Erogenous Zone: Part of the body that is a source of pleasure such as the lips, mouth, genitals, and anus.

Excitement Phase: First phase of the human sexual response cycle in which vasocongestion builds in the man and woman.

Gender: A psychosocial construct that changes over time and is distinct from sex, which is an individual's biological state of maleness or femaleness.

Gender Dysphoria: An intense, persistent discomfort resulting from one's own perception of the inappropriateness of sex assignment made at birth.

Human Sexual Response Cycle: Encompasses four distinct stages in which the body responds to sexual arousal.

Orgasm Phase: Third phase of the human sexual response cycle in which men and women experience rhythmic contractions followed by extreme pleasure.

Plateau Phase: Second phase of the human sexual response cycle marked by vasocongestion and myotonia.

Resolution Phase: Fourth phase of the human sexual response cycle in which the body returns to an unaroused state.

Sexual Attitude Reassessment (SAR): An intensive 2-day workshop to assist participants in reevaluation of sexual attitudes.

Sexual Desire: One's internal psychological state of pleasure governed by sexual pleasure centers in the brain.

Sexual Health: Refers to a state of physical, emotional, psychological, and social well being in regard to sexuality. This state of health extends beyond the absence of disease and dysfunction and ensures the sexual rights of all persons to be respected, protected, and fulfilled (WHO, 2004).

Sexual Orientation: Sexual preference for intimate partners of the same, opposite, or either sex. An individual may be heterosexual, homosexual, lesbian, bisexual, or asexual.

Transgendered: Arching term that describes transsexuals, whose sense of themselves clashes with their original biological sex: cross-dressers, and others whose appearance is at odds with traditional gender expectations.

Transsexual: An individual who is profoundly unhappy in the sex assignment made at birth, and who seeks to change or has changed the body to be as much as possible like that of the opposite sex.

World Association for Sexology (WAS): An international association of sexologists, researchers, and policy makers who develop international policies related to sex.

COMPETENCIES

Upon completion of this chapter, the learner should be able to:

1. Generalize and apply the definition of sexual health for a client experiencing a sexual disorder.

2. Make inferences as to why this time period is referred to as the "third sexual revolution."

3. Synthesize the various theories of sexual development and relate them to sexual health for clients.

4. Identify two different factors that health care professionals use to define sexual problems.

5. Analyze the components of a comprehensive sexual history and formulate a model for use with clients.

6. Discuss sexual disorders across the life span.

7. Analyze the professional nursing roles in relation to sexual themes and issues.

8. Cite clinical examples of and relevant research in sexual health care.

9. Assess the sexual health of a client.

10. Analyze the data obtained in the assessment to determine appropriate diagnoses.

11. Formulate a plan of care for the client with a sexual disorder.

12. Make a referral to an appropriate health care provider if the client is unable or unwilling to execute necessary interventions.

13. Evaluate the plan of care for its effectiveness and revise it if necessary.

CHAPTER OUTLINE

Third Sexual Revolution

Definitions of Sexual Health

The Nurse's Attitude Toward Sexuality

Self-Awareness

Reactions Toward Others

Human Sexuality

Physiology of Human Sexuality

Love

Sexual Orientation

Sexuality: Theories and Perspectives

    Psychoanalytical Theory

    Behavioral Theory

    Social Learning Theory

    Self-Actualization Theories

    Sociological Theories

Psychosocial Causes of Sexual Disorders

Lack of Knowledge

Lack of Communication

Body Image Disturbance

History of Abuse

Fear

Women's Cultural Positions

Homophobia

Aggression

Neurobiological Factors

Depression

Bipolar Disorders

Substance-Use Disorders

Stress and Coping Patterns

Sexuality and Sexual Disorders across the Life Span

Childhood

Adolescence

Young Adulthood

Adulthood

Middle Adulthood

Older Adulthood

Specific Sexual Disorders and Treatment Modalities

Gender Identity Disorders

Sexual Dysfunctions

    Arousal Disorders

    Desire Disorders

    Orgasmic Disorders

    Sexual Pain Disorders

    Sexual Dysfunction Caused by a General Medical Condition

    Substance-Induced Sexual Dysfunction

Paraphilia

The Role of the Nurse

The Generalist Nurse

The Advanced-Practice Psychiatric Registered Nurse

The Nursing Process

Assessment

    Sexual Dysfunction

    Ineffective Sexual Patterns

    Other NANDA Diagnoses

Outcome Identification and Planning

Implementation

Evaluation

Research on Sexual Issues Relevant to Psychiatric Nursing

Sexuality is a basic human right. All human beings are sexual beings. It has been said that people learn about sex from five basic resources: family, friends, school, spiritual centers, and the media. And yet culture also affects sexual development, answering what is and what is not sexually appropriate. On a more personal level, sexual experimentation expands one's knowledge base. Being unable to reach one's sexual potential can have long-lasting effects, not only on personal well-being and health, but also on relationships.

Sexual health is a lifelong process of awareness, exploration, growth, and development. Sexual relationships can propel an individual into new growth potential, create an ongoing laboratory for adventure and satisfaction, or at times become boring and lackluster. When the "sexual connection" is off balance, partners need to use communication skills to explore the lack of interrelatedness and create new opportunities for growth and sexual satisfaction. This chapter challenges the nurse's knowledge of sexuality, attitudes, and biases related to sexual function and assists them in providing a nonjudgmental and respectful environment for their relationships with clients.

THIRD SEXUAL REVOLUTION

Various research professionals in the sexology community believe that people are in the middle of a third sexual revolution with a new mind-set. At the core of the mind-set is the belief that sexual health is a basic human right. Emerging from that belief comes the challenge to all societies to accept and celebrate diversity. This bold challenge is the outcome of the World Association for Sexology (WAS) meeting in Hong Kong in August 1999. Members proposed a Declaration of Sexual Rights and challenged all societies to examine their laws and policies for compliance, not only with universal human rights, but also sexual rights.

Dr. Eli Coleman, president of the WAS in 1999, stated that the third sexual revolution (Williams, 1999) would make the women's emancipation movements of the 1930s and the sexual revolution of the 1960s pale by comparison. The last sexual revolution of the 1960s pushed mankind to acknowledge women's issues, gay and lesbian rights, contraception, and medical advances. One advance was the advent of penicillin for sexually transmitted diseases (STDs). Today's sexual revolution changes at diverse levels: *biological, pharmacologic, social, religious,* and *legal aspects* of living.

Biologically, the sexual life cycle has expanded, thanks to earlier onset of puberty and an increase in average life expectancy. Improved contraception technology, along with better methods of treating infertility, have given people more control over their reproductive lives. Advances on the biomedical front, such as introduction in 1998 of Viagra (sildenafil citrate) to treat erectile dysfunction, have opened up the vast arena of pharmacotherapies for treatment of sexual disorders.

The human immunodeficiency virus (HIV) epidemic has forced communication among public policy makers, sex researchers, educators, and the public to focus on sexual behaviors, new vaccines, and sexual health. Protease inhibitors and other new drugs for the treatment of HIV will cause mother/infant transmission of the virus to decline and will allow people who are HIV positive to live long, productive lives.

On a societal level, all communities are challenged to deal with the impact of the "age of the Internet." Information and relationships have been expanded. It is commonly known that chat rooms, E-mail, cybersex, and Internet dating provide new freedom. Yet new freedoms require new responsibilities.

The revolution is also the result of legal and religious changes. As the influence of organized religion declines throughout the world (Williams, 1999), international law has begun to accommodate same-gender partnerships and to extend legal rights and protections to people, regardless of their sexual orientation. Every revolution puts the present populations to a test, and this third sexual revolution is no different. Each person and community will be required to revisit old notions, beliefs, and behaviors and become more adaptable to future possibilities. In this chapter, a variety of theories on sexual development and health are presented. Sexual issues and themes that the professional nurse will encounter are explored, along with the classification system for specific sexual disorders and treatment modalities. The roles of the generalist and the advanced-practice nurses are then described. Before going any further discussing theories and the like, there is a need to define sexual health and the nurse's responsibility.

DEFINITIONS OF SEXUAL HEALTH

According to World Health Organization, ([WHO], 1975), sexual health is the "integration of the somatic, emotional, intellectual and social aspects of sexual being, in ways that are positively enriching, and that enhance personality, communication and love" (p. 3). The WHO is describing a whole person, in which the sexual self cannot be separated. A sense of unity within the individual thus reflects sexual health as well as nonsexual health. Sexual health is personal. Each person within the context of his physical, emotional, intellectual, social, cultural, and spiritual environment defines it.

The WAS in August 1999 adopted the *Declaration of Sexual Rights* (Williams, 1999). This document identifies 11 human rights and states, "Sexuality is an integral part of the personality of every human being. Its full development depends upon the satisfaction of basic human needs such as the desire for contact, intimacy, emotional expression, pleasure, tenderness and love. Sexuality is constructed through the interaction between the individual and social structures. Full development of sexuality is essential for individual, interpersonal, and societal well being."

THE NURSE'S ATTITUDE TOWARD SEXUALITY

Nursing has traditionally recognized and appreciated humans' holistic nature. However, in spite of a fundamental belief in the importance of the total health of the person, until recently, sexual aspects of health care have been overlooked. There are a number of reasons for this. Human sexuality has traditionally been ignored and its importance downplayed in Western health care in general. In addition, the field of nursing emerged during the Victorian era; when one considers the attitudes and values of that era, along with the religious undertones and traditions of nursing, one can readily grasp why nurses had conflicts with sexual aspects of health. However, nursing professionals have also typically supported knowledge as a method to empower individuals and groups. For example, in the early 1900s, Margaret Sanger led the fight to educate women about their bodies and birth control. In spite of controversy, the American Nurses Association (ANA) has resolved in the 1980s and 1990s to (1) support birth control knowledge and access for men and women, even adolescents; and (2) work to preserve the availability of various alternatives to unwanted pregnancy. Today more nurses are choosing to specialize in sexology. The psychiatric nursing community, in particular the advanced-practice psychiatric registered nurse, in private practice focus on the care given to this population. But they do this using a wide body of knowledge and collaborating within professional associations that provide standards for care and a credentialing process.

In the late 1990s the ANA spoke of the crisis in today's health care system resulting from high costs, limited access, and concerns about quality (ANA Position Statement, p. 2). In response to the crisis, development of the role of the Psychiatric Mental Health-Nurse Practitioner (PMH-NP) began to offer mental health clients an affordable, accessible, quality provider. PMH-NPs are in a position to provide a broad array of services, due to their educational background, expertise in primary mental health care delivery, and ability to collaborate and refer to appropriate providers. In addition to psychotherapeutic skills, the curriculum includes physical diagnosis; health promotion; pharmacology; pathophysiology; and management of acute, episodic, and chronic health care problems with practicums in these areas. The educational endeavor prepares the clinician to offer holistic services including diagnosis, treatment, and prescriptive therapy.

American Association of Sex Educators, Counselors, and Therapists (AASECT) is a multidisciplinary, national association for sexology professionals. AASECT, along with Sexuality Information Education Council of the United States (SIECUS), have become one center for sexual public policy issues in the United States. AASECT provides standards and a credentialing process for professionals to advance their knowledge and skill levels, thus providing quality sexual care to clients.

SELF-AWARENESS

Self-awareness and awareness of others regarding sexual issues or themes are key attributes nurses need to be most effective in their role of client advocate. First, nurses need to be aware of their own attitudes, values, and beliefs regarding sexual health. Second, nurses need to be aware of their clients' sexual issues. Third, nurses need to be aware of how their personal attitudes, values, and beliefs affect their ability to recognize and react to clients' sexual issues and themes. The nurse who has self-awareness is able to do quality checks on the nursing care he delivers. The unaware nurse is unable to do this.

REACTIONS TOWARD OTHERS

A word of caution is appropriate here. Untoward reactions have been observed in nurses faced with sexual issues and themes. Strong reactions may indicate the need for the nurse to seek help to address personal issues that prevent his own sexual health. Seeking outside help to work through and resolve sexual issues and themes is strongly encouraged. Both the nurse and the client will benefit from resolving issues that prevent self-awareness in the nurse.

Throughout history and across cultures, many standards for sexual behavior have been accepted. One current standard for human sexual behavior is that pleasure should be maximized, whereas the coercion of others and giving and receiving of pain is minimized. Thus a wide range of human sexual behavior exists. It is often unsettling and even upsetting to nurses who have not examined their own sexual attitudes, values, and beliefs to be faced with the diversity of sexual behaviors that human beings exhibit from person to person and culture to culture. As in various aspects of nursing care, the nurse is expected to be nonjudgmental in delivering sexual health care. Being nonjudgmental does not imply agreement with others' values and beliefs.

The World Association for Sexology Declaration of Sexual Rights

Adopted August 26, 1999

Sexual rights are universal human rights based on the inherent freedom, dignity, and equality of all human beings. Since health is a fundamental human right, so must sexual health be a basic human right. In order to assure that human beings and societies develop healthy sexuality, the following sexual rights must be recognized, promoted, respected, and defended by all societies through all means. Sexual health is the result of an environment that recognizes, respects, and exercises these sexual rights.

1. *The right to sexual freedom.* Sexual freedom encompasses the possibility for individuals to express their full sexual potential. However, this excludes all forms of sexual coercion, exploitation, and abuse at any time and situations in life.

2. *The right to sexual autonomy, sexual integrity, and safety of the sexual body.* This right involves the ability to make autonomous decisions about one's sexual life within a context of one's own personal and social ethics. It also encompasses control and enjoyment of our own bodies free from torture, mutilation and violence of any sort.

3. *The right to sexual privacy.* This involves the right for individual decisions and behaviors about intimacy as long as they do not intrude on the sexual rights of others.

4. *The right to sexual equity.* This refers to freedom from all forms of discrimination regardless of sex, gender, sexual orientation, age, race, social class, religion, or physical and emotional disability.

5. *The right to sexual pleasure.* Sexual pleasure, including autoeroticism, is a source of physical, psychological, intellectual and spiritual well being.

6. *The right to emotional sexual expression.* Sexual expression is more than erotic pleasure or sexual acts. Individuals have a right to express their sexuality through communication, touch, emotional expression and love.

7. *The right to sexually associate freely.* This means the possibility to marry or not, to divorce, and to establish other types of responsible sexual associations.

8. *The right to make free and responsible reproductive choices.* This encompasses the right to decide whether or not to have children, the number and spacing of children, and the right to full access to the means of fertility regulation.

9. *The right to sexual information based upon scientific inquiry.* This right implies that sexual information should be generated through the process of unencumbered and yet scientifically ethical inquiry, and disseminated in appropriate ways at all societal levels.

10. *The right to comprehensive sexuality education.* This is a lifelong process from birth throughout the lifecycle and should involve all social institutions.

11. *The right to sexual health care.* Sexual health care should be available for prevention and treatment of all sexual concerns, problems and disorders.

CRITICAL THINKING

Mary Ann has come to the clinic in marital crisis. She and her husband, Mike, have been married for 3 years. They recently had a baby, and Mary Ann finds herself exhausted, with no sexual desire for Mike. You are the assessing nurse at the clinic. As Mary Ann states her history, you empathize and begin to identify with her symptoms of hypoactive sexual desire. Since entering nursing school you find your own desire to wax and wane in your relationship. Which of the following would be appropriate interventions?

a. Tell Mary Ann you know exactly how she feels, telling her about your own dilemma.

b. Help her identify options to decrease her stress and discuss communication interventions with her husband to expand their understanding in the relationship.

c. Make an appointment to talk with the psychiatric clinical nurse specialist at the clinic and discuss your countertransference issue.

d. Talk with your husband about the case, hoping he will understand your dilemma through the similarities.

If the nurse cares about the client, the client's experience is worthy of concern, regardless of how it differs from the nurse's. To assist in this process of understanding one's sexual attitudes, AASECT promotes Sexual Attitude Reassessment (SAR) seminars. SAR is an intensive 2-day workshop. It provides a process-oriented, structured group experience in which participants are exposed to a wide spectrum of topics and sexually explicit media presentations with discussions throughout the seminar. This multidisciplinary workshop can enhance the sexual awareness of the neophyte to the expert nurse in all practice arenas.

HUMAN SEXUALITY

The concept of human sexuality and response is a mind and body experience that involves a cascade of biological responses to sexual stimulation. The *DSM-IV-TR* (APA, 2000) describes this cascade as a four-phase response cycle: desire, excitement, orgasmic, and resolution. Psychiatric nurses are more likely to respond appropriately and effectively to questions and concerns about human sexuality when they understand the concept of human sexuality and its impact on quality of life. The following section depicts the human sexual response cycle.

PHYSIOLOGY OF HUMAN SEXUALITY

A brief review of normal human sexuality helps the nurse understand and compare behaviors and symptoms in the client with a sexual disorder. The classic work of Masters and Johnson (1966) set the stage for our current understanding of the four stages in the human sexual response cycle. The contributions of this research team in the 1950s and 1960s opened the science of sexology. They observed more than 700 men and women in approximately 10,000 cycles of sexual arousal and orgasm. On the basis of their observations, they identified the following stages of sexual response: excitement, plateau, orgasm, and resolution. The physiological processes of vasocongestion (increased blood flow to the genital area) and myotonia (muscle contraction throughout the body) occur during sexual activity.

The excitement phase begins with arousal. Vasocongestion produces an erection in the male sex organ, the penis, and lubrication in the female's vaginal canal. During the excitement phase, the woman's clitoris and breast tissue swell. The inner and outer lips, or labia, of the vagina swell and flatten out, while the vagina balloons out and the cervix pulls up internally to accommodate the penis. The clitoris has been compared to the man's penis in that it is made of spongy tissue that fills with blood during arousal. Like the penis the clitoral hood retracts as excitement builds. Recent studies reveal the true size of the clitoris to be about 3 to 4 inches long, with approximately 2 inches hidden inside the body.

Both the man and woman may develop a sexual flush that resembles a measles rash on the upper abdomen and chest.

Pulse and blood pressure increase in both sexes. The skin of the man's scrotum thickens, the scrotal sac tenses, and the contents of the sac pull up closer to the body. The spermatic cord shortens, elevating the testes.

Plateau phase is marked by involuntary contractions in the man's and woman's genitals. The man's penis is completely erect, testes become engorged, and a few drops of fluid appear at the tip of the penis. This fluid may contain live sperm. In the woman, the outer third portion of the vagina swells and thickens. The vagina becomes smaller; the clitoris retracts into the body, becoming more sensitive to touch and increasing the levels of arousal. Vasocongestion and myotonia continue to build until the resultant tension produces an orgasm.

Orgasm phase in the man is characterized by rhythmic contractions. Ejaculate is forced into a bulb at the end of the urethra, and then the urethra bulb and the penis itself contract rhythmically to force semen out. In the woman the process is similar. Some women who have very strong pubococcygeal (PC) muscles expel fluid from the urethra during orgasm. They describe the fluid as watered-down skim milk, tasting sweet and usually about a teaspoon in volume. Alice Ladas, Marilyn Whipple, and John Perry (1983) developed a device to measure uterine muscle strength in addition to PC muscle strength. Their study revealed that women who experienced ejaculation possessed stronger uterine and PC muscles. In analyzing the contents of ejaculate, they found a significant difference between urine and female ejaculate in terms of glucose, fructose, prostatic acid phosphatase, urea, and creatinine.

Rhythmic contractions of the muscles occur in the man and woman about 0.8-second intervals during orgasm. Both the woman and the man experience sudden increases in pulse rate, blood pressure, and breathing. Muscles contract throughout the body, including the anal sphincter.

In the resolution phase, the body returns to the unaroused state. The processes of vasocongestion and myotonia are reversed. In the woman, breast swelling and sex flush disappear rapidly, and the genital changes that occurred during arousal disappear. Resolution occurs in 15 to 30 minutes, unless the woman did not reach orgasm, in which case resolution can take up to 1 hour. Many women have the ability to have multiple orgasms with additional clitoral stimulation. Sexologists remain in debate over male multiorgasmic experiences. In both the man and woman, pulse rate, blood pressure, and breathing gradually return to normal. In the man, penile erection is lost immediately. A refractory period occurs in which the man is incapable of arousal. The length of the refractory period varies with age and other individual differences. In older men, it may last up to 24 hours, whereas in some younger men it lasts only a few minutes. A refractory period is not present in women.

Kaplan (1974) suggested an alternative to the Masters and Johnson model based on her work as a sex therapist. This biphasic model was divided into vasocongestion and muscular contractions. Later, a third phase—sexual desire—was added. Because vasocongestion and muscular contraction are controlled by separate parts of the nervous system, the parasympathetic and sympathetic nervous systems, respectively, this approach has merit. In clients with sexual problems, treatment depends on the part of the central nervous system affected. Sexual desire also has a neurophysiological component.

The nervous system and sex hormones are important parts of sexual desire and behavior. The sex hormones, testosterone, an androgen secreted by the male testes, and progesterone, an estrogen secreted by the female ovaries, are regulated by the anterior lobe of the pituitary gland and the hypothalamus, located on the lower side of the brain. The hypothalamus, pituitary, gonads, testes, and ovaries work together in sexual functions such as the menstrual cycle, pregnancy, puberty, and sexual behavior (Georgiadis et al., 2006; Sisk & Zehr, 2005). The human sexual response is complex. Sexual disorders and difficulties can arise from multiple sources within this cycle. Some of these are discussed in the remainder of this chapter.

There are more than 25 infectious diseases that can be transmitted through sexual activity, STDs, and can lead to female infertility and life-threatening pregnancy complications. The Centers for Disease Control and Prevention (CDC) in Atlanta, Georgia state that sexually transmitted diseases remain a major threat in the United States and estimate 19 million STD infections occur annually (CDC, 2005); almost half among youth ages 15 to 24. Three reportable diseases are chlamydia, gonorrhea, and syphilis. And yet, many more are not reportable including human papillomavirus (HPV), and herpes. Of the reportable STDs there are over 4 million cases of chlamydia in the United States each year making it the most common treatable STD. In its early stages, chlamydia causes no symptoms in 75 percent of women and half of men. According to the CDC (2005), approximately 25 percent of the estimated 1 million persons living with human immunodeficiency virus (HIV) in the United States are unaware that they are infected with HIV and are at risk for transmitting the virus to others. Recent findings from a study using rapid HIV testing in emergency departments implicate the importance of integrating HIV testing in clients seeking help in emergency rooms to ensure early treatment and prevention (CDC, 2007). Knowing a partner's sexual history—previous partners, STDs, what form of birth control and protection are used—are critical areas of communication in today's sexual climate.

Two lesser-known diseases are responsible for two thirds of all new cases of sexually transmitted diseases in the United States. Human papillomavirus (HPV) and trichomoniasis are not as notorious as syphilis, herpes, chlamydia, gonorrhea, or HIV, but they can cause serious health problems.

According to the CDC (2004) Fact Sheet, genital human papillomavirus (HPV) is the most common sexually transmitted infection in the United States, and more than 20 million people are presently infected. Women are at the highest risk of being infected. Women have an 80 percent chance of getting HPV by the time they are 50. Annual estimates indicate that about 6.2 million people get a new HPV infection each year. Young people who are in their late teens and early 20s are most likely to be infected. HPV refers to a group of viruses that includes more than 100 strains or types, of which 30 are sexually transmitted and generally infect the genital areas of men and women. Although the majority of HPV infections cause no clinical symptoms and are self-limited, persistent infection with oncogenic types is associated with cervical cancer. The American Cancer Society estimates that more than 11,000 women will be diagnosed with cervical cancer, of which 3,600 will die, in the United States. The first HPV quadrivalent vaccine, Gardasil, formulated to prevent cervical cancer and genital warts caused by HPV, was introduced in 2007. This vaccine works by protecting against four types of HPV commonly noted to cause these diseases. Medical recommendations suggest administering the vaccine to girls 11 and 12 years of age and also to older girls and women who did not receive it when they were younger (Markowitz et al., 2007). Controversy about the vaccination of girls ages 11 and 12 continues to be debated by states in which vaccinations are mandatory.

As many as 5 million Americans get the parasitic infection trichomoniasis every year, but many do not know they have it. Men are often asymptomatic. In women it can cause a discharge with an unpleasant odor, which lead many to mistake it for a yeast infection. If left untreated, trichomoniasis can lead to preterm labor. This STD can be cured with antibiotics.

LOVE

Love is a very human trait that is not mentioned often in nursing or sex education textbooks. Romantic love and sexual activities appear to go together and yet there is discomfort in talking about the relationship between them. These concepts are elusive. A major component that enhances the love connection and moves a relationship to new levels is intimacy. At the heart of intimacy is self-disclosure, feeling safe enough in a relationship to be vulnerable and share oneself.

Janet Woitiz (1985) states, "intimacy means you have a love relationship with another person where you offer, and are offered, validation, understanding and a sense of being valued intellectually, emotionally and physically." Thus intimacy gives an individual the freedom to be oneself, not to walk on eggshells, have a fear of being judged, or make a mistake. More about the relationship between love and sex is offered in the section on helping people change their sexual behavior.

SEXUAL ORIENTATION

The American Psychiatric Association (APA, 2000) considers variations in sexual orientation, that is, homosexuality and bisexuality, as healthy sexuality. No one knows why a person becomes gay, lesbian, or bisexual. Theories that have posited that nonheterosexual sexual orientations result from disturbed family relationships, labeling of opposite-gender-linked behavior (boys playing with dolls), or an unpleasant sexual experience have not been supported through scientific study.

Although it seems plausible that there is a biological basis for differences, there is little evidence to support this premise. Controversy surrounding the precise basis of sexual orientation continues, indicating the underpinning of sexual orientation requires additional research. The complex interactions between sexual development—within the context of neurodevelopmental factors—social and familial systems, and individual traits may play key roles in sexual orientation (Bogaert, 2007; Rahman, 2005).

Researchers have used positron emission tomography (PET) scans of the brain to study one particular part of the hypothalamus, called the central division of the bed nucleus of the stria terminalis (BSTc). This area, which is thought to influence sexual behavior, is on average 44 percent larger in men than in women. Other studies are under way to further understand brain function, physiology, and their role in sexual orientation.

SEXUALITY: THEORIES AND PERSPECTIVES

It is important to know the different theoretical perspectives on sexuality. No theory can claim to be the real truth. This chapter, while acknowledging the different viewpoints of theorists, focuses on the here-and-now problem of the client, the perception and awareness of both the client and nurse, and the nurse's role in helping the client solve the identified problem. In sexual health care, as in all nursing activity, the nurse's therapeutic use of the self is expected. The therapeutic interaction between nurse and client should never be underestimated. The nurse's concern for and acceptance of the client and the problem can have a profound influence on the health care outcome.

Psychoanalytical Theory

In his theory of personality development, Sigmund Freud (1962) stated that parts of the personality are unconscious. This theory has become most influential in Western thought. Freud developed an idea of sexual energy or drive that he called *libido*. Libido is the major motivating force behind human behavior, according to Freud.

In psychoanalytical theory, the personality is subdivided into three sections: the id, ego, and superego. The *id* is the source of psychic energy; it contains the libido and operates on the pleasure principle. The *ego* helps keep the id's energy under control. It acts in concert with the reality principle. The *superego*, or conscience, operates in response to an ideal principle. For example, if left on its own, the id would seek out pleasure without regard to social mores or consequences of its behavior. The id must have a functioning ego to keep it from doing what is unacceptable to others in public, such as masturbating while riding on the subway. The superego checks both pleasure and reality-oriented behavior by adhering to ideal behavior as taught within the context of a particular culture. For example, a person has been taught that it is wrong to let another person believe a relationship will be ongoing when sexual intercourse is really all that is

sought. The id wants intercourse, the ego knows the potential sexual partner wants involvement as well as intercourse, and the superego prevents the ego and id from promising a commitment that is not really felt. As other examples, a person's superego may believe that one must not receive pleasure by giving another person pain or that one should not engage in sexual intercourse before marriage. See Chapter 2 for an in-depth discussion of psychoanalytic concepts.

Freudian theory has had a profound influence on how society, particularly, views human development and behavior. Even though Freud has fallen into disfavor in recent years, this theory of personality remains the standard against which we hold all others accountable. In terms of psychosexual development, Freud believed the child passed through developmental stages, each focused on a different erogenous zone. An erogenous zone is a part of the body—such as the lips and mouth, genitals, anus, and rectum—that is a source of pleasure. Sucking and defecating cause pleasure, as does rubbing the genitals. According to Freud, a person could become fixated, or stuck, in a stage if passage through it was blocked. Nail biting or thumb sucking might be considered evidence of being fixated at the oral stage, for instance.

Freud's perception of women and sexuality reflected his era. Nowadays, feminists support the notion that he was speaking and acting on his own biased Victorian viewpoint of women, rather than on scientific evidence (Donovan, 1988).

Behavioral Theory

Learning theories are based on the notion that the frequency with which a behavior is enacted is related to reinforcement or punishment from something or someone within the individual's internal or external environment. Some rewards, like food and sex, are considered primary. That is, they are intrinsically rewarding. If a person is hungry, food decreases the hunger, rewarding the person. See Chapter 2 for a discussion of behavioral theories.

Behavior modification is a common modality used in treatment of male orgasmic disorders or premature ejaculation. Clients are taught to identify the "point of inevitability"—that moment in time when one knows orgasm is imminent. Masturbation exercises are the framework in which the man identifies the point of inevitability, withholds further stimulation, desensitizes his body to acute pleasure, and choreographs a new pleasure threshold for sexual activity with his partner.

Life experiences and learning influence sexual behavior. A person whose first experience with sex-related activities was positive is more likely to increase the frequency of these activities than is a person whose first sex-related experience was not positive. If the first encounter with sex involves punishment, like the pain of rape or the guilt of being caught and severely punished for masturbating, the behavior is less likely to occur later or may occur in an altered form. An example of sex of an altered form is a woman's becoming sexually promiscuous or a prostitute after undergoing prolonged sexual abuse as a child. Perhaps as a child, she received extra spending money for keeping silent about the abuse and now associates sex with money or comfort, not love.

Punishment and reward must be immediate to shape behavior. If a person does something "bad" and is not caught and punished until time passes or is not punished every time the behavior is enacted, chances are the frequency of the behavior will not decrease. In fact, it may increase. Behavior modification, the use of operant conditioning to change behavior, has become popular in educational as well as therapeutic settings. Aversion therapy, or punishing the behavior until it no longer occurs, has also been used in sex therapy.

Aversion therapy was used years ago in work with sex offenders. In extreme cases, castration was seen as an option. Today castration is seen as a violation of our sense of civilization. Relapse prevention treatment strategies and the "no cure" mind-set are predominate forms of treatment for sex offenders.

Social Learning Theory

In the dominant American culture, social learning of sexual behaviors is not direct. Sexual activities occur behind closed doors and on the screen in movie theaters. Consequently, much learning about sex is through indirect example and innuendo, which open up the possibility of misunderstanding and lack of information. Children have five general resources for sexual learning: parents, spiritual centers, school, peers, and the media. Parents have the opportunity to be the primary sex educator for children and yet, all too often, because of poor or no role modeling, they abdicate this role (Dumas, 1996; Lou, Zhao, Gao, Shah, 2006; Macdowall et al., 2006).

Self-Actualization Theories

Humanistic psychologists, notably Maslow (1970) and Rogers (1951), view humans as growth oriented. Sex is viewed as one of many means of achieving self-actualization, one's human potential. Sex is not merely for reproduction, but rather a means of having fun, giving and receiving pleasure. For many, accepting pleasure can be difficult outside as well as inside the bedroom. Often an individual is more comfortable giving than receiving and may consistently place the needs of others before his own (Hooper, 1992). Feeling that one deserves pleasure is an essential element in a healthy sexual relationship and leads to higher levels of self-actualization. Learning to be comfortable with pleasure and pleasuring can be a challenge. It requires several things; first, one must learn what satisfies; second, one must have the ability to communicate this information to one's partner; third, be specific about sexual preferences; and last, learn to accept pleasure from a partner.

Impersonal sex, in which another human being is treated as a sex object, is incongruent with the tenets of self-actualization. The goal of being an authentic person cannot be achieved through using another for sexual gratification or abusing the sexual relationship.

Sociological Theories

The structural-functional theory of families addresses sexual behavior. According to this point of view, sex roles are fixed and oriented toward maintaining the structure of society. The belief is that society regulates sexuality in an effort to preserve order and prevent chaos. Regulation occurs through laws, religious teaching, accepted behaviors of the group, and division of labor.

The Internet has had a major impact on sexuality from a sociological basis. People use sex-related Internet sites for entertainment and recreation, much as they would use other materials such as magazines and videos. Men accessed sexual content more than women, and they tended to prefer visual stimuli, whereas women spent more time at interactive, communication-oriented sites, specifically chat rooms. It has been noted that for those predisposed to sexually compulsive behavior, online sexual content is a more powerful trigger than traditional materials owing to the Internet's "Triple A"— access, affordability, and anonymity.

PSYCHOSOCIAL CAUSES OF SEXUAL DISORDERS

As previously discussed, causative factors associated with sexual disorders are complex and multidimensional and include a host of causes. Of particular interest is the role of psychosocial causes and the role of the nurse in promoting healthy resolution of signs and symptoms of sexual disorders and an optimal level of functioning.

LACK OF KNOWLEDGE

People's lack of knowledge about sex can give them problems. There has been great debate in America over the last several decades as to what children should be taught about sex, when, and by whom it should be taught. One segment of the population views sex and reproduction education as a private family matter, whereas another faction views sex and reproduction as a social issue that affects the population as a whole, thereby requiring public education. Some people believe that if adolescents have knowledge of sex and birth control, they will be promiscuous, leading to the breakdown of the social fabric of society. And yet, the opposite is true; when children have sexual information, can ask parents questions, and sexual conversations are given at different times about different subjects, they make wiser choices for themselves (Lou et al., 2006).

Comprehensive sexuality education versus abstinence-only education has been debated widely in this country and others. In June 1999, a survey sponsored by Advocates for Youth and SIECUS reported wide support among American adults for broad-based sexuality education. However, under the

Nurse Leslie is admitting John, a 49-year-old man, into the care unit for chest pain. As part of her nursing history she will include a sex history. Some options for this discussion are listed below. Which is the most appropriate?

a. "Now, I need to ask you some questions about your sexuality."

b. "After a heart attack, many people have questions about resuming sexual relations. What are your present concerns?"

c. "I understand you were in bed with your wife when the chest pain began. Were you having sex?"

d. "A normal part of the assessment is taking a sexual history. Describe your present sexual relationship with your wife. What are your current concerns?"

rubric of preventing teen pregnancy, the welfare reform legislation passed by Congress in 1996 included a provision that made $50 million a year available to the states for abstinence education for 5 years through 2002.

There are currently three federal programs dedicated to funding restrictive abstinence-only education: Section 510 of the Social Security Act; the Abstinence Family Life Act, teenage pregnancy prevention component; and the Special Projects of Regional and National Significance program (SPRANS).

Even with the federal funding for these restrictive programs, evidence shows that comprehensive sexuality education

Findings from the 2007 DHHS study *Impacts of Four Title V, Section 510 Abstinence Education Programs* Final Report, April 2007, revealed the following:

◆ Overall, the programs had no effect on the sexual abstinence of youth.

◆ Youths in these programs were no less likely to have unprotected sex, a concern that has been raised by some critics of these programs.

◆ Youngsters in the four evaluated programs were no more likely than youth not in the programs to have abstained from sex in the four to six years after they began participating in the study.

◆ Youths in both groups who reported having had sex also had similar numbers of sexual partners and had initiated sex at the same average age.

This document can be downloaded at http://www.mathematica-mpr.com/publications/pdfs/impactabstinence.pdf

programs that provide information about both abstinence and contraception can help delay the onset of sexual activity in teenagers, reduce their number of sexual partners, and increase contraceptive use when they become sexually active. These findings were part of *Call to Action to Promote Sexual Health and Responsible Sexual Behavior*, issued by former Surgeon General David Satcher in June 2001 (Satcher, 2001).

Parents and grandparents by virtue of their relationship to children and the importance of their message are the primary sexuality educators for children. Schools teaching abstinence-only sex education limit the information children receive. In fact, sex education in schools may provide helpful curriculum, but experience shows it can only supplement the information and attitudes gained at home.

Nursing has traditionally supported knowledge as a method to empower individuals and groups. Sex education has become a part of nursing practice, whether the nurse works in a school, birth control clinic, and hospital or community system. Nurses need to be knowledgeable about sex and aware of a client's need for information. Getting in the habit of asking clients about sex-related issues or whether they have any questions about sex issues is a good idea. The nurse who cannot or is unwilling to address the client's sex-related questions is obligated to make a referral to a specialized sex educator or sex therapist.

LACK OF COMMUNICATION

Communication is an integral part of all relationships and provides the venue to resolve problems and address issues. Sexual satisfaction is positively correlated with effective communication and marital harmony. This is particularly important when individuals fail to openly communicate their sexual needs to their partners. Researchers submit that long-term sexual relationships and sexual satisfaction are positively correlated with several intimacy issues, the partner's ability to perform sexually, and negatively correlated with marital or couple discord (Haning, et al., 2007; Litzinger & Gordon, 2005). Poor communication is often the reason couples seek sex and marital therapy.

Relationship and intimacy satisfaction are also linked to communication and receptiveness to one's partner's unmet intimacy needs. Poor communication is likely to interfere with intimacy and a willingness to share feelings or discuss unmet sexual needs. In comparison, effective communication engenders trust, empathy, and a willingness to respond to the partner's concerns and unmet needs, and ultimately promotes intimacy satisfaction. When working with couples presenting with ineffective or poor communication skills, it is imperative to thoroughly assess how feelings are expressed, the level of intimacy, and the quality of relationships. Collectively, these factors affect sexual satisfaction and must be addressed as target interventions and outcome measures when couples present with sexual problems. Psychiatric nurses can help couples improve their communication through psychoeducation concerning ways to express their feelings appropriately and develop effective problem-solving skills. See Chapter 28 for a detailed discussion of marital and couples therapy.

BODY IMAGE DISTURBANCE

A person's body image may be the source of his sexual problems. We all have in our minds an ideal body image that has been shaped by our culture. Both male and female Americans have been found to be dissatisfied with some aspects of their bodies.

Body image disturbances also result from medical conditions and surgical procedures that affect one's perception of body, including certain cancers and medical conditions. Surgical procedures, including mastectomy, ileostomy, colostomy, and hysterectomy, often affect self–body image, quality of life, and sexual function. Sexual function is also impacted by reproductive cycles across the life span, including dysmenorrhea and menopause. Psychiatric nurses play key roles in helping women and men cope with physical and emotional distress associated with these conditions. In addition, people with disabilities may suffer from body image problems that affect their sexual function. Similar to other clients with body image disturbances, these individuals can gain a more meaningful and quality sexual function with the help of sex therapists and nurses.

HISTORY OF ABUSE

Past experience of abuse can lead to sexual problems. Sexual abuse in childhood, inappropriate parent-child relationships, rape (both in and out of marriage), and other traumas can have lasting effects on sexuality. Sometimes, the experience of past abuse has been repressed to such degree that the abuse survivor has no awareness or memory of it. Sexual problems may appear bizarre and unexplainable or understandable. The following clinical example reflects these issues.

FEAR

Fear is yet another cause of sexual problems. For example, fear of pregnancy or STDs such as HIV infection can interfere with sexual satisfaction. Although nurses must encourage and explicitly teach clients avoidance of risky sexual practices, giving the idea that sex is dangerous and that all aspects of human closeness should be avoided is shortsighted and irresponsible. Sex is a basic human need that involves much more than intercourse. Nonrisky behaviors such as cuddling, necking, petting, and mutual masturbation can be encouraged as alternatives to risky behaviors. To encourage unattainable standards like total abstinence may lead to hopeless, helpless feelings that end in the client's abandoning any effort to control unsafe sex practices.

David Schnarch, a sex therapist (1997), described the concept of "wanting." One partner may "not want to want" the other, thus equating sexual closeness with fear. "Wanting to be wanted" demonstrates one's ability to experience sexual closeness as a positive aspect of the relationship, neither too close to fear engulfment by the other nor too far apart to feel rejected. This concept is helpful in working with clients to assist them in disclosing their feelings about sexual desire in relationship to their partner.

WOMEN'S CULTURAL POSITIONS

Cultural factors influence women's positions and roles within societies. In societies in which women are devalued and experience sexual violence and risk of HIV infection, women are less likely to experience sexual freedom or even control over their bodies. The World Health Organization and other human rights organizations are working to improve the health of women exposed to violence and focus on sexual and reproductive health and the prevention of HIV infection. In Western societies, women also face many challenges related to being in the workforce and maintaining their roles as homemakers, partners in relationships, and parents. Oftentimes, women find themselves too tired and busy to have a quality sexual relationship with their spouse or partner.

HOMOPHOBIA

Homophobia, the irrational fear of homosexuality, is a common occurrence in American life. Groups as varied as

CLINICAL EXAMPLE

The Client with a Sexual Desire Disorder

One couple who entered therapy, Sally and Mike complained of discrepancies of desire. Mike's desire was greater than Sally's. He felt rejected and awkward in their sexual relationship. Sally had been sexually abused by her father from the age of 7 until age 12, when she told him "no." She had become Dad's surrogate wife. Yet, when confronted, Dad left home, married a younger woman, and totally avoided Sally and her mother. This left Sally feeling responsible for the ending of family life, even as turbulent as it had been. She experienced a "sexual stall-out" at age 12, leaving her unable to tap into her full potential of sexuality in her marital relationship.

In therapy she was able to acknowledge her grief associated with sexual abuse and understand that she was not responsible for her parents divorce. As a couple they worked together to establish a reasonable sexual climate and the ability to pleasure one another through romantic connections.

Nurses need to ask about past and present sexual abuse. Many clients in substance abuse units, inpatient and outpatient, have histories of abuse. It is more difficult to assess the prevalence of history of abuse among clients in general psychiatric wards; however, sexual abuse is thought to be widespread.

political campaigns, spiritual centers, and the APA (2000) have studied homosexuality in our culture. Opinions range from homosexuality is immoral to a normal sexual variation. In 1974, the APA voted that homosexuality is not a mental disorder. In spite of this, gay men and lesbian women continue to experience discrimination, ridicule, and hate crimes.

AGGRESSION

Aggression can be played out sexually in our culture. Rape is an example of using sex as a weapon in an aggressive act. According to the Alan Guttmacher Institute (1999), there are at least four types of rapists. There is the one whose assault is the explosive expression of a pent-up sexual impulse. The sadistic rapists comprise a second group. They are motivated by an impulse to punish and hurt the victim. The impact of suffering seems to fuel their sexual satisfaction. A third type is the aggressive criminal out to pillage and rob. Last are those whose offenses appear entirely dissociated from sex impulse but that actually are in the nature of symbolic sex acts (such as kleptomaniacs).

Sadomasochism is another form of aggressive sexuality practiced by some couples. For some individuals, prior emotional, sexual, or physical abuse can contribute in some cases to a person's need to engage in this self-destructive behavior. There are two roles in the sadomasochistic setting. The dominant person (sadist) who derives sexual pleasure by degrading, humiliating, binding, or inflicting pain on the sex partner, and the submissive partner (masochist) who receives this treatment, and in the process, claims to derive sexual pleasure. At the 2002 national conference in Miami, Florida, the AASECT provided several workshops to assist sex therapists owing to client increase of interest in bondage-dominance-sadomasochistic (BDSM) behaviors. Unfortunately, death can result from this form of sex play. A cardinal rule of BDSM is that everything that happens in the sex play is consensual. Individuals engaged in this process who feel unsafe then have the responsibility to stop the process and protect themselves.

NEUROBIOLOGICAL FACTORS

As mentioned earlier, sexual activity is a complex endeavor that involves many factors. The neurobiological aspects of sexuality are affected by age, genetic makeup, disease, use of mood-altering substances, nutrition, and many other variables.

DEPRESSION

Underlying depression may lead to fatigue and feelings of unworthiness. Lack of libido from dysregulation of various neurochemistry processes is probable. Depressed people often report no interest in sexual activity. The selective serotonin uptake inhibitor (SSRI) medications available in the marketplace have led to speedy resolution of depressive symptoms. Examples of SSRIs include Citalopram (Celexa) and escitalopram (Lexapro). The serotonin-norepinephrine reuptake inhibitors (SNRIs), such as venlafaxine (Effexor) and duloxetine (Cymbalta), are also associated with sexual side effects similar to SSRIs. These drugs tend to be the first line of treatment for depressive and anxiety disorders because of their safer side effects profile and efficacy. However, a major drawback are the sexual side effects of these medications—for some individuals a decrease in sexual desire, for many, orgasmic retardation. Sexual side effects are a major reason for nonadherence to antidepressant medications and the major reason for nonadherence to medications in general. In addition, other medications, such as bupropion (Wellbutrin), should also be considered because of fewer sexual side effects. Nurses working with clients who are depressed and are experiencing sexual problems need to inform them of these side effects and assist them in their decision making.

BIPOLAR DISORDERS

Bipolar disorders, both depressed and manic episodes, along with medications used to treat them, can cause sexual problems. During manic episodes, the client is more likely to be hypersexual and impulsive and engage in high-risk behaviors, such as unprotected sex or substance use. Depressed episodes are similar to unipolar depression, and clients often complain of reduced libido, reduced sexual responsiveness, and fatigue (Lam, Donaldson, Brown, & Malliaris, 2005). Common medications used to treat bipolar disorders include lithium, novel mood stabilizers such as lamotrigine (Lamictel), and conventional agents such as valproic acid (Depakote) and carbamazepine (Tegretol). Sexual problems associated with these agents stem from sedation and reduced libido.

SUBSTANCE-USE DISORDERS

Use of mood-altering substances changes the neurochemistry of the brain and the rest of the nervous system (Crenshaw & Goldberg, 1996). Lack of libido, arousal disorders, and impotency in males have been noted with both short- and long-term substance use. Sexual themes and issues often emerge during recovery from addiction. See the Substance-Induced Sexual Dysfunction section in this chapter for more information.

STRESS AND COPING PATTERNS

Emerging evidence links the perception of stress and physiologic responses to multidimensional brain regions, including the prefrontal lobe, the hippocampus, and amygdala (McEwen, 2007). Together these brain regions determine the nature of stress, and when a threat is perceived, they activate a cascade of neuroendocrine and biochemical problems to maintain homeostasis. Of particular importance is the effect stress and coping patterns have on biological, social, and behavioral responses, including sex drive and performance.

Myths to Overcome about Sexuality

Myth	Fact
1. In a couple relationship, each partner is responsible for the other's level of sexual desire.	1. Sexual desire is an internal psychological mechanism. Individuals are responsible for their own level of desire. In the course of life, one's sexual desire waxes and wanes owing to physical, hormonal, environmental, and relationship experiences.
2. Children will ask parents or guardians questions about sexuality when the time is right.	2. Children are often uncertain how to bring up sexual issues with parents. If they mature in a home with "askable" parents, parents who consider any question appropriate, the likelihood of asking sexual questions increases. It is a mistake to wait for children to ask for information. There are predictable questions to be asked about body parts, such as differences between the sexes, and these issues need to be addressed at different times and not in one discussion.
3. Older adults lose sexual function after they reach the age of 65.	3. Individuals can remain sexually healthy for a lifetime. Sexual desire, sexual pleasure, and sexual function are based on the person's individual needs and wants, not on age.
4. Gay men are pedophiles.	4. Pedophilia is a sexual disorder in which an individual has fantasies and activities with prepubescent children. Gay men have sexual desire for other men, not children. Homosexuality is not a sexual paraphilia.

An individual's ability to modulate and cope with stressful situations is based on early life events that influence coping patterns of emotional and stress responsiveness. Adaptive responses stem from mobilizing internal and external resources to mitigate and cope with stress. Maladaptive responses limit the individual's ability to mobilize resources to dampen stress responses and often place the individual at risk for medical and psychiatric conditions. Nurses can empower clients to develop adaptive coping behaviors by exploring the meaning of current stressful events and their impact on overall health and quality of life.

SEXUALITY AND SEXUAL DISORDERS ACROSS THE LIFE SPAN

Sexual themes and issues are present throughout the life span. Nurses need to incorporate sexual histories in their assessments. See Table 24–1 for a summary of sexual issues across the life span.

Discussing sexuality provides a glimpse of the client's psychological and mental health makeup. It offers psychiatric mental health nurses information about the client's capacity to love and be loved, receive and reciprocate pleasure, to form meaningful and intimate relationships, and to adapt to changes across the life span. Performing a sexual assessment and fielding sexual questions may be uncomfortable due to personal reactions or getting in touch with one's own sexuality and sexual concerns; uncertainty about which questions to ask; and body language that conveys personal

moral repugnance concerning specific sexual practices and orientation. It is imperative to explore personal reactions, both verbal and nonverbal (body language), to questions that generate anxiety and uncertainty to establish healthy nurse-client relationships. Clients observe facial expressions, voice tone, and evidence of discomfort or embarrassment (e.g., blushing) during these personal discussions. Even if the nurse does not condone or agree with certain sexual practices, it is imperative to convey empathy and acceptance of the client as an individual.

TABLE 24–1
Sexual Issues across the Life Span

Childhood:	Identification with gender
Adolescence:	Identity development vs. role confusion
Young Adulthood:	Intimate relationship development
Adulthood:	Generativity, guiding children
Middlescence:	Redefinition of identity and roles
Old Age:	Changing physical and mental conditions

Awareness of life span issues is equally important in understanding individual wishes, needs, and cultural and religious beliefs about sexuality and intimacy. For instance, adolescents may express concerns about gender identity or birth control, and younger single adults may complain of orgasmic and desire or arousal difficulties, and/or infidelity. Middle-aged clients may complain of erectile dysfunction, anorgasm, and coping difficulties with their sexuality after a death, infidelity, divorce, or separation. Physiological changes associated with menopause and middle to older adulthood also increase the risk of sexual difficulties. Health education is an invaluable nursing intervention that offers insight to physiological changes associated with aging. It is imperative to dispel the myth that sexuality (desire and arousal) dissipates during older adulthood. Nurses must assess individual wishes, preferences, and concerns.

CHILDHOOD

Sexuality is a lifelong phenomenon that begins with birth, when the nurse midwife or physician announces, "It's a girl" or "It's a boy." Gender identity is defined by whether someone identifies as male or female. The culture in which the child grows up and relationships define and limit boundaries of sexual behavior. By the time the child reaches 3 years old, he or she proclaims to be a boy or a girl. Psychologists believe "gender constancy"—knowing one will always be a male or a female is developed by ages 5 to 7. There are some children who have gender disorders and for a variety of hormonal, prenatal, and, possibly, environmental factors, they do not feel that their actual physical sexual anatomy matches their gender. About 1 in 100,000 men and 1 in 130,000 women are transsexual. Remember, transsexuals are not the same as transvestites, who are people who like to dress as the other gender for sexual arousal.

The following clinical example illustrates a potential problem that arises in childhood—the gender identity disorder known as gender dysphoria.

ADOLESCENCE

Erikson (1964) described a theory of ego development that was based on Freud's work. Erickson conceptualized ego development as occurring in eight stages over a life span. Adolescence is characterized as the years from 12 to 20, when a person tackles the task of creating an identity in the midst of confusion. If the goal of identity development is not achieved, unresolved conflicts will result in behavioral disorders.

Today's adolescents face many challenges concerning their sexuality due to the media blitz of sexual behaviors on the Internet, iPods, movies, and open discussions with peers. Biological and psychosocial changes during this period of rapid growth and exposure to sexual materials make relationships with families and friends, along with cultural and religious beliefs, even more significant in helping the adolescent discover his own sexuality and

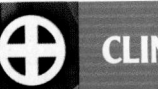

CLINICAL EXAMPLE

Gender Identity Disorder

At his kindergarten teacher's insistence, Frank's mother brought him to the clinic. Frank, now 5 years old, had insisted that he was a girl for as long as his mother could remember. He often played quiet games with stuffed animals or dolls. He liked to wear nightshirts and long tee shirts, which he pretended were dresses. Frank refused to stand to urinate; he preferred to sit down for this activity. Once, his estranged father, who was currently not living at home, showed him the "correct" way to urinate. During this demonstration, Frank screamed, fell on the floor, and yelled, "I am a girl and this (pointing to his penis) will fall off soon." Frank's teacher complains that Frank will not line up with the boys, plays alongside the girls, and refuses to enter the boys' restroom.

The nurse needs to encourage the parents not to respond to Frank in a negative way that could harm his self-esteem. The nurse could work collaboratively with the child psychiatric treatment team to develop a plan for behavioral therapy aimed at helping Frank fit in with his peers. Behaviors such as going to the boys' bathroom would be expected, while the nurse and teacher remain aware that Frank may be taunted and possibly abused by his peers. His safety and self-esteem are of utmost importance.

The parents also need to be aware that in later years Frank would benefit from therapy to identify transsexual issues and options. Some transsexual men choose to live the life of a woman, taking hormones and ultimately having gender reassignment surgery. Transgendered is an arching term that describes transsexuals, whose sense of themselves clashes with their original biological sex, cross-dressers, and others whose appearance is at odds with traditional gender expectations.

sexual behaviors. Several studies implicate the importance of the youth-parent relationship in having frank discussions and answering questions about sex, expectations, and responsibilities (Kao, Guthrie, & Loveland-Cherry, 2007). Historically, researchers reported that communication between parents and adolescents about sex, particularly in minority families, has been understudied and that additional data are necessary for which sex-related topics are discussed and how the subject matter is communicated. Major parent-adolescent topics included HIV and STDs, rather than birth control, sexual behavior, or physical development (Miller, Kotchick, Dorsey, Forehand, & Ham, 1998). Findings from a 2006 study of non–sexually active African American and Hispanic girls demonstrated that parents and peers are mutually strong influences within the dynamic social context of the adolescent's life, but despite the negative effects that sexually active peers have on adolescent sexual delay, responsive parent-adolescent sex discussions can buffer or mitigate these influences (Fasula & Miller, 2006). These findings strengthen earlier findings that implicated the importance of strong parent-adolescent communication about sex. (See Research Abstract.) Psychiatric nurses must work with parents and adolescents

CLINICAL EXAMPLE

Identity versus Role Confusion

Eighteen-year-old Ann Marie has raised the concern of her family, the faculty at the community college she attends, and her co-workers at the fast-food restaurant where she works. The source of this concern is her impulsive and sometimes self-destructive behavior. Ann Marie is not doing well in school; she is indecisive about her career goals, as indicated by her changing majors every semester. Co-workers complain that she is late for work and say she appears not to care that she might be fired. Along the same line, Ann Marie's parents worry because their daughter goes out with a different boyfriend every night. There is reason to believe that she is having sex with these various boys. Drinking behavior is suspected.

Ann Marie needs for the nurse to help her set limits on her behavior while improving her sense of self-worth. The college counselor can help with career goal development. Marie needs to learn the dangers in her present course; alcohol use that lowers inhibition coupled with a number of sexual contacts can result in sexually transmitted diseases including HIV and unplanned pregnancy.

CLINICAL EXAMPLE

Isolation as a Result of Failure to Develop Intimacy

Jay, age 28, avoids social interactions in his work as a computer programmer. He lives with his parents, as he always has done. His older sister worries that he is "not doing what 28-year-old men do." She has tried involving Jay in her life by inviting him to parties to meet her friends. He has refused her efforts. Jay fears he will say or do the wrong thing. He becomes anxious and extremely sensitive to questions that family acquaintances ask him about his social life.

Any help the nurse can give that breaks down Jay's isolation is essential. Intimacy is difficult for Jay so that pushing him to do too much too fast will fail. Small steps toward socialization might include getting involved in a computer network, a computer interest group, or anything that moves him toward people at a pace he can tolerate.

through psychoeducation that helps parents develop the knowledge and communication skills necessary to discuss sexual topics with their adolescents effectively.

YOUNG ADULTHOOD

The major task of young adulthood is development of an intimate relationship. Erickson (1964) identified isolation as the outcome of the failure to develop intimacy.

ADULTHOOD

The task of adulthood is generativity, that is, guiding children and being constructive and creative at work. Failure results in stagnation and self-indulgence. In recent years, infertility has become a problem of adulthood.

MIDDLE ADULTHOOD

Middle adulthood is the period around the middle of the life span heralded by hormonal changes in both sexes that lead to gradual decline in reproductive function.

RESEARCH ABSTRACT

African-American and Hispanic Adolescents' Intentions to Delay First Intercourse: Parental Communication as a Buffer for Sexually Active Peers

Fasula, A., & Miller, K. S. (2006). *Journal of Adolescent Health, 38,* 193–200.

Study/Problem

The purpose of the study was to assess the modulating effects of mothers' responsiveness during discussions about sex on the negative relationship between their adolescents' sexually active peers and delay among African American and Hispanic populations.

Method

Researchers reviewed interview data from 530 adolescents who were not sexually active to determine the effects of mother-adolescent sex talks and peers on intentions to delay or become sexually active within the next year. Logistic regression was performed to test the moderating effects of adolescents' reports of mothers' openness, support, and understanding during discussions about sex on the relationship between perceived peer sexual activity and adolescent sexual delay.

Findings

Researchers concluded that mothers' responsiveness had a buffering effect on the negative effects of sexually active peers. Despite their peers being sexually active, non–sexually active adolescents whose mothers scored above-average responsiveness were 1.6 times more likely to postpone intercourse than were adolescents who reported that their mothers had average responsiveness.

Implications for Psychiatric Nurses

These findings strengthen the importance of working with parents and adolescents to ensure they have effective communication skills that convey support and education about the sexual issues confronting today's adolescents. Providing psychoeducation about sexual issues also strengthens the bond between parents and adolescents during a turbulent developmental period.

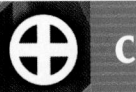

CLINICAL EXAMPLE

Stress of Infertility on a Relationship

George and Annie began seeking treatment for infertility 3 years ago without success. All of their sexual activities have revolved around Annie's fertile periods and attempts to conceive. The stress has resulted in marital problems, and the couple has discussed divorce. During this ordeal, many couples begin to lose feelings of love and closeness and begin to doubt the commitment of marriage.

An infertility support group led by a nurse with knowledge and experience in this area will help this couple share their experiences with others and learn they are not alone. It is important that a knowledgeable health professional be the group leader because misinformation is a real danger in leaderless support groups or psychotherapy groups led by someone who does not understand infertility and its treatment.

During midlife, both sexes begin to redefine themselves, their needs, and their wants. Because our culture idolizes youthful sexuality, the perception of lost youth may cause anxiety. Most people succeed in making the transition to middle adulthood in a healthy manner. Some do not. Those who are unwilling to accept this transition may face a crisis situation with a variety of possible outcomes.

CLINICAL EXAMPLE

Desire and Sexual Function

Matt and Sybil are a dual career couple in their 50s with two children ages 16 and 12. They have both worked to develop successful careers. The children are the second success they have invested in. Their home is a comfortable place for family and friends to gather. And yet, their marriage and sexual connection seem to be relegated to the back burner. Matt's sexual desire is low. He wonders if it will ever get better. Sybil enjoys sex with Matt, but lately has felt rejected because he rarely initiates. Both would like more time together to nurture the relationship but do not make the time.

The nurse in the clinic could suggest sex therapy with an AASECT-certified sex therapist. The nurse therapist would assist the couple to share their concerns and perspectives. Helping them identify their successes during the marriage would be of value, while refocusing time and attention to their sexual connection. What are the various turn-ons and turn-offs? What have they tried in the past to nurture the relationship? How do their sexual styles complement each other? Assisting the couple to invest daily in the intimate connection and romance is often the first step back to a loving, sexually satisfying relationship.

OLDER ADULTHOOD

Older adulthood is now divided into young old and old old. Sexuality and sexual function vary according to the person's gender and physical and mental conditions. Sexual activity may decline somewhat in old age, but many people remain sexually active into their 80s and 90s. Decline in sexual activity may have more to do with attitudes about aging and the death of a spouse than with sexual dysfunction. Although physical changes do occur that make sex in old age different from sex in other periods of life (women experience less lubrication and elasticity and declining estrogen levels, resulting in thinner vaginal walls; men produce less testosterone, take longer to achieve an erection, and experience a longer refractory period), adjustments can be made for all of these changes so that sexual activity need not stop in old age.

SPECIFIC SEXUAL DISORDERS AND TREATMENT MODALITIES

Table 24–2 lists the sexual disorders recognized by the APA's (2000) *Diagnostic and Statistical Manual of Mental Disorders* (4th edition Revision) *(DSM-IV-TR)*. These disorders are described next.

GENDER IDENTITY DISORDERS

Sexuality is an integral part of a person's life; it is not limited to sexual intercourse. Gender identity is inborn and culturally defined. At various times, the average male or female may contemplate what it would be like to be the opposite sex. At times, for example, at Halloween or at a masquerade party,

---

TABLE 24–2
Sexual and Gender Disorders

Gender Identity Disorders

Sexual Dysfunctions

Sexual Arousal Disorders

Sexual Desire Disorders

Orgasmic Disorders

Sexual Pain Disorders

Sexual Dysfunction due to General Medical Condition

Substance-Induced Sexual Dysfunction

Paraphilias

Note. Data from *Diagnostic and Statistical Manual of Mental Disorders* (4th edition, Text Revision) *(DSM-IV-TR)*, by American Psychiatric Association, 2000, Washington, DC: Author. Adapted with permission.

Aging and Sexuality

Mary and James, 76 and 80 years of age, respectively, had always had a satisfying sex life in their marriage. Sexual intercourse has decreased in frequency to twice a month because James has difficulty achieving an erection. Both Mary and James view this as an acceptable change in behavior. Neither one wants to lose the closeness of sexual expression. For this reason, the regularity of cuddling and touching has remained constant. The couple continues to experience sexual satisfaction in their marriage.

It is possible that James' erection problems have a physiological source that can be treated. The nurse can suggest a medical work-up with a urologist if it has not been done recently. Due to the popularity of Viagra (sildenafil citrate) medication to increase the firmness of erections, men with impotency do have other options in their later years to sustain sexual function. The urologist would probably discuss this and other options, such as a penis ring, a vacuum pump, or even penis implants, with James and Mary. Acknowledging that people in old age still need and have sex is essential to good nursing care for this group.

Although Viagra (sildenafil citrate) offers new options to enhance sexual function, within the first year on the market, about 130 Americans who took Viagra died. The Food and Drug Administration issued warnings recommending that clinicians be cautious about prescribing Viagra. The new label states men who have had a heart attack, stroke, or life-threatening arrhythmia in the last 6 months, or who have significantly low blood pressure, significantly high blood pressure, a history of cardiac failure or unstable angina, or the eye disease, retinitis pigmentosa, not receive the drug. Research is also underway to evaluate the effectiveness of Viagra for women.

Since the advent of Viagra, two other medications are now available in the marketplace for Erectile Dysfunction—vardenafil HCL (Levitra) and tadalafil (Cialis). Cialis has a 36-hour window for erectile enhancement thus taking the time worry out of quality sexual activity.

---

a person of either sex may try on the role of the other sex by putting on gender-identified clothing or adopting gender-typical mannerisms.

Gender identity disorder is not allowing oneself to experience the role of the other; rather, it is a pervasive distress over being a boy or a girl. A child with a gender identity disorder may be preoccupied with the dress and behavior stereotypical of the opposite sex. In addition, the child persists in asserting that he or she will develop the sex organs of the other sex. In adulthood, this condition is referred to as transsexualism. The person is persistently (for at least 2 years) preoccupied with getting rid of current primary and secondary sexual characteristics.

Other identity problems are seen in children and adults who cross-dress, that is, wear culturally appropriate dress of the opposite sex. This cross-dressing is not to be confused with wearing clothes of the opposite sex for the purpose of feeling sexual arousal known as transvestic fetishism.

SEXUAL DYSFUNCTIONS

Understanding human sexuality and responses often help the cognize sexual dysfunction. Because of the tremendous stress that often results from sexual dysfunction, nurses must assess their impact on the client's sense of well-being and self-esteem. In addition, the nurse needs to collaborate with the client and significant others and develop holistic interventions that reduce stress and facilitate adapting an optimal level of health.

Arousal Disorders

Sexual arousal disorders are primary disorders in people who have an inadequate physiological response during the period of sexual arousal. In women, the problem is a persistent or recurrent inability to attain or maintain lubrication and swelling of the vagina during the excitement phase. In men it is a persistent or recurrent inability to attain or maintain an erection. For a diagnosis of sexual arousal disorder in both men and women, no other Axis I diagnosis should be evident. For example, major depression, substance abuse, and sexual dysfunction related to a medical condition (e.g., spinal cord injury) all cause changes in a person's physiological ability for sexual arousal.

Desire Disorders

Disorders in sexual desire are primary problems as identified by the person experiencing them or by the clinician during assessment. The disturbance must cause marked distress or difficulty in interpersonal relationships. Sexual desire may be hypoactive, or there may be an aversion to all sexual activity. Hypoactive desire disorder is marked by low or absent sexual fantasy or activities. The person's age, sex, and life context (culture, relationship, etc.) must be taken into account.

Sex therapists state that desire difficulties are often the major reason people seek "sex therapy." They have coined the term "discrepancies of desire" to describe the disequilibrium between partners relative to their desire for sexual activity. Desire is a personal experience and can be dampened by many factors. The therapist assists the couple to review relationship issues, self-image issues, and time factors which may hinder desire. Enhancing desire usually is multifaceted and requires that both partners engage in behavior adjustments to promote sexual well-being.

An aversion to sexual activity is a persistent and extreme avoidance of all or almost all genital sexual contact with a partner. The individual reports anxiety, fear, or disgust when confronted by a sexual opportunity with a partner. The presence of another Axis I diagnosis, such as depression or obsessive-compulsive disorder, must be ruled out before a sexual desire disorder diagnosis is made.

Orgasmic Disorders

Both men and women can suffer from orgasmic disorders. In the *DSM-IV-TR*, the APA (2000) has made an effort to account for the variations in normal female functioning. The APA assumes that women have more frequent orgasms as they age, become more experienced, and are less fearful of becoming pregnant. The type of stimulation also plays an important role in female sexual response.

An orgasmic disorder for both men and women is a persistent or recurrent delay in or absence of orgasm following a normal sexual excitement phase. The disorder may be further categorized as generalized (occurs every time) or situational (orgasm may occur with self-stimulation or occurs with only a particular partner) (APA, 2000).

Premature ejaculation is another type of orgasmic disorder. The condition can be persistent in nature or recurrent, in that ejaculation may occur with minimal sexual stimulation before, on, or shortly after penetration and before the person wishes it. The nurse must consider issues like the duration of the excitement phase, age, medications, novelty of the sexual partner or situation, and recent frequency of sexual activity.

Sexual Pain Disorders

Persistent or recurrent genital pain in men or women before, during, or after intercourse that cannot be explained by other medical or psychiatric conditions is called dyspareunia. Vaginismus refers to an involuntary spasm of the musculature of the outer two thirds of the vagina that interferes with vaginal penetration with penis, finger, tampon, or speculum. Like other sexual conditions identified in the *DSM-IV-TR* (APA, 2000), the sexual pain disorders must be persistent or recurrent to warrant diagnosis and treatment. Both sexual pain disorders must cause a problem for the person individually and interpersonally.

Sexual Dysfunction Caused by a General Medical Condition

There are times when a general medical condition such as hypertension interferes with sexual function, thus causing a great deal of distress, disruption of sexual functioning, and interpersonal problems (Fogel & Lauver, 1990; Lubkin, 1986). The sexual dysfunction may result in secondary male erectile disorder, secondary dyspareunia, secondary vaginismus, or another secondary sexual dysfunction. Table 24–3 lists nonpsychiatric medical conditions that affect sexual functioning.

Substance-Induced Sexual Dysfunction

Substance-induced sexual dysfunction is associated with an array of drugs including over-the-counter and prescrip-

TABLE 24–3	
Medical Conditions That Affect Sexual Function	

Neurological	**Genital Disease in Females**
Spinal cord injury	
Cervical disc problems	Infections
Multiple sclerosis	Cancers
Vascular	Allergies to spermicide
Atherosclerosis	**Genital Disease in Males**
Sickle cell anemia	Prostatitis
Endocrine	Orchitis
Addison's disease	Tumor
Cushing's syndrome	Trauma
Hypothyroidism	**Surgical Procedures**
Diabetes mellitus	**Systemic Conditions**
Systemic Disease	Chronic renal failure
Liver disease	HTN
Renal disease	Chronic pain syndromes
Pulmonary disease	Fibromyalgia
Arthritis	Chronic fatigue syndrome
Cancer	

tion drugs, illicit substances, and alcohol. Questions about current medications and recent or history of substance use (including alcohol) must be an integral part of the nursing assessment. Data from this assessment provide information necessary to make a differential diagnosis of primary or secondary sexual dysfunction. Table 24–4 lists drugs associated with drug-induced sexual dysfunction.

PARAPHILIA

Paraphilia is an umbrella term for variations in sexual behavior. Sex is abnormal when it (1) is uncomfortable for the person doing it, (2) is inefficient in that it causes problems in that person's life (e.g., results in arrest), (3) is viewed by the person's culture as bizarre, and (4) does harm to the person and others.

The *DSM-IV-TR* (APA, 2000) delineates sexual variations that are problematic to the individual. The problem may be viewed as mild (the person is distressed by the urge but does not act on it), moderate (occasionally the urge is acted on), or severe (the person repeatedly acts on the urge). In all cases the individual has symptoms over a period of at least 6 months, which are recurrent and intense. Table 24–5 presents a list of the paraphilias and their definitions.

Compulsive sexual behavior (CSB) is a serious psychosexual disorder that can be identified and treated successfully.

TABLE 24–4
Drugs That Affect Sexual Function

Prescription Drugs	
Antianxiety agents	Antiarrhythmic agents
Alprazolam (Xanax)	Disopyramide (Norpace)
Diazepam (Valium)	Antihypertensive agents
Doxepin (Sinequan)	Beta blockers
Anticholinergic agents	Diuretics
Homatropine methyl-bromide (Homapin)	Sympatholytics
Mepenzolate bromide (Cantil)	Others
Methantheline bromide (Banthīne)	Cimetidine (Tagamet)
Propantheline bromide (Pro-Banthīne)	Sulfasalazine (Azulfidine)
Anticonvulsant agents	Over-the-counter drugs with anticholinergic properties
Phenytoin (Dilantīn)	**Social Drugs**
Antidepressant agents	Alcohol
Most can cause changes	Amyl nitrate
Antipsychotic agents	Cocaine
Most can cause changes	Lysergic acid
	Marijuana
	Heroin
	Methadone

CSB does not always involve strange and unusual sexual practices. Many conventional behaviors can become the focus of an individual's obsessions and compulsions. Some examples are the compulsive use of masturbation (self-stimulation) and pornography (magazines, books, videos, and Internet surfing). The exact mechanism of CSB is still under debate, and various treatment approaches have been developed. Research is needed to further clarify the nature of the disorder, the mechanisms involved, and to test the most effective treatment approach. In the meantime, individuals suffering from CSB should not hesitate to seek professional guidance to properly assess their problem and to find help through counseling and treatment.

THE ROLE OF THE NURSE

Any time a nurse and client interface, sexual concerns may be addressed. In dealing with any client, from the client who comes to a teen clinic with a complaint of acne to the client who comes to a geriatric clinic for treatment for hyperten-

sion, the nurse can take a sexual history and open up the topic for the client to express any concern. Regardless of practice setting, nurses need to create a safe and therapeutic environment that enables the client to express feelings and ask questions about sexual issues. For example, "One part of the nursing assessment is the sexual assessment. Are you sexually active? (If yes, then proceed. If no, ask what the concerns are for not having an active sex life at this time.) Often people describe their sexual relationship as unfulfilling. It may be caused by stress, exhaustion, disinterest, or even

TABLE 24-5
Definitions of Paraphilia

Exhibitionism: exposure of one's genitals to strangers

Fetishism: sexual fixation on an object to which erotic significance is attached

Frotteurism: sexual fantasies involving touching and rubbing against a nonconsenting individual

Pedophilia: sexual fantasies and activities with prepubescent children

Sexual masochism: sexual fantasies comprising being humiliated, beaten or bound, or made to suffer

Sexual sadism: sexual fantasies, behaviors, or acts that generate psychological or physical suffering of another person

Transvestic fetishism: recurrent and intense sexual urges and sexual fantasies involving cross-dressing

Voyeurism: sexual arousal at secretly viewing the nude body

Paraphilia not otherwise specified include the following:

  Telephone scatalogia: obscene phone calls

  Necrophilia: sexual fantasies and acts involving corpses

  Partialism: exclusive sexual focus on a part of the body, for example, the feet

  Zoophilia: sexual fantasies and acts with animals

  Coprophilia: feces hold sexual meaning for the individual

  Klismaphilia: sexual fantasies and arousal involving enemas

  Urophilia: urine produces sexual response

Note. From *Diagnostic and Statistical Manual of Mental Disorders* (4th edition, Text Revision) *(DSM-IV-TR),* by American Psychiatric Association, 2000, Washington, DC: Author. Reprinted with permission.

difficulties in the relationship. What concerns do you have in your sexual relationship?" Then the nurse must be willing to listen or must refer the client to someone who will. In this way, sexual issues and themes can be addressed openly in a way that gives comfort to the client.

The psychiatric-mental health nurse is in a key position to support sexual behavior changes in groups at risk for HIV infection. More effort in developing effective client-centered counseling and educational programs is needed. Psychiatric-mental health nurses are uniquely qualified to provide holistic care, counseling, and education to clients at risk for HIV infection. In addition, in an administrative role, the nurse can ensure that groups at risk are targeted for appropriate and effective services. In a scientific role, the nurse researcher can generate and test theories regarding interventions that may be used in clinical settings to support behavior changes in people at risk for HIV infection.

American Nurses Association's (ANA) *Scope and Standards of Psychiatric-Mental Health Nursing Practice* (2000) states that every nurse should own and use three essential documents: a copy of the nurse state practice act, the legal source that defines the scope and privileges of practice in which the nurse practices; the American Nurses Association Code for Nurses, which describes the ethical responsibilities for conduct by nurses; the previously mentioned document because it sets the standards for a particular nursing specialty. The first attempt to define standards of practice for psychiatric nurses was begun in 1961. Revisions were made and published in 1976, 1982, 1994, and 2000.

THE GENERALIST NURSE

The role of the generalist nurse varies with each practice setting. Clients often confide in the generalist nurse information of an intimate nature. The generalist nurse uses the therapeutic relationship to listen and express caring concern to the client. The listening and caring activities of the generalist nurse are vital to the client's healing process.

The generalist nurse addresses sexual themes and problems in the same way the nurse addresses other problems: through the nursing process. The nurse needs to feel comfortable asking about clients' sexual concerns and listening to their problems. After assessment, the nurse develops methods to increase the client's awareness of the problems and potential solutions. Increasing awareness involves education and counseling skills. The generalist nurse is responsible for knowing his personal limitations, be they lack of knowledge of sexual issues, or lack of skill in these areas. The nurse can overcome limitations in knowledge, skills, and differences in values and beliefs by assisting the client through referral, consulting with appropriate professionals, and seeking continuing education opportunities or further education.

THE ADVANCED-PRACTICE PSYCHIATRIC REGISTERED NURSE

The advanced-practice psychiatric-mental health nurse (e.g., clinical nurse specialist, nurse practitioner) uses psychotherapy and may or may not specialize in sex therapy. Regardless of whether the advanced-practice nurse is a certified sex therapist, effort to determine the appropriate intervention is necessary for the client with a sexual problem. The psychiatric generalist nurse may seek wise counsel from these clinicians or choose to refer for client follow-up.

Advanced practice as outlined in the ANA's *Standards of Psychiatric and Mental Health Nursing Practice* (2000) requires at least a master's degree in the specialty. The advanced-practice psychiatric registered nurse functions as a psychotherapist with individuals, families, and groups. The advanced-pratice psychiatric registered nurse who specializes in sex therapy should be recognized by the state in which he practices as an APRN. In addition, in-depth training in sex therapy should be evident. The AASECT identifies qualifications for practice in this area and issues a directory of certified professionals.

The advanced practice psychiatric nurse is poised to offer consumers vast options to cope with and manage sexual disorders. Psychotherapies and pharmacotherapies provide a cadre of treatment options for the client with a sexual disorder.

THE NURSING PROCESS

Sexual health promotion requires the client's active participation and, ultimately, assumption of responsibility for care. The client must use an organized, systematic process to choose a specific course of action for behavior change. Psychiatric clients may have difficulty with decision making. Being faced with choices for behavior change may create conflict within the person and the family. Feelings of helplessness in the client may encourage unnecessary dependence on the nurse. It is the nurse's job to enable the client to operate free of help as quickly as possible, while ensuring the client's self-care potential.

Facilitating changes in sexual behavior begins with the nurse assessing the meaning that the client attaches to sexual behavior. Interventions are then developed to help the client identify alternative sexual methods or nonsexual methods of finding meaning. For example, if John, a late adolescent, is engaging in sexual activities in order to satisfy the need for touch, then safe-sex ways of touching can be explored. Hochhauser offers that simply pointing out the dangers of an activity does not bring about change (Hochhauser & Greensweig, 1992). The nurse needs to be willing to discuss openly and nonjudgmentally the meaning of John's desire for sexual activity, instead of simply reciting its dangers.

A sexual history includes all aspects of sexuality and therefore is holistic. Sexual influences are part of the evaluation—role modeling by parents; messages by parents, early exploration, masturbation, initial experiences with intercourse and religious influences encompass the assessment. In addition, levels of desire, arousal, orgasmic function, pain, and frequency of sexual activity should be discussed with the client. An overall health assessment, including a thorough physical examination, is basic to good problem identification, because sexuality includes neurological, vascular, muscular, biochemical, hormonal, psychosocial, and other components. A sexual history should include the context in which the problem emerged and the context in which it currently exists, awareness of both the nurse's and client's underlying anxieties and prejudices, a description of the experience as it is lived by the client, the meaning of the problem from the client's perspective, and the support currently available to the client and the nurse. See Table 24–6, Comprehensive Sexual History.

ASSESSMENT

The North American Nursing Diagnosis Association (NANDA, 2007) lists the following diagnoses with human sexuality as the phenomenon of concern.

Sexual Dysfunction

Sexual dysfunction is the person's experience of change in sexual function. The person views this change as unsatisfying, unrewarding, inadequate, or socially inappropriate.

Sexual dysfunction can arise from various etiologies across the spectrum of human sexual response. Numerous examples emerge from individual human response to stress, surgery, value conflicts, body image changes, loss

TABLE 24–6
Comprehensive Sexual History

The nurse can formulate client questions related to the following categories: sexual development, current sexual function, and current sexual relationship to provide a comprehensive sexual history.

Sexual Development

Parental messages

Childhood experiences

Significant relationships

History of sexual abuse/trauma

Initial sexual experience

Religious influences

Current Sexual Function

Desire (how often felt)

Masturbation frequency

Ability to be aroused

Use of erotic material—video, books, magazines, Internet, iPod

Use of fantasy

Orgasmic function with partner

Orgasmic function with self

Sexual pain

Unpleasant sexual experiences

Sexually transmitted diseases

Birth control

Medical conditions

Medications

Alcohol, substance use

Reproductive history, including menarche, pregnancies, menopause

Current Sexual Relationship

Who initiates

Foreplay

Frequency of sexual activity

Frequency of intercourse

Satisfaction with intercourse

Affairs

Repertoire of sexual behaviors

Ability to communicate sexual needs with partner

of meaning, as well as many other sources. Disruption within the body, the family, or community can create this problem.

Ineffective Sexuality Patterns

Expression of concerns regarding one's sexuality often underlies ineffective sexual patterns. Defining characteristics include difficulties, limitations, and alterations in sexual performance. Related factors comprise lack of an intimate partner, conflicts about sexual orientation or variant practices, a lack of intimacy with a significant other, and fear of pregnancy or STD (NANDA, 2007).

Other NANDA Diagnoses

Other NANDA diagnoses that may apply are Interrupted Family Processes, Process, Ineffective Coping, Spiritual Distress, Anxiety, Fear, Acute Pain, Disturbed Personal Identity, and Disturbed Body Image.

OUTCOME IDENTIFICATION AND PLANNING

Working in partnership with the client, family, and interdisciplinary team to enable the client's sexual behavior change involves open communication and cooperation. All parties need to be aware of the nature of the problem and how to work toward a satisfactory change. This involvement is not always easy; conflict and discomfort may arise. Encouraging participants' expression of differences in values and beliefs while advocating acceptance of the client's wish to change should be the focus of nursing interventions.

Nursing Care Plan 24–1 identifies the nursing diagnoses and desired outcomes for the case study of Mary O. and specifies the nursing actions needed to achieve these outcomes and the rationales for these actions.

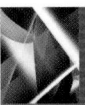

CASE STUDY

The Client with Sexual Problems (Mary O.)

Mary is a 32-year-old with a history of bipolar II disorder. During her admission, she confides in the nurse concerning her lack of interest in sexual desire for her husband. She also reports that during the past few months, since she began taking medications for bipolar disorder, her energy level has waned along with decreased libido. Her history also reveals that she has been married 2 years and that prior to getting married, her husband knew about her bipolar disorder. She further describes her lack of interest in sex as feeling less attracted to her husband, Mark. Before their marriage she was an aggressive real estate agent and well known in the community. She also reports that Mark has become more controlling and emotionally distant. During the discussion she questions if she made a mistake marrying and moving away from her job and support systems. This scenario depicts the impact of multiple stressors on an individual with bipolar II disorder, including having decreased sexual desire.

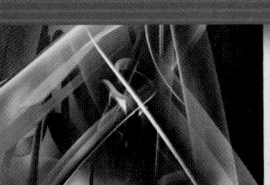

NURSING CARE PLAN 24–1

The Client with Sexual Problems (Mary O.)

Nursing Diagnosis: Sexual Dysfunction related to lack of desire

Outcome Identification	Nursing Actions	Rationales	Evaluation
1. By (date), Mary will state her sexual needs to her partner using a scale of 1–10 to prioritize the need (1 is low level need, 10 is high).	1a. Introduce a topic of sexuality with client and partner.	1a. To enable client and partner to share concerns and improve communication.	*Goal met:* Mary discusses sexual concerns. Mary identifies preexisting concerns.
	1b. Determine what sexual problems existed before depression.	1b. Preexisting problems may not be related to depression.	

(continues)

Nursing Care Plan 24–1 (continued)

Outcome Identification	Nursing Actions	Rationales	Evaluation
	1c. Explain to couple that sexual desire usually returns with resolution of the depression.	1c. Lack of sexual desire is a symptom of depression, knowing that can decrease guilt feelings and inadequacy.	Mary identifies lack of desire as symptom. Mary reviews sexual-enhancing options to increase sexual desire.
	1d. Explore options to improve sexual functioning and enhance sexual desire toward husband.	1d. Sexual-enhancing techniques offer the client more options and control.	
	1e. Explore other sexual options with couple- touch, and foreplay options, and sexual lubricants.		

Nursing Diagnosis: Dysfunctional Family Processes related to marital distance and conflicts

Outcome Identification	Nursing Actions	Rationales	Evaluation
1. By (date), Mary will report an increase of satisfaction in marriage using a 1–10 scale (1 = low, 10 = high).	1a. Help client identify needs and wants in marriage.	1a. Knowledge of self can enhance ability to get needs met.	*Goal met:* Mary is willing to explore self. Mary is able to tolerate conversation with partner. Mary and husband will use session for growth.
	1b. Assist client in sharing needs with partner and exploring his needs and wants.	1b. Enhanced couple communication enhances marriage.	
	1c. Arrange couples sessions with therapist to prepare for discharge.	1c. The nurse psycho-therapist can facilitate talks and resolution of conflicts.	

Nursing Diagnosis: Situational Low Self-Esteem related to guilt and negative self-evaluation

Outcome Identification	Nursing Actions	Rationales	Evaluation
1. By (date), Mary will report greater self-acceptance.	1a. Identify early warning signals for hypomanic symptoms.	1a. Awareness leads to effective coping options.	*Goal met:* Mary will understand her illness and report symptoms. Mary will verbalize positive self-statements. Mary will identify her successes.
	1b. Assess negative self-thoughts for validity, determine distortions and positive cognitions to replace them with.	1b. Negative cognitions distort one's reality.	
	1c. Identify three positive attributes.	1c. To remotivate and encourage self-acceptance.	

TABLE 24–7
Reports of Medical and Surgical Risk Factors in Women with Sexual Function Complaints

Sexual Complaints	Hysterectomy	Menopause with HRT	Menopause without HRT	SSRIs
Lack of sensation	100%	57%	50%	67%
Inability to reach orgasm	100%	75%	75%	50%
Lack of sexual desire	52%	45%	45%	40%
Lack of lubrication	67%	50%	17%	17%
Pain or discomfort	68%	67%	67%	75%

HRT = hormone replacement therapy. SSRIs = selective serotonin reuptake inhibitors.

IMPLEMENTATION

Interventions should be aimed at (1) removal of the cause of the problem, (2) symptom management for problems that cannot be readily treated because their etiology is unknown or effective treatment is unavailable, (3) case management for the client with chronic problems, and (4) family support. Of course, intervention varies with each condition and client system.

EVALUATION

The outcome of nursing interventions should be that the client reports satisfactory and socially appropriate sexual functioning within the context of his situation. Concern for the sexual partner if there is one is also an expected client outcome (NANDA, 2007).

RESEARCH ON SEXUAL ISSUES RELEVANT TO PSYCHIATRIC NURSING

Nurses are expected to provide sex education and counseling to various groups of clients across the life span and cultural arenas. Nurses have often been frustrated by issues of motivation for change and the traditional approach to client health education, that is, to tell the client what the risk is and what to change to decrease that risk and then presume that the client will change the behavior to avoid it. This model of health education often does not work and creates conflict in the nurse-client relationship when it fails.

"New view" is an approach to treating women who present with sexual problems. It emerged from a group of clinicians, sex therapists, and social scientists responding to what they saw as a growing medicalization of sexuality in clinical settings. Assessment and treatment incorporate psychosocial, sociocultural, and socioeconomic contexts of human sexuality and sexual problems as well as understanding of the physiologic and biologic aspects. The foundation of the approach is the consideration of the relational and sociocultural factors that contribute to women's expressions about their sexual problems. A thorough sexual history questionnaire and diagnostic and treatment grid lend to the effectiveness of this approach.

SUMMARY

- Clients, alone or with their partners, seeking help with a sexual problem challenge the nurse to form a therapeutic relationship that offers a safe and accepting atmosphere that promotes expression of feelings and concerns about sexuality.

- Self-awareness about one's own sexuality is crucial to understanding those inherent in the client with a sexual problem.

- During the course of generalist and advanced-nursing practice, sexual themes and issues are present.

- The prudent nurse asks questions about the client's sexual health, gives permission for the client to discuss problems or concerns of a sexual nature, and seeks appropriate interventions for the client and family.

- Appropriate interventions must be guided by the nature of the problem and within the cultural context. Education, advice, therapeutic intervention, and referral are possible actions the nurse may take in promoting the client's sexual health.

SUGGESTIONS FOR CLINICAL CONFERENCES

1. Create a client scenario and role model sexual history taking with classmates; use the comprehensive sexual history model.

2. Present case histories of clients and develop plans of care across the life span with sexual disorders. For each case, identify the (a) psychosocial issues, (b) treatment options, (c) client and family teaching needs, and (d) issues raised for the nurse.

3. Discuss ways in which children are taught about sexual identity by their families, culture, schools, and other institutions.

4. Bring to the conference and discuss items from the media that stereotype men and women in particular ways.

5. Think of various words (slang, profanity, words from foreign languages) that are used to describe male and female genitalia and sexual activities. Write these words on the board. Keep track of the feelings these words provoke in you. As a group, discuss the emotional effects of the words.

6. Invite gay, heterosexual, bisexual, and transsexual men and women to a panel discussion on sexual orientation.

STUDY QUESTIONS

1. A and B have been socialized in a culture where young people engage in sexual activity at the beginning of puberty. In this context, A's desire to wait until marriage would be likely to be considered:
   a. unusual
   b. maladaptive
   c. a cultural variation
   d. an individual choice

2. L. M. is a 40-year-old banker with a drinking problem who recently separated from his wife of 16 years. His typical alcohol consumption is two gin martinis at lunch, two vodkas on the rocks before dinner, and a bottle of wine with dinner. Recently, his day has begun with an "eye opener" of a shot of vodka. L. M. is in for a checkup for stomach pain. He mentions that his sexual desire has declined, and he has had one or two episodes of impotence. The nurse attributes L. M.'s problems to:
   a. stress
   b. marital discord
   c. alcohol consumption
   d. underlying general medical conditions

3. In an effort to help L. M., the nurse:
   a. enrolls him in a stress management class
   b. schedules a meeting with his estranged wife to open up lines of communication
   c. gives L. M. the meeting times for the local Alcoholics Anonymous
   d. waits for results of a differential diagnosis prior to making a referral

4. A. L., age 21, and B. L., age 25, have been dating for several months. B. L. has been pressing A. L. to have sexual intercourse with him. A. L. has not experienced sexual intercourse before and had planned on waiting for marriage. One cause of A. L.'s reluctance is her belief about sex outside of marriage. From Freud's perspective, the part of this personality that contains this belief is:
   a. ego
   b. id
   c. superego
   d. none of the above

5. According to Erikson, B. L. is attempting to:
   a. reproduce
   b. resolve aggressive issues
   c. fulfill his intimacy needs
   d. gain respect from his peers

6. Taking a sexual history is often difficult and generates fears and anxiety in the nurse. The nurse can allay some of these feelings by doing which of the following?
   a. Avoiding discussions with the client concerning sensitive sexual behavior
   b. Disclosing personal sexual issues with the client to open communication
   c. Learning about the broad range of sexual expression
   d. Referring the client to a sex therapist

7. A 55-year-old client presents in the outpatient ambulatory care clinic. During the assessment he remarks, "I am having a lot of sexual problems and I am concerned my wife will look for a younger man." The most appropriate nursing response is which of the following?
   a. "Please tell me more about your sexual problems."
   b. "Have you thought about taking Viagra?"
   c. "What makes you think your wife will look for a younger man?"
   d. "Let me refer you to a sex therapist to discuss your concerns."

8. Performing a detailed psychiatric history helps determine if there is an underlying psychiatric basis for sexual dysfunction. Which of the following is the *least* helpful psychiatric data from the client with a sexual disorder?
   a. Ask about current substance use and treatment
   b. Inquire about recent stressors, history of trauma, and quality of interpersonal relationships
   c. Assess the client's cultural beliefs about sexual health
   d. Inquire about family history of sexual problems

9. During a visit to the woman's health clinic one of your clients reports that she has no interest in being intimate

with her spouse. Which of the following is an inappropriate nurse response?
   a. "Has this happened before?"
   b. "Have you started any new medications or changed dosages?"
   c. "How long have you had this difficulty?"
   d. "Do you suspect your spouse of having an affair?"

10. A 20-year-old man is seen in the community mental health clinic because of acute anxiety. During your assessment he mentions that he is gay and his parents, who are very religious, would just die if they knew about his sexual orientation. What is the most appropriate nurse response?
   a. "I can see you are pretty anxious right now. Tell me more of your concerns about being gay."
   b. "If I were your parents I would be upset too."
   c. "I can arrange for a meeting between you and your parents so you can share your concerns with them."
   d. "What is your religious affiliation?"

RESOURCES

Please note that because Internet resources are of a time-sensitive nature and URL addresses may change or be deleted, searches should also be conducted by association or topic.

Internet Resources

1. Investigate recent sites for information on women's sexuality, advances, and research.

2. Review sex educational material available for clients at SIECUS, AASECT, and other sites.

3. Explore sites regarding sexual pharmacology and other biological interventions.

4. Identify themes related to homosexuality on the Internet—acceptance, hate crimes, social networks, and so on.

http://www.cdc.gov/hiv/stats   Centers for Disease Control and Prevention (CDC)

http://www.cdc.gov/print.do?url=http://www.cdc.gov/vaccines/vpd-vac/hpv/hpv-vacsafe-effic.htm   CDC website with additional information about the HPV vaccine

Other Resources

American Nurses Association (ANA)
   8515 Georgia Avenue
   Suite #400
   Silver Springs, MD 20901
   1-800-274-4ANA
   http://www.nursingworld.org

American Association of Sex Educators, Counselors, and Therapists (AASECT)

P.O. Box 1960
Ashland, VA 23005-1960
(804) 752-0026

American Psychiatric Nurses Association (APNA)
   1555 Wilson Blvd., Suite 602
   Arlington, VA 22209
   1-866-243-2443
   http://www.apna.org

Sexuality Health Network
   3 Mayflower Lane
   Shelton, CT 06484
   http://www.sexualhealth.com

Sexuality Information Education Council of the United States (SIECUS)
   130 W. 42nd St., Suite 350
   New York, NY 10036
   (212) 819-9770
   http://www.siecus.org

REFERENCES

Alan Guttmacher Institute. (1999). *Adolescents and STDs.* Retrieved June, 2002, from http://www.agi-usa.org

American Nurses Association. (2000). *A statement on psychiatric-mental health nursing practices and standards of psychiatric-mental health practice.* Washington, DC: Author.

American Psychiatric Association. (2000). *Diagnostic and statistical manual of mental disorders* (4th edition, Text Revision) (*DSM-IV-TR*). Washington, DC: American Nurses Publishing.

Bogaert, A. F. (2007). Extreme right-handedness, older brothers, and sexual orientation in men. *Neuropsychology, 21,* 141–148.

Centers for Disease Control and Prevention. (1999). *Mortality L285 slide series* (through 2000). Retrieved June 21, 2002, from http://www.cdc.gov/hiv/graphics/mortalit.htm

Centers for Disease Control and Prevention. (2004). *Genital HPV Infection.* CDC Fact Sheet. Available at http://www.cdc.gov/std/HPV/default.htm

Centers for Disease Control and Prevention. (2005). STD Surveillance 2005. National Profile. http://www.cdc.gov/std/stats/toc2005.htm.

Centers for Disease Control and Prevention. (2007). Rapid HIV testing in emergency departments—three U.S. sites, January 2005–March 2006. *Morbidity and Mortality Weekly Report, 56,* 597–601.

Crenshaw, T. L., & Goldberg, J. P. (1996). *Sexual pharmacology.* New York: W.W. Norton.

Donovan, J. (1988). *Feminist theory.* New York: Continuum.

Dumas, L. S. (1996). *Talking with kids about tough issues.* Menlo Park, CA: Kaiser Family Foundation.

Erikson, E. (1964). *Childhood and society.* New York: W.W. Norton.

Fasula, A. M., & Miller, K. S. (2006). African-American and Hispanic adolescents' intentions to delay first intercourse: Parental communication as a buffer for sexually active peers. *Journal of Adolescent Health, 38,* 193–200.

Fogel, C. I., & Lauver, D. (1990). *Sexual health promotion.* Philadelphia: W.B. Saunders.

Freud, S. (1962). *Three essays on the theory of sexuality.* New York: Avon.

Georgiadis, J. R., Kortekaas, R., Kuipers, R., Nieuwenburg, A., Pruim, J., Reinders, A. A., et al. (2006). Regional cerebral blood flow changes associated with clitorally induced orgasm in healthy women. *European Journal of Neuroscience, 24,* 3305–3316.

Haning, R. V., O'Keefe, S. L., Randall, E. J., Kommor, M. J., Baker, E., & Wilson, R. (2007). Intimacy, orgasm likelihood, and conflict predict sexual satisfaction in heterosexual male and female respondents. *Journal of Sex and Marital Therapy, 33,* 93–113.

Hochhauser, M., & Greensweig, E. (1992). *Why do people have sex? Implications for AIDS education.* Paper presented at the Sixth International Conference on AIDS Education, Washington, DC.

Hooper, A. (1992). *The ultimate sex book: A therapist's guide to sexual fulfillment.* New York: Dorling Kindersley Limited.

Kao, T. S., Guthrie, B., Loveland-Cherry, C. (2007). An intergenerational approach to understanding Taiwanese American adolescent girls' and their mothers' perceptions about sexual health. *Journal of Family Nursing, 13,* 312–332.

Kaplan, H. S. (1974). *The new sex therapy.* New York: Brunner/Mazel.

Klingman, L. (1999). Assessing the female reproductive system: A guide through the gynecologic exam. *American Journal of Nursing, 99,* 37–43.

Ladas, A., Whipple, B., & Perry, J. (1983). *The G spot and other discoveries about human sexuality.* New York: Dell.

Lam, B., Donaldson, C., Brown, Y., & Malliaris, Y. (2005). Burden and marital and sexual satisfaction in the partners of bipolar patients. *Bipolar Disorders, 7,* 431–440.

Laumann, E., Paik, A., & Rosen, R. (1999). Sexual dysfunction in the United States: Prevalence and predictors. *Journal of the American Medical Association, 281,* 537–544.

Litzinger, S., & Gordon, K. C. (2005). Exploring relationships among communication, sexual satisfaction, and marital satisfaction. *Journal of Sex and Marital Therapy, 31,* 409–424.

Lou, C. H., Zhao, Q., Gao, E. S., & Shah, I. H. (2006). Can the Internet be used effectively to provide sex education to young people in China? *Journal of Adolescent Health, 39,* 720–728.

Levine, S. B. (1998). Sexuality in mid-life. New York: Plenum.

Lubkin, I. M. (1986). *Chronic illness: Impact and interventions.* Boston: Jones & Bartlett.

Macdowall, W., Wellings, K., Mercer, C. H., Nanchahal, K., Copas, A. J., McManus, S., et al. (2006). Learning about sex: Results from Natsal 2000. *Health Education and Behavior, 33,* 802–811.

Markowitz, L. E., Dunne, E. F., Saraiya, M., Lawson, H. W., Chesson, H., & Unger, E. R. (2007). Quadrivalent human papillomavirus vaccine: Recommendations of the Advisory Committee on Immunization Practices (ACIP). *Morbidity and Mortality Weekly Reports, 56,* 1–24.

Maslow, A. H. (Ed.). (1970). *Motivation and personality* (2nd ed.). New York: Harper & Row.

Masters, W. H., & Johnson, V. E. (1966). *Human sexual response.* Boston: Little, Brown.

Masters, W. H., & Johnson, V. E. (1970). *Human sexual inadequacy.* Boston: Little, Brown.

McEwen, B. S. (2007). Physiology and neurobiology of stress and adaptation: Central role of the brain. *Physiology Review, 87,* 873–904.

Miller, K. S., Kotchick, B. A., Dorsey, S., Forehand, R., & Ham, A. V. (1998). Family communication about sex: What are parents saying and are their adolescents listening? *Family Planning Perspectives, 30,* 218–222, 235.

North American Nursing Diagnoses Association (NANDA). (2007). *Nursing diagnoses: Definitions and classification 2007–2008.* Philadelphia: Author.

Rahman, Q. (2005). The neurodevelopment of human sexual orientation. *Neuroscience and Biobehavioral Reviews, 29,* 1057–1066.

Rogers, C. R. (1951). *Client-centered therapy: Its current practice, implications, and theory.* Boston: Houghton Mifflin.

Satcher, D. (2001). Call to action to promote sexual health and responsible behavior. Washington, DC: Health Services Technology Assessment Text. Can be accessed at: http://www.ncbi.nlm.nih.gov/books/bv.fcgi?rid=hstat (Accessed March 17, 2007).

Schnarch, D. (1997). *Passionate marriage.* NY: WW Norton & Co. Inc.

Sisk, C. L., & Zehr, J. L. (2005). Pubertal hormones organize the adolescent brain and behavior. Frontiers in *Neuroendocrinology, 26,* 163–174.

Von Sadovsky, V., Keller, M. L., & McKinney, K. (2002). Image. *Journal of Nursing Scholarship, 34,* 133–138.

Williams, M. A. (1999a, September). *Revolution.* Paper presented at the meeting of Contemporary Sexuality: The International Resource for Educators, Researchers and Therapists.

Woitiz, J. G. (1985). *Struggle for intimacy.* Deerfield Beach, FL: Health Communications, Inc.

World Association for Sexology (WAS). (1999). *Declaration of sexual rights*. Paper presented at the meeting of the World Association for Sexology, Hong Kong.

World Health Organization (WHO). (1975). *Education and treatment in human sexuality: The training of health professionals*. (Tech. Rep. No. 572). Geneva, Switzerland: Author.

SUGGESTED READINGS

Barbach, L. (1975). *For yourself: The fulfillment of female sexuality*. New York: Anchor Books.

Barback, L. (1984). *For each other: Sharing sexual intimacy*. New York: Signet Books.

Boston Women's Health Book Collective. (1998). *Our bodies, ourselves for the new century*. New York, NY: Touchstone.

Castleman, M. (2004). *Great sex: A man's guide to the secret principles of total-body sex.* New York, NY: St. Martins Press.

Dodson, B. (1987). *Sex for one: The joy of self-loving.* New York, NY: Harmony Books.

Heiman, J., & LoPiccolo, L. (1998). *Becoming orgasmic: A sexual growth program for women.* New York, NY: Prentice-Hall.

Kashak, E., & Tiefer, L. (2001). *A new view of women's sexual problems.* Binghamton, NY: Haworth Press.

Louden, J. (1992). *The woman's comfort book.* San Francisco: Harper Books.

Louden, J. (1994). *The couple's comfort book.* San Francisco: Harper Books.

Maltz, W. (1992). *The sexual healing journey: A guide for survivors of sexual abuse.* New York, NY: Harper Collins.

Northrup, C. (1995). *Women's bodies, women's wisdom: Creating physical and emotional health and healing.* New York, NY: Bantam.

Zilbergeld, B. (1992). *The new male sexuality.* New York: Bantam Books.

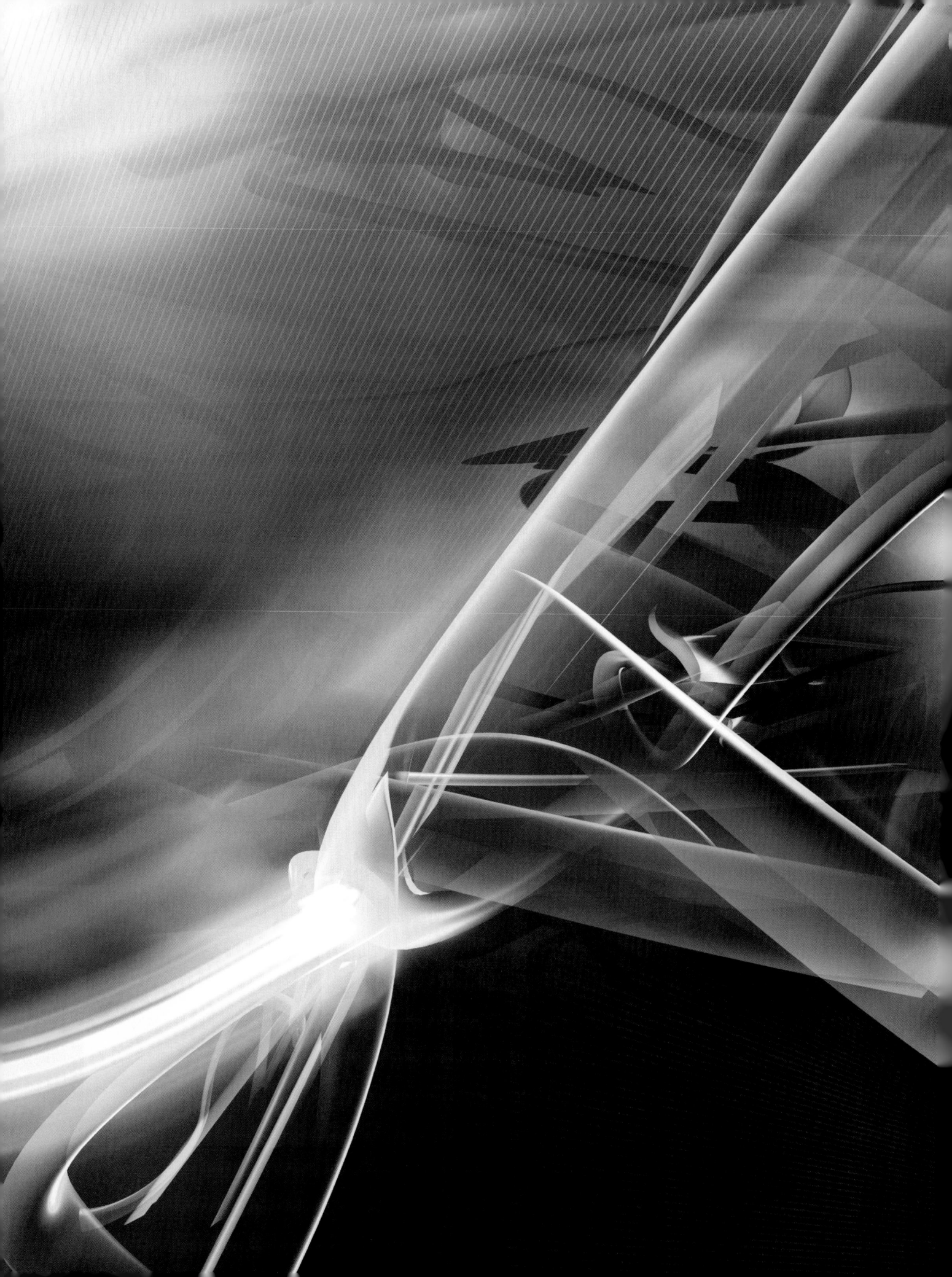

CHAPTER 25

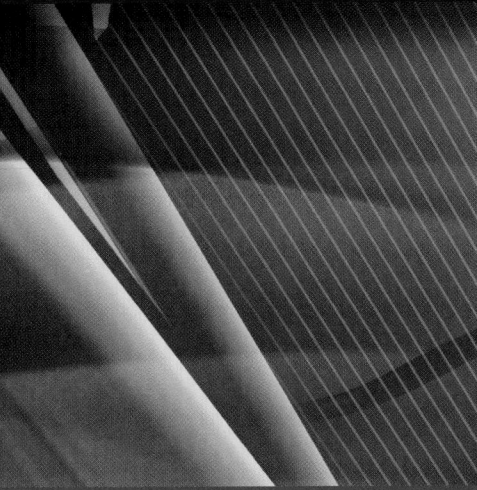

The Client Who Survives Violence

Deborah Antai-Otong, MS, APRN, BC, FAAN
Laura Smith-McKenna, RN, MS, DNSc
Christine Grant, PhD, RN

KEY TERMS

Child Maltreatment: Refers to actions and behaviors that result in serious physical injury, neglect, sexual abuse, and serious mental injury to a child.

Cycle of Violence: A dynamic described by some survivors of intimate partner abuse. The cycle begins with low levels of abuse, which build to an acutely abusive incident involving levels of violence higher than that of the abuse experienced on a regular basis. Following the acute violence, the perpetrator engages in actions designed to keep the relationship from ending, creating an "ideal" dynamic to keep the survivor involved. If there is no change in the abusive behaviors, the tension building stage begins again, leading to another cycle of acute violence.

Elder Abuse: Abuse of a person over 60 years of age, which may include physical abuse but also sexual, emotional, or financial abuse and abandonment.

Intergenerational Transmission of Violence: Describes the phenomenon of violent behaviors being learned and repeated by subsequent generations of abusive families.

Intimate Partner Violence: Physical, sexual, or emotional and psychological abuse of men or women occurring in past or current intimate relationships, cohabiting or not, and including dating relationships.

Neglect: The failure to provide for the individual's basic needs for subsistence, including food, housing, clothing, education, medical care, and emotional care. At its most extreme, neglect results in death, especially in the older adults and in very young children.

Pedophile: An adult who is sexually attracted to children and who abuses them sexually.

Perpetrator: A person who inflicts abuse or injury on another.

Physical Abuse: Involves the intentional use of physical force against another person, including but not limited to, pushing, slapping, biting, choking, punching, beating, and using a gun, knife, or other weapon.

Psychological Abuse: Usually verbal abuse designed to control another through use of intimidation, degradation, or fear.

Sexual Abuse: Abusive sexual contact, completed or attempted, against the will of the other, or in circumstances in which the other is unable to understand, refuse, or communicate unwillingness to engage in the sexual activity.

Sexual Assault: Abusive sexual contact, completed or attempted, against the will of the other, or in circumstances in which the other is unable to understand, refuse, or communicate unwillingness to engage in the sexual activity.

Shaken Baby Syndrome: A form of child abuse depicted by a compilation of signs and symptoms associated with the violent shaking of an infant or small child.

COMPETENCIES

Upon completion of this chapter, the learner should be able to:

1. Analyze the client as a survivor of violence and abuse across the life span.

2. Assess factors related to the client's risk for violence or abuse.

3. Differentiate the immediate and long-term effects on clients of experience with violence or abuse, or both, across the life span.

4. Discuss ethical and legal issues related to the nurse's role in assessing for and reporting the client's experience with violence or abuse, or both.

5. Formulate a plan of nursing care for clients who survive or perpetrate violence or abuse, or both.

6. Apply the nursing process to survivors and perpetrators of violence

7. Analyze cultural factors that influence the incidence of violence and the client's response to violence or abuse, or both.

8. Discuss one's own attitudes about violence and abuse and the effects of violence and abuse on one's own life.

CHAPTER OUTLINE

Violence is a leading worldwide public health problem (World Health Organization [WHO], 2005). Violence is also an inescapable public health problem, with an estimated 1.9 million women and 3.2 million men being physically assaulted each year (Tjaden & Thoennes, 2000b). Prevalence of some types of violence varies based on race, ethnicity, and culture, with some minority women and men reporting more frequent and more violent victimization. Violence accounts for the death of 1.6 million people and is among the foremost causes of death for people aged 15 to 44 years worldwide, accounting for 14 percent of deaths among males and 7 percent of deaths among females. For every homicide that results from violence, millions more are injured and suffer from a broad range of physical, sexual, reproductive, and mental health problems (WHO, 2002, 2006). Nurses and other health care providers must guard against insensitivity when working with survivors of violence.

Although violence is prevalent in most societies, the concepts of violence and abuse are complex, and definitions vary. Nurses, physicians, and health care providers from other disciplines may not share common concepts and definitions of violence and abuse. Competing frameworks can create controversy and lack of understanding. The statistics and consequences of violence and abuse require nurses to prepare for collaboration necessary to the coordination of effective interventions with survivors and perpetrators of violence and abuse.

Nurses are mandated reporters of many types of violence and abuse. They will encounter survivors and perpetrators of violence and abuse in all health care settings. The *Diagnostic*

and Statistical Manual of Mental Disorders (4th edition Revision) *(DSM-IV-TR)* (American Psychiatric Association [APA], 2000), includes a section categorizing severity of mistreatment (Table 25–1). Knowledge of the incidence, dynamics, and risk factors related to violence and abuse is essential. In addition, nurses need to be aware of their own feelings regarding violence and abuse to interact with clients using nursing process skills. (Chapter 6 discusses therapeutic relationships with these clients.) This chapter focuses on the effects of violence on the individual client who survives, on the family context, and on the nursing process with individuals and families experiencing violence and abuse across the life span.

DEFINITIONS AND INCIDENCE OF VIOLENCE

Because definitions of abuse vary, clarification of common definitions are necessary. Variation in the definition of abuse is one factor contributing to inaccurate statistics of incidence of violence and abuse.

CHILD MALTREATMENT

Child maltreatment refers to actions and behaviors that result in serious physical injury, neglect, sexual abuse, and serious mental injury to a child. The WHO World Report on Violence and Health indicates that child abuse is a major, unrecognized problem affecting the formative years and welfare of children throughout their life span. According to the WHO, approximately 57,000 children were victims of homicide in 2000. Due to a lack of routine investigation or autopsies of child deaths, it is difficult to discern the true extent of this problem (WHO, 2002). During their meeting in Geneva in 1999 a consensus of recommendations was made. See Figure 25–1, Major Recommendations on the Prevention of Child Abuse.

According to U.S. Department of Health and Human Services (DHHS) 2005 Fact Sheet concerning the 2002

TABLE 25–1
Problems Related to Abuse or Neglect as Defined by *DSM-IV-TR*

The focus of clinical attention is harsh abuse of one person by another (e.g., physical and sexual abuse or child neglect).

Specify whether the client is a victim or perpetrator.

The following categories apply:

1. Physical abuse of child
2. Sexual abuse of child
3. Neglect of child
4. Physical abuse of adult (e.g., intimate partner violence, elder abuse)
5. Sexual abuse of adult

Note. From *Diagnostic and Statistical Manual of Mental Disorders* (4th edition, Text Revision) *(DSM-IV-TR)*, by the American Psychiatric Association, 2000, Washington, DC: Author.

- Research (evidence-based to approach child abuse prevention)

- Data collection (standardized assessment tools for prevalence, consequences, and cost using a data bank)

- Good practices to identify and initiate various preventive measures—primary, secondary, and tertiary

- Advocacy to promote international awareness and concern for child abuse as a public health problem (global electronic discussion network)

- Policy that defines the WHO's definition of child abuse, using a multidisciplinary and collaborative approach, and legislative issues

- Training to develop and integrate educational systems

Figure 25–1 Major Recommendations on the Prevention of Child Abuse.
(Note. From Child Abuse and Neglect, by the World Health Organization, 1999, retrieved June 24, 2000, from http://www.who.int/violence_injury_prevention/main.cfm.)

national child abuse and statistics reported by states, there was a slight increase in the number of survivors nationwide, from 900,000 in 2002 to about 906,000 in 2003. Almost 61 percent of survivors suffered neglect, whereas 19 percent suffered physical abuse, 10 percent were sexually abused, and 5 percent suffered emotional and psychological abuse. Fatalities resulting from child abuse rose slightly at 1,500. The prevalence of shaken baby syndrome remains unchanged at about 1,200 to 1,600 (DHHS, 2005).

Concerns about the global prevalence of maltreatment of children continue to be echoed by world organizations. The *United Nation's Secretary General Study of Violence Against Children*, published in 2006 (United Nations, 2006), concluded that violence against children occurs everywhere, in every country and across all social groups. The purposes of this study were to galvanize and depict the global nature, prevalence, and causes of violence against children; propose preventive measures; and respond to it. The secretary concluded that violence against children is never justifiable. There is urgency for societies to end violence against children and recognize child maltreatment as multidimensional and requiring multifaceted responses.

Although child abuse takes many forms, some types of violence against children by parents or guardians are unrecognized and characterized as "discipline" rather than abuse. This section focuses on serious physical injury, neglect, sexual abuse, and serious mental injury.

Physical Abuse and Injury

According to the Department of Human Health Services Fact Sheet (2005) on Child Maltreatment from child protective service agencies' data, which is considered underestimates, nearly a million children in this country experienced or were at risk for child abuse, neglect, or both. Head trauma, which often results from shaking, accounted for the leading cause of death and disability among maltreated infants and children. The physical abuse of a child is any intentional injury inflicted by the child's caretaker. Physical abuse can be a single episode or repeated events and involves inflicting physical injury by punching, beating, kicking, shaking, or otherwise harming a child. Shaken-baby syndrome (SBS) affects about 1,200 to 1,600 children annually. SBS is a compilation of signs and symptoms resulting from violently shaking an infant or child (see Table 25–2). Depending on the severity of the injury, the child's physical functioning is either permanently or temporarily impaired. The harm causes severe pain to the child and may be accompanied by a pattern of separate, unexplained injuries (see Table 25–3 for forms of child physical abuse).

Nurses must always consider physical abuse when the child has bruises or other injuries that are difficult to explain or inconsistent with the given explanation. Oftentimes, these children are withdrawn, overly aggressive, or exhibit delay in developmental tasks. A child who has frequent visits to the hospital emergency room or other practice settings for the treatment of bizarre or strange complaints

with overly doting parents or guardians may be a victim of Munchausen syndrome by proxy. Characteristics of this syndrome involve a parent or guardian asking or forcing the child to take substances that induce signs of physical illnesses (e.g., dehydration, diarrhea) and seeking medical attention to manage them (Stirling & American Academy of Pediatrics Committee on Child Abuse and Neglect, 2007) (see Chapter 12).

TABLE 25–2
Shaken Baby Syndrome

- Lethargy, decreased or poor muscle tone
- Marked agitation and irritability
- Feeding and appetite disturbances, vomiting without apparent cause
- Poor sucking and swallowing reflexes
- Failure to thrive
- Seizures
- Breathing difficulties
- Changes in head circumference, bulging fontanels
- Difficulty lifting head
- Unequal pupils, dilated pupils, difficulty tracking

TABLE 25–3
Forms of Child Physical Abuse

- Skin and soft tissue injury (i.e., bruises, hematomas, and abrasions
- Internal injuries
- Dislocations and fractures
- Loss of teeth caused by shaking, slapping, punching, kicking, striking, and hitting
- Throwing of child or throwing objects against the child
- Branding or loop or restraint marks made by belt buckles, handprints, electric cords, ropes, or ligatures
- Hair loss caused by pulling the child by the hair
- Burns caused by spills, immersions, flames, and branding
- Wounds caused by gunshots, knives, razors, or other sharp objects

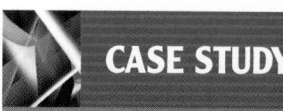

CASE STUDY

The Child Experiencing Physical Abuse (Charlie)

Charlie, an 8-year-old boy, is transferred to the child psychiatry unit after a court-ordered psychiatric evaluation. Charlie has a known history of being abused by his natural mother. A recent attempt to reunite mother and son ended when Charlie reported to the school nurse that his mother was beating him.

See Nursing Care Plan 25–1.

NURSING CARE PLAN 25–1

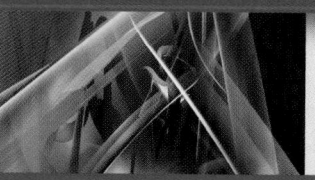

The Child Experiencing Physical Abuse (Charlie)

Nursing Diagnosis: Situational Low Self-Esteem related to physical abuse

Outcome Identification	Nursing Actions	Rationales	Evaluation
1. By [date], Charlie will identify feelings of self-worth.	1a. Encourage Charlie to verbalize his thoughts and feelings related to his mother and her abusive actions.	1a. Understanding of the client's perception of abuse and role in the experience is essential to validate the client's feelings.	*Goals met:* Charlie is able to express one positive attribute about himself. Charlie is able to demonstrate trust in his relationship with the nurse by continuing to discuss feelings.
	1b. Offer acceptance to Charlie. Do not use direct confrontation, yet support Charlie in his attempts to verbalize.	1b. Clients need to be viewed as worthwhile persons regardless of their experiences. Positive feedback gives clients the recognition they need to experience success.	
2. By [date], Charlie will express fears related to abuse.	2a. Support Charlie's ventilation of feelings.	2a. Memories of the abuse may evoke distress in Charlie.	
	2b. Create situations to discuss feelings in a safe manner.	2b. Indirect explorations of fears through play, storytelling, and board games can alleviate feelings of anxiety and fear.	
	2c. Anticipate Charlie's stress related to fears and provide problem-solving techniques.	2c. Increased stress interferes with a child's ability to cope. Teaching the child to handle fears will decrease anxiety of relating abuse.	

(continues)

Outcome Identification	Nursing Actions	Rationales	Evaluation
3. By [date], Charlie will demonstrate improved ability to deal with the effects of physical abuse.	3a. Spend time with Charlie to help him with full expression of a range of feelings.	3a. The child's ability to express feelings is critical to successful healing.	Charlie verbalizes his feelings and thoughts freely and openly.
	3b. Accept all feelings Charlie expresses as valid.	3b. Successful emotional processing of abuse must occur in a wide variety of expressions.	
	3c. Encourage Charlie to explain his feelings.	3c. Clients' distortions and misperceptions need to be corrected.	
	3d. Continually expose Charlie to the realities of his abuse and legal proceedings that may be occurring.	3d. Realization of future outcomes will help clients grieve their losses.	

Neglect

Legal definitions of neglect vary by individual states. On a practical basis **neglect** is nebulous and encompasses a continuum of behaviors. The CDC (2001) defines neglect as a failure to provide for the child's basic needs, including food, housing, clothing, education, medical care, and emotional care. There are many variations of the term "healthy growth and development," and situations involving neglect are not easily identified. Neglect (see Table 25–4 for types of neglect and behaviors indicating neglect), at its most extreme, results in death, especially in very young children.

Emotional or Psychological Abuse

Emotional or *psychological abuse* refers to acts or behaviors or omissions by primary caregivers that result in or increase the risk of serious behavioral, cognitive, emotional, and mental disorders. This definition includes, but is not limited to, psychological, verbal, and mental injury. The relationship

TABLE 25–4
Types of Neglect and Behaviors Indicating Neglect

Type of Neglect	Behavior Indicating Neglect
Failure to protect	Ingestion of poison, accidents (including falls, electric shocks, and burns), and disregard for the child's safety. Lack of appropriate supervision.
Physical neglect	Failure to provide food, clothing, and shelter. Failure to provide adequate heating, diet, and hygiene. Indicators include diaper dermatitis, lice, odors, scabies, dirty appearance, inappropriate clothing for the season, lack of adequate bedding, and a living environment infested with insects or rodents. Other signs include failure to immunize, poor dental hygiene, malnutrition, and failure to provide the child with hearing and seeing aids.
Medical neglect	Failure to provide for the medical needs of the child, including failure to seek timely intervention or failure to comply with prescribed medical treatment. Indicators include repeated urgent health care visits, delayed diagnosis, physical incapacity, and avoidable complications.
Emotional neglect and nonorganic failure to thrive	Failure to provide nurturing and psychological support. Indicators include delayed growth and development; depression; poor school performance; acute, psychiatric manifestations (withdrawal, phobias, hyperactivity, and acting out); and difficulties with relationships (inability to trust, attention-seeking behaviors, or suspiciousness).

between childhood maltreatment and mental disorders is well documented (Kaplow & Widom, 2007; Widom, DuMont, & Czaja, 2007). Recent studies also implicate child maltreatment and neglect as markers for other factors that make an impact on the developing child and increase the risk of lifelong maladaptive behaviors. Examples of mental disorders associated with childhood maltreatment and abuse include post-traumatic stress disorder (PTSD) and other anxiety disorders, depression, and antisocial behaviors. Risk factors for emotional abuse and other forms of maltreatment include poverty, parental substance misuse, or inadequate social and family functioning (DHHS, 2005). The ultimate emotional scar of maltreatment lies in its impact on the child's perception of self and others within the social context. Sadly, the children often recognize the hatred implied by the caregiver's behavior and are forced to perceive selves as worthless or unlovable.

The potential negative impact of emotional and other forms of maltreatment require nurses to recognize high-risk groups and clinical signs of maladaptive behaviors in both the child and caregiver. For instance, a child who appears overly anxious or frightened or a caregiver who fails to provide basic needs such as safety and nutrition may imply emotional abuse. Nurses must be careful and document observations and signs of maltreatment and report them according to state and federal laws. Health education is also pivotal in reducing child maltreatment and provides opportunities for nurses to teach parenting classes, anger management, and make appropriate community referrals to strengthen caregivers' coping skills.

Sexual Abuse

Sexual abuse is defined as abusive sexual contact, completed or attempted, against the will of the other, or in

---

DSM-IV Diagnostic Criteria for Pedophilia

302.2 Pedophilia

A. Over a period of at least 6 months, recurrent, intense sexually arousing fantasies, sexual urges, or behaviors involving sexual activity with a prepubescent child or children (generally age 13 years or younger).

B. The fantasies, sexual urges, or behaviors cause clinically significant distress or impairment in social, occupational, or other important areas of functioning.

C. The person is at least 16 years and at least 5 years older than the child or children in Criterion A.

Note. Do not include an individual in late adolescence involved in an ongoing sexual relationship with a 12- or 13-year-old.

Specify if:

Sexually attracted to males.

Sexually attracted to females.

Sexually attracted to both.

Specify if:

Limited to incest.

Specify type:

Exclusive type (attracted only to children).

Nonexclusive type.

TABLE 25–5
Types of Sexual Abuse Behaviors

- Penile penetration of the anus and/or vagina
- Insertion of object into the anus and/or vagina (e.g., finger)
- Fellatio and cunnilingus
- Masturbation of the victim
- Masturbation of self in front of the victim
- Manipulation of the genitals (e.g., touching, caressing)
- Exposure of the perpetrator's genital to the victim
- Exposure of pornography to the victim (e.g., sexually explicit magazines, books, videos, DVDs, or on the Internet)

---

circumstances in which the other is unable to understand, refuse, or communicate unwillingness to engage in the sexual activity. In addition, it refers to sexual contact with a person 5 or more years older than the child victim, whether by force or consent. The sexual contact includes a wide variety of sexual behaviors such as touching and exposing of the child's sexual parts for the sexual gratification of the perpetrator; sexual intercourse, oral and anal penetration; rape; the prostitution of children; and the use of children in pornography. The sexual contact can also be observed contact (i.e., exposing the genitals to the child or having the child view sexually explicit activity). (Table 25–5 lists types of sexual abuse behaviors.) Some adults who sexually abuse children are attracted to them sexually. The term for such a person is pedophile. The fourth edition of the *DSM-IV-TR* (APA, 2000) defines pedophilia under the paraphilias category of the sexual and gender identity disorders (see the display on the *DSM-IV-TR* diagnostic criteria for pedophilia).

Often overlooked, unrecognized, and undertreated is the sexual abuse of boys. In a meta-analysis of 166 studies representing 149 sexual abuse samples, Holmes and Slap (1998) found the prevalence of sexual abuse of boys common and ranged from 4 to 76 percent. The highest risk were younger boys less than 13 years, nonwhite, of low socioeconomic status, and not living with their fathers. Perpetrators were non-male relatives known by the children. The long-term effects of sexual abuse of boys were similar to girls and included psychological problems, substance abuse, mental illness, and sexual disturbances. These data also included a discussion about treatment considerations. A barrier to timely and appropriate interventions involved the reluctance of boys to discuss sexual abuse. This reluctance to discuss the abuse was identified as wanting to forget the event, wanting to protect the perpetrator, and fearing retaliation. Unfortunately, these data indicated that actions to help the abused males were limited. Nurses working with the sexually abused boy need to recognize the hesitancy of males to discuss these issues and, like females, must create an accepting and safe environment that promotes disclosure. Contemporary findings support these data indicating the emotional and physical impact of sexual abuse of boys (Dube et al., 2005).

Sexual abuse is differentiated from incest in that sexual abuse of children can involve a wide variety of perpetrators, not just blood relatives. Incest is a legal term describing a form of sexual abuse and is defined by each state's civil and criminal code. Incest is illegal in all states, but the behaviors that are considered incestuous may vary from state to state. For example, in Pennsylvania, the state code considers incest as sexual intercourse with a blood relative or a relative by adoption, including whole or half relations. Incest encompasses a wide variety of sexual behaviors and enormous effects on the victims.

Child abuse recognition and reporting has increased dramatically since the creation of the Society for the Prevention of Cruelty to Children in New York City in 1874, in response to the plight of one little girl, Mary Ellen Wilson.

Nurses are responsible for reporting suspected child maltreatment as mandated by these state reporting laws. All states and U.S. territories have laws and statutes requiring the reporting of child abuse and neglect to designated agencies or officials. Nurses who care for children and their families are in key positions to identify possible incidents of child abuse and neglect. Each state's reporting laws specify how to report, to whom, when, and the contents of the report. Most states have legal provisions to protect nurse reporters from civil lawsuits and criminal prosecution resulting from the reporting made in "good faith." Failure to report abuse by a designated mandated reporter, such as a nurse, could result in criminal penalties and loss of licensure. All nurses are urged to obtain copies of their state's reporting laws.

INTIMATE PARTNER VIOLENCE

Intimate partner violence (IPV), or domestic violence, is the most common type of violence perpetrated toward women. Violence against women encompasses intimate partner; sexual violence by any perpetrator, and various forms of violence against women, such as physical violence perpetrated by friends or strangers. Perpetrators of

 CLINICAL EXAMPLE

Recognizing and Reporting Child Abuse

Mary Ellen Wilson was abandoned as an infant and was taken in and raised by Mary McCormack Connolly. In the winter of 1873, Etta Wheeler, a missionary from St. Luke's Methodist Church in New York City, became aware that Mary Ellen was being beaten, starved, and imprisoned by her stepmother. Mrs. Wheeler contacted the police, who declined to get involved with the case, even though Mary Ellen was being beaten daily with a whip and locked in a dark, unventilated room. Mrs. Wheeler then approached the president of the Society for the Prevention of Cruelty to Animals and enlisted his aid. The child's court testimony reads as follows (Lazoritz, 1990, p. 143):

My name is Mary Ellen. I don't know how old I am. My mother and father are both dead. I have had no shoes or stockings this winter. I have never been allowed to go out of the rooms except in the night time . . . my bed at night is only a piece of carpet on the floor underneath a window. Mamma has been in the habit of whipping and beating me almost every day with a rawhide-twisted whip. The whip always left black and blue marks on my body. The cut on my head was made by a pair of scissors in mamma's hand. I have never been kissed by mamma. Whenever she went out she locked me in the bedrooms. I do not want to go back to live with mamma because she beats me so.

IPV include current or former spouse, boyfriend, or girlfriend (American Association of Colleges of Nursing [AACN], 2000). High-risk groups of IPV include young, childbearing women who are 16 to 24 years old (U.S. Department of Justice, 2006). Unfortunately, 30 percent of female homicide victims are killed by their spouses, boyfriends, or former partners, resulting in women being likely to be killed five times more than men because of IPV (U.S. Department of Justice, 2006).

It is commonly accepted that men underreport their own assaults and may also tolerate a certain level of violence from their intimate partner as a result of traditional cultural norms. Survivors of IPV are likely to be faulted for their abuse and are less likely to seek professional guidance or mention the abuse than survivors assaulted by strangers. A conservative estimate is that 1.3 million women and 835,000 men experience physical assault at the hands of an intimate partner each year (Tjaden & Theonnes, 2000b). Intimate partner violence is the foremost cause of injury to women, and as many as 45 percent of battered women report sexual abuse or rape in addition to repeated physical and psychological abuse. Studies consistently reveal that about 64 percent of women raped, physically assaulted, or stalked were the victims of a current husband, former husband, partner, boyfriend, or date (Tjaden & Thoennes, 2000b).

Major types of IPV include actual or threatened physical abuse, sexual assault, emotional abuse, or verbal abuse.

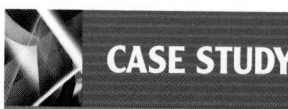

The Child Experiencing Sexual Abuse (Kerrie)

Kerrie, age 5, reveals to her mother that she doesn't like being touched. On questioning, Kerrie reveals that when she visits her father on the weekends, he crawls into her bed, lifts up her nightgown, and fondles her. Kerrie's mother contacts the local counseling center and is referred to an advanced-practice psychiatric-mental health nurse.

See Nursing Care Plan 25–2.

NURSING CARE PLAN 25–2

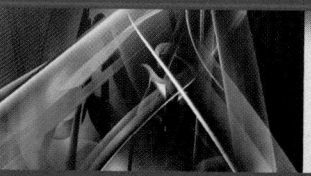

The Child Experiencing Sexual Abuse (Kerrie)

Nursing Diagnosis: Fear

Outcome Identification	Nursing Actions	Rationales	Evaluation
1. By [date], Kerrie will engage in discussions/therapeutic play sessions about sexual abuse.	1a. Assess post-traumatic stress response.	1a. Specific behavioral affective and cognitive responses correlate with post-traumatic stress disorder (see text).	*Goals met:* Kerrie participates in therapeutic plan.
	1b. Reassure Kerrie that she is not to blame.	1b. Children do not understand the concept of consent and the motives of the offender.	Kerrie verbalizes that she is not responsible for abuse. Kerrie experiences a full range of emotions through self-expression.
	1c. Encourage Kerrie to express feeling about abuse through play, the use of puppets or dolls for reenactment, stories or role play, or artwork.	1c. Developmentally appropriate interventions facilitate children's expression of trauma and associated memories.	Kerrie expresses appropriate physical boundaries within relationships. Family provides empathy to Kerrie and reinforces responsibility of abuser.
	1d. Record Kerrie's disclosure and clarify with mother the child's use and meaning of unfamiliar words (e.g., "pee pee" may mean vagina to the child).	1d. Contributions by family members can provide corrective information and an accurate understanding of the events. Family participation can assist the child's recovery.	Kerrie perceives parental figures as protective and available. Family is receptive to educational and supportive approaches.

(continues)

Outcome Identification	Nursing Actions	Rationales
2. By [date], Kerrie will express feelings of fear, guilt, and anger.	2a. Provide nurturant behaviors.	2a. Enhances trust and models positive behaviors for parents.
	2b. Guide mother to offer love and support to Kerrie.	2b. Fears of blame and retaliation can emerge in the child without continuous parental support.
3. By [date], Kerrie's mother will develop a plan to assist in Kerrie's recovery.	3. Identify Kerrie's coping skills and assess her educational needs.	3. The parent and child require an accurate understanding of abuse dynamics.

Physical abuse involves the intentional use of physical force against another person, including, but not limited to, pushing, slapping, biting, choking, punching, beating; and use of a gun, knife, or other weapon (U.S. Department of Justice, 2006).

Sexual assault is defined as abusive sexual contact, completed or attempted, against the will of the other, or in circumstances in which the other is unable to understand, refuse, or communicate unwillingness to engage in the sexual activity. Sexual assault is likely to have a profound psychological effect on the client and result in an array of mental health problems, such as depression, sexual dysfunction, anxiety disorders, substance-related disorders, and post-traumatic stress disorder (PTSD). In addition, these clients may suffer medical problems related to acute injuries and stress-related health problems (Suris, Lind, Kashner, & Borman, 2007). (See Research Abstract.)

Because the nurse is likely to be the first non-family member whom women encounter in emergency departments, battered women's shelters, college health clinics, primary care and office settings, or telephone crisis hotlines, she must be aware of symptoms that indicate acute stress reactions and

---

My Experience with Intimate Partner Violence

I used to think that abuse was normal because my father was abusive to my mother. I remember when he used to come home from work—we were terrified because we did not know what he was going to do. No one spoke and we all crept around talking in low voices for fear that he would be upset and hit someone. The first time my husband hit me, I did not know what happened. I was taken to the emergency room and I discovered that my arm was broken. I was afraid to tell the nurse that my husband twisted my arm so hard he broke it. I told her that I slipped and fell down the stairs. I could not tell her anything else because my husband answered most of the questions and he never left the room.

I was so frightened, and memories of my childhood surfaced. I married a man just like my father. The last incident of abuse was 5 years ago. It took me a long time to feel confident in myself or believe that I could make it on my own. I am now attending classes at a junior college. I was one of the lucky ones—to get out of the abusive relationship before I lost my life and dignity.

CRITICAL THINKING

1. Discuss the following statements:
   a. Men beat women to gain control and power.
   b. A survivor who stays in the abusive intimate relationship has a personality disorder or defect.
2. The world is violent. Discuss the factors that contribute to the high incidence of violence in the United States and other parts of the world, including handguns, drugs, poverty, sexism, and racism.
3. The intergenerational transmission of violence theory proposes that a child learns to be violent. What factors contribute to a person's expressing herself through violent means?
4. Blaming the survivor is a powerful force in cases of sexual assault, particularly in cases of teenage survivors of incest. Discuss this phenomenon.
5. Discuss how you would evaluate a caretaker's stress in regard to caring for an elderly dependent parent. How would you plan to evaluate the older adult?
6. Discuss how violence may differentially affect various cultures:
   a. Homicide is the leading cause of death in African American men.
   b. Family is all-important in the Hispanic culture.
   c. Divorce is shameful in Asian cultures.

- Advocating on behalf of survivors and their children
- Acknowledging the importance of making changes in the health care system to improve appropriate responses to violence

Psychological or emotional **abuse** is usually verbal abuse designed to control another through use of intimidation, degradation, or fear (AACN, 2000). Stalking may be included in the definition of psychological abuse. Nurses need to be aware of the reality that men are also survivors of intimate partner violence and that screening for exposure to violence must include all clients, not only women and girls presenting themselves for health care.

Overall, because survivors of IPV are less likely to disclose the abuse to nurses, it is important to create a supportive and empathetic environment that promotes expression of feelings. In addition, when the client reports IPV, the nurse needs to validate the client's feelings and grief and refrain from minimizing the emotional impact of violence. The nursing assessment needs to include questions about abuse and violence, both as survivor and perpetrator. Issues concerning perpetrators of violence are crucial to the prevention of future violence. Inquiring about history of consequences of violence, such as legal issues, needs to be assessed along with appropriate referrals to batterers intervention programs. In addition, the client's spiritual needs must be assessed. By providing emotional support and spiritual care the nurse is likely to strengthen internal resources and coping patterns and buffer the client against emotional and psychological distress. Spiritual care offers the survivor a greater understanding of self and mental connection with a higher power.

provide immediate emotional support. The nurse also needs to screen for sexual, physical, and psychological abuse. Information about the survivor must be kept confidential, and discussions with the perpetrator concerning IPV should never be done in the presence of the survivor. Once IPV is discussed, the nurse needs to use a direct and calm approach and focus on the abuser's behavior rather than the survivor's. Appropriate referrals to batterers intervention programs are important in dealing with IPV. Most states require participation in these programs as a stipulation of battering even when survivor objects or drops charges.

Initially, the client may be distant and untrusting, appear to be in a daze or state of shock, have problems answering questions spontaneously, and be emotionally distraught and tearful. Others may be overly compliant and exhibit very little emotion. Although the latter client appears less distraught than the former, the nurse must assess the emotional impact of this stressful situation. Nurses should also focus on the impact of the violence on the survivor's daily life, considering the social context and the degree to which the violence alienates the client from others. It is imperative for the nurse to assess the survivor's coping responses and offer help in resolving acute symptoms.

Warshaw (1998) delineates the following guiding principles when working with survivors of IPV:

- Providing safety of the survivors and their children must be a priority
- Respecting the woman's right and ability over her life choices
- Holding perpetrators responsible for the abuse and stopping it

ELDER ABUSE

Each year an estimated 10 percent of adults 65 years and older are abused, and 4 percent experience moderate-to-severe abuse. By 2030, the U.S. population will comprise about 70 million people, thereby increasing the risk of elder abuse (Greenberg, 1996; Program Resources Department, American Association of Retired Persons [AARP] and Administration on Aging [ADA], U.S. Department of Health and Human Services, 1993). Findings from the ADA's *National Elder Abuse Incidence Study: Final Report* (1998) support this trend and show that as many as 787,027 elders may have been abused or neglected in domestic settings in 1996. Findings from these data also indicate that almost four times as many new incidents of elder maltreatment were underreported than those reported and substantiated by the Adult Protective Services. In 1987, the American Medical Association's Council on Scientific Affairs defined elder abuse as an act or omission that results in harm or potential harm of an older adult (Council on Scientific Affairs, 1987). **Elder abuse** is abuse of a person over 60 years of age, which includes physical, sexual, financial, emotional, or psychological abuse; neglect; abandonment; material exploitation; and self-neglect. Self-neglect often manifests as an older adult's refusal or failure to provide self with basic needs (e.g., adequate food, water, clothing, shelter, and medication).

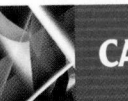

CASE STUDY

Kendra is a 30-year-old mother of two who has been seen in the emergency room several times the past six months with various injuries that indicate intimate partner violence. You notice that your co-workers question why she continues to return to her spouse and display little empathy during this visit. You are assigned to her and realize you have mixed feelings about her situation. While taking her blood pressure you notice she has several bruises on her arm and neck.

NURSE: Kendra, tell me what caused the bruises on your arm and neck.

CLIENT: I was in the pool with the kids and slipped as I got in.

NURSE: Slipped in the pool?

CLIENT: Yes.

NURSE: I noticed this is your third visit to the emergency room the past few months and each time you have different injuries.

CLIENT: I guess I am just accident prone.

NURSE: Are you and your children safe at home?

CLIENT: Of course we are. (She stops and becomes tearful.)

NURSE: (Silent and offers a tissue.)

CLIENT: Thank you.

NURSE: It sounds like you and your children are not safe.

CLIENT: My husband would kill me if I discussed anything with you or anyone else.

NURSE: I understand this is difficult to discuss, but I want to help. I want you and your kids to be safe.

CLIENT: How can you protect me?

NURSE: I can't protect you, but I can offer help in getting you and your kids in a safe place. You and your kids deserve to live free of fear and abuse.

CLIENT: I appreciate your offer, but I just can't leave now, but I will think about our talk.

NURSE: I respect your right to make your own decision. Please let me know if I can be of any assistance when you decide.

Discussion

This nurse took an extra step in assessing this client's situation. Although she had a lot of ambivalence concerning this client, she chose to express concern and offer support. Data indicate that women in abusive relationships stay in the relationship for many reasons and it is imperative for the nurse to respect her right to leave or return. She will know when it's safe to leave. It was important for the nurse to inquire if she and her kids were safe. It indirectly asks if she is in a violent or abusive relationship. It also helped the client look at her situation from a different perspective. Although she did not directly admit she was dealing with intimate partner violence it was inferred by the pattern of injuries from past visits and the current emergency room visit and expressed fears if she discussed them with the nurse. Nurses working with women in abusive relationships must put aside their own values and beliefs and support the client's decision, while offering hope or protection when she chooses it.

CASE STUDY

The Woman Experiencing Battering (Shelley)

Shelley, a 34-year-old mother of four, has been married to Jay for 9 years. Jay, an executive, demands perfection in his job and in his family. Over the past 3 years, since the birth of their fourth child, Jay has become increasingly hostile, belligerent, and abusive. Shelley has repeatedly been to her family physician with vague physical complaints. On New Year's Day, she went to the emergency department for a head injury she claimed occurred when she fell on the ice. In reality, Jay beat her during one of his angry rages. Shelley contacted the Victim Resource Center for counseling with an advanced-practice psychiatric-mental health nurse.

See Nursing Care Plan 25–3.

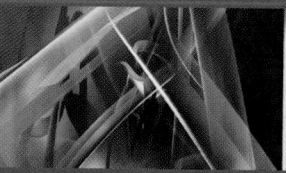

The Woman Experiencing Battering (Shelley)

Nursing Diagnosis: Fear and Anxiety
related to physical threat to self by batterer

Outcome Identification	Nursing Actions	Rationales	Evaluation
1. By [date], Shelley will describe the abuse and identify her fears.	1a. Approach Shelley nonjudgmentally. Ensure privacy and confidentiality.	1a. Conveying respect and empathy supports the client's self-worth.	*Goals met:* Shelley reports the extent of her abuse and her need for protection.
	1b. Assess level of danger to her by assessing her home situation and available resources. Inquire of Jay's escalating violence.	1b. Enhances the client's awareness of the potential for further injury.	Shelley is knowledgeable about community resources. Shelley identifies supportive family members and enlists their help.
2. By [date], Shelley will express the need for external resources.	2a. Provide Shelley with information on services available for battered women.	2a. The client's ability to be autonomous and in control is increased through knowledge, education, and outside resources.	
	2b. Explore with Shelley whether she can disclose her situation to trusted family members.	2b. Disclosure of abuse to others facilitates the potential for ending the abuse.	
	2c. Explore Shelley's fears related to contacting resources and informing supportive family members.	2c. The client may be afraid of retaliation by her husband's family and fear that her disclosure of abuse will not be believed. Survivors of battering may hold incorrect beliefs about their "causing" the abuse. Allowing Shelley to freely discuss her fears will provide the nurse with the opportunity to provide information and education about the dynamics of battering	

(continues)

Nursing Care Plan 25–3 *(continued)*

Outcome Identification	Nursing Actions	Rationales	Evaluation
3. By [date], Shelley will devise a plan to leave the home if needed.	3. Provide local service information, and refer Shelley to a support group if she desires. Allow Shelley to verbalize an escape plan.	3. Information gathering provides client with opportunities for increased self-awareness and facilitates control of self.	Shelley verbalizes a plan of action to ensure the safety of herself and her children.

During the Second Assembly on Aging held in Madrid Spain, April 2002, United Nations Secretary-General Kofi Annan reported data from a 20-year study of global elder abuse. Data from the survey identified three broad categories of elder abuse:

◆ *Neglect*—isolation, abandonment, and social exclusion

◆ *Violation*—of human, legal, and medical rights

◆ *Deprivation*—of choices, decisions, status, finances, and respect

These data also indicated that as a result of elder abuse, older adults may suffer from a loss of respect within the family, which can result in behavior that is disrespectful, dishonoring, isolating, or condescending. Researchers also concluded that oftentimes the perpetrators of elder abuse are family members, friends, or acquaintances (United Nations, 2002).

Elder abuse is underreported, and the ambiguous definitions used by both legal and social service agencies contribute to the variation in estimating the occurrence of elder abuse. While narrowly defined in the past as physical abuse only, a broader definition of elder abuse might include *physical abuse* but also *sexual abuse, emotional* or *psychological abuse, financial abuse,* and *abandonment* (Smith-McKenna, 1997). Typically, the profile of the abused older adult is female, isolated socially and perhaps geographically, and economically and physically dependent on a family system, without skills to deal with long-standing intergenerational conflict. The perpetrator may be a close relative, highly stressed, and dependent on the abused older adult financially or psychologically, or both (Schiamberg & Gans, 2000; Vandeweerd et al., 2006).

Caregiver's Stress

Caring for overly dependent older adults increases the risk of caregiver stress, particularly when the caregiver is unprepared for the duties or lacks resources. When assessing an older adult for abuse or neglect, the nurse needs to also assess the caregiver's ability to care for the client and available resources. In the case of a caregiver feeling ill-prepared to care for the older client, referrals for community resources and respite care must be considered.

CAUSATIVE FACTORS OF ABUSE: THEORIES AND PERSPECTIVES

Theoretical perspectives concerning causes and correlates of violence and abuse are vast. Many factors contribute to abuse and violence across the life span. Research shows that survivors of abuse and violence are also likely to become perpetrators. Similarly, inadequate family functioning contributes to neglect and child psychopathology. Psychological perspectives focus on individual characteristics and personality as key factors in aggression. Certain personalities, such as the antisocial, suspicious, paranoid, and sadistic types, appear to play a role in perpetuating violence and abuse.

PSYCHOANALYTICAL THEORY

Psychoanalytical theories suggest that aggression is a basic instinct that is expressed or suppressed as a result of a wide variety of interpersonal and intrapersonal factors. When a basic need of the person is not met, the person instinctively responds in an aggressive manner. This instinctivist theory proposes that aggression is an innate drive and that humans are fundamentally motivated by aggression (Ardrey, 1966; Lorenz, 1966).

NEUROBIOLOGICAL THEORY

Studies on aggression or violence indicate dysregulation in neurochemical, neuroendocrine, and neuroanatomical structures and genetic-environmental factors. Clients with an underlying brain disorder are likely to exhibit aggressive, explosive, and assaultive behaviors across the life span (Coccaro, McCloskey, Fitzgerald, & Phan, 2007). Biological theorists suggest that the limbic system and neurotransmitters play a role in the development of violent behavior. The limbic system influences memory storage, information interpreting and processing, and the autonomic functions of the nervous system. Within the limbic system's influence is the mediation of the aggressive sexual and emotional responses (Oquendo, Krunic, Parsey, Milak et al., 2005). Interference with the processing of information through brain lesions, substance use, head injury, malnutrition, and medical conditions such as epilepsy may contribute to the expression of aggression (Coccaro et al., 2007).

Additionally, research has suggested that exposure to trauma can evoke persistent biological abnormalities (Coccaro et al., 2007). PTSD, often diagnosed in survivors of sexual and physical trauma, has been associated with a hyperadrenergic state, hypofunctioning of the hypothalamic-pituitary-adrenocortical system, and dysregulation of the endogenous opioid system (Simeon et al., 2007). Physiological changes include sympathetic hyperarousal, excessive startle reflex, abnormalities in sleep physiology, and traumatic nightmares.

SOCIAL LEARNING THEORY

Social learning theory relies on role modeling, identification, and social interactions. Social learning theorist, such as Bandura (1973), postulated that behavior occurs as a result of cognitive and environmental factors and that aggression may be simulated and become a learned behavior. Children raised in abusive families are at risk of mimicking abuse or violent behaviors. Nurses need to identify high-risk groups and maladaptive coping behaviors and initiate adaptive coping behaviors that enable the child to manage stress and feelings effectively. Teaching the family adaptive coping skills provides opportunities for the child to model healthy and appropriate behaviors.

SOCIOLOGICAL THEORIES

Sociological theories of violence address cultural attitudes toward aggression, societal structures that permit aggression, and social frustration and fragmentation. Violence as a cultural attitude is reflected in the glorification of violent behavior in movies, song lyrics, and television, degradation of women, and in the acceptance of aggression or violence as part of daily living. In addition, social psychologists focus on the social learning that contributes to violence. When people grow up in a family context of violence, they learn that violence is a legitimate form of communication, often resulting in intergenerational transmission of violent behaviors (Fonagy & Target, 2005; Fonagy, Gergely, & Target, 2007).

An issue that is often overlooked but sharply criticized involves concerns about survivors either returning to the abusive relationship or maintaining close ties with the perpetrator. Researchers suggest that abused women view leaving violence as a form of loss and grief associated with their sense of security (Constantino, Sekula, Lebish, & Buehner, 2002; Theran, Sullivan, Bogat, & Stewart, 2006). Hence, severing ties with the perpetrator may have a profound impact on the survivor's sense of security and self-worth. Understandably, a social support system is a basic human need that satisfies the need for close bonds and intimacy. Oftentimes if a woman's sense of self-worth is defined by relationships, subsequently severing emotional ties, even

when they are abusive or violent, generates emotional distress or mental health problems (Constatino et al., 2002; Theran et al., 2006).

Implications for the nurse caring for the client in an abusive relationship must begin with understanding the emotional ties associated with the perpetrator. It is also important to understand that the survivor will leave the relationship when it feels safe. Acceptance and support of the client's decisions and feelings are critical elements of treatment planning and must be the foundation of the nurse-client relationship. Self-awareness about the client's decision enables the nurse to recognize the importance of client preferences and choices in dealing with abuse and violence.

PSYCHOSOCIAL FACTORS

The psychosocial factors or characteristics of abusive families have also been identified. The U.S. DHHS (2005) has identified a set of risk factors or correlates for child abuse that includes the following:

◆ Isolation from family and friends

◆ High ratio of negative to positive interactions with various family members

◆ High level of expressed anger and impulsivity

◆ Inappropriate expectations of the child

◆ Relatively high rate of both actual and perceived stress

Irrespective of the theoretical account of child abuse, there are certain factors that are consistently mentioned in the literature. Impulse control, anger control, conditioned emotional arousal, immature personality development, and emotion-focused coping are examples of the factors cited in the child abuse literature (Kaplow & Widom, 2007; Widom et al., 2007). In addition, the family unit has changed considerably over the past century. It has been redefined and includes single parents or guardians, stepfamilies, and grandparents. In addition to redefining families, societies are more mobile, and close proximity with extended families is minimal, resulting in a loss of support and increasing isolation during stressful periods. If there is abuse in the family, the family may respond by becoming even more isolated.

Yet families' increased isolation is only one factor and in itself does not explain the abuse of children. In the 1970s, the popular belief was that abusive parents had personality disorders that predisposed them to aggressive impulses and acting out. However, that view discounts social and cultural factors. Violence against children is better seen as an interaction of various factors, including psychological, sociological, cultural, situational, and societal influences.

GENERAL SYSTEMS THEORY

The psychological perspective looks for causes of violence within the individual, whereas the sociological view looks at

RESEARCH ABSTRACT

Women's Experiences with Violence: A National Study

Moracco, K. E., Runyan, C. W., Bowling, J. M., & Earp, J. A. (2007). *Womens Health Issues, 17,* 3–12.

Study Problem

The aim of this study was to examine women's experiences with violence and determine national lifetime estimates of victimization of women from diverse backgrounds including stalking behaviors.

Method

Researchers used a population-based national sample of noninstitutionalized women ages 18 years of age and older (*n* = 1,800), using a telephone survey on women's experiences with six types of violence, including being stalked and repeatedly contacted and physical and sexual assault by intimate partners and others. They examined the lifetime and previous-year prevalence of violent experiences based on bivariate differences in experiences among subjects and used a logistic regression to model the odds of adult lifetime and previous-year victimization.

Findings

Researchers demonstrated that 60 percent of the women experienced at least one type of violence since age 18; 10 percent reported violence in the previous year. Adult lifetime and prior-year prevalence varied by types of violence and by socioeconomic and demographic factors. Risk factors for experiencing violence in their adult lifetimes include women under age 55, those receiving public assistance, and lesbian/bisexual life preferences. In comparison, women age 18 to 24 had increased risks of victimization in the previous year.

Implications for Psychiatric Nurses

The prevalence of violence against women is well documented. Data from this study strengthen this premise and require psychiatric nurses to identify women at risk for violence across the life span. Psychiatric nurses must work with women who survive violence to determine their experiences and formulate a plan of care to address their needs.

the structure of the family. Straus, Gelles, and Steinmetz (1980) claimed that the family is society's most violent social institution. Straus (1973) presented the following eight propositions to illustrate how general systems theory relates to family violence:

1. Violence among family members has many causes and roots. Normative structures, personality traits, frustrations, and conflicts are only some of them.

2. More family violence occurs than is reported.

3. Most family violence is either denied or ignored.

4. Stereotyped family violence imagery is learned in early childhood from parents, siblings, and other children.

5. Family violence stereotypes are continually reaffirmed for adults and children through ordinary social interactions and the mass media.

6. Violent acts by violent persons may generate positive feedback—that is, these acts may produce desired results.

7. Use of violence, when contrary to family norms, creates additional conflicts over ordinary violence. The conflict now becomes the use of violence, not the behavior, that elicited that response in the first place.

8. Persons who are labeled violent may be encouraged to play out a violent role, either to live up to others' expectations of them as violent or to fulfill their own concept of themselves as violent or dangerous.

FEMINIST THEORY

Abuse of partners has been discussed from several theoretical vantage points, all of which vary considerably. The feminist perspective holds that female or partner abuse is the result of attitudes in our patriarchal society that support the inequality of women (Yodanis, 2004). Other literature has focused on the psychological nature of the interactions between the partners and emphasizes the dyadic patterns in the relationships (for a discussion of dyads, see Chapter 28).

Feminists (Ferree, 1990; Goldner, Penn, Sheinberg, & Walker, 1990; Schechter, 1982) refer to domestic violence as wife battering and assert that it is a means of keeping women in a subordinate position. Feminist theory goes on to explain that although only some men batter, others may benefit from the atmosphere of intimidation that it creates (Kilpatrick, 2004).

ROLE OF COPING AND ADAPTATION

Determining the proclivity for violence involves looking beyond pathology to maladaptive coping patterns. Role disturbance, power imbalance, and marital dissatisfaction all are correlates of abuse. Families with members who engage in maltreatment tend to exhibit a pattern of coping characterized by a low level of social exchange, low responsiveness to positive behaviors, and high responsiveness to negative behaviors. These families cope ineffectively and demonstrate inconsistent punishment and discipline. Failure to cope with or adapt to stress leads to low frustration tolerance, which, in turn, can escalate a situation to a crisis level. The resolution to the perceived crisis is often violence or abuse.

The relationship between specific psychosocial roles of family factors, such as substance misuse, is likely to result in ineffective coping patterns in the offspring. Alcohol abuse and substance abuse also play a role in abuse in the family. Maladaptive coping in the form of substance abuse can interfere with the person's ability to parent. Normally, family deficits in managing or coping with stress involve maltreatment and harsh and inconsistent interactions that result in transgenerational maladaptive coping patterns (Harris, Lieberman, & Marans, 2007).

Inadequate parenting skills, difficulties with intimacy, and ineffective interpersonal skills may result in a proclivity for abusive behaviors. Yet none of these characteristics has direct causation. There is no single cause of violence, and violence occurs in all socioeconomic, cultural, religious, and ethnic groups. Child abuse, for example, is an exceedingly complex problem. To characterize the problem as stemming from one underlying cause, no matter what the theoretical viewpoint, would be an oversimplification. Child abuse in the twenty-first century is the result of complicated interplay of several factors: poor parenting skills, social isolation, poverty, substance abuse, or a combination of these things. Family members' methods of coping, ineffective communication, and their ability to adapt to stress is but one influence in the development, escalation, or intervention of violence.

When working with families exhibiting maladaptive coping patterns, it is imperative for the nurse to assess their coping style, disciplining patterns, and cultural factors. Acting-out behaviors in the child or adolescent may indicate inadequate parenting or a mental or physical problem. When the nurse suspects child or elder abuse, the nurse must report it according to state laws governing abuse. Nursing interventions may include family crisis intervention, appropriate community referrals, or legal referrals.

For the most part, survivors of violence may also exhibit a pattern of behaviors, particularly in the presence of the perpetrator. Issues around control may surface as answering questions rather than allowing the survivor to respond to the nurse's questions or overt fearfulness and quietness.

CULTURAL FACTORS

Cultural factors may also influence abuse or violence. Cultural norms define social relationships and religious practices and are often transmitted by each generation. Transcultural factors may influence the clients' behavior in two different cultures. The challenge for psychiatric nurses is grasping the scope of violence or abuse on the individual. For instance, if a client comes with her partner and the partner is very controlling and refuses to allow her to answer questions, is this abuse or a cultural norm? Western culture might interpret this behavior as controlling and possibly covering up an abusive relationship. In comparison, some cultures condone this behavior and the woman is comfortable with the control, which has little do to

with abuse. It is also essential for nurses to assess and understand the culture in which the survivor resides before assuming that abuse or violence exists. It is important for nurses to assess and understand the differences between and within various cultural groups so that assessment can be structured to identify the unique needs of the clients from various cultural groups. Interventions also need to take into consideration the barriers that exist and limit access to culturally appropriate services (Yoshioka & Dang, 2005).

ABUSE AND VIOLENCE ACROSS THE LIFE SPAN

Although there are known immediate effects of violence that include physical, psychological, emotional, and spiritual harm, long-term consequences can be serious.

CHILDHOOD

The impact of abuse across the life span is well documented. Most data indicate that developmental coping skills and available resources have a profound impact on these effects. Psychiatric nurses play key roles in identification and prevention of abuse regardless of the client's age and provide interventions that facilitate adaptive resolution.

Acute Effects of Child Maltreatment

The immediate effects of child abuse on the survivor and the family are enormous. Regardless of the type of abuse a child sustains, research suggests that maltreated children demonstrate the following effects at varying levels of severity: disruptions in relationships, behavioral symptomatology, and developmental deficits (Fonagy & Target, 2005; Kaplan & Widom, 2007; Widom et al., 2007).

Disruptions in relationship can be observed in children through their interactions with their primary caregivers. Abused and neglected children may have difficulties in exploring and coping with the demands of new relationships and may demonstrate distortions in their relationships with their caregivers. These distortions include a tendency to be passive with the abusing parent or guardian rather than being either difficult or compliant. Some abused children may exhibit excessive dependency, wariness, and an inability to form interpersonal relationships.

Critical to an understanding of the effects of abuse on the child and adolescent is an appreciation of the components of the abuse. The nature of the act; the relationship of the perpetrator to the child; the response of other caregivers to the abuse; the frequency of the abuse; the duration and the severity of the abuse; and child-specific factors such as gender, coping and adaptation ability, and developmental level must be taken into account.

Children who are abused and neglected often present with varied acute symptoms. The nurse needs to consider the

TABLE 25–6
Immediate Effects of Abuse on the Child and Adolescent

Behavioral

- Acting out
- Aggression
- Hyperactivity
- Self-destructive acts
- Antisocial and delinquent behaviors (e.g., cruelty to animals, fire setting, and fecal smearing)
- Sexual acting out (promiscuity, prostitution, or sexualization)
- Somatic complaints and psychosomatic symptomatology

Emotional

- Depression
- Anxiety
- Anger
- Fears and phobias
- Psychotic processes
- Self-depreciating thoughts

Cognitive

- Distractability
- Concentration difficulties
- Memory impairment
- Poor judgment

Interpersonal

- Poor peer relationships
- Conflictual family relationships
- Disrespect and disregard for authority

Although the immediate effects of childhood victimization vary, an overriding effect is the erosion of trust. Without the ability to trust, a child cannot develop healthy relationships or meet the daily challenges of life. Children who are abused also have a confused sense of self. The loss of self-esteem directly related to the abuse often results in self-doubt, self-blame, and self-hatred. The nurse may recognize the immediate effects of child abuse through the child's expression of shame, embarrassment, guilt, and a sense of being different from other children.

The effect of child abuse on the family can be disruptive and reflective of the child's adaptation. Family members may respond to the disclosure of abuse with disbelief, minimization, denial, anger, hostility, and feelings of revenge.

Long-Term Effects of Child Maltreatment

The long-term aftermath of child abuse is complex and insidious. The human cost of the mistreatment of children is staggering. Children who are abused inherit a litany of psychological effects, poor interpersonal relationships, cognitive and developmental deficits, and low self-esteem. Over time, many of these children present with behavioral problems and psychopathology, some of which persist for a lifetime.

Children who are physically abused, neglected, or sexually victimized grow up with fundamental deficiencies in forming healthy relationships, independence, and motivation (Kaplan & Widom, 2007; Widom et al., 2007). The challenges of adulthood, such as achieving independence and forming intimate relationships, are compromised. The child may exhibit delayed developmental tasks such as trusting others or gratification in life experiences. Without early and effective intervention, these children grow up haunted by the fear of abandonment or exploitation (Oquendo et al., 2007). Oftentimes, these children develop dyscontrol behaviors, characterized by aggression, impulsivity, and agitation. In response to these fears, it is not unusual for the adult to seek out powerful authority figures who appear to be special caretakers. The adult survivor of child abuse has difficulty maintaining personal safety in the context of intimate relationships and may experience intense, unstable relationships. The adult survivor is also at risk of repeated victimization later in life.

ADOLESCENCE AND ADULTHOOD

Adolescents and adults, like children, are likely to experience acute and chronic effects of abuse or violence. Understanding age-related responses to these situations is crucial to the nurse caring for these clients.

Acute Effects of Intimate Partner Violence

Women's response to repeated acts of IPV has been described in the nursing literature in great depth. Researchers submit that the acute impact of abuse or violence generates an array of responses, including biological, physical, psychosocial, and behavioral (Constantino et al., 2002; Simeon et al., 2007). During the initial assessment process, the survivor

various defense mechanisms children may use to cope with the reality of the abuse. Like adults, children need to protect themselves from the emotional pain of the abuse. Common defense mechanisms used by children include denial, regression, projection, dissociation, and repression. Nurses also need to be aware of the immediate effects seen in children who are abused and neglected, some of which are delineated in Table 25–6. Nurses need to be very careful not to draw conclusions without a thorough assessment. Special educational preparation is necessary to perform a thorough assessment of a child who is suspected of being abused. Accurate documentation of social interactions with primary caregivers and the physical and mental status examinations is crucial to appropriate treatment planning.

may attribute physical wounds or diseases to something other than IPV.

Acute biological responses include intense anxiety, hyperarousal, elevated heart rate and blood pressure, muscle tension, sleep and concentration disturbances, and panic reactions. Physical symptoms may include bruises; swellings; burns; lacerations; fractures; abdominal injuries (especially during pregnancy); unwanted pregnancies; miscarriage; sexually transmitted diseases (STDs), including HIV; and homicide. Survivors may also develop stress-related conditions such as headaches, asthma, pelvic pain, irritable bowel syndrome, or other gastrointestinal disturbances.

Psychological responses include feeling embarrassed or fearful to disclose the abuse or sometimes feeling fearful that the nurse will not believe these clients. They may feel the need to protect the perpetrator, may excuse the abusive behavior, or may cover for the perpetrator in an attempt to be viewed favorably by either the abuser or others. Additional psychological responses include intense fear, anxiety, sexual dysfunction, eating problems, sleep disorders, suicide, PTSD, depression, and alcohol and other drug abuse. Many women who have experienced IPV develop a recognized pattern of psychological symptoms called *battered woman syndrome* (Walker, 1993). These symptoms are usually transient but are observed in a recognizable pattern in women who have been physically, sexually, or seriously psychologically abused by their partner. Components of battered woman syndrome are consistent with PTSD. For example, it is common for abused women to experience flashbacks to the violent incidents, and when the intrusive memories are too overwhelming, it is not uncommon for abused women to dissociate from the memories. Abused women experience avoidance of thoughts about the abuse, depression, and anxiety-based symptoms (see Chapter 11 for more information on PTSD). These effects are directly related to the destructiveness, unpredictability, and uncontrolled nature of the violence. The attacks—verbal, physical, and sexual—typically occur without warning or can be in response to some minor infraction that the perpetrator uses as an excuse to assault the survivor. Walker (1984) defines this recurrent violence as cycle of violence. The cycle of violence begins with low levels of abuse, which builds to an acutely abusive incident involving levels higher than that of the abuse experienced on a regular basis. Following the acute violent episode, the perpetrator engages in actions designed to keep the relationship from ending, generating an "ideal" dynamic to keep the survivor involved. If there is no change in the abusive behaviors, the tension building stage emerges again, resulting in another cycle of violence. The abused woman realizes that she cannot reason with her abuser and is helpless to resist the attacks. It is during these acute battering incidents that the woman feels psychologically trapped (Walker, 1989, 1993).

Behavioral responses of the survivors are a direct result of the abuse. For example, many survivors learn that to respond to the violence with physical fighting serves only to escalate the perpetrator's violence. Survivors of IPV endure abuse to

TABLE 25–7
Effects of Abuse on the Family

Acute Effects	Chronic Effects
• Yelling, screaming, verbal outbursts	• Psychopathological/ mental disturbances
• Erratic discipline	• Separation or divorce
• Corporal punishment	• Running away
• Isolation of members	• Court intervention
• Unrealistic expectations	• Social service involvement
• Disengagement or enmeshment	• Disturbances in school and work
• Role disruption	• Health problems
• Power struggles	• Drug or alcohol misuse
	• Intrafamilial homicide

protect their children, to protect other relatives, and in some instances, to protect their lives. Survivors often assume responsibility for the marriage or relationship and believe that to end the relationship indicates personal failure. One of the extreme behavioral responses to IPV is the realistic fear of homicide. This can involve the death of the abused partner, children, and the perpetrator.

Long-Term Effects of Intimate Partner Violence

The consequences of violence against intimate partners are enormous. The physical injuries survivors experience can be severe and disabling. The psychological effects can include passivity, lowered self-esteem, inability to deal with anger, and failure to nurture the self (Humphreys & Lee, 2005). The high correlation of post-traumatic stress disorder in women and men survivors of interpersonal violence is well documented (Duxbury, 2006). Psychiatric nurses are poised to identify behavioral, psychological, and neurobiological signs of trauma-related disorders. Survivors may become socially isolated, financially unstable, and engage in self-blame. IPV creates feelings of terror, constant anxiety, apprehension, and lingering self-doubt about the survivor's ability to cope. Other long-term effects from IPV include marital rape, sexual dysfunction, confusion regarding intimacy, and negative feelings toward and fear of the opposite sex.

See Table 25–7 for a summary of the general immediate and long-term effects of violence and abuse on the family.

OLDER ADULTHOOD

Abuse of older adults, similar to other age groups, can have profound emotional and physical effects. Recognizing high risk groups and behaviors enable the nurse to prevent abuse and promote safety in older adults.

Acute Effects of Elder Abuse

Older adults who survive abuse may present with unexplained physical injuries, such as fractures, bruises, abrasions, or hematomas, and may appear dehydrated, untidy, malnourished, or oversedated. The abused older adult may be in need of hearing, vision, and walking appliances, indicating that basic physical needs are not being met. Commonly, the psychological effects present in the abused older adult are withdrawal, passivity, hopelessness, and nonresponsiveness. The survivor of elder abuse may resist talking about the injuries, especially if the older adult is dependent on the perpetrator for her livelihood. The abused older adult is often embarrassed, humiliated, and defensive and protective of the perpetrator.

Long-Term Effects of Elder Abuse

The long-term physiological and psychological effects of elder abuse are similar to the immediate effects of abuse and include permanent injuries, such as fractures, dehydration, or electrolyte imbalances, and possibly death. Feelings of helplessness, hopelessness, and persistent despondency and depression often evolve over time. Elder abuse also increases the risk of suicide, particularly when coupled with depression. As previously mentioned, the older adult may be dependent on the perpetrator and reluctant to discuss circumstances surrounding injuries.

TREATMENT MODALITIES

The specific type of intervention used with a family or individual experiencing abuse is determined by the family's or survivor's current situation, ability to verbalize feelings, and willingness to effect change.

CRISIS INTERVENTION

Crisis intervention provides the family with immediate emotional support and facilitates adaptive coping responses and effective problem-solving skills. Initially, the child and parents or guardians may be seen separately and then together to assess family stressors, strengths, and coping patterns. It is important for the nurse to validate the survivor's feelings and provide safety. Parents or guardians who abuse their children may present with issues of chronic low self-esteem, depression, dependency, immaturity, impulsiveness, suspiciousness, and lack of empathy. Environmental stresses include financial problems, intergenerational transmission (i.e., parents usually raise their children the way they were brought up), or difficulties with family structures (i.e., single-parent families, large families, or blended families). These stressors can contribute to serious family dysfunction, resulting in child maltreatment. The nursing interventions include interventions that facilitate healthy parenting skills, stress management, improve communication, foster positive parent-child interactions, and to help

parents or guardians manage their conflicts. The nurse also needs to coordinate psychosocial services that link the family with necessary resources to reduce fragmented health care.

INTENSIVE HOME-BASED SERVICES

Intensive home-based (family preservation) services are becoming increasingly popular. This provides short-term, intensive interventions aimed at preventing the necessity of removal of the children from the home. Short-term concrete behavioral objectives that stop the violence or abuse are jointly contracted with the family and the professional.

Individual Therapy

Individual therapy ranges from insight-oriented psychotherapy to behavioral treatment. The following are some of the issues discussed in individual therapy:

- ◆ Past history of abuse
- ◆ Attitudes toward violence
- ◆ Cultural considerations
- ◆ Meaning ascribed to events
- ◆ Anger/impulse control
- ◆ Safety plan
- ◆ Sexuality and intimacy
- ◆ Stress
- ◆ Coping skills
- ◆ Substance misuse

Therapy for abusive parents or guardians focuses on the parents' ability to protect their children and meet their developmental needs. See Chapter 26 for further description of individual psychotherapy.

Couples/Marital Therapy

In families experiencing child maltreatment, couples therapy can be beneficial when parents or guardians realize that their anger toward and frustration with each other are being redirected onto the children. Couples can be taught direct and effective styles of communication that encourage expression of their feelings, listening techniques, and effective verbalizations.

In families in which incest is occurring, the focus of couples therapy is on the effect of the incest on the dyad. Issues in therapy include the couple's capacity for intimacy, sexual relations, communication, respect, and an examination of roles and responsibilities.

Couples therapy is not advised in IPV until the abusive partner has demonstrated an ability to control the dangerous physically abusive behaviors (see Chapter 28).

Family Therapy

Family therapy can also be a productive intervention if the family members are verbal, the children are old enough to participate, and the behavior related to anger in the family is controlled. The goal of intervention is to prevent further maltreatment. The following are examples of family therapy objectives:

◆ Confrontation of the abuse

◆ Identification of the pattern of abuse

◆ Setting of short- and long-term goals for the family in relation to the abuse

◆ Discussion of family roles and rules

Issues discussed with abusive families include the following:

◆ Impulse control

◆ Judgment errors (life choices)

◆ Conflicts with authority

◆ Manipulative behaviors, scapegoating, mixed or incongruent messages

◆ Tendency to act out rather than talk

◆ Blurred boundaries

◆ Role dysfunction

◆ Imbalance of power

◆ Communication skills

◆ Trust and intimacy

See Chapter 28 for further discussion of family and couples therapy.

Group Therapy

Group therapy interventions provide unique opportunities for family members to work on issues of trust, differentiation, and responsibility. It enhances interpersonal communication and provides safe opportunities for social relationships. Group therapy reduces isolation by bringing parents together, and improve self-esteem by introducing parents to other families who are struggling. Groups help parents learn to trust and receive and give support. During the group process, members confront their use of denial, projection, and rationalization defenses.

Group therapy is often the treatment of choice for child sexual offenders. Interestingly enough, in some cases of severe pedophilia, group therapy may reinforce the fantasies of the perpetrators. Some researchers suggest that the most promising treatment of sex offenders is a comprehensive cognitive-behavioral approach and antiandrogens (Hall & Hall, 2007). It may also be the treatment of choice for adult survivors of childhood sexual abuse. Chapter 27 provides more information on group therapy.

ACUTE PSYCHIATRIC HOSPITALIZATION

Psychiatric assessment should be considered when clients are chronically depressed, suicidal, or express affective or thought disorders. Crisis situations require immediate management when the client is a danger to self and others. Short-term inpatient stabilization is usually the treatment of choice in these cases (see Chapter 9).

PHARMACOLOGIC INTERVENTIONS

Pharmacologic interventions are useful in treating affective (mood) disorders, psychosis, acute anxiety reactions, and biological responses. A comprehensive physical and psychosocial assessment is necessary before beginning medication. These examinations provide information about differential diagnoses and the current health status.

SUBSTANCE ABUSE THERAPY

Substance abuse therapy provides medical treatment, addictions treatment, and support services for nonabusers. Most communities have services for drug and alcohol abusers, including:

◆ Detoxification programs

◆ Inpatient hospital programs

◆ Outpatient programs

◆ Health services

◆ Parent education classes

◆ Employment training or retraining

◆ Self-help or support groups (e.g., Parents Anonymous, Narcotics and Alcoholics Anonymous, Al-Anon) (see Chapter 21 for discussions of types of self-help groups)

◆ Educational support (i.e., high school graduate equivalent degree [GED] courses)

◆ Legal referrals and resources

BATTERERS INTERVENTIONS

Most batterers' intervention programs are based on the Duluth model which focuses on an educational process for perpetrators who batter their partners and involves a theoretical framework. This approach focuses on the issue of gender, blaming others for violence, common beliefs about batterers, and a process by which the batterer can examine his or her actions in light of self as a person. Oftentimes treatment is court ordered and nurses working with batterers often find them resistant to change and unwilling to accept their role in the cycle of violence. Major treatment includes weekly sessions with a theme per week focus, which include:

◆ Nonviolence

◆ Non-threatening behavior

◆ Respect, trust, and support

◆ Honesty and accountability

◆ Sexual respect, partnership

◆ Negotiation and fairness

The number of meetings is decided in advance and often parallels court order for treatment (Pence & Paymar, 1993).

TREATMENT FOR CHILDREN

Depending on the abuse experienced, the age, and verbal skills of the child, various therapies may be used to assist the child to deal with the violence.

Art Therapy

Art therapy allows children to express their feelings and thoughts rather than verbally expressing themselves. Art therapy is helpful as both a diagnostic and therapeutic tool (see Chapter 6).

Group Therapy

Group therapy allows abused children to regain their status as children. The group provides peer interactions and age-appropriate tasks. If both sexes are in a group, the co-leaders need to be a male and a female. Survivors are validated for their feelings and reinforced that they are not at fault. For example, if the child comments about being sad or upset, these feelings are accepted and validated by the group leader(s). Sometimes children from abusive families have been taught that expressing their feelings is not acceptable, and they begin to doubt their significance. By encouraging expressing of feelings, the child begins to feel worthwhile and positive about self. Groups for sexually abused children can help correct the distortions in the parent-child relationship. Groups should be in a safe place for children to talk and play out their feelings. The group leaders are role models who help the children learn to relate to peers who have also been abused.

Individual Therapy

Individual therapy is suggested for children who can verbalize their feelings and needs. Therapy is directed toward their fears, conflicts, and the disclosure of the trauma associated with the abuse. Therapy helps the child process the abuse.

Play Therapy

Play therapy is indicated for children too young to have the capacity for introspection and verbalization (toddler to 6 years old). Play therapy allows children to demonstrate their feelings through their actions. The abusive behaviors are observed in their play.

Special Education Programs

Special education programs for physically, developmentally, or emotionally disabled children should be considered by the nurse when these children present with maltreatment.

Therapeutic Day Schools

Therapeutic day schools are also available for maltreated children. These programs provide a safe environment in which children can develop the ability to trust. The consistent routine

with professionals allows children to test their feelings and actions, such as anger and fear, in an accepting environment.

Other Services

Other services for children include early childhood intervention programs, supportive services such as community or church groups, and, when indicated, out-of-the-home placement.

THE ROLE OF THE NURSE

Because violence and abuse are prevalent in our society, nurses will encounter survivors and perpetrators of violence and abuse in a variety of health care settings. It is important for nurses to prepare for assessment and intervention with survivors, perpetrators, and witnesses of this widespread health problem (Smith-McKenna, 1997).

PREPARING FOR THE NURSE'S ROLE

Certain competencies will help nurses to prepare for effective interventions with survivors, perpetrators, and witnesses of violence and abuse.

1. The nurse needs to recognize that interpersonal violence is a serious social problem worldwide that has persistent and severe physical and mental health consequences. Although violence and abuse are endemic, they are still not openly discussed in some families, communities, and cultures. The incidence is high and the consequences of some types of violence and abuse affect the remainder of the survivor's life.

2. The nurse needs to become familiar with the dynamics of abusive relationships and with the physical and mental health effects of ongoing and previous violence or abuse across the life span. In most states with legislation designed to protect survivors of violence, the nurse is expected to assess for and to report suspected abuse of children, women, and older adults, whether or not actual abuse can be documented. Ideally, the nurse's report activates a complex system, which not only furthers the assessment, but also, in the event of actual abuse, coordinates intervention activities from various agencies. These interventions are designed to provide safety for the individual being abused and, if possible, maintain the integrity of the family.

3. The nurse needs to be aware of the various resources in the community that can provide the supportive services needed by both survivors and perpetrators of violence. The nurse is less likely to blame the survivor, avoid the problem, or use denial if she is aware of the resources available in the community to meet the needs of those involved in the violent situation.

4. The nurse must make a practice of assessing every client seen in any health care setting for experience with violence. The question must be asked directly, in a

private setting, and in a manner that is comfortable for the nurse. Instruments developed by nurses can be incorporated into health history protocols to collect assessment data related to exposure to violence and abuse across the life span (MacFarland, 2007).

5. It is important for the nurse to recognize the effect that violence has had on her own life. Because interpersonal violence is endemic, the nurse's life has also been affected by violence and abuse. The nurse's experience with violence will influence her attitude and response to experiences of violence of her clients. Introspection and processing of her own feelings regarding caring for survivors and perpetrators are important exercises for the nurse.

6. The nurse must identify a support network to assist in dealing with the feelings engendered by working with this truly vulnerable population. Sadness, rage, anger, fear, vulnerability, and frustration are just a few of the emotional consequences of working with survivors and perpetrators of violence and abuse. Self-care by the nurse will allow this important work to continue in the face of these stressful emotions.

LEGAL AND ETHICAL ISSUES

Violence is clearly a significant global health problem. Nurses are in a key position to prevent and identify violence and abuse and to intervene on behalf of both survivors and perpetrators. Nurses need to remain alert to women's and children's increased risk of abuse. Nurses have a mandate to question the health care system's response to survivors of violence and to explore alternate ways in which the needs of these special populations can be met.

Questions and statements that can encourage discussion include the following:

◆ What behaviors should be defined as violent?

◆ What behaviors, including aggressive communication, should be defined as morally intolerable?

◆ What specific personality traits are associated with violence?

◆ What are the criteria for abused children to be placed in foster care?

◆ What are your thoughts about corporal punishment?

◆ Is abuse of children not recognized or underreported by professionals because many fear the consequences of recognition?

◆ What are children's rights?

◆ What responsibilities do women have in staying in an abusive relationship?

◆ What are your thoughts about violent offenders and rehabilitation?

◆ How do nurses' attitudes toward violence impede the progress of survivors?

THE NURSE'S ROLE IN THE LEGAL SYSTEM

Nurses have a mandated responsibility to report suspected abuse and neglect of children, adolescents, and older adults. In some states, nurses are also mandated reporters of IPV. Nurses need to be aware of the state statutes directing mandatory reporting and ensure that the protocols established in the practice setting are consistent with those legal statutes (Table 25–8).

Policies and protocols for reporting are well established. Typically, the following are specified:

◆ Roles and responsibilities of the professional nurse

◆ Definition of abuse and neglect

◆ Type and specificity of information needed

◆ Descriptions of necessary documentation

◆ Legal rights of the nurse

◆ Coordination and collaboration procedures

TABLE 25–8
Child Abuse: How the Nurse Fits into the Reporting and Intervention Process

Steps 1 Through 3: The Nurse's Role

1. The nurse suspects reportable child abuse. A case conference is convened as indicated.

2. Reports are made to the state authority (child protective services or law enforcement) by telephone or in person.

3. A written report may be required. The content should include the following:

   a. Demographics of the child and the family

   b. Nature and content of injuries, in detail

   c. Caretaker information

Steps 4 Through 7: The State's Role

4. The state agency initiates an investigation: High-risk assessments require response within 24 to 48 hours.

5. Family assessment takes place.

6. Case management ensues. If abuse is indicated, the child protective service worker may initiate any or all of the following:

   a. Treatment

   b. Referrals

   c. Court intervention

7. Close case.

THE GENERALIST NURSE

The generalist nurse is integral to the mental health team that intervenes on behalf of the survivors and their families. The generalist nurse has the skill and expertise to provide client interventions at all junctures, and in all practice settings implements the nursing process to assist clients to explore feelings related to the abuse. The generalist nurse acts as an advocate while helping clients negotiate the many systems (such as health care and protective services; schools; the workplace; community agencies' grassroot service organizations, food banks, day care centers, shelters, self-help or support groups; fraternal organizations; ethnic, cultural, and religious organizations; and social and recreational groups) that may affect them. The generalist nurse uses the nursing process to assess the clients' physical and mental health status, to determine the diagnoses and expected outcomes individual to the clients, to develop a plan of care and implement nursing interventions, and to evaluate client response and progress. In addition, the generalist nurse collaborates and coordinates the client care with other health professionals.

Nurses are in a key position to assess the survivors' emotional responses following traumatic experiences with interpersonal violence and abuse. They have the skill to develop and implement the therapeutic relationship that is so important for the clients' optimal functioning.

THE ADVANCED-PRACTICE PSYCHIATRIC REGISTERED NURSE

Advanced-practice psychiatric registered nurses conduct psychiatric evaluations of children and families, provide treatment for survivors and perpetrators, and provide clinical consultation to other professionals. They may provide testimony in court, either as expert or as fact witnesses. The expert nurse witness offers an opinion about the particular case. The opinion is based on the nurse's education, training, and experience and is in a substantive area (e.g., IPV or sexual abuse). Expert testimony involves offering factual material about the case and the methodology used to analyze the information.

THE NURSING PROCESS

The family who is experiencing violence requires careful assessment and intervention. Because interpersonal violence is the result of multiple interacting factors, the nurse's intervention needs to address as many issues as possible.

ASSESSMENT

The initial assessment of the survivor or the family includes a careful history of the violence or abuse. In obtaining the history, the nurse needs to pay close attention to the following factors:

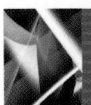

CASE STUDY

The Older Adult Experiencing Physical Abuse (Ms. Morgan)

Ms. Morgan, a frail 85-year-old woman, was referred to the psychiatric nursing consultation service after she appeared in the emergency department with signs of being overmedicated and with unexplained bruises on her back. Her 54-year-old daughter, who stated to the psychiatric nurse, "You don't know what I have been through," accompanied Ms. Morgan. "She's always wetting herself. I can't do it all!"

See Nursing Care Plan 25–4.

Family structure and function

Sex role socialization and role strain

Social functioning of each member

Ability of each member to fulfill task performance

Coping style of each member

Resources available to the family in the home and community

Daily stresses experienced by the family

Expression of frustration and anger

Belief about aggression and violence

Health status of the family

Quality of family relationships

Each factor needs to be explored in depth with the family members. The psychiatric nurse needs to develop a style of interviewing that is comfortable but adaptive to each individual or family. Table 25–9 presents guidelines for assessing patterns of physical abuse of a child.

TABLE 25–9
Guidelines for Assessing Physical Abuse of a Child

- History of injury given by the parent or guardian does not match the injury observed
- Delay in seeking treatment for the child
- Past history of unexplained injuries
- Concealment of injuries by parents or guardian
- Recurrent injuries
- Failure to gain appropriate weight

NURSING DIAGNOSES

The following are possible nursing diagnoses that may be applied to families and individuals who have experienced violence. The list is not comprehensive but may serve as a reminder.

◆ Anxiety

◆ Compromised Family Coping

◆ Ineffective Coping

◆ Delayed Growth and Development

◆ Interrupted Family Processes

◆ Fear

◆ Hopelessness

◆ Impaired Parenting

◆ Post-Trauma Syndrome

◆ Powerlessness

◆ Rape Trauma Syndrome

◆ Chronic Low Self-Esteem

◆ Risk for Trauma

◆ Risk for Self-Directed Violence

◆ Risk for Other-Directed Violence

OUTCOME IDENTIFICATION AND PLANNING

The nursing care plan for a family or individual who has experienced violence is derived from the nursing diagnoses, which are made on the basis of careful data gathering during assessment. The plan contains the outcome measures and objectives for the care. Outcome measures are individualized and set within realistic time frames and prioritized. For example, the survivor of IPV needs a plan that is mutually derived, one that is specifically sensitive to the survivor's desire to end or leave the violent relationship. A short-term goal of separating from the intimate partner would be unrealistic if the survivor had not thought through the consequences of pending actions. The point of leaving a violent partner is the most dangerous time for the survivor, with great potential for homicide.

During the planning stages, the nurse collaborates with the client and family and develops the outcome criteria, or anticipated results, by which to determine whether the goals of the nursing care plan were met. The outcome criteria reflect the client's behavior and are extremely individualized.

See Nursing Care Plans 25–1 through 25–4 for examples of how to document the plan of care for survivors of child sexual abuse, child physical abuse, intimate partner abuse, and elder abuse.

IMPLEMENTATION

The implementation phase is the individualized application of the plan of care to the client and the client's unique experience. During the implementation phase, the nurse accepts a variety of roles to help the client achieve his or her goals. The nurse responds to the client as counselor, educator, advocate, therapist, and health promoter.

NURSING CARE PLAN 25–4

The Older Adult Experiencing Physical Abuse (Ms. Morgan)

Nursing Diagnosis: Hopelessness
related to being a survivor of violence (battering)

Outcome Identification	Nursing Actions	Rationales	Evaluation
1. By [date], client will recognize the abusive behavior she has experienced.	1a. Assure the client of confidentiality.	1a. Assurance is essential for the client to feel comfortable opening up because denial is a common defense mechanism when one is abused by a loved one.	*Goal met:* Client verbalizes knowledge about abusive behaviors.

(continues)

Outcome Identification	Nursing Actions	Rationales	Evaluation
	1b. Respect her right to make her own decisions.	1b. Allowing the client to make her own decisions will restore a sense of self-worth and being in control.	
	1c. Interview the client to ensure she does not experience pressure by abuser.	1c. The client may not feel safe in the presence of her daughter, especially to disclose abusive events that are painful to recall, are humiliating, and are embarrassing. The client may feel disloyal to her daughter and because of the perceived disruption she is creating in the family, she may feel pressure to recant.	
2. By [date], client will express feelings of fear, anxiety, and helplessness related to the abuse.	2a. Spend time with the client to promote expression of feelings. Understand meaning of present stressors (recent MI).	2a. Abusive experiences by her daughter may be perceived by the client as a loss of an important relationship; therefore, the client will need to re-establish trust through her relationship with the nurse to feel comfortable in revealing her feelings.	*Goal met:* Client verbalizes acceptance of her feelings about the abuse as valid. Client develops adaptive coping skills. Client's self-esteem increases.
	2b. Be nonjudgmental and aware of personal feeling.	2b. A nonjudgmental approach is critical, because the client may be reluctant to disclose her feelings if she senses blame by the nurse. Issues of abuse may evoke ambivalent, confusing feelings in the nurse and may interfere with the therapeutic relationship.	
	2c. Accept the client's ability to reveal abuse and pace interview accordingly.	2c. Acknowledgment of the reality of the abuse can be frightening and painful.	

(continues)

Nursing Care Plan 25–4 *(continued)*

Outcome Identification	Nursing Actions	Rationales	Evaluation
3. By [date], the client will not present as a danger to herself [potential for self-injury].	3a. Assess client's potential for suicide and any suicide ideation or plan.	3a. Disclosure and discussion of the abuse may trigger feelings of worthlessness and hopelessness. The client may believe she is a burden to her family and therefore deserves to die.	*Goal met:* The client expresses anger and hopelessness appropriately.
	3b. Refer the client for counseling if she verbalizes suicidal ideations or plan.	3b. Referral is necessary to protect the client from herself and any suicidal impulses	
4. By [date], the client will be provided with alternative methods of care.	4a. Investigate need for complete physical assessment of the client.	4a. A client's health status is affected by abuse. Basic needs in terms of hydration, nutrition, and elimination may not be met	*Goal met:* The client and her family participate in community programs designed for the family and caretakers.
	4b. Enlist assistance from other family members.	4b. Additional assistance will provide stress relief to the caregiver.	
	4c. Refer the client and her family to an adult day center for older adults and respite care.	4c. Alternative programs will relieve stress on the family and provide the client with maximum attention to her needs.	

EVALUATION

The final phase of the nursing process is the evaluation phase. The nursing care is evaluated in the context of the stated outcome criteria. The evaluation phase is not a discrete entity but rather occurs throughout the nursing process. When the nurse examines the outcome criteria, she also examines her own behavior and feelings in relation to the client and the care that is offered. The nursing process is an important and significant part of the client's total care, especially when the client has been traumatized by violence.

SUMMARY

◆ Violence is a significant health problem worldwide.

◆ Psychiatric nurses are in a key position to identify; intervene; and treat the survivors, witnesses, and perpetrators of violence.

◆ It is imperative for psychiatric nurses to have an understanding of the complexities of violence that are a family context and to appreciate the cues signifying that violence is occurring and the events that trigger it.

◆ Nurses need careful preparation to identify and intervene with individuals and families at risk for violence and abuse.

◆ Nurses need to recognize their role in case finding because they are in the forefront of the effort to identify and assess victims.

◆ The therapeutic relationship between the psychiatric nurse and the client is a powerful force, and it is within this relationship that survivors can learn to trust and provide physical safety for themselves and their families.

SUGGESTIONS FOR CLINICAL CONFERENCES

1. Invite volunteers from local women's shelter to share experiences

2. Provide several scenarios involving various forms of abuse and encourage students to discuss their feelings about survivor and perpetrator

3. Invite rape crisis counselor to discuss the role of these services and potential volunteer opportunities

4. Set up scenario and encourage students to role play interviewing a survivor

STUDY QUESTIONS

1. Increases in reporting of child maltreatment and abuse are attributed to:
   a. improved investigations
   b. greater awareness of the problem, resulting in a willingness to report
   c. the frequency of witnessing abuse
   d. more child protective service workers in the hospital

2. Nurses working with families at risk for violence can assess family members by:
   a. caring for the infant individually
   b. interviewing mothers or guardians individually
   c. interviewing all members about their contributions to the child's care
   d. interviewing extended family members

3. Of the following categories of young children, which is most at risk of violence?
   a. Emotionally stable children
   b. Premature and colicky infants
   c. Highly intelligent children
   d. Physically and mentally disabled children

4. A mother of two small children has decided to remain with her spouse even though she has experienced 2 years of battering. A desirable response is:
   a. "Let's discuss a plan of safety."
   b. "You'll leave when you're ready."
   c. "I think you are at risk. Please reconsider."
   d. "I can't work with you any more."

5. To effectively plan for the care of an older abused client, the nurse needs to appreciate that older adults:
   a. have diminished cognitive capacity
   b. are often disoriented
   c. are prone to reminiscing about past events
   d. are often humiliated and defensive when asked about abusive experiences

6. A 20-month-old has been admitted for second-degree burns surrounding his genital area. His mother told the nurse the child grabbed for the hot cocoa cup and spilled it on himself. The nurse is required by law to do which of the following?
   a. Testify in court on the injuries.
   b. Report suspected child abuse.
   c. Have the mother arrested.
   d. Refer the mother for counseling.

7. A toddler was admitted for second-degree burns on her back. Her mother told the nurse the child accidentally turned on the hot shower and burned herself.

The toddler's mother is 16 years old. In which of the following areas would the nurse provide health teaching?
   a. Normal growth and development
   b. Bonding techniques
   c. How to childproof the apartment
   d. Parenting skills

8. The nurse is caring for a young woman who has been sexually assaulted. Which of the following is indicative of successful adjustment to the trauma?
   a. She moves to another town.
   b. She resumes her work and activities.
   c. She takes classes in martial arts.
   d. She remains silent about the assault.

9. Which of the following statements made by a survivor of intimate partner violence (IPV) would indicate to the nurse that the woman was admitting that she was a survivor of intimate partner violence?
   a. "It would be nice to be out of the situation, but I cannot afford to leave. I have no skills."
   b. "My husband has never visited me when I've been in the hospital. He even said he will take me out more often."
   c. "Last time it happened I tried to talk to his mother. She said he was never like this growing up."
   d. "I have the shelter number and I've decided to work on my high school diploma while the children are in school each day."

10. The nurse is caring for a 3-month-old infant after he was brought to the emergency department with a grand mal seizure. His mother and her boyfriend report he has not been eating well and he has problems breathing. Physical findings from the nursing assessment reveal lethargy, breathing difficulties, underweight, bulging fontanels, and unequal pupils. The most probable cause of the infant's symptoms is which of the following?
    a. Shaken baby syndrome
    b. Hydrocephalus
    c. Dehydration and failure to thrive
    d. Developmental disorder

RESOURCES

Please note that because Internet resources are of a time-sensitive nature and URL addresses may change or be deleted, searches should also be conducted by association or topic.

Internet Resources

1. Family Violence Prevention Fund (FVPF). Contact the FVPF online and go to "legislative updates." Review recent legislation related to health care providers' responsibilities related to mandatory reporting of violence against children, women, and elders. http://www.fvpf.org

2. Role of the Nurse. Contact your state's Board of Registered Nursing (BRN) website, and review the Nurse Practice Act

sections that describe mandatory reporting regulations (child abuse, elder abuse, intimate partner violence) for nurses in your state. http://www.BRN.org

3. Domestic Violence Continuing Education. Complete this domestic violence module to give you ideas on how to elicit information from a client about intimate partner violence. Share this website and information with a nurse in practice. http://www.nurseweek.com/ce/ce261a.html

http://www.aacn.nche.edu/Publications/positions/ violence.htm American Association of Colleges of Nursing (AACN). (1999). *Position statement: Violence as a public health problem.* (Accessed June 1, 2006)

www.acf.hhs.gov/programs/cb/pubs/cm03/ index.htm Department of Health and Human Services (DHHS) (U.S.). (2005). Administration on Children, Youth, and Families (ACF). Child maltreatment 2003 [online]. Washington, (DC): Government Printing Office; 2005

http://www.dontshake.com/ National Center on Shaken Baby Syndrome (Accessed June 1, 2006)

http://www.mincava.umn.edu Batterer Intervention State Standards, Minnesota Center Against Violence and Abuse

http://www.sfms.org.org/domestic.html Domestic Violence: A Practical Approach for Clinicians

http://www.who.int/violence_injury_prevention/ violence/world_report/factsheets/en/ childabusefacts.pdf World Health Organization— Child Abuse and Neglect (Fact Sheets)

http://www.xq.com.com/cuav/domviol.htm Same-Sex Domestic Violence

Other Resources

Asian Task Force Against Domestic Violence, Inc.
P.O. Box 120108
Boston, MA 02112
(617) 338-2350
Hotline: (617) 338-2355
http://www.atask.org

famvi.com
P.O. Box 17186
Indianapolis, IN 46217
(530) 831-5506
http://www.famvi.com/

Family Violence Prevention Fund (FVPF)
383 Rhode Island Street, Suite #304
San Francisco, CA 94103
(415) 252-8900
http://www.fvpf.org

International Federation on Aging
380 St. Antoine Street West, Suite 3200
Montreal, Quebec, Canada H2Y3X7
(514) 987-8191
http://www.ifa-fiv.org

National Coalition Against Domestic Violence (NCADV)
P.O. Box 18749
Denver, CO 80218
(303) 839-1852
http://www.mcadv.org/

National Domestic Violence Hotline
P.O. Box 161810
Austin, TX
(800) 799-SAFE
TTY: (800) 787-3224
http://www.ndvh.org/

Nursing Network on Violence Against Women,
International (NNVAWI)
1801 H Street, B5
Modesto, CA 95354
(888) 909-9993
http://www.nnvawi.org

United Nations
Division for the Advancement of Women
2 UN Plaza, DC2-12th Floor
New York, NY 10017
http://www.un.org/womenwatch/dav

World Health Organization
Women's Health and Development Programs (WHD)
1211 Geneva 27
Switzerland
41-22-791-21-11
http://www.who.int-whd/WHD/activities/whd-vaw.htm

REFERENCES

Administration on Aging. *The national elder abuse incidence study: Final report.* (1998, September). Retrieved June 24, 2002, from http://aoa.gov/abuse/report/default.htm

American Association of Colleges of Nursing. (2000). Position statement: Violence as a public health problem. *Journal of Professional Nursing, 16*(1), 63–69.

American Psychiatric Association. (2000). *Diagnostic and statistical manual of mental disorders* (4th edition, Text Revision) *(DSM-IV-TR)*. Washington, DC: Author.

Ardrey, R. (1966). *The territorial imperative.* New York: Antheneum.

Bandura, A. (1973). *Aggression: L A social learning analysis.* Englewood Cliffs, NJ: Prentice-Hall.

Centers for Disease Control. National Center for Injury Prevention and Control. (2001). Press Release: *Study finds school-associated violent deaths rare, fewer in events, but more deaths per event.* Retrieved October, 2002, from http://www.cdc.gov/od/oc/media/pressrel/ro11204.htm

Coccaro, E. F., McCloskey, M. S., Fitzgerald, D. A., & Phan, K. L. (2007). Amygdala and orbitofrontal reactivity to social threat in individuals with impulsive aggression. *Biological Psychiatry, 62,* 168–178.

Constantino, R. E., Sekula, K., Lebish, J., & Buehner, E. (2002). Depression and behavioral manifestations of depression in female survivors o f the suicide and their significant other and female survivors of abuse. *Journal of the American Psychiatric Nurses Association, 8,* 27–32.

Council on Scientific Affairs. (1987). Elder abuse and neglect. *Journal of the American Medical Association, 257,* 966–971.

Dube, S. R., Anda, R. F., Whitfield, C. L., Brown, D. W., Felitti, V. J., Dong, M, et al. (2005). Long-term consequences of childhood sexual abuse by gender of victim. *American Journal of Preventive Medicine, 28,* 430–438.

Duxbury, F. (2006). Recognising domestic violence in clinical practice using the diagnoses of posttraumatic stress disorder, depression and low self-esteem. *British Journal of General Practice, 56,* 294–300.

Ferree, M. M. (1990). Beyond separate spheres: Feminism and family research. *Journal of Marriage and the Family, 52,* 866–884.

Fonagy, P., & Target, M. (2005). Bridging the transmission gap: An end to an important mystery of attachment research? *Attachment and Human Development, 7,* 333–343.

Fonagy, P., Gergely, G., & Target, M. (2007). The parent-infant dyad and the construction of the subjective self. *Journal of Child Psychology and Psychiatry, 48,* 288–328.

Goldner, V., Penn, P., Sheinberg, M., & Walker, G. (1990). Love and violence: Gender paradoxes in volatile attachments. *Family Process, 29,* 343–364.

Greenberg, E. M. (1996). Violence and the older adult: The role of the acute care nurse practitioners. *Critical Care Nursing Quarterly, 19,* 76–84.

Hall, R. C., & Hall, R. C. (2007). A profile of pedophilia: Definition, characteristics of offenders, recidivism, treatment outcomes, and forensic issues. *Mayo Clinic Proceedings, 82,* 457–471.

Harris, W. W., Lieberman, A. F., Marans, S. (2007). In the best interests of society. *Journal of Child Psychology and Psychiatry, 48,* 392–411.

Holmes, W. C., & Slap, G. B. (1998). Sexual abuse of boys: Definition, prevalence, correlates, sequelae and management. *Journal of the American Medical Association, 280,* 1855–1862.

Humphreys, J., & Lee, K. (2005). Sleep disturbance in battered women living in transitional housing. *Issues in Mental Health Nursing, 26,* 771–780.

Kaplow, J. B., & Widom, C. S. (2007). Age of onset of child maltreatment predicts long-term mental health outcomes. *Journal of Abnormal Psychology, 116,* 176–187.

Kilpatrick, D. G. (2004). What is violence against women: Defining and measuring the problem. *Journal of Interpersonal Violence, 19,* 1209–1234.

Lazoritz, S. (1990). Whatever happened to Mary Ellen? *Child Abuse and Neglect, 14,* 143–149.

Lorenz, K. (1966). *On aggression.* New York: Harcourt, Brace, & World.

MacFarland, J. (2007). Pregnancy following partner rape: What we know and what we need to know. *Trauma and Violence Abuse, 8,* 127–134.

Oquendo, M. A., Krunic, A., Parsey, R. V., Milak, M., Malone, K. M., Anderson, A., van Heertum, R. L., & Mann, J. (2005). Positron emission tomography of regional brain metabolic responses to a serotonergic challenge in major depressive disorder with and without borderline personality disorder. *Neuropsychopharmacology, 30,* 1163–1172.

Oquendo, M. A., Bongiovi-Garcia, M. E., Galfalvy, H., Goldberg, P. H., Grunebaum, M. F., Burke, A. K., et al. (2007). Sex differences in clinical predictors of suicidal acts after major depression: A prospective study. *American Journal of Psychiatry, 164,* 134–141.

Pence, E., & Paymar, M. (1993). *Education groups for men who batter: The Duluth Model.* New York: Springer Publishing.

Program Resources Department, American Association of Retired Persons (AARP), and Administration on Aging (AOA), U.S. Department of Health and Human Services. (1993). *A profile of older Americans.* Washington, DC: American Association of Retired Persons.

Schechter, S. (1982). *Women and male violence: The visions and struggles of the battered women's movement.* Boston: South End.

Schiamberg, L. B., & Gans, D. (2000). Elder abuse by adult children: An applied ecological framework for understanding contextual risk factors and the intergenerational character of quality of life. *International Journal of Human Development, 50,* 329–359.

Simeon, D., Knutelska, M., Yehuda, R., Putnam, F., Schmeidler, J., & Smith, L. M. (2007). Hypothalamic-pituitary-adrenal axis function in dissociative disorders, post-traumatic stress disorder, and healthy volunteers. *Biological Psychiatry, 61,* 966–973.

Smith-McKenna, L. (1997). Elder abuse: Preparing to identify and intervene in healthcare. *Home Care Provider, 2*(1), 30–33.

Stirling, J., & American Academy of Pediatrics Committee on Child Abuse and Neglect. (2007). Beyond Munchausen syndrome by proxy: Identification and treatment of child abuse in a medical setting. *Pediatrics, 119,* 1026–1030.

Straus, M. A. (1973). A general systems theory approach to a theory of violence between family members. *Social Science Information, 12,* 105–125.

Straus, M. A., Gelles, R. J., & Steinmetz, S. K. (1980). *Behind closed doors: Violence in the American family.* Garden City, NJ: Anchor/Doubleday.

Suris, A., Lind, L., Kashner, T. M., & Borman, P. D. (2007). Mental health, quality of life, and health functioning in women veterans: Differential outcomes associated with military and civilian sexual assault. *Journal of Interpersonal Violence, 22,* 179–197.

Theran, S. A., Sullivan, C. M., Bogat, G. A., & Stewart, C. S. (2006). Abusive partners and ex-partners: Understanding the effects of relationship to the abuser on women's well-being. *Violence Against Women, 12,* 950–969.

Tjaden, P., & Thoennes, N. (2000a). *Extent, nature and consequences of intimate partner violence: Findings from the National Violence Against Women Survey.* Report for grant 93-IJ-CX-0012, funded by the National Institute of Justice and the Centers for Disease Control and Prevention. Washington, DC: National Institute of Justice.

Tjaden, P., & Thoennes, N. (2000b). *Full report of the prevalence, incidence, and consequences of violence against women.* Washington, DC: National Institute of Justice and the Centers for Disease Control and Prevention.

United Nations General Assembly. (2006). *Rights of the child. Report of the independent expert for the United Nations on violence against children.* Available online at http://www.unicef.org/violencestudy/reports/SG_violencestudy_en.pdf

United Nations Second World Assembly on Aging. (2002). United Nations Department of Public Information. DPI/2264.

U.S. Department of Health and Human Services (DHHS). (2005). *Administration on children, youth, and families (ACF). Child maltreatment 2003.Washington, DC:* Government Printing Office. Available online at www.acf.hhs.gov/programs/cb/pubs/cm03/index.htm

U.S. Department of Justice: Toolkit to End Violence against Women http://toolkit.ncjrs.org/ (Accessed June 1, 2006).

Vandeweerd, C., Paveza, G. J., & Fulmer, T. (2006). Abuse and neglect in older adults with Alzheimer's disease. *Nursing Clinics of North America, 41,* 43–55.

Walker, L. (1984). *The battered woman syndrome.* New York: Springer.

Walker, L. (1989). *Terrifying love.* New York: Harper & Row.

Walker, L. (1993). The battered woman syndrome is a psychological consequence of abuse. In R. J. Gelles & D. R. Luseke (Eds.), *Current controversies on family violence* (pp. 133–153). Newbury Park, CA: Sage.

Warshaw, C. (1998). Identification, assessment, and intervention with victims of domestic violence. In C. Warshaw & A. Ganley (Eds.) *Improving the health care response to violence: A resource manual for health care providers* (2nd ed., pp. 49–86). San Francisco: Family Violence Fund.

Widom, C. S., DuMont, K., & Czaja, S. J. (2007). A prospective investigation of major depressive disorder and comorbidity in abused and neglected children grown up. *Archives of General Psychiatry, 64,* 49–56.

World Health Organization. (1999). *Child abuse and neglect.* Retrieved June 24, 2002, from http://www.who.int/violence_injury_prevention/main.cfm

World Health Organization. (2002).Child abuse and neglect (Fact Sheets). http://www.who.int/violence_injury_prevention/violence/world_report/factsheets/en/childabusefacts.pdf.

World Health Organization. (2005). *Milestones of a Global Campaign for Violence Prevention 2005: Changing the face of violence prevention.* Geneva, Switzerland: WHO Press. http://whqlibdoc.who.int/publications/2005/9241593555_eng.pdf.

World Health Organization. (2006). *Preventing child maltreatment: A guide to taking action and generating evidence.* Geneva: Author. Available online at http://www.crin.org/docs/who_maltreatment_guide.pdf

Yodanis, C. L. (2004). Gender inequality, violence against women, and fear: A cross-national test of the feminist theory of violence against women. *Journal of Interpersonal Violence, 19,* 655–675.

Yoshioka, M. R., & Choi, D. Y. (2005). Culture and interpersonal violence research: Paradigm shift to create a full continuum of domestic violence services. *Journal of Interpersonal Violence, 20,* 513–519.

SUGGESTED READINGS

Becker, R. A. (1991). *Don't talk, don't trust, don't feel.* Deerfield Beach, FL: Health Communications, Inc.

Evans, P. (1993). *Verbal abuse: Survivors speak out.* Holbrook, MA: Bob Adams, Inc.

Miller, A. (1990). *The untouched key.* New York: Random House.

Nicarthy, J. (1986). *Getting free.* Seattle: Pepper Vine.

HOTLINE

National Domestic Violence Hotline
1-800-799-SAFE (7233) or 1-800-787-3224 (TDD)

UNIT 3

Therapeutic Interventions

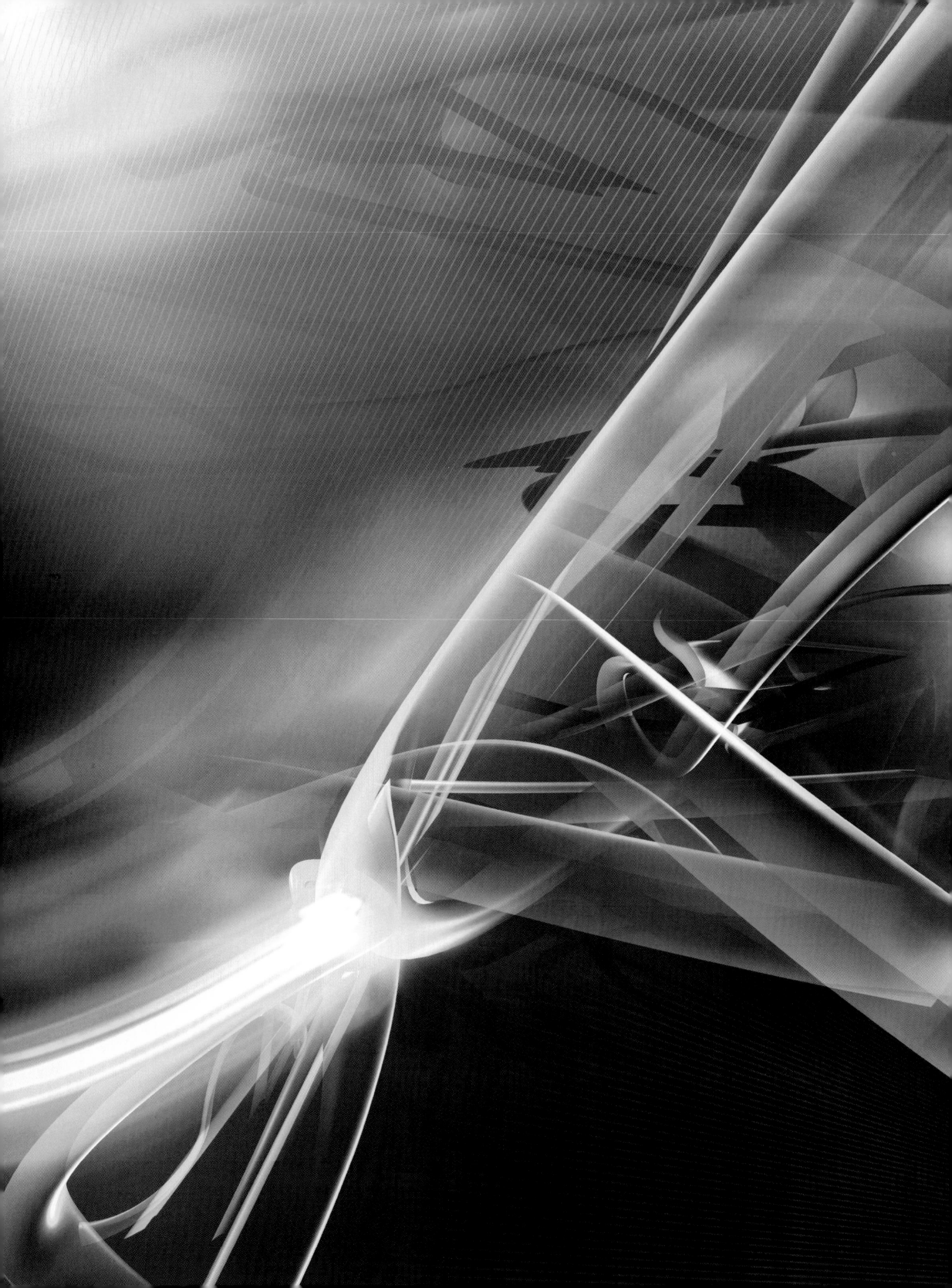

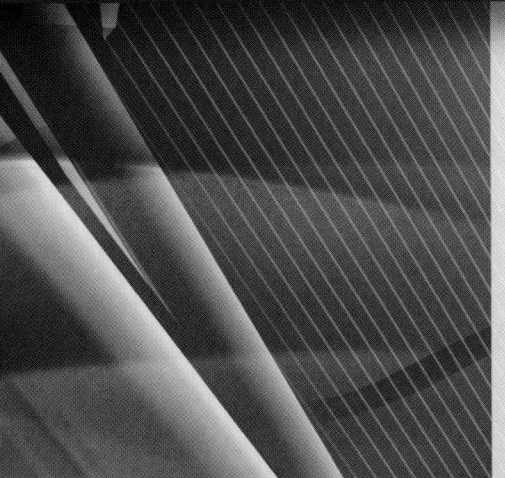

CHAPTER 26

Individual Psychotherapy

Deborah Antai-Otong, MS, APRN, BC, FAAN

KEY TERMS

Catharsis: The healthy release of ideas that helps the client gain insight into conflicts and early developmental turmoil.

Confrontation: The act of pointing out contradictions or incongruencies among feelings, thoughts, and behaviors, specifically pointing out parts of the assessment or treatment process that are contradictory or confusing.

Countertransference: Refers to intense emotional reactions to the client stemming from the therapist's early childhood experiences.

Eclecticism: Implies that the therapist uses two or more theories to develop an effective treatment to meet a client's needs.

Free Association: The client's spontaneous expression of thoughts.

Insight: Refers to the client's self-awareness and understanding of the meaning and reason for his behavior or motives.

Play Therapy: An individualized intervention that offers children a symbolic way to express feelings, anxiety, aggressions, and self-doubt.

Psychoanalysis: A form of psychodynamic psychotherapy in which the therapist and client explore the client's conscious and unconscious conflicts and coping patterns.

Psychotherapy: A global process in which people seek professional help to resolve problems, promote personal growth, and reduce or eliminate maladaptive responses.

Self-Disclosure: Exposing oneself to others; to make publicly known.

Termination: The final phase of psychotherapy. This process involves exploring areas of accomplishment, goal attainment, and feelings generated by ending the relationship.

Therapeutic Alliance: Refers to a trusting relationship that helps the client explore interpersonal and intrapersonal conflicts and gain insight into maladaptive behaviors.

Therapeutic Use of Self: An intervention that involves self-awareness, empathy, acceptance, self-disclosure, and other means of facilitating a therapeutic relationship.

Transference: Refers to unconscious displacement or reenactment of feelings and attitudes from the client to the psychotherapist.

COMPETENCIES

Upon completion of this chapter, the learner should be able to:

1. Describe major theoretical concepts of individual psychotherapy.
2. Assess the significance of psychotherapy across the life span.
3. Appraise the essential qualities of nurse psychotherapists.
4. Analyze the influence of psychotherapy on facilitating adaptive behaviors.
5. Gain self-awareness of reactions to specific clients.

CHAPTER OUTLINE

Historical Perspectives

Cultural Considerations

Theories and Concepts of Individual Psychotherapy

Psychoanalytic and Psychodynamic Therapies

    Goals

    Treatment Techniques

Psychotherapy refers to a global term for the use of professional help to resolve problems, promote personal growth, and reduce maladaptive responses. Achieving an understanding of their feelings and behaviors is a major goal for people who undertake psychotherapy. Psychotherapy is within the scope of the advanced-practice psychiatric registered nurse. The nurse psychotherapist has a master's degree and is nationally certified as an advanced-practice psychiatric-mental health registered nurse. Nurse psychotherapists offer a broad range of cost-effective mental health care that is distinct from other mental health professionals, specifically a focus of the whole person *within a social and interpersonal context* (Lego, 1997, p. 193). In addition, the nurse psychotherapist is likely to integrate principles of health promotion, holism, and health education that facilitate health and illness prevention.

Psychotherapy is an invaluable form of treatment in which the nurse and client engage in an interactional relationship that promotes adaptive behavioral changes, encourages insight, and facilitates optimal functioning. Psychotherapy begins with a therapeutic relationship that facilitates adaptive behavioral changes and improves interpersonal relationships. Adaptive behavioral changes are likely to occur as the client understands and modifies maladaptive coping behaviors and develops effective coping, problem-solving, and social skills that promote health. This chapter focuses on major concepts of individual psychotherapy and its usefulness in improving interpersonal relationships, promoting adaptive behavioral changes, and strengthening communication across the life span.

HISTORICAL PERSPECTIVES

Psychotherapy has its roots in the early works of Sigmund Freud. His early work with Josef Breuer involving the use of hypnosis with a client named Anna O. generated much data that advanced the understanding and treatment of neurosis. Although the term *neurosis* is obsolete, it is relevant to a discussion about the history of psychotherapy. Dramatic changes in her symptoms were noted while under hypnosis. Freud's works with Breuer as well as his other clinical experiences with clients with neurosis such as Anna are the basis of psychoanalysis. Psychoanalysis is a form of psychodynamic psychotherapy in which the therapist and client explore the client's conscious and unconscious conflicts and coping patterns. The major techniques used in psychoanalysis include free association, transference, and therapeutic alliance.

Psychoanalytic concepts have been integrated into other forms of psychotherapy. Corsini (1984) described psychotherapy as a process that focuses on changing the client's cognitions (thought processes), affect (feelings), and behaviors. Clients' ability and willingness to change help them explore the meaning of maladaptive behaviors and develop effective coping behaviors. Many clients seek treatment because they want to change.

Hildegarde Peplau, a pioneer in psychiatric nursing, believed that clients with sociopsychological and emotional problems are appropriate candidates for psychotherapy. She described individual psychotherapy as an interpersonal process between a therapist and a client that consists of three phases: orientation, working through, and termination (Peplau, 1968). See Chapter 2 for Peplau's Interpersonal Theory.

Another noted nurse, June Mellow (1967) developed a form of nursing psychotherapy on the basis of her extensive work with a woman experiencing an acute psychotic schizophrenic episode. She used the nurse-client relationship to establish trust, provide safety, and to assess and meet the client's psychosocial needs.

CULTURAL CONSIDERATIONS

Recent data from the U.S. Census Bureau (2000) indicate that the United States is undergoing enormous demographics that are resulting in a more culturally diverse society. In view of these dramatic societal changes, psychiatric nurse therapists must continue to offer mental health services that are client centered and culturally sensitive. Major treatment issues that promote culturally sensitive mental health care include establishing rapport, making an accurate diagnosis of symptom expression, and developing an appropriate treatment plan. In addition, nurse therapists must recognize their personal responses and perception of diverse populations. In many cultures, facilitating family and community involvement and valuing sociocultural factors, such as spiritual and religious affiliations, are crucial to positive client outcomes. See Chapter 7 for further discussion about cultural and ethnic treatment considerations.

THEORIES AND CONCEPTS OF INDIVIDUAL PSYCHOTHERAPY

The success of helping relationships is influenced by the client's ability to form open, trusting interactions. The client brings an array of present and past experiences into psychotherapy that affects his perception of the nurse and present stressors and motivation to modify or change. The nurse also brings past and present experiences into this relationship, and the nurse's theoretical orientation and self-awareness influence the meaning of the client's responses to stressors. Many therapists use an eclectic approach to psychotherapy. The term eclecticism in psychotherapy implies that the therapist uses two or more theories to develop an effective treatment to meet a client's needs (Norcross, 1991). An eclectic approach increases the likelihood that psychotherapy will be successful and provides the client with an assortment of interventions. An important factor that influences the outcome of individual psychotherapy is ego function or integrity.

Ego is a psychoanalytical term that refers to the part of the personality that mediates and controls basic biological urges by trying to gratify them within socially acceptable domains. The significance of ego structure in psychotherapy is its influence on the client's ability to form therapeutic interactions, tolerate frustration, and motivation to make adaptive behavioral changes. Predictably, clients with healthy ego function have high self-esteem, have good impulse control, adapt positively to stress, tolerate frustration, manage anxiety effectively, and form healthy meaningful interpersonal relationships. In contrast, those with poor ego function, have low self-esteem, poor impulse control, low tolerance for stress and frustration, distorted perceptions of themselves and others, and difficulty forming healthy interactions. See Chapters 2 and 15 for an in-depth discussion of ego function.

Several factors contribute to the lack of a therapeutic relationship. Major factors include non-ahherence, inability to form trusting relationships, and premature termination (Frank & Gunderson, 1990). Likewise, the nurse's attitude about the client's ability to change, cultural or belief system conflicts, and a lack of empathy predictably interfere with a therapeutic nurse-client relationship.

There is no single determinant of successful or unsuccessful psychotherapy. The effectiveness of psychotherapy varies. A number of studies dating back to the 1950s confirm the success of psychotherapy in helping clients in distress (Piper, Azim, Joyce, & McCallum, 1991; Stevenson & Meares, 1992; Wolpe, 1958). However, in other studies there were few differences in the outcome found between therapy and control groups who did not receive treatment (Seeman, Barry, & Ellinwood, 1964; Truax, 1963).

Research consistently demonstrates the cost-effectiveness and quality of psychotherapy provided by nationally certified advanced-practice psychiatric nurses. Advanced-practice psychiatric nurses, particularly clinical nurse specialists, offer cost-effective and quality psychotherapy that is comparable or superior to other licensed mental health professionals (Reasor & Farrell, 2005). Given that client-centered, quality, cost-effectiveness, resource allocation, and positive clinical outcomes are major goals of psychotherapy, advanced-practice psychiatric nurses often seek various strategies to enhance these processes. Forming collaborative relationships with psychiatrists is often a condition of prescriptive authority in most states.

In a small exploratory study, characteristic activities and outcomes of collaborative relationships between psychiatric-mental health clinical nurse specialists (CNSs) with prescriptive authority and their collaborating psychiatrists researchers were identified. Findings from this study indicated that effective communication, trust, shared treatment goals for clinical outcomes, mutual professional values, and respect for clinical competency are essential characteristics for successful collaboration. Major benefits of this nurse-psychiatrist collaborative relationship for nurses were enhanced professional development and job satisfaction—for psychiatrists, shared workload responsibilities and for the client, increased access to mental health services and continuity of health care. Although this study was limited to nurses from the Minnesota state board of nursing with prescriptive authority and collaborative relationships with psychiatrists, inference concerning the importance of these relationships and potential benefits to nurses, psychiatrists, and clients is difficult to dispute (Kaas, Dehn, Dahl, Frank, Markley et al., 2000).

Overall, psychotherapy is a facilitative process in which the therapeutic relationship is used to promote the client's health, growth, and development of adaptive coping behaviors. Successful client outcomes depend on accurate assessment of complex client needs and the integration of various psychotherapy concepts into treatment and evaluation.

Table 26–1 lists some individual psychotherapies and their goals, duration, and techniques, along with disorders in which these therapies may be used.

PSYCHOANALYTIC AND PSYCHODYNAMIC THERAPIES

Psychoanalytic psychotherapy has its roots in hypnosis that stems from Josef Breuer's and Sigmund Freud's work with a young neurotic woman named Anna O. This woman, who showed alterations in perceptions during consciousness, was observed under hypnosis to be free of symptoms. Sigmund Freud's later work and collaboration with Breuer on hysteria provided the foundation of the major concepts of psychoanalytical theory. Breuer and Freud's (1955) work became the foundation of their publication, *Studies on Hysteria.*

Freud eventually developed the technique of free association, in which the client says the first thing that comes to mind, without restrictions, in response to something the therapist says. Free association is the heart of psychoanalytical psychotherapy. It provides verbal catharsis, the healthy release of ideas that helps the client gain insight into conflicts and early developmental turmoil (Karasu, 1990). The goal of free association is to minimize the conscious screening of thoughts or verbal expressions. This intervention allows clients to present rational, logical, and relevant explanations of things. Because clients are free to say the first thing that comes to mind, regardless of whether it is appropriate or embarrassing, their unconscious censorship is reduced. This technique facilitates a deeper understanding of maladaptive behaviors and conflicts. Like other psychoanalytic techniques, it brings areas of conflict into the conscious, or here and now, and enables the client to resolve them (English & Finch, 1964).

The therapist who uses psychoanalytical psychotherapy is called an analyst. An analyst is usually a psychiatrist or other mental health professional who has been trained in psychoanalysis. Treatment focuses on creating an environment that

TABLE 26–1
Psychotherapies: Theoretical Approaches

Type	Goal	Specific Illness	Duration	Techniques
Psychoanalytic	• Personality restructure	• Oedipal conflict	3 to 6 years	• Free association • Therapeutic alliance • Transference interpretation • Defense analysis
Supportive therapy	• Support reality testing • Promote adaptation and restoration of coping skills	• Ego deficits • Overwhelming stress • Cognitively impaired	days to years	• Strengthen ego • Reality-based interactions • Administration of psychotropics
Brief psychotherapy	• Assess nature of defense mechanisms	• Anxiety, impulsivity • Resolution of childhood conflicts	<12 months	• Interpretation of transference • Exploration of defenses
Interpersonal psychotherapy	• Improve interpersonal skills and communication	• Depression	12 to 16 weeks	• Reassurance • Assess meaning of feelings • Empathy • Emotional support

promotes regression, interpreting free association, dreams, and transference. Ideally, analysts have been through psychoanalysis as part of their training and are able to maintain neutrality. Duration of treatment may range from at least four sessions per week, lasting up to 3 to 4 years (Falkenstrom, Grant, Broberg, & Sandell, 2007).

Goals

The goals of psychoanalytical psychotherapy include (1) facilitating resolution of tension generated by repressed memories of traumatic childhood psychosexual issues to achieve reorganization of client's personality, (2) settling unconscious discord, and (3) increasing insight. Psychoanalytic psychotherapy is a long-term treatment that involves a gradual integration of repressed conflicts into the personality.

Treatment Techniques

The following are the major treatment techniques of psychoanalytical psychotherapy:

- ◆ Therapeutic alliance
- ◆ Interpretation of transference
- ◆ Resolution of countertransference
- ◆ Free association
- ◆ Neutrality

Refer to Chapters 2 and 15 for a discussion of psychoanalytic theory.

Therapeutic Alliance

Therapeutic alliance is the trusting relationship in which the therapist and client feel free to explore interpersonal and intrapersonal conflicts and gain insight into the client's maladaptive behaviors. Purposes of this relationship involve developing trust, assessing, and resolving the client's presenting symptoms.

Transference

The hallmark of psychoanalysis is transference. Transference refers to unconscious displacement or reenactment of feelings and attitudes from the client to the psychotherapist. Transference may be positive or negative in tone. In positive transference, the client displaces his feelings of warmth, esteem, or love for someone else onto the therapist. In negative transference, the client reacts to the therapist with hate, anger, or rage he feels toward some other particular person. Regardless of what feelings, thoughts, or attitude are expressed, they reveal the client's need to resolve infantile conflicts (Piper et al., 1991).

In interpreting the client's transference, the therapist helps him examine and understand the origins and meaning of specific transference reactions and their relationship to early childhood experiences. The interpretation of the transference link the "here-and-now disturbance" with the client's "there-and-then experience" (Kernberg, 1984, p. 9). A client's expression of anger and rejection after a session is canceled is an example of transference. The therapist's pointing out that the client expressed similar reactions when dealing with feelings of abandonment by a mother who worked all the time is an example of interpretation of transference.

Countertransference

Psychotherapy tends to evoke strong reactions in not only the client, but also the therapist. Countertransference refers to intense emotional reactions to the client stemming from the therapist's early childhood experiences. Like the client's transference, the therapist's countertransference may be positive or negative and may stem from feelings toward early childhood figures. Freud (1958) suggested that countertransference should be overcome or minimized because it interferes with the therapeutic relationship. In contrast, others suggested that it is a significant part of the therapeutic process (Heimann, 1950). Countertransference, like transference, has unconscious components stemming from unresolved conflicts. Singer (1970) delineated three categories of countertransference as:

- ◆ Overly kind and concerned
- ◆ Overly hostile and angry
- ◆ Intense anxiety

In addition, Singer (1970) asserted that the therapist's countertransference reactions may occur during sessions or they may occur in fantasies or dreams. Resolution of countertransference is crucial to therapists understanding themselves and their clients. Professional supervision or psychoanalysis are forums for resolving these conflicts. Dombeck and Brody (1995) define *clinical supervision* for psychotherapy as a forum for nurse therapists and other mental health professionals to reflect feelings about certain client situations and to create a balance between self-awareness and formal learning. Effective supervision requires an atmosphere of motivation, empowerment, support, and mutual respect.

Neutrality

Neutrality is another psychoanalytic technique that places the therapist in a passive and permissive role. It enables the client to project onto the therapist certain feelings or attitudes from early childhood relationships (Kernberg, 1984). Like other psychoanalytic techniques, it evokes feelings and thoughts that can be explored and understood in terms of the need to develop adaptive coping behaviors.

BRIEF PSYCHOTHERAPIES

Brief or short-term psychotherapy stems from Franz Alexander and Thomas French's work in the 1940s with clients suffering from psychosomatic illnesses. They found that brief psychotherapy helped their clients resolve emotional problems that affected biological processes.

During a time when cost containment and quality health care are treatment priorities, brief psychotherapy continues to offer clients brief, focused interventions to cope with present stressors or crises. This client-centered approach continues to gain widespread popularity because it enables mental health professionals to curb treatment costs while offering the client quality care.

Brief psychotherapy refers to any treatment in which the number of sessions is limited, usually 15 or fewer, which helps clients relate present stressors to past experiences. It is useful in treating acute distress, such as grief reactions, but not severe symptoms that require immediate resolution, such as suicidal ideations or acute psychosis. The client with a spastic colon can benefit from brief psychotherapy. This individual may present with "acute" gastrointestinal symptoms and have a negative diagnostic workup. Brief psychotherapy can alleviate acute physical and emotional symptoms and help the client gain insight into past experiences and current stressors. Positive client outcomes are influenced by an ability to form a meaningful relationship with the therapist, motivation to understand the meaning of present symptoms, and willingness to make adaptive behavioral changes.

Goals

The major goals of brief psychotherapy begin with collaboration with the client to determine treatment goals and termination dates. Likewise treatment goals are to assess the client's problems, remove distressful symptoms, support adaptive coping behaviors, and promote optimal functioning. Therapeutic interactions evolve through the use of trust, patience, and flexibility (Davanloo, 1978).

Interpersonal Psychotherapy

Interpersonal psychotherapy is one type of short-term psychotherapy. It is based on the assumption that a person's mental processes and behaviors stem from his relations with others. A person's interpersonal style is the foundation of his coping patterns and is based on early interactions with primary caregivers, evolves over time, and is inherent in one's interactions with others (Klerman, Weissman, Rounsaville, & Chevron, 1984; Millon, 1969).

Goals

The primary goals of interpersonal psychotherapy are to assess maladaptive interactions and teach adaptive coping skills. Providing guidance, clarifying areas of interpersonal difficulties, facilitating problem solving, and helping the client gain insight into maladaptive behaviors are major interventions. Clients with impaired social skills and depression can benefit from interpersonal psychotherapy.

Stress-Reducing Therapy

Supportive, or stress-reducing, psychotherapy is used to strengthen clients' adaptive coping behaviors and promote homeostasis (Rogers, 1942). People who are experiencing stress often feel inadequate, helpless, and isolated. Stress-reducing therapy provides them with emotional and biological support during crisis or stressful events.

Goals

The major treatment goals of supportive therapy are to promote restoration of health, maintain adaptive coping behaviors, strengthen ego function, improve coping behaviors or patterns, enhance problem-solving skills, and mobilize resources and options.

Creating a supportive climate begins with the establishment of a therapeutic nurse-client relationship that initially encourages dependence and, later, independence. Supportive therapy reduces stress that interferes with optimal functioning. Clients with schizophrenia or dementia can benefit from supportive therapy because it provides an empathetic and encouraging relationship that facilitates reality testing or ego functioning and monitoring of clients' responses to treatment. Ongoing emotional support increases social interaction and promotes growth and independence. Crisis intervention and administration of psychotropics can enhance supportive psychotherapy.

Behavioral Therapy

Behavioral therapy originated in 1920, at which time Watson and Rayner described their renowned case with Little Albert. This experiment involved a child who was fearful of a white mouse and all furry objects. They surmised that conditioning could help the youngster deal with his fears of these objects, but they were unable to test these strategies because the child was discharged from the hospital. However, several years later, Jones (1924) used Watson and Rayner's strategies to treat children with phobias.

Behavioral therapy is based on the assumption that complex human behaviors or responses are learned and therefore may be unlearned. Similarly, adaptive and maladaptive responses are influenced by a stimulus-response that is mediated by the nervous system. Wolpe (1958, 1973) asserted that a behavior is a response, the stimulus occurs before the response, and the activation of the afferent nerves is modulated by sensory stimuli. For example, the client who walks into a crowd (stimulus) and "panics" (response) and experiences dizziness, heart palpitations, and dry mouth (arousal of sympathetic nervous system) is experiencing a stimulus-response mediated by the autonomic nervous system.

Clients with anxiety disorders, phobias, and depression can reduce their distress through various behavioral therapies such as systematic desensitization, flooding, participant modeling, aversion therapy, positive reinforcement, assertiveness and social skills training, and various psychotropics. Table 26–2 describes these behavioral therapy techniques. See Chapters 11 and 29 for specific psychosocial and psychopharmacologic interventions.

Cognitive Therapy

The term *cognitive* stems from the Latin word *cogitare*, meaning "to know." *Cognitive therapy* refers to a collaborative relationship between the nurse psychotherapist and the client who assumes that depression or anxiety stems from faulty or

TABLE 26–2
Behavioral Therapy Techniques

Type	Definition	Techniques
Systematic desensitization	Client is exposed to stimulus that produces anxiety	• Relaxation training • Hierarchy construction desensitization of stimulus (Wolpe, 1958, 1973)
Flooding	Increased exposure to anxiety-producing stimulus	• Expose to specific phobia, both real and imagined
Participant modeling	New behavior learned through observation	• Behavioral rehearsal
Assertiveness and social skills training	Teaches client how to behave appropriately in confident manner	• Role modeling • Positive reinforcement • Desensitization
Aversion therapy or conditioned reflex therapy	Association of abstinence responses with behavior that has offensive consequences (exposure to noxious stimulus)	• Administration of Antabuse in a client who has alcoholism disorder is an example • Expose to specific phobia
Positive reinforcement	Reward for desired behavior change	• Token economies • Positive feedback

Note. From *The Practice of Behavior Therapy* (2nd ed.), by J. Wolpe, 1973, New York: Pergamon Press.

distorted cognitions or maladaptive coping responses. Major treatment goals focus on modifying these thoughts or behaviors by helping clients recognize their distorted cognitions and maladaptive behaviors. Major strategies include homework assignments, interruption and reversal of irrational beliefs and attitudes, and reduction of feelings generated by

distorted cognitions (Beck, 1976; Beck, Rush, Shaw, & Emery, 1979). All in all, these interventions teach clients how to make adaptive cognitive and behavioral changes to improve their anxiety or mood and level of functioning.

The benefits of cognitive therapy are illustrated in the clinical example, in which the nurse psychotherapist carefully questions the client's overgeneralization and negative self-talk.

Dialectical Behavior Therapy

Dialectical Behavior Therapy (DBT) was introduced in 1987 by Marsha Linehan. The primary aim of DBT is to help individuals with borderline personality disorder develop coping skills rather than enable them to effectively manage intense emotional states. Similar to other behavioral therapies, a compassionate and accepting approach is used to improve insight into maladaptive behaviors. Similar to other cognitive behavioral therapies, DBT is used to challenge distorted cognitions or schemata associated with intense anxiety and distress in clients with borderline personality. Skills' training is the core feature of DBT in which the psychotherapist focuses on behavioral control and master skills to resolve trauma issues; integrate positive concept and self-respect, develop adaptive behavioral changes, experience sustained joy, and attain client-centered goals (Ebner-Priemer et al., 2007; Linehan, 1999; Linehan, Heard, & Armstrong, 1993).

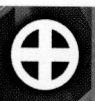

CLINICAL EXAMPLE

Using the Cognitive Therapy Techniques with a Depressed Client

Phil, a depressed client, complains that "today has been a terrible day and everything has gone wrong." After questioning Phil, the nurse discovers that only one negative thing has transpired: a co-worker turned down Phil's invitation to lunch. After questioning by the nurse, Phil was able to identify several positive occurrences, including an outstanding job appraisal. The nurse pointed out a lack of congruency between Phil's negative thoughts and feelings and events at work. The nurse gave Phil a "homework assignment" of keeping a log or diary of events and thoughts that occurred before feeling "depressed and down." Follow-up sessions allowed the nurse to confront or challenge Phil's overgeneralization and negative self-talk and the lack of congruency between his thoughts and feelings and reality.

Johnston (1990) asserted that the capacity to form a collaborative nurse-client relationship and the client's motivation to change determine the success of cognitive therapy. The nurse's ability to establish a working alliance is crucial to the success of cognitive therapy. It enables the nurse to establish a nonthreatening climate, which helps the client recognize irrational belief systems that distort reality and thereby generate distress. Cognitive therapy has been helpful in treating clients with anxiety, personality, and depressive disorders (Beck et al., 1979; Beck, Brown, Berchick, Stewart, & Steer, 1990; Beck & Freedman, 1990; Beck, Skodol, Clark, Berchick, & Wright, 1992; Patience, McGuire, Scott, & Freeman, 1995; Persons, 1998). Chapters 9, 10, and 11 describe the use of cognitive therapy to treat anxiety and depressive disorders.

INDIVIDUAL PSYCHOTHERAPY ACROSS THE LIFE SPAN

Numerous studies attest to the efficacy of psychotherapy at different stages in the life span. Approaches to individual psychotherapy are based on individual needs and vary with clients' developmental stage, cognitive abilities, ego integrity, and motivation for treatment. See Table 26–3 for a summary of effective techniques of individual psychotherapy for clients of different ages.

CHILDHOOD

The practice of child psychotherapy dates back to 1909, when Freud published his famous work with a 5-year-old boy with phobia (1959a, 1959b). Erikson (1959) and Piaget (1969) contributed to the understanding of the normal developmental stages of childhood and adolescence. Later, the child guidance clinic model (Kanner, 1955) specified that while one therapist works with a child, a second therapist works with the parents, legal guardian, or primary caregivers. Successful outcomes required focusing on maladaptive interactions in the child and the family system. Currently, child psychotherapists lean toward increasing information about adaptive and maladaptive developmental responses, developing adept assessments and effective treatment, and understanding the cause of childhood mental disorders (Chambless & Hollon, 1998; Curry, 2001).

Protecting children from profound distress and facilitating adaptive coping patterns are germane to the mental health of future generations. Presently, mental health care for children and adolescence is lacking and in turmoil. Epidemiological data show that as high as 20 percent of children up to the age of 18 years have one or more mental disorders during some period of their lifetime. Of this number, about 50 percent will have serious childhood mental disorders, approximately 8 million children and adolescents (Roberts, Attkisson, & Rosenblatt, 1998). In

TABLE 26–3
Individual Psychotherapy across the Life Span

	Effective Psychotherapeutic Techniques	Nursing Challenges
Childhood	• Supportive therapy • Play therapy • Behavioral modification • Cognitive therapy	• Client's immature ego function and inability to express feelings • Motivation for treatment • Establishment of trust
Adolescence	• All types	• Establishment of working relationship with client
Young and middle adulthood	• All types	• Role transitions • Developmental stress (marriage, divorce, parenthood) • Financial concerns • Careers
Older adulthood	• All types	• Understanding of aging process, role of medications, presenting symptoms, and coping patterns • Motivation for treatment

addition, the global emotional and behavioral impact of violence and war on youth and their families are on the rise. Major barriers to mental health care for youth include economic, cultural, and racial factors. Efforts to address these issues are articulated in the surgeon general's report (Satcher, 2000).

The following are predictors of psychosocial and neurobiological health in children and adolescents (Compas, 1987; Mallinckrodt, 1992):

◆ The capacity to use various support systems
◆ A sense of self-worth and competence
◆ A sense of belonging
◆ The ability to respond to developmental crises
◆ Parents, legal guardian, or primary caregiver's competence

Treatment strategies are determined by the child's developmental stage, severity of symptoms in the child, and the parents', legal guardian's, or primary caregiver's coping skills. Establishment of a therapeutic relationship is the basis of all psychotherapies. A climate that fosters trust, safety, and growth is the major goal of child psychotherapy.

Types of Child Psychotherapy

Child psychotherapy includes supportive, play, behavioral modification, and cognitive therapies. Regardless of treatment approaches, they must be family based, conducted in a culturally competent manner, and enhance social and emotional well-being and development in primary schools (Scahill, 2001).

Supportive Psychotherapy

Supportive psychotherapy enables children with normal developmental stress to maintain and improve their adaptive coping behaviors.

Play Therapy

Play therapy is an individualized intervention that offers children a symbolic way to express feelings, anxiety, aggressions, and self-doubt. In play therapy, a simple playroom can be used as a therapeutic tool. The premise behind play therapy is that because their verbal skills are inadequate, children usually communicate better through play than verbally (Axline, 1947, 1955).

Playrooms are an essential part of psychotherapy with children. These rooms usually have an array of playthings and toys that allow children to communicate fantasies and express feelings. The typical playroom contains special drawers or storage space; multigenerational families of dolls of various races and cultures; anatomically correct dolls for assessment of sexual and abuse issues; toy soldiers and policeman; dollhouse furnishings; crayons and clay; puppets; sponge-like balls; tools such as hammers; rubber knives; building blocks; cars, trucks, and airplanes; and cooking and eating utensils (Everstine & Everstine, 1993).

Behavior Modification

Behavior modification teaches children how to modify maladaptive target behaviors through positive reinforcement or a token system. Modeling plays a vital role in behavior modification, and success is contingent on training the parents, legal guardian, or primary caregivers to provide positive reinforcement, so that behavior modification occurs at home (Gordon, Lerner, & Keefe, 1979).

Cognitive Therapy

Cognitive therapy has been shown to be effective for modifying childhood disorders, including enuresis, depression, and anxiety (Ronen & Abraham, 1996; Rosenbaum & Ronen, 1997). Recent studies indicate that cognitive therapy is superior to alternative psychosocial interventions during acute treatment of childhood and adolescent depressive disorders (Brent, Kolko, Birmaher, Baugher, & Bridge, 1999; Cohen, Mannarino, & Staron, 2006; Deblinger, Mannarino, Cohen, & Steer, 2006) (see Research Abstract). Cognitive therapy enables the impulsive child to correct negative, distorted cognitive process and improve self-image.

The success of treating children and adolescents experiencing distressful physical and psychological symptoms requires collaboration with families and the youth's network. Cognitive behavioral therapy along with diverse approaches have been extensively adapted to use with children and families based on developmental stage and capacity and willingness to participate in psychotherapy. The appropriateness of CBT in children ages 5 to 8 due to their cognitive developmental level is questionable and age-appropriate approaches must be considered when working with this age group (Connolly & Bernstein, 2007; Freeman, et al., 2007).

Psychotherapy Issues Unique to Children

The success of any treatment requires active parent-child participation. Parents, legal guardians, or primary caregivers act as role models, and in some cases as therapists, and reinforce and encourage adaptive coping behaviors. Various forms of psychotherapy are appropriate for all age groups.

The major differences between child psychotherapy and adult psychotherapy relate to specific developmental needs and tasks. There are four principal differences in children and adult seeking treatment. First, children have immature ego function and defense mechanisms. Childhood traumas and problems can result in permanent impairment of personality and physical development. Second, children typically do not seek treatment voluntarily. They are usually brought in by their parents, legal guardian, or primary caregivers, who want them to be "fixed" after having exhausted their coping and problem-solving skills. Unfortunately, children may also be identified as the "problem" in dysfunctional families. This challenges the nurse to encourage the children to participate in treatment while attempting to establish trust. Third, children tend to externalize internal conflicts to work through their distress. They have difficulty problem solving and verbalizing their feelings except through changing things in the environment. Finally, children are inclined to reenact their feelings in new situations and eagerly engage in new experiences (Mishne, 1986). The nurse can use these attributes to engage children in the therapeutic relationship and facilitate adaptive changes.

Because children's problems are complex and their abilities and level of understanding differ from those of adults, play therapy, parental behavioral modification programs, and the various psychotherapies must be tailored to meet the unique needs of each child and his parents, legal guardian, or primary caregivers.

ADOLESCENCE

Adolescence is a time of biological and psychosocial turmoil and transition. Adolescents have to balance feelings generated by their needs for both separation and dependence, cope with underlying feelings of poor self-esteem and inadequacy, and determine an identity. Typical adolescent behaviors include poor impulse control, mood swings, and poor frustration tolerance. This developmental stage also includes identification with peers and a sense of belonging. Erikson (1959) described adolescence as the final stage of childhood and a time during which personal identity is formed. Piaget (1969) defined adolescence as a period in which abstract thinking and intellectual development are achieved. Adolescence is further influenced by cultural, ethnic, neurobiological, and psychosocial factors.

Assessment Foci

The assessment of adolescents, like the assessment of children, is based on age-appropriate behaviors and mastery of developmental tasks. The assessment process is complicated by the turbulence of adolescence, but Kessler (1966) suggested that assessment of the adolescent should address the following:

1. Behaviors appropriate to the youth's chronological age
2. Duration, frequency, and number of symptoms
3. The degree of social dysfunction
4. Severity of behavior
5. Adaptive and maladaptive responses (personality traits)
6. The degree of subjective distress

Transference Issues

The transference reactions of children and adolescents differ from those of adults because they still live with their significant primary caregivers or early objects. As a rule, they do not displace their feelings toward and perceptions of these significant figures onto other objects. Instead, their behavior and attitude usually relate to their parents, legal guardian, or primary caregivers in the here and now. They perceive the therapist as an extension of their parents. Transference reactions provide the therapist with opportu-

nities to explore impaired thought processes and distorted cognitions (Sandler, Kennedy, & Tyson, 1980).

Countertransference Issues

Countertransference, like transference, emerges in psychotherapy with adolescents. Because adolescence is often a period of turmoil, teenage clients have a natural ability to evoke strong reactions in the therapist because of their need to express feelings generated by neurobiological and psychosocial stressors. Their tendency to express feelings through acting out rather than words frequently generates stress in the therapist (Giovacchini, 1985). The therapist can use interpretations of their countertransference reactions to enhance self-awareness and understanding of adolescent clients' symptoms.

Establishing a Working Relationship with an Adolescent

Successful identification of the adolescent client's needs and development of effective interventions depend on the nurse-client relationship. The nurse's first task is to establish alliance with the adolescent and the parents, legal guardian, or primary caregivers. Initially, adolescents presenting for treatment are likely to be more provocative, more intense, and cruder than adults seeking treatment. They are less trusting and open during the early stages of treatment, frequently denying their problems and blaming their parents. Acting out may include self-destructive behaviors such as substance abuse, truancy, promiscuity, self-mutilation, or suicide attempts.

Establishing a *working* relationship with adolescents challenges nurses to use patience and draw on their understanding of adaptive and maladaptive developmental tasks. The major desirable client outcomes include enhancing and maintaining of self-esteem; developing adaptive coping skills; and forming healthy, meaningful relationships.

Similar to other age groups, adolescents may also benefit from various psychotherapies such as cognitive, behavioral, and psychodynamic approaches to manage depressive, anxiety, and other mental disorders (Birmaher et al., 2000; Brent & Birmaher, 2002; Brent et al., 1999; Curry, 2001). Major treatment goals for adolescents include modifying distorted cognitions or maladaptive coping behaviors; facilitating adaptive coping behaviors that enable them to engage in pleasant activities, social skills, problem-solving, and assertive communication. Cognitive therapy empowers adolescents to establish goals that use self-monitoring to modify and challenge distorted cognitions. It also helps the youth control emotional states by using various interventions such as deep abdominal breathing and other relaxation techniques.

ADULTHOOD

The transition from adolescence to adulthood generates tremendous stress. Primary adult transitions include establishing a career, entering into marriage or other meaningful relationships, divorce, managing financial problems, parenting, and caring for aging parents. Stressful life events often generate crises or maladaptive coping patterns. Psychotherapy can be used to identify individual strengths and limitations that enable clients to develop adaptive coping patterns and interactions. Psychotherapy provides an atmosphere of trust, empathy, acceptance, and opportunity for growth.

Clients seeking treatment have complex needs and experience vast forms of distress such as depression, anxiety, and physical complaints. Psychotherapy may be used alone or in conjunction with a case management approach to meet complex client needs. The case management approaches include psychotherapy, prescribing medications, monitoring client responses to an array of interventions such as medications, other somatic therapies, and psychosocial interventions (American Nurses Association [APA], 2000). Initial contact with the client often begins in an acute or ambulatory care setting, such as the emergency department, and continues for an expanded period in the community. Collaboration with various community health care professionals such as advanced-practice registered nurses (APRN), psychiatrists, psychologists, and social workers, is important to ensure seamless comprehensive care.

OLDER ADULTHOOD

Older adults represent the fastest growing segment of the American population. They constitute 12 percent of the population, or approximately 25 million people, and it is estimated

that by 2050, this figure will more than double (U.S. Census Bureau, 2000). Furthermore, in the United States, the proportion of adults 85 years or older is growing so fast that in the next few decades, 1 in 4 persons older than 65 will be among the oldest old (Agree & Freedman, 1999). These statistics suggest a need for theory development and research regarding the effectiveness of psychotherapy in meeting the needs of older adults.

Historically, the effectiveness of working with older adults has been debated. Freud (1959b) suggested that older adults were not appropriate for psychoanalysis, but his colleague, Abraham, disputed this notion and suggested that they could benefit from treatment (Fenichel, 1945). In spite of early debate, the number of older adult clients who seek treatment continues to lag behind other age groups, with only 4 percent of mental health clinic workloads and 3 percent of private practitioners treating them (Hunkeler et al., 2006; Reynolds et al., 2006). Various explanations account for these figures, including older adult's hesitancy to confide in younger therapists, older adult's self-reliance, and therapists' hesitancy to work with them. Older adults are more likely to be misdiagnosed and mismanaged when they present with psychiatric symptoms and psychosocial stressors. Accurately diagnosing their distress is further compromised because they are more likely than younger individuals to report phy-sical symptoms than emotional distress, further making it difficult for a differential diagnosis of medical and psychiatric problems. Older adults tend to feel more comfortable seeking help for psychiatric problems from their primary care provider than a mental health professional (Hunkeler et al., 2006). Another challenge for nurse

RESEARCH ABSTRACT

A Follow-up Study of a Multisite, Randomized, Controlled Trial for Children with Sexual Abuse–Related PTSD Symptoms

Deblinger, E., Mannarino, A. P., Cohen, J. A., & Steer, R. A. (2006). *Journal of the American Academy of Child and Adolescent Psychiatry, 45,* 1474–1484.

Study/Problem

To determine if the distinct responses previously associated with trauma-focused, cognitive behavioral therapy (TF-CBT), and child-centered therapy (CCT) for treating post-traumatic stress disorder (PTSD) and related problems in children with a history of sexual abuse would persist following treatment and to assess potential predictors of treatment outcome.

Method

The sample consisted of 183 children 8 to 14 years old, and their primary caregivers were assessed 6 and 12 months following their posttreatment evaluations. Researchers used mixed-model repeated analyses of covariance to evaluate PTSD symptoms in children and their caregivers who had been previously treated with TF-CBT.

Findings

Data demonstrated that children and their caregivers exhibited fewer symptoms of PTSD and described less shame than the children who had been treated with CCT at both 6 and 12 months. Researchers also found that posttreatment outcomes and predictors of PTSD symptoms were positively correlated with multiple traumas and higher levels of depression at pretreatment in children assigned to the CCT condition only.

Implications for Psychiatric Nurses

Trauma-related responses in children and families are complex and multidimensional. This study offers an evidence-based approach using cognitive behavioral therapy to treat children and their families exposed to traumatic events. Advanced-practice psychiatric nurses can use cognitive behavioral therapy to identify and treat children and families at risk for PTSD and other stress disorders.

psychotherapists is working with older adults presenting with concomitant dementia. Because dementia affects the client's ability to participate in psychotherapy, there are questions about the appropriateness of psychotherapy in these clients. The decision to provide psychotherapy to clients with dementia must be thoroughly assessed and based on individual needs and capacity to participate in treatment.

Even though the number of older adult clients seeking treatment is less than that of other age groups, this population is at risk. Older adults experience numerous losses such as the deaths or debilitating illnesses of loved ones, decline in socioeconomic well-being, and mental and physical functioning. The high prevalence of completed suicides, particularly among older European American white males, suggests that nurses need to identify stressors and formulate effective interventions that support adaptive coping behaviors and relieve physical and mental distress.

Individual psychotherapy is a useful treatment strategy for older adults. Understanding of the normal aging process, the role of medications, presenting symptoms, coping patterns, and motivation for treatment are major elements of psychotherapy with this age group.

Teri and Logsdon (1992) stated that the following are essential qualities for psychotherapists working with the older adult:

1. An interest in the older adult and a perception of working with the older adult as a challenge, rather than a hopeless endeavor
2. Specialized training on the aging process
3. A caring attitude toward older adults
4. Ability to set realistic and individual treatment goals

They described work with the older adult client as challenging and rewarding and an opportunity to appreciate the uniqueness and complexity of the human aging process. Psychotherapy with this age group "maximizes the full spectrum of human knowledge," Teri and Logsdon (1992, p. 86) stated, integrating theories and research findings toward the development of effective interventions. Growing evidence supports these assertions and points out that older adults benefit from psychotherapy as evidenced by better functional and emotional status and improved quality of life. Researchers also submit that depressed older adults also benefit from holistic approaches that integrate psychotherapy and antidepressants (Hunkeler et al., 2006; Reynolds, et al., 2006).

SUMMARY

Individual psychotherapy across the life span challenges nurses to understand and appreciate the uniqueness of each developmental stage. It reveals a full spectrum of human development and people's methods of coping with the daily stress of living. Individual psychotherapy is a treatment modality that uses the nurse-client relationship to facilitate effective coping responses and promote optimal health. It also encourages self-awareness and growth in clients, which are necessary for them to understand their behaviors and maximize their resourcefulness.

THE ROLE OF THE NURSE

Individual psychotherapy focuses on changing personality structure and maladaptive behaviors. The outcome of psychotherapy is determined by the quality of the therapeutic use of self, the client's perception of presenting symptoms or behaviors and motivation for change, and neurobiological and psychosocial factors. Therapeutic use of self involves self-awareness, empathy, acceptance, self-disclosure, and other means of facilitating a therapeutic relationship. Certain conditions must exist to facilitate a positive outcome. A key player in the psychotherapy process is the psychotherapist.

THE GENERALIST NURSE

Psychotherapy is limited to nurses who at least have a master's degree and are clinically competent to assess and oversee complex client needs. Conducting psychotherapy requires an in-depth understanding of human behaviors and various psychosocial, psychiatric, and biological theories and their application to complex client problems. Generalist nurses are educationally and clinically unprepared to conduct psychotherapy. However, they can provide other therapeutic interventions, such as telecare, crisis intervention, or grief counseling to clients and families, and support them during stressful periods. These are effective strategies that provide immediate emotional support, mobilize resources and adaptive coping behaviors, and foster problem solving during crisis or disaster situations.

Generalists may use theories and principles as guides for safe care and develop care plans that are theory- and evidence-based. Knowledge of the client's underlying mental health problems can assist the nurse in designing and implementing interventions such as providing consistency, setting limits, and establishing clear boundaries, and encouraging experimentation with new coping strategies. Although individual psychotherapy lies outside the scope of generalist nursing practice, the therapeutic relationship is the cornerstone of all professional nursing alliance. Trust, empathy, and advocacy, essential to nursing care rendered in all practice settings, must be grounded in establishing and maintaining caring therapeutic nurse-client relationships. (See Chapter 6 for additional discussions about boundaries and the caution of therapeutic touch.)

THE ADVANCED-PRACTICE PSYCHIATRIC REGISTERED NURSE

The American Nurses Association (ANA, 2000) defines the nurse psychotherapist as an advanced-level (master's degree), clinical nurse specialist or psychiatric-mental health nurse practitioner, who is educated and clinically prepared and certified to provide psychotherapy. The nurse psychotherapist independently performs various forms of psychotherapy and is accountable for his practice and health care delivery. ANA (2000) specifies that the nurse psychotherapist is responsible for the following:

1. Structuring a therapeutic nurse-client agreement
2. Collaborating with health professionals to facilitate effective treatment
3. Maintaining and refining his professional skills through continuing education and collaboration with other psychotherapists
4. Providing continuity of care in the therapist's absence
5. Providing clinical supervision and role modeling for nurses and other mental health students, and offering continuing education
6. Integrating biological concepts into practice through prescriptive authority within state regulations
7. Evaluating the client's progress in attaining expected outcomes

PHASES OF THE THERAPEUTIC RELATIONSHIP

Psychotherapy is a powerful treatment modality that enables the nurse to form a therapeutic relationship with the client to assess and relieve distress, change maladaptive coping patterns, prevent mental illness, promote growth and development, and enhance mental and functional status (ANA, 2000).

Psychotherapy is an interactive process that evolves over time between the nurse therapist and the client. Patience and genuine interest are crucial to successful outcomes, because they facilitate verbal and nonverbal communication that promotes a greater understanding of the complex process of client responses.

Professional Supervision

The multifacet basis of psychiatric disorders necessitates nurse psychotherapists to engage in life-long learning opportunities and monitor and manage their own reactions to difficult or challenging nurse-client situations through various venues. Strong emotions or reactions to clients' situations and problems, when left unresolved, often interfere with one's ability to maintain an objective perspective, healthy boundaries, and therapeutic relationships (Ferro & Basile, 2004; Lauro et al., 2003; Townsend, 2005). *Clinical supervision* offers a venue to resolve such situations and develop professional skills necessary to address and maintain healthy nurse-client relationships. Clinical supervision helps the nurse psychotherapist maintain and advance psychotherapeutic skills, deal with complex client situations, such as personality disorder and treatment-resistant depression, and review ethical concerns and difficult dealings

with other clinical situations. This collaborative relationship is based on mutual respect and may involve supervision between the nurse psychotherapist and a peer or peer group that provides a confidential forum to present and review difficult cases, analyze personal reactions (e.g., countertransference issues), and provides opportunities to use evidence-based strategies to facilitate personal and professional development (Betan, Heim, Conklin, & Westen, 2005). Additional benefits of clinical supervision include a forum to:

◆ Employ emotional support to identify strengths, abilities, and areas to improve clinical skills
◆ Validate clinical skills and interventions, especially for difficult or complicated cases
◆ Improve and maintain healthy interactions with clients
◆ Enhance personal awareness and insight and facilitate professionals and clinical growth
◆ Make diagnostic and therapeutic use of personal responses to the client
◆ Develop and implement evidence-based strategies based on individual needs, wishes, preferences, and cultural, age, and gender-specific needs
◆ Maintain a standard of practice for the advanced practice psychiatric registered nurse

THE NURSING PROCESS

The nursing process is an integral part of psychotherapy. A theoretical framework is used to guide the evaluation and data collection process and determine diagnoses. Diagnoses determine outcome identification and evaluation.

ASSESSMENT AND DIAGNOSIS

In the initial stage of psychotherapy, the client's symptoms and present stressors are assessed. Present and past coping patterns are assessed in a manner that conveys a caring and concerned attitude. Clients are often reluctant to discuss their problems with a stranger because of shame, guilt, or distrust. Active listening, which helps the nurse identify common themes, can allay these feelings, both verbal and nonverbal, in the client's presenting symptoms. A common theme among depressed clients is the feeling of being a failure or a loser, suggesting a lack of control or feelings of helplessness.

The specific theoretical framework being followed determines how the client is approached, how information is elicited, how treatment strategies are developed, and how responses to interventions are evaluated. In addition, theoretical concepts determine the focus of observation, such as here-and-now rather than past events, and the data collection process. Data collection helps in the development of the nursing and medical diagnoses.

Client education is a major component of psychotherapy. During the assessment process, the nurse educates the client about psychotherapy and the specific roles and expectation of each of them. This discussion addresses boundary issues and the collaborative nature of psychotherapy. The client is encouraged to play an active role in psychotherapy and share responsibility for outcome identification and response to treatment.

OUTCOME IDENTIFICATION AND PLANNING

Outcome identification or goal setting is a collaborative endeavor between the nurse and client. This involves problem identification and expected outcomes from interventions. Active client participation in this process fosters independence and responsibility in treatment.

IMPLEMENTATION

The client's problems or diagnoses, motivation for treatment, cognitive processes, and developmental stage, as well as the time frame for treatment determine the specific interventions used. In addition, the nurse's theoretical perspective for psychotherapy influences interventions. For instance, if the client has cognitive distortions that have activated maladaptive responses, a cognitive-behavioral approach may be helpful in facilitating adaptive coping behaviors. This eclectic approach (i.e., both cognitive and behavioral therapies) is more flexible because it integrates several theories that are based on client needs, ability to learn, and developmental stage.

As the nurse-client relationship evolves, several treatment issues may arise. Countertransference, client resistance, client insight, confrontation, self-disclosure by the nurse, and confidentiality are integral aspects of psychotherapy (Table 26–4).

Countertransference has already been discussed in this chapter.

Resistance

Resistance is a phenomenon that occurs during early treatment, and clients use it to ward off uncomfortable feelings,

TABLE 26–4
Therapeutic Techniques

Issue	Interventions
Countertransference: interferes with the nurse's ability to provide objective client interventions	Recognize personal reactions to specific clients (i.e., anger, hostility, rescuing, or overprotectiveness).
Resistance: maintains the client's status quo and interferes with working through the therapeutic process and building adaptive coping	Assess the meaning of this phenomenon to the client. • Prescribe no change in resistance (paradoxical intent or asking the client to do the opposite of what the nurse wants)
Insight: basis for motivation/understanding the course of illness and treatment outcome	Provide the client and significant others with education regarding the illness, treatment outcome, and course/outcome of interventions. • Encourage ventilation of feelings and concerns regarding illness/treatment • Clarify client and family's feelings • Avoid interpreting behaviors too quickly
Self-disclosure: based on the nature of the nurse-client relationship; excessive use interferes with the therapeutic process	Limit information to what the nurse is comfortable with sharing such as "yes, I am married."
Confidentiality: absolute is unrealistic with children/adolescents; it is the basis of trust	Discuss record-keeping with the client and family. • Maintain computerized records • Follow legal and ethical protocols for duty to warn and duty to protect • Discuss specific issues with the client and significant others
Confrontation: interferes with clear communication and understanding of incongruencies	Point out incongruencies among the client's thoughts, feelings, and behaviors

particularly anxiety, generated by underlying repressed conflicts. Symptoms of resistance include missed appointments, tardiness, or refusal to do homework assignments.

Insight

Insight refers to the client's self-awareness and understanding of the meaning and reason for his behavior or motives. This term generally means that the client or significant other has knowledge of the illness and is aware of behaviors that contribute to remission or exacerbation of symptoms. An example of a client with insight is the man who comes to the emergency department or nurse's office requesting a refill of lithium because he knows that he will become manic or psychotic and require hospitalization if he stops taking the drug. In contrast, an example of the client with poor insight is seen in the man who stops taking lithium, becomes manic, and requires an involuntary admission. Poor insight in psychotherapy interferes with restoration of health and optimal functioning.

Nurses cannot instill insight into clients, but they can provide therapeutic climates that increase its likelihood. Resisting the temptation to interpret clients' behaviors and helping them understand the relationship between maladaptive behaviors and persistent distress can be therapeutic. Insight often overwhelms the client with feelings and ideas that need to be backed up with adaptive behavioral changes. If insight does not exist, the client experiences little change (Carkhuff & Berenson, 1967).

Resistance and poor insight often require nursing interventions that facilitate clients' understanding of their persistent maladaptive responses.

Confrontation

Confrontation refers to the act of pointing out contradictions or incongruencies among feelings, thoughts, and behaviors, specifically pointing out parts of the assessment or treatment process that are contradictory or confusing. It also reduces vagueness and incongruencies in client affect, behavior, or communication. Trust, patience, and empathy are prerequisites to confrontation and requires patience and empathy (Kernberg, 1984). Its effectiveness lies in its potential to help clients develop adaptive coping responses by clarifying the meaning of resistance, distortions, and poor insight.

Self-Disclosure

Self-disclosure on the part of the nurse therapist is an important part of the nurse-client relationship. Self-disclosure has some therapeutic value. Psychotherapy is an interactive process that would become stagnant unless the client felt some connectedness with the nurse therapist. Judith Simon (1988) described self-disclosure as the antithesis of detachment or neutrality advocated by psychoanalytic theory. She noted that self-disclosure can enhance the therapeutic alliance and the therapist's self-awareness and enable the

nurse to role model appropriate behaviors and responses, validate reality for the client, and increase the therapist's satisfaction with a case. Some degree of self-disclosure is a natural part of the nurse-client relationship; in the course of therapy, for example, nurses may reveal their marital status, professional specialty, and family. For example, a picture of a child or spouse provides information about the nurse's family, and certificates or diplomas indicate the nurse's professional education and formal instruction. Knowledge of the nurse's education and clinical expertise is important to most clients seeking psychotherapy, because it informs them of the nurse's competency.

The degree of self-disclosure by the nurse depends on the nature of the nurse-client relationship, the nurse's comfort in sharing personal information with clients, and the appropriateness of clinical situations. Too little self-disclosure reduces the opportunities for reality testing, slowing the development of a trusting relationship and making the client feel less comfortable disclosing pertinent information about himself. On the other hand, too much self-disclosure may have negative consequences, which may blur boundaries between the nurse therapist and the client, particularly if it is done to meet the nurse's needs rather than the client's. An example of blurred boundaries between the nurse and the client is sexual involvement. Avoiding discussions of emotionally provocative and very personal subjects can decrease negative consequences of self-disclosure. Ultimately, the decision to self-disclose must be in the client's best interest and the nurse must recognize the benefits and perils of this treatment issue (Guetheil & Gabbard, 1998).

Confidentiality

Clients must feel that information shared with the nurse psychotherapist remains private and confidential. Concerns such as sexual orientation, mental and physical illness, and participation in psychotherapy are personal matters. Respecting and appreciating the significance of information divulged by the client are critical to maintaining a trusting relationship. Discussing and maintaining client records are additional aspects of confidentiality.

Confidentiality is affected by several factors, including legal and ethical matters and the client's developmental stage. The complexity of legal and ethical dilemmas associated with confidentiality challenges psychotherapists to create environments of trust and maintain open communication with clients and significant others about information that remains in therapy and which has to be shared with others when appropriate. The client who comes into therapy threatening to shoot his wife is an example of a situation that affects confidentiality, which cannot be maintained for several reasons. First, the therapist has a legal and ethical duty to warn and protect the client's wife, to notify the police, and to use sound judgment to intervene appropriately (*Tarasoff v. Regents of University of California*, 1976). Second, the client must understand that this information is deemed imminently dangerous.

Even though confidentiality is the basis of trust, it is unrealistic to maintain it completely with children and adolescents. For instance, it is imperative to inform the child that confidentiality will be maintained to promote trust, except when the youth is a danger to self or others. Parents, the legal guardian, or primary caregivers, must be informed when the need for protection, structure, and safety exist, such as acting out, self-destructive behaviors, or threats to harm self or others.

EVALUATION

Nurses can evaluate the effectiveness of psychotherapy by comparing client outcomes with their own and the client's expectations. Evaluation is a continuous process in which objective and subjective data are integrated.

Termination

Termination is an integral aspect of psychotherapy and the evaluation process. It is a painful process for most clients, and they must be encouraged to verbalize their feelings about it. The ending of psychotherapy is just as crucial as the beginning or working phases. It must begin as soon as possible and can be initiated with a discussion of the duration of treatment. Often, terminating practices, including summarizing therapy, reviewing client outcomes, dealing with anxiety and fears associated with the loss of the relationship, and identifying benefits of treatment, should be performed over a period of months, if feasible.

Premature termination occurs when a client leaves intensive psychotherapy before the agreed-upon time frame. Frayn (1992) stated that the following factors increase the likelihood of premature termination:

- ◆ Extreme anxiety
- ◆ A lack of trust
- ◆ Denial or lack of insight
- ◆ Negative therapeutic alliance
- ◆ Substance abuse
- ◆ Personality disorder
- ◆ Negative reactions to the therapist
- ◆ Poor ego functioning manifested by poor impulse control, low tolerance for frustration, and poor social adaptation

Early identification of these behaviors helps the nurse assess their appropriateness for individual psychotherapy, rather than other treatment modalities.

Premature termination can be a highly stressful experience for therapists, generating anxiety, anger, or a sense of powerlessness (Searles, 1986). Frayn (1992) reassured therapists that premature termination does not reflect a failure of treatment outcome. Professional assistance in managing countertransference reactions can help nurses effectively explore intense reactions to clients who terminate treatment prematurely.

CASE STUDY

Individual Psychotherapy for a Client with Borderline Personality Disorder (Mrs. Lively)

Mrs. Lively is admitted with a diagnosis of borderline personality disorder. Her history reveals present and past hospitalizations associated with recurrent suicidal ideations and prescription drug abuse. She is very demanding and goes into rage episodes with little provocation. The mental health team has recommended individual psychotherapy because she has been disruptive in group therapy during past hospitalizations.

Theory

Personality Disorder: Borderline Personality Disorder (APA, 2000). (See Chapter 15 for a discussion of borderline personality disorder.) Major psychodynamic issues include intense fear of abandonment and dependency needs, poor ego functioning (poor impulse control, fluid boundaries, poor self-esteem, and distorted cognitions), and intense affect (rage, anger).

Theoretical Approach

The theoretical framework is eclectic (cognitive, interpersonal, and supportive).

Assessment

The assessment process is continuous and begins during the initial contact with client during which time the nurse collects data. The nurse analyzes the data and determines diagnoses that guide holistic outcome identification, interventions, and evaluation.

Data Collection

The advanced-practice psychiatric-registered nurse interviews Mrs. Lively. The client and nurse discuss the therapeutic contract, which specifies the purpose, time, place, and confidentiality of sessions. Issues such as the client's expectations of treatment, problem identification, and the client's perception of her role in therapy are addressed. During the initial session, Mrs. Lively denies having a problem.

(continues)

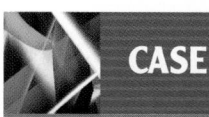

Data collection is an ongoing process. Mrs. Lively has been seen in individual psychotherapy twice a week for several weeks and she has continued to deny having problems or difficulty coping with present stressors. Information from the mental health team and her record suggest that Mrs. Lively is noncomplaint. Assessment findings are as follows:

- Poor ego functioning manifested by poor impulse control, clinging behaviors
- Self-destructiveness manifested by substance abuse, suicidal ideations
- Impaired ability to form trusting interpersonal relationships
- Nonadherence
- Poor insight
- Anger and rage

Nursing Diagnoses

- Violence, Risk for Self-Directed
- Ineffective Coping
- Chronic low self-esteem
- Noncompliance

Planning

A care plan is drawn up to achieve the following desired client outcomes:

- Client develops adaptive, long-term coping behaviors as evidenced by a decrease in anger outbursts
- Client identifies one to two positive attributes
- Client verbalizes feelings rather than acting on them

See Nursing Care Plan 26–1.

Interventions

The determination of nursing interventions is a dynamic process between the nurse and the client. This process begins with discussion concerning the therapeutic contract, involves collaboration and partnership with the client. Clinical supervision is part of this process and may be used when a difficult situation arises and to promote professional development as a psychotherapist.

Therapeutic Contract

The nurse meets with Mrs. Lively twice per week at 9:00 A.M. for 45 minutes. The client and nurse's roles in treatment are clearly delineated.

Collaboration

Client's progress will be discussed with the client and the mental health team.

Clinical Supervision

The nurse consults with the clinical supervisor to deal with transference and countertransference issues, enhance clinical skills, and promote personal and professional growth.

Partnership with Client

The nurse and client agree on an eclectic approach using cognitive, interpersonal, and supportive therapies.

Evaluation

Evaluation is an ongoing process, with feedback on progress toward the outcome criteria in the nursing care plan provided to Mrs. Lively during each session. For example:

- The client's present adaptive coping responses are difficult to assess this early in treatment, but her anger outbursts have decreased from two to three times a week to once a week.
- She is able to identify one positive attribute.
- She is able to recognize reasons for feeling angry.
- She uses adaptive coping skills, such as calling a friend when she felt stressed, rather than self-destructive behaviors during current treatment, and she denied having suicidal ideations on discharge.

Discharge Planning

Mrs. Lively will continue weekly sessions with the nurse psychotherapist.

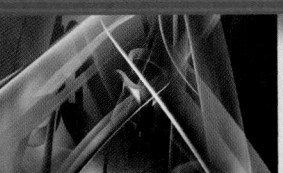

Individual Psychotherapy for a Client with Borderline Personality Disorder (Mrs. Lively)

Nursing Diagnosis: Ineffective Coping; Chronic Low Self-Esteem; High Risk for Self-Directed Violence

Outcome Identification	Nursing Actions	Rationales	Evaluation
1. By [date], Mrs. Lively will develop adaptive, long-term coping behaviors.	1. Meet with Mrs. Lively twice per week for 45 minutes.	1. Enables nurse to form intensive and therapeutic relationship with client.	*Goal met:* Mrs. Lively's angry outbursts have decreased from 2–3 times per day to once per day.
2. By [date], Mrs. Lively will identify several positive attributes.	2. Clearly delineate client and nurse roles.	2. Enables client to take responsibility in treatment process.	Mrs. Lively is able to identify one positive attribute.
3. By [date], Mrs. Lively will verbalize feelings rather than acting on them.	3. Discuss Mrs. Lively's progress with mental health team.	3. Provides ongoing feedback about areas of improvement/change.	Mrs. Lively did not try to harm herself during this hospitalization and denied having suicidal ideations on discharge.
	4. Use cognitive, interpersonal and supportive therapies with Mrs. Lively's agreement.	4. Eclectic approach provides client with diverse treatment to meet complex needs.	

SUMMARY

◆ Psychotherapy lies within the domain of the advanced-practice psychiatric-registered nurse.

◆ Individual psychotherapy is helpful in exploring the meaning of the client's maladaptive responses, collaborate with clients to identify desired outcomes, and evaluate clients' response to interventions.

◆ Although both the nurse and the client are players in this interactive process, the client is ultimately responsible for resolving adaptive coping behaviors. Psychotherapists facilitate this process through therapeutic relationship, promoting insight, and increasing self-esteem.

SUGGESTIONS FOR CLINICAL CONFERENCES

1. Invite a psychiatric clinical nurse specialist or psychiatric mental nurse practitioner to provide a case history of a psychotherapy client, discussing treatment goals, interventions, and evaluation.

2. Discuss the theoretical perspective(s) of the nurse therapist.

3. Identify the maladaptive behaviors in the case history.

4. Identify the role of the generalist and the clinical nurse specialist in facilitating adaptive behavioral changes.

5. Role-play confrontation and self-disclosure with other nursing students.

STUDY QUESTIONS

1. Mary, a 15-year-old girl, is admitted to the acute psychiatric unit because of problems controlling her temper and striking her mother during a heated argument. Developmentally, what are her main stressors?
   a. Dealing with her need to control her temper
   b. Learning how to develop adaptive coping behaviors
   c. Dealing with issues associated with dependency
   d. Staying out of trouble at school and with her parents

2. As her nurse, you are responsible for gathering information to assist in making a provisional diagnosis. She has been shouting at other clients off and on over the past few days. What is the initial step in assessing this client?
   a. Keeping her calm
   b. Approaching her in a calm, nonjudgmental manner
   c. Inquiring about her hobbies and school activities
   d. Setting limits and informing her that yelling is unacceptable

3. Which of the following reflects an adolescent treatment issue in psychotherapy?
   a. "It is so easy to talk to you during this first meeting."
   b. "I do not know you so why should I answer your question?"
   c. "My parents are having a pretty tough time with me."
   d. "Why are people so concerned about me?"

4. Self-disclosure is an important part of psychotherapy. Which of the following nurse statements has the greatest risk for negative consequences of self-disclosure?
   a. "I have been married about 15 years."
   b. "I have been in recovery about 10 years."
   c. "My wife left me 2 months ago and I am very stressed."
   d. "My oldest child attends one of the local universities."

5. The success of psychotherapy is influenced by several qualities in the client and nurse psychotherapist. Which comment suggests that the client might terminate treatment prematurely?
   a. "I need to cancel my appointment today."
   b. "I do not have a drinking problem!"
   c. "I really enjoy these sessions and hope we can meet several more times."
   d. "I am not sure if my insurance will pay for these sessions."

6. Which of the following statements indicates a therapeutic alliance?
   a. "I really look forward to these sessions."
   b. "Your style is different from my previous therapist."
   c. "I disagree with your diagnosis."
   d. "I really need something to calm my nerves."

7. The nurse psychotherapist is providing care for a young client who was recently hospitalized with a diagnosis of borderline personality disorder. The main treatment goal in caring for her is to do which of the following?
   a. Facilitate coping and behavioral skills to manage intense emotional states
   b. Prevent suicidal and other self-destructive behaviors
   c. Promote adherence to antidepressant medications
   d. Become less dependent on the nurse

8. A 15-year-old client is referred to the nurse psychotherapist because of anger problems in school. The most important consideration for the nurse psychotherapist is which of the following?
   a. Establish alliance with the adolescent and his parents or legal guardian
   b. Promise him that everything he shares is confidential
   c. Inform the client what he needs to do to manage his temper
   d. Point out his negative habits and replace them with positive ones

9. Ini, a 3-year-old is seen in the women's health clinic and the nurse notices that she has drawn a picture of waves of water. When questioned, the toddler states she misses her little sister and that her mother cries "all the time." When her mother returns the nurse shares the toddler's picture and informs her of the toddler's remarks. Her mother informs the nurse that her youngest child recently died and she does feel sad and cries a lot. Which best describes the toddler's behavior?
   a. Art or play therapy, a form of communication, is a normal expression of the toddler's sadness and grief.
   b. The picture is insignificant due to the toddler's immature cognitive development and poor understanding of grief.
   c. The child is experiencing pathological grief and needs to be referred to a psychotherapist.
   d. The mother has overburdened her child and both need to be referred to a psychotherapist.

10. Dialectical behavioral therapy shows great promise in the treatment of borderline personality disorder. Which of the following statements made by the client with borderline personality disorder would indicate the client understands her condition?
    a. "I am going to the gym and exercise because I am so stressed."
    b. "I want to kill myself and need to go to the emergency room."
    c. "You are responsible for me feeling so bad!"
    d. "If you had not said what you said I wouldn't be so mad!"

RESOURCES

Please note that because Internet resources are of a time-sensitive nature and URL addresses may change or be deleted, searches should also be conducted by association or topic.

Internet Resources

http://www.nursingworld.org   *The American Nurse* Online Journal of Issues in Nursing

http://www.AACAP.org   American Academy of Child and Adolescent Psychiatry

http://www.AAMFT.org   American Association for Marriage & Family Therapy

http://www.agpa.org   American Group Psychotherapy Association

http://www.agpa.org/group/ethicalguide.html   American Group Psychotherapy Association-Ethical Guide

http://www.psych.org   American Psychiatric Association

http://www.NMHA.org   National Mental Health Association

http://www.NAMI.org   National Alliance for the Mentally Ill

http://www.nimh.gov   National Institute of Mental Health. Report of the National Advisory Mental Health Council's Clinical Treatment and Services Research Workgroup (1998) *Bridging Science and Service.*

http://www.nami.org   National Alliance for the Mentally Ill (NAMI)/Advocate

REFERENCES

Agree, E. M., & Freedman, V. A. (1999). Implications of population aging for geriatric health. In J. J. Gallo, J. Busby-Whitehead, P. V. Rabins, R. Silliman, & J. Murphy (Eds.), *Reichel's care of the elderly: Clinical aspects of aging* (pp. 659–669). Baltimore: Williams & Wilkins.

American Nurses Association. (2000). *Scope and standards of psychiatric-mental health nursing practice*. Washington, DC: Author.

American Psychiatric Association. (2000). *Diagnostic and statistical manual of mental disorders* (4th edition, Text Revision) *(DSM-IV-TR)*. Washington, DC: Author.

American Psychiatric Association. (2000). Practice guideline for the treatment of patients with major depressive disorder, revised. *American Journal of Psychiatry, 157*(Suppl.), 1–45.

Axline, V. M. (1947). *Play therapy: The inner dynamics of childhood*. Boston: Houghton Mifflin.

Axline, V. M. (1955). Play therapy procedures and results. *American Journal of Orthopsychiatry, 25,* 618–626.

Beck, A. T. (1976). *Cognitive therapy and emotional disorders*. New York: International Universities Press.

Beck, A. T., Brown, G., Berchick, R. J., Stewart, B. L., & Steer, R. A. (1990). Relationship between hopelessness and ultimate suicide: A replication with psychiatric outpatients. *American Journal of Psychiatry, 147,* 190–195.

Beck, A. T., & Freedman, A. (1990). *Cognitive therapy of personality disorders*. New York: The Guilford Press.

Beck, A. T., Rush, A. J., Shaw, B. F., & Emery, G. (1979). *Cognitive therapy of depression*. New York: Guilford Press.

Beck, A. T., Skodol, L., Clark, D. A., Berchick, R., & Wright, F. (1992). A crossover study of focused cognitive therapy for panic disorders. *American Journal of Psychiatry, 149,* 778–783.

Betan, E., Heim, A. K., Conklin, C. Z., & Westen, D. (2005). Countertransference phenomena and personality pathology in clinical practice: An empirical investigation. *American Journal of Psychiatry, 162,* 890–898.

Birmaher, B., Brent, D. A., Kolko, D. J., Baugher, M., Bridge, J., Holder, D., et al. (2000). Clinical outcome after short-term psychotherapy for adolescents with major depressive disorder. *Archives of General Psychiatry, 57,* 29–36.

Brent, DA & Birmaher, B. (2002). Clinical practice. Adolescent depression. *New England Journal of Medicine, 29,* 347, 667–671.

Brent, D. A., Kolko, D. J., Birmaher, B., Baugher, M., & Bridge, J. (1999). A clinical trial for adolescent depression: Predictors of additional treatment in the acute and follow-up phases of the trial. *Journal of the American Academy of Child and Adolescent Psychiatry, 37,* 906–914.

Breuer, J., & Freud, S. (1955). *Studies in hysteria*. New York: Basic Books.

Carkhuff, R. R., & Berenson, B. G. (1967). *Beyond counseling and therapy*. New York: Holt, Rinehart, & Winston.

Chambless, D. L., & Hollon, S. D. (1998). Defining empirically supportive therapies. *Journal of Consulting and Clinical Psychology, 66,* 7–18.

Cohen, J. A., Mannarino, A. P., & Staron, V. R. (2006). A pilot study of modified cognitive-behavioral therapy for childhood traumatic grief (CBT-CTG). *Journal of the American Academy of Child and Adolescent Psychiatry, 45,* 1465–1473.

Compas, B. E. (1987). Coping with stress during childhood and adolescence. *Psychological Bulletin, 101,* 393–403.

Connolly, S. D., Bernstein, G. A., & Work Group on Quality Issues. (2007). Practice parameter for the assessment of children and adolescents with anxiety disorders. *Journal of the American Academy of Child and Adolescent Psychiatry, 46,* 267–283.

Corsini, R. J. (1984). *Current psychotherapies* (3rd ed.). Itasca, IL: F. E. Peacock.

Curry, J. F. (2001). Specific psychotherapies for childhood and adolescent depression. *Society of Biological Psychiatry, 49,* 1091–1100.

Davanloo, H. (1978). *Basic principles and techniques in short-term psychotherapy*. New York: Spectrum.

Deblinger, E., Mannarino, A. P., Cohen, J. A., & Steer, R. A. (2006). A follow-up study of a multisite, randomized, controlled trial for children with sexual abuse-related PTSD symptoms. *Journal of the American Academy of Child and Adolescent Psychiatry, 45,* 1474–1484.

Dombeck, M. T., & Brody, S. L. (1995). Clinical supervision: A three-way mirror. *Archives of Psychiatric Nursing, 9,* 3–10.

Ebner-Priemer, U. W., Welch, S. S., Grossman, P., Reisch, T., Linehan, M. M., & Bohus, M. (2007). Psychophysiological ambulatory assessment of affective dysregulation in borderline personality disorder. *Psychiatry Research, 150,* 265–275.

English, O. S., & Finch, S. T. (1964). *Introduction to psychiatry*. New York: W. W. Norton.

Erikson, E. (1959). *Childhood and society*. New York: Norton.

Everstine, D. S., & Everstine, L. (1993). *The trauma response*. New York: W. W. Norton.

Falkenstrom, F., Grant, J., Broberg, J., & Sandell, R. (2007). Self-analysis and post-termination improvement after psychoanalysis and long-term psychotherapy. *Journal of American Psychoanalysis Association, 55,* 629–674.

Fenichel, O. (1945). Neurotic acting out. *Psychoanalytic Review. 39,* 197–206.

Ferro, A., & Basile, R. (2004). The psychoanalyst as individual: Self-analysis and gradients of functioning. *Psychoanalytic Quarterly, 73,* 659–682.

Frank, A. F., & Gunderson, J. G. (1990). The role of the therapeutic alliance in the treatment of schizophrenia: Relationship to course and outcome. *Archives of General Psychiatry, 47,* 228–236.

Frayn, D. H. (1992). Assessment factors associated with premature psychotherapy termination. *American Journal of Psychotherapy, 46,* 250–261.

Freeman, J. B., Choate-Summers, M. L., Moore, P. S., Garcia, A. M., Sapyta, J. J., Leonard, H. L. & Franklin, M. E. (2007). Cognitive behavioral treatment for young children with obsessive-compulsive disorder. *Biological Psychiatry, 61,* 337–343.

Freud, S. (1958). The dynamics of transference. In J. Strachey (Ed. and Trans.), *The standard edition of the complete psychological works of Sigmund Freud* (Vol. 12, pp. 97–108). London: Hogarth Press. (Original work published 1910.)

Freud, S. (1959a). Analysis of a phobia in a five-year-old boy. In A. Strachey & J. Strachey (Trans.), *Collected papers* (Vol. 3, pp. 149–289). New York: Basic Books.

Freud, S. (1959b). On psychotherapy. In J. Riviere (Trans.), *Collected papers* (Vol. 1, pp. 249–263). New York: Basic Books.

Giovacchini, P. (1985). Introduction: Countertransference responses to adolescents. In S. Feinstein, M. Sugar, A. Esman, J. Looney, A. Schwartzberg, & A. Sorosky (Eds.), *Adolescent psychiatry, vol. 12: Developmental and clinical studies,* (pp. 447–448). Chicago: University of Chicago Press.

Gordon, S. B., Lerner, L. L., Keefe, F. J. (1979). Responsive parenting: An approach to training parents of problem children. *American Journal of Community Psychology, 7,* 45–56.

Gutheil, T. G., & Gabbard, G. O. (1998). Misuses and misunderstandings of boundary theory in clinical and regulatory settings. *American Journal of Psychiatry, 155,* 409–414.

Heimann, P. (1950). On countertransference. *International Journal of Psycho-Analysis, 31,* 81–84.

Hunkeler, E. M., Katon, W., Tang, L., Williams, J. W. Jr, Kroenke, K., Lin, E. H. B., et al. (2006). Long- term outcomes from the IMPACT randomized trial for depressed elderly patients in primary care. *British Medical Journal,* doi:10.1136/bmj.38683.710225.BE (Online).

Johnston, N. E. (1990). Cognitive therapy. In A. Baumann, N. E. Johnston, & D. Antai-Otong (Eds.), *Decision-making in psychiatric and psychosocial nursing* (pp. 108–109). Philadelphia: B. C. Decker.

Jones, M. C. (1924). Elimination of children's fears. *Journal of Experimental Psychology, 7,* 382–390.

Kaas, M. J., Dehn, D., Dahl, D., Frank, K., Markley, J., & Hebert, P. (2000). A view of prescriptive practice collaboration: Perspectives of psychiatric-mental health clinical nurse specialists and psychiatrists. *Archives of Psychiatric Nurses, 14,* 222–234.

Kanner, L. (1955). *Child psychiatry* (3rd ed.). Springfield, IL: Charles C Thomas.

Karasu, T. B. (1990). Toward a clinical model of psychotherapy for depression I: Systematic comparison of three psychotherapies. *American Journal of Psychiatry, 147,* 133–147.

Kernberg, O. F. (1984). *Severe personality disorders.* New Haven, CT: Yale University Press.

Kessler, J. (1966). *Psychopathology of childhood.* Englewood Cliffs, NJ: Prentice-Hall.

Klerman, G. L., Weissman, M. M., Rounsaville, B. J., & Chevron, E. S. (1984). *Interpersonal psychotherapy for depression.* New York: Basic Books.

Lauro, L., Bass, A., Goldsmith, L. A., Kaplan, J. A., Katz, G., & Schaye, S. H. (2003). Psychoanalytic supervision of the difficult patient. *Psychoanalytic Quarterly, 72,* 403–438.

Lego, S. (1997). Point of view: Top ten reasons why psychiatric nurses are a great resource. *Journal of the American Psychiatric Nurses Association, 3,* 191–195.

Linehan, M. M. (1999). *Understanding borderline personality disorder: The dialectical approach.* New York: Guilford.

Linehan, M. M., Heard, H. L., & Armstrong, H. E. (1993). Naturalistic follow-up of a behavioral treatment for chronically parasuicidal borderline patients. *Archives of General Psychiatry, 50,* 971–974.

Mallinckrodt, B. (1992). Childhood emotional bonds with parents, development of adult social competencies, and availability of social support. *Journal of Counseling Psychology, 39,* 453–461.

Mellow, J. (1967). Evolution of nursing through research. *Psychiatric Opinion, 4,* 15–21.

Millon, T. (1969). *Modern psychopathology.* Philadelphia: W. B. Saunders.

Mishne, J. M. (1986). *Clinical work with adolescents.* New York: The Free Press.

Norcross, J. C. (1991). Prescriptive matching in psychotherapy. An introduction. *Psychotherapy, 28,* 439–443.

Patience, D. A., McGuire, R. J., Scott, A. I., & Freeman, C. P. (1995). The Edinburgh primary care depression study: Personality disorders and outcome. *British Journal of Psychiatry, 167,* 324–330.

Peplau, H. E. (1968). Psychotherapeutic strategies. *Perspectives in Psychiatric Care, 6,* 264–289.

Persons, J. B. (1998). Indications for psychotherapy in the treatment of depression. *Psychiatric Annals, 28,* 80–83.

Piaget, J. (1969). The intellectual development of the adolescent. In G. Caplan & S. Levovici (Eds.), *Adolescence: Psychosocial perspective* (pp. 22–26). New York: Basic Books.

Piper, W. E., Azim, H. F., Joyce, A. S., & McCallum, M. (1991). Transference interpretation, therapeutic alliance, and outcome in short-term individual psychotherapy. *Archives of General Psychiatry, 48,* 946–953.

Reasor, J. E., & Farrell, S. P. (2005). The effectiveness of advanced practice registered nurses as psychotherapists. *Archives of Psychiatric Nursing, 19,* 81–92.

Reynolds, C. F. III, Dew, M. A., Pollock, B. G., Mulsant, B. H., Frank, E., Miller, M. D., et al. (2006). Maintenance treatment of major depression in old age. *New England Journal of Medicine, 354,* 1130–1138.

Roberts, R. E., Attkisson, C., & Rosenblatt, A. (1998). Prevalence of psychopathology among children and adolescents. *American Journal of Psychiatry, 155,* 715–725.

Rogers, C. R. (1942). *Counseling and psychotherapy.* Boston: Houghton Mifflin.

Ronen, T., & Abraham, Y. (1996). Retention control training in the treatment of younger versus older enuretic children. *Nursing Research, 45,* 78–92.

Rosenbaum, M., & Ronen, T. (1997). Parents and children's appraisals of each other's anxiety while facing a common threat. *Journal of Clinical Child Psychology, 26,* 43–52.

Sandler, J., Kennedy, H., & Tyson, P. L. (1980). *The technique of child psychoanalysis: Discussion with Anna Freud.* Cambridge, MA: Harvard University Press.

Satcher, D. (2000). *Mental health: A report of the surgeon general.* Rockville, MD: U.S. Department of Health and Human Services.

Scahill, L. (2001). Surgeon general's conference on children's mental health: Developing a national action agenda. *Journal of the American Psychiatric Nurses Association, 7,* 51–56.

Searles, H. F. (1986). *My work with borderline patients.* London: Jason Aronson.

Seeman, J. A., Barry, E., & Ellinwood, C. (1964). Interpersonal assessment of play therapy outcome. *Psychotherapy Theory, Research, and Practice, 1,* 64–66.

Simon, J. (1988). Criteria for therapist self-disclosure. *American Journal of Psychotherapy, 43,* 404–415.

Singer, R. (1970). *Key concepts in psychotherapy.* New York: Basic Books.

Stevenson, J., & Meares, R. (1992). An outcome study of psychotherapy for patients with borderline personality disorder. *American Journal of Psychiatry, 149,* 358–362.

Tarasoff v Regents of the University of California. (1976). 17 Cal 3d 425, 131; Cal Reporter 14, 551 P 2d.

Teri, L., & Logsdon, R. C. (1992). The future of psychotherapy with older adults. *Psychotherapy, 29,* 81–87.

Townsend, M. (2005). Interprofessional supervision from the perspectives of both mental health nurses and other professionals in the field of cognitive behavioural psychotherapy. *Journal of Psychiatric Mental Health Nursing, 12,* 582–588.

Truax, C. B. (1963). Effective ingredients in psychotherapy: An approach to unraveling the patient-therapist interactions. *Journal of Clinical Psychology, 10,* 256–263.

U. S. Census Bureau. (2000). *Census 200 redistricting (Pub. L. No. 94–171) Summary File, table PL I.* Washington, DC: U. S. Government Printing Office.

Watson, J. B., & Rayner, R. (1920). Conditioned emotional reactions. *Journal of Experimental Psychology, 3,* 1–4

Wolpe J. (1958). *Psychotherapy by reciprocal inhibition.* Stanford, CA: Stanford University Press.

Wolpe, J. (1973). *The practice of behavior therapy* (2nd ed.). New York: Pergamon Press.

SUGGESTED READINGS

Antai-Otong, D. (2000). Continued professional development. In C. A. Shea, L. R. Pelletier, E. C. Poster, G. S.

Stuart, & M. P. Verhey (Eds.), *Advanced practice nursing in psychiatric-mental health care* (pp. 467–480). St. Louis, MO: Mosby.

Basch, M. F. (1980). *Doing psychotherapy.* New York: Basic Books.

Mirkin, M. P., Suyemoto, K. L., & Okun, B. F. (2005). *Psychotherapy with women.* New York: Guilford Publications, Inc.

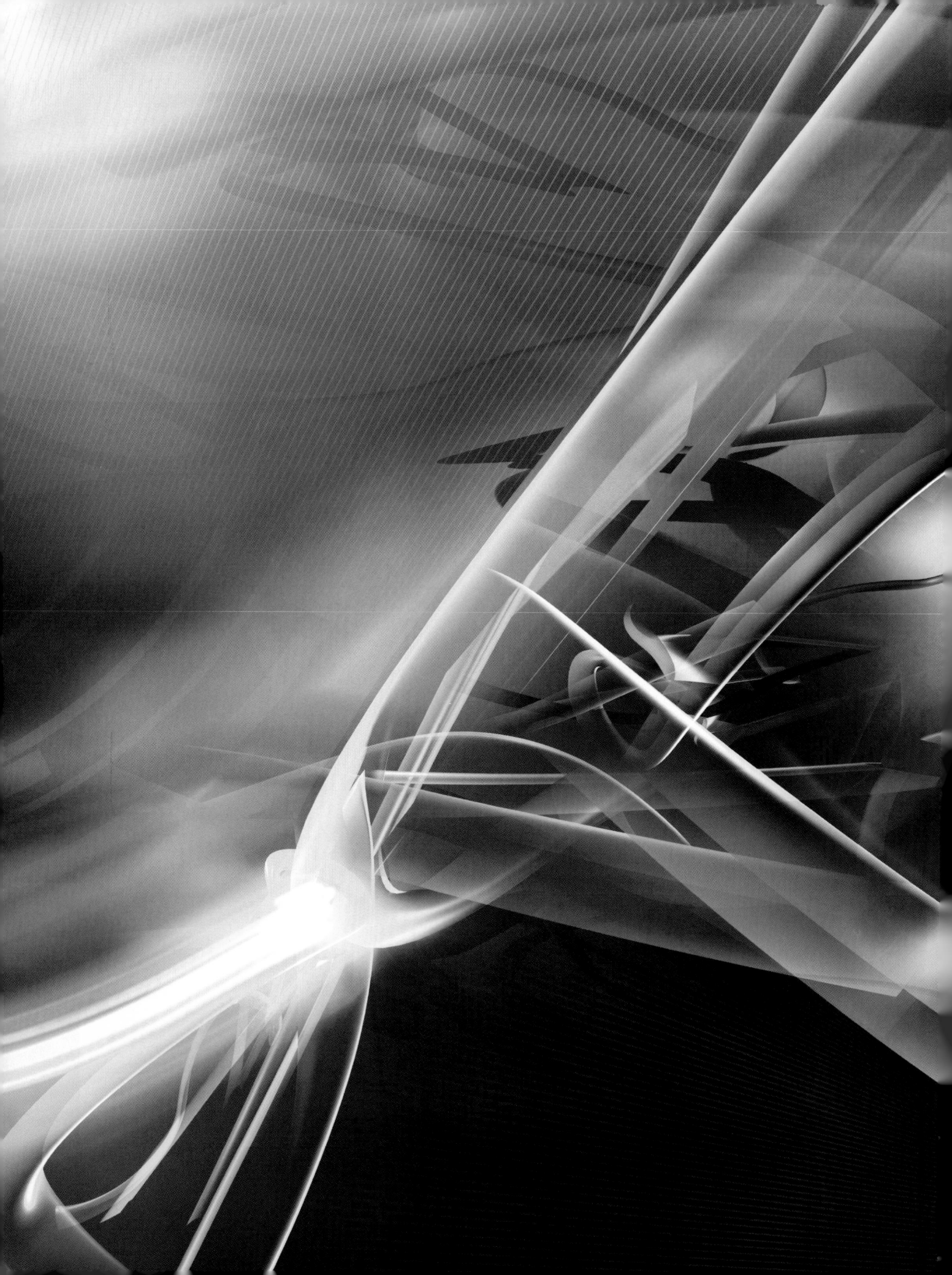

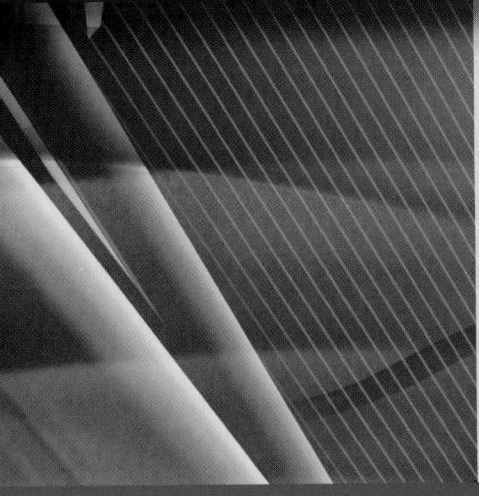

CHAPTER 27

Group Therapy

Martha Buffum, DNSc, APRN, BC, CS

Erika Madrid, DNSc, RN, CS

KEY TERMS

Behavioral/Cognitive Model: Combines behavioral and cognitive therapies. That is, the behavioral model focuses on behaviors that present in the here and now, identification of maladaptive behaviors that will become targets for change, motivation for the behaviors, and reinforcers of the behaviors.

Communication/Systems Model: Communication theory applied to group therapy that considers both the content of messages of the group members and the method of transmission of these messages. The systems model aspect of this type of group considers subgroups, boundaries, and communication within and between these groups in relation to the whole group.

Content Analysis: The evaluation of themes and specifics about what was said during the group therapy session. Examples of content themes are sadness, loneliness, leisure time activities, and relationship issues.

Existential/Gestalt Model: Facilitates people's self-actualization processes by helping them become more aware of their full potential, their alternatives or choices, and their feelings and emotions. The primary goal in this model is to help individual members take responsibility for their emotions and behaviors through the process of support and feedback.

Group Therapy: In mental health, a modality of treatment for more than one person that provides therapeutic outcomes for each individual.

Insight-Oriented or Process-Oriented Groups: For individuals with high levels of cognitive functioning. Insight-oriented

groups focus on the development of intellectual awareness, thinking patterns, and emotional factors influencing behavior.

Process: Refers to the manner in which clients talk about themselves and the way the group responds. Analysis of group process provides assessment of the therapy's effects on individual group members.

Psychodynamic Model: A model of group therapy in which the problems of the members of a group are viewed as similar to the problems a person would present in individual therapy. That is, the problems of the people in the group are conceptualized to center on unconscious conflicts and basic love-hate instincts (constructive versus destructive forces). Freudian theory of psychoanalysis is the underlying foundation for psychodynamic therapy.

Psychoeducational Group: Group that offers information to a large number of people simultaneously, providing both information and emotional support. Persons who are motivated to learn about their illness or to develop self-awareness benefit from this type of group.

Therapeutic Factors: The standards for the conduct of group therapy. They include the following: imparting of information, instillation of hope, universality, altruism, corrective recapitulation of the primary family group member, development of socializing skills, imitative behavior, interpersonal learning, group cohesiveness, catharsis, and existential factors.

COMPETENCIES

Upon completion of this chapter, the learner should be able to:

1. Define major components of group therapy.

2. Explain the contributions of various group therapists, such as Pratt, Metzel, Adler, Moreno, and Slavson, to group therapy.

3. Discuss Yalom's therapeutic factors.

4. Describe the different theoretical models of group therapy.

5. Explain the differences between group process and content.

6. Identify the function of the psychiatric-mental health nurse in the role of group leader, therapist, and cotherapist.

7. Describe the psychiatric-mental health nurse's involvement on an assigned psychiatric unit and in the community.

8. Describe issues that are the focus of groups for specific populations such as children, adolescents, psychiatric clients, medically ill persons, and older adults.

9. Formulate outcome measures for evaluating the effectiveness of groups.

A **group is two** or more people who are together for a purpose or a common reason (Crenshaw, 1989). Therapy is a treatment used for its beneficial effects. In mental health, group therapy is a modality of treatment for more than one person that provides therapeutic outcomes for each individual. This chapter discusses the history of group therapy and its evolution in the psychiatric-mental health arena, the theoretical foundations on which group therapy is based, the specific role of the psychiatric nurse in group therapy, the application of the nursing process to group therapy, types of groups relevant to particular people and needs, and current trends in research on group therapy.

HISTORICAL PERSPECTIVES

There is disagreement about the exact origins of group therapy (Dreikurs, 1959; Mullan & Rosenbaum, 1967). Although therapeutic group interaction may have occurred throughout the world, such as in Greek drama, medieval plays, and Franz Mesmer's hypnotic institute, no documentation acknowledged the beneficial effects or therapeutic intentions of such interactions. Modern group therapy has been documented as beginning in 1905 with Joseph Hersey Pratt, a Boston internist (Mullan & Rosenbaum, 1967). See Table 27–1 for a summary of researchers' contributions.

TUBERCULOSIS AND THE HOME SANATORIUM (EARLY 1900s)

Pratt worked with clients with tuberculosis who were living at home. He recognized the social as well as physical elements of the disease, noting that the clients felt discouraged about their plight. His treatment regimen involved weekly meetings of a small class of 15 to 20 clients. All of the members of the class had tuberculosis, were poor, and were from varied racial and religious backgrounds. Selection for the class depended on a client's and her family's willingness to follow strict guidelines regarding the need for open air, no work, a particular diet, rest, and hygiene. All levels of illness were included. The class meetings continued over 1 year.

Pratt lectured at each class about the care and treatment of tuberculosis. He had each client keep a record book in which she documented the details of her life, including daily temperature, diet, and rest periods. Pratt noted the camaraderie that developed. The clients did not talk about their symptoms. They were supportive and encouraging, as was Pratt. Symptom improvement was more encouraging than in the tuberculosis sanatoriums.

Part of Pratt's treatment regimen included nurse visits to clients' homes. These additional acts of caring and reinforcement of education most likely contributed to clients' feelings about themselves, their illness, and their membership in the class. Pratt's (1906) philosophy was that his clients improved because a large amount of care was given to a small number

of clients. His work continued, evolving in the area of emotional reeducation on the basis of the philosophy that group therapy has a beneficial effect because of the interpersonal dynamics involved and group members' influence on each other.

ALCOHOL TREATMENT (1920s)

Dr. Julius Metzl, a police physician in Vienna, developed a method of group counseling for persons with alcoholism. Metzl's groups involved persons who had undergone individual counseling, who acknowledged their alcoholism, who were accepted into the group by fellow members, and who were from the same socioeconomic level. Some of the principles he used were later adopted by Alcoholics Anonymous. His work was published in an obscure journal on alcoholism in 1927 and later by a colleague, Rudolf Dreikurs, in 1928 in a psychiatric journal. At that time, persons with alcoholism were considered psychiatric clients. Metzl's work pioneered a systematic approach to the group treatment of psychiatric clients (Dreikurs, 1959).

Metzl's work also pioneered the distinction between individual and group or collective counseling (Dreikurs, 1959). With these clients, group methods appeared to be more successful than individual counseling. In individual counseling, limited time was allowed per person, and only one counselor shared observations with the client. The counselor's intellectual ability was assumed to be a powerful force against one individual's reasoning. In contrast, group or collective counseling afforded the group the benefit of any one individual's confrontation by the counselor or any group member. The group approach offered a forum in which the achievement of sobriety could be displayed, the belief that one could accomplish what another did was generated, and members were convinced that successful sobriety was possible. The power of suggestion, then, was a force that each member could bring to the group, and each member was influential. In the alcoholic groups, all members were expected to participate, and all members voluntarily promised after their first session not to drink for 1 week.

COLLECTIVE COUNSELING AND GROUP PSYCHOTHERAPY (1920s AND 1930s)

The term *collective counseling* was established in Vienna by Adler and his coworkers in 1921 at the Counseling Center for Parents and Children (Dreikurs, 1959). Psychiatric thinking in the Adlerian sense included the group as a natural setting. That is, the whole family was in treatment when a child was emotionally disturbed.

PSYCHODRAMA (1930s)

Jacob Moreno claimed that he used group therapy in Vienna as early as 1910, and in 1932 he presented his findings to the

TABLE 27-1
Summary of Researchers' Contributions

Researcher	Time Period	Focus of Group Work	Description of Group	Treatment	Contributions
Pratt	1900s	Tuberculosis (TB) and the home sanatorium	15–20 poor clients representing a variety of racial and religious backgrounds	Education on care and treatment of TB. Each client kept a record of temperature, diet, rest, etc. Nurse visited clients' homes.	Noted camaraderie, support, and encouragement among clients. Symptom improvement was greater than in sanatorium.
Metzl	1920s	Treatment for alcoholism	Clients had individual counseling, acknowledged their alcoholism, and were of the same socioeconomic background	Group members used power of suggestion that sobriety was possible. Members promised not to drink for 1 week.	Pioneered systematic approach to group treatment of psychiatric clients and made distinction between individual and group counseling.
Moreno	1930s	Psychodrama	Clients were actors and audience, therapist was a director, and staff served as auxiliary egos.	Client acted the role emphasizing the problem and the rest of the group provided the sounding board of public opinion.	Coined terms *group psychotherapy* and *group therapy*. Established connection between group therapy and psychiatry.

American Psychiatric Association. This presentation may have established the connection between group therapy or group psychotherapy and psychiatry.

Moreno came to the United States in 1925, and he is credited with coining the terms *group psychotherapy* and *group therapy*. Moreno's specific method of therapy was known as psychodrama—the exploration of the truth through dramatic means. The five instruments used in the group setting included the following (Moreno, 1946):

1. The stage, which gave the client the opportunity of expression

2. The subject or client, who enacted a role emphasizing a past or present problem

3. The director, who was the therapist and producer of the drama

4. The staff of therapeutic aides (auxiliary egos), who were responsive to the producer and acted as real or imagined persons in the client's life

5. The rest of the group, who acted as an audience and sounding board of public opinion

For further discussion of psychodrama, see the Psychodrama and Role-Playing Techniques section.

Moreno's contributions also included the publishing of the first journal devoted to group therapy, *Impromptu*. For 18 years, he edited *Sociometry*, which he founded in 1937. In 1944, he turned this journal over to the American Sociological Association, which devoted it to social psychology. In 1947, Moreno founded the publication *Sociatry*, the name of which he later changed to *Group Psychotherapy*.

Other individuals were applying group methods to specific populations during the 1930s. Samuel Slavson, originally an engineer, began an activity group therapy at the Jewish Board of Guardians. This type of therapy combined group work, education, and psychological analysis. He emphasized the use of the group setting for the acting out of impulses, conflicts, and behavior patterns. Primarily, the activity group therapy was for children from 8 to 15 years. He practiced this therapy for 9 years, presenting it in 1943 and calling it *situational therapy* (Mullan & Rosenbaum, 1967). This was the forerunner of children's group play therapy.

INFLUENCE OF COMMUNICATION BEFORE WORLD WAR II

In contrast to the United States, many physicians in Europe in the early 1900s did not present or publish their experiences with groups. Freud was interested in the group mind and the influence of the group on the individual, but he did not work with groups. The field of psychiatry was new and busy defining itself. Thus internists' work in the area of group therapy methods went unnoticed by psychiatrists. To the Adlerian psychologists, use of group methods with families was part of individual counseling and went undocumented. According to Dreikurs (1959), German, Austrian, Russian, and Danish psychotherapists had been using group methods before 1930. All public forms of group therapy ceased during the period of fascism in Austria between 1927 and 1934 (Dreikurs, 1959). Furthermore, the lives and work of Metzl and other pioneers in group therapy became obscured by the Holocaust.

AFTER WORLD WAR II (1940s TO 1960s)

There was much growth in the use of group therapy at the end of World War II because there was a shortage of trained personnel and many clients needed treatment. New methods that required briefer treatment periods were explored. Group therapies now included support, education, inspiration, emotional expression, and reconstruction.

Therapy groups began to be observed for research in the 1950s (Whitaker & Lieberman, 1969). These included psychiatric clients at the Veterans Administration Hospital in Chicago and the Department of Psychiatry at the University of Chicago. Different therapeutic approaches and styles were observed in short-term groups of hospitalized veterans who suffered from acute states of anxiety or severe character pathology.

Interest in the group method extended beyond therapy and problem-oriented work during the 1950s. An understanding of group dynamics was an objective of the training of group therapists. The T-group, or basic skills training group, was specifically designed for the experience of being in a group, understanding the group process, studying leadership style, and examining group functions for efficient problem solving. The first T-groups met in Bethel, Maine, in 1948 and 1949 (Goldberg, 1970). Feedback and training for leadership in human relations were part of the education of the participants, who included businesspersons, community workers, and members of the armed forces (Bradford, Gibb, & Benne, 1964). The groups were so successful in training and educating therapists in group dynamics and interpersonal communication that the National Training Laboratories was established in 1950 within the National Education Association (Yalom, 1985). T-groups led to a desire for intensity of interpersonal interactions, which led to therapy groups for the general population in the form of encounter groups and marathons.

Encounter groups and *intensive T-groups*, were studied in college students. Results of studies of 12-week encounter groups in college students demonstrated some change in most participants; specifically, some were able to maintain a positive change, and some suffered from negative sequelae (Yalom, 1995). Different groups had different experiences, and the role of the leader emerged as a vital element influencing individuals' outcomes. Although generalizations to the general population could not be made from these studies, these investigations helped develop leadership styles for improving the evolving group therapy movement. That is, the most successful leaders of these groups provided emotional stimulation, established limits and rules, were empathetic and caring, and offered clarification and explanations for translating feelings into ideas (Yalom, 1995).

According to Fromm (1957), humans exist in a social context and need to feel related to fellow humans. Furthermore, he asserted that people have a strong need to know themselves and other humans. This philosophy was the basis of the approach in the innovative groups of the 1950s and 1960s, which were developed in a sensitivity-group movement that occurred throughout the United States. Encounter groups provided a type of therapy to the interested population at large. For example, the Esalen Institute in California, founded on Perls's (1969) gestalt psychology, devoted itself to group training and group workshops wherein the marathon group was practiced.

The power of group suggestion is strong. The Synanon community, originally a residential treatment program designed for persons addicted to drugs, opened to growth movement individuals who believed in group process. All aspects of life were managed communally, with decisions made by group process. Members learned genuine assertion of expression and recognition that the group's power was greater than that of any individual.

FAR EAST WAR EXPERIENCES AND BEYOND (1970s TO PRESENT)

Postwar traumas have emerged in soldiers who had been prisoners of war during World War II, the Korean War, the Vietnam War, the Gulf War in the 1990s, and Afganistan and the war in Iraq in the 2000s. *Post-traumatic stress disorder* (PTSD) became an evermore frequently used term in the 1980s, when veterans began revealing the devastation of their lives owing to the reliving of trauma and the extreme difficulty they have had adjusting to civilian life. The Veterans Health Administration has attended to veterans' needs for PTSD treatment through group therapy and group psychoeducational methods (Britvić,

Radelić, & Urlić, 2006; Kingsley, 2007; Ljubotina, Pantić, Franciskovié, Mladić, & Priebe, 2007). These groups address issues such as anger management, coping strategies, stress reduction, interpersonal communication, support, and childhood trauma. From successes with veterans, other types of PTSD groups have been described for civilian prisoners of war, older veterans, and partners of combat veterans (Britvić, et al., 2006; Kingsley, 2007; Ljubotina et al., 2007).

PTSD group therapy treatment in the 1990s has expanded to other trauma victims (Amir, Weil, Kaplan, Tocker, & Witztum, 1998). Psychotherapeutic modalities for PTSD occur in individual and group settings and include behavioral, cognitive, and psychodynamic approaches (Sherman, 1998). Cognitive-behavioral group therapies for PTSD have been used for various traumas and concomitant psychiatric illness in groups of women, children, and adolescents (Lau & Kristensen, 2007; Stacciarini, O' Keefe, & Mathews, 2007; Storch, Geffken, et al., 2007).

During this same period, group therapy approaches also were used in drug and alcohol treatment programs as well as in behavioral medicine treatment approaches. The 1980s brought a greater focus on the integration of the mind-body approaches to health and wellness and the use of group approaches to dealing with the psychological aspects of physical diseases, both in prevention and treatment. With this change, behavioral medicine established itself as a legitimate component of overall medical care. Behavioral medicine addresses the psychological factors of illness and seeks to complement the medical model and help the person cope. Its preventive focus emphasizes health-promoting benefits of stress management and pain control measures to help prevent the onset of illness.

ISSUES FROM 1990 TO 2000: HEALTH CARE REFORM, MANAGED CARE

The 1990s in the United States was the era of health care reform because of the rising costs of health care and the inability of the political structure to enact any form of national health insurance or health care reform. Managed care, with it usual capitation system that determines in advance the cost of health care, has provided a means for cost containment. It has all but replaced the old fee-for-service system that existed in both medical and psychiatric treatment. Managed care and economic-market-driven forces have a greater influence than ever on how health care is delivered and by whom. Mental health services have not been immune to this trend. Mental health managed care plans that were in existence have expanded, and group therapy approaches have become more popular because they are seen as being able to effectively and efficiently treat individuals for a wide range of mental health disorders (Chou, Wallace, Bloom, & Hu, 2005).

ISSUES EMERGING IN THE TWENTY-FIRST CENTURY: DISASTER RESPONSE

The events of September 11, 2001 brought the United States into an era involving fear of terrorism, grief over substantial loss of life, anger at being attacked and vulnerable, and preparation for disasters and crises on a global scale. Both professional and volunteer responders to traumatic and horrifying events have advocated and trained for rapid mental health responsiveness. For example, the critical incident stress debriefing (CISD) method has been frequently utilized with trauma victims and their rescuers in varying settings and circumstances. This technique involves a structured interactive approach enabling brief discussion about a critical incident—any type of event that triggers unusually strong feelings in the afflicted individuals—designed to respond to severe psychological trauma within hours after a traumatic event. CISD is crisis-oriented and is not a replacement for professional psychotherapy. Many public health, fire, police, and airline agencies have employee training programs for CISD so that they can respond to emergencies (Miller, 2006). Interventions can include any number of sessions with an individual or groups. Some researchers report minimal or even negative effectiveness in reducing risk or improving recovery from PTSD (Jacobs, Horne-Moyer, & Jones, 2004; Wagner, 2005). Others support the use of CISD as a valid and beneficial rapid emergency response to urgent human needs (Riddell & Clouse, 2004). Some see it as psychological first aid, others see the technique as helpful for an entire community that shares the trauma (Macy, Behar, Paulson, Delman, Schmid, & Smith, 2004). Still other recent findings about PTSD risk reduction suggest better CISD effectiveness with the rescuers (secondary victims of trauma) than with the actual victims of trauma (Jacobs et al., 2004).

In addition to disaster response, other disorders received renewed attention and more innovative approaches. Borderline personality disorders, which in the past had not been amenable to most group techniques, are now responding favorably to Dialectical Behavior Therapy (DBT). DBT is an approach that has a group as well as individual component and is based on behaviorist and cognitive theory. The group therapy part consists of weekly meetings and focuses on four modules of skill building; core mindfulness, emotion regulation, interpersonal effectiveness, and distress tolerance skills (Linehan, 1993).

Despite these innovations, the United States health care system in the new millennium faces many challenges that impact group and other psychological therapies. An increasingly inadequate and dysfunctional United States health care system and rising health care costs have resulted in a 15 to 20 percent rate of uninsured persons without medical or psychiatric coverage (Sullivan, 2000). According to a recent press release by the Census Bureau (2007), it has revised estimates of the number of uninsured people for 2004 and 2005. The number and percentage of people who were uninsured in 2005 changed from 46.6 million (15.9 percent of the population) to 44.8 million (15.3 percent) (Lu, 2007). The strained rising costs and governmental programs have not filled the gap. As a result, support groups addressing the management of chronic diseases have become more important as patients take more control of their health. Medical treatments, especially for chronic disorders, are frequently augmented by support group participation. These groups have improved clients' coping strategies and outcomes of treatment (Lipscomb & Snyder, 2002; Till, 2003). Additionally, information technology and the use of the Internet have created a more knowledgeable consumer of the limited health care resources.

Unfortunately chronic mental illness, addictive disorders/substance dependence, and associated homelessness continue to be problematic especially in United States urban areas (Crane, 2007; Schmidt et al., 2007). Although approaches to successfully treat these problems are available, the commitment to allocate the needed resources has not materialized. Dwindling financial resources at the federal, state, and local level brought about by tax cuts and the costs of military actions in the Middle East and elsewhere compound the situation and offer little hope of improvement in the near future.

CULTURAL CONSIDERATIONS

Cultural sensitive health care became more evident in the mental health field in the United States starting in the 1990s. Because of the growing and changing demographics occurring in the United States, mental health services have begun identifying and formulating culturally sensitive mental health care. Some of the issues that relate to providing effective group therapy services to different ethnic and racial groups involve the goals of the group therapy, the types of therapists leading the groups, and the advantages of heterogeneous groups and homogeneous groups (Verkuyten, 2005; White, Gibbons, & Schamberger, 2006). These issues are addressed next.

IMPACT AND INFLUENCES OF DIVERSITY ON GROUP THERAPY

With the growing diverse populations in the United States, nursing competency in cultural sensitivity is essential. The two major goals of group therapy that are especially important in the treatment of minorities and interracial groups are:

1. Increasing the capacity of the individual member to relate to the group

2. Fostering authenticity, autonomy, and the ability to resist group pressures in the group members

These goals help the individual and society in general because they address the fundamental issues of acculturation and integration into American society that many racial and ethnic minorities face.

Another crucial aspect of the success of group treatment with ethnically diverse clientele involves the characteristics of the therapist. Although bilingual, bicultural therapists are frequently preferred, the nurse therapist, to be effective, does not have to be of the same ethnic or racial group as the clients. The nurse therapist does have to be culturally competent, however, and able to avoid the problems of stereotyping and counter-transference. Self-awareness is a crucial part of providing culturally competent mental health care. Nurses need to recognize their values, beliefs, and own culture and their potential impact on interpreting the client's symptoms, diagnosing, and formulating a treatment plan.

As to whether to use heterogeneous or homogeneous groups with culturally diverse clients, this would depend on how much acculturation exists in the individual group members from the minority group. Heterogeneous groups are preferred because they are richer in context and accomplish the acculturation goals. However, they only work where different ethnic groups have ongoing contact in school, work, and socially rather than in parallel societies. Homogeneous groups are preferred when the minority members are not acculturated or when strong religious, sociocultural, or political views necessitate it.

Gender issues also continue to be addressed. Specifically, the feminist perspective in interpersonal group therapy provides an opportunity for women to look at their interpersonal problems in a sociopolitical context. The group as social microcosm with its here and now focus assists participants in keeping their experiences within context, which is a less self-blaming approach. This approach helps women to confront gender-specific injustice and inequity and formulate new relationships with others that are healthier and less deferential (Rogers, 2006).

THERAPEUTIC FACTORS OF GROUP THERAPY

All therapy groups are designed to benefit the members. Insight-oriented or process-oriented therapy groups are for individuals with high levels of cognitive functioning. Insight-oriented groups focus on the development of intellectual awareness, thinking patterns, and emotional factors influencing behavior. Process-oriented groups focus on developing individuals' awareness of the patterns of behaviors and interactions occurring within the group. Yalom (1985, 1995) proposed 11 therapeutic factors of insight-oriented or process-oriented group therapy, which are presented in Table 27–2. They can also be applied to education, activity, and task groups, which may be more beneficial for people with cognitive impairments. However, because no two individuals view one event in the same manner, these

---

TABLE 27–2
Yalom's Therapeutic Factors for Group Therapy

- Imparting of Information. Information is presented through lecture or teaching aids, or information is shared among members.

- Instillation of hope. The therapist and group have the attitude that the client will get better and that the treatment modality is beneficial.

- Universality. Problems, thoughts, feelings are shared by other group members—no one is alone or isolated with one's own issues.

- Altruism. Each group member gives to another within the group; this process is therapeutic and increases the giver's self-esteem.

- Corrective recapitulation of the primary family group member. The members' responses are influenced by past family experiences. Members gain insight into their behavior when they learn that their reactions to others are similar to their reactions to their own family members.

- Development of socializing techniques. By accepting feedback about their interpersonal communication and behavior, members become more socially skillful in relationships.

- Imitative behavior. Growth is demonstrated when the client identifies with other members. Imitating the healthy aspects of other members of the group.

- Interpersonal learning. Interpersonal learning results from feedback from others and insight into oneself. This learning is transferable to other situations, enabling clients to assert themselves, trust others, test reality, give to others, and expect caring from others.

- Group cohesiveness. There is a feeling of connectedness among group members. Cohesiveness is demonstrated when positive as well as negative feedback can be given in an atmosphere of acceptance without group disintegration.

- Catharsis. Clients express their deeply felt emotions.

- Existential factors. Clients realize that loneliness, death, and the meaning of existence are issues for all men and women; that there is a limit to how much control humans have over these issues; and that there is universal learning about human existence.

Note. Data from *The Theory and Practice of Group Psychotherapy* (4th ed.), by I. Yalom, 1995, New York: Basic Books. Adapted with permission.

---

therapeutic factors may not be of equal value to all participants of all groups. Each person has unique needs, wants, and life experiences. The therapeutic benefits of group participation vary with participants' perceptions, levels of functioning, degree of experience with groups, insights into problems, duration of psychological treatment, and relationships with others in the group. According to Yalom (1985, 1995), any group experience offers potential benefit or harm or may be important or meaningless. Nurses need to be comfortable using this powerful modality when working with clients.

ADVANTAGES AND DISADVANTAGES OF GROUP THERAPY

The advantages of group therapy are based on the purpose of the group and the motivation of the participants. For example, a psychoeducational group that provides information and emotional support can benefit families of persons with Alzheimer's disease. They are eager to learn and are experiencing problems that others in the group face. An inspirational group, such as Alcoholics Anonymous, is a similar type of group because it helps those afflicted learn from others in a safe setting. Both types of groups can be effective with large groups (from 20 to 50 persons or more). Usually, the members of such groups are motivated to learn, to participate, and to help others in the process of helping themselves.

Group therapies offer people a chance to help each other (altruism), to feel less alone in the world, to learn about themselves and other people, to practice new behaviors, to practice problem-solving skills to improve communication, and to foster better relationships. In an atmosphere of mutual helping, self-esteem is enhanced as a result of feeling important and worthwhile. Persons in group therapy can feel strengthened and hopeful from the process of sharing, from feeling accepted and supported, and through helping others.

A major disadvantage is that a participant's individual needs may not be addressed to her satisfaction. Attention to individual problems is not the focus of group therapy as it is in individual therapy. Persons who need more attention from the therapist may feel frustrated with feedback only from peers. Also, each person's problems may not get addressed in every session. A person may get overlooked for many sessions in a group environment. Talkative members may monopolize the group meetings, and shy persons may not know how to interject their concerns. A person's needs may be incongruent with those of other group members, so there may not be "goodness of fit" for every member in the group. The therapist's style and skills need to blend with the purpose of the group, the experiences and needs of the members, and the personalities of the individuals.

TYPES OF CLIENTS APPROPRIATE FOR GROUP THERAPY

Not all individuals profit from group therapy. That is, persons undergoing an acute psychotic episode, an acute manic phase of bipolar illness, or confusion related to dementia are examples of persons who could probably not participate productively in an insight-oriented group. Moreover, during these acute phases of illness, these persons would be disruptive to a group session focused on verbal expression. For these individuals, exercise or task-centered groups are more useful, helping them discharge energy and focus attention on physical activities. The nurse should consider influential factors when determining appropriateness for groups such as psychosis, medication, and cultural (ethnic or religious) needs.

Clients with psychotic disorders can participate in some groups once their thoughts are cleared, verbalizations are mostly coherent, and perceptual distortions are diminished. Usually, regulation on antipsychotic medication facilitates such improvement. Some clinicians report that medication interferes with expression of feelings because of sedation. It is unclear whether the newer, less-sedating antipsychotics result in clients' increased alertness for participating in groups. The nurse needs to remember that even if the client is sedated, involvement in interaction can be beneficial. As a result of medication, clients can attend group therapy and often stay for the entire session. Furthermore, the group method offers an opportunity to conduct medication teaching, which is definitely in the nursing domain. The challenging issue is timing—the client should not be undersedated or oversedated if she is to gain any benefit from the group.

Cultural, racial, and ethnic diversity raises issues in group therapy, as it does in all aspects of health care. That is, group leaders must be attentive to the potential vulnerabilities, interpretations, sensitivities, and feelings of isolation associated with being from a minority in a group composed of a recognized majority. Likewise, gender minorities can feel similarly in groups. People of diverse cultures and ethnicities may benefit from group psychotherapy, depending on the interaction of multiple factors such as the following: their own personality characteristics; psychopathology; the other group members' personalities, psychopathologies, past experiences; the therapists' style, skill, comfort level with cultural diversity, and ability to create a safe environment. Recent authors emphasize therapist education about cultural differences and the role that culture, ethnicity, or race plays for individuals and groups (Verkuyten, 2005; White, Gibbons, & Schamberger, 2006). Most importantly, group therapists must confront transference and countertransference within the group to work on discrimination and be able to understand clients' issues representing pathology or racial concerns (prejudice or discrimination). Excess focus on racial issues can prevent all members from feeling cohesion, a sense of belonging, and the freedom to self-disclose (Verkuyten, 2005; White, Gibbons, & Schamberger, 2006).

GROUP THERAPY AND PSYCHIATRY

Moreno (1946) first brought group therapy to the attention of psychiatrists. Today, most psychotherapists are trained in group therapy. Psychotherapists' disciplines include psychiatry, psychology, nursing, social work, and marriage and family counselors. The American Group Psychotherapy Association (AGPA) is the organization within psychology that is dedicated exclusively to group therapy. Members of this organization include psychologists, psychiatrists, nurses, social workers, and other mental health professionals.

GROUP THERAPY: THEORIES AND PERSPECTIVES

Theoretical frameworks that are the foundations for group therapy practice are derived from the behavioral sciences of psychology, social psychology, and sociology. These sciences seek to understand individual and group behavior, the two often being quite different. Individuals have been observed to act differently when they are part of a group rather than alone. Different motivations for their behavior are at work when they are part of a group, making it necessary to apply different explanatory theories.

Group theory, in general, focuses on both the treatment of people in groups and on the properties of groups themselves (Corey, 2000). Group behavior theories describe and predict the behavior of members of groups as a function of their being in a group. Group therapy theories prescribe interventions that effect positive change in the group members.

Psychoanalytical theory and group dynamics theory were the main models of group therapy practice 70 years ago, when group therapy began. Currently, there are several group therapy theoretical models (Roller, 2006; Scheidlinger, 2004). The six main theoretical models are the psychodynamic/psychoanalytic model, the interpersonal/interactional model, the communication/systems model, the group process/group analysis model, the existential/gestalt model, and the behavioral and cognitive models.

PSYCHODYNAMIC/PSYCHOANALYTIC MODEL

The psychodynamic model of group therapy has its origins in Freud's psychoanalytical theory of human behavior and shares some of the same basic assumptions as Freudian theory (Rutan, 1992). Psychoanalytical theory assumes the existence of the id (pleasure principle), the superego (internalized parent or conscience), and the ego (reality principle that mediates between the id and the superego) as the psychological determinants of human behavior (Breuer & Freud, 1957). In the psychodynamic model of group therapy, the problems of the members of a group are viewed as similar to the problems a person would present in individual therapy. That is, the problems of the people in the group are conceptualized to center on unconscious conflicts and basic love-hate instincts (constructive versus destructive forces).

The nurse group leader needs to keep in mind a main principle of Freudian theory as applied to group therapy; that is, the existence of unconscious motives, referred to as latent content in groups, underlies group behavior. This implies that the group as a collective body has unconscious fears and desires, as if the group as a whole had a psyche of its own (Rutan, 1992). The unconscious conflicts have meaning to all the members, but they are not fully aware of them. Frequently, the group simultaneously experiences a wish (a disturbing motive) and a fear (a reactive motive).

Whitaker and Lieberman (1969) examined the process of the development of the group unconscious. They used the term *nuclear conflicts* to refer to conflicts from earlier life experiences that individuals bring to and manifest within the group. These nuclear conflicts differ from group focal conflicts, whereby individual and total group concerns become interdependent. Focal conflicts consist of shared desires, fears, and agreed-upon solutions. Both nuclear and focal conflicts are frequently unconscious. The nurse group leader's job is to tailor the group interventions so that the group members become aware of and discuss these unconscious conflicts.

Another important principle of psychoanalytic theory that is applied to group therapy is the symbolic reenactment of the past in present relationships, a phenomenon known as transference. Transference, normally manifested as a distortion of present relationships with others and originates from disturbed early formative relationships (frequently those with parents and siblings), can take various forms, depending on the object of the transference. The clue to the existence of transference is the existence of strong emotions by one member of the group toward another member or the leader of the group. Transference can be successfully examined in the group setting, assisting clients to gain insight into their feelings and behaviors through the process of consensual validation or ongoing agreement and feedback by the other group members. Reenactment provides the opportunity to work through past conflicts.

INTERPERSONAL/INTERACTIONAL MODEL

The interpersonal model of group psychotherapy is similar to the psychodynamic model, but it emphasizes peer interactions and interpersonal learning, rather than insight (Leszcz, 1992). Founded on the theories of Harry Stack Sullivan (1953), the model views clients' current emotions and behaviors as reflecting clients' past relationships with significant others, in particular, parental figures. This transference is evident in the client's one-to-one relationships with other members in the group, the client's relationship to the group as a whole, and the client's relationships in other group settings. Although the group focuses on present relationships, it may replicate family dynamics.

The goal of interpersonal therapy is the reconstruction of the person's personality. Because people have a strong need for interpersonal security, anxiety is viewed as the chief disruptive force in interpersonal relationships. In groups, the members manifest their problems in relating to others, and the leader serves to protect the members from feeling insecure and to boost their self-esteem. Relief from anxiety is found in interactions that increase members' self-respect and self-esteem. Distortions in perceptions of current interpersonal relationships can occur because of earlier experiences. These distortions hinder mutual understanding. In interpersonal therapy groups, learning can occur when the group leader assists the process of consensual validation of group members' feelings, thoughts, behaviors, and interactions with one another.

Transactional analysis, originated by Berne (1961), is theoretically the closest to the interpersonal model. Transactional analysis views the client's interactions with others as being influenced by her adult, parent, and child ego states; these ego states are similar to Freud's ego, superego, and id, respectively (Gladfelter, 1992). Interactions among the group members in transactional analysis groups are analyzed on the basis of the ego states that clients display in their games, scripts, and transactions. Games are interchanges between people that result in bad feelings or blaming others. Scripts are life plans chosen early by the child ego state that may be maladaptive for the adult. Transactions are communicative interchanges between the ego states of two or more persons. People frequently change ego states in their interactions with others. This ability to switch ego states contributes to a healthier adaptation to life, whereas rigidity in maintaining just one ego state can be associated with personality dysfunction.

COMMUNICATION/SYSTEMS MODEL

In the communication/systems model of group therapy, the group is considered as a whole. The group is viewed as more than the sum of its parts or individual members, with boundaries and change mechanisms taking on great importance. Systems theory applied to group therapy focuses on subgroups and boundaries and communications between these subgroups (Azarian, 1992).

Communication theory applied to group therapy considers both the content of messages of the group members and the method of transmission of these messages. Communication is both verbal and nonverbal, and messages can be misinterpreted if they are unclear. Communication contains both manifest elements and latent elements. The manifest elements are in the overt message; they are the feelings, thoughts, and opinions that are in the awareness of the sender. The latent elements are in the covert, or hidden, message and are the feelings and thoughts of which the sender is not aware. Therefore, there can be double message communications. The group leader is responsible for pointing out these double messages when they occur in the group and for teaching members the difference between clear and vague communication. The group leader also functions as a role model of clear and congruent communication. The nurse group leader, being aware of clear communication, will be sure to function as a good role model regardless of the type of group she leads.

Dysfunctional communication, unclear or confusing communication, is a result of not learning to communicate properly or of not taking responsibility for messages being sent (Marram, 1978). In groups, dysfunctional communication usually allows the sender to avoid responsibility for saying what she really wants to say or means. The sender's avoidance of responsibility may manifest as blaming, projection of anger, denial of feelings, withdrawal, or other defensive behaviors. The group leader needs to confront this phenomenon. The timing and the participation of the other group members in this confrontation are important because group members need to feel supported and secure if they are to change their dysfunctional patterns. The leader also models effective communication and works on building group members' self-esteem.

GROUP PROCESS/GROUP ANALYSIS MODEL

Most group practitioners use the group process model, which originated in the 1940s, and its principles along with other individually focused theoretical models, such as the psychodynamic model or the interpersonal model. The group process framework sees groups as being in a constant state of flux, with the goal of the group being to find a state of equilibrium (Cartwright & Zander, 1960). Individual interactions in the group create tensions, and the group as a whole seeks ways to reduce these tensions. Group norms or acceptable ways of acting evolve from interactions between people and crystallize into the group culture.

According to the group process model, groups typically go through the following stages: the introductory phase, the established or working phase, and the termination phase. The main issues groups deal with during all these phases

relate to dependence (the handling and distribution of power) and interdependence (members' feelings about closeness with others). Healthy groups are able to resolve anxieties concerning dependency and interdependency (authority and intimacy issues), whereas unhealthy groups cannot. Successful group leaders are able to mobilize the capacity of the group members to resolve these authority and intimacy issues without conflict. This process happens gradually as trust develops among the group members. If these issues of authority and intimacy are not at least partially resolved, the group is unable to move on to other tasks.

EXISTENTIAL/GESTALT MODEL

The application of existential and gestalt theoretical frameworks to group therapy began in the 1960s with the Human Potential Movement, and its main proponents were Fritz Perls (1969), Abraham Maslow (1962), and Carl Rogers (1961). These similar frameworks all have a here-and-now focus, with the goal of increasing people's awareness of their feelings. A person's feelings are thought to be suppressed by the person's own constraints or the constraining expectations of others. Self-actualization is a secondary goal of existential or gestalt therapy. A self-actualized person assumes responsibility for herself and makes choices about feelings, thoughts, and behaviors. Clients are free to define themselves and become self-actualized, but this process is impeded by their own self-imposed limitations caused by fear or emotional pain.

The existential/gestalt model of group therapy facilitates people's self-actualization processes by helping them become more aware of their full potential, their alternatives or choices, and their feelings and emotions. Although most types of groups have the goal of helping individual members take responsibility for their emotions and behaviors through the process of support and feedback, in existential/gestalt groups this is the preeminent goal. The group functions as a microcosm of the real world of social interactions for the members. After focusing on the here and now of the social interactions demonstrated in the group, individual members can apply what they learned to their personal social interaction problems outside the group.

According to these frameworks, insight into the "why" of behavior is less important than insight into the "what" of behavior. Dealing with personal problems through increased awareness is viewed as a growth process, not a corrective process. Individuals can deal adequately with their own life problems if they know what these problems are; they do not necessarily have to know why they exist. The group experience provides an environment in which people can identify with and accept the forming self through experiences of awareness.

BEHAVIORAL AND COGNITIVE MODELS

Behavioral therapy also focuses on the "what" of behavior—that is, specific behaviors that present themselves in the here and now. The behavioral model further focuses on the motivation for these behaviors, or the reinforcers of the behaviors. Behaviors are viewed as adaptive or maladaptive, and maladaptive behaviors become the targets for change. Behavioral change is brought about through punishment of maladaptive acts and the positive reinforcement of adaptive behaviors. The goal of behavioral therapy is to change specific behaviors and determine how this change will be achieved.

The **behavioral/cognitive model** of group therapy conceptualizes group membership as a reinforcer. The social climate of the group is seen as the source of positive social reinforcement. The group offers the members a feeling of belonging and offers interactions that allow members to be heard and appreciated by others. The ways other members and the group leader respond to the behavior of an individual member can be reinforcing or extinguishing and therefore the stimulus for change. For example, the positive response of group members to a member's behavior contributes to the reinforcement of that member's behavior. On the other hand, a negative response from any member contributes to extinguishing the behavior.

Cognitive therapy is similar to behavioral therapy in that it focuses more on changing behavior than on obtaining insight into the reasons for that behavior. This form of therapy examines the cognitions (thoughts) and related feelings that contribute to maladaptive behaviors. People's cognitions are believed to result from goals, standards, and values that are mainly learned from families and culture. These can become maladaptive when they become unrealistic rules of "shoulds," "oughts," and "musts" and internalized commands that are often projected onto others (Ellis, 1992).

In cognitive group therapy, clients are helped to change their thoughts, feelings, and behaviors through the use of confrontation and homework assignments. During the group therapy session, the members share their homework assignments, along with their problems, with the group, with the purpose of identifying their core dysfunctional beliefs. The other group members and the leader help the member identify these dysfunctional, irrational beliefs and dispute them, helping the person to change them and the accompanying dysfunctional behaviors (Heldt et al., 2006; Rosenberg & Hougard, 2005).

Cognitive behavioral approaches are finding more applications than ever (Beck & Lewis, 2000; Ryle, 2004). For example, in substance abuse treatment, cognitive behavior group therapy has been combined with contingency management to produce the favorable outcome of prolonged abstinence for cocaine addicts (Poling et al., 2006).

PSYCHODRAMA AND ROLE-PLAYING TECHNIQUES

Psychodrama and role playing are specific techniques used in group therapy that involve action rather than conversation, but they are not separate theoretical models. Psychodrama has its roots in the theater and is used by the group members to reenact conflictual situations or interactions. The object is to gain an understanding of the behavior of oneself or the other person involved in the actual situation. Psychodrama is based on spontaneity, reality testing, catharsis, and role reversal. Alter egos are used in psychodrama. The purpose of the alter egos is to enact roles that require the client to explore the meaning of feelings and behaviors that maintain her present problems. Members of the group act out the conflictual situation while other members serving as alter-ego representatives ("doubles") stand beside them and indicate what they might be thinking or feeling. The individual involved in the actual situation frequently reverses roles in the psychodrama to gain a better understanding of the other person who was involved in the interaction (Moreno, 1946).

Role playing is similar to psychodrama. It uses role reversal but not alter egos. The members of the group must guess what the actors in the role-play are thinking, feeling, or trying to convey. The group as a whole discusses the interactions of the actors. These techniques work best when a member has experienced an actual situation that may serve as the basis of the psychodrama or the role-play (Marram, 1978).

SUMMARY OF THEORETICAL FOUNDATIONS

This brief overview of the theoretical models of group therapy practice has attempted to provide a beginning understanding of the concepts that underlie the dynamics and processes that occur in all groups, not just therapeutic groups. Which theory the clinician or group therapist uses depends on the goals and purposes of her group. For example, an outpatient support group for substance abusers will have quite different goals from an inpatient grief process group. Frequently, group therapists will use a combination of models, that is, an eclectic approach, to guide their work.

Even if they do not acknowledge using an eclectic approach, most group therapists use principles from various models:

◆ Transference/countertransference (transference is the client reacting to the therapist or other group members as if the person were someone from the client's past; countertransference is when the therapist experiences this reaction toward a client)

◆ Group resistance (group members are angry, uncooperative)

◆ Here-and-now focus (present-day issues rather than the past)

◆ Underlying group process themes (naming the issues of group interaction)

◆ Boundary management and cohesiveness (clarity about structure, rules, and relationships among group members; group holding together)

- Facilitation of feedback and self-disclosure (using communication skills to provide own and others': [1] feedback within the group and [2] to provide safety, comfort, relevance in self-disclosure of the group members)

- Process versus content focus (examining the message through the issues presented by interactions within the group versus the actual meaning of the words that comprise the content; this examination is more briefly referred to as metamessage versus message)

These concepts come from the psychodynamic, interpersonal, communication/systems, and group process models.

What is most important is that the nurse group therapist uses some theoretical concepts and principles to guide her work, thereby providing a secure structure for the group. Otherwise, because of the complexity and rapidity of group interactions, the group therapist or leader can quickly lose control and the group may fail in its therapeutic mission, that is, for the members to be of benefit to each other. Some examples of when the nurse should recognize and act on the need for clear communication to describe boundary issues and maintain group cohesion include: (1) when one group member consistently talks about her own symptoms whenever another group member talks about hers; (2) when one person always offers to fill the need voiced by another group member (e.g., child-care, elder care, transportation). Examples of questions the nurse leader should ask when wondering when to intervene in a group are as follows:

- What should I say when Ms. S. is undergoing an experience similar to one that I've had? Or, should I say anything about myself?

- What should I say when Mr. T. and Ms. J. keep talking while others are talking and it is clear that they are angry?

- Mr. Z. continuously brings up past events and his feelings about them. How should I gently guide him to the present time?

THE ROLE OF THE NURSE

Nurses have the unique opportunity to work with clients in numerous health care settings. During the current length of hospital stays of only a few days to 1 or 2 weeks, nurses learn about clients' needs, disease process, recovery from crises, and resources after discharge. Because most units offer many groups, nurses usually participate with clients in some aspect of this treatment modality. Staff nurses may be leaders of activity, psychoeducation, task, or support groups. They can also be therapists and co-therapists. Although groups in inpatient settings may have diminished, their utilization in outpatient psychiatric and medical settings has expanded.

The American Nurses Association (ANA) *Scope and Standards of Psychiatric-Mental Health Nursing Practice* (2000)

specifies that nurses must provide structure and maintain a therapeutic environment, and that advanced clinical expertise is required for functioning as a psychotherapist in individual and group treatment modalities.

THE GENERALIST NURSE

Staff nurses on psychiatric units participate in and lead groups based on needs of clients for education, support, recreation, task, exercise, symptom management, medication, and problem solving. In the community, nurses conduct groups based on specific needs and issues for clinic, medically ill, mentally ill, or homeless persons with psychosocial aspects of their situations.

THE ADVANCED-PRACTICE PSYCHIATRIC REGISTERED NURSE

Group therapy, like other psychotherapies, requires graduate preparation. Graduate preparation and clinical expertise as an APRN enables the nurse to analyze complex client problems and apply various theories that facilitate adaptive coping behaviors.

Educational Preparation

Psychiatric nurses practicing as therapists (or psychotherapists) in group therapy need to have at least a master's degree in psychiatric-mental health nursing. Curricula at the master's level include psychodynamic education about group process, group therapy training, and supervision of therapeutic groups. Preparation for the master's degree can lead to a clinical specialty in psychiatric-mental health nursing, and certification opportunities are also provided by the ANA. Current preparation may include education as a nurse practitioner or a clinical nurse specialist, each focused on psychiatric-mental health nursing. At this advanced-practice level of expertise, nurses can offer counseling and conduct groups in settings that are part of in- and outpatient psychiatric services. Also, other psychiatric settings where nurses can lead groups include intensive outpatient psychiatric services such as partial hospitalization or day treatment services. Some advanced-practice psychiatric registered nurses are also involved in their own private practices.

Because the nurse is often the coordinator of the assessments by other professionals, the presence of a nurse in inpatient group therapy is optimal. Much overlap exists between the disciplines involved in inpatient psychiatry, and each professional offers a different perspective. For example, the social worker, who may be more aware than other professionals of rehabilitation opportunities in the community, provides the client with specifics about appropriate placement options for discharge. The occupational therapist may provide the most realistic appraisal of the client's functional abilities. The nurse, on the other hand, may be most aware of the client's physical conditions, medication requirements, and social skills. The nurse who is a group therapist may also be one of the nursing staff who works daily with all clients. Nurses also participate in groups as co-therapists. Because nurses have 24-hour responsibility for client care, their participation in group therapy facilitates the continuity of care.

Supervision

Supervision is one professional's guiding the practice of another professional. For example, a clinical nurse specialist, social worker, psychologist, or psychiatrist may supervise a nurse, or an experienced nurse may supervise a new nurse. In group therapy, supervision includes the ongoing evaluation of the leader's behavior, emotions, and interventions. The goal of this process is self-awareness through self-evaluation. Constructive criticism and feedback on performance are essential components of learning effective group leadership. All practitioners of group therapy need professional supervision to gain insight into their motives for their own interactions and to gain awareness of possible countertransference reactions. Supervision, then, is for both the novice and the expert group leader; it can be done in individual sessions or in group sessions, as in peer supervision.

Supervision works best when the supervisor has no authority over the supervisees. Bonnivier (1992) described a peer supervision group established for nurses to explore their countertransference reactions to clients. The goals of the group were (1) to recognize countertransference reactions, which are unconscious by nature; (2) to explore and examine the basis and meaning of the reactions; and (3) to develop, collaboratively, interventions that would help the nurses behave therapeutically rather than angrily. After 1 year, the group of nurses felt that they could manage their countertransference therapeutically. As a result, the group became incorporated into nursing education on a yearly basis. The absolute requirement was that no one with administrative responsibilities over any of the members could participate in supervision. Hence, participants were free to examine their thoughts and feelings without fear of repercussions. Contemporary studies support these findings and the importance of clinical supervision, particularly in clients with a propensity to engender strong emotions and interfere with objective treatment planning, such as those with borderline personality disorder (Chatziandreou, Tsani, Lamnidis, Synodinou, & Vaslamatzis, 2005; Davidson, 2006).

An important aspect of supervision is understanding the group therapist's own reactions. When the focus of the group involves PTSD or critical incident stress debriefing techniques, the group leader may begin having nightmares or intrusive images of atrocities or terrifying events mentioned during group interactions. This is a common occurrence, described most recently in mental health professionals serving combatant soldiers in the military in Iraq (Jaffe, 2005). Therapists are "secondary" trauma victims similar to rescuers of traumatized victims and often need assistance coping with their own reactions.

Co-Therapy

Co-therapy is joint or dual leadership of a group. Sometimes an experienced therapist is the leader and the co-therapist is a less-experienced practitioner. This type of co-therapy is a strategy for training the new leader (Yalom, 1983). However, both therapists may share the leader role equally. Co-therapy is advantageous for those who like to work with others, to discuss each other's roles and participation within the group, and to explore the relationship they share with each other. More attention and interaction are available to clients when the leaders have distinctly different personalities. Clients witness the co-therapists actively solving problems and resolving conflicts. Ideally, such exposure provides clients role modeling of healthy, assertive, and successful relationships. When co-therapists are of different genders, clients can benefit optimally from the two therapists' resolution of gender-related issues, that is, identification with one sex and conflict resolution with the opposite sex. Most groups lend themselves to co-therapy.

GROUP THERAPY ON PSYCHIATRIC UNITS

Some of the purposes of group therapy in the hospital setting include encouraging social involvement, developing rapport between clients and staff, enabling clients to demonstrate support for each other and participate in mutual problem solving, and promoting the development of a sense of solidarity as a group of individuals in the hospital situation. Groups offer clients opportunities to explore new communication skills, make use of social contacts, obtain peer feedback on individual problems, resolve interpersonal conflicts occurring within the group, and experience group support for evaluating behaviors. Clients sometimes accept confrontation or criticism better from other clients than from staff. Psychotic process manifested in hallucinations or delusions, mania, or depression cannot be resolved in group therapy (Yalom, 1995).

Groups on inpatient units are limited by shortened hospital stays. Hence, each group must be considered as lasting for only one meeting. Nurse group leaders might focus these groups on establishing commonality between clients who are at different functional levels, decreasing anxiety, decreasing social isolation, and providing opportunity to work onday-to-day interpersonal problems. These groups must provide a feeling of safety for clients to feel comfortable with self-disclosure (Reeve, 2006; Winship & Hardy, 2007).

Styles of Group Leadership

Historically, physicians or nurses primarily filled the group leadership role. In the past 40 years, nurses, social workers, psychologists, and psychiatrists have filled the role. There are many styles of and theoretical approaches to conducting insight- or process-oriented groups, but, according to Rogers (1971), a client-centered philosophy is the basic foundation of all of them. Accordingly, the specific functions of the group leader are to:

◆ Facilitate interactions within the group
◆ Respond to the feelings and meanings inherent in each member's statements
◆ Accept the group and its members
◆ Understand each person's verbal contribution
◆ Identify how those statements relate to the member
◆ Use self-disclosure and expression thoughtfully and professionally
◆ Provide feedback
◆ Avoid excessive planning or use of games or gimmicks
◆ Limit the use of interpretations

Rogers' style is a reflective, as opposed to authoritarian, style. Thus, rather than directing, confronting, and controlling the direction of the group, the nurse group leader would encourage the expression of feelings and convey emotional comfort. In contrast, a confrontive style might be used with groups of persons with substance-related disorders, whose defensive posture is detrimental to their recovery. The styles of group leadership are summarized in Table 27–3.

One of the functions listed above is exemplified in an example of a nurse group leader who acknowledges both a member's verbal contributions without allowing the person to monopolize or to be targeted by others and provides opportunity to refocus the statement on the member. Specifically, when a person verbalizes feelings of dislike of another member's actions, the nurse should nonjudgmentally acknowledge that person's statement and focus the conversation quickly on what the angered person needs.

The group leader sets the tone of the group. She is responsible for providing structure in terms of the time and place of sessions, establishing rules for safe self-expression and confidentiality, and facilitating expression of feelings and participation by all members. The group leader establishes a climate of comfort relatively free of tension and anxiety, balances the needs of the group against those of any member, and intervenes to promote safety and self-awareness (Pasquali, Arnold, & DeBasio, 1989). Clearly, the nurse group leader needs the skills for identifying and using different styles based on client need.

Nurses as Group Leaders

Although nurses were involved with group therapies since the tuberculosis psychoeducation experiments, it was not until the 1960s that nursing education included group dynamics and process. Advanced education and training in group leadership were offered at the graduate nursing level. However, in the psychiatric units, nurses were often the only

TABLE 27–3
Summary of Characteristics of Group Leadership

Reflective

Facilitation

Empathic listening

Responsiveness

Acceptance

Identification of relevance of one member's statements to other member

Thoughtful use of self-disclosure

Ability to confront

Provision of feedback

Limited use of interpretation

Avoidance of excessive planning, games, or gimmicks

Authoritarian

Directiveness

Confrontation

Control of members' participation

Control of choice of topics

Planning methods for conduct of group sessions without allowing input from others

staff available to hold group meetings, regardless of their education or preparation. Thus, psychiatric nurses have probably been doing group work for educational and communicative purposes longer than has been documented.

Ken Kesey's (1963) *One Flew over the Cuckoo's Nest* is a negative demonstration of the nurse's role in group psychotherapy. Nurse Ratched is a malevolent, controlling, and domineering woman in a starched, white uniform. Her efforts to facilitate clients' self-disclosure are humiliating experiences for the clients, and group support is thwarted as she verbally threatens to reveal private material to the clients' families. Her tactics, far from being therapeutic, reveal unethical use of staff authority and a distinct lack of communication skills and group therapy training.

Yalom (1983) reported that a particular nurse-run inpatient group in 1974 provided clients with social learning experiences and open discussion of feelings that facilitated ward functioning. Clients reported that the group experience enhanced their use of other ward group activities. The negative aspect was the formality of the group, which was manifested in, among other things, the nurses' starched, white uniforms. Not surprisingly, nurses on most psychiatric units abandoned these white uniforms more than 20 years ago.

PROCESS AND CONTENT

Discussion about group sessions includes analysis of both process and content. Process refers to the manner in which clients talk about themselves and the way the group responds. Analysis of group process provides assessment of the therapy's effects on individual group members. The assessment involves evaluation of individual clients' responses to each other, to the group as a whole, and to the leader. Group process can be described by the degree of the group's openness, cohesiveness, and responsiveness to particular individual concerns and the degree of consistency of individual behavior within the group. For example, a consistent tendency of older group members to act as parents or rescuers may influence the contributions of younger members who perceive them as parental figures. Questions that the leader may ask to evaluate group process include the following:

- ◆ Who started the group today?
- ◆ What happened when Ms. X. told her story?
- ◆ Did Mr. T. try to rescue as he always does?
- ◆ Did Mr. I. fall asleep?
- ◆ What precipitated Ms. Z.'s departure from the room?
- ◆ Who responded when Mr. Q. started crying?

Group process varies with each session and with the current moods of or events specific to individual members and to the group as a whole. Sometimes, the therapist may share her process comments with the group to stimulate insight or to teach group dynamics.

Content analysis is the evaluation of what was said during the group therapy session. Content includes overall themes of the group session. Examples of content themes are sadness, loneliness, leisure time activities, and relationship issues. The therapist's own content, as a group member, is included in this discussion. What is not said is often discussed also. Topics may be avoided because they can evoke painful or conflict-ridden emotions.

Content and process are interrelated and are often discussed together. In a co-therapy situation, a helpful method for examining both is for one therapist to focus on process while the other focuses on content. Questions that could be asked include the following:

- ◆ Under what conditions did Ms. X. say what she said? And to whom?
- ◆ What was the person's response and what did that trigger in Ms. Z., Mr. Q., and Ms. S.?
- ◆ When Mr. J. left the room, what did Ms. X. say, and how did the mood in the room change?

Like process, content varies within the group according to individual members' differences in moods, events, and relationships with each other.

In the psychiatric unit, or community-based settings, some groups may lend themselves better than others to process and content discussions. That is, a group of people who are verbal, self-aware, and high functioning will talk and react, solve problems, and seek personal change. In contrast, less reaction to one another in problem solving occur in activity-oriented groups, in which clients are performing tasks and are moving at different paces. Certainly, the focus of the group determines the kind of activities that might occur in the session. Nevertheless, there is always information to assess and discuss about what was said, who said it and how, who did what activity, and what the themes of the session were.

TABLE 27–4
Nursing Diagnoses That May Be Applied to a Group as a Whole or to Individual Members within a Group

Ineffective Health Maintenance

Ineffective Role Performance

Anticipatory Grieving

Anxiety

Body Image Disturbance

Caregiver Role Strain

Decisional Conflict

Defensive Coping

Dysfunctional Grieving

Family Processes, Dysfunctional Alcoholism

Grieving

High Risk for Self-Mutilation

Hopelessness

Ineffective Denial

Disabled Family Coping

Ineffective Coping

Deficient Knowledge (of medication)

Ineffective Therapeutic Regimen Management

Noncompliance

Parental Role Conflict

Post-Trauma Response

Powerlessness

Rape-Trauma Syndrome

Risk for Loneliness

Risk for Low Self-Esteem

Social Isolation

Sorrow, Chronic

Spiritual Distress

Note. From: *Carpenito-Moyet, L. J. (2006).* Nursing diagnosis: Application to clinical practice (10th ed.). New York: Lippincott Williams & Wilkins.

Psychiatric units are well-suited to task or activity groups, particularly for all ages of lower functioning clients. Horticultural group therapy is described as a beneficial activity for promoting the relationships between student nurses and clients in a psychiatric inpatient setting (Smith, 1998). In groups lasting 30 to 90 minutes, clients were productive and interested in the activities involving nature. Students described how clients became trusting, disclosing concerns, feelings, and frustrations about their mental illness.

THE NURSING PROCESS

The nursing process—assessing, diagnosing, planning, intervening, and evaluating the plan—is applied to individuals within a group as well as to the group as a whole. For example, 10 clients who have the same problem may be in one group. In this manner, specific interventions can be used for all of the members. Klose and Tinius (1992) developed a group for clients with low self-esteem, teaching them and having them practice specific strategies for enhancing self-esteem. The group's particular focus combined insight-oriented therapy and education, creating the opportunity for group members to provide constructive social interaction, trust, and support. Studies that use group therapy to enhance self-esteem and reduce depression continue to demonstrate the efficacy of this approach (Stinson & Kirk, 2006). Nursing diagnoses that might be applied to a whole group or to persons within a group are listed in Table 27–4.

Occasionally, an entire group can be viewed as the client and the nursing process applied. For example, the group may face a recently discharged member's suicide. The entire group may be avoiding or denying the reality of the event, and a nursing diagnosis such as ineffective coping or dysfunctional grieving might be considered. Similarly, a group for clients with schizophrenia may be given a diagnosis of ineffective health maintenance because all members are currently unable to procure and prepare food for themselves as a result of preoccupation with internal stimuli. A nursing diagnosis with plan and interventions can be applied to the group when all of the members support problematic or destructive behaviors by any one, several, or all members.

GROUPS THAT FOCUS ON STRESS-RELATED ISSUES

Various types of groups exist to help the client deal with the stresses of life. The most common ones are task groups, teaching groups, self-awareness/personal growth groups, therapy groups, and social groups. These groups differ in focus, their goals, and the functions of the leader and members. Table 27–5 identifies several types of groups.

Self-awareness groups focus on the interpersonal concerns (the here and now) of the members, with the goal of developing interpersonal strengths. Therapy groups are

TABLE 27–5
Types of Groups, Their Purposes, and Examples

Type	Purpose	Example
Task	Performance of particular task	Occupational therapy group; poetry group
Focus Group	Sharing of thoughts and experiences on a specific topic	Focus groups with school-age children; health disparities; strategic planning
Social	Recreation; comfort; mutual meeting of needs	Recreational outings, e.g., bowling
Teaching	Imparting of information	Medication group
Psychoeducational	Imparting of information; processing of emotional concerns	Dual diagnosis (combination of psychiatric diagnosis and substance abuse) groups
Support/Therapeutic	Coping with particular stresses and concerns	Cancer support group; Alzheimer's disease caregiver support groups
Self-Help/Mutual Support	Peer support (no professional leader)	Overeaters Anonymous; Alcoholics Anonymous; online support groups
Psychotherapeutic	Interpersonal concerns; present problems; past experiences; self-understanding; insight oriented	Inpatient or outpatient groups
Symptom Management	Specific target (psychosis); coping strategies; stress management; not insight oriented	Persons with schizophrenia group; exercise group; reminiscence group

also member focused, but past experiences are also taken into consideration. The goal of therapy groups is to help the members gain self-understanding and find more satisfactory ways of relating to others. Social groups focus on enjoyment and mutual meeting of needs, the purpose being to allow members to find recreation, relaxation, and comfort. The goal of teaching groups is to impart information.

Although all types of groups are important, nurses are generally more interested in the groups in which they can use their professional skills to bring about educative or therapeutic effects on clients. Therefore, nurses are frequently involved in teaching, therapy, and support groups.

TASK GROUPS

Task groups focus on the performance of a specific task agreed on by the group. This task is usually important to the members of the group, and the group stays together only long enough to accomplish it. In mental health treatment centers, these groups are sometimes conducted by occupational therapists, but nurses also lead groups that have specific purposes, such as collage making, poetry writing, or planning of an outing.

Focus Groups

Focus groups need to be mentioned as a subtype of task groups. Focus groups or group interviews, which started off as tools in market research, have expanded to health care–related areas (Kelly, Caldwell, & Henshaw, 2006; Patterson & Kelley, 2005). Typically data is collected from a group discussion among four to ten participants who share their thoughts and experiences on a topic set by the investigator/facilitator. The advantage of a group interview is that it is more time efficient than individual interviews and the group process may trigger additional ideas as well as more discussion and clarity on the topic. Ruff, Alexander, & McKie (2005) used focused group interviews in their work with black menopausal women to help understand the needs of this population to help decrease health disparities.

TEACHING GROUPS

Medication groups, an example of teaching groups, are an important aspect of psychiatric care usually provided by nurses or clinical pharmacists. Antipsychotics and antidepressants have unpleasant side effects that often result in clients' nonadherence with medication regimens. In groups, members at varying stages of illness help each other by sharing coping strategies for managing side effects. They problem-solve and evaluate whether the side effects outweigh the benefits of the drugs for their illnesses. The group leader offers education about purposes, dosage, safe and unsafe side effects, metabolism, drug or food interactions, and the usual length of time necessary for the medication to start taking effect. Overall, groups encourage awareness of symptoms of illness, side effects of medications, and resources for obtaining information.

PSYCHOEDUCATIONAL GROUPS

Educative or teaching groups are those in which the nurse usually acts as the leader and imparts some health-related information. Psychoeducational groups are a variation of this type of group and are those in which the nurse imparts some information but also facilitates discussion of the related psychosocial issues. An example of this is a group run by public health nurses that provides information on the treatment and management of sexually transmitted diseases but also encourages discussion of self-esteem and social issues related to these diseases (Madrid & Swanson, 1995).

Dual diagnosis groups are becoming popular for people with psychiatric diagnoses who become involved with alcohol and substance abuse or addiction. The nurse leader is challenged to provide education and promote insight, enabling clients to acknowledge the abuse of substances as personally problematic. In addition to use with dual diagnosis clients, psychoeducational groups are used successfully for social skills training for schizophrenics. This usually unresponsive population benefits the most when psychoeducation is combined with supportive group processes, thereby enhancing the effect of both approaches (Bäuml, Pitschel-Walz, Volz, Engel, & Kessling, 2007; Rummel, Hansen, Helbig, Pitschel-Walz, & Kissling, 2005) (see Research Abstract).

SUPPORTIVE/THERAPEUTIC GROUPS

Supportive/therapeutic groups help members cope with the sources of stress in their lives and focus on existing strengths (Kim & Kim, 2001). This stress may be related to physical, psychological, or social problems. Support groups focus on thoughts, feelings, and behaviors. The group provides a safe environment for clients to share with others who are often in the same situation or dealing with the same stressors. Examples of these types of groups are cancer support groups, divorce support groups, and impaired health professional support groups. The nurse may act as the facilitator or initiator of these groups .

A new phenomenon related to diminishing health care resources and the advent of the information age is the use of online (via personal computer) support groups. Finfgeld (2000) reports on the two forms of on-line groups that exist. The comprehensive version offers a variety of services in addition to interactive support, including educational materials and expert professional advice, whereas the other version is merely an interactive support group where individuals can ventilate and offer support to each other. Typical topics are depression, substance abuse, cancer, eating disorders, coping with AIDS and HIV, and caretaking of family members who have Alzheimer's disease. The advantages of online support groups are convenience and anonymity. Disadvantages are

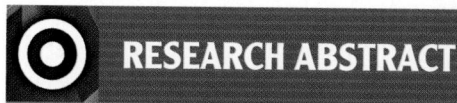
Psychoeducation and Compliance in the Treatment of Schizophrenia: Results of the Munich Psychosis Information Project Study

Pitschel-Walz, G., Bauml, J., Bender, W., Engel, R. R., Wagner, M., & Kissling, W. (2006). *Journal of Clinical Psychiatry, 67,* 443–452.

Study Problem/Purpose

The aim of this study was to examine whether psychoeducational groups for clients with schizophrenia and for their families could reduce rehospitalization rates and improve adherence to treatment.

Methods

The sample consisted of 236 inpatients who met *DSM-III-R* criteria for schizophrenia or schizoaffective disorder and who had regular contact with at least one relative or other key person. They were randomly assigned to one of two treatment conditions. In the intervention condition, clients and their relatives were encouraged to attend psychoeducational groups over a period of 4 to 5 months. Researchers separated the clients from their relatives in the psychoeducational programs and each consisted of eight sessions. Clients in the other treatment condition received routine care. Outcomes were compared over 12-month and 24-month follow-up periods. The study was conducted from 1990 to 1994.

Findings

Data revealed a significant reduction in hospitalization rates after 12 and 24 months in clients who attended the psychoeducational groups compared with clients involved in the routine care without psychoeducational care (p < 0.05). In addition, clients who participated in the psychoeducation groups demonstrated increased adherence to treatment compared with clients under routine care without psychoeducation.

Implications for Psychiatric Nursing

These data indicate that in the short-term, eight psychoeducational sessions with clients and family involvement in separate groups can significantly enhance the treatment of schizophrenia. Psychoeducation is within the scope of psychiatric nurses and strengthens the importance of client and family education in improving client outcomes as evidenced by reduced hospitalization and adherence to treatment.

transient memberships, leaderless groups, a delay in seeking professional help, and an absence of physical contact (Goldkaramnay, Bauer, Haug, Wolf, & Kordy, 2007).

SELF-HELP/MUTUAL-HELP GROUPS

Self-help groups and mutual-help groups for individuals with psychiatric-mental health problems are peer support groups that are run by the members and have no professional leader. However, they usually do adhere to a prescribed structure. Alcoholics Anonymous (AA) and other substance abuse or codependency groups modeled on the twelve-step program are the best known of these mutual-help groups. Groups such as Overeaters Anonymous and Recovery Inc. are also becoming more prominent. Medical self-help groups, which more commonly do have a professional leader, have followed the lead of the psychiatric-mental health groups and also have become commonplace.

Although medical self-help groups have anecdotal evidence regarding their effectiveness, research has not substantiated remarkable improvements in clients with this intervention, only small to moderate ones (Barlow, Burlingame, Nebeker, & Anderson, 1999). In spite of this they remain very popular, especially among females, and are obviously a source of support for those individuals coping with physical illness and psychiatric problems (Wituk, Shepherd, Slavich, Warren, & Meissen, 2000).

In general, self-help groups have arisen in populations that have conditions that cause them to exhibit some behaviors that are unacceptable to or stigmatized by society and for which effective treatment has not yet been found. The focus of self-help groups is not on insight into behavior or the reconstruction of personality, the traditional focuses of psychiatric practitioners. Instead, the focus is on controlling members' dysfunctional behavior, decreasing stress by giving advice and sharing coping strategies, and maintaining members' self-esteem and legitimacy in the face of societal pressure. In addition, self-help groups focus on socialization of members. The socialization process goes beyond meeting individual members' needs for social contact to include instillation of the perspectives and values of the entire group, which are usually more in accord with societal norms (Marram, 1978).

People abusing substances have turned to mutual-help groups to assist them with their recovery process. Mutual-help groups are associations that are voluntarily formed, are not professionally led, and operate through face-to-face supportive interaction focusing on a mutual goal. The first of the mutual-help groups was AA, founded officially in 1935. Early AA members developed what they called the Twelve Steps to guide the recovery process (Brown, 1985; Kurtz, 1979).

Alcoholics Anonymous has been viewed as relatively successful in helping people abusing alcohol to remain sober. Because it is nonprofessional, cost sparing, and an ongoing source of assistance, it is an invaluable resource to the community. Nurses frequently refer clients misusing substances to this type of group. AA meetings may be geared to special-interest groups (e.g., homosexual persons, professionals, or students).

Other Twelve Step programs have developed through adaptation of AA's approach. Narcotics Anonymous, Gamblers Anonymous, Debtors Anonymous, Cocaine Anonymous, Overeaters Anonymous, and Sex and Love Addicts Anonymous are examples. The Twelve Steps have also been applied to syndromes of compulsive behavior and other difficulties encountered in the children, partners, and close associates of substance abusers. Al-Anon, Codependents Anonymous, and Adult Children of Alcoholics are examples of these groups. The goals of these groups in addition to support involve promoting psychological and behavior change in their members (Humphreys, 1996).

The proliferation of mutual-help groups is one of the important social developments of this century. The reason for this social development is not completely understood, but the structure is relatively straightforward. In general, Twelve Step meetings follow one of these general formats:

◆ Uninterrupted talk(s) by one or more speakers about "what it was like, what happened, and what it is like now"

◆ A discussion in which each person at the meeting has the opportunity to speak briefly

◆ Some combination of the preceding two options

The format and choice of a particular step (of the Twelve Steps) of meetings vary according to the group's size, the region of the country in which the group meets, the ethnic and gender composition of the group, and other cultural characteristics of the members (Fuller & Hiller-Sturmhofel, 1999).

PSYCHOTHERAPEUTIC GROUPS

The biological basis for illness and symptoms provides a rationale for conducting groups made up of clients who suffer from the same ailments and problems. Having the same nursing diagnosis increases the likelihood that clients can be helpful to one another as they learn together to cope with their illness. An advantage of common-illness groups is that the rapid client turnover in the hospital provides ongoing membership of persons in different phases of the same illness. Denial becomes more difficult when people view the same symptoms in others.

Pollack (1990) began an inpatient group for people with bipolar disorder who were knowledgeable about their diagnosis, voluntarily took their medication, were sufficiently stabilized on their medication that they could attend meetings, and were motivated to attend. The group met weekly, incorporating new members. Yalom's 11 therapeutic factors were the therapists' goals for this group (see Table 27–2). After 9 months, three goals emerged as most prominent: sharing information, coping with bipolar disorder, and improving interpersonal relationships. Clients recognized similar experiences, such as needing to be the center of attention, experiencing high-energy levels or euphoric moods, and feeling the despair of depressive episodes. Skillful group leadership was required at these meetings because of the need for behavioral limits.

Other groups offered on the psychiatric unit might include groups for stress reduction, suicide prevention, intellectual discussion, occupational therapy, movement or dance therapy, current events, discharge issues, sexual health concerns, cooking, leisure activity, and entertainment.

SYMPTOM MANAGEMENT GROUPS
Medical Diagnoses

Medically ill clients benefit from groups that combine education, support, and symptom management. Gregoire, Kalogeropoulos, and Corcos (1997) described how 54 men with prostate cancer and some family members experienced reassurance, decreased anxiety, and a positive outlook from participating in 10 weekly group sessions with a nurse and a psychologist. Acquisition of new coping strategies is an anecdotal outcome of such groups that encourage interaction between members.

Clinicians in many health care environments conduct groups focused on specific conditions. For example, "Easy Breathers Club" is an ongoing symptom management and peer support group for clients with chronic obstructive lung disease at one VA hospital. Other examples are listed on the Kaiser Permanente website and include symptom management for conditions such as asthma and lung disease, cancer, fibromyalgia, diabetes, and heart disease, and for self-improvements such as weight management, and stress reduction (http://members.kaiserpermanente.org/kpweb/classes/list.do). Still another example includes the chronic disease self-management model that partners patients with health care providers, involves lay leaders who also have chronic disease, and offers a full curriculum and a focus on a personalized action plan (Linnell, 2005).

Rossi and colleagues (1997) describe 22 meetings over two years with five female and two male adolescents with epilepsy. Their sessions focused on improving comprehension and acceptance of epilepsy and consequences of the condition for all aspects of their lives. The aims were to assist these young people to interact with each other and to gain an improved sense of self. Different from self-help groups, the authors concluded that the participants benefited from sharing their suffering, anxiety, and feelings about shame or avoidance by peers. Also, the adolescents learned about their condition and demonstrated less denial by choosing to be more compliant with medication.

Psoriasis is a dermatologic condition that affects social and psychological effects, and the resulting emotional stress tends to worsen the condition. Seng and Nee (1997) describe 7 sessions with 10 clients where the focus was on knowledge, acceptance, stress management, and coping. On evaluation, the patients reported that their improved knowledge helped them cope and manage stress, that they learned from each other, and that they felt more self-confident.

An 8-session weekly program of cognitive behavioral group treatment was done with 19 menopausal women with hot flashes. The treatment included education, relaxation training and cognitive restructuring. Though the sample was small, the findings revealed moderate success in reducing the frequency of vasomotor symptoms that were measured by daily diaries (Keefer & Blanchard, 2005).

In a study that addressed the importance of a supportive group experience for clients with life-threatening illnesses who need palliative care interventions, Miller and colleagues (2005) conducted a group therapy approach with 69 clients randomly assigned to intervention or control groups; there were 12 distinct groups over 12 months. The intervention group received specific facilitated support with the opportunity to express their experience while the control group received standard care. While 51 clients completed the study, intervention clients, as compared with controls, had less distress with depressive symptoms and death-related feelings of meaninglessness and better spiritual well-being.

Attention has been focused on the possibility of prolonging survival with group therapy for women with metastatic breast cancer. Goodwin and colleagues (2001) conducted a multi-center study with 235 women with a life expectancy of at least three months, randomly assigning them to either a weekly supportive-expressive group of 8 to 12 women for up to one year or a control group without any group intervention. All of the women were monitored at frequent intervals for up to one year, during which time they all received educational materials and any needed medical attention. The supportive-expressive group fostered support, encouraged emotional expression about cancer and its impact on all aspects of their lives, the treatments, their relationships with others, communication with each other outside of the group, and their strategies for coping. While this type of group did not significantly prolong survival (17.9 months in the intervention group and 17.6 months in the control group), the authors report that the women who were initially the most distressed improved their mood, their perception of pain, and feelings of distress. Contemporary findings continue to support the importance of supportive groups to clients with medical conditions and offer psychiatric avenues to mobilize psychosocial support, strengthen coping skills, and optimize treatment planning.

While pharmacologic treatments provide benefit, group therapies are used for improving psychosocial needs in transplant patients with conditions such as alcoholism or obesity. For example, cognitive behavioral groups that target risk factors for transplantation patients, at both pre- and post-transplant, offer promise in reducing distress and depression and improving compliance with behavioral changes and overall quality of life (Jowsey, Taylor, Schneekloth, & Clark, 2001).

Psychiatric Diagnoses

Group therapy is a helpful treatment method with clients with schizophrenia. Kanas (1991) described a short-term approach of nine meetings. The therapeutic goals include teaching clients how to cope with their psychotic experiences and improve their interpersonal relationships. Members learn from one another's content and from the practice of interaction. The purposes of the group include providing safety, avoiding anxiety, promoting trust, and decreasing isolation and loneliness. This approach is used *in conjunction with antipsychotic medication.*

Homelessness is fraught with problems, including mental illness. Some clinicians have addressed psychiatric treatment for homeless persons through groups. McCracken and Black (2005) describe a therapeutic community in a shelter resulting in improvements in psychiatric symptoms, social functioning, and substance abuse after six months. Berger (2000) reported conducting twice weekly groups with veterans in an urban men's shelter that focused on problem-solving, coping strategies, self-improvements and change, and peer support. Symptoms associated with homelessness are problems such as: feelings of powerlessness and humiliation; being without food, clothing, shelter, hygiene, and money; having to stand in lines; dangers of living on the street; substance abuse; family; holidays; life in the shelter and the community. The men reported that these groups, which were process-oriented, topically focused, educational, or cognitive-behaviorally structured, were helpful and appreciated (S. Berger, personal communication, May 13, 2000).

Kehoe (1999) describes a therapy group about spiritual issues for clients with chronic mental illness in a day treatment center. Group rules maintaining tolerance of diversity, respect for other persons' beliefs, and a ban on proselytizing served to promote tolerance, self-awareness, and a satisfying exploration of value systems. Contrary to myth, a spiritual focus did not increase delusional thinking or strengthen defenses. Recent findings from Mohr and colleagues (2006) support this notion and demonstate the high prevalence and interest of discussing spiritual and religious issues among clients with schizophrenia. Results from this study emphasize the clinical importance of spirituality in the care of clients with schizophrenia and that the relationship between religion and mental illness requires a distinctly sensitive response to each client's unique experience.

Buccheri, Trygstad, Kanas, Waldron, and Dowling (1996) combined symptom management, psychoeducation, and support in their study of nurse-led groups for clients with schizophrenia in an outpatient day treatment program at a VA Medical Center. To manage auditory hallucinations, the symptom management classes met 12 weekly times and were structured to include discussion of strategies, opportnities to practice strategies, evaluation in sessions of new strategies, and question-and-answer period. Participants described a positive experience such as: (1) feeling less alone in symptoms, (2) validated, (3) chance to learn from others how to manage hallucinations, (4) opportunity to be or find a role model, (5) feeling hope because others experienced a decrease in frequency and intensity of the symptom. The majority of these clients were still using individualized strategies that lessened the intensity of their auditory hallucinations 12 months later (Buccheri, Trygstad, Kanas, & Dowling, 1997). Findings were replicated in a larger study and participants sustained improvements for 12 months (Buccheri et al., 2004).

STRESS MANAGEMENT GROUPS

The basis of several stress management groups is a biological approach to coping with stress. Relaxation groups teach slower breathing, deep muscle relaxation, elimination of distraction, and achievement of a calm mind and a peaceful mood. Exercise groups provide for the discharge of energy without demanding fine motor coordination. Exercise stimulates the whole body and can create a peaceful, relaxed, and satisfied mood. Similarly, music groups produce relaxation. Humor groups promote enjoyment of social interaction and feelings of well-being while discharging excess physical and emotional tension. Art groups promote creative expression and self-satisfaction. (Leardi et al., 2007; Storch, Gaab, Küttel, Stüssi, & Fend, 2007).

GROUP THERAPY ACROSS THE LIFE SPAN

Table 27–6 summarizes the issues that may be addressed by group therapy across the life span.

CHILDHOOD

Emotional disturbances and psychiatric disorders in children often present as conduct and affective disorders (Reeve, 2006; Webster-Stratton, Reid, & Hammond, 2004). Assessment is frequently made through observations of children in group activities at school, on the hospital unit, with their peers, and with their families. Providing a safe environment for emotional expression is paramount in working with children. Developmental tasks must also be considered, so that feelings are expressed in age-appropriate activities. Some nonverbal group activities include play therapy, art therapy, movement or dance therapy, and sand tray therapy. Depending on the family, the therapist, the child, and the group, ages 8 to 10 years may be appropriate for verbal therapy groups. Childhood issues that might be amenable to group therapy include traumas such as accidents and natural disasters, grief over the death of a parent or other family member, and poor social adjustment. Many concerns, such as sexual abuse, neglect, battering, or parental substance and alcohol abuse, may be best managed in one-to-one therapy. However, successful group models exist for dealing with these problems.

Group therapy appears to be particularly useful in assisting children to improve their social skills (Edwards, Céilleachair, Bywater, Hughes, & Hutchings, 2007; Webster-Stratton et al., 2004). In a study of 102 elementary school children ages 8 to 10 years, Shechtman (1991) tested the hypothesis that small-group therapy would be effective in enhancing intimate friendships with same-sex peers. All of these children had been referred for counseling, and they were divided according to the similarity of their problems

TABLE 27–6
Group Therapy across the Life Span

Age Range	Issues That Are the Focus of Group Work
Children	Social skills, emotional expression, behavioral expression of feelings, adult support, protection from unsafe environment
Adolescents	Peer relationships, sexual feelings, appropriate expression of feelings, social pressures, school performance, vocation and future plans, drugs, autonomy, relationships with parents
Adults	Gender support (for heterosexual and homosexual clients), parental roles, substance abuse, addiction, post-traumatic stress disorder, survivors of physical and/or sexual violence, incest survivors, dysfunctional relationships, marital discord, chronic illness
Older Adults	Adjustment to aging, loneliness, widowhood, chronic illness, peer relationships, family relationships, financial adjustments, changes in housing, grieving of losses of friends and health, life review, preparation for end of life
Confined Older Adults	Adjustment to health deterioration, adjustment to environment, loss of autonomy, change in family role, family relationships, caregiver relationships, grieving of losses, preparation for end of life, life review

into control (no therapy) and experimental (group psychotherapy) groups. Recognizing the value of Yalom's therapeutic factors (see Table 27–2), the experimental group's therapy emphasized self-expression, support, freedom within stated limits, caring, and group cohesion. Enriching experiences included puppetry, drama, and social games. By the end of the study, the experimental group had demonstrated significant increases in the development of close relationships, supporting the hypothesis. Shechtman concluded that group therapy is a viable method for helping children to cope and feel secure, wanted, and loved in a society that can produce disruption, personal loss, and detachment in children's lives.

Childhood obesity is a major health problem worldwide. Young and colleagues (2007) conducted a meta-analysis that compared the mean effect sizes of family-behavioral and other treatment and control weight-loss groups for children, in which this approach demonstrated a positive correlation between family participation and weight loss in children. These findings are consistent with other findings that demonstrated decreased obesity and associated medical problems in childhood obesity (Jiang, Xia, Greiner, Lian, & Rosenqvist, 2005; Young, Northern, Lister, Drummond, & O'Brien, 2007).

ADOLESCENCE

Adolescents are struggling with autonomy and independence from their parents and other authorities. As they establish their own identity, they are particularly vulnerable to peer pressure. Their problems are often reflective of social pressures and the concern they feel about their actions and physical appearance. Despite their need for independence, they are dependent and require a great deal of emotional support from parents. Teenage issues include same- and opposite-sex peer relationships, sexually transmitted diseases, pregnancy, drug abuse, sexual abuse, aggression, social adjustment to school, depression, and suicide.

Adolescent tobacco, drug, and alcohol use/abuse, in particular, are ineffective ways of coping with the problems of this age group (Faden & Goldman, 2004). Life skills training, which is a school-based approach using cognitive behavioral techniques in group discussion and educational classes, has been effective in prevention of use of these substances. In addition to providing information about the effects of alcohol, tobacco, and other drugs, life skills training focuses on personal self-management skills and social skills (Seal, 2006).

The combination of a strong desire for peer acceptance and rebellion toward authority makes adolescents optimal candidates for group therapy. Education groups, such as on prevention of infection by the human immunodeficiency virus (HIV), are effective with this age group. Alateen is effective for teenagers, particularly when alcoholic family members fail to support the adolescent. Peers coping with similar problems can be helpful and informative, strengthening one another's self-esteem. On the other hand, peers can also be cruel, scapegoating, and rejecting of each other. Group leadership skills are important with this age group to foster group cohesion, peer support, constructive behavior, and effective communication (Möhlen, Parzer, Resch, & Brunner, 2005). Nurses are in a good position to provide educational and emotional support to teens. Skillful nurse group leaders can facilitate peer support and role model effective communication.

ADULTHOOD

Adults dealing with the stressors of modern life use a variety of support and therapy groups related to specific psychological or social concerns. Women's self-actualization groups and support groups began in the 1970s as part of the women's movement. Men's support groups are a more recent phenomenon, starting in the mid- to late 1980s (Kipnis, 1991). These groups allow the members to deal with the general issues that are thought to be relevant to each gender and their social roles and expectations. Some of these groups are geared specifically toward homosexual persons.

There are also women's groups that address specific problems such as incest and molestation or physical abuse. These groups may be mutual-support groups modeled on the Twelve Step AA structure or they may be leader-facilitated therapy groups (Lau & Christensen, 2007; Stacciarini et al., 2007).

Group approaches are also very effective in substance abuse prevention and treatment with adults. At-risk adults who are children of alcoholics are a group that responds well to these approaches, which helps to break the intergenerational chain of alcohol and drug dependence. To maximize effectiveness, tobacco cessation programs rely heavily on group support to supplement medical measures such as nicotine replacements and antidepressants (Stead & Lancaster, 2005).

Pressures from social roles and transitions have spawned a variety of other types of support groups. For example, there are couples groups, multiple-family groups, parenting groups, new mothers groups, single parents groups, divorce groups, and bereavement groups. These groups are frequently short term (10 to 12 sessions) and have a brief therapy and psychoeducational structure. Ongoing support and social groups, such as Parents without Partners and Resolve (for infertility), are helpful when problems or concerns are not easily or quickly resolved.

Chronic medical conditions also frequently require ongoing support groups. Support groups for conditions such as cancer, HIV infection, acquired immunodeficiency syndrome (AIDS), multiple sclerosis, Parkinson's disease, and ostomies help people to adapt to the physical and psychological changes associated with shared maladies (Grande, Myers, & Sutton, 2006). Members of these groups share emotions and adaptation strategies with each other in an effort to gain and give comfort and hope. Because family members also are affected by the medical and psychological conditions of their loved ones, there are support groups to address their concerns. Alzheimer's disease support groups and the Alliance for the Mentally Ill are but two examples of these family support groups (Gallagher-Thompson & Coon, 2007).

OLDER ADULTHOOD

Persons over 65 years of age are considered elderly in American society. Because it is genetically and environmentally influenced, the aging process differs in each person. Regardless of individual differences, mental health may decline as health problems resolve. Participation in peer support groups, activity groups, religious or cultural organizations, volunteer centers, and senior citizens' centers may contribute to the maintenance of mental health. Older adults have rich past experiences, and opportunities to share and reminisce can provide benefit to others' mental health (Plastow, 2006).

Mental health problems of older adults that may be amenable to group therapy include depression, social isolation, and grief. Grieving often occurs in response to adjustment to retirement, widowhood, loss of physical health and independence, loss of role in the family, and loss of family support. Inpatient and outpatient group therapy might focus on the maintenance of self-esteem through support and peer acceptance. Skills that might be taught in groups include problem solving, coping, and confrontation of negative beliefs. Creative expression through literature, poetry, music, art, and humor can emphasize the universality about each individual's depth of the human experience.

Persons caring for their relatives with a dementing illness often suffer from depression. Coon and colleagues (2003) studied small groups of women (n = 169) over four months who were distressed caregivers and randomly assigned them to either anger management, depression management, or a wait-list control group. While the pretreatment level of depression and anger impacted mood and coping, women in the two treatment groups had significant reductions in anger and depression compared to the control group. The authors concluded that skills training is most effective for caregivers when their pretreatment characteristics are considered and group treatment is tailored to individual needs.

Many older adults must care for their spouses. Debilitating and progressive diseases take physical, emotional, and financial tolls on individuals and families. For example, elderly persons caring for a spouse with Alzheimer's disease suffer from more depression and anxiety than do noncaregiving spouses (Buffum, 1992). In a study of 96 elderly spouse caregivers of community-residing persons with Alzheimer's disease, Buffum and Brod (1998) found that the use of humor was significantly correlated with a sense of well-being. Indeed, caregivers of persons with advanced symptoms used less humor and had more psychological distress than those caring for persons with mild symptoms. To assist families in caring for their loved ones and for their own mental health, local chapters of the Alzheimer's Association offer regular and frequent support groups. These groups are educational as well as supportive. For some members, these groups are useful because they provide time away and a social network of understanding, new friends. Contemporary studies confirm the significance of support groups for caregivers of loved ones with Alzheimer's disease and other dementias (Gallagher-Thompson & Coon, 2007; Rabinowitz et al., 2006). Major outcomes from this research include reduced caregiver's distress and depression, self-efficacy, and improved coping and problem-solving skills. Psychiatric nurses are in key positions to identify signs and symptoms of caregiver's distress, involve families in the decision-making process, and make appropriate referrals for inpatient and community-based support groups.

CONFINED OLDER ADULTS

At retirement homes and nursing homes, groups provide residents with social opportunities. These include, but are not limited to, arts and crafts groups, day weekend outings, hobby clubs, dances, dinners, newspaper publications, exercise clubs, spiritual practices, and current events groups. Depending on the elders' level of functioning and motivation, the staff's creativity, and the financial resources of the facility, the possibilities are endless.

An example of staff creativity is the "Living in the Moment" group for patients with dementia who are residents of a nursing home. In one VA long-term care hospital, a social worker and nurse conduct a 90-minute, twice weekly group for patients with all levels of dementia. The group aims to stimulate, socialize, and actively engage the patients in meaningful activity. The structure involves introductions, saying the pledge of allegiance, orienting to the day and season, reviewing current events that include sports and reading horoscopes, chair exercises often with a ball, a special activity of the day (e.g., musical instruments, "name that tune," reminiscing about a holiday, favorite foods), hand-washing and snack, and summarizing the day's events before ending. According to the staff conducting the groups, the patients—despite their limitations—appear to enjoy the group, as evidenced in their facial expressions or verbalizations.

In a rehabilitation environment, Yaretzky, Levinson, and Kimchi (1996) described benefits of art therapy in a group of eight hospitalized older clients with stroke or femur neck fractures. Using clay and specific themes, the authors combined sensorimotor activities, social interaction, and future direction in leisure time activity. Art therapy is a way to promote verbal and nonverbal communication, self-disclosure, support, cognitive therapy, and physical and sensorimotor therapy.

Zerhusen, Boyle, and Wilson (1991) studied depressed older residents in an intermediate care nursing home in Ohio. Their cognitive group therapy program consisted of a 10-week program that met for two 1-hour sessions each week. Leaders offered education about depression, information about cognitive therapy, and expectations about the group and the roles of the members. Behavior change was taught through planning desired activities, and cognitive change was taught by confronting members' negative thoughts and providing alternatives. Zerhusen and colleagues found significant differences between pre- and postintervention scores on the Beck Depression Inventory (BDI) in persons who attended the cognitive therapy group. No improvement in BDI scores was seen in clients who attended music therapy groups or in control groups.

Jones (2003) tested two types of reminiscence interventions with 30 women with depression in a long-term care facility. The women were randomly assigned to either the facility's standard reminiscence group or to the "Nursing Interventions Classification" reminiscence group. Using

Brink's Geriatric Depression Scale, the level of depression at pretreatment was comparable between the groups. After a (3-week, six-session group treatment, the posttest scores indicated significantly lower depression levels in the nurse-initiated intervention, the "Nursing Interventions Classification" reminiscence treatment, than in the standard treatment.

The cognitively impaired older adults who reside in nursing homes or who attend senior day care centers also profit from group experiences. The focus of these groups is on the maintenance of self-esteem through supportive interaction. Often, this is done with reminiscence groups or with telling of humorous stories from the past. In cases of mild or nonprogressive impairment, groups can assist the individual to mourn loss of function and establish new goals in accord with decreased abilities (Snyder, Jenkins, & Joosten, 2007). Chao and colleagues (2006) reported additional benefits of reminiscence therapy for focusing on promoting strengths and abilities and increasing self-esteem and life satisfaction in older adults with depression residing in nursing homes.

VETERANS

Much of the group therapy research has come from the Department of Veterans Affairs hospitals. Many of the hospitals are teaching hospitals associated with universities. Also, veterans of military service are often accustomed to working in groups and helping each other as buddies. Problems that veterans of wars have in common include adjustment to civilian life and PTSD resulting from the trauma of combat or prisoner-of-war experiences. Currently, Vietnam War veterans use PTSD groups for support, spiritual development, management of anger, development of coping skills for living with others, and socialization. PTSD has been diagnosed in about 15 percent of the veterans who served in Vietnam and the 1991 Gulf War. Recent findings of returning combat veterans from Afghanistan and Iraq who have sought help at VA facilities have shown about a 10 percent incidence of PTSD. Those serving in ground units who are continuously or repetitively exposed to combat are at highest risk for PTSD or other mental disorders (Kang & Hyams, 2005). Likely, VA research will test new group modalities in efforts to prevent devastating long-term effects of PTSD.

Phases of treatment for PTSD include group therapy. Current research implicates the long-term efficacy of group therapy for clients with PTSD mitigates the intensity of PTSD symptoms (Gray, Elhai, & Frueh, 2004). Some researchers assert that although the intensity of PTSD symptoms are decreased with group therapy, changes in the personality of veterans with PTSD are deeply rooted and they continue to maintain some symptoms (Britvić, Radelić, & Urlić, 2006). Therapeutic interventions in groups include education, supportive confrontation, communication training, social skills training, relaxation training, stress management, problem solving, and goal setting. Other group treatment models have included veterans

suffering from the double trauma of war and childhood abuses, older veterans (Creamer, Elliott, Forbes, Biddle, & Hawthorne, 2006; Gray et al., 2004), group trauma reexposure therapy, trauma-focused group psychotherapy, and anger management.

Loo, Ueda, and Morton (2007) conducted a group therapy study that focused on race-related stressors among Vietnam veterans. They used an eclectic group intervention that integrated psychosocial education, identity reframing, cognitive differentiation, and cognitive restructuring, which focused on "depersonalizing discrimination" and rejection of faulty beliefs. Major outcomes from this study demonstrated this approach was effective in treating and reducing the psychological aftermath associated with adverse race-related events.

CURRENT RESEARCH ON GROUP THERAPIES/INTERVENTIONS

Nurses have been researching groups as part of their professional practice since the 1970s. They examine the uses of education groups, therapy groups, and support groups as interventions to help clients cope with physical and psychological conditions. The researchers either describe the process of using group interventions or evaluate the effectiveness of group interventions over other types of interventions.

Group treatment evaluation studies address the application of theory, varying populations, methods and styles of group therapy, and varying research methods. Based on Peplau's theory, Sorenson (2003) evaluated short-term cognitive group therapy to ameliorate distress that women felt from traumatizing provider interactions in their childbearing experience. The intervention was monthly for five 4-hour meetings and involved a curriculum for the telling of stories, a cognitive-behavioral program for depressed women, and a cognitive enhancement program with a workbook and exercises. The nine participants improved markedly from pre- to post-intervention, felt that group discussions helped them to validate their experience, and wanted more content related to trauma resolution.

An important theoretical work applies Hildegard Peplau's Interpersonal Theory of Nursing to group psychotherapy (Lego, 1998). Just as the nurse-client relationship produces improvement in clients' interpersonal relationships, the nurse fulfills many roles within a group context that parallel the one-to-one relationship. In a group setting the nurse moves the clients through phases known as orientation, identification, exploitation, and resolution. The nurse, known to the clients in their individual therapy prior to group, takes on new roles to foster improvements for clients to interrelate in group psychotherapy. Specifically, the nurse is a stranger, resource person, teacher, leader, surrogate parent, and counselor.

Another nurse researcher used a "Gruen" model of Postpartum Depression Group Therapy for a 10-week intervention combining education, stress reduction, support system development, and cognitive restructuring (Ugarriza, 2004). While depression decreased in the six participants in the treatment group compared with the eight participants in the no-treatment controls, the women felt education was most helpful. Most women had difficulty attending sessions related to childcare responsibilities.

Some researchers have focused on different therapies for depression in older women. Jones (2003) found that specific interventions for reminiscence based on the Nursing Interventions Classification system in six sessions over 3 weeks reduced depression better than the women's long-term facility standard program. Phoenix, Irvine, and Kohr (1997) utilized a unique nursing program of 10 weekly sessions with depressed women in a psychogeriatric clinic to improve coping, enhance learning, and promote insight. A major feature of their program was the opportunity for the women to share their stories.

Other nurse researchers study group therapy for symptoms associated with mental illness in in- and out-patient psychiatric settings. Miller, Eisner, and Allport (1994) have created the Creative Coping Group for patients during a short-term hospitalization for borderline personality disorder. Based on Linehan's Dialectical Behavior Therapy that addresses emotional control issues, interpersonal relationship effectiveness, and tolerance of distress, Miller and colleagues focused on precursors to chronic suicidal behavior. They used education, group exercises, discussion, and homework assignments to foster insight and awareness into symptoms, feelings, and behaviors. Buccheri and colleagues (2004), who have been teaching behavioral strategies to groups of persons with schizophrenia who have persistent auditory hallucinations, have found that participants have been able to sustain reduction in the intensity of voices for 12 months and anxiety for 9 months after completion of 10 classes.

Some researchers focus on research reviews. One nurse researcher group conducted a meta-analysis of 20 randomized clinical trials to evaluate the effectiveness of cancer support groups (Zabalegui, Sanchez, Sanchez, & Juando, 2005). They found that participation significantly improved participants' depression and anxiety and concluded that the positive impact warrants nurses' promotion of support groups to their patients. Weber and Sherwill-Navarro (2005) conducted a comprehensive literature review of psychosocial consequences of prostate cancer and included a review of support groups. They found large variation in types of groups, mens' perceptions of stigma in attending them, reluctance of men to seek emotional support through groups, and less use of groups by African-American men despite their higher prevalence of prostate cancer as compared to Caucasian counterparts. Those who attended support groups tended to be retired, Caucasian, well-educated professionals, and they reported fewer somatic symptoms than nonparticipants.

Several researchers acknowledge the benefits of groups specifically attuned to ethnic groupings. Jones, Brazel, Peskind, Morelli, and Raskind (2000) developed a group therapy program for African-American veterans with PTSD

and found that participants were more open and communicative with each other than when they were in racially mixed groups. Similarly, Hsiao, Lin, Liao, and Lai (2004) developed a therapy group for inpatients in Taiwan that incorporated traditional Chinese cultural values. Specifically, they established "pseudo-kin" relationships among participants and therapists, did warm-up exercises and structured activities, and used methods to focus on interpersonal issues—all in keeping with the value of maintaining harmonious relationships.

Qualitative studies provide the best description of group process and experiences. Gance-Cleveland (2004) conducted a school-based support group for adolescents with an addicted parent and found that participants generally felt empowered; they increased knowledge, improved coping, grew more resilient, improved interpersonal relationships, and improved school performance. Coggins and Bullock (2003) conducted focus groups to explore sexual and fertility challenges women face in abusive relationships; their analyses provide information about these women's reality and their thought processes for coping, survival, and staying in their relationships.

Qualitative studies offer the best details for replicating the types of groups they describe. Marzen-Groller and Bartman (2005) identify how to create a successful support group for new amputees that incorporates a peer visitation process for inpatients and future group members. Lanza, Demaio, and Benedict (2005) describe a support group for health care staff who have been violently assaulted. Both of these studies provide details about their program content and about participants' experiences.

Nurse researchers describe innovative approaches within groups. For example, Washington and Moxley (2004) describe methods for increasing self-efficacy in chemically dependent women in recovery through the use of scrapbooks and portfolios. DeMarco, Roberts, and Chandler (2005) conducted a pilot study to test a group writing intervention for decreasing nurses' negative behaviors in the workplace and found that cohesion and supportive relationships developed that enabled discussion of important topics. Similarly, Dellasega and Haagen (2004) conducted a pilot study to test the use of narrative writing within traditional group therapy methods with caregivers of older adults and found that participants improved their physical and mental health and established additional coping strategies.

Psychoeducational groups are often nurse researchers' focus for managing patients and their family responses to chronic conditions. Dysvik, Vinsnes, and Eikeland (2004) evaluated an 8-week multidisciplinary pain management program in 76 chronic pain patients using a cognitive-behavioral group approach to provide dialogue, education, and physical activity. Findings revealed improvements in coping and health-related quality of life; however, those who dropped out tended to be older and sicker.

Larson, Franzen-Dahlin, Billing, von Arbin, Murray, and Wredling (2005) conducted a randomized trial with 100 spouses of caregivers of stroke patients over 6 months. Fifty persons were assigned in groups of ten to the intervention and received six sessions about the nature of stroke, treatment and recovery, psychological and social effects, prevention of recurrence, followed by group discussion of these topics. The control group received only information during the patients' hospitalization and at discharge. Both groups were followed for 12 months. The authors found that caregivers who attended 5 to 6 times had a significant decrease in their negative well-being and an increase in quality of life.

In sum, nurses study the groups they develop and facilitate in efforts to improve all types of health outcomes. Earlier publications by van Servellen and colleagues (1991, 1992) have emphasized the importance of describing the purpose, process, and outcomes of groups led or co-led by nurses. They proposed a standardized protocol for documenting and evaluating studies of nurse-led groups on inpatient psychiatric units so that effectiveness can be systematically established; this protocol is presented in Table 27–7. Providing documentation of research findings will lead to evidence-based practice improvements and better patient outcomes.

SUMMARY

◆ The types of group therapies vary and include process, psychoeducation, task, self-help, and support groups.

◆ Group therapy began in the early 1900s with groups designed to provide education and emotional support.

TABLE 27–7
Protocol for Planning and Evaluation of Nurse-Led Groups on Inpatient Units

- Title of group
- Staff involved in design, study of the group, and leadership of the group
- Purpose and goals of the group
- Theoretical foundations for the group
- Group composition: client population, content, methods
- Outcome measures: evaluation methods, frequency of evaluation, group process, and documentation of individual progress

Note. Data from "Nursing-Led Group Modalities in a Psychiatric Inpatient Setting: A Program Evaluation," by G. van Servellen, E. Poster, J. Ryan, and J. Allen, 1991, *Archives of Psychiatric Nursing, 5,* 128–136. Adapted with permission.

Pratt, Metzl, Adler, and Moreno were the pioneers of group therapy.

◆ Yalom's 11 therapeutic factors are the aims for most groups today. Some work has been done to operationalize the factors for evaluating groups and exploring the relationship between the factors and client outcomes.

◆ Theoretical perspectives on group therapy come from psychology, social psychology, and sociology. Group behavior theories describe and predict people's behavior in groups and group settings, whereas group therapy theories prescribe interventions that promote positive change in group members.

◆ Theories of group therapy include six models: psychodynamic/psychoanalytic, interpersonal/interactional, communication/systems, group process/group analysis, existential/gestalt, and behavioral/cognitive. Different groups may be based on different perspectives; however, some groups are based on components of many theories. It is most important that the group therapist base her work on some theoretical foundation, lest the group lose its therapeutic mission.

◆ Evaluation of groups include discussion and analysis of the process and content of each session. Process is the patterns of interaction and the methods of communication. Content is the verbal and nonverbal themes of the session. Communication of each member and each therapist is looked at in relation to the whole group.

◆ Psychiatric nurses lead groups in many capacities. Advanced education and training are required for the role of therapist. Supervision and co-therapy are among the roles filled by the clinical specialist in psychiatric-mental health nursing.

◆ Staff nurses on psychiatric units participate in and lead groups based on needs of clients for education, support, recreation, task, exercise, symptom management, medication, and problem solving. In the community, nurses conduct groups based on specific needs and issues for clinic, medically ill, mentally ill, or homeless persons with psychosocial aspects of their situations.

◆ Many groups exist to help people with specific problems. Persons under stress may seek groups for support, education, and coping strategies. Most communities also provide group therapies for children, adolescents, and the elderly. Some groups are of the self-help type, having no professional leaders. *The Internet is a recent resource for self-help.*

◆ Nursing research has been focused on description, content, and effectiveness of group therapies offered to ill persons. Outcomes have included client satisfaction, symptom management, social interaction, and use of resources. Further outcome measurement research is needed to demonstrate specific results of group therapies.

SUGGESTIONS FOR CLINICAL CONFERENCES

1. Conduct a 1-hour, task oriented group with your peers. Record your observations at the end of the session. Explore group process and content regarding (a) who took the leadership position and how the group members responded; (b) how conflicts were resolved; (c) how problems were resolved; (d) the nature of each member's participation; and (e) members' satisfaction with the task accomplished.

2. Attend a group on the psychiatric unit or community based setting to which you are assigned. Identify the type and purpose of the group, theoretical perspective(s) of the leader(s), the characteristics of the leader(s) and the outcomes of the group.

3. Compare two groups. For example, attend an Alanon meeting and an Alzheimer's disease family support group. How are the groups similar? How are they different? Identify the type of group (task, activity, psychoeducation, or process oriented) and the theoretical perspective.

4. Explain how you would evaluate the effectiveness of the group.

STUDY QUESTIONS

1. Which is the most important composition for creating a therapy group?
   a. The clients are cognitively intact and do not abuse substances.
   b. The persons are of similar backgrounds and educational level.
   c. All clients have the same problem and same severity of illness.
   d. The persons are motivated to learn about themselves, their problems, and their interactions with others.

2. What is it called when a client leaves his group therapy session describing how he now knows he is not alone in his symptoms?
   a. Altruism
   b. Transference
   c. Interpersonal learning
   d. Universality

3. What term describes group leaders' discussion of the patterns of behavior of group members?
   a. Content
   b. Transference
   c. Countertransference
   d. Process

4. What term describes group leaders' discussion about what was said in the group?
   a. The nursing process
   b. Transference
   c. Group leadership
   d. Content

5. What activities best describe the nurse's role in group therapy?
   a. Assist the psychiatrist to conduct inpatient groups.
   b. Lead, co-lead, and plan in-patient psychotherapeutic groups.
   c. Set up medication classes and assist the clinical pharmacist in conducting the groups.
   d. Take notes during the group.

6. Theoretical frameworks that are the foundations of group therapy are derived from which three disciplines?
   a. Anatomy, physiology, and neurology
   b. Psychiatry, sociology, and neurology
   c. Psychology, social psychology, and sociology
   d. Group behavior theory, psychiatry, nursing

7. What might be the best outcomes for evaluating group therapy effectiveness?
   a. Client satisfaction, cost-effectiveness, and phone calls to leaders
   b. Client satisfaction, symptom improvement, coping skills
   c. Phone calls to leaders, complaints to agency director, attendance
   d. Complaints about group members, direct dialogue with leaders, attendance

8. During a medication group one of the clients expresses concerns about the new client's appearance. The new client was admitted to the unit several days ago. As the nurse group leader what is the most appropriate response to the client's comments?
   a. "You wouldn't want anyone attacking you, so leave Mr. J alone!"
   b. "What concerns you about his appearance?"
   c. "Are you concerned about his clothes or grooming?"
   d. "What do the rest of you think about Mr. J's appearance?"

9. You are the nurse leader of a dual diagnosis group and one of the clients attends the meeting smelling of alcohol and marijuana. The most appropriate response to the client is which of the following?
   a. "Have a seat and we will discuss this after the meeting."
   b. Ask members how they want to handle this situation.
   c. Remind the client about the rules concerning sobriety and ask him to leave.
   d. "Please go to the lab and submit a drug test."

10. While leading a stress debriefing group one of the staff point out a co-worker who is not participating. Which statement indicates another member understands the basis of stress debriefing group?
   a. "Members are here voluntarily and participants can remain silent if they wish."
   b. "All members are expected to participate in the group process."

c. "I am going to take notes and will share them at the end of the meeting if you like."

d. "Maybe she is just overwhelmed and unable to express her feelings at this time."

11. Two nurses are discussing plans for their client group. What should be in the plan to promote group cohesiveness?

a. Let the group know which clients are behaving in ways approved by the nurses.

b. Help the group identify group goals that are consistent with the individual members' goals.

c. Make most decisions about the group in advance and each group member aware of the nurses' decisions.

d. Seat the most talkative members nearest the nurse where they can be more clearly heard by the group.

12. The nurse is the leader of a client group. The members relate superficially, test each other and the group rules, and compete for the nurse's attention. This behavior is typical of which stage of group development?

a. Orientation

b. Working

c. Feedback

d. Termination

CRITICAL THINKING

1. How can the therapist demonstrate cultural competence in group therapy with ethnically diverse clientele?

2. What determines when you would refer a client to a support group versus an insight-oriented therapy group? How would you decide on the type of group?

3. What would be the advantages and disadvantages of using an eclectic model versus one particular model of group therapy?

4. What are the challenges in the nursing role in co-leading group therapy? What are some ways to address these challenges?

5. What are the unique contributions that nurses bring to group therapy?

6. What principles would guide your responses to feedback during clinical supervision about your interactions that occurred during group therapy?

7. When is it more therapeutic to address process than content in group therapy?

8. How would you determine the need for a group on an inpatient psychiatric unit?

9. What factors would you consider in establishing a group in an outpatient setting?

10. When would you think clients would benefit from a self-help group for substance abuse?

11. What determines when it is appropriate to refer adolescents to group therapy?

12. What are particular age-related benefits for older adults participating in groups?

RESOURCES

Please note that because Internet resources are of a time-sensitive nature and URL addresses may change or be deleted, searches should also be conducted by association or topic.

Internet Resources

1. Go to the website http://www.health.org, which is the national clearinghouse for drug and alcohol. Find information about Alcoholics Anonymous, Al-Anon, Alateen, Narcotics Anonymous.

2. Go through a search engine and find an online support group or chat room for depressed men and women.

3. Go to a website for group therapy about healing from a loss, such as http://www.losscounseling.com/about.html and determine what could be useful to share with a grieving person.

REFERENCES

American Nurses Association. (2000). *Scope and standards of psychiatric-mental health clinical nursing practice.* Washington, DC: Author.

Amir, M., Weil, G., Kaplan, Z., Tocker, T., & Witztum, E. (1998). Debriefing with brief group psychotherapy in a homogenous group of non-injured victims of a terrorist attack: A prospective study. *Acta Psychiatrica Scandinavica, 98*(3), 237–242.

Armstrong, M. A., & Rose, P. (1997). Group therapy for partners of combat veterans with post-traumatic stress disorder. *Perspectives in Psychiatric Care, 33*(4), 14–18.

Azarian, Y. (1992). Contemporary theories of group psychotherapy: A systems approach to the group-as-a-whole. *International Journal of Group Psychotherapy, 42,* 177–203.

Barlow, S., Burlingame, G., Nebeker, R. S., Anderson, E. (1999). Meta-analysis of medical self-help groups. *International Journal of Group Psychotherapy, 50*(1), 53–69.

Bäuml, J., Pitschel-Walz, G., Volz, A., Engel, R. R., & Kessling, W. (2007). Psychoeducation in schizophrenia: 7-year follow-up concerning rehospitalization and days in hospital in the Munich Psychosis Information Project Study. *Journal of Clinical Psychiatry, 68,* 854–861.

Beck, A., & Lewis, C. (2000) *The process of group psychotherapy: Systems for analyzing change.* Washington DC: American Psychological Association.

Berne, E. (1961). *Transactional analysis in psychotherapy.* New York: Grove.

Bonnivier, J. (1992). A peer supervision group: Put counter-transference to work. *Journal of Psychosocial Nursing and Mental Health Services, 30*(5), 5–8.

Bradford, L., Gibb, J., & Benne, K. (1964). *T-group theory and laboratory method: Innovations in re-education.* New York: Wiley.

Breuer, J., & Freud, S. (1957). In J. Strachey (Ed. and Trans.), *Studies on hysteria.* New York: Basic Books.

Britvić, D., Radelić, N., & Urlić, I. (2006). Long-term dynamic-oriented group psychotherapy of posttraumatic stress disorder in war veterans: Prospective study of five-year treatment. *Croatian Medical Journal, 47,* 76–84.

Brown, S. (1985). *Treating the alcoholic: A developmental model of recovery.* New York: Wiley.

Buccheri, R., Trygstad, L., Dowling, G., Hopkins, R., White, K., Griffin, J. J., Henderson, S., Suciu, L., Hippe, S., Kaas, M. J., Covert, C., Hebert, P. (2004). Long-term effects of teaching behavioral strategies for managing persistent auditory hallucinations in schizophrenia. *Journal of Psychosocial Nursing and Mental Health Services, 42*(1), 18–27.

Buccheri, R., Trygstad, L., Kanas, N., & Dowling, G. (1997). Symptom management of auditory hallucinations in schizophrenia. Results of 1-year follow up. *Journal of Psychosocial Nursing and Mental Health Services, 35*(12), 20–28.

Buccheri, R., Trygstad, L., Kanas, N., Waldron, B., & Dowling, G. (1996). Auditory hallucinations in schizo-phrenia. Group experience in examining symptom man-agement and behavioral strategies. *Journal of Psychosocial Nursing and Mental Health Services, 34*(2), 12–26.

Buffum, M. (1992). *Burden and humor: Relationships to men-tal health in spouse caregivers of Alzheimer's disease.* Ann Arbor, MI: University Microfilms International.

Buffum, M., & Brod, M. (1998). Humor and well-being in spouse caregivers of patients with Alzheimer's disease. *Applied Nursing Research, 11*(1), 12–18.

Carpenito-Moyet, L. J. (2006). *Nursing diagnosis. Application to clinical practice* (10th ed.). New York: Lippincott Williams & Wilkins.

Cartwright, D., & Zander, A. (1960). *Group dynamics research and theory* (2nd ed.). New York: Elmsford, Row & Peterson.

Chatziandreou, M., Tsani, H., Lamnidis, N., Synodinou, C., & Vaslamatzis, G. (2005). Psychoanalytic psychotherapy for severely disturbed borderline patients: Observations on the supervision group of psychotherapists. *American Journal of Psychoanalysis, 65,* 135–147.

Chao, S. Y., Liu, H. Y., Wu, C. Y., Jin, S. F., Chu, T. L., Huang, T. S., et al. (2006). The effects of group reminiscence therapy on depression, self esteem, and life satisfaction of elderly nursing home residents. *Journal of Nursing Research, 14,* 36–45.

Chou, A. F., Wallace, N., Bloom, J. R., & Hu, T. W. (2005). Variation in outpatient mental health service utilization under capitation. *Journal of Mental Health and Policy Economy, 8,* 3–14.

Coggins, M., & Bullock, L. F. (2003). The wavering line in the sand: The effects of domestic violence and sexual coer-cion. *Issues in Mental Health Nursing, 24*(6–7), 723–738.

Coon, D. W., Thompson, L., Steffen, A., Sorocco, K., & Gallagher-Thompson, D. (2003). Anger and depression management: Psychoeducational skill training interven-tions for women caregivers of relative with dementia. *The Gerontologist, 43,* 678–689.

Corey, G. (2000). *Theory and practice of group counseling* (5th ed). Pacific Grove Ca: Brooks/Cole.

Crane, D. R. (2007). Research on the cost of providing fam-ily therapy: A summary and progress report. *Clinical Child Psychology and Psychiatry, 12,* 313–320.

Creamer, M., Elliott, P., Forbes, D., Biddle, D., & Hawthorne, G. (2006). Treatment for combat-related posttraumatic stress disorder: Two-year follow-up. *Journal of Traumatic Stress, 19,* 675–685.

Crenshaw, B. G. (1989). Groups and group therapy. In B. Johnson (Ed.), *Psychiatric-mental health nursing* (2nd ed., pp. 199–221). Philadelphia: J. B. Lippincott.

Davidson, L. (2006). Supervision and mentorship: The use of the real in teaching. *Journal of the American Academy of Psychoanalysis and Dynamic Psychiatry, 34,* 189–195.

Dellasega, C., & Haagen, B. (2004). A different kind of caregiving support group. *Journal of Psychosocial Nursing and Mental Health Services, 42*(8), 46–55.

DeMarco, R. F., Roberts, S. J., & Chandler, G. E. (2005). The use of a writing group to enhance voice and connection among staff nurses. *Journal of Nurses Staff Development, 21*(3), 85–90.

Dreikurs, R. (1959). Early experiments with group psy-chotherapy: A historical review. In H. M. Ruitenbeck (Ed.), *Group therapy today* (pp. 18–27). New York: Atherton.

Drozdek, B., DeZan, D., & Turkovic, S. (1998). Short-term group psychotherapy of ex-concentration camp prisoners from Bosnia-Herzegovina. *Acta Medica Croatica, 52*(2), 119–125.

Dysvik, E., Vinsnes, A., & Eikeland, O. (2004). The effectiveness of a multidisciplinary pain management program managing chronic pain. *International Journal of Nursing Practice, 10,* 224–234.

Edwards, R. T., Céilleachair, A., Bywater, T., Hughes, D. A., Hutchings, J. (2007). Parenting programme for parents of children at risk of developing conduct disorder: Cost effectiveness analysis. *British Medical Journal, 334,* 682. Available online at http://www.bmj.com/cgi/content/full/334/7595/682

Ellis, A. (1992). Group rational-emotive and cognitive-behavioral therapy. *International Journal of Group Psychotherapy, 42,* 63–80.

Faden, V., & Goldman, M. (2004). Interventions for alcohol use and alcohol use disorders in youth. *Alcohol Research and Health 28*(3), 163–174.

Finfgeld, D. (2000). Therapeutic groups online: The good, the bad, and the unknown. *Issues in Mental Health Nursing, 21,* 241–255.

Fromm, E. (1957, March 16). Man is not a thing. *Saturday Review,* pp. 9–11.

Fuller, R., & Hiller-Sturmhofel, S. (1999). Alcoholism treatment in the United States: An overview. *Alcohol Research and Health 23*(2), 69–86.

Gallagher-Thompson, D., & Coon, D. W. (2007). Evidence-based psychological treatments for distress in family caregivers of older adults. *Psychology and Aging, 22*, 37–51.

Gance-Cleveland, B. (2004). Qualitative evaluation of a school-based support group for adolescents with an addicted parent. *Nursing Research, 53*(6), 379–386.

Gladfelter, J. (1992). Redecision therapy. *International Journal of Group Psychotherapy, 42*, 319–333.

Goldberg, C. (1970). *Encounter: Group sensitivity training experience*. New York: Science House.

Golkaramnay, V., Bauer, S., Haug, S., Wolf, M., & Kordy, H. (2007). The exploration of the effectiveness of group therapy through an Internet chat as aftercare: A controlled naturalistic study. *Psychotherapy and Psychosomatics, 76*, 219–225.

Goodwin, P. J., Leszcz, M., Ennis, M., Koopmans, J., Vincent, L., Guther, H., Drysdale, E., Hundleby, M., Chochinov, H. M., Navarro, M., Speca, M., & Hunter, J. (2001). The effect of group psychosocial support on survival in metastatic breast cancer. *New England Journal of Medicine, 345*, 1719–1726.

Grande, G. E., Myers, L. B., & Sutton, S. R. (2006). How do patients who participate in cancer support groups differ from those who do not? *Psychooncology, 14*, 321–334.

Gray, M. J., Elhai, J. D., & Frueh, B. C. (2004). Enhancing patient satisfaction and increasing treatment compliance: Patient education as a fundamental component of PTSD treatment. *Psychiatric Quarterly, 75*, 321–332.

Gregoire, I., Kalogeropoulos, D., & Corcos, J. (1997). The effectiveness of a professionally led support group for men with prostate cancer. *Urologic Nursing, 17*(2), 58–66.

Heldt, E., Blaya, C., Isolan, L., Kipper, L., Teruchkin, B., Otto, M. W., et al. (2006). Quality of life and treatment outcome in panic disorder: Cognitive behavior group therapy effects in patients refractory to medication treatment. *Psychotherapy and Psychosomatics, 75*, 183–186.

Hsiao, F-H., Lin, S-M., Liao, H-Y., & Lai, M-C. (2004). Chinese inpatients' subjective experiences of the helping process as viewed through examination of a nurses-focused, structured therapy group. *Journal of Clinical Nursing, 13*, 886–894.

Humphrey, K. (1996). World view change in adult children of Alcoholics/Al-Anon self-help groups: Reconstructing the alcoholic family. *International Journal of Group Psychotherapy, 46*(2), 255–263.

Jacobs, J., Horne-Moyer, H. L., & Jones, R. (2004). The effectiveness of critical incident stress debriefing with primary and secondary trauma victims. *International Journal of Emergency Mental Health, 6*(1), 5–14.

Jaffe, G. (2005, November 28). In Iraq's war zones, therapists take on soldiers' trauma. The Wall Street Journal, Al. http://www.WSJ.com, accessed 11/28/2005.

Jiang, J. X., Xia, X. L., Greiner, T., Lian, G. L., & Rosenqvist, U. (2005). A two year family based behaviour treatment for obese children. *Archives of Disease in Children, 90*, 1235–1238.

Jones, E. D. (2003). Reminiscence therapy for older women with depression: Effects of a nursing intervention classification in assisted-living long-term care. *Journal of Gerontological Nursing, 29*(7), 26–33.

Jones, L., Brazel, D., Peskind, E. R., Morelli, T., & Raskind, M. A. (2000). Group therapy program for African-American veterans with posttraumatic stress disorder. *Psychiatric Services, 51*(9), 1177–1179.

Jowsey, S. G., Taylor, M. I., Schneekloth, T. D., & Clark, M. M. (2001). Psychosocial challenges in transplantation. *Journal of Psychiatric Practice, 7*(6), 404–414.

Kaiser Permanente Members Website, http://members.kaiserpermanente.org/kpweb/classes/list.do, accessed December 31, 2005.

Kanas, N. (1991). Group therapy with schizophrenic patients: A short-term, homogeneous approach. *International Journal of Group Psychotherapy, 41*, 33–48.

Kang, H. K., & Hyams, K. C. (2005). Mental health care needs among recent war veterans. *New England Journal of Medicine, 352*(13), 1289.

Keefer, L., & Blanchard, E. B. (2005). A behavioral group treatment program for menopausal hot flashes: Results of a pilot study. *Applied Psychophysiological Biofeedback, 30*(1), 21–30.

Kehoe, N. C. (1999). A therapy group on spiritual issues for patients with chronic mental illness. *Psychiatric Services, 50*(8), 1081–1083.

Kelly, L., Caldwell, K., & Henshaw, L. (2006). Involving users in service planning: A focus group approach. *European Journal of Oncology Nursing, 10*, 283–293.

Kesey, K. (1963). *One flew over the cuckoo's nest*. New York: New American Library.

Kim, S., & Kim, J. (2001). The effects of group intervention for battered women in Korea. *Archives of Psychiatric Nursing, 15*, 257–264.

Kingsley, G. (2007). Contemporary group treatment of combat-related posttraumatic stress disorder. *Journal of the American Academy of Psychoanalysis and Dynamic Psychiatry, 35*, 51–69.

Kipnis, A. (1991). *Knights of armor*. Los Angeles: Jeremy Torcher.

Klose, P., & Tinius, T. (1992). A self-esteem group at an inpatient psychiatric hospital. *Journal of Psychosocial Nursing and Mental Health Services, 30*(7), 5–9.

Kurtz, E. (1979). *Not God: A history of AA*. Center City, MN: Hazelden Educational.

Lanza, M. L., Demaio, J., & Benedict, M. A. (2005). Patient assault support group: Achieving educational objectives. *Issues in Mental Health Nursing, 26*(6), 643–660.

Larson, J., Franzen-Dahlin, A., Billing, E., von Arbin, M., Murray, V., & Wredling, R. (2005). The impact of a nurse-led support and education programme for spouses of stroke patients: A randomized controlled trial. *Journal of Clinical Nursing, 14,* 995–1003.

Lau, M., & Kristensen, E. (2007). Outcome of systemic and analytic group psychotherapy for adult women with history of intrafamilial childhood sexual abuse: A randomized controlled study. *Acta Psychiatrica Scandinavica, 116,* 96–104.

Leardi, S., Pietroletti, R., Angeloni, G., Necozione, S., Ranaletta, G., & Del Gusto, B. (2007). Randomized clinical trial examining the effect of music therapy in stress response to day surgery. *British Journal of Surgery, 94,* 943–947.

Lego, S. (1998). The application of Peplau's theory to group psychotherapy. *Journal of Psychiatric and Mental Health Nursing, 5,* 193–196.

Leszcz, M. (1992). The interpersonal approach to group psychotherapy. *International Journal of Group Psychotherapy, 42*(1), 37–61.

Linehan, M. (1993). *Cognitive behavioral treatment of borderline personality.* New York: Guilford Press.

Linehan, M. (1993). *Skills training manual for treating borderline personality disorder.* New York, NY: Guilford Press.

Linnell, K. (2005). Chronic disease self-management: One successful program. *Nursing Economics, 23*(4), 189–198.

Lipscomb, J., & Synder, C. F. (2002). The outcomes of cancer outcomes research: Focusing on the National Cancer Institute's quality of care initiative. *Medical Care 2002, 40*(6 suppl): III 3–10.

Ljubotina, D., Pantić, Z., Franciskovic, T., Mladić, M., & Priebe, S. (2007). Treatment outcomes and perception of social acknowledgment in war veterans: Follow-up study. *Croatian Medical Journal, 48,* 157–166.

Loo, C. M., Ueda, S. S., & Morton, R. K. (2007). Group treatment for race-related stresses among minority Vietnam veterans. *Transcultural Psychiatry, 44,* 115–135.

Lu, L. (2007). Census reverses estimates of the number of underinsured population. *Center on Budget Policy and Priorities.* Available online at http://www.cbpp.org/4-5-07health.pdf

Macy, R., Behar, L., Paulson, R., Delman, J., Schmid, L., & Smith, S. (2004). Community-based, acute posttraumatic stress management: A description and evaluation of a psychosocial-intervention continuum. *Harvard Review of Psychiatry, 12*(4), 217–228.

Madrid, E., & Swanson, J. (1995). Psycho-educational groups for young adults with Genital Herpes: Training group facilitators. *Journal of Community Health Nursing, 12*(4), 189–198.

Marram, G. (1978). *The group approach in nursing practice* (2nd ed.). St. Louis, MO: C. V. Mosby.

Marzen-Groller, K., Bartman, K. (2005). Building a successful support group for post-amputation patients. *Journal of Vascular Nursing, 23,* 42–45.

Maslow, A. (1962). *Toward a psychology of being.* Princeton, NJ: Van Nostrand.

McCracken, L. M., & Black, M. P. (2005). Psychiatric treatment of the homeless in a group-based therapeutic community: A preliminary field investigation. *International Journal of Group Psychotherapy, 55*(4), 595–604.

Miller, C. R., Eisner, W., & Allport, C. (1994). Creative coping: A cognitive-behavioral group for borderline personality disorder. *Archives of Psychiatric Nursing, 8*(4), 280–285.

Miller, D. K., Chibnall, J. T., Videen S. D., & Duckro, P. N. (2005). Supportive-affective group experience for persons with life-threatening illness: Reducing spiritual, psychological, and death-related distress in dying patients. *Journal of Palliative Medicine, 8*(2), 333–343.

Miller, L. (2006). Critical incident stress debriefing for law enforcement: Practical models and special applications. International *Journal of Emergency Mental Health, 8,* 189–201.

Möhlen, H., Parzer, P., Resch, F., & Brunner, R. (2005). Psychosocial support for war-traumatized child and adolescent refugees: Evaluation of a short-term treatment program. *Australian and New Zealand Journal of Psychiatry, 39,* 81–87.

Mohr, S., Brandt, P. Y., Borras, L., Gilliéron, C., & Huguelet, P. (2006). Toward an integration of spirituality and religiousness into the psychosocial dimension of schizophrenia. *American Journal of Psychiatry, 163,* 1952–1959.

Moreno, J. (1946). Psychodrama and group therapy. *Sociometry, 9,* 249–253.

Mullan, H., & Rosenbaum, M. (1967). *Group psychotherapy.* New York: Free Press.

Pasquali, E., Arnold, H., & DeBasio, N. (1989). *Mental health nursing—A holistic approach* (3rd ed.). St. Louis, MO: C. V. Mosby.

Patterson, B. J., & Kelley, L. E. (2005). Lessons learned: One experience with focus groups in a school setting. *Journal of School Nursing, 21*(3), 158–163.

Perls, F. (1969). Gestalt therapy verbatim. Lafayette, CA: Real People Press.

Phoenix, E., Irvine, Y., & Kohr, R. (1997). Sharing stories. Group therapy with elderly depressed women. *Journal of Gerontological Nursing, 23*(4), 10–15.

Plastow, N. A. (2006). Libraries of life: Using life history books with depressed care home residents. *Geriatric Nursing, 27,* 217–221.

Poling, J., Oliveto, A., Petry, N., Sofuoglu, M., Gonsai, K., Gonzalez, G., et al. (2006). Six-month trial of bupropion with contingency management for cocaine dependence in a methadone-maintained population. *Archives of General Psychiatry, 63,* 219–228.

Pollack, L. (1990). Improving relationships—Groups for inpatients with bipolar disorder. *Journal of Psychosocial Nursing and Mental Health Services, 28*(5), 17–22.

Pratt, J. H. (1906). The "home sanitorium" treatment of consumption. In H. M. Ruitenbeck (Ed.). *Group therapy today* (pp. 9–17). New York: Atherton.

Rabinowitz, Y. G., Mausbach, B. T., Coon, D. W., Depp, C., Thompson, L. W., & Gallagher-Thompson, D. (2006). The moderating effect of self-efficacy on intervention response in women family caregivers of older adults with dementia. *American Journal of Geriatric Psychiatry, 14*, 642–649.

Reeve, J. (2006). Group psychotherapy with children on an inpatient unit: The MEGA group model. *Journal of Child and Adolescent Psychiatric Nursing, 19*, 3–12.

Riddell, K., & Clouse, M. (2004). Comprehensive psychosocial emergency management promotes recovery. *International Journal of Emergency Mental Health, 6*(3), 135–145.

Rogers, C. (1961). *Client centered therapy.* Boston: Houghton Mifflin.

Rogers, C. (1971). Carl Rogers describes his way of facilitating encounter groups. *American Journal of Nursing, 7*, 265–279.

Rogers, W. A. (2006). Feminism and public health ethics. *Journal of Medical Ethics, 32*, 351–354.

Roller, B. (2006). Group psychotherapy in psychiatric hospitals and clinics passes the 70-year mark. *International Journal of Group Psychotherapy, 56*, 501–504.

Rosenberg, N. K., & Hougaard, E. (2005). Cognitive-behavioural group treatment of panic disorder and agoraphobia in a psychiatric setting: A naturalistic study of effectiveness. *Nordic Journal of Psychiatry, 59*, 198–204.

Rossi, G., Bonfiglio, S., Veggiotti, P., & Lanzi, G. (1997). Epilepsy: A study of adolescence and groups. *Seizure, 6*, 289–295.

Ruff, C. C., Alexander, I. M., & McKie, C. (2005). The use of focus group methodology in health disparities research. *Nursing Outlook, 53*(3), 134–140.

Rummel, C. B., Hansen, W. P., Helbig, A., Pitschel-Walz, G., Kissling, W. (2005). Peer-to-peer psychoeducation in schizophrenia: A new approach. *Journal of Clinical Psychiatry, 66*, 1580–1585.

Rutan, J. C. (1992). Psychodynamic group psychotherapy. *International Journal of Group Psychotherapy, 42*, 19–35.

Ryle, A. (2004). The contribution of cognitive analytic therapy to the treatment of borderline personality disorder. *Journal of Personality Disorders, 18*(1), 3–35.

Scheidlinger, S. (2004). Group psychotherapy and related helping groups today: An overview. *American Journal of Psychotherapy, 58*, 265–280.

Schmidt, U., Lee, S., Beecham, J., Perkins, S., Treasure, J., Yi, I., et al. (2007). A randomized controlled trial of family therapy and cognitive behavior therapy guided self-care for adolescents with bulimia nervosa and related disorders. *American Journal of Psychiatry, 164*, 591–598.

Seal, N. (2006). Preventing tobacco and drug use among Thai high school students through life skills training. *Nursing and Health Sciences, 8*, 164–168.

Seng, T. K., & Nee, T. S. (1997). Group therapy: A useful and supportive treatment for psoriasis patients. *International Journal of Dermatology, 36*, 110–112.

Shechtman, Z. (1991). Small group therapy and preadolescent same-sex friendship. *International Journal of Group Psychotherapy, 41*, 227–243.

Sherman, J. J. (1998). Effects of psychotherapeutic treatments for PTSD: A meta-analysis of controlled clinical trials. *Journal of Traumatic Stress, 11*(3), 412–435.

Smith, D. J. (1998). Horticultural therapy: A garden benefits everyone. *Journal of Psychosocial Nursing and Mental Health Services, 36*, 14–21.

Snyder, L., Jenkins, C., & Joosten, L. (2007). Effectiveness of support groups for people with mild to moderate Alzheimer's disease: An evaluative survey. *American Journal of Alzheimer's Disease and Other Dementias, 22*, 14–19.

Sorenson, D. S. (2003). Healing traumatizing provider interactions among women through short-term group therapy. *Archives of Psychiatric Nursing, 17*(6), 259–269.

Stacciarini, J. M., O'Keefe, M., & Mathews, M. (2007). Group therapy as treatment for depressed latino women: A review of the literature. *Issues in Mental Health Nursing, 28*, 473–488.

Stead, L. F., & Lancaster, T. (2005). Group behaviour therapy programmes for smoking cessation. *Cochrane Database Systematic Reviews, 18*, CD001007.

Stinson, C. K., & Kirk, E. (2006). Structured reminiscence: An intervention to decrease depression and increase self-transcendence in older women. *Journal of Clinical Nursing, 15*, 208–218.

Storch, M., Gaab, J., Küttel, Y., Stüssi, A. C., & Fend, H. (2007). Psychoneuroendocrine effects of resource-activating stress management training. *Health and Psychology, 26*, 456–463.

Storch, E. A., Geffken, G. R., Merlo, L. J., Mann, G., Duke, D., Munson, M., et al. (2007). Family-based cognitive-behavioral therapy for pediatric obsessive-compulsive disorder: Comparison of intensive and weekly approaches. *Journal of the American Academy of Child and Adolescent Psychiatry, 46*, 469–478.

Sullivan, H. S. (1953). *The interpersonal theory of psychiatry.* New York: Norton.

Sullivan, K. (2000). On the efficiency of managed care plans. *Health Affairs, 19*(4), 129–148.

Till, J. (2003). Evaluation of support groups for women with breast cancer: Importance of the navigator role. *Health and Quality of Life Outcomes, 1*, 16.

Trygstad, L., Buccheri, R., Dowling, G., Zind, R., White, K., Griffin, J., Henderson, S., Suciu, L., Hippe, S., Kaas, M., Covert, C., & Hebert, P. (2002). Behavioral management of persistent auditory hallucinations in schizophrenia: Outcomes from a 10-week course. *Journal of the American Psychiatric Nurses Association, 8*, 84–91.

Ugarriza, D. N. (2004). Group therapy and its barriers for women suffering from postpartum depression. *Archives of Psychiatric Nursing, 18*(2), 39–48.

van Servellen, G., Poster, E., Ryan, J., & Allen, J. (1991). Nursing-led group modalities in a psychiatric inpatient setting: A program evaluation. *Archives of Psychiatric Nursing, 5,* 128–136.

van Servellen, G., Poster, E., Ryan, J., Allen, J., & Randell, B. (1992). Methodological concerns in evaluating psychiatric nursing care modalities and a proposed standard group protocol format for nurse-led groups. *Archives of Psychiatric Nursing, 6,* 117–124.

Verkuyten, M. (2005). Ethnic group identification and group evaluation among minority and majority groups: Testing the multiculturalism hypothesis. *Journal of Personality and Social Psychology, 88,* 121–138.

Wagner, S. L. (2005). Emergency response service personnel and the critical incident stress debriefing debate. *International Journal of Emergency Mental Health, 7,* 33–41.

Washington, O. G., & Moxley, D. P. (2004). Using scrapbooks and portfolios in group work with women who are chemically dependent. *Journal of Psychosocial Nursing and Mental Health Services, 42*(6), 42–53.

Weber, B. A., & Sherwill-Navarro, P. (2005). Psychosocial consequences of prostate cancer: 30 years of research. *Geriatric Nursing, 26*(3), 166–175.

Webster-Stratton, C., Reid, M. J., & Hammond, M. (2004). Treating children with early-onset conduct problems: Intervention outcomes for parent, child, and teacher training. *Journal of Clinical Child and Adolescent Psychology, 33,* 105–124.

Whitaker, D., & Lieberman, M. (1969). *Psychotherapy through the group process.* New York: Atherton.

White, T. M., Gibbons, M. B., & Schamberger, M. (2006). Cultural sensitivity and supportive expressive psychotherapy: An integrative approach to treatment. *American Journal of Psychotherapy, 60,* 299–316.

Winship, G., & Hardy, S. (2007). Perspectives on the prevalence and treatment of personality disorder. *Journal of Psychiatric Mental Health Nursing, 14,* 148–154.

Wituk, S., Shepherd, M. D., Slavich, S., Warren, M. L., & Meissen, G. (2000). A topography of self-help groups: An empirical analysis. *Social Work, 45*(2), 157–165.

Yalom, I. (1983). *Inpatient group psychotherapy.* New York: Basic Books.

Yalom, I. (1985). *The theory and practice of group pscyhotherapy* (3rd ed.). New York: Basic Books.

Yalom, I. (1995). The theory and practice of group psychotherapy, 4th ed. New York: Basic Books.

Yaretzky, A., Levinson, M., & Kimchi, O. L. (1996). Clay as a therapeutic tool in group processing with the elderly. *American Journal of Art Therapy, 34*(3), 75–82.

Young, K. M., Northern, J. J., Lister, K. M., Drummond, J. A., & O'Brien, W. H. (2007). A meta-analysis of family-behavioral weight-loss treatments for children. *Clinical Psychology Reviews, 27,* 240–249.

Zabalegui, A., Sanchez, S., Sanchez, P. D., & Juando, C. (2005). Nursing and cancer support groups. *Journal of Advanced Nursing, 51*(4), 369–381.

Zerhusen, J. D., Boyle, K., & Wilson W. (1991). Out of the darkness: Group cognitive therapy for depressed elderly. *Journal of Psychosocial Nursing and Mental Health Services, 29*(9), 16–21.

SUGGESTED READINGS

Klein, R. H., & Schermer, V. L. (2000). *Group psychotherapy for psychological trauma.* New York: Guilford Press.

Rutan, J. S., & Stone, W. N. (2001). *Psychodynamic group psychotherapy* (3rd ed.). New York: Guilford.

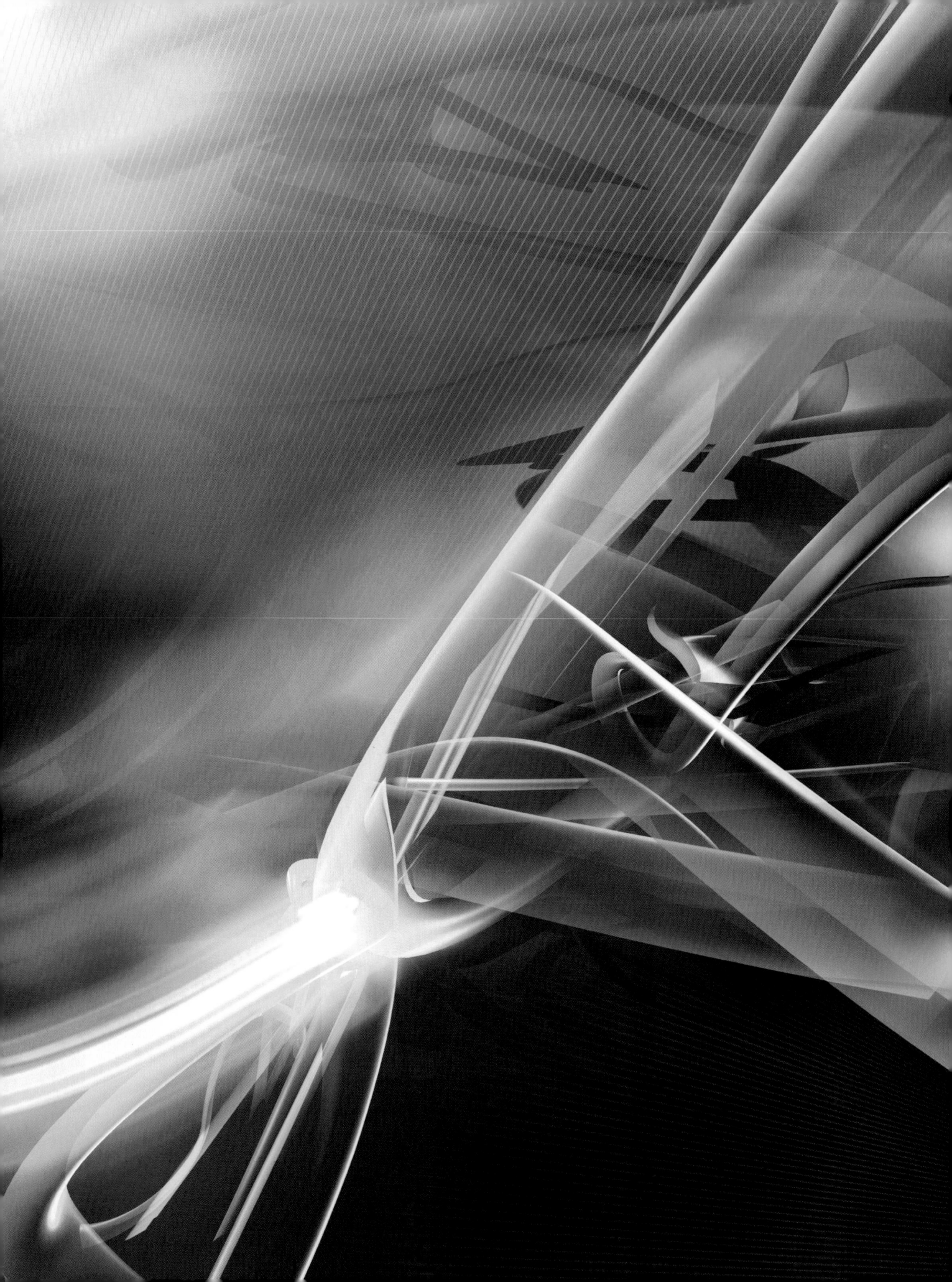

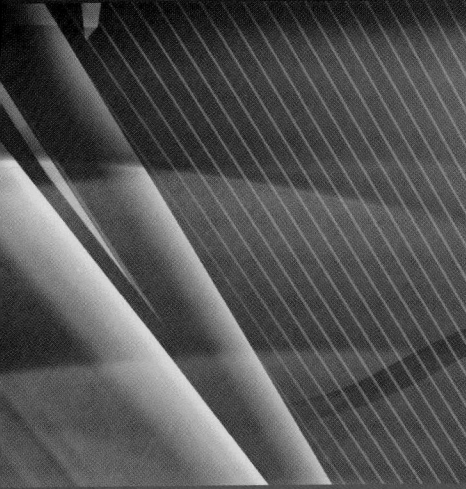

CHAPTER 28

Familial Systems and Family Therapy

Deborah Antai-Otong, MS, APRN, BC, FAAN

KEY TERMS

Boundaries: Rules that define who and how members participate in a subsystem or relationship.

Closed System: In system's theory, this refers to a limited exchange of energy and information about the environment. Boundaries are often rigid and impermeable.

Congruent Communication: Refers to messages that do not contradict each other. Normally, these messages promote clear and consistent boundaries and roles and effective problem solving.

Disengagement: Implies that family boundaries are rigid or impermeable and distant.

Double-Bind Messages: Refers to transactions that involve a binder and a victim.

Dyad: A two-person relationship, such as husband-wife and father-child.

Enmeshment: Implies overinvolvement or lack of separateness of family members.

Equilibrium: Refers to the capacity of a system to use available resources to manage and reduce tension and stress.

Family: Refers to a dynamic system of people living together who are united by meaningful emotional bonds.

Family Roles: Expected patterns or specific behaviors within a social context.

Family Structure: The manner in which a family adapts and maintains itself.

Family Therapy: Also a specialized intervention that is used to treat clients within a social context, rather than individually.

Feedback Mechanism: A process that permits exchange of energy and matter across various boundaries.

Functional Family System: Refers to open systems composed of individuals, couples, children, and communities who are able to adapt to change or crisis.

Genogram: A family assessment tool that maps pictorial illustration of family history (generations).

Identified Client: Refers to the client whose symptoms are the focus and serve as the reasons for seeking treatment.

Incongruent Communication: Occurs when more than one message is sent and the messages contradict each other.

Marital Schism: A term used to describe intense marital conflict in which a parent attempts to enlist a child as an ally against the other parent.

Marital Skew: Severe marital discord arising from acceptance of maladaptive behaviors in one partner by the other partner.

Open System: In systems' theory, a term used to imply that members or parts are interrelated and responsive to each other's needs.

Pseudomutuality: A transaction that infers a sense of relatedness and emotional connectedness; in reality, it represents shallow and empty relationships.

Relational Resilience: Refers to the family's ability to mobilize resources and confront psychosocial and biological stresses effectively using adaptive coping responses.

Scapegoating: A form of displacement that involves blaming a member for the actions of others.

Subsystem: A smaller system within larger systems.

Transactional: Refers to a set of pattern interactions among family members.

Triangulation: A term that describes a maladaptive triad transactional pattern.

COMPETENCIES

Upon completion of this chapter, the learner should be able to:

1. Recognize societal trends and their impact on family structure
2. Discuss family roles and structures.
3. Compare the functional family system and the dysfunctional family system.
4. Analyze major maladaptive family communication patterns.
5. Discuss the role of culture on family roles and functioning.
6. Describe the evolution of families across the life span.
7. Develop a nursing care plan for the family experiencing crisis.

CHAPTER OUTLINE

The American family is transforming and this transformation parallels immense societal changes. Since the early 1960s, young adults have delayed marriage and chosen to use effective birth control. The result of this is that fewer children are being born and parents are older than the typical couples of decades ago. In addition, over the past few decades there has been a surge in the divorce rate, and the number of single-parent families has increased. This trend has remained stable the past two decades. Two-parent homes declined from 81 percent in 1980 to 72 percent in 1999 (U.S. Bureau of the Census, 2001). Households headed by a single parent grew from just under 6.1 million in 1980 to nearly 7.8 million in 1999 and accounted for 20 percent of family households (U.S. Bureau of the Census, 2001). Of these data single fathers comprised 2 percent of family households with their own children under 18 in 1980 and 5 percent in 1999, while single mothers comprised 18 percent of these households in 1980 and 23 percent in 1999 (U.S. Bureau of the Census, 2001).

Furthermore, family structures have evolved from the traditional couple with 2.4 children to single-parent families, gay and lesbian couples, grandparents functioning as parents, and single-person households. Traditional couples and families still exist, however, and for many people it is the only definition of a "real" family. Nurses are challenged to work with people in various relationships as familial systems.

Regardless of its composition, the family serves numerous purposes within a society. Early family interactions serve and provide the foundation of lifelong relationships and adaptive processes such as effective problem-solving and communication skills. Likewise, families provide a sense of identity through cultural transmission, safety, belongings, and social parameters (Minuchin, 1974).

This chapter explores familial interactions and their influence on the development of adaptive and maladaptive behaviors in social contexts. The major concepts of family therapy are discussed, drawing on the work of pioneers such as Salvador Minuchin, Jay Haley, Carl Whitaker, and others. These family therapists' contributions are the foundation of current approaches to family and marital therapy.

CHARACTERISTICS OF FAMILIAL SYSTEMS

Numerous societal changes have made it difficult to define the term *family*. This term stems from the Latin word, *familie*, meaning "household or dwelling place." Simply speaking, a family is a dynamic system of people living together who are united by meaningful emotional bonds. The family has two major functions: It ensures survival of the species and transmits culture. Families are complex systems. Their ability to integrate biological, psychosocial, spiritual, and cultural factors is determined by family structure and roles (Ackerman, 1958; Baumann & Beckingham, 1990; Robinson, 1997; Satir, 1967; Tay & McCubbin, 2002).

FAMILY STRUCTURE

Family structure refers to the forms a family takes in adapting and maintaining itself (Minuchin, 1974). The heart of the family structure is the dyad. A dyad is a two-person relationship, either adult-adult relationship or adult-child relationship. Dyads determine roles, culture, and function. The increase in the divorce rate, single-male parents, and gay couples with children have contributed to a change in the definition of family structure. Thus, there is an increased need for nurses to understand family interactions and function and their role in promoting the health of family members.

Table 28–1 lists some types of family structures. The nuclear and extended families are two examples. The extended family normally consists of a nuclear family and three generations (Walsh, 1982). Historically, extended families have been a vital source of caring for the young, older adults, and the sick. Less traditional family structures, such as stepfamilies, unmarried couples, and single-parent families, have gained acceptance over the past decade.

Overall, the family structure determines how family members interact and carry out their functions in the family. Specifying what constitutes a family is a complex process that is greatly influenced by societal trends and tolerance of diversity.

TABLE 28–1
Major Family Structures

Type	Composition
Nuclear Family	Parents and children (adopted or conceived)
Blended or Stepfamilies	Remarried members with children from a previous marriage or relationship
Extended Family	Multigenerational—at least two generations consisting of nuclear family, which include children, aunts, uncles, cousins, and others who reside together
Single-Parent Family	One-parent family (widowed, divorced, separated, never married male or female)
Other Familial Systems	Individuals living together because of common bonds, loyalties, and goals

FAMILY ROLES

Family roles are the behavioral patterns or specific behaviors that are expected of persons within the family context. These roles are learned, goal directed, and transmitted within the family. Roles help the family fulfill its functions. Moreover, they are the foundation of children's early interactions with primary caregivers, who provide a repertoire of responses to children's needs. People's roles and relationships with others in adulthood are built on their early interactions with their primary caregivers (Spiegel, 1957). Industrialization conferred traditional family roles to institutions such as nursing homes, extended care, and day care centers.

Women's gender role has evolved from staying at home and raising children to working to bring a second paycheck into the household. Furthermore, women have the freedom to pursue various careers that were traditionally held by men. These societal changes have resulted in increased responsibilities for women. For example, by desire or default, they are the primary caregivers of children and housekeeping, as well as employees outside of the home. Role overload can affect their emotional closeness with partners. Reductions in quality time, intimacy, and emotional support increase the likelihood of marital and family stress. Family crisis often erupts under these conditions (Fauchier & Margolin, 2004; Kaczynski, Lindahl, Malik, & Laurenceau, 2006).

Men, like women, face societal and family stress involving the changing role of parenthood. This is particularly evident with seriously ill children. Research indicates that fathers are often less prepared to cope with the child's illness and spouse's distress. Furthermore data indicate that the fathers' responses to family stress can be explained as impacted by gender roles, and the perceptions of access to quality of support systems, work, and health care providers. Interventions provide fathers and families with the parenting skills training that enhance coping with stresses and challenges of taking care of a seriously ill child (Pelchat, Lefebvre, & Levert, 2007; Sullivan-Bolyai, Rosenberg, & Bayard, 2006).

Epstein and Bishop (1981) divided family roles into two categories: necessary family functions and other family functions.

Necessary Family Functions

Necessary family functions refer to those family roles that are critical to the health and well-being of family members. Epstein and Bishop (1981) identified the following as necessary family functions:

- Allocation of resources (e.g., food, water, shelter, and financial)
- Nurturance and emotional support (e.g., validation, reassurance, and comfort)
- Sexual gratification of marital partners or couples (e.g., initiating and responding to each other's sexual needs)
- Development of life skills (e.g., academia and personal development)
- Maintenance and management of family systems (e.g., negotiating and problem-solving skills, managing finances)

Other Family Functions

Epstein and Bishop (1981) defined *other family functions* as roles that are not essential for adaptive functioning but are part of the family developmental process. These functions may be maladaptive or adaptive. Maladaptive functions are related to parental conflict and subsequent family turmoil. In contrast, adaptive functions involve healthy families to allocate roles, use authority, and deal with conflicts effectively, and are flexible in adapting to role changes. These qualities maintain and promote health among family members. See Table 28–2 for a description of additional family functions.

THEORETICAL CONSIDERATIONS

Distinguishing theoretical considerations that play roles in functional and dysfunctional family interactions is both interesting and necessary for the psychiatric nurse. The following section focuses on various theories and concepts of family dynamics and human interactions.

HEALTHY FAMILY SYSTEMS

Defining a healthy family system is difficult. Most family theory research focuses on maladaptive responses in members. Over the past 30 years, research has identified healthy family patterns and strengths. Family strength has been delineated as healthy familial interactions and relationships that foster self-esteem and a positive outlook on life (Otto, 1962). Moreover, healthy family systems are capable of withstanding and rebounding from crisis and distress because of their relational resilience. Relational resilience refers to the family's ability to mobilize resources and confront psychosocial and biological stresses effectively using adaptive coping responses to foster a

---

TABLE 28–2
Duvall's Major Family Tasks

- Physical maintenance
- Allocating resources
- Division of labor
- Socialization of members
- Procreation and separation of family members
- Maintaining order
- Placement of members into society
- Maintenance of motivation and morale

Note. From *Family Development* (3rd ed.), by E. Duvall, 1977, Philadelphia: J. B. Lippincott. Adapted with permission.

sense of collaboration, competence, and confidence in its members (Beitlin & Allen, 2005; Walsh, 1996, 2003; Walters, McDonough, & Strohschein, 2002).

In systems theory, healthy or functional family systems are open systems composed of individuals, couples, children, and communities. Cultural factors are an integral aspect of open systems and govern system members' behavior inside and outside the family system. In functional families, members' biological, psychosocial, and cultural needs are met. Health is correlated with adaptation to change or crisis generated by developmental stages. Ultimately, the manner in which the family manages and copes with a crisis or stressful event and reorganizes and resolves these events has a far-reaching impact on its members' immediate and future adaptation (Walsh, 1996, 2003). The McMaster Model of Family Function (Epstein & Bishop, 1981; Epstein, Bishop, & Baldwin, 1982) is based on systems theory and defines six areas of family function that influence healthy outcomes in times of crisis or change:

◆ *Problem solving* that provides basic human needs
  Example: Parents talk to the teenager about the mother's promotion and need to relocate. The teenager expresses feelings about the move, with encouragement from the parents. All agree that this is a difficult choice, but the move is necessary.

◆ *Communication* that is clear, congruent, and direct
  Example: Parents are clear about the necessity of relocating and expressing their concerns and feelings. The teenager is able to understand the basis of the move while expressing feelings about leaving friends. Each member is allowed to express feelings in a clear, direct, and congruent manner.

◆ *Role allocation* that suits family members' interests and is otherwise appropriate and allows for role sharing
  Example: In this scenario, the father has to quit his job and seek new employment. In the meantime, the family accepts that the father may have difficulty finding employment and he may have to reverse roles with the mother (i.e., household chores previously performed by the mother).

◆ *Affective responsiveness,* wherein emotions are expressed freely, are validated, and are accepted
  Example: The members of this family have been able to share their feelings and concerns, with validations from the parents and the teenager about the family's relocation plans.

◆ *Affective involvement,* in that family members are sensitive to each other's needs
  Example: Family members in this scenario feel sadness and disappointment about moving because of their close ties with the community. Individual expression of feelings and concerns enable the family members to resolve their problems as an open system.

◆ *Behavioral control,* in the form of flexible rules and feedback mechanisms

Example: Although the family members have limited choices about the move, they are able to make a decision about neighborhoods and possible employment plans concerning the father's job and adolescent's choice of school.

Family function evolves throughout the life span. Societal and technological changes continue to shape family norms. Each generation perpetuates the former generation's culture and adaptive processes. Nurses' personal family experiences and perception of the family are critical to their understanding of the role of family dynamics and their role in modeling family members' behavior, responding to change, and promoting health.

GENERAL SYSTEMS THEORY

In their classic works, von Bertalanffy (1968) and Miller (1965) surmised that the human organism is part of a system and critical to its maintenance. Systems theory delineates the major components of systems and hierarchy of subsystems that comprise the whole. A number of theorists have described families as systems that function as interdependent parts or members. Furthermore, families are subsystems within larger social systems and within a suprasystem composed of individual members and their biological systems (Bronfenbrenner, 1979; Haley, 1962).

As a dynamic social system, the family provides intimacy for the mates, opportunities for procreation, economic well-being of members, cultural transmission, education on both verbal and nonverbal communication, and modulation of emotions. Family structure determines the rules, roles, and communication patterns of the family (Napier & Whitaker, 1978).

According to the general systems theory, the major components of a system are (1) interrelatedness of parts, (2) boundaries, (3) modulation of tension and stress, (4) equilibrium, and (5) feedback mechanisms. Systems require continuous feedback and resist major changes to ensure maintenance of homeostasis.

Interrelatedness of Parts

Interrelatedness, or wholeness, infers that change in one part affects the entire system.

Boundaries

Its members, social interactions, and boundaries determine system identification. Boundary delineation is the basis of family function, the family, and the roles and hierarchy of the members of the family, all of which govern the action and participation of members (Minuchin, 1974). Moreover, boundaries maintain the individuality of the system's members, that is, the separateness between and within subsystems. The family defines the role and hierarchy of its members through boundaries that govern their action and participation in the system. Furthermore, boundaries protect certain aspects of the system members' roles, expectations, and communication patterns. Clearly defining boundaries, which serve as the mechanism for transmitting data (energy), and maintaining some degree of freedom for the system are capabilities of functional family systems. Predictable family environments provide safety, security, and growth. Conversely, blurred, rigid, or inconsistent rules and boundaries increase the likelihood of crisis or symptoms in members. Blurred or undefined boundaries include triangulation, disengagement, and enmeshment (Minuchin, 1974). Triangulation refers to a three-person or triad emotion interaction. For instance, parents argue often and one of them enlists one of the neighbors by asking, "Sean, what do you think about your Harry being out all night?" By bringing the neighbor (third person) into the argument, the couple is unable to resolve "their" issues. When working with families who use this form of communication, it is imperative for the nurse family therapist to avoid becoming the "third person" in the triangle. Disengagement implies that family boundaries are rigid, impermeable, and distant. For example, one of the children asks a question concerning the upcoming family outing because of a project at school. Rather than asking the child about his project, the parents distance themselves from the child and refuse to discuss this issue. Enmeshment implies overinvolvement or a lack of separateness of family members. Blurred boundaries are seen in the case of incest. A sexual relationship between a child and a parent is unacceptable and inappropriate because it involves crossing intergenerational boundaries between the adult (parent) and child. Incest may be acceptable or tolerated within the family, but society shuns it and considers it unacceptable and illegal.

Modulation of Tension and Stress

Tension and stress are inherent in systems because of the individuality among system members, which manifests itself in interactions, actions, and reactions. The regulation of system pressures is vital to sustaining equilibrium. Families who are experiencing tension and stress must respond effectively to reduce the likelihood of maladaptive responses or crisis.

Scenario

A female gang member physically assaulted the Carter family's oldest daughter after a football game. She returned home emotionally distressed. Her parents called the police to have the gang member arrested. The daughter had difficulty coping with the situation and was initially emotionally withdrawn and depressed. Her parents became upset because they were unable to help their child. Tension in the family mounted as members became irritable and agitated. The school nurse referred them to an advanced-practice psychiatric-mental health nurse for family psychotherapy.

During their initial sessions, the nurse psychotherapist inquired about the event and asked each member to discuss his or her feelings about the recent event and what they needed from each other to resolve this family crisis. The marital dyad and family dynamics were assessed, including family strengths, resources, and communication and coping patterns. Questions concerning treatment outcomes and family preference helped the family develop a sense of control and treatment strategies that facilitated healthy crisis resolution. After several sessions, they began to express feelings about the incident and pulled together as a family. The daughter began to interact with family members in the sessions and at home. Tension and stress were lowered and the family returned to a precrisis level of function.

This scenario demonstrates several system components. The family's ability to seek help from each other indicates that the Carter family is an open system. In open systems, members are interrelated and are responsive to each other's needs (Miller, 1965; von Bertalanffy, 1968). In addition, open systems nurture self-worth, value, and appreciation of change (Satir, 1967). Mr. and Mrs. Carter exhausted their coping skills, but they recognized the need to help their daughter through a stressful ordeal. Family psychotherapy provided crisis intervention, which represented an exchange of energy or feelings across boundaries and information about the environment or trauma. It mobilized resources, supported adaptive behaviors, and encouraged the formation of new coping skills.

In contrast, closed systems limit the exchange of energy and information about the environment. Had the Carter family ignored their daughter's feelings and behavior, she may have become seriously disturbed, depressed, or suicidal. Likewise, if they had been unable to discuss their own feelings and be open to family therapy, the family would have remained stagnant or "stuck" at this stage unable to resolve the crisis and grow as a family. Closed systems are normally chaotic, destructive, and dysfunctional because members have distorted perceptions of themselves and the world (Satir, 1967).

Fortunately, the Carter family was able to restore equilibrium by using internal and external resources. Their coping skills were adequate psychosocial and biological resources, which allowed them to effectively manage and reduce family tension and stress.

Equilibrium

A system's equilibrium is sustained when sufficient resources are available for the system to manage and reduce tension and stress. Maximizing resources reduces the risk of maladaptive responses and illness and act as buffers to restore and maintain homeostasis.

As living systems, families evolve and change throughout the life cycle. Family evolution is a complex process that involves biological, psychosocial, and developmental components. Living systems are maintained by organization, competence, and coherence, which continuously create and sustain life (Maturana & Varela, 1991; Slesnick, Bartle-Haring, & Gangamma, 2006). Developmental crises such as the birth of a child require families to use adaptive coping processes to facilitate growth and maintain equilibrium in members and the system.

Feedback Mechanisms

Feedback mechanisms permit the exchange of energy and matter across various boundaries. Systems are influenced by and affect their environments. Feedback mechanisms enable systems to modify their structure, encourage growth, and change within acceptable parameters. Feedback mechanisms determine if a system is open or closed.

People are social beings who continuously interact within social contexts and have experiences that are psychological, biological, and sociocultural in nature. Humans function within social systems or families that have expectations, roles, communication patterns, and rules that maintain equilibrium. The advanced-practice psychiatric-mental health nurse must be able to work with families and communities with sociocultural and emotional contexts. Working with families requires assessing their strengths, resources, communication patterns, and willingness to change. The level of change often parallels the family system's health. The role of the nurse family therapist offers a wealth of opportunities for families to use adaptive coping skills that facilitate and restore health to each member.

COMMUNICATION OR TRANSACTION THEORY

The word *communication* stems from the Latin word, *communicatus*, which means to "impart, participate, or share." Communication is verbal and nonverbal and involves the conveying and receiving of thoughts, feelings, and ideas within a social context. Communication is more than simply sending a message and is "qualified, modified, reinforced, contradicted, and specially framed" (Weakland, 1976, p. 117). Clear communication patterns facilitate healthy interactions and interpersonal relationships. Healthy family interactions arise from clear communication patterns. In contrast, unclear, incongruent, or impaired communication patterns interfere with social interaction and increase the risk of maladaptive responses that lead to unhealthy family interactions. See Chapter 6 for an in-depth discussion of therapeutic communication.

INCONGRUENT COMMUNICATION

Incongruent communication occurs when more than one message is sent and the messages contradict each other. Incongruence between what is said and what is meant produces confusion. Normally, these messages accompany inconsistent smiling, frowning, or tone of voice (Satir, 1967). The mother who slaps her child while saying "I love you" and the husband who, with a smile, tells the wife that he hates her are examples of incongruent communication. Family members often make statements that are contradictory or qualified. Early in the history of family therapy, impaired communication was considered the sole basis for serious mental illnesses such as schizophrenia and was related to family chaos and confusion (Haley, 1959). Recent advances in neurobiological research have dispelled this myth and indicate a relationship among neurobiology, genetic, and psychosocial factors as the cause of mental illness. Although biological advances explain and modulate family transactions, other factors such as

psychosocial stressors continue to play a vital role in creating and maintaining system function. Healthy family transactions involve various roles and processes that foster problem solving, negotiating, and effective communication.

The nurse therapist must be a resource person, active observer, and effective educator, and teach families how to achieve clear communication. Through observations and interpretation of family transactions, the nurse therapist affords the family adaptive and effective techniques in communication (Smoyak, 1975). The burden of deciphering communication rests on the receiver. Effective communication is vital to healthy family function and is particularly important during infancy and early childhood because the members' perceptions of themselves and the world are based on their early interactions with primary caregivers. Communicating trust and love during formative years is crucial to developing healthy adult relationships. In addition, family roles, function, and culture are transmitted by verbal and nonverbal communication. Furthermore, impaired communication patterns interfere with problem solving, self-esteem, coping, and negotiating, subsequently increasing stress and tension among members.

IMPAIRED COMMUNICATION

Ineffective communication patterns play major roles in family crisis. A number of theorists have defined impaired communication patterns. They include scapegoating, marital schism, marital skew, double-bind messages, and pseudomutuality.

Scapegoating

Scapegoating involves blaming a family member for the actions of another family member. It is a form of displacement whereby more threatening issues may be shunned. An example of scapegoating is the adolescent whose mother yells at him for his tardiness at school when she is really angry at her husband for being out all night. Scapegoating tends to keep the marital dyad or couple from focusing on their problems. In this case, the wife focused on problems with the adolescent to divert attention from marital conflict.

Marital Schism

Marital schism occurs when one spouse consistently belittles the other, there is chronic and severe marital discord (Lidz, Fleck, & Cornelison, 1965), and one or both parents actively secure a child as an ally in marital conflict. This concept is similar to triangulation, which enlists a third person, but not necessarily a child. An example is the father who criticizes his wife in front of the children, seeking an alliance against her. Serious parental conflicts are minimized or discounted by marital schism, but intimacy is compromised, and the parents fail to provide the children's emotional, social, and cultural needs.

Marital Skew

Marital skew happens when the dominant or controlling parent exhibits maladaptive behaviors and the other submits or accepts them without question. For instance, a husband feels powerless because his wife is sexually aloof and cold. Dependency and masochism are major themes in this marital or couple dyad. Emotional and physical abuses within the dyad are examples of dependency and masochism. Lidz and colleagues (1965) surmised that these conflicts contribute to distortions, denial, and irrationality in children.

Double-Bind Messages

Double-bind messages are transactions that involve a binder and a victim. The victim cannot escape the binding and is "caught up in an ongoing system which produces conflicting definitions of the relationship and consequent distress" (Bateson, Jackson, Haley, & Weakland, 1962, p. 157). In other words, the conflicting messages cause the person to question relationships with the family. The victim is unable to respond to or get out of the situation. A clinical example is the adolescent who attempts to separate from family by forming relationships with his peers. The parents express dismay and use guilt to keep the youth from becoming autonomous. Bowing to pressure, he cancels a date and stays home with his parents. The parents' overprotectiveness and smothering focus on the youth rather than on marital conflict. The youth perceives unclear communication of affection generated by his parents, evoking guilt and punishment for seeking autonomy or separation. Double-bind messages represent incongruent communication patterns, which is discussed next.

Pseudomutuality

Pseudomutuality is a transaction that implies a sense of relatedness and emotional connectedness, but in reality represents shallow and empty relationships. This term is synonymous to "fitting together as a family at the expense of self differentiation". A distorted, superficial, or an inflated sense of unity tends to prevent intimacy and creates distance and turmoil in the family. Deluded family transactions hinder change because they maintain the status quo. The child learns that there is inconsistency between what is real (e.g., her parents are always fighting) and what is said (e.g., "We don't disagree or argue about anything because we have a perfect marriage"). Confusion and chaos are sustained because making changes would force parents to admit they are denying marital conflict.

CONGRUENT COMMUNICATION

Congruent communication patterns afford members with clear and consistent boundaries and roles and effective problem-solving skills. Like incongruent communication, congruent communication involves more than one message, but in this case, the messages do not contradict each other. An example is the man who looks at his child and says "I love you" then reaches out and gently caresses her on the head. The verbal and nonverbal messages are congruent because both convey warmth and caring.

At the heart of healthy family interactions is the communication ability of the marital or couple dyad. Clear, open, direct, and honest communication between the two members of the dyad is crucial to healthy family function. Healthy communication also includes spontaneity, validation, and responsiveness to new input or new ideas (Lewis, Beavers, Gassett, & Phillips, 1976). Differences and disagreements are perceived as acceptable and valued rather than threatening to the health of the system. The health of family members often parallels the family's ability to tolerate, value, and encourage individuality. Family conflicts are inherent and essential for individual and family system growth and development. Problem solving, negotiation, and conflict resolution are skills passed on by healthy couples. Healthy, stable dyads provide family members with psychosocial and biological support that fosters autonomy and self-esteem. These behaviors are critical to the family's ability to manage crisis and maintain health.

Families often seek therapy because of crises stemming from impaired communication or transactional patterns and family tension. Nurse psychotherapists can help families improve their communication patterns that facilitate healthy crisis resolution. Family therapy involves identifying maladaptive transactions between members, focusing on family and individual strengths, and facilitating effective problem-solving skills that promote health in members and the system.

CULTURAL CONSIDERATIONS

Culture provides people with a repertoire of values, beliefs, traditions, rituals, and a perception of themselves and the world. The characteristics of culture are that (a) it is learned or conveyed through generations, (b) it is adaptive and evolving, and (c) it is composed of unique components and patterns (Mead 1955; Young, 1944). Understanding ethnicity is pertinent for individuals working with families because ethnicity determines cultural norms and values associated with family function, problem solving, and the methods of caretaking. Moreover, ethnicity and cultural factors also affect nurses' therapeutic approaches to care (Abernethy, Houston, Mimms & Boyd-Franklin, 2006; McGoldrick, Giordano, & Garcia-Preto, 2005). Culture links intergenerational values, beliefs, and rituals. Intergenerational "connectedness" also generates a sense of belonging, comfort, and self-validations within family systems. Because family development is influenced by cultural factors as well as psychosocial and biological ones, nurses' understanding of individuals and families can be strengthened by appreciating cultural needs and uniqueness.

In addition to understanding the family's psychosocial, biological, and cultural needs, the nurse must also be aware of his culture and ethnicity and their potential impact on the nurse's perception of the family's symptoms and needs. The nurse therapist must be able to assess the family's cultural and psychosocial needs and implement a culturally sensitive plan of care. See Chapter 7 for a discussion of cultural and ethnic considerations.

CULTURAL INFLUENCES ON FAMILY ROLES

Family roles are usually determined by cultural factors related to access to community systems. For instance, being able to provide for the basic needs of family members has a profound effect on a person's self-concept and place within the family and society.

To cite one segment of the population, the African American man's provider role recurrently depends on his access to community systems or the workforce. Those who access these systems are viewed the same as other ethnic groups. They have financially enabling factors—social, economical, and emotional resources—that help them provide for themselves and their families. The quality of the *provider role* affects decision making, child rearing, and the quality of marital relationship. However, barriers that reduce access to community systems, such as education and financial equity, often inhibit African Americans and other ethnic groups from filling their role of family provider (McAdoo, 1993).

ASSESSING THE ROLE OF CULTURE ON FAMILY FUNCTIONING

The American society is a diverse population made up of a number of cultures. Assessing families' cultural needs involves approaching them with awareness that each family has unique needs. Stereotyping perceptions of families can interfere with objective data collection and formulation of interventions. Assessing the role of the influence of culture on health is complex and must take into account such things as dietary restrictions, health practices, management of stress, and roles (Abernethy et al., 2006; Antai-Otong, 2002; Boyd-Franklin, 1989; Chung, Kim, & Abreu, 2004).

The definition of family varies among cultural groups. African Americans often refer to families as a wide network of kin and community. Italian Americans' family values imply a strong, tightly knit three- or four-generation system. Asian American families place tremendous value on solidarity in their community and connectedness but are reluctant to expose family conflict to outsiders because it reflects disloyalty. The traditional Chinese family system includes ancestors and descendants (Chung et al., 2004). Regardless of culture, the definition of family is diverse and the nurse therapist must establish its meaning with each family encounter to provide individualized family interventions and facilitate adaptive behavioral changes (Hodge, 2005; Mitrani, Feaster, McCabe, Czaja, & Szapocnik, 2005).

Family theorists and advanced-practice psychiatric nurses and other psychotherapists increasingly attend to the cultural factors embedded within the family context. Family therapists also recognize the impact of the therapeutic process and treatment outcomes of their own culture. In addition, nurse therapists need to be cognizant of their own values and beliefs implicit in their theoretical framework. Understanding the family's sociocultural and environmental contexts are vital for interpreting the meaning and function of family behavior and developing culturally sensitive interventions (McGoldrick, Giordano, & Garcia-Preto, 2005).

Regardless of culture or ethnicity, when families seek therapy, they share a story, which contains a choice of aspects told and those left untold (Rothbaum, Rosen, Ujiie, & Uchida, 2002). Stories emphasize some issues, while other issues remain obscure. What the family shares rests on the *culture of the therapy*. When the nurse psychotherapist and family meet, each brings their separate culture (i.e., values, beliefs, religion, stories, and expectations). During the sessions, a new culture evolves that blends the two cultures (those of the nurse and family). The nature of the new culture of therapy depends on the family's previous experiences in therapy, initial contact with the nurse, and the nature of communication between the two (Pare, 1996; Tuyn, 2003). Pare (1996) adds that the culture of therapy gives meaning to or frames the phenomena and transactions that transpire throughout family therapy.

Nurse family therapists can facilitate the culture of therapy through self-awareness and knowledge of cultural diversity. Self-awareness and understanding diverse cultures are pivotal to establishing a therapeutic relationship and understanding the family's experiences and needs. Likewise, nurses must understand their own culture and ethnicity and their impact on clinical practice. Odell, Shelling, & Young (1994) suggested several ways for health care providers to develop culturally sensitive family interventions:

- ◆ Understand the effect of ethnicity and culture on family roles and functions.
- ◆ Avoid stereotyping by recognizing the variability of normative family structures and functioning within and among diverse cultures.
- ◆ Be aware of subtle cultural variation in language, such as nonverbal expression of distress.
- ◆ Adapt therapeutic approaches to the family's cultural patterns.
- ◆ Be flexible and innovative to facilitate adaptive behavioral changes within the family system.
- ◆ Use family support systems inherent with specific family cultures and communities.

By integrating these concepts into their practice, nurse therapists can respond proactively to the increased emphasis on multiculturalism in the United States. Working with families requires sensitivity to the family's cultural heritage and awareness of their unique transactional or communication patterns, attitudes, rituals, and behaviors. See Chapter 7 for a detailed discussion of cultural issues.

EVOLUTION OF FAMILIES ACROSS THE LIFE SPAN

The evolution of families is both intriguing and multifaceted. Numerous influences determine how the family evolves over time, deals with individuality, responds to crisis, and nurtures its members.

FAMILY DEVELOPMENT

The concept of family cycle refers to the evolution of family systems. This process is influenced by functional and dysfunctional coping styles that affect the provision of basic needs, interactional patterns, and procreation. Historical patterns, maintenance of behaviors, and survival describe the evolution of a family in terms of a three-generation concept that unites older and younger generations.

Persons, like families, evolve over time. Families depict persons in stages across the life span. Developmental stages are marked by enormous energy and potential for growth and change, according to Erikson's (1963) description of normal developmental (adaptive) and abnormal (maladaptive) responses of growth and development. Duvall's (1977) work identified various stages of the family cycle and their role in creating and maintaining culture and meeting members' needs (see Table 28–2). Her work provides a classic explanation of expected family developmental tasks. Like Erikson, she asserted that each stage is predictable and parallels individual and family development. Other family theorists have described families in terms of changing family cycles. These stages are based on family patterns that parallel societal shifts (e.g., decreased birth rates and increased aging population) and are referred to as

1. the individual
2. the couple
3. families with children
4. families with adolescent children
5. middle-aged couples (contraction and partnership stages)
6. older couples (disappearance stage) (Carter & McGoldrick, 1988; Howells, 1975).

Mastery of each stage affects subsequent stages of adaptation and is modulated by internal and external demands on the system, which maintains continuity and growth.

THE INDIVIDUAL

Securing a place in society, sexual gratification, and a sense of intimacy are major developmental issues for young adults. Adults normally enter relationships at various developmental stages, seeking to separate from their family of origin and form a sense of identity. Identity often integrates professional goals and sexuality. Biological, psychosocial, cultural factors, as well as ego function, are crucial to this developmental task. The effort to prove that one is capable of independent living and using effective decision making produces stress. Mastering intimacy depends upon successful resolution of previous developmental crises. Whether one received trust, love, and acceptance from one's primary caregivers is at the heart of whether one achieves intimacy (Erikson, 1963).

Self-assuredness and the ability to form meaningful relationships enable young adults to take responsibility for their general well-being. Joining the workforce, finding an apartment, or buying a new car promote a sense of accomplishment and strengthen self-esteem and independence. Managing daily household chores and negotiating boundaries with the family of origin facilitate separateness and individuation in extended families. These transitions are the foundation of intimate relationships. Intimate relationships can meet psychosocial, cultural, and physical needs (Thomas, 1992).

THE COUPLE (DATING/COURTSHIP AND EARLY MARRIAGE STAGES)

Two people may be brought together by complementary needs and a sense of completeness, commitment, belonging, and sharing. Creation of a viable union involves negotiating one's relationship with one's family of origin. Separation issues play a key role in this success. Successful mastery of intimacy is vital to healthy intimate interpersonal relationships. Delineation of roles and boundaries, negotiation of differences, and acceptance of each other's limitations and strengths are key transactions during courtship. Later, negotiation of differences and conflicts is undertaken and continues during early marriage (Skynner, 1976).

Satir (1988) noted that people in successful relationships:

1. Believe that people are human (i.e., imperfect)
2. Understand and know themselves (i.e., identity, self-differentiation)
3. Are responsible for their behavior and able to stand on their own feet (i.e., independent and have clear boundaries)

Marriage is usually the culmination of these relationships; however, couples may choose to remain unmarried. Commitment to the new family challenges the couple to develop a sense of self-worth, risk taking, and potential for growth (Satir, 1988). Many cultures perceive marriage as a bond and commitment between two people. Each person brings a repertoire of biological, psychosocial, and cultural qualities that affects their perception of themselves and the world and their ability to manage stress and maintain meaningful relationships. Individual and couple strengths are linked to the management of conflicts and adaptation to change across the life span (Thomas, 1992).

When two people fall in love and decide to marry, there is hope that life will be happier. Love between two people is generally considered to be one of the most rewarding human experiences (Erikson, 1968). Self-worth is often tied to the quality of the relationship. People with high self-esteem are inclined to need less validation from their partners than do those with low self-esteem. People with low self-esteem are more likely to depend on their partners for fulfillment of emotional needs, a sense of self-worth, and survival. Satir (1988) claimed that couples have three parts: "you, me, and us" (p. 145). The development of each is crucial to a healthy marriage or meaningful relationships. These terms imply self-differentiation, which fosters healthy adult relationships.

As the relationship evolves, couples learn how to relate to each other and appreciate similarities and differences. These qualities are pertinent to formation of meaningful relationships. Trust promotes autonomy and effective problem solving. Healthy couples have a clear sense of identity, independence, and intimacy. The developmental tasks of early marriage are (1) formation of particular dyad boundaries, (2) initiation of relationships with in-laws, (3) formation of a satisfactory sexual relationship, (4) planning for children, and (5) formalizing of careers (Thomas, 1992).

BLENDED AND STEPFAMILIES

America's divorce rate has risen over the past two decades and has played a role in the increased prevalence of blended families, or stepfamilies. Major conflicts in stepfamilies arise from members' attempts to adjust to different roles and rules and their sense of family loyalty. The person who marries someone with children from a previous marriage has the monumental task of adjusting to a ready-made family. The problems are compounded when both persons have children. Children often feel loyal to their natural parents and perceive the new marriage as betrayal (Whiteside, 1983).

The major tasks of the stepfamily are listed in Table 28–3. Time is a key aspect in the resolution of stepfamily issues.

Psychiatric mental health nurses who work with families must be cognizant of their own definition of families to ensure their values and beliefs do not interfere with those of clients and their families. (See Myths about Stepfamilies.) Stepfamilies and blended families are complicated systems and require time to establish new rituals and traditions. Typically it takes 4 to 7 years for individuals to get acquainted; create positive relationships; and develop new rituals, traditions, and family history. Similar to other developmental issues the age in which stepfamilies or blended families form is governed by numerous factors, but the age of the child or children plays a

---

Myths about Stepfamilies

Myth: The only real family involves biological parents.

Reality: Today the definition of family has changed and it varies among people. Since 50 percent of all marriages end in divorce, stepfamilies are more the norm than the exception. There are single-parent, foster, step, and blended families—each family has its own uniqueness and each is worthwhile.

---

key role in how well they adapt to new families. It is imperative for the parents and nurse to understand normal developmental behaviors unique to age group to determine normalcy versus difficulty adapting or resistance or hostility. Younger children (e.g., less than 10 years of age) adjust easier due to their need to bond and have close and stable family relationships. They are also more accepting of a new sibling or parent, especially when the parent displays warmth and caring. Depending upon the nature of the child's relationship with biological factors, abandonment issues may surface during the transition. Adolescents have the most difficult time dealing with stepfamilies and blended families. Developmental issues concerning independence and opposition to authority figures coupled with these changes make it difficult to accept and adapt to the new family system (Grych, Raynor, & Fosco, 2004). It is important for the family to understand these issues and allow time for the youth to adjust to the new family. It is important to maintain normal rules and expectations and provide consistent and firm limits during adolescence and this transition. Encourage the biological (custodial) parent to remain mainly responsible for limit setting and discipline of the children until the stepparent forms a strong bond with them (Cheng, Dunn, O'Connor, & Golding, 2006; Dunn, O'Connor, & Cheng, 2005).

THE FAMILY WITH CHILDREN (EXPANSION AND CONSOLIDATION STAGES)

This life cycle involves moving from dating, early courtship, and early marriage. Normally, this involves a couple without children. The subsequent stage involves expanding the dyad and expanding it to include pregnancy, the birth experience, and young children. Similarly, to other developmental stages it challenges the family to mobilize resources and cope with inherent stressors.

The Family with Young Children

Pregnancy and the birth experience precipitate major developmental changes. Anticipation of the new arrival places tremendous stress on the couple and other children already in the family. Major stressors include uncertainty of their competency as parents, the need to provide adequate caretaking, and the need for stable employment. The birth of and bonding with a child are major developmental tasks for the new parents. Appreciation of parental roles and support for

---

TABLE 28–3
Major Tasks of Stepfamilies

- Mourn loss or resolve issues from the previous relationship or marriage.
- Establish new family traditions and rituals.
- Develop a stable relationship with spouse or partner (give enough time to restructure roles and functions).
- Form new relationships.

Note. From "Late-Life Marriages, Older Stepfamilies, and Alzheimer's Disease," by D. R. Kuhn, D. J. Morhardt, and G. Monbrad-Framburg, 1993, *Families in Society: The Journal of Contemporary Human Services, 74,* pp. 154–162; and "Families of Remarriage: The Weaving of Many Life-Cycle Threads," by M. Whiteside, 1983, in *The Family Life-Cycle: Implications for Therapy* (pp. 100–110), by H. A. Liddle (Ed.), Rockville, MD: Aspen Systems.

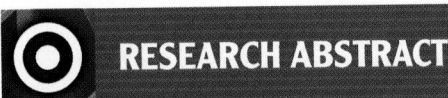

RESEARCH ABSTRACT

Spiritual Experiences of Parents and Caregivers Who have Children with Disabilities or Special Needs

Speraw, S. (2006). *Issues in Mental Health Nursing, 27,* 213–230.

Study Problem/Purpose

The purpose of this phenomenological study was to highlight personal experiences of parents and caregivers who sought to provide formal religious education for their children with special needs or disabilities.

Methods

Researchers used applied phenomenology described by Thomas and Pollio (2002) and Merleau-Ponty's existential philosophy to assess the nature of human experience from a personal perspective. Researchers used face to face, 1- to 3-hour taped interviews in the clients' homes to gather data with a goal of obtaining the fullest quality of the phenomenon using transcripts, assessing contextual underpinnings, and synthesis of key themes. Subjects included 26 parents/caregivers and 44 children with special needs and 15 different faiths.

Findings

Data analysis revealed that a lack of recognition from religious leaders and members of faith communities of spirituality of children with special needs generated a sense of helplessness or disillusionment and feelings of alienation and lack of emotional support. Caregivers and families who felt their children were accepted and welcomed expressed feeling support and strengthened by their faith.

Implications for Psychiatric Nurses

Spirituality and religious beliefs offer caregivers/parents a source of acceptance and support when caring for children or family members with special needs. They often represent the basis of the family's coping skills and source of support. Nurses are poised to perform a spiritual assessment and inquire about the caregiver's quality of support and strengths when dealing with challenging situations. Developing quality nurse-client relationships provides a venue to understand the client and family's experience.

each other buffer couples against feelings of inadequacy and promote healthy interactions and growth.

Emerging changes of men's gender roles place them in active parental roles. Men are discovering the emotional and biological rewards of forming intimate relationships with their children. Fathers who willingly accept their role functions in the process of child rearing gain self-esteem and fulfillment (Garfield & Isacco, 2006). The arrival of a child has a profound effect on the marital and family relationships. The couple moves from nurturing each other to caring for a human being totally dependent on them for maintenance of biological and psychosocial needs (Skynner, 1976). As the child becomes mobile and more independent, the healthy couple encourages and validates the child's autonomy. The toddler's newfound independence promotes self-esteem and separateness. The emergence of identity begins as the child realizes that boundaries exist between himself and his parents. Parents' tolerance of autonomy is critical to the child's mastery of this developmental stage. Resolution of attachment or bonding aids the child in moving from his relationships with his parents to society (Bowlby, 1969).

The child's progression through various developmental stages coincides with the family cycle. Adaptation and mastery of developmental milestones maintain homeostasis. The phase of consolidation centers on managing stress generated by problems of adolescence, independence in children, and conflicts between parents and siblings. Conflicts create tension and stress within the family system. Change fosters growth, spontaneity, and health.

The Family with Adolescent Children

Each developmental phase places enormous stress on families. Adolescence is one of the most stressful times in the family cycle. The adolescent tests the issues of control and autonomy with family renegotiation. As the adolescent's cognitive abilities mature, a search for identity begins, and the youth starts to integrate and evaluate his relationships with peers and question parental authority. Developmentally, adolescence generates tension and intensifies family turmoil. This developmental stage is represented by the maturation of the adolescent-parent relationship. Inevitably, parents and adolescents develop a balance of autonomy and closeness (Diamond & Liddle, 1999). Functional parents support, reinforce, and favor the adolescent's autonomy, self-direction, and independence. Increased family involvement in decision making increases internal motivation and positive self-esteem. Flexible family boundaries empower adolescents with some form of freedom in moving back and forth across them (Beveridge & Berg, 2007).

The family's successful mastery of transitions is determined by its repertoire of biological, psychosocial, and cultural resources. Developmental stages challenge parents to provide safe, caring, and open systems that promote trust, autonomy, initiative, industry, and identity (Erikson, 1963). Chapters 2 and 15 present detailed descriptions of developmental tasks.

Functional and Dysfunctional Families

Table 28–4 lists the characteristics of functional and dysfunctional familial systems. Functional, or healthy, families adapt to changes effectively, promoting developmental transitions. Boundaries remain well defined and predictable,

TABLE 28-4
Characteristics of Functional and Dysfunctional Familial Systems

Components	Functional Families	Dysfunctional Families
Family structure	Provides for basic needs (i.e., biological, psychosocial, cultural), clear role delineation	Neglects basic needs, irrational, and confused role delineation
Differentiation (refers to the degree of individuality and togetherness)	Parents are well differentiated with sense of identity, loyal to nuclear family, and separation from family of origin	Lack of identity, fusion, enmeshment, lack of autonomy, lack of separation from family of origin
Communication patterns	Spontaneous, congruent, clear, direct, and honest	Distorted, superficial, vague, exaggerated, contradictory, incongruent communication (i.e., scapegoating, marital skew, double-bind messages)
Boundaries (refer to rules defining and maintaining individuality between subsystems)	Clearly delineated between members and subsystems, flexible and adaptable to change	Blurred, lack of clarity, rigid, inconsistent, and fail to adapt to change and tension
Emotional/affective responsiveness	Genuine warmth and affection expressed between subsystems (i.e., parents, parent-child, sibling-sibling)	Distant, hostile, cold, aloof, and superficial

yet flexible, and have adequate feedback mechanisms to sustain the open system.

In dysfunctional families, boundaries are rigid or blurred. The marital dyad is the heart of family health or dysfunction. When parents fail to adapt to their children's changing developmental needs, the risk of maladaptation increases (Atwood & Stolorow, 1984). Biological and psychosocial factors such as mental illness, impaired nutrition, safety, and coping skills play key roles in maladaptation. Distant alliances with extended families or exhausted social networks compromise access to larger social systems, increasing the risk of crisis (Saulnier & Rowland, 1985).

An example of maladaptive coping behaviors is in the case of a mother who has not separated from her family of origin and who subsequently has difficulty tolerating autonomy and independence in her children because they represent extensions of her family. When children attempt to separate, the mother experiences enormous anxiety. Normal childhood behaviors (e.g., autonomy and independence) are perceived as threatening and unacceptable. To minimize this distress, the mother may punish children by emotional withdrawal and abandonment or by physical abuse or neglect (Mahler, 1968; Masterson, 1988).

Chaos and turmoil are common themes in dysfunctional families, increasing the risk of maladaptive responses throughout the life span. The intensity of maladaptation or symptoms, such as inadequate or impaired communication or conflict resolution skills, is influenced by the family's ability to solve problems, manage stress, and cope with life span transitions. Biological and psychosocial factors also play key roles in the couple's ability to manage family tension. Biological factors in-

clude depression in a parent or poverty that contributes to a parent's ability to provide for his family's basic physical needs. The significance of a parent's failing to meet biological needs is seen in the example of a father who is severely depressed and therefore unable to work and provide for his family. He is emotionally inaccessible to his wife and children. His wife feels neglected and angry, and she triangles one of the children into the parental dyad to diffuse her feelings. The children in this family are likely to feel fearful and uncertain about their wellbeing. Symptoms of maladaptation may take the form of poor academic performance, depression, delayed growth and development, and substance abuse. Increased tension and crisis are likely to result when dysfunctional family patterns fail to reduce tension and mobilize internal and external resources that restore stability (Lewis et al., 1976).

THE MIDDLE-AGED COUPLE (CONTRACTION AND FINAL PARTNERSHIP STAGES)

The major developmental tasks of middle adulthood include creating and guiding the next generation. As the last child leaves home, the couple is once again alone and their relationship is highlighted. During this period the couple recognizes reduced involvement with their children and the need for new interests. Couples who have renewed their relationships throughout the years see this developmental transition as an opportunity to spend time together, solidifying the intimacy of their relationship.

Physiological changes such as mood swings and fluctuation in weight related to menopause may affect a woman's perception of herself and her relationship with her spouse

(Deeks, 2004). Women's perceptions of biological changes that occur during menopause transition vary. A 2007 qualitative study of 20 women going through menopause transition demonstrated various concepts of menopause transitions. Major themes from this study include different physical changes with both positive and negative psychological changes, along with viewing it as a natural part of the reproductive cycle (Lindh-Astrand, Hoffman, Hammar, & Kjellgren, 2007).

Watching their waistline and hairline change may make men increasingly concerned about their body image and thus experience reduced self-esteem. Alterations in body image caused by the aging process challenge couples to reassess their assets and strengths. Aging is inevitable and most people eventually reconcile themselves to it over time. The healthy couple recognizes that they cannot stay young forever and accept biological changes occurring in each other. A sense of contributing to society and satisfaction with overall accomplishment are important psychosocial factors affecting this transition. Positive self-esteem is crucial to a successful mastery of this developmental task. Transmission of generational traditions and cultural values to grandchildren is another rewarding experience for the middle-aged couple.

Failure to master previous developmental tasks increases the risk of maladaptive responses to the aging process. The evidence of growing older may threaten the couple's self-esteem, limiting their ability to recognize lifelong strengths and assets. A negative self-image compromises their ability to move through the life span realistically. Grandchildren may remind them that they are growing old, rather than engaging them in activities that contribute to the next generation. Longstanding maladaptive coping responses, such as substance abuse, self-destructive behaviors, and ineffective coping skills, further increase the likelihood of depression and suicide. Short-term marital therapy can be very helpful in defusing stressful situations, improving communication, and promoting a healthier adaptation to the couple's changing lifestyle.

Some middle-aged couples are now experiencing the dilemma of caring for aging parents and also coping with adult children who have returned home. These stressors often compromise the couple's financial stability and newly found freedom.

THE OLDER COUPLE (DISAPPEARANCE STAGE)

Older couples are faced with the task of retirement. Retirement presents couples with opportunities to explore lifestyles other than those of a worker. Couples who are fortunate enough to own their own businesses or have careers that are not affected by forced retirement have the option of continuing their job or developing other hobbies and fun endeavors. Healthy couples often have little difficulty coping with aging and retirement. Active family involvement with grandchildren, great grandchildren, and other members is important.

Aging also confronts couples with significant losses. Possible losses during this developmental stage include

TABLE 28–5
Evolution of the Family

Developmental Stages of Families

Stages	Tasks
Individual	Identity and separation
Dating/courting	Intimacy
Early marriage	Separation from family of origin
Expansion	Parenting
Consolidation	Conflict resolution and adaptation to parent-child conflict
Contraction	Last child leaves home
Final partnership	Renewal of couple's relationship; caring for aging parents; adaptation to changes in body image
Phase of disappearance	Adjustment to retirement, losses, and new generation

Note. From *Principles of Family Psychotherapy*, by J. G. Howells, 1975, New York: Brunner/Mazel. Adapted with permission.

loss of one's spouse, independence, income, and health. Dependency on other family members challenges the older adult to preserve autonomy in the face of extensive reliance on the family as caregivers. The death of the couple means that the original family has disappeared, but the couple lives on through other family systems (Howells, 1975). Perpetuation of families is maintained through the legacy of family members who have died.

The 2000 Census reveals that approximately 1.2 million persons over age 50 are currently cohabiting. About 90 percent of these individuals were previously married (Brown, Lee, & Bulanda, 2006). Given the structure of families has transformed over the past few decades along with parallel societal changes and economic pressures, some older adults are seeking relationships to ensure emotional support, financial security, and quality companionship. Despite these benefits, some researchers submit major disadvantages of cohabitation in this age group include higher levels of depression than their married counterparts, perhaps due to less stability and interpersonal conflicts with adult children compared to those married (Brown, 2000).

SUMMARY OF FAMILY EVOLUTION

Families evolve over time. They are established when individuals enter relationships and end with the death of a spouse or couple. Milestones include marriage, the births of children, graduations, the marriages of children, and the arrival of grandchildren. Transitional stages challenge families to adapt to and manage stress generated by necessary changes within and outside the system that involve biological, psychosocial, and cultural factors. Functional or healthy families resolve crises effectively and grow and mature over time. Members from these systems tend to develop adaptive coping behaviors. Conversely, dysfunctional families are more likely to impede change when they use maladaptive coping responses in managing stress. Family members from these systems often develop maladaptive coping behaviors. See Table 28–5 for a summary of the developmental stages of families.

THE ROLE OF THE NURSE

When do families seek family or couple's therapy? The psychiatric nurse can answer this question by exploring and assessing the meaning of the client's symptoms and how they maintain dysfunctional family interactions. Families seeking treatment for a symptomatic child or adolescent usually require immediate help to deal with maladaptive coping responses. Because of the complexity of a dysfunctional family system, the psychiatric nurse must develop innovative assessment skills and interventions. Recognition that families are *not* the sole cause of mental illness is vitally important. Vulnerable individuals are at risk for responding in maladaptive ways, not only by how they communicate with their family systems, but also by the combination of genetic, biological, environmental, and psychosocial factors.

THE GENERALIST NURSE

Family therapy lies within the scope of advanced-practice nursing practice. However, the role of the generalist nurse may involve case management, health education, crisis intervention, crisis hot lines, and referrals. The generalist nurse is likely to be involved with families as a case manager in the home, community, and acute inpatient settings. In these roles the generalist nurse may be involved in data collection that facilitates recognition of a family crisis and need for referral for therapy and other health care resources. Frequently, the psychiatric nurse recognizes the urgency of a referral of families for acute management of a crisis and later to a nurse therapist to facilitate healthy crisis resolution. Health education is an integral part of nursing. It offers the nurse an opportunity to work with families and clients to understand basic information about their illnesses and manage their care. Interventions often include teaching families how to administer or monitor the clients' response to medications and other treatment. The psychiatric nurse also provides crisis intervention, assesses the family's involvement in treatment, and provides referrals for support groups and other community and Internet resources. During psychiatric home visits, the generalist nurse works with families and provides health education, medication monitoring (i.e., adherence issues), and observes for adverse side effects and response to treatment. Although generalist nurses do not provide family therapy, their interventions are crucial to successful treatment outcomes concerning familial systems.

THE ADVANCED-PRACTICE PSYCHIATRIC REGISTERED NURSE

Family and marital therapies are forms of psychotherapy that require a minimum of a master's degree in the behavioral or social sciences, nursing, or psychology. Professional supervision and ongoing training are crucial aspects of a career working with families and couples in crisis.

The advanced-practice psychiatric registered nurse (i.e., clinical nurse specialist) has a master's degree, with special training in psychotherapy. The behavioral, biological, and social sciences serve as the bases of assessment, identification of client outcomes, and development of interventions to address maladaptive familial interactions and impaired communication patterns. The nurse often plays an active role in therapy sessions; otherwise, family turmoil escalates and minimizes the nurse's effectiveness (Smoyak, 1975; Whitaker, 1976). Most nurses use an array of theories, or an eclectic approach, and tailor them to meet the complex needs of each family.

Co-Therapy

Family interactions and processes are multifaceted and can be emotionally exhausting. They require that the nurse be actively engaged in the family system as well as an observer of interactions. Co-therapy, one approach of which involves one therapist actively interacting with the system while the other observes verbal and nonverbal family-therapist interactions, is an effective strategy. Other approaches involve more dynamic interactions between both therapists and family members. This approach is particularly effective when working with large families or multigenerational issues. It provides a parental subsystem and role model for functional interactions. In addition, co-therapists provide each other professional and emotional support to deal with the anxiety and perplexities of therapy. Co-therapy can be extremely useful in the assessment of the active therapist's verbal and nonverbal transactions with the family (Olds, 1977).

The disadvantages of co-therapy are that it is a complex process, it is time consuming, it is expensive, and the coordination of the two therapists' schedules is difficult. There is no consensus on the usefulness of co-therapy, but it is wise to terminate a co-therapy relationship when an impasse exists. This reduces the effectiveness of a co-therapy relationship and compromises the treatment process (Olds, 1977). Proponents of co-therapy assert that it provides a major source of support (Napier & Whitaker, 1978), whereas critics contend that it is unnecessary because therapists should be able to handle families alone (Friedman, 1971; Kuehn & Crinella, 1969).

Nurses should consider the feasibility and usefulness of co-therapy because it can be very helpful with severely dysfunctional families. Co-therapy can also be a rewarding and fulfilling experience between two family therapists.

A Family in Crisis

Nurse therapist: "Mrs. Marshall, tell me about your reasons for seeking treatment today."

Mother: "Larry has been getting into a lot of trouble at school lately. If you could just straighten him out we would not have all of these problems."

Identified client (Larry): "Mom, you and dad are always blaming me!"

Nurse therapist: "Larry, tell me what it's like to be blamed all the time."

Larry: "Well, it doesn't feel good because no matter what I do, it's never right."

Nurse therapist: "What do you mean by 'its never right'?"

Larry: "Well, I used to work real hard trying to make good grades, but even when I do pretty good, I always hear, 'Your sister has always brought home all A's.' They also tell me that if I did better in school, things would be less stressful at home."

Nurse therapist: "I see that you are pretty upset. What do you need from your mother right now?"

Larry: "Mom, I just want to hear some positive things from you and dad sometimes. You are always yelling at me and each other and this really bothers me. I wish you and dad would stop fighting so much."

Nurse therapist: "Mrs. Marshall, how was the decision made for you and your son to seek treatment today?"

Mother: "Well, we have been having a lot of problems with Larry lately concerning his grades."

Nurse therapist: "Mrs. Marshall, tell me a little bit about what is going on in the family."

Mother: "Well, Larry's father and I have been going through some rough things lately. He is never home and when he comes home he is so negative towards me and the kids."

Nurse therapist: "Where is he today?"

Mother: "He said that he did not need help and that if someone could fix Larry, we would not be so stressed out."

Nurse therapist: "Tell me what you see as the family problem."

Mother: "I see now that it isn't Larry's problem. I have serious marital problems that seem to be affecting me and the kids."

Nurse therapist: "How has the family dealt with this problem in the past?"

Mother: "We haven't done a very good job."

Nurse therapist: "What do you need from therapy at this point?"

Mother: "I need to learn how to stop yelling at the kids, especially Larry, and stop blaming him for problems between his dad and me."

Nurse therapist: "Larry, what would help you the most right now?"

Larry: "If mom and dad would stop fighting and blaming me for everything. It's scary and upsetting to see the two people I love the most tearing each other apart."

Mother: "Larry, I am so sorry because the problems between your dad and me are our problems, not yours."

Marital Therapy and Family Therapy

Marital therapy and family therapy are useful, specialized interventions that focus on maladaptive interactions within the family system. Couples and families usually seek therapy when they are unable to resolve stress using their usual coping skills.

Marital therapy is a therapeutic approach that alters the marital or couple dyad. Major goals are to help couples understand maladaptive interactions and to modify how they satisfy mutual needs. Recent studies suggest that couples in which one spouse is depressed can affect family function. Marital therapy, family-focused psychosocial interventions, and pharmacotherapy are effective in alleviating bipolar depression and improving role task performance (Miklowitz et al., 2007).

Family therapy is also a specialized intervention that is used to treat clients within a social context, rather than individually. The advantage of this approach over individual psychotherapy, is its effectiveness in changing a system and the behaviors of its individual members. In essence, family therapy is a realistic perspective of a client's world, because input from various members decreases distortions or hearsay information. In addition, interactions with family members facilitate an in-depth assessment of family structure and development of family outcomes (Bandler & Grindler, 1975; Grindler & Bandler, 1976).

Families often present for therapy with what has been called the identified client. The client's symptoms are the focus and serve as the reasons for seeking treatment. Theoretical frameworks that target maladaptive behaviors define interventions. The maladaptive behaviors of one member, such as an adolescent's abuse of alcohol, are seen as representing a family problem. Framo (1982) noted that the most effective way to promote health in children is to help the parents. Symptomatic children mirror the quality of the parental subsystem. The following clinical example ("A Family in Crisis") illustrates the dynamics of families who focus on the identified client (Larry, a 15-year-old boy) rather than on family issues. This clinical example demonstrates how important it is to assess reasons for seeking treatment and facilitate understanding of each member's perspective. The nurse therapist initially focused on the identified client (Larry), but quickly shifted the focus from him to the marital dyad. Ideally, the father would have been part of this session, but he was absent from this initial session. Obviously, the adolescent's behavior stemmed from conflicts between his parents. By refocusing attention on the couple, the nurse was able to protect the youth and encourage him to express his feelings and gain a realistic picture of the real family problems.

Structural Family Therapy

One approach the advanced-psychiatric nurse may take in treating families in crisis is Minuchin's (1974) structural family therapy. Structural family therapy involves systems and various subsystems. This approach is based on the premise that certain family structures or arrangements affect transactional and communication patterns. Family transactions are the bases of rules that organize the way members relate to each other while modulating behavior. The family's adaptability to change within and outside the systems affects homeostasis.

The major concepts of structural family therapy are boundary, alignment, and power. Identified clients or members cannot relinquish or change family dynamics without modification of family structure or function. Impaired family transactions maintain symptoms in the identified client. Therapy aims to modify impaired family transactions.

Structural therapy focuses on the here and now, rather than on the past. Assessment data are obtained from inspection of family transactions and interpersonal processes. Successful outcomes are based on alleviation or reduction of symptoms and feedback from family members.

THE NURSING PROCESS

The major concepts of structural family therapy are demonstrated in the following case study.

ASSESSMENT

Parental conflict and divorce often affect children's well-being. The risk of maladaptive responses in adolescents increases with family turmoil, which is a severe stressor for children and adolescents and interferes with competent parenting and marital performance. Bringing children into the marital conflict further compromises the parent-child relationship (Amato & Keith, 1991).

The following are major treatment goals of structural family therapy:

◆ Reduce tension

◆ Facilitate effective communication

◆ Clarify family rules and roles

◆ Improve problem-solving skills

◆ Delineate clear boundaries between family members

Ultimately, family structures should be changed, in that maladaptive transactions are altered into adaptive ones.

The nurse begins to establish a therapeutic alliance by joining the family and positioning himself as the leader to accommodate transactional patterns. *Joining* allows the nurse to orchestrate and relate to the family system. *Accommodation* necessitates adjusting to facilitate the joining process. These family dynamics underscore an appreciation of family function and structure rather than condoning the maladaptive interactions. In essence, the nurse psychotherapist becomes a part of the family structure and thus part of the status quo, which enables family themes, areas of support, and strength to be assessed (Minuchin, 1974).

Assessment involves exploring areas in the family structure that are unable to maintain function. The nurse observes the client's behavior and maladaptive responses other than the presenting symptoms. This can be seen in the man who feels inadequate (presenting symptom), but avoids closeness (behavior) with his wife because he fears rejection. Data gathered during assessment provide the basis of therapeutic interventions and outcomes. Pertinent data include interactions of parent-child subsystems and of the couple. *Family mapping* is an assessment tool used to illustrate here-and-now interactions between members of the system and its subsystems (Minuchin, 1974). Table 28–6 summarizes the components of family assessment.

The genogram is another tool that elicits invaluable historical generational data of families (Bowen, 1978). It offers invaluable data about mental and medical conditions and their potential role on the family system and level of functioning (see Figure 28–1).

Nurses need to collect as much information about the child's presenting symptoms as possible, including recent stressors and changes. Observing interactions of the couple and parent-child subsystems during the initial interview provides vital information about the family structure and function. Family members need to speak for themselves and avoid

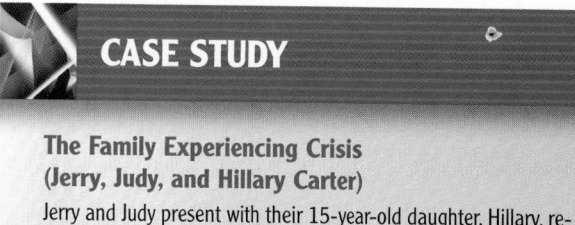

CASE STUDY

The Family Experiencing Crisis (Jerry, Judy, and Hillary Carter)

Jerry and Judy present with their 15-year-old daughter, Hillary, reporting that her grades have fallen over the past semester and that she has had a weight gain of 15 pounds. She is rebellious and frequently argues with her mother. The advanced-practice psychiatric nurse gets the referral from the school counselor, who reports that Hillary has become increasingly despondent and is sleeping in class.

TABLE 28–6
Components of Family Assessment in Structural Therapy

Component	Intervention
1. Establish Therapeutic Alliance	Nurse is an active participant and directs his own behavior to communication and to influence specific family transactions
2. Major Aspects of Assessment	Helps the family understand interactional patterns. Assesses family patterns such as: • Communication • Decision making • Boundaries • Coping behaviors/patterns • Developmental stage of couple/parents
3. Major Tasks (Outcome Identification)	Develop rational social context that encourages changes in social interactional patterns around issues associated with identified problems (family members and nurse are active participants)
4. Interventions	• Facilitate transactions • Discourage family interaction by promoting interactions between the therapist and family members • Escalate stress, which encourages members to adapt or restructure interactions • Assign family tasks (during session and homework) • Use symptoms to restructure (e.g., exaggerating, minimizing focus, relabeling) • Clarify the meaning of behavior or symptoms • Support the family system • Provide psychoeducation • Empower members
5. Evaluation	Based on family outcomes and feedback from members, and nurse's observation

Note. Adapted from *Families and Family Therapy*, by S. Minuchin, 1974, Cambridge, MA: Harvard University Press. Adapted with permission.

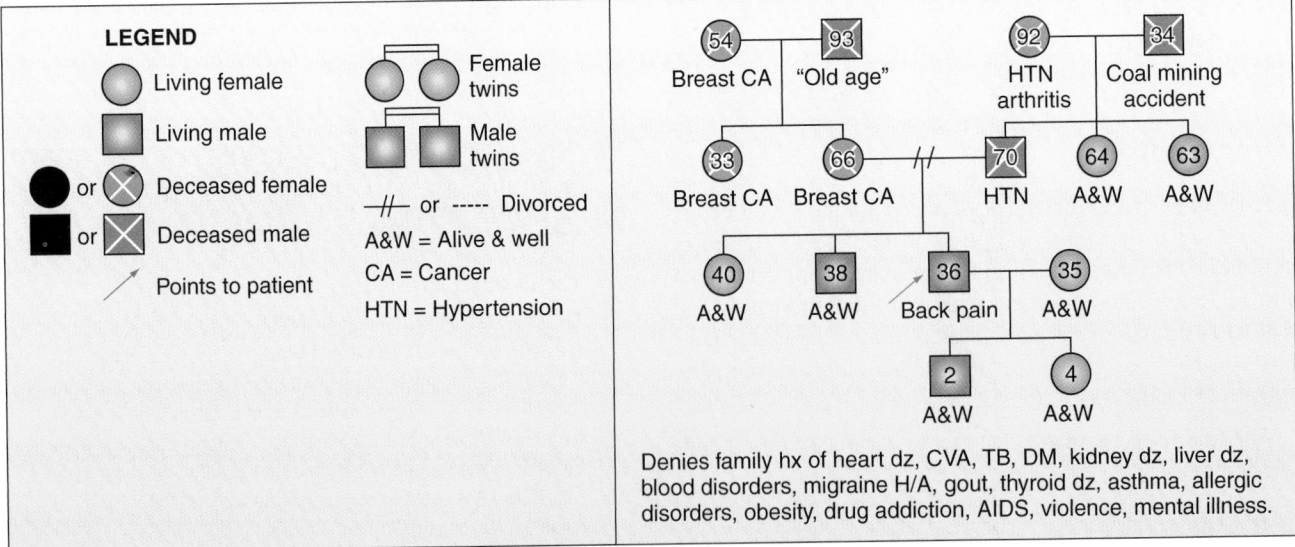

Figure 28–1 Family health history and genogram.

speaking for other members. Data are generally collected within sessions in which the family assessment of its transactions and of its members' attempts to maintain status quo positions are observed (Minuchin, 1974).

In the case study involving Jerry, Judy, and Hillary, Hillary was the identified client, and her major symptoms were failing grades, altered eating patterns, and increased social isolation. The problem extends beyond rebelliousness and arguments with her mother, but more importantly, how these symptoms maintain the couple dyad or subsystems. In cases such as this, the child should not be approached immediately, because this reinforces the family label of the sick role. However, if the child is scapegoated, the nurse needs to align with her to minimize this process.

Several areas were identified during the assessment of Hillary's family:

◆ Arguments were increasing between Jerry and Judy over Jerry's long work hours.

◆ Jerry spent most of his free time with Hillary rather than with Judy.

◆ Judy expressed anger and resentment toward Hillary.

◆ Judy frequently criticized Hillary's weight gain.

NURSING DIAGNOSES

The major nursing diagnoses for the Hillary case study are:

Compromised Family Coping related to inability to express feelings, directly, to get needs met

Situational Low Self-Esteem related to feelings of inadequacy and lack of trust (couple)

Situational Low Self-Esteem related to parental criticism and disturbed body image

Violence, Risk for Self-Directed (adolescent)

PLANNING

Therapeutic interventions are based on problem identification and strategies that reduce or alleviate symptoms in the identified client. Restructuring interventions, such as joining and accommodation modify impaired transactions address developing modified transactions. "Joining" and "accommodation" refer to the therapist's entering and conforming to a family system with the goal of initiating a therapeutic relationship. This relationship is used to identify maladaptive transactional or communication patterns and help family members form adaptive ones (Minuchin, 1974).

The following client outcomes (outcome identification) were identified for Hillary's family:

◆ Hillary's family develops adaptive and coping skills to manage stress.

◆ Boundaries between marital and parental-child subsystems are clearly defined and maintained.

◆ Hillary avoids engaging implicitly or explicitly in her parents' conflict.

◆ Subsystems clarify and communicate feelings and thoughts appropriately.

◆ Hillary identifies at least two positive assets and develops adaptive coping skills.

◆ Hillary expresses feelings, rather than acting on them.

Nursing Care Plan 28–1 identifies the nursing actions needed to achieve these outcomes, along with the rationales for these actions.

IMPLEMENTATION

Alternative transactions are explored when the nurse enters alliances with family subsystems and develops a therapeutic contract. Therapeutic techniques preserve family members' self-identity and support mutuality, or the sense of belonging. The major techniques of structural family therapy are:

◆ Dissuade present members from talking about or for each other in session.

◆ Encourage the family to discuss strengths and competence.

◆ Support the scapegoated or identified client.

◆ Maintain age-appropriate behaviors associated with independence.

The nurse psychotherapist actively interacts with family members. This process begins with discussing options to disengage from maladaptive transactional patterns and pointing out adaptive ones. Asking the adolescent to talk to a parent and vice versa, rather than talking through the nurse psychotherapist creates new scenarios. This is an experiential (emotions generated by specific interactions between members and the nurse) process that centers on the family's presenting symptoms. Focusing on the adolescent's concerns also decreases his negativity, promotes engagement into treatment, and increases the potential of a more meaningful conversation with parents (Diamond & Josephson, 2005; Diamond & Liddle, 1996, 1999).

EVALUATION

As family members change, their transactions also change. The degree of family restructure is assessed throughout treatment. Client outcomes and the family's and nurse's perceptions regarding adaptive coping behaviors are the basis for evaluation. Structural family therapy involves meeting with the child and couple for 6 months. Response to family therapy depends on reasons for seeking treatment, insight, economic factors, and severity of symptoms.

Termination begins during the initial stage of therapy and involves assessing problem areas, identifying outcome

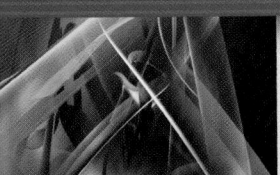

The Family Experiencing Crisis (Jerry, Judy, and Hillary)

Nursing Diagnosis: Ineffective Coping

Outcome Identification	Nursing Actions	Rationales	Evaluation
1. By [date], Hillary's family will develop adaptive coping skills to manage present crisis.	1a. Establish rapport and assess reasons why Hillary's family is seeking treatment at this time.	1a. Alliance is developed and basis and duration of crisis are determined.	*Goal met:* Alliance and therapeutic contract are established.
	1b. Assess transactional patterns and coping behaviors of Hillary's family.	1b. Jerry begins to focus on present marital problems.	Jerry focuses primarily on concerns for Hillary's behavior.
	1c. Direct questions to Jerry and Judy.	1c. Communication patterns improve in the marital dyad.	Jerry answers most questions, Judy is silent.

Nursing Diagnosis: Interrupted Family Processes Related to Situational Stressors

Outcome Identification	Nursing Actions	Rationales	Evaluation
1. By [date], Hillary's family will share their feelings appropriately	1a. Encourage Hillary's family to express their feelings and thoughts regarding present stressors.	1a. Hillary is able to express anger appropriately toward her mother.	*Goal met:* Hillary expresses anger towards Judy. Judy remains silent while Jerry inquires about meaning of Hillary's anger.
	1b. Encourage Judy and Jerry to express their feelings.	1b. Judy is able to express her anger to Jerry, specifying her reasons, and Jerry is able to share his feelings about family and marital stress.	Judy angrily tells Jerry that he is never home and that she is lonely most of the time.
2. By [date], Hillary's family will recognize their family roles.	2. Assess what Judy and Jerry want from their relationship.	2. Attention turns to dyad conflict.	Jerry states he was not aware of Judy's anger and that it was being taken out on Hillary.

Nursing Diagnosis: Low Self-Esteem Related to Present Crisis

Outcome Identification	Nursing Actions	Rationales	Evaluation
1. By [date], Hillary's family members will identify positive assets and qualities.	1. Encourage Hillary, Judy, and Jerry to talk about positive qualities and assets.	1. Family can identify their strengths.	*Goal met:* Hillary, Jerry, and Judy identify positive attributes and qualities.

(continues)

Nursing Care Plan 28–1 (continued)

Nursing Diagnosis: High Risk for Violence: Self-Directed (Adolescent)

Outcome Identification	Nursing Actions	Rationales	Evaluation
1. By [date], Hillary will express feelings, rather than acting on them.	1. Observe Hillary for signs and symptoms of depression.	1. Adolescents are at risk for acting out.	*Goal met:* Hillary verbalizes feelings and denies suicidal ideations. She interacts more with family/friends. Communication between Jerry and Judy, and Hillary and her parents improves. The family's coping skills improve.

measures, establishing interventions, and evaluating outcomes. In the last session, the nurse helps family members discuss their role in attaining treatment goals, supporting and accepting each other, and recognizing strengths that will help maintain the family structure during a crisis.

RESEARCH AND FAMILIAL SYSTEMS

Familial systems mediate clients' responses across the life span. Research is needed for all levels of the nursing process. Research on the effectiveness of the advanced-practice psychiatric nurse psychotherapist is sparse. Advanced-practice psychiatric nurses are playing key roles of primary mental health care providers. Primary prevention of high-risk groups is the prime focus of health care delivery models. High-risk families include those with a mentally ill parent and those in which substance abuse or poverty is present.

Methods that increase understanding of the relationship between developmental stages and various roles and patterns in different ethnic and cultural groups are crucial to identifying high-risk groups and promoting primary prevention. Interdisciplinary research can also assist nurses and other mental health professionals in developing qualitative and quantitative methods to examine the roles of fathers in diverse populations.

Nurses have always been a major force in health care delivery. Families enter health care systems through numerous portals. The child with hemophilia, the pregnant woman with acquired immune deficiency syndrome (AIDS), and the middle-aged couple dealing with a parent with Alzheimer's disease all bring familial roles in the health care arena. Nurses can collaborate with families and other health professionals to explore factors that affect family function. Psychoeducation, crisis intervention, supportive therapy, and psychopharmacology are a few areas in which nurses can evaluate family involvement.

SUMMARY

- ◆ Families are important aspects of the health care system, and the nurse's daily interactions with them submits the need to understand how they function and manage stress.

- ◆ Recognizing the influence of family roles on maintenance and promotion of the client's adaptive and maladaptive behaviors is vital to outcome identification.

- ◆ Family and marital therapies are invaluable approaches to managing clients' crises and maintaining health.

- ◆ Through family therapy, families members learn effective communication patterns, grow, express feelings, and clarify boundaries. Boundaries are a barometer of family function.

- ◆ Understanding systems theory helps nurses assess clients as a whole rather than a part.

- ◆ Research is needed to identify the effectiveness of nursing interventions and assess the impact of factors such as cultural diversity, changing roles of fathers and mothers across the life span, and age-specific factors.

- ◆ The effectiveness of various family therapy techniques needs to be explored by advanced-practice psychiatric nurses.

SUGGESTIONS FOR CLINICAL CONFERENCES

1. Present and discuss a history of a family in crisis
2. Role-play functional and dysfunctional family systems
3. Identify current societal trends that influence mental health and family structure
4. Role play congruent and incongruent communication patterns

5. Develop and present a family psychoeducational program that addresses psychopharmacological and psychotherapeutic interventions

STUDY QUESTIONS

1. General systems theory can be applied to families. Which of the following represents an open system?
   a. Johnny is not allowed to play with neighborhood children his age.
   b. Mrs. Jones waits for her daughter at least 30 minutes before school ends.
   c. Judy brings home a new friend who wants to play dolls.
   d. Mr. Lind visits his mother everyday.

2. Which system's theory concept allows an exchange of energy and matter across boundaries?
   a. Feedback mechanism
   b. Steady state or equilibrium
   c. Input mechanism
   d. Hierarchy of subsystems

3. The couple dyad is the basis of effective family transactions. Which of the following represents pseudo-mutuality?
   a. Parents report that they have a perfect marriage after the child attempts suicide.
   b. A child is admitted to the hospital for the fourth time in 2 weeks with asthma attack.
   c. The couple argues and resolves dispute over who will take the children to the soccer game.
   d. An adolescent expresses anger toward his father when he is grounded for staying out late.

4. The *best* definition of congruent communication is:
   a. clear, direct, and honest
   b. conveys verbal cues
   c. confusing and contradictory
   d. contributes to maladaptive coping behaviors

5. Functional families manage change by:
   a. perceiving it as a threat
   b. mobilizing resources within and outside the system
   c. minimizing resources to cope with stress
   d. decreasing permeability of boundaries

6. The most important aspect of a culturally sensitive family assessment is which of the following?
   a. Recognizing one's own ethnicity and its impact on the client's
   b. Applying common cultural stereotypes on similar cultural groups
   c. Confronting inappropriate behaviors, such as quietness and other nonverbal behavior
   d. Challenging family support systems, particularly maladaptive ones

7. Mrs. Jones' adult children, who are expressing concerns about their mother's isolation, bring in an 80-year-old with recent crying spells. The family reports that Mr. Jones recently died. Which of the following best describes the evolution of this family?
   a. The contraction and final partnership stage
   b. Disappearance stage
   c. Expansion and consolidation stage
   d. The sandwich generation stage

8. Evaluation, the efficacy of family therapy or interventions, is an important part of the nursing process. Which of the following is not a part of the evaluation process?
   a. The family makes adaptive behavioral changes.
   b. The family reports that goals have been met.
   c. The nurse perceives that his goals have been met for the family.
   d. The nurse encourages the family members to discuss their role in attaining treatment goals.

9. A family was referred to family therapy after their teenager son experienced behavioral problems in school. Which statement by the father indicates that he understands the purpose of family therapy?
   a. "Our son will realize the consequences of his actions and try harder to behave."
   b. "It will help us learn to communicate and problem solve better as a group."
   c. "I expect the therapist to tell my wife to quit babying my son."
   d. "The therapist will tell us how to make our son behave better in school."

10. An adolescent and her family are referred for family therapy. As part of the process you need to evaluate the adolescent initially separate from the family. During the initial evaluation of the adolescent she asks if you will keep everything she shares confidential. Which of the following statements indicates the nurse's knowledge about working with adolescents?
    a. "I promise I will keep everything confidential only if you agree to be honest with me."
    b. "I am unwilling to make this promise, but I can assure you confidentiality about personal discussions except information that indicates you are a danger to yourself or others."
    c. "This is family therapy. Everything you share with me I have to share with your parents."
    d. "What concerns you the most about talking to me?"

RESOURCES

Please note that because Internet resources are of a time-sensitive nature and URL addresses may change or be deleted, searches should also be conducted by association or topic.

American Association for Marriage and Family Therapy
112 South Alfred Street
Alexandria, VA 22314-3061
(703) 838-9808
http://www.aamft.org/index_nm.asp

American Family Therapy Academy
2020 Pennsylvania Ave. NW, #273
Washington, DC 20006
(202) 333-3690
http://www.afta.org

http://www.kidscount.org/ (Accessed April 8, 2006)
KIDS COUNT, a project of the Annie E. Casey Foundation, is a national and state-by-state effort to track the status of children in the United States. The organization works with policymakers and communities with benchmarks of child well-being.

National Alliance for the Mentally Ill
Colonial Place Three
2107 Wilson Blvd, Suite 300
(703) 524-7600
Helpline (800) 950-6264
http://www.nami.org

REFERENCES

Abernethy, A. D., Houston, T. R., Mimms, T., Boyd-Franklin, N. (2006). Using prayer in Psychotherapy: Applying Sue's differential to enhance culturally competent care. *Cultural Diversity & Ethnic Minority Psychology, 12*, 101–114.

Ackerman, N. W. (1958). *The psychodynamics of family life.* New York: Basic Books.

Amato, P. R., & Keith, B. (1991). Marital conflict, the parental-child relationship, and child self-esteem. *Family Relations, 35*, 103–110.

Antai-Otong, D. (2002). Culturally sensitive treatment of African Americans with substance-related disorders. *Journal of Psychosocial Nursing, 40*, 1–6.

Atwood, G. E., & Stolorow, R. D. (1984). *Structures of subjectivity: Explorations in psychoanalytic phenomenology.* Hillsdale, NJ: Analytic Press.

Bandler, R., & Grindler, J. (1975). The structure of magic. Palo Alto, CA: Science and Behavior Books.

Bateson, G., Jackson, D. D., Haley, J., & Weakland, J. H. (1962). A note on double bind. *Family Process, 2*, 154–161.

Baumann, A., & Beckingham, A. C. (1990). Blended families. In A. Baumann, N. E. Johnston, & D. Antai-Otong (Eds.), *Decision-making in psychiatric and psychosocial nursing* (pp. 166–167). Philadelphia: B. C. Decker.

Beitin, B. K., & Allen, K. R. (2005). Resilience in Arab American couples after September 11, 2001: A systems perspective. *Journal of Marital and Family Therapy, 31*, 251–267.

Beveridge, R. M., & Berg, C. A. (2007). Parent-adolescent collaboration: An interpersonal model for understanding optimal interactions. *Clinical Child and Family Psychology Review, 10*, 25–52.

Bowen, M. (1978). *Family theory in clinical practice.* New York: Aronson.

Bowlby, J. (1969). *Attachment and loss* (Vol. 1). New York: Basic Books.

Boyd-Franklin, N. (1989). *Black families in therapy: A multisystems approach.* New York: Guilford Press.

Bronfenbrenner, U. (1979). *The ecology of human development.* Cambridge, MA: Howard University Press.

Brown, S. L. (2000). The effect of union type on psychological well-being: Depression among cohabitors versus marrieds. *Journal of Health and Social Behavior, 41*, 241–255.

Brown, S. L., Lee, G. R., & Bulanda, J. R. (2006). Cohabitation among older adults: A national portrait. *Journal of Gerontology. Series B, Psychological Sciences and Social Sciences Behavior Psychology Science, 61*, S71–S79.

Carter, B., & McGoldrick, M. (1988). *The changing family cycle.* New York: Gardner Press.

Cheng, H., Dunn, J., O'Connor, T. G., & Golding, J. (2006). Factors modulating children's adjustment to parental separation: Finding from a community study in England. *Journal of Abnormal Psychology, 34*, 239–250.

Chung, R. H., Kim, B. S., & Abreu, J. M. (2004). Asian American multidimensional acculturation scale: Development, factor analysis, reliability, and validity. *Culture, Diversity and Ethnic Minority Psychology, 10*, 66–80.

Deeks, A. A. (2004). Is this menopause? Women in midlife—psychosocial issues. *Australian Family Physician, 33*, 889–893.

Diamond, G., & Josephson, A. (2005). Family-based treatment research: A 10-year update. *Journal of the American Academy of Child and Adolescent Psychiatry, 44*, 872–887.

Diamond, G. S., & Liddle, H. A. (1996). Resolving therapeutic impasses between parents and adolescents in multidimensional family therapy. *Journal of Consulting and Clinical Psychology, 64*, 481–488.

Diamond, G. S., & Liddle, H. A. (1999). Transforming negative parent-adolescent interactions: From impasse to dialogue. *Family Process, 38*, 5–26.

Dunn, J., O'Connor, T. G., & Cheng, H. (2005). Children's responses to conflict between their different parents: Mothers, stepfathers, nonresident fathers, and nonresident stepmothers. *Journal of Clinical Child and Adolescent Psychology, 34*, 223–234.

Duvall, E. (1977). *Family development* (3rd ed.). Philadelphia: J. B. Lippincott.

Epstein, N. B., & Bishop, D. S. (1981). Problem centered systems therapy of the family. *Marital and Family Therapy, 7*, 23–31.

Epstein, N. B., Bishop, D. S., & Baldwin, L. W. (1982). McMaster model of family functioning: A view of the normal family. In E. Walsh (Ed.), *Normal family processes* (pp. 115–141). New York: Guilford Press.

Erikson, E. H. (1963). *Childhood and society* (2nd ed.). New York: Norton.

Erikson, E. H. (1968). *Identity: Youth and crisis.* New York: W. W. Norton.

Fauchier, A., & Margolin, G. (2004). Affection and conflict in marital and parent-child relationships. *Journal of Marital and Family Therapy, 30*, 197–211.

Framo, J. L. (1982). *Explorations in family and marital therapy: Selected papers of James L. Framo*. New York: Springer.

Friedman, A. S. (1971). Co-therapy as family therapy and as a training model. In A. S. Friedman (Ed.), *Therapy with families of sexually acting-out girls*. New York: Springer Publishing.

Garfield, C. F., & Isacco, A. (2006). Fathers and the well-child visit. *Pediatrics, 117,* e637–e645. Available online at http://pediatrics.aappublications.org/cgi/content/full/117/4/e637

Grindler, J., & Bandler, R. (1976). *The structure of magic II*. Palo Alto, CA: Science and Behavior Books.

Grych, J. H., Raynor, S. R., & Fosco, G. M. (2004). Family processes that shape the impact of interparental conflict on adolescents. *Developmental Psychopathology, 16,* 649–665.

Haley, J. (1959). Family of the schizophrenia client: A model system. *Journal of Nervous and Mental Disorders, 129,* 357–374.

Haley, J. (1962). Whitaker family therapy. *Family Process, 1,* 69–100.

Hodge, D. R. (2005). Social work and the house of Islam: Orienting practitioners to the beliefs and values of Muslims in the United States. *Social Work, 50,* 162–173.

Howells, J. G. (1975). *Principles of family psychotherapy*. New York: Brunner/Mazel.

Kaczynski, K. J., Lindahl, K. M., Malik, N. M., & Laurenceau, J. P. (2006). Marital conflict, maternal and paternal parenting, and child adjustment: A test of mediation and moderation. *Journal of Family Psychology, 20,* 199–208.

Kuehn, J., & Crinella, F. M. (1969). Sensitivity training: Interpersonal "overkill" and other problems. *American Journal of Psychiatry, 126,* 841–845.

Kuhn, D. R., Morhardt, D. J., & Monbrad-Framburg, G. (1993). Late-life marriages, older stepfamilies, and Alzheimer's disease. *Families in Society: The Journal of Contemporary Human Services, 74,* 154–162.

Lewis, J. M., Beavers, R. W., Gassett, J. T., & Phillips, V. A. (1976). *No single thread: Psychological health in family systems*. New York: Brunner/Mazel.

Lidz, T., Fleck, S., & Cornelison, A. (1965). *Schizophrenia and the family*. New York: International Universities Press.

Lindh-Astrand, L., Hoffman, M., Hammar, M., & Kjellgren, K. I. (2007). Women's conception of the menopausal transition—a qualitative study. *Journal of Clinical Nursing, 16,* 509–517.

Mahler, M. (1968). *On human symbiosis and the vicissitudes of individuation, Vol. I: Infantile psychosis*. New York: International Universities Press.

Masterson, J. F. (1988). *The search for the real self*. New York: Free Press.

Maturana, H. R., & Varela, F. J. (1991). *The tree of knowledge* (2nd ed.). Boston: New Science Library.

McAdoo, J. L. (1993). The roles of African-American fathers: The ecological perspective. *Journal of Contemporary Human Services, 74,* 28–35.

McGoldrick, M., Giordano, J., & Garcia-Preto, N. (2005). *Ethnicity & family therapy*, 3rd edition. New York: Guilford Publication, Inc.

Mead, M. (1955). *Cultural patterns and technical change*. New York: New American Library Mentor Books.

Miklowitz, D. J., Otto, M. W., Frank, E., Reilly-Harrington, N. A., Wisniewski, S. R., Kogan, J. N., et al. (2007). Psychosocial treatments for bipolar depression: A 1-year randomized trial from the Systematic Treatment Enhancement Program. *Archives of General Psychiatry, 64,* 419–426.

Miller, J. G. (1965). Living systems: Basic concepts, structures, and process: Cross-level hypothesis. *Behavioral Sciences, 10,* 193–237, 337–411.

Minuchin, S. (1974). *Families and family therapy*. Cambridge, MA: Harvard University Press.

Mitrani, V. B., Feaster, D. J., McCabe, B. E., Czaja, S. J., & Szapocnik, J. (2005). Adapting the structural family systems rating to assess the patterns of interaction in families of dementia caregivers. *Gerontologist, 45,* 445–455.

Napier, A. Y., & Whitaker, C. (1978). *The family crucible*. New York: Harper & Row.

Odell, M., Shelling, G., & Young, K. S. (1994). The skills of marriage and family therapist in straddling multicultual issues. *American Journal of Family Therapy, 22,* 145–155.

Olds, V. (1977). Use of co-therapist in family therapy. In J. Buckly, J. J. McCarthy, & M. A. Quaranta (Eds.) *New directions in family therapy* (pp. 132–137). Oceanside, New York: DABOR Science.

Otto, H. A. (1962). What is a strong family? *Marriage and Family Living, 24,* 77–81.

Pare, D. A. (1996). Culture and meaning: Expanding the metaphorical repertoire of family therapy. *Family Process, 35,* 21–42.

Pelchat, D., Lefebvre, H., & Levert, M. J. (2007). Gender differences and similarities in the experience of parenting a child with a health problem: Current state of knowledge. *Journal of Child Health Care, 11,* 112–131.

Robinson, D. L. (1997). Family stress theory: Implications for family health. *Journal of the American Academy of Nurse Practitioner, 9,* 17–23.

Rothbaum, F., Rosen, K., Ujiie, T., & Uchida, N. (2002). Family systems theory, attachment theory, and culture. *Family Process, 41,* 328–350.

Satir, V. (1967). *Conjoint family therapy*. Palo Alto, CA: Science and Behavior Books.

Satir, V. (1988). *The new peoplemaking*. Mountain View, CA: Science and Behavior Books.

Saulnier, K. M., & Rowland, C. (1985). Missing links: An empirical investigation of network variables in high-risk females. *Family Relations, 34,* 557–560.

Skynner, A. C. R. (1976). *Systems of family and marital psychotherapy*. New York: Brunner/Mazel.

Slesnick, N., Bartle-Haring, S., & Gangamma, R. (2006). Predictors of substance use and family therapy outcome among physically and sexually abused runaway adolescents. *Journal of Marital and Family Therapy, 32,* 261–281.

Smoyak, S. (1975). *The psychiatric nurse as a family therapist.* New York: John Wiley & Sons.

Spiegel, J. (1957). *The resolution of conflict within the family. Psychiatry, 20,* 1–16.

Sullivan-Bolyai, S., Rosenberg, R., & Bayard, M. (2006). Fathers' reflections on parenting young children with type 1 diabetes. *American Journal of Maternal and Child Nursing, 31,* 24–31.

Tay, Y. R., & McCubbin, M. (2002). Family stress, perceived social support and coping following the diagnosis of a child's congenital heart disease. *Journal of Advanced Nursing, 39,* 190–198.

Thomas, M. B. (1992). *An introduction to marriage and family therapy.* New York: Merritt.

Thomas, S. P. & Pollio, H. R. (2002). *Listening to Patients: A phenomenological approach to nursing research and practice.* New York: Springer.

Tuyn, L. K. (2003). Metaphors, letters, and stories: Narrative strategies for family healing. *Holistic Nursing Practice, 17,* 22–26.

U. S. Bureau of the Census. (2001). *Statistical Abstract of the United States, 2000* p. 58, Table 68. http://www.census.gov/prod/2001pubs/statab/sec01.pdf. (Accessed April 8, 2006).

von Bertalanffy, L. (1968). *General systems theory: Foundations, development, applications* (rev. ed.). New York: George Braziller.

Walters, V., McDonough, P., & Strohschein, L. (2002). The influence of work, household structure, and social, personal and material resources on gender differences in health: An analysis of the 1994 Canadian National Population Health Survey. *Social Science Medicine, 54,* 677–692.

Walsh, F. (1982). *Normal Family Process.* New York: Guilford Press.

Walsh, F. (1996). The concept of family resilience: Crisis and challenge. *Family Process, 35,* 261–281.

Walsh, F. (2003). Family resilience: A framework for clinical practice. *Family Process, 42,* 1–18.

Weakland, J. (1976). Communication theory and clinical change. In P. J. Guerin (Ed.), *Family therapy* (pp. 111–128). New York: Gardner Press.

Whitaker, C. (1976). The hindrance of theory in clinical work. In P. J. Guerin (Ed.), *Family therapy* (pp. 154–164). New York: Gardner Press.

Whiteside, M. (1983). Families of remarriage: The weaving of many life-cycle threads. In H. A. Liddle (Ed.), *The family life-cycle: Implications for therapy* (pp. 100–110). Rockville, MD: Aspen Systems Corporation.

Young, K. (1944). *Social psychology* (2nd ed.). New York: F. S. Crofts.

SUGGESTED READINGS

Asaro, M. R. (2001). Working with adult homicide survivors, part II: Helping family members cope with murder. *Perspectives in Psychiatric Care, 37,* 115–124.

Butler, M. H., & Wampler, K. S. (1999). Couple-responsible therapy process: Positive proximal outcomes. *Family Process, 38,* 27–54.

Doornbos, M. M. (2002). Family cargivers and mental health care system: Reality and dreams. *Archives of Psychiatric Nursing, 16,* 39–46.

Freeman, J., Epston, D., & Lobovitz, D. (1997). *Playful approaches to serious problems: Narrative therapy with children and their families.* New York: W. W. Norton.

Glick, I. D., Berman, E. M., Clarkin, J. F., & Rait, D. S. (2000). *Marital and family therapy* (4th ed.). Washington, DC: American Psychiatric Press.

Minuchin, S., Lee, W-Y., & Simon, G. M. (1996). *Mastering family therapy: Journeys of growth and transformation.* New York: John Wiley & Sons.

North American Nursing Diagnosis Association (NANDA). (2001). *Nursing diagnoses: Definitions and classification, 2001–2002.* Philadelphia: Author.

Pruett, K. (1987). *The nurturing father.* New York, NY: Warner Books.

Rouf, W. C. (1994). *Generation of seekers: The spiritual journey of the baby boomers.* New York: Harper Collins.

Walzlawick, P., Weakland, J. H., & Fischm R. (1974). *Change: Principles of problem formation and problem resolution.* New York: W. W. Norton.

Wynne, L. C. (1984). The epigenesis of relational systems: A model for understanding family development. *Family Process, 23,* 297–318.

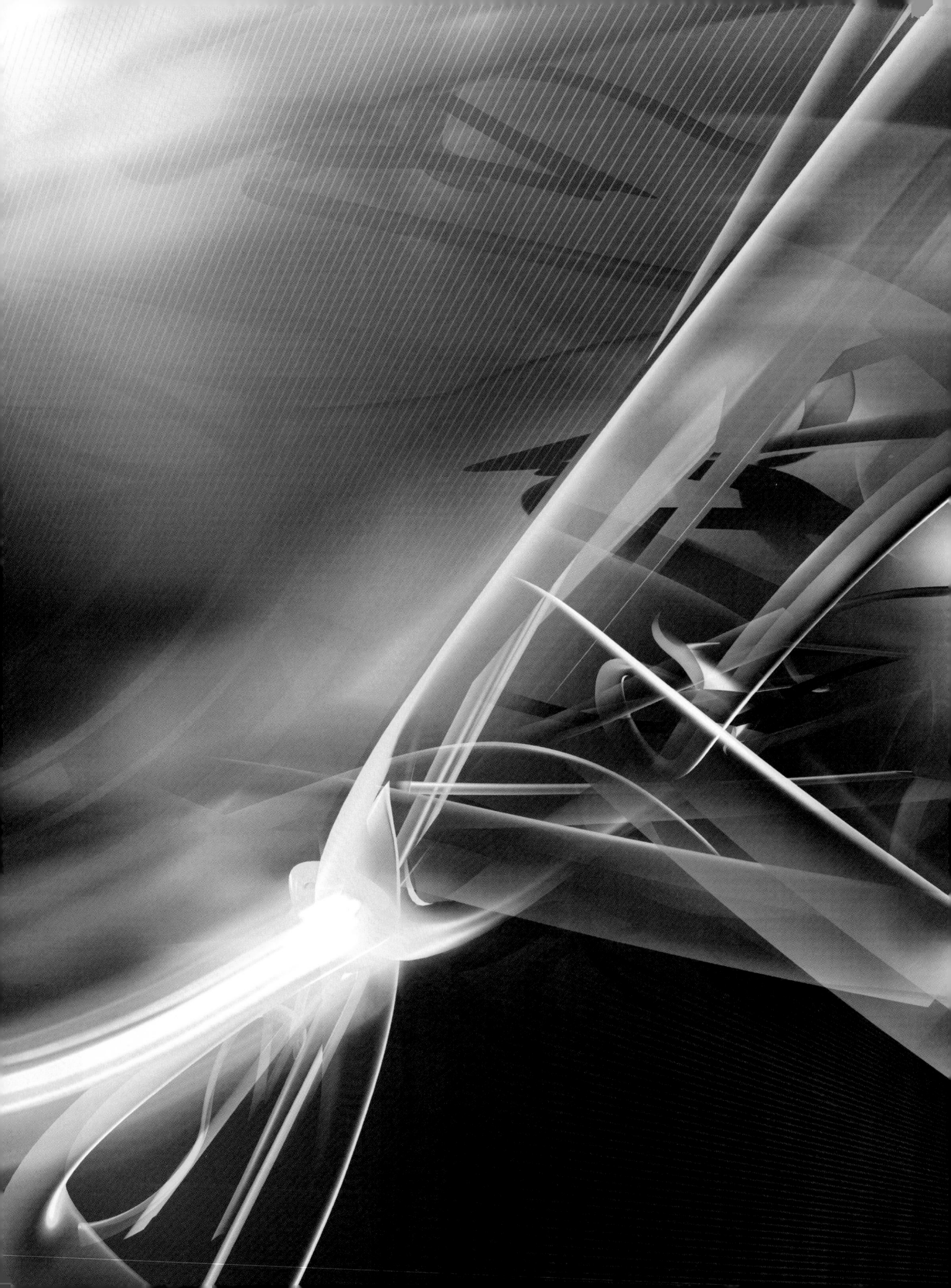

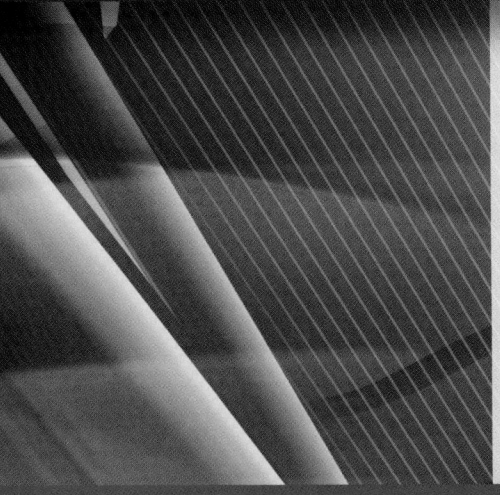

CHAPTER 29

Psychopharmacologic Therapy

Valerie Levi, Pharm D
Deborah Antai-Otong, MS, APRN, BC, FAAN
Duane F. Pennebaker, PhD, FNAP, FRCNA
Joy Riley, DNSc, RN, CS

KEY TERMS

Akathisia: Subjective feelings of restlessness and an inability to sit still resulting from dopamine blockade by certain antipsychotics; part of the extrapyramidal side effects.

Akinesia: A condition characterized by the inability to make voluntary movements.

Antipsychotics: Psychotropic medications used to treat acute and chronic psychotic disorders; agitation and aggression. These agents are divided into newer atypical and conventional or typical agents.

Anxiolytic: Drug used to reduce anxiety, and is synonymous to the term sedative. Examples include benzodiazepines such as diazepam, lorazepam, and clonazepam.

Cogwheeling: Refers to rigidity or rhythmic contractions noted on passive stretching of muscles, as occurs in Parkinson's disease.

Cytochrome P450 (CYP) Enzymes: Enzymes primarily located in the liver, which play a key role in the metabolism of most psychotropic medications.

Dopaminergic Pathway: Nerve fibers in the mesocortical area that project to the cortex and hippocampus regions of the limbic system.

Dystonia: Slow sustained muscle spasms of the trunk, neck, or limb; the result of dopamine blockade from antipsychotic medications.

Exponential Kinetics: A pharmacokinetic model in which a constant fraction of a drug is eliminated in a set unit of time.

Extrapyramidal Side Effects (EPS): Involuntary motor movements; and muscle tone side effects that result primarily from dopamine blockade by neuroleptic medications.

Genomics: The study of the human genome sequencing and its contributions to disease and treatment.

Human Genome: The entire genetic information present in a human cell.

Linear Kinetics: A pharmacokinetic model in which a constant amount of drug is eliminated in a set unit of time.

Neuroleptic Malignant Syndrome (NMS): A rare and potentially life-threatening syndrome primarily caused by antipsychotic medications and characterized by marked muscle rigidity, high fever, altered consciousness or delirium, tachycardia, hypoxia, hypertension, and diaphoresis.

Neurotransmitters: Nervous system biochemicals involved in facilitating neurotransmission of impulses across synapses between neurons. Examples include serotonin, norepinephrine, and dopamine.

Off-label medication: Denotes a prescribed medication to use for a purpose other than the parameters of the approved label.

Paradoxical Reactions: A response to a drug that is opposite to what would be predicted by the drug's pharmacology.

Pharmacodynamics: The study of biochemical and physiological actions and effects of drugs.

Pharmacogenetics: The study of molecular genetic variation that explains individual drug responses and may help identify biological predictors of adverse effects.

Pharmacokinetics: The study of a drug's absorption, distribution, metabolism, and excretion or elimination.

Pharmacology: The scientific study of chemical formulations (drugs), including their sources, properties, uses, actions, and effects.

Sedatives: Drugs that are virtually synonymous to anxiolytics; used to calm nervousness, irritability, or excitement; these agents depress the central nervous system and tend to cause lassitude and reduced mental activity.

Serotonin Syndrome: A condition characterized by serotonergic hyperstimulation that includes restlessness, hyperthermia, myoclonus, hypertension, hyperreflexia, diaphoresis, lethargy, confusion, and tremor and which may cause death.

Steady State: The state whereby the amount of drug eliminated from the body equals the amount being absorbed.

Synaptic Transmission: The process of nerve impulse transmission through the generation of action potentials from one neuron to another.

Tardive Dyskinesia: A complex range of involuntary movements associated with long-term and usually high-potency antipsychotic treatment. A chronic, progressive, and potentially fatal syndrome from prolonged dopamine blockade by antipsychotic medications. Major manifestations include choreiform movements of the face, tongue, upper and lower extremities, such as tongue movement or protrusion, lip sucking, chewing, and smacking; other symptoms include puffing of cheeks and pelvic thrusting.

Teratogenic: A substance or medication that can interfere with normal embryonic development and results in malformations or anomalies.

COMPETENCIES

Upon completion of this chapter, the learner should be able to:

1. Describe current knowledge about the brain and behavior as it relates to the clinical and pharmacokinetics of the major psychopharmacologic agents.

2. Describe the clinical and pharmacologic properties of the major psychopharmacologic agents and the use of these agents in the treatment of mental illness.

3. Apply knowledge about the pharmacokinetic properties of the major psychopharmacologic agents to individualized client care.

4. Explain the nurse's role in the administration and prescription of psychopharmacologic agents within the treatment regime.

5. Describe the importance of client and family education in the use of psychopharmacologic agents in the treatment of mental illness.

6. Comprehend the nurse's responsibilities and the ethical issues confronting the nurse in the use of psychopharmacologic agents.

CHAPTER OUTLINE

The Human Genome and Pharmacology

The Brain and Behavior

Neuroanatomical Structures Relevant to Behavior

Cortical Structures
  The Cerebral Cortex
  The Four Lobes and Their Functions
  The Association Cortices
  The Basal Ganglia
  The Hippocampus and the Amygdala

Subcortical Structures
  The Brainstem
  The Cerebellum
  The Diencephalon

Neurophysiology and Behavior

Neurons
  Synaptic Transmission

Neurotransmitters
  Biogenic Amines
  Acetylcholine
  Amino Acids
  Peptides
  Neurotransmitter Action

Pharmacokinetic Concepts

Pharmacology

The past three decades of research in the neurosciences has dramatically increased our understanding of the neurobehavioral aspects of mental illness to the extent that the 1990s were referred to as the *Decade of the Brain* and more recent discoveries of the human genome and bioinformatics in 2000. Scientists predict that the discovery of the human genome or human genetic blueprint offers incredible promise for the treatment of diseases, including mental illness. Historically, the advent of the first psychotropic medications in the 1950s significantly changed the treatment of the mentally ill. Part of the role of the psychiatric-mental health nurse has evolved in tandem with the unfolding success of psychotropic medications. The psychiatric-mental health nurse's knowledge of psychopharmacology and its associated therapeutic agents is a significant factor in contemporary practice. The psychiatric nurse has a critical role in assisting clients to incorporate the psychopharmacologic agents into their efforts to recover and maintain mental health and prevent negative sequel and relapse. In addition, the psychiatric-mental health nurse is responsible for assessing the therapeutic effects of the drugs. Monitoring adverse reactions, knowing therapeutic dosages, documenting administration, and educating the client and family members about the psychopharmacologic agents being used in the treatment regime. At the advanced-practice level in many states, psychiatric-mental health nurses also have prescriptive authority. This chapter presents an overview of current major concepts that relate brain and behavioral response to the major psychopharmacologic agents used in the treatment of mental illness.

Recommended treatments and drug therapies are changed as clinical and scientific findings are made available. In this chapter, we provide the most current information available at the time of this writing about the pharmacotherapeutic agents covered herein. The information provided, however, is not intended to replace sound clinical judgment or individualized client care. Nurses are legally and ethically responsible for being familiar with information such as the action, dosage, adverse effects, and drug interactions of the medications they administer. The reader is advised to check product information before administering any drug, especially new or infrequently ordered drugs. Unless otherwise noted, all information concerning the pharmacokinetic and clinical properties of the psychopharmacologic agents discussed in this chapter is based on adult oral dosages. It is assumed that the student has had a prerequisite to the materials in this chapter's introduction to pharmacology and the anatomy and physiology of the brain and central nervous system (CNS).

THE HUMAN GENOME AND PHARMACOLOGY

Tremendous technological advances in bioinformatics and the human genome or genetic mapping discovery have propelled the study of pharmacology into a new era. Drugs are believed to exert their curative effects by modifying the molecular structure of target proteins in the body. Today's researchers are bypassing lengthy animal studies and turning to a fast-growing new era of computer science known as bioinformatics. Bioinformatics are being used to fuel scientists' quest for newer drugs and better targets. Bioinformatic algorithms are being used to help pharmaceutical companies predict the future of proteins encoded by newly discovered genes.

Scientists have conducted the most extensive analysis of the human genetic blueprint, or human genome. This analysis of the human genome sequencing has provided scientists with an access to the 3 billion letters of DNA code arranged in 23 chromosomes. These findings have also revealed that the genome is the same from person to person, except those of identical twins who have some differences that make it unique. Virtually every cell in the body, except red blood cells (RBCs), carries a copy of the genome.

Researchers believe that once these genetic sequences are decoded, they will gain a better analysis of the molecules within human cells and dysregulation of vast body functions. Experts also expect these data to usher in an era of medications tailored to people's unique genetic profiles and provide health care providers the ability to predict, early in life, the risk of disease. Renowned scientist, Francis Collins, submits that understanding the genetic basis of a disease helps predict what protein it produces and provides opportunities to develop a drug to block it. Predictably, the discovery of the human genome has revolutionized medicine and the way drugs are used to fight diseases. Before the human genome discovery, diseases were treated by intervening at the level of symptoms—the final phase in a complex cascade of biochemical processes. Treating symptoms usually involved guessing which medications would work to treat individual people.

In the present era of the human genome discovery, scientists predict that diseases such as cancer and diabetes, obesity, heart disease, Alzheimer's disease, Parkinson's disease, and various psychiatric disorders, such as schizophrenia and bipolar and major depressive disorders, will be treated before symptoms occur. The basis of genomics is the ability to use medication to bolster or neutralize the effects of the person's proteins with fine precision by destroying unhealthy cells and leaving healthy cells alone. More importantly genomics allow health care providers from the onset to know the best medicine for the individual.

Pharmacogenetics is the study of molecular genetic variation that explicates divergent responses to medication and offers the prospect of identifying biological predictors of drug responses. Researchers also believe pharmacogenetics may clarify the means of determining the molecular substrates of drug efficacy and drug-related side effects. Molecular genetics offer a fresh approach to explaining the variance of psychotropic drug response. Biological predictors of drug response pave the way to determine the molecular substrates of drug efficacy and drug-induced adverse events (Howland, 2006; Malhotra, Murphy, & Kennedy, 2004). Advances in molecular biology, human genomics, and bioinformatics are ongoing and are bringing promise to people suffering diverse illnesses. Scientists also predict that over the next few years, genome-based drugs will become the accepted standard of care.

THE BRAIN AND BEHAVIOR

The brain is a unique mass of tissue consisting of approximately 10 billion neurons. These neurons coordinate all of a person's entire behavior by means of unceasing electrochemical activity (Ganong, 2005). The brain's high metabolic rate enables it to continually process, sort, analyze, integrate, score, and retrieve information from the environment. Because of its energy needs, the brain demands a constant supply of oxygen and glucose, approximately 20 percent of the body's total needs. These and small amounts of other nutrients (e.g., amino acids, vitamins, and minerals) are provided by a continuous supply of blood, 15 percent of the total cardiac output.

The brain stores energy mainly in the form of glucose, which is used to fuel the ion pump that maintains a resting state or propagates impulses. However, it stores only enough to last about 30 seconds (Ganong, 2005). Thus, the brain metabolism is quickly and severely altered when cerebral blood flow is compromised.

Behavior is the expression of brain function and represents a complex interplay between the person and the environment. Although certain characteristics of human behavior are universal in nature, many more are specific to the individual. Recent research indicates that genetics and neuroendocrine mechanisms may influence behavior; however, theories arising from this research remain controversial.

NEUROANATOMICAL STRUCTURES RELEVANT TO BEHAVIOR

The brain can be divided into cortical and subcortical structures. The *cortical structures* (right and left cerebral hemispheres) make up the outer and largest portion of the brain and include the cerebral cortex, or gray matter; the underlying white matter; and the basal ganglia, hippocampus, and amygdala. The *subcortical structures* include the brainstem, which is made up of the midbrain, the pons, and the medulla; the cerebellum; and the diencephalon, which consists of the thalamus and the hypothalamus (see Figure 2–4). Although each area performs highly specified functions, all areas are connected by an elegant network of nerve pathways that enables the brain to perform complex interactions and associations that result in appropriate psychomotor responses.

CORTICAL STRUCTURES

Cortical structures of the brain consist of the cerebral cortex, which is vastly convoluted, and deep fissures that divide the cerebral hemispheres into several distinct regions, called lobes. Different functions lie within the domain of each area ranging from higher brain functions associated with intelligence and reasoning to vision and perceptions. The role of these regions to psychiatric nursing is vast; they provide for human behaviors and target sites for pharmacologic agents.

The Cerebral Cortex

The cerebral cortex, or surface layer, of the brain (also called the gray matter) is composed almost exclusively of nerve cell bodies. It is divided by gyri (ridges) and sulci (grooves), which greatly multiply the surface area and potential for function. Localized areas of the cerebral cortex either have specific functions or serve as integration areas referred to as *association areas* (Pierri & Lewis, 2005). Association serves as intermediates to assimilate and integrate multiple and diverse sensory stimuli from the specialized cortices. These areas enable the brain to generate complex responses involving more than one behavioral domain.

The Four Lobes and Their Functions

The cerebral hemispheres each have four lobes: frontal, parietal, temporal, and occipital (see Figure 2–4). The occipital lobes are primarily visual areas. They receive impulses from the retina and interpret visual stimuli for recognition and identification. The *occipital areas* also connect with the areas of the cortex involved with perception, recall, and optically induced reflexes. The interactions between these cortices provide three-dimensional vision and recognition.

The *parietal lobes* perform a variety of sensory functions. The anterior portions are specialized in somatic sensation and perception. The more posterior parietal areas integrate visual and auditory stimuli useful for the sense of body position and movement in three-dimensional space.

The *temporal lobes* perform primarily auditory processing and, on a basic level, detect sound and tone intensity. Wernicke's area, which is responsible for recognition and interpretations of words and letters for speech, is located here. Long-term memory storage areas are thought to be stored in the temporal lobes, as is the ability to add affective perception to experience.

The *frontal lobes* are vital for cognition. Virtually all other areas of the brain provide information to and receive it from the frontal lobes. These are the areas of highest intellectual function, such as judgment, reasoning, and abstract thinking. The frontal lobes also organize more complicated motor responses and initiate complex voluntary and reflex movements. Psychomotor activity is also generated in the frontal lobes, including the inhibition of emotional impulses. Broca's area, located in the frontal temporal lobe junction, is responsible for speech articulation and lies close to the Wernicke's area. Interaction between speech and hearing centers is the foundation of communication in human beings.

The Association Cortices

Three main association areas lie between the primary functional cortices: the prefrontal motor association cortex, the limbic (affective) association cortex, and the sensory (parietal-temporal-occipital) association cortex (Pierri & Lewis, 2005). These association cortices enable a person to assimilate and integrate input from all sensory experiences and formulate effective response patterns such as assessment and problem solving followed by appropriate movement and speech. The *prefrontal association cortex* integrates sensory and intellectual information as well as correction in the planning of movement. The *limbic association cortex* adds affective tone to responses, and the *parietal-temporal-occipital association cortex* processes sensory information to enhance perception and language (Pierri & Lewis, 2005).

The Basal Ganglia

The basal ganglia are centralized collections of neuron cell bodies (nuclei) lying within the white matter (see Figure 2–4). These nuclei include the caudate nucleus, the putamen, which are sometimes called the striatum; and the globus pallidus, sometimes called the lenticular nucleus (Pierri & Lewis, 2005). Their principal function is the modulation of impulses for movement from the motor cortex to provide the smooth sequencing and execution of complex response. They also play a role in some cognitive processes, particularly the caudate nucleus (Pierri & Lewis, 2005).

The Hippocampus and the Amygdala

The amygdala and the hippocampus are structures generally considered being part of the *limbic system*; they are often referred to as the *limbic lobe* (see Figure 9–1 and Figure 10–1). Other structures included in the limbic system are the parahippocampal gyrus and the circulate gyrus. In general, the limbic system has a primary role in the behavioral responses of mood, memory, and learning. Dysfunction in these areas results in the inability to form new memory (Pierri & Lewis, 2005).

The amygdala, located in the temporal lobes, is composed of many nuclei with connecting tracts to the hypothalamus, hippocampus, cerebral cortex, and thalamus (Pierri & Lewis, 2005). The amygdala is involved in short-term memory and its conversion to long-term memory. In addition, the amygdala is believed to be involved in learning through assimilation and integration of information from different modalities. It is also involved with the hippocampus in encoding emotional memories. In animal studies, direct stimulation of the amygdala has produced aggressive behavior, suggesting that this structure may play a major role in adding affect tone to human responses (Pierri & Lewis, 2005). Recent studies indicate that dysregulation of the hippocampus and amygdala may play a role in exaggerated stress responses found in various anxiety disorders such as posttraumatic stress disorder (PTSD).

SUBCORTICAL STRUCTURES

Subcortical structures are located in the lower part of the brain and comprise the brainstem, medulla, midbrain, cerebellum, and diencephalon. Similar to cortical or higher brain regions, these structures play key roles in human behavior and regulation of diverse homeostatic processes including metabolism, sleep, wakefulness, temperature regulation, blood pressure, and motor function.

The Brainstem

The brainstem, which connects the brain to the spinal cord and peripheral nervous system, is composed of the medulla, the pons, the midbrain, and its reticular formation. These structures have specialized neural and physiological-regulating functions such as regulation of the heart, breathing patterns, and circadian rhythms. The brainstem also contains nuclei (clusters of nerve cell bodies) that secrete important neurotransmitters that influence brain activity and response. Biofeedback mechanisms that measure oxygen levels and blood pressure within the brain maintain the blood flow required for normal brain demands (Pierri & Lewis, 2005).

The *medulla* is the origin of adrenergic (adrenaline) pathways that project to the hypothalamus, the locus ceruleus, and vagus nerve. The locus ceruleus, a cluster of neurons located in the pons, is the source of noradrenergic (norepinephrine) pathways projecting to the spinal cord, cerebellum, and brainstem but largely converging in the thalamus and hypothalamus (see Figure 10–1). The *reticular formation* is a diffuse network of nuclei known to integrate motor, sensory, and visceral functions but, more importantly, it is involved in regulation of arousal and consciousness. This network is responsive to the presence of norepinephrine, serotonin, acetylcholine, and dopamine — neurotransmitters that mediate brain function on the most basic level (Pierri & Lewis, 2005).

The *midbrain* lies between the pons and the diencephalon. Structures in the midbrain include the tectum, the tegmentum, the red nucleus, and substantia nigra. These nuclei synthesize dopamine, a neurotransmitter important in movement and memory. The tectum mediates whole body movements in response to visual and auditory stimuli. The ventral portion of the tegmentum is the origin of a network of fibers known as *mesolimbic dopaminergic pathway*, which projects to the limbic system. Another set of fibers,

the mesocortical dopaminergic pathway, projects to the cortex and hippocampal regions of the limbic system. The substantia nigra gives rise to another set of dopaminergic fibers, associating with the nigrostriatal pathway, between the striatum, the subthalamic nucleus, and the cortex (Pierri & Lewis, 2005).

The Cerebellum

The cerebellum lies dorsal to the pons and medulla and actually wraps around the brainstem. It resembles the cerebral cortex in that it has distinct lobes and a foliated surface. The cerebellum receives afferent somatosensory pathways from the spinal cord, efferent motor relays from higher cortical areas, and input about balance from the vestibular system of the inner ear. The body integrates all this information to plan and coordinate movement and posture.

The Diencephalon

The thalamus and the hypothalamus must lie in the area called the *diencephalon*. It is the primary synaptic relay center of the brain for different sensory modalities, including somatic sensation, audition, and visual information. The *thalamus* distributes sensory information to the sensory cortex and also mediates motor functions by acting as a conduit for information from the cerebellum and the basal ganglia to the motor cortex.

The *hypothalamus* lies beneath the thalamus, with numerous afferent and efferent pathways to and from the other areas of the brain and the pituitary gland. The hypothalamus plays a vital role in the control of the endocrine system, the autonomic nervous system, and the limbic system through the release of hormones (see Figure 2–4). Functions and activities regulated by the hypothalamus include temperature regulation, eating and drinking (appetite), metabolism, glucose utilization, blood pressure and fluid balance (osmolarity), sexual behavior, and emotional responses.

NEUROPHYSIOLOGY AND BEHAVIOR

All behavior is generated and controlled by the nervous system. Nerve tissue is the most fragile of all tissue types and does not have regenerative and restorative abilities — injury to neurons within the brain and the spinal cord is permanent. Protective bone structures such as the skull and spinal column exist to prevent injury from external sources. Physiological mechanisms exist as well to shield the fragile brain tissue from chemical or mechanical injury. One of these mechanisms is a type of nerve cell called *glia*, or "nerve glue." Microglia and macroglia hold the conducting neurons in place and sequester extracellular potassium, thereby protecting neighboring neurons from inappropriate depolarization.

A particular type of glia, the astrocyte, wraps around penetrating capillaries and arterioles to stabilize them but, more importantly, to create a barrier between the blood vessels and the nervous tissue. This *blood-brain barrier* is impermeable to many substances that circulate in the bloodstream yet are toxic to brain tissue. The blood-brain barrier prohibits molecules of low lipid solubility and strongly ionized agents from leaving the blood and entering the brain tissue. Most drugs do not cross this barrier but neither do large molecular bodies, such as bacteria or blood cells, which would contaminate the neural tissue. Phagocytic microglia act as scavengers to remove by-products and other debris from the brain tissue and are the basis of scar formation in injured brain tissue.

NEURONS

The most abundant type of nerve cell is the conducting neuron, which generates and transmits nerve impulses. Dendrites are projections from the neuron cell body that receive impulses from adjacent neurons. The axon, another projection from the cell body, is responsible for impulse propagation to other cells (see Figure 2–3).

Synaptic Transmission

Synaptic transmission, the propagation of electrochemical impulses from neuron to neuron, is the basic mechanism for all nervous system activity. The transfer of ionic charge along the cell membrane of the conducting neuron to the targeting receiving neuron accomplishes this process, known as synaptic transmission. Ion channels (microscopic water-filled tunnels that perforate the cell membrane) open and close, depending on cellular demands, and allow ions such as sodium, potassium, and calcium to diffuse into or out of the cell. As ions flow across the cell membrane, the voltage charge increases to a critical threshold and an impulse is generated. This electrochemical impulse is called an *action potential*. As the action potential moves toward the end of the axon (terminal button), the voltage change triggers the release of neurochemicals called neurotransmitters from their storage vesicles into the extracellular space (synaptic cleft). These neurochemicals diffuse across the synaptic cleft and attach to specific receptor sites to initiate the impulse at the next neuron (see Figure 2–4). After the impulse is transferred, some of the neurotransmitters remain in the synaptic cleft and are either broken down by enzymatic processes or reabsorbed into the presynaptic membrane by a process of reuptake. These processes of neurotransmitter degradation of reuptake can be altered by the action of psychotropic medications (Tecott & Smart, 2005). The psychopharmacologic agent may increase or decrease the degradation or reuptake of the transmitter to alter its activity and "normalize" the transmitter levels. This regulation serves to alleviate the symptoms of mental illness.

NEUROTRANSMITTERS

Neurotransmitters in the brain play an important role in normal function and survival. Many neurological diseases and virtually all medications that act on the nervous system influence the neurotransmitter systems in some way.

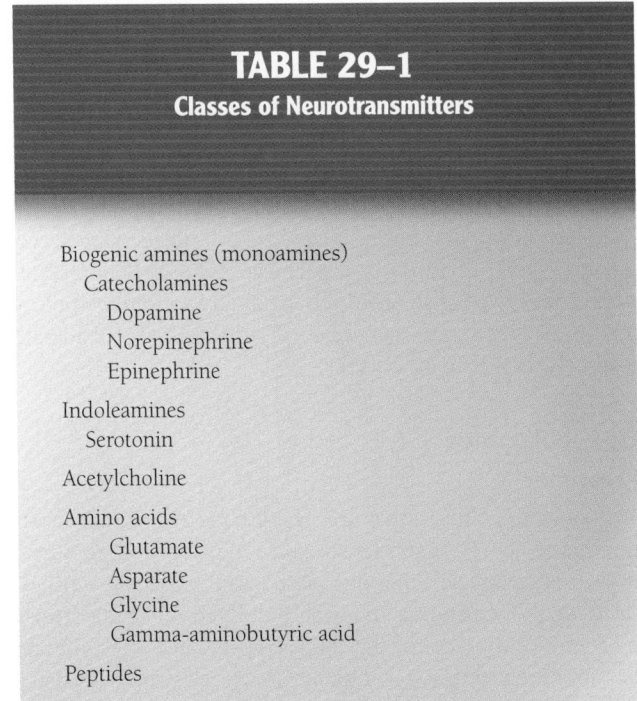

TABLE 29–1
Classes of Neurotransmitters

Biogenic amines (monoamines)
    Catecholamines
        Dopamine
        Norepinephrine
        Epinephrine
Indoleamines
    Serotonin
Acetylcholine
Amino acids
    Glutamate
    Asparate
    Glycine
    Gamma-aminobutyric acid
Peptides

Neurotransmitters have either excitatory or inhibitory abilities. Only a few have both, depending on the nature of the postsynaptic membrane. Excitatory transmitters generate an action potential in the receiving neuron, whereas an inhibitory neurotransmitter dampens or stops the activity of the receiving neuron.

There are four classes of neurotransmitters: the biogenic amines, acetylcholine, the amino acids, and the peptides (Table 29–1).

Biogenic Amines

The first class of neurotransmitters is known as the biogenic amines, or monoamines. This class is divided into two subclasses: indoleamines and catecholamines. Serotonin is an indoleamine. Dopamine, norepinephrine, and epinephrine are catecholamines.

Indoleamines

Serotonin, also known as 5-hydroxytryptamine (5-HT), is hypothesized to play a significant role in states of consciousness, mood, depression, anxiety, and, possibly, schizophrenia (see Chapter 9). Its highest concentrations are found in blood platelets and in the gastrointestinal tract. Serotonin is synthesized from the amino acid L-tryptophan. It is metabolized by monoamine oxidase (MAO) to yield 5-hydroxyindoleacetic acid (5-HIAA), which can be assayed by 24-hour urine collection. Specialized nuclei, the upper and caudal raphe nuclei located within the pons, secrete 5-HT to the serotonergic pathways and their target brain areas: the upper brainstem, the limbic system, and the hypothalamic-pituitary axis (Esposito, 2006; Tecott & Smart, 2005) (see Figure 9–1).

There are at least three different receptors and a number of subreceptors for 5-HT. Lysergic acid, a commonly abused hallucinogen, is an agonist of 5-HT in that it mimics its actions at receptor sites. The selective serotonin reuptake inhibitors (SSRIs) are potent inhibitors of 5-HT; 5-HT reuptake into the presynaptic cleft, and have a low affinity for cholinergic, norepinephrine, and histamine receptors. SSRIs produce somewhat fewer adverse side effects (Tecott & Smart, 2005). In essence, the efficacy and antidepressant properties of SSRIs stem from their ability to inhibit the reuptake of 5-HT and increase 5-HT in the brain (Saddock, Saddock, & Sussman, 2006).

Catecholamines

Dopamine

The catecholamine dopamine is perhaps the single most important neurotransmitter, because it affects a large number of neurological functions. Dopamine is largely synthesized in the substantia nigra and the ventral tegmentum. It is concentrated in the nigrostriatal and mesolimbic dopaminergic tracts (see Figure 14–1). It is used particularly in the limbic system but also diffusely throughout the brain, and it is believed to play a role in the initiation and execution of movement and regulation of emotional responses. Overactivity of dopamine is hypothesized to play a central role in many symptoms of schizophrenia (see Chapter 14 and Figure 14–1). It also plays a role in the regulation of the endocrine system by altering the hypothalamus to manufacture hormones for storage and release by the pituitary (Sadock, Sadock, & Sussman, 2006).

Dopamine is synthesized from the amino acids phenylamine and tyrosine and metabolized by MAO and catechol O-methyltransferase. There are currently six known postsynaptic dopamine receptors: D_1, D_{2A}, D_{2B}, D_3, D_4, and D_5 (Tecott & Smart, 2005). Each of these receptors may exert different dopaminergic influences; thus abnormalities in the dopaminergic system can cause various mental illnesses that respond to different treatments.

Norepinephrine and Epinephrine

Norepinephrine is believed to play a role in learning and memory. Neurons in the locus ceruleus and the lateral tegmentum produce norepinephrine and supply the noradrenergic pathways to the cerebral cortex, limbic system, brainstem, and spinal cord (see Figure 11–1).

Norepinephrine is depleted in clients with Alzheimer's disease and Korsakoff's syndrome, contributing to characteristic symptoms of compromised short-term and long-term memory and limited learning ability (see Chapter 16). Norepinephrine is also thought to play a role in mood stabilization, depression, drive, and motivation. Tricyclics, at one time the most commonly prescribed class of antidepressants, act by increasing levels of norepinephrine in the limbic system. Norepinephrine and epinephrine are also secreted by the adrenal glands and play important roles in the arousal of the autonomic nervous system and the stress response (see Figure 11–1).

Norepinephrine is synthesized from dopamine, and it is metabolized in the same manner; however, its distribution in the brain is not as widespread. There are four known norepinephrine receptors in the brainstem and midbrain: alpha-1, alpha-2, beta-1, and beta-2. These receptors appear to provide evidence that norepinephrine plays a key role in blood pressure regulation and skeletal muscle flexion and that it influences the thalamus, hypothalamus, and cerebral cortex (Tecott & Smart, 2005).

Acetylcholine

Acetylcholine is believed to be the main transmitter responsible for intellectual functioning. It is heavily concentrated in the anterior thalamic nucleus, the septal nuclei, and the association pathways that connect all primary and association areas with the frontal lobe (see Figure 16–1). Acetylcholine transfers the impulses that convey calculations, problem analysis, recognition, learning, and recall. Acetylcholine levels have been found to be low in clients with Alzheimer's disease and other forms of dementia (Tecott & Smart, 2005). Also critical to skeletal and cardiac muscle excitation, acetylcholine is released at the motor end plate to initiate the contraction of the muscle fibers. Interference with acetylcholine at this peripheral location is the underlying pathology of myasthenia gravis, a neuromuscular disease characterized by gradual weakness and wasting of muscle.

Amino Acids

A third class of neurotransmitters is the amino acids. They include glutamate, aspartate, glycine, and gamma-aminobutyric acid (GABA). Glutamate and aspartate are excitatory in nature. They are rapid acting and serve as intermediate neurotransmitters to regulate ionic conditions along the axon membrane before the release of other transmitters in the synaptic cleft. A receptor common to both glutamate and aspartate is the N-methyl-D-aspartate (NMDA) receptor. This specialized receptor records new experiences for learning and future use as memory. NMDA receptors are particularly sensitive to the effects of alcohol and are the first receptors to be destroyed in chronic alcohol use. Glutamate and aspartate also participate in the motor impulses initiated in the cerebellum and the spinal cord.

Glycine and GABA are inhibitory in nature. Glycine can be found mainly in the corticohypothalamic projection pathway through the reticular activating system in the brainstem. It serves as the impulse modulator for messages going to the spinal cord and the peripheral nervous system. GABA is synthesized from glutamate, and it is present in much higher concentrations throughout the brain than all of the other neurotransmitters described here. GABA pathways exist between the cortex and the hypothalamic-pituitary axis (see Figure 11–1). It serves as the brain's modulator and limits the effects of excitatory transmitters. GABA inhibits neuronal transmission by hyperpolarizing the receptor site to render it less sensitive to continual stimulation. GABA acts in the basal ganglia to regulate sensorimotor impulses for smooth and controlled movement. Low levels of brain GABA predispose a person to convulsions and disorganized sensorimotor function. The choreatic movements that characterize Huntington's disease are associated with a loss of the intrastriatal GABA activity and basal ganglia dysregulation, which contribute to the emergence of the hyperkinetic features of this disease (Ganong, 2005). Benzodiazepines enhance GABA binding to receptor sites and are effective in treating anxiety. Anticonvulsants work in a similar manner to modulate hyperstimulation by their anti-kindling properties and prevent seizures. Perhaps the efficacy of anticonvulsants as mood stabilizers stem from these properties.

Peptides

Another class of neurotransmitters, the peptides, is involved in the activation and regulation of response to stress and injury such as pain perception and reflex function. Peptides are produced in the neuronal cell body and are mediated by genetic coding. The actions of enzymes, amino acid residues, and other chemical actions regulate the activity of peptides (Sadock, Sadock, & Sussman, 2006). Some families of neuroactive peptides are the endogenous opioids, including endorphins and enkephalins. These neurotransmitters are believed to play a role in the modulation of stress, pain, and mood. Substance P is primarily found in afferent sensory motor neurons in the striatonigral pathway and are believed to be at the first synapse of slow pain. High concentrations are found in the nigrostriatal system and the hypothalamus, where it plays a role in neuroendocrine regulation. Dysregulation of Substance P is hypothesized to contribute to symptoms found in Alzheimer's disease and mood disorders (Ganong, 2005).

Neurotransmitter Action

Much of the current knowledge about mental illness, neurological diseases, and the medications that treat them is based on the understanding of the role of neurotransmitters in synaptic transmission. Recall that the process of synaptic transmission by axons of neurons is accomplished by an increase in sodium and potassium permeability across the cell membrane. The flow of ions creates an action potential that travels to the end of the axon, where the voltage change triggers the release of neurotransmitters from the presynaptic membrane into the synaptic cleft (Tecott & Smart, 2005) (see Figure 2–4).

The neurotransmitter diffuses across the synaptic cleft to the postsynaptic receptor site on the receiving neuron. The neurotransmitter attaches to each of these chemical structures in a manner similar to a key fitting a lock: the chemical structure makes an exact close fit with the receptor site. Once attached, the neurotransmitter activates the postsynaptic receptor by opening the ion channels, changing the membrane potential, and initiating another action potential at the next neuron (Tecott & Smart, 2005). An excitatory transmitter generates an action potential in the receiving neuron (depolarization), whereas an inhibitory neurotransmitter dampens or prohibits the activity of the receiving neuron (hyperpolarization).

Once the transmitter has performed its function, it must be removed to terminate its action; otherwise, the action potential is abnormally prolonged, inhibited, or exaggerated. The production and release of excess neurotransmitter or the excessive sensitivity of the receptor site to the action of the neurotransmitter also produce an exaggerated effect. For example, excessive norepinephrine secretion could be a cause of anxiety disorders (see Figure 11–1). Conversely, deficient synthesis or insufficient release of the neurotransmitter, or decreased sensitivity of the receptor site produces abnormal results; for example, low dopamine levels could be a factor in depression (Tecott & Smart, 2005). The action of neurotransmitters is ended by one of two mechanisms: reuptake or enzymatic deactivation. The postsynaptic potential produced by almost all transmitter substances are terminated by *reuptake*, in which the transmitter is rapidly pumped from the synaptic cleft back into the presynaptic terminal bouton. Enzymes (frequently MAO) that metabolize the transmitter accomplish enzymatic deactivation. Acetylcholine, dopamine, and norepinephrine activity are terminated in this manner (Tecott & Smart, 2005).

This description of synaptic transmission is greatly oversimplified. In reality, the surface of receptor sites in any individual neuron may have 2,000 to 3,000 receptor sites that may be highly specialized or that may perform a variety of functions.

Behavior is the manifestation of the combined actions of potentials emerging from masses of neurons in the primary and association areas in the response to a person's thoughts. It stands to reason that many behaviors and neurological symptoms of underlying general medical conditions are a manifestation of disruption to the transmission of processes described earlier. Brain injury from trauma or hypoxia or abnormal cell formation in tumor interferes with normal neural function and metabolism. With aging, the brain undergoes changes more gradually. Its plasticity is reduced as neurons die, and glia becomes more rigid with scar tissue. The blood-brain barrier becomes increasingly permeable, which compromises neural tissue integrity. The overall brain metabolic rate slows, and mentation may become cloudy as transmitter activity becomes sluggish or levels become suboptimal. Brain water is decreased, which lessens the absorbability of neuropharmacologic agents. All of these factors have significant pharmacokinetic implications for the effective treatment of abnormal neural processes present in mental illness.

PHARMACOKINETIC CONCEPTS

The efficacy of pharmacologic agents parallels its ability to reach appropriate concentrations at sites of actions. It is crucial for the psychiatric nurse to understand major concepts associated with general principles of pharmacologic actions and drug efficacy.

PHARMACOLOGY

Pharmacology is the scientific study of chemical formulations (drugs), including their sources, properties, uses, actions, and effects. Two areas of concern for the psychiatric-mental health nurse are pharmacodynamics and pharmacokinetics. Pharmacodynamics refers to the actual biochemical and physiological effects on living tissue that are caused by the interaction of drugs with tissue receptors. In other words, the pharmacodynamic principles focus on what the drug does to the body. Pharmacokinetics, on the other hand, is the study of the absorption, distribution, metabolism, and elimination of drugs. In other words, it is concerned with what the body does with the drug.

Pharmacodynamic and pharmacokinetic concepts are important, because they provide the psychiatric-mental health nurse with an understanding of the relevant properties of psychopharmacologic agents. These concepts also explain the therapeutic properties of drugs, their potential adverse effects, their use in the treatment of mental illness, their interactions with other pharmaceutical agents, and these interactions on human responses. Of continued interest is the potential role that race and ethnicity play in the pharmacokinetics of psychotropic drugs. Pharmacokinetic principles are emphasized in the pharmacodynamic discussions of the psychotropic drugs described in this chapter.

FACTORS THAT INCLUDE DRUG INTENSITY AND DURATION

The first set of concepts is concerned with the general pharmacokinetic effects of psychopharmacologic agents. There are four factors that influence the intensity and duration of drug effect: absorption, distribution, metabolism, and elimination.

ABSORPTION

Absorption is the process by which drug molecules pass from the site of administration into the systematic circulation. Absorption is affected by route of administration (e.g., oral,

intramuscular, or intravenous), drug formulation, and such factors as food and antacids in the case of oral administration.

DISTRIBUTION

Distribution is the movement of the drug from the site of administration throughout the body and dilution in body fluids. The volume of distribution is an indicator of the degree of distribution a drug undergoes. A drug with low volume is limited to intravascular space. Medium distribution means the drug appears in most extracellular fluid, and high distribution means drug concentration occurs inside the cell and body fats. Factors that affect the body-fat-water ratio such as age, sex, and weight also affect drug distribution (Sadock, Sadock, & Sussman, 2006).

METABOLISM

Metabolism is the formulation of active and inactive metabolites through the conversion of a drug into a new, usually less active and more water-soluble compound and also by-products or waste products. The enzyme system is responsible for metabolism of most drugs and it is located in the endoplasmic reticulum of the liver (known as the microsomal fraction). Other areas of metabolism are the epithelium of the gastrointestinal tract, the kidneys, the lungs, and the skin. The first-pass effect refers to the site of the initial drug metabolism. As mentioned, the liver is the principal organ of drug metabolism. However, some drugs (e.g., clonazepam and chlorpromazine) are metabolized in the intestine. Thus the intestinal metabolism can contribute to first-pass effect. First-pass effects, then, may limit the bioavailability of orally administered drugs such that alternate routes may be needed to be used to achieve the desired therapeutic blood levels (Sadock, Sadock, & Sussman, 2006).

ELIMINATION

Elimination is the removal of the drug, drug by-products, and inactive metabolites from the body, usually through urine or feces, perspiration, and respiration (Sadock, Sadock, & Sussman, 2006).

 THE MORE YOU KNOW

Mixed Result in Drug Trial on Pretreating Schizophrenia

The long-awaited study supported by Eli Lily and the National Institute of Mental Health raised more questions than answers in the first long-term trial of early drug treatment. Positive results from the study were deemed marginally significant and the negative results were much clearer. Ethical concerns about the daily use of the antipsychotic drug Zyprexa of individuals not yet diagnosed with schizophrenia were raised along with stigma-

tization, particularly for adolescents. The study encountered numerous obstacles including recruitment problems and a high drop-out rate from the beginning in 1997. Toward the end of the study two-thirds of the young people in both groups had dropped out, making it difficult to analyze differences between them. Significant weight gain (a median of 20 pounds) occurred during the study.

Benedict Carey, *The New York Times*, Monday, May 1, 2006, A12.

STEADY STATE, HALF-LIFE, AND CLEARANCE

There are three important concepts in the pharmacokinetics of drugs: steady state, half-life, and clearance.

Steady State

Steady state is the condition that occurs when the amount of drug removed from the body equals the amount being absorbed. The steady state is important because it represents the amount of drug required to achieve the desired therapeutic effects. Not all drugs have linear kinetics (a linear relationship between dose and plasma concentration) in steady state. Linear kinetics is a pharmacokinetic model in which a constant amount of a drug is eliminated in a set unit of time. It depicts the relationship between a drug's absorption and elimination necessary to a steady state. In linear kinetics, the drug half-life is *dose dependent*.

For certain drugs and for most drugs in large doses, however, the relationship is nonlinear. In this model, called exponential kinetics, the half-life of a drug is independent of dose. For example, this occurs with imipramine (Tofranil) in older adults and in the long-term use of carbamazepine (Tegretol) or chlorpromazine (Thorazine). Caution is required, therefore, in increasing dosages into the upper range of acceptable prescribed dosages or using these drugs in special populations, such as older adults or clients with comorbid illnesses, in whom the likelihood of toxicity is high (Sadock, Sadock, & Sussman, 2006).

Half-Life

A drug's half-life is the time in hours needed for the amount of drug in the body (as measured by plasma concentration) to decrease by one half, or 50 percent. The half-life of a drug is important for predicting the length of time necessary for the drug to be totally eliminated from the body. Drugs with long half-lives have slow rates of egress from the body. This information is useful, for example, when the advanced-practice psychiatric nurse is waiting for one antidepressant to be eliminated from the body before starting another. Such is the case when switching from treatment with a monoamine oxidase inhibitor (MAOI) to an SSRI. For untoward effects to be avoided, drugs with short half-lives, such as the benzodiazepine triazolam (Halcion), may require tapering off of the dose rather than abrupt discontinuation (Sadock, Sadock, & Sussman, 2006). The half-life of a drug is also important for determining the time required for achieving the stable concentration (or steady state) of a drug. In general, drugs require four to five half-lives to achieve steady state. Knowledge about the drug's half-life is also important for determining the frequency of dosing. Drugs with short half-lives require more frequent dosing. Drugs with long half-lives can be administered in a once-a-day dose.

Clearance

Clearance is the volume of blood in millimeters per minute from which all of the drug is removed per unit of time. Clearance determines the magnitude of the steady-state concentration and therefore the dosage required achieving the desired steady state of a drug. Drugs that are efficiently eliminated by renal excretion and hepatic metabolism require higher dosage regimen than do those that are inefficiently eliminated.

Protein Binding

Another important factor in understanding the pharmacokinetic properties of drugs is *protein binding*. Once the drug is absorbed into the vascular system, protein molecules transport it, usually albumin, to the site of action (Sadock, Sadock, & Sussman, 2006). The plasma proteins are generally unable to exit the vascular beds because of their molecular size. Similarly, protein-bound drugs are unable to exit unless they are freed from their binding sites. The stronger the binding site, the slower the freeing of drugs, resulting a longer duration of action. As the drug is metabolized, more of the drug is released from the binding sites. Occasionally, two or more drugs compete for the same binding sites. When this occurs, the drug with the strongest affinity for the binding site displaces the other drug. When this interaction occurs, the displaced drug usually produces a toxic effect because a large concentration is free in the vascular bed (Sadock, Sadock, & Sussman, 2006).

Active Metabolites

Active metabolites play an important role in pharmacokinetics. With the exception of lithium, most of the psychopharmacologic agents produce active metabolites during the process of metabolism. In general, metabolites are more water soluble than the parent compound. The half-life of a metabolite is equal to or longer than that of its parent compound. The cyclic antidepressants, the antipsychotics, and some anxiolytics have major active metabolites. These drugs may require a longer time to reach a steady state. Therefore, active metabolites complicate conclusions about the clinical effects of psychopharmacologic agents based solely on serum levels and steady-state phenomena (Sadock, Sadock, & Sussman, 2006).

CULTURAL CONSIDERATIONS

The field of pharmacogenetics has exploded over the past 10 years. Findings from current research indicate that most of the genes governing the expression and function of enzymes that modulate the metabolism of psychotropic agents have been sequenced and differentiated (Vandel, Talon, Haffen, & Sechter, 2007). Researchers have discovered that common mutations at the genetic and cellular levels are responsible for cross-ethnic variations in the response to psychotropic medications. In addition, these findings indicate that gene-encoding proteins (e.g., transporters and receptors) modulate and mediate the action of neurotransmitters and target sites of various psychotropic drugs. Extensive data also show that pharmacokinetics—absorption, distribution, metabolism, and excretion—modulate the fate and nature of most medications and that culture and ethnicity substantially affect the variability of metabolism and drug responses (Vandel et al., 2007).

As previously mentioned the P-450 enzymes, which recently have been studied extensively, seem to control the rate-limiting stages in the metabolism of most psychotropics. Interestingly enough, the activity of these enzymes is greatly modulated by genetic polymorphisms (e.g., number of alleles [alternative forms of a gene] and gene frequencies), whose distribution varies considerably among ethnic groups (Vandel, Talon, Haffen, & Sechter, 2007). Recent gene studies indicate that some individuals' enzyme systems are nonfunctional (poor metabolizers), less-efficient functioning (intermediate metabolizers), and enhanced action (extensive metabolizers). The extensive metabolizer group is further broken down into normal functioning and ultrarapid metabolizers (Vandel et al., 2007). An important clinical implication for psychiatric nurses is linking culture to the client's response (e.g., poor, desired, adverse reactions), rather than assuming that a poor response is a nonadherence problem. Other clinical issues include the necessity of increasing or decreasing the drug because the client is an ultrarapid or poor or ultra metabolizer. Overall, the role of culture and ethnicity on gene expression is complex and interesting. Understanding the influence of culture and ethnicity on client responses throughout treatment planning enables the psychiatric nurse to appreciate their significance in all areas of care, including psychosocial and other biological interventions. Psychiatric nurses need to assess the client and family's perception of mental illness and the role of medication. Issues regarding psychoeducation concerning desired and adverse drug reactions along with psychosocial interventions play key roles in medication adherence. By linking culture and ethnicity to client responses, the psychiatric nurse can develop a more holistic and individualized plan of care that enhances the client's response to pharmacologic and other treatment modalities.

PSYCHOPHARMACOLOGIC THERAPEUTIC AGENTS

Compelling evidence of the role of intricate biological, genetic, and neuroanatomical influences on signs and symptoms of psychiatric disorders explains the significance of pharmacologic agents in promoting mental health. Psychiatric nurses play pivotal roles in symptom management and facilitating an optimal level of functioning in the client with a mental disorder. The following section provides an overview of pharmacologic agents and their role in providing hope and a quality of life for clients and their families experiencing various psychiatric disorders.

MEDICATION ADMINISTRATION

Historically, the responsibility of the nurse regarding medications was limited to the principles of medication administration, specifically, the *correct drug* to the *correct client* in the *correct dose* by the *correct route* at the *correct time*. The nurse needs to follow facility protocol for medication administration procedures. As with any client treated on inpatient or outpatient settings, documentation and reporting of procedures must be followed with the client with a mental disorder. Although these basic principles are essential, much more is required if the therapeutic purpose is to be attained.

Advanced-practice psychiatric-mental health nurses, similar to generalist psychiatric-mental health nurses are responsible for safe medication administration. Their responsibilities extend beyond direct administration although they may prescribe medications for administration. Advanced-practice mental health nurses must prescribe based on evidence-based data, clinical practice guidelines, and state and federal regulations. They must attain and maintain knowledge of psychopathology, neurobiology, and physiology. In addition the nurse recommends or prescribes pharmacotherapy based on the client's mental health problem, psychiatric and medical conditions, and the individual uniqueness, such as age, gender, physical condition, religious and cultural beliefs, health practices, and potential side effects on the client or unborn child. Prescriptive privileges and responsibilities also require knowledge of expected therapeutic actions, anticipated side-effect profile, course of action, and benefit-risk ratio. The advanced-practice psychiatric-mental health nurse also evaluates pharmacotherapy outcomes by employing standardized clinical instruments and client reports to determine efficacy of treatment. Finally, advanced-practice psychiatric–registered nurse collaborates with the client and mental health team, primary care and specialty clinic providers to address complex and difficult clinical situations.

Presently, psychiatric nurses must be able to integrate basic and complex principles into their understanding of medications; client responses, both desired and adverse; and recognize the role of families and health teaching into appropriate treatment planning. Psychiatric nurses play key roles in making accurate diagnoses, prescribing a plan of care that includes pharmacologic and nonpharmacologic treatment planning, and monitoring client responses. Understanding the effects of various pharmacologic agents involves knowing actions of specific agents and promoting safe and appropriate care for clients with assorted mental disorders and medical conditions.

Antidepressants

Depression is a common, disabling illness with enormous social and economic consequences; it is estimated that 18 to 23 percent of women and 8 to 11 percent of men experience at least one serious depression in their lifetime (see Chapter 9). Untreated, depression can be a dangerous illness; approximately 15 to 20 percent of clients with a primary affective illness (depression or bipolar disorder) die from suicide (Mann & Currier, 2007). Historically, depression has been described as either endogenous or exogenous. Endogenous depressions were assumed to result from biological alterations and thus treatable with medications. Reactive or exogenous depressions were thought to occur in reaction to an environmentally caused event, such as the loss of a family member or a job. These depressions were "worked through" and not treated with medication. This dichotomy is currently generally rejected. The decision to use medication is now based on the severity of the presenting symptoms and *not* on presumed causality.

Antidepressants, as their name suggests, are medications prescribed to treat depression. In addition, antidepressants are used in the treatment of dysthymia; anxiety disorders, including obsessive-compulsive disorder, panic disorder, PTSD; somatoform disorders; eating disorders; and childhood enuresis. Like the antipsychotics, most antidepressants have been categorized by their chemical structures. The newer antidepressants are being categorized by their chemical actions. The clinical and pharmacokinetic parameters of the antidepressants are presented in Table 29–2).

Heterocyclics

The largest group of antidepressants can be described as heterocyclic, indicating their common structural characteristic: carbon rings. The most familiar type of antidepressant is a subgroup of the heterocyclic compounds called tricyclic antidepressants, or TCAs, so named because of the three carbon rings that characterize all the medications in this subclass. Maprotiline (Ludiomil) is considered a tetracyclic. Clomipramine (Anafranil) is an effective antidepressant, which is the first-line drug of choice in the treatment of obsessive-compulsive disorder. This drug may be useful in the treatment of the depressed client with marked obsessive features. It also shows promise to clients experiencing chronic pain, other anxiety disorders, and phobias (Sadock, Sadock, & Sussman, 2006).

Mechanism of Action

Until recently, the heterocyclics were thought to work by inhibiting the presynaptic reuptake of norepinephrine (a catecholamine) and 5-HT (an indoleamine). Currently, however, several other hypotheses are being advanced. One approach focuses on the slower adaptive changes in norepinephrine and 5-HT systems and reregulation of an abnormal receptor-neurotransmitter relationship. It is thought that this regulatory action speeds up the client's natural recovery process from a depressive episode by normalizing neurotransmission efficacy (Tecott & Smart, 2005). One specific reregulation hypothesis is the down-regulation theory, which suggests that depression occurs concomitantly with increased norepinephrine activity. According to this theory, antidepressants promote a down-regulation of activity by decreasing beta-adrenergic receptor sensitivity to norepinephrine (Tecott & Smart, 2005).

The heterocyclics are equally effective clinically, and many have similar metabolic pathways. These drugs are often divided into subgroups according to potency and reactions (Sadock, Sadock, & Sussman, 2006). As an example of grouping by secondary properties, the TCAs are grouped into secondary and tertiary amines. Secondary amines are considered activating antidepressants, whereas tertiary amines are considered sedating antidepressants. Thus, an activating secondary amine, desipramine (Norpramin), may be a useful choice for the client whose depression has retarded (slowed) her mental and physical activity, whereas imipramine (Tofranil), a commonly used tertiary sedating amine, may be a better choice for an agitated client who is not sleeping well.

Side Effects, Dosage, and Drug Interactions

Heterocyclic antidepressants usually take 2 to 4 weeks to have any significant antidepressant effect. Side effects, however, can occur within 24 hours and can continue throughout the course of treatment. A comparison of the relative degree of side effects for the antidepressants is presented in Table 29–3. Some side effects are beneficial to the client; for example, sedation is a benefit to a client suffering from insomnia. More frequently, however, side effects such as dry mouth, constipation, orthostatic hypotension, blurred vision, and impaired sexual arousal (erectile function and orgasm) are annoying at best and can seem debilitating at worst. To a person already suffering from depression these side effects can seem like too great a burden to bear. The nurse is in an excellent position to listen and offer hope by pointing out that the side effects will lessen and may disappear with time, whereas the antidepressant effects will increase.

It may take longer than 4 weeks to find the optimum dose of an antidepressant. Although 70 percent of clients respond positively to the first antidepressant prescribed, it is not unusual for a client to have to switch to another medication. This can be discouraging for the client. Again, the nurse can provide needed encouragement and perspective during this period. All these medications can cause side effects to some degree in all clients. The associated symptoms of adverse effects of the antidepressants are presented in Table 29–4.

Other possible side effects from heterocyclics include the following:

◆ Risk of seizures: All heterocyclics can lower the seizure threshold and must be used with caution in clients with a history of seizures. Moreover, bupropion, maprotiline, and clomipramine, even at therapeutic levels, have been associated with seizures in clients without a history of seizures.

◆ Psychiatric disorders: Tricyclic and heterocyclic antidepressants can precipitate a manic episode in clients with bipolar I disorder with and without a prior diagnosed manic episode. These drugs may also exacerbate psychotic disorders. Therefore, it is imperative to make an accurate distinction between unipolar and bipolar depression. It is practical to begin with a low dose in these clients and monitor them for signs of mania or psychosis, or consider another antidepressant.

◆ Cardiac effects: Caution must be used when administering heterocyclics to clients with cardiovascular disease. In high doses, TCAs may produce arrythmias, sinus tachycardia, flattened T waves, and depressed ST segments and QT intervals. Because the result of these arrythmias prolongs conduction time, preexisting conduction defects contraindicate the use of these antidepressants.

TABLE 29-2

Clinical and Pharmacokinetic Parameters of Antidepressant Medications

Generic Name	Brand Name	Dosage Range (mg/Day)	Half-Life (Hours)	Onset of Clinical Effects	Elimination Period after Last Dose	Amine Blocking Activity*
Tertiary Amines						
Amitriptyline	Elavil	75–200	31–46 (18–44 for nortriptyline)	2–4 weeks for all tertiary amines	≥2 weeks for all tertiary amines	NE (2), 5-HT (4)
Clomipramine	Anafranil	75–300	19–37			NE (2), 5-HT (5)
Doxepin	Sinequan, Adapin	75–300	8–24 (desmethyline)			NE (1), 5-HT (2)
Imipramine	Tofranil	75–200	11–25 (12–24 for desipramine)			NE (2), 5-HT (4)
Trimipramine	Surmontil	75–200	7–30			NE (1), 5-HT (1)
Secondary Amines						
Amoxapine	Asendin	150–300	8–30 (30 for 7-hydrox and 8-hydrox)	2–4 weeks for all secondary amines	2–4 weeks for all secondary amines	NE (3), 5-HT (2), DA (2)
Desipramine	Norpramin	75–200	12–24			NE (4), 5-HT (2)
Nortriptyline	Aventyl	75–150	18–44			NE (2), 5-HT (3)
Protriptyline	Vivactyl	20–40	67–89			NE (4), 5-HT (2)

	Brand	Dosage (mg)	Half-life			Neurotransmitter effect*
Tetracyclic						
Maprotiline	Ludiomil	75–300	21–25	3–7 days 2–3 weeks	2 weeks	NE (3), 5-HT (1)
Triazolopyridine						
Trazodone	Desyrel	50–600	4–9	1–4 weeks	2 weeks	5-HT (3)
Nefazodone	Serzone	300–600	3.5–5			5-HT₂ (3), NE (1)
Bicyclics						
Fluoxetine	Prozac, Prozac Weekly	20–80, 90	2–5 days (7–9 days for norfluoxetine)	1–4 days	4 weeks	NE (1), 5-HT (5)
Paroxetine	Paxil, Paxil CR	10–60, 25–62.5	5–21	Up to 8 weeks	2 weeks	NE (1), DA (1), 5-HT (5)
Sertraline	Zoloft	50–200	24 N-desmethylsertraline (62–104 hours)	Up to 8 weeks	2 weeks	NE (1), DA (1), 5-HT (5)
Citalopram	Celexa	20–60	35	Up to 8 weeks	2 weeks	NE (1), DA (1), 5-HT (5)
Escitalopram	Lexapro	5–20	27–32	Up to 8 weeks	2 weeks	NE (1), DA (1), 5-HT (5)
Fluvoxamine	Luvox	50–300	15	Up to 8 weeks	2 weeks	
Bupropion	Welbutrin	200–300	8 days (4 weeks for active metabolites)	1–4 weeks	2 weeks	NE (1), 5-HT (1), DA (1)
Mirtazapine	Remeron	15–30	20–40	6–8 weeks		NE (2), 5-HT₂, (5) 5HT₃, (5), H2 (5)
Venlafaxine	Effexor/Effexor, XR	75–375/75–225	4–10	6–8 weeks	2 weeks	NE (1), DA (1), 5-HT (5)
Duloxetine	Cymbalta	60–100	12	Up to 8 weeks	2 weeks	NE (1), DA (1), 5-HT (5)

*NE, norepinepherine; DA, dopamine; 5-HT, serotonin. 0 = none, 1 = very weak, 2 = weak, 3 = moderate, 4 = strong, 5 = strongest.

TABLE 29–3
Incidence of Adverse Effects for Antidepressants

Medications	Anticholinergic Effects	Sedation	Orthostatic Hypotension
Amitriptyline (Elavil)	***	***	**
Clomipramine (Anafranil)	***	***	**
Doxepin (Adapin, Sinequan)	**	***	**
Imipramine (Tofranil)	**	**	***
Trimipramine (Surmontil)	**	**	**
Amoxapine (Asendin)	***	**	*
Desipramine (Norpramin)	*	*	*
Nortriptyline (Aventyl, Pamelor)	**	**	*
Protriptyline (Vivactil)	***	*	*
Maprotiline (Ludiomil)	**	**	*
Trazodone (Desyrel)	*	**	**
Nefazodone (Serzone)	**	**	*
Fluoxetine (Prozac)	*	0	*
Fluvoxamine (Luvox)	*	0	**
Paroxetine (Paxil)	*	0	*
Sertraline (Zoloft)	*	0	*
Citalopram (Celexa)	*	0	*
Escitalopram (Lexapro)	*	0	*
Bupropion (Wellbutrin)	**	**	*
Venlafaxine (Effexor)	**	**	*
Mirtazapine (Remeron)	*	**	*
Duloxetine (Cymbalta)	**	*	0

0, minimal or no sedation. * low; ** moderate; *** high incidence of adverse effects.

◆ Risk of overdose: Drug overdoses with these agents can be lethal, especially when combined with alcohol. Because the risk of suicide is also a consideration with depressed clients, until stabilized, they should not be given more than 1 week's supply at a time. In addition, because of the prolonged half-lives of these agents, particularly with overdosing, the risk of cardiac arrythmias is high, requiring cardiac monitoring in the intensive care unit for 3 to 4 days after the overdose attempt (Sadock, Sadock, & Sussman, 2006).

◆ Metabolites: One of the breakdown products of the antidepressant amoxapine (Asendin) is loxapine (Loxitane). Because loxapine is an antipsychotic, it carries the risk of extrapyramidal side effects (EPS) and tardive dyskinesia (TD). Many prescribers are reluctant to prescribe this medication for this reason.

Heterocyclics have the potential to produce the following:

1. Increase serum levels with concomitant use of fluoxetine (Prozac) or cimetidine (Tagamet)
2. Decrease therapeutic blood levels for some smokers
3. Increase pressor response to norepinephrine and intravenous epinephrine
4. May reduce the serum levels with concomitant use of birth control pills through induction of hepatic enzymes

Selective Serotonin Reuptake Inhibitors (SSRIs)

SSRIs have become the first-line treatment of major depression because of the favorable side effect profile and efficacy. As their name implies, SSRIs potently and selectively inhibit the neuronal reuptake pump of 5-HT in the synaptic cleft and increase 5-HT transmission with little effect on the reuptake of norepinephrine or dopamine. SSRIs share this property with

TABLE 29–4
Symptoms Associated with Adverse Effects of Tricyclics and Related Antidepressants

System	Common Side Effects	Less Common Side Effects
Cardiovascular	Orthostatic hypotension, tachycardia	Palpitations
	Hypertension for SSRIs such as fluoxetine, and SNRIs such as venlafaxine	
Central Nervous	Drowsiness, weakness, fatigue, dizziness, tremors	Confusion, disturbed concentration, decreased memory, electrocardiographic changes
	Maprotiline: headaches, restlessness	
	Fluoxetine: headaches, insomnia, anxiety, sexual disturbances	
	Bupropion: agitation, headache, confusion, involuntary movements, ataxia, insomnia, seizures	
	SSRIs and other antidepressants have been associated with an increased risk of suicide among adolescents and adults. On October 15, 2004, the FDA directed pharmaceutical companies of antidepressant medication to include a "black box" warning that informs health care providers and consumers about the increased risk of suicidal thoughts and behaviors in youth being treated with these medications. In addition, psychiatric-mental health nurses and other health care providers must provide closer monitoring of children and adolescents prescribed these agents. Health education that includes the risks and precautions must also be afforded to mitigate these risks.	
Neurological	Risk of seizures have been associated with bupropion, especially in individuals with a history of seizures, at-risk (e.g., alcohol withdrawal); and history of an eating disorder	Numbness, tingling, paresthesias of extremities, akathisia, ataxia, tremors, extrapyramidal side effects, neuropathy, seizures
Autonomic	Dry mouth, blurred vision, constipation, urinary retention	
	Fluoxetine: excessive sweating	
Gastrointestinal	Maprotiline: nausea	
	Trazodone: vomiting	
	Fluoxetine/sertraline: nausea, diarrhea, weight loss, dry mouth	Vomiting, nausea, diarrhea, flatulence
	Bupropion: nausea, vomiting, abdominal cramps, constipation, dry mouth	
Allergic	Paroxetine	Skin rash, pruritus, urticaria, photosensitivity, edema
Respiratory		Pharyngitis, rhinitis, sinusitis
Genitourinary	Sexual side effects, such as desire, arousal, and erectile and orgasmic disorders	

Note. The U.S. Food and Drug Administration has issued a "black box" warning for suicide risk associated with all antidepressants.

TCAs. Fortunately, their actions avoid the vast actions of TCAs, including blockage of histamine, cholinergic, and alpha₁ adrenergic receptors, and their adverse effects (Sadock, Sadock, & Sussman, 2006; Tecott & Smart, 2005). Thus their action appears to be more specific and their side effect profile more narrow. Examples of SSRIs include fluoxetine (Prozac Weekly), sertraline (Zoloft), paroxetine (Paxil), citalopram (Celexa), and escitalopram (Lexapro). Fluvoxamine (Luvox), another SSRI, has shown efficacy in the treatment of obsessive-compulsive disorder (see Table 29–2).

The SSRIs have diverse structures. Paroxetine, for example is a phenylpiperidine derivative, whereas sertraline is a naphthaleneamine derivative. The efficacy of paroxetine and sertraline for the management of major depression has been established by controlled studies of 6 to 8 weeks, principally in outpatient settings (Sadock, Sadock, & Sussman, 2006). Paroxetine's metabolism through the cytochrome P450 (cyp) 2D6 suggests potential drug interactions and dosage adjustments.

Drug Interactions and Side Effects

The SSRIs are eliminated by extensive hepatic biotransformation involving the P450 enzyme system, and all are involved in varying degrees in mediating the effects on the metabolism of other drugs (e.g., inhibition of cytochrome P450). Thus, caution should be used with other coadministration of SSRIs and other drugs metabolized by this isoenzyme, including MAOIs, phenothiazines, alprazolam, triazolam, and type IC antiarrythymics (e.g., flecainide, encainide, and propafenone) or drugs that inhibit this enzyme (e.g., quinidine) (Sadock, Sadock, & Sussman, 2006).

SSRIs are generally well absorbed and have a more rapid onset of action than do other classes of antidepressants— 1 to 3 weeks, rather than the 2 to 4 weeks suggested for the heterocyclics. Of note, fluoxetine has a significantly longer half-life (e.g., 2 to 3 days; metabolite norfluoxetine, 7 to 9 days) than do most other antidepressants, which means that it will take much longer to clear out of the client's system on discontinuation of the medication. Due to the long half-life of fluoxetine, Prozac Weekly was developed for the ease of administration and to improve client adherence. It is recommended for all the SSRIs that an MAOI not be used concomitantly and that at least 5 weeks should lapse between discontinuation of an SSRI and initiation of treatment with an MAOI because of potential life-threatening drug interactions (i.e., 5-HT syndrome, hypertensive crisis). Similarly, at least 2 weeks should be provided from the discontinuation of MAOI therapy and the initiation of therapy with an SSRI (Sadock, Sadock, & Sussman, 2006).

The side effect profile for SSRIs differs from those of the heterocyclics and MAOIs. Common side effects include restlessness, insomnia, nausea, diarrhea, headache, dizziness, dry mouth, and tremor; ejaculatory delay may also occur in males. Unlike most other antidepressants, fluoxetine does not stimulate the appetite or cause carbohydrate craving. On the contrary, there is some evidence that SSRIs decrease appetite and can lead to weight loss initially. The SSRIs rarely appear to affect the electrocardiogram and have only minimal cardiovascular effects (Sadock, Sadock, & Sussman, 2006).

The SSRIs appear to be much safer in overdose than other antidepressants and are not potentiated by alcohol. These features are attractive when one is prescribing to a population with a higher than average risk of suicide. Finally, the SSRIs need less dosage titration than do the heterocyclic or MAOI antidepressants. In general, this makes them easier to prescribe and easier to take.

A potential problem that can arise for clients taking medications that affect serotonin is called serotonin syndrome, a condition of serotonergic hyperstimulation. Various combinations of medications can cause it, but it most commonly results from the combination of MAOIs with serotonergic agents. These serotonergic agents include L-tryptophan (an amino acid precursor of 5-HT) as well as fluoxetine, clomipramine, and paroxetine. The possibility of serotonergic syndrome provides additional rationale for the waiting period between antidepressant therapies involving MAOIs.

Classic features of 5-HT syndrome are changes in mental status, restlessness, myoclonus, hyperreflexia, diaphoresis, shivering, and tremor. Obviously, though, these symptoms are not specific to 5-HT syndrome. Careful observation of clients on medications and an understanding of 5-HT syndrome enable the nurse to be alert to this possibility. The treatment of choice is to discontinue the involved medications and provide supportive measures.

Dopamine-Norepinephrine Reuptake Inhibitors (DNRIs)

Bupropion (Wellbutrin) is a unicyclic antidepressant that is unrelated to heterocyclic antidepressants or MAOIs. This drug is metabolized to hydroxybupropion. As its name implies, bupropion is a dopamine-norepinephrine reuptake inhibitor (DNRI) whose primary action involves inhibiting the reuptake of norepinephrine and dopamine. Major uses for bupropion include the treatment of major depression and attention-deficit hyperactivity disorder. It has a favorable side effect profile, and it is often used as a first-line drug for the treatment of major depression (Sadock, Sadock, & Sussman, 2006). The most common side effects of bupropion include headache, anxiety, diaphoresis, and gastrointestinal disturbances. The incidence of seizures is 0.4 percent, which is four times that of major antidepressants. Nurses must administer bupropion with extreme caution to clients with a history of seizure disorders or who are taking medications that lower the seizure threshold (e.g., antipsychotic agents) and history of eating disorders. Combining bupropion with an MAOI is potentially dangerous and must be avoided (Sadock, Sadock, & Sussman, 2006).

Serotonin-Norepinephrine Reuptake Inhibitors (SNRIs)

Venlafaxine (Effexor) and duloxetine (Cymbalta) are structurally distinct but have similar properties in that they both block the reuptake of norepinephrine (NE), 5-HT, and to a lesser degree, dopamine. Their dual action on NE and 5-HT may be of use in alleviating the painful physical symptoms associated with depression and diabetic peripheral neuropathy. At lower doses they act is a potent 5-HT reuptake inhibitor. Higher doses of venlafaxine act as a potent norepinephrine inhibitor. The once-daily dosing and prolonged duration of absorption of venlafaxine extended release (XR) offer the advantage of enhancing client treatment adherence, facilitating administration, and improving the side-effect profile. Primary uses for venlafaxine include major depression, chronic pain syndromes, generalized anxiety disorder, and attention-deficit hyperactivity disorder.

Duloxetine (Cymbalta) is marketed in a 2-hour delayed-release enteric-coated capsule to obviate severe nausea associated with this medication. Maximum concentration occurs within 6 hours. Duloxetine is classified as a balanced selective serotonin and norepinephrine reuptake inhibitor. It is approved for the use of major depressive disorder (MDD) and diabetic peripheral neuropathic pain (DPNP). It has also been used in stress urinary incontinence (SUI). Common side effects of duloxetine include insomnia, headache, somnolence, nausea, diarrhea, and dry mouth. Caution should be taken when duloxetine is coadministered with CNS depressants and serotonergic agents. In renally impaired clients, duloxetine should be initiated at a lower dose and increased gradually. It is not recommended for clients with severe renal impairment (creatinine clearance <30 mL/min) or end stage renal disease (requiring dialysis). Duloxetine is also not recommended for use in clients with hepatic dysfunction (Wernicke, Gahimer, Yalcin, Wulster-Radcliffe, & Viktrup, 2005; Westanmo, Gayken, & Haight, 2005). Common side effects of SNRIs are similar to SSRIs and include headache, early stimulation, gastrointestinal disturbances, nervousness, ejaculatory disturbances, anxiety, sleep disturbances, and modest dose-related hypertension. Venlafaxine should not be combined with MAOIs because of the risk of 5-HT syndrome (Sadock, Sadock, & Sussman, 2006). Venlafaxine can be a beneficial antidepressant if titrated properly to avoid adverse effects.

Serotonin Modulators

Trazodone (Desyrel) is structurally unrelated to the tricyclics or tetracyclics but they have many similar properties. Trazodone is a potent antagonist at postsynaptic 5-HT$_2$ receptor sites and a weak inhibitor of 5-HT reuptake. These features are postulated to enhance 5-HT$_{1A}$ neuronal transmission. Common clinical indications of trazodone are major depression, sleep disturbances, and premenstrual dysphoric syndrome. Trazodone is structurally unrelated to the tricyclics or tetracyclics but they have many similar properties. Trazodone is a potent antagonist at postsynaptic 5-HT$_2$ receptor sites and a weak inhibitor of 5-HT reuptake. These features are postulated to enhance 5-HT$_{1A}$ neuronal transmission and account for its antidepressant and anxiolytic properties (Odagaki, Toyoshima, & Yamauchi, 2005). Recent studies implicate trazodone as an effective sleep agent for psychotropic-induced sleep disturbances with some success. However, further clinical experience is needed to confirm these preliminary data (Mendelson, 2005). It has the benefit of having more sedative and anxiolytic properties and fewer anticholinergic side effects than other secondary amines, particularly desipramine and nortriptyline. Common clinical implications of trazodone are major depression, sleep disturbances, and premenstrual dysphoric syndrome.

Major side effects of trazodone include sedation, nausea, and blurred vision. A significant concern about trazodone is the side effect of priapism—it is the only antidepressant associated with this adverse reaction. Trazodone is also associated with orthostatic hypotension and changes in cardiac conduction (Sadock, Sadock, & Sussman, 2006).

Norepinephrine-Serotonin Modulator

Mirtazapine (Remeron) is a novel antidepressant whose primary efficacy stems from its ability to facilitate 5-HT and norepinephrine transmission. This antidepressant is the first of a new class of agents that are presynaptic alpha-2 adrenoreceptor antagonists as well as 5-HT$_2$ and 5-HT$_3$ antagonists. Structurally, mirtazapine is a tetracyclic compound unrelated to TCAs. However, like TCA antidepressants, this antidepressant possesses varying degrees of anticholinergic, antihistaminic, antiadrenergic, and dopamine reuptake blocking properties and are responsible for a wide range of side effects. It is a member of a class known as piperazinoazepines and is unrelated to any known class of psychotropic agents. Major clinical implications for mirtazapine include depression and some anxiety disorders (Sadock, Sadock, & Sussman, 2006). Mirtazapine has also been shown to shorten sleep latency and deepen sleep, which is useful in treating insomnia associated with depression (Sadock, Sadock, & Sussman, 2006). An orally disintegrating table is also available, Remeron SolTab®, for the use in clients who check their medication or have swallowing difficulties.

Common side effects of mirtazapine include sedation, weight gain, and dizziness. Other side effects include anticholinergic effects, hypertension, increased serum lipid levels, and agranulocytosis. Few drug interactions have been reported between mirtazapine and other agents; however, caution should be used when combining it with other CNS depressants and MAOIs.

Despite the efficacy of the SSRIs and novel antidepressants, 10 to 30 percent of clients experiencing depression fail to respond to these therapies, and 12 to 25 percent respond but have recurrent depressive episodes (Antai-Otong, 2007a; Dunner et al., 2006; Trivedi et al., 2006).

Monoamine Oxidase Inhibitors (MAOIs)

MAOIs are no longer considered first-line treatment for depression because of the improved tolerability and safety of new-generation antidepressants. Developed and prescribed in the early 1950s, the MAOIs were the first effective antidepressants as well as the first drugs that gave neuropharmacologists an opportunity to study the relationship between neurotransmitters and mood (Kennedy, Holt, & Baker, 2005). MAO is an enzyme that catalyzes the breakdown of various amines, including epinephrine, norepinephrine, 5-HT, and dopamine. Inhibition of MAO results in an increased concentration of these amines in the synaptic cleft. Thus, the MAOI antidepressant effects are thought to result from the increased availability of CNS norepinephrine and 5-HT (Sadock, Sadock, & Sussman, 2006). MAOIs are also useful in the treatment of personality disorders, hypochondriasis, agoraphobia with panic attacks, PTSD, pain syndromes, obsessive-compulsive disorder, and phobias. The clinical and pharmacokinetic parameters are presented in Table 29–5.

Side Effects, Dietary Precautions, and Drug Interactions

As Table 29–6 indicates, the side effects of MAOIs are similar to those produced by the heterocyclics. The most troublesome common side effect is orthostatic hypotension. Furthermore, MAOIs, when combined with tyramine-rich food or some medications, can cause a hypertensive reaction, a potentially life-threatening condition. Tyramine is a monoamine present in some foods such as chocolates, beer, and aged cheeses. Because MAOIs prevent the body from breaking down this monoamine, tyramine can provoke the release of norepinephrine from endogenous stores in the body, causing an increase in blood pressure (Kennedy et al., 2005). Most hypertensive reactions are quite mild, with a 20 to 30 mm Hg rise in systolic blood pressure accompanied by headache, flushing, or sweating. An undetected severe reaction, although rare, can result in a cerebrovascular accident (CVA). The fear of hypertensive crisis prevents many prescribers from using any medication from this class.

The general advice that can be given regarding dietary precautions with MAOI therapy is that any food subjected to fermentation during its processing or storage may be rich in tyramine and thus may present the risk of a hypertensive crisis. Foods that are very high in tyramine include cheeses such as Camembert, cheddar, Emmenthaler, and Stilton; meats such as fermented sausages (bologna, pepperoni, salami, and summer sausage); fish (especially herring); overripe fruits such as avocados and bananas; and Chianti wine. Other foods that have vasopressors and should be used in moderation include beers, wine, chocolate, and coffee.

Some drugs must be avoided as well. Phenlyethylamine compounds, including amphetamines, phenylpropanolamine, ephedrine, phenylephrine, and related stimulants; decongestants; and bronchodilators all may provoke severe reactions in clients treated with MAOIs. The narcotic meperidine (Demerol) must be avoided. Persons taking MAOIs must also avoid concomitant use of heterocyclics and SSRIs. There must be an antidepressant-free period when the client stops an MAOI before beginning another class of antidepressants, and vice versa (Sadock, Sadock, & Sussman, 2006). Any nurse involved in health education is urged to consult a more detailed source. The list of foods and medicines to avoid can appear intimidating to both the prescriber and the client. This probably explains why MAOIs are rarely initially prescribed as first-line treatment for depression. However, it should be emphasized that these can be very useful medications, especially in clients with

---

TABLE 29–5
Clinical and Pharmacokinetic Parameters of Monoamine Oxidase Inhibitor

Generic Name	Brand Name	Dosage Range (mg/Day)	Half-Life (Hours)	Onset (Weeks)	Duration (Weeks)
Isocarboxazid	Marplan	30–50	?	1–4	2
Phenelzine	Nardil	45–90	?	4	2
Tranylcypromine	Parnate	30–60	1.5–3.2	2–12 days	3–4 days

TABLE 29–6
Symptoms Associated with Adverse Effects of Monoamine Oxidase Inhibitors

System	Common Side Effects	Less Common Side Effects
Cardiovascular	Orthostatic hypotension	Palpitations, tachycardia, peripheral edema
Central Nervous	Dizziness, headache, confusion, fatigue, drowsiness	Akathisia, ataxia, neuritis, chills, vertigo, memory impairment, weakness, restlessness, hyperreflexia, tremors
Gastrointestinal	Constipation, nausea, vomiting	Dysuria, diarrhea, urinary retention, incontinence, weight gain
Miscellaneous	Dry mouth, blurred vision	Excessive sweating, nystagmus

serious, difficult-to-treat, or refractory depression. Many clients are willing to live with the prescriptions if they can experience relief from depression.

Mood Stabilizers

Historically, lithium has been recognized as the drug of choice for the treatment of bipolar disorders. Contemporary research suggests that other drugs, specifically anticonvulsant agents such as valproic acid (Depakene) and carbamazepine (Tegretol) are more effective than lithium in the treatment of acute mania and rapid-cycling episodes. In general, these drugs are referred to as mood stabilizers because of their ability to stabilize the mood despite the etiology (Table 29–7).

Lithium

Lithium is a naturally occurring alkali metal that shares some characteristics with other monovalent cations such as sodium and potassium. In 1949, Cade, in Australia, was the first to report the therapeutic effects of lithium to treat mania. However, lithium was not approved for use in the United States until 1970 because of reported severe and sometimes fatal cases from uncontrolled use as a substitute for sodium chloride. Lithium is used to treat acute hypomanic or manic episodes

and recurrent affective disorders. Table 29–8 presents the clinical and pharmacokinetic parameters of lithium. Seventy to ninety percent of clients with "typical" bipolar illness respond to lithium (Sadock, Sadock, & Sussman, 2006). Although lithium has been shown to have mild antidepressant properties, it is not as effective as antidepressants. Sometimes it is used to treat schizoaffective disorders, often in conjunction with an antipsychotic agent. Lithium is also useful in preventing recurrent depressive episodes and as an adjunct to antidepressants in the treatment of major depression when the illness is partially refractory to antidepressants alone. Lithium has also been found to be effective in the treatment of aggressive or impulsive behaviors.

Mechanism of Action

Lithium remains one of the most effective treatments for depression and mania in bipolar I and II disorders (Jefferson & Greist, 2005), yet despite extensive research, its biological therapeutic efficacy remains obscure. Lithium is less effective than other antimanic agents in the treatment of rapid-cycling bipolar disorders. Researchers speculate that membrane transport systems and ion channels play key roles in the regulation of intracellular lithium. Lithium is a monovalent cation with intricate physiological and pharmacologic effects by the brain. By virtue of the ionic properties, it shares other monovalent

TABLE 29–7
Clinical and Pharmacokinetic Parameters of Mood Stabilizers (Antimanic Agents)

Generic Name	Brand Name	Dosage Range (mg/Day)	Half-Life (Hours)	Onset (Days)	Duration	Effective Blood Level
Lithium	Eskalith Lithobid	Acute: 1,800 Maintenance: 900–1,200	21–30	5–14 days	2 weeks	0.8–1.2 mEq/L
Topiramate	Topamax	Maintenance: 400–1,300	21 (Serum monitoring unnecessary)			
Lamotrigine	Lamictal	Maintenance: 300–500	29 (Serum monitoring unnecessary)			
Valproic acid*	Depakene	1,200–2,500	5–20			50–125 µg/mL
Divalproex sodium	Depakote	1,200–2,500	5–20			
Carbamazepine						4–12 µg/mL

Atypical Antipsychotics

Olanzapine-fluoxetine (Symybax) for bipolar depression [dose range 6/25 mg/day; 6/50 mg/day and 12/50 mg/day] ½ life for Olanzapine/Fluoxetine is 21–54 hours/1–3 days active metabolite (norfluoxetine) is 4–16 days, respectively.

*Note: Atypical antipsychotics, such as olanzapine, quetiapine, aripiprazole, and risperidone are FDA approved to treat bipolar disorder as monotherapy and adjunct with mood stabilizers for mania. Further discussions about dose and half-lives are forthcoming.

TABLE 29–8
Adverse Effects Associated with Lithium Therapy

Plasma Level (mEq/L)	Common Side Effects	Less Common Side Effects
<1.5	Initial treatment: fine hand tremors, polyuria, mild thirst, transient and mild nausea, and discomfort	Twitching, muscular weakness, restlessness, dry mouth, and thinning hair
	Afterwards: fatigue, acne, electrocardiographic changes, hypothyroidism	
1.5–2.0	Diarrhea, vomiting, nausea, drowsiness, muscle weakness, lack of coordination (may be early signs of toxicity)	
2.0–3.0	Giddiness, ataxia, blurred vision, tinnitus, vertigo, increasing confusion, slurred speech, blackouts, incontinence, fasciculation, myoclonic twitching, hyperreflexia, hypertonia	
>3.0	Seizures, arrhythmias, hypotension, peripheral vascular collapse, stupor, spasticity, coma	

and divalent ions such as sodium, magnesium, and calcium. Its transport across the cellular membrane enables it to modulate an array of enzymatic processes (Jefferson & Greist, 2005).

Although lithium may cross cell membranes and replaces sodium in support of a single-action potential, it cannot replace the action of sodium in the sodium pump and therefore cannot maintain cellular membrane potential. Lithium's effect on transmembrane ion pumps can possibly alter the distribution of sodium, potassium, and calcium ions. However, these effects appear to occur at higher than therapeutic concentrations of lithium (Jefferson & Greist, 2005).

Other evidence suggests that lithium's effects are caused by its action on the second-messenger system. One of the second-messenger systems involves lithium's inhibition of receptor-mediated activation of adenyl cyclase. Because this effect occurs at lithium levels outside the therapeutic concentration levels, it is an unlikely mechanism. However, the inhibition of adenyl cyclase may contribute to some lithium toxic effects, such as an increase in urine concentration and antithyroid effects. Lithium blocks the ability of neurons to restore normal levels of the membrane phospholipid phospharidylinositol 4,5-biphosphate (PIP_2) after it is hydrolyzed post activation of receptors. PIP_2 is hydrolyzed into two second messengers: diacylglycerol and inositol 1, 4, 4-triphosphate (IP_3). IP_3 acts to release calcium from intracellular stores, which sets off a cascade of events in many cellular processes. Because the IP_3 cannot cross the blood-brain barrier, the brain must regenerate its own IP_3. Depletion of PIPs from cells may reduce the responsiveness of neurons to muscarinic cholinergic, alpha-adrenergic, or other stimuli. Thus, lithium could modulate the hyperactive neurons that contribute to the manic episode (Jefferson & Greist, 2005).

Effects, Side Effects, and Adherence

When used to treat acute hypomanic or manic episodes, lithium can begin to be effective within 1 to 2 weeks, but it may take as long as several months to stabilize the mood totally. Antipsychotics and benzodiazepines are often used to manage the behavioral excitement and psychotic symptoms during the early stages of lithium therapy (Hirschfeld, 2006; McIntyre et al., 2005; Tohen et al., 2006). Lithium is used for maintenance therapy, with the goal of decreasing the severity and frequency of affective episodes. Even with regular lithium, some clients can experience symptoms, periods of distress, and unpleasant side effects (Jefferson & Greist, 2005).

About 20 to 30 percent of clients discontinue lithium therapy on their own. The reasons vary. Some clients deny their need for lithium because they deny they have an illness. Some stop taking it after the episode is resolved, believing that prophylactic use of the medication is unnecessary. Others enjoy the euphoria associated with manic episodes, and others report that lithium decreases their creativity and productivity. Finally, some clients stop taking lithium because of its side effects. The nurse needs to assess clients' reasons for discontinuing medication before confronting or educating them about adherence issues.

The common side effects of lithium can include polydipsia, polyuria, tremor, gastric irritation, diarrhea, sexual disturbances, a lack of spontaneity, and weight gain. Many of these side effects appear only in the first days. However, though possibly transient and clinically benign, these side effects can be so bothersome to clients that they stop taking the drug. Sometimes, reducing the dose or using a slow-release form or medications such as propranolol (Inderal) or primidone (Mysoline) may be given to alleviate lithium-induced tremor. Coarser, more severe tremors may be caused by lithium toxicity.

Clinically adverse cardiovascular reactions are rarely seen in lithium at therapeutic levels, although serious cardiovascular effects can occur in overdose (Jefferson & Greist, 2005).

A second category of side effects may result from either chronic administration of an inappropriately high dose or acute overdose of lithium (see Table 29–8). These toxic reactions usually occur at normal serum levels higher than 2 mEq/L, although they can occur at serum levels, especially in older adults. Gastrointestinal symptoms may appear, followed by CNS depression, which can include somnolence, sluggishness, ataxia, dysarthria, seizures, increased muscle tone, and increased deep tendon reflexes. At serum levels of 3 mEq/L or higher, cardiovascular collapse can occur. Changes in the client's status in such areas as decreased serum sodium levels, use of diuretics, decreased renal function, and pregnancy can result in the accumulation of lithium and result in toxicity (Jefferson & Greist, 2005; Sadock, Sadock, & Sussman, 2006).

The kidneys excrete lithium almost entirely. Thus, effective regulation of lithium depends in part on the sodium and fluid balance of the body. As an example, sodium depletion can lead to marked lithium retention and possible toxicity. Conversely, high levels of lithium can lead to sodium excretion. Because diuretics affect kidney action, they can also affect lithium levels. Thiazide diuretics commonly cause increased levels of lithium by decreasing clearance; this can happen quite quickly. Potassium-sparing diuretics may also cause moderate increases in lithium levels over time. Osmotic drugs and carbonic anhydrase inhibitors such as an acetazolamide (Diamox) can decrease lithium levels by increasing excretion (Jefferson & Greist, 2005).

Long-term lithium therapy can have serious consequences for clients. It can cause a decrease in thyroid hormone. Transient and mild disturbances in thyroid function testing are common during early treatment. Women and clients with preexisting thyroid abnormalities are at risk of this thyroid-related complication. Researchers submit that lithium impedes the secretion of hormone from the gland. Approximately 4 percent of clients taking lithium develop hypothyroidism and require supplemental hormone replacement treatment, such as levothyroxine (Synthroid). Because hypothyroidism mimics depression, the clinician needs to consider both possibilities (Jefferson & Greist, 2005).

The second serious adverse reaction that can occur with long-term lithium therapy is permanent structural changes in the kidneys. These changes result in chronic tubulointerstitial nephropathy. Because both the thyroid and renal changes are potentially serious side effects, several guidelines need to be followed:

1. Thyroid and renal studies must be performed before lithium is prescribed, and then it must be ordered on a regular follow-up basis.

2. Regular lithium levels must be obtained.

3. The client should be always maintained on the lowest effective level of lithium.

4. Because dehydration may increase renal damage, adequate fluid intake must be maintained.

5. Clients and family members must be educated about conditions that increase the risk of lithium toxicity, including sodium diet restrictions, profuse sweating, or diarrhea and vomiting.

Nonsteroidal anti-inflammatory drugs (NSAIDS) such as ibuprofen (Motrin), naproxen (Naprosyn), diclofenac (Voltaren), ketoprofen (Orudis), and celecoxib (Celebrex) can increase lithium levels. Risk factors for adverse reactions to these agents include high doses, older age, and renal impairment (Jefferson & Greist, 2005).

Finally, an encephalopathic syndrome similar to neuroleptic malignant syndrome has occurred in a few clients treated with an antipsychotic and lithium. Although rare, the possibility of this syndrome increases the necessity of monitoring clients for neurological toxicity (Jefferson & Greist, 2005).

Dosage and Toxicity

Lithium is available as a carbonate (pills, tablets, or Eskalith) and as a citrate (liquid). It is usually ordered two or three times a day, although some prescribers believe a once-daily dosing is effective. Lithium has a rather narrow range of effectiveness; too little lithium has little therapeutic value, but only a little too much can produce toxicity. Because of this narrow range, clients need to be well educated about signs of toxicity. It is for this reason also that clients on lithium are required to have serum lithium levels obtained. Initially, these are required frequently as the correct dosing regimen is sought. When stable, lithium levels are required every 1 to 3 months. The lithium levels need to be determined 12 hours after the client's last dose to be interpreted correctly. Although values may differ among laboratories, the usual therapeutic range is 0.5 to 1.5 mEq/L. When clients with bipolar disorders do not respond to lithium or cannot tolerate it, other agents can be used (Jefferson & Greist, 2005).

All medications, including lithium and various anticonvulsants that have been documented to be effective agents for clients with bipolar disorder, are potentially teratogenic. Llewellyn, Stowe, and Strader (1998) suggest that the treatment plan for women with bipolar disorder, who are of reproductive age or potential, should include several strategies, regardless of the antimanic agent:

1. Assess and document the client's birth control method.

2. Order a pregnancy test.

3. Document informed consent regarding the risks for pregnancy exposure.

Emerging research concerning lithium use during pregnancy cautions women to make informed decisions with their providers and obstetricians to ensure appropriate and safe medication management that often focuses on risk versus benefit of any psychotropic use during pregnancy and lactation. Research indicates adverse effects, including postpartum depression and failure to bond with the infant when relapse occurs. A recent study that aimed at quantifying lithium exposure in nursing infants concluded that serum lithium levels in nursing infants were low and well-tolerated and there were no significant adverse physical or behavioral effects observed in the infants (Viguera et al., 2007).

Nonresponding Clients

Although lithium is considered the mainstay of pharmacologic intervention for most clients with bipolar disorders, it is recognized that some clients with classic bipolar disorder and a significant number of clients with bipolar variants do not respond to lithium therapy. This subgroup of nonresponders may include those with rapid-cycling bipolar disorder (four or more affective episodes per year), schizoaffective disorder, or dysphoric or mixed mania (defined as a state that simultaneously has both manic and depressive features); older adults; and those with manias arising from underlying general medical conditions, such as CNS diseases, conditions caused by strokes, tumors, traumatic brain injury, and infections. It is also evident that some persons whose symptoms are controlled with lithium cannot tolerate its short- or long-term side effects.

Anticonvulsants

The three most common alternatives to lithium for the treatment and prophylaxis of bipolar I disorders are carbamazepine (Tegretol), valproic acid (Depakene), and lamotrigine (Lamictal). Like lithium, these agents exert some antidepressant effects prophylactically, but they are not effective as primary agents for treating major depression.

Valproic Acid and Its Derivatives

This group includes valproic acid, its sodium salt valproate, and divalproex sodium (Depakote). Regardless of the form, the dosage is expressed as valproic acid equivalents. Valproic acid is prescribed as an anticonvulsant and has been found effective in the treatment of a host of mental illnesses such as bipolar disorder, anxiety and psychotic disorders, drug withdrawal and dependence, TD, agitation associated with dementia, and borderline personality disorder (Frye & Post, 2005). Its mechanism of action remains unclear, but it is thought to be a GABA-ergic drug. The mechanism of action may also involve the monoamines, specifically by enhancing serotonergic and reducing dopaminergic function. The results of valproic acid's actions on these neurotransmitters is believed to be the basis of its efficacy in exerting antimanic effects, particularly in the treatment of bipolar disorder I in the acute manic phase (Frye & Post, 2005).

As with lithium and valproic acid, serum blood monitoring is necessary. The most common side effects of valproic acid are the gastrointestinal disturbances, which can be reduced by using the enteric-coated divalproex sodium preparation. The most serious adverse reactions include hepatic failure, pancreatitis, endocrine disturbances, and teratogenesis, although the incidence is low. Children younger than 2 years of age and clients with severe seizure disorders accompanied by mental retardation are among the higher-risk groups for serious adverse side effects (Frye & Post, 2005). Hence, liver function tests are necessary before initiating valproic acid medication. The nurse can review with the client the potential signs and symptoms of liver failure (malaise, weakness, lethargy, facial edema, anorexia, jaundice, and vomiting) as well as monitoring for them throughout treatment. A complete blood count, including platelets, is also recommended because thrombocytopenia has been reported. These diagnostic tests, along with valproic acid serum levels, need to be performed regularly while the client is on valproic acid.

Initial treatment with valproic acid may be associated with drowsiness, tremor, and nausea. Other side effects of this medication include hair loss, weight gain, and headache. As previously mentioned pure valproic acid is very *poorly* tolerated by clients; the enteric-coated form is preferred. Valproic acid's most significant drug interactions involve its effects on other anticonvulsants; otherwise, it has few significant drug interactions.

Overall, valproic acid is well tolerated and its enteric-coated form, divalproex sodium (Depakote) is more easily tolerated than valproic acid. Because of valproic acid's tendency to inhibit hepatic enzymes, there is a possibility for increases in the levels of other medications. It is also highly protein bound and may displace other highly bound drugs from protein-binding sites. Although both valproic acid and carbamazepine are prescribed as single-agent medications, it is not unusual to see both of them used in combination with lithium. As is true of lithium, both carbamazepine and valproic acid are dangerous in overdose and are contraindicated during pregnancy due to their teratogenic properties. Because valproic acid and carbamazepine are anticonvulsants, neither should be stopped abruptly because they may precipitate status epilepticus.

Carbamazepine

Carbamazepine is prescribed for a host of conditions, including seizure disorder, trigeminal neuralgia, phantom limb pain, alcohol withdrawal, and restless leg syndrome (see Table 29–7). An off-label medication indication is neuronal diabetes insipidus. An off-label medication involves prescribing a medication for a medical use other than the one approved by the FDA. The example of off-label medication is when the atypical antipsychotic agent, quetiapine, is used to treat insomnia rather than schizophrenia (Fountoulakis et al., 2004; Post & Frye, 2005). Off-label medication prescribing is legal, common, and necessary with the caveat of the following therapeutic bases:

◆ The client has a psychiatric condition for which no medication is labeled
◆ Client lies outside parameters of labeled demographics (e.g., child, adolescent, pregnant women)
◆ Lack of symptom remittance with labeled medication

Psychiatric-mental health nurses who prescribe, dispense, or administer off-label medications must have a full understanding of the basis for such use along with legal and ethical consideration and potential adverse consequences of their action to minimize legal litigation. As client advocates, it's imperative for the nurse to ensure safe medication by obtaining informed consent from the client and/or guardian or surrogate; understanding and documenting reasons for prescribing the medication and closely monitoring client responses—both desired and adverse effects to off-label medications, particularly among vulnerable populations (Zito, Safer, Gardner, Soeken, & Ryu, 2006). Carbamazepine has also been found to exert potent antimanic effects. It has recently been used for treating intermittent explosive behavior disorder, which is associated with undiagnosed temporal lobe epilepsy. Although its exact mechanism remains unknown, there has been a focus on carbamazepine's ability to inhibit kindling. *Kindling* refers to a neurophysiological response that eventually produces a progressive sensitization of a neuron. Some researchers link kindling to mood disorders, including bipolar I disorder and major depression (Mazza et al., 2007).

Side Effects, Toxicity, and Drug Interactions

As with lithium, monitoring serum blood levels are necessary. Carbamazepine can cause aplastic anemia and agranulocytosis. Although the incidence of these adverse reactions is low, a complete blood count, including platelets, reticulocytes, chemical screen, and electrolytes, is suggested before initiating treatment and should be repeated regularly while the client continues on carbamazepine. In addition, regular testing is also required to check serum levels. The nurse can explain the rationale for this required blood study as well as provide encouragement around the sometimes frustrating need for regular venipuncture. The nurse can remind the client of the importance of reporting any signs and symptoms of possible hematological problems such as fever, sore throat, mouth ulcers, easily bruising, petechiae, or purpural hemorrhage. Any rash needs to be reported immediately.

Initial treatment with carbamazepine may be associated with mild degrees of sedation, tremor, slurred speech, nausea, vomiting, vertigo, ataxia, and blurred vision. The client is encouraged to take carbamazepine with food to decrease any nausea. Generally, these side effects lessen over time. If they persist or worsen, toxicity should be considered, the medication discontinued, and a serum level obtained.

Carbamazepine is a pharmacologically complicated drug with several drug interactions that should be kept in mind. Besides inducing its own metabolism, it induces the metabolism of other drugs. For example, the concentration of antipsychotic medication (especially haloperidol [Haldol]) is decreased when carbamazepine is coadministered. This means that a client with previously well-controlled symptoms may experience a worsening of symptoms when carbamazepine is administered. The nurse can help the client monitor the symptoms during this initial period. Carbamazepine may reduce the effect of birth control pills, and it can cause birth defects. Both the clients and their prescribers need to be aware that a higher dose of birth control pills may be required. Erythromycin can inhibit carbamazepine metabolism and lead to carbamazepine toxicity. Some additional medications that interact with carbamazepine metabolism and lead to toxicity are cimetidine (Tagamet), verapamil (Isoptin), and isoniazid (INH). Conversely, carbamazepine may increase the risk of isoniazid-induced hepatoxicity (Post & Frye, 2005).

Lamotrigine

Another anticonvulsant agent, lamotrigine (Lamictal), is also being used to treat treatment-refractory bipolar depression II.

Lamotrigine acts at voltage-sensitive sodium channels. Presumably, this effect stabilizes neuronal membranes and modulates the presynaptic release of glutamate and aspartate. Like other antimanic agents, this drug is contraindicated during lactation and pregnancy.

Side Effects, Toxicity, and Drug Interactions

Common side effects of lamotrigine include dizziness, ataxia, headache, tremor, depression, somnolence, rash, vomiting, memory disturbances, diarrhea, and rash. One of the most alarming side effects of lamotrigine is a life-threatening rash known as Stevens-Johnson syndrome. Most rashes appear within 2 to 8 weeks of the initiation of lamotrigine therapy, but some occur after long-term treatment. The incidence is considerably higher in pediatric clients, with a reported incidence of 1 in 50 to 1 in 100 (Ketter, 2005). Nurses must assess clients for this rash and provide health education about desired and potential adverse drug reactions. Informed consent and health teaching are a necessary part of treatment planning. The rash is also likely to occur during prolonged treatment (e.g., 6 months), and there is an increased risk when this drug is combined with valproic acid. Nurses must instruct the client to discontinue this medication at the first sign of a rash and seek medical attention. High-risk groups for this life-threatening rash include children, women, and those using valproic acid (Antai-Otong, 2005; Alvestad, Lydersen, & Brodtkorb, 2007). The importance of assessment and psychoeducation is indicated in the following Research Abstract, Rash from Antiepileptic Drugs: Influence by Gender, Age, and Learning Disability.

Major drug interactions with lamotrigine include those drugs that inhibit the *hepatic cytochrome P450* system, including carbamazepine. Serum blood levels are not required with lamotrigine.

Topiramate

Inconsistent findings implicate the efficacy of topiramate in the treatment of bipolar disorders. Topiramate's efficacy lies with inhibition of sustained repetitive firing and its enhancement of GABA effects. It blocks the adenosine monophosphate (AMP)-type glutamate receptor (Keller, 2005). This medication is well tolerated with slow titration. Major side effects of topiramate are CNS related and include sedation, diplopia, cognitive blunting, parethesias, and a distinct word-finding difficulty in about 15 percent of clients (Keller, 2005). Additional effects include weight loss and formation of kidney stones because of its weak carbonic anhydrase inhibitor properties. Serum monitoring is not required.

A final note about novel anticonvulsant agents used as mood stabilizers: Although it is too early to discern their long-efficacy and side effect profile, preliminary findings indicate that tiagabine has more efficacy in treating co-occurring psychiatric and substance-related disorder, sleep problems, and chronic pain syndromes than treating core symptoms of bipolar disorder (Pollack et al., 2005; Yatham, 2004). Likewise, oxcarbazepine (Trileptal) has never demonstrated significant efficacy in the treatment of bipolar disorder in large-scale studies. Oxcarbazepine is a derivative of carbamazepine,

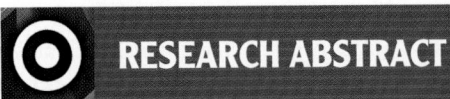

RESEARCH ABSTRACT

Rash from Antiepileptic Drugs: Influence by Gender, Age, and Learning Disability

Alvestad, S., Lydersen, S., & Brodtkorb, E. (2007). *Epilepsia, 48,* 1360–1365.

Study Problem/Purpose

The aim of this retrospective study was to evaluate the incidence of skin reactions of current antiepileptic drugs (AEDs) and to explore their correlation with clinical parameters such as gender, age, and learning disability.

Methods

Consecutive subjects with epilepsy were studied retrospectively. A detailed survey of medical records concerning all treatment with AEDs was evaluated ($n = 663$).

Findings

Skin reactions were found in 14 percent of the subjects and in 5 percent of the exposures. Ninety-seven percent of the reactions occurred to either carbamazepine (CBZ, 11 percent), phenytoin (PHT, 8 percent), lamotrigine (LTG, 8 percent), oxcarbazepine (8 percent), or phenobarbital (2 percent). Females demonstrated a significantly higher incidence of skin reactions than males (19 percent versus 8 percent), and this incidence was significantly less often in subjects with learning disabilities than other groups (7 percent versus 16 percent). These differences were significant for CBZ, PHT, and LTG when analyzed separately. Researchers found that females had a higher rash frequency during the reproductive years, whereas men demonstrated less frequent rash in the same phase of life.

Implications for Psychiatric Nursing

Although this study involved clients with epilepsy, anticonvulsant agents are a mainstay treatment for clients with various psychiatric disorders, such as bipolar disorders, both depressed and manic episodes, impulsivity disorders, and agitation. Psychiatric nurses are compelled to stay abreast of reasons for administering and prescribing these agents along with potentially adverse side effects. Data from this study strengthened the importance of health education about cutaneous rashes associated with lamotrigine, carbamazepine, oxcarbazepine, and other anticonvulsants and identification of high-risk groups. It also indicated the importance of nursing assessment of clients on these agents for signs of serious rashes that must be reported and immediately evaluated.

without its serious anemia side effects. Further studies are necessary before newer anticonvulsants can be recommended as a first-line treatment or routine use to treat bipolar disorder. Major side effects of oxcarbazepine are fatigue, GI, CNS, serious dermatological reactions, reduced T_4, without alterations in T_3, and TSH and hyponatremia. Close monitoring of sodium levels, particularly in the presence of fatigue is required. Health education about serious skin reactions is equally important. In comparison, tiagabine is believed to produce less dose-related cognitive disturbances than older drugs. The most common side effects of tiagabine are CNS and are GI related (Keller, 2005). Fluoxetine and olanzapine (Symbyax) is FDA approved for depressive episodes associated with bipolar disorder. Fluoxetine (Prozac), an antidepressant, and olanzapine (Zyprexa), an antipsychotic, were the first combination approved for the use in bipolar depression.

Antipsychotics

The term antipsychotic refers to a group of drugs classified as *dopamine receptor antagonists*. The efficacy of agents in treating psychotic symptoms lies in their ability to decrease dopamine activity. Researchers submit that psychotic disorders, including schizophrenia, substance-induced and other psychiatric illnesses are linked to increased dopamine activity.

Typical or Conventional Antipsychotics

The advent of antipsychotic agents in the early 1950s revolutionized psychiatric care. Many clients who had been institutionalized indefinitely, often in inhumane conditions, were afforded symptom relief. The antipsychotic medications are divided into families based on their chemical structures. These structures also determine the mechanism of action of the medications. The clinical and pharmacokinetic parameters of the antipsychotics are presented in Table 29–9. Table 29–10 lists receptor sites and side effects of antipsychotics.

Phenothiazines

Before the advent of atypical antipsychotics, the most commonly prescribed antipsychotics belonged to the *phenothiazine* family. There are three distinct classes in this family. The *apiphatic phenothiazines* include chlorpromazine (Thorazine), promazine (Sparine), and triflupromazine (Vesprin) (Sadock, Sadock, & Sussman, 2006). The apiphatic phenothiazines are relatively low in antipsychotic potency and high in sedation effects. The *piperidine phenothiazines* include thioridazine (Mellaril) and mesoridazine (Serentil). These medications are of medium potency in antipsychotic actions, sedation, and EPS. The third class of phenothiazines is the *piperazines*. Commonly prescribed medications in this class include trifluphenazine, fluphenazine (Prolixin), prochlorperazine (Compazine), and perphenazine (Trilafon) (Sadock, Sadock, & Sussman, 2006). These medications were once considered to be first-line treatment of schizophrenia and other psychotic disorders. They are considered to be effective in controlling psychotic symptoms with little or no sedation, but they are more likely than atypical antipsychotics to produce acute and chronic adverse reactions, such as EPS and TD.

TABLE 29–9
Pharmacokinetic Properties of Antipsychotics

Medications	Dosage Range (mg/Day)	Onset (Minutes)	Duration of Action (Hours)	Half-Life (Hours)
Typical Antipsychotic Agents				
Chlorpromazine (Thorazine)	30–800	30–60	4–6	10–20
Promazine (Sparine)	40–1,200	30–60	4–6	
Triflupromazine (Vesprin)	60–150	15–30	12	
Thioridazine (Mellaril)	150–800	30–60	4–6	9–30
Mesoridazine (Serentil)	30–400	30–60	4–6	
Acetophenazine (Tindal)	60–120	30–60	4–6	
Perphenazine (Trilafon)	12–64	30–60	4–6	8–21
Prochlorperazine (Compazine)	15–150	30–60	3–4	
Fluphenazine (Prolixin)	0.5–40	30–60	6–8	14–153
Trifluoperazine (Stelazine)	2–40	30–40	4–6	
Chlorprothixene (Taractan)	75–600	30–60	4–6	
Thiothixene (Navane)	8–30	Slow	12–24	34
Haloperidol (Haldol)	1–15	Erratic	24–72	12–38
Molindone (Moban)	15–225	Erratic	36	1.5
Loxapine (Loxitane)	20–250	20–30	12	5–19
Pimozide (Orap)	1–10	Varies	>24	53–55
Atypical Antipsychotic Agents				
Clozapine (Clozaril)	300–900	Varies		4–66
Risperidone (Risperdal)	2–6			20–30
Olanzapine (Zyprexa)	5–40			21–54
Quetiapine (Seroquel)	50–750			6
Ziprasidone (Geodon)	20–160			2–5
Aripiprazole (Abilify)	10–30			75

Butyrophenones

A second class of antipsychotic medications is butyrophenones. The most commonly prescribed drug in this class is haloperidol. Haloperidol is considered similar in potency to the phenothiazine piperazines. It is also related to EPS, particularly acute dystonic reactions (Sadock, Sadock, & Sussman, 2006).

Thioxanthenes

A third class of antipsychotics is the thioxanthenes, which includes chlorprothixene (Taractan) and thiothixene (Navane). These medications are chemically similar to the phenothiazines and act in similar manners. Molindone (Moban), an indole, and loxapine are also examples of antipsychotics.

Mechanism of Action

All antipsychotic medications just discussed act by blocking the actions of dopamine in the nigrostriatal area of the mesolimbic area of the brain. A comparison of the degree of side effects of the various antipsychotics is presented in Table 29–11. It is currently believed that these medications have an affinity for the subtype dopamine receptors known as D_2 receptors. The nigrostriatal area and the mesolimbic areas of the brain are rich in these receptors. The action in the mesolimbic area is surmised to decrease the psychotic symptoms of hallucinations and delusions. Additional actions of these drugs include decreasing hostility and agitation, increasing organization in thought processes, and decreasing withdrawal behavior owing to high anxiety and sensory overload associated with psychosis.

Side Effects

The action in the nigrostriatal area precipitates a cascade of side effects known as extrapyramidal side effects (EPS). These side effects include akathisia, a subjective feeling of restlessness (Table 29–12). Clients experiencing this side effect appear

TABLE 29–10
Receptor Affinity for Atypical Antipsychotics

Medication	D_1	D_2	5-HT$_{2A}$	M_1	α_1	H_1
Clozapine	High	Low	High	High	High	High
Risperidone	Low	High	High	Low	High	Low
Olanzapine	High	High	High	High	High	High
Quetiapine	Low	Low	Moderate	Moderate	Moderate	Moderate
Sertindole	Moderate	High	High	Low	High	Low
Ziprasidone	Moderate	High	High	Low	High	Low
Aripiprazole	Low	High	High	Low	Moderate	Moderate

5-HT$_{2A}$: greater blockade in reference to D_2 leads to fewer EPS.
M_1: dry mouth, constipation, blurred vision, urinary retention, memory deficits, and sinus tachycardia.
a_1: orthostatic hypotension, sexual dysfunction, dizziness, and reflex tachycardia.
H_1: sedation and weight gain.

TABLE 29–11
Incidence of Adverse Effects for Antipsychotics

Medication	Anticholinergic Effects	Sedation	Extrapyramidal Symptoms	Orthostatic Hypotension
Chlorpromazine (Thorazine)	**	***	**	***
Promazine (Sparine)	***	**	**	**
Triflupromazine (Vesprin)	**	***	**	**
Thioridazine (Mellaril)	***	***	*	***
Mesoridazine (Serentil)	***	***	*	**
Acetophenazine (Tindal)	*	**	**	*
Perphenazine (Trilafon)	*	*	**	*
Prochlorperazine (Compazine)	*	**	**	*
Fluphenazine (Prolixin)	*	*	***	*
Trifluoperazine (Stelazine)	*	*	***	*
Chlorprothixene (Taractan)	**	***	**	**
Thiothixene (Navane)	*	*	***	*
Haloperidol (Haldol)	*	*	***	*
Molindone (Moban)	*	*	***	*
Loxapine (Loxitane)	*	**	***	**
Pimozide (Orap)	**	*	***	*
Clozapine (Clozaril)	***	***	rare	***
Risperidone (Risperdal)	*	**	*	*
Olanzapine (Zyprexa)	**	**	*	**
Quetiapine (Seroquel)	*	**	*	**
Ziprasidone (Geodon)	*	*	*	**
Aripiprazole (Abilify)	*	*	*	*

* Low; ** Moderate; *** High incidence of adverse effects.

TABLE 29–12

Extrapyramidal Side Effects from Antipsychotic Medications

	Acute Dystonia	Akathisia	Dyskinesia	Dystonia	Tardive Dyskinesia	Pseudo-Parkinsonism
Manifestations	Painful and frightening to the client Rapid-onset oculogryic crisis Opisthotonos Torticollis	Subjective feelings of restlessness Tenseness or jumpiness Inability to sit still Rocking back and forth on feet Crossing legs frequently Inability to relax	Masklike face No swinging of arms Hesitancy of speech Decreased muscle strength Shuffling gait Pill-rolling motion Drooling	Involuntarily muscular activity shown by tic, spasm, tremor of face, arms, legs, and neck Resting tremor Rabbit syndrome	Tongue protrusion Rigidity Cogwheeling Complaints of feeling stiff or inability to move easily Numbness of limbs Hyperflexia Tight feeling in throat	Protrusion of tongue Chewing movement Puffing of cheeks Pelvic thrusting	Muscle rigidity and stiffness, resting tremors, drooling, flat facies
Onset (days)	Hours to 5 days	4–72	5–30	1–5	1–5	Months up to 2 or more years after treatment was begun	30–90 days
Treatment	Anticholinergic agents Symptoms disappear when antipsychotic is discontinued or dosage is reduced	Anticholinergic agents Symptoms disappear when antipsychotic is discontinued or dosage is reduced	Anticholinergic agents Symptoms disappear when antipsychotic is discontinued or dosage is reduced	Anticholinergic agents Symptoms disappear when antipsychotic is discontinued or dosage is reduced	Anticholinergic agents Symptoms disappear when antipsychotic is discontinued or dosage is reduced	No effective treatment Prevention is essential	Anticholinergic agents (symptoms may persist despite discontinuation of antipsychotic agent)

restless and move constantly. It is important to assess for akathisia, because it is often mistaken for agitation.

Parkinsonian-like or pseudoparkinsonism extrapyramidal side effects include akinesia, which is slowed or no movement. Manifestations of this side effect include hesitant speech; decreased blinking; and a slow, shuffling gait. Clients display a mask-like facial expression not unlike that of a client with Parkinson's disease. This side effect may contribute to an appearance of flattened or blunt affect. Closely allied to akinesia is dyskinesia, which is an abnormal, involuntary movement disorder. These movements are spastic, tic-like, or tremorous. They are particularly noticeable in the hands, tongue, and nose.

Still another extrapyramidal side effect is dystonia—abnormal tension or muscle tone. Clients with dystonia often appear rigid and exhibit cogwheeling, a deep tremor of the muscles when a limb is moved while in a flaccid state. Clients may also have acute dystonic reactions, which have a rapid onset and are frightening and embarrassing. An acute dystonic reaction usually begins with a tightening of the jaw and thickening of the tongue. If untreated, acute dystonia may progress to impairment of the intercostal muscles and compromised respiration. Other symptoms of acute dystonia are oculogyric crisis (eyes roll back), opisthotonos (neck contracts backward), and torticollis (neck contracts laterally) (Sadock, Sadock, & Sussman, 2006).

Anticholinergic Agents

Extrapyramidal side effects (EPS) are treated with a group of medications known as anticholinergic agents (Table 29–13). These agents include benztropine (Cogentin), diphenhydramine (Benadryl), and trihexyphenidyl (Artane), and their mechanism of action is anticholinergic. Amantadine (Symmetrel) is another commonly used antiparkinsonian agent, which acts by dopaminergic mechanisms. Benztropine and diphenhydramine are both well absorbed and therefore act rapidly when administered intramuscularly, making them particularly useful in the treatment of acute dystonic reaction. Clients may be placed on these medications prophylac-

tically, although whether this practice is safe and efficacious is controversial. Table 29–14 presents the symptoms associated with the adverse effects of the medications for EPS.

Other side effects of antipsychotic medications include orthostatic hypotension, sedation, and endocrine and anticholinergic effects (Table 29–15). Endocrine effects are probably caused by the action of the medication on the hypothalamus. Included in the metabolic changes are weight gain, abnormal glucose levels, amenorrhea, and galactorrhea. In addition, men may experience an inability to maintain erections and retrograde ejaculation, and women may experience inhibition of orgasm. Anticholinergic side effects include dry mouth, blurred vision, urinary difficulties, and constipation. The anticholinergic side effects, in particular, tend to decrease over time. However, all of these adverse reactions should be considered for purposes of client and family education.

Another consequence of antipsychotic medications is tardive dyskinesia. Initially, tardive dyskinesia was thought to occur only after prolonged use of antipsychotics, but current research is showing an increased prevalence of this side effect after short-term administration, particularly in the older adult (Jeste, 2004). Researchers now believe that TD represents stimulation of dopamine transmission in the basal ganglia and up-regulation of dopaminergic receptors (Casey, 2004). Interestingly, when conventional antipsychotic agents are compared to the atypical antipsychotic agents, the latter are associated with a significantly lower incidence of developing tardive dyskinesia, especially in older adults (Chou & Friedman, 2006; Correll, Leucht, & Kane, 2004; Jeste, 2004). Using atypical antipsychotics at the lowest effective dose may prevent symptoms of TD. Older adults have a four- to five-time incidence of TD than clients ages 25 to 35 (Chou & Friedman, 2006; Jeste, 2004). The American Psychiatric Association (APA) Task Force on TD estimated an incidence of 5 percent annually of exposure in young adults and 30 percent incidence after 1 year of treatment among older adults (APA, 1992). TD is irreversible and severely debilitating. In addition, there is no known treatment except to decrease antipsychotic medication to the absolute minimal level that will still afford symptom control. The most important factor in treating TD is that the antipsychotic medication should never be abruptly stopped or the symptoms will quickly, and possibly irreversibly, exacerbate. Therefore, it is imperative that the nurse distinguishes these symptoms from those of EPS. Major symptoms of TD begin with orofacial dyskinetic manifestations such as mouth smacking, frequent blinking and frowning, chewing movements, protrusion of tongue, and puffing of cheeks, and later accompanied by limb and truncal movements.

Early detection of TD is essential. The nurse is often involved in routine screening and monitoring of clients for the presence of abnormal movements. Although standard neurological examinations can be used for this purpose, the Abnormal Involuntary Movement Scale (AIMS), designed by the National Institute of Mental Health (NIMH), is more often used (Table 29–16). The client should be screened before any antipsychotic is begun and every 2 weeks to monthly and

My Experience with Extrapyramidal Side Effects

"My mouth is so dry. I feel like I can't swallow. Why is my mouth tight? Why are my eyes so dry? Even when I blink a lot they are still very dry. I do not know why you are giving a medication that makes me feel so bad. I thought that the medication was supposed to make me feel better. I do not hear voices, but I do not like the way I feel. I am having a hard time sitting still and feel like my legs are moving on their own. I feel so jumpy and strange; in fact, it feels like I am not inside my own body. Please give me something to calm me down and make me sit still and feel 'like a normal person again.'"

TABLE 29–13
Clinical and Pharmacokinetic Parameters of Extrapyramidal Side Effect Medications

Generic Name	Brand Name	Dosage Range (mg/Day)	Half-Life (Hours)	Onset Oral	Onset Intra-muscular	Duration (Hours)
Dopaminergic						
Amantadine	Symmetrel	100–300	9–37	4–48 hours*	NA	12–24
Anticholinergics						
Benztropine mesylate	Cogentin	0.5–6	?	1–2 hours	15 minutes	24
Biperiden	Akineton	2–16	18–24	60 minutes	15 minutes	6–10
Diphenhydramine	Benadryl	10–400	4–15	30–60 minutes	15–30 minutes	4–6
Procyclidine	Kemadrin	7.5–20	11–12	30–45 minutes	NA	4–6
Trihexyphenidyl	Artane	1–10	5.6–10	60 minutes	NA	6–12

*Response takes 2 weeks.

TABLE 29–14
Adverse Effects Associated with Antiparkinsonian Medications for Extrapyramidal Side Effects (EPS)

System	Common Side Effects	Less Common Adverse Side Effects
Cardiovascular		Orthostatic hypotension, tachycardia, palpitations
Central Nervous	Dizziness, drowsiness, blurred vision	Confusion, headache, disorientation
	Amantadine: anxiety, confusion, irritability, difficulty concentrating	Amantadine: fatigue, insomnia, weakness, visual disturbances
Gastrointestinal	Dry mouth	Amantadine: dry mouth, increased frequency of urination
	Amantadine: nausea, vomiting, anorexia, constipation	
Miscellaneous	Amantadine: urinary retention	Amantadine: skin rash, dyspnea

every 12 months thereafter (APA, 1992). The NIMH shows areas to be screened and includes the examination procedure.

A rare, but potentially fatal syndrome associated with antipsychotic medication is neuroleptic malignant syndrome (NMS). The exact cause of this syndrome is unknown, but it may be associated with effects on the hypothalamus and medulla. The symptomatology of NMS is similar to that of malignant hyperthermia. This syndrome can occur anytime during treatment with antipsychotics, including the novel antipsychotics. NMS has a rapid onset and constitutes a medical emergency. Symptoms include:

◆ Hyperpyrexia (up to 107°F)
◆ Severe muscle rigidity that precipitates elevated blood creatinine phosphokinase (CPK) and white blood cells
◆ Changes in consciousness (agitation or delirium)
◆ Elevated or labile pulse and blood pressure
◆ Profuse diaphoresis

TABLE 29–15
Adverse Effects Associated with Antipsychotics

System	Common Adverse Effects	Less Common Adverse Effects	Mechanism
Autonomic Nervous	Dry mouth, blurred vision, constipation, orthostatic hypotension	Urinary retention, weight gain, dyspepsia, priapism, incontinence	Blockage of muscarinic cholinergic receptors
Cardiac	Ziprasidone: cardiac arrhythmias (some potentially fatal)	Tachycardia	
	Clozapine	Cardiac arrhythmias	
Central Nervous	Sedation, extrapyramidal symptoms, headache, tardive dyskinesia		Blockage of alpha-adrenoreceptors
			Blockage of dopamine receptors
			Supersensitivity of dopamine
Endocrine		Galactorrhea, changes in libido, impotence in men, amenorrhea	Blockage of dopamine receptors, resulting in hyperprolactinemia
Hepatic	Jaundice at 2–4 weeks of medication		Unknown
Gastrointestinal	Nausea, vomiting	Diarrhea	Unknown
Ocular	Photophobia, blurred vision	Miosis	Unknown
Dermatological	Skin rashes	Urticaria, petechiae, erythema, hyperpigmentation	Unknown
Respiratory		Nasal congestion	Unknown
Hemic/Lymphatic		Clozapine: leukopenia, may cause agranulocytosis in up to 3% of clients	Unknown

- ◆ Incontinence
- ◆ Mutism
- ◆ Hypoxia
- ◆ Myoglobinuria and acute renal failure (in severe cases)

Treatment includes supportive care and symptomatic relief of hyperpyrexia; dantrolene (Dantrium) to decrease muscle rigidity and spasm, fever, and tachycardia; and bromocriptine (Parlodel), a centrally active dopamine agonist (Strawn, Keck, & Caroff, 2007).

Atypical Antipsychotics

With prevailing evidence for the efficacy and benefit of novel or atypical antipsychotics over traditional antipsychotics, the standard of practice has changed rapidly over the past few years. During the late 1990s, conventional antipsychotics were considered the first-line treatment for schizophrenia and were considered equivalent to the efficacy of atypical antipychotics for the treatment of positive symptoms. However, by the turn of the century, the APA as first-line treatment for schizophrenia (Currier, 2000; Ho, Miller, Nopolous, & Andreasen, 1999), recommended the atypical antipsychotics. In addition, the advent of the atypical antipsychotics represents an advancement in the treatment of schizophrenia and other psychotic disorders. Historically, treatment of these clients centered on managing their symptoms with little regard for their quality of life. The novel antipsychotics offer the client with schizophrenia an improved quality of life with fewer side effects that interfere with a higher level of functioning. With atypical neuroleptics, symptom relief occurs with fewer EPS, or at doses below those that precipitate EPS. Common atypical agents include clozapine (Clozaril), risperidone (Risperdal), olanzapine (Zyprexa),

TABLE 29–16
Abnormal Involuntary Movement Scale and Examination Procedure for Evaluating Tardive Dyskinesia

Instructions: Complete examination procedure before making ratings. Asterisk (*) denotes activated movements.

Examination Procedure

Either before or after completing the Examination Procedure, observe the client unobtrusively, at rest (e.g., in waiting room).
The chair to be used in this examination should be a hard, firm one without arms.

1. Ask the client whether there is anything in his or her mouth (gum, candy, etc.) and, if there is, to remove it.
2. Ask the client about the *current* condition of his or her teeth. Ask the client if he or she wears dentures. Do teeth or dentures bother the client *now*?
3. Ask the client whether he or she notices any movements in mouth, face, hands, or feet. If yes, ask the client to describe them and to what extent they *currently* bother the client or interfere with his or her activities.
4. Have the client sit in the chair with hands on knees, legs slightly apart, and feet flat on floor. (Look at entire body for movements while client is in this position.)
5. Ask the client to sit with hands hanging unsupported (if male, between legs; if female and wearing a dress, hanging over knees). (Observe hands and other body areas.)
6. Ask the client to open his or her mouth. (Observe tongue at rest within mouth.) Do this twice.
7. Ask the client to protrude his or her tongue. (Observe abnormalities of tongue movement.) Do this twice.
*8. Ask the client to tap his or her thumb with each finger, as rapidly as possible for 10 to 15 seconds, first with right hand, then with left hand. (Observe facial and leg movements.)
*9. Ask the client to stand up. (Observe the client's profile. Observe all body areas again, hips included.)
*10. Ask the client to extend both arms outstretched in front with palms down. (Observe trunk, legs, and mouth.)
*11. Have the client walk a few paces, turn, and walk back to chair. (Observe hands and gait.) Do this twice.

Abnormal Involuntary Movement Scale (AIMS)

Movement Ratings: Rate highest severity observed. Rate movements that occur upon activation less than movements that occur spontaneously.

Codes:

0 = None

1 = Minimal; may be extreme normal

2 = Mild

3 = Moderate

4 = Severe

		(Circle one)				
Facial and Oral Movements	1. Muscles of facial expression, e.g., movements of forehead, eyebrows, periorbital area, cheeks; include frowning, blinking, smiling, grimacing.	0	1	2	3	4
	2. Lips and perioral area, e.g., puckering, pouting, smacking.	0	1	2	3	4
	3. Jaw, e.g., biting, clenching, chewing, mouth opening, lateral movements.	0	1	2	3	4
	4. Tongue Rate only increase in movement both in and out of, NOT inability to sustain movement.	0	1	2	3	4

(continues)

TABLE 29–16
Abnormal Involuntary Movement Scale and Examination Procedure for Evaluating Tardive Dyskinesia *(continued)*

		(Circle one)				
Extremity Movements	5. Upper (arms, wrists, hands, and fingers). Include choreic movements (i.e., rapid objectively purposeless, irregular, spontaneous), athetoid movements (i.e., slow irregular, complex, serpentine). Do NOT include tremor (i.e., repetitive, regular, rhythmic).	0	1	2	3	4
	6. Lower (legs, knees, ankles, and toes), e.g., lateral knee movement, foot tapping, heel dropping, foot squirming, inversion and eversion of foot.					
Trunk Movements	7. Neck, shoulders, hips, e.g., rocking, twisting, squirming, pelvic gyrations.	0	1	2	3	4

Global Judgments	8. Severity of abnormal movements.	None, normal	0
		Minimal	1
		Mild	2
		Moderate	3
		Severe	4
	9. Incapacitation due to abnormal movements.	None, normal	0
		Minimal	1
		Mild	2
		Moderate	3
		Severe	4
	10. Client's awareness of abnormal movements. Rate only client's report.	No awareness	0
		Awareness, no distress	1
		Aware, mild distress	2
		Aware, moderate distress	3
		Aware, severe distress	4
Dental Status	11. Current problems with teeth and/or dentures.	No	0
		Yes	1
	12. Does client usually wear dentures?	No	0
		Yes	1

Note. Adapted from *ECDEU: Assessment Manual for Psychopharmacology (DHEW)*, Publ. No. 76-338, by W. Guy, 1976, Washington, DC: Department of Health, Education, and Welfare, Psychopharmacology Research Branch.

---

quetiapine (Seroquel), ziprasidone (Geodon), and aripiprazole (Abilify) (see Table 29–10, Receptor Affinity for Atypical Antipsychotics).

Mechanism of Action

The efficacy of the newer antipsychotic agents are also associated with their well-documented control of positive and negative symptoms of schizophrenia along with their favorable side effect profile. Pharmacologically, novel antipsychotics differ from traditional neuroleptics. Traditional neuroleptic agents have D_2 antagonism without 5-HT_2 antagonism, whereas the novel agents are serotonin-dopamine-2 (D_2) antagonists. Theoretically, this explains the improved efficacy of atypical antipsychotic agents over conventional agents in the treatment of negative symptoms of schizophrenia. The D_2 and 5-HT_{2A} antagonism properties confer a lower incidence of EPS and TD, which are the most troublesome side effects of the conventional antipsychotics. Atypical antipsychotics do not raise prolactin levels, which every conventional agent does. These newer agents are more effective than traditional agents in reducing negative symptoms; improving cognitive, sexual, and mood

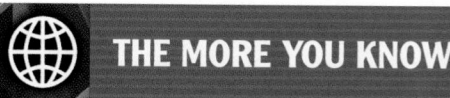
function; and controlling agitation and aggression. Overall, atypical neuroleptics are more likely to improve the client's quality of life and function and experience fewer acute and chronic adverse drug reactions seen in traditional antipsychotic agents (Van Kammer & Marder, 2005).

Side Effects

Atypical antipsychotics, such as olanzapine, clozapine, and risperidone, generally do not produce neurological side effects. Newer antipsychotic agents tend to have a different side effect profile, with a lower risk of motor symptoms, but often, additional undesired adverse reactions. Despite the lower side effect profile of these agents, nurses must thoroughly assess the client's response to them and potential side effects. The nursing assessment should include careful observation of the client's movements and asking her to describe any problems throughout antipsychotic treatment. Common side effects of novel antipsychotic agents include sedation, weight gain, insomnia, orthostatic hypotension, agitation, constipation, hypersalivation, and dry mouth.

Many of the side effects associated with atypical antipsychotic agents are dose related. At high doses they have similar side effect profiles as the conventional agents. Although, there is limited evidence of EPS or TD, clozapine does produce a potentially life-threatening agranulocytosis. Therefore, clients on this medication must comply with routine blood monitoring. The cost of clozapine remains high. However, this medication and others in this family have brought dramatic symptom relief to clients who have been labeled treatment resistant.

Sedatives and Hypnotic Agents

Sedatives or anxiolytic agents are used primarily to treat anxiety disorders or anxiety-provoking situations. In comparison, hypnotics are used to promote sleep. Sedatives and hypnotic agents offer limited use and are often used as adjunct therapy with other nonpharmacologic interventions such as cognitive behavioral therapy and sleep hygiene. The following section focuses on both groups of drugs.

Anxiolytics

An anxiolytic is any medication used to treat anxiety. Whether to treat anxiety is often a difficult and controversial decision. Anxiety is a universal experience, a common response to daily stress and conflict. Psychiatric nurses must assess the distress and disabling effects of anxiety and collaborate with the client and treatment options. Health education is an integral part of treatment planning and must include both pharmacologic agents and nonpharmacologic approaches such as stress management and deep abdominal breathing exercises.

Anxiety manifests psychologically as anything from uneasiness and irritability to a frightful feeling of doom. It can present physically in a variety of autonomic nervous system manifestations: tachycardia, palpitations, irregular heart rhythm, dizziness, tremor, excessive sweating, dry mouth, diarrhea, abdominal pain, or headache. More commonly, it presents with a combination of physiological and psychological symptoms. Anxiety can underlie other psychiatric conditions (e.g., depression) as well as many medical conditions such as endocrine disorders. Clearly, the diagnosis and assessment of anxiety are important and challenging initial tasks. Like other psychiatric conditions, anxiety can be treated with environmental, social, psychological, and nonbiological interventions. These interventions should be considered along with medications (see Chapter 11).

Current nomenclature divides anxiety disorders into three major subtypes: phobic disorders (agoraphobia, social phobia, and simple phobia), anxiety states (panic disorder, generalized anxiety disorder, and obsessive-compulsive disorder), and PTSD.

Benzodiazepines, antianxiety agents, are the most widely used and prescribed drugs in the world. Other classes of drugs that are used to treat anxiety disorders include antidepressants, antihistamines, barbiturates, propanediols, beta blockers (e.g., propranolol), nonbenzodiazepines (buspirone), and the antipsychotic drugs (Table 29–17). Although the general use of antidepressants has been discussed, their use in treating anxiety can be considered here. Clients with a history of anxiety are likely, even with optimal medication response, to require long-term pharmacologic intervention. Because prolonged administration of benzodiazepines may be associated with drug dependence, it is particularly important to assess the particular type of anxiety disorder the client has. Some anxiety disorders, such as agoraphobia, panic disorder, and PTSD, often respond well to antidepressants. Buspirone

TABLE 29–17
Clinical and Pharmacokinetic Parameters of Antianxiety Medications

Generic Name	Brand Name	Dosage Range (mg/Day)	Half-Life (Hours)	Onset (Minutes)	Duration (Hours)
Benzodiazepines					
Alprazolam	Xanax	0.75–4	12–15	15–60	Varies by age,
Chlordiazepoxide	Librium, et al.	15–100	5–30	15–45	illness, and dosage
Clorazepate	Tranxene	15–60	30–100	30–60	
Diazepam	Valium, et al.	4–40	20–80	15–45	
Halazepam	Paxipam	60–160	14	30–60	
Lorazepam	Ativan	2–4	10–20	15–45	
Oxazepam	Serax	30–120	5–20	15–90	
Prazepam	Centrax	20–60	30–100	?	
Clonazepam	Klonopin	1–6 mg	30–100	15–45	
Other Drugs					
Buspirone	BuSpar	15–60	2–11	3–4 weeks	Varies by age, illness, and dosage
Chlormezanone	Trancopal	300–800	24	15–30	6
Diphenhydramine	Benadryl, et al.	75–200	2.4–4.3	30–60	4–10
Hydroxyzine	Atarax, Vistaril	50–100	3	15–30	4–6
Meprobamate	Miltown, Equinil	1,200–1,600	6–48	60	6–17

and venlafaxine and SSRIs such as paroxetine appear useful in generalized anxiety (Antai-Otong, 2007b; Rickels, Rynn, Iyengar, & Duff, 2006; Stein, van der Kolk, Austin, Fayyad, & Clary, 2006).

The antianxiety agents were introduced with the promise that they were effective, safe, and nonaddicting. Experience with benzodiazepines and other antianxiety agents have shown otherwise. They can all produce tolerance, dependence, and withdrawal symptoms.

Benzodiazepines

Chlordiazepoxide (Librium), the first benzodiazepine, was marketed in 1960, and diazepam (Valium), 3 years later. Presently, there are more than three dozen benzodiazepines available. They are the mainstays of treatment for anxiety, insomnia, alcohol withdrawal, stimulant drug intoxication, and psychosis. Benzodiazepines are highly effective for the alleviation of acute anxiety and retain at least a portion of their efficacy over time. They are relatively safe in an overdose situation, although the combination of a benzodiazepine with alcohol or another sedative-hypnotic agent can be hazardous (Dubovsky, 2005). Overall, the safety profile of benzodiazepines is unparalleled.

The anxiolytic potency of a benzodiazepine correlates with its affinity for benzodiazepine receptors. The efficacy of benzodiazepines is their ability to modulate the GABA system. GABA is a large neurotransmitter system that constitutes about 30 percent of the cortical and thalamic inhibitory system. Benzodiazepines raise the seizure threshold and increase the frequency and activity of the brain waves. Other sedative-hypnotics, such as barbiturates, also produce these effects. The benzodiazepines, especially diazepam, cause skeletal muscle relaxation. Again, it appears that the GABA-ergic action of benzodiazepines may at least account for the anticonvulsant and muscle relaxant effects. The effects on other organ systems appear to be minimal (Dubovsky, 2005).

As with all CNS depressants, the most common adverse effects of the benzodiazepines are drowsiness and ataxia. The older adult may be more vulnerable to these reactions, because they usually achieve higher blood and tissue drug levels for a given dose and also because the aging brain is more sensitive to the effects of sedatives. Although complications of benzodiazepines during pregnancy are uncertain, some data indicate that these agents can produce palate abnormalities and should be used with caution during pregnancy (Dubovsky, 2005).

Reports of paradoxical reactions, or disinhibition, are not infrequent. An increased tendency to express hostility, rage, or aggression, even in persons with no previous history of these feelings, has been reported with diazepam (Valium), alprazolam (Xanax), and chlordiazepoxide (Librium). Benzodiazepines have well-documented amnestic properties. Certainly, this effect can be used to the client's advantage. For example, benzodiazepines can be given during painful or unpleasant procedures in part because they cause anterograde amnesia. However, the untoward effects of amnesia in regular doses of benzodiazepines must also be assessed.

Tolerance to the sedative effects of benzodiazepines develops; whether it also develops to the sleep-maintaining or antianxiety effects is unclear. Although benzodiazepine drugs have been used recreationally, most clients have not abused these drugs. The possibility of addiction must be considered, though, because there are some exceptions. First, most prescribers believe that these agents should not be prescribed to clients with substance-related disorders, except when used as part of a detoxification protocol. Second, if a client takes more of a benzodiazepine than is prescribed, this behavior needs to be carefully examined. Third, it should be recognized that the type of anxiolytic prescribed, the dosage used, and the duration of the agent's effect all can affect the possibility of a problem in compliance. As an example, the shorter the half-life of the drug prescribed, which increases the frequency of dosing, the greater the risk of dependency and addiction.

Benzodiazepine withdrawal can lead to reactions much like those observed with other sedative-hypnotic compounds, such as barbiturates and alcohol. Whereas withdrawal reactions from cessation of benzodiazepine use were once thought to be rare, clinicians now believe that clients taking benzodiazepines for long periods, even at standard doses, are vulnerable to withdrawal reactions if the drug is discontinued abruptly. Therefore, clients need to consult with their prescriber and taper off the medication gradually.

Mild symptoms of withdrawal include insomnia, dizziness, headache, anorexia, tinnitus, blurred vision, and shakiness. These symptoms may also indicate a returning anxiety. If these symptoms begin to wane after several weeks, a withdrawal reaction seems unlikely.

Severe signs of withdrawal may include hypotension, hyperthermia, neuromuscular rigidity, psychosis, and seizures. Short-acting benzodiazepines may have a higher risk of withdrawal symptoms because longer-acting agents are self-tapering.

Buspirone

Buspirone (BuSpar) is structurally and pharmacologically unrelated to benzodiazepines. It has no direct effect on $GABA_A$ receptors, is not a CNS depressant, and lacks the sedative action of the benzodiazepines. It is speculated that buspirone exerts its anxiolytic effect by acting as a partial agonist at $5\text{-}HT_{1A}$ receptors, particularly in the hippocampus and other limbic structures. It also increases the norepinephrine metabolism in the locus ceruleus. Buspirone does not appear to produce tolerance or dependence and has neither anticonvulsant nor muscle relaxant properties. The most common side effects are dizziness, nausea, headache, nervousness, lightheadedness, and excitement. Unlike any of the benzodiazepines, buspirone is effective only when taken regularly. It takes 1 to 2 weeks to show initial effects; maximal effectiveness may be reached after 4 to 6 weeks (Dubovsky, 2005).

Antihistamines

Because of their sedative effects, drugs that block central and peripheral histamine receptors (primarily H_1) are sometimes used to calm anxious clients. Hydroxyzine (Vistaril) and diphenhydramine (Benadryl) are frequently prescribed examples of this class. Besides sedation, these medications also have antiemetic and antihistamine properties. Unlike most antianxiety agents, antihistamines depress the seizure threshold and must be used cautiously in clients with seizure disorders. They have more anticholinergic action than the benzodiazepines do, which limits their use, particularly in older adults (Dubovsky, 2005).

Barbiturates

Benzodiazepines have largely replaced the once popular barbiturates. There are several reasons for this. First, benzodiazepines appear to be more effective than the barbiturates in treating anxiety. Second, barbiturate overdose can be extremely dangerous. Third, barbiturates interact pharmacologicly with a greater number of agents.

Propranolol

Propranolol blocks beta-noradrenergic receptors in the peripheral sympathetic nervous system and probably centrally as well. Although drugs specific to beta-1 (cardiac) and beta 2 (pulmonary) receptors have recently been developed, propranolol itself blocks receptors competitively and without discrimination. Propranolol has extensive effects on the cardiovascular system, the pulmonary bronchi, and carbohydrate and fat metabolism. Although propranolol is probably not as effective an antianxiety agent as other medications, clients with somatic complaints may find it useful. It should be noted that propranolol has not been approved for the treatment of anxiety or other psychiatric conditions. Propranolol is sometimes given to alleviate lithium-induced tremors (Dubovsky, 2005).

Propanediols

The propanediols (e.g., meprobamate [Equanil]) were extremely popular in the 1950s, but controlled studies have failed to demonstrate their superiority over barbiturates in the treatment of anxiety. Neither class of drugs is used today.

Antipsychotics

The significant negative side effect profile of the antipsychotics, particularly the conventional agents, makes them a poor choice to treat anxiety. Only when psychosis is the cause of the anxiety are they considered.

Hypnotics

Almost 20 percent of clients who visit physicians complain of difficulty sleeping, and half of these clients are prescribed hypnotics. Insomnia is a symptom with diverse causes, including medical, psychological, and situational. It is important to search for a specific treatable cause before prescribing a nonspecific therapy such as a hypnotic. The client's normal sleeping patterns need to be assessed and reviewed; non-pharmacologic interventions, or sleep hygiene measures, should be implemented whenever possible (Wang, Wang, & Tsai, 2005). Sleep hygiene measures are practices that promote sleep such as drinking warm milk; taking a warm bath; reading; developing a regular routine for preparing for sleep; and avoiding food or fluids high in caffeine such as chocolates, coffee, tea, or colas (see Chapter 23).

There are many substances, differing widely in their chemical structure, that can be considered sedative-hypnotics in that they produce dose-dependent CNS depression. The more commonly used agents are presented in Table 29–18 and the symptoms of adverse effects of their use are listed in Table 29–19. There can be cross-reactivity between these diverse compounds. For example, a client who has developed tolerance to a benzodiazepine not only will be tolerant to other benzodiazepines but will also be tolerant to barbiturates and other CNS depressants. Abrupt discontinuation of any of these medications is associated with a withdrawal syndrome. All clients, regardless of whether they have a history of a substance-related disorder, who are regularly using small amounts of sedative-hypnotics may gradually develop tolerance and experience a withdrawal syndrome if the drug is suddenly stopped or significantly decreased. Note that the features of withdrawal syndrome (tremulousness, irritability, and sleep disturbance) may be mistaken for the initial target symptoms. The nurse may be able to explore this in a careful interview.

In summary, it is important to remember (1) the need for careful evaluation before any medication is prescribed or administered; (2) the importance of short-term use if these medications are chosen; (3) the relevance of educating the client on sleep hygiene measures.

Benzodiazepines and Other Hypnotic Agents

Should a hypnotic (sedative or sleeping pill) be prescribed, the most likely choice would be a benzodiazepine. Examples of major hypnotics or sedatives are flurazepam (Dalmane), temazepam (Restoril), and zolpidem (Ambien), a nonbenzodiazepine but within the same schedule as hypnotics. It is likely that most, if not all, of the benzodiazepines used to treat anxiety could also be used to induce sleep at the appropriate dosage. It is a corporate decision whether to market benzodiazepines as anxiolytics or hypnotics; FDA labeling approval is based almost entirely on information supplied by the manufacturer.

The two major concerns in choosing a benzodiazepine hypnotic are rapidity of onset and half-life. For clients who report difficulty falling asleep, the rate at which the drug achieves its hypnotic effects is important. Two benzodiazepines that have rapid onset are diazepam (Valium) and flurazepam (Dalmane). Benzodiazepines with long half-lives decrease sleep latency (the time required to fall asleep), decrease early morning awakenings, and usually increase the total amount of sleep. However, the trade-off may be daytime drowsiness and related unwanted effects. Over time, their use must be assessed in terms of the benefits for the client (Dubovsky, 2005).

The second important consideration is half-life. Benzodiazepines with short half-lives do not accumulate, but they may cause rebound insomnia. Benzodiazepines decrease the length of sleep in stages 3 and 4 and their effect on rapid eye movement (REM) sleep varies, depending on the client, the illness, and the type and dosage of the drug. Rebound insomnia may occur when a benzodiazepine with a short half-life is used on several consecutive nights.

Flurazepam is a long-acting drug that resembles diazepam. Its half-life of 50 to 100 hours means that the blood level on the eighth morning after a consecutive week of nightly flurazepam is likely to be 4 to 6 times that found on the first morning. A long half-life can have positive consequences: it may be useful for clients who are anxious and have rebound insomnia. Rebound insomnia is less likely with long-acting agents. Negative consequences may include morning hangover (residual sedation and impaired cognitive and motor skills). In addition, potential interactions with other sedatives, including alcohol, may be prolonged.

Temazepam (Restoril), with its shorter half-life, may reduce the hangover, but increase rebound insomnia. Zolpidem (Ambien) is a hypnotic that acts at the GABA-benzodiazepine complex, similarly to benzodiazepines, but it is not a benzodiazepine. This short-acting sleep agent does not produce tolerance. Zolpidem is useful to decrease sleep latency, increase total sleep time, and decrease the number of nighttime awakenings. Zaleplon (Sonata) also has a short half-life. It decreases sleep latency but does not increase total sleep time or decrease the number of awakenings. Although zolpidem and zaleplon are structurally not benzodiazepines, the differences are subtle and thus claims to safety and efficacy need to be carefully evaluated over time.

Eszopiclone (Lunesta), is a novel nonbenzodiazepine hypnotic, used to treat symptoms of insomnia. Its pharmacokinetic and pharmacodynamic makeup are similar to zolpidem and zaleplon. However, unlike zolpidem and zaleplon, eszopiclone is not restricted to short-term use, unlike both zolpidem and zaleplon. Eszopiclone is well-tolerated, and similar to other nonbenzodiazepines. Its major side effects include a bitter and unpleasant taste, headache, and dizziness (Scharf, 2006).

Other Agents

The caveats mentioned regarding the prescription of barbiturates for anxiety apply equally to the prescription of hypnotics. Because of problems with tolerance, abuse, dependency, adverse effects, rebound, and the danger of overdose, barbiturates are rarely prescribed. Other agents formerly widely used and now much less frequently prescribed, for many of the same reasons, are chloral hydrate, glutethimide (Doriden), methaqualone (Quaalude), paraldehyde, and bromides.

TABLE 29-18

Clinical and Pharmacokinetic Parameters of Sedatives and Hypnotics

Generic Name	Brand Name	Dosage Range (mg/Day) Hypnotic	Sedative	Onset (Minutes)	Half-Life (Hours)	Duration of Action (Hours)
Nonbarbiturate						
Acetylcarbromal	Paxarel	—	250–500 bid or tid	15–60	?	
Chloral hydrate	Noctec	0.5–1g	250 tid	30–60	7–10	4–8
Ethchlorvynol	Placidyl	500	100–200 tid	15–60	10–20	5
Ethinamate	Valmid	—	500–1,000	20	2.5	3–5
Glutethimide	Doriden	250–500	—	30	10–12	4–8
Methyprylon	Noludar	200–400	—	45	3–6	5–8
Paraldehyde	Paral	10–30 ml	5–10 ml	10–15	3.4–98	8–12
Propiomazine	Largon	—	10–20			
Benzodiazepines						
Estazolam	Prosom	1–2	NA	30–60	10–24	
Flurazepam	Dalmane	15–30	NA	15–45	50–100 (2–100 for metabolites)	7–8
Quazepam	Doral	15	NA	45–120	25–41	
Temazepam	Restoril	15–30	NA	20–30	10–17	6–8
Triazolam	Halcion	0.125–0.5	NA	15–30	1.5–5.5	6–8
Barbiturates						
Long acting						
Phenobarbital	Barbital, Luminal	100–320	30–120	≥ 60	53–118	10–12
Mephobarbital	Mebural	—	90–400		11–67	
Intermediate acting						
Amobarbital	Amytal	65–200	30–480	45–60	16–40	6–8
Aprobarbital	Alurate	40–160	120		14–34	
Butabarbital	Butisol, Butratan	50–100	45–120		66–140	
Talbutal	Lotusate	120	60–80		15	
Short acting						
Secobarbital	Secondal	100	—	10–15	15–40	3–4
Pentobarbital	Nembutal	100	40–120		15–50	

TABLE 29–19
Adverse Effects Associated with Sedatives and Hypnotics

System	Common Adverse Effects	Less Common Adverse Effects
Benzodiazepines		
Cardiovascular	Palpitations	Tachycardia
Central Nervous	Sedation, lack of concentration, dizziness, drowsiness	Tremors, apprehension, nervousness, confusion, headaches, lethargy, weakness, paradoxical excitation, euphoria, coordination disorders
	Estazolam: somnolence, asthenia	
Gastrointestinal		Nausea, vomiting, heartburn, constipation, diarrhea
Nonbarbiturates		
Cardiovascular		Hypotension
Central Nervous	Dizziness, drowsiness	Ataxia, headache, paradoxical excitation, blurred vision
		Methyprylon: vertigo, nightmares
Gastrointestinal	Glutethimide: skin rash	Heartburn, constipation, diarrhea, flatulence, offensive breath, dry mouth
Barbiturates		
Cardiovascular		Hypotension, bradycardia, syncope
Central Nervous		Ataxia, confusion, hyperkinesia, paradoxical excitation, agitation, vertigo
Gastrointestinal		Nausea, vomiting, constipation, diarrhea
Dermatological		Skin rash, urticaria (with asthma)
Respiratory		Hypoventilation, apnea

Antihistamines

Sedating antihistamines, many of which are available over the counter, can be effective hypnotics for some adults. Diphenhydramine is probably the most commonly used drug in this class. It may suppress REM sleep, and REM rebound occurs following its discontinuation. Because of its anticholinergic effects, confusion and delirium can develop in susceptible clients, older adults, and persons taking drugs with anticholinergic activity.

Psychostimulants: Used in the Treatment for Attention Deficit/Hyperactivity Disorder

The most commonly prescribed medications for clients with attention deficit/hyperactivity disorder (ADHD) are methylphenidate (Ritalin) and dextroamphetamine (Dexedrine) which are class II (controlled) substances. Methylphenidate is prescribed more often than dextroamphetamine, because it has been extensively studied (Greenhill et al., 2002; McMaster University, 1999; Castle, Aubert, Verbrugge, Khalid, & Epstein, 2007). The use of stimulant drugs results in an immediate and often dramatic improvement in behavior-attentiveness, and enhanced academic and occupational performance.

Mechanism of Action

Methylphenidate and amphetamine are the most frequently prescribed pharmacological treatments of ADHD. Methylphenidate, like other psychostimulants, blocks dopamine and increases dopamine by releasing it from the terminal. Psychostimulants increase dopamine in the nucleus accumbens, which is thought to be the basis of the reinforcing effects of drug addiction. The dopamine transporter (DAT) is a chief target site for amphetamine and methylphenidate, used in the treatment of ADHD. The efficacy of methylphenidate and amphetamine lies in their ability to increase extracellular dopamine in the striatum and cortical brain regions (Iversen, 2006; Volkow et al., 2004). More specifically, stimulant-induced dopamine increases in the nucleus accumbens, modulates incentive and motivation and enhances the saliency of a task by increasing the interest and improving attention and performance. Methylphenidate and amphetamine's capacity to expand dopamine is also posited to enhance their reinforcing properties, and perhaps be one of the primary underpinnings associated with their abuse. Whilst abuse of these agents is possible, the incidence is inconsequential. Scientists submit that steady state and stable and increased dopamine levels parallel the therapeutic range of stimulant medications, whereas, abrupt and rapid increases in dopamine enhance their reinforcing effects (Volkow, 2006). During the past decade researchers have developed a newer preparations that decrease the rate of brain uptake and unlike older preparations cannot be injected or snorted and result in rapid release of dopamine (Spencer et al., 2006). For these reasons, newer preparations of psychostimulants are mainly controlled-release and have less addictive properties and hence less likely to be abused.

Implications for Psychiatric Nurses

Pretreatment must involve a comprehensive physical and psychiatric evaluation that includes mental status exam; differential diagnosis; diagnostic studies, such as thyroid function, liver panel, and chemistries; ECG; and cardiac work up. Baseline blood pressure and pulse, along with height and weight, must also be assessed during pretreatment and regularly throughout treatment. Due to the risk of abnormal movements, such as tics, using standardized tools, such as the Abnormal Involuntary Movement Scale and Angus-Simpson scale must be performed for baseline data and to monitor for this side effect. Assessing the client and family's understanding of the youth's condition, health practices, preferences, and cultural needs must be part of the initial and ongoing treatment plan.

Dosage

The therapeutic dose of stimulants varies and must be individualized. The initial dose of standard methylphenidate or dextroamphetamine is 2.5 to 5 mg once daily. The dose may be increased every three to five days while adverse effects, behavior, and academic function are assessed through reports from parents and teachers. Once the lowest effective dose is determined, the duration of behavioral efficacy can be determined and used to assess the need for and timing of additional doses. Additional daily doses of methylphenidate should be similar to the first dose, whereas for dextroamphetamine, a smaller dose (2.5 to 5 mg less) may be adequate to extend efficacy.

Side Effects/Toxicity

Common side effects of psychostimulants include: irritability, sleep disturbances or insomnia, dry mouth, dizziness, headaches, nausea, stomachache, tachycardia, precipitation or exacerbation of tics, and appetite suppression. These side effects tend to be short lived and diminish over time. Eating small meals rather than three large meals often curtails any appetite disturbances and nausea. Shorter-acting agents are more likely to increase the risk of rebound hyperactivity—consider using long-acting agents. Dizziness may also be associated with orthostatic hypotension and indicate the importance of monitoring blood pressure and heart rate. Increased agitation may indicate co-occurring psychiatric conditions, such as bipolar disorder or the dose may need to be lowered. High doses are also associated with agitation, irritability, psychosis, bruxism, and dilated pupils.

Like all health teaching involving medication, information concerning persistent and distressful side effects must be

reported to the primary care giver. Stimulants are also habit forming or addictive. Clients with a history of substance use are especially susceptible to addiction and these agents should be avoided or used cautiously when there is a positive family history of substance abuse. Clients taking psychostimulants must also be cautioned about stopping medications suddenly to avert rebound hyperactivity. These agents are also contraindicated in clients presenting with heart disease, agitation, motor tics, diagnosis of or positive family history of Tourette's syndrome, glaucoma, pregnancy, taking an MAOI in the last 2 weeks, seizure disorder, thyroid disease, or marked anxiety. More serious side effects associated with psychostimulants include hallucinations of which auditory hallucinations are the most common. Liver damage, irritation, increased heart rate, and tics along with other serious side effects must be reported immediately (Hechtman, 2005; Stein, 2004). Clients should be monitored for increased blood pressure, tachycardia, GI disturbances, mania, and hyperthyroidism throughout treatment. Although rare, severe liver damage may occur when taking atomoxetine and pemoline, making it essential to monitor the client's liver enzymes and educate family about symptoms to report such as malaise, jaundice, or abdominal pain.

PSYCHOPHARMACOLOGIC THERAPY ACROSS THE LIFE SPAN

It is crucial for the psychiatric nurse to understand the influence of age-related pharmacokinetic and pharmacodynamic processes and their impact on side effect profiles and indication for health education. This section focuses on these issues and the role of the nurse in providing safe drug administration, symptom management and drug response monitoring.

SEDATIVE AND ANTIANXIETY AGENTS

Because the metabolism of benzodiazepines is slowed in the older adult client, these drugs are likely to remain in the body at higher concentrations than they would under comparable conditions in a younger person. Agents that are not recommended owing to active metabolites are chlordiazepoxide, clorazepate, diazepam, halazepam, and flurazepam. Likewise, barbiturates with longer half-lives and meprobamate should be avoided in this age group. Regardless of the antianxiety or sedative changes, their effects on the older adults, especially on their mental status, must be regularly assessed.

ANTIPSYCHOTICS

The side effects of primary concern in the older adult population are anticholinergic effects, parkinsonian effects, TD, orthostatic hypotension, cardiac abnormalities, reduced bone density, sedation, and cognitive impairment (Van Kammer & Marder, 2005). Antipsychotics, especially the conventional agents, with greater hypotensive and anticholinergic effects such as mesoridazine (Serentil) and thioridazine should be avoided. The novel antipsychotic agents, such as olanzapine and quetiapine, have favorable side effect profiles that make them the first-line treatment for older adults with psychotic disorders (Sadock, Sadock, & Sussman, 2006).

CHILDREN AND ADOLESCENTS

Indications for the use of psychotropic medications in children and adolescents have been revolutionized for more than a decade. However, the use of these agents in children presents philosophical, ethical, legal, and diagnostic problems. A nurse who is working with children who have been prescribed psychotropic medication needs to consider the following points:

◆ Developmental factors such as age, gender, weight, and physical health play major roles in how children and adolescents react to drugs. Hepatic metabolism appears to be greatest during infancy and childhood, approximately two times the adult rate in prepuberty and equivalent to adult by age 15 (Sussman, 2005). The clinical significance of this premise suggests that younger children might need higher milligram-per-kilogram dosages than older youth or adults (Sussman, 2005).

◆ Drug pharmacokinetics differ in children and adults. For example, a child's liver represents a proportionally larger amount of the total body weight; children often metabolize agents more quickly (Prasad, 2005; Sussman, 2005). Although drug absorption for most medications is similar in children and adults, children tend to have a faster absorption rate and reach peak plasma levels earlier (Sussman, 2005). A lower level of protein binding and lower percentage of body adipose tissue result in smaller depots for drug storage, which means quicker onset of action and decreased duration of effect. Therefore, children may often require relatively higher and more frequent doses than adults, but they tend to develop fewer side effects (Sadock, Sadock, & Sussman, 2006).

◆ When unwanted reactions do occur, they are generally less severe and respond more readily to a decrease or discontinuation of the medication. Children should be systematically and repeatedly questioned about the development of untoward reactions, because they volunteer this information less readily than adults (Sussman, 2005). Most of the untoward effects that children do develop are similar to those in adults.

◆ As previously discussed, children's distinct physiology may affect the way medications are absorbed, distributed, metabolized, and eliminated. For example, the hepatic P450 cytochrome enzyme system in younger children (less than 2 years old) appears to work slower, resulting in higher blood levels of some medications along with risk of serious side effects. Side effects may differ in younger children making it necessary for nurses to carefully assess risk factors (Prasad, 2005).

◆ Children are still *developing* physically (height and weight and reproductive), socially, neurologically, and cognitively (Prasad, 2005). Nurses must use the nursing process to ensure that all medications administered to youngsters and adolescents, particularly long-term use, *do not harm* or produce injurious results.

◆ Tremendous progress has been made in formulating effective psychopharmacologic strategies for children and adolescents. In addition, advances in the ability of making appropriate psychiatric diagnoses of childhood and adolescent conditions and subsequent development of psychotropic medications have paved the way for treatment. Despite these developments, with the exception of stimulants, there is a dearth of rigorous studies of psychotropic conditions in children and adolescents. The increase in reported cases of suicide resulted in the FDA issuing a black box warning on all antidepressants used by adolescents and adults (see Internet Resources for a list of specific antidepressant medications). Research in children is justified based on the need to ensure adequate psychoeducation on the efficacy and safety of promising pharmacologic agents (Harpaz-Rotem & Rosenheck, 2006).

◆ When administering or prescribing psychotropics to children and adolescents it is imperative to weigh the risk-benefit ratio and balance it against the clinical need. Medication risks in children and adolescents can be reduced by carefully choosing the appropriate dose and thoroughly monitoring for potential side effects, including increased suicidality. Controversy concerning the association between antidepressants and suicide risk continue to be debated. Findings from a recent study conducted by Simon and colleagues (2006) found that during the first 6 months of treatment, the risk of suicide in children and adolescents was one in 3,000, and the risk of serious suicide attempt was one in 1,000. They concluded that the risk of serious suicide attempt increased more during the initial month of treatment than during the following 5 months. However, they asserted that the risk was highest during the month prior to treatment (see Research Abstract, Suicide Risk During Antidepressant Treatment).

Antipsychotics

Once a diagnosis has been established that indicates the need for a dopamine receptor antagonist, such as the phenothiazines or serotonin-dopamine antagonists, such as olanzapine, an antipsychotic agent may be prescribed or administered. Major indications for these drugs include psychoses, Tourette's disorder, and self-injurious behaviors. Side effects produced by these agents are similar to those produced in adults. Young clients may be at a higher risk for EPS. It may be safer to initiate therapy with an atypical antipsychotic. If pediatric clients fail atypical agents, then a typical antipsychotic may be tried. Doses are initiated at half the recommended adult dosage and titrated every 3 to 4 days. Because of the potential for weight gain with the

RESEARCH ABSTRACT

Suicide Risk During Antidepressant Treatment

Simon, G. E., Savarino, J., Operskalski, N., Wang, P. S. (2006). *American Journal of Psychiatry, 163,* 41–47.

Study Problem/Purpose

The purpose of the study was to evaluate the risk of suicide death and serious suicide attempt and its association with the initiation of antidepressant treatment.

Method

The researchers conducted a population-based study to evaluate data from computerized records of antidepressant prescriptions filled from January 1, 1992, through June 30, 2003, of individuals of a prepaid health plan in Washington state and Idaho. Approximately 65,103 clients with 82,285 episodes of antidepressant treatment were identified during this period. Approximately 70 percent of the subjects were women, with a mean age of 44 years old.

Findings

Researchers found that the risk of suicide attempt was 314 per 100,000 in children and adolescents, compared to 78 per 100,000 in adults. They also concluded that the risk of death by suicide was not significantly greater during the month postinitiation of antidepressant therapy, but asserted that the risk of suicide attempt was greatest in the month preceding antidepressant treatment and a progressive decrease after starting medication. Finally, they submitted that when the 10 newer antidepressants (included on the FDA black box list) were compared to older antidepressants, an increased risk was only associated with the initiation of the older drugs. Based on these data there was no significant increase in suicide risk postinitiating newer antidepressant medications.

Implications for Psychiatric Nurses

Suicide risk exists with the diagnosis of most psychiatric disorders, especially depression. Regardless of age group all clients must be assessed for suicide risk prior to, during, and after antidepressant and nonpharmacotherapy treatment. Health education must be an integral part of all treatment across the life span, particularly with children and adolescents. Adolescents must assent to participate along with informed consent from parents, family members, and significant others. Close monitoring for worsening symptoms, increased suicidality (e.g., thoughts, plan), and despondency is essential during these vulnerable periods.

agents, encourage low-calorie snacks and exercise. It is recommended to monitor for TD every 3 months by evaluating clients with the AIMS (Findling, Schulz, Reed, & Blumer, 1998).

Antidepressants

Although the FDA has not approved the use of antidepressants in children younger than 12 years of age, the ultimate decision to medicate rests with the physician or advanced-practice psychiatric nurse and parents. Because hepatic metabolism of TCAs is more rapid in children, they may require adult doses of antidepressants. However, the nurse should closely observe as well as closely question young children who are taking antidepressants, because they may not report adverse effects and may develop serious toxicity at relatively low doses. More rapid metabolism may also mean that the therapeutic response may take longer in children than adults.

TCAs have been approved for use in children and adolescents with enuresis, attention-deficit hyperactivity disorders, and depression. Imipramine (Tofranil), desipramine (Norpramine), and nortriptyline (Aventyl) have been studied most extensively in children and adolescents. Major side effects are similar to those in adults, but cardiovascular ones pose the most significant concern. Because of the safety concerns about cardiovascular side effects, TCAs are not the first-line treatment for depression in children and adolescents. Before being placed on a tricyclic antidepressant, Coffey (2000) recommends the following:

◆ A thorough history of health that includes individual and family history of cardiovascular, neurological, and other medical conditions

◆ Baseline electrocardiogram (ECG) before initiating medication

◆ Serum blood monitoring with specified parameters

The SSRI antidepressants are being used extensively in the treatment of depression, obsessive-compulsive disorder, panic disorder, and selective mutism. Overall, these agents are the first-line treatment of specified psychiatric disorders in youth because of their reduced risk of cardiovascular toxicity (Coffey, 2000). SSRIs may be more effective, although caution must be used in clients with other psychiatric disorders. With the use of SSRIs, there is the potential for inducing mania and irritability. Whatever agent is chosen, therapy in pediatric population clients should be initiated at half the recommended adult dosage and titrated at a minimum of 2 weeks.

Stimulants and Nonstimulants

Stimulant drugs are also called psychostimulants, because of their sympathomimetic properties. Stimulants used to treat attention deficit/hyperactive disorder (ADHD) will be the scope of this discussion. Pharmacologic treatment demonstrated the most efficacious results are central nervous system stimulants, such as methylphenidate hydrochloride (Ritalin; Ritalin SR, Concerta), dextroamphetamine, and amphetamine salts combinations (Adderall, Adderall XR). Second-line medications include stimulants, such as pemoline (Cylert) and nonstimulants, such as atomoxetine (Strattera), both of which can cause rare, but severe liver damage. Modafinil (Provigil) has recently been introduced as a new medication for ADHD. Its clinical profile is akin to conventional stimulants such as methylphenidate, despite an apparently different mode of action. Historically, this medication was used primarily to treat narcolepsy. Recent data from three large, drug company–sponsored trials of a film-coated formulation of modafinil (modafinil-ADHD; Sparlon) in children and adolescents with ADHD demonstrated consistent improvements in ADHD symptoms compared with placebo (Swanson et al., 2006; Turner, 2006). Major benefits of modafinil in the therapies for ADHD are that it can be administered once daily and has less reinforcing properties compared to conventional stimulants.

Among the stimulants, methylphenidate hydrochloride (Ritalin) by far has been the most commonly used psychotropic medication in child psychiatry. Stimulants carry FDA indications for treatment of ADHD (Greenhill et al., 2002). From 1987 to 1996 stimulant use increased fourfold from 0.6 to 2.4 percent among subjects 18 years old and younger in the United States. In a recent study, researchers explored trends in pediatric use of stimulants in the United States. Zuvekas and his colleagues (2006) discovered that stimulant use among youth under 19 years of age was 2.7 percent in 1997 and 2.9 percent in 2002 and concluded there was no statistically significant change during these 6 years. They also discerned that stimulant use was greatest among 6- to 12-year-olds, 4.8 percent in 2002, as compared with 3.2 percent among 13- to 19-year-olds and 0.3 percent among children under 6-years of age. Findings from this study also revealed that about 2.2 million children received stimulant medication in 2002 when compared to 2.0 million in 1997 (Zuvekas, Vitiello, & Norquist, 2006). The significance of these data indicate the complexity of treating children and adolescents with ADHD, particularly with co-occurring psychiatric conditions, such as conduct disorders, anxiety, and depression.

Clinical trials of adequate design have demonstrated strong evidence that short-acting stimulants are relatively effective in reducing core symptoms of ADHD and that adverse effects are predictable and rarely serious (American Academy of Pediatrics, 2001; Charach, Ickowicz, & Schachar, 2004; McMaster University, 1999; The MTA Cooperative Group, 1999). Despite evidence of efficacy in treating ADHD, limitations associated with current short-acting stimulants are well documented (Greenhill et al., 2002; National Institute of Mental Health, 2004). Major limitations of short-acting agents include short duration and multiple dosing, including dosing at school, risk of ridicule by peers, and adult supervision, and risk of abuse. Historically, stimulants were short acting and more recently intermediate-acting and sustained-released formulas have been developed. Intermediate-acting and sustained-released agents have not demonstrated superiority to short-acting

agents in efficacy. Dramatic changes have occurred over the past few years in the treatment of ADHD. Long-acting, once-a-day dosing medications have mostly become the most common pharmacological treatment of ADHD in children and adolescents due to their substantial clinical and regimen convenience. Major clinical benefits of the long-acting agents include therapeutic dosing, less peer ridicule, since once-a-day dosing allows for home administration and parental supervision, and lower risk of addiction or abuse.

Dosing

Short-acting stimulants are generally divided into twice-a-day dosing, four 4-hour intervals and administered in the morning and midday, whereas long-acting agents may be administered every 8 to 12 hours. Newer agents, such as atomoxetine (Strattera), a nonstimulant, may be taken once a day. Dextroamphetamine (Dexedrine) has been approved by the FDA in children with ADHD, 3 years of age and older. Ritalin SR and LA (Concerta) have FDA approval to treat ADHD in children 6 years and older. (See Table 29–20.)

Nonstimulants: Treatment of ADHD

The first nonstimulant atomoxetine (Strattera) was approved by the FDA in 2002 for the treatment of school-aged children and adolescents with ADHD. In comparison to stimulants, whose actions primarily regulate dopamine, atomoxetine is a selective inhibitor of the presynaptic noradrenaline transporter with minimum affinity for other receptors or transporters. It increases both norepinephrine and dopamine levels, primarily in the prefrontal cortex (Hechtman, 2005). The clinical development of this medication was conducted mainly using pediatric subjects and included a provision for school-aged children and adolescents who completed short-term studies, usually 6 to 12 weeks to maintain long-term treatment for up to 5 years (Biederman, Gao, Rogers, & Spencer, 2006; Michelson et al., 2004). Atomoxetine is metabolized primarily by the cytochrome P450 enzyme system. Major drug interactions include SSRIs, which may increase atomoxetine levels. Although it is a nonstimulant, its side-effect profile is similar to stimulants, including mild increase in blood pressure. A serious side effect associated with atomoxetine is severe liver damage. Therapeutic dosing varies and must be tailored to the child or adolescent. Typically, administering 10-mg dose to 30-kg dose per child, the maximum serum concentration occurs in about 1.5 to 2 hours and results in concentrations of generally 10 µg/ml in plasma after administration, decreasing by 50 percent in about 2 hours. The FDA recently issued a new warning for atomoxetine concerning the potential risk of severe liver damage. Two cases of liver damage were reported in an adolescent and adult who took this medication several months. Both individuals regained normal liver function after discontinuing the drug. The United States Food and Drug Administration (FDA, 2005) has stipulated discontinuance of this medication when there is evidence of jaundice, such as yellowing of the skin or whites of eyes, or laboratory studies indicate liver damage (e.g., increased liver enzymes): http://www.fda.gov/fdac/departs/2005/205 upd.html#adhd

TABLE 29–20
Clinical and Pharmacokinetic Parameters of Stimulants and Nonstimulants for ADHD

Generic Name	Brand Name	Dosage Range (mg/Day)	Peak Plasma Concentration (Hours)	Half-Life
Stimulants				
Methylphenidate (MPH) OROS MHP MPH hydrochloride	Ritalin, Ritalin LA (short acting, typically given at 8 a.m. and 12 noon) Concerta (Ritalin XR)	10–60 mg/day or up to 0.5 kg/per dose *Child:* *Adolescent:* not to exceed 2 mg/kg/day (maximum 72 mg/day)	2–3 hours Immediate release (1–2 hours) Sustained release (4–5 hours)	6 hours (BID dosing) 2–3 hours (multiple dosing) 8–12 hours
Dextroamphetamine	Dexedrine		Extended release (6–8 hours) 2–4 hours	12 hours 12 hours
Pemoline	Cylert		2–4 hours	15 hours (once a day dosing)
Mixed-amphetamine salts	Adderall Adderall XR	Usually ½ dose or MPH		
Nonstimulants				
Atomoxetine	Strattera	Start slow: 0.5 mg/kg/day (*initial dose* [3–5 days]; not more than 100 mg/day in adolescents over 70 kg and adults); *Target dose:* 1.2–1.4 mg/kg/day (100–300 mg/day) Once- or twice-a-day dosing	1–2 hours	5 hours

Contraindications

Contraindications for stimulants and nonstimulants include comorbid seizures disorders, tics, Tourette's syndrome, mania or anxiety symptoms, and use of MAOIs within 15 days of treatment. Considerable caution must be used when treating the youth with co-occurring or positive history of substance-related disorders. Side effects are frequently associated with treatment adherence (Charach, Ickowicz, & Schachar, 2004). Most adverse side effects experienced by children treated with stimulants for ADHD are relatively mild and resolve with dose adjustment and include appetite suppression, nausea, irritability, sleep disturbances, abdominal pain/stomachache, motor tics, headache, dizziness, fatigue, and listlessness. Serious side effects, such as hallucinations, are rare. (Greenhill et al., 2002; McMaster University, 1999). Debate continues concerning the duration of long-term stimulant use of long-acting stimulants in children due to their potential effect on height and weight (MTA Cooperative Group, 2004; Spencer, Newcorn, Kratochvil, Ruff, Michelsen, & Biederman, 2005).

Psychiatric nurses play key roles in working with children and adolescents with ADHD, and their families, teachers, school nurses, and others. Working with the client, parent, teachers, and mental health team requires close scrutiny of data during the evaluation and assessment period. It is imperative to distinguish between ADHD and bipolar disorder in children and adolescents. This process includes asking questions about family history of psychiatric conditions, such as bipolar disorder and mood disorders and substance abuse history. Pharmacological interventions using stim-ulants and nonstimulants are an integral part of treatment. Psychoeducation is a critical component of pharmacological and nonpharmacological intervention, in which the nurse must be knowledgeable of medication regimens, administration, and prescription of these agents. Understanding the child and family's experience about taking medication, health practices, wishes, and preferences enables the nurse to work effectively to enhance treatment adherence. It is imperative to perform a comprehensive nursing assessment and ascertain a careful family history of substance abuse. Working with other disciplines and specialties including pediatric providers, school nurses, teachers, and primary care providers makes it necessary to understand and educate them about current guidelines for the assessment of children with ADHD. (See Chapter 17, The Client with Attention-Deficit Disorder. See Table 29–20, Clinical and Pharmacokinetic Parameters of Stimulants and Nonstimulants for ADHD.)

Mood Stabilizers

Mood stabilizers or antimanic agents are used alone or as adjunct medications in the management of bipolar and other psychiatric disorders. Because of the complexity of bipolar disorder and the range of symptoms that fluctuate and cycle between depressions and mania, psychiatric nurses must understand the role of mood stabilizers in symptom management. In addition, they must be able to work with clients and their families and develop holistic treatment planning that integrates these agents with other interventions to facilitate an optimal level of functioning.

Lithium

Although lithium has not been approved by the FDA in the treatment of bipolar disorders in children, it has been used successfully to manage bipolar I and bipolar II disorders. Because the renal clearance of lithium is higher in children than in adults, children and adolescents may require higher doses to achieve therapeutic blood levels. In addition, renal, thyroid, and cardiac function must be monitored regularly (Jefferson & Greist, 2005).

Valproic Acid (Depakene)

Although the anticonvulsant valproic acid (Depakene) has not been approved by the FDA for the treatment of psychiatric disorders in children and adolescents, recent study results are promising, and, in some cases, it is being used as first-line treatment for bipolar I and bipolar II disorders. Side effects from this drug are the same in children and adolescents as those in adults (Frye & Post, 2005).

Sedative and Antianxiety Agents

SSRIs are considered the first-line agents for children and adolescents. TCAs and benzodiazepines may be used when the child has not responded to SSRIs. Before initiating TCAs in children and adolescents, the nurse must order or obtain a baseline ECG because of the potential cardiotoxic effects of these agents. Third-line agents would include MAOIs, antihistamines, and beta-adrenergic antagonists. With the pediatric population it is efficacious to implement cognitive-behavioral therapy. Interventions include illness education, support, relaxation training, and parent behavior management training (Dubovsky, 2005).

The Pregnant Client

Women with psychiatric disorders requiring medications are challenged to manage and control their symptoms while ensuring the safety of their unborn child. Studies indicate that women with recurrent depression have a high prevalence of relapse when they discontinue antidepressants and indicate being depressed during pregnancy poses greater risks than medication (Cohen et al., 2006). Data implicate that 75 percent of women who stop antidepressant medications during pregnancy relapse, usually in the first trimester. This is the strongest predictor of postpartum depression during 9 months prior to delivery (Altshuler et al., 2001; Freeman et al., 2002; Hendrick & Altshuler, 2002). A plethora of research concerning issues of using psychotropic medication during pregnancy continues to grow, indicating the importance of reducing relapse during pregnancy and postpartum due to potentially adverse effects on the mother and infant (Cohen et al., 2006).

Caution must be exercised in the administration and prescription of pharmacotherapy in pregnant women. Although there are inconsistent findings regarding the safety of some psychotropic medications, there is growing evidence that demonstrates the necessity to manage psychiatric symptoms ranging from major depression to mania in bipolar disorder. It is understandable for women to take and for mental health providers to prescribe medications during pregnancy, but there may be circumstances when a failure to provide adequate and appropriate treatment may pose a danger or even be life-threatening. A failure to treat psychiatric disorders, such as major depression during pregnancy can be detrimental (Altshuler et al., 2001; Cohen et al., 2006; Freeman et al., 2002) and include:

◆ Preterm labor

◆ Low birth weight

◆ Maternal stress

◆ Postpartum depression

◆ A failure to bond and thrive

◆ Negative impact on relationship with significant other and other children (Bonari et al., 2004)

Despite the importance of treating women during pregnancy, psychiatric nurses must fully understand potential adverse effects of psychotropics. For instance, certain medications, such as the SSRI paroxetine, have been implicated in serious cardiac anomalies in children exposed to the medication during pregnancy. The FDA has issued a black box warning for paroxetine use during pregnancy. It is now a category D risk for pregnant women. A major prenatal complication associated with paroxetine use during pregnancy is persistent pulmonary hypertension. Data concerning this serious complication indicate that the risk of persistent pulmonary hypertension is sixfold in women who took paroxetine than women who did not (FDA, 2006). Equally disconcerting is the use of mood stabilizers, such as lithium, valproic acid, and carbamazepine during pregnancy. Notable side effects from these agents include a higher incident of heart defects and birth anomalies in infants of women who used lithium during the first trimester. However, recent studies suggest that lithium poses fewer dangers for the fetus than previously thought (Yonker et al., 2004). Findings from other studies indicate valproic acid and carbamazepine are implicated in the risk of physical malformations, development delay, and spina bifida (Yonker et al., 2004).

The decision to prescribe or administer medications during pregnancy must be based on a risk-benefit ratio, informed consent from both the mother and spouse or significant other, and understanding of consequences of untreated psychiatric conditions. To help nurses and other health care providers understand underlying dangers of certain medications, the FDA has established categories (e.g., A, B, C, D, X). These categories provide information about the teratogenic risk of psychotropic agents (see Table 29–21). It behooves the psychiatric nurse to be familiar with these categories and administer and prescribe medications accordingly. Health education about untreated psychiatric conditions, risks and benefits, and documentation of informed consent are important nursing interventions during this vulnerable period (Suppaseemanont, 2006).

OLDER ADULTS

Although people age 65 and older make up more than 12 percent of the U.S. population, they receive 25 percent of the prescriptions written for psychotropic medications and 22 percent of all other prescriptions. Older adults are more likely to be receiving multiple medications and thus are at a greater risk for drug interactions; psychotropic medications place older adults at particular risk for cardiac effects. Polytherapy that includes psychotropic drugs with anticholinergic action is the greatest precipitant of adverse reactions. When the older adult experiences changes in mental status functioning, such as confusion, restlessness, irritability, depression, or psychosis, medications should be suspected as the cause. Because of age-related changes older adults are also more likely to metabolize and eliminate drugs slower, thus requiring *lower* dosages of medications (Sussman, 2005). The following are some of these age-related changes:

- Decreased renal flow, glomerular filtration, and renal tubular secretions of 50 percent by age 80 mean that medication may stay in the body longer.
- Gastric motility is decreased.
- An increased ratio of adipose tissue to lean body mass results in increased retention of fat-soluble drugs, including psychotropics such as sedatives, antidepressants, and antipsychotics.
- Many drugs are bound to plasma proteins, which are synthesized in the liver. With age, there may be fewer plasma-binding sites and fewer drug-metabolizing enzymes, leading to prolonged, sustained serum drug concentrations. In addition, all psychotropic medications (except lithium) bind extensively to plasma albumin. Because albumin levels decrease with age, older adult clients may be more susceptible than middle-aged clients to toxic responses and may thus require smaller doses of medications.
- Decreased liver function limits drug metabolism and contributes to drug accumulation and overdose.
- Cardiac output may decrease with age, delaying circulation time and thus affecting the distribution of drugs to tissue.

An *adverse drug effect* may be much more significant to an older adult than a younger one. The postural hypotension and dizziness that can be produced by some psychotropics may be merely annoying to a younger person but can predispose an older person to falling.

TABLE 19–21
Current FDA Categories for Drug Use in Pregnancy

Category	Description
A	Adequate, well-controlled studies in pregnant women have not shown increased risk of fetal abnormalities
B	Animal studies have revealed no evidence of harm to the fetus. However, there are inadequate and well-controlled studies in pregnant women. **Or** Animal studies have shown an adverse effect, but adequate and well-controlled studies in pregnant women have failed to demonstrate risk to the fetus.
C	Animal studies have shown an adverse effect and there are no adequate and well-controlled studies in pregnant women. **Or** No animal studies have been conducted and there are no adequate and well-controlled studies in pregnant women.
D	Studies, adequate well-controlled or observational, in pregnant women have demonstrated a risk to the fetus. However, the benefits of therapy may outweigh the potential risk.
X	Studies, adequate well-controlled or observational, in animals or pregnant women have demonstrated positive evidence of fetal abnormalities. The use of the product is contraindicated in women who are or may become pregnant.

http://www.fda.gov/fdac/features/2001/301_preg.html#categories (Accessed October 4, 2006)

Many psychotropic medications produce anticholinergic side effects such as blurred vision, dry mouth, urinary retention, constipation, and tachycardia. Older adult clients, especially those with some underlying cognitive disorder, may also experience an acute toxic delirium secondary to these anticholinergic effects. Excessive sedation in the older adult client is possible with most psychotropic medications. Oversedation may not only be mistaken for depression, but may also reduce the client's personal contact with the surroundings, impair cognitive capacities, and decrease self-esteem. Signs of CNS depression may include ataxia, dysarthria, diplopia, blurred vision, confusion, dizziness, vertigo, nystagmus, muscle weakness, incoordination, somnolence, and (rarely) respiratory depression (Sussman, 2005).

There is also increased risk of cardiac effects from antipsychotics and heterocyclics. These risks include tachycardia, increased incidence of premature ventricular contractions, heart block, and atrial and ventricular arrhythmias. Alcohol and drug use must be carefully assessed in the older adult client. The use of these agents significantly complicates prescribing for this population.

Antidepressants

The side effects profile of SSRI antidepressants make them the drug of choice for older adult clients experiencing depression and anxiety disorders. The SSRI antidepressants cause fewer troublesome side effects, including anticholinergic and cardiac, and are therefore the first-line treatment for older adult clients. Other antidepressants with lower anticholinergic potential, such as amoxapine, desipramine, and trazodone, are also preferred for this population over more strongly anticholinergic antidepressants such as amitriptyline, doxepin, imipramine, and protriptyline. The MAOIs are useful in that they lack anticholinergic effects, but they can produce significant hypotension. The sedative effects of cyclic antidepressants may be useful in treating sleep disturbances, but they may be problematic in that they produce daytime drowsiness. For older clients it is recommended to use the XR formulation of venlafaxine (because of the potential for hypertension with the regular release) and SR formulation of bupropion (because of the increased risk of seizures).

Mood Stabilizers

Valproic acid is the first-line mood stabilizer in the older adult. However, it is contraindicated in clients with hepatic disease or severe hepatic dysfunction. Lithium can be used safely in the older adult client, but it is generally used in lower dosages, maintaining blood levels in the range of 0.4 to 0.6 mEq/L. Even these dosages may produce signs that appear toxic. Diuretics must be cautiously administered because they may cause increased lithium levels or hypokalemia (Sussman, 2005). The dose of lithium may need to be decreased significantly in elderly clients with renal dysfunction.

Sedative and Antianxiety Agents

Because the metabolism of benzodiazepines is slowed in the older adult client, these drugs are likely to remain in the body at higher concentrations than they would under comparable conditions in a younger person. Agents that are not recommended owing to active metabolites are chlordiazepoxide, clorazepate, diazepam, halazepam, and flurazepam. Likewise, barbiturates with longer half-lives and meprobamate should be avoided in this age group. Regardless of the antianxiety or sedative changes, their effects on the older adults, especially on their mental status, must be regularly assessed.

Antipsychotics

The side effects of primary concern in older adults are anticholinergic effects, parkinsonian effects, TD, orthostatic hypotension, cardiac abnormalities, reduced bone density, sedation, and cognitive impairment (Van Kammer & Marder, 2005). Antipsychotics, especially the conventional agents, with greater hypotensive and anticholinergic effects, such as mesoridazine (Serentil) and thioridazine, should be avoided. The novel antipsychotic agents, such as olanzapine and quetiapine, have favorable side effect profiles that make them the first-line treatment for older adults with psychotic disorders (Sadock, Sadock, & Sussman, 2006).

Acetylcholinesterase Inhibitors (Cognitive Enhancers)

For the purpose of this discussion it is important for the nurse to understand target sites for medication used to enhance cognitive function in individuals with mild to moderate dementia in Alzheimer's disease (AD). The cholinergic system originates in the basal forebrain and projects diffusely to the cerebral cortex; the limbic and paralimbic regions receive the most abundant cholinergic projections. The basal forebrain nuclei interface with the limbic system and cerebral cortex, where they play an important role in mediating emotional responses. The basal forebrain nuclei are atrophic in Alzheimer's disease, producing to a widespread cholinergic deficit. The cholinergic disturbance may contribute to neuropsychiatric manifestations of the disease. An explanation for the cholinergic deficit found in AD stems from several premises. The depletion of the neurotransmitter acetylcholine (Ach), particularly in individuals with mild to severe forms of AD, stems from decline in choline acetyltransferase activity—this enzyme produces Ach. The loss or deficit of this enzyme reduces cholinergic neurons and decreases in acetylcholinesterase (AChE), an enzyme that breaks down Ach. Deficits in these chemicals also increase butyrylcholinesterase, which is another enzyme that degrades Ach. Due to their important role in cognition and executive functioning, these neurotransmitters and neural pathways are target sites for pharmacologic interventions for cognitive impairment in AD.

A group of drugs classified as acetylcholinesterase inhibitors (AChEIs), Donepezil (Aricept), galantamine (Reminyl), and rivastigmine (Exelon), have been approved in many countries for the treatment of AD, despite a lack of clarity that the efficacy, in the short term, was modest, symptomatic, and apparent only in a subgroup of clients (Sadock, Sadock, & Sussman, 2006). They delay the breakdown of released acetylcholine, increase synaptic concentration of AcH, particularly in the hippocampus and cerebral cortex, hence preserving executive functioning and slowing further deterioration in the cognitive impairment in mild-to-moderate dementia of the Alzheimer's type (Behl, Lanctôt, Streiner, Guimont, & Black, 2006).

A newer agent used in the treatment of cognitive disturbances of AD is memantine (Namenda). Unlike its other cognitive enhancers, memantine is an N-methyl-d-asparate (NMDA) partial antagonist and is indicated in the treatment of moderate to severe stages of AD. Overactivation of NMDA is believed to contribute to cellular death found in AD and the efficacy of memantine is believed to stem from the protection of cells by partially reducing NMDA hyperactivity. Currently, it is the only drug approved for moderate to severe AD (Reisberg et al., 2006; Sadock, Sadock, & Sussman, 2006).

Side Effects, Toxicity, and Drug Interactions

The AChEIs are relatively safe and well-tolerated. These agents have a low incidence of sedation and orthostatic hypotension. In clinical trials, these agents were associated with transient and dose-related adverse effects during initiation of treatment (Wilkinson et al., 2002). GI disturbances include nausea, diarrhea, loss of appetite, vomiting, and in rare cases weight loss. GI disturbances can be reduced by slow titration, low doses, and administering the medication with meals. The most frequent CNS side effects include syncope, dizziness, abnormal dreams, fatigue, muscle cramps, and headache. Abrupt discontinuation leads to abrupt cognitive decline. Donepezil and galantamine have been associated with bradycardia in clients with cardiac disease (Birks, 2006; Cummings, 2004).

The side-effect profile of memantine is similar to AChEIs and includes both GI and CNS disturbances. This medication is contraindicated in clients with severe renal disease. Memantine is eliminated partly via tubular secretion and when administered with other drugs that use the same cationic system, such as hydrochlorothiazide (HCTZ), cimetidine (Tagamet), ranitidine (Zantac), it may alter serum levels of both agents. Alkaline urine is also significantly reduced (e.g., 80 percent) in alkaline urine and results in accumulation of the medication and heightened risk of side effects (Sadock, Sadock, & Sussman, 2006).

Implications for Psychiatric Nurses

As with all medications, it is imperative for the nurse to participate in the evaluation, diagnosis, and treatment of AD. Ruling out medical and psychiatric conditions is part of this process, which involves performing a comprehensive psychosocial history that includes history of symptoms; current prescribed and over-the-counter medication; mental status examination; physical, functional, and neurological status; and findings from diagnostic studies.

THE ROLE OF THE NURSE

Pharmacotherapy is an integral aspect of caring for clients with psychiatric disorders. Psychiatric nurses have major responsibilities in administering and ordering various psychopharmacologic agents. Information concerning the purpose, side effect profiles, client preferences, cultural, age-related issues, and health education are pivotal to safe medication administration and adherence to treatment. Specific roles and responsibilities of the generalist and advanced-practice registered psychiatric nurse will be discussed in this section.

THE GENERALIST NURSE

Psychopharmacology today requires that nurses, clients, physicians, pharmacy specialists, and significant others collaborate by designing quality management strategies that promote optimal benefits and minimal harm. Because nurses are most likely to be the primary team members to administer, observe, assess pharmacologic responses, and intervene when appropriate, they must anticipate responses that the medications are likely to produce. In essence, the psychiatric-mental health nurse has a professional responsibility to comprehend basic knowledge of pharmacology and be able to anticipate drug responses, rather than simply reacting to them later.

The nurse must understand basic processes underlying the client's symptoms and behaviors and reasons for administering specific psychopharmacologic agents. The initial step in pharmacotherapy involves gathering baseline data and assessing the client's mental and physical status and capacity for self-care. Assessment information is critical to the client's safety because it guides the decision to prescribe and evaluate therapeutic and adverse responses to medication. Nurses need to assess the significance of the medication to the client related to family sick role issues and concerns about control and stigma. In addition, nurses are ethically and legally responsible for ensuring that the client and significant others have the information necessary for them to make an informed consent regarding the purpose, desired effects, and potential adverse or interactive effects of these agents and to achieve and maintain an optimal level of health (American Nurses Association [ANA], 2000). The nurse is responsible for (ANA, 2000):

- Providing opportunities for the client and significant others to explore their feelings and concerns related to the medications
- Assessing the client health teaching needs and using them as a guide to individualized health education and include information about delayed beneficial or optimal effects
- Collaborating with the client's health care provider to assess and individualize the client's medication and treatment needs
- Applying current research findings to guide nursing actions related to medications
- Using nursing interventions to minimize or alleviate adverse effects of medications

- Monitoring the client's responses to all medications and include such actions as monitoring applicable diagnostic and laboratory studies, vital signs, and drug levels
- Evaluating the client's holistic response to medications and document the response

THE ADVANCED-PRACTICE PSYCHIATRIC REGISTERED NURSE

Advanced-practice psychiatric-mental health nurses have even greater responsibilities that extend beyond basic pharmacology. They include prescribing pharmacologic agents and ordering and interpreting diagnostic studies. Other responsibilities require additional expertise and knowledge of diagnosis and treatment of mental disorders and the ability to plan a pharmacotherapy regimen. The client's past history, current mental and physical status, preferences, and outcome-based treatment plan should guide the nurse's role in pharmacology. Explanations regarding the treatment plan should be given to the client and significant others, and their ideas about it should be respected (ANA, 2000; Sadock, Sadock, & Sussman, 2006).

Educational preparation for the advanced role begins at the master's degree level and progresses through clinical experience, leading to certification as an advanced-practice registered nurse psychiatric-mental health (APRN-PMH [i.e., clinical nurse specialist, psychiatric-mental health nurse practitioner]). Concerning the use of pharmacologic agents, the role of the certified psychiatric-mental health specialist often includes prescriptive authority. Responsibilities inherent in prescriptive authority involve ordering medications and interpreting relevant diagnostic and laboratory tests. Additional responsibilities of the APRN-PMH with prescriptive authority include seeking to effect desired therapeutic responses and anticipating and minimizing adverse drug interactions.

The inclusion of prescriptive authority in the advanced-practice role is guided by federal and statutory regulations governing prescriptions. The APRN-PMH applies neurobiological, psychopharmacologic, and physiological knowledge of all aspects of the therapeutic process. Of particular significance is the use of this knowledge to make differential diagnoses of mental disorders and medical conditions, develop therapeutic strategies based on clinical indicators, and to treat the mental disorders with pharmacologic agents (ANA, 2000). Health teaching is also an integral aspect of pharmacologic interventions and must focus on educating other nurses and health care providers about pharmacologic agents and consulting about their use and management.

TREATMENT ADHERENCE

A major challenge to nurses in psychiatric-mental health nursing practice is medication adherence. *Adherence* refers to the extent that a client follows treatment recommendations. It also results when clients have insight into their illness and make informed choices that help them master the challenges. The outcome of clients' nonadherence with a medication regimen is often recurrence or exacerbation of symptoms (relapse) and rehospitalization. Nonadherence relapse rates are estimated to be 50 percent in the first year and 70 percent in the second year after treatment (Cooper et al., 2007; Copper, Moisan, & Grégoire, 2007; Valenstein et al., 2006). Factors that contribute to medication adherence and poor treatment outcomes may be partly related to a lack of integration of services, failure to meet the client's needs, and medication side effects. Additional factors include stigma and cultural factors concerning ambivalent attitudes about drugs that often reflect a knowledge deficit about drug treatment for mental disorders. Most researchers submit that enhancing medication adherence during the early course of psychiatric disorders, such as schizophrenia, is likely to have a substantial impact on positive treatment outcomes (Cooper et al., 2007; Valenstein et al., 2006). Psychiatric nurses must actively involve themselves in coordinating holistic health care that facilitates symptom management and positive treatment outcomes. Clients often believe that taking psychotropic medications deprives them of control over their lives or that these agents are addictive and they will never be able to stop taking them (Sadock, Sadock, & Sussman, 2006).

Age-related factors also play a role in adherence, particularly in older adults. Approximately 40 percent or more of older adults fail to take their medications as prescribed. Because of the stigma of mental illness and taking medications, some clients may refuse to adhere to medication regimens. Researchers assert that several factors contribute to nonadherence in older adults:

- failure to refill prescriptions
- failure to follow correct dosing schedule
- forgetfulness
- failure to understand instructions owing to sensory or cognitive impairment
- inadequate finances to pay for medication
- detailed dosing schedules
- side effects
- stigma
- beliefs that drugs are unnecessary or dosage is too much
- inability to afford the cost of medication(s)
- fatalistic beliefs about health
- distrust of mental health systems, providers (Cooper et al., 2007; Cooper, Moisan, & Grégoire, 2007; Valenstein, 2006)

Another overlooked factor that contributes to adherence is *culture*. Because culture shapes beliefs and prospects that govern the client's attitudes and responses about medication, adherence may be a serious problem in cross-cultural clinical settings. Primary reasons for ethnic differences stems from communication dilemmas and disagreements between the client and nurse (Vandel et al., 2007). Nurses need to appreciate the impact of the client's culture, individual needs, and beliefs about health care and integrate them into treatment planning.

The nurse also needs to be mindful of a number of principles of medication use that are important to ensure the desired therapeutic effects. First, no person should be seen as only a medical client or only a psychiatric client. Nurses should afford all clients a comprehensive examination that contributes to making a differential diagnosis of medical, mental, or substance-related disorders. For instance, treating a medical condition such as hypothyroidism may cure a client's depression, whereas treating a psychiatric illness such as depression may improve the client's irritable bowel syndrome.

Second, psychosocial or alternative options should always be considered first. Crisis intervention, sleep hygiene, counseling, substance-related treatment, and stress management techniques are alternatives to medication.

Third, medications alone are rarely indicated in the treatment of any psychiatric disorder; medication in combination with psychotherapy is almost always more effective than medication alone. Psychiatric illnesses, including depression or anxiety disorders, can be best understood and treated by using a biopsychosocial model.

Finally, the nurse should consider the following points:

- The smallest possible effective dose should be used for the shortest effective period. This principle must be balanced against the knowledge that failure to use an inadequate dosage and to continue medication long enough are significant contributors to treatment failures. As a rule, older adults should be started on lower doses than younger clients.

- Whenever possible, medication dosing should be simplified (i.e., once-a-day dosing). Avoid midday dosing if possible.

- The simpler the drug regimen, the higher the compliance. In most instances, a once-a-day dosing schedule is possible. An obvious exception is lithium; most prescribers believe that its short half-life necessitates more frequent dosing.

- Polypharmacy should be avoided when possible. Combinations of psychoactive drugs generally are not more effective than a single dose (Sadock, Sadock, & Sussman, 2006). The more medications a client takes, the higher the risk of side effects she experiences, making compliance more difficult.

- Overall, the safety of using most psychiatric medications during pregnancy and lactation has not been established. The prescriber and the client must carefully assess the use of these medications. The basic rule is to avoid administering any drug to pregnant women, particularly during the first trimester or lactation. The most teratogenic drugs in psychopharmacology are lithium and anticonvulsants such as valproic acid, carbamezepine (Sadock, Sadock, & Sussman, 2006; Spratto & Woods, 2000). See Table 29–22, Guidelines for Enhancing Medication Adherence.

TABLE 29–22
Guidelines for Enhancing Medication Adherence

- Help the client develop insight about his illness through the nurse-client relationship and impart psychoeducation, encourage family involvement and support. Integrating the client's wishes, preferences, culture, and health practices is crucial to this process. Insight is reflected in the client's willingness to understand and accept his illness and treatment options to manage symptoms, behaviors, and improve quality of life.

- Assist client in acquiring knowledge about medications, including actions, precautions, side effects, signs of toxicity, drug interactions, and food and drug interactions.

- Explore client's beliefs about medications and their effects.

- Explain nature of and time span for onset of therapeutic results.

- Help client develop strategies for dealing with common side effects and missed doses of medication.

- Relate medications to the target symptoms associated with client's illness, fucntional status, and quality of life.

- Explore with client any differing expectations regarding barriers and facilitators for medication adherence and medication effects.

- Provide written and verbal instructions to reinforce adherence to treatment.

- Develop strategies to help client incorporate medication taking into daily routine.

- Include family members or significant others in education about client's medications and illness and their own needs as caregivers.

- Explain complications that can result from use of alcohol and other drugs that can lead to establishment of a maladaptive pattern of coping.

LEGAL AND ETHICAL ISSUES

Psychiatric nurses must have a strong commitment to the health of their clients and families concerning medications and other treatment modalities. This process involves initiating treatment planning that protects the rights of clients and assures safe, culturally-sensitive and holistic health care.

CLIENT ADVOCACY

Another invaluable role of the mental health nurse is *client advocate*. Nurses are first-line advocates for clients receiving psychotropic medications because they often administer the medication and are the first to detect errors, potential drug interactions, or changes in the client's mental and physical status.

The administration of psychotropic medications presents unique challenges to nurses. Medications themselves are often quite potent, and individual responses are relatively unpredictable. To complicate the matter further, clients have difficulty complying with the medication regimen, giving informed consent, recognizing and reporting therapeutic and adverse effects, and applying psychoeducational material. The first and foremost responsibility of psychiatric nurses is client advocacy (ANA, 2000). With respect to pharmacologic interventions, nurse advocacy activities include a strong commitment to the client's health and overall welfare and well-being. Additional responsibilities comprise actions to protect the client from harm, while taking appropriate actions on behalf of the client to ensure the use of the least restrictive environment. This is particularly salient in ethical dilemmas created by the use of chemical restraints in some situations. (See Chapter 8.)

RIGHT TO REFUSE

As mentioned, obtaining informed consent from the client with a mental disorder can be difficult. Many clients in these settings, perhaps because of their respective illnesses, their beliefs and culture, or their fears, are reluctant to comply with medication administration. Except in unusual circumstances, a client with a mental disorder has the *right to refuse* medication. First, a client may have been involuntarily committed to a hospital because she was judged to be gravely disabled and harmful to herself or others. States vary in their statutes regarding medicating these clients against their will, and it is imperative that the nurse be familiar with the laws of the state in which she practices. In addition, in certain cases, a court may order clients to be medicated against their wishes. This usually happens to clients with long histories of nonadherence who have shown clear improvement when their symptomatology is under the control of medication. In clients without such legal support, however, exceptions may still need to be made. For example, in some cases, it may be believed that the client is so severely endangered by her behavior that a life-threatening crisis is imminent. It may be advisable for the nurse to collaborate and consult with the interdisciplinary team and significant others. If a decision is made to medicate a client against her will, it is imperative that documentation be clear, descriptive, and inclusive of other interventions that were tried.

Obviously, assessing the client's capacity to comprehend information is challenging. However, the nurse also has a legal and ethical obligation to inform the client to the best of her ability to understand what a medication is, what symptoms can be expected to be treated, and its potential risks (ANA, 2000; Antai-Otong, 2006; Sadock, Sadock, & Sussman, 2006). Information should be provided that will enable the client and family members to recognize signs of symptom

remittance as well as adverse effects. Clients and significant others should receive written and verbal information about methods, any contraindications, and particularly any adverse effects that could precipitate an emergency (such as the development of neuroleptic malignant syndrome). See Chapter 8 for an in-depth discussion of the right to refuse treatment.

PSYCHOEDUCATION

Antai-Otong (2007b) asserts that the most effective ways to improve adherence are communication and health education. Interventions such as providing the client with written instructions and verbal communication are particularly helpful when the client is on several medications or has instructions for drug titration.

This notion is consistent with the role of the psychiatric nurse in psychopharmacology. Perhaps one of the challenges most enjoyed by the psychiatric-mental health nurse is the development of creative psychoeducational strategies for medications. Common strategies include medication education groups, Internet sites, printed instructions, and self-medication programs. It is also crucial for the client's family or significant others to be involved in the educational and treatment process. A frequent problem cited by mental health advocacy groups is that families are often uninformed about the treatment itself and its risks and potential benefits. This process should also be documented. Other factors such as the Internet and telemental health are making an impact on the mental health consumer's understanding about mental illness, the role of neurobiology, technological advances, psychoeducation, and treatment options.

MEDICATION MONITORING

A final area of particular interest in the legal and ethical administration of psychotropic agents is medication monitoring. The nurse must be thoroughly familiar with both the expected outcomes of the medication and the potential adverse effects. These include physical, affective, and behavioral sequelae. For instance, the nurse should know which medications would affect blood pressure or sexual function. See Table 29–23 for a list of these medications. Many psychiatric settings use some sort of formalized system of symptom documentation, whether checklists for adverse effects or abbreviated mental status report for affective, motor, and behavioral assessment. It is imperative that the nurse develops excellent assessment skills for this purpose.

IMPLICATIONS FOR RESEARCH

The evolution of psychopharmacology is phenomenal. As more and more clinical trials of new agents are studied and receive FDA approval, psychiatric nurses must be able to discern empirical data that provides the basis of administering and prescribing psychotropic agents. Ethical issues continue to impact how we treat individuals across the life span. Fortunately more clinical trials include children and adolescents in attempts to

Antidepressants	Antipsychotics	Alpha-Antagonists
Amitriptyline (Elavil)	Acetophenazine (Tindal)	Doxepin (Sinequan) >150 mg/day
Imilpramine (Tofranil)	Chlorpromazine (Thorazine)	Trifluoperazine (Stelazine >5 mg/day)
Protriptyline (Vivactyl)	Chlorprothixene (Taractan)	
Perphenazine and amitriptyline (Triavil)	Thloridazine (Mellaril)	
	Haloperidol (Haldol)	

understand pharmacokinetics and pharmacodynamics to ensure appropriate dosing, safety, and efficacy in the treatment of psychiatric disorders in this age group. As more older adults live longer and experience developmental and degenerative brain disorders it is imperative for psychiatric nurses to ensure safe medication administration through knowledge of appropriate dosing, careful monitoring for side effects, and efficacy in the treatment of psychiatric disorders.

SUMMARY

◆ Recent advances in research on the brain have created virtual explosion of knowledge of the relationship between the brain and human behavior.

◆ As a result, health care professionals' understanding of the neurobiological basis of many mental illnesses has been enhanced dramatically, and more efficacious pharmacologic agents for the treatment of mental illness have been developed.

◆ Technological advances in the study of genetics and human behavior offer promise and hope to clients and their families regarding improved quality of life.

◆ This chapter has provided the reader with a review of areas of neuroanatomy and neurophysiology related to the pharmacokinetics of psychopharmacologic agents used across the life span.

◆ Principles of psychopharmacokinetics and pharmacodynamics that are germane to an understanding of the complexity of psychopharmacologic management of mental illnesses have been discussed.

◆ The nurse's roles in the use and administration of these agents and health education of clients and their families have been described.

◆ The legal issues related to psychopharmacology and the ethical considerations in the management of pharmacotherapy treatment have been highlighted.

SUGGESTIONS FOR CLINICAL CONFERENCES

1. Role-play one of your clients on medication and describe its effects, both positive and negative. Then discuss nursing interventions that could help the client and family cope with the drug's side effects and adhere to therapy.

2. Review your clinical area's policy concerning client refusal to take medications. Does it conform to legal and ethical standards? How is the client's freedom of choice supported and maintained? Interview a nurse in your clinical area about strategies he or she uses to assist clients with decisions about taking medications. Discuss whether these strategies conform with the clinical unit's policy and with legal and ethical standards.

3. Differentiate the signs and symptoms of tardive dyskinesia, extrapyramidal side effects, and neuroleptic malignant syndrome. Identify factors that place clients at risk for each. Then discuss interventions that can help clients prevent these side effects or remedy their severity.

4. Invite an advanced-practice registered psychiatric-mental health nurse from your clinical setting to talk about her role in psychopharmacologic therapy. Discuss this role in relation to ANA's (2000) *Scope and Standards of Psychiatric-Mental Health Nursing Practice.*

5. Select a client you are working with who is taking medication. Explain what the client and her family need to know about the medication, and what teaching strategies you have been using to convey this information. Evaluate the effectiveness of your teaching at subsequent clinical conferences and discuss what should be done if the client is not adhering or complying with the medication regimen.

STUDY QUESTIONS

1. The neurological blood-brain barrier is composed of:
   a. histaminic receptors in the stomach
   b. endothelial cells in the small intestine
   c. endothelial cells in the brain
   d. noradrenergic neurons in the brain

2. Which of the following structures is considered part of the limbic system?
   a. The frontal lobe
   b. The thalamus
   c. The pons
   d. The amygdala

3. Parkinson's disease involves a depletion of which neurotransmitter in the basal ganglia of the brain?
   a. Norepinephrine
   b. Dopamine
   c. Gamma-aminobutyric acid
   d. Glycine

4. Which of the following structures associated with the reception of speech is located in the temporal lobe?
   a. Wernicke's area
   b. Broca's area
   c. Korsakoff's area
   d. Hippocampus

5. The concept of drug half-life time is important to determine:
   a. the dosage necessary to achieve therapeutic effects
   b. toxicity
   c. how often a drug needs to be administered
   d. side effects of the drug

6. A client experiencing akathisia most likely displays:
   a. a tremor on resting
   b. orthostatic hypotension
   c. chewing, puffing movements around the mouth
   d. agitation and restlessness

7. Pseudoparkinsonism is caused by which of the following mechanisms?
   a. A sudden increase in serotonin in the limbic system
   b. A depletion of gamma-aminobutyric acid in the striatum
   c. An increase in norepinephrine in the termporal lobe
   d. A depletion of dopamine in the basal ganglia nigrostriatum

8. Which of the following is an important issue in using medications in older adults?
   a. Aging alters the ability to metabolize and excrete medications.
   b. Older adults may have difficulty managing a number of medications at once.
   c. Older adults have a higher rate of nonadherence.
   d. Older persons are more susceptible to the cardiovascular effects of drugs.

9. Which of the following statements indicates the client understands side effects associated with taking valproic acid for bipolar disorder?
   a. "My nurse asked me to report signs of fatigue, abdominal pain, clay-colored stools, and yellow eyeballs immediately."
   b. "My nurse said to call if I develop diarrhea, a metallic taste, and excessive sweating."
   c. "I now have a rash, hair loss, and difficulty walking."
   d. The patient requires sedation and is experiencing ataxia and hair loss.

10. In teaching a client about her new antianxiety medication, alprazolam (Xanax), the nurse should include which of the following?
    a. Caution the client to avoid foods containing tyramine.
    b. Caution the client not to drink alcoholic beverages.
    c. Instruct the client to take alprazolam 1 hour after meals.
    d. Instruct the client to double up a dose if she forgets to take her medication.

11. The nurse realizes that a client taking buspirone (Buspar) needs additional medication teaching when he says which of the following?
    a. "I'll take my drugs as soon as I feel anxious."
    b. "I won't drink any alcohol."
    c. "I'll report any troubles with my heart or vision."
    d. "I'll have my blood checked every month."

12. In teaching a client for whom clozapine has been prescribed, the nurse would include which of the following?
    a. The drug will be given every four weeks by intramuscular injection.
    b. The drug will probably cause weight reduction.
    c. There is a high incidence of extrapyramidal side effects.
    d. The signs and symptoms of blood dyscrasias.

13. A 23-year-old client has been admitted to the psychiatric unit with a diagnosis of bipolar disorder, manic episode. Her current medication is haloperidol and lorazepam to treat acute psychosis. Lithium has been ordered. Which of the following indicate your understanding about this medication?
    a. Check results of a pregnancy test, CBC with differential, chemistries, and thyroid panel.
    b. Check results of liver enzymes, CBC with differential, and ECG.
    c. Check results of liver enzymes, thyroid panel, and pregnancy test.
    d. Check results of CBC with differential, drug screen, and electrolytes.

14. Which statement indicates a need for more teaching by the nurse concerning fluoxetine therapy?
    a. "I will take this medication in the morning."
    b. "I will use calamine lotion if I get a skin rash."
    c. "It will take a month before I feel better."
    d. "I will check with my physician before I take any other medications."

RESOURCES

Please note that because Internet resources are of a time-sensitive nature and URL addresses may change or be deleted, searches should also be conducted by association or topic.

Internet Resources

Agency of Health Care Policy and Research. *Treatment of attention deficit/hyperactivity disorder.* Rockville (MD): The Agency; 1999. AHCPR Publication no. 99-E017. Available: http://www.ahrq.gov/clinic/adhdsum.htm (Accessed April 21, 2006)

American Academy of Pediatrics Committee on Drugs http://aappolicy.aappublications.org/cgi/reprint/pediatrics;110/1/181.pdf (Accessed April 2, 2006)

http://www.apna.org American Psychiatric Nurses Association

Committee on Quality Improvement, Subcommittee on Attention-Deficit/Hyperactivity Disorder (2000). Clinical Practice Guidelines: Diagnosis and Evaluation of the Child with Attention-Deficit/Hyperactivity Disorder. *Pediatrics, 105,* 1158–1170

FDA List of Drugs Receiving a boxed warning, other product labeling changes and a medication guide pertaining to pediatric suicidality (2.3.2005) http://www.fda.gov/cder/drug/antidepressants/MDD_alldruglist.pdf (Accessed April 2, 2006)

http://www.fda.gov/cder/drug/antidepressants/PI_template.pdf FDA Public Health Advisory (2005). Suicidality in adults being treated with Antidepressant Medications. (Accessed October 6, 2006).

Food and Drug Administration. Regulations requiring manufacturers to assess the safety and effectiveness of new drugs and biological products in pediatric patients: final rule. *Federal Register.* 1998;63(Dec 2):66631-66672

Safety: Antidepressant Use in Children, Adolescents, and Adults

Food and Drug Administration (FDA) asks manufacturers of all antidepressant drugs to include in their a black box warning to alert advanced practice psychiatric nurses and other clinicians to a heightened risk of suicidality in children and adolescents being treated with antidepressants along with the results of pediatric studies.

http://pediatrics.aappublications.org/cgi/reprint/105/5/1158?ijkey=0ba0c640a054d4d3bd480135c8a41b3f33c34fal (Accessed April 20, 2006)

Public Health Advisory: Suicidality in Adults Being Treated with Antidepressant Medications (issued 6/30/2005) (Accessed April 2, 2006)

Hirschfeld, RMA (2006). *Practice guideline for the treatment of patients with bipolar disorder, 2nd edition.* Available at: http://www.psych.org/psych_pract/treatg/pg/Bipolar2ePG_05-15-06.pdf (Accessed March 24, 2007)

http://www.fda.gov/cder/drug/antidepressants/antidepressantList.htm U.S. Food and Drug Administration (2005). Antidepressant drugs that have health care professional and patient information sheets. (Accessed October 6, 2006).

http://www.fda.gov/cder/drug/antidepressants/default.htm U.S. Food and Drug Administration (2005). Antidepressant use in children, adolescents, and adults. (Accessed October 6, 2006).

REFERENCES

Alpert, J. E., Berstein, J. G., & Rosenbaum, J. F. (1997). Psychopharmacological issues in the medical setting. In N. H. Cassem, T. A. Stern, J. F. Rosenbaum, & M. S. Jellinek (Eds.), *Massachusetts General Hospital handbook of general hospital psychiatry* (4th ed., pp. 249–303). St. Louis: Mosby.

Altshuler, L. L., Cohen, L. S., Moline, M. L., Kahn, D. A., Carpenter, D., Docherty, J. P., & Ross, R. W. (2001). The expert consensus guidelines series. Treatment of depression in women. *Postgrad Med, (Spec No)*, 1–107.

Alvestad, S., Lydersen, S., & Brodtkorb, E. (2007). Rash from antiepileptic drugs: Influence by gender, age, and learning disability. *Epilepsia, 48,* 1360–1365.

American Academy of Pediatrics. (2001). Clinical practice guideline: Treatment of the school-aged child with attention-deficit/hyperactivity disorder. *Pediatrics, 108,* 1033–1044.

American Nurses Association. (2000). *The scope and standards of psychiatric-mental health practice.* Washington, DC: Author.

American Psychiatric Association Task Force. (1992). *Tardive dyskinesia.* Washington, DC: Author.

Antai-Otong, D. (2005). Mitigating cutaneous side effects of lamotrigine. *Perspectives in Psychiatric Care, 41,* 193–196.

Antai-Otong, D. (2006). Psychiatric patients and ethical issues. In V. D. Lachman (Ed). *Applied Ethics in Nursing* (pp. 133–144). New York: Spinger Publishing Company.

Antai-Otong, D. (2007a). The art of prescribing monotherapy antidepressant: A thing of the past? Implications for the treatment of major depressive disorder. *Perspectives in Psychiatric Care, 43,* 142–145.

Antai-Otong, D. (2007b). Pharmacologic management of posttraumatic stress disorder. *Perspectives in Psychiatric, 43,* 55–59.

Behl, P., Lanctôt, K. L., Streiner, D. L., Guimont, I., & Black, S. E. (2006). Cholinesterase inhibitors slow decline in executive functions, rather than memory, in Alzheimer's disease: A 1-year observational study in the Sunnybrook dementia cohort. *Current Alzheimer Research, 3,* 147–156.

Biederman, J., Gao, H., Rogers, A. K., & Spencer, T. J. (2006). Comparison of parent and teacher reports of attention-deficit/hyperactivity disorder symptoms from two placebo-controlled studies of atomoxetine in children. *Biological Psychiatry, 60,* 1106–1110.

Birks, J. (2006). Cholinesterase inhibitors for Alzheimer's disease. *Cochrane Database of Systematic Review, Issue 2*, CD005593, DOI: 10. 1002/146/51858.

Bonari, L., Pinto, N., Ahn, E., Einarson, A., Steiner, M., & Koren, G. (2004). Perinatal risks of untreated depression during pregnancy. *Canadian Journal of Psychiatry, 49*, 726–735.

Casey, D. E. (2004). Pathophysiology of antipsychotic drug-induced movement disorders. *Journal of Clinical Psychiatry, 65*, Suppl 9, 25–28.

Castle, L., Aubert, R. E., Verbrugge, R. R., Khalid, M., & Epstein, R. S. (2007). Trends in medication treatment for ADHD. *Journal of Attention Disorder, 10*, 335–342.

Charach, A., Ickowicz, A., & Schachar, R. (2004). Stimulant treatment over 5 years: Adherence, effectiveness and adverse effects. *Journal of the American Academy of Child and Adolescent Psychiatry, 43*, 559–567.

Chou, K. L., & Friedman, J. H., (2006). Tardive syndromes in the elderly. *Clinics in Geriatric Medicine, 22*, 915–933.

Coffey, B. J. (2000). Pediatric psychopharmacology. In B. J. Sadock & V. A. Sadock (Eds.), *Kaplan & Sadock's comprehensive textbook of psychiatry* (7th ed., Vol. II., pp. 2831–2840). Philadelphia: Lippincott Williams & Wilkins.

Cohen, L. S., Altshuler, L. L., Harlow, B. L., Nonacs, R., Newport, D. J., Viguera, A. C., et al. (2006). Relapse of major depression during pregnancy in women who maintain or discontinue antidepressant treatment. *JAMA, 295*, 599–507.

Cooper, C., Bebbington, P., King, M., Brugha, T., Meltzer, H., Bhugra, D., et al. (2007). Why people do not take their psychotropic drugs as prescribed: Results of the 2000 National Psychiatric Morbidity Survey. *Acta Psychiatrica Scandinavia, 116*, 47–53.

Cooper, D., Moisan, J., & Grégoire, J. P. (2007). Adherence to atypical antipsychotic treatment among newly treated patients: A population-based study in schizophrenia. *Journal of Clinical Psychiatry, 68*, 818–825.

Correll, C. U., Leucht, S., & Kane, J. M. (2004). Lower risk for tardive dyskinesia associated with second-generation antipsychotics: A systematic review of 1-year studies. *American Journal of Psychiatry, 161*, 414–425.

Cummings, J. L. (2004). Treatment of Alzheimer's disease: Current and future therapeutic approaches. *Reviews in Neurological Diseases, 1*, 60–69.

Currier, G. W. (2000). Atypical antipsychotic medications in the psychiatric emergency service. *Journal of Clinical Psychiatry, 61*(Suppl. 14), 21–26.

Dubovsky, S. (2005). Benzodiazepine agonists and antagonists. In B. J. Sadock & V. A. Sadock (Eds.), *Kaplan and Sadock's comprehensive textbook of psychiatry, Vol. II* (3rd ed., pp. 2781–2791). Philadelphia: Lippincott Williams & Wilkins.

Dunner, D. L., Rush, A. J., Russell, J. M., Burke, M., Woodard, S., Wingard, P., et al. (2006). Prospective, long-term, multicenter study of the naturalistic outcomes of patients with treatment-resistant depression. *Journal of Clinical Psychiatry, 67*, 688–695.

Esposito, E. (2006). Serotonin-dopamine interaction as a focus of novel antidepressant drugs. *Current Drug Targets, 7*, 177–185.

Findling, R. L., Schulz, S. C., Reed, M. D., & Blumer, J. L. (1998). The antipsychotics. A pediatric perspective. *Pediatric Clinics of North America, 45*(5), 1205–1232.

Fountoulakis, K. N., Nimatoudis, I., Iacovides, A., Kaprinis, G. (2004). Off-label indications for atypical antipsychotics: A systematic review. *Annals of General Hospital Psychiatry, 3*, 4.

Freeman, M. P., Smith, K. W., Freeman S. A., et al. (2002). The impact of reproductive events on the course of bipolar disorder in women. *J. Clin Psychiatry, 63*, 284–287.

Frye, M. A., & Post, R. M. (2005). Valproate. In B. J. Sadock & V. A. Sadock (Eds.), *Kaplan and Sadock's comprehensive textbook of psychiatry, Vol. II* (3rd ed., pp. 2756–2766). Philadelphia: Lippincott Williams & Wilkins.

Ganong, W. F. (2005). *Review of medical physiology*. New York: McGraw-Hill.

Greenhill, L. L., Pliszka, S., Dulcan, M. K., Bernet, W., Arnold, V., Beitchman, J., Benson, R. S., Bukstein, O., Kinlan, J., McClellan, J., Rue, D., Shaw, J. A., Stock, S., & American Academy of Child and Adolescent Psychiatry. (2002). Practice parameter for the use of stimulant medications in the treatment of children, adolescents and adults. *Journal of the American Academy of Child and Adolescent Psychiatry, 41*, (2 Suppl), 26S–49S.

Harpaz-Rotem, I., & Rosenheck, R. A. (2006). Prescribing practices of psychiatrists and primary care physicians caring for children with mental illness. *Child Care and Health Development, 32*, 225–237.

Hechtman, L. (2005). Attention-deficit disorders. In B. J. Sadock & V. A. Sadock (Eds.), *Kaplan and Sadock's comprehensive textbook of psychiatry, Vol. II* (3rd ed., pp. 3183–3204). Philadelphia: Lippincott Williams & Wilkins.

Hendrick, V., & Altshuler, L. (2002). Management of major depression during pregnancy. *American Journal of Psychiatry, 159*, 10, 1667–1673 (Clinical Case Conference).

Ho, B. C., Miller, D., Nopoulos, P., & Andreasen, N. C. (1999). A comparative effectiveness study of risperidone and olanzapine in the treatment of schizophrenia. *Journal of Clinical Psychiatry, 60*, 658–663.

Howland, R. H. (2006). Personalized drug therapy with pharmacogenetics—part 2: Pharmacodynamics. *Journal of Psychosocial Nursing and Mental Health Services, 44*, 13–16.

Iversen, L. (2006). Neurotransmitter transporters and their impact on the development of psychopharmacology. *British Journal of Pharmacology, 147*, Suppl 1, S82–S88.

Jefferson, J. W., & Greist, J. H. (2005). In B. J. Sadock & V. A. Sadock (Eds.), *Kaplan and Sadock's comprehensive textbook of psychiatry, Vol. II* (3rd ed., pp. 2839–2851). Philadelphia: Lippincott Williams & Wilkins.

Jeste, D. V. (2004). Tardive dyskinesia rates with atypical antipsychotics in older adults. *Journal of Clinical Psychiatry* 65 (Suppl 9), 21–24.

Keller, T. A. (2005). Topiramate. In B. J. Sadock & V. A. Sadock (Eds.), *Kaplan and Sadock's comprehensive textbook of psychiatry, Vol. II* (3rd ed., pp. 2753–2756). Philadelphia: Lippincott Williams & Wilkins.

Kennedy, S. H., Holt, A., & Baker, G. B. (2005). Monoamine oxidase inhibitors. In B. J. Sadock & V. A. Sadock (Eds.), *Kaplan and Sadock's comprehensive textbook of psychiatry, Vol. II* (3rd ed., pp. 2854–2862). Philadelphia: Lippincott Williams & Wilkins.

Ketter, T. A. (2005). Lamotrigine. In B. J. Sadock & V. A. Sadock (Eds.), *Kaplan and Sadock's comprehensive textbook of psychiatry, Vol. II* (3rd ed., pp. 2749–1253). Philadelphia: Lippincott Williams & Wilkins.

Lehne, R. A., Moore, L. A., Crosby, L. J., & Hamilton, D. B. (1998). *Pharmacology for nursing care* (3rd ed.). Philadelphia: W.B. Saunders.

Llewellyn, A., Stowe, Z. N., & Strader, J. R. (1998). The use of lithium and management of women with bipolar disorder during pregnancy and lactation. *Journal of Clinical Psychiatry, 59*(Suppl. 6), 57–64.

Malhotra, A. K., Murphy, G. M. Jr., & Kennedy, J. L. (2004). Pharmacogenetics of psychotropic drug response. *American Journal of Psychiatry, 161*, 780–796.

Mann, J. J., & Currier, D. (2007). A review of prospective studies of biologic predictors of suicidal behavior in mood disorders. *Archives of Suicide Research, 11,* 3–16.

Mazza, M., Di Nicola, M., Marca, G. D., Janiri, L., Bria, P., & Mazza, S. (2007). Bipolar disorder and epilepsy: a bidirectional relation? Neurobiological underpinnings, current hypotheses, and future research directions. *The Neuroscientist, 13,* 393–404.

McIntyre, R. S., Brecher, M., Paulsson, B., Huizar, K., & Mullen, J. (2005). Quetiapine or haloperidol as monotherapy for bipolar mania-1 12-week, double-blind, randomised parallel-group, placebo-controlled trial. *European Neuropsychopharmacology, 15,* 573–585.

McMaster University. (1999). *The treatment of attention deficit hyperactivity disorder. Agency for Healthcare Research and Quality. Evidence Based Report/Technology Assessment No. 11 AHRQ. Pub No. 00-E005.* Rockville, MD: U.S. Department of Health and Human Services.

Mendelson, W. B. (2005). A review of the evidence for the efficacy and safety of trazodone in insomnia. *Journal of Clinical Psychiatry, 66*, 469–476.

The MTA Cooperative Group. (1999). Multimodal Treatment Study of Children With ADHD. A 14-month randomized clinical trial of treatment strategies for attention-deficit/hyperacticvity disorder. *Archives of General Psychiatry, 56*, 1073–1086.

Michelson, D., Buitelaar, J. K., Danckaerts, M., et al. (2004). Relapse prevention in pediatric patients with ADHD treated with atomoxetine: A randomized, double-blind, placebo-controlled study. *J Am Academy of Child and Adolescent Psychiatry, 43*, 896–904.

National Institute of Mental Health. (2004). Multimodal treatment study of attention deficit hyperactivity disorder. Follow-up at 24-month outcomes of treatment strategies for attention deficit hyperactivity disorder. *Pediatrics, 113*, 754–762.

Odagaki, Y., Toyoshima, R., & Yamauchi, T. (2005). Trazodone and its active metabolite m-chlorophenylpiperazine as partial agonists at 5-HT1A receptors assessed by [35S]GTPgammaS binding. *Journal of Psychopharmacology, 19*, 235–341.

Pierri, J. N., & Lewis, D. A. (2005). Functional neuroanatomy. In B. J. Sadock & V. A. Sadock (Eds.), *Kaplan and Sadock's comprehensive textbook of psychiatry, Vol. II* (3rd ed., pp. 3–32). Philadelphia: Lippincott Williams & Wilkins.

Pollack, M. H., Roy-Byrne, P. P., Van Ameringen, M., Snyder, H., Brown, C., Ondrasik, J., & Rickels, K. (2005). The selective GABA reuptake inhibitor tiagabine for the treatment of generalized anxiety disorder: Results of a placebo-controlled study. *Journal of Clinical Psychiatry, 66*, 1401–1408.

Post, R. M., & Frye, M. A. (2005). Carbamazepine. In B. J. Sadock & V. A. Sadock (Eds.), *Kaplan and Sadock's comprehensive textbook of psychiatry, Vol. II* (3rd ed., pp. 2732–2746). Philadelphia: Lippincott Williams & Wilkins.

Prasad, S. (2005). A new paradigm for developing drugs in children: Atomoxetine as a model. *Archives of Disease in Childhood 90* (Suppl 1), il3-il6.doi: 10.1136/adc.2004.059378.

Reisberg, B., Doody, R., Stoffler, A., Schmitt, F., Ferris, S., & Mobius, H. J. (2006). A 24-week open-label extension study of memantine in moderate to severe Alzheimer disease. *Archives of Neurology, 63*, 49–54.

Rickels, K., Rynn, M., Iyengar, M., & Duff, D. (2006). Remission of generalized anxiety disorder: A review of the paroxetine clinical trials database. *Journal of Clinical Psychiatry, 67*, 41–47.

Sadock, B. J., Sadock, V. A., & Sussman, N. (2006). *Kaplan & Sadock pocket handbook of psychiatric drug treatment*, 4th ed. Philadelphia: Lippincott Williams & Wilkins.

Scharf, M. (2006). Eszopiclone for the treatment of insomnia. *Expert Opinion Pharmacotherapy, 7*, 345–356.

Simon, G. E., Savarino, J., Operskalski, N., Wang, P. S. (2006). Suicide risk during antidepressant treatment. *American Journal of Psychiatry, 163*, 41–47.

Spencer, T., Newcorn, J. H., Kratochvil, C. J., Ruff, D., Michelson, D., & Biederman, J. (2005). Effects of atomoxetine on growth after 2-year treatment among pediatric patients with attention deficit hyperactivity disorder. *Pediatrics, 116*, e74–e80. www.pediatrics.org.cgi/doi/10.1542/peds.2004-0624.

Spencer, T. J., Biederman, J., Ciccone, P. E., Madras, B. K., Dougherty, D. D., Bonab, A. A., Livni, E., Parasrampuria, D. A., & Fischman, A. J. (2006). PET Study examining pharmacokinetics, detection and likeability, and dopamine transporter receptor occupancy of short- and long-acting oral methylphenidate. *American Journal of Psychiatry, 163,* 387–395.

Spratto, G. R., & Woods, A. L. (2000). *PDR nurse's drug handbook.* Montvale, NJ: Delmar and Medical Economics Company, Inc.

Stein, M. A. (2004). Innovations in attention-deficit/hyperactivity disorder pharmacotherapy: Long-acting stimulant and nonstimulant treatments. *American Journal of Managed Care, 10:* 589–598.

Stein, D. J., van der Kolk, B. A., Austin, C., Fayyad, R., & Clary, C. (2006). Efficacy of sertraline in posttraumatic stress disorder secondary to interpersonal trauma or childhood abuse. *Annals of Clinical Psychiatry, 18,* 243–249

Strawn, J. R., Keck, P. E. Jr., & Caroff, S. N. (2007). Neuroleptic malignant syndrome. *American Journal of Psychiatry, 164,* 870–876.

Suppaseemanont, W. (2006). Depression in pregnancy: Drug safety and nursing management. *MCN. The American Journal of Child Nursing, 31,* 10–15.

Sussman, N. (2005). General principles of psychopharmacology. In B. J. Sadock & V. A. Sadock (Eds.), *Kaplan and Sadock's comprehensive textbook of psychiatry, Vol. II* (3rd ed., pp. 2676–2699). Philadelphia: Lippincott Williams & Wilkins.

Swanson, J. M., Greenhill, L. L., Lopez, F. A., Sedillo, A., Earl, C. Q., Jiang, J. G., & Biederman, J. (2006). Modafinil film-coated tablets in children and adolescents with attention-deficit/hyperactivity disorder: Results of a rendomized, double-blind, placebo-controlled, foxed dose study followed by abrupt discontinuation. *Journal of Clinical Psychiatry, 67,* 137–147.

Tecott, L. H., & Smart, S. L. (2005). Monoamine neurotransmitters. In B. J. Sadock & V. A. Sadock (Eds.), *Kaplan and Sadock's comprehensive textbook of psychiatry, Vol. II* (3rd ed., pp. 49–60). Philadelphia: Lippincott Williams & Wilkins.

Tohen, M., Calabrese, J. R., Sachs, G. S., Banov, M. D., Detke, H. C., Risser, R., Baker, R. W., Chou, J. C.-Y., & Bowden. C. L. (2006). Randomized, Placedbo-controlled trial of olanzapine as maintenance therapy in patients with bipolar I disorder responding to acute treatment with planzapine. *American Journal Psychiatry, 163,* 247–256.

Trivedi, M. H., Rush, A. J., Wisniewski, S. R., Nierenberg, A. A., Warden, D., Ritz, L., et al. (2006). Team: Evaluation of outcomes with citalopram for depression using measurement-based care in STAR*D: Implications for clinical practice. *American Journal of Psychiatry, 163,* 28–40.

Turner, D. (2006). A review of the use of modafinil for attention-deficit hyperactivity disorder. *Expert Review of Neurotherapeutics, 6,* 455–468.

United States Food and Drug Administration. (2006). Alert: Increased risk of neonatal persistent pulmonary hypertension. This alert can be found at http://www.fda.gov/cdr/drug/infosheets/HCP/paroxetine.HCP.htm. (Accessed October 4, 2006).

United States Food and Drug Administration. (2005). *FDA Consumer Magazine, 39,* November-December. http://www.fda.gov/fdac/departs/2005/605_upd.html

Valenstein, M., Gaboczy, D., McCarthy, J. F., Myra Kim, H., Lee, T. A., & Blow, F. C. (2006). Antipsychotic adherence over time among patients receiving treatment for schizophrenia: a retrospective review. *Journal of Clinical Psychiatry, 67,* 1542–1550.

Vandel, P., Talon, J. M., Haffen, E., & Sechter, D. (2007). Pharmacogenetics and drug therapy in psychiatry—the role of the CYP2D6 polymorphism. *Current Pharmaceutical Design, 13,* 241–250.

Van Kammer, D. P., & Marder, S. R. (2005). Serotonin-dopamine agonist (atypical or second generations antipsychotics). In B. J. Sadock & V. A. Sadock (Eds.), *Kaplan and Sadock's comprehensive textbook of psychiatry, Vol. II* (3rd ed., pp. 2714–2738). Philadelphia: Lippincott Williams & Wilkins.

Viguera, A. C., Newport, D. J., Ritchie, J., Stowe, Z., Whitfield, T., Mogielnicki J., et al. (2007). Lithium in breast milk and nursing infants: Clinical implications. *American Journal of Psychiatry, 164,* 342–345.

Volkow, N. D. (2006). Stimulant medications: How to minimize their reinforcing effects? Editorial. *American Journal of Psychiatry 163,* 359–361.

Volkow, N. D., Wang, G., Fowler, J. S., Telang, F., Maynard, L., Logan J., Gatley, S. J., Pappas, N., Wong, C., Vaska, P., Zhu, W., & Swanson, J. M. (2004). Evidence that methylphenidate enhances the saliency of a mathematical task by increasing dopamine in the human brain. *American Journal of Psychiatry, 161,* 1173–1180.

Wang, M. Y., Wang, S. Y., & Tsai, P. S. (2005). Cognitive behavioural therapy for primary insomnia: A systematic review. *Journal of Advanced Nursing, 50,* 553–564.

Wernicke, J. F., Gahimer, J., Yalcin, I., Wulster-Radcliffe, M., & Viktrup, L. (2005). Safety and adverse event profile of duloxetine. *Expert Opinion Drug Safety, 4,* 987–993.

Westanmo, A. D., Gayken, J., & Haight, R. (2005). Duloxetine: A balanced and selective norepinephrine-

and-serotonin-reuptake inhibitor. *American Journal of Health System Pharmacology, 62,* 2481–2890.

Wilkinson, D. G., Passmore, A. P., Bullock, R., Hopker, S. W., Smith, R., Potocnik, F. C., Maud, C. M., Englebrecht, L., Hock, C., Ieni, J. R., & Bahra, R. S. (2002). A multinational, randomised, 12-week comparative study of donepezil and rivastigmine in patients with mild to moderate Alzheimer's disease. *International Journal of Clinical Practice, 56,* 441–446.

Yatham, L. N. (2004). Newer anticonvulsants in the treatment of bipolar disorders. *Journal of Clinical Psychiatry, 65,* Suppl 10, 28–35.

Yonkers, K. A., Wisner, K. L., Stowe, Z., et al. (2004). Management of bipolar disorder during pregnancy and the postpartum period. *American Journal of Psychiatry, 161,* 608–620.

Zito, J. M., Safer, D. J., Gardner, J. F., Soeken, K., & Ryu, J. (2006). Anticonvulsant treatment for psychiatric and seizure indcations among youths. *Psychiatric Services, 57,* 681–688.

Zuvekas, S. H., Vitiello, B., & Norquist, G. S. (2006). Recent trends in stimulant medication use among U.S. children. *American Journal of Psychiatry, 163,* 579–585.

SUGGESTED READINGS

Kaas, M. J., Dahl, D., Dehn, D., & Frank, K. (1998). Barriers to prescriptive practice for psychiatric/mental health clinical nurse specialists. *Clinical Nurse Specialist, 12,* 200–204.

Menzies, V., & Farrell, S. P. (2002). Schizophrenia, tardive dyskinesia and the abnormal involuntary scale (AIMS). *Journal of the American Psychiatric Nurses Association, 8,* 51–56.

Okpaku, S. O. (1998). *Methods in transcultural psychiatry.* Washington, DC: American Psychiatric Press.

Pfeffer, C. Pediatric depression and its treatment, www.fda.gov/ohrms/dockets/ac/04/slides/4006S1_02_Pfeffer_files/outline.htm (Accessed April 6, 2006) [slide show].

Sadock, B. J., Sadock, V. A., & Sussman, N. (2006). *Kaplan & Sadock pocket handbook of psychiatric drug treatment,* (4th ed.). Philadelphia: Lippincott Williams & Wilkins.

Smith, M. W., Mendoza, R. P., & Lin, K. M. (1999). Gender and ethnic differences in the pharmacogenetics of psychotropics. In J. M. L. Herrera (Ed.), *Cross-cultural psychiatry,* 323–341. New York: John Wiley & Sons.

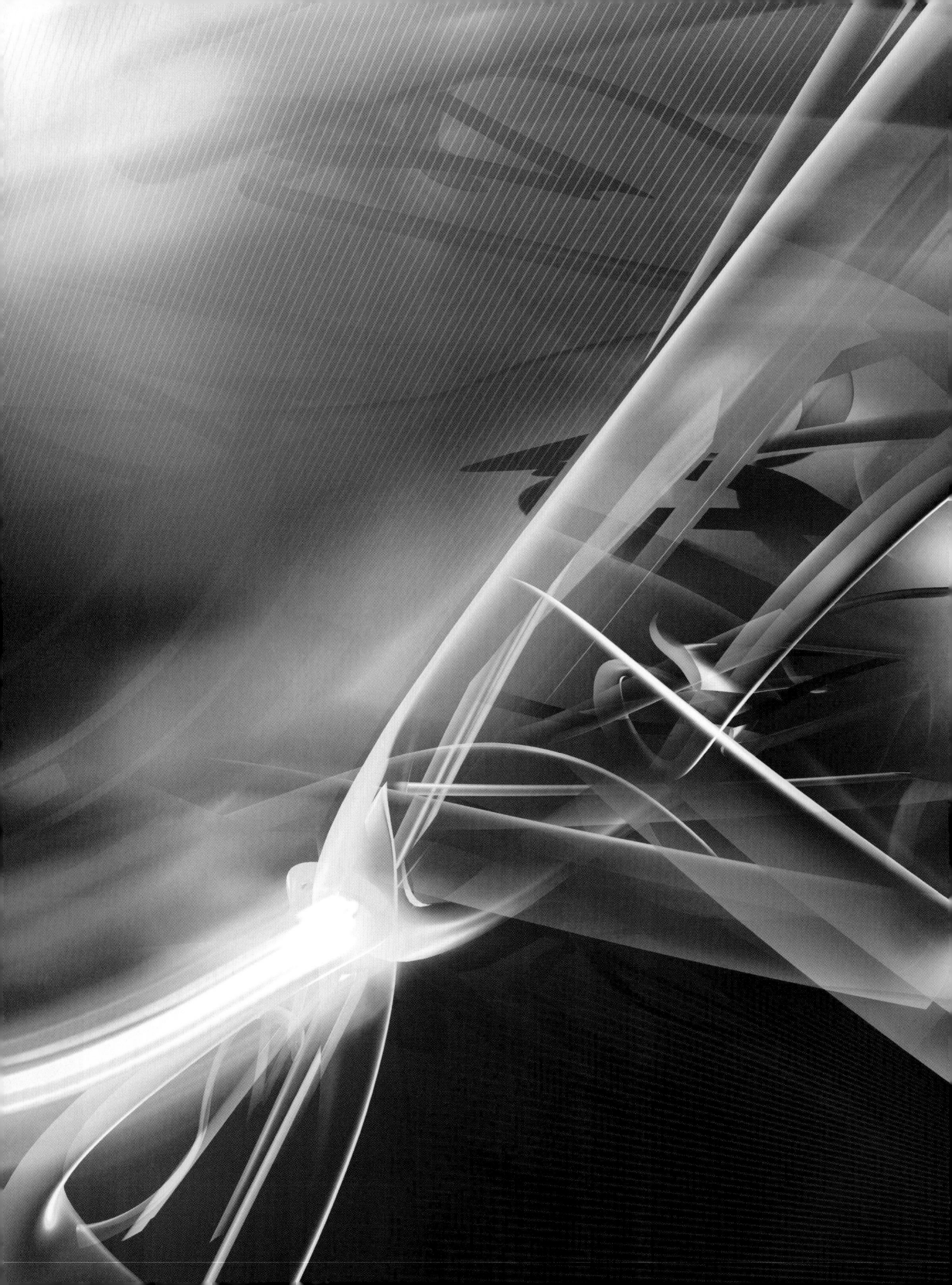

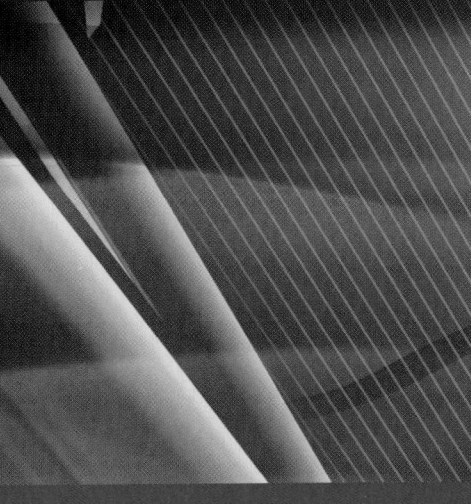

CHAPTER 30

Electroconvulsive, Other Biological (Somatic), and Complementary Therapies

Deborah Antai-Otong, MS, APRN, BC, FAAN

KEY TERMS

Aromatherapy: The practice of using essential oils, the pure volatile aspects of aromatic plant products, for therapeutic purposes, including ameliorating anxiety, stress, and depression.

Chronobiology: Field of science and medicine that explores the many bodily changes governed by hours and the seasons; includes studies of cellular rhythms all the way through those populations and ecosystems.

Circadian Rhythms: Biological cycles occurring over an approximate 24-hour period and influencing biochemical, biological, and behavioral processes.

Deep Brain Stimulation (DBS): A surgical procedure involving implantation of a medical device called a brain pacemaker used to treat various disabling neurological symptoms, such as Parkinson's disease and intractable or treatment-resistant depression.

Electroconvulsive Therapy: Electric current induction of seizures, primarily for treatment of mental disorders; used most frequently in depression.

Hydrotherapy: Refers to the continuous baths and cold wet-sheet packs used to produce a calming effect to control emotional and mental disturbances.

Insulin-Shock Therapy: Refers to administering large doses of insulin to induce marked hypoglycemia, which produces a coma or seizure.

Light Therapy: A biological intervention that increases exposure to artificial light, whose intensity is equivalent to outdoor levels, more than 2,000 lux. The aim of therapy is to suppress melatonin secretion and produce phase shifts of melatonin production.

Melatonin: A metabolite of serotonin produced by the pineal gland. It is produced during darkness and is involved in the feedback loop that is regulated according to the degree of environmental light. Melatonin is implicated in the regulation of seasonal and circadian variance and in the body's adjustment to time zones, and it is a biological marker for the effects of light therapy in SAD.

Phase Advancing: A response to a light stimulus that is intentionally presented hours before the expected onset of solar or wavelength of environmental light.

Phase Delaying: Refers to a response elicited by a light stimulus presented hours later than expected.

Psychosurgery: Surgical or chemical alteration involving severing brain fibers with the purpose of modifying behavioral disturbance, thoughts, or mood.

Seasonal Affective Disorder: Recurrent depression that occurs during winter months and remits in the spring. Major symptoms include depressive mood, hypersomnia, tiredness, increased appetite, and cravings for carbohydrates.

Sleep-Wake Cycle: One of the body's biological rhythms normally determined by the day-night cycle.

Transcranial Magetic Stimulation (TMS): A noninvasive and relatively safe stimulation of the dorsa lateral prefrontal area used to rapidly change magnetic fields to induce electrical current to flow in the brain. Its antidepressant properties may involve induction to get electrical current across the insulating tissues of the scalp and skull without discomfort. It has recently been indicated as an effective treatment for depression. Repetitive transcranial magnetic stimulation is known as rTMS.

Vagus Nerve Stimulation (VNS): A surgical procedure involving subcutaneous implantation of a pace-maker-like generator, which sends electric pulses to the left vagus nerve. It is used to treat refractory depression and epilepsy. It is used as the last resort when clients fail to respond to traditional treatment.

COMPETENCIES

Upon completion of this chapter, the learner should be able to:

1. Discuss major indications for electroconvulsive therapy (ECT).

2. Describe the nursing care of the client undergoing ECT.

3. Recognize major contraindications for ECT.

4. Describe the role of the melatonin in seasonal affective disorder (SAD).

5. Review adverse effects of phototherapy.

6. Describe the biological basis of acupuncture.

7. Discuss causative factors of sleep-wake cycle disturbances.

Somatic therapies, also called biological therapies, have evolved since the 1930s and are becoming increasingly helpful in enabling mental health professionals to understand the neurobiology of brain functions. Numerous researchers have described the relationship between neurobiology and mental disorders. Historically, psychiatrists have explored vast treatment modalities on the assumption that the biological and psychological components of mental illness affect human behavior. Psychiatry is shifting from primarily behavioral to primarily biological paradigms.

Advances in research on the brain, genetic, neuroimaging and other neuroscientific studies show distinct parallels between cellular and molecular processes that result in psychiatric disorders. These discoveries are increasingly narrowing the abyss between the mind and body by linking client experiences with complex brain processes (Peled, 2006).

The complexity of brain function and the brain's role in sustaining health or well-being are the bases of biological therapies. Somatic therapies used in the past include continuous baths, cold sheets, psychosurgery, and convulsive therapies. Some of these interventions were inhumane and their effectiveness was questionable, but they were effective in calming clients. Technological advances have spawned new biological therapies such as psychopharmacology, electroconvulsive therapy (ECT), light therapy, and sleep cycle alterations.

This chapter focuses on the impact of biological therapies on psychiatric-mental health nursing. The evolution of biological therapy, insulin-shock therapy, psychosurgery, ECT, and newer biological therapies is discussed. Other somatic therapies are discussed in Chapters 9 and 29. The terms *somatic therapy* and *biological therapy* are used interchangeably in this chapter.

HISTORICAL ASPECTS OF BIOLOGICAL THERAPIES

Somatic therapies evolved as researchers in the nineteenth century directed their energies toward improving ways to treat the mentally ill. The U.S. Congress's proclamation of the 1990s as the Decade of the Brain renewed interest in biological therapies as viable treatment modalities. In issuing this proclamation, Congress wished to draw attention to the growing number of people afflicted with disorders and disabilities involving the brain (U.S. Congress, 1989). Technological advances in neurobiology have increased scientists' understanding of the brain's role in mental illness and other neurological disorders such as Alzheimer's disease. As scientists seek to understand the complexity of mental disorders and to develop innovative treatments for them, psychiatric-mental health nursing continues to play a vital role in reducing symptoms in the mentally ill.

PSYCHOSURGERY

Ergas Moniz (1936), a Portuguese neurologist, introduced modern psychosurgery as prefrontal lobotomy. In prefrontal lobotomy, the nerve fibers that connect the thalamus with the frontal lobe of the brain are severed. Moniz surmised that the frontal lobe played a crucial role in formation of mental illness and that by modifying various pathways or fibers joining the frontal lobe and the thalamus, emotional and mental disturbances could be relieved. Initial surgical techniques involved drilling burr holes into the top or side of the skull and injecting alcohol at these sites; wires were used to sever the frontal lobe. This procedure was blind in nature because the surgeon could not depict the surgical location. The American physicians Walter Freeman and James Watts introduced a modified version of this procedure in the United States the same year.

Psychosurgery never gained overwhelming popularity, and its use eventually waned because its effectiveness was questionable and was supported by little research. Charges of abuse by neurosurgeons and accusations of social control and racial suppression added to the lack of acceptance of psychosurgery as a viable treatment for mental disorders. In addition, severe complications from this procedure consisted of motor dysfunction, seizures, and cognitive impairment (Kalinowsky & Hoch, 1950; Millon, 1969).

Historically, the nursing interventions required by clients undergoing prefrontal lobotomies were the same as those required by clients undergoing any neurosurgical procedure, including monitoring neurological and vital signs, seizure activity, mental status changes, vomiting, and hemorrhaging. Major postoperative complications from psychosurgery included infection, seizures, and hemorrhaging (Kalinowsky & Hoch, 1950; Steele & Manfreda, 1959).

Since its advent more than 60 years ago, psychosurgery has been refined and restricted to specific destruction of modest regions of brain tissue. Major procedures include radioactive implants, cryoprobes, electrical coagulation, proton beams, ultrasonography, and bilateral cingulotomies (Rauch & Cosgrove, 2000). Currently, alteration of fronto-limbic pathways that alter emotional disturbances, such as chronic debilitating mental disorders that fail to respond to traditional treatment and chronic intractable depression, are the chief reason for psychosurgery (Flaherty et al., 2005). Overall, psychosurgery has been the least acceptable of the somatic therapies and has been used only as a last resort when clients fail to respond to other treatments.

HYDROTHERAPY: CONTINUOUS BATH AND COLD WET-SHEET PACK

Other procedures that were once used to control emotional and mental disturbances included two forms of hydrotherapy: the continuous bath and cold wet-sheet pack. The continuous bath was used to control agitation and erratic emotional disturbances and induce sleep. This procedure was used before bedtime and consisted of lying on a hammock dangling in a warm, continuous bath for extended periods. The client was constantly watched and assessed for signs of overheating, dizziness, convulsions, behavioral changes, and drowning (Steele & Manfreda, 1959).

Cold wet-sheet packs produced a sedative effect, promoting sleep and reducing agitation, anxiety, and irritability. This procedure consisted of removing the client's clothes, asking the client to void, and enclosing him into the wet-sheet pack. In a room that was dim and quiet to facilitate relaxation, the client was literally wrapped in at least two sheets that had been soaked in cold water and wrung out. A blanket was used to reduce chilling. The rationale behind the cold wet-sheet pack was the constriction of blood vessels. Chilling for 5 to 10 minutes was intended to dilate blood vessels, thereby increasing cerebral flow and blood volume. The warmth subsequently produced a calming effect (Steele & Manfreda, 1959).

CONVULSIVE THERAPIES

Convulsive therapies were a major discovery during the twentieth century. A pioneer in convulsive therapies was Manfreda Sakel, a German psychiatrist, who realized that a coma could be induced by administering large amounts of insulin. He noted recovery from an insulin-induced, coma-produced calmness in clients who were formerly confused, delirious, and agitated. He therefore surmised that repeated doses of insulin could produce remission of schizophrenic symptoms. His work was soon embraced by the psychiatric community (Sakel, 1938).

Insulin-Shock Therapy

In insulin-shock therapy large doses of insulin were administered to induce marked hypoglycemia in clients. The hypoglycemic state produces a coma that may or may not induce a seizure. Insulin-shock therapy was used in clients with catatonia and paranoid forms of schizophrenia, but its exact psychotherapeutic effect was unknown. Major complications of this treatment modality were shock and death. Insulin-shock therapy lost its popularity years ago and disappeared from psychiatric treatment because of its questionable efficacy and potential danger.

Metrazol

Sakel's work stirred the interest of Ladislau von Medunna, a Hungarian neuropsychiatrist. In 1935, von Medunna postulated that schizophrenia and epilepsy rarely occurred concurrently. Von Medunna injected camphor in oil intramuscularly to induce seizures, but because of numerous side effects, such as pain and unreliable response, he resorted to using tylenetetrazol (Metrazol). Metrazol, a potent synthetic stimulant, was used to produce electrical stimulation of the brain and induce seizures. This treatment, like others, was not free of side effects. Major disadvantages were unreliable seizure activity, intense feelings of doom between injections, and loss of consciousness lasting approximately 3 to 30 seconds (Kalinowsky & Hoch, 1950). In spite of these side effects, treatment with Metrazol gained popularity because it successfully induced remission of psychosis and depression. Its use declined with the emergence of electroshock therapy (EST).

Electroshock Therapy

Researchers continued search for the ideal approach to mental and emotional illnesses. In 1938, Italian physicians Ugo Cerletti and Luciano Bini discovered they could produce seizures with an electric current rather than a chemical stimulus. Cerletti (1950) surmised that seizures were biochemical drives that mobilized protective responses capable of improving adaptation and producing therapeutic results in the mentally ill. Cerletti and Bini reported the first successful application of EST in a client with catatonic schizophrenia. Clients often experienced profound anxiety and fear during the interval between the application of EST and loss of consciousness. They were given drugs such as amobarbital and thiopental sodium to allay these feelings. Other common complications included lumbar and dorsal spine fractures (Cerletti, 1950; Steele & Manfreda, 1959).

EST became the dominant somatic therapy for mental disorders during the 1940s. However, several researchers observed that only a few clients with schizophrenia benefited from EST and only those who were acutely ill, agitated, catatonic, or those with affective symptoms found relief (Pacella, Barrera, & Kalinowsky, 1942).

The term electroshock therapy was later changed to electroconvulsive therapy, or ECT. Modifications of this technique have emerged over the years, reducing its dangers. In 1940, Bennett, an American psychiatrist, improved ECT when he introduced a new method of anesthesia derived from the curare plant. He suggested that inducing paralysis during ECT reduced the risk of fractures. In 1951, succinylcholine was introduced to psychiatry and eventually became the most widely used muscle relaxant during this procedure. ECT remained in favor among psychiatrists until the advent of psychotropics in the 1950s. Antidepressants and antipsychotics were the primary psychotropics, and they also curtailed the use of barbiturates, wet packs, and restraints. Recent years have seen a resurgence of ECT, but controversy about its effectiveness remains.

Vagus Nerve Stimulation, Transcranial Magnetic Stimulation, and Deep-Brain Stimulation

Three relatively new somatic treatments for psychiatric disorders are vagus nerve stimulation (VNS), transcranial magnetic stimulation (TMS), and deep brain stimulation (DMS). Clinical studies indicate that clients with severe or retractable mood disorders, such as mania, depression, severe Tourette's syndrome, and Parkinson's disease may benefit from these somatic therapies (Dannon, Lowengrub, Gonopolski, & Kotler, 2006; Flaherty et al., 2005; Husain, Montgomery, Fernandes, & Morrow, 2002; Rush et al., 2000; Steward, Desaloms & Sanghera, 2005). The efficacy of VNS lies in its ability to produce minute currents that activate various brain regions. Normally, a device is implanted in the upper left side of the chest and a stimulating lead is attached to the left vagus nerve in the carotid sheath. A handheld magnet is used to activate the device that produces a seizure supposedly in the cortical region of the brain (Schachter & Saper, 1998). Preliminary studies indicate this procedure produces negligible cognitive and autonomic side effects. Major side effects include local irritation, hoarseness, cough, headache, neck pain, dysphagia, and a low risk of infection at the implantation side. TMS is thought to be a more precise method of seizure induction than ECT. Supposedly its electrophysiologic effects involve inducing currents into the prefrontal cortex through rapidly magnetic fields and results in mild antidepressant effects (Sackeim et al., 2001).

The precise mechanism linked to the effectiveness of DMS continues to be studied, but most research indicates it stems from using electrical impulses from the neurostimulator via the extension wire and lead which goes into the brain and blocks electrical signals from targeted brain regions, such as the thalamus and inferior thalamic peduncle. Supposedly, alterations in serotonin, norepinephrine, and other neurotransmitters in the frontal lobes results in overactivity of the orbitofrontal cortex and subsequent depression. Researchers postulate that the use of chronic high-frequency electrical stimulation activated by TMS stabilizes these regions and produces antidepressant effects (Velasco, Velasco, Jimenez, & Salin-Pascual, 2005). See Figure 30–1. Preliminary data demonstrate that TMS affects genetic activity, various neurotransmitter activity, such as serotonin and dopamine, and the formation of proteins

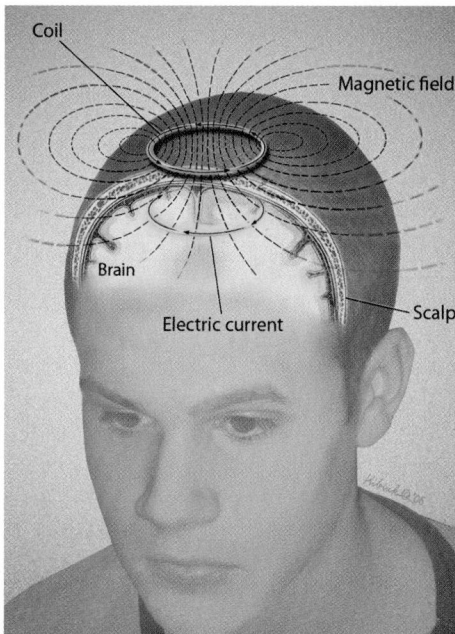

Figure 30–1 Transcranial magnetic stimulation *(From Gage, F. H., Akil, H., & Price, D. L. [2002]. Transcranial Magnetic Stimulation. Society for Neuroscience. http://www.sfn.org/index.cfm?pagename=brainBriefings_transcranial_MagneticStimulation [Accessed December 11, 2006]. Illustration by Linda Kibuik. Copyright © 2002 Linda Kibuik. Artist for Society for Neuroscience.)*

necessary for cellular signaling, all of which may play a role in obviating treatment-resistant depression. A primary disadvantage of TMS is its lack of therapeutic potency when compared to unilateral ECT (Abrams, 2002). However, recent data shows greater promise in the level of therapeutic potency. A recent 6-week double-blind, randomized, sham-controlled trial in 50 patients with treatment-resistant depression, conducted by Fitzgerald and his colleagues, indicated that sequential application of both high-frequency left-side rTMS and low-frequency rTMS to the right prefrontal cortex has considerable treatment efficacy in treatment-resistant depression. Findings from this trial demonstrated significant effectiveness during 4 to 6 weeks of active treatment (Fitzgerald et al., 2006).

Major side effects include:

◆ Transient cognitive deficits

◆ Temporary hearing loss due to loud clicking associated with electrical energy discharge into the coil

◆ Pain and irritation in the scalp, face, and neck due to repetitive muscle contraction

◆ Risk of seizures in clients with preexisting neurological conditions (Cohen et al., 2004; Fitzgerald et al., 2003).

ELECTROCONVULSIVE THERAPY

The historical aspects of somatic therapies are the foundation for contemporary advances in the treatment of mental disorders. This section discusses the historical aspects of ECT, its clinical indications, risks, theories, and effectiveness as a treatment modality for serious mental disorders.

HISTORICAL ASPECTS

The misconceptions held by neuropsychiatrists early in the twentieth century that epilepsy and schizophrenia rarely occurred simultaneously provided the rationale for the use of ECT. Its use climaxed in the 1940s and 1950s, when it was considered the treatment of choice for severe mental illness such as schizophrenia and manic-type bipolar disorder. As mentioned, the use of ECT promptly declined with the advent of psychotropics in the 1950s. Today, ECT continues to be a controversial treatment modality. The controversy stems from the debate about whether its psychotherapeutic effect on the brain is worth its perceived invasiveness and brain-damaging aspects (Fink, 1991).

Black (1993) noted that ECT parallels psychosurgery as one of the least accepted forms of treatment. However, recent years have seen an increased acceptance of ECT as a safe, effective, and economical form of treatment, yet it is rarely used as the first line of treatment (Olfson, Marcus, Sackeim, Thompson, & Pincus, 1998). While the effectiveness of ECT continues to be researched, this intervention is gaining approval for treating neurological disorders such as refractory parkinsonism and neuroleptic malignant syndrome.

MAJOR CLINICAL INDICATIONS

Coffey and Weiner (1990) identified the major indications for ECT as major depression, psychosis, the need for a swift onset of action, and certain medical conditions. In 90 percent of cases, ECT is used to treat *major depressive episodes*. A number of researchers investigating its effectiveness contend that it is better than placebo in sustaining remission of depressive symptoms in at least 80 percent of the time (Coffey & Weiner, 1990; Gagné, Furman, Carpenter, & Price, 2000). The extent of improvement parallels the severity of illness. Other studies comparing the efficacy of antidepressants with that of ECT have revealed a marked improvement in depressed clients with ECT (Dannon, Lowengrub, Gonopolski, & Kotler, 2006).

Recent studies indicate the effectiveness of ECT in clients with Parkinson's disease (Strome, Zis, Doudet, 2007). Target symptoms for ECT include motor signs and symptoms and depression in clients without psychiatric comorbidity. Studies show that depression occurs in about 40 percent of clients with Parkinson's disease (Lieberman, 2006).

Clients experiencing acute mania, delirium, and schizophrenia, particularly those with catatonia and affective symptoms, have exhibited a good response to ECT (Greenhalgh, Knight, Hind, Beverley, & Walters, 2005). Catatonia refers to a complex syndrome manifested by marked stupor and muscle rigidity or overactivity. This disorder is generally seen in clients with schizophrenia or affective disorders. ECT continues to be a controversial treatment for psychosis. Indications for ECT during psychotic episodes include ineffective response or contraindication to other therapies. In one study, some clients were found to show improvement when antipsychotic medications were added to this treatment modality (Chanpattana, et al., 1999).

One advantage of ECT is its ability to produce a rapid onset of action in severely depressed clients who need immediate treatment to alleviate life-threatening conditions such as suicidal risk, catatonia, or profound malnutrition and dehydration (Lalitanatpong, 2005).

Welch (1997) delineated the following groups as good candidates for ECT regardless of diagnosis:

1. Severely malnourished depressed clients at risk for medical complications

2. Medically ill clients with cardiac arrhythmias or coronary artery disease who cannot tolerate antidepressants or antipsychotics (i.e., older adult clients)

3. Psychotically depressed clients whose symptoms are not relieved by traditional antidepressant regimens

4. Clients who did not respond to medications during previous depressive episodes

5. Clients with catatonia, which may be a symptom of schizophrenia, endocrine disorders, or brain lesions

6. Clients with delusional depression

Welch (1997) noted that in 50 percent of cases, untreated catatonia increases the likelihood of pulmonary complications, venous embolus, contractures, and impaired skin integrity. Table 30–1 summarizes the indications for ECT.

TABLE 30–1
Indications for Electroconvulsive Therapy

Psychiatric	Medical
Major depression (80%)*	Catatonia secondary to medical conditions
Schizophrenia (10–20%)†	Neuroleptic malignant syndrome (NMS) secondary to neuroleptic use
Acute mania (3%)	Hypopituitarism
	Intractable seizure disorder
	Parkinsonism

*Primary indicator.
†Secondary role.

Note. Data adapted from *The Practice of Electroconvulsive Therapy: Recommendations for Psychiatric Training and Privileging*, by the American Psychiatric Association Task Force on Electroconvulsive Therapy, 2001, 2nd ed., Washington, DC: Author.

MECHANISM OF ACTION: NEUROBIOLOGICAL THEORIES

The efficacy of ECT is linked with the production of grand mal seizures. The exact neurobiological effect of seizures elicited by ECT remains unknown. Current animal studies suggest that seizures elicited by ECT create alterations in neurochemical, neuroendocrine, and neurophysiological processes that are similar to those produced by antidepressants (Black, 1993). Other researchers surmise that the relationship between seizures and decreased mental disturbance is associated with neurochemical and neurophysiological processes. Grover, Mattoo, and Gupta (2005) postulated that ECT produces alterations in several neurotransmitter receptors such as acetylcholine, norepinephrine, dopamine, and serotonin. This process is the same as that produced by long-term antidepressant use. Contemporary findings from positron emission tomography consistently demonstrate that there is increased blood flow in the thalamus and decreased cerebral blood flow in the anterior cingulate and medial frontal cortex shortly post ECT compared with that before ECT (Grover et al., 2005; Takano et al., 2007).

Neurophysiological theories suggest that certain regions in the brain are hyperactive during seizures and hypoactive after ECT. Marangell, Silver, and Yudofsky (1999) noted that the electrical stimulus generated by kindling, or persistent stimulation, calms hyperactive brain circuits. Other theories about the effectiveness of ECT suggest that it increases levels of some neuropeptides, which stabilize the mood and modify regional cerebral blood flow (Jimenez-Vasquez, 2007).

Imaging technology is another avenue through which researchers are attempting to understand the effects of ECT on the brain. Imaging techniques include computed tomography (CT); magnetic resonance imaging (MRI); regional cerebral blood flow (RCBF); positron emission tomography (PET); and single photon emission computed tomography (SPECT). Findings are inconclusive that morphological changes do occur in the brain after a course of ECT. Other research data suggest that there are marked global increases during ECT. It is estimated that the cortical RCBF increases about 300 percent during generalized seizures, while the cerebral metabolic rate (CMR) for glucose and oxygen increases approximately 200 percent.

RISKS

ECT is generally considered a very safe treatment, and technical advances in its study show decreasing risk of this therapy. Abrams (2002) describes ECT as a low-risk procedure, whose safety is associated with a greater understanding of neurobiological processes and increased proficiency in monitoring. In addition, there is a lack of conclusive evidence that ECT produces brain damage or that it worsens dementia.

Initial risks, such as fractures, decreased with the advent of effective muscle relaxants and short-acting anesthetics, the use of supported oxygen perfusion, improvements in equipment, and increased competence of staff. As a result of these advances, the mortality rates have dropped tremendously and this rate has remained constant the past 2 decades (Kramer, 1999). Reports indicate 2 deaths per 100,000 treatments (Kramer, 1999). Today ECT is considered one of the safest somatic interventions that uses general anesthesia. Morbidity and mortality generally result from secondary complications from cardiovascular factors such as arrhythmias, myocardial infarction, or hypertension (Nuttall, Bowersox, Douglass, McDonald, Rasmussen, et al., (2004).

Clients with impaired cardiovascular and cerebral function have the greatest risk for adverse effects from ECT. Cardiovascular workload increases rapidly during the onset of the seizure or ECT because of the initial sympathetic arousal. This stimulation generally persists throughout the seizure and is intensified by circulating catecholamines that peak after 3 minutes after the start of the seizure (Grover et al., 2005). When the seizure ceases, the parasympathetic response persists, producing a transient hypotension and bradycardia. The client's baseline physiological function normally returns within 5 to 10 minutes (Welch, 1997). The major biological responses to ECT are listed in Table 30–2.

The major cardiovascular complications from ECT include:

◆ Acute myocardial infarction

◆ Coronary arrhythmias

◆ Myocardial rupture

◆ Cardiac arrest

◆ Congestive heart failure

◆ Hypertension

Cerebral responses to ECT arise from the tremendous amount of oxygen used during the procedure. The rate of oxygen consumption doubles during ECT, producing increased cerebral blood circulation, with a subsequent rise in intracranial pressure and increased permeability of the blood-brain barrier. These cerebral responses place the client at risk for neurological complications. Major neurological contraindications for ECT include space-occupying brain lesions, which have been related to decompensation and death. In spite of these risk factors, some clients with these lesions have been successfully treated with ECT.

CONTRAINDICATIONS

Most researchers contend that contraindications for ECT have diminished since the advent of the use of brief pulse stimulation, rather than the traditional sine wave stimulus, to initiate a grand mal seizure. The principal advantage of the brief pulse stimulation is that it uses significantly less electrical energy than the sine wave stimulation. Another factor that reduces cognitive impairment and adverse reactions to ECT

TABLE 30–2
Major Biological Responses to ECT

Major Physiological Responses to ECT

Cardiovascular (Hyperdynamic State)
- Cerebral vascular accidents (CVA) [stroke]
- Hydrocephalus
- 25% Increase in heart rate with induction of anesthesia
- Vagal stimulation—transient bradycardia during and after administration of electrical stimulus
- Increased heart rate at the end of seizure
- Increased blood pressure rate parallels heart rate
- ↑ Arterial hypertension

Cerebral
- Seizure increases EEG activity
- Transient memory and cognitive impairment
  disorientation
  confusion
  forgetfulness
  retrograde and anterograde amnesia
  headaches
  ↑ cerebral blood flow and velocity

Theories of Neurobiological Effects of ECT

Neurochemical
- Dysregulation of postsynaptic beta-adrenergic receptors
- Alterations in transmitter sites (e.g., acetylcholine, norepinephrine, dopamine, and serotonin)
- Increase of cerebrospinal fluid calcium levels

Neurophysiological
- Subdues kindling sites in the brain
- Increases neuropeptides
- Affects cerebral blood flow

ECT, electroconvulsive therapy; EEG, electroencephalogram.

TABLE 30–3
Contraindications to ECT

- Intracranial lesions (e.g., tumors)
- Acute myocardial infarctions
- Severe hypertension

ECT, electroconvulsive therapy.

is unilateral placement of electrodes on the nondominant hemisphere (Abrams, 2002).

At one time, clients with various neurological conditions such as space-occupying brain lesions, hydrocephalus, arteriovenous malformations, and clients recovering from strokes, were absolutely contraindicated for ECT. Studies consistently indicate that ECT can be administered safely and efficaciously to these clients, however (Kang & Passmore, 2004; Rasmussen, Perry, Sutor, & Moore, 2007). At one time, pregnancy was also considered a contraindication for ECT. However, recent studies indicate that severely depressed pregnant women who are at risk for malnutrition and suicide may be candidates for ECT and need to be closely monitored (i.e., fetal cardiac monitoring and avoidance of hyperventilation) during and after treatment. The usefulness of administering ECT to a pregnant client must outweigh potential dangers of this procedure before it can be implemented (Pinette, Santarpio, Wax, & Blackstone, 2007; Richards, 2007).

Table 30–3 lists the contraindications to ECT.

OUTPATIENT ECT

The number of clients receiving ECT has risen in recent years. Treatment in outpatient settings is possible because ECT is a short, relatively safe and well-tolerated procedure with a low risk for adverse reactions (Abrams, 2002). Outpatient ECT is usually coordinated by a registered nurse who engages the client and family in the education process that prepares them for treatment. Preparation for outpatient ECT is the same as inpatient treatment. (See Client and Family Health Teaching.)

MAINTENANCE ECT

In spite of its effectiveness in managing mood disorders, early relapse is common in ECT unless maintenance treatment is used. Good candidates for maintenance ECT are clients who

have responded favorably as inpatients or those who have not responded to traditional medication regimens. The principal goal of maintenance is relapse prevention. Relapse is relatively common after 6 months after ECT treatment; the relapse rate is 30 to 60 percent. An antidepressant or lithium has been used as an adjunct to ECT to sustain its therapeutic effects for about 6 months. Some researchers have challenged this notion, however, arguing that continuation of psychotropics may not be efficacious in clients who did not respond to antidepressants before ECT (Abrams, 2002; Kho, Zwinderman, & Blansjaar, 2005).

Various psychotherapies are surmised to enhance the effectiveness of ECT. Studies show that psychotherapy and psychotropics can reduce relapse between 6 and 12 months after ECT. ECT is only one component of the treatment for depression. Psychiatric-mental health nurses can promote clients' health by actively working with them and their families to identify psychosocial factors that may precipitate depressive episodes. Collaborating with ECT team members allows nurses to mobilize resources and support the client at risk for relapse. Treatment approaches must incorporate psychosocial and biological therapies to meet clients' needs during vulnerable periods.

LIFE SPAN ISSUES

ECT remains a controversial form of treatment for psychiatric disorders. This is particularly relevant to treating children and adolescents. This section encompasses the management of ECT across the life span.

ECT IN CHILDREN AND ADOLESCENTS

The use of ECT in children and adolescents is limited to the same conditions suggested for adult populations. Its use is rare, and research supporting its efficacy is scarce. Guidelines for the administration of ECT to children 12 years of age or younger are delineated by the American Psychiatric Association Task Force on Electroconvulsive Therapy (2001) and include the following:

1. It should be confined to those cases when other treatments are infeasible or unsafe.

2. Recommendations for ECT must come from two psychiatrists who are experienced in working with this population and are not involved in the case.

3. The anesthetist must be adept in working with this age group.

Other suggestions include developing policies that parallel state and federal guidelines for the administration of ECT to this age group.

Electroconvulsive therapy continues to generate moral, practical, and ethical debate when performed on children and adolescents. A dearth of published data related to clinical indications, use, clinical outcomes, and complications of ECT in

CLIENT AND FAMILY HEALTH TEACHING

Major Components of a Health Education Plan for Clients Undergoing ECT

Your physician has ordered electroconvulsive therapy (ECT) as a treatment for your depression. This teaching plan will help you understand the procedure, including desired and potential adverse effects.

Purpose of ECT: To rapidly relieve your depressive symptoms and alleviate your suicidal ideations.

Pretreatment

1. Your physician will be asked to voluntarily sign an informed consent, giving permission to perform ECT and sedate you during the procedure.

2. Other orders to prepare you for this procedure include:
   - a complete physical examination
   - laboratory studies that include drawing your blood, gathering a urine specimen, x-rays of your skull and back, and electrocardiogram (ECG). These tests will ensure that it is safe to receive ECT.

3. It is important to know about your current medications, including over-the-counter drugs and herbs.

Do not drink or eat anything by mouth 6 to 8 hours before your scheduled procedure (if you are taking routine cardiovascular medication, you may be allowed to take it with sips of water several hours before your procedure).

The Procedure Day

You will be asked to wash your hair and avoid using hairspray or creams to reduce the risk of burns.

You will be asked to do the following shortly before being taken to the procedure room:

Remove dentures, eye glasses, or contact lenses.

Empty your bladder.

Your doctor has ordered a premedication that will be given as an injection (shot)—it will make your mouth dry, but this is essential to reduce the risk of aspiration.

You will be asked to put on a gown.

Your blood pressure, pulse, respirations, and temperature will be checked before and after the procedure.

A blood pressure cuff will be placed on your arm so your vital signs can be continuously monitored.

You will have an oral airway and oxygen mask to maintain your oxygen level, and electrodes that are connected to an ECG machine will be used to monitor your heart during the procedure.

A pulse oximeter will be clipped to your finger to monitor your oxygen levels (saturation).

You will be placed on a stretcher and a nurse will accompany you to the procedure room.

Your forehead or temples will be wiped with a cool solution to remove skin oils, so the electrodes will stay attached and reduce burns.

An intravenous line will be placed in your arm or hand so that medications can be administered.

Medications will be used to sedate you in preparation for the procedure (the effects of these medications will last until the procedure is completed.)

You will be monitored very closely throughout the procedure and recovery period.

When you awaken you will feel drowsy and may experience some temporary memory loss (difficulty recalling events before the procedure), mild confusion, and a headache.

---

this population makes controlled data difficult to gather (Segal, Szabo, & du Toit, 2004). Despite evidence to support clinical indications for ECT in children and adolescents, researchers from the American Academy of Child and Adolescent Psychiatry developed practice parameters for use of ECT with adolescents. In addition to those delineated by the APA (2001) guidelines, researchers believe ECT should be considered in adolescents when the youth fails two or more trials of pharmacotherapy or when severity of symptoms preclude waiting for a response to medications. As with other biological therapies, consent from parents or legal guardian is mandatory, and the adolescent's needs to concur with or assent to the procedures. Statutory regulations and institutional procedures must also be followed (Ghaziuddin et al., 2004).

ECT IN ADULTS AND OLDER ADULTS

The management of mental disorders in older adults has received increased attention in the past decade. Concern regarding the treatment of people 65 years of age and older arises from the enormous growth of this population, which comprises 12.8 percent of the U.S. population. The older population is expected to grow in future decades, with the most rapid increase between 2010 and 2030, when the baby boomer generation reaches 65 years (U.S. Census Bureau, 2000).

Another concern for older adults is their vulnerability to a host of psychosocial and neurobiological stressors generated by the aging process. Psychosocial stressors include loss of health, loved ones, and financial security. The brain is affected by the aging process in that levels of neurotransmitters and precursors, such as dopamine and norepinephrine, are lowered, increasing the likelihood of depression. Lowered levels of these biochemicals are caused by neuroendocrine function of the thyroid and pituitary glands in the older adult.

Depression in the older adult is often defined in terms of chronicity and disability. High mortality rates suggest the need for aggressive efforts to identify high-risk groups and accurately diagnoses and treat mood disorders in the older adult client. These efforts may be compromised because of changes in drug metabolism and medical conditions that contraindicate the use of antidepressants.

ECT is considered a viable treatment option for the severely depressed older adult. Predictors of a hopeful outcome include neurovegetative symptoms such as sleep, appetite, energy, and cognitive disturbances. Less favorable outcomes are predicted in the client with coexisting mental disorders such as dementia or somatization disorders. The somatization disorders refer to physical complaints such as headaches, nausea, or vomiting that have no physical or underlying general medical basis (American Psychiatric Association [APA], 2000, 2001).

Major complications from ECT among older adults fall into several categories: cardiovascular, respiratory, cognitive impairment, and falls (Huuhka, Seinela, Reinikainen, & Leinonen, 2003). Clients 75 years of age and older who have coexisting medical conditions such as ventricular arrhythmias or recent myocardial infarctions present the greatest risk for serious complications from ECT. General anesthesia significantly increases the risk of cardiovascular complications in the older adult client who has experienced a myocardial infarction in the last 3 months, and ECT is contraindicated during this period (Baldwin, Jeffries, Jackson, Sutcliffe, & Thacker et al., 2004; Huuhka et al., 2003). In spite of these

risks, older adult clients can benefit from the therapeutic effects of ECT.

The psychiatric nurse reduces these complications by collaborating with members of the treatment team. Collaboration is enhanced when the nurse:

◆ Establishes a therapeutic relationship with the client and family

◆ Participates in the pre-ECT evaluation process by gathering pertinent physical assessment data such as blood pressure, heart and respiratory status, and present medications and medical conditions

◆ Assesses current medications and treatment regimens (see Table 30–4 for a list of medications that interact with ECT)

◆ Documents, reports, and discusses these findings with the treatment team

THE ROLE OF THE NURSE

Nursing care of the client undergoing ECT challenges the nurse to assess client's needs and concerns and develop holistic interventions that reduce anxiety, provide health education, and provide safe recovery. This section focuses on these issues along with the role of the nurse in the

---

TABLE 30–4
Medication Interactions with ECT

Agents That Increase Seizure Activity	Agents That Decrease Seizure Activity	Other Drug Interactions	Prolong Seizure Activity
Theophyllin	Benzodiazepines	*MAOs (phenelzine) (potent pressor agents that increase or decrease blood pressure)	CNS stimulants (also ↑ risk of dysrhythmias and B/P)
Caffeine	Anticonvulsants		Calcium channel blockers ↑ cardiovascular depression
Lithium	Barbiturate anesthetic	†Lithium increases severity of post-ECT cognitive impairment and may increase length of hospital stay	*Carbamazepine prolongs action of suxamethonium (succinylcholine)
Tricyclic antidepressants	Propofol anesthetic		
Trazodone (Desyrel)	Herbs		
Fluoxetine (Prozac)	CNS stimulants prolong seizures; increase dysrhythmias; increase BP	Delirium CBZ, LMG, Topiramate inhibit seizure activity CBZ—prolong action of suxamethonium	
Bupropion (Wellbutrin)			
Antipsychotic agents			

ECT, electroconvulsive therapy; MAO, monoamine oxidase.

*Need to be discontinued two weeks prior to ECT.

†Needs to be discontinued a week prior to ECT because it enhances action of neuromuscular blocking agent.

implementation of treatment protocols and legal and ethical considerations.

PSYCHOSOCIAL CONSIDERATIONS

Clients and family members anticipating ECT frequently feel anxious because they have misconceptions about the procedure. Common misconceptions about ECT are that it will result in electrocution, permanent brain damage, memory loss, and death. Several studies suggest that in spite of modifications in technique and pretreatment instructions, these misconceptions prevail (Brodaty, Berle, Hickie & Mason, 2003; Dowman, Patel, & Rajput, 2005). Another study disputes this notion, suggesting that only a small percentage of clients actually dislike ECT and are unwilling to submit to more treatment (Nelson, 2005).

Historically, nurses have supported clients' decisions about ECT, provided education, and assessed psychosocial and biological needs. Assessing and responding to psychosocial needs of clients and families are responsibilities of the psychiatric-mental health nurse. Psychiatric nurses can allay fears and anxiety by providing environments that encourage expression of feelings, thoughts, and concerns regarding the procedure. Various educational media are useful in describing the ECT process, including videos, tours of the facility, and discussion of responsibilities of the ECT team (APA, 2001).

ECT PROTOCOLS

Several organizations, including the American Nurses Association ([ANA], 2000); APA, and the Royal College of Nursing (1987) have developed protocols for ECT.

The ANA defined the role of the nurse in caring for the client undergoing ECT or other psychobiological interventions as follows. The nurse:

1. Provides educational and emotional support for the client and family

2. Assesses the client's baseline or pretreatment level of function

3. Prepares the clients for the ECT process

4. Monitors and evaluates the client's response to psychobiological treatment, shares it with the health team, and modifies treatment as needed (see Nursing Care Plan 30–1 for the client undergoing ECT)

In 1987, the Royal College of Nursing formulated guidelines that delineated the nurse's role in the ECT process and suggested that nursing functions should include coordinating the process, attending educational programs on ECT, participating on interdisciplinary teams, and developing educational programs.

Practical training that enables the nurse to participate as a team member in the ECT procedure is critical to increasing the nurses' confidence in how to set up equipment,

monitor client responses, assist with resuscitation, and how to use a defibrillator. Competency in these areas is linked to quality and safe post-ECT care (Munday, Deans, & Little, 2003).

The APA (2001) Task Force on ECT recommends that nurses are responsible for:

1. Educating clients and families about ECT

2. Organizing care, including tending to the treatment area to ensure that equipment is available and working (e.g., emergency equipment, monitoring devices, and ECT equipment)

3. Carrying out various nursing interventions to ensure clients' safety and understanding before and after ECT

Overall, various ECT protocols emphasize the significance of nurses in teaching, ensuring safety, and providing emotional support for the client undergoing ECT.

ETHICAL AND LEGAL CONSIDERATIONS

Controversy over the advantages and disadvantages of ECT continues to be widespread among mental health advocates, clients, families, and mental health professionals. The persistent fears and myths affect the public's perception of this treatment modality, which uses electricity to change behavior. Clients and their families need to be informed of the benefits and potential risks of all treatment, particularly somatic interventions. The informed-consent process is a mechanism that encourages dynamic interactions among clients, families, and health professionals. In these interactions, the team considers ethical and legal issues, and psychosocial factors are addressed.

Informed Consent

Clients must be informed of the purpose of ECT and other somatic treatment and the benefits and risk factors associated with them. This information needs to be integrated into individualized treatment plans that encourage the client's, family's, and other health care professionals' active participation in the decision-making process. These interactions convey to the clients and their families that they are respected and are essential in decisions about treatment.

The term *informed consent* refers to a legal standard that claims the client has been given information that enables him to make an educated decision whether to accept the treatment planned for him. The process of informed consent is an active process that begins, not ends, with the signing of the written consent form. It evolves among clients, families, and members of the ECT team throughout treatment (Abrams, 2002; Black, 1993). Three critical measures must exist within this process:

1. Voluntary consent

2. Competency of client

3. Information exchange

Furthermore, informed consent implies that the individual has the capacity to make informed decisions and voluntarily submits to treatment after being presented adequate information about the procedure by the physician and other members of the ECT team.

Initially, the physician evaluates the client for appropriateness for ECT and then, medically, to determine risk factors. An anesthesia evaluation addresses the nature and extent of anesthetic risk and need for modification of medications or anesthetic procedures (APA, 2001). The physician and client together, with the client actively participating in the informed-consent process, determine the decision for treatment. Client competency is an essential part of the informed-consent process and nurses must be aware of hospital and state policy regarding involuntary treatment for an incompetent client. The presence of a life-threatening situation, along with a lack of appropriate treatment options, plays a major role in the decision to perform ECT on an incompetent client. See Chapter 8 for an in-depth discussion of informed consent.

THE NURSING PROCESS

This section discusses client assessment, nursing diagnoses, outcome criteria, implementation and planning, and evaluation of a client undergoing ECT.

ASSESSMENT

Any procedure conducted under general anesthesia requires a medical and physical evaluation. In addition, the effects of ECT place enormous stress on the cardiovascular, respiratory, musculoskeletal, and neurological systems. Pretreatment diagnostic tests and examinations provide vital information about the client's physical and mental ability to undergo the procedure (Abrams, 2002; APA, 2001).

Abrams (2002) suggests a number of pre-ECT procedures:

1. Thorough medical history
2. Physical examination
3. Routine blood and urine examinations (complete blood count, electrolytes, chemistries, urinalysis)
4. ECG
5. Skull radiographs or use of imaging technique to rule out brain tumor (i.e., CT scan, MRI when a tumor is suspected)
6. Pseudokinesterase testing (the absence of this enzyme, which is responsible for catalyzing succinylcholine, a muscle relaxant used in ECT, increases the risk of apnea after ECT)

The electroencephalogram (EEG), brain CT, or MRI are not considered a good screening tool for ECT and should be used only when other diagnostic findings show structural changes.

Nursing assessment must also include performing a mental status exam with a particular focus on the client's cognitive, neurological, and functional status, in which orientation and memory involving recent, remote, and past memory is assessed as baseline data. Neurological data includes, but is not limited to size of pupils, reaction to light, gait, quality of hand grasps, quality of speech, evidence or absence of tremors and other abnormal movements, and nystagmus. Questions about the client's expectations from the procedure, current events, and the capacity to participate in informed decision making help the nurse monitor pre- and post-ECT cognitive and functional status.

Another concern of clients undergoing ECT is the interaction of ECT with a host of drugs. Most medications affect a person's seizure threshold and may need to be increased, decreased, or stopped if the client is undergoing ECT. The use of psychotropics, such as monoamine oxidase inhibitors (MAOIs), antidepressants, and lithium, needs to be suspended 2 weeks before ECT (Naguib & Koorn, 2002).

Using a psychosocial assessment tool that elicits the following information can enhance assessment of the client:

◆ Duration of presenting symptoms
◆ Identification of present stressors
◆ Reasons for seeking treatment
◆ Current treatment, including all medication (e.g., prescribed and over the counter), herbs, and diet regimen
◆ Past treatment, including ECT and response
◆ Risk of dangers toward self or others (i.e., presence of suicidal or homicidal ideations, intent, plan, past attempts)
◆ Past psychiatric treatment
◆ Current and past substance misuse
◆ Present physical and mental status

Pretreatment Preparation

After the client is assessed to be appropriate for ECT, pretreatment preparation begins. Pretreatment nursing care varies, but it generally includes preparing the client both physically and psychologically for ECT. To prepare the client physically for the procedure, the nurse:

◆ Assists the physician with the medical examination
◆ Educates the client and family on, for example, the preoperative protocol
◆ Instructs the client to take nothing by mouth at least 6 to 8 hours before treatment (clients receiving routine cardiovascular medications may be allowed to take these agents with sips of water several hours before treatment)
◆ Asks the client to remove dentures, eyeglasses, or contact lenses
◆ Asks the client to void
◆ Confirms that the client's hair is shampooed and dry (and especially free of hairspray or creams) to reduce risk of burns

Psychological preparation includes encouraging expression of feelings and thoughts regarding ECT (see the nurse-client dialogue) and preoperative teaching (APA, 2001; Royal College of Nursing, 1987).

The next part of pretreatment is premedication. Premedication normally consists of an intramuscular injection of an anticholinergic agent, such as atropine, to produce a mild tachycardia to minimize vagal stimulation produced by ECT and to reduce oral secretions. ECT induces a powerful vagal stimulation both during the procedure and promptly after it (Abrams, 2002; APA, 2001).

NURSING DIAGNOSES

Major nursing diagnoses identified for the client undergoing ECT include the following:

◆ Deficient Knowledge

◆ Anxiety

◆ Risk for Injury

◆ Decreased Cardiac Output

◆ Disturbed Thought Processes

◆ Self-Care Deficit

◆ Activity Intolerance

◆ Risk for Aspiration

OUTCOME IDENTIFICATION

Outcome criteria for the client undergoing ECT include the following:

1. The client makes an informed decision about ECT.

2. The client experiences minimal anxiety and fears about the procedure.

3. The client maintains vital signs within selected parameters during and after ECT.

4. The client remains free of injury.

IMPLEMENTATION AND PLANNING

The ECT team generally consists of a psychiatrist, an anesthesia specialist, a registered nurse, and other nursing staff. The psychiatrist is normally responsible for coordinating the ECT team and managing medical treatment. The anesthesia specialist is responsible for providing anesthesia, maintaining a patent airway, and initiating emergency interventions if adverse reactions such as cardiac arrhythmias or respiratory distress occur.

The registered nurse is usually responsible for overseeing the general nursing care, including affirming that appropriate drugs are available and that all emergency and resuscitation equipment are working properly, including oxygen and suction equipment. General nursing care before the procedure consists of (a) ensuring that the client is wearing comfortable attire to allow for placement of monitoring electrodes, (b) asking the client to void to minimize bladder distention and incontinence, (c) taking and recording the client's vital signs, and (d) escorting the client to the treatment room. Reassurance and explanation throughout treatment will allay the client's fears and anxiety.

After the client is assisted to the cart or stretcher, the nurse continues client education by explaining the placement of the blood pressure cuff and intravenous line. Later, the forehead or temples will be cleansed with alcohol or saline solution to reduce skin oils. Removal of skin oil ensures proper and ideal electrode contact and minimizes skin burns (APA, 2001). Once the client is on the stretcher and the intravenous line is in place, the nurse continues to reassure by standing close by and explaining what is happening. The next step in preparation for ECT is electrode placement.

Recent modifications have been made in the location of the electrode placements. Historically, electrodes were placed bilaterally, but unilateral placement or stimulation has recently gained popularity. Bilateral ECT refers to placement on both sides of the head about 1 inch above the ear opening and outer seam of the eyelid. Unilateral ECT refers to electrode placement over the nondominant cerebral hemisphere, usually the right side of the head and the right ear in right-handed persons to facilitate EEG monitoring. Additionally, the nondominant side of the brain possibly involves nonverbal responses and emotions rather than memory and language functions. Unilateral electrode placement is preferred because it reduces cognitive side effects such as confusion, disorientation, and abnormal EEG changes (Abrams, 2002; APA, 2001). Abrams (2002) asserted that the location of electrode placement is prompted by the variety of treatment.

Once the electrodes are in place, further monitoring is vital to safe administration of ECT. The monitoring equipment used includes the following (Abrams, 2002):

◆ Pulse oximeter (clipped to the finger to monitor oxygen saturation)

◆ Cardiac monitoring

◆ Blood pressure measurement (manual or automatic cuff)

◆ Peripheral nerve stimulator (placed over the ulnar nerve to assess muscle relaxation)

Anesthesia Administration

The purposes of general anesthesia during ECT are as follows:

- To modulate the motor activity generated by the seizure activity
- To facilitate rapid induction and recovery
- To reduce adverse effects such as musculoskeletal injury
- To expand the therapeutic effects of ECT

The major anesthetic agents used in ECT are short-acting anesthetics and muscle relaxants that are given intravenously shortly before induction of seizures or ECT. The neurobiological effects of ECT are closely monitored to appraise its effects and prolonged seizure activity. Seizure activity arises from application of controlled electrical stimulus to the scalp. The client's cardiovascular, respiratory, and systemic status is steadily monitored for adverse reactions (Abrams, 2002; APA, 2001).

Frequency of Treatment

ECT is normally given three times a week until therapeutic response is achieved, approximately after 6 to 12 treatments, or 200 to 600 seizure seconds, and generally not exceeding 20 treatments. Typically, ECT is administered every other day. Less frequent treatment has been associated with less cognitive disturbances, but it also delayed onset of action (Lerer et al., 1995). The number of treatments administered is usually based on the following:

- Diagnosis
- Client's response to treatment
- Client's response to past treatment
- Severity of illness
- Quality of response

It is common for seriously ill clients to have up to two treatments per session, usually administered 1 to 2 minutes apart. Conditions that indicate two treatments include life-threatening mental disorders such as severe depression with suicidal preoccupation, catatonia, lethargy, and mania. Clients experiencing depression or psychotic disorders usually exhibit signs of improvement after several treatments, frequently reaching maximum therapeutic response after 5 to 10 treatments (Kho et al., 2005).

EVALUATION

The nursing care of clients recovering from ECT is the same as for those recovering from general anesthesia. Initially, the client is placed in a supine position to facilitate drainage of secretions. Major systems assessed during the recovery period are the respiratory, cardiovascular, and neurological systems. Maintaining stability is the major goal of recovery.

Once the client fully recovers from anesthesia, as evidenced by regained consciousness and stable vital and neurological signs within designated parameters, and remains free of injury, the client can be discharged from the recovery area to the postrecovery area. The client needs continued reassurance, emotional support, and frequent reorientation to encourage full recovery from ECT.

After an ECT treatment, most clients experience confusion, transient memory or cognitive deficits, and headaches. Cognitive impairment is manifested by difficulty recalling new information (anterograde amnesia) and in remembering events before treatment (retrograde amnesia) (Squire, 1986). Transient memory impairment may endure from minutes to hours, depending on the type, number, and spacing of treatments. Transitory memory deficits are normal responses to ECT and are not considered complications (Abrams, 2002). Clients receiving bilateral ECT are more likely to experience significant loss of old information than those receiving unilateral ECT (Dannon et al., 2006).

Post-ECT agitated delirium is another adverse reaction that needs to be assessed and treated, usually with a benzodiazepine such as diazepam (Valium) or lorazepam (Ativan).

CASE STUDY

The Client Undergoing Electroconvulsive Therapy (Mrs. Moser)

Mrs. Moser is 48 years old and has been unsuccessfully treated with several antidepressants for the past 3 months. Her depression has worsened over the past month. Her husband accompanies her to the ambulatory care area for outpatient ECT. She and her husband express concern about the procedure. Mrs. Moser's history is negative for present suicidal ideations or suicidal gestures in the past. She is dressed and groomed appropriately, but her mood is depressed. She is distant and her speech is monotone and lacks spontaneity. Her husband is supportive and expresses an interest in his wife's care. Mrs. Moser is anxious about the procedure.

The nurse completes the assessment, including Mrs. Moser's understanding about ECT. The nurse reinforces instructions provided by the physician and encourages Mrs. Moser to express her feelings about the procedure. The Mosers admit they are very anxious about the procedure, but they understand its benefits and possible adverse reactions. Mrs. Moser signs the informed-consent form and reports that she has not drunk or eaten anything since midnight as instructed. She also reports that she shampooed her hair last night and has not used hairspray or creme on it. She is instructed to put on a hospital gown and empty her bladder. She is given a preoperative injection and instructed to remain in bed with the siderails up. Mr. Moser is allowed to stay in the room until she is escorted to the ECT treatment room. See Nursing Care Plans 30–1 and 30–2.

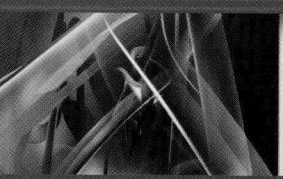

The Client Undergoing Electroconvulsive Therapy (Mrs. Moser)—Pretreatment

Nursing Diagnosis: Deficient Knowledge

Outcome identification	Nursing Actions	Rationales	Evaluation
1. By [date], Mrs. Moser will understand the ECT procedure, including its purpose, benefits, and risks.	1. Have Mrs. Moser actively participate in the informed-consent process. 2. Encourage Mrs. Moser to express her feelings, thoughts, and fears regarding ECT.	1. Enables client to make an informed decision. 2. Enables client to cope with feelings and anxiety effectively.	*Goal met:* Mrs. Moser verbalizes her understanding of ECT and voluntarily participates in informed-consent process.

Nursing Diagnosis: Anxiety

Outcome identification	Nursing Actions	Rationales	Evaluation
1. By [date], Mrs. Moser will experience minimal anxiety.	1. Approach Mrs. Moser in a calm, confident, and reassuring manner. 2. Teach Mrs. Moser relaxation techniques. 3. Continuously assess Mrs. Moser's anxiety levels.	1. Allays anxiety by providing a calm environment. 2. Reduces anxiety. 3. Provides information on clients response to stress/tension.	*Goal met:* Mrs. Moser experiences minimal anxiety regarding procedure.

Approximately 10 percent of clients develop delirium shortly after treatment. Symptoms of delirium include restlessness, disorientation, blank starring, confusion, and difficulty following instructions. Delirium normally lasts 10 to 45 minutes (Abrams, 2002). For further discussion of the symptoms of delirium, see Chapter 16.

The following are other adverse reactions to ECT:

◆ Mania

◆ Aspiration

◆ Ruptured bladder

◆ Nausea and vomiting

◆ Headaches (generally occur in one third of clients and relieved with aspirin)

Clients recovering from ECT require close monitoring to assess for return to pre-ECT mental and physical status.

Client education is an essential aspect of preparing the client and family for adverse reactions.

OTHER BIOLOGICAL THERAPIES

The efficacy and relevancy of ECT and other somatic therapies to psychiatric nursing is well documented. Recent years have heralded in other biological therapies whose efficacy are still being tested and proven to provide alternative therapies that bring relief to clients with various psychiatric conditions. The following discussion integrates complex biological processes that provide the bases of biological therapies.

BIOLOGICAL CYCLES

Major nursing interventions for the newer biological therapies are based on the client's presenting symptoms, duration

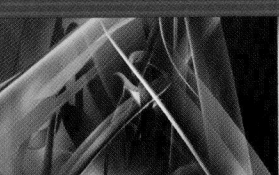

The Client Undergoing Electroconvulsive Therapy (Mrs. Moser)—Posttreatment

Nursing Diagnosis: High Risk for Injury

Outcome Identification	Nursing Actions	Rationales	Evaluation
1. By [date], Mrs. Moser will undergo ECT safely and be free of injury. Vital and neurological signs will remain within specific parameters.	1. Monitor Mrs. Moser's neurological signs.	1. Provides information on physical status and response to treatment.	*Goal met:* Mrs. Moser remains free of injury. Her vital signs return to pretreatment level (stable). She is oriented to person, place, date, and time. She is taking fluids and diet and is free of nausea and vomiting. No seizure in activity observed. She denies suicidal ideations.
	2. Put siderails up and bed in low position.	2. Reduces falls and promotes safety.	
	3. Monitor changes or adverse reaction.	3. Provides information on physical status.	
	4. Maintain quiet environment.	4. Promotes rest and facilitates return to previous level of function.	
	5. Reorient Mrs. Moser as needed.	5. Promotes cognitive function and orientation.	
	6. Observe Mrs. Moser for delirium or agitation.	6. Clients who have undergone ECT are at risk for these behaviors.	
	7. Offer Mrs. Moser oral fluids and diet as tolerated.	7. Promotes hydration/nutrition.	
	8. Maintain seizure precautions.	8. Reduces risk of injury.	
	9. Assess for symptoms of suicidality.	9. Depressed clients are at risk for this behavior. Promotes safety.	

of symptoms, level of dangerousness, and past treatment responses. In addition, nursing interventions also arise from the client's present mental and physical status and treatment preferences. Because most of the new biological interventions occur in the client's home, daily documentation is crucial to assessing the client's response and compliance.

All organisms are affected by environmental cues that modulate their biological rhythms; examples of these cues are the length of day (circadian rhythm) and the seasons. Biological rhythms are the innate pacemakers or timekeepers that mediate an organism's interpretation of its surroundings and its behavioral and biological responses. Biological rhythms are natural, expected, and vital to homeostasis and survival. Human cycles, such as the light-dark, rest-activity, reproductive, and metabolic cycles are examples of biological rhythms that are affected by environmental cues (Higashimoto et al., 2007).

Aging and certain conditions, such as shift work, sleep deprivation, and jet lag, affect the stability of biological rhythms (Higashimoto et al., 2007). The study of biological rhythms and regulation is chronobiology.

The hypothalamus is the central regulator of the circadian cycle. Environmental cues are transmitted via neural pathways of the retinohypothalamic tract (RHT). This neural pathway begins in the retina and is essential for the modulation of the circadian rhythms by light. Furthermore, certain genetic influences arise from various components, such as c-fos in the suprachiasmatic nuclei (SCN) of the hypothalamus, that regulate the circadian oscillations of a number of body functions such as temperature, sleep, and seasonal mood responses. The SCN is the primary pacemaker of the circadian system. It lies in the anterior of the hypothalamus directly above the optic chiasm, allowing it to receive visual input from the retina. The

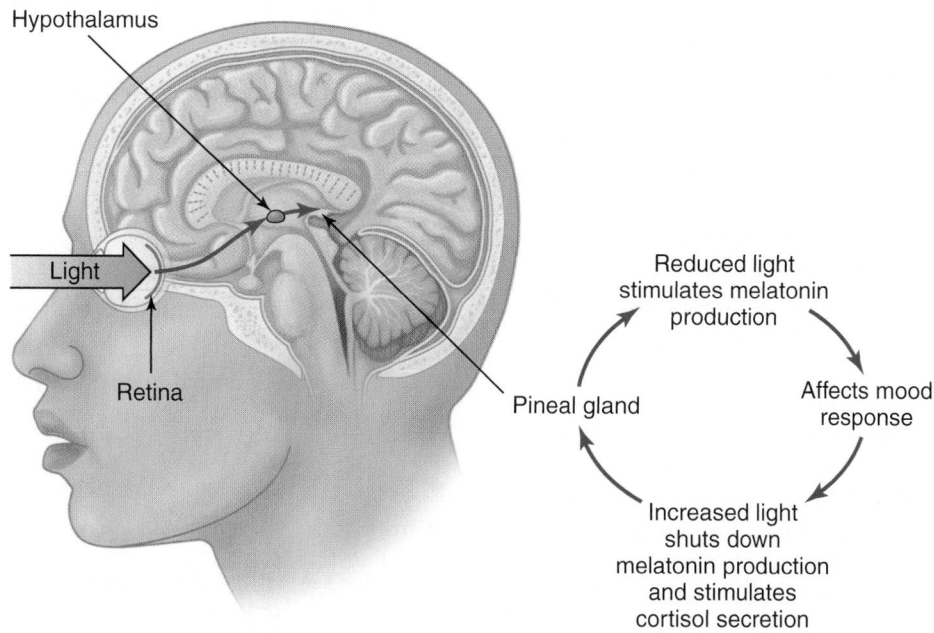

Figure 30–2 Retino-hypothalamic-pineal mechanism.

retina, through the SCN to the pineal gland, where melatonin is produced, conveys environmental cues. **Melatonin** is a chemical mediator of seasonal changes that is released during the night and reduced by light (Evans, Elliott, & Gorman, 2007) (Figure 30–2).

Conditions capable of activating the SCN include heat, dehydration, electrical stimulation, and light. The hormonal and metabolic components of the brain and body function according to a daily cycle of 24 to 25 hours in length. For example, high corticosteroid secretion occurs in the morning and high melatonin secretion from the pineal gland occurs at night. Normally, the decreased light conveyed through the retina at the end of the day leads to production of melatonin in the pineal gland. Melatonin is influenced by solar light or wavelengths of light linked with circadian phase modulation (Glickman, Byrne, Pineda, Hauck, & Brainard, 2006). Recent molecular, genetic, and behavioral research implicates individual genes as biological markers that govern circadian rhythms in mood regulation (McClung, 2007).

All biological cycles are influenced by seasonal changes linked to the timing of wavelength light, hormones and metabolism, available light, and components of the sleep-wake cycle. **Phase advancing** is a response to a light stimulus that is intentionally presented hours before the expected onset of solar or wavelength of environmental light. **Phase delaying** refers to a response elicited by a light stimulus presented hours later than expected.

New biological therapies are based on directing specific aspects of the circadian cycle to reduce symptoms of **seasonal affective disorder** (SAD). SAD is a mood disorder that occurs primarily during the fall and early winter months and remits in the spring. Symptoms often include hypersomnia; fatigue; irritability; increased appetite, especially sweet food; and atypical depression (Lewy, Lefler, Emens & Bauer, 2006). Symptoms of SAD usually occur at the same time each year. Hypersomnia refers to the need for at least 1 additional hour of sleep during the winter months than in the summer months. This symptom may represent an underlying alteration in the phase-delayed circadian rhythm, differing from terminal insomnia, which usually manifests as a phase-advanced rhythm. Light therapy or phototherapy and sleep cycle alterations are examples of methods of manipulating the circadian cycle. See Chapter 9 for more information about SAD and Chapter 23 for an in-depth discussion of sleep disorders.

LIGHT THERAPY (PHOTOTHERAPY)

Light therapy was introduced as a treatment for SAD in the 1980s (Rosenthal et al., 1984). **Light therapy** is a biological treatment that involves increased exposure to artificial light whose intensity is equivalent to outdoor levels. The goal of this treatment modality is to suppress melatonin secretion and produce phase shifts of melatonin secretion. The biological effects of light therapy make it an accepted treatment modality for SAD (Michalak et al., 2007; Terman & Terman, 2006). The effectiveness of light therapy is based on the premise that neuronal pathways that transmit light from the eye to the hypothalamus and, ultimately, to the pineal gland affect seasonal rhythms. Pineal melatonin secretion is altered by light. Light therapy suppresses nocturnal melatonin secretion, suggesting a relationship between seasonal changes and the mood of clients with SAD. Its effectiveness is linked with phase advancing and normalizing melatonin levels (Terman & Terman, 2006).

The typical process of light therapy consists of exposure to light that is about 2500 lux or 200 times stronger than usual indoor lighting. A lux is a unit of illumination equal to 1 lumen per square meter. The client is advised to establish a sleeping pattern (baseline) between 10:00 A.M. and 6:00 A.M. during the first week, during which no light treatment is given. Over the next few weeks, the client is exposed to several hours of light treatment. This normally consists of sitting 3 feet from the lights in either the morning or evening and looking at the lights every 1 or 2 minutes for 2 hours. Furthermore, the client is instructed to avoid exposure to natural morning light (Avery et al., 1991).

Dawn stimulation differs from traditional light therapy because it occurs earlier during the sleep cycle, with a gradual increase in exposure to dim light exposure. In an earlier study, Avery et al. (1993) compared the effects of dawn stimulation with placebo, using a dimmer form of light therapy introduced by Terman and Schlager (1990). The findings supported earlier research that demonstrated the effectiveness of dawn stimulation in alleviating winter depression (Avery et al., 1993).

The exact mechanism of the psychotherapeutic effects of light therapy is unknown. Clients usually show improvement within 7 days; however, the full response often occurs within several weeks. Combining light therapy with an antidepressant may also enhance the efficacy of each treatment modality.

The nursing care for the client undergoing light therapy consists of engaging the client in the informed-consent process and educating him and his family about the protocol of light therapy. The protocol for light therapy varies, but timing must be designed to secure treatment compliance.

The following is the protocol for dawn stimulation (Avery et al. (1993):

◆ Ask the client to sleep between the hours of 10:00 P.M. and 6:00 A.M.

◆ Ask the client to keep a daily log of sleeping patterns.

◆ The first week provides baseline information (no light therapy is used).

◆ Beginning with the second week, gradually expose the client to a 75-watt incandescent reflector flood light positioned 4 feet from the pillow.

◆ Gradually increase (2.2 log/lux/hour) dawn stimulation over a 2-hour period from 4:00 to 6:00 A.M. to a maximum of 250 lux.

◆ Instruct the client to avoid sunlight before 8:00 A.M.

◆ Instruct the client to avoid looking directly into the light.

The major side effects of light therapy include headaches; insomnia; agitation; eyestrain; and in clients with bipolar I disorder, recurrent mania. These symptoms may emerge after the average 2-week course of therapy (Avery et al., 1993; Levitt et al., 1993). Clients need to be assessed throughout the course of treatment for these side effects, particularly for ocular symptoms, because this is the site of entry for this form of treatment. Some question has been raised about the safety of light therapy, but most researchers agree that this is a rare occurrence even with light therapy at 10,000 lax. However, they suggested a careful ophthalmological history be taken and an ophthalmologist be consulted if retinal damage is believed to be indicated. Manifestations of retinal damage include blurred vision, glare, and floaters in red blood cells in the

RESEARCH ABSTRACT

Controlled Trial of Bright Light and Negative Air Ions for Chronic Depression

Goel, N., Terman, M., Terman, J. S., Macchi, M. M., & Stewart, J. W. (2005). *Psychological Medicine, 35,* 945–955.

Study Problem/Purpose

The aim of this study was to examine the efficacy of two nonpharmacologic treatments, bright light and high-density negative air ions for nonseasonal chronic depression.

Methods

Researchers used a randomized controlled trial that consisted of 24 women and 8 men with major depression and single episode and chronic depression. Subjects were randomly assigned to exposure to bright light (10,000 lux) or high-density or low-density placebo control (negative air ions). Blinded raters evaluated symptom severity weekly with the Structured Interview Guide for the Hamilton Depression Rating Scale—Seasonal Affective Disorder (SIGH-SAD) version. Saliva samples were collected in the evening before and after treatment for ascertainment of circadian melatonin rhythm phase.

Findings

Data revealed that the SIGH-SAD score improvement was 53.7 percent for bright light and 51.1 percent for high-density ions versus 17.0 percent for low-density ions. Researchers also found that the remission rates were 50 percent, 50 percent, and 0 percent respectively. They concluded that both bright light and negative air ions were effective for treatment of chronic depression; and remission rates were similar to those for SAD, although unrelated to seasonal patterns or mediation by circadian rhythm phase shifts.

Implications for Psychiatric Nursing

Although the traditional use of light therapy has proven efficacy in the treatment of SAD, these findings indicate it may also be useful in some clients with major depression unrelated to seasonal patterns or circadian rhythms.

vitreous humor. Other high-risk groups that may be sensitive to light therapy are clients with retinal disease, photosensitivity, systematic lupus erythematosus, and history of skin cancer. Clients with these conditions require the attention and consultation with the appropriate specialist if light therapy is to be used. Light therapy can be used as an adjunct to traditional biological therapies such as antidepressants or lithium.

SLEEP CYCLE ALTERATIONS

Altering sleep cycles is based on the premise that certain mood disorders include alterations in the 24-hour circadian cycle. Sleepiness occurs at the low point of the body temperature in the circadian rhythm. Normally, sleeping occurs in two phases: rapid eye movement, or REM, and non-REM. REM sleep is characterized by vivid dreaming and a consistently high level of brain activity. Non-REM, or slow wave, sleep is characterized by diminished brain activity. Sleep deprivation is an example of an alteration in the sleep cycle. Clients experiencing depression usually have more REM sleep and are sensitive to the timing of lightness and darkness (Gottesmann & Gottesman, 2007).

Sleep deprivation is a biological therapy that consists of depriving clients of 1 hour of REM sleep. A typical sleep deprivation regimen occurs by advancing or delaying the time the client retires for bed. Varying the sleep-wake cycle facilitates reestablishment of normal sleeping patterns. The sleep-wake cycle refers to one of the body's biological rhythms normally determined by the day-night cycle. See Chapter 23 for an in-depth discussion of sleep cycles and disorders.

COMPLEMENTARY THERAPIES

Alternative therapies are becoming increasingly popular and it is estimated that one in three people seeking conventional health care may also be using complementary therapies (Eisenberg et al., 1993). Because of the advent and prevalent use of complementary therapies, psychiatric nurses need to familiarize themselves with a basic understanding of complementary approaches and their outcome.

During the early 1990s the National Institutes of Health (NIH) formed the Office of Alternative Medicine (OAM) to evaluate an array of unconventional or alternative therapies, their usefulness, and scientific explication for their efficacy. In 1995, the OAM developed a database for disseminating data on alternative-complementary research, networking with NIH on initiative that included grant writing, organizing conferences, and clinical research projects (OAM, 1998).

The OAM changed its name to the National Center for Complementary and Alternative Medicine in the 1990s and continues to use its database to disseminate information about complementary therapies (http://nccam.nih.gov/). During the twenty-first century, various therapies, including omega-3 fatty acids, have been researched in the treatment of depression and Alzheimer's disease with inconclusive results and with implications for additional research to determine efficacy. It is imperative for psychiatric nurses to educate

themselves about these therapies, although conclusive evidence of their efficacy requires thorough investigation. Discussing these therapies with clients does not indicate that the nurse endorses these therapies, but it supports the client's decision to use complementary therapies and answers questions about side effects or potential risk associated with these therapies.

The following therapies are examples from this classification of alternative therapies, including acupuncture, aromatherapy, and massage.

ACUPUNCTURE

Acupuncture has been a part of traditional China medicine over five thousand years, and its healing techniques dates back to ancient medicine. The premise of acupuncture is that health is determined by of the balance of qi or chi, the essential life energy in all living beings. According to the acupuncture theory, chi circulates in the body along 12 major energy pathways named channels or meridians. Each meridian is linked to specific internal organs and systems. Acupuncture specialists submit that each meridian system contains over one thousand acupoints that can be stimulated to enhance the flow of chi. Acupuncture involves insertion of thin, solid, usually stainless steel needles into these acupoints (under the skin). The premise of acupuncture stems from its ability to restore and rebalance the flow of energy, thereby relieving pain and restoring health.

Acupuncture has proven to be effective in the treatment of pain by stimulating the release of the body's normal pain-killing chemicals, endorphins and enkephalins. Needle manipulation or the stimulation of cutaneous or subcutaneous tissue produces its therapeutic effects by activating strong muscle contractions and subsequent numbness, heaviness, and radiating paresthesia. This sensation resembles deep muscle pain. Both acupuncture and muscle exercise release endogenous opioids and oxytocin. Endorphins exert effects by binding to opioid receptors (Basbaum & Fields, 1984). Other researchers attribute relief to stimulation of vast neurotransmitters and neuromodulators, thereby altering the perception of pain. Similar effects are believed to play a role in mood disorders and substance abuse. Acupuncture has also been used to treat headaches (Cabyoglu, Ergene, & Tan, 2006), dysmenorrhea, and mood and anxiety disorders (Manber, Schnyer, Allen, Rush, & Blasey, 2004). Acupuncture is thought to promote a sense of well-being, calmness, and improved sleep in clients with mood and anxiety disorders (Cabyoglu, Ergene, & Tan, 2006).

AROMATHERAPY

The use of oils for religious and healing purposes dates back to biblical and historical times and famous seductions, such as Cleopatra. Aromatherapy was coined by French chemist Rene-Maurice Gattefosse in 1928 and has become one of the most popular alternative therapies throughout the world. Aromatherapy is a unique form of herbal medicine that uses the healing properties of essential oils of various plants. Through a process of steam distillation or cold-pressing, the volatile essences of the plant's oil are extracted. In aromatherapy, plant or herbal oils are inhaled using atomizers or they are readily absorbed through the skin through baths, hot or cold compresses, massage, or topical application of diluted oils. Aromatic molecules interact with various body surfaces that are modified by vast biological processes before affecting the limbic system. Global effects of aromatherapy are believed to produce an array of healing or therapeutic effects by interacting with the body's immune system, central nervous system, and gastrointestinal and circulatory systems, modulating mood and emotional states. Researchers showed that several essential oils altered brain wave activity. These data show that oils such as basil, rosemary, jasmine, peppermint, rose, and cloves work by heightening or stimulating energy levels. Essential oils that produce a calming or tranquilizing effect include orange, lavender, neroli, lemon, lavender, sandalwood, and chamomile (Hur et al., 2007; Lin, Chan, Ng, & Lam, 2007).

MASSAGE THERAPY

Massage therapy, along with other alternative therapies, was part of ancient Chinese culture of maintaining health. Massage therapy is believed to produce calming effects on the central nervous system and promote muscle relaxation. Ultimately, these effects increase circulation, improve the flow of lymph, and have metabolic and visceral effects (Soden, Vincent, Craske, Lucas, & Ashley, 2004).

In conclusion, alternative therapies are used to treat vast medical, addictive, and mental disorders. Psychiatric nurses must familiarize themselves with various alternative therapies and, when appropriate, integrate them with conventional therapies and develop individualized care to restore holistic health care. If clients choose alternative therapies, nurses need to caution them about potential side effects and discourage them from abandoning traditional treatment unless they consult with their primary care provider.

NURSING RESEARCH AND BIOLOGICAL THERAPIES

Historically, psychiatric-mental health nursing research has paralleled psychiatric paradigms. The Decade of the Brain prompted a shift from a primarily psychological-behavioral paradigm, based on interactions with the client, to the study of the impact of neurological process on behavior. The vast interest in the science of neurobiology and advances in technological studies of the brain has resulted in expanded opportunities for psychiatric-mental health research by nurses.

The psychiatric nurse's involvement in research varies according to his interest, educational level, and expertise in the research process. Some nurses may be able to collaborate with others to develop treatment research protocols. Other psychiatric nurses may prescribe or administer research medication or other biological therapies. Regardless of their role, nurses involved in research use the nursing process to assess client needs, formulate client outcomes and interventions, and evaluate and modify client responses to protocols. Aromatherapy, massage therapy, manipulation of circadian or sleep-wake cycles, or light therapy are examples of biological therapies that nurses can use to modify distressful behaviors.

SUMMARY

- ◆ The emergence of biological therapies in the 1930s laid the foundation of many of today's interventions.

- ◆ One of the earliest and continually controversial therapies is ECT.

- ◆ Advances in neurobiology and neuroimaging studies have increased the legitimacy of ECT for treating specific client populations.

- ◆ Nurses play a vital role in educating and providing emotional comfort to clients undergoing ECT.

- ◆ Psychiatric nurses must familiarize themselves with alternative therapies and be able to integrate them into conventional treatment.

- ◆ Newer biological therapies are innovative strategies designed to help clients suffering from SAD and sleep cycle disturbances.

- ◆ Numerous research and educational opportunities have emerged for nurses as a result of the advent of newer biological therapies.

SUGGESTIONS FOR CLINICAL CONFERENCES

1. Invite a nurse who is experienced in massage therapy or aromatherapy to demonstrate various techniques and relate them to the treatment of various psychiatric disorders. Encourage students to discuss benefits and potential adverse effects of these techniques.

2. Present a case history of a client undergoing ECT.

3. Present case histories of clients who were treated with ECT.

4. Divide group into groups on the basis of their feelings and thoughts about ECT and debate issues.

5. Discuss ethical and legal considerations related to somatic therapies.

6. Explain the nursing care of a client undergoing light therapy.

STUDY QUESTIONS

1. Mrs. Watson is a 54-year-old recently widowed client who is seen in the community mental health center complaining of depression. Which of the following

comments makes her a good candidate for electroconvulsive therapy?

  a. She expresses fears of her dead spouse returning to seek revenge.

  b. She reports thoughts of not wanting to get up some mornings.

  c. She states that she really misses her spouse.

  d. She states that she needs to spend time alone to deal with her grief.

2. Mr. Jones has signed a release form for ECT. An important nursing intervention for pre-ECT is which of the following?

  a. Ask if he has shampooed and removed all creams and oils from his hair.

  b. Instruct him to take several sips of water to reduce oral dryness.

  c. Explain that he will probably have to spend several days in the hospital post-ECT.

  d. Instruct him not to remove his dentures.

3. A major contraindication for ECT is hypertension. The major reason for this condition is:

  a. ECT produces cardiovascular overload and increases circulating catecholamines.

  b. ECT reduces oxygen consumption and increases the risk of a stroke.

  c. When the seizure ceases, the client may experience transient hypotension and tachycardia.

  d. Anesthesia induction decreases the heart rate and produces bradycardia.

4. Mary is a 26-year-old woman who complains of depression and increased appetite during the winter months. She asks the nurse why this happens. What is the best explanation for this disorder?

  a. Decreased exposure to sunlight decreases melatonin production and depression.

  b. Depression during winter months stems from holiday stress.

  c. Winter months often contribute to people staying inside, thereby increasing isolation.

  d. Decreased exposure to sunlight increases the production of melatonin.

5. Markie has been diagnosed with seasonal affective depression and is in her third week of phototherapy. As her nurse you have informed her to report which of the following reactions?

  a. Rhinorrhea and nasal stuffiness

  b. Eye redness and burning

  c. Alopecia or hair loss

  d. Difficulty swallowing

6. The efficacy of acupuncture in treating mood and anxiety disorders involves activation of which of the following?

  a. Norepinephrine

  b. Endorphins

  c. Monoamine oxidase

  d. Serotonin

7. Mr. Carlos is an airline pilot and he presents complaining of difficulty sleeping. An important approach that assists in restoring his normal sleeping patterns involves phase advancing. Which of the following best describes this intervention?

  a. Instruct him to go to bed late and wake up later than usual.

  b. Instruct him to go to bed early and wake up earlier than usual.

  c. Instruct him to stay awake as long as possible until he falls asleep.

  d. Instruct him to avoid caffeine or excessive exercise before going to bed.

8. One of your depressed clients is scheduled for transcranial magnetic stimulation (TMS). Which of the following statements indicates her understanding of this procedure?

  a. "I am so glad I will be awake because being put to sleep is frightening."

  b. "I am very nervous about being put to sleep."

  c. "I understand that permanent memory loss is a potential side effect of this procedure."

  d. "I am going to be depression-free after the procedure."

9. The nurse is caring for a client with depression who is scheduled for ECT. Which of the following is essential for the nurse to include in his post-ECT plan?

  a. Ask the client to repeat his name and DOB post-procedure

  b. Explain to the family that the waiting time is about 5 hours.

  c. Encourage the client to breathe deeply when awakening post-ECT.

  d. Ask the client to be careful when getting up the first time after the procedure.

10. A client with major depression is scheduled for ECT tomorrow. The nurse would plan for which of the following activities?

  a. Force fluids 6 to 8 hours before treatment.

  b. Administer succinylcholine (Anectine) during pretreatment care.

  c. Encourage the client's spouse or partner to accompany him.

  d. Reorient the client frequently during posttreatment care.

11. A severely depressed client received ECT this morning. Which of the findings listed below would the nurse *least* expect to assess posttreatment?

  a. Headache

  b. Memory loss

  c. Paralytic ileus

  d. Disorientation

RESOURCES

Please note that because Internet resources are of a time-sensitive nature and URL addresses may change or be deleted, searches should also be conducted by association or topic.

Internet Resources

http://www.acupuncture.com/ Acupuncture resources for patients, practitioners, and students.

http://www.life.uiuc.edu/jeff/alextech.html Alexander technique

http://www.nice.org.uk/ pdf/59ectenglishfp.pdf National Institute for Clinical Excellence (2003). *Guidance in the Use of Electroconvulsive Therapy.* (Accessed February 24, 2006)

http://www.nice.org.uk/page.aspx?o=68305 National Institute for Clinical Excellence NICE (2003). Guidance on the Use of Electroconvulsive Therapy—Full Guidance. (Accessed March 30, 2006).

http://www.mum.edu/TM_Research_home.html Scientific Research on the Transcendental Meditation Program

Other Resources

Tao of Wellness
A Professional Acupuncture Corp.
1131 Wilshire Blvd. #300
Santa Monica, CA 90401
(310) 917-2200
Fax: (310) 917-2205

Tianyou Hao
Case Western Reserve School of Medicine, "Chinese Qigong"
Cleveland, OH
(216) 368-2229

Biofeedback Training Associates
255 West 98th St.
New York, NY 10025
(212) 222-5665

REFERENCES

Abrams, R. (2002). *Electroconvulsive therapy,* 4th ed. New York: Oxford University Press.

American Nurses Association. (2000). *Scope and standards of psychiatric-mental health nursing practice.* Washington, DC: American Nurses Publishing.

American Psychiatric Association Task Force on Electroconvulsive Therapy 2nd ed. (2001). *The practice of electroconvulsive therapy: Recommendations for psychiatric training and privileging.* Washington, DC: American Psychiatric Press.

American Psychiatric Association. (2000). *Diagnostic and statistical manual of mental disorders* (4th ed., Text Revision). Washington, DC: Author.

Avery, D. H., Bolte, M. A., Dager, S. R., Wilson, L. G., Weyer, M., Cox, G. B., et al. (1993). Dawn stimulation treatment of winter depression: A controlled study. *American Journal of Psychiatry, 150,* 113–117.

Avery, D. H., Khan, A., Dager, S. R., Cohen, S., Cox, G. B., & Dunner, D. L. (1991). Morning or evening bright light treatment of winter depression? The significance of hypersomnia. *Biological Psychiatry, 29,* 117–126.

Baldwin, R., Jeffries, S., Jackson, A., Sutcliffe, C., Thacker, N., Scott, M., & Burns, A. (2004). Treatment response in late-onset depression: Relationship to neuropsychological, neuroradiological and vascular risk factors. *Psychology Medicine, 34,* 125–136.

Basbaum, A. I. & Fields, H. L. (1984). Endogenous pain control pathways: Brain-stem pathways and endorphin circuitry. *Annual Review of Neuroscience, 7,* 309–338.

Black, J. L. (1993). ECT: Lessons learned about an old treatment with new technologies. *Psychiatric Annals, 23,* 7–14.

Brodaty, J., Berle, D., Hickie, I., & Mason, C. (2003). Perceptions of outcome from electroconvulsive therapy by depressed patients and psychiatrists. *The Australian and New Zealand Journal of Psychiatry, 37,* 196–199.

Bullock, M. L., Kiresuk, T. J., Pheley, A. M., Culliton, P. D., Lenz, S. K. (1999). Auricular acupuncture in the treatment of cocaine abuse: A study of efficacy and dosing. *Journal of Substance Abuse Treament, 16,* 31–38.

Cabyoglu, M. T., Ergene, N., & Tan, U. (2006). The mechanism of acupuncture and clinical applications. *International Journal of Neuroscience, 116,* 115–125.

Cerletti, U. (1950). Old and new information about electroshock. *American Journal of Psychiatry, 107,* 87–94.

Chanpattana, W., Chakrabhand, M. L., Sackeim, H. A., Kitaroonchai, W., Kongsakon, R., Techakasem, P., et al. (1999). Continuation of ECT in treatment-resistant schizophrenia: A controlled study. *Journal of ECT, 15,* 178–192.

Coffey, C. E., & Weiner, R. D. (1990). Electroconvulsive therapy: An update. *Hospital and Community Psychiatry, 41,* 515–521.

Cohen, H., Kaplan, Z., Kotler, M., Kouperman, I., Moisa, R., & Grisaru, N. (2004). Repetitive transcranial magnetic stimulation of the right dorsolateral prefrontal cortex in posttraumatic stress disorder: A double-blind, placebo-controlled study. *American Journal of Psychiatry, 161,* 515–524.

Dannon, P. N., Lowengrub, K., Gonopolski, Y., & Kotler, M. (2006). Current and emerging somatic treatment strategies in psychotic major depression. *Expert Review of Neurotherapeutics, 6,* 73–80.

Dowman, J., Patel, A., & Rajput, K. (2005). Electroconvulsive therapy: Attitudes and misconceptions. *Journal of ECT, 21,* 84–87.

Eisenberg, D. M., Kessler, R. C., Foster, C., Norlock, F. E., Calkins, D. R., & Delbanco, T. L. (1993). Unconventional medicine in the United States: Prevalence, costs and patterns of use. *New England Journal of Medicine, 328,* 246–252.

Evans, J. A., Elliott, J. A., & Gorman, M. R. (2007). Circadian effects of light no brighter than moonlight. *Journal of Biological Rhythms, 22,* 356–367.

Fink, M. (1991). Impact of the antipsychiatry movement on the revival of electroconvulsive therapy in the United States. *Psychiatric Clinics of North America, 14,* 793–801.

Fitzgerald, P. B., Benitez, J., de Castella, A., Daskalakis, Z. J., Brown, T. L., & Kulkarni, J. A. (2006). A randomized, controlled trial of sequential bilateral repetitive transcranial magnetic stimulation for treatment-resistant depression. *American Journal of Psychiatry, 163,* 88–94.

Fitzgerald, P. B., Brown, J., Marston, N. A., Daskalakis, Z. J., de Castella, A., & Kulkarni, J. A. (2003). Transcranial magnetic stimulation in the treatment of depression: A double-blind, placebo-controlled trial. *Archives of General Psychiatry, 60,* 1002–1008.

Flaherty, A. W., Williams, Z. M., Amirnovin, R., Kasper, E., Rauch, S. L., Cosgrove, G. R., & Eskandar, E. N. (2005). Deep brain stimulation of the anterior internal capsule for the treatment of Tourette syndrome: Technical case report. *Neurosurgery, 57* (4 Suppl.), E403.

Gagné, G. G., Furman, M. J., Carpenter, L. L., & Price, L. H. (2000). Efficacy of continuation ECT and antidepressant drugs compared to long-term antidepressants alone in depressed patients. *American Journal of Psychiatry, 157,* 1960–1965.

Ghaziuddin, N., Kutcher, S. P., Knapp, P., Bernet, W., Arnold, V., Beitchman, J., Bensent, R. S., et al., (2004). Practice parameter for use of electroconvulsive therapy with adolescents. *Journal of the American Academy of Child and Adolescent Psychiatry, 43,* 1521–1539.

Glickman, G., Byrne, B., Pineda, C., Hauck, W. W., & Brainard, G. C. (2006). Light therapy for seasonal affective disorder with blue narrow-band light emitting diodes (LEDS). *Biological Psychiatry, 59,* 502–507

Gottesmann, C., & Gottesman, I. (2007). The neurobiological characteristics of rapid eye movement (REM) sleep are candidate endophenotypes of depression, schizophrenia, mental retardation and dementia. *Progress in Neurobiology, 81,* 237–250.

Greenhalgh, J., Knight, C., Hind, D., Beverley, C., & Walters, S. (2005). Clinical and cost-effectiveness of electroconvulsive therapy for depressive illness, schizophrenia, catatonia and mania: Systematic reviews and economic modelling studies. *Health Technology Assessment, 9,* 1–156, iii–iv.

Grover, S., Mattoo, S. K., & Gupta, M. (2005). Theories on the mechanism of electrovulsive therapy. *German Journal of Psychiatry, 8,* 70–84.

Higashimoto, M., Homma, Y., Umetsu, M., Konno, Y., Ono, K., Yoshimoto, N., et al. (2007). Circadian rhythm of apoprotein H (beta2-glycoprotein-1) in human plasma. *Biochemical and Biophysical Research Communications, 360,* 418–422.

Hur, M. H., Oh, H., Lee, M. S., Kim, C., Choi, A. N., & Shin, G. R. (2007). Effects of aromatherapy massage on blood pressure and lipid profile in Korean climacteric women. *International Journal of Neuroscience, 117,* 1281–1287.

Husain, M. M., Montgomery, J. H., Fernandes, P., & Morrow, L. (2002). Safety of vagus nerve stimulation with ECT. *American Journal of Psychiatry, 159,* 1243 [Letter].

Huuhka, M. J., Seinela, L., Reinikainen, P., & Leinonen, E. V. (2003). Cardiac arrhythmias induced by ECT in elderly psychiatric patients: Experience with 48-hour Holter monitoring. *Journal of ECT, 19,* 22–25.

Jimenez-Vasquez, P. A., Diaz-Cabiale, Z., Caberlotto, L., Bellido, I., Overstreet, D., Fuxe, K., et al. (2007). Electroconvulsive stimuli selectively affect behavior and neuropeptide Y (NPY) and NPY Y(1) receptor gene expressions in hippocampus and hypothalamus of Flinders Sensitive Line rat model of depression. *European Neuropsychopharmacology, 17,* 298–308.

Kalinowsky, L. B. & Hoch, P. H. (1950). *Shock treatment and other somatic treatments in psychiatry.* New York: Grune & Stratton.

Kang, N., & Passmore, M. J. (2004). Successful ECT in a patient with an orbital cavernous hemangioma. *Journal of ECT, 20,* 267–271.

Kho, K. H., Zwinderman, A. H., & Blansjaar, B. A. (2005). Predictors for the efficacy of electroconvulsive therapy: Chart review of a naturalistic study. *Journal of Clinical Psychiatry, 66,* 894–899.

Kramer, B. A. (1985). Use of ECT in California, 1977–1983. *American Journal of Psychiatry, 142,* 1190–1192.

Kramer, B. A. (1999). Use of ECT in California, revisited: 1984–1994. *Journal of ECT, 15,* 245–251.

Lalitanatpong, D. (2005). The use of electroconvulsive therapy and the length of stay of psychiatric inpatients at King Chulalongkorn Memorial Hospital, Thai Red Cross Society. *Journal of the Medical Association of Thailand, 88*(Suppl. 4), S142–S148.

Lerer, B., Shapira, C., Calev, A., Tubi, N., Drexler, H., Kindler, S., et al. (1995). Antidepressant and cognitive effects of twice-versus three-times-weekly ECT. *American Journal of Psychiatry, 152,* 564–570.

Levitt, A. J., Joffee, R. T., Moul, D. E., Lam, L. W., Teicher, M. H., Lebegue, B., et al. (1993). Side effects of light therapy in seasonal affective disorders. *American Journal of Psychiatry, 150,* 650–652.

Lewy, A. J., Lefler, B. J., Emens, J. S., & Bauer, V. K. (2006). The circadian basis of winter depression. *Proceedings of the National Academy of Science of the United States of America, 103,* 7414–7419.

Lieberman, A. (2006). Depression in Parkinson's disease—A review. *Acta Neurologica Psychiatrica, 113,* 1–8.

Lin, P. W., Chan, W. C., Ng, B. F., & Lam, L. C. (2007). Efficacy of aromatherapy (Lavandula angustifolia) as an intervention for agitated behaviours in Chinese older persons with dementia: A cross-over randomized trial. *International Journal of Geriatric Psychiatry, 22,* 405–410.

Manber, R., Schnyer, R. N., Allen, J. J., Rush, A. J., & Blasey, C. M. (2004). Acupuncture: A promising treatment for depression during pregnancy. *Journal of Affective Disorder, 83,* 89–95.

Marangell, L. B., Silver, J. M. & Yudofsky, S. C. (1999). Psychopharmacology and electroconvulsive therapy. In R. E. Hales, S. C. Yudofsky, & J. A. Talbott, *Textbook of Psychiatry,* (3rd ed. pp. 1025–1132). Washington, DC: American Psychiatric Press Inc.

McClung, C. A. (2007). Circadian genes, rhythms and the biology of mood disorders. *Pharmacology and Therapeutics, 114,* 222–232.

Michalak, E. E., Murray, G., Levitt, A. J., Levitan, R. D., Enns, M. W., Morehouse, R., et al. (2007). Quality of life as an outcome indicator in patients with seasonal affective disorder: Results from the Can-SAD study. *Psychological Medicine, 37,* 727–736.

Millon, T. (1969). Modern psychopathology: A biosocial approach to maladaptive learning and functioning. Philadelphia: W. B. Saunders.

Moniz, E. (1936). Prefrontal leucotomy in the treatment of mental disorder. *American Journal of Psychiatry, 93,* 1379–1385.

Munday, J., Deans, C., & Little, J. (2003). Effectiveness of a training program for ECT nurses. *Journal of Psychosocial Nursing and Mental Health Services, 41,* 20–26.

Naguib, M., & Koorn, R. (2002). Interactions between psychotropics, anaesthetics, and electroconvulsive therapy: Implications for drug choice and patient management. *CNS Drugs, 16,* 229–247.

Nelson, A. I. (2005). A national survey of electroconvulsive therapy use in the Russian Federation. *Journal of ECT, 21,* 151–157.

Nuttall, G. A., Bowersox, M. R., Douglass, S. B., McDonald, J., Rasmussen, L. J., Decker, P. A., et al. (2004). Morbidity and mortality in the use of electroconvulsive therapy. *Journal of ECT, 20,* 237–241.

Office of Alternative Medicine. (1998). Mission Statement *Complementary and Alternative Medicine in NIH, 5,* 8.

Olfson, M., Marcus, S., Sackeim, H. A., Thompson, J., Pincus, H. A. (1998). Use of ECT for the inpatient treatment of recurrent major depression. *American Journal of Psychiatry, 155,* 22–29.

Pacella, B. L., Barrera, E. S., & Kalinowsky, L. (1942). Variations in the electroencephalogram associated with electroshock therapy in patients with mental disorders. *Archives of Neuro-Psychiatry, 47,* 367–384.

Peled, A. (2006). Brain profiling and clinical-neuroscience. *Medical Hypotheses, 67,* 941–946.

Pinette, M. G., Santarpio, C., Wax, J. R., & Blackstone, J. (2007). Electroconvulsive therapy in pregnancy, *Obstetrics & Gynecology, 110,* 465–466.

Rasmussen, K. G., Perry, C. L., Sutor, B., & Moore, K. M. (2007). ECT in patients with intracranial masses. *Journal of Neuropsychiatry and Clinical Neuroscience, 19,* 191–193.

Rauch, S. L., & Cosgrove, G. E. (2000). Neurosurgical treatments. In B. J. Sadock & V. A. Sadock (Eds.), *Comprehensive textbook of psychiatry,* (7th ed. Vol. 1, pp. 2516–2520). Philadelphia: Lippincott Williams & Wilkins.

Richards, D. S. (2007). Is electroconvulsive therapy in pregnancy safe? *Obstetrics & Gynecology, 110,* 451–452.

Rosenthal, N. E., Sack, D. A., Gillin, J. C., Lewy, A. J., Goodwin, F. K., Davenport, Y., et al. (1984). Seasonal affective disorder: A description of the syndrome and preliminary findings of light therapy. *Archives of General Psychiatry, 41,* 72–80.

Royal College of Nursing. (1987). RCN nursing guidelines for ECT. *Convulsive Therapy, 3,* 158–160.

Rush, A. J., George, M. S., Sackeim, H. A., Marangell, L. B., Husain, M. M., Giller, C., et al. (2000). Vagus nerve stimulation (VNS) for treatment resistant depressions: A multicenter study. *Biological Psychiatry, 47,* 276–286.

Sackeim, H. A., Rush, A. J., George, M. S., Marangell, L. B., Husain, M. M., Nahas, Z., et al. (2001). Vagus nerve stimulation (VNS) predictors for treatment-resistant depression: Efficacy, side effects, and predictors of outcome. *Neuropsychopharmacology, 25,* 713–728.

Sakel, M. (1938). *The pharmacological shock treatment of schizophrenia.* New York: Nervous and Mental Disease.

Schachter, S. C., & Saper, C. B. (1998). Vagus nerve stimulator. *Epilepsia, 39,* 677–686.

Segal, J., Szabo, C. P., & du Toit, J. (2004). Child and adolescent electroconvulsive: A case report. *World Journal of Biological Psychiatry, 5,* 221–229.

Soden, K., Vincent, K., Craske, S., Lucas, C., & Ashley, S. (2004). A randomized controlled trial of aromatherapy massage in a hospice setting. *Palliative Medicine, 18,* 87–92.

Squire, L. R. (1986). Memory functions as affected by electroconvulsive therapy. *Annals of New York Academy of Science, 462,* 307–314.

Steele, K. M., & Manfreda, M. L. (1959). *Psychiatric nursing* (6th ed.). Philadelphia: F. A. Davis.

Steward, R. M., Desaloms, J. M., & Sanghera, M. K. (2005). Stimulation of the subthalamic nucleus for the treatment of Parkinson's disease: Postoperative management, programming, and rehabilitation. *Journal of Neuroscience Nursing, 37,* 108–111.

Strome, E. M., Zis, A. P., & Doudet, D. J. (2007). Electroconvulsive shock enhances striatal dopamine D1 and D3 receptor binding and improves motor performance in 6-OHDA-lesioned rats. *Journal of Psychiatry and Neuroscience, 32,* 193–202.

Takano, H., Motohashi, N., Uema, T., Ogawa, K., Ohnishi, T., Nishikawa, M., et al. (2007). Changes in regional cerebral blood flow during acute electroconvulsive therapy in patients with depression: Positron emission tomographic study. *British Journal of Psychiatry, 190,* 63–68.

Terman, M., & Schlager, D. S. (1990). Twilight therapies, winter depression, melatonin and sleep. In J. Montpaisir & R. Godbout (Eds.). *Sleep and biological rhythms: Basic mechanisms and application to psychiatry* (pp. 113–128). New York: Oxford University Press.

Terman, M., & Terman, J. S. (2006). Controlled trial of naturalistic dawn simulation and negative air ionization for seasonal affective disorder. *American Journal of Psychiatry, 163,* 2126–2133.

U.S. Census Bureau, Population Estimates Program. (2000). Resident population estimates of the United States by sex, race, and Hispanic origin: April 1, 1990, to July 1, 1999, with short-term projection to November 1, 2000. http://www.census.gov/population/estimates/nation/intfile3-1.txt

U.S. Congress. (1989). *Decade of the brain proclamation*. Public Law 101–158 (HJ Res. 174). July 25, 1989, 130 STAT. 152–154.

Velasco, F., Velasco, M., Jimenez, F., & Salin-Pascual, R. (2005). Neurobiological background for performing surgical intervention in the inferior thalamic peduncle for the treatment of major depression disorders. *Neurosurgery, 57,* 439–448.

Welch, C. A. (1997). Electroconvulsive therapy in the general hospital. In N. H. Cassem, T. A. Stern, J. F. Rosenbaum, & M. S. Jellinek (Eds.), *Massachusetts General Hospital handbook of general hospital psychiatry* (4th ed., pp. 89–99). St Louis: Mosby–Year Book.

SUGGESTED READINGS

Birch, S., Hammerschlag, R. (1996). *Acupuncture efficacy: A compendium of controlled clinical trials*. Tarrytown, NY: National Academy of Acupuncture and Oriental Medicine.

Encyclopedia of complementary practices. (1999). New York: Springer.

Holmes, C., Hopkins, V., Hensford, C., MacLaughlin, V., Wilkinson, D., & Rosenvinge, H. (2002). Lavender oil for agitated behavior in severe dementia: A placebo-controlled study. *International Journal of Geriatric Psychiatry, 17*(4), 305–308.

Ottosson, J. O., & Fink, M. (2005). *Ethics in electroconvulsive therapy*. New York: Brunner-Routledge.

Snyder, M., & Lindquist, R. (1998). *Complementary/alternative therapies in nursing* (3rd ed.). New York: Springer.

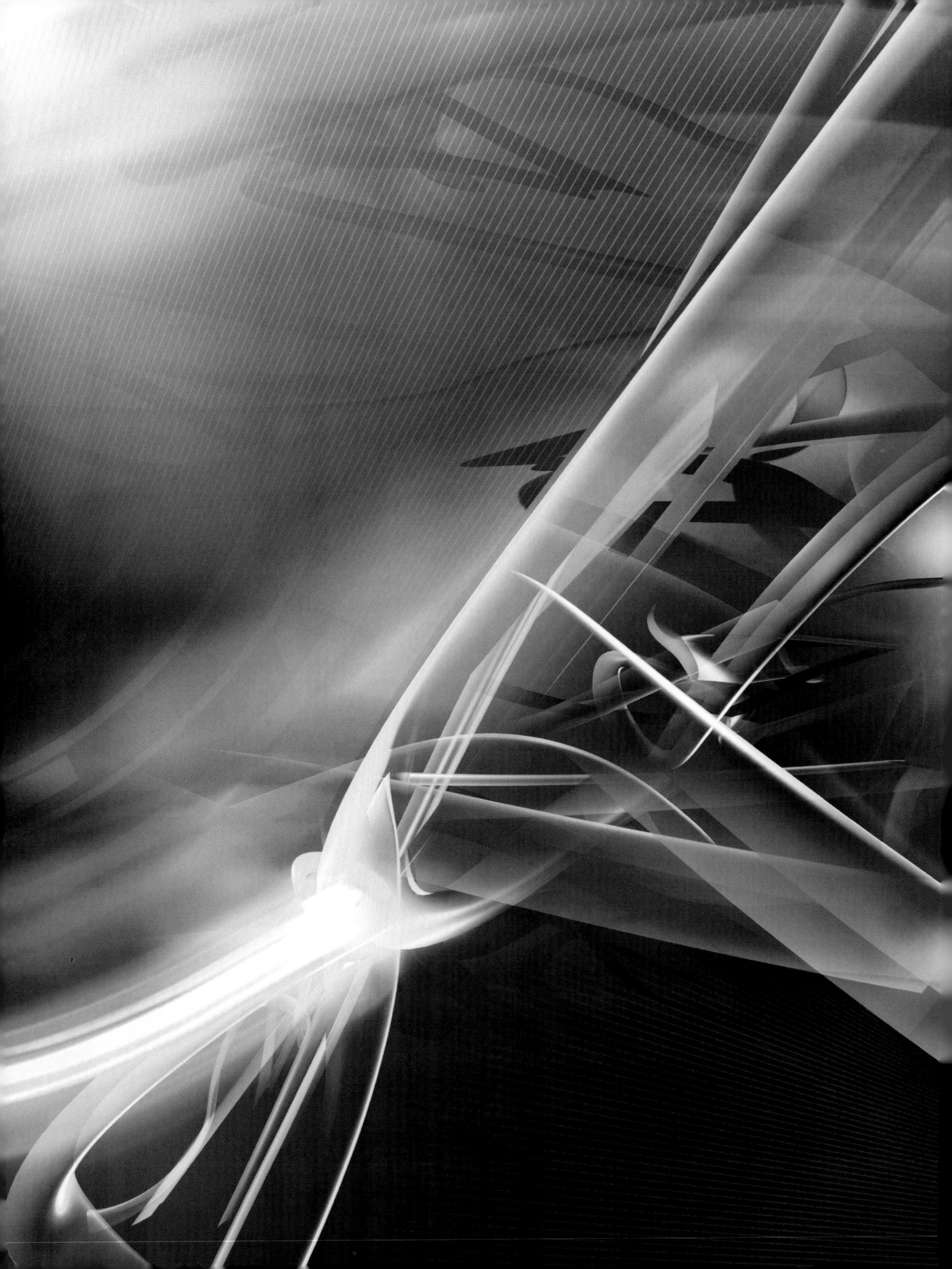

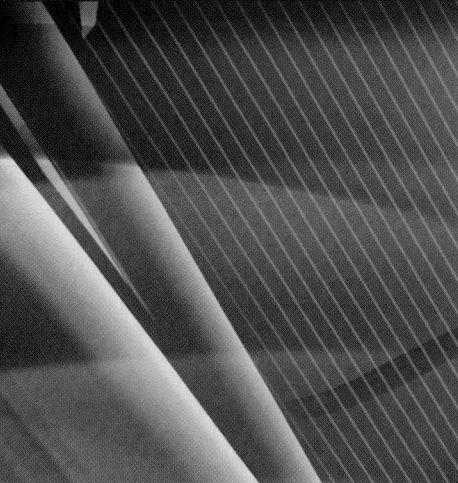

CHAPTER 31

Crisis Intervention Management: The Role of Adaptation

Deborah Antai-Otong, MS, APRN, BC, FAAN

KEY TERMS

Adaptation: Refers to sustaining homeostasis; the ability to mobilize resources and adjust to demands of internal and external environments.

Crisis: A turning point, or acute emotional turmoil, that stems from developmental, biological, situational, or psychosocial stressors that momentarily render the person's normal coping mechanisms inadequate.

Crisis Intervention: Short-term, here-and-now focus intervention that alleviates the impact of crisis-generated stress, enhances coping and problem-solving skills, and mobilizes resources of affected clients.

Disaster: Refers to a sudden, unexpected, and calamitous event that leads to great loss, damage, or destruction.

Grief: A normal profound response to loss.

Maturational Crisis: Refers to developmental stages marked by biological, psychosocial, and social transitions that generate predictable and characteristic disturbances in behavior and emotional responses.

Situational Crisis: Refers to unexpected crisis that arises from several sources, including environmental, physical or personal, or psychosocial.

Stress: A stimulus or demand that generates disruption in homeostasis or produces a reaction.

Stress Debriefing: A crisis intervention technique that relies on three therapeutic modalities: provide an opportunity to express one's feelings in the context of group support, facilitate normalization of reactions to an abnormal event, and learn about postdisaster reactions.

COMPETENCIES

Upon completion of this chapter, the learner should be able to:

1. Discuss major components of crisis intervention.
2. Differentiate between normal and abnormal grief reactions.
3. Compare maturational and situational crises.
4. Describe major factors that affect the response to disasters.
5. Recognize factors that affect the outcome of crisis situations.
6. Describe factors that influence the outcome of family crises.
7. Differentiate the role of the generalist nurse and the advanced-practice nurse in crisis management.

CHAPTER OUTLINE

Crisis

Stress

Adaptation

Perspectives and Theories

Legislative Influences: The Community Mental Health Movement

Crisis Theory
> Origins of Crisis Theory

Psychoanalytical Theories
> Sigmund Freud
> Erik Erikson's Maturational Crisis

Grief Theory
> Erik Lindemann
> Management of Grief Reactions

Crisis is an integral aspect of human growth and development. Successful resolution of crisis is a complex process shaped by one's repertoire of adaptive coping behaviors. The core of coping behaviors parallels ego function, developmental stage, and neurobiological and psychosocial factors.

The terms crisis and *stress* are often used interchangeably and are related to adaptation. Delineating the meaning of these terms is important to understanding the concept of crisis.

This chapter discusses the historical aspects of crisis theory, analyzes major concepts of crisis management, and defines the role of the psychiatric-mental health nurse in helping clients experiencing crises across the life span.

CRISIS

The concept of crisis is often associated with the potential for adaptive responses and usually not akin to illness. It is a symbol of danger or opportunity. In contrast, the concept of stress is often associated with negative connotations or potential for

illness (Rapoport, 1965). People are constantly adapting to internal and external changes that are critical to survival, health, and growth. Adaptation to these demands depends on mobilization of psychological and physiological resources.

What is a crisis and how is it different from stress? Caplan (1961, p. 18) defined a crisis as a situation "when a person faces an obstacle to important life goals that is, for a time, insurmountable through the utilization of customary methods of problem-solving. A period of disorganization ensues, a period of upset, during which many abortive attempts at solutions are made." In other words, crisis refers to acute emotional turmoil that stems from developmental, biological, situational, or psychosocial stressors that momentarily render the person's normal coping mechanisms inadequate.

Successful resolution of crisis is a complex process and represents adaptive responses to stressful encounters. Crises evolve when normal coping mechanisms fail to abate anxiety. Failure to reduce stress using normal coping behaviors often results in an increase in anxiety and tension and feelings of helplessness, unfolding into a state of turmoil. A crisis situation is also a time in which individual ego defenses are amenable to growth and adaptive change (Caplan, 1961, 1964; Davanloo, 1978).

STRESS

Stress involves a reaction to a stressful event and circumstances that precipitated it. No two people respond to stressors in the same manner. A stressor can be psychological or physiological, and its source can be both internal or external. Selye (1976) described stress as the body's nonspecific response to demand in terms of potential illness or disequilibrium. Stressful events are potential sources of crises if they are not handled effectively.

Lazarus (1966) disputed the notion that stress only depicts illness or potential for maladaptation. He suggested that stress is a complex phenomenon that influences adaptation and that it is associated with stimulus or response. In simple terms, stress is a relationship between the person and the environment that is appraised as taxing or surpassing available resources and threatening one's well-being (Lazarus & Folkman, 1984).

Other investigators minimize the impact of stress and refer to it as meaningless and insignificant. They contend that this term is outdated and its uses should be limited to catastrophes or disasters (Dimsdale, Keefe, & Stein, 2000; Weiner, 1985). Despite this early notion, the adverse impact of acute and chronic stress on mental and physical health is well documented. It challenges psychiatric nurses to understand the complexity and role of stress in adaptation and health and remains an integral part of psychiatric-mental health nursing.

ADAPTATION

The term *adaptation* stems from the Latin word *adaptare*, which means to adjust, and it is defined as a turning point in which adaptive coping responses are used to manage stressful situations. Adaptive responses are those that maintain homeostasis or health, such as survival, maturity, procreation, and mastery of developmental tasks (Andrews & Roy, 1986).

PERSPECTIVES AND THEORIES

This section describes the major changes in American psychiatry and explains crisis, psychoanalytical, and grief theories.

LEGISLATIVE INFLUENCES: THE COMMUNITY MENTAL HEALTH MOVEMENT

The Joint Commission on Mental Health and Mental Illness introduced the modern concepts of the community mental health delivery services in 1961. President Kennedy's communication to the U.S. Congress and the passage of the Mental Health Act of 1963 underscored prevention, treatment, and rehabilitation of the mentally ill. The president stressed the community's responsibility in providing care for this

population. As a result of Kennedy's messages, major changes in American psychiatry emerged (Caplan, 1964) and the new principles became the bases of a comprehensive community and preventive approach to mental health care. The U.S. Congress responded to this need by decreeing that each mental health center has a minimum of five essential services:

1. 24-hour emergency care
2. Outpatient services
3. Partial hospitalization
4. Inpatient services
5. Consultation and education

Subsequent legislation stipulated additional services for children and older adults, as well as services such as screening before hospitalization, aftercare, transitional housing, substance abuse treatment, and victim programs. Crisis centers were crucial to the community mental health model. Efforts to expend energy on removing conditions that contribute to mental illness became a major focus of community mental health care. The levels of preventive care provided through these centers include primary (health promotion), secondary (early case-finding), and tertiary (rehabilitation).

Overall, the major objectives of the community mental health centers are to maximize resources, provide various levels of prevention, and evaluate interventions and research. However, recent legislative and socioeconomic factors have curtailed funding and interest in supporting community mental health services. Dramatic changes in health care delivery systems and managed care and decreased access to care have contributed to the marked rise in the number of homeless persons with mental illness. Consequently, many of these clients seek care through emergency departments, community shelters, and the penal system (Antai-Otong, 2004; Kaskie, Wallace, Kang, & Bloom, 2006; Redlich, Steadman, Robbins, & Swanson, 2006).

CRISIS THEORY

Crisis theory is an integral part of nursing and provides a foundation of various preventive and health promotion activities. A discussion of the origins of crisis theory follows.

Origins of Crisis Theory

Historically, crisis theory stems from various concepts of human growth and development. The commonality of these theories lies in their relationship to adaptive and maladaptive responses to stress. Adaptive behaviors are shaped by neurobiological and psychosocial factors that contribute to ego and personality development. Early theorists such as Freud, Erikson, Lindemann, and Caplan contributed to the evolution of crisis theory.

Crisis intervention is a relatively new approach to preventing mental illness. Its primary focus is early case finding, assessment, and prevention of deleterious effects of stress (Caplan, 1961). Its interdisciplinary roots highlight the significant role of psychiatric-mental health nurses in prevention and health promotion.

PSYCHOANALYTICAL THEORIES

This section includes a discussion of Freud's theory on psychosexual development and Erikson's theory of maturational crisis.

Sigmund Freud

Freud's (1961) theory on psychosexual development emphasized the influence of conscious and unconscious conflicts on adaptation. These developmental periods are marked by normal neurobiological and psychosocial stresses. The capacity to master these tasks depends on the person's developmental stage, ego function, and personality traits. These influences represent one's repertoire of coping skills.

Freud and other psychoanalytical theorists stressed the importance of early childhood experiences on adaptive and maladaptive coping responses throughout the life span. They also postulated the impact of these experiences on the progression of growth and development and coping patterns during normal and maturational crises. An in-depth discussion of ego and personality development is found in Chapter 15.

Erik Erikson's Maturational Crisis

Erik Erikson's theory of maturational crisis (1963) concurred with that of Freud and other psychoanalysts, paralleling stages of psychosocial growth and development with Freud's psychosexual tasks. Erikson's theory stressed the relevance of the individual's ability to master normal developmental tasks. He asserted that "psychosocial survival is safeguarded only by vital virtues which develop in the interplay of successive and overlapping generations" (Erikson, 1964, p. 114). Additionally, he clarified the notion that "life-cycle is an integrated psychosocial phenomenon" based on early childhood milestones (Erikson, 1964, p. 114).

Early childhood experiences are the bases of ego function or strength. Healthy ego function is determined by mastering the initial task of trust, which fosters a sense of self-worth (Erikson, 1964). These early beginnings serve as the foundation for confronting subsequent developmental tasks. In other words, the person's ability to adapt to crisis effectively begins at birth and progresses throughout the life span. The ego governs this entire process.

Erikson's (1963) eight stages of development encompass specific tasks or maturational crisis. Resolution of each stage is determined by resolution of the previous developmental task. These stages are discussed in detail in "Life Span Issues: Maturational Crises" in this chapter and are displayed in Table 31–1.

Maturational or developmental crises are predictable and anticipated responses to developmental tasks. People with

TABLE 31–1
Maturational Crises: Erikson's Eight Stages of Development

	Primary Developmental Task	Sources of Maladaptive Response to Crises
Infancy	Basic trust vs. mistrust	Birth ("the most radical change of all"); unreliable provision of basic needs by caregiver
Toddler Period	Autonomy vs. shame and doubt	Overcontrolling, smothering, neglectful, or rejecting parents
Preschool Period	Initiative vs. guilt	Failure to develop trust; impaired self-esteem
Middle Childhood	Industry vs. inferiority	Entering school: dealing with criticism, authority figures, working with others
Adolescence	Identity vs. role confusion	Endocrine changes; social pressures; divorce; lack of empathy and consistent limit setting from family; acceptance of own inadequacies ("apt to suffer more deeply" than at any other stage)
Early Adulthood	Intimacy vs. isolation	Formation of intense interpersonal relationships; clarifying sexuality; lack of validation from early caregivers
Middle Adulthood	Generativity vs. stagnation	Divorce; empty nest syndrome; aging/menopause; major illness; retirement; self-absorption; isolation
Late Adulthood	Integrity vs. despair	Prospect of death

Note. Adapted from *The Life Cycle Completed: A Review* by Erik H. Erikson, with the permission of W. W. Norton & Company, Inc. Copyright © 1982 by Rikan Enterprises, Inc. All rights reserved.

healthy ego function tend to respond to developmental crises effectively using adaptive coping skills. In contrast, people with poor or inadequate ego function tend to become overwhelmed by stress and are vulnerable to developmental arrest. Developmental arrest increases the risk or vulnerability of illness and other maladaptive responses.

Internal and external coping resources influence individual responses to crisis. Internal coping resources constitute innate and acquired processes. Genetic, ego function, and neurobiological factors influence innate processes; they are presumed to be unconscious. Acquired processes evolve through life experiences (Roy & Andrews, 1991). External resources involve psychosocial and cultural factors, such as the number and meaning of stressors, and available support systems. External resources allow people to adapt and cope with stress effectively.

Erikson's (1963) delineation of adaptive and maladaptive responses to developmental tasks provides nurses with parameters for assessing healthy coping behaviors. Psychiatric-mental health nurses can support and reinforce adaptive behaviors by recognizing normal and abnormal responses to developmental tasks.

GRIEF THEORY

This section discusses Lindemann's study of classic grief and bereavement. It also includes a discussion of grief management.

Erik Lindemann

Lindemann's (1944) contribution to crisis theory arises from his classic grief and bereavement study with loved ones of the victims of the Boston Coconut Grove Club Fire in 1942 that killed 491 people. His studies focused on the phenomenon of the mourning process and its impact on health. He delineated the normal bereavement process and described predictable stages that people may go through after emotional disturbances. Grief refers to a normal response to loss. He surmised that the grief process takes 4 to 6 weeks and involves a progression of psychological stages. Caplan (1964) contended that Lindemann's work provided the foundation of the crisis theory as a conceptual framework for preventive psychiatry.

In his studies, Lindemann found that most people who were mourning resolved their grief effectively and recovered from emotional and biological distress within 4 to 6 weeks. Additionally, he found a smaller group of mourners who did not resolve their grief as well as the former group; people in the smaller group exhibited severe psychiatric and psychosomatic disturbances, including depression and gastrointestinal problems. He then compared characteristics of people in each group and found that those who were able to work through their grief tended to manifest several reactions, such as withdrawal from daily activities, feelings of emotional pain and loneliness, crying spells, and loss of appetite. They focused primarily on the loss and the memories of their loved one. Lindemann believed that the latter symptoms were the basis of the phenomenon of mourning. Moreover, he noted

that reliving the memory of loved ones allowed people to gain a sense of reality of their loss.

Lindemann (1944) stated that the time frame of healthy grief reaction rests on the mastery of grief work, particularly freedom from intense emotional ties with the deceased, adaptation to the loss of the loved one, and establishment of new meaningful relationships. Furthermore, he postulated a relationship between the absence of mourning and the formation of maladaptive responses, and he noted the following characteristics of those who fail to mourn:

◆ They continue to live their lives as usual.
◆ They fail to cry or express emotional pain.
◆ They complain of feeling numb.
◆ They lack preoccupation with loved ones.
◆ They deny feelings regarding their loss.
◆ They experience alterations in their social interactions.

These people are likely to develop an illness and express anger or resentment toward health professionals. Lindemann stressed the need for health care professional to facilitate the grief process by recognizing adaptive and maladaptive behaviors in the mourning client. See Chapter 9 for a discussion of normal and abnormal grief.

Appreciation of the grief process involves understanding the meaning of grief, bereavement, and mourning. See Table 31–2 for the *Diagnostic and Statistical Manual of Mental Disorders* (4th edition Revision) (*DSM-IV-TR*) description of bereavement). The term *grief* arises from the Latin word *gravis* and is a normal, profound emotional response to loss. It promotes mental health by allowing the client to work through and cope with loss and

---

TABLE 31–2
DSM-IV-TR Concepts on Bereavement

- Focus of clinical attention is a "normal" response to the loss of a loved one and includes the following:
  1. Individuals who present with symptoms illustrative of major depressive disorder, such as alterations in sleep, appetite, and cognitive function.
  2. Individuals who perceive symptoms as a natural part of the grief process.
  3. Individuals who seek professional treatment for relief of associated appetite and sleep disturbances.
- Symptoms may vary among various culture groups.
- If symptoms persist longer than 2 months, a diagnosis of Major Depressive Disorder may be considered.

Note. From *Diagnostic and Statistical Manual of Mental Disorders* (4th edition, Text Revision) (*DSM-IV-TR*), by American Psychiatric Association, 2000, Washington, DC: Author. Adapted with permission.

accept its reality. Additionally, it facilitates social processing and sharing of feelings and emotional pain generated by loss. Grief reactions are actual, anticipatory, unresolved, or pathological.

Anticipatory grief refers to experiencing grief before it occurs. For example, an 18-year-old boy who knows that he has to leave home to live on a college campus may grieve the loss of his youth and the security of his parents' taking care of his major needs. Another example is that of a young woman who is diagnosed with acquired immunodeficiency syndrome (AIDS), who, along with her family, grieve over her eventual death.

People experiencing anticipatory or actual grief may feel angry, sad, or guilty. *Unresolved* or *pathological grief reaction* has been discussed earlier. Depression and perceptual disturbances are possible negative or maladaptive outcomes of grief reactions. Bereavement occurs when loss is inevitable. Mourning is the process in which grief is resolved.

Management of Grief Reactions

The aim of grief management is to prevent chronic and deleterious reactions to loss. The impact of loss may leave the client bewildered and experiencing immense emotional pain. Grief work is a process that helps the client accept and resolve the pain of sorrow. This process begins when clients free or release themselves from the bondage of their loved one; readjust to living without the deceased; and form new, meaningful relationships. Grief work can be enhanced by:

1. Coping with painful experiences

2. Reliving experiences and times with one's loved one

3. Experiencing and trying out rewarding relationships

Eventually, the intensity of emotional pain dissipates and becomes more tolerable as the client masters and embraces the loss of a loved one (Lindemann, 1944, 1979). Symptoms of acute stress or trauma responses are similar to grief reactions. Psychiatric nurses must assess the client's symptoms by inquiring about the time of the event, onset of symptoms, and previous coping patterns. See the following dialogue.

NURSE: Mr. Ruth, when did your wife die?

CLIENT: She died a month ago.

NURSE: Describe what it's been like without your wife.

CLIENT: I am not doing a very good job because I have spent a lot of time alone.

NURSE: I understand the sadness you must be going through, but it is important to spend time with friends or family who care about you.

CLIENT: I do not know what to say and I feel so awkward going without my wife (alone).

NURSE: Your reactions and feelings are pretty normal, but it is important to avoid being alone.

Grief work is strengthened by spiritual beliefs that often provide emotional comfort, promote healthy discussions of life, and reduce guilt. Nurses play a critical role in assessing spiritual needs and mobilizing resources that provide emotional support during stressful periods. Some clients may feel uncomfortable asking for spiritual support. Nurses can minimize discomfort by directly asking the client about interests or preferences she may have for spiritual support. Approaching the client in a caring and nonjudgmental manner allows the nurse to assess spiritual needs. Furthermore, understanding the meaning of one's own personal spiritual beliefs and grief reactions enhances the nurse's understanding of those of the client.

PREVENTIVE PSYCHIATRY

Caplan's early work with Lindemann in 1946 at the Harvard-Wellesley Project established early crisis intervention concepts. Numerous so-called suicide prevention centers were established in this country in the 1960s. The quality of services provided varied with each center's role and function and paralleled the national mental health movement, which included suicide prevention and crisis intervention (McGee, 1974).

Gerald Caplan

Caplan's (1964) renowned work, *Principles of Preventive Psychiatry*, was the foundation of most literature and research associated with crisis theory. A number of nurse theorists have modified his work and made notable contributions to nursing practice, but the principal nursing contributors have been Aguilera (1990, 1994, 1998), Aguilera and Messick (1978), and Hoff (1989).

Caplan's (1964) definition of preventive psychiatry referred to a comprehensive perspective that integrated theoretical and clinical concepts used to decrease the prevalence of mental illness (primary prevention), the duration of symptoms (secondary prevention), and the deleterious effects of disorders (tertiary prevention).

Caplan described primary prevention from a life span perspective noting that people have various basic needs that parallel with developmental stages. He sorted these needs into three groups: biological, psychosocial, and sociocultural. Biological needs include nourishment, safety, sensory stimulation, and exercise. Psychosocial needs refer to interactions with significant others that promote cognitive and affective maturation. Sociocultural needs arise from customs, rituals, values, and social structure that influence personality maturity and ego function. Social norms and expectations have a profound effect on behavior, feelings about one's self, and one's role in the world. Furthermore, culture influences language, beliefs, traditions, and endeavors.

Caplan (1961) also linked mental health, or successful crisis resolution, with ego function. He listed three criteria used to assess ego function. The first criterion is the capacity to modulate affect, such as anger, anxiety, or frustration, during stressful periods. People with healthy ego function tend to mobilize internal and external resources to maintain health or homeostasis. The second criterion is the use of adaptive problem solving. Does the person cope effectively with stress, or does the person become ill or use maladaptive problem solving to reduce the overwhelming effects of stress?

The third criterion is the ability to maintain reality testing. People who use adaptive coping behaviors have a repertoire of internal and external resources that maintain reality testing. In face of a threat or loss, the person handles the crisis effectively. People with inadequate coping skills tend to regress when faced with a crisis situation in which internal and external resources are overtaxed. Regression is a primitive defense mechanism used to revert to an earlier stage of development or childlike thinking to deal with crisis. Impaired reality testing may range from severe anxiety reactions to psychosis (Caplan, 1961). The impact of crisis is based on complex processes that determine how anxiety is modulated, how problem-solving skills are mobilized, and how reality testing is maintained.

ORIGINS OF CRISIS

People interact with their environment constantly. Normally, stress challenges people to maintain a steady state or equilibrium using a repertoire of innate and acquired coping skills. An array of habitual problem-solving mechanisms is constantly called on to minimize the effects of uncomfortable feelings and thoughts. These mechanisms are primarily unconscious. A crisis evolves when the usual coping behaviors fail to maintain integrity (Caplan, 1961). What conditions contribute to crisis situations?

Parad and Caplan (1965) described three interrelated conditions that produce a state of crisis:

a. A hazardous event that poses a threat
b. An emotional need that denotes earlier threats and increased vulnerability
c. An inability to respond adaptively

Understanding the human response to crisis requires clarifying its origins and meanings to the individual (Hoff, 1989). Crisis originates from various sources and complex processes such as life events (situational) and developmental or maturational events.

Situational Crisis

Situational, or unexpected, crisis originates from three sources (Hoff, 1989):

1. Environmental, such as tornadoes, fires, riots, and outbreak of disease
2. Physical or personal, such as amputations, disfiguring, debilitating, or terminal illness
3. Interpersonal or psychosocial, such as the death of a loved one or divorce

MATURATIONAL CRISIS

Maturational, or developmental, crisis is described as normal crisis because it is expected in association with normal growth and development. This period is marked by biological, psychosocial, and social transitions that generate characteristic disturbances in behavior and emotional responses. The basis of maturational crisis is depicted in Freud's psychosexual theory and Erikson's eight developmental tasks, which delineate human development and associated biological and cognitive behaviors evolving throughout the life span. Each state generates enormous stress and the need to master developmental crises. Erikson (1968) believed that each developmental stage is a turning point that provides opportunities for both adaptation and maladaptation.

MANIFESTATIONS OF CRISIS

Caplan (1964) listed major characteristics of crisis as follows:

◆ A state of increased tension and feelings of helplessness are present.
◆ Emergency coping or problem-solving mechanisms are needed.
◆ A state of disorganization may ensue.
◆ The situation is self-limiting and it usually lasts from 1 to 6 weeks.

Crisis situations frequently render individuals more dependent on external resources than at other times of their lives. This has been depicted as situational dependency or an adaptive response. Clients are responsive to the possibility of constructive changes during this period, and nurses are in pivotal positions to facilitate a return to a higher level of function.

CRISIS: THE ROLE OF ADAPTATION

Crisis situations confront people with novel experiences that frequently exhaust their usual coping mechanisms. Crisis resolution is a complex process that is affected by appraisal of the event or stressor, available support systems, sociocultural and neurobiological factors, and ego function.

COPING MECHANISMS

Coping mechanisms are both conscious and unconscious and determine how one adapts to environmental demands. The aim of coping is homeostasis or adaptation. Internal and external resources are the basis of adaptation.

Lazarus and Folkman (1984, p. 141) defined coping as "constantly changing cognitive and behavioral efforts to manage specific external and/or internal demands that are appraised as taxing or exceeding the resources of the person." Additionally, they defined coping as a dynamic process that is mobilized by continuous appraisals and reappraisals of environmental transactions.

Cognitive appraisal underscores the perception of stressful events and threats to one's well-being. Appraisals pertain to value or appreciation, which, in terms of coping, refer to the significance of internal and external events that are linked to health and adaptation. Events may be perceived as irrelevant, benign or nonthreatening, or threatening or harmful. Lazarus (1966) identified two forms of appraisals: primary and secondary.

Primary Appraisal

Primary appraisal refers to the initial response to a stressor and the ultimate goal of prevailing over a situation. Lazarus (1966) delineated three types of primary appraisals, including (1) irrelevant (events that do not pose a threat to the person); (2) benign positive (events that are positive and enhance adaptation or stimulate a sense of well-being); and (3) stressful.

Stress appraisals are regarded as (1) injurious; (2) hazardous; or (3) demanding or challenging (Lazarus, 1966). Life events that have negative connotations or cause damage, such as physical illness, injury to self-esteem, and loss of normal functioning, are defined as *injurious*. *Hazardous* threats are anticipated occurrences that encourage people to use coping skills and reduce anticipated risks. This form of appraisal normally arouses negative feelings and thoughts, such as anger, grief, and helplessness (Lazarus, 1991). This premise suggests that there are no universal stressors and that danger and threats are determined by individual perception of situations. The potential for adaptive as well as maladaptive responses exists with hazards. For example, the woman who discovers that her husband is having an affair with another woman perceives this situation as a threat to her marriage and livelihood. She is determined to keep her marriage together by seeking marital therapy. Initially, her husband is reluctant to seek treatment, but later he agrees and discovers the basis of marital discord and attempts to work things out.

Demanding or challenging situations also provide opportunities for using and enhancing coping and adaptive responses, but responses differ from hazardous form, because they generate positive feelings such as enthusiasm, motivation, and excitement. For example, the couple anticipating the birth of triplets is challenged to manage multiple births with enormous parental responsibilities. A challenge form of appraisal normally produces positive thoughts, such as "We've been through a lot worse times. We can make it on one income." The implication is that challenge appraisals represent healthier adaptive and coping skills that promote a sense of well-being.

Secondary Appraisal

Secondary appraisal emerges with any form of perceived threat or harm if primary appraisals are ineffective or maladaptive. The rationale of secondary appraisal is to

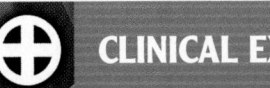

CLINICAL EXAMPLE

An Adolescent Using Secondary Appraisal Coping Skills

An example of secondary appraisal of coping options is seen in the adolescent who became angry with his parents after he was grounded for failing a class. He expressed anger to his parents, and he later got into a heated argument with his sister. He shouted and reminded her of a recent breakup with a boyfriend, who is now dating someone else. The boy felt guilty because his sister began to cry. He realized that he was responsible for the argument and for being grounded. He later apologized to his sister and parents for yelling and arguing when he realized that this was not the best way to handle his frustration and anger. His self-esteem had been threatened because of poor grades and being grounded.

assess coping resources, options, and choices. Lazarus (1966) emphasized the significance of secondary appraisals as follows:

◆ They are the basis of coping mechanisms.

◆ They enhance or promote a positive outcome of primary appraisals.

◆ They strengthen coping resources and options.

The outcome of the coping process depends on individual efforts to alter threatening events and attempts to change the person's appraisal of the stress to minimize the threat (Hansen & Johnson, 1979). *Reappraisal* refers to alteration in appraisal based on new information from the individual and the environment. Reappraisal is a form of cognitive processing that differs from other appraisals because it occurs after the initial appraisal (Lazarus & Folkman, 1984).

Overall, three forms of appraisals—primary, secondary, and reappraisal—determine the scope of stress and emotional reactions to stressful situations. Cognitive appraisal is an evaluation of the environment, perception of stress, and use of coping mechanisms. Stressful events or crises provide opportunities to improve adaptation and coping skills (Lazarus & Folkman, 1984).

SUPPORT SYSTEMS

Social support is crucial to everyday living because it affords people with a sense of value, security, and self-esteem. Studies show that individuals with adequate support systems are resilient, they develop a sense of well-being, and they respond more adaptively to stressful events. Furthermore, social networking provides a feedback mechanism that maintains social identity, security, a sense of belonging, and validation (Picardi et al., 2007; Ward-Griffin, Schofield, Vos, &

Coatsworth-Puspoky, 2005). Typically, support systems comprise families and friends, who feel their needs are addressed during crises. Crisis situations can present individuals with distressful experiences, and families are the most significant resource promoting effective and adaptive coping mechanisms. Families validate members' feelings and facilitate the mourning process.

Quality support systems also provide positive, life-sustaining beliefs and shared values, expectations, and enrich the meaning and purpose of life and ultimately create a sense of connectedness and coherence. Aaron Antonovsky's (1987) concept of sense of coherence infers that this phenomenon consists of three components which contribute to overall well-being and coping: comprehensibility, manageability, and meaningfulness. *Comprehensibility* involves the extent in which the environment is structured and understood (promotes a sense of predictability and security). *Manageability* refers to degree of resilience and the individual's ability to mobilize resources and adapt to stressful situations. *Meaningfulness* is the degree in which life difficulties or stressors are perceived as worthwhile and challenging rather than overtaxing or onerous. Antonovsky (1987) further submitted that of the three components, *meaningfulness* has the greatest impact on coping and adaptation and overall health.

In contrast, people with inadequate support systems are more likely to use maladaptive responses during crises. These clients are vulnerable to the deleterious effects of crisis. In this situation, crisis intervention is useful in assessing client needs, promoting a sense of well-being and mastery, reinforcing adaptive coping behaviors, and mobilizing resources through feedback and validation of feelings.

In summary, social support is vital to effective coping. Close and caring relationships provide a protective buffer during crisis situations. Furthermore, social networking fosters a sense of sharing, validates feelings, and provides reassurance and acceptance. People experiencing crises often isolate themselves when they most need to turn to others for support. Isolation or inadequate support systems increase the likelihood of deleterious effects of crisis and mental illness. Crisis intervention is a useful strategy that helps clients, mobilizes resources, enhances support systems, and facilitates formation of adaptive coping mechanisms.

SOCIOCULTURAL FACTORS

As previously discussed, people normally do not face a crisis alone, but within a social network composed of a spouse, family, friends, community, or religious affiliations. Social systems typically comprise common bonds such as values, traditions, and beliefs systems. Close ties afford people with resources that support and reinforce adaptive problem-solving skills.

Sociocultural factors interact with the life cycle at each maturational crisis of individual and family development. Cultural factors define the character, timing, and rituals of developmental stages and life passages (McGoldrick, Giordano, & Garcia-Preto, 2005; Utsey, Hook, & Stanard, 2007) and the nature of support systems.

Social support systems determine the perception of a crisis and one's ability to master it. Social functioning is related to individual roles, relationships, and cultural factors. An example of the impact of sociocultural factors is the family faced with coping with an unmarried pregnant adolescent. One family may perceive this situation as devastating and insist that the daughter consider having an abortion, whereas another family may decide to keep the child within the family although they may perceive the same situation as being undesirable. Each family resolves crisis situations based on its common beliefs, values, and traditions. The outcome really depends on their ability to express feelings and receive support during the crisis.

The concept of coping involves a host of factors, including sociocultural influences. Psychiatric-mental health nurses need to assess client needs, incorporating their uniqueness into interventions that facilitate adaptive coping responses to stressful events. Self-awareness of one's own culture enables psychiatric nurses to assess the client's experience, make an accurate diagnosis, and initiate an appropriate plan of care. See Chapter 7 for an in-depth discussion of cultural and ethnic considerations.

EGO FUNCTION

The ego is the core of the personality, and it modulates the social function of cognition (perceptions), behavior, anxiety, problem solving, and reality testing. Its role in adaptation arises from its ability to mediate between the person and reality through the use of defense mechanisms (internal and external environments). The ego uses defense mechanisms to protect or buffer itself against impulses and affects such as guilt, anxiety, and shame. *Ego strength* refers to the ability to modulate these functions in the face of numerous stimuli or stress. The principal goal of ego function is to maintain equilibrium or adaptation (Caplan, 1961).

NEUROBIOLOGICAL FACTORS

Historically, neurobiological responses to emotions were considered a critical part of coping and adaptation because they influence an array of responses to stressful situations. This premise has been well documented by researchers such as Cannon and Selye. Cannon (1914) coined the term *fight or flight* response. This response activates physiological processes in the form of anger or fear, arousing the sympathetic nervous system. Cannon studied the role of the adrenal medulla in mediating the biological response generated by strong emotions and pain.

Selye's (1946) studies supported Cannon's theory; he referred to the physical reaction to stress as *general adaptation syndrome* (Selye, 1946) and, later, *stress response* (Selye, 1956). Both theorists surmised that strong emotions, such as anxiety and fear, activate the release of cortisol from the adrenal cortex.

Selye (1976) also postulated that illnesses such as allergies and collagen diseases arise from abnormal or prolonged stress responses. Others supported this notion and linked life events to illness (Holmes & Rahe, 1967; Squire, 1987).

Stein (1986) noted that four decades have failed to produce evidence to support the premise that prolonged stress destroys any tissues. Several researchers have disputed the assertion and demonstrated that stress adversely affects health (e.g., immune and cardiovascular systems) and places people at risk for other illnesses such as coronary artery disease (Rohleder & Karl, 2006). Prolonged stress has a potentially deleterious affect on immune cellular function, such as natural killer (NK) cells and lymphokine-activated killer (LAK) cell (Sakami et al., 2004). Research indicates that individuals with healthy coping behaviors have increased immune cellular function, whereas those with ineffective or inadequate coping skills have decreased immune cellular function and increased vulnerability to immune system disorders including certain cancers, autoimmune disorders, skin disorders, and coronary artery disease (Morikawa et al., 2005). Researchers continue to assert that neurobiological and psychosocial factors represent complex nonspecific aspects of stress response and that specific components involve external (control and anticipation) and internal resources (coping mechanisms and perception of stressor).

The neurobiological basis of coping has been linked with the immune response, neurotransmitters, neuroendocrine systems, and genetics. (These factors are discussed in Chapters 11 and 13.)

Adaptation to stress and healthy outcomes are based on the integration of the appraisal of process, available support system, sociocultural factors, ego function, and neurobiological factors. Assessing coping patterns, reinforcing adaptive responses, and mobilizing resources are critical nursing interventions that facilitate adaptation to crisis situations.

LIFE SPAN ISSUES: MATURATIONAL CRISES

The human experience is stressful. Everyday living presents people with potential crises, and their ability to mobilize internal and external resources determines the impact of stressful encounters. This process begins in utero and continues until death. Life span crises include moving through developmental stages and events such as becoming a parent, getting married, being a victim of violence, and developing a terminal illness.

Erikson's (1963) eight developmental stages (see Table 31–1) represent maturational crises. As previously cited, these stages are anticipated and present people with normal disturbances or crises. Each stage challenges people to master specific tasks that are based on successful resolution of previous stages. He described each stage as a crisis state generated by radical changes that provide the potential for growth. Additionally,

developmental crises are turning points manifested by "increased vulnerability . . . and are a source of generational strength" (p. 96) and maladaptation (Erikson, 1968).

INFANCY: TRUST VERSUS MISTRUST

Erikson (1968) asserted that the most radical change of all begins with the birth experience, as the infant evolves from intrauterine to extrauterine existence. This period represents a crisis not only for the newborn but also for the new parents. Interactions with primary caregivers serve as the basis for the child's emotional and biological well-being.

Bowlby's attachment theory (1969) emphasized the importance of bonding and its effects on the child's sense of trust and validation. The role of primary caregivers in this process involves accessibility and responsiveness to the infant's needs (e.g., nurturance, nutritional, and protection). Bowlby further believed that attachment behaviors or affectional bonds are vital to survival and the ability to form meaningful relationships throughout the life span.

The primary developmental task during this period is trust versus mistrust. Trust emerges as the primary caregivers meet the infants' basic need through consistent, affectionate and caring environments. Early trusting interactions provide the foundation of personality development and self-concept. (The attentive mother who responds to a crying infant by holding and feeding the infant provides an example of a positive bonding experience. In contrast, the mother who ignores the cries of the infant provides an example of an abusive and neglectful experience.) Bonding enables parents to communicate love, warmth, safety, and validation to the infant. When the infant develops and gains a sense of well-being and trust, anxiety and sadness are generated by the normal separation-individual process (Erikson, 1963).

In contrast, impaired early affectional bonding compromises healthy parent-child interactions, increasing the likelihood of mistrust. Mistrust usually evolves when the infant is unable to rely on primary caregivers to have their basic needs met. Events that affect the early bonding process include serious illnesses, socioeconomic concerns, and impaired family interactions. Disturbances in this process contribute to formation of maladaptive behaviors throughout the life span (Erikson, 1963).

Early interactions with primary caregivers affect how the child adapts to subsequent developmental stages. Newly found mobility and need for autonomy challenges the child and parents to master the stress of the second stage of autonomy versus shame and doubt.

TODDLER PERIOD: AUTONOMY VERSUS SHAME AND DOUBT

Accelerated motor and intellectual growth mark the second year. The child experiences a newly found sense of mobility, autonomy, and early speech. The major developmental task is autonomy versus shame and doubt (Erikson, 1963). The toddler develops a sense of mastery over self and impulses. Major sensorimotor developments during this stage are feeding oneself, controlling anal sphincter (toilet training), tolerating delays, variable reasoning, listening and concentration (Piaget, 1952, 1969), and exploring the environment.

Successful resolution and mastery of autonomy and independence depend on the primary caregivers' parenting skills. Parents who encourage, reward, and set consistent limits regarding acceptable behaviors provide environments that promote autonomy, independence, and self-esteem in the toddler. The toddler continues to separate and individuate from primary caregivers, who support this newly found independence. Parents continue to provide safety and assist with encounters that the child is unable to handle. The child learns that even with newly found freedom, the parents are accessible for emotional "refueling."

In comparison, parents who are overcontrolling, smothering, neglectful, or rejecting provide climates that discourage autonomy and separateness. Feelings of shame and self-doubt arise, laying the foundation for maladaptation manifested by poor self-concept, depression, and self-destructive behaviors in adolescence and adulthood.

PRESCHOOL PERIOD: INITIATIVE VERSUS GUILT

The child with a sense of self-worth and independence has the capacity to initiate motor and intellectual activities. Children who are 3 to 5 years old begin to play with peers and interact with others. An understanding of right or wrong (moral sense or superego) evolves during this stage. The child who successfully resolves the task of initiative is conscientious, dependable, and exhibits some self-discipline. These attributes emerge as part of the child's personality.

The child who fails to develop a sense of trust often feels shame and experiences doubt about herself. Impaired self-esteem interferes with the confidence needed to endure independence and initiative. As a result, guilt and feelings of inadequacy arise as symptoms of unsuccessful resolution of this developmental stage.

MIDDLE CHILDHOOD: INDUSTRY VERSUS INFERIORITY

Entering school is a crisis for the youngster and family. School places customary demands for academic performance associated with learning and proficiency. Additionally, school provides socialization that involves dealing with acceptance, criticism, authority figures, and working effectively with others. The child with a positive self-concept is challenged by these demands and participates in traditional learning and masters and fulfills goals. Active parental participation in school and home endeavors plays a critical role in enhancing the child's well-being and self-esteem.

Furthermore, physical and cognitive development enable the child to perform complex motor tasks such as ballet, gymnastics, and soccer. Concrete thought processes become more organized and logical (Piaget, 1969). Successful resolution of industry permits the child to actively share and interact with others while experiencing a sense of companionship.

In contrast, children with a negative self-concept and who feel socially alienated may find school overwhelming. These children tend to feel lonely, depressed, or extremely anxious. These responses often reflect impaired family-child relationships that are overprotective, indifferent, or rejecting.

ADOLESCENCE: IDENTITY VERSUS ROLE CONFLICT

Adolescence is a critical stage of development because it represents a time of turmoil that places the youth at risk for crisis. Kaplan (1984) described adolescence as "an inner emotional upheaval, a struggle between the eternal human wish to cling to the past and the equally powerful wish to get on with the future" (p. 19). Erikson (1968) noted that the pressures of adolescence are associated with the "final stage of identity formation" and the youth is "apt to suffer more deeply" (p. 163) than at any previous stage or any stage thereafter. Resolution of this developmental crisis is built on successful resolution of previous stages. The major developmental task of adolescence is identity versus role confusion (Erikson, 1963).

Early Adolescence

Early adolescence challenges the youth to master drastic role changes precipitated by tremendous neurobiological and psychosocial demands. Neurobiological demands are activated by endocrine changes connected with maturation of the cells of the hypothalamus and stimulation of gonadal hormones. These endocrine changes affect the mood and behavior of the adolescent and produce the major physical changes of secondary sex characteristics.

Psychosocial demands include negotiating the transition from elementary school to middle school. Academic demand is clearly increased, with an emphasis on achievement. Biological and psychosocial demands or puberty changes affect the adolescent's self-image, contributing to fears of insecurity and failure.

Early adolescence also represents a period when peers are important because they facilitate the process of separating from parents (Mishne, 1986). Parents continue to play vital roles in the adolescent's life, but separation from them increases *cathexis* (concentration of psychic energy of self) (Mishne, 1986). Parent-child relationships validate the youth through emotional support and acceptance. Parental coalitions also buffer the youth against negative feelings, behaviors, and choices. Furthermore, parents are challenged to deal with the youth's mood swings and defiance against them. Adolescents can benefit from healthy parental alliances that respond to these behaviors with love, understanding, and consistent limit setting. Healthy and predictable parental behaviors are critical to successful resolution of crisis during adolescence. Family turmoil, the death of a parent, marital discord, or divorce can be devastating to adolescents.

Middle Adolescence

Middle adolescence finds the youth constantly seeking and forming new relationships apart from the family to displace early close family ties (Blos, 1962). Additionally, this stage denotes maturation of sexual identity. Self-absorption and self-awareness impart self-reliance and separation from significant others, which are the basis of identity. Adolescents attempt to individuate in terms of sexual changes and societal demands as adults. Heterosexual relationships become important and lay the foundation for the subsequent stage of intimacy versus isolation.

Adolescent confusion frequently arises from struggles with independence versus dependence, separation issues, and gaining a sense of who one is. The term *identity* is used to describe the ability to experience one's uniqueness and relevance. Successful resolution of this task is confirmed during subsequent developmental stages.

Late Adolescence

Integration of the personality to promote stable work and intimate relationships and a personal value system are aspects of crisis resolution in late adolescence. The older adolescent often experiences a sense of mourning coupled with depression or anxiety connected with acceptance of her limitations and inadequacies (Erikson, 1963; Mishne, 1986).

The adolescent who unsuccessfully resolves the crisis of this state develops *role confusion*. This individual is unable to form adult identity and has difficulty responding to societal expectations. This adolescent has failed to resolve crises related to trust, autonomy, initiative, and industry, which are the foundations of identity. Families that lack empathy or consistency and predictable limit setting produce chaotic environments that increase vulnerability to maladaptive responses in their members.

EARLY ADULTHOOD: INTIMACY VERSUS ISOLATION

The young adult comes of age representing another generation in a family system. The ability to define an identity of self and form intense interpersonal relationships provides the basis of this developmental crisis. *Identity* in this life stage refers to the capacity to make adult decisions and manage adult stress. Resolution of previous developmental crises prepares the young adult to embark on the path of defining her place in society. The crisis of this stage is intimacy versus isolation (Erikson, 1963).

Intimacy refers to the capacity to form close, meaningful relationships with others and to clarify one's sexuality. Basic qualities of intimacy are a proficiency in the sharing of feelings, mutual understanding, commitment, responsibility, and love. Erikson (1968) defined love as the most vital human quality and the basis of trust and successful resolution of all developmental tasks.

A lack of love or validation by early caregivers interferes with the capacity to form close, warm, and intimate relationships. The young adult with this experience is often distrustful or interacts with others superficially. Moreover, this individual has a heightened sense of self-absorption that interferes with self-awareness, which is gained through feedback and perceptions from others (Erikson, 1963). The withdrawn and isolated person is likely to use maladaptive responses to cope with crisis situations.

Endeavors that facilitate resolution of this stage include pursuit of careers and jobs and the formation of meaningful relationships. Careers and jobs are pursued through higher academic institutions or technical or other training. Proficient social skills are essential aspects of this process, which help young adults make realistic adult decisions.

Marrying or forming other long-term relationships affect sexuality, fidelity, and loyalty that affect the capacity to master shared identity or intimacy. Intimate relationships and careers lay the foundation for future crises and resolution of developmental tasks. An inability to establish intimacy interferes with self-understanding and self-actualization. Parenthood ushers in a new generation and enhances further growth and maturity of the young adult.

MIDDLE ADULTHOOD: GENERATIVITY VERSUS STAGNATION

The developmental crisis for middle adulthood is generativity versus stagnation. Generativity is concerned with "establishing and guiding" (Erikson, 1968, p. 138), enhancing productivity and creativity and contributing to the next generation. Bearing and raising children, establishing pastimes outside the family, and sustaining meaningful relationships are examples of generativity. Generativity arises from the need to participate and promote continuity and heritage for subsequent generations. Caring for others and self is the basis of this developmental task. People begin to look over their lives and examine family, community, and social accomplishments and contributions.

Successful resolution of this challenge arises from adaptive responses to previous developmental crises. Various crises affect the middle-aged adult, including divorce, empty nest syndrome, biological changes related to aging and menopause, major medical illnesses, and retirement. Factors such as a positive self-concept and the capacity to form meaningful relationships promote effective resolution of this developmental crisis.

In contrast, people concerned about themselves rather than others are less likely to function interdependently. They tend to experience boredom, a sense of emptiness, and lack the capacity to contribute to subsequent generations. A sense of *stagnation* compromises the ability to feel needed or loved. Self-absorption and increased isolation pose threats to self-concept and create a vulnerability to maladaptation.

LATE ADULTHOOD: INTEGRITY VERSUS DESPAIR

The final developmental crisis is integrity versus despair (Erikson, 1963). Successful resolution of this crisis, like other maturational crises, depends on a sense of trust, autonomy, initiative, industry, identity, intimacy, and generativity. Each generation is responsible for maintaining wisdom and mature judgment. The members sustain and share the integrity of experience while fostering the needs of the next generation. Vigor, productivity, and stamina wane with aging, but the gift of wisdom and knowledge provide the new generation with a sense of closure, connectedness, and appreciation of life.

Integrity refers to soundness and completeness. It fosters a sense of wholeness and acceptance that minimizes the *despair* and disgust of completing the life cycle and experiencing a sense of powerlessness generated by the prospect of death. The person who unsuccessfully resolves this crisis often feels life has been too short and finds it difficult to accept psychosocial and biological changes. Death is not perceived as life's finite boundary (Erikson, 1968).

In summary, Erikson (1968) delineated developmental tasks in terms of the whole life cycle process, including the sequence of generations and interactions with society. Developmental stage or maturational crises are anticipated, and predictable responses evolve throughout the life cycle; each stage lays the foundation of subsequent adaptation. Factors such as characteristics of early caregivers, socioculture considerations, and neurobiology play major roles in the formation of self-concept and the capacity to adapt to crises. Crisis situations provide opportunities to form adaptive coping behaviors and to promote growth.

FAMILIES IN CRISIS

The present socioeconomic climate of this country places people and families at risk for crises. Tremendous stress on families stems from responses to psychosocial factors such as deterioration of family systems, variable unemployment rates, and violence. Other societal stressors include the explosion of youth violence, increasing substance misuse, and dementias such as Alzheimer's disease.

Families seeking help are often referred for treatment after a member exhibits symptoms of self-destructive behaviors such as suicide attempt or threat of running away from home. Other reasons for seeking help include the inability to care for a loved one with a debilitating illness such as Alzheimer's disease. A crisis occurs when individuals or families encounter stressful situations and normal coping mechanisms fail to resolve the disruption (Caplan, 1964). Additionally, families in crisis experience impaired or ineffectual interactional patterns, which generate disruptive coping responses.

What factors determine how families handle crisis situations? Caplan (1961) described the following five interpersonal

requisites for maintenance of the well-being or health in individuals and families. They are:

1. *Love* (unconditional)—the need to love and be loved
2. *Support*—related to the need to "depend" on others
3. *Impulse control*—psychological and biological control of gratification of needs
4. *Feel part of a group*—a sense of security, belonging, and identity
5. *Personal achievement and recognition* (culturally determined)—need to feel content and good about personal accomplishments and validation

Families who integrate these attributes provide environments that foster trust, independence, initiative, and industry. Each crisis challenges children and families to use previously successful and resourceful coping behaviors to grow and sustain well-being and health.

Healthy families take care of the needs of their members and support each other during crises (Caplan, 1964). Additional adaptive qualities of healthy families include strong parental leadership qualities, effective communication patterns, clear boundaries and roles, and flexibility. Healthy family interactions facilitate formation of close, meaningful relationships within and outside of the family system. Family activities are directed toward helping members master problems rather than avoiding or restricting activities to relieve tension. Specific behaviors, such as the child who easily expresses feelings and relates to others effectively, often mirror the parents' sense of well-being and health.

In comparison, unhealthy families fail to integrate Caplan's attributes and instead create climates with inconsistent leadership, sometimes placing children in adult roles during crises. These families also tend to use impaired communication patterns and unclear, blurred, or rigid boundaries and roles. Children are often scapegoated and experience various forms of abuse. Children and adolescents exhibiting maladaptive behaviors such as substance abuse, depression, or suicide attempts must be assessed as soon as possible to reduce the deleterious effects of stressful events. Maladaptive behaviors in the young often arise from chaotic family systems and reflect inner feelings of helplessness, low self-esteem, and frustration.

Family responses to crisis situations are time limited and increase responsiveness to external influences to facilitate adaptive responses. Theories on crisis intervention with families surmise that the family is the core of the crisis and has the greatest influence on maintaining or resolving the situation (Greef & Holtzkamp, 2007). Crisis intervention needs to focus on the child's behavior as a symptom of family disruption (Caplan, 1961).

THE ROLE OF THE NURSE

Crisis intervention is an effective treatment modality that facilitates adaptation and health restoration. Psychiatric-mental health nurses can use crisis intervention in all clinical settings in which clients experience distress or crises. Client situations may range from disasters, such as a hurricane, to the developmental task of parenthood.

THE GENERALIST NURSE

The primary goal of the generalist nurse in crisis intervention is to collaborate with other members of the crisis team to resolve the immediate crisis or emergency. The generalist nurse uses interventions that foster health, enhance coping skills, and decrease disability (American Nurses Association, 2000).

THE ADVANCED-PRACTICE PSYCHIATRIC REGISTERED NURSE

In comparison, the advanced-practice psychiatric registered nurse incorporates basis crisis intervention techniques with various other approaches, such as psychotherapy and prescriptive authority, to strengthen coping skills and minimize the deleterious effects of crisis. Additionally, the advanced-practice nurse provides direct and independent clinical care, including differential diagnoses, to assess and manage complex client problems.

DISASTERS: RESPONSE TO MASSIVE STRESS

Disasters have been described as calamities or adversities that create vast stress. The catastrophic events of September 11, 2001, remind us of the unpredictable nature of tragedy and disaster. Tragically, almost 3,000 people lost their lives in the September 11 events, and these estimates fail to capture the profound emotional, psychological, and economical impact on family members, friends, communities, and societies. The impact of these tragic events continues to haunt survivors and those who witnessed the events from afar. Psychiatric nurses are often on the front line working with survivors and must provide interventions, ranging from critical incident stress debriefing to consultation with other health care providers working in non-mental health settings. In the event of a disaster, psychiatric nurses must use a spectrum of interventions that involve early identification of high-risk groups, mobilize resources that strengthen client coping skills, and facilitate adaptive resolution.

One of the most devastating natural disasters occurred August 29, 2005 at which time Hurricane Katrina made landfall southeast of New Orleans, Louisiana. Prior to the arrival of Katrina, residents of New Orleans and surrounding parishes were ordered to evacuate. Because of this order and subsequent flooding, approximately 400,000 residents became displaced (CDC, 2006a). According to unpublished data from the American Red Cross, on August 28, an estimated 50,000 individuals began moving into evacuation centers throughout the state of Louisiana (American Red Cross, unpublished data, 2005).

Survivors of Hurricane Katrina have experienced tremendous physical, mental, emotional, and socioeconomic challenges (CDC, 2006a). Results from a recent report conducted by the CDC (2006b) indicate that approximately 2 months after Hurricane Katrina made landfall, 20.2 percent of housing units lacked water, 24.5 percent had no electricity, 43.2 percent had no telephone service, and 55.7 percent of households contained one or more members with a chronic health condition. The most unsettling health conditions involved people with chronic diseases complicated by dehydration, physical exhaustion, and heat exhaustion and concerns about contaminated water. Apart from these hardships, almost 50 percent of adults displayed intense emotional distress, suggesting the possible need for mental health services. The devastation of Katrina has been especially difficult for children. A report from the Children's Defense Fund (CDF) indicates after 7 months post-Katrina, tens of thousands of children are left to wrestle with their profound losses without adequate mental resources. Recommendations from the CDF suggest a need to create emergency mental health services, mobile health clinics, school-based clinics, and emergency relief services to address these issues. In addition, community assessments after natural disasters can evaluate and identify health-related emotional needs and facilitate public health support and interventions (CDC, 2006b). Overall, communities and countries that encounter the wrath and devastation from natural disasters, such as hurricanes and Tsunamis, require immediate physical and emotional support to maintain basic life needs and cope with the adversities of catastrophic events.

Disasters are overwhelming, stressful events that generate feelings of profound fear, panic, horror, and doom. Disasters disrupt normal patterns of living and force people to respond to crisis situations without the use of their normal coping mechanisms. When entire communities are ravaged, people also lose their roots or frame of reference and sense of safety, control, and closeness (Norris, Baker, Murphy, & Kaniasty, 2005; Rogers & Lawhorn, 2007).

Disasters occur in varied forms and include both natural and man-made types, war atrocities, childhood abuse, factory explosions, and school shootings. Unfortunately, these events have become a part of life.

RESEARCH ON PSYCHOLOGICAL RESPONSES TO DISASTERS

The 1972 flood disaster of Buffalo Creek, West Virginia, left 125 people dead and nearly 5,000 homeless. Everyone exposed to this disaster experienced some form of psychological manifestation of survivors described by Lifton & Olson (1976). Psychological impact included the following five constellations:

1. *Death and imprint and death anxiety:* Consists of vivid memories and images of the disaster and its destructiveness. People experienced sleeplessness, a fear of crowds, and recurring nightmares.

2. *Death guilt (survivor's guilt):* Manifests by preoccupation with persistent thoughts of dead relatives or friends. These

feelings were frequently part of their nightmares. Survivors often had problems forgiving themselves for surviving.

3. *Psychic numbing:* Refers to an impaired capacity to feel, and this was shown by distancing, social withdrawal, aloofness, and limited interpersonal relationships. Survivors of the Buffalo Creek flood exhibited apathy, confusion, and indifference. Numbing is a defense mechanism used to deny or protect the survivor from confronting or reliving the horrible experience. Biological aspects of numbing are associated with activation of endorphins, which results in "emotional numbing" (van der Kolk, McFarlane, & Weisaeth, 1996).

4. *Impaired interpersonal relationships:* Refers to the enormous need for survivors to seek love and affection while being unable to accept available resources. Survivors tend to be suspicious of closeness and affection during times that they really need them. Anger and unexpressed rage often emerge, putting more distance in relationships. These responses tend to disperse and increase when survivors fail to adequately externalize rage and anger.

5. *Struggle for significance:* Refers to efforts to make sense of almost dying and then surviving a traumatic experience.

Other disasters stem from war atrocities and traumatic experiences. Several investigators have demonstrated a relationship between the intensity of combat exposure and the evolution of post-traumatic stress disorder (PTSD) (Breslau, Reboussin, Anthony, & Storr, 2005). These studies explored the severity of psychopathology, both PTSD and depression, and level of function in clients exposed to war atrocities and traumatic combat. A number of survivors of the Nazi holocaust suffer symptoms of PTSD and exhibit similar symptoms as those of veterans from the Vietnam War (Reeves, Parker, & Konkle-Parker, 2005; Yehuda, Golier, & Kaufman, 2005). (See Chapter 11.)

More recent tragedies and disasters include the 2007 Virginia Tech shootings, which stunned the community, country, and world because of the catastrophic impact on the lives of victims, survivors, health care providers, and disaster workers. The magnitude of destruction and the media exposure brought these horrific events into the homes of millions. These traumatic events, along with other disasters, reminded people of their vulnerability to violence and its global impact on individuals, families, communities, and society.

People exposed to disasters, both survivors and disaster workers, are at risk for developing acute and chronic stress-related disorders such as acute stress disorder and PTSD (DeSalvo et al., 2007; Fullerton, Ursano, & Wang, 2004). Some researchers also submit that the development of these disorders may result from a biological response in the immediate aftermath of a traumatic incident, which consequently leads to a maladaptive psychological response (Delahanty & Nugent, 2006). Historically, studies exploring the meaning and responses to disasters date back to Lindemann's renowned study of the Coconut Grove Fire of 1944. Clinical and empirical research was also generated by the Buffalo Creek flood disaster that destroyed an entire community

(Erikson, 1976). Major findings from these studies suggest widespread and persistent personality and behavioral changes in survivors, such as maladaptation and bereavement.

FACTORS INFLUENCING RESPONSE TO DISASTERS

Disasters place immense stress on individuals, families, and communities, taxing resources and compromising adaptive responses. Sarason and Sarason (1984) surmised that the outcome of disasters is influenced by several factors such as predictability, duration, intensity, locus of control, and state of self-concept.

Predictability

Predictability affects stress reactions, which may be of low or high intensity. It affects the ability of the person and community to cope or prepare for the disaster.

Duration

Examples are the severe flooding in Texas in 2007 and Hurricane Katrina in 2005. Stress responses to Hurricane Katrina were complicated by persistent lack of government support for safe and timely rescue and adequate housing and shelter. Survivors of these disasters lost their homes, property, dignity, and sense of well-being and safety. In spite of the destruction of the hurricane and flooding, communities were able to deal with their immediate needs by banding together to seek shelter, food, water, and safety. The disasters were forecast in advance, but their intensity and duration were so profound that victims attempted to cope with their losses for an extended period after the disaster had occurred.

Intensity

Intensity or severity varies with the degree of loss, type of injury, repertoire of coping mechanisms, and appraisal of the event.

Locus of Control

The nature of disasters makes it difficult to predict or have control of their impact on the lives of people and communities. Recent hurricane and severe flooding disasters left many victims feeling helpless, with little control over recovering their losses or finding temporary food and living quarters. Loss of control frequently generates feelings of powerlessness, helplessness, frustration, and depression.

State of Self-Concept

Impaired self-confidence or low self-esteem results in inadequacy or ineffectiveness in handling stressful situations. For example, in a natural disaster in which families have lost their possessions, a man may feel that his family relies on him for shelter, food, and safety. The man who feels confident is likely to remain calm within himself and his family by seeking support from other victims and other community resources. Even though he is unable to locate immediate shelter, his confident response promotes a sense of safety and security in his family. In contrast, the man who is fearful and uncertain about himself and his family members will lack confidence in managing the situation and will not cope as well.

THE NURSING PROCESS

Disasters and crises have a profound and unpredictable effect on people, families, and communities (see the Research Abstract). Nurses are challenged to identify high-risk groups and assess the impact of the disaster and crisis on survivors and to recognize maladaptive responses. Survivors show the resilience of the human spirit and survival instinct. Nurses play a major role in mobilizing internal and external resources that facilitate a sense of control, confidence, and that reinforce support systems. Restoration and maintenance of health and adaptation are basic to the survivors' well-being. Lifton and Olson (1976) suggested that psychological health can be improved in survivors by the following:

◆ Recognizing their profound agony

◆ Identifying causes of the disaster or trauma

◆ Encouraging the desire to live and rebuild

◆ Educating people about the meaning of disaster and strength as a survivor

Psychiatric triage is often an initial intervention that prioritizes care and enables survivors to receive immediate emotional support through crisis intervention or critical incident stress debriefing (CISD) (Mitchell, 1988). Stress debriefing is a crisis intervention technique that relies on three therapeutic modalities: provide an opportunity to express one's feelings in the context of group support, facilitate normalization of reactions to an abnormal event, and learn about postdisaster reactions (Knobler, Nachshoni, Jaffe, Peretz, & Yehuda, 2007). Finally, crisis intervention is used to mobilize resources by identifying viable options, such as shelter, food, water, and safety, during the early stages of emotional, social, and physical turmoil. Several treatment modalities, such as crisis intervention, family therapy (see Chapter 28), and psychotherapy, can facilitate health promotion.

The efficacy of stress debriefing is currently the basis of much controversy. Several meta-analyses and randomized controlled trials (RCTs) demonstrate that this intervention is ineffective in the prevention of PTSD after a traumatic event. In fact, several studies report potential worsening of stress-related symptoms in clients and emergency personnel receiving stress debriefing (Sijbrandij, Olff, Reitsma, Carlier, & Gersons, 2006 Wagner, 2005). Some researchers submit that CISD should be reduced or employed only with extreme caution as a crisis intervention until more studies can confirm its usefulness (Bledsoe, 2003). Based on these findings, CISD should never be mandatory. A lack of evidence that shows the ineffectiveness of CISD does not preclude the usefulness of providing education of normal stress reactions and providing emotional support from being used during the aftermath of traumatic incidents.

An area often forgotten when disasters occur is the impact of these events have on nurses and other disaster workers, stemming from exposure to catastrophic events. Perhaps the most difficult aspect of disaster work is exposure to dead bodies and violent death (Morgan et al., 2006). An effort to reduce and relieve stress reactions in disaster workers also includes CISD. The psychiatric nurse's role in CISD includes

RESEARCH ABSTRACT

The Inspiration of Hope in Bereavement Counseling

Cutliff, J. R. (2004). *Issues in Mental Health Nursing, 25,* 165–190.

Aim/Purpose of the Study

Attempted to answer the question, Do bereavement counselors inspire hope in their clients, and if so, how?

Method

The researchers used a modified grounded theory to glean the nature of hope and hope inspiration under the auspices of bereavement counseling. Data collection involved unstructured interviews collected in a quiet room, either in the client's home or a counseling center. The interviews were 1 to 2 hours using a loose structure. Due to the process of the constant comparison method, data were collected and coded in a nonlinear process.

Findings

Data analysis revealed an implicit projection of hope and hopefulness, a core variable, and three subcore variables, such as using the relationship as a venue to express feelings (catharsis) and facilitating healthy closure. The theory also indicated that this hope inspiration may be subtle and an unobtrusive process between the counselor and client produced an environment of inspiration and hope.

Implications for Psychiatric Nurses

More and more there is evidence that supports the role of hope and spirituality in coping and resilience. Working with clients with psychiatric conditions and establishing healthy, supportive, and empathic nurse-client relationships inspire hope in many clients. Psychiatric nurses, like other nurses, are poised to integrate interventions that promote strength, hope, and resilience across the life span.

helping survivors normalize their responses to abnormal situations. As members of the CISD team, psychiatric nurses can work with various populations and assist them in normalizing their responses to disasters by providing immediate emotional support, educating them about normal stress reactions, monitoring their symptoms, and making appropriate mental health referrals.

The following case study points out areas that must be assessed and addressed when a family presents with a crisis.

How can this family be helped? Crisis intervention is a useful strategy in which families and children can find relief from overwhelming circumstances such as those in the case study. It is a mechanism that furnishes immediate emotional support, feedback, and clarification of incongruencies.

Langsley & Kaplan (1968) pointed out that family crisis-intervention has several advantages. It enhances self-awareness, clarifies the roles of members in sustaining it, develops fresh coping skills, and gains a sense of competency to manage the situation. Some families may benefit from family therapy. (See Chapter 28 for in-depth discussion of family therapy.)

ASSESSMENT

The assessment process begins with establishing rapport and assessing members from a here-and-now approach and the present crisis to determine the existing stressors and reasons for seeking treatment at this time. The following questions are useful in eliciting information regarding the nature of the family crisis:

◆ What specific event or circumstances have brought you in today?

◆ How did this occur?

◆ How has the family dealt with it?

◆ What has made it difficult for you to deal with it at this time?

Inquiring about present and past coping patterns provides invaluable information about the family's level of function, communication patterns, developmental stage, and problem-solving skills. When there is risk for injury, levels of danger must be assessed and dealt with immediately. In the case of Edet, it is imperative to resolve the following questions:

◆ How long has he had thoughts of dying?

◆ What does dying mean to him?

◆ What has stopped him from acting on those thoughts?

◆ Does he have a plan or means to kill himself?

◆ Has he made attempts in the past?

◆ Have other family members tried to kill themselves or made previous attempts?

Additionally, Edet's parents must be assessed for potential for injury to themselves or others, including present and past behaviors.

NURSING DIAGNOSES

The major nursing diagnoses of family crises are:

◆ Disabled Family Coping

◆ Anxiety

◆ Interrupted Family Processes

The family is at least temporarily unable to mobilize adequate resources and effective problem solving to resolve a crisis situation.

PLANNING

Nursing Care Plan 31–1 identifies the desired outcomes for the nursing diagnoses listed earlier and delineates the nursing actions needed to achieve these outcomes, along with the rationales for these actions.

CASE STUDY

The Family Experiencing a Crisis Situation (Edet, Mother, Father)

Ten-year-old Edet was seen in the emergency department (ED) after he sustained several dog bites from a neighbor's pet. Edet was quiet and withdrawn. He refused to discuss the incident and stated that he wished he were dead. His statement disturbed his mother. She informed the nurse that her son has been behaving differently for several months (he had begun to sleep in class, and his grades had been falling the past 6 weeks), and that she was concerned about his safety. Additionally, she commented that she is unsure if the child let the dog bite him on purpose. Later, Edet's father came to the ED after parking the car, and his mother discussed her concerns with his father. The child and his parents were referred to the psychiatric nurse liaison-consultant for evaluation and crisis intervention. The nurse discovered that the family had been experiencing major financial problems since the father was laid off his $120,000-a-year job. He had been unable to find gainful employment over the past 6 months. He is a 49-year-old aerospace engineer who feels pessimistic about a comparably paying job because of his age and reduction in government spending on defense. He and Edet's mother admitted that this had been devastating to the family, particularly because they have two older children in college. They also admit they have been ignoring their 10-year-old son. Other family stressors included the parents' concerns about maintaining their current lifestyle and frequent arguments that have created a distancing in their relationship. Edet stated that he feels responsible for the family problems and he cries a lot during the night. Furthermore, he is frightened by the arguments between his parents, and feels like no one cares about him.

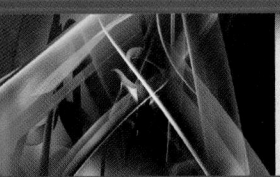

NURSING CARE PLAN 31–1

The Family Experiencing a Crisis Situation (Edet, Mother, Father)

Nursing Diagnosis: Ineffective Coping

Outcome Identification	Nursing Actions	Rationales	Evaluation
1. By [date], family will identify realistic perception of stressors or crisis.	1a. Assist family in identifying precipitating event.	1a. Identifying precipitating event facilitates identification of the problem (crisis situation).	*Goal met:* Family members are able to identify recent changes or stressors.
	1b. Explore and assess meaning of major lifestyle change or stressor.	1b. Assessing the meaning of lifestyle changes and stress helps the family gain insight into the present crisis.	
2. By [date], family will develop adaptive coping patterns.	2. Assess family's current and past coping skills.	2. Assessing the family's past coping skills assists in identifying the present level of functioning and coping skills.	

Nursing Diagnosis: Anxiety

Outcome Identification	Nursing Actions	Rationales	Evaluation
1. By [date], family will learn how to decrease anxiety effectively.	1a. Assess level of anxiety.	1a. Family gains an understanding of present level of anxiety.	*Goal met:* Family gains an understanding of ineffective problem solving. Anxiety is reduced by effective communication skills.
	1b. Teach members adaptive stress-reducing measures.	1b–d. Problem solving mobilizes resources and reduces stress and decreased feelings of helplessness.	
	1c. Encourage problem solving.		
	1d. Confront self-defeating behaviors.		
	1e. Teach effective communication skills.	1e. Effective communication of feelings promotes understanding and insight into the family's response to stress.	

(continues)

Nursing Care Plan 31–1 (continued)

Nursing Diagnosis: Interrupted Family Processes

Outcome Identification	Nursing Actions	Rationales	Evaluation
1. By [date], family will express and share their feelings regarding present crisis.	1. Encourage sharing of feelings.	1. Sharing feelings allows members to support each other and to clarify the crisis situation.	*Goal met:* Family develops effective coping skills and resolves crisis effectively.
2. By [date], family will maintain functional system.	2a. Identify the family's strengths and weaknesses.	2a–c. Identifying strengths and options and reorganizing roles decrease feelings of powerlessness and problem areas.	
	2b. Provide and offer the family options and resources.		
	2c. Assist the family in reorganizing their roles around decisive concerns.		

IMPLEMENTATION

Nursing interventions are based on the assumption that a family crisis is time limited and responsive to adaptive changes. This process begins when the nurse suggests several options for handling the crisis. The nurse-client relationship is used to focus on reasons for the present crisis, to identify recent coping responses and strengths, and to explore ways to reduce symptoms and distress. Encouraging family participation reduces feelings of helplessness and encourages problem solving.

EVALUATION

In this case study, it is important for Edet's parents to take charge of the present situation by providing safety for the child. Their concerns for his safety and willingness to seek help promoted a sense of security in the child. Children often feel frightened and confused when sudden life changes occur. Edet's parents also had difficulty handling their fears and uncertainty about the situation, and this heightened his sense of helplessness. Edet's expression of wanting to die symbolized these feelings. In consultation with the nurse, the parents expressed their feelings and identified the reasons for the present crisis. This discussion clarified and dispelled the notion that the child was responsible for his parents' present crisis. His parents were encouraged to tell the child how important he was and to spend quality time with him.

SUMMARY

◆ A crisis is a turning point that stems from an imbalance between a stressful event and inability to mobilize resources to adapt to it.

◆ A period of disorganization often ensues, providing an opportunity for formation of improved coping skills and potential growth.

◆ Ideally, people emerge from a crisis situation functioning at a precrisis or higher level.

◆ Caplan's and Lindemann's contributions to the crisis theory and crisis management have prevailed for almost half a century, providing nurses with a practical and effective approach to helping clients in crises.

◆ Crisis intervention mobilizes internal and external resources, which promote adaptive coping responses.

◆ Crisis resolution is governed by nature and duration of stressor and psychosocial, neurobiological, and behavioral factors. Psychiatric nurses are well suited to facilitate adaptation and healthy resolution across the health continuum.

SUGGESTIONS FOR CLINICAL CONFERENCES

1. Invite an advanced-practice psychiatric registered nurse to discuss several case histories of clients in crisis and discuss the generalist and advanced practice role

2. Present several disaster scenarios and the role of stress debriefing

3. Encourage students to select and present several cases involving grief and express their feelings about the clients feelings and their responses

4. Discuss attitudes of students regarding death and dying issues.

STUDY QUESTIONS

1. Several members of a family are brought to the emergency department with severe burns and smoke inhalation caused by a neighborhood fire. The mother is found crying in the waiting area with her 5-year-old daughter. As a member of the psychiatric triage unit, what is your initial response to this family?
   a. Approaching them in a calm, reassuring manner
   b. Inquiring about the events surrounding the fire
   c. Encouraging the mother to express feelings about the fire
   d. Letting the mother know that her crying will upset her daughter

2. After spending time with her daughter, the mother leaves the room and continues to cry. The *best* nursing intervention at this time is to:
   a. Leave her alone until she seeks your assistance.
   b. Assess her thoughts and feelings about the situation.
   c. Acknowledge her pain and provide emotional support.
   d. encourage her to stay strong for the family.

3. Crisis intervention may be used in this situation to:
   a. identify and mobilize resources
   b. identify past psychiatric treatment
   c. assess past responses to stress
   d. Recognize the impact of early childhood traumas

4. One of your colleagues participated in stress debriefing of a group of high school youth who witnessed one of their schoolmates shoot himself. After the debriefing you notice that you have an overwhelming sense of sadness and need to be alone. Based on your understanding of stress reactions, how do you describe your responses?
   a. Admit that you should avoid traumatic events because of your inability to handle them.
   b. Recognize that these are normal reactions to an abnormal situation.
   c. Seek professional counseling because your reactions are abnormal.
   d. Avoid discussing your reactions with others.

5. Mrs. Mertz recently lost her husband of 46 years. Her family brought her to the mental health clinic because she has become increasingly despondent and isolative over the past few weeks and cries all the time. She denies needing psychiatric help, but she admits missing her husband. Mrs. Mertz's symptoms suggest that she is experiencing:
   a. a normal grief reaction
   b. an abnormal grief reaction
   c. physical problems that require attention
   d. major depressive episode symptoms

6. Mrs. Mertz may benefit from grief work. The major goals of grief work include all of the following *except:*
   a. establishment of a therapeutic alliance
   b. mobilization of resources
   c. assessment of coping patterns
   d. Provision of psychotropic medications

7. Marty is a generalist nurse who works in the psychiatric triage unit. One of his clients is complaining of feeling overwhelmed by his present crisis. Which of the following interventions is not within the scope of Marty's role as a generalist nurse?
   a. Offer short-term psychotherapy because of his present distress.
   b. Assess his level of dangerousness to himself or others.
   c. Encourage the client to express his feelings and identify his strengths.
   d. Offer him options for dealing with his present situation.

8. Nicole, a 15-year-old girl, is brought into the adolescent crisis unit with her mother who is expressing concerns about her daughter's adamant requests to get a tattoo because all of her friends have one. Nicole is cooperative and relaxed. She also states that she does not understand her mother's reasons for bringing her in today. Nicole's mother explains that her daughter has never argued with her in the past and has been pretty compliant with family rules. As her nurse, your response to Nicole's mother will be based on which of the following?
   a. This mother-daughter conflict represents a maturational crisis.
   b. Nicole's behavior reflects a situational crisis.
   c. This is a family crisis and requires a referral for extensive family therapy.
   d. If Nicole's maladaptive behavior persists, a referral for medications should be considered.

9. Which of the following statements is true about critical incident stress debriefing?
   a. There is empirical evidence of its efficacy in the prevention of PTSD.
   b. It is mandatory and must be used by anyone exposed to a critical incident.
   c. There is no evidence of its efficacy in the prevention of PTSD.
   d. It offers participants psychotherapy, emotional support, and education about normal stress responses.

10. You are working with a family who has experienced a major family crisis, the sudden death of a family member. Which of the following is an indicator of how the family will cope with this situation?
    a. "We have been through tougher times; we'll get through this one."
    b. "What are we going to do? We just can't go on without her."
    c. "How could she die on us like this? I am so mad at her."
    d. "Our family must be cursed. Bad things keep happening to us."

11. A client walks into the mental health outpatient center and states, "I've had it. I can't go on any longer. You've got to help me." The nurse asks the client to be seated in a private interview area. Which action should the nurse take next?
    a. Reassure the client that someone will help him soon.
    b. Assess the client's insurance coverage.

c. Find out more about what is happening to the client.

d. Call the client's family to come and provide support.

CRITICAL THINKING

Ms. Jones is seen in the emergency room after witnessing a serious MVA. She has not sustained any physical injuries except for a lacerated knee. She is crying and distraught. Which of the following statement is a *normal stress reaction?*

a. "I feel perfectly fine and would like to go home."

b. "I cannot remember anything."

c. "I need to call my job because I have an important meeting tomorrow."

d. "I need to talk to you about my family."

RESOURCES

Please note that because Internet resources are of a time-sensitive nature and URL addresses may change or be deleted, searches should also be conducted by association or topic.

Internet Resources

http://www.ffcmh.org   Federation of Families for Children's Mental Health

http://www.ncptsd.org/facts/disasters/fs_grief-disaster.html   National Center for PTSD—resources for post disasters

http://www.ncvc.org/   National Center for Victims of Crime, for more information about violence and resources

http://www.mentalhealth.org/child   Center for Mental Health Services, for information regarding Family Guide Systems for Care of Children with Mental Health Needs

http://www.cdc.gov/mmwr/preview/mmwrhtml/mm5502a5.htm   Centers for Disease Control and Prevention (2006). *Assessment of Health-Related Needs After Hurricanes Katrina and Rita—Orleans and Jefferson Parishes, New Orleans Area*, Louisiana, October 17–22, 2005 (Accessed April 29, 2006)

Other Resources

CMHS National Mental Health Services
   Knowledge Exchange Network (KEN)
   P.O. Box 42490
   Washington, DC 20015
   (800) 749-2647
   http://www.mentalhealth.org/child
Center for Mental Health Services, Child, Adolescent, and
   Family Branch
   P.O. Box 42490
   Washington, DC 20015
   (301) 443-1333 (Spanish is spoken)

REFERENCES

Aguilera, D. C. (1990). *Crisis intervention: Theory and methodology* (6th ed.). St. Louis: C. V. Mosby.

Aguilera, D. C. (1994). *Crisis intervention: Theory and methodology* (7th ed.). St. Louis: C. V. Mosby.

Aguilera, D. (1998). *Crisis intervention: Theory and methodology* (8th ed.). Philadelphia: C. V. Mosby.

Aguilera, D. C., & Messick, J. M. (1978). *Crisis intervention: Theory and methodology* (3rd ed.). St. Louis: C. V. Mosby.

American Nurses Association. (2000). *Scope and standards of psychiatric-mental health nursing practice.* Washington, DC: Author.

Andrews, H., & Roy, Sr., C. (1986). *Essentials of the Roy adaptation model.* Norwalk, CT: Appleton-Crofts.

Antai-Otong, D. (2004). *Psychiatric emergencies: How to accurately assess and manage the patient in crisis.* Eau Claire, WI: Professional Educational Systems Inc.

Antonovsky, A. (1987). *Unraveling the mystery of health: How people manage stress and stay well.* San Francisco: Jossey-Bass.

Bledsoe, B. E. (2003). Critical incident stress management (CISM): Benefit or risk for emergency services? *Prehospital Emergency Care, 7,* 272–279.

Blos, P. (1962). *On adolescence.* New York: The Free Press.

Bowlby, J. (1969). *Attachment and loss: Vol. 1, attachment.* New York: Basic Books.

Breslau, N., Reboussin, B. A., Anthony, J. C., & Storr, C. L. (2005). The structure of posttraumatic stress disorder: Latent class analysis in 2 community samples. *Archives of General Psychiatry, 62,* 1343–1351.

Cannon, W. B. (1914). The function of the adrenal medulla. *American Journal of Physiology, 33,* 356–377.

Caplan, G. (1961). *An approach to community mental health.* New York: Grune & Stratton.

Caplan, G. (1964). *Principles of preventive psychiatry.* New York: Basic Books.

Centers for Disease Control and Prevention. (2006a). Surveillance in hurricane evacuation centers—Louisiana, September-October 2005. *MMWR Morbidly and Mortality Weekly Report, 20,* 32–35.

Centers for Disease Control and Prevention. (2006b). Assessment of health-related needs after Hurricanes Katrina and Rita—Orleans and Jefferson Parishes, New Orleans area, Louisiana, October 17–22, 2005. *MMWR Morbidly and Mortality Weekly Report, 55,* 38–41.

Davanloo, H. (1978). *Basic principles and techniques of short-term psychotherapy.* New York: Spectrum Publications.

Delahanty, D. L., & Nugent, N. R. (2006). Predicting PTSD prospectively based on prior trauma history and immediate biological responses. *Annals of New York Academy of Sciences, 1071,* 27–40.

DeSalvo, K. B., Hyre, A. D., Ompad, D. C., Menke, A., Tynes, L. L., & Muntner, P. (2007). Symptoms of posttraumatic stress disorder in a New Orleans workforce following Hurricane Katrina. *Journal of Urban Health, 84,* 142–152.

Dimsdale, J. E., Keefe, F. J., & Stein, M. B. (2000). Stress and psychiatry. In B. J. Sadock & V. A. Sadock (Eds.), *Comprehensive textbook of psychiatry* (7th ed., pp. 1835–1846). Philadelphia: Lippincott Williams & Wilkins.

Erikson, E. (1963). Childhood and society, (Rev. ed.). New York: W. W. Norton.

Erikson, E. (1964). *Insight and responsibility*. New York: W. W. Norton.

Erikson, E. H. (1968). *Identity: Youth and crisis*. New York: W. W. Norton.

Erikson, K. T. (1976). Loss of community at Buffalo Creek. *American Journal of Psychiatry, 133*, 302–325.

Freud, S. (1961). The ego and the id. In J. Strachey (Ed. & Trans.), *The standard edition of the complete psychological works of Sigmund Freud* (Vol. 19, pp. 3–66). London: Hogarth Press. (Original work published 1923.)

Fullerton, C. S., Ursano, R. J., & Wang, L. (2004). Acute stress disorder, posttraumatic stress disorder, and depression in disaster or rescue workers. *American Journal of Psychiatry, 161*, 1370–1376.

Greef, A. P., & Holtzkamp, J. (2007). The prevalence of resilience in migrant families. *Family and Community Health, 30*, 189–200.

Hansen, D. A., & Johnson, V. A. (1979). Rethinking family stress theory: Definitional aspects. In W. R. Burr, R. Hill, F. I. Nye, & I. L. Reiss (Eds), Contemporary theories about the family: Research-based theories (Vol. I, pp. 582–603). New York: Free Press.

Hoff, L. A. (1989). *People in crisis* (3rd ed.). Redwood, CA: Addison-Wesley.

Holmes, T. H., & Rahe, R. H. (1967). The social readjustment rating scale. *Journal of Psychosomatic Research, 11*, 213–218.

Joint Commission on Mental Health and Mental Illness. (1961). *Action for mental health science edition*. New York: Basic Books.

Kaplan, L. J. (1984). *Adolescence: The farewell to childhood*. New York: Simon & Schuster.

Kaskie, B., Wallace, N., Kang, S., & Bloom, J. (2006). The implementation of managed behavioral healthcare in Colorado and the effects on older Medicaid beneficiaries. *Journal of Mental Health Policy and Economics, 9*, 15–24.

Knobler, H. Y., Nachshoni, T., Jaffe, E., Peretz, G., & Yehuda, Y. B. (2007). Psychological guidelines for a medical team debriefing after a stressful event. *Military Medicine, 172*, 581–585.

Langsley, D., & Kaplan, D. (1968). *Treatment of families in crisis*. New York: Grune & Stratton.

Lazarus, R. S. (1966). *Psychological stress and the coping process*. New York: McGraw-Hill.

Lazarus, R. S. (1991). *Emotion and adaptation*. New York: Oxford University Press.

Lazarus, R. S., & Folkman, R. (1984). *Stress, appraisal, and coping*. New York: Springer Publications.

Lifton, R. J., & Olson, E. (1976). The human meaning of total disaster: The Buffalo Creek experience. *Psychiatry, 39*, 1–18.

Lindemann, E. (1944). Symptomatology and management of acute grief. *American Journal of Psychiatry, 101*, 141–148.

Lindemann, E. (1979). *Beyond grief: Studies in crisis intervention*. New York: Jason Aronson.

McGee, R. K. (1974). *Crisis intervention in the community*. Baltimore: University Park Press.

McGoldrick, M., Giordano, J., & Garcia-Preto, N. (2005). Ethnicity & Family Therapy, 3rd ed. New York: Guilford Publication, Inc.

Mishne, J. M. (1986). *Clinical work with adolescents*. New York: The Free Press.

Mitchell, J. T. (1988). The history, status and future of critical incident stress debriefing. *JEMS Journal of Emergency Medical Services, 13*, 47–52.

Morgan, O. W., Sribanditmongkol, P., Perera, C., Sulasmi, Y., Van Alphen, D., & Sondorp, E. (2006). Mass fatality management following the South Asian tsunami disaster: Case studies in Thailand, Indonesia, and Sri Lanka. *PloS Medicine, 3*, e195.

Morikawa, Y., Kitaoka-Higashiguchi, K., Tanimoto, C., Hayashi, M., Oketani, R., Miura, K., Nishijo, M., & Nakagawa, H. (2005). A cross-sectional study on the relationship of job stress with natural killer cell activity and natural killer cell subsets among healthy nurses. *Journal of Occupational Health, 47*, 378–383.

Norris, F. H., Baker, C. K., Murphy, A. D., & Kaniasty, K. (2005). Social support mobilization and deterioration after Mexico's 1999 flood: Effects of context, gender, and time. *American Journal of Community Psychology, 36*, 15–28.

Parad, H. J., & Caplan, G. (1965). Framework for studying families in crisis. In H. J. Parad (Ed.), *Crisis intervention: Selected readings* (pp. 53–72). New York: Family Service Association of America.

Piaget, J. (1952). *The origins of intelligence in children*. New York: International Universities Press.

Piaget, J. (1969). *The early growth of logic in the child*. New York: W. W. Norton.

Picardi, A., Battisti, F., Tarsitani, L., Baldassari, M., Copertaro, A., Mocchegiani, E., et al. (2007). Attachment security and immunity in healthy women. *Psychosomatic Medicine, 69*, 40–46.

Raphael, B., & Wooding, S. (2004). Debriefing: Its evolution and current status. *Psychiatric Clinics of North America, 27*, 407–423.

Rapoport, L. (1965). The state of crisis: Some theoretical considerations: In H. J. Parad (Ed.), *Crisis intervention: Selected readings* (pp. 22–31). New York: Family Service Association of America.

Redlich, A. D., Steadman, H. J., Robbins, P. C., & Swanson, J. W. (2006). Use of the criminal justice system to leverage mental health treatment: Effects on treatment adherence and satisfaction. *Journal of the American Academy of Psychiatry and Law, 34*, 292–299.

Reeves, R. R., Parker, J. D., & Konkle-Parker, D. J. (2005). War-related mental health problems of today's veterans: New clinical awareness. *Journal of Psychosocial Nursing and Mental Health Services, 43,* 18–28.

Rogers, B., & Lawhorn, E. (2007). Disaster preparedness: Occupational and environmental health professionals' response to Hurricanes Katrina and Rita. *AAOHN Journal, 55,* 197–207.

Rohleder, N., & Karl, A. (2006). Role of endocrine and inflammatory alterations in comorbid somatic diseases of post-traumatic stress disorder. *Minerva Endocrinology, 31,* 273–288.

Roy, Sr., C., & Andrews, H. (1991). *The Roy adaptation model: The definitive statement.* Norwalk, CT: Appleton-Crofts.

Sakami, S., Maeda, M., Maruoka, T., Nakata, A., Komaki, G., & Kawamura, N. (2004). Positive coping up- and down-regulates in vitro cytokine productions from T cells dependent on stress levels. *Psychotherapy and Psychosomatics, 73,* 243–251.

Sarason, I. G., & Sarason, B. (1984). *Abnormal psychology* (4th ed.). Englewood Cliffs, NJ: Prentice-Hall, Inc.

Selye, H. (1946). The general adaptation syndrome and the diseases of adaptation. *Journal of Clinical Endocrinology, 6,* 117–196.

Selye, H. (1956). *The stress of life.* New York: McGraw-Hill.

Selye, H. (1976). *The stress of life* (Rev. ed.). New York: McGraw-Hill.

Sijbrandij, M., Olff, M., Reitsma, J. B., Carlier, I. V., & Gersons, B. P. (2006). Emotional or educational debriefing after psychological trauma. Randomised controlled trial. *British Journal of Psychiatry, 189,* 150–155.

Stein, M. (1986). A reconsideration of specificity in psychosomatic medicine: From olfaction to the lymphocyte. *Psychosomatic Medicine, 48,* 3–22.

Squire, L. R. (1987). *Memory and the brain.* New York: Oxford Press.

Utsey, S. O., Hook, J. N., & Stanard, P. (2007). A re-examination of cultural factors that mitigate risk and promote resilience in relation to African American suicide: A review of the literature and recommendations for future research. *Death Studies, 31,* 399–416.

van der Kolk, B. A., McFarlane, A. C., & Weisaeth, L. (1996). *Traumatic stress: The effects of overwhelming experience on mind, body, and society.* New York: Guilford Press.

Wagner, S. L. (2005). Emergency response service personnel and the critical incident stress debriefing debate. *Internal Journal of Emergency Mental Health, 7,* 33–41.

Ward-Griffin, C., Schofield, R., Vos, S., Coatsworth-Puspoky, R. (2005). Canadian families caring for members with mental illness: A vicious cycle. *Journal of Family Nursing, 11,* 140–161.

Weiner, H. (1985). The concept of stress in light of studies on disasters, unemployment, and loss: A critical analysis. In M. R. Zales (Ed.), *Stress in health and disease* (pp. 24–94). New York: Brunner/Mazel.

Yehuda, R., Golier, J. A., & Kaufman, S. (2005). Circadian rhythm of salivary cortisol in Holocaust survivors with and without PTSD. *American Journal of Psychiatry, 162,* 998–1000.

SUGGESTED READING

Armstrong, K., Zatzick, D., Metzler, T., Weiss, D. S., Marmar, C., Garma, S., et al. (1998). Debriefing of American Red Cross Personnel: Pilot study on participants' evaluations and case examples from the 1994 Los Angeles Earthquake relief operation. *Social Work in Health Care, 27,* 33–50.

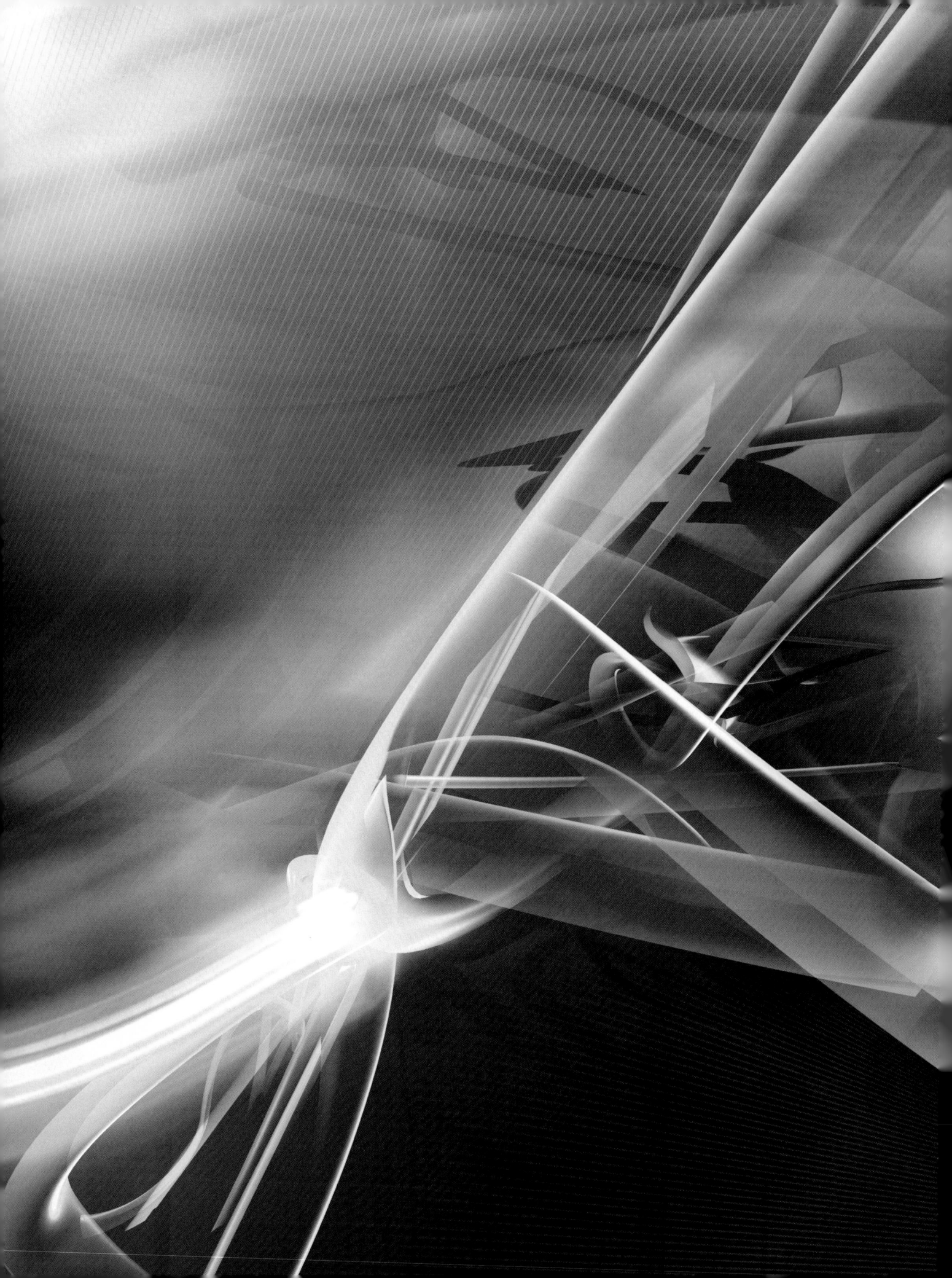

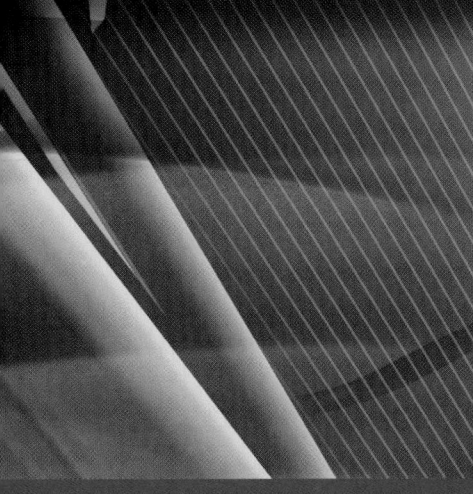

CHAPTER 32

Milieu Therapy/ Hospital-Based Care

Johnnie Bonner, MS, RNCS

KEY TERMS

Assertive Community Treatment (ACT): Refers to a model of mental health care that provides the client and family with many case management functions, including ongoing assessments, treatment planning, and monitoring of mental, physical, and social functioning. The precise approach varies, but an individual is generally designated as the *broker of care* or treatment coordinator.

Containment: A term for safety, food, shelter, and medical care issues in milieu therapy.

Continuum of Mental Health Care: Refers to a model that is distinct from one area of treatment planning and encompasses a comprehensive or multisystem perspective mental health care delivery model.

Holding Environment: A descriptive term for a therapeutic milieu that incorporates traditional milieu therapy variables. The term *healing environment* is sometimes used interchangeably with holding environment.

Intensive Case Management: A concept similar to ACT that has shown to be cost-effective and efficacious in the treatment of serious mental illnesses.

Involvement: Includes the basic milieu therapy concept of the client's responsibility to participate actively in treatment and other decision making.

Milieu: A French term for middle space, or a safe place and environment.

Milieu Therapy: A treatment modality that uses the total physical and social environment as a therapeutic agent to provide psychosocial rehabilitation for psychiatric clients. Traditionally, milieu therapy includes key variables or components that are also defined here. The term is sometimes used interchangeably with the term *therapeutic milieu*.

Open Communication: Active and honest sharing of feelings, thoughts, and information. Confidentiality is unit based and unhealthy secret keeping is discouraged, but privacy is respected.

Validation: Affirmation of the client's individuality and right to be treated with respect and dignity.

COMPETENCIES

Upon completion of this chapter, the learner should be able to:

1. Analyze the eight components or variables of traditional milieu therapy.
2. Describe the client's role in a therapeutic community.
3. Identify key components of the nurse's role in the therapeutic milieu.
4. Describe the nursing process in the management of the therapeutic milieu.
5. Implement developmentally appropriate approaches to milieu interventions.

CHAPTER OUTLINE

Traditional Aspects of Milieu Therapy

Concepts and Principles of Milieu Therapy in a New Era

Containment

Support

Validation

Structure

TRADITIONAL ASPECTS OF MILIEU THERAPY

Historically, the term milieu referred to an inpatient and structured environment that facilitated stabilization and psychosocial rehabilitation. Inpatient treatment was the primary mode of treatment, which normally included extended lengths of stay. Before the advent of psychotropic agents in the 1950s, treatment of persons with serious mental illnesses was primarily confined to isolation and restraints. On discharge, the clients often received inadequate access to mental health services, resulting in high relapse rates and, thus, recidivism and poor client outcomes. This traditional model of milieu therapy eventually became a pink elephant and was extremely costly and virtually ineffective in managing complex client needs. During the 1950s milieu therapy played a significant role in the treatment of serious mental disorders because it integrated major biological, social, and behavioral concepts into treatment planning. Limitations of earlier psychotropic medications were their lack of management of disabling negative symptoms. The advent of psychotropics during this period reduced lengths of stay and relapse rates by managing some of the positive symptoms that further advanced the role of deinstitutionalization.

Mental health care delivery models paralleled socioeconomic changes, technological and neurobiological advances, and treatment options. During the 1980s the new drug clozapine (Clozaril) was introduced into the market and used to treat refractory symptoms in clients with schizophrenia, offering hope for clients and their families. The 1990s have brought in a plethora of new treatment modalities for these clients. Specifically, these drugs are managing positive and negative symptoms and have fewer risks than their predecessors although they have a host of side effects too. Because the newer drugs have produced significant cognitive changes, clients with serious mental illnesses have become more functional and their quality of life has substantially improved.

The continuum of mental health care services continues to evolve and redefine the concept of milieu therapy. This model represents a comprehensive mental health care delivery system. Important aspects of this continuum include community-based mental health services. Furthermore, there is mounting evidence that supports the efficacy and cost-effectiveness of community-based mental health services (Kasprow & Rosenheck, 2007; Perfas & Spross, 2007). The treatment of serious mental illness has gone from isolation and restraints to psychosocial rehabilitation and living in a community or home setting, contributing to the community and society. Researchers submit that multiple-system psychoeducational family groups and improvements in medication adherence partly mediate the efficacy and cost-effectiveness of these approaches (Bauml, Pitschel-Waltz, Volz, Engel, & Kessling, 2007). Psychosocial rehabilitation that includes various treatment modalities, such as family and client psychoeducation, assertive community treatment, and intensive case management continue to bring hope to persons with serious mental illnesses (see Chapter 33). The two approaches have similar characteristics: both focus on the need for intensive help for the client in the community and various clinical settings, and both center on the client's complex health needs involving medication, housing, and finances. Nowadays, milieu therapy is an integral part of this continuum. It extends beyond the walls of an acute psychiatric inpatient unit and is part of the continuity of care, which may be accomplished by consistency of care, maintenance of a healing environment, and interactive communication between the client and staff. Redefining the milieu therapy concept has to be evidence based, empirically sound, client centered, and culturally sensitive. The role of the nurse is less hands on with this new model of milieu therapy and more client centered. Major nursing responsibilities include creating a safe environment, administering and monitoring treatments and client responses, health teaching, and promoting independence and psychosocial skills that facilitate quality of life and an optimal level of functioning.

In today's health care arena there is a greater focus on client-centered, cost-contained, and evidence-based care that addresses complex client needs along a continuum of services. Nurses and other mental health professionals are rapidly developing less-intensive and more cost-effective and innovative services. The continuum of services is naturally linked to milieu therapy and outpatient services, which offer the client structure and continuity of care to facilitate an optimal level of functioning and improved quality of life (Granholm et al., 2007).

Regardless of the setting, therapeutic environments or milieu therapy facilitate stabilization and improved cognitive processes and behaviors, strengthen social interactions between staff and other clients, and require and enhance the client-nurse partnership. The continuum of mental health care is shaped by staff practices and attitudes, human nature, and group dynamics. It is a dynamic and continuous process that involves commitment in order to maintain and promote therapeutic effects within a social context (Edelen et al., 2007; Kennard 2004).

The purpose of this chapter is to discuss major concepts of milieu therapy and its role in the continuum of mental health care. It also focuses on the role of the nurse in stabilization and management of acute symptoms and behaviors and initiating nursing interventions that facilitate psychosocial rehabilitation, symptom management, and promote an optimal level of functioning. A major challenge for today's psychiatric nurse is integrating traditional milieu therapy concepts into a contemporary mental health care continuum that extends from acute psychiatric units to the community and home.

CONCEPTS AND PRINCIPLES OF MILIEU THERAPY IN A NEW ERA

Dramatic changes in the health care system and a greater focus on cost containment and evidence-based mental health care require a new approach to milieu therapy. Greater emphasis must be placed on symptom management as well as functional improvement among clients with severe mental illness.

Clearly it is important to respond to pressures to reduce lengths of stay and to develop programs that address the client's needs, ranging from a structured hospital setting to manage acute symptoms and to offer safety and stabilization, to community services such as assertive community to facilitate psychosocial rehabilitation and assist the client in reaching an optimal level of functioning. Hospitalization is an important part of milieu therapy. It provides a safe, structured, and supervised environment and reduces stress in the client and family members. During this period, the nurse and other members of the interdisciplinary team can closely monitor the client's symptoms, reactions to treatment, level of functioning, and adverse treatment reactions. Antipsychotic agents are used extensively during hospitalization, which facilitate rapid resolution of acute symptoms. During this acute period, nurses must anticipate the client's anxiety and fears and initiate proactive interventions such as verbal de-escalation and medication management to reduce the client's stress and facilitate uneventful symptom management. Because of shorter lengths of stay, the client's acute symptoms may not completely resolve before a transfer to a partial or day hospital or home care referral is made.

Presently, milieu therapy focuses on the mental health continuum and emphasizes wellness and adaptation in the community and within a social and cultural context. In addition, advances in neurobiology and the advent of safer, more effective pharmacologic and psychosocial treatment offer renewed hope for clients and their families in attaining quality of life (Lanza, 2000). These transitions in the mental health care continuum offer psychiatric nurses numerous opportunities to use various resources of institutional and community-based services that enhance the restoration of the clients' optimal level of functioning (American Nurses Association [ANA], 2000).

Today's client with a severe mental illness is likely to receive this care in a community or home-based setting (see Chapter 33). Milieu therapy is part of the mental health continuum that enables nurses and other health care providers to provide seamless mental health care that includes vast treatment interventions such as case management, ACT, partial hospitalization and acute admissions for acute symptoms, and medication stabilization (Keshavan, Roberts, & Wittmann, 2006).

Although the traditional model of milieu therapy is less applicable today than it was more than 50 years ago, its basic concepts are useful in reframing today's version. Today's version of milieu therapy is part of the mental health continuum rather than a stand-alone model of care. Major benefits of this model have been previously discussed in this chapter. The traditional model of milieu therapy involved five key variables, namely, containment, support, validation, structure, and involvement (Gunderson, 1978). These concepts are applicable in today's contemporary milieu therapy, and, like the traditional approach, provides the client with interventions that facilitate an optimal level of functioning and improved quality of life (Kingsley & Bloom, 2004; Norton & Bloom, 2004).

CONTAINMENT

Containment deals with the client's basic needs and includes safety, food, and shelter, and medical care issues of a unit. It includes locked doors, seclusion, and restraints when necessary for clients to feel safe and assured that their illness will not harm them, the hospital, or the staff (LeCuyer, 1992). The newer version is likely to focus on less restrictive containment measures, including "time outs," verbal de-escalation, and chemical restraints. The role of the psychiatric nurse is pivotal during the containment period when the client's risk of danger and harm to self and others are imminent, and for medication stabilization. During this period, new medications may be ordered and administrated, requiring titration and close monitoring for desired and adverse drug reactions. Throughout the stabilization period, the nurse monitors the client's physical and mental status by checking the vital and neurologic signs and providing 24-hour care, which includes maintenance of physical and mental integrity, ongoing assessment, medication administration, and monitoring (Sullivan, Barron, Bezman, Rivera, & Zepata-Vega, 2005). As the client's symptoms abate and cognitive processes improve, and as the client gradually returns to a higher level of functioning, the nurse and other team members reassess the client's needs. Each part of the mental health continuum must have identifiable outcomes that guide treatment, progression and reassessment of the client's condition to ensure the plan depicts a true picture of his overall health. As implied, the containment concept is dynamic, and it is not limited to an acute inpatient setting. The client's symptoms may exacerbate in any setting. Nursing interventions depend on the client's clinical presentations, level of functioning, available support system, and preferences.

During the containment period, the care of clients who are acutely ill must also include medical tests and mental status examination to rule out physical or mental conditions that may be contributing to the client's presentation. Nurses need to perform a complete mental status examination and inquire about support systems, suicide risk, substance-use history, cultural factors, and assessment of physical and sexual abuse. In addition, a comprehensive

treatment plan that designates a treatment coordinator who will manage the mental health continuum is crucial to client outcome and continuity of care. Additional areas, including documentation of care, management of co-occurring substance-related disorders, psychoeducation, and discharge planning, are pivotal aspects of containment and treatment coordination (Royal Australian and New Zealand College of Psychiatrists Clinical Guidelines Team for the Treatment of Schizophrenia and Related Disorders, 2005).

The containment aspect milieu therapy, like other dimensions, continues to evolve and meet the needs of today's client with a serious mental illness.

SUPPORT

A supportive and therapeutic milieu is an integral part of healing and restoration of mental health. Supportive nursing interventions include establishing a healthy and therapeutic nurse-client relationship. The nurse-client relationship offers encouragement, attention, reassurance, praise, education, direction, and other techniques to enhance self-esteem and self-worth. Similar to containment, supportive and self-care activities are an integral part of mental health care continuum and milieu, extending from the acute management phase throughout psychosocial rehabilitation and treatment planning. Supportive and self-care activities include psychoeducation about the client's mental illness, medication regimes, symptom management, enhancing recreational or leisure activities, and facilitating social skills that enable the client to make life skills decisions (ANA, 2000; Bauml et al., 2007). Furthermore, a supportive climate fosters competence, adequacy, autonomy, and, ultimately, strengthens coping and interpersonal skills. Support, like containment, is part of the mental health continuum and is relevant in today's health care arena.

Assertive community treatment (ACT) and intensive case management have become an integral part of the mental health care continuum for helping people with severe mental illness achieve optimal levels of reintegration into the community. This approach, like other aspects of this continuum and milieu therapy, center on everyday issues such as medication, housing, and finances. This model provides *supportive* mental health care that facilitates the coordination, integration, and allocation of client-centered (Thornicroft, 1991) and holistic care within designated resources that provide ongoing contact with a treatment coordinator. In addition, the ACT and intensive case management models have been implemented in various mental health care systems in an effort to increase appropriate and adequate community care, namely, by reducing fragmented services and promoting seamless and continuum of care. Data from a meta-analysis of 44 studies of the effectiveness of mental health case management over 20 years (Ziguras & Stuart, 2000) and others (Draine, 1997; Mueser, Bond, Drake, & Resnick, 1998) indicate that the models of mental health care are effective and cost saving. In addition, clients receiving these services have *improved* treatment outcomes as evidenced by:

- symptom management
- clients' level of social functioning
- client and family satisfaction
- family burden of care

In addition to these findings, Ziguras and Stuart (2000) concluded that both types of case management resulted in a small-to-moderate improvement in the effectiveness of mental health care services. ACT actually had some demonstrable advantages over intensive case management in reducing hospitalization. Findings from this study validate perception that ACT and other intensive case management models should target clients who are at risk of hospitalization.

Obviously, any model that improves client outcomes, reduces health care costs, enhances client and family satisfaction, and reduces hospitalization, offers hope for clients with serious mental illnesses. The role of the nurse is very clear and pivotal in successful treatment planning because the nurse is an integral part of the mental health continuum. The nurse is often a case manager involved in stabilization, creating a supportive environment, and initiating interventions that reduce symptoms. As a clinical case manager or broker of care, the nurse is responsible for conducting psychosocial and physical assessment, developing a plan of care, coordinating access to necessary services, and monitoring mental status and social functioning. This model transcends practice settings and is an integral part of the mental health care continuum. Symptom management promotes independence and self-efficacy. In addition, the psychiatric nurse prescribes and administers various forms of treatment, ranging from pharmacologic agents to supportive and medication groups, all of which are crucial components to health promotion and the mental health care continuum. Finally, because the nurse is working intimately with the client and family, the nurse monitors for treatment responses and documents and communicates clinical findings to various team members.

As the client and family move through the mental health continuum from containment, followed by supportive and healing environments, other components must be considered and integrated into the milieu, namely, validation.

VALIDATION

Successful mastery of daily living and psychosocial rehabilitation skills fosters a sense of independence and validates self-efficacy. Throughout the treatment process, validation of the client as a unique individual is intrinsic to the mental health treatment model. Nurses play key roles in initiating and maintaining a respective relationship with the client and family members, which begins with initial social interactions, and remains throughout treatment. Encouraging the client to identify preferences, cultural needs, and health teaching concerns is a basic nursing responsibility. Affording privacy of communication, documentation, and respect for the client's wishes and needs requires active listening skills. Understanding and appreciation of the client's uniqueness and holistic needs promote a sense of self-worth, personal respect, and models health relationship behaviors that promote social skills development and independence.

STRUCTURE

Historically, the meaning of structure was generally associated with restraints and excessive environmental control of the nursing staff. The concept of structure is important in any healthy relationships and must be used appropriately to enable the client to regain control in situations in which controls are lacking, such as worsening agitation, yelling, and throwing things during an acute exacerbation. Obviously, the client cannot be allowed to exhibit violent behaviors, and the nurse and other staff need to offer structure that protects the client from self and others. Nursing interventions in this case require verbal de-escalation and limit setting to help the client regain control that has obviously been lost as evidenced by violent behaviors. As the nurse maintains control, so shall the client when these techniques are used. If the client continues to escalate, it is imperative to have a mechanism to muster up support and help the client regain control. This often involves chemical or physical restraints when the client fails to respond to less-structured approaches with verbal de-escalation.

Recently, there has been an outcry from various client advocacy groups and mental health professions about the use of physical control with the client with a mental illness. This stems from abuse of these interventions in the past rather than using less-aggressive means to provide structure or control. This chapter has focused primarily on acute management and short lengths of stay, but another area that requires a brief discussion is the structure component of milieu therapy in long-term mental health facilities. Basically, clients in these settings must receive the same level of respect, holistic health care, and an environment that helps them reach an optimal level of functioning. Issues such as control or structure are perceived differently in these settings than those found in the mental health continuum definition of structures. An example is found in the following research review.

A study conducted by Vittengl (2002) concerning structure of temporal regularities in physical control in a state psychiatric hospital found that physical control varied with the time of day and often coincided with unit activities and resultant violent incidents. Findings from Vittengl's study indicate that nurses working in long-term care facilities, such as state mental health facilities, need to understand and discern the appropriate timing of physical control (e.g., mechanical restraint and locked seclusion), develop preventive measures during high-risk times and activities, and recognize implementation choices. Furthermore, these data suggest that nurses in these institutions are in pivotal positions to recognize high-risk patterns and activities associated with violence in long-term care facilities and initiating preventive measures and structure to address these concerns.

In a 2005 study of restraint and seclusion use in the Pennsylvania State Hospital system from 1990 to 2000 and relationship to staff injuries from client assault from 1998 to 2000, researchers found that the average rate of restraint decreased from 3.5 episodes to 1.2 episodes per 1,000 hospital days, and average seclusion fell from 10.8 to 1.3 hours (Smith et al., 2005). Clients from culturally diverse groups were more likely to be put in seclusion for longer lengths of time than whites. Seclusion and use of restraint was less likely to occur during the night tour of duty; but if restraints were used, it would be for longer periods. Younger clients were more likely to be secluded and restrained than older adults. There were no significant changes in staff injuries. Researchers concluded that the staff's ability to reduce use of seclusion and restraints was associated with several factors, including client advocacy, increased nurse-client staffing ratios, accessibility to response teams, and atypical antipsychotic medications (Smith et al., 2005). (See Research Abstract, A Pennsylvania State Hospital System's Seclusion and Restraint Reduction Program.)

Other client populations that providers thought benefited from the traditional "structured" model of milieu therapy were those with personality disorders (e.g., borderline). In the past, their self-destructive behaviors often intensified on discharge, resulting in longer hospitalization without empirical evidence that the longer stay was beneficial. Amazingly, as cost containment and need to provide evidence-based care became the mainstay of health care, other innovative interventions were found to be more effective than the structure inherent in long-term psychiatric treatment. One such model is dialectical behavior therapy (DBT). This highly structured treatment approach has proven effective in treating chronically suicidal clients with borderline personality traits. In addition, unlike prolonged hospitalization and structured milieu environments that often fostered dependence and negative staff countertransference, DBT fosters independence and control over their maladaptive behaviors. This model also addresses issues of self-respect and increases the capacity to modulate emotions and sustain positive feelings (Comtois & Linehan, 2006; Rizvi & Linehan, 2001; Swenson, Torrey, & Koerner, 2002). DBT requires special graduate-level preparation, and for many advanced-practice psychiatric-mental health nurses, it is a dramatic change of reworking one's therapeutic beliefs and acquiring new skills. Apart from the specialized training, the nurse therapist needs to participate in professional supervision to deal with countertransference and self-destructive issues inherent in working with clients with a borderline personality disorder (see Chapters 15 and 26).

RESEARCH ABSTRACT

A Pennsylvania State Hospital System's Seclusion and Restraint Reduction Program

Smith, G. M., David, R. H., Bixler, E. O., Lin, H. M., Altenor, R. J., Hardenstine, B. D., et al. (2005). *Psychiatric Services, 56,* 1115–1122.

Study Problem/Purpose

The purpose of this study was to examine the use of seclusion and mechanical restraint at a state hospital from 1990 to 2000 and the prevalence of staff injuries from patient assaults from 1998 to 2000.

Methods

Researchers reviewed and analyzed the records of clients older than 18 years of age who were committed to one of the nine state hospitals in Pennsylvania. Two databases were used in each of the nine hospitals: one identified date, time, duration, and justification for each episode of seclusion or restraint; and the other identified when a client was hospitalized, the demographic characteristics, and the client's diagnosis. Rate and duration of seclusion and restraint were analyzed. The prevalence of staff injuries from client assaults was determined by reports from compensation claims.

Findings

The rate and duration of seclusion and mechanical restraint decreased significantly from 1990 to 2000. Researchers found that the rate of seclusion decreased from 4.2 to 0.3 episodes per 1,000 client-days and that the average duration of seclusion decreased from 10.8 to 1.3 hours. The rate of restraint decreased from 3.5 to 1.2 episodes per 1,000 patient-days. The average duration of restraint decreased from 11.9 to 1.9 hours. Clients from racial or ethnic minority groups had a higher rate and longer duration of seclusion than whites. Seclusion was less likely to occur during the night shift. Although restraints were used less during the night shift, they were left on longer. The rate of restraint was higher during the week than during weekends and holidays, and older clients were less likely to be secluded or restrained than younger clients. There were no significant changes in the rates of staff injuries from 1998 to 2000. Researchers concluded that many factors were associated with the success of this effort, such as advocacy efforts, state policy change concerning the use of seclusion and restraint, increased nurse-to-client ratios, and the use of atypical antipsychotic medications.

Implications for Psychiatric Nursing

Although these findings did not demonstrate reduced staff injuries due to client assaults, they do implicate the importance of limitation of the use of restraints and seclusion, policy that addresses these issues, and the prudent use of nursing interventions, including atypical antipsychotic medications, to ensure a safe environment to manage acute psychiatric symptoms. It is also imperative for nurses to participate in annual training and use teams to reduce workplace violence and ensure a safe environment for staff.

Other examples of structure include written guidelines or expectations for conduct, a schedule of suggested activities and therapies, a process for orienting new clients, and contingency plans for nonadherence with routines and expectations (Royal Australian and New Zealand College of Psychiatrists, 2005). Historically, this type of structure was useful in treating clients who had lengthy hospital stays. They can still be used with some modification that takes into consideration client and family preferences, cultural factors, and symptomatology. For instance, if the client lives in a residential home, orientation of the new client is essential, whereas if the client lives at home with family, this rule is not applicable. Structure also refers to additional activities, including psychotherapies, community meetings, staff meetings, and treatment planning processes. Again community meetings are relevant in residential extended care settings but less appropriate for a 3-day acute admission or home setting. Ultimately, the decision to provide various forms of structure often parallels several factors. These factors include the timing and frequency of interventions within constraints of the client's length of stay, place of care, cost containment, and the client's preferences and level of functioning. Structure, like other components of milieu therapy and the mental health continuum, also focuses on involvement.

INVOLVEMENT

Involvement, like other components of milieu therapy, is intrinsic to positive treatment outcomes. Historically, the concept of involvement was limited to long-term inpatient mental health care with a focus on the client's responsibilities in treatment participation. The client's participation or involvement in treatment remains crucial to positive treatment outcomes. However, in today's health care arena, involvement is often synonymous with self-efficacy. ANA (2000) links this concept with self-care activities, which is a major dimension of direct nursing care within the therapeutic milieu.

Nursing interventions that promote involvement include focusing on activities of daily living that promote symptom management, medication adherence, hygiene, adequate nutrition, and safety. In addition, the nurse needs to assess health teaching needs, foster recreational or stress management activities, and facilitate development of social skills training in various areas of the community such as shopping, banking, and paying for an apartment or home. These important experiences and attainment promote a sense of competency and move clients from dependent to independent and interdependent behavioral changes (ANA, 2000; Bauml et al., 2007). Supportive family members need to be part of involvement; in fact, to exclude them often contributes to poor treatment outcomes.

OPEN COMMUNICATION

Open communication is a necessary component of successful treatment planning. This process involves effective communication, active listening, consultation with other services, and appropriate and timely documentation. Enhancing negotiation and social and group interaction skills is an integral aspect of open communication and milieu therapy. During an era when information is readily accessible from various sources, including the Internet and computer, nurses and other mental health care professionals are openly communicating with clients, families, communities, and other providers and share relevant information that guides treatment planning and offers feedback about the clients' responses and adherence to treatment. Many systems have computerized databases, including progress notes, that ease information retrieval. Issues such as confidentiality and other legal and ethical issues must be respected.

Regardless of the practice settings, the nurse is responsible for establishing a process for disseminating information about client preferences, adherence to treatment, and medication side effects or desired responses. Clients and families have a right to know about their diagnosis, prognosis, and treatment options. At the same time nurses must maintain open communication with the client, ensure confidentiality, and adhere to Health Insurance Portability and Accountability Act (HIPPA) guidelines. Open communication is a crucial part of the process and requires patience, empathy, and a therapeutic nurse-client relationship (see Chapter 6).

FAMILY AND COMMUNITY

More and more studies are linking family involvement with positive client outcomes. To exclude family and community from the client's care limits the nurse's perspective about the client's experiences and cultural concerns. Family and community often link the client to diverse health care services in various aspects of the mental health continuum. Families and other support systems involved in the care of the client with a serious mental illness often provide needed emotional support, case management, financial support, advocacy, and housing for their loved one. Although the family willingly provides these resources to the client, over time they impose considerable burden. Because of the chronic nature of mental illness and its potential impact on the client and family, involving them in treatment is crucial to positive treatment outcomes. During the assessment and treatment process nurses must assess the level of the caregiver's burden and strengthen resources to reduce their stress. They must also develop evidence-based interventions that address the needs of families. The healthier the family, the more likely their support will improve client outcomes. Family involvement enables them to understand their loved one's conditions, symptoms, and treatment options that promote an optimal level of functioning. Active family participation reduces their stress and anxiety and offers an opportunity to discuss their caregiver issues. Family support groups enable them to work with other families and share their feelings and concerns and therefore feel less isolated.

PHYSICAL ENVIRONMENT

Although today's health care system changes have moved the client from long-term care to community and home settings, the client's physical environment is part of the therapeutic milieu. A safe and comfortable physical environment that is found lacking in the homeless or incarcerated population of clients with mental illness is a right that every client deserves. A physical environment is a basic need that helps the client feel safe, proud, and capable of a better life. A therapeutic physical environment enriches other therapies by strengthening the client's self-efficacy and self-esteem.

CULTURAL CONSIDERATIONS

Tremendous variations exist across cultures and family practices, perceptions of illness, stigma, and expectations of health care providers. Figures from the U.S. Census Bureau (2000) also confirmed a more diverse society. Because of a Western-based mental health treatment system, various cultures have a mistrust of the mental health community. Nurses and other interdisciplinary team members must assess cultural needs and integrate these considerations into milieu therapy. Nursing interventions that integrate cultural factors and encourage family involvement are likely to produce culturally sensitive mental health care services. Considering the complexity of cultural factors in client and family behaviors, along with stigma and adherence to traditional health practices and healing methods, it is imperative to work with the client and family to develop client- and family- centered mental health care governed by perceptions of mental health and illness. Cultural factors are equally influenced by religious and spiritual beliefs, quality of family support systems, coping styles, and indigenous culture-bound traits. Researchers submit that treatment should comprise a structured, culturally sensitive, comprehensive approach that respects individual differences along with the cultural milieu (Barnard, 2007; Chan, Hsiung, Thompson, Chen, & Hwu, 2007; Sanchez & Gaw, 2007).

A multicultural study (Guarnaccia, 1998) of family caregivers demonstrated that about 75 percent of Latino clients and 60 percent of African American clients reside with their families, relative to 30 percent of European American clients. Many minority populations from this study had large support systems and religious organizations for help, whereas the European American clients relied more on professional help and had fewer social networks. African Americans and Latino clients also expressed greater hope, optimism, and faith about long-term outcomes of their family member's mental illness. Researchers felt these qualities played a role in one's resilience and adaptation within a social context (Guarnaccia, 1998; Pickett, Cook, & Heller, 1998). Emerging research continues to support these assertions and implicates the importance of assessing the needs of clients and their families to ensure culturally sensitive mental health care (Chan et al., 2007; Roberts, Alegria, Roberts, & Chen, 2005). African Americans had more effective and adaptive coping skills and a higher level of self-worth than other minority groups. Major barriers to mental health care included lower socioeconomic status and educational preparation. In addition, minority populations

were hesitant to seek help outside of the family or community owing to stigma and attitude toward caregivers.

Implications for psychiatric nurses providing milieu therapy include self-awareness about one's own culture and its potential impact on how one perceives others. Nurses also need to include the client, family, and other community networks in the treatment plan to strengthen the client's social support systems. It is also imperative for nurses to distinguish symptoms unique to each culture from diagnostic criteria. Performing a spiritual assessment of all clients is relevant to understanding the role of spirituality and religion in the clients' life and perception of illness. Assessing health practices, family attitudes about the client's symptoms, treatment and the mental health care system, and client preferences can facilitate a culturally sensitive plan of care. Culturally sensitive milieu therapy must be effectively coordinated to ensure continuity of care (see Chapter 7).

MILIEU THERAPY ACROSS THE LIFE SPAN

The nurse planning the day-to-day management of a therapeutic milieu must consider developmental issues across the life span and for special diagnostic populations. The traditional milieu therapy approach may be adapted to treat children, adolescents, adults, and older populations, whereas the contemporary approach using the mental health care continuum offers an array of evidence-based treatment that provides services to clients and their families across the life span. Treatment issues and modalities for adult treatment are well covered elsewhere, so this section focuses only on considerations and adaptation of milieu therapy for the child, adolescent, and older adult. Table 32–1 summarizes examples.

CHILDHOOD

Children who are treated in a variety of settings for a wide range of symptoms and diagnoses present some common needs and developmental issues. An obvious set of needs for children is providing age-related safety and supervision. This may occur on an acute inpatient unit, long-term residential facility, day hospital, or home-based care. These requirements differ from adult needs on the basis of children's lack of judgment, immature cognitive development, impulsivity, and short attention span. Regardless of when the child enters the continuum of health care, successful treatment outcomes require active parental or guardian participation (Delaney, 2006; Jaffee, Caspi, Moffitt, Polo-Tomas, & Taylor, 2007).

An interesting study by Irwin, Kline, and Gordon (1992) described a milieu therapy program that focused on the primary problem among disturbed children: the inability to form meaningful, trusting relationships with peers and adults. The program fostered the formation of *discriminating attachments*: children were encouraged to select and work out treatment issues with a specific staff member. Limit setting and consequences for problem behaviors were handled within the context of these special relationships. The purpose of this strategy was to avoid the message that all adults are interchangeable. Nursing implications from this study structure is an essential component of milieu and that children, like adults with impulse control, benefit from firm and consistent limit settings regardless of where they enter the mental health continuum.

In addition to firm and consistent limit setting, Irwin and colleagues (1992) stressed the importance of discharge rituals. Special attention was made so that the child could acknowledge attachments and work through separation and abandonment issues. Having the child and family maintain some contact with hospital staff smoothed the transition from hospital to outpatient treatment. Thus separation was not so abrupt and the child did not feel abandoned by his special staff member (Irwin et al., 1992).

Behavioral interventions are important in treatment milieus for children. Children's short attention span requires putting a consequence as close as possible to the behavior it is intended to modify. Peer relationships and coping skills can be improved by implementing consequences for the entire group and therapy assignments for certain kinds of acting-out behavior. In a 2007 study involving the impact of a milieu-based behavioral management program on the frequency of aggressive behaviors in a child and adolescent mental health inpatient unit, researchers concluded that aggression in these units can be reduced by implementing a comprehensive behavioral management program. This approach involved client-centered treatment plans, reinforcement of appropriate behaviors, early detection and prevention, staff training, and interventions using the least restrictive option (Dean, Duke, George, & Scott, 2007).

An old approach that has worked in traditional milieus is token economics. This behavioral approach allows clients to earn reinforcements in the form of tokens for engaging in designated or appropriate behaviors. Ultimately, the tokens are traded for a favorite item or privilege. The process of token economics involves a learning experience that facilitates behavioral changes. Children engaging in this activity require parental involvement and monitoring. Special efforts must be set up to avoid using expensive items and rewards. Proper planning and a focus on facilitating positive behavioral changes are primary goals of this token economics (LePage, 1999; Liberman, 1997).

ADOLESCENCE

Healthy adolescents normally share some needs such as those of younger children across the developmental continuum; adolescents in treatment may also have special problems with advanced or delayed development. Safety and supervision continue to be issues, and the possibility of sexual acting out increases. Adolescents with acute mental disorders need a therapeutic environment or milieu that integrates collaborative interventions that encourage a sense of responsibility for self and

strengthen their social, problem-solving, and coping skills. Effective coping skills enable the youth to manage stressful situations and interpersonal relationships through formation of self-awareness and self-efficacy (Edelen et al., 2007). In addition, the nurse has to assess the client for mental illness, level of danger to self and others, substance-related disorders, and medical problems such as juvenile-onset diabetes.

School issues are an important aspect of treatment for all school-age groups. Both behavioral problems and educational needs must be addressed. Neuropsychological and psychoeducational testing are technological and theoretical advances in the school-hospital partnership. Structure varies with the setting and local education systems, but a close collaboration between classrooms, family, and community is often part of milieu therapy for the adolescent. Adolescents, like adults, are more likely to be treated along the mental health continuum, ranging from a short-stay hospitalization for acute management and crisis resolution, to partial hospitalization for continued stabilization, and back into the community or home to work on family issues. Family therapy must be an integral part of milieu therapy and may even involve the parent staying home to monitor the child's suicidal behavior in the event hospitalization is not approved.

Another issue concerning adolescence is the need for autonomy and separation from the family of origin. Developmentally, adolescents are sensitive to issues of autonomy, peer pressure, privileges, and responsibility. The treatment milieu often deals with these issues through a behavioral reinforcement and privilege system that ties progress to individual treatment goals (Hall & DeJong, 2006).

ADULTHOOD

Issues affecting the adult participating in milieu therapy have been previously discussed. However, it is important to note that client-centered and holistic care must be part of all health care.

OLDER ADULTHOOD

Depending on the older adult's functional and mental status, treatment is consistent with other adults. Special consideration about age-related changes, including pharmacokinetics and sensory changes such as those affecting the client's hearing or sight, must be considered when establishing a plan of care. Like other age groups, milieu therapy needs to be individualized and culturally sensitive. A comprehensive evaluation is necessary to rule out medical and psychiatric conditions that affect functional status. Suicide risk, cognitive and sensory deficits, social losses, limited income, physical changes, and health problems must be addressed in the therapeutic environment for the older adult. Wandering, severe withdrawal, agitation, verbal abusiveness, and aggressive behaviors must be thoroughly assessed to rule out neurological or psychiatric disorders or drug interactions. Clear communication may be difficult because of hearing, visual, and memory problems; nonverbal aspects of communication, including touch and positive affect, need to be used purposefully to enhance communication and support.

TABLE 32-1

Milieu Elements and Interventions across the Life Span

	Child	Adolescent	Adult	Geriatric
1. Containment (Safety) (Continuum of mental health services)	• Close supervision • Time out • Seclusion • Mental and physical status exams • Health education/parenting classes as needed • Discharge planning • Identify cultural needs and integrate into treatment planning	• Flexible supervision • Quiet time • Seclusion • Suicide alert • Mental and physical status exams • Discharge planning • Identify cultural needs and integrate into treatment planning	• Flexible supervision • Quiet time • Medication • Mental and physical status exams • Discharge planning • Identify cultural needs and integrate into treatment planning	• Close supervision • Suicide alert • Provide medical care • Emotional support • Mental and physical status exams • Discharge planning • Identify cultural needs and integrate into treatment planning
2. Support (Continuum of mental health services)	• Give attention • Reassure • Direct • Redirect • Praise • Touch* • Hug* • Use ACT, intensive case management • Facilitate psychosocial rehabilitation	• Give attention • Reassure • Encourage • Educate • Praise • Use ACT, intensive case management • Facilitate psychosocial rehabilitation	• Reassurance • Encouragement • Educate • Praise • Give feedback • Use ACT, intensive case management • Facilitate psychosocial rehabilitation	• Give attention • Reassure • Encourage • Give direction • Provide comfort measures • Use ACT, intensive case management • Facilitate psychosocial rehabilitation
3. Structure (Continuum of mental health services)	• Schedule activity: short time periods Enhance activities of daily living skills	• Schedule activity: + free time DBT model for personality disorders	• Schedule activity: + free time DBT model for personality disorders	• Schedule activity: with rest periods DBT model for personality disorders

4. Involvement (Continuum of mental health services)	• Allow choices • Teach problem solving Focus on symptom management and medication adherence Foster recreational activities and social skills training in community	• Expect active participation • Teach decision making Focus on symptom management and medication adherence Foster recreational activities and social skills training in community	• Expect the client to participate in treatment planning Focus on symptom management and medication adherence Foster recreational activities and social skills training in community	• Encourage social activity Focus on symptom management and medication adherence Foster recreational activities and social skills training in community
5. Open Communication (Continuum of mental health services)	• Teach to name feelings • Encourage verbal expression of feelings • Develop trust Consultation with various services Timely and accurate documentation	• Avoid secret keeping • Discourage manipulation • Encourage verbal sharing with peers	• Explain that confidentiality is unit based • Encourage appropriate self-disclosure	• Encourage to share memories • Encourage to acknowledge loss and adaptation
6. Family and Community (Continuum of mental health services)	• Avoid abrupt separations • Provide emotional support ACT and intensive case management models Integrate cultural considerations	• Strong school–unit collaboration ACT and intensive case management models Integrate cultural considerations	• Assist with return to work ACT and intensive case management models Integrate cultural considerations	• Assist with placement/home care decisions ACT and intensive case management models Integrate cultural considerations
7. Physical Environment (Continuum of mental health services)	• Age-sized furniture • Client rooms easily observed • Pleasant sensory stimulation	• Group activity areas • Quiet areas • Music areas	• Group activity areas • Quiet areas • Attractive furniture	• Safe mobility aids • Many orientation cues

*Only with client consent.

Note. Data adapted from "Behavioral Management Leads to Reduction in Aggression in a Child and Adolescent Psychiatric Inpatient Unit," by A. J. Dean, S. G. Duke, M. George, and J. Scott, 2007, *Journal of the Academy of Child and Adolescent Psychiatry, 46,* pp. 711–720; "Top 10 Milieu Interventions for Inpatient Child/Adolescent Treatment," by K. R. Delaney, 2006, *Journal of Child and Adolescent Psychiatric Nursing, 19,* pp. 203–214; "Level 1 Therapeutic Model Site," by P. S. Hall and J. A. DeJong, 2006, *American Indian and Alaskan Native Mental Health Research, 13,* pp. 17–51; and "Royal Australian and New Zealand College of Psychiatrists Clinical Practice Guidelines for the Treatment of Schizophrenia and Related Disorders," by Royal Australian and New Zealand College of Psychiatrists Clinical Guidelines Team for the Treatment of Schizophrenia and Related Disorders, 2005, *Australia and New Zealand Journal of Psychiatry, 39,* pp. 1–30.

The continuum of mental health milieu therapy may involve the client's home or an extended care facility. Nurses must assess each client's needs and create a warm, accepting, and safe environment that promotes mental health rather than regression. Normally, the nurse is part of an interdisciplinary team that addresses these issues in facilities and home settings. Working with the family and community is essential to the client's mental health and a part of the therapeutic environment that restores health and facilitates quality of life.

Regardless of where the client resides, modification of the environment promotes comfort and integrity and environmental ambience (Yao & Algase, 2006). Uncluttered, wide, well-marked passageways that are provided with support devices and resting places are needed within rooms and along corridors to accommodate weaker, slower, less-agile clients. Boundaries to rooms and special areas need to be distinctly marked; for example, color changes assist orientation for the visually and cognitively impaired. For the disoriented client who is prone to wander, indoor and outdoor areas, which provide safe containment without restricting activity and movement, can provide sensory and social stimulation. The environment must also be rich in orientation cues for cognitive challenges such as family pictures and personal items. Social involvement can be encouraged by structured interactions such as reminiscence groups, group leisure activities, or comfortable group living areas, where spontaneous socialization can occur. Major nursing interventions for the older adult may include respite care for the caregiver, adult day care services, crisis intervention, health education, empowerment, psychotherapy, recreational therapy, and grief work.

In today's changing and evolving health care system, nurses are in pivotal positions to develop innovative treatment models such as the mental health care continuum milieu therapy approach. Regardless of where the client enters this continuum, nurses can offer unique interventions that enhance stabilization and symptom management; monitor the client's safety, response to treatment, and treatment adherence; and facilitate independence and self-efficacy. Milieu therapy is a critical component in the mental health care continuum, and the nurse has numerous opportunities to develop and use evidence-based interventions to help the client reach an optimal level of functioning and quality of life.

THE ROLE OF THE NURSE

Milieu therapy continues to evolve and occur in vast practice settings. Nurses must collaborate with the client, family, and other members of the health care team and implement treatment that facilitates stabilization, recovery, and maintenance. The ultimate goal of milieu is to return the client to an optimal level of functioning and reduce relapse.

THE GENERALIST NURSE

Nurses have long had a very responsible role in the establishment, maintenance, and evaluation of the therapeutic environment of mental health care facilities. Nurses are unique on the interdisciplinary team in terms of the large number of their ranks and the amount of time they spend with clients. Considering these circumstances, nurses have a vital opportunity and responsibility to be the broker of care for clients in various clinical settings on the mental health care continuum.

In addition, nurses are natural leaders in the creation and management of the therapeutic milieu. As valued members of the treatment team, nurses collaborate with the client, other members of the team, and consultants to create and manage a therapeutic environment. Nurses are also excellent case managers and must use these skills to extend milieu therapy beyond the acute psychiatric unit. This also requires education about case management and community resources. As a broker of mental health care in the case management role, the nurse links the client to important community resources that facilitate recovery, strengthen social skills and rehabilitation, and, when indicated, back to the emergency department, to treat medical and psychiatric conditions.

Major responsibilities of the nurse on an acute psychiatric unit or emergency department involve stabilization, safety, medication management, and monitoring. Stabilization requires astute observational and decision-making skills. A thorough and comprehensive biopsychosocial assessment is crucial and helps the nurse with a differential diagnosis of medical and psychiatric conditions. Appropriate laboratory and diagnostic studies are a part of the comprehensive assessment. Once stabilization occurs, the generalist nurse may use major components of milieu therapy to address, monitor, and manage the client's condition. Crisis intervention, medication administration, monitoring side effects and level of danger to self and others, and psychoeducation are crucial during this acute period.

THE ADVANCED-PRACTICE PSYCHIATRIC REGISTERED NURSE

The advanced-practice psychiatric nurse is likely to share responsibilities with the generalist nurse, but provides a complex level of care. Advanced-practice mental health care requires graduate-level preparation and experience to address the needs of complex client populations. Examples of treatment include prescribing medications, medication management, monitoring treatment responses, providing psychotherapies, intensive case management, and psychiatric liaison consultation.

THE NURSING PROCESS

In the therapeutic milieu, nursing assessment, diagnosis, planning, intervention, and evaluation must reflect recognition of the collective and individual needs of a group of clients, depending on care setting and simultaneous consideration of each client's individual needs. Insight and competence are required to weigh individual needs against collective needs. The milieu therapy approach offers the flexibility and mechanisms for conflict resolution that the nurse needs to make therapeutic clinical judgments that best serve both the client and milieu.

ASSESSMENT

In the case study, it is important for the nurse to analyze the children's behaviors, duration of symptoms, and past treatment. It is also important to determine the meaning of hitting in each child's family. Are they merely mocking behaviors seen in the home? What other places do these behaviors occur? Additional assessment data may be the reasons for seeking treatment. The nurse performs a biopsychosocial assessment that includes data concerning the clients' physical problems, current medications, medical problems, risk of dangerousness, and mental status examination. A comprehensive history of the family dynamics, ability to care for the child, history of mental illness and medical problems, substance misuse, legal problems, and level of functioning need to be assessed throughout treatment. In addition, the social context in which behaviors occur must be assessed to determine their role in the family.

NURSING DIAGNOSES

The nursing diagnoses in the case study include (children and their families):

◆ Risk for Other-Directed Violence

◆ Ineffective Coping

◆ Interrupted Family Process

◆ Compromised Family Coping

◆ Situational Low Self-Esteem

OUTCOME IDENTIFICATION

Major nursing interventions in milieu therapy include crisis management and health teaching through various modalities, including case management. Case management in both inpatient and outpatient settings enables the nurse to provide a mental health continuum of care that supports each client and family in reaching their highest level of functioning. In the case of potential violence, the nurse is responsible for monitoring the clients' safety, improving problem solving, and coordinating a holistic treatment plan.

PLANNING

Establishing a plan of care for the client in milieu therapy often involves collaboration with the nurse and other providers in diverse community and inpatient settings. In the case of the child and family, it is imperative for the nurse to work with local mental health agencies and schools to assist the child in forming and maintaining adaptive coping skills, while assisting the parents or guardians to address couple and family issues that contribute to the child's acting-out behavior.

CASE STUDY

Clients with Aggressive Behavior Toward Peers (Bobby and Ellen)

Bobby and Ellen, 10-year-old clients are on a short-stay unit in which a milieu approach is used to treat children with severe behavioral problems. Each has a problem with hitting others when he or she becomes frustrated. The treatment team was interpreting the behavior to them as a problem in relating to peers ("making and keeping friends"). Hitting is a common behavior among children so the treatment team has clarified the expected conduct in community meeting: that the children will learn to express feelings with appropriate words, not hitting.

As the group left the unit classroom this morning, Bobby and Ellen each started pushing and hitting children next to them in line. Other children in the group also began yelling and pushing each other. The staff immediately implemented the preplanned group consequences and therapy activities for this type of behavior, with spontaneous adaptations to fit the situation. Interventions from the group plan can be incorporated into individual nursing care plans or master treatment plans where applicable. See Nursing Care Plan 32–1.

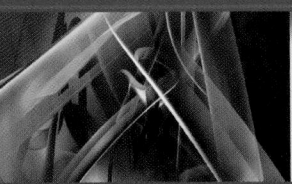

NURSING CARE PLAN 32–1

Clients with Aggressive Behavior Toward Peers (Bobby and Ellen)

Nursing Diagnosis: Risk for Other-Directed Violence

Outcome Identification	Nursing Actions	Rationales	Evaluation
1. By [date], clients learn alternative ways to express feelings other than hitting or shoving others.	1a. Establish rapport. Encourage expression of feelings.	1a. Establishes therapeutic interaction. Conveys empathy, caring, and interest.	*Goal met:* Nurse forms therapeutic relationship. Clients express feelings. Clients do not express suicidal ideations or act on thoughts.
	1b. Maintain a safe environment. Assess level of dangerousness.	1b. Provides safety and control and decreases acting-out behaviors.	
	1c. Observe for mood changes.	1c. Change in mood or anxiety level increases risk of dangerousness.	
	1d. Assign each child to a provider.	1d. Provides some security for the child, and enables the staff to monitor the child for signs of escalation.	
	2. Encourage each child to describe feelings.	2. Enables the child to identify choices and consequences.	
	3. List and discuss alternative behaviors to cope with present stressors.	3. Listing behaviors introduces new coping behaviors.	

Nursing Diagnosis: Ineffective Coping

Outcome Identification	Nursing Actions	Rationales	Evaluation
1. By [date], clients develop enduring adaptive coping skills (age-specific).	1a. Explore meaning of present hitting behaviors in group.	1a. Helps the clients understand self and present responses.	*Goal met:* Clients return to pre-hospitalization level of functioning. Clients develop adaptive coping skills. Clients' self-esteem increases.
	1b. Encourage dialogue with the roommate in group.	1b. Validates understanding of meaning of present symptoms. Processing with roommate is a manageable small step toward group processing within a safe social context.	
2. Clients form a healthy relationship with roommate.	2. Assist each child in identifying strengths, resources, and coping skills.	2. Places focus on positive attributes and increases self-esteem.	

(continues)

Nursing Care Plan 32–1 *(continued)*

Nursing Diagnosis: Interrupted Family Processes and Compromised Family Coping

Outcome Identification	Nursing Actions	Rationales	Evaluation
1. By [date], each family will be able to develop adaptive coping behaviors and parenting skills.	1a. Set up family conference to assess family dynamics, needs, and problem areas.	1a. By focusing on the children's behavior in the context of the family, the children are less likely to feel responsible for family-related problems.	*Goal met:* The couple acknowledges their marital problems and role in children's behavior. Parents develop adequate parenting skills.
	1b. Focus on childen's behavior as a family problem rather than targeting the children.	1b. Provide health education about the children's behaviors and parenting skills.	The children hits are reduced to one time per month. Couples participate in marital therapy.
2. The children's hitting will be reduced to once a month.			

Nursing Diagnosis: Situational Low Self-Esteem

Outcome Identification	Nursing Actions	Rationales	Evaluation
1. By [date], clients verbalize 2–3 positive attributes and show increased self-esteem.	1a. Provide successful experiences. 1b. Convey acceptance and empathy. 1c. Encourage active participation in treatment.	1a–c. Successful experiences increase confidence, mastery, and personal competence.	*Goal met:* Clients' self-esteem increases. Clients are able to explore options to deal with present stressors.

IMPLEMENTATION

Implementing a plan of care stems from the diagnosis, outcome identification, and nursing interventions using a milieu model of care that integrates various modalities, including ACT, intensive case management, family's and couple's therapy, and psychoeducation. Self-promotion activities for each child may include learning how to express feelings or writing them down rather than hitting. For the couples, it may involve strengthening their parenting skills and attending AA meetings for alcohol use.

EVALUATION

The evaluation of these children and families depends on established treatment outcomes. In the case study the children reduced the number of times they hit and learned alternative ways to express frustration and anger. Each couple participated in parenting classes and marital therapy. The successfulness of these outcomes is highly contingent on the efficacy of case management resulting from the role of the nurse as a case manager or psychotherapist in the mental health continuum of milieu therapy.

SUMMARY

◆ Milieu therapy continues to evolve and respond to societal, legislative, and economical changes.

◆ The pressure to provide holistic, client-centered, and cost-effective mental health care services along a continuum provides nurses with vast opportunities to play a role in the mental health continuum that defines the importance of milieu therapy.

◆ There is growing evidence that clients with mental illness require intensive case management and a broker of care who coordinates, organizes, and advocates for client-centered mental health care.

◆ The psychiatric-mental health nurse is in a prime position to meet these challenges and play a role in positive treatment outcomes by implementing evidence-based mental health care as a case manager and provider of milieu therapy across the life span.

◆ Adaptations of the milieu therapy approach are applicable across the life span and for all diagnostic populations.

◆ Milieu therapy refers to the social environment of treatment and psychosocial rehabilitation.

SUGGESTIONS FOR CLINICAL CONFERENCES

1. Depending on your clinical rotation setting, observe one of the following:

   a. Client interactions in a community meeting: Describe the behavior of clients in the early, middle, and late phases of treatment.

   b. Client/client and client/staff interactions in an outpatient mental health care waiting room: Do the clients seem at ease? Are interactions pleasant? How does the secretary respond to clients?

   c. Therapist style of interaction in group therapy or psychoeducation: Does the therapist encourage members to support and communicate with peers, or take a more identified expert role? Are you encouraged to participate or only observe?

2. Ask a client to describe how other clients in the program have contributed to his treatment progress.

3. Give examples that you have observed in the clinical setting of nursing staff using the following interventions:

   a. Setting limits

   b. Giving support for risk taking

   c. Coaching clients in practicing new behaviors

4. Using the steps of the nursing process, identify an actual or potential problem in the unit milieu and discuss effective problem solving for that issue with the interdisciplinary treatment team.

5. Discuss how a research tool such as the Ward Atmosphere Scale might be used in the clinical setting where you are rotating.

STUDY QUESTIONS

1. The goal of support in milieu therapy is to:
   a. suppress aggressive behavior
   b. accept feelings of regression and dependence
   c. gain client compliance
   d. promote growth and competence

2. Adolescents and clients with substance-related problems benefit from which of the following aspects of milieu therapy?
   a. Peer feedback and support, client responsibility for self
   b. Strong external control of behavior
   c. Didactic educational groups
   d. Isolation from old community

3. A client tells you that you are the only staff member she can talk to, then mentions that something has been bothering her that she does not want everyone else to know. In formulating your response to the client, you will consider which of the following principles of milieu therapy?
   a. Therapeutic trust has been established.
   b. Confidentiality is unit based in a therapeutic milieu.
   c. Secret keeping is a way to gain rapport with clients.
   d. Open communication will occur.

4. Characteristics of a therapeutic community (milieu) include:
   a. well-defined authority based on discipline-specific expertise
   b. encouraging the client to separate from family and community responsibilities
   c. client participation in treatment and responsibility for self
   d. relieving the client of the stress of treatment plan decisions

5. Telemental health offers clients with medical and psychiatric conditions self-care management skills that enable them to manage their conditions. A major issue for using telehealth technology in the clients home is all but which of the following?
   a. Maintaining confidentiality between the nurse and client and data security
   b. Monitoring co-occurring medical and psychiatric conditions is difficult to manage in the home
   c. Establishing secure websites for group dialogues and chat rooms
   d. Selecting the appropriate client for home telemental health services

6. The nurse is meeting a new client on the unit. Which action, by the nurse, is most effective in initiating the nurse-client relationship?
   a. Introduce self and explain the purpose and the plan for the relationships
   b. Describe the nurse's family and ask the client to describe his/her family.
   c. Wait until the client indicates a readiness to establish a relationship.
   d. Ask the client about reasons he was brought to the hospital.

7. A client on the inpatient psychiatric unit refuses to eat and states that the staff is poisoning her food. Which action should the nurse include in the client's treatment plan?
   a. Explain to the client that the staff can be trusted.
   b. Show the client that others eat the food without harm.
   c. Offer the client factory sealed foods and beverages.
   d. Institute behavior modification with privileges dependent on intake.

8. A 78-year-old woman was recently admitted to a nursing home because of confusion, disorientation, and negativistic behavior. She has had difficulty sleeping since admission. Which of the following would be the best intervention?
   a. Provide her with a glass of warm milk.
   b. Ask the physician for a mild sedative.

c. Do not allow her to take naps during the day.

d. Ask the family what they prefer.

9. A 26-year-old client with a diagnosis of schizophrenia is sitting alone in his room. He alternates quiet, listening behaviors with agitated talk. The nurse enters his room and observes his behavior. What should the nurse say first?

a. "You need to come out to the day room area with the group now."

b. "Why are you hearing voices again?"

c. "You appear to be listening to something."

d. "I know you hear something, but there is no one here."

10. The nurse is making a home visit to a client with chronic schizophrenia. During the visit the client asks the nurse to leave. What is the most appropriate initial response from the nurse?

a. "I just got here after driving miles to your home."

b. "Ok. I will leave as you like, but tell me your reasons for wanting me to leave."

c. "You need your medication and since I am already here, please roll up your sleeve."

d. "Let me speak to your mother about this."

RESOURCES

Please note that because Internet sources are of a time-sensitive nature and URL addresses may change or be deleted, searches should also be conducted by association or topic.

Internet Resources

1. Run a search with a general search engine like Google or Yahoo for the term "milieu therapy." Scan through three to five pages of hits of the thousands available to note descriptions of treatment programs claiming to use milieu therapy.

2. Find a study guide at http://www.harding.edu/spollard/CHAPTER_15. Scan the questions and answer those relevant to this chapter.

3. Look for a directory of therapeutic communities for 2001 at http://www.therapeuticcommunities.org for an idea of the current prevalence of this treatment modality. For some thoughts on how this term is used by substance treatment programs, go to http://www.ncbi.nlm.nih.gov to find an article on residential therapeutic communities.

REFERENCES

American Nurses Association. (2000). *Scope and standards of psychiatric-mental health nursing practice.* Washington, DC: American Nurses Publishing.

Barnard, A. G. (2007). Providing psychiatric-mental health care for Native Americans: Lessons learned by a non-Native American PMHNP. *Journal of Psychosocial Nursing and Mental Health Services, 45,* 30–35.

Bauml, J., Pitschel-Waltz, G., Volz, A., Engel, R. R., & Kessling, W. (2007). Psychoeducation in schizophrenia: 7-year follow-up concerning rehospitalization and days in hospital in the Munich Psychosis Information Project Study. *Journal of Clinical Psychiatry, 68,* 854–861.

Chan, S. W., Hsiung, P. C., Thompson, D. R., Chen, S. C., & Hwu, H. G. (2007). Health-related quality of life of Chinese people with schizophrenia in Hong Kong and Taipei: A cross-sectional analysis. *Research in Nursing & Health, 30,* 261–269.

Comtois, K. A., & Linehan, M. M. (2006). Psychosocial treatments of suicidal behaviors: A practice-friendly review. *Journal of Clinical Psychology, 62,* 161–170.

Dean, A. J., Duke, S. G., George, M., & Scott, J. (2007). Behavioral management leads to reduction in aggression in a child and adolescent psychiatric inpatient unit. *Journal of the Academy of Child and Adolescent Psychiatry, 46,* 711–720.

Delaney, K. R. (2006). Top 10 milieu interventions for inpatient child/adolescent treatment. *Journal of Child and Adolescent Psychiatric Nursing, 19,* 203–214.

Draine, J. (1997). A critical review of randomized field trials of case management for individuals with serious and persistent mental illness. *Research on Social Work Practice, 7,* 32–52.

Edelen, M. O., Tucker, J. S., Wenzel, S. L., Paddock, S. M., Ebener, P., Dahl, J., et al. (2007). Treatment process in the therapeutic community: Associations with retention and outcomes among adolescent residential clients. *Journal of Substance Abuse Treatment, 32,* 415–421.

Granholm, E., McQuaid, J. R., McClure, F. S., Link, P. C., Perivoliotis, D., Gottlieb, J. D., et al. (2007). Randomized controlled trial of cognitive behavioral social skills training for older people with schizophrenia: 12-month follow-up. *Journal of Clinical Psychiatry, 68,* 730–737.

Guarnaccia, P. J. (1998). Multicultural experiences of family caregiving: A study of African Americans, European Americans, and Hispanic American families. *New Directions for Mental Health Services, 77,* 45–62.

Gunderson, J. (1978). Defining the therapeutic processes in psychiatric milieus. *Psychiatry, 41,* 327–335.

Hall, P. S., & DeJong, J. A. (2006). Level 1 Therapeutic Model site. *American Indian and Alaskan Native Mental Health Research, 13,* 17–51.

Irwin, M., Kline, P. M., & Gordon, M. (1992). Adapting milieu therapy to short-term hospitalization of children. *Child Psychiatry and Human Development, 21*(3), 193–201.

Jaffee, S. R., Caspi, A., Moffitt, T. E., Polo-Tomas, M., & Taylor, A. (2007). Individual, family, and neighborhood factors distinguish resilient from non-resilient maltreated children: A cumulative stressors model. *Child Abuse and Neglect, 31,* 231–253.

Kahn, E. M., & White, E. M. (1989). Adapting milieu approaches to acute inpatient care for schizophrenic patients. *Hospital and Community Psychiatry, 40,* 609–614.

Kasprow, W. J., & Rosenheck, R. A. (2007). Outcomes of critical time intervention case management of homeless veterans after psychiatric hospitalization. *Psychiatric Services, 58,* 929–935.

Kingsley, N., & Bloom, S. (2004). The art and challenges of long-term and short-term demographic communities. *Psychiatric Quarterly, 75,* 249–261.

Kennard, D. (2004). The therapeutic community as an adaptable treatment modality across different settings. *Psychiatric Quarterly, 75,* 295–307.

Keshavan, M. S., Roberts, M., & Wittmann, D. (2006). Guidelines for clinical treatment of early course schizophrenia. *Current Psychiatry Reports, 8,* 329–334.

Lanza, M. L. (2000). The community meeting: Review, update, and synthesis. *International Journal of Group Psychotherapy, 50*(4), 473–485.

LeCuyer, E. A. (1992). Milieu therapy for short stay units: A transformed practice theory. *Archives of Psychiatric Nursing, 6*(2), 108–116.

LePage, J. P. (1999). The impact of token economy on injuries and negative events on an acute psychiatric unit. *Psychiatric Services, 50,* 941–944.

Liberman, R. P. (1997). Schizophrenia practice guideline [letter]. *American Journal of Psychiatry, 154,* 1792–1793.

Mueser, C. D., Bond, G. R., Drake, R. E., & Resnick, S. G. (1998). Models of community care for serious mental illness: A review of research on case management. *Schizophrenia Bulletin, 24,* 37–74.

Norton, K., & Bloom, S. L. (2004). The art and challenges of long-term and short-term democratic therapeutic communities. *Psychiatric Quarterly, 75,* 249–261. Special section: The therapeutic community in the 21st century. Introduction. *Psychiatric Quarterly, 75,* 229–231.

Perfas, F. B., & Spross, S. (2007). Why the concept-based therapeutic community can no longer be called drug-free. *Journal of Psychoactive Drugs, 39,* 69–79.

Pickett, S., Cook, J., & Heller, T. (1998). Support group satisfaction: A comparison of minority and white families. *New Directions for Mental Health Services, 77,* 63–73.

Rizvi, S. L., & Linehan, M. M. (2001). Dialectical behavior therapy for personality disorders. *Current Psychiatry Reports, 3,* 64–69.

Roberts, R. E., Alegria, M., Roberts, C. R., & Chen, I. G. (2005). Concordance of reports of mental health functioning by adolescents and their caregivers: A comparison of European, African and Latino Americans. *Journal of Nervous and Mental Disorders, 193,* 528–534.

Royal Australian and New Zealand College of Psychiatrists Clinical Guidelines Team for the Treatment of Schizophrenia and Related Disorders. (2005). Royal Australian and New Zealand College of Psychiatrists clinical practice guidelines for the treatment of schizophrenia and related disorders. *Australia and New Zealand Journal of Psychiatry, 39,* 1–30.

Sanchez, F., & Gaw, A. (2007). Mental health care of Filipino Americans. *Psychiatric Services, 58,* 810–815.

Smith, G. M., David, R. H., Bixler, E. O., Lin, H. M., Altenor, R. J., Hardenstine, B. D., et al. (2005). A Pennsylvania State Hospital system's seclusion and restraint reduction program. *Psychiatric Services, 56,* 1115–1122.

Sullivan, A. M., Barron, C. T., Bezman, J., Rivera, J., & Zepata-Vega, M. (2005). The safe treatment of the suicidal patient in an adult inpatient setting: A proactive approach. *Psychiatric Quarterly, 76,* 67–83.

Swenson, C. R., Torrey, W. C., & Koerner, K. (2002). Implementing dialectical behavior therapy. *Psychiatric Services, 53,* 171–178.

Thornicroft, G. (1991). The concept of case management for long-term illness. *International Review of Psychiatry, 3,* 125–132.

U.S. Census Bureau. (2000). *Census 2000 Redistricting,* Pub. L. No. 94–171 (Summary File, Table PL 1). Washington, DC: U.S. Government Printing Office.

Vittengl, J. R. (2002). Temporal regularities in physical control at a state psychiatric hospital. *Archives of Psychiatric Nursing, 16,* 80–85.

Whitley, S. (2004). The evolution of the therapeutic community. *Psychiatric Quarterly, 75,* 233–248.

Yao, L., & Algase, D. (2006). Environmental ambiance as a new window on wandering. *Western Journal of Nursing Research, 28,* 89–104.

Ziguras, S. J., & Stuart, G. W. (2000). A meta-analysis of the effectiveness of mental health case management over 20 years. *Psychiatric Services, 51,* 1410–1421.

SUGGESTED READINGS

Antai-Otong, D. (2001). *Psychiatric emergencies.* Eau Claire, WI: Professional Educational Systems.

Barrio, C. (2001). The cultural relevance of community support programs. *Psychiatric Services, 51,* 879–884.

Bloom, S., & Kingsley, N. (2004). The therapeutic community in the 21st century. *Psychiatric Quarterly, 75,* 229–231.

Kennard, D. (2004). The therapeutic community as an adaptable treatment modality across different settings. *Psychiatric Quarterly, 75,* 295–307.

Kingsley, N., & Bloom, S. (2004). The art and challenges of long-term and short-term demographic communities. *Psychiatric Quarterly, 75,* 249–261.

Sullivan, A. M., Barron, C. T., Bezman, J., Rivera, J., & Zepata-Vega, M. (2005). The safe treatment of the suicidal patient in an adult inpatient setting: A proactive approach. *Psychiatric Quarterly, 76,* 67–83.

Sullivan, A. M., Bezman, J., Barron, C. T., Rivera, J., Curley-Casey, L., & Marino, D. (2005). Reducing restraints: Alternatives to restraints on an inpatient psychiatric service—utilizing safe and effective methods to evaluate and treat the violent patient. *Psychiatric Quarterly, 76,* 51–65.

Whitley, S. (2004). The evolution of the therapeutic community. *Psychiatric Quarterly, 75,* 233–248.

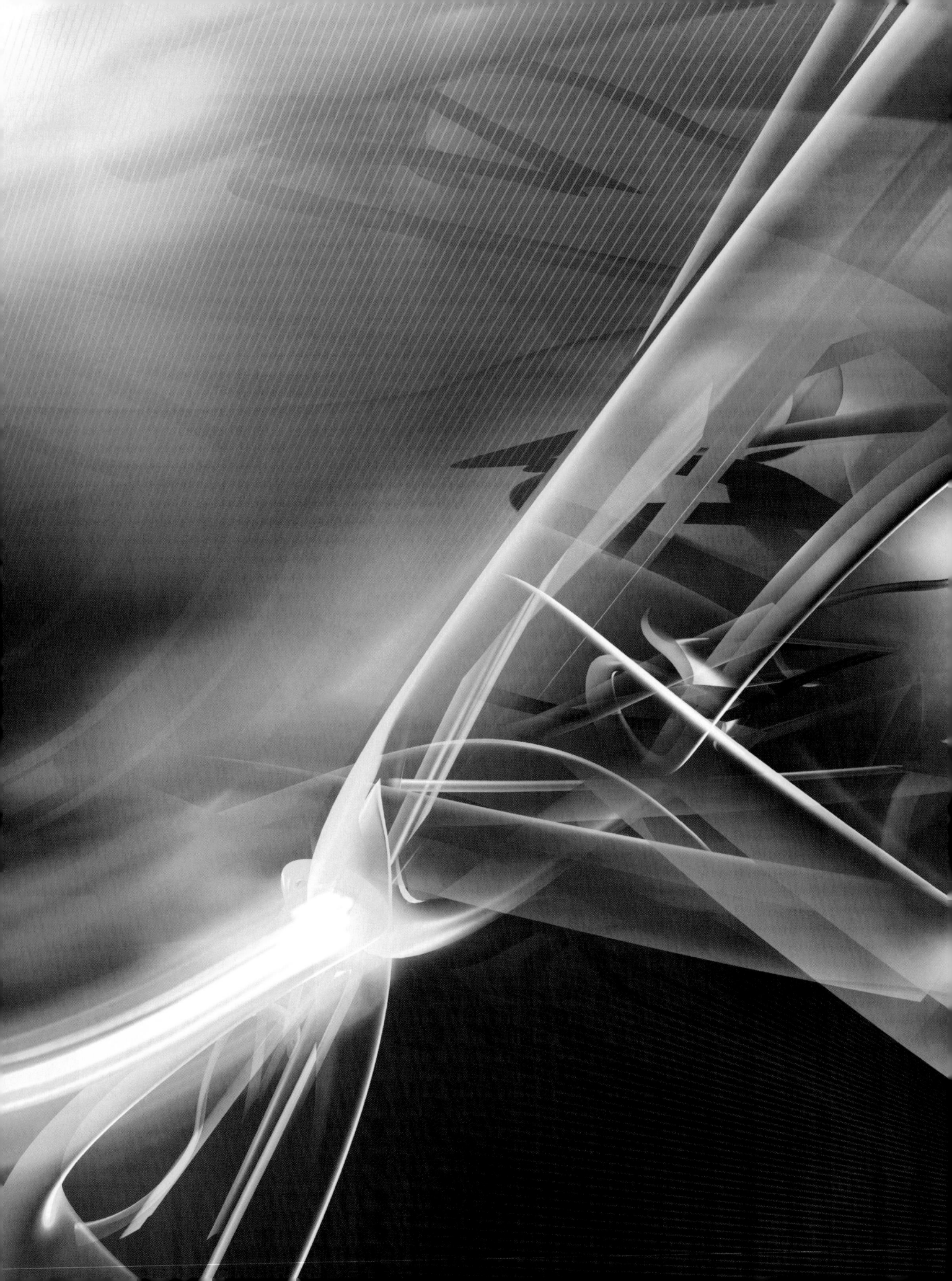

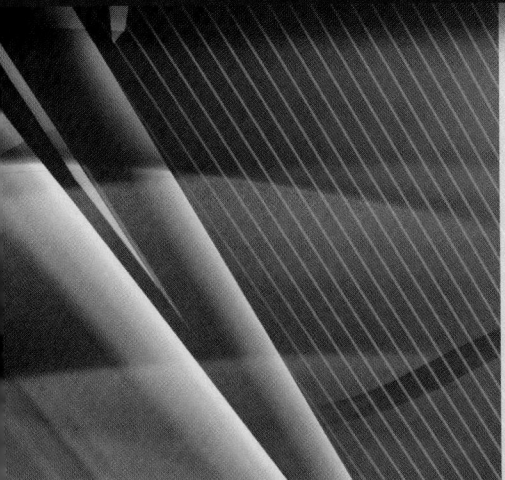

CHAPTER 33

Home- and Community-Based Care

Barbara Jones Warren, PhD, RN, CNS, CS

KEY TERMS

After-Care: Involves that care occurring after a person's discharge from the hospital.

Case Manager: A collaborative director with a consumer in the management of her holistic care.

Community Mental Health: A treatment approach that provides various levels of mental health, wellness, and illness services to individuals living within various community settings.

Community Mental Health Centers: Treatment facilities located within the community that provide different specialized levels and varieties of mental health care as well as coordination of physical and mental health care to any person needing mental health treatment.

Community Support Systems (CSS): Integrative approaches to quality mental health care for consumers that combine various types of mental health at the primary, secondary, and tertiary levels of care.

Decompensation: The exacerbation of mental disorder symptomatology that affects a person's everyday functioning ability.

Deinstitutionalization: The release of clients from public state mental health hospitals into the general community settings (e.g., group homes, residential facilities, with their families).

Dual Diagnosis: Refers to the condition of a person who has been diagnosed with a mental disorder and substance use or abuse. The term *dual diagnosis* may also be used to describe a person who has a mental disorder and mental retardation or developmental disability diagnosis. May also be known as a co-occuring diagnosis.

Extended Care: Involves long-term, more intensive care for someone who has been discharged from the hospital.

Foster Care: An alternative living arrangement for underage persons who legally cannot or choose not to live with their biological families or guardians.

Group Home Treatment: A structured living environment in which persons live with other individuals who are at various stages of their recovery process.

Hospice: Refers to end-of-life health care for clients.

Palliative Care: Combines the use of culturally competent, compassionate, therapeutic, and supportive therapies for persons who are diagnosed with a life-threatening disorder and for their families or significant others.

Partial Hospitalization/Day Treatment: A specific time-defined, outpatient, active psychiatric treatment program that is grounded in therapeutic communication and structured clinical services.

Phase-Specific Community-Oriented Interventions: Those that target specific symptoms during various stages of treatment within an intensive case management model, specifically persons with first-episode psychosis.

Primary Prevention: Includes those strategies and interventions that reduce a person's risk to develop mental illness.

Program for Assertive Community Treatment (PACT): Refers to an intensive case management approach involving careful monitoring of clients, access to mobile mental health teams, and aggressive holistic client-centered treatment planning. PACT programs are available 24 hours a day.

Psychosocial Rehabilitation: Refers to health services whose goal is to restore the client's ability to function in the community through social interaction, independent living, and vocational enhancement.

Recovery: Refers to a state of wellness or function characterized by symptom management and attaining an optimal level of function and quality of life. It is client-centered and based on principles of hope, healing, and optimism. In substance-use treatment, it refers to a state of physical and psychological health in which abstinence from dependency-producing drugs is complete and comfortable.

Secondary Prevention: Involves nurses' use of strategies and interventions that help reduce the progression of a mental illness.

Serious Disabling Mental Disorders (SDMD): A term used to describe serious and chronic psychiatric disorders such as schizophrenia, bipolar disorders, and major depressive disorder.

Short-Term Hospitalization: A structured, inpatient admission that involves providing safety for individuals at risk of harm to self or to others, evaluating acute psychiatric symptoms, facilitating medication and psychiatric stabilization, and providing psychosocial and pharmacological interventions to restore overall functioning.

Telemental Health: Live interactive videoconferencing used to provide an array of psychiatric-mental health services to clients and families residing in remote or rural areas. Major services provided through this venue include medication management, counseling, psychiatric liaison consultation among providers, and emergency psychiatric assessment.

Tertiary Prevention: Refers to measures that minimize relapse and chronic disability and restore the client to an optimal level of functioning.

COMPETENCIES

Upon completion of this chapter, the learner should be able to:

1. Describe the historical events that led to the development of community mental health services.

2. Describe how the concepts of recovery and culture can be incorporated into the nursing process.

3. Identify the types of mental health services available for persons within the community.

4. Describe the roles of the nurse as a clinician, consultant, and educator in community mental health settings.

5. Analyze the community mental health services that are needed for persons across the life span.

6. Discuss the role of the nurse in home health and telemental health care.

CHAPTER OUTLINE

The History of Community Mental Health

The Role of the Psychiatric-Mental Health Nurse

Levels of Care in Community Mental Health

Community Mental Health Centers

Types of Services and Populations Served

    Care of the Incarcerated Client

Community Mental Health across the Life Span and Special Populations

Infancy, Childhood, and Adolescence

Adulthood and Older Adulthood

Persons with Developmental Disorders

Persons Requiring Palliative and Hospice Care

Social Issues in Community Settings

Homelessness

Alcohol and Other Substance Misuse

The Role of the Nurse

The Generalist Nurse

The Advanced-Practice Psychiatric Registered Nurse

The Nursing Process

Assessment

Nursing Diagnoses

Outcome Identification and Planning

Implementation

Evaluation

Community mental health is a treatment approach that provides various levels of mental health, wellness, and illness services to individuals living within various community settings (Jerrell, 1999). The purpose of the community mental health treatment approach is to provide quality treatment to persons in the least restrictive settings possible (Department of Health and Human Services [DHHS], 1999). This approach helps to minimize disruption in an individual's life and, thus, facilitate her ability to continue everyday activities and normal functions. It is important to understand that persons may receive mental health within a variety of settings. Examples of community mental health care include short-term hospitalization, partial hospitalization, group home treatment, rehabilitative treatment, and support treatment programming.

Community mental health treatment has been in existence for approximately 40 years, and it continues to evolve as the needs of clients and the mental health system change. The purpose of this chapter is to explain the types of mental health, wellness, and illness services that are available within community settings for persons across the life span. The roles of the generalist nurse and advanced-practice nurse will also be delineated. In addition, barriers to mental health care and implications for psychiatric-mental health nursing practice are discussed throughout the chapter.

THE HISTORY OF COMMUNITY MENTAL HEALTH

Persons with mental illness were treated inhumanely until the mid-nineteenth century. Dorothea Dix, a schoolteacher, was instrumental in improving care within public mental hospitals. Before this time, persons were relegated to large institutions in order to rid society of a "contamination." A current development in community mental health involves the work of Dr. Hildegard Peplau, the founder of psychiatric-mental health nursing. Dr. Peplau (1988, 1991) describes psychiatric-mental health nursing as an "art and science." According to Dr. Peplau, the nurse uses her professional knowledge, skill, and therapeutic communication techniques in order to develop interventions and strategies that will maximize the person's mental health and wellness in various settings. Guided by Dr. Peplau's work, psychiatric nurses have been and continue to be instrumental in the development of cost-effective, quality mental health care outcomes through the use of their nursing "art and science" (Peplau, 1988).

Today's community mental health services evolved out of several other historical occurrences. Among these are the Mental Health Act of 1963, deinstitutionalization of clients from public mental health hospitals, an increase in public awareness of different mental health treatments, development of mental health prevention programs, and pharmacologic treatment advances. The need for these services intensified as persons with serious disabling disorders moved into community locations. Previously used coping resources and strategies were no longer available. In addition, individuals were unfamiliar and often uncomfortable with navigation within the community. Subsequently, many persons with mental health disorders were unable to access existing community physical or mental health care systems.

Persons were living in the community but were not part of the community structure. Exacerbation of illness often occurred because the safety community mental health centers' net was not in place. Hence, persons often sought refuge from their families in nursing homes or homeless shelters. Some became part of the forensic system when decompensation occurred and when symptoms, such as confusion, inappropriate social behaviors, and psychosis, occurred or intensified. Originally, it was estimated that community care of persons with mental illness would be less expensive than hospital care. It was proposed that these persons could use existing physical care facilities for all their care. However, later statistics indicated that care costs were the same or even higher when persons had exacerbations of their illness. Community mental health was examined more closely during the advent of managed health care. Outcomes were closely monitored. Case management has evolved into an important component within today's community mental health system (Kasprow & Rosenheck, 2007; Perfas & Spross, 2007).

Case management and other psychiatric treatment are enhanced by quality nurse-client relationships in which the nurse assesses individual needs, wishes, and preferences and health practices. Culturally sensitive care requires the nurse to integrate culture, ethnicity, and health practices through active decision making to enhance the client's willingness to access community and home-based care (Yamashita, Forchuk, & Mound, 2005).

Case management along with other psychiatric treatment is part of the continuum of care proven to enhance clinical outcomes and client-centered chronic disease management. In a small Dutch treatment intervention study of clients with first psychotic episodes of schizophrenia, Linszen and colleagues (2001) describe the concept of continuum or continuity of care as an ongoing therapeutic and professional relationship, support for the family, and the management of illness and adherence to medication. Coping skills and stress management play critical roles in advancing recovery during the first 5 years after the onset of psychosis in schizophrenia. They further noted that early recognition of schizophrenia and other major psychiatric disorders and appropriate intervention may be less important to positive clinical outcomes as continuity in care with the client and caregivers. Data from this study indicate that mental health referrals are inadequate to serve the complex needs of clients, particularly first episode schizophrenia and families with major psychiatric disorders (Linszen, Dingemans, & Lenior, 2001). Current practice and treatment include the following as critical to effective management of first episode schizophrenia and related disorders:

- Early detection and comprehensive treatment
- Comprehensive and continual intervention—assured during the initial 3 to 5 years following because the course of illness is governed by treatment afforded during this vulnerable period

- Antipsychotic medication is the mainstay treatment; atypical agents should be used as first-line medications along with close monitoring for adverse side effects

- Holistic and client-centered psychosocial interventions should be routinely afforded to all clients and their families

- Appropriately trained mental health professionals must be involved in care across the mental health continuum and include management of co-occurring conditions, such as substance abuse, depression, and anxiety

- Culturally sensitive and age-specific care and treatment environments must be an integral part of mental health care

- Active participation in decision making and treatment planning must be available to clients, families, and communities

- Maintenance of good physical health and prevention and early interventions of serious medical illness must be part of the comprehensive and holistic treatment plan (Royal Australian and New Zealand College of Psychiatrists, 2005)

Social awareness regarding the need for mental health services and changing health care finances have continued to create a climate for new developments in community mental health. By the early 1990s, clients from the state hospitals had become clients within the community mental health system. The conceptual process of recovery was born during this time. Anthony (1993) describes recovery as a process by which someone regains a sense of self as a person who has strengths, abilities, options, and possibilities, despite having a mental disorder. This process of recovery may occur at any level of symptomatology or care that a person is experiencing. A person's recovery may be facilitated when mental health providers incorporate the concepts of empathy, affirmation, encouragement, and acceptance into their professional practices. However, the societal problem of stigma regarding mental illness exists today and continues to present challenges for persons with mental illness (Crisp, Gelder, Goddard, & Meltzer, 2005; Griffiths, et al., 2006).

Major treatment goals of home based and community mental health include improving client functioning by increasing accessibility to health services, focusing on psychosocial and physical treatment and identifying and responding to complex client and family problems (Malla, Norman, Scholten, Manchanda, & McLean, 2005). Recent studies indicate that successful treatment of persons with serious mental illnesses in the community requires a comprehensive and holistic early maintenance program to enhance outcomes, particularly those with first episode psychosis (American Psychiatric Association, 2004; Royal Australian and New Zealand College of Psychiatrists, 2005; Malla et al., 2005). Improvements and modifications of health care delivery in community settings must be client centered, phase specific, involve families, and integrate pharmacologic, psychosocial, and cultural interventions.

THE ROLE OF THE PSYCHIATRIC-MENTAL HEALTH NURSE

The psychiatric-mental health (PMH) nurse has been instrumental in the evolution of community mental health. PMH nurses are often the case managers or collaborative directors with a consumer in the management of her holistic care. In

RESEARCH ABSTRACT

An Exploration of Factors Affecting Implementation of a Randomized Controlled Trial of a Transitional Discharge Model for People with Serious Mental Illness

Sharkey, S., Maciver, S., Cameron, D., Reynolds, W., Lauder, W., & Veitch, T. (2005). *Journal of Psychiatric and Mental Health Nursing, 12,* 51–56.

Study Problem/Purpose
The purpose of this study was to explore process and contextual factors encountered during the implementation of a randomized controlled trial in a mental health setting.

Methods
Researchers explored the quality systems during the trial using a mixed design that included group meetings, diaries, field notes, and feedback conducted within the context of perspectives about program implementation (*n* = 16). Content, data, and thematic analysis were used to analyze the data (e.g., meeting notes and diaries).

Findings
Findings related to the context of the study, specifically organizational, practitioner, and trial preparation issues. Key themes from these data reflected positive and negative experiences linked to the implementation, including organizational issues, roles and relationships, and communication. Researchers concluded that there are several key areas concerning how to conduct randomized controlled trials involving people as part of the intervention. Of particular interest is research that uses people-based trials to obtain quantitative data concerning particular events to guide psychiatric nursing practice.

Implications for Psychiatric Nursing
Research is an important part of psychiatric nursing. Understanding various research methodologies and their impact on client care enables psychiatric nurses to participate in data collection and apply findings to nurse interventions.

addition, PMH nurses conduct physical, spiritual, psychological, and cultural assessments on consumers. They also collaborate with the client and family and develop individualized psychoeducation regarding holistic needs for both consumers and other clinicians. As providers of a host of mental health services, PMH nurses are also responsible for prescribing medications, monitoring client responses, and coordinating health services throughout the continuum of care.

Today's PMH nurses are also part of an interdisciplinary team that provides comprehensive and holistic care through various treatment modalities, including crisis mental health teams, crisis hot lines, and mental health home care. As members of the mental health community-based team the nurse provides care to clients across the life span and must understand age-specific issues and appreciate the role of culture and families and treatment outcomes. Finally, PMH nurses conduct and participate research studies and implement clinical guidelines that enhance positive client outcomes.

LEVELS OF CARE IN COMMUNITY MENTAL HEALTH

Prevention and wellness are important concepts in the delivery of community mental health nursing care. Preventive care and nursing theorists have described three levels of psychiatric care. These include primary, secondary, and tertiary prevention levels. Primary prevention includes those strategies and interventions that reduce a person's risk to develop mental illness. Examples of primary prevention include the person's use of stress management techniques and alcohol, substance, and depression awareness programs. Secondary prevention involves nurses' use of strategies and interventions that help reduce the progression of a mental illness. For example, counseling techniques for a person who has experienced a traumatic life event (e.g., death of a person close to her, multiple negative life events) may prevent a further psychiatric illness such as depression. Tertiary preventive strategies refer to those methods nurses use to help persons return to a higher level of health and functioning. Nurses may use this approach with an individual with schizophrenia who needs to learn activities of daily living or how to take her antipsychotic medication correctly. The illness is not eliminated; however, the person is at a higher level of health and therefore can function more comfortably.

Additional levels of mental health care include after and extended care. After-care involves that care occurring after a person's discharge from the psychiatric hospital. Examples of after care include a person's attendance in substance abuse or support group programs. Extended care involves long-term, more intensive care for someone who has been discharged from the hospital. Persons receiving this care may attend everyday mental health care facilities or live in mental health group homes.

Psychosocial rehabilitation refers to a system's approach to health services whose goal is to restore the client's ability to function in the community through social interaction, independent living, and vocational enhancement (Barton,

1999). Ultimately, the program hopes to reintegrate the client back into the community successfully. Clients are actively involved in their treatment plan and collaborate with psychiatric nurses and other team members. Vocational and social skills building interventions facilitate this transition. Vocational counselors are part of the team and assist in placing the clients in an appropriate work or vocational setting that fosters independence, self-esteem, and interpersonal skills. As more and more clients are served in the community, the need for psychiatric nurses as team members is greater.

COMMUNITY MENTAL HEALTH CENTERS

Community mental health centers were initially developed in different catchment or geographic (e.g., north, south, east, and west) areas of cities. Persons received treatment at the center in catchment areas where they resided. Community mental health centers are those treatment facilities that provide different specialized levels and varieties of mental health care as well as coordinate physical and mental health care to any person needing mental health treatment. These centers are quite similar to the preventive and primary managed health care facilities that individuals use for routine, physical health care needs. However, providers within mental health facilities specialize in treatment issues for persons with mental health needs. In addition, providers are often credentialed or board certified in their specialty discipline areas (PMH nursing, psychiatry, psychology, or social work).

TYPES OF SERVICES AND POPULATIONS SERVED

There are different types of services that may be provided to clients needing community mental health treatment that corresponds to their recovery process. These include short-term hospitalization, partial hospitalization, group and foster home treatment, rehabilitative treatment, and support treatment programming. These types of services were initially and formally established in 1987 when the National Institutes of Mental Health developed community support systems for persons with serious disabling mental disorders (SDMD). Serious disabling mental disorders (SDMD) is a term used to describe serious, chronic, and potentially disabling psychiatric disorders, such as schizophrenia, major depressive disorder, and bipolar disorders (Wykes, Reeder, Corner, Williams, & Everitt, 1999). (See Table 33–1.)

Community support systems (CSS) are integrative approaches to quality mental health care for consumers that combine various types of mental health at the primary, secondary, and tertiary levels of care (Jerrell, 1999).

Short-term hospitalization refers to a structured inpatient admission that involves providing safety for individuals at risk of harm to self or to others, evaluating acute psychiatric symptoms, facilitating medication and psychiatric stabilization, and providing psychosocial and pharmacologic interventions to restore overall functioning. This type of mental health treatment is for individuals who are in crisis and

TABLE 33-1
Partial Hospitalization across the Life Span

	Common Diagnoses	Therapeutic Modalities
Early childhood (ages 2–5) **Childhood** (ages 6–9) **Preadolescence** (ages 10–12) **Adolescence** (ages 13–17)	Conduct disorders, chemical dependency, developmental delays, and pervasive personality disorders Substance-use disorders, bipolar disorder, ADHD, major depression	Play therapy; self-esteem–enhancing activities; parenting skills; problem solving; family living skills training; academics; individual, group, and family therapy
Adulthood (ages 18–64)	Depression, bipolar disorder, chemical dependency, anxiety disorder, personality disorder, schizophrenia	Individual, group, and family therapy; stress management; psychodrama; psychoeducation; family living skills training; men's and women's groups
Older adulthood (ages 65+)	Depression, mild to moderate dementia, adjustment disorder, paranoia	Individual, group, and family therapy; stress management; medication group; psychoeducation; community living skills training; occupational/recreational therapy; grief groups; coping with illness, disability, and loss

require rapid stabilization of their mental and physical status back to a higher level of their recovery process. Short-term and partial hospitalization are often combined to provide stability for those persons who are experiencing more incapacitating mental disorders. For example, individuals with treatment-resistant serious disabling mental disorders (SDMD), mental retardation, developmental disabilities, or alcohol or substance abuse are primary candidates for this holistic treatment approach.

Malla and colleagues (2002) developed a model similar to the ACT that specifically targets the prevention and early phase-specific community-oriented interventions for clients and families experiencing *first-episode psychosis*. The strength of this model is its focus on *early identification* of this high-risk group and implementation of early interventions to reduce recidivism and facilitate positive outcomes. Major concerns about these clients include (Malla & Norman, 1999):

◆ Most clients are young and lack experience with mental health services.

◆ They are unlikely to comply with treatment designed for clients in the chronic stage of their illnesses.

Interventions are based on the stress-vulnerability model of the development and course of psychotic disorders and includes low-dose, atypical antipsychotic agents [e.g., risperidone (Risperdal), olanzapine (Zyprexa), aripiprazole (Abilify), quetiapine (Seroquel), and ziprasidone (Geodon)] and diverse psychosocial interventions. One of the psychosocial interventions, called "recovery through activity and participation," or RAP, is used during inpatient and outpatient transition. Major goals of RAP are similar to ACT and include

enhancing basic life skills, communication, and psychosocial support during the period of recovery from acute psychosis. Family involvement is crucial to the success of community mental health treatment. Family interventions include psychoeducation during the engagement period, crisis intervention, and social support. This model offers psychiatric nurses another treatment modality that targets the client's phase of illness. (Additional information about the family psychoeducation can be obtained from the authors on the author's program website, http://www.pepp.ca)

Partial hospitalization/day treatment is a specific time-defined, outpatient, active psychiatric treatment program that is grounded in therapeutic communication and structured clinical services (Jerrell, 1999). Partial hospitalization works especially well for those clients who need more than traditional outpatient care but less than 24-hour-a-day care (Jerrell, 1999). It is also advantageous for persons who have difficulty stabilizing without the presence of a structured treatment process. Partial hospitalization is an alternative to inpatient hospitalization, transitional and rehabilitative. In addition, it helps persons with SDMD to maintain or improve the state of their recovery process. Partial hospitalization may also be referred to as "day treatment" because individuals participate in the program during the day and return to their regular living environment at night (Karterud & Wilberg, 2007).

Researchers have developed and implemented additional models of community mental health services that are cost-effective, client- and family-centered, and integrate pharmacologic and psychosocial interventions. One such model is the assertive community treatment (ACT). Similarly to the *phase-specific community-oriented model* previously mentioned, the Program for Assertive Community Treatment (PACT) is an intensive case management approach that has been shown to reduce hospitalization and result in cost-effective mental health care (Stein, 1993). Key aspects in PACT lie in its focus on client strengths in adapting to community life (instead of mental illness); affording support and consultation to clients and their natural support systems, including families; intensive case management to ensure active participation in treatment, medication adherence, and access to appropriate health professionals to address holistic needs (APA, 2004). PACT programs that demonstrate the strongest evidence of positive clinical outcomes include those with client-staff ratio of 10 to 1 and creative allocation of community resources (Taube, Morlock, Burns, & Santos, 1990). A lack of community, state, and federal funding allocated to mental health services is a major barrier to implementing PACT and other intensive case management programs. Its cost-effectiveness lies in its focus on client-centered and holistic care, which involves intensive monitoring and accessibility of mobile mental health teams. Reduced hospitalizations enhance the clients' quality of life. This community-based program also uses psychoeducation, living skills training, and strengthens the clients' social networks and support systems. In addition, supported work settings, such as sheltered workshops, are an integral part of this program.

Group home treatment is a structured living environment in which persons live with other individuals who are at various stages of their recovery process. In addition, there are mental health professionals and aides who live within the home and provide guidance, counseling, and therapeutic treatments for the residents. Group home treatment is another option for persons who do not require hospitalization but need a structured living environment as opposed to living independently. Group homes need to meet certain criteria in order to protect the persons who reside within them. License criteria vary from state to state.

Telemental health is a form of live interactive videoconferencing used to provide an array of psychiatri-mental health services to clients and families residing in remote or rural areas. Major services provided through this venue include medication management, counseling, psychiatric liaison consultation among providers, and emergency psychiatric assessment. Telemental health has its roots in telemedicine (Stevens & Rasmussen, 1982). The first documentation of telemedicine was in 1920 at Haukland Hospital in Norway, during which time radio links were used to provide health care support to ships at sea. In 1968 the National Institute of Mental Health funded a project to develop closed-circuit microwave relay stations between the Department of Psychiatry at Dartmouth Medical School and a rural hospital in New Hampshire. Recent advances since the 1990s have produced a plethora of inexpensive, consumer friendly telecommunication systems, such as videoconferencing, that enable psychiatric nurses and other clinicians to interact with clients living in remote or rural areas; to provide consultation to colleagues; and to conduct psychiatric assessments. It also provides an array of services to groups of clients in their homes, community-based clinics, or group homes (Shore, Hilty, & Yellowlees, 2007). Some researchers submit that telemental health or telepsychiatry is just as effective as face-to-face client interactions (Frueh, Monnier, Yim, Grubaugh, Hamner, & Knapp, 2007; O'Reilly, Bishop, Maddox, Hutchinson, Fisman, & Takhar, 2007).

Emerging evidence supports telemental health in the treatment of psychiatric disorders, such as post-traumatic stress disorder (PTSD). Findings from a randomized trial that compared the efficacy of telemental health and same-room treatment for combat-related PTSD using cognitive behavioral therapy in 14 weekly, 90-minute sessions demonstrated no group differences in clinical outcomes at 3-month follow-up (Frueh et al., 2007). The study consisted of 97 clients of which 38 were randomized (17 into telemental or telepsychiatry, 21 into the same room) and about 25 had at least one post-baseline evaluation. Client satisfaction between the two groups was similar. The same-room group reported greater comfort in talking with their therapist at post-intervention and demonstrated better treatment adherence. Findings from this study support other studies that implicate comparable outcomes and equivalent levels of client adherence, satisfaction, and health cost using telemental health in the treatment of PTSD, depression, and other psychiatric disorders (Frueh et al., 2007; O'Reilly et al., 2007; Ruskin et al., 2004).

Care of the Incarcerated Client

There are growing concerns about the criminalization of individuals with severe mental illness. A reported 10 to 15 percent of clients in jails and state and federal prisons have psychiatric disorders as well as treatment provided in these facilities and postrelease (National Commission on Correctional Health Care, 2002; Teplin, McClelland, Abram, & Weiner, 2005). Factors including deinstitutionalization; shortage of acute psychiatric beds, co-occurring substance use disorders, homelessness, poor access to community services; gaps between criminal justice, health care, and community support systems; limited civil commitment criteria; and the role of the police (Lamb & Weinberger, 2005; Lamb, Weinberger, & Gross, 2004; Weisman, Lamberti, & Price, 2004). Recent studies indicate the need to create innovative and creative approaches to provide care to individuals who are incarcerated and at risk of incarceration. One such approach is the *Sequential Intercept Model* (Munetz & Griffin, 2006). This approach offers a conceptual model for communities to create an interface between the criminal justice and mental health systems to address issues about the criminalization of people with mental illness. The multipoint integration service model provides a comprehensive diversion program that forges linkages at various points along the criminal justice continuum. Major linkages between the client and criminal justice system include interface with health care and community support. Similar to the sequential intercept model the multipoint integration approach offers an array of options and opportunities to interface various services with the criminal justice system and link incarcerated persons with psychiatric disorders with mental and physical health care and community support services (Munetz & Griffin, 2006; Weisman, Lamberti, & Price, 2004).

COMMUNITY MENTAL HEALTH ACROSS THE LIFE SPAN AND SPECIAL POPULATIONS

The previously described levels of care and types of treatments are applicable for individuals of all ages. However, children, adolescents, adults of all ages, persons with mental retardation and developmental disabilities, and persons with life-threatening illnesses may require additional types of services.

INFANCY, CHILDHOOD, AND ADOLESCENCE

Residential levels of treatment may be combined for infants, children, and adolescents living in foster care environments. Foster care is an alternative living arrangement for underage persons who legally cannot or choose not to live with their biological families or guardians. Foster care may be temporary or permanent until children or adolescents become of legal age and are released from court system supervision. Children and adolescents who are diagnosed with mental retardation or developmental disorders have the right to live in safe family environments. In cases of abuse or neglect, family and child protective services assume guardianship of vulnerable children and adolescents and make decisions regarding approved foster care environments for them. Infants, children, and adolescents may be in foster care in single family, group, or residential homes. Persons or organizations that run these homes are licensed according to strict state and deferral guidelines.

The availability of residential facilities for children and adolescents is shrinking because of constraints in funding and the changing environment regarding the institutionalization of these populations. However, one of the current concerns of PMH nurses is the remanding of children and adolescents who have mental disorders into juvenile and adult prison systems. Mental health and wellness treatment is often not addressed for these populations. In addition, children and adolescents with mental disorders may exhibit antisocial, impulsive, violent, and alcohol and other substance abuse behaviors. Children and adolescents' symp-tomatology may exacerbate in conjunction with the appearance of abuse and violence when it is not treated or therapeutically managed.

ADULTHOOD AND OLDER ADULTHOOD

Mental health care for adults should be tailored to their particular psychosocial, physical, and cultural needs. Among these are mental disorder diagnosis, community environment, physical status, gender, sexual orientation, class, age, race, ethnicity, and employment and career needs as well as any other self-identified need that the client may have (Barnard, 2007; Chan, Hsiung, Thompson, Chen, & Hwu, 2007; Lutz & Warren, 2001). (Please refer to Chapter 7 regarding these cultural issues.)

One in five older adults has a mental illness. Projected figures involving older adults with mental illness are expected to more than double, from 7 million in the year 2000 to 15 million by the year 2030 (Jeste, et al., 1999).

Older adults with severe and persistent mental illness are defined as individuals 65 years and older with lifelong or late-onset mental disorders with residual impairment. Diagnoses among this age group include psychotic disorders, bipolar disorders, recurrent major depression substance-use disorders, and dementia (Trollor, Anderson, Sachdev, Brodaty, & Andrews, 2007). In addition, older clients experience age-related issues such as considerable functional decline, medical comorbidity, and cognitive deficits. Although home care is an alternative to institutional care for older adults, it is not covered under Medicare and most predict that current budget constraints will further compromise access to this service (Van Citters & Bartels, 2004).

Psychiatric nurses must identify these issues plaguing older adults and collaborate with the client, family, and other community health care services and implement interventions such as home health care, meals-on-wheels, respite care that promotes functional status, increase access to health care services, and contend with their long-term mental health needs.

There are some additional needs that older adults have besides the needs for adults in general. Therapeutically based foster, day, and residential living care facilities often assist in the older adult's individual management of the symptomatology associated with their mental disorder diagnoses. Various levels of mental health care may be available in each one of these facilities. In addition, these facilities can provide temporary or permanent housing and are licensed according to strict state and federal guidelines and regulations.

The purpose of any treatment facility is to provide additional structure for older adults while promoting their independence and safety and maintaining their integrity. In addition, these persons have multiple needs. These include among others monitoring of their mental illness symptomatology, physiological needs, and cultural and spiritual needs. Group homes often provide the type of environment that will nurture older adults and meet their need for social interaction and self worth.

PERSONS WITH DEVELOPMENTAL DISORDERS

Individuals who are diagnosed with mental retardation or developmental disabilities (MR/DD) have a variety of special needs that may be met within residential and group home facilities. Within this environment, individuals are helped to learn social and vocational skills. These facilities are often structured according to the mental and developmental level of the persons who live within them. For example, some individuals may require more assistance with their activities of daily living as opposed to learning vocational skills. In addition, monitoring of physical, psychological, cultural, and spiritual needs by health care professionals is another therapeutic aspect of residential and group home environments.

PERSONS REQUIRING PALLIATIVE AND HOSPICE CARE

PMH nurses are often instrumental in the development and delivery of palliative and hospice, or end-of-life care for clients because these nurses have knowledge regarding holistic client needs. Palliative care combines the use of culturally competent, compassionate, therapeutic, and supportive therapies for persons who are diagnosed with a life-threatening disorder, and hospice, or end-of-life care is available for clients and their families or significant others (Gazelle, 2007; Willis, Demiris, & Oliver, 2007). This care may be provided in clients' homes or in home-like facilities if they are extremely incapacitated or debilitated and require medical treatment in conjunction with their palliative care. Nurses may provide the direct care or coordinate the delivery of palliative or end-of-life care with other health care professionals. (See Table 33–2, Hospice Care Issues across the Life Span.)

As more and more end-of-life care occurs in the home and community-based settings it is imperative for psychiatric nurses to evaluate the impact of palliative home care on the client and caregiver. The emotional and physical impact of caregiving is well documented (Orner, 2006; Seoud et al., 2007). The caregiver's needs must be assessed initially when caring for clients requiring palliative and hospice care and throughout care. Providing emotional support, making community referrals, and providing respite care to caregivers enables them to care for their loved ones themselves in their homes and communities.

SOCIAL ISSUES IN COMMUNITY SETTINGS

Homelessness, violence, trauma, abuse, and the presence of increasing societal substance misuse have created a new set of challenges for PMH nurses. Society often stigmatizes persons who incur these situations. In fact, this may create a double jeopardy situation if persons concomitantly experience these occurrences and mental illness. In addition, clients often experience an exacerbation of mental and physical illness symptomatology when they experience violence, trauma, abuse, and lack of access to health care and mental health services. These persons may not receive treatment for their mental or physical illnesses because they may lack health insurance. Adding to the problem is that early abuse and trauma may lead to the development of borderline personality disorder with symptoms of mood swings, poor impulse control, somatic distress, poor interaction skills, and self-destructive behaviors (Hunt, 2007). Finally, persons who are abused or traumatized often have multiple physical complaints and lack an ability to discriminate between destructive and perilous activities.

HOMELESSNESS

Factors leading to homelessness are manifold and include lack of economic resources, poor support systems, co-occurring psychiatric and substance-related disorders; incarceration, and failure to adhere to treatment. Psychiatric nurses are challenged to identify and link high-risk clients to appropriate health care services. The homeless had a shorter length of inpatient stay. Additional solutions to reducing homelessness in persons with mental disorders is working with members of comprehensive community-based programs that work with agencies to find low-income housing, supportive income (Caton et al., 2005; Desai & Rosenheck, 2005; Reid, Berman, & Furchuk, 2005). In addition, homeless persons often develop chronic physical problems that are exacerbated by poor living conditions, stress, mental illness disorders, and alcohol and other substance use. It is estimated that over 50 percent of homeless persons have psychiatric problems (Caton et al., 2005). Furthermore, there is a growing population of persons under 40 years old who have chronic and severe mental illness symptomatology and yet have not accessed or received appropriate treatment (Caton et al., 2005).

Homelessness may occur at any life span, affecting school-age children, adolescents, and different ages of adults, including older adults. Especially salient is the fact that there is a growing population of women and their children who have mental health problems and are not being treated. It is estimated that approximately 12 percent or 7.5 million youths have a mental disorder (Hunt, 2007). Women from racial and ethnic cultural groups are more susceptible to homelessness because they often have fewer economic and social support resources (Wenzel, Tucker, & Elliott, et al., 2004). Hence, they are more prone to develop physical and emotional problems.

ALCOHOL AND OTHER SUBSTANCE MISUSE

Persons who experience mental illness symptomatology often use alcohol and other substances as self-treatment approaches for their mental distress. Partial treatment and residential facilities are often beneficial treatment approaches for persons who have "dual diagnoses" challenges. Dual diagnosis refers to the condition of a person who has been diagnosed with a mental disorder and substance use or abuse. However, the term *dual diagnosis* may also be used to describe a person who has a mental disorder and mental retardation or developmental disability diagnosis. Emergency shelter clinics as well as community support programs may provide clients with additional treatment options for their addiction(s) and mental illness. Group work is another valuable treatment approach for chemical dependency. There are also a variety of 12-step community approaches for cocaine, methamphetamine, heroin, and alcohol that are grounded on clients' learning of the steps toward recovery from their addiction(s). In addition, there are support groups for family members or other significant persons.

The PMH nurse needs to use holistic techniques in the development and implementation of treatment approaches for persons with chemical dependency and mental illness. There is a physical, emotional, and psychological component to the addictive process. Current addiction literature

TABLE 33–2
Hospice Care Issues across the Life Span

	Response to Death and Dying	Nursing Implications
Childhood	Young children perceive death as separation, lacking a cognitive understanding of death. Factors that affect a child's reaction to death include • Family reactions • Cultural-ethnic-religious influences • Availability of emotional support	• Assess family and child's perception of illness (younger children may express feelings through behavior or other activities.) • Teach parents and child (age appropriate) about medications and other palliative measures. • Assess child and family members' emotional, physical, social, and spiritual needs. • Assess child's reaction to and perception of death. • Encourage child and family to express the meaning of child's impending death. • Facilitate the grief process. • Instruct family and parents how to institute various comforting measures, such as pain medication, touching, hugging, music, and other relaxation measures. • Encourage mobilization of social support systems.
Adolescence	Adolescents recognize that death is part of living, but they have difficulty accepting their own death.	• Encourage mobilization of support systems. • Assess for self-destructive behaviors, such as substance abuse and suicidal behaviors. • Encourage youth to express feelings. • Encourage independence and self-care. • Help youth cope with fears, anxiety, grief, and anger. • Encourage family to participate in grief process. • Encourage social interactions with peers as long as possible. • Provide comfort and relaxation measures. • Assess coping skills
Adulthood	Young adults may be struggling with leaving young children and spouse. Middle-aged adults may struggle with similar issues and concerns about body image if illness involves mutilation (e.g., mastectomy, colostomy, or prostatectomy).	• Assess client's and family's coping patterns. • Assess past reactions to death. • Assess understanding of impending death. • Teach family members comfort and relaxation measures. • Encourage self-care as long as possible. • Encourage client to express feelings. • Assess client's level of dangerousness, especially when depression or cognitive impairment is present.
Older Adulthood	Older adults often struggle with leaving a spouse but may be resigned to impending death, depending on age and resolution of developmental task of integrity, severity of pain, and physical disability.	• Assess coping patterns. • Teach family members comfort and relaxation measures. • Assess level of dangerousness, especially when depression or cognitive impairment is present.

Note. Data from *Clinical Work with Adolescents,* by J. M. Mishne, 1986, New York.: Free Press.

indicates that persons diagnosed with schizophrenia have brain receptors that are especially sensitive and responsive to nicotine and other addictive substances. Appropriate treatment for clients' mental illness often reduces their need to use substances as well. A combination of brief, motivational, and long-term therapies promote recovery for dually diagnosed clients. (See Chapter 21.)

Successful treatment of dually diagnosed clients with substance-related disorders and major psychiatric conditions involves an integrated approach that focuses on mental health and substance use issues by an interdisciplinary treatment team. Psychiatric mental health nurses play important roles in the care of clients who are dually diagnosed by providing health education, coordinating mental and physical care, and administering medication (Pawsey & Castle, 2006).

THE ROLE OF THE NURSE

It is important that generalist and advanced-practice (APRN) PMH nurses coordinate their nursing practice within community settings in order to provide quality, cost-effective mental health care for persons who have mental disorder and/or addictive diagnoses.

THE GENERALIST NURSE

The generalist nurse uses a firm grounding in the nursing process to access and develop the initial treatment intervention, strategies, protocols, outcomes, and evaluation for the client. The nurse incorporates assessment of cultural needs into the nursing process. It is also important for the generalist nurse to have knowledge of differences between mental illness and MR/DD and the effect that homelessness, violence, abuse, trauma, and addictions have on the client's mental and physical health. The generalist nurse is also likely to be part of a comprehensive mental health care team that assesses acute and chronic symptoms of mental illnesses and comorbid physical problems, implements interventions that reduce the risk of danger to self and others, and enhances treatment responses and outcomes. Other interventions include administering medications, monitoring client responses to treatment, providing crisis intervention and psychoeducation, and facilitating access to various community services. (See Table 33–3, Education Programs Provided by Community Mental Health Centers.)

THE ADVANCED-PRACTICE PSYCHIATRIC REGISTERED NURSE

The APRN coordinates the initial treatment program with the generalist nurse as they determine the feasibility, availability, and referral for community mental health and addiction programs for the client. In addition, the APRN PMH nurse often has additional expertise in the area of cultural competence for specific diverse cultural groups. The APRN may be the case manager for several treatment teams and will coordinate care for multiple clients. The generalist nurse is often one of the treatment team members responsible for the monitoring of medication, psychological, and physical issues of clients within that team. Finally, it is imperative that the generalist and the APRN PMH nurses be the advocates for clients as they promote the clients' themes for recovery.

TABLE 33–3
Education Programs Provided by Community Mental Health Centers*

Populations	Programs
Child	Developmental assessments
	Referral to educational services
	Referral to psychiatric services
	Stress management
Adolescent	Teen parenting classes
	Individual and family therapy
	Vocational-educational counseling
	Referral for psychiatric chemical dependency services
	Psychological testing
Older Adults	Respite care
	Senior centers
	Educational program for caregivers
	Medication management
	Referral for housing options
	Transportation coordination
	Referral to volunteer agencies
	Coordination of home health visits
	Referral to psychiatric services
Clients with acquired immune deficiency syndrome	Individual, marital, and family counseling
	Medication management
	Support groups for clients and families
	Client, family, and community education
	Screening for the human immunodeficiency virus
	Crisis intervention
Chemical dependency	Referral to chemical dependency services
	Laboratory services
	Medication management
	Support groups (such as Alcoholics Anonymous, Narcotics Anonymous)

*This is not a comprehensive list, but samples of what a community mental health center may offer.

THE NURSING PROCESS

Caring for persons in community-based and home mental health care settings offers the psychiatric nurse diverse opportunities to facilitate an optimal level of functioning and quality of life. The nursing process provides the basis of client-centered and holistic treatment planning.

ASSESSMENT

Assessment data from this case study indicates the need for intensive case management that involves the client, family, psychiatric nurse, and other members of the treatment team. During his early treatment post discharge, the nurse must assess his mental and functional status, self-care needs, interactions with others, and risk of danger to self and others. Assessing health educational needs must also be an integral part of this process and guide the nurse in interventions that promote understanding of mental illness, client preferences, and treatment options. (See the Case Study.)

NURSING DIAGNOSES

During early post discharge the nurse must identify nursing diagnoses that guide outcome identification. The following nursing diagnoses were identified from the assessment:

- ◆ Disturbed thought processes
- ◆ Self-care deficit
- ◆ Chronic low self-esteem
- ◆ Deficient knowledge related to medication and community services

OUTCOME IDENTIFICATION AND PLANNING

The nurse works with the client, family, and members of the treatment team to determine goals consistent with the assessment and nursing diagnoses. Major goals for this client include promoting symptom management to improve thought processes, enhancing self-efficacy and self-esteem, and increasing the client and family's understanding of mental illness and treatment options.

1. Client will learn and define reality testing and control behaviors negatively affected by thought disturbances.
2. Client will maintain appropriate hygiene and grooming and participate in activities of daily living (ADLs).
3. Client will attend sessions with the nurse and develop a therapeutic relationship.
4. Client will be able to identify two to three positive attributes by a specified date.
5. Client will identify the medication, its purpose, the schedule, and potential side effects.

IMPLEMENTATION

Community and home-based mental health care involve coordinating health services that are consistent with the plan of care. Psychiatric nurses must implement interventions that prevent mental and physical illness and facilitate symptom management, health promotion, and maintenance. Psychiatric nurses must involve the client and family members in the plan of care to assist them in coping with the daily demands of living with someone with a mental illness. Various strategies, including intensive case management and psychosocial rehabilitation, offer the nurse an array of innovative strategies that promote health and enhance the client and family's strengths and coping skills. (See Nursing Care Plan 33–1.)

EVALUATION

Evaluation of the client's treatment responses parallel treatment goals and involve monitoring symptom management and the client's functional status and quality of life. This also includes assessing the family ability to cope and manage their stress. (See Nursing Care Plan 33–1.)

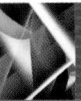

CASE STUDY

The Client with Schizophrenia in a Community Mental Health Center (CMHC) (Fred)

Fred is a 32–year-old man who was recently discharged from an acute inpatient unit where he received treatment for schizophrenia. He was to continue living at home with his parents but was required to obtain follow-up services from the community mental health center. During assessment, he was fearful of the nurse, but he later shared that he felt the microwave oven was sending him mental messages and that he saw foreign spies lurking in his closet and behind the furniture at home. He had poor eye contact, his speech was hesitant, he made periodic upward glances, and he was mildly anxious. Although his clothes were clean, his hair was unkempt. The nurse at the community mental health center developed the initial care plan for Fred on the basis of the assessment. See Nursing Care Plan 33–1.

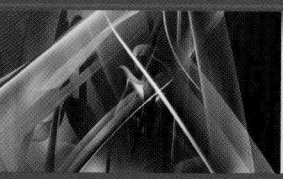

The Client with Schizophrenia in a Community Mental Health Center (CMHC) (Fred)

Nursing Diagnosis: Chronic Low Self-Esteem related to inability to trust and withdrawal from contact with others

Outcome Identification	Nursing Actions	Rationales	Evaluation
1 By [date], Fred will attend sessions with the nurse and will tolerate the nurse–client relationship and actively participaate in his plan of care.	1a. Set up appointments that are convenient to Fred and his family. Meet Fred at these times and demonstrate an accepting attitude.	1a. When a nurse follows through with meetings, the client learns that the nurse is trustworthy. An accepting attitude promotes a positive self-esteem.	*Goal met:* Fred freely engages in nurse–client interactions and actively participates in his plan of care. Fred attends three other CMHC activities this month. Fred begins to express his feelings through painting and clay.
	1b. Observe Fred's pattern of interaction and attendance.	1b. The nurse must assess and gather data on which to base interventions and goals.	
	1c. Encourage Fred to use a variety of media to express his feelings, such as painting, clay, and magazine pictures.	1c. The use of a variety of media may promote the client's self-expression in a non-threatening manner.	
	1d. Provide positive reinforcement to Fred for talking.	1d. Reinforcement increases the probability that the client will talk more in the future.	
	1e. Discuss with Fred ways he might spend his day.	1e. Discussion helps the client develop problem-solving abilities.	
	1f. Give Fred information about other CMHC programs.	1f. This provides him with several community resources and support systems.	
	1g. Explore Fred's difficulty in trusting people and his progress in this area.	1g. Discussion identifies obstacles and facilitates problem solving. Identifying progress reinforces positive behaviors.	

(continues)

Nursing Care Plan 33–1 (continued)

Outcome Identification	Nursing Actions	Rationales	Evaluation
	1h. Meet with Fred and his family to assess his ability to trust and socialize away from the CMHC.	1h. Meetings help to develop and reinforce the client's support system and provide data from the family. The nurse should meet with the family exclusively only when necessary, because the client may become suspicious and stop trusting the nurse.	

Nursing Diagnosis: Disturbed Thought Processes related to inability to evaluate reality

Outcome Identification	Nursing Actions	Rationales	Evaluation
1 By [date], Fred will learn to define and test reality and control behaviors negatively affected by thought disturbance.	1a. Support reality: remind Fred of session times and location, what was discussed last session, etc.	1a. Reinforcement and validation of reality helps the client learn to distinguish between reality and nonreality.	*Goal met:* Fred demonstrates reality testing, controls impulsive and socially inappropriate behaviors, and identifies adaptive ways to cope.
	1b. Listen attentively and tell Fred when you do not understand what he is saying.	1b. Clarifying helps the nurse identify the thoughts of the client that are not reality based. It also helps the client develop more effective communication techniques.	
	1c. Reinforce reality-based behaviors and beliefs.	1c. Enhances reality testing.	
	1d. Validate reality by saying that you believe that Fred sees and hears hallucinations but that you do not see and hear the same things.	1d. The nurse acknowledges the client's experience with hallucinations without validating their reality.	

Nursing Diagnosis: Deficient Knowledge regarding medication and community services

Outcome Identification	Nursing Actions	Rationales	Evaluation
1. By [date], Fred will identify medication name, schedule, and possible side effects.	1a. Teach Fred the name of the medication he is taking, his medication schedule, and possible side effects of the medication.	1a. The client will learn to take medications correctly, which will help to alleviate symptoms. Increased knowledge promotes self-efficacy, independence, and self-esteem	*Goal met:* Fred is able to state the name of his medication, the importance of taking it, how to obtain it, the dosage, and side effects.

(continues)

Nursing Care Plan 33–1 (continued)

Outcome Identification	Nursing Actions	Rationales	Evaluation
	1b. Encourage Fred to ask questions and then answer them.	1b. Increase understanding of his responsibilities in his treatment plan.	Fred reports a plan to maintain social activities. Fred attends outside activities and discusses his reaction to them.
2. By [date], Fred will take medications as prescribed.	2a. Teach Fred about the necessity of taking medications daily.	2a. Discussing adherence to medication regimen promotes learning and behavior.	
3. By [date], Fred will use community resources.	3a. Discuss with Fred how he may obtain medication from the CMHC.	3a. Psychoeducation about medication promotes adherence to medication regimen.	
	3b. Plan for daily opportunities for positive activity.	3b. Promotes independence and socialization and increases self-esteem.	
	3c. Give Fred information on CMHC activities and services.	3c. Reinforces positive behavioral changes.	
	3d. Arrange for transportation to these activities.	3d. Same as above.	

Nursing Diagnosis: Self-Care Deficit (Hygiene)
related to lack of interest in body and appearance

Outcome Identification	Nursing Actions	Rationales	Evaluation
1 By [date], Fred will be maintaining good personal hygiene.	1a. Teach Fred the importance of good hygiene.	1a. Helps the client identify positive consequences of his behaviors.	*Goal met:* Fred demonstrates good personal hygiene at each session. Fred is able to discuss any difficulties he is having tending to hygiene.
	1b. Teach Fred how to tend to personal hygiene: washing, laundry, bathing, combing hair, going to barber, etc.	1b. Promotes self-efficacy and responsibilities in daily hygiene and grooming.	
	1c. Reinforce when client attends session neatly groomed.	1c. Reinforcement increases positive behaviors.	
	1d. Reassess and monitor grooming and hygiene practice.	1d. Provides immediate feedback and reinforces positive behavioral change.	

SUMMARY

◆ Home- and community-based mental health care are critical elements of the continuum of mental health care.

◆ Persons with mental disorders can direct their recovery process and be collaborative partners with the health care professionals who provide health care services.

◆ PMH nurses must be knowledgeable regarding the process of recovery as it relates to the interaction of the availability of treatment programs for clients diagnosed with mental and substance abuse disorders, homelessness, violence, abuse, and trauma.

◆ Palliative and hospice care are other areas in which PMH nursing expertise may be used because therapeutic holistic care is needed within these levels of care.

◆ Finally, the collaborative work among generalist and APRN PMH nurses, the client, family, and the community mental health team is the basis of holistic, quality, appropriate, cost-effective mental health care. These endeavors support the evolution of clients' recovery processes.

SUGGESTIONS FOR CLINICAL CONFERENCES

1. Invite members of an ACT team to discuss their roles in working with various client groups in the community, highlighting the role of the psychiatric nurse

2. Invite psychiatric nurses/staff from local Veterans Affairs facility to discuss and demonstrate their telemental health program.

3. Identify community mental health needs in your area and how you can contribute to meeting these needs

4. Identify community referral agencies in your area that do or could use community psychiatric nurses

5. As a small group activity, develop a partial hospitalization program for depressed high-functioning adults and one for adolescents with developmental disorders (e.g., mental retardation)

STUDY QUESTIONS

1. An example of a rehabilitative service is:
   a. palliative
   b. foster
   c. hospice
   d. vocational

2. An intricate component of a client's recovery process includes all of the following components *except*:
   a. self-awareness
   b. inner strength
   c. acceptance of the presence of a mental illness
   d. talking with others about failures

3. An 81-year-old male was recently admitted to a local nursing home because of confusion and disorientation. Which activity would you engage the client in at the nursing home?
   a. Reminiscence groups
   b. Sing-a-longs
   c. Discussion group
   d. Exercise class

4. The community mental health nurse is making an initial home visit for an older adult. During the visit, the nurse must assess the client's ability to provide self-care in the home. Which of the following areas of concern should be assessed for determining the client's ability to remain at home?
   a. Elimination
   b. Cognitive abilities
   c. Exercise
   d. Metabolism

5. The mother of a 2-year-old tells the nurse that her son has temper tantrums, demanding cookies at the supermarket, and asks how she can best handle these temper tantrums. The nurse should suggest to the mother that she should do which of the following?
   a. Buy one box of cookies for each shopping trip
   b. Leave him home while she goes shopping
   c. Remain calm and ignore his behavior
   d. Discipline the child immediately when he demands cookies

6. The nurse is planning nursing interventions for parents who abuse their children. It is important for the nurse to recall which of the following regarding these parents?
   a. Plan ahead as to when and how to abuse their children
   b. Ask for help generally only after feeling overwhelmed with the problem
   c. Lack of remorse or guilt concerning the abuse
   d. Are always products of abuse themselves

7. When working with groups of older clients in a day care setting, the nurse can promote socialization best by implementing which of the following interventions?
   a. Grouping clients together by age and gender to encourage the development of friendships based on common characteristics
   b. Assign a different nurse to group activities each day to familiarize clients with staff
   c. Avoid discussion of client's life outside the day care setting to encourage participation in current activities.
   d. Get to know the clients and accompany them to group events such as singing, crafts, communal meals, etc.

8. Which of the following clients is most likely to benefit from telemental health?
   a. The client with Alzheimer's disease
   b. Clients living in remote or rural areas
   c. Clients with post-traumatic stress disorder
   d. b and c

9. Mr. Linsey is 40 years old and lives in a residential home with several clients diagnosed with schizophrenia and bipolar disorder. The caregiver noticed that he did not take his psychiatric medication during breakfast and questioned him about this. Which of the following responses indicates a lack of insight into his illness?

a. "I forgot to take it. Thanks for the reminder."
b. "I usually take it several times a week because it makes me too sleepy."
c. "I have an upset stomach. I will take it shortly."
d. "I want to talk to my nurse practitioner because I am having side effects."

RESOURCES

Please note that because Internet resources are of a time-sensitive nature and URL addresses may change or be deleted, searches should also be conducted by association or topic.

Support Groups and Organizations

National Alliance for the Mentally Ill (NAMI)
2107 Wilson Blvd. 3rd Floor
Arlington, VA 22201
(703) 524-7600
http://www.nami.org

The Attention Deficit Information Network, Inc.
475 Hillside Ave.
Needham, MA 02194
(781) 455-9895
http://www.addinfonetwork.com

Internet Resources

http://www.nami.org/Content/NavigationMenu/Inform_Yourself/NAMI_en_espa%Flol/NAMI_en_espa%Flol.htm. NAMI (Spanish website) (Accessed May 31, 2006)

http://www.ncptsd.org/disaster.html Resources about disaster mental health service.

http://familydoctor.org/e266.xml Schizophrenia: New Medications (Spanish) (Accessed May 31, 2006)

http://www.psych.org/psych_pract/treatg/quick_ref_guide/Schizophrenia_QRG.pdf Treating Schizophrenia: A Quick Reference Guide (Accessed May 31, 2006)

http://www.surgeongeneral.gov/library/mentalhealth/toc.html The Surgeon General provides information about mental health across the continuum.

REFERENCES

American Psychiatric Association. (2004). *American Psychiatric practice guidelines for the treatment of patients with schizophrenia,* 2nd ed. Washington, DC: American Psychiatric Press Inc. http://www.psych.org/psych_pract/treatg/pg/Schizophrenia2ePG_05-15-06.pdf. (Accessed May 31, 2006).

Anthony, W. A. (1993). Recovery from mental illness: The guiding vision of the mental health services in the 1990s. *Psychiatric Rehabilitation, 2*(3), 17–24.

Barnard, A. G. (2007). Providing psychiatric-mental health care for Native Americans: Lessons learned by a non-Native American PMHNP. *Journal of Psychosocial Nursing and Mental Health Services, 45,* 30–35.

Barton, R. (1999). Psychosocial rehabilitation services in community support systems: A review of outcomes and policy recommendations. *Psychiatric Services, 50,* 525–534.

Caton, C. L., Dominguez, B., Schanzer, B., Hasin, D. S., Shrout, P. E., Felix, A., McQuistion, H., Opler, L. A., & Hsu, E. (2005). Risk factors for long-term homelessness: Findings from a longitudinal study of first-time homeless single adults. *American Journal of Public Health, 95,* 1753–1759.

Chan, S. W., Hsiung, P. C., Thompson, D. R., Chen, S. C., & Hwu, H. G. (2007). Health-related quality of life of Chinese people with schizophrenia in Hong Kong and Taipei: A cross-sectional analysis. *Research in Nursing & Health, 30,* 261–269.

Crisp, A., Gelder, M., Goddard, E., & Meltzer, H. (2005). Stigmatization of people with mental illnesses: A follow-up study within the Changing Minds campaign of the Royal College of Psychiatrists. *World Psychiatry, 4,* 106–113.

Department of Health and Human Services, U. S. Public Health Service (DHHS). (1999). *Mental health: A report of the surgeon general.* Retrieved September, 2002, from http://www.surgeongeneral.gov/library/mentalhealth.html

Desai, M. M., & Rosenheck, R. A. (2005). Perceived reasons for loss of housing and continued homelessness among homeless persons with mental illness. *Psychiatric Services, 56,* 172–178.

Frueh, B. C., Monnier, J., Yim, E., Grubaugh, A. L., Hamner, M. B., & Knapp, R. G., (2007). A randomized trial of telepsychiatry for post-traumatic stress disorder. *Journal of Telemedicine and Telecare, 13,* 142–147.

Gazelle, G. (2007). Understanding hospice—an underutilized option for life's final chapter. *New England Journal of Medicine, 357,* 321–324.

Griffiths, K. M., Nakane, Y., Christensen, H., Yoshioka, K., Jorm, A. F., & Nakane, H. (2006). Stigma in response to mental disorders: A comparison of Australia and Japan. *BMC Psychiatry, 6,* 21. doi:10.1186/1471-244X-6-21.

Hunt, M. (2007). Borderline personality disorder across the lifespan. *Journal of Women and Aging, 19,* 173–191.

Health Resources and Services Administration (HRSA), Bureau of Health Professions, Division of Nursing. (2004). *Moving toward elimination of health disparities in the United States.* Retrieved May 12, 2006, from http://www.hrsa.gov/OMH/OMH/disparities/.

Jepson, C., McCorkle, R., Adler, D., Nuamah, I., & Lusk, E. (1999). *Image: Journal of nursing scholarship, 31,* 115–120.

Jerrell, J. M. (1999). Skill, symptom, and satisfaction changes in three service models for people with psychiatric disability. *Psychiatric Rehabilitation Journal, 22*(4), 342–348.

Jeste, D. V., Alexopoulos, G. S., Bartels, S. J., Cummings, J. L., Gallo, J. J., Gottlieb, G. L., Halpain, M. C., Palmer, B. W., et al., (1999). Consensus Statement on the upcoming crisis in geriatric mental health: Research agenda for the next 2 decades. *Archives of General Psychiatry, 56,* 848–853.

Karterud, S., & Wilberg, T. (2007). From general day hospital treatment to specialized treatment programmes. *International Review of Psychiatry, 19,* 39–49.

Kasprow, W. J., & Rosenheck, R. A. (2007). Outcomes of critical time intervention case management of homeless veterans after psychiatric hospitalization. *Psychiatric Services, 58,* 929–935.

Lamb, H. R., & Weinberger, L. E. (2005). The shift of psychiatric inpatient care from hospitals to jails and prisons. *Journal of the American Academy of Psychiatric Law, 33,* 529–534.

Lamb, H. R., Weinberger, L. E., & Gross, B. H. (2004). Mentally ill persons in the criminal justice system: Some perspectives. *Psychiatric Quarterly, 75,* 107–126.

Linszen, D., Dingemans, P., & Lenior, M. (2001). Early intervention and a five-year follow-up in young adults with a short duration of untreated psychosis: ethical implications. *Schizophrenia Research, 51,* 55–61.

Lutz, W. J., & Warren, B. J. (2001). Symptomatology and medication monitoring for public mental health consumers: A cultural perspective. *Journal of the American Psychiatric Nurses Association, 7*(4), 115–124.

Malla, A. K., & Norman, R. M. G. (1999). Facing challenges of intervening early in psychosis. *Annals of the Royal College of Physicians and Surgeons of Canada, 32,* 394–397.

Malla, A. K., Norman, R. M. G., Manchanda, R., McLean, T. S., Harricharanm, R., Cortese, L., et al. (2002). Status of patients with first-episode psychosis after one year of phase-specific community-oriented treatment. *Psychiatric Services, 53,* 458–463.

Malla, A., Norman, R., Scholten, D., Mancanda, R., & Mclean, T. (2005). A community intervention for early identification of first episode psychosis: Impact on duration of untreated psychosis (DUP) and patient characteristics. *Social Psychiatry and Psychiatric Epidemiology, 40,* 337–344.

Mishne, J. M. (1986). *Clinical work with adolescents.* New York: Free Press.

Munetz, M. R., & Griffin, P. A. (2006). Use of the sequential intercept model as an approach to decriminalization of people with serious mental illness. *Psychiatric Services, 57,* 544–549.

National Commission on Correctional Health Care. (2002). *The health status of soon-to-be-released inmates: A report to Congress.* Washington, DC: National Commission on Correctional Health.

O'Reilly, R., Bishop, J., Maddox, K., Hutchinson, L., Fisman, M., & Takhar, J. (2007). Is telepsychiatry equivalent to face-to-face psychiatry? Results from a randomized controlled equivalence trial. *Psychiatric Services, 58,* 836–843.

Orner, P. (2006). Psychosocial impacts on caregiving of people living with AIDS. *AIDS Care, 18,* 236–240.

Pawsey, B., & Castle, D. (2006). Substance use and psychosis. *Australian Family Physician, 35,* 110–112.

Peplau, H. (1988). The art and science of nursing. *Nursing Science Quarterly, 1,* 8–15.

Peplau, H. (1991). *Interpersonal relations in nursing.* New York: Springer.

Perfas, F. B., & Spross, S. (2007). Why the concept-based therapeutic community can no longer be called drug-free. *Journal of Psychoactive Drugs, 39,* 69–79.

Reid, S., Berman, H., Forchuk, C. (2005). Living on the streets in Canada: A feminist narrative study of girls and young women. *Issues in Comprehensive Pediatric Nursing, 28,* 237–256.

Royal Australian and New Zealand College of Psychiatrists. (2005). Royal Australian and New Zealand College of Psychiatrists clinical practice guidelines for the treatment of schizophrenia and related disorders. *Australian and New Zealand Journal of Psychiatry, 39,* 1–30.

Ruskin, P. E., Silver-Ayalian, M., Kling, M. A., Reed, S. A., Bradham, D. D., Hebel, J. R., et al. (2004). Treatment outcomes in depression: Comparison of remote treatment through telepsychiatry to in-person treatment. *American Journal of Psychiatry, 161,* 1471–1476.

Seoud, J., Nehme, C., Atallah, R., Zablit, C., Yeretzian, J., Levesque, L., Giroux, F., & Ducharme. F. (2007). The health of family caregivers of older impaired persons in Lebanon: An interview survey. *International Journal of Nursing Studies, 44,* 259–272.

Shore, J. H., Hilty, D. M., & Yellowlees, P. (2007). Emergency management guidelines for telepsychiatry. *General Hospital Psychiatry, 29,* 199–206.

Stein, L. (1993). A system approach to reducing relapse in schizophrenia. *Journal of Clinical Psychiatry, 54*(Suppl. 3), 7–12.

Stevens, I., & Rasmussen, W. T. (1982). Remote Medical Diagnosis System (RMDS) concept. *Journal of Medical Systems, 6,* 519–529.

Taube, C. A., Morlock, L., Burns, B. J., & Santos, A. B. (1990). New directions in research on assertive community treatment. *Hospital and Community Psychiatry, 41,* 642–647.

Teplin, L. A., Abram, K. M., & McClelland, G. M.(1996). Prevalence of psychiatric disorders among incarcerated women. *Archives of General Psychiatry, 53,* 505–512.

Teplin, L. A., McClelland, G. M., Abram, K. M., & Weiner, D. A. (2005). Crime victimization in adults with severe mental illness: Comparison with the National Crime Victimization Survey. *Archives of General Psychiatry, 62,* 911–921.

Trollor, J. N., Anderson, T. M., Sachdev, P. S., Brodaty, H., & Andrews, G. (2007). Prevalence of mental disorders in the elderly: The Australian National Mental Health and Well-Being Survey. *American Journal of Geriatric Psychiatry, 15,* 455–466.

U.S. Department of Health and Human Services (DHHS). (1999). *Mental health: A report of the surgeon general—executive summary*. Rockville, MD: U.S. Department of Health and Human Services, Substance Abuse and Mental Health Services Administration, Center for Mental Health Services, National Institute of Health, National Institute of Mental Health.

Van Citters, A. D., & Bartels, S. J. (2004). A systematic review of the effectiveness of community-based mental health outreach services for older adults. *Psychiatric Services, 55,* 1237–1249.

Weisman, R. L., Lamberti, J. S., & Price, N. (2004). Integrating criminal justice, community healthcare, and support services for adults with severe mental disorders. *Psychiatric Quarterly, 75,* 71–85.

Wenzel, S. L., Tucker, J. S., Elliott, M. N., Hambarsoomians, K., Perlman, J., Becker, K., Kollross, C., & Golinelli, D. (2004). Prevalence and co-occurrence of violence, substance use and disorder, and HIV risk behavior: A comparison of sheltered and low-income housed women in Los Angeles County. *Preventive Medicine, 39,* 617–624.

Willis, L., Demris, G., & Oliver, D. P. (2007). Internet use by hospice families and providers: A review. *Journal of Medicine Systems, 31,* 97–101.

Wykes, T., Reeder, C., Corner, J., Williams, C., & Everitt, B. (1999). The effects of neurocognitive executive processing in patients with schizophrenia. *Schizophrenia Bulletin, 25*(2), 291–307.

Yamashita, M., Forchuk, C., & Mound, B. (2005). Nurse case management: Negotiating care together within a developing relationship. *Perspectives in Psychiatric Care, 41,* 2, 62–70.

SUGGESTED READINGS

American Psychiatric Association (APA). (1997). *Practice guidelines for the treatment of patients with schizophrenia.* Washington, DC: American Psychiatric Press.

Borson, S., Bartels, S. J., Colenda, C. C., Gottlieb, G. L., & Meyers, B. (2001). Consensus statement: Geriatric mental health services research: Strategic plan for an aging population. Report of the Health Services Work Group of the American Association for Geriatric Psychiatry. *American Journal of Geriatric Psychiatry, 9,* 191–204.

Carey, K. B., Carey, M. P., Maisto, S. A., & Purnine, D. M. (2002). The feasibility of enhancing psychiatric outpatients' readiness to change their substance use. *Psychiatric Services, 53,* 602–608.

Fischer, E. P., Shumway, M., & Owen, R. R. (2002). Priorities of consumers, providers, and family members in the treatment of schizophrenia. *Psychiatric Services, 53,* 724–729.

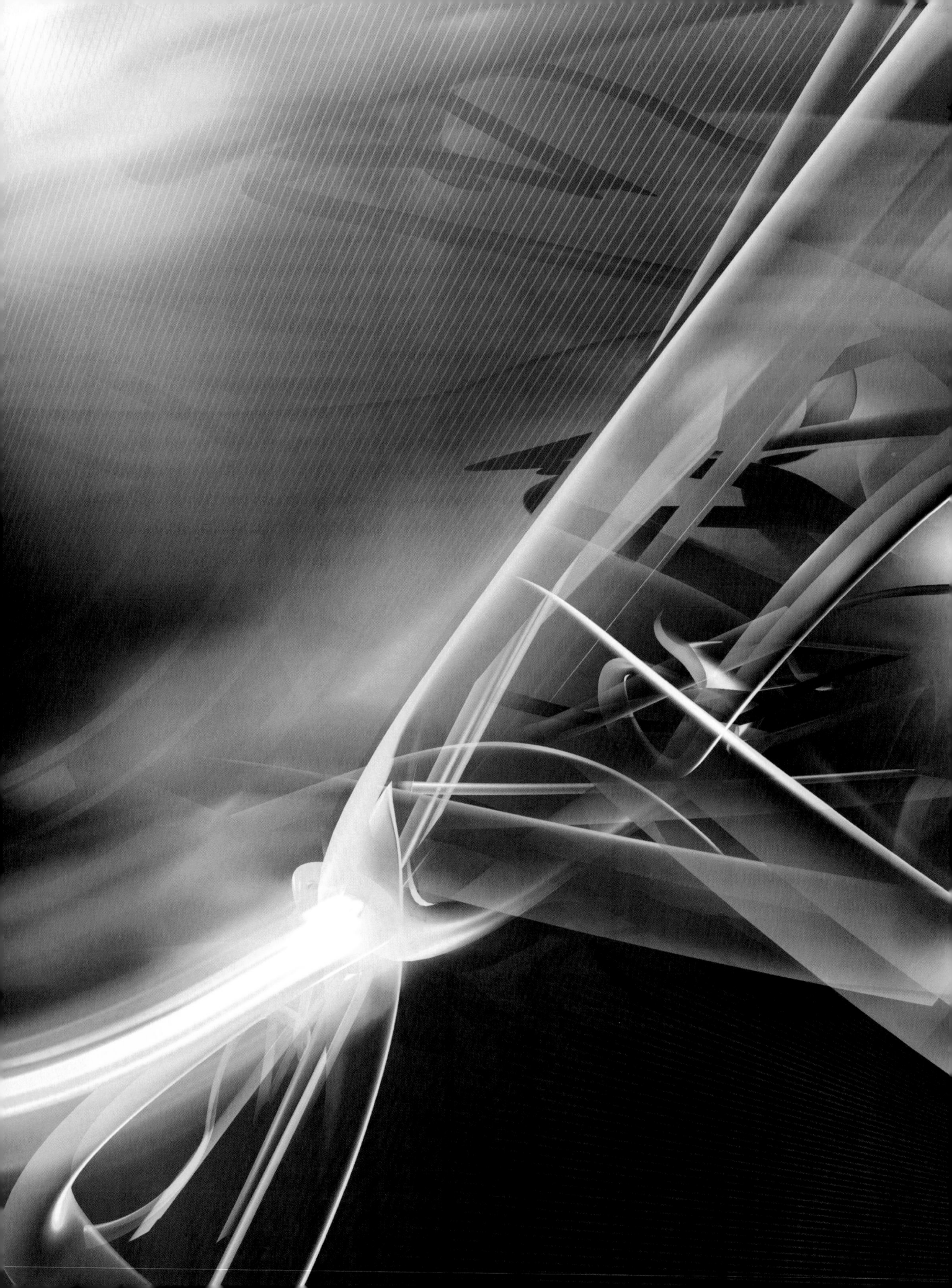

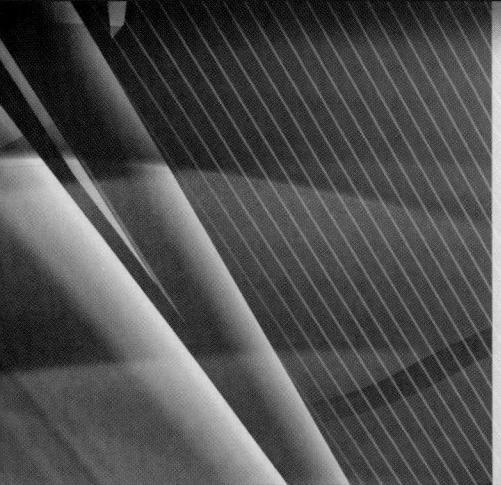

CHAPTER 34

Psychosocial Care in Medical-Surgical Settings

Sheryl A. Innerarity, RN, PhD, FNP, CS
Deborah Antai-Otong, MS, APRN, BC, FAAN

KEY TERMS

Body Image: One's physical perception, sense of identity, strengths, and limitations.

Mental Status Examination: The part of the clinical assessment that compiles nursing observations and impressions of the client during the interview. Data from this examination include general appearance, mood and affect, speech patterns, perception, thought content and processes, level of consciousness and cognition, impulsivity, ability to abstract, judgment and insight, and reliability.

Spiritual Assessment: Process involving gathering data concerning the client's belief system, affirmation coping mechanisms, and psychosocial resources.

Spirituality: A dynamic phenomenon that enables a person to discover meaning and purpose in life, particularly during stressful life events..

COMPETENCIES

Upon completion of this chapter, the learner should be able to:

1. Analyze the relationships among biological, psychosocial, and spiritual factors in medical-surgical settings.

2. Recognize symptoms of psychosocial stress in clients who are experiencing medical and surgical conditions.

3. Integrate psychosocial, spiritual, and physiological interventions in clients with medical-surgical conditions.

4. Discuss the psychosocial and spiritual needs of the client across the life span.

CHAPTER OUTLINE

Clients' and Their Families' Psychosocial Responses in the Medical-Surgical Setting

The Angry Client

The Demanding Client

The Depressed Client

The Dying Client

    Psychosocial Interventions

    Biological Interventions

    Spiritual Interventions

Specific Medical Conditions in the Medical-Surgical Setting: Life Span Issues

Hospitalization during Childhood and Adolescence

Hospitalization during Early and Middle Adulthood

    The Client with a Spinal Cord Injury

    The Client with AIDS

    The Client with Breast Cancer

Hospitalization during Late Adulthood

The Role of the Nurse

The Generalist Nurse

The Advanced-Practice Psychiatric Registered Nurse

The Nursing Process

Assessment

Nursing Diagnoses

Outcome Identification/Planning

Implementation

Evaluation

Research in Medical-Surgical Settings

The client entering the hospital and other institutional facilities often experiences enormous stress generated by fear of the unknown, loss of privacy, autonomy, and dependency on others. The client's response to his illness and hospitalization is affected by psychosocial, cultural, spiritual, and biological factors. Developmental stage, personality traits, coping behaviors, support systems, and the nature of illness also influence it. Hospitalization can increase feelings of helplessness, anxiety, and stress. The client surrenders control over the time he eats, sleeps, bathes, and performs activities of daily living. Additional stressors include impaired personal identity, which is affected by removal of personal clothing and other items, and the staff's insistence on traditional hospital clothing. The capacity to handle stress is a complex process and the person's response to the stress of hospitalization may be unpredictable.

When coping with their fears and concerns, some clients may become demanding, angry, and uncooperative as a means of maintaining control over some aspect of their lives. When the nurse's perception of the client's situation differs from the client's, misunderstanding evolves. Understanding the meaning of the clients' behaviors helps nurses maximize and promote adaptive coping responses in clients in the medical-surgical settings.

Evidence also suggests that a lack of support systems and close ties to family and friends compromises the immune system's responses, consequently increasing the risk of infections and serious illness, impairing the wound-healing process, and decreasing responses to vaccines. Other studies suggest a link between psychiatric disorders and an increased risk of medical conditions. For instance, natural killer T-cell function is decreased in depression, as well as the total number of T cells, hence increasing the risk of medical illness in these clients (York et al., 2007). Accordingly, many medically ill clients may be in the institutional environment because they lack adequate and quality support systems and resources that healthier people have. This premise may also explain the high utilization of health care resources by people who are mentally ill.

Loss of individuality, increased feelings of helplessness, and dependency are elements of dehumanization. Nurses can provide humane care by approaching clients in an empathetic and caring manner. Therapeutic alliances foster autonomy and decrease feelings of powerlessness. Clients must be active participants in their care. Clients demand quality care that involves informed consent, some control over their environment, and safe humane treatment. This chapter focuses on stress generated by hospitalization or institutionalization in a nonpsychiatric setting and discusses the effects of biological and psychosocial factors on the medically ill in various clinical settings. In addition, it discusses ways in which every nurse can help clients identify their emotional responses to physical illness and develop adaptive coping skills.

CLIENTS' AND THEIR FAMILIES' PSYCHOSOCIAL RESPONSES IN THE MEDICAL-SURGICAL SETTING

Illness and hospitalization place tremendous stress on clients and families. Anger, depression, and anxiety are common responses to illness. The 45-year-old man who is diagnosed with multiple sclerosis or the child hospitalized for cystic fibrosis experience similar feelings—fear of the unknown, sadness as a result of separation from significant others, and annoyance over the disruption in their lifestyle. Regardless of the source of these feelings, clients need emotional support, opportunities to express their feelings, and assistance in maintaining a sense of well-being. Nurses play major roles in helping clients cope with illness and hospitalization, including transitions to rehabilitation facilities and long-term care facilities.

Most clients have difficulty conforming to the daily hospital or facility routine. The psychological trauma stems from changes related to major medical illnesses and treatment. In addition to the change in their daily routines, clients must cope with other major stressors such as changes in personal and professional roles to which they have strong emotional ties. People's self-esteem, value systems, and sense of self-worth are linked to their roles. Debilitating, life-threatening, or chronic illnesses such as renal failure, breast cancer, diabetes, heart disease, and acquired immunodeficiency syndrome (AIDS) also threaten people's livelihood. Anger, depression, and demanding behaviors are normal reactions to these situations. Staff reactions frequently set the tone for client reactions. Understanding the need for clients to express their feelings and maintain some control and dignity is crucial to the effectiveness of treatment.

Like adults, children find hospitalization and illness highly stressful. Developmental stage, previous life experiences, family dynamics, history, and seriousness of illness play important roles in the children's response and adaptation to stress. The earlier the illness, the greater is the risk of injury and emotional, social, and academic deficits. Younger children tend to experience attachment and separation anxiety. Healthy child-parental relationships can buffer the deleterious effects of stress on infants. Separation, pain, loss of control, body image changes, and family dynamics influence the youth's response to hospitalization and illness.

Childhood and adolescent illnesses place overwhelming stress on families, often resulting in immense parental guilt and emotional and physical strain. These responses increase the risk of overprotectiveness by parents and of dependency in the chronically ill child. In addition, as the family attempts to cope with the child's illness and feelings, adaptive coping behaviors are taxed, generating anger, frustration, depression, and the likelihood of complications of severe physical and emotional stress.

Nurses play a key role in assessing and identifying clients at risk for maladaptive responses to illness and participating in crisis intervention. Demanding and angry clients are often labeled as problem clients because they disrupt the daily routine of the unit. All behavior has meaning and needs to be thoroughly assessed. Control and dependency factors tend to trigger intense feelings and behaviors.

Working in medical-surgical or extended care settings is often frustrating and stressful. Clients have numerous physical and emotional needs that require immediate or eventual attention. Numerous factors contribute to stressful work environments such as increased workloads and sicker and more demanding, depressed, suicidal, and dying clients. Nurses need to use innovative treatment modalities that enable them to establish meaningful relationships, which mobilize clients' adaptive coping responses, strengthen resilience, and promote mental and physical health.

THE ANGRY CLIENT

Angry and demanding clients often generate feelings of helplessness and frustration in the nurse. These feelings can be effectively managed by recognizing the meaning of the client's responses and maintaining composure in the most stressful situations. Anger typically symbolizes feelings of inadequacy, fear, and helplessness, and should not be personalized.

Major interventions include approaching the client in a calm and firm manner, and using direct eye contact, a normal voice tone, and active listening skills. These responses validate the client's feelings and convey empathy, yet provide verbal limit setting. It is critical that the nurse be able to assess verbal and nonverbal cues to detect imminent physical aggression in the client. The likelihood of aggression increases when a client feels he is ignored or discounted. Hurried and unconcerned responses to the client may create or increase his feelings of anger, powerlessness, fear, and dependency. Setting firm limits on the appropriate manner in which anger can be expressed is indicated if the client strikes out or throws things. Speaking to the client in a firm, accepting, and caring tone is crucial to minimizing acting-out behaviors. Normally, physical or verbal aggression indicates that the client is feeling out of control. Nurses can help the client regain control by remaining calm and accepting and using firm, consistent limit setting. In addition, the client's emo-

tional needs can be assessed by encouraging verbalization of feelings and providing a safe environment that reduces stress and enhances adaptive coping skills (Antai-Otong, 2004a, 2007). Table 34–1 lists the Dos and Don'ts for coping with angry clients.

THE DEMANDING CLIENT

Demanding clients, like angry ones, often generate intense emotional reactions in the nurse. They are usually time conscious and self-absorbed and lack concern for others. Clients with chronic obstructive pulmonary disease (COPD) can be very demanding. These clients routinely experience intense anxiety, particularly during an extreme dyspneic episode. Their lack of control over their illness, their fear of being unable to breathe, and the stimulant effects of bronchodilators increase their anxiety. As anxiety increases, feelings of dependency and helplessness and fears of dying ensue.

Major interventions for clients with COPD include encouraging activities that promote optimal ventilation; maintaining a calm, concerned approach; encouraging expression of feelings; and staying with the client during anxious periods. Anxiety and demanding behaviors can be further reduced by encouraging participation in stress reduction and breathing exercises.

Overall, the nurse can help clients maintain control by speaking in a confident and caring voice to reduce escalation of negative responses. Keeping promises is necessary to establishing trust and establishing rapport. Managing demanding behavior requires active listening skills and patience to understand the meaning of the client's complaints and frustration. Accordingly, simple explanations regarding treatment procedures and daily routine and encouragement to participate in treatment reduces clients' fears and enhances a sense of control. Ignoring demanding clients or responding indifferently increases anxiety and fears (Antai-Otong, 2007). Maintaining therapeutic interactions is the key to establishing rapport and facilitating adaptive coping behaviors. Table 34–2 lists dos and don'ts for coping with demanding clients.

THE DEPRESSED CLIENT

Feelings of helplessness and anger often precede depression. The prevalence of depression is 10 percent in the general population, and untreated depression places clients at risk for complications and death (Lahlou-Laforet et al., 2006). Moreover, recent research data suggest that women have a worse prognosis than men following acute myocardial infarction (Garavalia, 2007). Lack of motivation, adherencce to treatment, and hope are major themes of depressed clients (Beck, Brown, Berchick, Stewart, & Steer, 1990; Das & O'Keefe, 2006). The following illustrates how the nurse can respond to the psychological needs of the depressed client.

First, recognizing symptoms of depression can help nurses develop effective interventions that help clients develop adaptive coping behaviors. See Chapters 9 and 10 for a detailed

TABLE 34–1
Dos and Don'ts for Coping with the Angry Client

What to Do	Why
Keep your own emotions in check, speak in a calm, reassuring way.	Gaining control over your feelings lets you think rationally. Only then can you help the client. If you become angry, you'll probably incite the client even more.
Watch the client's body language	The client's body language gives you clues to his or her potential for physical aggression. Pacing indicates agitation, for example; a clenched fist may mean imminent physical violence.
Let the client air feelings.	When the client airs his or her feelings, anger and tension decrease, enabling the client to deal with the situation rationally.
Determine the source of the client's anger.	Knowing the source of anger enables you to recognize that the anger is not directed toward you.
Involve the client in his or her treatment.	Involving the client in daily care decreases his or her feelings of helplessness and dependency.
Provide controls or limits as needed.	Setting limits on the client's behavior provides some controls. The client often welcomes these limits.

What Not to Do	Why
Don't shout or argue with the client. Avoid touching the client or invading the client's space.	Shouting, arguing, and touching the client can escalate anger. These behaviors prevent you from dealing effectively with the client and can make him or her become physically violent. Touching the client or invading his or her space can be threatening to the client and make him or her feel cornered. This may result in retaliation toward you.
Don't let the client stand between you and the door.	Maintain easy access to the door in case the client becomes violent and you need to get out quickly.
Don't patronize or talk down to the client.	Patronizing the client increases anger and potential for aggression.
Don't discount the client's feelings.	Dismissing the client's feelings interferes with establishing a therapeutic nurse-patient relationship.
Don't take it personally.	This is not about you. Becoming defensive interferes with your ability to focus on the client.

Note. From "When Your Patient Is Angry," by D. Antai-Otong, 1988, *Nursing, 18,* pp. 44–45.

discussion of depression and bipolar disorder. The following manifests depression (American Psychiatric Association [APA], 2000):

- Depressed or sad mood
- Changes in appetite, concentration, and sleeping patterns
- Social isolation
- A lack of interest or motivation, particularly things that were once valued
- Expressed feelings of hopelessness
- Decreased libido and energy

Second, assessing the client's history and duration of depressive symptoms and identifying recent stressors or major lifestyle changes, such as recent losses or illness, is necessary.

TABLE 34–2
Dos and Don'ts for Coping with the Demanding Client

Do	Rationale
Realize that the demanding client likely feels fearful, anxious, or angry and may even feel guilty.	Fearful people need control. Determine what the client can control and share control when appropriate. The client will feel that you are trying to meet his or her needs.
	You can then understand the client's demands. Also, it keeps you from taking what the client says personally.
Keep promises. If you say you'll be there in 20 minutes, be there.	Keeping promises increases the client's trust in you and decreases his or her fear of losing control.
Set limits. Reassure the client that you'll check on him or her regularly and be there immediately in an emergency. Strive for continuity of care.	Limit setting gives the client structure and decreases feelings of helplessness because he or she knows what to expect.
Listen to the client's complaints. If the client is frustrated by hospital procedures, let him or her express their concerns and then explain why things run as they do.	The client gains insight into his or her feelings.

Don't	Rationale
Make excuses for not being immediately available to the client.	Demanding clients are self-absorbed. They won't feel sympathy for other clients.
Argue with the client.	The client will think you are losing control and will feel more anxious and angry.
Ignore call lights or respond to them *slowly*.	The client will feel more fearful and anxious and that he or she is unimportant.

Note. From "Dealing with Demanding Patients," by D. Antai-Otong, 1988, *Nursing, 19*, pp. 94–95 .

For example, the 50-year-old business executive who recently suffered a myocardial infarction is at risk for depression because of potential lifestyle changes and because depressed individuals are at higher risk for cardiovascular disease. The client has generally worked more than 60 hours a week, and his life has centered primarily on advancing his career. His wife expresses concern that he refuses to talk to her or other family members and barely eats. He also admits having thoughts of dying and feeling "less than a man" because he cannot take care of his family.

Emerging research indicates that people who lack emotional well-being are more likely to suffer from cardiovascular disease (Citrome & Yeomans, 2005). This client may have had long-standing stress and depression before this physical event, which further damages self-esteem. Individuals with long-standing anxiety or depression are at a significantly higher risk of developing hypertension (Alkadhi & Alzoubi, 2007).

The assessment process involves gathering information from the client and from his family members who provide invaluable data about the client's level of functioning and emotional state. It also involves performing a spiritual assessment. Performing a spiritual assessment offers the client an opportunity to talk about this aspect of his life if desired. If the client expresses a need to talk about his spiritual or religious life, nurses must listen and integrate this datum into the assessment. If the client does not wish to talk about this part of his life, nurses must also honor the request while maintaining an open mind for other important dimensions of the client's life.

A spiritual assessment provides useful information about the client's values and beliefs and enables the nurse to gain a better perspective of the client's individual needs. Expressing feelings and thoughts to the nurse helps clients and families understand the meaning and normality of present responses.

Third, assessing depressive symptoms is critical to reducing complications, such as associated impaired nutrition; biological complications, such as hypertension, hyperglycemia, or cardiac arrhythmias related to nonadherence to treatment; and suicide. A psychiatric consultation-liaison nurse (PCLN) should be consulted when a client is assessed to be suicidal or homicidal and the nurse feels in need of assistance in formulating an effective treatment plan. See Chapter 35 for more information on the role of the PCLN and Chapter 19 for a detailed discussion of the suicidal client.

Overall, medical-surgical clients experiencing major role or lifestyle changes often feel helpless, hopeless, and depressed. Nurses can minimize these feelings and potential complications by assessing early depressive symptoms and reducing stress and suicidal risk.

THE DYING CLIENT

Death and dying issues frequently arouse feelings of helplessness, anger, and frustration in the nurse. Exploring the meaning of these feelings can help the nurse understand those of the dying client. Establishing rapport and conveying concern and empathy are vital to forming a therapeutic relationship. Death completes the cycle of the life span and its certainty frequently generates feelings of hopelessness, guilt, and helplessness in the dying client, his family, and the nurses who are caring for him (Kubler-Ross, 1969).

Coping skills, developmental stage, and cultural, spiritual, psychosocial, and biological factors all influence the client's response to death. Exploring one's early memories of these events is critical to understanding the client's feelings and attitudes about death and to self-awareness. Self-awareness strengthens healthy responses to dying clients. Crisis ensues when the dying client is unable to mobilize available resources to reduce anxiety and stress. Nurses can mobilize resources by collaborating with clients, their families, and chaplains to ensure active participation and enhance independence and self-esteem.

The response to death and dying varies among children and adolescents. Their perception of death is influenced by factors that affect adults' perceptions of death, that is, developmental stage and cultural, spiritual, biological, and psychosocial influences. Some children may perceive death as magical and believe that the dead will eventually wake up and return to life. For example, many cartoon characterizations, such as the Road Runner, that are shown splattered on the pavement later jump up and spring back to life, reinforcing this perception. The child's perception of death needs to be explored. This process can be facilitated by play therapy, art, and support groups, which encourage the child or adolescent to express feelings about death. Anxiety and fears often stem from fear of abandonment. Explanations can help the child understand death and facilitate the grief process (McCaffrey, 2006).

In general, death and dying concerns generate various emotional reactions, which include depression, helplessness, hopelessness, guilt, anger, and hostility. Some clients may even deny their feelings and experience difficulty grieving. Understanding the emotional reactions and related somatic interventions, such as chemotherapy, irradiation, dialysis, or life-support systems, is important when caring for the dying client. Clients with cancer and their caregivers have increased levels of insomnia and depression. It is important for the nurse to assess the caregiver and family needs when caring for the dying client. Frequently manifestations of loss and grief precede the death of the client (Carter, 2005; Penson et al., 2005).

When a depressed or anxious dying client refuses further treatment, the nurse should realize that there are therapeutic options remaining that are beneficial. One such approach is cognitive behavioral therapy (CBT). CBT is a psychotherapy approach that is used to help the client deal with distorted perceptions of self, others, and his/her future that generate anxiety and depression. The PCLN uses this approach to challenge these distortions, hence reducing anxiety and depression and facilitating adaptive coping behaviors. CBT has proven to be a helpful approach to treating these clients. Although CBT will not change the course of the disease process, it enables the client to develop adaptive coping skills and a healthier perspective about personal responses and behaviors (Watson, 2000). There are also factors that increase the risk of depression in clients with cancer, including advanced stage of the disease, female gender, low socioeconomic status, and social isolation (Kick, 1999).

An individualized care plan that incorporates psychosocial, biological, and spiritual components is critical to caring for the dying client. Emotional comfort and physical comfort are essential client outcomes. Assessing the needs of the dying client begins with identifying present stressors, present and past coping mechanisms, spiritual needs, and available support systems.

Psychosocial Interventions

Empathy and compassion are vital to *psychosocial* interventions and the grief process. Kubler-Ross's (1969) dynamic five stages of grief (Table 34–3) are useful in assessing the client's and family's response to loss and death. Therapeutic interactions convey compassion, concern, value, and respect of the client's uniqueness. Active listening, therapeutic use of

---

TABLE 34–3
Kubler-Ross's Five Stages of Grief Applied to the Medical–Surgical Client

Stage	Client Behavior
Denial	Client refuses to acknowledge limits and comply with treatment.
Anger	Client is demanding, nonadherent, argumentative, and critical of his or her care and of others.
Bargaining	Client seeks new or questionable treatment modalities.
Depression	Client exhibits social withdrawal, agitation, impaired eating, sleep disturbance, and altered concentration patterns.
Acceptance	Client participates in care and verbalizes feelings; appetite, concentration, and sleeping patterns improve.

Note. From *On Death and Dying*, by E. Kubler-Ross, 1969, New York: McMillan. Reprinted with permission.

touch, and silence are the basis of nursing interventions. Encouraging clients and their families to express their feelings and thoughts facilitates their grief process and helps them maintain their individuality (Antai-Otong, 2007).

Focusing on positive aspects of the client's life strengthens self-esteem and coping mechanisms. Additional psychosocial interventions include encouraging the client to participate actively in care and increasing his social interactions. Participation in daily care fosters independence and a sense of control over some aspects of the client's life. Social interaction decreases feelings of alienation and despair. Nurses can seek out the client at regular intervals during each shift. Regular visits by the chaplain service should also be available as part of social and spiritual interaction. In community settings, visiting nurses need to make regular visits to ensure access to nursing staff and to decrease the client's loneliness and depression. Support groups and structured community programs also enhance social interactions and self-worth.

Biological Interventions

Biological interventions such as chemotherapy, irradiation, and surgery can increase clients' feelings of helplessness and anxiety, further compromising their ability to cope and adapt. Nurses need to assess these needs and collaborate with other members of the treatment team to promote comfort and maintain clients' integrity, quality of life, and dignity. Providing pain medication and privacy, supporting the client's spiritual needs, explaining all procedures, and involving the client in daily care are critical nursing interventions.

The client's emotional and biological stamina is often compromised by various biological interventions. One might wonder why some clients handle their illness better than others. Continued assessment of various attributes that allow different clients to deal with death and dying should shed some light on this question.

Spiritual Interventions

There is a growing interest in the relationship of spirituality to medicine and overall health care (Unruh, 2007). **Spirituality** is defined as a dynamic phenomenon that enables clients to discover meaning and purpose in life, particularly during agonizing life events (Howard, Balneaves, & Bottorff, 2007; Shiff & Moore, 2006). The essence of spirituality transcends language and is often expressed in symbols, myths, and stories universally, and involves a personal relationship with a higher being or power (Underwood & Powell, 2006). Spiritual and religious beliefs provide strength and hope. Researchers also submit that spirituality plays a key role in health maintenance, well-being, and coping with illness (Narayanasamy, 2006; Wilding, Muir-Cochrane, & May, 2006). Performing a **spiritual assessment** involves obtaining personal data about the client's belief system, affirmation, coping behaviors, and psychosocial resources. Nurses can use spirituality to reinforce coping mechanisms and facilitate grieving (Power, 2006). In various populations, religious beliefs and rituals are often the basic means by which 20 to 40 percent of clients cope with life

stressors (Howard, Balneaves, & Bottorff, 2007; Shiff & Moore, 2006).

Grieving helps nurses connect with clients and their families and appreciate their experience while exploring personal reactions to death and dying. Exploring one's early memories of these events is critical to understanding the client's feelings and attitudes about death and self-awareness. Self-awareness strengthens healthy responses to dying clients. Regular visits by the priest, minister, or rabbi need to be available to clients and families. Table 34–4 outlines the role of spirituality in coping. (See Chapter 9.)

The following clinical example portrays a client undergoing irradiation treatment and the nursing interventions that reinforce his coping behaviors and promote his emotional and physical comfort.

SPECIFIC MEDICAL CONDITIONS IN THE MEDICAL-SURGICAL SETTING: LIFE SPAN ISSUES

Life span factors play a major role in people's adaptation and response to physical and emotional stressors. Medical-surgical conditions affect clients and families throughout the life span and can affect clients' developmental mastery. Understanding and integrating life span factors is critical in developing individualized care.

HOSPITALIZATION DURING CHILDHOOD AND ADOLESCENCE

Physical illness that occurs in early life poses more stress than physical illness occurring in later years. Long-term effects of

TABLE 34–4
Role of Spirituality in Coping

- Allows client to feel bonded with others and higher being
- Provides client with sense of worth and affirmation
- Generates resourceful energy
- Helps client find significance and aim in life
- Stems from client's belief system, values, and perception of illness and stressors
- Strengthens resilience and family ties
- Facilitates a realistic perspective about life
- Reduces stress
- Mobilizes adaptive coping resources

CLINICAL EXAMPLE

The Dying Client

The nurse greets Mr. Jones and his wife before his radiation therapy. He has had a "bad night," he says, describing it as painful and restless. The nurse approaches the client in a caring and concerned manner, extending his hand, using good eye contact, and inquiring about pain medication. Mr. Jones says he does not feel like he needs pain medication, even though it was prescribed for him on a p.r.n. basis. Further exploration of Mr. Jones's feelings about pain medication reveals that his reluctance to ask for pain medication is associated with feeling less than a man. He is a World War II veteran who prides himself as being strong and in control of his life.

The nurse spends about 10 minutes explaining that Mr. Jones's condition warrants using p.r.n. pain medication and that he can control his pain by using it. The nurse further assures the client that taking an analgesic is not a sign of weakness and that it is ordered to relieve his pain. Encouraging Mr. Jones to take the medication alleviates feelings of helplessness generated by severe pain. He and his wife express appreciation for the nurse's thoughtfulness and time. This clinical example demonstrates how the nurse can use therapeutic interactions, such as compassion, active listening, education, and acceptance, to maximize the coping behaviors, promote comfort, increase self-esteem, and maintain integrity in the dying client.

childhood debilitating illnesses can disrupt psychosocial, biological, and academic development and generate family turmoil.

The child or adolescent with a chronic or acute physical illness requires that the nurse use biological and psychosocial interventions to help the client and family cope with tremendous stress. The emotional impact of physical illness is influenced by numerous factors such as the nature and cause of the injury, developmental stage, family coping patterns, and nature of medical treatment.

The influence of family on the health and treatment of children and adolescents dealing with hospitalization and serious medical conditions is well documented. Researchers submit that the family function and structure, family circumstances, coping patterns, resources, values, beliefs, roles, and relationships with the child predict clinical outcomes. Family circumstances reflect the emotional climate in which the child resides both in and outside the home. Nurses working with children and their families must assess cultural and ethnical factors that govern health practice, childrearing, and perception of the child's illness. This process also includes assessing the quality of parent-child relationship, health, and behaviors. Depending upon the reasons for the child's hospitalization or seeking treatment, the nurse is poised to assess the family and child's unique needs and provide client-centered care that addresses their emotional, physical, spiritual, and psychological needs (Postovsky & Ben Arush, 2004; Schor & American Academy of Pediatrics Task Force on the Family, 2003).

Younger children tend to suffer from separation anxiety generated by hospitalization, unfamiliar people, pain, and distressful treatment modalities. They usually feel abandoned during hospitalization because of special care that often involves reverse isolation to reduce infection. Because family members are the most significant people to the child, he may cry when family members leave. Helping the child and family cope with hospitalization is critical to restoration of mental and physical health.

Adolescents are struggling to gain independence, identity, and separation from families. Hospitalization and chronic illness place the youth in a dependent position that increases their anxiety and feelings of powerlessness and inadequacy. Personal appearance, athletic abilities, and acceptance by peers are major components of the youth's self-concept. A threat to or change in body image can have a profound effect on the adolescent's self-image and concept. The physically ill adolescent may be faced with disfigurement, limitation in body movements, and poor academic performance, which intensify feelings of alienation and isolation among peers. Limited social interactions also threaten self-esteem and increase the risk of depression. Acceptance, positive affirmation, and support are vital to helping the adolescent adapt to serious and long-term illnesses.

The following are major nursing interventions that promote optimal level of function and restoration of health in the child and adolescent:

◆ Assessing developmental stage

◆ Explaining procedures and treatment

◆ Spending quality time to listen and assess the youth's concerns and emotional and physical status

◆ Encouraging expression of feelings and thoughts of present illness

◆ Encouraging age-appropriate participation in treatment

◆ Providing positive feedback and affirmation through encouragement and compliments

◆ Observing for symptoms of depression and suicidal risk (i.e., change in appetite, apathy, sad or irritable mood, self-depreciating statements, isolation)

◆ Encouraging parent-child interactions and participation in care

◆ Arranging for academic work to be brought to the hospital or for a teacher to work with the student when possible

Families of hospitalized children and adolescents also experience tremendous stress because of the youth's condition. Families often experience guilt, anxiety, and fears about their child's condition. Moreover, they feel powerless and helpless, which is manifested in detachment, extreme anger, or overprotectiveness. Siblings often feel overlooked and resentful because of the attention given to the sick child's immense needs. Siblings of children with cancer and serious medical conditions experience a more somber responsibility burden from the illness overlooked by their parents. Because the parents are more engrossed on the child's physical health and emotional needs, the siblings' physical complaints and emotional problems often go unnoticed. Nurses must assess the needs of siblings who frequently experience tremendous stress and ineffective coping responses (Houtzager, Grootenhuis, Caron, & Last, 2005). A recent study using quantitative and qualitative methodologies to assess quality of life in siblings of children with cancer demonstrated significant improvements pre- to postcamp (Houtzager et al., 2005; Packman, et al., 2005). Researchers submit beneficial effects of camp as a psychological intervention and demonstrate the significance of these methodologies in discerning the impact of serious medical conditions on the lives of their siblings. An implication for nurses is the value of assessing the needs of the entire family when working with children and adolescents experiencing life-threatening or serious medical conditions. A failure to address the needs of siblings and relatives living with the child can have a negative impact on the emotional climate in which the family lives. Fears of the unknown, financial strain, physical exhaustion, and intense guilt and anxiety often compromise the parents' coping skills and adaptation to the child's injuries or illness.

To mobilize the family's resources and maximize their coping mechanism, the nurse first establishes a therapeutic relationship that involves approaching the parents in a nonjudgmental and understanding manner, reassuring them that everything possible is being done to provide for the child's well-being. Next, the nurse provides health education about the child's condition and actively involves the parents in the child's care. Throughout treatment the nurse encourages them to express their feelings and supports the family in crisis. The family and youth need to be informed of treatment procedures and progress. These interventions can decrease their feelings of powerlessness and helplessness, thereby strengthening the parent-child relationship and facilitating the adaptation process.

Emotional responses to physical illness vary among children, adolescents, and their families. Exploring the meaning of the client's responses helps the nurse and other treatment team members develop an effective treatment plan that restores health and promotes optimal function.

Nurses caring for children with serious medical conditions must provide family-centered care. Shelton, Jepperson, and Johnson (1987) recommend the following strategies for children with special health care needs:

1. Recognize that the family is the constant in the youth's life, whereas nursing staff varies.

2. Facilitate collaboration between parents or caregivers and health care staff.

3. Share consistent information with parents/caregivers in a therapeutic and supportive manner.

4. Implement policies and programs that promote financial support for families.

5. Recognize family strengths and respect for individual and cultural coping patterns.

6. Integrate developmental and emotional needs of the youth and family into the health care system.

7. Encourage parent-to-parent support.

8. Provide holistic health care that is flexible, accessible and responsive to the family's needs.

HOSPITALIZATION DURING EARLY AND MIDDLE ADULTHOOD

Tremendous stress is generated during early adulthood as the person struggles to master intimacy, understand his sexuality, and identify career goals. Physical illness that interferes with accomplishing these tasks places severe stress on the young adult and impedes developmental progress. In this section, three medical conditions—spinal cord injury, AIDS, and breast cancer—are discussed because they place the individual and significant others at risk for emotional stress and turmoil. In addition, they challenge nurses to explore personal reactions to demanding situations and to develop effective interventions that facilitate adaptive coping skills in clients and in themselves.

The Client with a Spinal Cord Injury

Spinal cord injuries affect younger adults who are active and productive. Injuries range from transient numbness to permanent paralysis. Sensory and motor loss usually occur below the level of the spinal cord injury. The higher the injury, the greater is the risk of serious complications. Major treatment goals during the acute phase include maintaining life-support systems and preventing further spinal cord injury. Maximizing the level of function is a major treatment goal for the client with a spinal cord injury.

The psychological responses to spinal cord injuries are extensive and complex. Both biological and psychosocial factors affect client function. Intensive, long-term physical and psychosocial rehabilitation is required. Biological factors such as bladder and bowel control, immobility, skin care, sexuality, sensory deprivation, and change in body image and lifestyle, evolve from acute to chronic concerns for clients and significant others.

Psychosocial factors affecting the client's response to the injury include the client's coping skills and available support systems. Psychosocial factors associated with loss in clients with spinal cord injuries include:

◆ Loss of mobility

◆ Increased dependency secondary to job loss or career

◆ Alterations in body image and self-concept

◆ Loss of control over body functions, such as sexuality, bladder, and bowel

◆ Potential loss of close interpersonal relationships

Understanding how the client copes involves assessing the impact of the injury on his livelihood. The client with a spinal cord injury suffers intense loss and grief, the resolution of which can be facilitated by using an accepting and understanding approach. Normal grief reactions include crying spells, depression, anger, and intense hostility toward loved ones and staff. Exploring the meaning of these behaviors helps nurses understand the extent of the client's emotional pain and coping skills.

The client who has lost function of personal body function, such as bladder and bowel control, and who depends on others for self-care is likely to feel angry, helpless, and powerless. The client with a spinal cord injury tends to be very demanding in efforts to ward off these feelings and gain control of some aspects of his life. How the nurse responds to the client's intense emotional reactions is vital to the client's adaptation process. Demanding behaviors should not be construed as a personal attack, but as a way the client attempts to cope with dramatic lifestyle and body image changes. Nurses need to (1) avoid personalizing clients' negative reactions, (2) explore the meaning of these reactions, and (3) collaborate with the client and significant others to help him develop alternative adaptive coping skills.

The client's injuries also place enormous demands on significant others. The quality of available support systems during this critical period of emotional and physical recovery is vital to health promotion. Nurses can assess the quality of significant relationships by observing family member's interactions with the client and participation in the client's care. Active involvement promotes a sense of accomplishment and decreases feelings of inadequacy and helplessness in the client and family.

The Client with AIDS

AIDS or human immunodeficiency virus (HIV) infection remains a worldwide health problem and challenges nurses to treat the client with an illness that involves complex psychosocial and neurobiological processes note Goodkin et al., (2006). That HIV type 1 (HIV-1) often results in cognitive-motor impairment, which is the most prevalent type of dementia in this disorder. This form of dementia also has a higher mortality rate (Goodkin et al., 2007). Autopsy studies show that 80 percent of clients with AIDS had neurological changes, and approximately half exhibited neurological disorders before their death. Recent data support this notion and indicate that 20 to 25 percent of persons with AIDS had dementia (Goodkin et al., 2007). A number of clients with AIDS experience neurological and mental disorders such as dementia, delirium, and mood disorders arising from general medical conditions. Computerized tomography (CT) scans show a progressive cortical dementia and diffuse cortical atrophy in the client with the HIV and AIDS-related encephalopathy (Moore et al., 2006). In addition, the terminal nature of AIDS places enormous psychosocial stress on the client and significant others. See Chapters 9 and 10 for a lengthy discussion of depression and bipolar disorders.

The psychosocial consequences of AIDS, like other life-threatening conditions, are multifaceted and include major lifestyle changes and losses, death and dying issues, and exposure to numerous medical interventions. Other potential psychosocial stressors include alienation from loved ones, financial problems, social stigma, threat to self-integrity, and isolation. See Chapter 16 for an in-depth discussion of cognitive disorders.

Mood and anxiety disorders are prevalent in HIV infection. An estimated 4 to 22 percent of HIV-positive men and 2 to 25 percent of HIV-positive women experience major depressive and anxiety disorders (Mello & Malbergier, 2006). Data from recent studies indicate a high prevalence of mood, anxiety, and substance use disorders in this population (Pence, Miller, Whetten, Eron, & Gaynes, 2006). Other researchers support these findings and submit that as HIV progresses to AIDS, the manifestations of depressive symptoms persist after the onset of AIDS (Kopnisky, Bao, & Lin, 2007). Mood disorders, including major depression and bipolar disorder, often complicate the care of persons with HIV and require early identification and treatment to reduce deleterious medical and psychiatric outcomes.

Assessing the cognitive function and associated behaviors is an important aspect of caring for the client with AIDS. The progression and span of behavioral and mental status changes are basic components of assessing cognitive function.

The first step in assessing cognitive function is a comprehensive mental status examination. A mental status examination is an unstructured tool used to assess psychiatric and neurological function. This information may be gathered from the client, family, or significant others. Assessed in the mental status examination are attention, language, memory, and higher cortical function such as judgment and ability to abstract. The results of a mental status examination are used in conjunction with other diagnostic tests to determine a differential diagnosis of AIDS dementia (see Chapter 5). Other members of the treatment team order diagnostic studies that include neuroimaging, lumbar puncture, serum chemistries, functional status testing, and a comprehensive neuropsychiatric examination. Results from these studies provide important information required to rule out alternative causes of cognitive-motor symptoms, such as infections, endocrine-related encephalopathy, or CNS tumors (Goodkin et al., 2007).

AIDS Dementia

AIDS dementia has a progressive degenerative course. Its symptoms include decreased concentration; memory, language and motor difficulties; and an inability to abstract or the use of poor judgment. The degree of impairment reflects the nature of brain involvement. In fact, early neurological manifestations of AIDS dementia or encephalopathy are often subtle. The American Academy of Neurology AIDS Task Force (1991) delineates the following criteria for minor cognitive-motor disorder in clients with HIV.

- Attention and concentration
- Memory
- Motor function (slowed, abnormal gait incoordination or hyperreflexia)
- Mood (irritable)
- Behavioral (emotional lability, amotivation)
- Personality changes

Later symptoms suggest diffuse brain involvement and include:

- Delirium
- Delusions
- Hallucinations
- Severe headaches
- Fever
- Marked personality changes
- Severe cognitive involvement
- Motor signs (i.e., ataxia, spastic gait)

Delirium in HIV Associated–Dementia

Delirium in HIV associated–dementia is an acute general medical condition manifested by disorientation, alterations in sensorium and attention, recent memory difficulties, motor restlessness or agitation, and perceptual distortions. Life-threatening symptoms of delirium include elevated blood pressure, pulse rates, and neurological changes (i.e., ataxia, nystagmus, or pupillary abnormality). This medical emergency is often misdiagnosed as a psychiatric disorder because of agitation, aggressive or violent behavior, and visual hallucinations. The symptoms of delirium must be assessed and reported as soon as possible because it has a high mortality rate. Delirium in the client with AIDS is a poor prognostic sign. Nursing care for the client with AIDS must assess for signs of delirium and report them in a timely manner to ensure appropriate medical interventions (Udall, Ryan, Berghus, & Harris, 2000). (See Chapter 16.)

Major nursing interventions during this emergency situation include the following:

- Reassuring the client and significant others
- Referring the client for immediate medical evaluation
- Monitoring the client's mental and physical status constantly (someone must be with the client at all times)
- Reorienting the client
- Anticipating the client's anxiety and potential violent or aggressive behavior

The client may be treated with a combination of an anxiolytic, such as lorazepam (Ativan), and antipsychotic agents such as haloperidol (Haldol), to manage persistent agitation and aggressiveness. This combination tends to lower the need for high doses of antipsychotics and reduce the risk of extrapyramidal side effects (Tariot, 1999). Nurses need to assess the client for desired and adverse reactions to these agents (see Chapter 29).

The complexity of neurobiological and psychosocial components of AIDS increases risks of depression and suicidal behaviors. The client's responses must be assessed throughout treatment in an effort to identify and mobilize hospital and community resources that facilitate adaptive coping skills and promote the highest level of function. Assessing and strengthening support systems are keys to maximizing emotional and physical resources.

The Client with Breast Cancer

The woman with breast cancer who enters the medical-surgical setting for surgical treatment faces major changes in body image and also the fear of death. In 2002, the prevalence of breast cancer in the United States was 2,290,000 of which 12,000 cases were found in men and 2,278,000 found in women (National Cancer Institute, 2006). Although heart disease kills more women, there are few diseases that instill more fear. African American women are more likely to die from breast cancer, and also are more likely to have breast cancer when younger than age 45.

Boman, Andersson, and Bjordis (1997) conducted a study of 97 women with breast cancer during a short hospital stay and found that achieving client trust needed special attention after surgery. Findings from these data also suggest that establishing trust with this population is crucial, especially in the areas of communication, emotional support, personal treatment, and practical assistance.

Culturally, women are more afraid of breast cancer than of other diseases, such a heart disease, which are more lethal. The woman who is preparing for a lumpectomy, mastectomy, or more radical surgery is afraid of the loss of intimacy engendered by a change in body image. The stages of Kubler-Ross's death and dying theory fit well with the responses of many women with breast cancer. Initially, diagnosis may be put off because of a fear of actually having cancer; therefore denial is a large factor. This may even be a factor once the client is admitted for surgical procedures; it is not unusual for this client to be unusually cheerful before and after surgery.

Cultural factors also impact women's perception of early or annual breast screening. Issues such as perception of benefits to have annual breast mammography screening, fatalism, perceptions of general health, and psychosocial factors may interfere with preventive health care. Assessing health education about breast cancer and other health-related problems provides nurses enormous opportunities to participate in preventive screening. (See Research Abstract, Psychosocial Correlates of Mammography Screening in Older African American Women.)

Because women with breast cancer are likely to have a short stay on the medical-surgical unit, efforts to provide psychosocial support is compromised or overlooked by nurses. However, during this short stay and postsurgical care the client may vacillate between the five stages; therefore

RESEARCH ABSTRACT

Psychosocial Correlates of Mammography Screening in Older African American Women

Farmer, D., Reddick, B., D'Agostino, R., & Jackson, S. A. (2007). *Oncology Nursing Forum, 34,* 117–123.

Study Problem/Purpose

The aim of this study was to examine the psychosocial correlates of older African American women's adherence to annual mammography screening, including fatalism, dispositional optimism, social support, knowledge of breast cancer screening recommendations, perceptions of general health, and components of the Health Belief Model (HBM).

Methods

A cross-sectional survey of 198 African American women ages 50 to 98 years who lived in low-income housing in central North Carolina was conducted. Women participated in group sessions at low-income housing complexes and completed questionnaires. Differences between who did and did not have a mammogram during the previous years were examined using correlate variables associated with the HBM. Stepwise multivariable regression models were adjusted to explore factors that correlated with social support and relevant components of the HBM.

Findings

There were few differences in groups by age, education, marital status, having a friend or family member with breast cancer, ever having had a clinical breast examination, self-rated health, cancer fatalism, disposi-tional optimism, or feelings about the seriousness of and their suscepti-bility to breast cancer. However, there were significant group differences on mammogram-related variables, specifically concerning whether women should have clinical breast examinations, benefits and barriers to mammography screening, and social support. Stepwise multivariable regression analyses demonstrated that dispositional optimism and social support were related significantly to perception of benefits; education, dispositional optimism, and cancer fatalism were related to barriers; and dispositional optimism was related to social support. The researchers concluded that older African American women with low incomes per-ceived barriers to cancer screening, educational and cancer knowledge detriments, and a lack of health-related social support to decreased ad-herence to mammography screening.

Implications for Psychiatric Nursing

Perceptions about mammography screening differ among various pop-ulations. Psychosocial, gender, and cultural factors play key roles in health promotion activities and often depend on nurses in various set-tings to thoroughly assess health education needs, particularly about preventive measures to identify breast cancer through annual mam-mography screening.

the woman with breast cancer who returns for nursing care may be very angry if the surgery did not "get" all of the can-cer (Kubler-Ross, 1969). Anger may stem from the client's perceived "mutilation" of breast surgery. In a qualitative study by Colyer (1996), it was noted that women experience can-cer as "an additional stigma and therefore as a double burden of isolation, alienation, and loss of autonomy" (p. 500). In addition, the client's perception of breast cancer may be one of an "enemy that is absorbing the body's nutrients," and con-currently "mounting an assault on personal integrity" (Colyer, 1996, p. 500).

Because therapy for breast cancer varies, it is difficult for the nurse to discern the type of education and counseling the client needs. However, given a chance to counsel a client with breast cancer, nurses might ask if they are aware of cos-metic surgeries to re-create breast tissue. These surgeries can ease the pain of body image changes in women with good prognosis. Chantler and colleagues (2006) conducted a study ($n = 31$) to stimulate the longitudinal needs of clients treated for breast cancer. The subjects were divided into two groups—those seen within 6 months of diagnosis were con-sidered the early group, while those seen in 6 to 12 months of their diagnosis were classified as the late group. Clients were asked to identify effective and ineffective psychoso-cial support and how these needs changed over time. Participants in the early group identified psychosocial needs as surgery and chemotherapy. In comparison, women in the late group focused on menopausal symptoms. Psychosocial concerns found in each group were the fear of disease re-currence and death. The researchers also concluded that health education of disease and results of diagnostic findings were both comforting and engendered a sense of control. Transportation provided by their significant others and childcare with their female friends were also deemed impor-tant sources of psychosocial support (Chantler, Podbilewicz-Schuller, & Mortimer, 2006).

Cosmetic reconstruction often needs to be planned before the initial lumpectomy or mastectomy, so discussions need to begin as early as possible. Reconstruction surgery can also be planned later, but most evidence suggests that women who elect it may not fare any better with self-esteem needs or do better physically (Roth, Lowery, Davis, & Wilkins, 2005).

Of course, some women do not have timely diagnosis of their breast cancer. This may be because the client delayed seeking medical assistance after discovering a lump. There may be guilt and anger about these issues as well, and the client's family may also be angry.

In the later stages of breast cancer, metastasis to the brain is common, resulting in neurological and mental health changes for which the nurse should be careful to observe. Subtle changes in cognition might signal early metastasis, which might respond to excision or radiation therapy. There are also many new breast cancer therapies available and emerging, and nurses should encourage clients to seek these opportunities when the physician feels they are viable options.

HOSPITALIZATION DURING LATE ADULTHOOD

This life span discussion ends with a focus on a complex condition that primarily affects the older client: cerebral vascular accident (CVA). A CVA, or stroke, results from suspension of blood circulation to the brain. Blood clots, cerebral emboli, hypertension, narrowing or hardening of arteries that supply the brain, and cerebral aneurysm cause CVA.

It is well documented that direct brain injury causes episodic changes in mood that eventually progress to major depression. Studies show that clients who suffer injury to the left hemisphere and areas around the frontal-subcortical circuits (Vataja et al., 2004) are vulnerable to severe depression (Barker-Collo, 2007). More recent research indicates that up to 50 percent of all clients who have suffered a CVA have depression resulting from impaired neurotransmitter secretion, and increased secretion of damaging chemical substances related to the hypoxia, swelling, and ischemia within the areas of the brain that are damaged.

These direct chemical changes compound the psychosocial issues associated with changes in body image, dependency, impaired mobility, locus of control, and deficit in communication (Thomas & Lincoln, 2006). In addition, an estimated two thirds of poststroke clients eventually manifest severe symptoms of depression, and the other one third present with these symptoms by the sixth month. Clients with past and family histories of depression are also at risk for depression.

Major psychosocial stressors for poststroke clients include the following:

1. Loss of ability to perform self-care (depending on the area and severity of brain damage)
2. Compromised coping skills
3. Difficulty adapting to limited or residual functioning
4. Personality changes and impaired intellectual function
5. Labile mood
6. Loss of effective communication skills
7. Change in body image
8. Loss of livelihood and ability to work
9. Change in self image

Neurobiological and psychosocial changes are expected outcomes in clients who have experienced a CVA. The client's increased dependency and neurobiological limitations often overwhelm family members. Supporting the client can minimize these feelings and family by establishing therapeutic relationships that provide emotional support, crisis intervention, and education about expected psychosocial and neurobiological changes and expectations. Considering the relatively safe and effective antidepressant medications that are now available, the post-CVA clients who are depressed are good candidates for these medications (Antai-Otong, 2004b).

Major client outcomes during the rehabilitation phase include the following:

◆ Recovery from the associated depression
◆ Attainment of an optimal level of function
◆ Development of adaptive coping behaviors
◆ Restoration of independence in self-care
◆ Adjustment to limited neurobiological function (client and family)

The following case study illustrates the nursing process in the care of the client who has experienced a CVA. Also see Nursing Care Plan 34–1.

CASE STUDY

The Client Who Has Experienced a CVA (Mrs. Jaycee)

Mrs. Jaycee is a 67-year-old woman who was a practicing pediatrician until a month ago when she suffered a mild CVA. She is now actively involved in speech therapy. Her mood fluctuates from sad to normal but mainly the former. Her family has been very supportive, but they are frustrated by her inability to cope with her illness. Her family reports that even though she is making tremendous progress, her mood is sad and depressed. They are concerned about her inability to cope. A request for consultation is sent to the PCLN, who initially sees Mrs. Jaycee alone and later sees her with her spouse. Mrs. Jaycee communicates by writing notes and expresses frustration and a sense of loss because of her recent illness. She denies suicidal or homicidal ideations, but she admits feeling depressed at times.

It is not uncommon for clients who have experienced a CVA to undergo mood changes, particularly depression. Mrs. Jaycee responds to a new-generation antidepressant and individual psychotherapy that integrates grief work and other strategies to enable her to work through her sense of loss and increase her self-esteem and confidence. Later sessions with her spouse also enable him to deal with his grief and concern for his wife's well-being. After several months, Mrs. Jaycee is able to cope with her illness and gain the confidence for other aspects of her rehabilitation.

THE ROLE OF THE NURSE

This section discusses the roles of the generalist and advanced-practice psychiatric registered nurse in the psychosocial care of clients in medical-surgical settings.

THE GENERALIST NURSE

The medical-surgical generalist nurse plays several roles in helping clients cope with psychosocial stresses. The initial process involves the psychosocial assessment, which enables the nurse to assess present stressors, present and past coping behaviors, strengths, spiritual needs, quality of support systems, and available resources. Clients seen in the inpatient or ambulatory care setting experience similar alterations in self-esteem and body image.

The woman seeking a mammogram after finding a lump in her breast is just as stressed as the man who suffers acute chest pain. Inevitably, death and dying issues emerge in these circumstances. Medical-surgical nurses can help clients manage psychosocial stresses by using active listening skills and responding in a concern and nonjudgmental manner. Nurses can enhance this process by assessing the client's and family members' spiritual and educational needs and by working with the treatment team to provide individualized holistic health care. Nurse-client interactions provide opportunities to express feelings, assess verbal and nonverbal responses, offer support and empathy, reduce feelings of helplessness, and promote an optimal level of health.

THE ADVANCED-PRACTICE PSYCHIATRIC REGISTERED NURSE

Clients experiencing various psychosocial reactions in medical-surgical settings may be seen by the PCLN. This advanced-practice psychiatric nurse identifies complex psychosocial responses of clients in medical-surgical settings. Major interventions include a complete psychosocial assessment, grief work, prescription of medications, crisis intervention, case management, and individual and family psychotherapy. In addition, the PCLN collaborates with the generalist nurse, the client and family, and the members of the health care team in inpatient, ambulatory, and community settings to mobilize the client's resources and promote an optimal level of functioning. See Chapter 35 for a discussion of the PCLN.

NURSING CARE PLAN 34–1

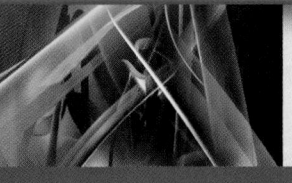

The Client Who Has Experienced a CVA (Mrs. Jaycee)

Nursing Diagnosis: Ineffective Coping
related to adaptation to alterations in physical function

Outcome Identification	Nursing Actions	Rationales	Evaluation
1. By [date], Mrs. Jaycee will adapt to and cope with limited physical function.	1a. Establish rapport with Mrs. Jaycee.	1a. Rapport conveys empathy and warmth.	*Goal met:* Therapeutic relationship with Mrs. Jaycee is established. Grief process is facilitated. Effective communication is established.
	1b. Assess Mrs. Jaycee's present/past coping behaviors.	1b–c. Strengths of previous coping patterns may be identified.	
	1c. Reorient Mrs. Jaycee as needed.		
	1d. Reassure Mrs. Jaycee that efforts will be made to help her communicate.	1d. Reassurance decreases anxiety and allows client to establish control over communication and care.	
	1e. Look directly at Mrs. Jaycee and use deliberate explanations and directions.	1e. Looking at the client conveys understanding and enhances communication.	

(continues)

Nursing Care Plan 34–1 (continued)

Outcome Identification	Nursing Actions	Rationales	Evaluation
	1f. Observe Mrs. Jaycee for signs of depression.	1f. Client is at risk for depression, grief reaction, and suicide risk.	

Nursing Diagnosis: Self-Care Deficit
related to cognitive impairment

Outcome Identification	Nursing Actions	Rationales	Evaluation
1. By [date], Mrs. Jaycee will participate in self-care activities.	1a. Assess Mrs. Jaycee's prestroke level of function (obtain this information from both Mrs. Jaycee and her family).	1a. Information about the client's baseline level of functioning is provided.	*Goal met:* Mrs. Jaycee and her family actively participate in her care. Family's initial attempts to do things for her that she was able to do for herself end after teaching begins. Mrs. Jaycee and her family are discharged to the rehabilitation program.
	1b. Encourage Mrs. Jaycee to participate in her daily care.	1b. Participation increases independence and restoration of function.	
	1c. Encourage Mrs. Jaycee's family to participate in her care.	1c. Family's sense of helplessness decreased, and grief process is facilitated.	
	1d. Teach Mrs. Jaycee's family about the mental status changes in her.	1d–f. Teaching facilitates rehabilitation process, promoting control and restoration of health to highest level.	
	1e. Adhere to discharge/rehabilitation treatment plan.		
	1f. Stress the importance of firmness, consistency, and support.		

THE NURSING PROCESS

The nursing process for the psychosocial care of clients in medical-surgical settings begins with assessment of the client's needs. Included in this section are the nursing diagnoses, outcome identification, implementation of nursing interventions, and evaluation of the client's response to treatment.

ASSESSMENT

Assessing the psychosocial needs begins with gathering data on the reason for seeking treatment, the nature and duration of symptoms, past and present medications, and substance use history. Inquiring how stress or similar events have been handled in the past assesses coping behaviors. This information helps the nurse develop an innovative plan of care to meet the client's present psychosocial needs.

Coping behaviors need to be assessed and strengthened throughout treatment. This includes identifying adaptive and maladaptive coping behaviors. Maladaptive coping responses include suicidal behaviors and substance misuse. It is imperative to inquire about present or past suicide attempts, circumstances, and treatment when assessing the client's coping behaviors. Furthermore, it is crucial to ask the client and family members about present and past substance abuse or dependence, because times of stress increase the likelihood of relapse or increased abuse of alcohol and other drugs.

NURSING DIAGNOSES

Major nursing diagnoses for clients experiencing psychosocial stressors include the following:

◆ Ineffective Coping
◆ Compromised or disabling Family Coping
◆ Self-care deficit, bathing, hygiene
◆ Low Self-Esteem
◆ Disturbed Body Image
◆ Anxiety

OUTCOME IDENTIFICATION/PLANNING

Clients in medical-surgical settings experience tremendous stress. Coping with physical illness challenges them to face a number of issues such as alterations in lifestyle, roles, and body image. Support systems are critical in helping them resolve crises generated by serious or life-threatening illnesses. Loss is a major concern for the client in the medical-surgical or rehabilitation setting. Nurses can facilitate the grief process by establishing therapeutic interactions that encourage expression of feelings and thoughts created by acute and chronic illnesses.

The following are the major client outcomes in medical-surgical settings:

1. Preservation of healthy physiological function
2. Reduction or cessation of the disease process
3. Resolution of the grief process
4. Strengthened adaptive coping behaviors
5. Maintenance of integrity, dignity, and quality of life
6. Participation in the treatment and rehabilitation process

IMPLEMENTATION

Different illnesses require different biological interventions. For example, the older adult client who experiences a CVA requires neurological monitoring, and the client with a spinal cord injury requires care for skin integrity.

Educating clients and families about the disease process, treatment modalities, and psychosocial responses is a major aspect of both the acute and rehabilitation phases. Support systems, community resources, and collaboration with nurses and other health care professionals are vital to the success of managing acute and chronic medication conditions.

The major nursing interventions for clients in medical-surgical settings and other institutions are as follows:

1. Establishment of rapport and therapeutic interactions with the client and family
2. Collaboration with the client, family, and interdisciplinary team to develop a comprehensive and holistic plan of care
3. Facilitation of the grief process
4. Reinforcement of the client's coping skills and mobilization of resources

EVALUATION

Evaluation of the client's responses to treatment is a continuous process that is based on observations of physical responses and verbal and nonverbal feedback from clients, families, and members of the treatment team.

RESEARCH IN MEDICAL-SURGICAL SETTINGS

The psychosocial needs of clients in the medical-surgical setting are immense, and there is a growing trend to measure the cost-effectiveness and quality of such nursing care. Evidence-based practice models must underlie nursing interventions. Nurses can address these demands by collaborating in research to explore the effectiveness of interventions that enhance coping behaviors, increase self-esteem, and promote comfort and healing. Medical-surgical clients tend to experience intense anxiety and depression. The severity of these symptoms can be measured by using standardized tools such as the Hamilton Anxiety and Depression Scales or Geriatric Depression Scale.

Medical research is ongoing related to the issues of stress, anxiety, depression, and the development of chronic illnesses as a result of mind-body interactions. Currently, there are researchers who are investigating the possibility that stress, anxiety, and depression actually precede the development of diabetes mellitus, particularly type 2. In individuals who have long-standing and chronic mental illness, it is not surprising that resultant disease occurs. Some estimates indicate that 40 percent of visits to gastroenterologists are related to the physical responses to depression.

Another area needing research includes the psychosocial responses to the diagnosis and treatment of breast cancer. Despite the trauma of this diagnosis, there is a lack of research in this area. With the issues discussed earlier related to stress and immune function (see Chapter 22, Sleep Disorders), it would benefit the woman with breast cancer to have decreased stress levels in order to have better immune function.

Nursing interventions can reduce symptoms and behaviors generated by acute and chronic medical conditions. Posttreatment scores and client feedback and responses can determine outcomes. The generalist nurse and the advanced-practice psychiatric nurse can develop a research project.

SUMMARY

◆ Medical-surgical conditions affect clients and families throughout the life span, and the individual responses to them are complex.

◆ Coping behaviors are taxed and compromised during illness and must be assessed on an ongoing basis so that support systems may be mobilized to reinforce them when needed.

◆ Often during acute or crisis events, the client has to depend on the nurse for survival. This process lays the foundation of therapeutic interactions that foster dependence and, later, independence.

◆ The client's psychological needs are immense and vary with developmental stage, the nature of the illness, personality traits, and coping skills.

◆ Assessing their special needs and collaborating with other team members to help clients meet them and attain their highest level of functioning maximize clients' resources.

◆ Clients in medical-surgical settings have tremendous psychosocial and biological needs.

- ◆ The discussion of physical conditions emphasizes the complexity of adaptation and the significance of the therapeutic process in mobilizing resources to promote clients' health and restore them to an optimal level of functioning.

- ◆ Self-awareness of the nurse's perceptions and experiences with death and dying promote a greater understanding of the client's experience.

SUGGESTIONS FOR CLINICAL CONFERENCES

1. Present the case histories of several clients with chronic and acute medical conditions and identify these clients' psychosocial and biological needs.

2. Present nursing care plans for angry, demanding, depressed, and dying clients

3. Role-play demanding, angry, and depressed clients.

STUDY QUESTIONS

1. Mrs. Lewis is admitted with a diagnosis of acute back strain. She is very demanding and frequently turns on the call light. The nurses expressed frustration and anger because the client criticizes them for taking too long to medicate her. What is the *best* approach to this client when she calls for pain medication?
   a. Take her the medication as soon as she can have a p.r.n.
   b. Set limits with her and explain the inappropriateness of her behavior.
   c. Explore her feelings about this hospitalization.
   d. Encourage her to talk about reasons for asking for pain medication.

2. Clients in medical-surgical settings are often overwhelmed by their illness. Which of the following indicates *ineffective coping* behaviors?
   a. The client is talkative and willing to participate in treatment.
   b. The client elicits assistance from family members in daily care.
   c. The client asks the nurse to assist in routine care.
   d. The client expresses anger because the call light was not answered.

3. Childhood responses to medical illnesses are influenced by all of the following *except:*
   a. developmental stage
   b. separation from parents
   c. nature of illness
   d. change in role

4. Adolescents with medical illnesses experience immense stress during hospitalization. Which is the best example of psychosocial stress for the medically ill adolescent?
   a. Fears of rejection by peers
   b. Loss of health

   c. Separation from parents
   d. Fears of academic failure

5. Clients who have had a stroke tend to become depressed. What is the best example of a depressed client who has suffered a stroke?
   a. Refuses to eat, isolates self, and is argumentative
   b. Demanding and critical of staff
   c. Argues with spouse and uncooperative with staff
   d. Frequently asks for assistance in managing daily care

6. The condition of a client diagnosed with chronic obstructive pulmonary disease (COPD) and cor pulmonale is deteriorating. The client is very hypoxemic, obtunded, and easily fatigued by any activity. The nurse who has been working with this client throughout this hospitalization is repositioning the client. Which of the following remarks made by the client indicates that the client has come to terms with death?
   a. "It is finally spring and that is my favorite time of the year."
   b. "Am I going to die?"
   c. "I'm very tired, but content and ready to go."
   d. "I'm feeling stronger by the moment."

7. A family member whose mother is terminally ill asks to speak to the nurse. Which of the following statements made by this child should indicate to the nurse that this family member understands the emotional response to death and dying?
   a. "Mother seems very comfortable; so we're able to recall some of our good times spent together."
   b. "My mother is irate because she says you all told her she had to have an advanced directive."
   c. "My mother is talking about redoing her bedroom when she's discharged. Doesn't she know she's dying?"
   d. "My mother is crying so much these days. Where's all this sadness coming from?"

8. The nurse is changing the dressing on a client who has had a modified radical mastectomy 2 days ago. The client refused to look in the direction of the nurse or the operative site. The nurse notices a tear running down the client's cheek. Which of the following responses would most appropriately facilitate the client's grief resolution?
   a. "You look very sad, it might help you feel better if you let yourself cry."
   b. "Tell me what the worst part of losing your breast is."
   c. "Everything is going to be all right; you can be fitted for a new bra and no one will notice."
   d. "Are you crying because you are concerned about how your partner will respond?"

RESOURCES

Please note that because Internet resources are of a time-sensitive nature and URL addresses may change or be deleted, searches should also be conducted by association or topic.

Internet Resources

http://www.cancer.org   American Cancer Society

Other Resources

The Knowledge Exchange Network (KEN)
    KEN Links-Children
    PO Box 42490
    Washington, DC 20015
    (800) 789-CMHS
    http://www.mentalhealth.org/links/children.htm

Depression and Related Affective Disorders (DRADA)
    Meyer 3-181
    600 North Wolfe St.
    Baltimore, MD 21287-7381
    (410) 955-4647
    http://www.drada.org

REFERENCES

Alkadhi, K., & Alzoubi, K. (2007). Role of long-term potentiation of sympathetic ganglia (gLTP) in hypertension. *Clinical and Experimental Hypertension, 29,* 267–286.

American Psychiatric Association. (2000). *Diagnostic and statistical manual of mental disorders* (4th edition, Text Revision) *(DSM-IV-TR)*. Washington, DC: Author.

Antai-Otong, D. (1988). When your patient is angry. *Nursing , 18,* 44–45. Springhouse, PA: Springhouse.

Antai-Otong, D. (2004a). *Psychiatric emergencies: How to accurately assess and manage the patient in crisis.* Eau Claire, WI: Professional Educational Systems Inc.

Antai-Otong, D. (2004b). Poststroke depression: Psychopharmacological considerations. *Perspectives in Psychiatric Care, 40,* 167–170.

Antai-Otong, D. (2007). *Nurse-client communication: A life-span approach.* Sudbury, MA: Jones and Bartlett Publishers.

Barker-Collo, S. L. (2007). Depression and anxiety 3 months post stroke: Prevalence and correlates. *Archives of Clinical Neuropsychology, 22,* 519–531.

Beck, A. T., Brown, G., Berchick, R. J., Stewart, B. L., & Steer, R. A. (1990). Relationship between hopelessness and ultimate suicide: A replication with psychiatric outpatients. *American Journal of Psychiatry, 147,* 190–195.

Boman, L., Andersson, K., & Bjordis, H. (1997). Needs as expressed by women after breast cancer surgery in the setting of a short hospital stay. *Scandinavian Journal of Caring Science, 11,* 25–32.

Carter, P. S. (2005). Bereaved caregivers' descriptions of sleep: Impact on daily life and the bereavement process. *Oncology Nursing Forum, 32,* E70–E75.

Chantler, M., Podbilewicz-Schuller, Y., & Mortimer, J. (2006). Change in need for psychosocial support for women with early stage breast cancer. *Journal of Psychosocial Oncology, 23,* 65–77.

Citrome, L., & Yeomans, D. (2005). Do guidelines for severe mental illness promote physical health and well-being? *Journal of Psychopharmacology, 19* (6 suppl.) 102–109.

Colyer, H. (1996). Women's perception of living with cancer. *Journal of Advanced Nursing, 23,* 496–501.

Das, S., & O'Keefe, J. H. (2006) . Behavioral cardiology: Recognizing and addressing the profound impact of psychosocial stress on cardiovascular health. *Current Atherosclerosis Reports, 8,* 111–118.

Garavalia, L. S., Decker, C., Reid, K. J., Lichtman, J. H., Parashar, S., Vaccarino, V., et al. (2007). Does health status differ between men and women in early recovery after myocardial infarction? *Journal of Women's Health, 16,* 93–101.

Goodkin, K., Vitiello, B., Lyman, W. D., Asthana, D., Atkinson, J. H., & Heseltine, P. N. (2006). Cerebrospinal and peripheral human immunodeficiency virus type 1 load in a multisite, randomized, double-blind, placebo-controlled trial of D-Ala1-peptide T-amide for HIV-1-associated cognitive-motor impairment. *Journal of Neurovirology, 12,* 178–189.

Houtzager, B. A., Grootenhuis, M. A., Caron, H. N., & Last, B. F. (2005). Sibling self-report, parental proxies, and quality of life: The importance of multiple informants for siblings of a critically ill child. *Pediatric Hematology Oncology, 22,* 25–40.

Howard, A. F., Balneaves, L. G., & Bottorff, J. L. (2007). Ethnocultural women's experiences of breast cancer: A qualitative meta-study. *Cancer Nursing, 30,* E27–E35.

Kopnisky, K. L., Bao, J., & Lin, Y. W. (2007). Neurobiology of HIV, psychiatric and substance abuse comorbidity research: Workshop report. *Brain, Behavior & Immunity, 21,* 428–441.

Kubler-Ross, E. (1969). *On death and dying.* New York: MacMillan.

Lahlou-Laforet, K., Alhenc-Gelas, M., Pornin, M., Bydlowski, S., Seigneur, E., Benetos, A., Kierzin, J. M., Scarabin, P. Y., et al. (2006). Relation of depressive mood to plasminogen activator inhibitor, tissue plasminogen activator, and fibrinogen levels in patients with versus without coronary heart disease. *American Journal of Cardiology, 97,* 1287–1291.

McCaffrey, C. N. (2006). Major stressors and their effects on the well-being of children with cancer. *Journal of Pediatric Nursing, 21,* 59–66.

Mello, V. A., & Malbergier, A. (2006). Depression in women infected with HIV. *Revista Brasileira de Psiquiatria, 28,* 10–17.

Moore, D. J., Masliah, E., Rippeth, J. D., Gonzalez, R., Carey, C. L., Cherner, M., et al. (2006). Cortical and subcortical neurodegeneration is associated with HIV neurocognitive impairment. *AIDS, 20,* 879–887.

Narayanasamy, A. (2006). The impact of empirical studies of spirituality and culture on nurse education. *Journal of Clinical Nursing, 15,* 840–851.

National Cancer Institute. SEER Cancer Statistics Review, 1975–2002. (2006). Available at: http://seer.cancer.gov/csr/1975_2002/sections.html. (Acessed April 30, 2006).

Packman, W., Greenhalgh, J., Chesterman, B., Shaffer, T., Fine, J., Van Zutphen, K., Golan, R., & Amylon, M. D. (2005). Siblings of pediatric cancer patients: The quantitative and qualitative nature of quality of life. *Journal of Psychosocial Oncology, 23,* 87–108.

Pence, B. W., Miller, W. C., Whetten, K., Eron, J. J., & Gaynes, B. N. (2006). Prevalence of DSM-IV-Defined mood, anxiety, and substance use disorders in an HIV clinic in the Southeastern United States. *Journal of Acquired Immune Deficiency Syndrome, 42,* 298–306.

Penson, R. T., Partridge, R. A., Shah, M. A., Goansiracusa, D., Chabner, B. A., & Lynch, T. J., Jr. (2005). Fear of death. *Oncologist, 10,* 160–169.

Postovsky, S., & Ben Arush, M. W. (2004). Care of a child dying of cancer: The role of the palliative care team in pediatric oncology. *Pediatric Hematology Oncology, 21,* 67–76.

Power, J. (2006). Spiritual assessment: Developing an assessment tool. *Nursing Older People, 18,* 16–18.

Roth, R. S., Lowery, J. C., Davis, J., & Wilkins, E. G. (2005). Quality of life and affective distress in women seeking immediate versus delayed breast reconstruction after mastectomy for breast cancer. *Plastic and Reconstruction Surgery, 116,* 993–1002.

Schiff, J. W., & Moore, K. (2006). The impact of the sweat lodge ceremony on dimensions of well-being. *American Indian and Alaskan Native Mental Health Research, 13,* 48–69.

Schor, E. L., & American Academy of Pediatrics Task Force on the Family. (2003). Family pediatrics: Report of the Task Force on the Family. *Pediatrics, 111,* 1541–1571.

Shelton, T., Jepperson, E., & Johnson, B. (1987). *Family-centered care for children with special health care needs* (pp. 34–49). Washington, DC: Association for the Care of Children Health.

Tariot, P. N. (1999). Treatment of agitation in dementia. *Journal of Clinical Psychiatry, 60*(Suppl. 8), 11–20.

Thomas, S. A., & Lincoln, N. B. (2006). Factors relating to depression after stroke. *British Journal of Clinical Psychology, 45,* Part 1, 46–61.

Udall, K. K., Ryan, R., Berghus, J. P., & Harris, V. L. (2000). Association between delirium and death in AIDS patients. *AIDs Patient Care STDS, 14*(2), 95–100.

Underwood, S. M., & Powell, J. (2006). Religion and spirituality: Influence on health/risk behavior and cancer screening behavior of African Americans. *Association of Black Nursing Faculty Journal, 17,* 20–31.

Unruh, A. M. (2007). Spirituality, religion, and pain. *Canadian Journal of Nursing Research, 39,* 66–86.

Vataja, R., Leppavuori, A., Pohjasvaara, T., Mantyla, R., Aronen, H. J., Salonen, O., Kaste, M., & Erkinjuntti, T. (2004). Poststroke depression and lesion location revisited. *The Journal of Neuropsychiatry and Clinical Neurosciences, 16,* 156–162.

Watson, M. (2000). What to do when a depressed or anxious cancer patient refuses further treatment. *Primary Care and Cancer, 20,* 19–24.

Wilding, C., Muir-Cochrane, E., & May, E. (2006). Treading lightly: Spirituality issues in mental health nursing. *International Journal of Mental Health Nursing, 15,* 144–152.

Working Group of the American Academy of Neurology AIDS Task Force. (1991). Nomenclature and research case definitions for neurologic manifestations of human immunodeficiency virus-type 1 (HIV-1) infection. *Neurology, 41,* 778-785.

York, K. M., Hassan, M., Li, Q., Li, H., Fillingim, R. B., & Sheps, D. S. (2007). Coronary artery disease and depression: Patients with more depressive symptoms have lower cardiovascular reactivity during laboratory-induced mental stress. *Psychosomatic Medicine, 69,* 521–528.

SUGGESTED READINGS

Brown, L. K., Lescano, C. M., & Lourie, K. J. (2001). Children and adolescents with HIV infection. *Psychiatric Annals, 31,* 63–68.

Centers for Disease Control and Prevention. (2000). U.S. HIV AIDS cases reported through June 2000. *HIV/AIDS Surveillance Report, 12.*

Gendelman, H., Lipton, S., Epstein, L., & Swindels, S. (Eds.). (1998). *Neurological and neuropsychiatric manifestations of HIV-1 infection.* Philadelphia: Chapman & Hall.

Meador, K. G., & Koenig, H. G. (2000). Spirituality and religion in psychiatric practice: Parameters and implications. *Psychiatric Annals, 30,* 549–555.

UNIT 4

Advancing Psychiatric Nursing Practice

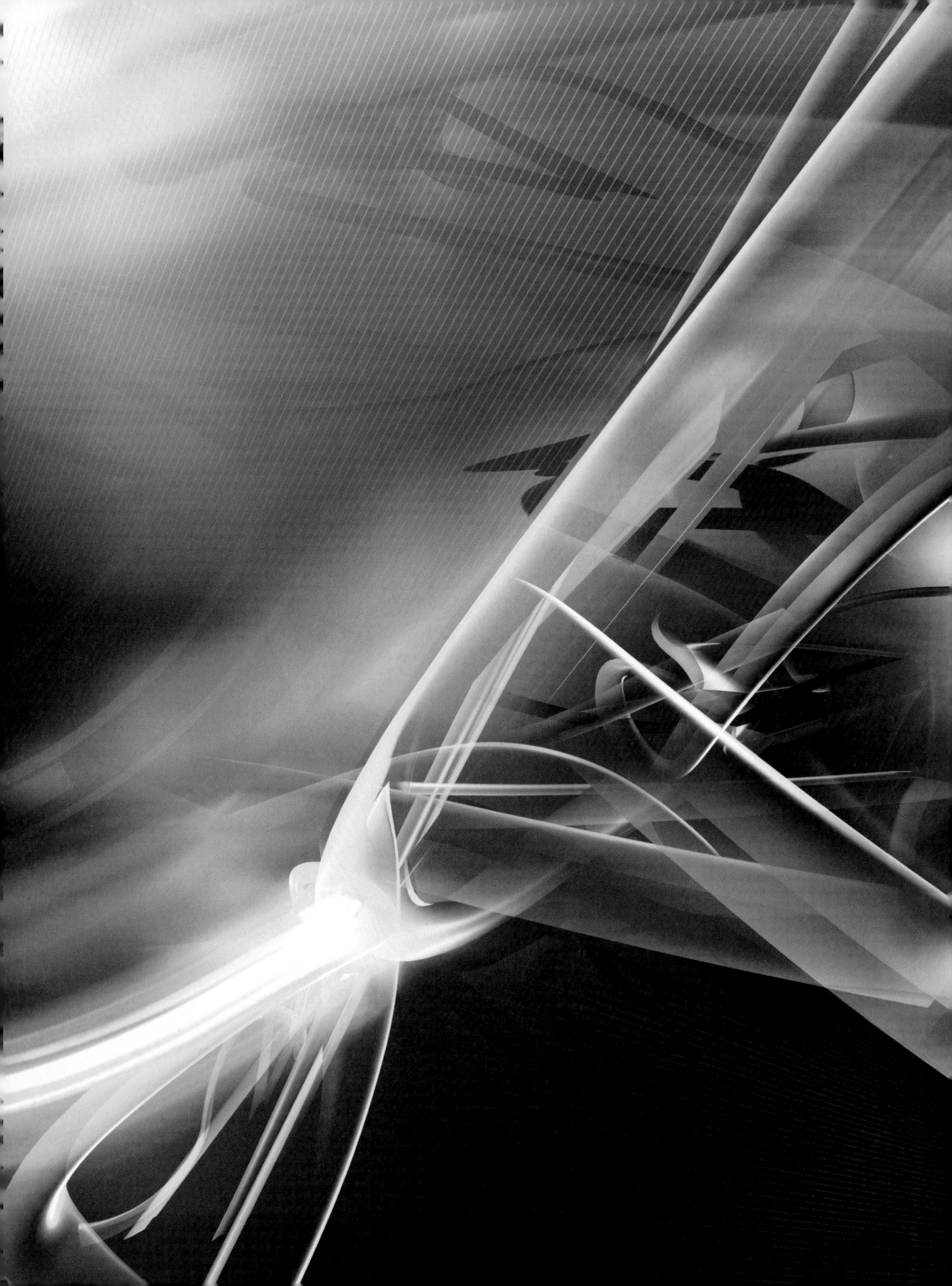

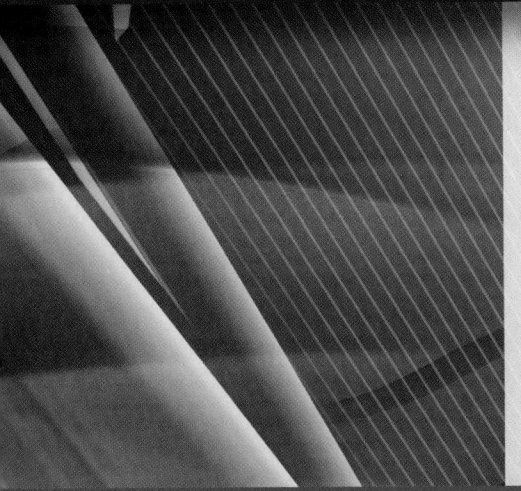

CHAPTER 35

Psychiatric Consultation-Liaison Nursing

Susan L. W. Krupnick, MSN, CARN, ANP, CS
Deborah Antai-Otong, MS, APRN, BC, FAAN

KEY TERMS

Consultation: Rendering of an expert opinion in response to a request.

Entrepreneur: An individual who organizes, manages, and risks assumption of a business venture or enterprise.

Intrapreneur: An individual who expands the traditional role as direct health care provider to that of creator of quality of care products and services within an institution or organization.

Liaison: The facilitation of the relationships between the client, the client's illness, the consultee, the health care team, and the environment.

Telemental health: The use of electronic technology like videoconferencing, telephone, secure messaging (e-mail), and the Internet to provide mental health care and consultation liaison services.

COMPETENCIES

Upon completion of this chapter, the learner should be able to:

1. Describe the historical development of psychiatric consultation-liaison nurse (PCLN) practice.

2. Analyze the traditional practice of PCLN within the health care delivery system.

3. Identify the expanding roles and functions of the PCLN within the changing health care delivery system.

4. Describe the goals of PCLN practice.

5. Analyze the steps in the consultation process.

6. Differentiate between direct and indirect models of consultation.

7. Describe the types of consultation in PCLN practice.

8. Discuss the educational preparation, professional experience, and clinical supervision necessary for PCLN practice.

9. Delineate future trends and opportunities for PCLN practice.

CHAPTER OUTLINE

History of PCLN Practice

Philosophy of PCLN Clinical Practice

Preparation for PCLN Practice

Education and Certification

The PCLN in the Health Care Delivery System

Evolution of Practice Models

Organizational Placement of the PCLN

Telemental Health PCLN Services

The Consultation Process

Entry: Request for Consultation

Diagnosis: Determining the Need for and Purpose of the Consultation

P sychiatric consultation-liaison nurse (PCLN) practice is a subspecialty of advanced-practice within the specialty of psychiatric-mental health nursing. The scope of PCLN practice is diverse and encompasses primary prevention, intervention, and rehabilitation strategies (American Nurses Association [ANA], 1990, 2000; Kurlowicz, 1998). This subspecialty emphasizes assessment, diagnosis, and treatment of behavioral, cognitive, developmental, emotional, and spiritual responses of clients and families with actual and potential physical dysfunction. PCLN practice, by definition, includes consultation and liaison activities.

Consultation is an interactive process between a consultant, who has expertise, and a consultee, who is seeking advice. It is an interpersonal educational process in which the consultant collaborates with a person or a group that influences and participates in health care delivery and has requested assistance in problem solving (Norwood, 1998). The recipient of PCLN services may be the client, family members, or health care providers. The term liaison is used to describe the linkage of health care professionals to facilitate communication, collaboration, and building of partnerships between clients and themselves (Hackett, Cassem, Stern, & Murray, 1997; Robinson, 1987). The liaison process is commonly used to explicate the teaching, or educative, component of the PCLN practice. The goals of consultation and liaison activities are mutually complementary and interdependent. The PCLN uses both processes in conjunction with specific theoretical knowledge, clinical expertise, and an ability to synthesize and integrate information to influence health care delivery systems and treatment outcomes.

HISTORY OF PCLN PRACTICE

Several significant forces have provided the impetus for the development of PCLN practice. These forces are multifaceted and include the general development of psychiatric-mental health nursing, the establishment and funding of psychiatric departments in university hospitals, and World War II, which ushered in the crisis intervention and brief psychotherapy models of treatment to address war-related mental health problems (see Table 35–1). The development, introduction, and expansion of psychopharmacology and the use of psychotropic medications in the 1950s and 1960s

increased the scope and impact of consultation-liaison services in the general hospital. The foundation was established, and PCLN practice emerged as a subspecialty of psychiatric nursing during the 1960s. During this period the nursing literature began to focus on the psychosocial assessment and management of the client with medical illness to advance therapeutic progress and positive outcomes (Dumas & Leonard, 1963; Elder, 1963; Johnson, 1963). However, Betty Sue Johnson of Duke University Medical Center was the first clinical nurse specialist (CNS) to describe her role as a psychiatric nurse providing consultation services to nurses in the general hospital. In an article published in 1963, Johnson described the concept of cross-service consultation and the implementation of a nurse-to-nurse consultation model. The goal was to promote a higher level of client care in conjunction with maximizing the use of available resources. The clinical consultant pool of nurses at Duke comprised head nurses, nursing supervisors, and instructors. Initially, they responded to requests from head nurses on medical-surgical units. The early PCLN work accomplished by these nursing pioneers focused on assessing and supporting the positive interpersonal relationship skills employed by the staff members and building on them with subsequent consultations. The medical-surgical unit staff members understood that the PCLN would not assume responsibility for the client care problem but would assist and support them in problem solving and comprehending the emotional impact of illness, suffering, and recovery of the client (Johnson, 1963).

The evolution of PCLN practice continued, and employing consultee-centered consultation was challenging the method of indirect intervention. The next stage of PCLN practice evolution involved acknowledging the need for an advanced practitioner to have direct involvement with the client. Comprehensive assessment of the client's psychological and behavioral responses required active, direct intervention by the PCLN using a client-centered consultation. This shift in the delivery of consultation services allowed PCLNs an opportunity to use their clinical expertise in direct assessment while collaborating with nursing staff members to formulate a holistic and relevant nursing care plan. In addition, with the expansion of consultation service into direct care, the complexity and intensity of client care was illuminated. In response to this increasing awareness and complexity, the PCLNs acknowledged their need to acquire additional theoretical

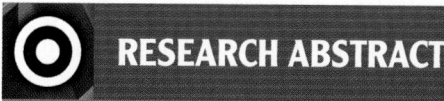

RESEARCH ABSTRACT

Rural versus Suburban Primary Care Needs, Utilization, and Satisfaction with Telepsychiatry Consultation

Hilty, D. M., Nesbitt, T. S., Kuenneth, C. A., Cruz, G. M., & Hales, R. E. (2007). *Journal of Rural Health, 23,* 163–165.

Study Problem/Purpose

The researchers examined rural and suburban primary care needs, utilization, and clinician satisfaction using telepsychiatry consultation.

Methods

Researchers used client demographics, reasons for consultation, diagnosis, and alternatives to telepsychiatric consultations of clients living in rural and suburban areas. Researchers collected 200 consecutive, first-time telepsychiatric consultations in these areas.

Findings

Primary findings from this study demonstrated higher satisfaction among clients living in rural settings than those living in suburban areas. Clients from rural or remote areas were more likely to be younger than age 18 years, use Medicaid, and require treatment planning compared with their suburban counterparts.

Implications for Psychiatric Nursing

Psychiatric consultation-liaison nursing (PCLN) is an important part of psychiatric-mental health nursing. Major implications from this study include the use of PCLN in telemental health to increase access consultation of clients living in rural and suburban areas. This cost-effective consultation process also implicates the unique opportunity PCLNs have to provide care along the health care continuum.

knowledge and clinical expertise in the realm of the consultation process and the psychophysiological approach to the care of clients in medical-surgical settings.

Enormous changes continue to impact the role of PCLN in inpatient, primary care, and communities and rural areas. This is particularly evident with the explosion of technology that has advanced telemental health. Telemental health or telepsychiatry may be used to replace face-to-face consultation with nurses and other providers, particularly those working in remote or rural practice settings. With the cost of health care and importance of advancing mental health services, access to psychiatric consultation liaison nursing provides an ideal opportunity to work with nurses and other health care personnel using vast technologies, such as secure messaging, videoconferencing, and the Internet (Hilty et al., 2006). A recent study conducted by Sharrock and colleagues (2006) demonstrated the usefulness of psychiatric liaison consultation to nonpsychiatric nurses seeking expertise in caring for clients with co-occurring medical and psychiatric conditions. This approach has helped nonpsychiatric nurses explore and develop direct client-centered interventions (Sharrock, Grigg, Happell, Keeble-Devlin, & Jennings, 2006).

PHILOSOPHY OF PCLN CLINICAL PRACTICE

The subspecialization of PCLN practice within psychiatric nursing is based on the synthesis, integration, and application of several theoretical models in nursing, psychiatry, psychology, and sociology. Specific models that are the foundations of PCLN practice include the consultation process, crisis intervention, systems theory, organizational behavior and dynamics, change and influence theory, problem-solving theory, cultural diversity and sensitivity, psychoneuroimmunology, and adult learning theory. The interrelationship of medical illness and its psychophysiological effects on hospitalized clients and their families is extremely intricate and requires sophisticated, multidimensional assessment and intervention by advanced-practice nurses. PCLNs become involved in these complex client care situations to perform comprehensive assessments, provide therapeutic interventions, collaborate with the client and family members, and strengthen the clinical skills of the primary care provider. PCLNs offer an array of services to clients and their support systems to reduce the incidence of distress, coping failure, and maladaptation in response to potential or actual physiologic dysfunction.

PREPARATION FOR PCLN PRACTICE

The PCLN is an advanced-practice nurse who has attained at least a master's degree in psychiatric-mental health nursing and has successfully completed a supervised graduate-level clinical program (ANA, 2000). Clinical knowledge and expertise in medical-surgical and critical care nursing enhance the PCLN's credibility as a role model and the ability to assess and understand the complexity of acutely ill clients. Administrative experience in a middle-management position, such as head nurse or nurse manager, assists the PCLN in comprehending the influence of health care organizations on clients and their families. In addition, management experience and administrative preparation can expand

TABLE 35–1
Psychiatric Consultation-Liaison Nurse (PCLN) Specialty Evolution: A Chronological Overview

Year	Event
1960s	Beginning emergence of the psychiatric nursing consultation process
1963	Publication of an article by Betty Sue Johnson of Duke University discussing cross-service nursing consultation with psychiatric nurses
1970s	First publication of PCLN research
1971	Initiation of the University of Maryland graduate program in PCLN practice
1973	Initiation of the Yale University graduate program in PCLN practice
1974	Publication of the first PCLN text, *Liaison Nursing: Psychological Approach to Patient Care*, by Dr. Lisa Robinson of the University of Maryland
1980s	A decade of practice expansion and innovation
1982	Publication of *Psychiatric Liaison Nursing: The Theory and Clinical Practice* by Anita Lewis and Joyce Levy
1987	Development of the initial proposal of standards of PCLN practice by PCLN regional task forces
1990s	Transitions and formal organizational structuring
1990	Formation of PCLNs as a special interest group within the Psychiatric-Mental Health Council of the American Nurses Association
1990	Publication of PCLN standards by the American Nurses Association
1992–1993	Organization of a national task force to develop a core curriculum for PCLN education
1993	Election of a governing board of the PCLN special interest group
1993	Celebration of 30 years of PCLN practice at the Annual National PCLN Conference and honoring PCLNs with excellence awards
1994	Formal beginning of the International Society of Psychiatric Consultation-Liaison Nurses on March 25, 1994, in Baltimore
1999	The organization merged with the Society for Education and Research in Psychiatric-Mental Health Nursing and Association of Child and Adolescent Psychiatric Nurses to form the International Society of Psychiatric-Mental Health Nurses
2000	Innovative uses for PCLN continue to emerge and include telemental and emental health consultation with clients, families, primary care providers, and specialty clinic providers living in remote or rural areas to improve access to mental health care.

the PCLN's knowledge of politics and the operations of health care organizations (Norwood, 1998). Management preparation can assist the PCLN in gaining the expertise necessary to participate in evaluating conditions, resources, and politics crucial to the effective management of nursing care.

The personal and professional attributes that are the cornerstone of successful PCLNs include an ability to be flexible, objective, innovative, and resilient and to interact with others in a mature and professional manner. PCLNs must acknowledge and manage intense levels of uncertainty and ambiguity while balancing their own emotional and physical sense of well-being. PCLNs need to possess an ability to practice independently and autonomously while establishing coalitions within their organizations. In addition, they must be able to network within and outside their organization to minimize their sense of isolation, which can accompany autonomous practice situations in which the practitioner is privileged to sensitive and confidential information. PCLNs must engage in self-exploration and sharing of feelings to alleviate the daily effects of vicarious traumatization or overwhelming emotional situations.

EDUCATION AND CERTIFICATION

Formal graduate education and preparation of PCLNs began in the 1960s at the University of Maryland under the direction of Dr. Lisa Robinson (1972) and at Yale University under the leadership of Jill K. Nelson and Diane Schilke Davis (1979) (see Table 35–1). In preparation for moving into the mid-1990s and the twenty-first century, PCLN graduate education began to be addressed by a national PCLN core curriculum task force. The purpose of the task force was to develop a comprehensive core curriculum to adequately prepare PCLNs to meet the challenges of health care.

Certification by the ANA in the subspecialty of PCLN practice does not exist during this period; however, certification as a CNS in psychiatric-mental health nursing is recommended as a prerequisite for PCLN practice and is necessary for third-party reimbursement (ANA, 1990). Professional certification combined with graduate nursing education may be used as qualification for a second licensure as an advanced-practice nurse (Minarik, 1992). PCLNs function in advanced-practice roles and therefore must constantly address their educational and learning needs in psychopharmacologic intervention. Presently, many advanced-practice nurses have prescriptive privileges and practice in accordance with state and federal laws and regulations.

THE PCLN IN THE HEALTH CARE DELIVERY SYSTEM

The evolution of the PCLN practice and placement of PCLNs within an organization are discussed in the following two sections.

EVOLUTION OF PRACTICE MODELS

The PCLN practice literature in the 1960s described how the early pioneers implemented the nurse-to-nurse consultation model in their practice (Johnson, 1963; Robinson, 1968) and became direct care providers of psychiatric services in general hospitals (Peterson, 1969). During this era, there was an increase in the number of publications that described diversity in the method of clinical practice from an autonomous position to a collaborative model between PCLNs and PCL physicians (Holstein & Schwab, 1965; Jackson, 1969). Several authors began to identify significant research in addressing the psychological needs of hospitalized clients (Dumas & Leonard, 1963; Elder, 1963; Elder & Diers, 1963; Peplau, 1964).

The 1970s ushered in a decade of proliferate role expansion (Table 35–2). The literature depicted this expansion into direct-care nurse consultation in general hospitals as well as emergency services and nursing homes (Faast & Elstun, 1979; Forhan-Andrianos, & Swain, 1979; Goldstein, 1979; Hedlund, 1978; Przepiorka & Bender, 1977). Some of the authors described collaborative practices in which the PCLN triaged clients in the emergency department before the PCL physician evaluated them. This groundbreaking practice portrayed a collaborative model among the client, nurse, and physician (Issacharoff, Goddahn, Schneider, Maysonett, & Smith, 1970; Robinson, 1974). Barton and Kelso (1971) also described how the nursing perspective enhanced the functioning of a collaborative PCL team.

Additional articles published in the 1970s described specific practice sites (e.g., the intensive care unit) or client populations (e.g., those with coronary disease or burns) for PCLN involvement (Baldwin, 1978; Davidson & Noyes, 1973; Pranulis, 1972). Several authors described their strug-

gles and successes with establishing these positions and implementing the PCLN practice. Studying the referral process came to the forefront and was beginning to be addressed in the literature (Nelson & Davis, 1980). A change in clinical practice was emerging as client-family situations became more complex. There was an increased level of sophistication needed by the PCLN to master these more complex and challenging consultations with somewhat diminishing resources.

This evolutionary process continued at a rapid rate during the 1980s with publication of more PCLN literature detailing specific roles, functions, and outcome evaluation of PCLN services. Advances in technology, diagnosis-related groups, and nursing shortages during the 1980s provided significant opportunities for the PCLN to be actively involved in developing strategies and programs to manage several sensitive clinical, organizational, and ethical situations that influenced the delivery of care (Alexander, 1985; Barbiasz et al., 1982; Fife, 1986; Fife & Lemler, 1983; Samter, Scherer, & Shulman, 1981). The PCLN is clearly a knowledgeable member of the interdisciplinary team in assessing the daily realities of a hospital or organization. The complex and sometimes provocative clinical issues that several PCLN authors described in the 1980s have led to the tumultuous health care environments of the 1990s. These include, but are not limited to, unexpected surgical incidents, addiction issues in clients in general hospitals, cultural assessments and the impact on care, acquired immunodeficiency syndrome (AIDS), and keeping aging clients in their homes (Campinha-Bacote, 1988; D'Affiliti, 2005; Fincannon, 1988; Grant, 1988; Sharrock & Happell, 2002; Wand, 2004).

Clients across the life span can benefit from psychiatric-liaison consultation. This is evident in both children and older adults. More and more nurses work with seriously ill

---

TABLE 35–2
Roles of PCLNs: Specialties and Subspecialties of Current Practitioners

Psychiatric and General Consultation

Acute confusional states	Cognitive therapy	Dissociative disorder
Addictive diseases	Combat stress counseling	Dysfunctional family systems
Adolescence/adolescent mental health	Community mental health nursing	Eating disorders
Adult children of alcoholics	Couples counseling	Ethics
Adult victims of domestic violence	Crisis intervention	Families in crisis
Alzheimer's caregivers	Cultural diversity	Generalized anxiety disorder
Alzheimer's disease	Death and dying	Geropsychiatry/aging
Behavioral medicine (mind–body)	Dementia diagnosis and family training	Homeless and unemployed
Bereavement/grief and loss counseling	Depression	Hospice/palliative care
Child and adolescent bereavement	Detoxification	Hypnosis/relaxation/imagery
Codependency	Developmentally impaired	Incest survivors and abuse

(continues)

TABLE 35–2
Roles of PCLNs: Specialties and Subspecialties of Current Practitioners *(continued)*

Psychiatric and General Consultation *(Continued)*

Marriage and family counseling

Milieu therapy

Minority mental health

Mood disorders

Multigenerational family therapy

Nephrology

Nonviolent crisis intervention

Panic disorders

Parent–family dynamics

Pediatrics

Perinatal bereavement

Phobias

Postpartum depression

Post-traumatic stress disorder

Pregnancy loss

Premenstrual syndrome (PMS) counseling

Psychiatric triage and emergency care

Psychoeducation for family members with a chronic mental illness

Psychological trauma

Psychopharmacology—monitoring mental status, medication management

Relationship and marital therapy

School health

Self-actualization

Sex therapy

Sexual abuse

Stepfamilies

Stress management

Suicide

Therapeutic touch

Time-limited psychotherapy

Transsexualism

Trauma/abuse

Trauma psychology (individuals and organizations)

Traumatic death

Women's health

Medical–Surgical Consultation

Advanced and terminal phase of illness counseling

Aggressive/difficult patients (inpatient management)

AIDS patients

Biofeedback

Cardiac comorbidity

Cardiology

Clients with automatic implantable cardioverter defibrillators

Clients with pituitary tumors

Coping with illness and hospitalization

Critical care

Cross-cultural nursing

Diabetes

Emotional response to physical illness

Nurses' support group for transplantation

Oncology

Oncology: hospice

Orthopedics

Pain management

Pain management in substance abusers

Psychoneuroimmunology

Pulmonary disease

Rehabilitation

Relaxation and guided imagery in hospitalized clients

Renal failure

Spinal cord injury

Spouses of clients in intensive care units

Support group for HIV and AIDS populations

Transplantation (cardiac, liver, bone marrow, other)

Trauma

Trauma: critical incident stress debriefing

Treatment planning

Administrative/Employee-Related Consultation

Administration

Assertiveness training

Career development

Circadian disorders in shift workers

Clinical ladder development

Communication skills development

Conflict management

Continuing education program development

Continuous quality improvement

Critical incident stress debriefing

Customer service in health care settings

Employee advocacy

Employee assistance

Health care ethics

Image enhancement

Inservice education

Management consultation

Management/counseling for chemically dependent nurses

Memorial service

Nurse's resiliency building

Nursing education/staff development

Organizational change process

Organizational communication

Organizational development

Peer assistance

Recruitment and retention

Research support

Retreat and workshop development

Staff stress management

Staff support groups

Team building

Total quality management

Work-related stress

Worker's compensation

Note. Data from *International Directory of Psychiatric Consultation-Liaison Nurses, 1993–1994* (2nd ed.), by S. Krupnick.

children in inpatient, primary pediatric care, and pediatrician's offices. PCLN nurses provide an invaluable service to nurses, other clinicians, children, and their families. Researchers submit studies that psychiatric-consultation liaison nursing is invaluable in supporting nonpsychiatric nurses, improving access to mental health services, and enhancing quality and cost-effective care (Canam, 2005). Despite the benefits of PCLN in caring for children and adolescents there remains a growing gap in addressing the needs of many children with co-occurring physical problems and psychosocial needs (Watson, 2006).

Robinson (1987) illuminated the similarities and differences in medical and nursing PCL practice. PCLNs and PCL physicians share many theoretical beliefs and practices. This intersection of practice can foster a duplication of services as well as produce gaps in practice. The demands of cost reduction facing administrators and clinicians in health care organizations during the 1990s led to an examination of all client services. PCLN and PCL physician services are being scrutinized for efficacy and efficiency. These efforts led to innovations in practice and were necessary to creative work design.

During the 1990s the PCLN faced many challenges caused by the threats and effects of workplace violence that was generated by clients and family members whose concerns have been addressed in the PCLN practice literature. Additionally, PCLNs are often instrumental in developing therapeutic approaches to identifying and treating violence and the emotional aftermath (Antai-Otong, 2001). Another health care issue that PCLNs have made contributions in is ethical decision making in relation to the level of care decisions that clients, families, and staff are faced with daily (Broom, 1991; Hart, 1990). PCLN authors are detailing their work with older depressed clients and the nurses who work with them (Kurlowicz, 1996, 2001) and recognizing the addictive processes in the health care professional (Krupnick, 1990).

The 1990s have produced some difficult times in the health care arena. PCLNs have been affected by downsizing or rightsizing, which has resulted in job loss for some PCLNs. This unfortunate situation produced opportunities for PCLNs to assist in improving work environments and diffusing work-related stress of those remaining staff members (Kane, 1992; Tommasini, 1992).

The literature of the 1990s also began to reflect the research that PCLNs were conducting or participating in. During this period there was limited writing about subspecialization within the PCLN practice, peer review for PCLNs to facilitate improvement, and the future of advanced-practice nursing practice (Minarik, 1992; Moschler & Fincannon, 1992; Titlebaum, Hart, & Romano-Egan, 1992).

The twenty-first century, like previous decades, continues to influence the role of the PCLN. Minarik and Neese (2002) submit that because of the dramatic changes in the health care arena, PCLN practice integrates the holistic needs of the client. In addition, this process is essential in addressing the client's psychiatric, psychosocial, and physical health care needs within a systems approach (Watson, 2006). An aging population and growing concerns about obesity and socio-economic issues, coupled with advances in neuroscience and medical technology, require PCLNs to make psychosocial diagnoses. In addition the PCLN has to implement an array of direct and indirect care interventions with clients presenting with co-occurring medical and psychiatric conditions and their families. Providing systems interventions is crucial to the role of the PCLN and requires expertise in collaboration and consultation with clients, families, and various health care providers (Meadows, Harvey, Joubert, Barton, & Bedi, 2007; Minarik & Neese, 2002).

ORGANIZATIONAL PLACEMENT OF THE PCLN

Traditional organizational placement for PCLNs in a health care environment has been either in the department of nursing, usually psychiatric nursing, or within the department of psychiatry. Historically, it has been proposed that clinical collaborations and alliances are best facilitated when the PCLN staff is in a staff position, rather than an administrative one. The premise is that no administrative authority (which means no direct influence over the evaluation of staff performance) facilitates the consultant's role. Therefore, the PCLN uses expert power rather than administrative, or line, "legitimate" power (Jimerson, 1986; Lewis & Levy, 1982). The movement of PCLNs into alternate practice settings such as home care, rehabilitation centers, outpatient clinics, and extended care facilities continues to be an arena of rapid expansion (ANA, 2000). These nurses have established themselves as intrapreneurs within workplaces and also entrepreneurs in designing and implementing practice programs as they function as independent contractors (Kurlowicz, 1998; Sharrock & Happell, 2001; Sharrock et al., 2006).

In today's transforming health care system, the prevalence of comorbid psychiatric and medical conditions is increasingly accepted. Unfortunately, mental conditions are more likely to go unrecognized and managed in nonmental health practice settings (Minarik & Neese, 2002; Yakimo, Kurlowicz, & Murray, 2004). A number of these conditions are chronic and debilitating and interfere with the client's level of functioning and quality of life (Kessler, Chiu, Demler, Merikangas, & Walters, 2005; Smith, 2003).

Changes in the health care system provide numerous opportunities for PCLNs. It is a natural transition for PCLNs to move into case management roles. Of particular importance for nurses is having a comprehensive understanding of the administrative role to traverse this transition smoothly. Administrative nursing experience can also advance the PCLN's knowledge of consultees and health care systems (Kurlowicz, 1998). Furthermore, some nurse administrators are trying to protect the PCLN's practice by work design. One approach has been to assign PCLNs in administrative positions to insulate them from possible job loss by assigning dual roles. Whether in a staff or line position within the health care organization, the PCLN's scope of power rests in expert authority based on extensive and specialized knowledge. The issue of including administration in the curriculum content for CNSs is beginning to be supported to adequately prepare them for future transitions in nursing care delivery. In addition to administrative expertise is the need to have expertise in performing a comprehensive psychiatric evaluation, including interviewing, history taking, mental status and health examinations, and family (Minarik & Neese, 2002). These recommendations are consistent with content from the ANA (1990, 2000) standards for PCLNs and commensurate with the advanced-practice registered psychiatric-mental health nurse.

The movement to case management systems and other innovative models such as nurse-managed centers and collaborative nurse case management fits well with the theoretical knowledge and clinical expertise of the PCLN in advanced-practice nursing practice. These nurses must competently negotiate organizational conflicts while effectively managing clinical situations and the health care staff to facilitate successful implementation of case management models in diverse practice settings (Minarik & Neese, 2002; Sharrock et al., 2006).

Finally, interdisciplinary psychiatric liaison teams have become a part of changing health care systems (Jorsh, 2006). The PCL nurse is an invaluable member of the team (Sharrock et al., 2006). Collectively the team is used in nonpsychiatric services to address the needs of clients with medical and psychiatric conditions. During an era when evidence-based practice, cost effectiveness, quality, and positive clinical outcomes are major drivers of health care decisions, psychiatric consultation-liaison nurses and team members are challenged to justify their value in complex health care systems (Yakimo, Kurlowicz, & Murray, 2004).

TELEMENTAL HEALTH PCLN SERVICES

The use of computers, videoconferencing, telephones, and other telecommunication in the delivery of health services is well-documented and not new to nursing or medicine (Frueh et al., 2007; Hilty, Marks, Urness, Yellowlees & Nesbitt, 2004; Hilty et al., 2004; Shore & Manson, 2004). Telemental health refers to the provision of consultation using telecommunications systems that facilitate PCLN-provider interactive "real-time" communication to address mental health needs. More and more the Internet, videoconferencing, telephone, and secure messaging (e-mail), are being used to provide consultation-liaison services, psychiatric evaluations to primary care, rural and remote practice settings. Remote interventions and consultations can be used to monitor the client's treatment plan, reduce client and health care system cost related to travel, cost savings and collaboration with providers. Services may range from reviews of general clinical issues, verbal case reviews, remote chart reviews to direct client observation.

THE CONSULTATION PROCESS

Each consultation is a unique experience that varies across practice settings. Consultation and liaison processes, which are

intertwined and represent an aspect of each consultation, are delineated in the following section. Generally, consultation is a marketing process in which the consultant provides recommendations adapted to the needs of the consultee (Rutherford, 1988; Sharrock & Happell, 2001). Caplan (1970) defined consultation as a process of communication between professionals that can be taught, applied, and analyzed systematically. The content of each consultation varies widely and is dependent on the specialized knowledge of the consultant. The skills and techniques are similar whether the focus is clinical or on process (Antai-Otong & Taylor, 1992).

The consultation process involves four processes: entry, diagnosis, response-intervention, and closure and evaluation. The major steps in the consultative process are outlined in Table 35–3. The goals of the consultation process are facilitated by the consultee's skills in managing a work-related problem and to advance the consultee's ability to master similar problems in the future.

PCLNs use several consultative activities. Lippitt and Lippitt's consultation model (1978) categorizes the various roles and corresponding activities used to actualize the consultation process (see Table 35–4).

ENTRY: REQUEST FOR CONSULTATION

Initially, the consultant must identify *who* is initiating the requesting consultation, for example, a nurse, physician, occupational or physical therapist, social worker, family member, client, or primary care administrator. The PCLN needs to consider the purpose and timing of the consultation request: *What* is the reason for the consultation? *Why* has it been requested at this time? Does the request relate to discharge, community-based follow-up, or medication management in

TABLE 35–4
Lippitt and Lippitt's Consultation Model

Role	Activities
Advocate	• Proposes guidelines • Persuades and directs in problem solving
Alternative identifier and linker	• Offers resources to the client • Collaborates to assess the possible consequences of choices
Fact finder	• Collects data
	• Stimulates thinking • Provides information requested or needed by consultant
Informational expert	• Provides policy or practice decisions
Joint problem-solver	• Identifies options and alternatives
	• Collaborates with consultee or team to solve problems
Objective observer/reflector	• Raises questions to be considered • Clarifies questions
Process counselor	• Observes and monitors problem-solving process • Raises issues • Provides feedback
Trainer/educator	• Provides instruction to the consultee

Note. Adapted from *The Consulting Process in Action,* by G. Lippitt and R. Lippitt, 1978, San Diego, CA: University Associates.

an extended care facility? Has something, such as a family member, visitor, or someone, perhaps a home health agency, changed recently? *What* else changed before the consultation was placed? The *who, what,* and *why now* are important areas to assess. Additionally, the affective, or emotional, tone of the communication by the consultee is equally relevant to understand and address. The consultant uses all of these factors to determine the immediacy of the consultation requested.

DIAGNOSIS: DETERMINING THE NEED FOR AND PURPOSE OF THE CONSULTATION

During the diagnosis stage of the consultation process, the consultant needs to ascertain the implications and appropriateness of this particular consultation request. The PCLN uses each consultation request as an opportunity to clarify and validate the psychological issues involved in the nursing care of clients. The PCLN provides an explanation of the PCLN role into each consultation. It is imperative to validate the involvement of the PCLN in the health care delivery team to facilitate making alliances and use of services. Additionally, each consultation provides an opportunity for the PCLN to be a role model and develop a clearer perspective of the consultee, treatment team, nursing practice setting, and client-family system.

The information of who, what, and why now that was obtained during the entry phase must be used to facilitate the diagnosis stage, and consultants need to discover the "hidden agendas," or covert reasons of the consultee before engaging themselves in the response stage of consultation. An exploration of the diverse perceptions as to the needs for and specific purpose of consultation must be illuminated so that the consultant can move into the response stage.

RESPONSE/INTERVENTION: ESTABLISHING A CONTRACTUAL AGREEMENT

The response or intervention stage involves the tasks of:

1. Establishing a contractual agreement between the consultee and consultant

2. Interacting between the consultee and consultant to seek and interpret information for accurate problem identification

3. Designing the "prescriptive" intervention

4. Evaluating the intervention and revision of plan (when necessary)

Establishing a contractual agreement between the consultee and the consultant is a necessary part of the consultation process. All aspects of the nurse-to-nurse consultation process must be discussed and mutually agreed on by the consultee and consultant. The decision-making process concerning the consultee's and consultant's responsibilities and roles in the plan of care is the primary focus of the contractual agreement. The primary nurse or health care provider or agency is responsible for contacting the consultant; collaborating with the consultant to negotiate the type and level of involvement, which is pivotal; and incorporating the consultant's recommendations into the plan of care. The consultant collaborates with the consultee to develop a plan of care, then conducts and writes an assessment with recommendations on the consultation form. In addition, the consultant makes follow-up contact with the consultee for evaluation of the plan's effectiveness and outcome (Sparacino, 1998).

If this recommendation is based on a fee for service, the issue of fees must be clearly defined, negotiated, and mutually agreed on. Some PCLN services are fee for service, and the consultee needs this information to be adequately informed about the fees that the client will be charged (Kennerly, 2006).

The consultant needs to enter the seeking and interpreting part of this stage of consultation with as few predetermined or set ideas as possible. It is important to keep an open mind while clarifying the nature of the request and listening for the explicitly as well as the hidden agendas for consultation. Explicit as well as hidden agendas for the consultation process need to be addressed for the consultation process to be complete and successful.

The issue that generated the consultation is initially conceptualized and defined by the consultee. The initial definition may be incomplete or inaccurate and become more coalesced throughout the information and interpretation stages. Exchanges between the consultee and consultant assist in clarifying the client-family issues relative to the needs and feelings of the consultee and how these issues intersect and affect each other. Lewis and Levy (1982) described the process of "dialoguing the total consultation." A comprehensive assessment of the client-family system, health care facility, community-based or home care setting, and the health care team must be addressed to obtain a complete analysis of the situation (see Table 35–5).

The next task is to collaborate with the consultee in recommending strategies for problem resolution. During this stage of response-intervention, the consultant and the consultee must determine the level and method of care to be provided by the PCLN. If the consultant is involved directly in the provision of care, individual roles, responsibilities, and accountability must be clearly negotiated and articulated by both consultation partners. In the direct consultation model, the PCLN assumes responsibility for interviewing the client and family, history taking, and performing mental and health status assessments; actively participates in the delivery of the psychosocial interventions; and collaborates in the evaluation and outcome of care. In the direct method, the consultant works with and through the health care professionals already involved in the client's and family members' care. Indirect consultation can be facilitated by using innovative approaches, including case or video conferences or telehealth that are consultee centered; scheduling time to focus on establishing mutual trust; and building alliances within the health care team. The PCLN uses indirect consultation to enhance support for both the consultee and family-client system, with the goal of a mutually rewarding and workable plan of care (see Table 35–6 for a further description of subtypes of consultation using direct and indirect models of consultation). Several significant factors must be addressed before the PCLN can decide whether the direct or indirect consultation method is appropriate for the situation (see Table 35–7 for a guide to determine which method is appropriate for the situation).

TABLE 35–5
Components of Consultation, Assessment, and Diagnosis

1. **Consultation request:** Who is requesting the consult? When is the request of consult placed? What is the purpose of the consult?

2. **Consultee:** Who is the consultee (nurse, client, family, physician, physical therapist, or other)? What is *your* relationship with this consultee? How experienced is the consultee? Is the consultee experiencing work-related or personal stress that is affecting this situation? Is this situation a *new* experience for this consultee or a repetitive pattern of consultation?

3. **Physician and health care team:** How does the physician view the problem? Is there conflict within the team? Is there any conflict with this patient and this physician? Does the physician value psychiatric nursing consultation? What is *your* relationship with this physician?

4. **Nursing staff members and the unit environment:** Is the unit a specialty setting (such as critical care, transplant, neonatal critical care)? Is the nursing staff experiencing significant stress from low staffing levels or cumulative patient losses? What type of leadership style does the nurse manager use? Is there a collaborative practice model on the unit between physicians and nurses, or are the relationships strained or conflictual?

5. **Family system:** Are any family members available to the client? Is the presence or absence of family members contributing to the distress? Are there family conflicts that are stressful for the client? Does the family have resources for support, or do they need additional support? What is this family's "usual" way of coping with health-related problems? What is the relationship between the family and the nursing and medical teams? How is the illness affecting the family system?

6. **Medical illness:** What are the most distressing signs and symptoms of the illness? What is the trajectory of the illness? How predictable or uncertain is the clinical course of this illness? Is the client's behavior possibly related to physiologic processes? Are treatments, tests and procedures, or medications contributing to the behavior?

7. **Chart review:** Has a psychosocial assessment been completed by nursing? Have there been numerous medical specialist consults with several changes in treatment? Has the client been moved from several units (e.g., critical care unit to medical or surgical units back to the critical care unit)? Is this client assigned a primary nurse or case manager? Are there inconsistencies in assessment of the client's condition, and uncertainty of a clear plan?

TABLE 35–6
Types of Consultation

Type	Focus	Purpose	Person or Group Primarily Responsible to	Example
Client				
Direct	Consultant works with client and the client's family, environment, and community	To actively intervene with mental health needs of the client, such as death and dying, anger, change in body image, grief and loss	Client and family	Client who has undergone a traumatic hemipelvectomy and is dealing with a change in body image and functional ability and loss; veterans from various wars with traumatic brain injury (TBI) and PTSD; family therapy strengthens individual and family coping skills
Indirect	Consultant works with client and caregiver	To facilitate interventions by client caregiver	Health care provider	Health provider responds to family members who are dealing with a chronically critically ill family member and are making level of care decisions, which is increasing their anxiety level
Consultee				
Staff—direct	Consultant works with staff member	To deal with mental health needs of staff member, such as adjustment to new role, stress of workload, and exposure to multiple deaths in unit	Staff member	Staff member who is considering leaving nursing because of workload demands and negative impact of work-related stress on family system
Staff—indirect	Consultant works with manager regarding a staff member	To facilitate interventions by manager for a professional staff member's growth and to help manager work with other staff in relation to a staff member having performance-related issues.	Manager	Assisting a staff member to directly confront peer who does not assume his share of the workload, and decrease overinvolvement of colleagues
Intragroup—direct	Consultant works directly with a staff group on their issues	To actively intervene in coping and group dynamic issues of a group of staff members	Group of staff members	Group discussion with staff members who are dealing with the death of a long-term client

(continues)

TABLE 35–6
Types of Consultation (continued)

Type	Focus	Purpose	Person or Group Primarily Responsible to	Example
Consultee (continued)				
Intragroup—indirect	Consultant works with a group of staff members to learn process for dealing with their own issues	To help a staff group learn to deal with group's mental health and group dynamics concerns	Group of staff members	Working with group of staff members to define group norms and role definitions
Intragroup—direct	Consultant works directly with two or more groups in relation to communication, collaboration, and conflict resolution	To actively intervene with two or more groups to develop or change patterns of communication, collaboration, or conflict resolution	Two or more groups	Physicians who desire research; nurses who desire clearly written protocols concerning the care of suicidal patients
Organizational or System				
Direct	Consultant works directly with administrators and managers on an administrative or organizational problem	To actively intervene in assessment, diagnosis, and change of organizational behavior	Administration manager	Provision of interventions needed for problems with absenteeism
Indirect	Consultant assists administrators and managers to develop proactive processes and programs to facilitate a mentally healthy organizational culture	To facilitate administrators and managers in the process of program development based on identified mental health needs of employees	Administration manager	Employee assistance programs, stress management programs

Note. Data from "Psychiatric Consultant Liaison Nursing," by V. M. Boyer and J. C. Kirsch, 1991, in N. L. Keltner, L. H. Schwecke, and C. E. Bostrom (Eds.), *Psychiatric Nursing: Psychotherapeutic Management Approach* (pp. 153–155), St. Louis: C. V. Mosby. Adapted with permission.

TABLE 35–7

Indications for Direct Versus Indirect Method of Consultation in Psychiatric Consultation-Liaison Nurse (PCLN) Practice

Direct	Indirect
• Problem identification is complex, unclear, and convoluted	• Problem identification is clear and straightforward
• Client request to speak with PCLN	• Consultee has established a "doable," effective plan and is requesting validation and support
• Special interest to PCLN or part of a specific program (e.g., trauma team, transplant team) that sees all these clients	• Consultee has adequate clinical skills and ability to establish and implement the recommended interventions
• Part or all of the planned interventions are beyond the consultee's clinical expertise	• Consultee feels comfortable with plan and is not experiencing anxiety over situation
• PCLN is new to the health care system and direct consultation would increase visibility	• Identified problem is with consultee, not client focused
• Consultee is overwhelmed with anxiety or anger over situation	• Physician or team does not want the client to be seen
• Alliances would be strengthened; systems networking would be enhanced	• Highly motivated consultee in agreement with plan
• Opportunity to model for consultee with a consultee-attended interview	• Consultee is user friendly and knowledgeable of PCLN role
• High-level resistance by consultee in relation to plan	• Low level of resistance by consultee in relation to plan
• Previously unsuccessful use of an indirect model with this consultee	• Previously successful use of an indirect model of consultation with this consultee

Throughout the response-intervention stage, follow-up reassessment and the evaluation of the outcomes based on the plan of care need to be negotiated, and both the consultee and consultant need to be involved in making revisions (see Table 35–8 for further clarification of responsibilities in the consultation process). The PCLN discusses the recommendations with the consultee; however, a formal written consultation report is necessary so that all members of the health care team have access to relevant information concerning the plan of care. The format for the consultation report may vary from facility to facility, but the following basic areas can serve as a blueprint (Ingersoll & Jones, 1992):

◆ Purpose of the consultation and problem identification

◆ Dates and activities throughout the consultation process

◆ Assessment of the present situation

◆ Specific interventions

◆ Recommendations on how to evaluate the outcomes of care

◆ Alternative plans for problem solving

Follow-up progress notes describing interventions are essential for an orderly and timely communication of relevant data.

TABLE 35–8

Responsibilities of Consultee and Consultant

Consultee	Consultant
• Identifies client care problem	• Contacts primary nurse
• Contacts appropriate consultant(s)	• Collaborates with primary nurse to negotiate level of involvement
• Incorporates recommendations into the nursing care plan	• Writes assessment and recommendations on consultation form
• Communicates plan of care with client, family, and colleagues	• Makes follow-up contact with consultee for evaluation of effectiveness

CLOSURE OF CONSULTATION

The closure stage of the consultation process is just as significant as the entry, diagnosis, and response stages. However, consultants periodically are remiss in establishing a formal closure phase that integrates disengagement, termination, and, equally important, evaluation of the consultation process.

Ideally, termination and disengagement naturally follow the resolution of the identified problem or completion of the project. Before disengagement and termination, an evaluation of the consultation process is negotiated. The outcome of the consultation process and the process itself are reviewed between the consultee and consultant. The evaluation process includes an assessment of the degree to which the desired or expected outcomes were achieved. A well-negotiated consultation includes time to explore whether the expectations of the consultant were met. This is a good idea for both the novice and the expert PCLN. However, this may be the one aspect of the closure stage that can "fall between the cracks," even if the consultation process appears to be successful. The evaluation process can be a time for professional growth for both the consultee and consultant. It is also anxiety provoking for both partners in the consultation process. Honest feedback about the clinical practice and interpersonal style can be an emotional challenge for both consultation partners. Included in this evaluation process itself is a self-appraisal by the PCLN of one's performance in the consultation process.

THE NURSING PROCESS

The PCLN provides consultation that strengthens the abilities of nurses and other staff to provide interventions and services for clients and effect change in the organization. The nursing process provides a systematic model that enables the nurse to gather data concerning clinicians and organizations, determine a problem or diagnosis, formulate outcome identification and planning, initiate interventions and evaluate outcomes. These dynamics are demonstrated using the following case study.

ASSESSMENT

The PCLN discussed the situation with the primary and associate nurses, the trauma nurse coordinator, and trauma service attending physician. After reviewing Mr. Charles's medical record and interviewing Mrs. Charles, the PCLN introduced herself briefly to the client, who was being administered a paralyzing agent, an amnestic benzodiazepine midazolam (Versed), and ventilator support. After completing an initial assessment, the PCLN negotiated with the health team to remain involved as a direct provider to the wife and the client, if he survived.

NURSING DIAGNOSES

- ◆ Anxiety—Mr. and Mrs. Charles
- ◆ Disturbed Body Image
- ◆ Anticipatory Grieving
- ◆ Pain—Mr. Charles
- ◆ Post-trauma Syndrome—Mr. Charles
- ◆ Powerlessness—Mr. and Mrs. Charles

OUTCOME IDENTIFICATION AND PLANNING

The PCLN and primary nurse collaborated on additional consultant referrals to the maternal-child CNS and the social worker to secure immediate housing for the spouse. PCLN

CASE STUDY

Direct, Client-Focused Consultation (Mr. Charles)

Mr. Charles is a 36-year-old married man. He is a construction worker who has been run over by a large truck. He suffered an immediate hemipelvectomy at the accident site, and he and his leg were transported by medical helicopter to the trauma center. Mr. Charles survived the initial trauma and was sent to the operating room. His wife was summoned and arrived at the hospital. When Mrs. Charles arrived in the surgical intensive care unit (SICU), the staff nurses learned that she was 7 months pregnant.

Mr. Charles's condition was very unstable the first 72 hours after the accident. He experienced two cardiac arrests, and Mrs. Charles fainted twice in the SICU. The PCLN was consulted on the fourth day of hospitalization during interdisciplinary trauma rounds by the trauma nurse coordinator, SICU staff nurse, and the trauma surgeon.

Consultation Request

The initial consultation request was for Mrs. Charles, to assess her ability to cope with the client's potential death. A secondary request for the consultation was to assist with the following:

- Mental status assessment for suspected delirium

- Pain management

- Anxiety management

- Disturbed body image related to traumatic hemipelvectomy with surgical revision, colostomy, and fractured extremity

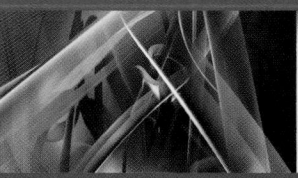

Direct Client-Focused Consultation
(Mrs. and Mr. Charles)

Nursing Diagnosis: Anticipatory Grieving
by Mrs. Charles related to the uncertainty of her husband's survival

Outcome Identification	Nursing Actions	Rationales	Evaluation
1. Within 24 hours, Mrs. Charles mobilized her family support to ensure another adult stays with her every day.	1a. PCLN will meet with Mrs. Charles daily for support and crisis intervention.	1a. Mrs. Charles required emotional support and assistance in problem solving during an intense crisis period in the early phase of this traumatic injury.	*Goal met:* Mrs. Charles discussed fears of husband dying before their first baby is born. Mrs. Charles activated her family and family support to have another adult with her every day.
	1b. Trauma team and critical care nurses will meet with Mrs. Charles to explore plans and possible outcomes.	1b. Mrs. Charles needed clear communication from the multidisciplinary trauma team to clarify confusion and assist her in problem solving.	
	1c. Social worker will assist Mrs. Charles in obtaining emergency housing.	1c. Mrs. Charles needed to be housed close to the medical center to facilitate her daily involvement in Mr. Charles's care.	

Nursing Diagnosis: Pain (Acute)
related to multiple orthopedic injuries and traumatic amputation

Outcome Identification	Nursing Actions	Rationales	Evaluation
1. Within 48 hours of admission to SICU, Mr. Charles will have effective pain control.	1a. PCLN recommended pain management consultation after 72 hours of inadequate pain control.	1a. To clarify assessment by nurses and client to improve pain management.	*Goal met:* Mr. Charles had a fluctuating pain control pattern for 8 days. When his mental status improved, he was able to use patient-controlled analgesia appropriately, and pain control was attained within 36 hours.
	1b. Streamlined pain medications with around-the-clock dosing instead of intermittent p.r.n. dosing.	1b. To decrease negative effect of polypharmacy and intermittent, p.r.n. dosing.	
	1c. Instruct Mr. Charles in correct use of patient-controlled analgesia pump after mental status improves.	1c. Incorporating Mr. Charles in his care and increasing his self-care concerning his pain will improve pain control.	

(continues)

Nursing Care Plan 35-1 (continued)

Nursing Diagnosis: Posttrauma Response

Outcome Identification	Nursing Actions	Rationales	Evaluation
1. Within 1 week, Mr. Charles will have diminished nightmares of traumatic event, improved sleep pattern, and fewer intrusive thoughts of the accident.	1a. PCLN will see client two or three times a week to begin debriefing from the accident.	1a. To allow Mr. Charles sufficient time to process feelings to diminish deleterious effects of posttrauma response and alleviate development of posttraumatic stress disorder.	*Goal met:* Mr. Charles was able to discuss his feelings of anger, disgust, and depression.
	1b. Exploration of client and wife's feelings related to the accident and disruption in their family, social, and occupational spheres of life.	1b. To encourage discussion of feelings (anger, fear, and depression) concerning significant body disruption and family function alterations.	Mr. Charles made a successful transition to a rehabilitation facility without developing posttraumatic stress disorder. Mr. Charles's symptoms of posttrauma response were controlled by the time of discharge to the rehabilitation center.
	1c. Multidisciplinary meetings to maintain a current, relevant plan of care to facilitate rehabilitation phase.	1c. To facilitate an effective discharge plan to minimize any distress related to discharge to a rehabilitation facility.	
	1d. Assist couple in normalizing posttrauma response vulnerability.	1d. To improve postaccident coping.	

involvement was maintained throughout Mr. Charles's 3-month hospitalization. Initially, the PCLN focused on Mrs. Charles and her parents. As the client's course became less tenuous after 2 weeks in the SICU, the PCLN provided direct care in collaboration with the trauma team members and SICU nursing staff.

Nursing Care Plan 35-1 identifies the desired outcomes for some of the nursing diagnoses listed earlier and delineates the nursing interventions necessary to achieve these outcomes, along with the rationales for each action.

IMPLEMENTATION

The PCLN saw Mrs. Charles for brief supportive therapy sessions three or four times a week and collaborated with the social worker, the pain management team, and the pastoral counselor to facilitate Mr. Charles's psychophysiological care. The maternal-child CNS remained involved—as Mrs. Charles moved into the end of her eighth month of pregnancy, she began to feel an increased level of anxiety, abandonment, and isolation as the birth was becoming imminent.

When the nursing staff suggested giving Mrs. Charles a baby shower to "normalize" her pregnancy experience, the PCLN and the SICU nurse manager conducted an explo-ration of the staff's need to be helpful and supportive. The decision was made to invite Mrs. Charles's parents and friends from her hometown (3 hours away). The baby shower was planned while Mr. Charles's condition improved, so the party was held in his SICU room. Additionally, the maternal-child CNS did joint teaching with both Mr. and Mrs. Charles to promote his inclusion in the pregnancy and childbirth education experience to facilitate a normal experience.

Mr. Charles was transferred from the SICU to a general medical-surgical unit; within weeks, he was admitted to the rehabilitation unit. Mrs. Charles went into labor and delivered a healthy daughter. The rehabilitation nursing staff, the PCLN, and the social worker arranged for Mr. Charles to travel to the hospital where his wife had delivered to visit her and their new baby. Mr. Charles was discharged to an extended care rehabilitation facility closer to his home with a positive feeling about his ability to adjust to his losses.

The strategies used by the PCLN throughout this consultation included:

◆ Providing immediate support for potential grief and mourning process by the wife

◆ Assessing, monitoring, and diminishing high levels of anxiety by the client and his spouse

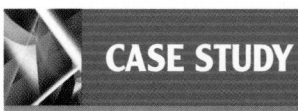

CASE STUDY

Indirect, Consultee-Focused Consultation (Assistant Nurse Manager (ANM))

Consultation Request

The PCLN received an urgent call from an assistant nurse manager (ANM) in the medical intensive care unit (MICU) asking the PCLN to come to the unit immediately to discuss an "overwhelming situation." The PCLN had an established relationship with the ANM and realized that her assessment of situations was usually accurate and not exaggerated. The PCLN also recognized the urgency in her voice. The PCLN met with the ANM to discuss the situation. The ANM had been caring for a young woman who had attempted suicide several days before, and now the MICU staff were saying that they felt like "air traffic controller." The ANM reported that the overwhelming number of visitors was "interfering with the nursing care."

Assessment

The ANM was upset about all the client's unrelated visitors. Throughout the ANM's description of this situation, it was apparent to the PCLN that she was extremely angry. The PCLN asked for validation about this assessment. The ANM said she was angry and upset because " I want to protect the client's privacy but I can't." She became tearful and was clearly distressed about this situation. The PCLN decided that further exploration of her strong, angry response to this situation was necessary. Discussion revealed that she was handling this clinical situation in the absence of the nurse manager, who was away for several weeks; at the same time she was dealing with a personal tragedy. Her brother had attempted suicide and was in a persistent vegetative state, somewhat similar to the possible outcome of this young client.

Nursing Diagnoses

- Anxiety
- Defensive Coping
- Powerlessness

Outcome Identification and Planning

The PCLN asked the ANM what would help her at this moment. She requested the PCLN's assistance in obtaining a list of who needed to visit this young woman. She also asked for some additional time to process her reaction to this particular situation.

Nursing Care Plan 35–2 identifies the desired outcomes from some of the nursing diagnoses listed earlier and delineates the nursing interventions necessary to achieve these outcomes, along with the rationales for these actions.

Implementation

Initially, the PCLN contacted another PCLN from the nearby children's medical center (where this young client had been followed) to facilitate information sharing with their staff. These staff members had provided care to this client for several years and were upset to hear that she had attempted suicide. Second, the PCLN spent time with the ANM listening to her describe the impact that this client's situation had on her. The PCLN made an agreement with the ANM to check with the MICU nurses daily to ascertain the level of anxiety over visitors. A case conference was planned to explore clinical issues, and a family meeting also occurred. A definitive visitor list was developed, and specific "point people" were determined to be "information disseminators" at the children's medical center.

The specific strategies that the PCLN used throughout this consultation included the following:

- Crisis intervention
- Values clarification
- Identification and resolution of ethical dilemmas
- Truth telling
- Advocacy

Evaluation

The ANM's level of anxiety and anger quickly diminished, and these feelings were replaced with guilt over her expressed anger. Within 24 hours the number of visitors had subsided and the staff members began to feel less overwhelmed and protective. The case conference illuminated the staff's feelings of sadness, loss, shock, and being out of control. Networking with the PCLN at the other health care facility decreased some of the tension that had developed. The family meeting was successful in providing the family and team members with an opportunity to discuss options in a client whose outcome was determined to be "medically futile." The family decided on withdrawal of life support and reported feeling supported throughout this overwhelming ordeal. The ANM used some additional scheduled time with the PCLN to share her feelings about this overwhelming situation and discuss specific alternative strategies for future stressful events.

- Facilitating information sharing
- Interpreting information given by the client and his wife
- Planning cross-service referral and consultation to facilitate a normal childbearing experience and pain management
- Implementing a mental status examination and cognitive improvement
- Reducing actual or potential problems in self-esteem, body image, grief, personal decision making, and quality of life

EVALUATION

An evaluation of the initial plan in relation to outcomes was positive. The outcomes of the initial period of care (the first week) resulted in an increase in the amount of information shared with the family members, which significantly reduced their anxiety. Cross-section consultation with the maternal-child CNS and PCLN support provided Mrs. Charles alleviated her fainting and confirmed a normal pregnancy with no deleterious effect on the fetus. At the end of 1 month, Mr. Charles's anxiety level began to diminish, his pain control management was dramatically improved, and the team considered weaning him from the ventilator. The client's mental status also improved, and he began to understand the impact of this traumatic event.

The PCLN collaborated with the primary nurse in planning for the client's transfer from SICU, and this well-planned transfer was successful in alleviating anxiety of the client and his family and in preparing the receiving nursing staff. This anticipatory guidance and planning reduced the client's anxiety response during his transfer.

Case conferences with the nursing staff in SICU assisted the nurse in successfully dealing with the impact of vicarious traumatization. In addition, the case conferences facilitated information sharing between the team members and the insurance nurse consultant, which facilitated comprehensive planning.

CONSULTATION PROCESS

The consultation is not without some potential problems, specifically of resistance, to the consultation process itself (Miller, 1983). Transferences and countertransference can also interfere with the consultation process. These consultation process issues can interfere with incorporation of the PCLN's recommendations into the plan of care.

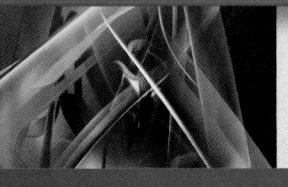

NURSING CARE PLAN 35–2

Indirect, Consultee-Focused Consultation (Assistant Nurse Manager [ANM])

Nursing Diagnosis: Anxiety

Outcome Identification	Nursing Actions	Rationales	Evaluation
1. Within 24 hours, the ANM's level of anxiety concerning the care of her young client will diminish.	1a. Explore with ANM feelings of anxiety in relation to visiting situation of client with suicide attempt.	1a. Identification of ANM's actual feelings of anxiety allowed her to redefine the situation and lessen her angry outburst.	*Goal met:* Client is able to identify feelings of anxiety and address competing situations that are increasing her anxiety.
	1b. Assist her in clarifying the interface of assuming leadership of the intensive care unit and responding to a personal tragedy that has similarities to the current situation.	1b. The ANM needed clarification and validation of her feelings to facilitate her problem-solving abilities.	

(continues)

Nursing Care Plan 35–2 *(continued)*

Nursing Diagnosis: Defensive Coping

Outcome Identification	Nursing Actions	Rationales	Evaluation
1a. Within 48 hours, the ANM's ego integrity, self-concept, and tolerable emotional level will be maintained. 1b. Within 48 hours the ANM will cope with a stressful situation in an adaptive problem-solving manner.	1a. Avoid direct confrontation of ANM's angry outburst. 1b. Examine the ANM's present coping behaviors and the consequences. 1c. Explore realistic interpretations and events with ANM and validate feelings. 1d. Develop mutually agreed-on goals to diminish ANM's increased defensiveness.	1a. Direct confrontation can increase anger and defensive coping. 1b. Clarifying the underlying reasons for behavioral responses assists in understanding the consequences, thereby facilitating behavioral changes. 1c. Establishing mutually agreed on goals and strategies helps promote behavioral changes and a concrete plan for continued personal growth for the ANM.	*Goal met:* ANM experiences less anger and hostility. ANM uses effective problem-solving strategies.

Nursing Diagnosis: Powerlessness

Outcome Identification	Nursing Actions	Rationales	Evaluation
1. Within 48 hours, the ANM's confidence, self-concept, and emotional resilience will be maintained.	1a. Determine the ANM's previous coping abilities and degree of mastery. 1b. Assist the ANM to identify feelings of powerlessness and the specific factors that contribute to these feelings.	1a. Reminding the ANM of previous success enhances self-confidence, acknowledges options, and promotes self-control. 1b. Awareness of these feelings and their causes can promote positive coping.	*Goal met:* ANM feels empowered and adequate. ANM uses resources to organize a workable plan and diminish feelings of being overwhelmed.

Resistance is a covert or overt force that is oppositional in nature and may originate from conscious or unconscious feelings. Resistance can be defined as behavior that protects a person from the psychological effects of change; it is not simply a rejection of ideas offered by the consultant. Resistance in the consultation process seems paradoxical because the relationship is engaged voluntarily.

There are several reasons for the resistance that occurs in the consultation process. Even though consultees may seek assistance, they may believe that they should have solved the problem themselves. Therefore, it may be difficult for the con-

sultees who feel inadequate to view a successful consultation as a positive, growth-producing experience. They may believe it is a personal defeat and become resistant to the consultant's ability to be successful, thereby "balancing the scales" and avoiding feelings of inadequacy because the consultant could not solve the problem either.

Resistance may also occur when consultees do not enter the consultation process in a completely voluntary manner. The supervisor or colleague may initiate or encourage the consultation process and then expect the "consultee" to use the consultant's services. Finally, resistance can develop when the consultee's workplace and personal issues become intertwined. A more complete description of specific resistance problems encountered in the consultation process is provided in Table 35–9.

There are several strategies that can be employed to manage resistance to the consultation process. Some interventions include the following:

◆ Provide accurate and complete information.

◆ Treat each consultee as an individual and with respect.

◆ Include all the case providers in the planning process.

◆ Allow time for exploration of feelings and the voicing of any objections to the proposed recommendations.

◆ Consider group, unit, or agency norms and routines during the consultation process.

◆ Provide feedback.

◆ Remain open to questions and revisions concerning recommendations for care.

◆ Design interventions that are within the expertise of the consultee

The PCLN can be most effective in alleviating resistance when considering all the possible reasons for the consultee's resistance.

The PCLN must carefully assess for the presence of transference and countertransference issues because they can affect all participants involved in the consultation process both positively and negatively (Marshall & Marshall, 1988). Transference can be a powerful force, involving the client's transfer of feelings and attitudes about a personal relationship with a significant other onto the nurse or the therapist. Unresolved conflicts and unmet expectations may be reactivated by illness and the hospital experience.

Countertransference refers to the health care provider's emotional and behavioral response generated by specific qualities in the client. Clients and families may stimulate conflicts in the nurse or other health care provider, including the PCLN involved in the consultation process. This can influence the delivery of psychological care. These feelings can be conscious or unconscious and can facilitate or interfere with the psychotherapeutic relationship.

PCLNs obviously are not immune to the effects of transference and countertransference. Hence, they need to be actively involved in a consistent clinical supervision relationship to learn and integrate problem-solving strategies to effectively manage their feelings. Clinical supervision affords PCLNs an opportunity to review their work with an experienced or senior clinician, a person with more experience and skills, to

TABLE 35–9
Types of Consultee Resistance

Type of Consultee	Description of Behavior
The eager consultee	This person experiences a great deal of anxiety about the situation and takes any recommendation(s) without determining whether it is appropriate to the particular situation
The "one-for-one" consultee	This assumes that the two people involved are on a reciprocal consultant–consultee basis. The consultee refers a case to the consultant as "payment" for a previous case consultation
The forgetful consultee	The consultee makes the initial request for consultation but then "forgets" and is remiss about appointments to discuss the situation, or forgets to read the consultation report and forgets the recommendations
The apologetic consultee	The consultant is asked to see the client; however, the consultee who requested the consult apologizes to the client and assures them that the consultant's assessment and recommendations need not be used
The expert consultee	The consultee already "knows" all the answers and is seeking agreement by the consultant. If disagreement occurs, the consultee may seek another opinion and not use the consultant again
The rejecting consultee	This consultee is angry at the client or family and tries to use the consultation process to punish the client

Note. Adapted from "Psychiatric Consultation in the General Hospital: An Exploration of Resistances," by A. J. Krakowski, 1975, *Diseases of the Nervous System, 36,* pp. 242–244.

facilitate an objective self-evaluation process (Kilminster, Cottrell, Grant, & Jolly, 2007). (See Chapter 26.) The use of either individual or peer group supervision can also enhance the PCLNs' ability to cope and adjust to this psychiatric specialty, which deals with clients' secrets and highly sensitive, potentially traumatizing physical and emotional material (Kilminster et al., 2007). PCLNs are at high risk for "compassion fatigue" as well as the effects of secondary exposure to traumatic events. They can become victims of these emotionally charged situations. The issues of parallel process (Deighton, Gurris, & Traue, 2007), vicarious traumatization, or contact victimization (Moulden & Firestone, 2007) all elaborate on the behavioral, cognitive, emotional, physical, and spiritual impact of nurses and other health care providers caring for clients who are survivors of atrocities and interpersonal violence (Antai-Otong, 2001).

PCLNs are requested to assist with several different types of intense and emotionally charged situations. Life-threatening illness and sudden and cumulative losses may contribute to the effects of disenfranchised grief for the consultee and PCLN (Doka, 1989, 1993). The PCLN must develop a self-care strategic plan that involves individual, group, personal, and work-setting strategies to counterbalance these effects. A few recommendations are offered in Table 35–10.

THE LIAISON PROCESS

The liaison process facilitates the relationship among the client and her response and adjustment to illness and suffering, the consultee, and the health care environment. Liaison work involves preventive measures and educative activities to support the collaborative relationship between the consultee and consultant. PCLNs engage in several liaison process activities (Table 35–11). The following clinical example is offered to illustrate the interface of consultation and liaison process.

PCLNS AND THE RESEARCH ROLE

The research aspect of any advanced-practice nurse is quite important to promote advances in nursing practice and treatment outcomes. The ANA's (2000) *Scope and Standards of Psychiatric-Mental Health Nursing Practice* delineates that the advanced-practice psychiatric-mental health nurse is responsible for advancing the field of mental health by engaging and collaborating with others in the research process to "discover, examine and test knowledge and theories" (p. 48) and integrate them into practice.

The actualization of this research into the practice is sometimes challenging. The PCLN who maintains accurate daily records and statistics of clinical consults and liaison activities is building a potential database to provide information for clinical investigation and validation of clinical practice (De Vito Dabbs, Curran, & Lenz, 2000). However, several restraining factors may inhibit the PCLN from developing an accurate database to facilitate the clinical research role. These restraining factors may include:

TABLE 35–10
Guidelines for Self-Care Plan

Individual
- Personal—psychophysical health, social supports, life balance, spiritual connections, creative expression, self-awareness, plans for getting help, community activism, relaxation, humor
- Professional—boundaries/limit setting, plans for emergency coping, variety of tasks, adequate training, replenishment, active and consistent participation in clinical supervision

Environmental
- Social—assessment and education of social supports
- Societal—educational strategies, coalition building, legislative reform social action
- Work environment—physical environment, articulated value system in concert with our value system, clear job tasks and personnel guidelines, supervisory and management support, collegial support

---

TABLE 35–11
Liaison Process Activities

Participating in discharge planning rounds on nursing units

Attending and participating in collaborative nursing and physician rounds

Unit-based educational programs

University teaching in nonpsychiatric programs concerning psychosocial issues

Teaching client education programs

Facilitating support groups for health care professionals

Facilitating client–family support groups

Forming a journal club on units

- Early stage of development of PCLN practice in the organization
- Organizational readiness
- No clear and easy method to organize, store, access, and retrieve records
- Organization that does not value or support the PCLN research role

CLINICAL EXAMPLE

The Client with Delirium: Direct Care Consultation

A unit-based CNS in the cardiothoracic SICU consulted the PCLN assigned to the unit. The request was to discuss a particular client who was "uncooperative, unmotivated, and refusing to following instructions." This client was a 60-year-old man who had undergone a lung transplantation. During the initial assessment by the PCLN, a mental status examination revealed that the client had severe delirium. The PCLN provided several recommendations in collaboration with the unit-based CNS. In addition, the PCLN recognized the persistent pattern of consult requests made in this particular SICU, which reflected a need for teaching the staff about clients' behavior in the presence of delirium.

This consultation involved direct delivery of care to the client and assessment of the staff's need to learn how to assess the mental status of posttransplant clients. The PCLN and the CNS collaborated to design an educational program to meet this learning need. This collaborative effort produced a successful outcome by increasing the staff's awareness and understanding about postoperative delirium. Initially, the number of PCLN consult requests actually increased, and the problem identified was correct for delirium instead of an "unmotivated or uncooperative" client.

◆ Lack of research mentor

◆ Overwhelming clinical workload

Many of these factors can be alleviated through networking with other PCLNs and other advanced-practice nurses within and outside the organization. Coalitions can be built to develop a group model to facilitate research (ANA, 2000). Additionally, developing collaborative relationships with doctorally prepared nurse researchers at nearby universities or within the organization can be a facilitative factor in developing collaborative research projects, especially for the novice researcher. PCLNs are in an excellent position to review and share relevant research findings with staff and integrate them into practice. Also, PCLNs encourage, support, and consult their nursing colleagues about research even if not directly in the project.

As health care resources dwindle, there is mounting pressure for the PCLN to demonstrate positive treatment outcomes. A recent study conducted by Kurlowicz (2001) demonstrated the benefits of medically ill older adults referred to the PCLN for symptoms of depression and delirium. Because of barriers previously discussed, this study provides an example of using an existing PCLN database as a cost-effective first step in development of PCLN interventions targeting a vulnerable population and their nursing staff.

The next step concerning research involves PCLNs sharing and communicating their findings at research conferences and in professional refereed journals to establish a research foundation that complements the strong practice base of the PCLN. Several important areas merit further research exploration by PCLNs, including the following:

◆ Cost analysis studies focusing on the cost-effectiveness of PCLN practice and service

◆ Employee access and utilization of PCLN services and their effect on staff emotional and physical well-being (e.g., stress, burnout, absenteeism)

◆ Impact of direct care interventions by a PCLN on client length of stay or nursing care hours

This evidence-based research may be crucial to the survival of the existing PCLN positions. Additionally, outcome-based research can be supported and validated by the expanding practice settings and moving from primarily client-based mental health issues to subspecialization and focusing more on organization-based issues.

FUTURE TRENDS AND ISSUES

PCLN practice continues to evolve and parallel changes within the nursing profession. Furthermore, changes in psychiatry, advances in neurobiology and genetics, along with a transforming health care system will significantly influence PCLN practice. Major forces driving health care delivery system include concerns for costs of service delivery, quality of life, and evidence-based practice. During a period of fiscal restraint, the psychosocial aspects of health care are vulnerable yet necessary. PCLNs must continue to make themselves visible, accessible, and marketable in the health promotion sphere of health care.

PCLNs possess advanced theoretical knowledge and clinical expertise ideal for health care promotion, wellness programs, and human resource management. PCLNs can be instrumental in assisting organizations to identify and modify the culture of the organization (Sharrock et al., 2006). Organizational consultations can propel the PCLN into higher visible positions. Participation by PCLNs on major organizational and community committees that have the legitimate power to have a positive impact on client and family care, focus on quality improvement, and address the well-being of the organization's workforce is of the utmost importance. By this activity, PCLNs can help shape the organization's culture with respect to clients and families and be a valuable asset to their employees (Sharrock et al., 2006).

The future viability of the PCLN practice is dependent on:

◆ Evidence-based research that validates the positive impact of the PCLN in the health care arena

- Marketing to nursing and medical services in traditional client-based mental health issues and contemporary practice of subspecialization and organizational-based practice

- Education of nurse colleagues to foster recognition, respect, and acknowledgment of the unique contributions of PCLN practice

- Third-party reimbursement and participation in political endeavors to educate consumers, third-party payers, and lawmakers

- Support current endeavors that support prescriptive authority and increase PCLN services in diverse practice settings

- Expand practice beyond traditional foci and integrate neuroscience, use data management strategies and informatics to develop databases; and track trends in outcome measures and cost savings and avoidance, telemental health, and other technologies; and provide services to nurses and other clinicians in primary care, rural, and remote practice settings

- Develop business skills and become more fiscally savvy in cost reduction, avoidance, and efficiency of services

- Telemental health and other technologies have generated cost-effective and quality approaches for PCLNs

The PCLN practice continues to expand into subspecialization; as it occurs, the issue of accountability becomes extremely important. An autonomous, independent practitioner such as the PCLN needs the support and feedback offered by a peer review system (ANA, 2000). Peer review is an organizational procedure that can provide quality improvement and empowerment for practitioners. It is a formal, objective, systematic exchange among professional colleagues.

PCLNs have significant opportunities to be on the cutting edge of health care delivery and strongly influence their own professional future by being proactive rather than reactive. Accessibility, accountability, and application of the PCLN practice are specific areas that need greater attention to ensure the continued presence of PCLN practice in a cost-containing health care environment.

SUMMARY

- PCLN has emerged as a subspecialty within the specialty of advanced-practice psychiatric-mental health nursing.

- This subspecialty has evolved in response to an increased awareness and recognition of the psychobiological interface and the significant role it plays in response to physical illness and recovery.

- Psychiatric-mental health consultation is defined as the provision of clinical expertise in relation to the delivery of psychological care in response to a specific request by nurses, other health care providers, and organizations.

- The liaison process links health care professionals and facilitates communication, collaboration, and establishing partnerships between clients and health care providers.

- PCLN practice has expanded from a traditional indirect health care delivery model of psychosocial care in the general hospital settings to diverse practice settings. PCLNs are now found in primary care, outpatient, home care, and mobile health delivery settings.

- PCLNs are employing both intrapreneurial and entrepreneurial skills as consultants to maintain their viability within a transforming health care system.

SUGGESTIONS FOR CLINICAL CONFERENCE

1. Discuss the extent to which the psychosocial dimension is incorporated into the plan of care for medical-surgical clients in the general hospital setting.

2. Write a PCLN assessment and intervention with a client who is agitated and disoriented in the surgical intensive care unit or home care setting.

3. Identify and discuss several situations in which you would request the involvement of a PCLN.

4. Differentiate PCLN practice from primary nursing practice.

5. Discuss innovative roles inherent in PCLN, such as informatics, building databases to trend outcome measures—both clinical and utilization—and their usefulness in advancing the role of an entrepreneur.

STUDY QUESTIONS

1. D. B., a 21-year-old female student, was in a motor vehicle accident 6 months ago. Although her injuries were minor, her friend was killed. She complains to the nurse in the trauma clinic of inability to concentrate, insomnia, and thoughts that she is "losing her mind." The nurse asks the PCLN to perform a psychosocial assessment. The most important information from the PCLN to obtain is:
   a. a complete physical and social history
   b. a complete drug and alcohol history, including reports from a drug screen
   c. a review of significant events of the past year
   d. an exploration of how she coped with the motor vehicle accident and her friend's death

2. The PCLN is in the emergency department dealing with a survivor of violence. The client has been medically stabilized and will be discharged. The first priority of the PCLN is to:
   a. encourage the client to express her feelings
   b. assess for physical trauma
   c. provide privacy and safety for the client during the interview
   d. help the client identify and mobilize resources and support systems

3. The nurse is caring for J. M., a 71-year-old man, with the following symptoms: temperature of 103.4°F, moderate dehydration, bilateral rales in the lower lobes of his lungs, disorientation to time and place, and severe agitation. The nurse contacts the PCLN to assist in developing an appropriate, least restrictive plan of care. The PCLN bases his recommendations on the understanding that:
   a. the client is experiencing delirium secondary to the infectious process
   b. the client is probably displaying early signs of Alzheimer's disease
   c. older people get confused as a normal part of the aging process
   d. a referral to a nursing home for continuing care will be necessary for this client

4. A medical intensive care unit nurse is caring for M. J., who overdosed on sertraline (Zoloft), lorazepam (Ativan), and acetaminophen (Tylenol). The nurse contacts the PCLN to assist in determining the client's level of care. M. J. is comatose and unresponsive to lifesaving and technological care. Which of the following actions is the first priority for the PCLN intervention during the first few days of M. J.'s ICU treatment?
   a. Complete a full psychiatric assessment.
   b. Get in touch with M. J.'s family and try to involve them in immediate decision making.
   c. Observe and record vital signs frequently, including neurological signs.
   d. Determine whether M. J. may need long-term therapy after hospitalization for overdose.

5. A. R. comes to the emergency department for an assessment of chest pain. As she is about to undergo an electrocardiogram, she says to the nurse, "I am so terribly afraid I am dying, even though I have had this pain before and the doctor can never find anything." Which of the following would be the best response for the nurse to make?
   a. "Our doctors here are the best. If there's something wrong, they'll find it."
   b. "Please be calm now so that your test will give use useful information."
   c. "You sound fearful. After the test is over, we can talk more about your feelings."
   d. "Do you think your pain is all in your head?"

6. One of your nurse practitioner colleagues who works in a rural area is concerned about her client who she has been treating for mild depression the past 2 months. The nurse practitioner reports that he has become distant and more agitated but is willing to allow her to perform a psychiatric evaluation using videoconferencing. She also reports he denies being suicidal at the present or in the past. Based on your understanding of your role as a PCLN, what is the most appropriate response to your colleague?
   a. Ask her to immediately go to the nearest emergency room because he is suicidal.
   b. Use telemental health teleconferencing and perform a psychiatric evaluation.

   c. Ask her to bring the client to your office for a complete psychiatric evaluation.
   d. Inquire about the client's medical condition.

RESOURCES

Please note that because Internet resources are of a time-sensitive nature and URL addresses may change or be deleted, searches should also be conducted by association or topic.

Internet Resources

http://www.apna.org   American Psychiatric Nurses Association

http://www.nacns.org   National Association of Clinical Nurse Specialists

http://www.ispn.org   International Society of Psychiatric Mental-Health Nurses

http://www.ispn-psych.org/html/ispcln.html   The International Society of Psychiatric Consultation-Liaison Nurses (ISPCLN)

REFERENCES

Alexander, S. (1985). The consultation role of the psychiatric nurse clinician: From general health care to the industrial setting. *Occupational Health Nurse, 33,* 569–571.

American Nurses Association. (1990). *Standards of psychiatric consultation-liaison nursing.* Kansas, MO: Author.

American Nurses Association. (2000). *Scope and standards of psychiatric-mental health nursing practice.* Washington, DC: American Nurses Publishing.

Antai-Otong, D. (2001). Critical incident stress debriefing: A health promotion model for workplace violence. *Perspectives in Psychiatric Care, 37,* 125–132.

Antai-Otong, D., & Taylor, R. (1992). Calling a psych consult. *American Journal of Nursing, 92,* 68–71.

Baldwin, C. A. (1978). Mental health consultation in the intensive care unit: Toward balance and precision of attribution. *Journal of Psychosocial Nursing and Mental Health Services, 161,* 17–21.

Barbiasz, J., Blandford, K., Byrne, K., Horvath, K., Levy, J., Lewis, A., et al. (1982). Establishing the psychiatric liaison nurse role: Collaboration with the nurse administrator. *Journal of Nursing Administration, 12,* 14–18.

Barton, D., & Kelso, M. T. (1971). The nurse as a psychiatric consultant team member. *Psychiatric Medicine, 2,* 108–115.

Boyer, V. M., & Kirsch, J. C. (1991). Psychiatric consultation liaision nursing. In N. L. Keltner, L. H. Schwecke, & C. E. Bostrom (Eds.), *Psychiatric Nursing: Psychotherapeutic man-agement approach* (pp. 153–155). St. Louis, MO: C. V. Mosby.

Broom, C. (1991). Conflict resolution strategies: When ethical dilemmas evolve to conflict. *Dimensions of Critical Care Nursing, 10,* 354–363.

Campinha-Bacote, J. (1988). Culturological assessment—an important factor in psychiatric consultation-liaison nursing. *Archives of Psychiatric Nursing, 2,* 244–250.

Canam, C. (2005). Illuminating the clinical nurse specialist role of advanced practice nursing: A qualitative study. *Canadian Journal of Nursing Leadership, 18,* 70–89.

Caplan, G. (1970). *The theory and practice of mental health consultation.* New York: Basic.

D'Affiliti, J. G. (2005). A psychiatric clinical nurse specialist as liaison to OB/GYN practice. *Journal of Obstetrics and Gynecological Neonatal Nursing, 34,* 280–285.

Davidson, S., & Noyes, R. (1973). Psychiatric nursing consultation on the burn unit. *American Journal of Nursing, 73,* 1715–1718.

Deighton, R. M., Gurris, N., & Traue, H. (2007). Factors affecting burnout and compassion fatigue in psychotherapists treating torture survivors: Is the therapist's attitude to working through trauma relevant? *Journal of Traumatic Stress, 20,* 63–75.

De Vito Dabbs, A., Curran, C. R., & Lenz, E. R. (2000). A database to describe the practice component of the CNS role. *Clinical Nurse Specialist, 14,* 174–187.

Doka, K. J. (1989). *Disenfranchised grief: Recognizing hidden sorrow.* Lexington, MA: Lexington.

Doka, K. J. (1993). *Living with a life-threatening illness: A guide for patients, their families, and caregivers.* New York: Lexington.

Dombeck, M. T., & Brody, S. L. (1995). Clinical supervision: A three-way mirror. *Archives of Psychiatric Nursing, 9,* 3–10.

Dumas, R., & Leonard, R. (1963). The effect of nursing on the incidence of postoperative vomiting. *Nursing Research, 12,* 12–15.

Elder, R. (1963). What is the patient saying? *Nursing Forum, 2,* 25–37.

Elder, R., & Diers, D. (1963). The patient comes to the hospital. *Nursing Forum, 2,* 89–93.

Faast, M., & Elstun, N. (1979). Psychiatric emergency service: A growing specialty. *Journal of Psychosocial and Mental Health Services, 16,* 13–19.

Fife, B. (1986). Establishing the mental health clinical specialist role in the medical setting. *Issues in Mental Health Nursing, 8,* 15–23.

Fife, B., & Lemler, S. (1983). The psychiatric clinical specialist: A valuable asset in the general hospital. *Journal of Nursing Administration, 13,* 14–17.

Fincannon, J. (1988). Meperidine addiction associated with amphotericin treatment in leukemia: Case study and staff reactions. *Archives of Psychiatric Nursing, 2,* 302–306.

Forhan-Andrianos, A., & Swain, C. R. (1979). Interfacing the role of the psychiatric clinical nurse specialist with a hospital emergency room setting. *Journal of Psychosocial and Mental Health Services, 4,* 24–26.

Frampton, D. B. (1998). Sexual assault: The role of the advanced-practice nurse in identifying and treating victims. *Clinical Nurse Specialist, 12,* 177–182.

Frueh, B. C., Monnier, J., Yim, E., Grubaugh, A. L., Hamner, M. B., & Knapp, R. G. (2007). A randomized trial of telepsychiatry for post-traumatic stress disorder. *Journal of Telemedicine and Telecare, 13,* 142–147.

Goldstein, M. J. (1979). Psychiatric clinical specialist in the general hospital. *Journal of Nursing Administration, 9,* 34–37.

Grant, S. M. (1988). The hospitalized AIDS patient and the psychiatric liaison nurse. *Archives of Psychiatric Nursing, 2,* 35–39.

Hackett, T. P., Cassem, N. H., Stern, T. A., & Murray, G. B. (1997). Beginnings: Consultation Psychiatry in a general hospital. In N. H. Cassem, T. A. Stern, J. F. Rosenbaum, & M. S. Jellinek (Eds.), *Massachusetts handbook of general psychiatry* (4th ed., pp. 1–9). St. Louis, MO: Mosby.

Hart, C. A. (1990). The role of the PCLN in the ethical decisions to remove life-sustaining treatments. *Archives of Psychiatric Nursing, 5,* 370–377.

Hedlund, N. (1978). Mental health nursing consultation in the general hospital. *Patient Counseling and Health Education, 1,* 85–88.

Hilty, D. M., Marks, S. L., Urness, D., Yellowlees, P. M. & Nesbitt, T. S. (2004). Clinical and educational telepsychiatry applications: A review. *Canadian Journal of Psychiatry, 49,* 1–3.

Hilty, D. M., Yellowlees, P. M., Cobb, H. C., Bourgeois, J. A., Neufeld, J. D., & Nesbitt, T. S. (2006). Models of telepsychiatric consultation-liaison service to rural primary care. *Psychosomatics, 47,* 152–157.

Holstein, S., & Schwab, J. (1965). A coordinated consultation program for nurses and psychiatrists. *Journal of the American Medical Association, 194,* 491–493.

Ingersoll, G. L., & Jones, L. S. (1992). The art of the consultation note. *Clinical Nurse Specialist, 6,* 218–220.

Issacharoff, A., Goddahn, J., Schneider, D., Maysonett, J., & Smith, B. (1970). Psychiatric nurses as consultants in a general hospital. *Hospital and Community Psychiatry, 21,* 361–367.

Jackson, H. (1969). Expanded practice in psychiatric nursing. *Nursing Clinics of North America, 4,* 527–540.

Jimerson, S. S. (1986). Expanded practice in psychiatric nursing. *Nursing Clinics of North America, 21,* 527–535.

Johnson, B. S. (1963). Psychiatric nurse consultant in a general hospital. *Nursing Outlook, 2,* 728–729.

Jorsh, M. S. (2006). Somatoform disorders: The role of consultation liaison psychiatry. *International Review of Psychiatry, 18,* 61–65.

Kane, J. (1992). Allowing the novice to succeed: Transitional support in critical care. *Critical Care Quarterly, 15,* 17–22.

Kennerly, S. (2006). Positioning advanced practice nurses for financial success in clinical practice. *Nurse Educator, 31,* 218–222.

Kessler, R. C., Chiu, W. T., Demler, O., Merikangas, K. R., & Walters, E. E. (2005). Prevalence, severity, and comorbidity of 12-month DSM-IV disorders in the

National Comorbidity Survey Replication. *Archives of General Psychiatry, 62,* 617–627.

Kilminster, S., Cottrell, D., Grant, J. & Jolly, B. (2007). AMEE Guide No. 27: Effective educational and clinical supervision. *Medical Teacher, 29,* 2–19.

Krakowski, A. J. (1975). Psychiatric consultation in the general hospital: An exploration of resistances. *Diseases of the Nervous System, 36,* 242–244.

Krupnick, S. (1990). Recognizing and avoiding negative addictions in your life. *Journal of Holistic Nursing Practice, 4,* 20–31.

Kurlowicz, L. H. (1996). Barriers to recognition of depression in hospitalized older adults. *Image: Journal of Nursing Scholarships, 29,* 96.

Kurlowicz, L. H. (1998). Psychiatric consultation-liaison nursing. In A. W. Burgess (Ed.), *Advanced-practice psychiatric nursing* (pp. 239–256). Stamford, CT: Appleton & Lange.

Kurlowicz, L. H. (2001). Benefits of psychiatric consultation-liaison nurse interventions for older hospitalized patients and their nurses. *Archives of Psychiatric Nursing, 15,* 53–61.

Lewis, A., & Levy, J. S. (1982). *Psychiatric liaison nursing: The theory and clinical practice.* Reston, VA: Reston.

Lippitt, G., & Lippitt, R. (1978). *The consulting process in action.* San Diego, CA: University Associates.

Marshall, R. J., & Marshall, S. V. (1988). *Transference-countertransference matrix.* New York: Columbia University Press.

Meadows, G. N., Harvey, C. A., Joubert, L., Barton, D., & Bedi, G. (2007). Best practices: The consultation-liaison in primary care psychiatry program: A structured approach to long-term collaboration. *Psychiatric Services, 58,* 1036–1038.

Miller, L. E. (1983). Resistance to the consultation process. *Nursing Leadership, 6,* 10–15.

Minarik, P. A. (1992). Second license for advanced-practice nursing practice? *Clinical Nurse Specialist, 6,* 221–222.

Minarik, P. A., & Neese, J. B. (2002). Essential educational content for advanced-practice in psychiatric consultation-liaison nursing. *Archives in Psychiatric Nursing, 16,* 3–15.

Moschler, L. B., & Fincannon, J. (1992). Subspecialization within psychiatric consultation liaison nursing. *Archives in Psychiatric Nursing, 6,* 234–238.

Moulden, H. M., & Firestone, P. (2007). Vicarious traumatization: The impact on therapists who work with sexual offenders. *Trauma, Violence and Abuse, 8,* 67–83.

Nelson, J., & Davis, D. (1979). Educating the psychiatric liaison nurse. *Journal of Nursing Education, 18,* 14–20.

Nelson, J., & Davis, D. (1980). Educating the psychiatric liaison nurses: Changes in characteristics over a limited time period. *General Hospital Psychiatry, 23,* 41–45.

Norwood, S. K. (1998). Psychiatric consultation-liaison nursing: Revisiting the role. *Clinical Nurse Specialist, 12,* 153–156.

Peplau, H. (1964). Psychiatric nursing skills and the general hospital patient. *Nursing Forum, 3,* 56–58.

Peterson, S. (1969). The psychiatric nurse specialist in a general hospital. *Nursing Outlook, 17,* 56–58.

Pranulis, M. A. (1972). A factor affecting the welfare of the coronary patient. *Nursing Clinics of North America, 7,* 445–455.

Przepiorka, K. M., & Bender, L. (1977). Psychiatric nursing consultation in a university medical center. *Hospital and Community Psychiatry, 28,* 755–758.

Robinson, L. (1968). Liaison psychiatric nursing. *Perspectives in Psychiatric Care, 6,* 87–91.

Robinson, L. (1972). A psychiatric nursing liaison program. *Nursing Outlook, 20,* 454–457.

Robinson, L. (1974). *Liaison nursing: Psychological approach to patient care.* Philadelphia: F. A. Davis.

Robinson, L. (1987). Psychiatric consultation-liaison nursing and psychiatric consultation-liaison doctoring: Similarities and differences. *Archives of Psychiatric Nursing, 1,* 73–80.

Rutherford, D. E. (1988). Consultation: A review and analysis of the literature. *Journal of Professional Nursing, 4,* 339–344.

Samter, J., Scherer, M., & Shulman, D. (1981). Interface of psychiatric clinical specialist in a community setting. *Journal of Psychosocial Nursing and Mental Health Services, 19,* 20–29.

Sharrock, J., Grigg, M., Happell, B., Keeble-Devlin, B., & Jennings, S. (2006). The mental health nurse: A valuable addition to the consultation-liaison team. *International Journal of Mental Health Nursing, 15,* 35–43.

Sharrock, J., & Happell, B. (2001). The role of the psychiatric consultation-liaison nurse in the improved care of patients experiencing mental health problems receiving care within a general hospital environment. *Contemporary Nursing, 11,* 260–270.

Sharrock, J., & Happell, B. (2002). The psychiatric consultation-liaison nurse: Thriving in a general hospital setting. *International Journal of Mental Health Nursing, 11,* 24–33.

Shore, J. H., & Manson, S. M. (2004). The American Indian veteran and posttraumatic stress disorder: A telehealth assessment and formulation. *Culture, Medicine & Psychiatry, 28,* 231–243.

Smith, G. C. (2003). The future of consultation-liaison psychiatry. *Australian and New Zealand Journal of Psychiatry, 37,* 150–159.

Sparacino, P. S. A. (1998). The advanced-practice nurse and measuring outcomes of care. *Clinical Nurse Specialist, 12,* 176.

Titlebaum, H., Hart, C. A., & Romano-Egan, J. (1992). Interagency psychiatric consultation-liaison nursing peer review and peer board: Quality assurance and empowerment. *Archives of Psychiatric Nursing, 6,* 125–131.

Tommasini, N. R. (1992). The impact of a staff support group on work environment of a specialty unit. *Archives of Psychiatry Nursing, 6,* 40–47.

Wand, T. (2004). Mental health liaison nursing in the emergency department: On-site expertise and enhanced coordination of care. *Australian Journal of Advanced Nursing, 22,* 25–31.

Watson, E. (2006). CAMHS liaison: Supporting care in general paediatric settings. *Paediatric Nursing, 18,* 30–33.

Yakimo, R., Kurlowicz, L. H., & Murray, R. B. (2004). Evaluation of outcomes in psychiatric consultation-liaison nursing practice. *Archives of Psychiatric Nursing, 18,* 215–227.

SUGGESTED READINGS

Antai-Otong, D. (2004). *Psychiatric emergencies*. Eau Claire, WI: PESI Healthcare.

Antai-Otong, D. (2007). *Nurse-client communication: A life span approach*. Sudbury, MA: Jones and Bartlett Publishers.

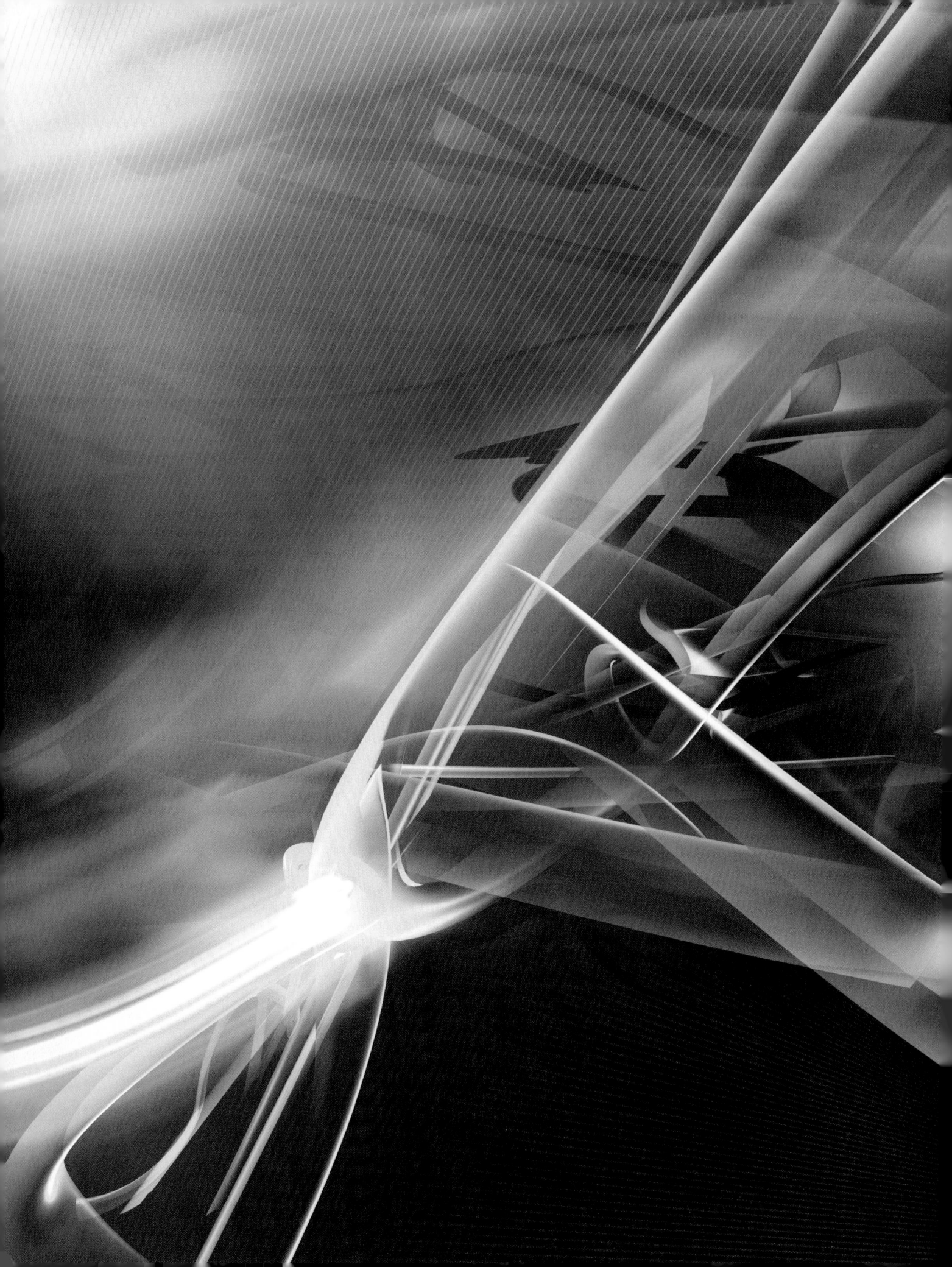

CHAPTER 36

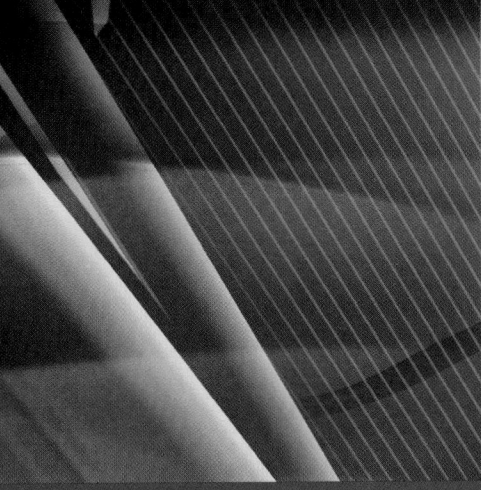

Psychiatric Nursing Research

Rose Nieswiadomy, PhD, RN
Deborah Antai-Otong, MS, APRN, BC, FAAN

KEY TERMS

Client Advocate: A person who tries to ensure that the rights of all prospective research subjects and actual subjects are adequately protected.

Critiquer of Research Findings: A person who evaluates research findings and determines the usefulness of these findings to nursing practice.

Data Collector: A person who gathers information for a research study, such as obtaining information from research subjects.

Principal Investigator: A person who takes the major role in the development and conduct of a research study.

Qualitative Research: Research that focuses on the meaning of the experiences (phenomena) to individuals rather than on the generalizability of study results.

Quantitative Research: Research that focuses on gathering numerical data, with the intent of generalizing the findings of the study.

Utilizer of Research Findings: A person who integrates research findings into clinical practice.

COMPETENCIES

Upon completion of this chapter, the learner should be able to:

1. Recall the steps in the scientific research process.
2. Analyze the roles of psychiatric nurses in research.
3. Discuss the results of some of the research studies across the life span that have been conducted by psychiatric nurses.
4. Explain barriers to research in psychiatric nursing.
5. Understand the need for quantitative and qualitative research in psychiatric nursing.
6. Describe the role of the National Institute of Mental Health in fostering psychiatric research.
7. Explain future needs for psychiatric nursing research.

CHAPTER OUTLINE

Issues in Research

Biological-Behavioral Factors

Stress and Coping

Technological Factors

Life Span Issues

Psychosocial Factors

Health Promotion and Disease Prevention

Steps in the Scientific Research Process

Identify the Problem to Be Studied

Survey the Literature on the Topic

Develop the Framework

Formulate Research Questions or Study Hypothesis

Operationally Define the Study Terms

Choose the Design for the Study

Select the Study Sample

Collect the Data

Analyze the Data

Communicate the Study Findings

The Role of the Nurse

The Generalist Nurse

The Advanced-Practice Registered Nurse

Principal Investigator

Member of a Research Team

Data Collector

Client Advocate

Critiquer of Research Findings

Utilizer of Research Findings

Published Research

Research across the Life Span

Childhood

Adolescence

Adulthood

Older Adulthood

Barriers to Psychiatric Research

Quantitative and Qualitative Research in Psychiatric-Mental Health Nursing

National Institute of Mental Health

National Institute of Nursing Research

Future Needs of Psychiatric Nursing Research

Nurses, like other health care providers, must define and promote their role in various health care settings, and research will help them accomplish this. As psychiatric nursing confronts challenges of this century, clinicians need to be continually apprised of technological and biological advances in treating mental disorders in the changing health care system. A host of issues present themselves as potential topics for psychiatric nursing research, such as the following:

◆ The link between biological interventions and behavioral responses

◆ The impact of health care trends (payment systems, lengths of stay, and community and primary-care provisions) on mental health systems

◆ Responses to demographic changes, such as increases in the number of older adults, people with varied cultural and ethnic backgrounds, and the number of people with chronic illness

◆ A comparison of complementary therapies and conventional therapies in the treatment of mental disorders

◆ Identification and assessment of high-risk populations and their needs

◆ The influence of culture, ethnicity, gender, and age on biological responses to pharmacologic agents

◆ Initiation and maintenance of preventive health care program

◆ Continuous rehabilitative care of persons with chronic mental illnesses

◆ Randomized controlled trials of nonpharmacologic interventions, such as cognitive behavioral therapy

◆ The influence of genetics on client symptoms and responses

◆ Outcomes of care based on nurse-centered interventions

Psychiatric nursing has long trailed other nursing specialties in conducting research. Poster, Betz, and Randall (1992) attributed this disparity to several factors: (1) a lack of psychiatric-mental health nursing coalition to help psychiatric nurses understand and employ research techniques; (2) a scarcity of nurses educationally and clinically prepared to conduct research; (3) a general lack of administrative support in the institutions where psychiatric nurses are employed; (4) a negative perception of research among psychiatric nurses. The authors found that positive attitudes toward research among psychiatric nurses paralleled the level of education these nurses possessed. Additionally, conducting research was found to be an expectation of advanced-practice psychiatric nurses, whereas the generalist nurse faced more barriers to research such as lack of administrative support and more focus on client care.

McCabe (2000) expressed the urgency of reframing the discipline of psychiatric nursing and bringing it into the twenty-first century. Major concerns included the current crisis in psychiatric-mental health nursing because leaders failed to respond to the realities of today's health care arena and its impact on the role of psychiatric nurses. Her solutions focused on a national consensus building process that included four critical components: redefining core concepts of psychiatric-mental health nursing; identifying clinical competencies that reflect these core components; matching and anticipating the realities of practice issues; and developing a research agenda that enables psychiatric nursing to expand its knowledge base. All of these components are significant to the survival of psychiatric-mental health nursing. However, of particular interest is the fourth component that addressed the development of a research agenda.

McCabe (2000) describes research as the portal to new knowledge because it enables psychiatric nurses to test theory and advances evidence-based practices. In addition, she recommended that psychiatric nursing needs a research agenda that reflects outcomes research, determinants of effective health care, nursing service models, and standards of practice for the chronically and persistently mentally ill. Likewise, the research agenda must also include positive aspects of mental illness and emotions, vulnerability factors, and a national psychiatric-mental health nursing research agenda (McCabe, 2000). These concepts were also supported by the American Nurses Association's (ANA) (2000) publication, *The Scope and Standards of Psychiatric-Mental Health Practice*. Overall, psychiatric nursing research must reflect realities of the present health care environment, identify vulnerable populations, and develop evidence-based research that advances mental health across the life span.

As psychiatric nursing moves further into the twenty-first century, various themes begin to emerge concerning an aging and diverse society; advances in technology, genetics, and telecommunication; and strong advocacy and demand for quality, safe, and client-centered mental health care. Mounting violence against children, families, older adults, and women offers opportunities for psychiatric nurses to explore and implement evidence-based interventions that reduce the acute and long-term effects of violence and restore dignity and normalcy across the life span. Moreover, growing casualties from global wars and terrorism challenge psychiatric nurses to carve out research agendas to address the needs of vulnerable populations. Demands from Congress to provide timely and quality care to war-injured veterans and their families suffering from a myriad of psychiatric, emotional, and physical losses will impact psychiatric nursing for many generations.

This chapter reviews further potential areas of psychiatric nursing research and the roles of the generalist nurse and advanced-practice nurse. In addition, it presents an overview of major steps in the research process and implications for psychiatric nursing practice.

ISSUES IN RESEARCH

Neurological factors, stress and coping, life span, and psychosocial factors are contributing issues in research that are discussed in the next sections.

BIOLOGICAL-BEHAVIORAL FACTORS

As previously stated, integrating biological and behavioral concepts into psychiatric nursing practice, education, and research

has become increasingly germane in the new millennium. Although explorations into the relationship between biological processes and behavioral responses is not new to medicine, nursing research in this area remains in its infancy. Historically, psychiatric nurses have been instrumental in research drug trials; there is a need to expand this role and explore further the behavioral changes brought about not only by psychotropic drugs but also by other biological interventions.

Apart from administrating psychotropic medications evidence-based research must be used to guide nursing practice. Data from these studies must be used to establish clinical parameters to monitor client responses, develop client-centered interventions to manage psychiatric symptoms and behavioral responses. Evidence-based psychiatric care enables the psychiatric nurse to integrate data that advances health promotion, self-care, disease management, and understand ethical and legal issues related to participation in research.

STRESS AND COPING

Stress often plays a major role in mental health. Research is needed to identify and help clients deal with distressful responses, including intense anxiety, grief reaction, depression, and maladaptive coping behaviors such as violence, substance-related disorders, and suicide attempt. Research can help practitioners develop strategies to promote comfort, reduce symptoms of anxiety, and reduce the deleterious courses of stress-related responses.

TECHNOLOGICAL FACTORS

Growing changes in the health care system require innovative strategies to enhance communication between the psychiatric nurse, clients, and their families. With society's growing use of the Internet, e-mails, and other telecommunication as a venue of nurse-client interactions, health education and health care need to receive care, psychiatric nurses must be prepared to respond to their needs. Despite the growing use of technologies, psychiatric nurses have been relatively slow with adoption of varied technologies to advance health care to monitor client responses to treatment and adherence to medications, increase access to care, provide health education, consultation to providers, advance screening processes and delivery interventions, apply telehealth and enhance self-care and disease management. Nursing research must explore strategies to integrate technology into mental health care and collaborate with the client to ensure quality, safe, and cost-effective health care.

LIFE SPAN ISSUES

Research into stress and coping in school-age children has produced useful tools such as the Schoolagers Coping Strategy Inventory, which arose from an examination of the type, frequency, and effectiveness of children's coping behaviors (Ryan, 1989). Research showed that the effects of stressful events such as loss and intimidation can have lasting effects on children

(Jacobson, 1994). Nursing research can explore these areas and provide guidance on how to help children reduce stress.

Research can offer unexpected solutions to common problems. For example, Melnyk's study (1994) reported how informational interventions can help children and their parents cope with hospitalization and home adjustment. Awareness of possible reactions in the hospitalized child helped parents cope with the child's illness so that they could support the child during various procedures by serving as buffer and lessening the negative impact of the hospitalization and illness.

A more recent study conducted by Li and Lopez (2005) confirm the importance of mitigating anxiety and other emotional responses in children during stressful medical procedures and tests. A convenience sample of 82 children admitted for day surgery was recruited in this study. Because of the dearth of objective tools to document children's emotional responses during stressful diagnostic and medical procedures the researchers used a panel of nurse experts to develop the Children's Emotional Manifestation Scale. Researchers submit that nurses can use this scale to assess stress levels in children preoperatively and use interventions to mitigate anxiety and improve coping skills in children undergoing surgical procedures (Li & Lopez, 2005).

Research can guide psychiatric nurses working with older adults experiencing depression. Depression in older adults is a growing concern due to its potential impact on quality of life and high incidence of suicide in this age group. Researchers also stress the importance of screening older adults for depression. Interventions that increase self-esteem and personal mastery lie within the domain of nursing. Group reminiscing in older adults is not a new concept, but a recent study further implicated it as a useful modality in the treatment—suggesting the significance of assessing older adults for depression (Stinson & Kirk, 2006).

From reading and performing such research, nurses can learn to develop and enhance age-appropriate coping patterns and preventive interventions to promote adaptation and reduce mental illness in all age groups.

PSYCHOSOCIAL FACTORS

A descriptive, qualitative study of adults with neural tubal defects (Nehring & Faux, 2006) using a naturalistic inquiry of 16 Caucasian, 11 African Americans, and 15 Mexican Americans explored the meaning of the past, present, and future life span and health concerns of adults with neural tubal defects. Findings from this study revealed three major themes: uncertainty about the future, concerns about access to health care, and concerns information and advocacy. Findings from this study provided information about adult trajectories concerning neural tubal defects across the life span and opportunities to provide anticipatory guidance and health care to individuals with psychosocial stressors. Researchers also concluded that individuals with lifelong health problems need health education to promote independence and self-advocacy (Nehring, & Faux, 2006).

HEALTH PROMOTION AND DISEASE PREVENTION

Research is greatly needed to address the needs of individuals, families, and communities from varied ethnicities, cultures, gender, and underserved and vulnerable groups such as seriously ill children, troubled adolescents, and frail older adults. Cultural sensitivity and research that ensures access and health parity are greatly needed to promote health and reduce disease and disability. Based on educational preparation psychiatric nurses are poised to develop holistic interventions that are client-centered, promote self-care management, and address the needs of caregivers. Research indicates that caregiving crosses all socioeconomic stratum and places enormous strain on the client, family, and communities (Chang & Horrocks, 2006). The high price of health care often contributes to the burden of caregiving and explains growing provision of informal care in homes and communities. Assessing the needs of caregivers and intervening to reduce stress and mobilize resources are critical to health promotion and disease management and quality of life.

Researchers continually seek strategies to improve the assessment of psychiatric symptoms and clinical outcomes. A convenience sample of psychiatric nurses rated descriptions of the Inventory of Voice Experiences (IVE) and their impact on the selection of interventions for the management of verbal auditory hallucinations (England, Tripp-Reimer, & Rubenstein, 2004). Verbal auditory hallucinations are an element of auditory hallucinations in which linguistic, dialogical characteristics of hearing and responding to inner voices are experienced (Rojcewicz & Rojcewicz, 1997). Data from the study provide nurses with opportunities to distinguish specific characteristics, antecedents, and consequences of voice hearing along with their implications for health and well-being. Researchers also submit that these data will facilitate identification of more explicit and meaningful treatment options for helping clients who hallucinate manage their voices (England et al., 2004; Nehring & Faux, 2006).

The remainder of this chapter reviews basic steps in the scientific research process and discusses various implications for psychiatric-mental health nursing.

STEPS IN THE SCIENTIFIC RESEARCH PROCESS

The steps in the scientific research process are generally similar for each study. Although the number of steps varies according to sources in the literature, the steps are fairly consistent. These steps are summarized in Table 36–1.

IDENTIFY THE PROBLEM TO BE STUDIED

Determining a problem to be studied can be challenging. The most difficult part is narrowing the subject down to a workable

TABLE 36–1
Steps in the Scientific Research Process

1. Identify the problem to be studied.
2. Survey the literature on the topic/problem.
3. Develop a study framework.
4. Formulate research questions or study hypothesis.
5. Operationally define the study terms.
6. Choose the design for the study.
7. Select the study sample.
8. Collect the data.
9. Analyze the data.
10. Communicate the study findings.

topic. The study topic may be based on personal experiences, previous research, or the suggestions provided by others in the literature.

Contributions of the psychiatric-mental health nurse at both the basic and advanced levels are vast and involve the use of research methods and application of findings to nursing practice. The ANA's (2000) publication, *The Scope and Standards of Psychiatric-Mental Health Practice*, denotes that the generalist nurse uses empirical data to improve clinical care and identifies practice problems for research study. In addition, this document describes the advanced-practice nurse's involving collaboration "with others in the research process to discover, examine, and test knowledge, theories and creative approaches to practice" (p. 48).

SURVEY THE LITERATURE ON THE TOPIC

Researchers do not want to "reinvent the wheel." Therefore, a review of the literature is necessary to determine what, if any, research has already been conducted on this particular topic. Other purposes of reviewing the literature are to help determine the study design and to discover if there are existing instruments available to measure the study variables (characteristics or attributes that differ among the people or objects that are being studied).

DEVELOP THE FRAMEWORK

The goal of research is to build a scientific knowledge base. The theoretical or conceptual framework for a study helps provide a knowledge base into which the study results can be placed. Theory and research are intertwined: Research can be used to test and refine theory, but studies without a theoretical basis provide a set of isolated facts. Research that is valuable in providing understanding of the study results. In other

words, the researcher can better explain why the study findings turned out as they did.

FORMULATE RESEARCH QUESTIONS OR STUDY HYPOTHESIS

Research questions allow the investigator to focus on specific aspects of the study problem. If the study framework is strong enough to make a prediction about the study results, a hypothesis is used to state the study prediction. Hypotheses should be based on theories or previous research.

Psychiatric nurses are in pivotal positions to identify research questions linked to improving client care. For instance, if the generalist nurse recognizes that a certain population of clients is exhibiting side effects from their medications resulting in nonadherence to treatment planning, efforts to understand the relationship between these factors is a research question. By working with the advanced-practice nurse, the generalist nurse can assist in looking for causal relationships and develop interventions that address these concerns.

OPERATIONALLY DEFINE THE STUDY TERMS

The study variables should be operationally defined, which means that the means of measuring or observing the variables must be specified. If anxiety were one of the study variables, the exact way of measuring this concept should be specified; for example, anxiety may be measured by pulse rate.

CHOOSE THE DESIGN FOR THE STUDY

The plan for how a study will be conducted is called the *study design*. Research designs also refer to the researchers' overall plan for answering the research questions or testing its hypotheses. Polit and Beck (2005) submit that in a quantitative paradigm, the design outlines strategies that are necessary to generate data that are factual and interpretable. Qualitative research focuses on the meaning of the experiences to individuals rather than on the generalizability of study results. Polit and Beck (2005) also submit that a quantitative research design comprises decisions pertaining to the following aspects of the study:

◆ Is an intervention necessary?

◆ What sorts of comparisons will be made?

◆ What procedures are necessary to control extraneous variables?

◆ When and how often will data be collected from study participants?

◆ In what setting will the study occur?

In essence, the research design integrates and guides methodological decisions and defines the direction that the research adopts.

Dimensions of quantitative designs vary and depend on the amount of control the researcher has over the independent variable, ranging from the greatest amount of control as seen in experimental designs to the least naturalistic and laboratory. For the purpose of this chapter, nonexperimental and experimental designs will be reviewed.

Designs can be broadly classified as experimental or nonexperimental. In an experimental study in nursing, the researcher usually carries out some type of intervention with a group of subjects and measures the outcomes. In nonexperimental studies, the researcher makes no interventions but rather collects data and records of what has been observed.

Qualitative research designs focus on several aspects that are usually post hoc characteristics of an event in the field rather than the designated features previously planned, as seen in quantitative research. The primary intent of qualitative research is to fully depict and explain a phenomenon. Domains of qualitative research range from cultural and lived experience perspective to environmental and social factors.

SELECT THE STUDY SAMPLE

A set of persons or objects that are of interest to the researcher must be selected. This is usually done by choosing a large group of interest, called the *population,* and then selecting a subset of this large group to study. Researchers can choose random or nonrandom samples. Most groups that have been studied by nurses are nonrandom convenience samples because they were chosen from a group that was convenient or available. This type of sampling process is not the most scientific; however, less time and money is involved in this type of sampling process.

COLLECT THE DATA

The data are the facts or pieces of information that the researcher collects in a study. The researcher decides what data to collect and how to collect them; who will collect the data; and where and when the data will be collected. Data collection may be a time-consuming task, but it is often considered the most enjoyable part of the research process.

ANALYZE THE DATA

Many nurses fear the step of analyzing the data because they believe that they must be able to compute statistical formulas. However, with today's computer technology, data analysis has become quite simple. A researcher can input large amounts of data and receive almost instantaneous results. In addition, statisticians are now available to help with data analysis. After the data are analyzed, the researcher must try to interpret the findings. The results of the study are co pared to the researcher's expectation that was stated in the hypothesis. Results are also compared with those of similar studies in the literature. After the findings have been interpreted, the researcher should suggest implications or changes that should be made in nursing practice, education, administration, and research as a result of the findings.

COMMUNICATE THE STUDY FINDINGS

Study results must be communicated to others before the research process is complete. There are a multitude of ways to communicate the results of nursing research, including oral presentations at research conferences, poster presentations, and publications of the results in professional journals and other publications.

THE ROLE OF THE NURSE

Psychiatric-mental health nurses claim that they are unqualified to conduct research and therefore believe that this relieves them of the responsibility of being involved in research. Although the role of the principal investigator is important, it is by no means the only role that nurses can play in research. Other roles include being a member of a research team, data collector, client advocate during the research study, critiquer of research findings, and utilizer of research findings.

THE GENERALIST NURSE

The generalist nurse, along with the advanced-practice nurse, is responsible for advancing the development of the field of mental health by participating in research. Typically, the generalist nurse uses research data to guide practice and provide evidence-based care. In addition, the generalist nurse must be able to demonstrate an awareness and value of research and be an intelligent consumer of research. For instance, a journal club that focuses on research pertaining to medication side effects, screening tools such as the Abnormal Involuntary Movement Scale (AIMS), health education, and family involvement offers a wealth of research concerning mental health care. Other areas of interests may include identifying clinical problems for research study, improving health care, and collaborating with members of the research team.

THE ADVANCED-PRACTICE REGISTERED NURSE

Research opportunities for the advanced-practice nurse vary with educational preparation and level of expertise. The role of the advanced-practice nurse who has a master's degree may involve collaborating with others in the research process to discover, examine, and test knowledge, theories, and develop innovative approaches to practice. Advanced-practice mental health nurses must be sophisticated consumers of research and active members of the research team. In addition, the advanced-practice nurse needs to develop research that is evidence based and initiates a plan of care that reflects clinical expertise to improve health and improve quality of life. The advanced-practice nurse who has a PhD is more likely to be involved in several areas concerning research such as appraising, designing, and conducting research.

Regardless of the role of the psychiatric-mental health nurse in research, the primary goal is to benefit people who are struggling with mental illness. Ultimately, nurses who participate in and conduct research improve the quality of care and the quality of life of the client.

PRINCIPAL INVESTIGATOR

The principal investigator of a research study is the person who has played a major role in the development and conduct of the research. Serving as principal investigator requires special research preparation, generally obtained in a master's or doctoral program. As the number of nurses with advanced educational preparation in research has increased, so has the number of research studies. However, many one-of-a-kind studies have been conducted as part of the requirement for an advanced degree, with few replication studies conducted thereafter. These isolated bits of knowledge have provided only slight advancement in the body of psychiatric-mental health nursing knowledge. Nurse researchers must be willing to continue their area of research after they complete their educational programs. The body of knowledge for psychiatric nurses will expand only as rapidly as there are nurses willing to conduct research studies.

MEMBER OF A RESEARCH TEAM

Each psychiatric nurse should consider becoming a member of the research team. The type of research preparation received in nursing school and the amount of clinical experience will dictate the nurse's ability to serve on a research team. Nurses with baccalaureate and higher degrees may be qualified for the role of coinvestigator. As nurses participate in research, it is quite likely that they will become interested in conducting their own studies.

DATA COLLECTOR

Data collectors are important to the success of a research project. Many research studies would never be completed without the assistance of data collectors. It is difficult for the principal investigator to do all the data collection that is required in a study.

Nurse researchers often point out the opportunity for the nurse, while collecting data, to educate consumers about risks factors in their daily lives. An example is that when the nurse is drawing blood, she can also discuss the benefits of exercise, the importance of nutritional habits, and stress-reduction techniques.

CLIENT ADVOCATE

The ethical aspects of a study are important. In the role of client advocate, the nurse can ensure that the rights of all prospective subjects and actual subjects are adequately protected. Nurses can answer questions about the study and make sure that the potential subjects fully understand the study before agreeing to participate. Nurses should also be available to subjects during the study if questions arise.

CRITIQUER OF RESEARCH FINDINGS

Nurses have to take responsibility for being informed about the most recent research findings in their areas of practice. When fulfilling the role of a critiquer of research findings, the nurse reviews and determines their applicability to nursing practice. The evaluation of research is not a simple task, but this skill can be attained by all nurses to some degree. It is beyond the scope of this book to present critiquing guidelines. For further information about critiquing, see Nieswiadomy (1998). For nurses lacking in formal preparation in critiquing, self-instruction, attending workshops, and joining critiquing groups at work are methods to obtain this skill. Malone (1990) stated that "the bridge between research and clinical application is based on an informed staff" (p. 4).

UTILIZER OF RESEARCH FINDINGS

It is not sufficient for the nurse to be informed about research findings; applicable findings should be integrated into the nurse's practice. As a utilizer of research findings, the nurse ensures that the latest knowledge is integrated into practice. However, nurses, just like other people, are reluctant to accept changes. Change is stressful and is frequently resisted. We want to do things "the way we have always done them."

Research findings are of little value if they are not used in practice. Nurses must be judicious in using the results of research studies, however. Therefore, it is extremely important that nurses know how to critique research results.

PUBLISHED RESEARCH

Research conducted by psychiatric-mental health nurses is not always easily identifiable in the literature. Because nurses in other specialty areas are also interested in mental health, the reader may be uncertain whether a particular study would qualify as psychiatric-mental health nursing research. If the research article concerns clients with a chronic mental illness, it is published in a nursing journal, and it is conducted by a nurse, the assumption can probably be made that the researcher is a psychiatric nurse.

McBride (1988) pointed out that nurses in the psychiatric specialty area have been more likely to study mental health than mental illness. Of the 400 psychiatric nursing references published between 1980 and 1989 that were reviewed by Fox (1992), fewer than 30 studies focused on chronic mental

TABLE 36–2
Examples of Studies on Chronic Mental Illness: 2000–2007

- Anders, R. L. (2000). Assessment of inpatient treatment of persons with schizophrenia: Implications for practice. *Archives of Psychiatric Nursing, 14,* 213–221.

- Kaas, M. J., Dehn, D., Dahl, D., Frank, K., Markley, J., & Hebert, P. (2000). A view of prescriptive collaboration: Perspectives of psychiatric-mental clinical nurse specialists and psychiatrists. *Archives of Psychiatric Nursing, 14,* 222–234.

- Matzkin, V. B., Geissler, C., Coniglio, R., Selles, J., & Bello, M. (2006). Cholesterol concentrations in patients with Anorexia Nervosa and in healthy controls. *International Journal of Psychiatric Nursing Research, 11,* 1283–1293.

- Schreiber, R., Stern, P. N., & Wilson, C. (2000). Being strong: How Black West-Indian Canadian women manage depression and its stigma. *Image: Journal of Nursing Scholarship, 32,* 39–42.

- Stinson, C. K., & Kirk, E. (2006). Structured reminiscence: An intervention to decrease depression and increase self-transcendence in older women. *Journal of Clinical Nursing, 15,* 208–218.

- Wagstaff, C. (2007). Towards understanding the self-perception of people with a psychotic illness who use illicit substances and have a history of disengagement from mental health services: Qualitative research. *International Journal of Psychiatric Nursing Research, 12,* 1503–1520.

illness. Fox discussed 24 of these studies in a chapter in the *Annual Review of Nursing Research* published in 1992. They are in Table 36–2.

Many published research studies that are classified as psychiatric-mental health nursing research are concerned with nurses themselves rather than clients. In Sill's classic research review article published in the 1977 issue of *Nursing Research*, the author indicated that one of the themes throughout the 1950s focuses on the personality characteristics, preferences, attitudes, and evaluation of learning of psychiatric nurses. One half of the studies discussed a book by Brooking entitled *Psychiatric Nursing Research*, published in England in 1986, which focuses on nurses. Although research concerning nurses themselves is important, a greater emphasis on psychiatric-mental health nursing research should be placed on clients.

For more information on the research that was published in the literature from 1952 to 1976, refer to Sills' excellent 1977 article, which discusses all types of psychiatric nursing research published during that period.

No other broad review of psychiatric-mental health nursing research since 1976 is available in the literature. However, in 1992, Fox presented a review of research specific to chronic mental illness that was published between 1980 and 1989. She surveyed general nursing research journals, such as *Nursing Research* and *Western Journal of Nursing*, and psychiatric nursing specialty journals, such as *Archives in Psychiatric Nursing, Issues in Mental Health Nursing,* the *Journal of Psychosocial Nursing and Mental Health Services,* and *Perspectives in Psychiatric Nursing.* She also reviewed issues of the *Community Mental Health Journal and Hospital and Community Psychiatry.* Research articles that were authored or coauthored by nurses (as determined by their published credentials) were included in this review.

The research was discussed under the following topics: community adjustment and intervention, recidivism, case management, client self-monitoring and client education, verbal and nonverbal communication, violence and seclusion, medication compliance, rural service use, and cultural compatibility. Fox (1992) reported that there is an increasing trend for psychiatric nurses to conduct qualitative rather than quantitative research. These two types of research designs are compared later in this chapter.

RESEARCH ACROSS THE LIFE SPAN

Life span issues continue to be an integral part of nursing research and parallel the current strategies goals of the NINR as more and more nurses explore the meaning of life experiences, develop cost-effective and evidence-based interventions, and collaborate with client, families, and communities to ensure holistic and culturally sensitive care and client-centered approaches. Research that focuses on acute and chronic illness across the life span is part of the mission of NINR. The following section discusses research literature across the life span. An example is presented of a clinical study for each age group.

CHILDHOOD

The role of the nurse in child psychiatry has been minimal, according to McBride (1988) because there are few graduate programs in this subspecialty, fewer nurses are entering this clinical specialty area, funding levels for children and youth are low, child psychiatric nurses are underutilized, and there is a lack of research and publications by nurses in this area. However, the enormous increase in psychotropic use in children and adolescents to manage psychiatric and behavioral disorders offers great opportunities for psychiatric nurses. The past two decades have revealed an alarming rise in prescriptions for stimulants for attention-deficit/hyperactivity disorder (ADHD) and antidepressants, particularly among 5- to 14-year-olds (Zito et al., 2003, 2006). Controlled clinical trials to determine the efficacy and safety of psychotropic use in children are rare (Greenhill, 1998). Data consistently demonstrate high psychotropic use, particularly stimulants in male gender, white race, 13 years of age, insured, Southerner, and functionally impaired (Cox, Motheral, Henderson, & Mager, 2003; Zito, et al., 2000). Concerns about this age group involve off-label (unlabeled) for treatment indications with a dearth of research that substantiates proven efficacy and approved use by the Food and Drug Administration (Alderman, Wolkow, & Fogel, 2006; Olfson, Marcus, Weissman, & Jensen, 2002). The paucity of randomized, double-blind controlled studies provide research initiatives to evaluate appropriate dosages, side-effect profiles, effectiveness, and safety of drug use in children.

The tremendous increase in psychotropic treatment in children and adolescents has also contributed to the development of reliable diagnostic tools tailored to children and adolescents to evaluate and monitor symptom management and quality of life during these developmental stages. One such study was conducted by Li and Lopez (2006). Researchers conducted a cross-sectional design to assess children's emotional responses to surgery. Children were asked to respond to the Chinese version of the State Anxiety Scale for Children. The researchers also monitored biological, behavioral, and emotional responses to stress. Findings from this study indicated that children's responses to stressful medical procedures vary and must be understood as a complex phenomenon (Li & Lopez, 2006).

Changing demographics in the U.S. population is also another area of interest for research. Research that enables the nurse to understand the impact of culture and ethnicity on the client's experience and improve the quality of nurse-client interactions is imperative to ensure client-centered care that integrates health practices, mores, religious and spiritual beliefs and preferences. In a study of communication skills and cultural awareness among health care professionals, Thomas and Cohn (2006) used an educational program to explore the impact of these variables on nurse-client interactions in clients with sickle cell disease. The results of the study demonstrated a positive and enduring impact on clinicians' ability to understand the clients' experience and communicate more effectively with clients with sickle cell disease.

One indication that psychiatric nurses may be showing more interest in children and adolescents was demonstrated by the publication in 1987 of the first issue of the *Journal of Child and Adolescent Psychiatric Nursing*. It is hoped that more research will be conducted with children in the future. However, the difficulty obtaining permission to conduct research with minors continues to limit research in this age group.

Jones and O'Brien (1990) described three unique child inpatient treatment techniques: (1) journal writing; (2) using clinical rounds with children; and (3) contracting for reduction in precaution levels. The child subjects were asked to rate the interventions. Journal writings were seen as helpful in sorting out and expressing feelings. The youth rounds helped the child inpatients to set daily goals. Finally, contracting for a change in precautions was rated high in helping the child inpatients keep their promises. Jones and O'Brien (1990) indicated that these three interventions provided the psychiatric nurses the opportunity to take a more active role in client treatment and promoted client involvement in the treatment process.

Examples of additional nursing research articles focusing on this and other age groups are found in Table 36–3.

ADOLESCENCE

Psychiatric nurses are increasingly conducting research with adolescents and publishing the results of these studies, although not as extensively as the research that is being conducted with adults. Again, it is important to mention the *Journal of Child and Adolescent Psychiatric Nursing*. The publication of this journal indicates psychiatric nurses' growing interest in this particular age group. However, obtaining permission to conduct research with this age group of minors is difficult, as is the case with children.

Yarcheski, Mahon, and Yarcheski (1999) examined three theories explaining state anger vis-à-vis among adolescents using hierarchical analysis. The stress theory, the differential emotions theory, and the personality trait theory were the basis of the development of explanatory theories of state anger for early adolescents. The sample consisted of 141 adolescents aged 12 to 14 years from an urban middle school. Approximately 77 percent were white and the remaining 23 percent were African American, Latino, or Asian American. The authors were surprised to find that the trait theory provided the strongest explanation for state anger in this population. That is, traits, such as trait anger and hostility, are generally enduring characteristics that eventually become integrated into the youth's personality and ultimately had greater weight in explaining anger than the relationship between person and environment. In comparison, anger responses to stress variables were the weakest and the authors attributed this to early adolescence, a time when complex cognitive processes are not fully developed.

Psychiatric nurses can use these data to develop preventive health promotion measures that involve assessing high-risk populations, such as prepuberty and early adolescence, for maladaptive coping skills and teaching or strengthening adaptive coping skills that enable them to manage their anger more effectively.

Other examples of recently published research articles on this age group are found in Table 36–3.

ADULTHOOD

Most research in psychiatric-mental health nursing has been conducted on adults. This is the largest group of clients seen by psychiatric nurses.

TABLE 36-3
Psychiatric Nursing Research across the Life Span: Published Studies

Childhood

Li, H. C. W., & Lopez, V. (2006). Assessing children's emotional responses to surgery: A multidimensional approach. *Journal of Advanced Nursing, 53*, 543–550.

Rice, M., & Broome, M. E. (2004). Incentives for children in research. *Journal of Nursing Scholarship, 36*, 167–172.

Brewer, S., Gleditsch, S. L., Syblik, D., Tietjens, M. E., & Vacik, H. W. (2006). Pediatric anxiety: Child life intervention in day surgery. *Journal of Pediatric Nursing, 21*, 13–22.

Speraw, S. (2006). Spiritual experiences of parents and caregivers who have children with disabilities or special needs. *Issues in Mental Health Nursing, 27*, 213–230.

Adolescence

Cotton, S., Zebracki, K., Rosenthal, S. L., Tsevat, J., & Drotar, D. (2006). Religion/spirituality and adolescent health outcomes: A review. *Journal of Adolescent Health, 38*, 472–480.

Jour Puskar, K. R., Sereika, S., Lamb, J., & Tusaie-Mumford, K. (2000). Substance abuse among high school students in rural Pennsylvania. *Journal of Addictions Nursing, 12*, 55–63.

Wong, Y. J., Rew, L., & Slaikeu, K. D. (2006). A systematic review of recent research on adolescent religiousity/spirituality and mental health. *Issues in Mental Health Nursing, 27*, 161–183.

Adults

Chang, K. H., & Horrocks, S. (2006). Lived experiences of family caregivers of mentally ill relatives. *Journal of Advanced Nursing, 53*, 435–443.

Irvine, F. E., Roberts, G. W., Jones, P., Spencer, L. H., Baker, C. R., & Williams, C. (2006). Communicative sensitivity in the bilingual healthcare setting: A qualitative study of language awareness, *Journal of Advanced Nursing, 53*, 422–434.

Sethabouppha, H., & Kane, C. (2005). Caring for the seriously mentally ill in Thailand: Buddhist family caregiving. *Archives of Psychiatric Nursing, 19*, 44–57.

Older Adulthood

Butler, F. R., & Zakari, N. (2005). Grandparents parenting grandchildren: Assessing health status, parental stress, and social supports. *Journal of Gerontonlogical Nursing, 31*, 43–54.

Ryan, R., Garlick, R., & Happell, B. (2006). Exploring the role of the mental health nurse in community mental health care of the aged. *Issues in Mental Health Nursing, 27*, 91–105.

Villaverde-Gutierrez, C., Araujo, E., Cruz, F., Roa, J. M., & Barbosa, W., et al. (2006). Quality of life of rural menopausal women in response to a customized exercise program. *Journal of Advanced Nursing, 54*, 11–19.

The growing number of caregivers across the life span makes caregiving research an important contribution to nursing practice. Young adults caring for a child with disabilities; the 21-year-old spouse who seeks to glean the meaning of her husband's traumatic brain injury on the quality of his and her life; the grandmother who raises her children; and the older adult caring for a loved one with Alzheimer's disease makes caregiving an integral part of today's society. Research that enables the nurse to design interventions that promote quality of life of informal caregivers and the client is sorely needed to address complex health care needs across the life span. Sethabouppha and Kane (2005) conducted a phenomenological study of 15 Thai Buddhist family caregivers of individuals with serious mental health problems to understand their perspectives about caregiving. Five themes emerged from this study, which included caregiving is a Buddhist belief, compassion, management, acceptance, and suffering. Nursing implications from this study included insights into the caregivers' experiences such as the degree of suffering, negative feelings associated with the role, and helping their loved ones manage their behavior and symptoms (Sethabouppha & Kane, 2005).

Examples of recently published research articles that the adult client are found in Table 36–3.

OLDER ADULTHOOD

The older adult population is a group in need of psychiatric-mental health nursing services (Fopma-Loy, 1989). Statistics indicate the great increase in the older adult population, and estimates suggest that by the year 2050, there will be more than 60 million people 65 years and older (Butler & Zakari, 2005; Fuller-Thomson & Minkler, 2000; U.S. Census Bureau, 2001). Although this group has needs for services similar to those of other adult groups, additional mental health services are needed because of the significant decline in physical status, loss of partners, and change in roles and lifestyles. These factors are expected to increase the risk of emotional distress and behavioral and social dysfunction (Puntil, 2005; Upton & Reed, 2005). The Coalition on Mental Health and Aging in 1995 proposed several strategies for dealing with their concerns, one of which was collecting data on late-life mental disorders. Older African Americans have higher rates of psychiatric disorders than other groups and are at higher risk for developing dementia and cognitive impairment. Depression and dementia are the most common mental health problems experienced by the aged.

Kurlowicz and colleagues (2005) conducted an exploratory study to determine the prevalence of depression among older African Americans attending an academic outpatient rehabilitation program using a depression with low somatic item content. Health records (n = 150) of the subjects seen during a 2-year period were examined, and depression was assessed by scores from the 30-item Geriatric Depression Scale (GDS). Findings from the study demonstrated that 30 percent of the sample scored positive for depression; 9 percent also reported having suicidal ideations within the previous week. The researchers concluded that six GDS items demonstrated difficulty discriminating between depressed and nondepressed—namely, being satisfied with life, getting bored easily, preferring to stay at home, finding life exciting, getting started on new projects, and being full of energy—and recommended additional testing of the GDS with like population of older, poor, and medically and functionally disabled older adults.

Examples of recently published research articles on the older adult client are found in Table 36–3.

BARRIERS TO PSYCHIATRIC RESEARCH

Historically researchers have identified the difficulties in studying clients with chronic mental disorders. Clients with the same psychiatric diagnosis vary—much more so than clients with the same medical diagnosis—in their degree of impairment and response to treatment. Laboratory values may provide a fairly reliable source of evaluation for a medical condition, but no similar methods for evaluating psychiatric conditions are available. The roles of genetics, culture, gender, and age challenge the generalizability of some data, particularly when drug trials or other treatments are limited to specific groups without consideration for variance in intricate neurobiological process, especially concerning drug metabolism. Apart from individual differences in response and

participation in clinical drug trials, a lack of consensus among researchers concerning diagnostic criteria and subject interpretations of findings from standardized research tools continues to be a barrier to psychiatric research.

There are ethical issues to be considered when conducting research with groups of people who may not be able to provide informed consent. Conducting research with clients experiencing psychological problems may be comparable to conducting research with children or the cognitively impaired older adults. The question arises as to whether informed can be met or if the client's symptoms interfere with the ability to understand a research study for which they volunteer. It is also difficult to obtain permission of institutional review boards to study clients with mental disorders. (See Chapter 8.)

QUANTITATIVE AND QUALITATIVE RESEARCH IN PSYCHIATRIC-MENTAL HEALTH NURSING

Most nursing research studies have been quantitative rather than qualitative in nature. Quantitative research focuses on gathering numerical data and making generalizations across groups of people. Qualitative research focuses on the meaning of experiences to people, and it is not as concerned about generalizing study results.

CRITICAL THINKING

1. What are the major characteristics of quantitative research?

2. Which of the following is an example of qualitative research?

   a. Reviewing recent studies on the National Institute of Nursing Research

   b. Developing a plan of care based on practice guidelines on depression

   c. Attending a nursing research workshop

   d. Discussing concerns about side effects concerning a psychotropic agent

3. Integration of nursing research in psychiatric-mental health nursing is demonstrated by:

   a. Reviewing recent studies on the National Institute of Nursing Research

   b. Developing a plan of care based on practice guidelines on depression

   c. Attending a nursing research workshop

   d. Discussing concerns about side effects concerning a psychotropic agent

TABLE 36–4
Quantitative and Qualitative Research Characteristics

Quantitative Research	Qualitative Research
• Generalizability often reflects quality of data	• Generalizability is sometimes challenged
• Focus: concise and specific concepts	• Focus: phenomenon
• Reductionistic	• Holistic, dynamic, and individual
• Objective	• Subjective
• Fixed design	• Flexible design
• Reasoning: logic, deductive	• Reasoning: dialectic, inductive
• Relationships: cause-and-effect, functional	• Patterns of association
• Tests theory	• Develops theory
• Control	• Shared interpretation
• Instruments	• Communication and observation
• Basic element of data analysis: numbers	• Basic element of data analysis: narrative descriptions
• Statistical analysis	• Individual interpretation
• Seeks generalizations	• Seeks patterns

Note. Adapted from *Essentials of Nursing Research* (5th ed.), by D. F. Polit, & C. T. Beck, 2005, Philadelphia: Lippincott.

Most research studies mentioned in this chapter have used quantitative methods. Qualitative studies may be distinguished from quantitative studies because qualitative ones have small sample sizes (possibly as small as eight or nine subjects), and few statistics are used. In contrast, quantitative studies will have large sample sizes and statistics—often lots of statistics! Table 36–4 presents other characteristics of qualitative and quantitative research.

For more than a decade, nurses have increasingly come to view qualitative research methods as appropriate for the development of nursing knowledge. Nurses have always considered individualized nursing care to be extremely important, but their research has generally followed the scientific method, which searches for proof and verification of study results. The focus is on groups and on the generalizability of findings. Qualitative research is typically used when little to nothing is known of a phenomenon and quantitative is used when information is readily available. An example of qualitative research is presented here:

Bernstein (2000) studied the "experience with acupuncture." A phenomenological investigation study was conducted to explore the meaning of women substance abusers' experiences while receiving acupuncture as part of the treatment for substance dependence. A method of data analysis, *Giorgi's modification of phenomenological method*, was used to discern the meaning of experiences by studying descriptions from subjects. The procedure for data analysis comprised five steps, one of which contained central themes and the natural meaning units. Analysis of the data after one treatment with acupuncture revealed seven major themes: anticipation of pain, anxiety about the new experience, mood elevation, inability to describe the experience, physical sensation, relaxation, and enhanced sleep. Conclusions from these data demonstrate that substance abusers' experiences with acupuncture indicated it as an acceptable new treatment modality with the potential for healing through integration and balance. Because this was only one study, other studies are needed to evaluate the effects of repeated treatments (Bernstein, 2000).

NATIONAL INSTITUTE OF MENTAL HEALTH

The National Institute of Mental Health (NIMH) has long considered psychiatric nursing to be one of the core mental health professional groups. The importance of nurses to the mission of this organization was greatly enhanced by the Task Force on Nursing that was appointed in 1985 by Dr. Shervert Frazier, the Director of the NIMH. Members of the task force included well-known nurses such as Joyce

Kilpatrick, Kathyrn Barnard, Jo Eleanor Elliott, and Ada Sue Hinshaw. The committee sought ways of increasing participation of nurses in the extramural activities of the NIMH, such as appointing nurses to advisory boards and increasing nurses' participation in grant-supported activities. The final report of the task group was presented in September 1987, and three major recommendations were made to the NIMH: (1) prepare psychiatric nurses to be researchers; (2) support the ongoing research careers of psychiatric nurses; (3) link psychiatric nurses with the existing system (McBride, Friedenberg, Babich, & Bush, 1992).

In regard to the first recommendation, the first NIMH institutional research training grant for psychiatric nurses was awarded in September 1989. The program emphasized geropsychiatric care (McBride et al., 1992). For the second recommendation, the support of ongoing research careers for psychiatric nurses has been fostered by several efforts. In October 1989, the NIMH cosponsored, with the National Institutes of Health, a conference entitled "Biological Psychiatry and the Future of Psychiatric-Mental Health Nursing." Several more research-building conferences for psychiatric nursing have been held since 1989. Additionally, funding for nursing research has increased a great deal, even though it is still low. Two research proposals submitted by nurse principal investigators were funded by the NIMH from 1985 to 1986 for a total of $98,138, whereas nine such proposals were funded from 1988 to 1989 for a total of $1,016,722 (McBride et al., 1992).

In regard to the third recommendation of the task force, McBride et al. (1992) discussed how nurses have become more linked to the NIMH system. In 1987, there were only four nurse members of the initial review groups (IRGs). This number increased to 10 nurses in 1990. For the first time, a nurse, Dr. Barbara Lowery, was appointed to chair an IRG (the Mental Health Behavior Research Review Committee).

NATIONAL INSTITUTE OF NURSING RESEARCH

The former NIMH initiatives contributed to the formation of the current National Institute of Nursing Research (NINR). On June 10, 1993, President Clinton enacted the National Institute of Health Revitalization Act of 1993, and later that year, Secretary of the Department of Health and Human Services (DHHS) Donna Shalala publicly changed the National Center for Nursing Research to the NINR.

Major goals of the NINR include supporting clinical and basic research to create and advance a scientific basis for the care of people across the life span. According to the broad mandate of NINR, the institute seeks to understand and lessen symptoms of acute and chronic illness, and prevent disease and its potential deleterious course. Moreover, the institute supports diverse research initiatives, including training and career development in nursing research in interdisciplinary practice areas.

As psychiatric nursing approaches the next decade it is imperative to integrate key issues addressed by the National Institute of Nursing Research. Historically, the NINR has guided nursing to reflect a state of the art research to promote and improve the health of individuals, families, communities, and populations across the life span. The Strategic Plan of the NINR 2006–2010 advances this mission and offers opportunities and support to nursing research initiatives in several ways:

- Integrate the biological-behavioral interface into nursing practice with a focus on sociocultural factors, genetics, life sciences, culture, and biologic and behavioral interventions that promote symptom management and disease prevention. Ethical issues, decision making, and health promotion are part of these intiatives.

- Adopt and adapt new technologies in vast areas including modification of technology to improve screening, monitoring and management of symptoms, and delivery of interventions. Telehealth and telemental health, and home monitoring using technologies are examples of technological approaches that advance NINR initiatives.

- Develop a cadre of nursing research investigators to address today's and future health care needs of individuals, families, communities, and populations across the life span.

- Advance health promotion and disease prevention.

- Eliminate health disparities associated with a growing national and global sensitivity of the impact of race, gender, genetics, socioeconomic, ethnicity and culture on individuals, families, and communities.

- Initiate caregiving research to address the needs of a growing number of caregivers across the life span.

- Manage symptoms in acute and chronic illness.

- Develop nursing science that promotes self-management in health and illness.

- Advance research in palliative care and respect for dying persons.

(See the entire NINR 2006–2010 Strategic Plan website in the Resources section at the end of this chapter.)

FUTURE NEEDS OF PSYCHIATRIC NURSING RESEARCH

Many nurse authors in psychiatric-mental health nursing have pointed out that this is the age of biological psychiatry. Some psychiatric nurses argued that the art of psychiatric nursing would be diminished if the focus shifted to biological issues. Others proposed that the new evidence of psychobiology must be integrated but psychosocial and interpersonal aspects that have been the foundation of practice should not be negated. It seems appropriate that psychiatric nurses be involved in neurobiological and psychopharmacologic treatment research but not lose sight of the benefits of other treatment modalities. Comparisons should be made between client responses to drugs and to other treatments. Nurses should examine and develop evidence-based treatment that integrates the relationship among the mind, the brain, and behavior.

Growing casualties from global wars in both Iraq and Afghanistan will have a far-reaching impact on American society and psychiatric nursing. Physical injuries (such as traumatic brain syndrome, loss of limbs, and functional decline) coupled with psychiatric conditions (such as PTSD, depression, suicide, and substance-use disorders) provide vast opportunities for psychiatric nurses to conduct and participate in research endeavors to maintain function and restore integrity, move clients from victims to survivors, strengthen social networks, and ensure access to health care (Busch, McBride, Curtis, & Vanderploeg, 2005). As psychiatric nurses move further into the twenty-first century, they must compete with other mental health professionals who will seize opportunities to be major advocates for veterans and other vulnerable populations and who will advanced self-care management across the life span.

The continued emphasis on evidence-based practice specifically, evidence-based research that compares the efficacy of two or more treatment modalities. Of even greater importance is the application of research data to nursing practice. The current emphasis on evidence-based practice in nursing and medicine is encouraging because clinicians are being encouraged to seek the latest research to improve and explore solutions to practice problems (McBride, 2007). Several organizations, including the National Association of Clinical Nurse Specialists (NACNS), Sigma Theta Tau International, and the Sarah Cole Hirsch Institute are offering grants for nurses to pursue and develop evidence-based and best practice models. The Hirsch Institute is poised to facilitate and accelerate research findings into practice. It has organized six focal areas: Maternity, Pediatrics, Gerontology, Cardiopulmonary, Oncology, and Home Health. A new focal area in Psychiatric-Mental Health is being developed. The Hirsch Institute also offers consultation services and educational support. (See Table 36–5, Research Questions for Psychiatric Nursing across the Life Span.)

The National Institute of Nursing Research/NIMH Mentorship Program was a response to the call of psychiatric-mental health nursing leaders to establish a cadre of researchers with a PhD and expand the number of funded psychiatric nursing researchers in the United States. A major focus on evidence-based practice and behavioral change was an integral part of this groundbreaking event (Cochrane, 2001). Over the next few years, the benefits of these efforts

TABLE 36-5
Research Questions for Psychiatric Nursing across the Life Span

Childhood

What is the most effective dose of antidepressants for a 12-year-old?

What are the most common adverse effects associated with stimulants during a 12-month period?

What is the most effective intervention for children and families coping with a serious family crisis?

What risk factors are associated with an increased risk of suicide in adolescents who take antidepressants?

What is the most effective treatment approach for the adolescent with a co-occurring substance-related disorder and a psychiatric disorder?

Adulthood

Is there a relationship between the nature of caregiving and caregiver distress?

What impact does individualized health education have on adherence to treatment?

What impact does martial discord have on childhood behaviors?

Older Adults

What factors increase the risk of depression in older adults?

What is the rate of relapse in older adults who discontinue antidepressants after 6 months?

What is the relationship between quality of support systems and suicide in older adults?

will flourish and be evidenced by improved health care and quality of life for the client with a mental illness.

SUMMARY

◆ Research has become an integral part of nursing.

◆ Every nurse should be familiar with the steps in the scientific research process.

◆ The roles of psychiatric nurses in research include those of (1) principal investigator; (2) member of the research team; (3) data collector; (4) client advocate; (5) critique of research findings; (6) utilizer of research findings.

◆ Much of the nursing research in psychiatric-mental health nursing has focused on nurses. However, the greatest emphasis should be on clients. Research that has been conducted on clients across the life span has focused on adults clients, but more research is needed on the other age groups.

◆ Quantitative research has been conducted more often than qualitative research.

◆ The NIMH considers psychiatric nursing as one of the core mental health professional groups. There has been an increasing interest in psychiatric-mental health research at the NIMH, and funding levels for this type of research continues to be increased at this agency.

◆ There is a great need for psychiatric-mental health research. Of particular relevance is the development of evidence-based models that advance mental health across the life span.

◆ Opportunities to advance the care and quality of life for individuals across the life span exist for nurses in all practice settings.

SUGGESTIONS FOR CLINICAL CONFERENCES

1. Identify research currently being conducted by or participated in by psychiatric-mental health nursing staff.

2. Discuss the role of the generalist and advanced-practice psychiatric registered nurse in clinical research.

3. Invite a psychiatric-mental health nurse researcher to discuss recent research findings and the associated nursing implications.

STUDY QUESTIONS

1. Which of the following statements is true concerning studies in psychiatric-mental health nursing?
   a. Most of these studies have used qualitative research designs.
   b. These studies are easily identifiable in the literature.
   c. Many of the studies have been concerned with nurses rather than clients.
   d. Psychiatric nurses have studied mental illness more than mental health.

2. Every psychiatric nurse is expected to carry out which of the following roles in research?
   a. Principal investigator
   b. Member of a research team
   c. Data collector
   d. Critiquer of research findings

3. Most research in psychiatric nursing has been conducted with which group of clients?
   a. Children
   b. Adolescents
   c. Adults
   d. Older adults

4. Future research in psychiatric nursing should focus on which of the following areas?
   a. Biological
   b. Psychosocial
   c. Interpersonal
   d. All of the above

5. Which of the following is a barrier to conducting nursing research with clients who have chronic mental illnesses?
   a. Clients with the same psychiatric diagnosis vary more in their impairment than do clients with the same medical diagnosis.
   b. The number of clients with chronic mental illnesses is decreasing every year.
   c. Nurses do not have access to client populations.
   d. Because of the large number of categories of mental disorders, nurses are unsure about which client group to study.

6. The nurse is caring for a client with schizophrenia on an acute inpatient unit. The client has been selected as a potential research subject in a study involving a new antipsychotic agent. Which of the following statements is the most accurate about clients with psychiatric disorders participating in research studies?
   a. They have the same legal and ethical rights as other research subjects.
   b. They are incompetent to make decisions; thus the nurse does need an informed consent.
   c. The client is incapable of making informed consent and should participate in treatment to study medications that can improve condition.
   d. The nurse must strongly encourage the client to provide informed consent.

7. Which of the following statements indicates the client comprehends the informed consent process?
   a. "Will I be paid to take this medication?"
   b. "I understand that I can withdraw from this research study at any time."
   c. "Will I lose my benefits if I refuse to participate in this research?"
   d. "What are the dangers in taking this medication?"

RESOURCES

Please note that because Internet resources are of a time-sensitive nature and URL addresses may change or be deleted, searches should also be conducted by association or topic.

Internet Resources

http://www.ninr.nih.gov/NR/rdonlyres/9021E5EB-B2BA-47EA-B5DB-1E4DB11B1289/4894/NINR_StrategicPlanWebsite.pdf   National Institute of Nursing Research. (2006). NINR strategic plan: Changing practice, changing lives. National Institute of Health, U.S. Department of Health and Human Services. (Accessed August 15, 2007)

http://www.iom.edu/   Institute of Medicine of the National Academies (Accessed April 10, 2006).

http://www.nih.gov/ninr   National Institute of Nursing Research (NINR)

http://www.nursingcenter.com   Nursing Research Journal

REFERENCES

Ahijevych, K., & Bernard, L. (1994). Health-promoting behaviors of African-American women. *Nursing Research, 43,* 86–89.

Alderman, J., Wolkow, R., & Fogel, I. M. (2006). Drug concentrations monitoring with tolerability and efficacy assessments during open-label, long-term sertraline treatment of children and adolescents. *Journal of Child and Adolescent Psychopharmacology, 16,* 117–129.

American Nurses Association. (2000). *The scope and standards of psychiatric-mental health practice.* Washington, DC: American Nurses Publishing.

Bernstein, K. S. (2000). The experience of acupuncture for treatment of substance dependence. *Image: Journal of Nursing Scholarship, 32,* 267–272.

Brooking, J. (1986). *Psychiatric nursing research.* Chichester, England: John Wiley.

Busch, R. M., McBride, A., Curtiss, G., & Vanderploeg, R. D. (2005). The components of executive functioning in traumatic brain injury. *Journal of Clinical and Experimental, 27,* 1022–1032.

Butler, F. R., & Zakari, N. (2005). Grandparents parenting grandchildren: Assessing health status, parental stress, and social supports. *Journal of Gerotonlogical Nursing, 31,* 43–54.

Chang, K. H., & Horrocks, S. (2006). Lived experiences of family caregivers of mentally ill relatives. *Journal of Advanced Nursing, 53,* 435–443.

Cochrane, C. (2001). The National Institute of Nursing Research/National Institute of Mental Health mentorship program: Building the capacity of psychiatric-mental health nurse researchers. *Journal of the American Psychiatric Nurses Association, 7,* 171–172.

Cox, E. R., Motheral, B. R., Henderson, R. R., & Mager, D. (2003). Geographic variation in the prevalence of stimulant medication use among children 5 to 14 years old: Results from a commercially insured U.S. sample. *Pediatrics, 111,* 237–243.

England, M., Tripp-Reimer, T., & Rubenstein, L. (2004). Exploration of the psychometric properties of an inventory of voice experiences. *Archives of Psychiatric Nursing, 19,* 58–69.

England, M., Tripp-Reimer, T., & Rubenstein, L. (2004). Nurse judgments of hallucinated voice descriptions: Relevance for intervention. *International Journal of Nursing Research, 9,* 1073–1091.

Fopma-Loy, J. (1989). Geropsychiatric nursing: Focus and setting. *Archives of Psychiatric Nursing, 3,* 189–190.

Fox, J. C. (1992). Chronic mental illness. In J. J. Fitzpatrick, R. L. Taunton, & A. K. Jacox (Eds.), *Annual review of nursing research* (Vol. 10, pp. 95–113). New York: Springer.

Fuller-Thomson, E., & Minkler, M. (2000). African American grandparents raising grandchildren: A national profile of demographic and health characteristics. *Health and Social Work, 25,* 109–118.

Jacobson, G. (1994). The meaning of stressful life experiences in nine- and eleven-year-old children: A phenomenological study. *Nursing Research, 43,* 95–99.

Jones, R. N., & O'Brien, P. (1990). Unique interventions for child inpatient psychiatry. *Journal of Psychosocial Nursing and Mental Health Services, 28,* 29–31.

Krach, P., & Yang, J. (1992). Functional status of older persons with chronic mental illness living in a home setting. *Archives of Psychiatric Nursing, 6,* 90–97.

Kurlowicz, L. H., Outlaw, F. H., Ratcliffe, S. J., & Evans, L. K. (2005). An exploratory study of depression among older African American users of an academic outpatient rehabilitation program. *Archives of Psychiatric Nursing, 19,* 3–9.

Li, H. C., & Lopez, V. (2005). Children's Emotional Manifestation Scale: Development and testing. *Journal of Clinical Nursing, 14,* 223–229.

Malone, J. A. (1990). Schizophrenia research update: Implications for nursing. *Journal of Psychosocial Nursing and Mental Health Services, 28,* 4–9.

McBride, A. B. (1988). Coming of age: Child psychiatric nursing. *Archives of Psychiatric Nursing, 2,* 57–64.

McBride, A. B. (2007). Mental health nursing today: A view from the USA. *International Journal of Nursing Studies, 44,* 335–337.

McBride, A. B., Friedenberg, E. C., Babich, K. S., & Bush, C. T. (1992). Nursing research in NIMH: An update. *Archives in Psychiatric Nursing, 6,* 138–141.

McCabe, S. (2000). Bringing psychiatric nursing into the twenty-first century. *Archives in Psychiatric Nursing, 14,* 109–116.

Melnyk, B. M. (1994). Coping with unplanned hospitalization: Effects of informational interventions on mothers and children. *Nursing Research, 43,* 50–55.

Nehring, W. M., & Faux, S. A. (2006). Transitional and health issues of adults with neural tubal defects. *Journal of Nursing Scholarship, 38,* 63–70.

Nieswiadomy, R. M. (1998). *Foundations of nursing research* (3rd ed.). Stamford, CT: Appleton & Lange.

Olfson, M., Marcus, S. C., Weissman, M. M., & Jensen, P. S. (2002). National trends in the use of psychotropic medications by children. *Journal of the American Academy of Child and Adolescent Psychiatry, 41,* 514–521.

Polit, D. F., & Beck, C. T. (2005). Essentials of Nursing Research: Methods, Appraisal, and Utilization, 5th ed. Philadelphia, PA: Lippincott Williams & Wilkins.

Poster, E. C., Betz, C. L., & Randall, B. (1992). Psychiatric nurses' attitudes toward and involvement in nursing research. *Journal of Psychosocial Nursing and Mental Health Services, 30,* 26–29.

Puntil, C. (2005). New graduate orientation program in a geriatric psychiatric inpatient setting. *Issues in Mental Health Nursing, 26,* 65–80.

Rojcewicz, S., & Rojcewicz, R. (1997). The "human" voices in hallucinations. *Journal of Phenomenological Psychology, 28,* 1–41.

Ryan, N. M. (1989). Stress-coping strategies identified from school-aged children's perspective. *Research in Nursing and Health, 12,* 111–122.

Sethabouppha, H., & Kane, C. (2005). Caring for the seriously mentally ill in Thailand: Buddhist family caregiving. *Archives of Psychiatric Nursing, 19,* 44–57.

Sills, G. M. (1977). Research in the field of psychiatric nursing—1952–1977. *Nursing Research, 26,* 201–207.

Stinson, C. K., & Kirk, E. (2006). Structured reminiscence: An intervention to decrease depression and increase self-transcendence in older women. *Journal of Clinical Nursing, 15,* 208–218.

Thomas, V. J., & Cohn, T. (2006). Communication skills and cultural awareness courses for healthcare professionals who care for patients with sickle cell anemia. *Journal of Advanced Nursing 53,* 480–488.

Upton, N., & Reed, V. (2005). Caregiver coping in dementing illness—implications for short-term respite care. *International Journal of Psychiatry Nursing Research, 10,* 1180–1196.

U.S. Census Bureau. (2001). The 65 years and older population: Census 2000 Brief. http://www.census.gov/prod/2001pubs/c2kbr01-10.pdf.

Yarcheski, A., Mahon, N. E., & Yarscheski, T. J. (1999). An empirical test of alternate theories of anger in early adolescents. *Nursing Research, 48,* 317–323.

Youngblut, J. M., & Brooten, D. (2000). Moving research into practice: A new partner. *Nursing Outlook, 48,* 55–56.

Zito, J. M., Safer, D. J., dosReis, S., Gardner, J. F., Boles, M., Lynch, F. (2000). Trends in the prescribing of psychotropic medications to preschoolers. *JAMA, 283,* 1025–1030.

Zito, J. M., Safer, D. J., dosReis, S., Gardner, J. F., Magder, L., Socken, K., Boles, M., Lynch, F., & Riddle, M. A. (2003). Psychotropic practice patterns for youth. *Archives of Pediatric Adolescent Medicine, 157,* 17–25.

Zito, J. M., Tobi, H., de Jong-van den Berg, L. T., Fegert, J. M., Safer, D. J., Janhsen, K., et al. (2006). Antidepressant prevalence for youths: A multi-national comparison. *Pharmacoepidemiology and Drug Safety, 15,* 793–798.

SUGGESTED READINGS

Dempsey, P. A., & Dempsey, A. D. (1996). *Nursing research: Text and workbook* (4th ed.). Boston: Little, Brown.

Frank-Stromborg, M. (1992). *Instruments for clinical nursing research.* Boston: Jones & Bartlett.

Hinshaw, A. S., Feetham, S. L., & Shaver, J. L. (1999). *Handbook of clinical nursing research.* Thousand Oaks, CA: Sage.

Polit, D. F. (1996). *Data analysis & statistics for nursing research.* Stamford, CT: Appleton & Lange.

Williams, S. J., & Torrens, P. R. (1999). Introduction to health services (5th ed.). Clifton Park, NY: Delmar Learning.

Wilson, H. S., & Hutchinson, S. A. (1996). *The consumer's guide to nursing research.* Clifton Park, NY: Thomson Delmar Learning.

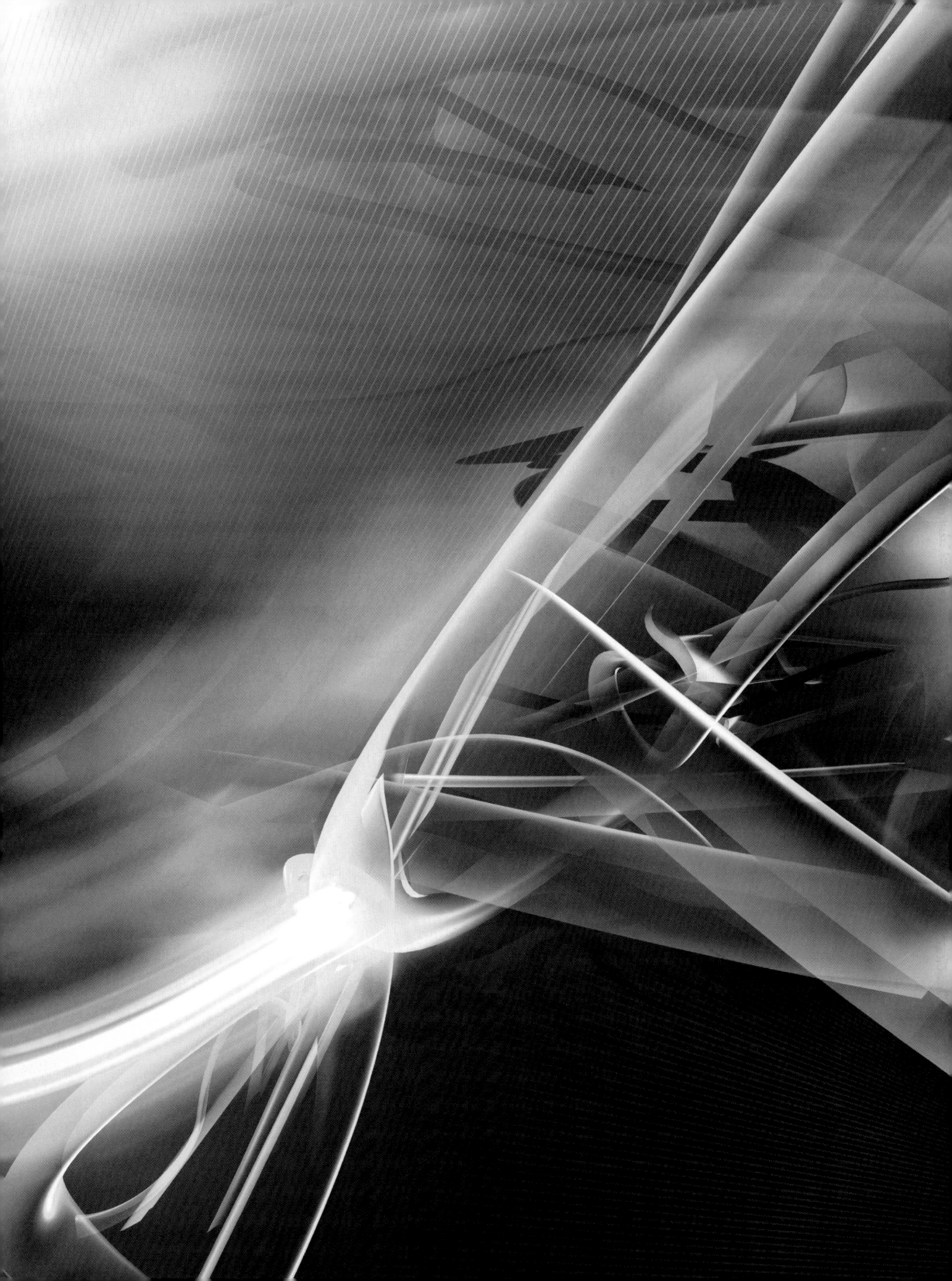

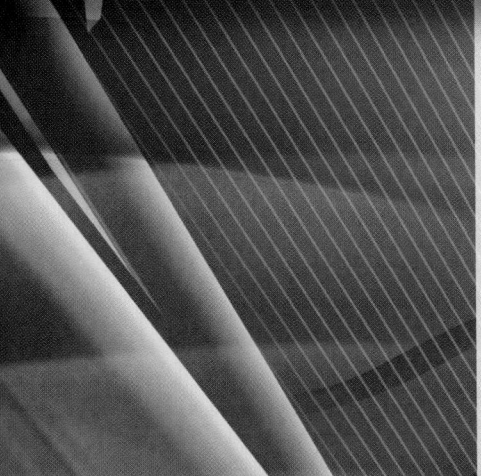

CHAPTER 37

The Future of Psychiatric Nursing

Deborah Antai-Otong, MS, APRN, BC, FAAN
Margaret Brackley, PhD, RN, CS

KEY TERMS

Assertiveness: Clearly communicating one's needs, desires, or beliefs directly and tactfully with self-confidence.

Case Management: A model of comprehensive and holistic health care delivery that concentrates the responsibility for all care given to a client in one person or agency.

Consumerism: A movement seeking to protect the rights of those acquiring a service (in this instance, mental health care) by requiring standards of effectiveness and safety.

Cultural Competence: Refers to the synthesis and modification of knowledge concerning people and groups into distinct standards, practices, and attitudes.

Evidence-Based Practice: Refers to interventions for which there is substantial empirical evidence that they improve client outcomes.

Leadership: The ability to lead and inspire others in a shared vision.

Nursing Informatics: The use of computers and information sciences to manage and process data, knowledge, and information in nursing practice and client care.

Performance Improvement: A method of ensuring the adequacy of care developed by Deming and adopted by health care systems.

Vulnerability: The potential susceptibility of a person, family, or group to a health deviation.

COMPETENCIES

Upon completion of this chapter, the learner should be able to:

1. Discuss the possible roles of the psychiatric nurse during this century.
2. Describe the leadership skills desired for psychiatric nurses.
3. Analyze the current trends and direction of psychiatric nursing.
4. Explore the impact of technology on psychiatric-mental health nursing practice.
5. Recognize the role of the psychiatric nurse in prevention and health promotion across the life span.
6. Analyze the basic principles of biological, psychosocial, and cultural factors into nursing practice.

CHAPTER OUTLINE

The Role of Psychiatric Nursing in the New Era

Psychiatric Nurse as a Provider of Care

Psychiatric Nurse as a Coordinator of Care

Psychiatric Nurse as a Member of a Profession

Leadership Skills in Psychiatric-Mental Health Nursing

Concepts of Empowerment

Political and Communication Savvy

Collaboration, Interdisciplinary Teams, and the Consumer

All nurses, regardless of their specialty area of practice, see clients with mental disorders. It makes no difference whether the nurse works in settings such as obstetrics, pediatrics, general medicine, primary care, or in the schools or community. Clients with psychiatric disorders are seen in every setting, specialty, or situation, and they deserve to receive the same quality of care as the rest of the population. The American Nurses Association (ANA), in conjunction with psychiatric specialty organizations, including the American Psychiatric Nurses Association (APNA), the International Society for Psychiatric Nurses (ISPN), set forth guidelines for basic mental health nursing. Clients with mental disorders should have health benefits equal to those of other citizens, including a wide range of services that are cost-effective, and allow for choice of health care provider.

General health care providers, registered nurses, school nurses, clinical nurse specialists, nurse practitioners, midwives, clinical nurse specialists, family practice and primary care physicians, internists, and pediatricians deliver most of the mental health care services. Although most clients with mental disorders are treated in community-based settings, most psychiatric nurses, including advanced-practice nurses, continue to work in hospital-based settings. Historically, researchers believed that these factors contribute to mental health care being provided by nonmental health care providers. Studies have demonstrated that 65 to 85 percent of mental health care provided by nonmental health care specialists is lacking in recognition of and appropriate treatment and referral for mental disorders. This situation must improve if all Americans are to have access to mental health care services under the auspices of managed health care.

Psychiatric-mental health nursing faces the arduous burden of balancing a practice in a rapidly evolving specialty. The history of psychiatric nursing is replete with distinct examples of philosophical changes that reflect socioeconomic, demographic, technological, and pharmacologic advances. Psychiatric nursing is guided by the philosophy of caring for the whole person, which includes biological, psychosocial and spiritual domains (Brimblecombe, Tingle, Tunmore & Murrells, 2007). Preparation for an explosion of demographic changes, advances in technology and information systems, an aging population, global violence, and health care disparities requires psychiatric nurses to examine their role in addressing the complexity of biological and behavioral responses to stress across the life span.

Psychiatric nursing is presently in the midst of another significant paradigm change that results from vast advances in neuroscience. Since the 1990s and the dawning of the Decade of the Brain, psychiatric nurses have embraced the impact of biological process on behavior and the role of pharmacologic and nonpharmacologic interventions. As neuroimaging studies continue to illuminate the biological basis of complex behaviors in mental health and mental illness, psychiatric nurses are challenged to understand the underpinnings of genomics, cellular and molecular processes associated with psychiatric symptoms, and the role of psychopharmacology (Gould & Manji, 2004; Swanson et al., 2005). For example, researchers continue to tweak clinical findings from molecular studies and link modulation of complex signaling pathways to higher-order brain functions and target sites that regulate mood, cognition, appetite, sexual arousal, sleep patterns, and weight, all of which are unique to mood disorders, implicating involvement of signaling pathways in the pathogenesis and treatment of mood disorders (Gould, Dow, O'Donnell, Chen, & Manji, 2007). Inferences from these findings further strengthen the need to use data to guide practice and implement evidence-based nursing interventions. Despite the explosion of neuroscience and its significant contributions to the care of clients with psychiatric disorders, psychiatric nursing practice has come full circle and provides a specialty that bridges biological underpinnings with psychosocial processes.

Apart from the biological and behavioral interface in psychiatric nursing, advances in information technology provide fertile ground for psychiatric nurses to create and implement client-centered and evidence-based interventions that sustain mental health and optimize function and recovery (Repique, 2007). An example is telemental health care, which allows psychiatric nurses to provide mental health services to clients and their families living in rural or remote areas. Telemental health care also gives these clients the ability to consult with nonmental health providers, as well as increased access to mental health care.

With more and more advanced-practice nurses working in community-based mental health and primary care settings, care is being delivered by psychiatric-mental health nurses. Despite the increase in advance-practice nurses practicing in community-based settings, a relatively large number of clients with depression and other psychiatric disorders seek mental health care from their primary care providers. Major drawbacks of receiving mental health care in primary care settings is the substantial variation in mental health services and a lack of evidence-based care (Dobscha, Leibowitz, Flores, Doak, & Gerrity, 2007; Weich, Nazareth, Morgan, & King, 2007).

This chapter further defines the role of the psychiatric nurse in the twenty-first century, assesses the impact of technology on practice, and aligns psychiatric-mental health nursing to the national goals as outlined in *Healthy People 2010* (U.S. Department of Health and Human Services [U.S. DHHS], 2000).

THE ROLE OF PSYCHIATRIC NURSING IN THE NEW ERA

The American Association of Colleges of Nursing (1986) issued a document on the essentials of nursing education and identified the three roles of the professional nurse as: provider of care, coordinator of care, and member of a profession. More recently, emphasis has been on recruitment of nurses into the profession with a greater emphasis on a diverse student population reflective of a diverse American

population. This chapter discusses future trends of health care and the way in which these trends are likely to influence roles in psychiatric-mental health nursing. Preparation for psychiatric nurse career development in this era must be instituted and maintained if adequate members of nurses with the necessary characteristics for future practice are to be available.

PSYCHIATRIC NURSE AS A PROVIDER OF CARE

The decade of the brain research continues to govern the understanding and treatment of mental illness, offering vast opportunities for psychiatric nurses to provide an array of interventions. The psychiatric nurse as a provider of care is expected to be more involved in primary care and preventive services in community-based settings. Care of clients with chronic mental illness, dementia and other cognitive disorders, dual diagnosis with substance abuse as one of the classifications, and violent and abusive behaviors occurs in hospital, home health, community, and correctional facilities. The psychiatric nurse must be prepared to work more autonomously than in the past as a result of the change in settings for mental health care. Psychiatric nurses must maintain diverse competencies such as initiating biological interventions, educating the client about mental illness, and observing for desired and adverse effects. Accordingly, they must understand the complexity of mental disorders, including genetic vulnerability, neurotransmitter dysregulation, physiological and psychological stress responses—acute and chronic—which guide in the development of evidence-based holistic mental health care.

PSYCHIATRIC NURSE AS A COORDINATOR OF CARE

As the coordinator of care, the psychiatric nurse will be a member of an interdisciplinary team or manage the care of a group of clients. Role changes include returning to more active involvement in milieu management, medication management, case management, managed care systems, psychosocial and rehabilitation services, and other approaches. Because of the various innovative models of care delivery, more attention must be given to nursing skills in critical thinking and self-learning strategies rather than those needed in traditional systems of client care.

PSYCHIATRIC NURSE AS A MEMBER OF A PROFESSION

One characteristic of a profession is reliance on a body of knowledge that is distinct from other disciplines. The chapter on research (see Chapter 36) addresses this issue; however, research is not the only source of knowledge. Knowledge comes from personal experience, an ethical system, and the artistic aspect of care (Watson, 1988). Psychiatric nurses must allow time for reflection and development of knowledge (Antai-Otong, 2007).

Nursing students should also develop the characteristics of a professional by the end of their educational program. As a member of a professional group, nurses must invest time and energy in activities that promote the preservation of psychiatric nursing as well as resources for clients and their families. Membership in appropriate professional organizations is essential for meeting the goals of the specialty. Providing input into the political process, thus ensuring adequate resource allocation not only for the nursing profession but also for underserved and stigmatized mental health consumer groups, is a professional responsibility. The Americans with Disabilities Act is helping to diminish some of the results of institutionalized stigma. Intensive education at all levels of society must be developed and implemented to address the stigma that the American culture associates with mental illness. Presently, there is no panacea to eliminate the stigma of mental illness. Unfortunately, despite increased knowledge of mental illness, stigma remains more intense, even though understanding improved. Broader knowledge that involves redressing the public's fears through involvement in advocacy, public education, and interactions with persons with mental illness in vast forums may eliminate stigma (Baumann, 2007).

LEADERSHIP SKILLS IN PSYCHIATRIC-MENTAL HEALTH NURSING

New nurses often ask what it takes to be a leader. The answer to this question lies in personal commitment and the willingness to take a risk. As members of a profession, nurses are expected to provide leadership within their potential sphere of influence. Leadership is the ability to lead and inspire others in a shared vision. Effective leaders optimize resources; support and guide the organization and others through modeling appropriate behaviors; understand relationships both with clients, families, colleagues and politicians; and create an environment of risk taking, recognition, empowerment, respect, learning, and creativity (Antai-Otong, 2007). In today's changing world, replete with challenging opportunities involving the advent of neuroimaging, genomics, informatics and alternative therapies, psychiatric nurses must be prepared to adapt to advances in instant communication, develop and maintain healthy interpersonal relationships, respond to global violence, understand the impact of the Internet and immediate access to knowledge on client care, and develop data-driven interventions to facilitate mental health across the life span. Collectively, effective leadership skills are critical to survival in the twenty-first century.

Psychiatric-mental health nurses often lead by modeling acceptance of stigmatized groups. Historically, psychiatric nursing has led the entire nursing profession in developing roles like the role of the clinical nurse specialist (McBride, 1990) and psychiatric nurse practioner. We have often led in reform of unjust practices through groups such as the National Alliance of the Mentally Ill (NAMI) and the American Mental Health Association. Psychiatric-mental health nurses have also forged the way for mental health care reform, for example, the work of the Society for Education and Research in Psychiatric-Mental Health Nursing (SERPN), to identify competencies and skills for psychiatric-mental health nursing education in nursing lobby groups that ensured adequate resources for mental health care reform. In addition, the American Psychiatric Nurses Association and ISPN have been leaders in forming coalitions with numerous organizations and influencing policies that affect mental health care, nursing practice, and advocacy for vulnerable populations.

Leadership skills are taught in basic programs of professional nursing. Nurses have the ability to influence various groups within health care. We try to influence clients and their families to adopt healthy lifestyles and health-promoting habits. We influence our peers, colleagues in other disciplines, policy makers, and clients through the use of power. Schutzenhofer (1992) concluded that students of nursing must learn early the significance of power and its impact on decision making and collaborative relationships. Too often we have thought of power as a negative quality that others have used against us. We must reframe this thinking to view power, especially power that is shared with others, as the means of exerting positive pressure to advance psychiatric-mental health nursing practice.

Collaboration with other disciplines is a leadership activity that will greatly increase our influence in health care. Schutzenhofer (1992) called for nurses to redefine ourselves as team players. We will be ahead in what some identify as the twenty-first century leadership style used by women, which is the leadership of collaboration instead of control. The power of one nurse is limited, whereas the power of many nurses in unison with other health care providers direct health care change. Another way we can use power effectively is by influencing policy makers through lobbying efforts, particularly through the efforts of other client advocacy groups, such as ANA and NAMI. In this manner, we can ensure that resources are made available to improve the quality of health care delivered.

CONCEPTS OF EMPOWERMENT

People in various settings and disciplines talk about empowerment in reference to federal workers, voters, consumers of health, and many other examples. To *empower* simply means to invest with power or authorize. We as nurses or voters are certainly authorized to provide good care for people or elect qualified representatives to government, so why should we discuss what we are already empowered to do? The truth is that "[we have not] educated nurses as full health caregiving professionals and have focused instead on how to prepare students to be institutionalized employees" (Watson, 1988).

As identified by Watson (1988), the traditional ways that schools of nursing have operated include the following:

◆ Treating students as objects

◆ Using mechanical or industrial terms such as products and aggregates

◆ Focusing on cognitive-technical outcomes alone, thereby creating competency without compassion or caring

◆ Restricting teaching and learning to behavioral objectives, factual information, and techniques

◆ Tolerating power and dependence roles for teachers and learners

◆ Separating doing from knowing and being

◆ Tolerating accreditation processes that are in direct conflict with nursing's moral and scientific beliefs and educational philosophies and theories

◆ Fixating on entry into practice and a degree rather than on how to educate thinking professional people in such a way as to prepare them for a role that is consistent with nursing's social, moral, and scientific mission to society

After defining the problem, Watson then suggested a "revolution" in nursing curricular practices. The National League of Nursing ([NLN], 1988, 1989) developed and published documents on curricular revolution in response to Watson's call. In this series, scholarly works are presented to increase the dialogue about the transition of educational practices. The impetus behind the need for change is the failure of nursing schools to empower its graduates to develop and deliver the kind of caring that is the essential aspect of nursing (Watson, 1988).

In a seminal article, Angela McBride (1999) outlined major issues facing the nursing profession in the first quarter and second quarter of the twenty-first century and submitted that drastic changes in academia reflect those of health care delivery. Increasingly, emphasis is being put on learning rather than teaching, and courses or programs are no longer taking place in traditional classrooms or bound by schedules. Student populations are more diverse in terms of gender, age, race, and learning styles. She predicted that in the future, nursing education will be a lifelong learning process and academic degrees will be an integral part of this process. Advances in distributed learning will have to compete with out-of-state universities and vie for students across state boundaries. The next quarter of the century is also likely to involve career counseling beyond disciplines, and schools will operate on principles of responsibility-centered management with an emphasis on economic modeling and benchmarking (McBride, 1999). Although these predictions reflect future trends in the nursing profession, Watson's (1988) are relevant to the future of nursing.

Psychiatric-mental health nursing has also addressed the issue of transforming nursing education. SERPN (1994) developed a position paper on essential competencies and skills for generalist and advanced-practice psychiatric-mental health nursing practice. The focus of this work is holistic care for clients with mental illness, which acknowledges the biological basis of mental illness and truly eliminates the destructive dualism of mind-body split.

A more recent response to educational needs of psychiatric nursing details the current crisis in this specialty that threatens its survival (McCabe, 2000). McCabe (2000) asserted that the current crisis has evolved from reduced enrollment in graduate programs and the danger of psychiatric nursing losing its identity and relevance in the nursing profession. Accordingly, she asserted that the survival of psychiatric nursing requires a renovation that involves reframing the specialty's uniqueness by clearly defining scopes of practice that fit into contemporary health care delivery models, or developing outcome measures that illustrate the impact of psychiatric nurses. McCabe (2000) described four critical components for renovating psychiatric nursing:

◆ Reconceptualize what constitutes educational content for all levels of nursing education.

◆ Identify core critical clinical competencies and practical clinical experiences.

◆ Develop and standardize outcome measures set forth by content and competencies

◆ Establish a national research agenda to expand and build on the knowledge base of the specialty.

Olson (2004) also pointed out concerns about the precipitous decline in psychiatric nursing graduate programs and the current crisis in advanced-practice psychiatric nursing. He also pointed out the following strategies to secure the future of this specialty:

◆ Formulate realistic educational expectations

◆ Standardize curricula

◆ Formulate an aggressive accreditation process

Other leaders support these earlier concerns and advocate that advanced-practice nurses must clearly articulate their role and contributions (Williamson, Webb, Abelson-Mitchell, & Cooper, 2006) as expert providers and coordinators of client care and quantify their contributions through data-drive outcomes. In an age when data drive everything and provide clear evidence of outcomes from treatment and interventions, psychiatric nurses are poised to advance their practice and elucidate their contributions to their clients, colleagues, and society.

In brief, efforts to advance the agenda and specialty of psychiatric-mental health nurses requires developing and implementing strategies in the practice and education to address these concerns. These efforts must also integrate principles of empowerment through healthy clinical and practice experiences, which enable nurses to respond effectively to the daily challenge of caring for persons with mental disorders (Bradbury-Jones, Irvine, & Sambrooke, 2007).

POLITICAL AND COMMUNICATION SAVVY

An essential aspect of empowerment is an understanding of the political process. The ANA (1993) has published a lobbying handbook to use at the local level to influence federal policy. Until recently, nurses remained outside the political process. This lack of involvement may have been a result of our military and religious origins or the position of women in contemporary society. Historically, organized nursing separated itself from struggles of equality probably in an effort to be nonthreatening to physicians, hospital administrators, and clients. Even during the suffrage movement for women, nursing did not take an official stand (Reverby, 1987). As our practice began to change because of pressures from other groups on legislators in the 1980s, nursing became involved in the political process. By this time women and minority rights had changed, and this may have influenced nurses to reevaluate their views on political involvement. Political activism has emerged in nursing as a positive force for change, and we continue to gain skill in coalition building to truly affect the legislative and social change process.

To effectively influence the public or individuals, nurses need to have exceptional communication skills (see Chapter 6). Psychiatric nurses have always been interested and skilled in communication, whether it involves listening to the client or family express feelings or being an advocate within large organizations and institutions. Awareness of one's communication style, strengths, and limitations is essential. Caring about the effect of the messages one conveys puts the responsibility to the sender for what the receiver of the message hears (Antai-Otong, 2007).

COLLABORATION, INTERDISCIPLINARY TEAMS, AND THE CONSUMER

As a member of the mental health care team, the nurse can exhibit leadership skills by advocating for the client and family while collaborating with both. The nurse acts as the cultural guide or interpreter of the mental health care facility. The nurse also serves in the "in-between" position in the group, which includes the client's family and health care team. Bishop and Scudder (1990) identified this position as privileged; that is, a position in which the nurse can minister to the client's needs, which demand extremely close contact; enter into the client's and family's experience of mental illness; and also act as an intermediary with all concerned participants in the care of this client. We also provide support and caring, sometimes covertly, as we empower people to take charge of their lives.

Before the consumer movement that began in the 1970s, health care professionals gave little thought to consumer concerns or demands. The general idea was that professionals knew what was best for the person with the mental illness; consumers and families had few avenues to question the decisions made in this paternalistic fashion (Hatfield, 1990). Consumers of mental health are now included in clinical decisions (treatment planning) as well as in programs that train mental health care professionals. The client's perception of the care she received is made available to students through direct interactions or panel discussions.

Models of care that include consumers, advocates, and significant others and families continue to grow. Most are based on redefining mental illnesses as illnesses that require treatment (Hatfield, 1990). Consumers and families often provide insight into the nature of these symptoms and their management by sharing their experiences with students and practicing nurses. The nurse must understand these experiences to grasp the profound meanings consumers and families have gleaned from their day-to-day life. Various family theorists have tried to describe families, some with the motivation of assigning cause for psychopathology to families. Hatfield (1990) wrote, "It is our view that while each of the traditional theorists of mental illness and the family provided new ways to label and describe families, they have contributed little to the understanding of these families" (p. 149).

When a family member is diagnosed with a mental disorder, both the client and family experience a great deal of stress. As members of the mental health care team, nurses often have the most direct contact with the client and her family because, as Virginia Henderson so aptly stated, the nurse is the "24-hour person" (1991). With the current changes in health care delivery, caring for persons with mental disorders is likely to occur in the community or home setting. Nurses must develop innovative strategies to assess the client's symptoms and experiences. To best assess how families cope with this distressful situation, the nurse must identify the meaning the client and family attach to the stress and whether or not they believe they can cope with it. Nurses must avoid assuming that the nurse's viewpoint is the same as the client's and family's.

The consumer of mental health services is a vital member of the mental health care team. The perspective introduced by this client is one that no outside consultant can provide.

My Experience with Brief Reactive Psychosis

I could hear someone saying they were only trying to help me. All I could feel was that I had to fight because I was tied down (restraints were being used) and being tortured (an intravenous catheter was being placed). I whispered to my husband to help. He told me to stop fighting. I felt hopeless. After several days, I decided to escape or kill myself. Someone was poisoning me; I could feel myself slipping away (antipsychotic medication was started). Then I heard your voice (nurse consultant's voice). You told me I was in the hospital, and you explained it all to me. I began to have hope that this torture would end—that I would be rescued. (At this point the medication had become effective and the psychiatric consultation-liaison nurse had begun the consultation process.)

Can an outside viewpoint describe the effects of psychoactive medications or what it is like to be placed in restraints? A client with brief reactive psychosis describes feelings in the accompanying display.

Nurses play major roles in the care of clients with serious mental illness. As new neurobiological and genetic-based treatments emerge, more nurses will need not only to initiate or monitor these therapies, but to design new nursing interventions as well. Families and clients need psychoeducation so they may participate in their care to the fullest extent. Mental health problems that do not fit into this category can be viewed as problems in living that need guidance and advice (Bäuml, Froböse, Kraemer, Rentrop, & Pitschel-Walz, 2006). Nurses have always assumed a major role in providing anticipatory guidance during periods of transitions such as the birth of a child or death of a loved one. In addition, nurses traditionally have provided counseling in vast health care settings and situations. This role of counselor will expand as the nation moves toward an emphasis on prevention of health problems.

ASSERTIVENESS AND CONFIDENCE IN PRACTICE SETTINGS

To provide health care in the ways previously discussed, the nurse needs to be assertive and able to resolve conflicts in the practice setting and confident in the necessary competencies and skills. Helping and caring for others are the essential cores of the professional nursing. Often this core is viewed to be in conflict with assertiveness, whose goals are achieved through direct and effective communication of one's needs, desires, and wishes; however, assertiveness is essential to nursing in that the nurse acts as protector of her own needs and is an advocate and consultant to the client and the family.

Assertiveness skills can be learned by the nurse and in turn taught to others. The results of such learning and teaching are increased self-worth and decreased helplessness and hopelessness in the nurse. Preservation of self-respect and dignity is inherent in assertion behavior.

INTEGRATING LEADERSHIP SKILLS IN NURSING CURRICULA

Nursing curricula contain both content and process. Educators have debated and written about what should be included as content in nursing programs, but until recently, little attention has been given to the process of educating nurses. A group of educators sponsored by NLN increased the dialogue about process in nursing education (NLN, 1988, 1989).

One factor that this group identified as being a barrier to the goals of creating nurses who are prepared to lead is the power relationship between the faculty and student previously mentioned by Watson (1988). Nursing has set up its model of teaching in much the same way health care has set up its power relationships. The client has the least knowledge and power, the physician has the most, and nurses are somewhere in between—sometimes they are powerless, and sometimes they are powerful, depending on the situation. These relationships are based on one person as the elite expert and the other as the powerless, unknowledgeable seeker. Students of nursing are treated as if they were powerless and lacked basic knowledge.

Tremendous changes in the health care system continue to influence the role of psychiatric nurses. These roles continue to reflect changes in mental health care delivery, specifically, movement from hospital-based settings to the more common community-based settings. Because of the present crisis in psychiatric-mental health nursing education, where content and clinical experiences in mental health settings are decreasing, educators must provide unique psychiatric nursing experiences to maintain realities in mental health care and the relevance of the specialty in nursing. Issues such as blurred roles with other health care providers who continue to thrive must be clearly delineated in an effort to carve out the role of psychiatric nurses in a changing health care system. This is particularly true among advanced-practice psychiatric nurses who must begin articulating their contributions to mental health care. Leaders submit that, as a profession, the present educational and practice trends are making it easier for nonmental health care providers to treat the mentally ill rather than advanced-practice psychiatric nurses (Perraud et al., 2006). This dilemma challenges educators and psychiatric nurses to rethink the relevance of traditional roles and respond to them by carving out innovative roles for the generalist nurse and advanced-practice psychiatric nurse.

Apart from addressing the present crisis in psychiatric nursing, leaders must also provide opportunities to develop leadership skills. Leadership skills must be an integral part of the curricula for undergraduate and graduate nursing students. Today's health care system requires that all involved persons become empowered to assume more responsibility for what they must do. This empowerment must be initiated at the beginning of the educational program with more democratic relationships between faculty and students. If all of those involved in education view each other as learners, with some more senior (faculty) than others (students), we can focus on the human development of both rather than on the development of the curriculum.

Finally, we must look at the effect of nursing education on students, faculty, and health care in general. If we fail to nurture our students, what kind of nurses will they become? This is particularly important today because most of today's nurses are middle aged and the profession is failing to attract younger nurses to a once highly regarded profession. Faculty must acknowledge that their mode of educating students is outdated and that there is a tremendous need to relinquish power over to students. Relinquishing this power offers opportunities to guide, nurture, and educate a new breed of nurses. Ultimately, a program can be judged only by the impact its graduates have had on the health of the community. To accomplish our goal of access to basic services, decreasing disparities among all people, and emphasizing the prevention of health problems, we must foster the empowerment of nurses, starting the day they decide to become a nurse.

TRENDS AND DIRECTIONS FOR RESEARCH IN PSYCHIATRIC-MENTAL HEALTH NURSING

Several trends in psychiatric-mental health nursing have been identified, including biological psychiatry, family partnerships, consumerism, evidence-based practice and the role of stress on illness. Evidence-based practice refers to interventions for which there is substantial empirical evidence that they improve client outcomes (Drake et al., 2001). These areas also warrant further research. In addition, most authors agree that (1) there is a substantial reduction in the number of hours in psychiatric-mental health content and clinical exposure for the undergraduate nursing student (McCabe, 2002); (2) there is an alarming decrease in the number of nurses who select psychiatric-mental health nursing as a specialty, especially graduate enrollment (Perraud et al., 2006; Williamson et al., 2006); (3) there is a lack of standardization among current graduate psychiatric-mental health nursing programs, hence making it difficult to articulate the role (Perraud et al., 2006; Williamson et al., 2006); (4) the explosion of knowledge in the area of neurobiology and genetics continues to transform psychiatric-mental health nursing practice; and (5) the setting and model of care are compelling psychiatric nurses to create and develop roles that meet the needs of their clients.

The growing complexity in nursing education has expanded and challenged academic institutions to meet the needs of diverse populations in rapidly evolving and highly technical health care environments. Suggestions for increasing enrollment in graduate programs include improving access to graduate programs using advances in information technologies. During the past 10 years there has been a plethora of online, distance, or web-based educational opportunities for psychiatric-mental health nurses and nurses from various backgrounds and locations to obtain graduate degrees in the specialty. In one study, researchers examined how one online program addressed educational preparation of psychiatric nurses seeking graduate degrees (Perraud et al., 2006). They concluded that this program indeed addressed complex psychiatric care while providing socialization as advance psychiatric-mental health nurse practitioners. They further submitted that online graduate programs in psychiatric-mental health are one solution to increasing the workforce and survival of this specialty. Findings from this study are consistent with others studies that indicate that online or web-based courses provide opportunities for undergraduate and graduate education that are parallel to societal needs and changes associated with obtaining higher education through innovative venues. Findings from these studies indicate that nursing students have demonstrated a relatively positive perception of their online or web-based educational experiences (Billings, Skiba, & Connors, 2005; Hall & Fabayo, 2006; Mahoney, Marfurt, daCunha, & Engebretson, 2005). (See Research Abstract, An Exploration of Scenario Discussion in a Web-Based Nursing Course.)

RESEARCH ABSTRACT

An Exploration of Scenario Discussion in a Web-Based Nursing Course

Hsu, L. L., & Hsieh, S. I. (2006). *Journal of Nursing Research, 14,* 155–165.

Study Problem/Purpose

The aim of this study was to design a nursing course on the basis of scenario discussion, web-based instruction (WBI), and the assessment of learning outcomes. Most of the students chose "good" for learning effectiveness.

Methods

The design of the study comprised two stages. First, the researchers developed the scenario discussion with the WBI system. Second, they evaluated learning outcomes within the context of a scenario discussion. A nursing-assessment score and learning-effectiveness survey were used in this study. The target population in this study was students who were enrolled in a 2-year nursing program and who were registered for the course Nursing I during the fall semester of 2002. Using simple random sampling, students (*n* = 43) were recruited and agreed to participate in the study.

Findings

Primary findings from this study demonstrated that students gave higher learning-effectiveness survey scores and nursing-assessment scores. Researchers attributed their lack of prior exposure to scenario discussion to frustration and anxiety while taking this course.

Implications for Psychiatric Nursing

Growing complexity in nursing education has increased the need to offer psychiatric nursing students innovative learning experiences. Educators must be in tune with these changes and work with students to ensure individualized and innovative educational methodologies to maintain and advance the role of psychiatric nursing in basic and advanced-practice nursing curricula.

The internet continues to open new research challenges. Typically, online studies involve participants accessing a specially designed Web page containing a survey or questionnaire. On completion of these tools, participants have the option of submitting their responses, which are automatically evaluated and scored or E-mailed back to the researcher. Primary advantages of online research involve access to a larger population, speed of data collection, and cost-effectiveness.

TECHNOLOGICAL ADVANCES IN NEUROBIOLOGY AND GENETICS

The previous decade of the brain research has provided remarkable changes in the perception and treatment of mental disorders. Of particular interest are recent genetic discoveries that promise to have an even greater impact on the treatment and prevention of mental illness. The influence of genetics is implicated by data that demonstrates a neurodevelopmental perspective of some psychiatric disorders, such as schizophrenia, bipolar disorder, and obsessive-compulsive disorder (Matsuzaki & Tohyama, 2007; Stewart et al., 2007). Major implications from these data include early diagnosis, risk of prevention, and psychoeducation concerning the course of illness and treatment options. The first Surgeon General's Report on Mental Health (DHHS, 1999) underscores these advances. This report became available at the end of 50 years, which reflects remarkable technological and genetic advances that help explain mental disorders and the brain. This report increases global awareness and recognition of the tremendous burden of disability associated with mental disorders. Scientific studies in mental health and mental illness are summarized in this report and delineate well-documented efficacious treatment modalities for persons across the life span. Other areas of interest include a focus on some psychiatric disorders from a developmental perspective that enhances understanding of mental illness in children and adolescents. This premise also suggests that factors that precipitate mental illness are complex and involve neuroscience, genetic vulnerability, culture, and psychosocial influences. Vulnerability to mental illness exists throughout the life span. Implications for psychiatric nurses include identifying high-risk groups, initiating preventive measures and health promotion, treating symptoms, and reducing the deleterious course of disease.

In 2005, the U.S. Surgeon General issued a Call to Action to Improve the Health and Wellness of Persons with Disabilities with the aim of improving the health status of individuals with disabilities across the life span. Major implications for psychiatric nurses include the following:

◆ Provide psychoeducation that optimizes function and quality of life

◆ Assess the client's individual needs by using active listening skills to identify and respond to the client's health concerns

◆ Communicate clearly and directly with the client to ensure understanding of information that is imparted

◆ Avoid using jargon and take the time to assess and understand the client's health care needs

◆ Be cognizant and patient of the extra time it may take the client to respond to questions

◆ Be the nurse that makes a difference

◆ Respect what the person with a disability (i.e., see the ability, strengths, and resilience in the disability)

Smeltzer (2007) noted that the 2005 U.S. Surgeon General's Call to Action was too important for nursing to ignore. She emphasized the need for nurse researchers, educators, leaders, and the profession as a whole to implement specific actions noted in this statement. Psychiatric nurse leaders, practitioners, educators, and researchers must respond to the Call to Action to facilitate the health and wellness of individuals with psychiatric disorders across the life span.

In addition, the report discussed the relevance of the dismantling of barriers, which previously interfered with availability and access of mental health care services to some citizens, despite disparities that still exist. Research data and experiences of millions of people, their families, and other advocates continue to tear down barriers, although the stigma of mental illness persists. Based on these data, mental disorders are believed to arise from health conditions that are manifested as alterations in thinking, mood, or behavior or a combination of all three that produce distress and impair functioning.

Advances in neurobiology continue to influence psychiatric-mental health nursing. Although the specialty is facing numerous challenges, nursing has a solid biopsychosocial foundation on which to address the interaction of vulnerable biological processes with environmental or psychosocial influences. Work in the area of genetics or psychoimmunology provides a foundation for nursing's value and belief of looking at the whole person within the environment (see Chapter 3).

BIOLOGICAL PSYCHIATRY

The interface among complex neurobiological process, genetics, and behaviors is well documented and strengthens the needs for psychiatric nurse educators to integrate these concepts into nursing curricula and learning experiences. The biological, genetic, and developmental aspects of human behavior interplay with the environmental, cultural, educational, and developmental aspects to create a multidimensional understanding of mental illness and treatment considerations. For a detailed explanation of this biobehavioral interface, see the causative factors sections of previous chapters in this book.

Faced with new knowledge, particularly data included in the Surgeon General's Report on Mental Health (DHHS, 1999), nurses must continue to broaden their views of biobehavior. New ways of thinking about mental illness and mental health necessitate new approaches to nursing care and practice roles. A cadre of nurses have been studying and writing about this problem. The number of such nurses must be increased through direct effort of the profession. Nurses in practice must become familiar with new knowledge and develop evidenced-based interventions to ensure appropriate care of their clients. Nursing interventions must also be tested to determine their efficacy. The psychiatric-mental health nurse of the future will be concerned about the psyche (mind) and soma (body). The major treatment for clients with mental disorders is pharmacologic and may include prescribed or over-the-counter products, such as herbs and dietary supplements. Psychiatric nurses must seek prescriptive authority and offer their clients an array of interventions. Offering an array of interventions will enable this specialty opportunity to reduce blurred roles between psychiatric nurses and other nonmental health care providers. Because of the present dilemma in psychiatric nursing, nurses must explore other avenues of providing services that promote mental health and reduce the chronicity of mental disorders. Psychiatric nurses need to focus on mental status, sleep-wake status, nutrition, the emotional aftermath of trauma and violence, and environmental manipulation to put the client in the best position to heal in the way first described by Nightingale in the last century.

Nurses have an advantage to do this than some of the other core disciplines of mental health because of their firm foundation on the biopsychosociocultural model of nursing care. They are further challenged to develop those skills and prescriptive authorization to compete with nonmental health professionals who are presently treating an exorbitant amount of clients with mental disorders. Technological advances in neurobiology and genetics confirm a biological basis of mental disorders, although psychosocial factors also play a role in exacerbation of symptoms. This knowledge allows for the discipline of nursing to realign psychiatric nursing into the mainstream of nursing, and with this alignment, old thinking about clients with serious, persistent mental disorders must be confronted and changed. The need to stigmatize people with mental disorders no longer exists if alterations in biology and genetic vulnerability play key roles in erratic behavioral responses.

PARTNERSHIPS IN HEALTH CARE: NURSES, CLIENTS, AND FAMILIES

A partner is one who is associated with another or others in an activity or a sphere of common interest. In the context of mental health care, the nurse enters into partnership with the client and family to work toward a common goal of alleviating troublesome symptoms and improving the quality of life for all involved. The most effective and efficient approach of achieving this goal is to decide what each person's role and responsibility is in the partnership. For example, if the nurse is working with a suicidal client, a "no suicide" contract is negotiated in which each person is assured of the role and responsibility of the other. The

client's responsibility is to report suicidal ideation in an agreed-on manner and not to act on the urge to commit suicide. The client's family's role and responsibility may be to ask the client about suicidal ideation, remove weapons from the home, and to call the mobile crisis team in case of emergency. The nurse will provide the necessary education on suicide, help the client and family develop a plan for intervention, see the client as indicated, and provide emergency care if needed. In this manner, each person knows the role and responsibility of the others and can live day to day with the knowledge that all that can be done for the client is being done. All parties must keep their part of the contract, and the contract is subject to renegotiation whenever any of the parties requests it.

Families are a major source of strength in the lives of clients with mental illness. Nurses who work with the client and family together can tap into their strength. To work effectively, the nurse must share power and knowledge with the client and family. Families have found satisfaction in collaborating with the mental health care professionals who respect the family's role in caregiving for the person with mental illness (Callahan, Boustani, & Unverzagt et al., 2006). The nurse can increase effectiveness by listening to the client and the family and learning about mental illness from them. From this dialogue, the nurse can glean information that can help in developing and implementing psychoeducation about topics the client and family may need clarified. In partnership, all parties can provide expertise and, in turn, each will benefit from the partnership and become more effective in alleviating symptoms and improving the quality of life for the client, the family, and the nurse.

Results from a survey of mental health professionals and consumer panelists that discussed what they wanted during a psychiatric emergency, revealed that consumers consistently emphasized the importance of client-centered care, respect, active listening, and involvement in treatment decisions (Allen, Carpenter, Sheets, Miccio, & Ross, 2003). Medications, such as haloperidol was perceived as a negative approach to managing psychiatric emergencies and greater acceptance of benzodiazepines in emergent situations was expressed. Twenty percent of the consumers ($n = 59$) attributed psychiatric emergencies to poor access to mental health care. Recommendations from the consumer panel about psychiatric emergency services included:

◆ Create innovative emergency room services
◆ Increase use of advance directives
◆ Provide more customer-friendly and comfortable physical environments while waiting for evaluation and treatment
◆ Use more peer support services
◆ Provide appropriate training of emergency staff to facilitate a humanistic and client-centered approach
◆ Establish collaborative clinician-nurse relationships
◆ Provide quality discharge planning and postdischarge follow-up

Mental health professionals similar to the consumer panelists recognized the value of collaborative relationships with clients and their families along with active participation in treatment decisions. A greater emphasis on consumer responsibilities in treatment decisions, collaboration with mental health professionals, and improved access to mental health services and using more nonpharmacological interventions to manage psychiatric emergencies are major themes for mental health care (Allen, Currier, Carpenter, Ross, & Docherty, 2005). These recommendations are consistent with other studies that indicate higher client satisfaction when they are listened to, respected by staff, and attention is given to their concerns and needs along with the provision of quality health care (Cleary, Horsfall, & Hunt, 2003). Implications for psychiatric nursing during an era when consumers and caregivers need to be involved in their care, adhere to treatment, and contribute to quality and positive clinical outcomes show that it is imperative to provided client-centered care in all health care settings.

On local, state, and national levels, nurses, clients, and families work in partnerships to ensure that adequate resources are available for clients with serious mental illness. Prevention of mental health problems is included in this partnership and is addressed in the final section of this chapter.

CONSUMERISM

The *American Heritage Dictionary of the English Language* (1992) defines a consumer as "one that acquires goods or services." Consumerism is the "movement seeking to protect and inform consumers by requiring such practices as honest packaging . . . and improved safety standards" (p. 405). The consumers of mental health services and their families have made policy makers and clinicians aware of their rights.

Consumers and their families had been quieter in the past when poor parenting skills, character flaws, and sinful behavior were thought to be the cause of mental illness (Flynn, 1993). Families feared judgment and censure if they dared to complain about the poor care and treatment of their relatives in institutions for the mentally ill. When biological bases for schizophrenia, major depression, and bipolar disorder were discovered, families eagerly educated themselves and began to feel more justified in demanding improved treatment for their loved ones.

Consumerism has had a profound effect on mental health services. The passage of Pub. L. 99-660 provided an avenue that ensured a variety of advocacy mechanisms to ensure quality of health care for clients with mental illness, and it mandated the states to develop comprehensive living arrangements for people with serious mental illness. Advisory councils oversee this effort in each state and are required to have consumers and families appointed to them (Flynn, 1993). Findings from a 2005 study that focused on identifying core competencies for community support providers working with individuals with psychiatric disabilities demonstrated that a range of personal characteristics, knowledge, and skills

influenced the quality of mental health community support (Aubry, Flynn, Gerber, & Dostaler, 2005). These researchers concluded that there is a need for specialized training and supervision and core competencies to identify and address the needs of clients with psychiatric disabilities.

The NAMI has played a pivotal role in advocating for clients and their families. They have continued to influence legislators and other policy makers in addressing issues that affect the care of persons with severe mental illnesses; for instance, several federal initiatives, such as the Ticket to Work and Work Incentives Act (TWWIIA, Pub. L. No. 106-170). Overall, the goals of these initiatives are to bring the perspectives of consumers to legislators and the private sector to improve the quality of health care (Bodenheimer, 2001).

Other laws have been enacted that appropriated funds to ensure health insurance for uninsured children. Pub. L. No. 105-33 provides funds to states to use to either supplement their existing Medicaid programs or as block grant monies under state programs to purchase health insurance for children. Most of the benchmark plans that states may select provide some coverage for mental health treatment, and all health plans must comply with the federal Mental Illness Parity Act of 1996 (Sperling, 1997).

In an effort to ensure consumer rights, President Clinton took the first step by appointing the Advisory Commission on Consumer Protection and Quality in the Health Care Industry. The appointment of this commission in 1997 (Advisory Commission on Consumer Protection and Quality in the Health Care Industry, 1997) issued a proposal that enumerates four categories of traditional consumer rights:

◆ The right to make informed medical decisions
◆ The right to confidentiality
◆ The right to emergency care
◆ The right to be treated with dignity and respect

Psychiatric-mental health nurses become consumer advocates by integrating quality management principles into their practice and helping the client assert all rights specified in the bill of rights.

In brief, consumerism involves numerous players who are invested in parity in treatment, housing, and employment of clients with serious mental illnesses. Efforts also involve client and family education and proactive political involvement, which ensure quality and accessible mental health care to all citizens.

PERFORMANCE IMPROVEMENT

Historically, quality improvement was left up to committees, which determined whether care met some designated standard. If care were found to be lacking, steps were taken to improve it. It was assumed that the people delivering the care could not be trusted to ensure its quality; hence, overseers brought in for periodic inspection were used to ensure that standards were met (Gilliam, 1988). This practice resulted in attention to quality issues just before and after inspection; it was not expected that ongoing efforts would be made to improve quality. This situation was not conducive to professional practice.

Because mental health care did not attune itself to the needs of the consumer and those with health insurance reached their policy limits, consumers of mental health services eventually became dependent on the state for their care. State services were usually underfunded and overburdened. Quality improvement in these institutions was more of a luxury rather than a necessity. The consumer and family suffered because of this situation.

Several years ago the Foundation for Accountability (FACCT) was created, and its approach to quality assessment differed from the National Committee for Quality Assurance, or NCQA. The NCQA has been involved in collecting extensive information to carry out efforts relevant to mental health care advocates because of its Medicaid measurement program and managed behavioral health care organization accreditation program. Endeavors of this newer FACCT involved the provision of consumer-friendly information and on consumer-focused quality measures in managed care environments. Several organizations, including NAMI and CMMS, are on the FACCT's board of directors (Hall, 1997). Psychiatric nurses need to form partnerships with their clients and mental health advocacy group to ensure access to quality mental health care by providing them with appropriate resources and referrals.

A newer approach to quality assurance is performance improvement. This concept is based on the notion that improvement is a continuous process based on tracking and trending health care performance and implementing action plans that resolve deficiencies and "close the loop." This premise also suggests that there is always room for improvement based on the dynamic nature of health care, client responses, and staff attributes and interactions. As data become the driving forces to measure or benchmark treatment outcomes, psychiatric nurses are poised to improve and provide quality health care. They must take the lead in redesigning processes to improve and implement quality health care; facilitate performance improvement processes to ensure client satisfaction and accurate medication management; maintain an environment of care that ensures client safety and delivery of age-specific health care; and collaborate with clients, families, and interdisciplinary team members to sustain high-quality care.

Pressure from outside groups, such as accreditation, makes health care institutions comply with a minimal standard of quality performance, thus increasing demands to improve. Publication of performance measures or report cards may maneuver consumers or employers away from health plans, medical groups, or hospitals, but health care providers employed at institutions who receive low marks on these report cards will be forced to improve the quality of care (Bodenheimer, 2001, 2005).

To avoid the loss of clients, hospitals and other agencies continue to explore ways to improve the quality of their care

and thus the perception of their customers. Many have adopted a system that empowers individuals directly involved in any activity to make changes to improve their work, which will result in customer satisfaction, whether the consumers are clients, physicians, nurses, or third-party payers of health care. Many have adopted continuous quality improvement, a method developed by Deming (1982), an American who consulted with the Japanese after World War II (his method is based on 14 points [Table 37–1]). Deming's recommendations for quality control were adopted and have contributed to the fact that, today, Japanese goods are known for their durability and quality.

NAMI has published several reports that are of interest here. The first, *Care of the Seriously Mentally Ill: A Rating of State Programs* (Torrey, 1990), uses various indicators to evaluate each state's mental health services, and it is published every 2 years. The second is a 1992 study funded by NAMI on the use of jails to contain people with serious mental illness entitled *Criminalizing the Seriously Mentally Ill: The Abuse of Jails as Mental Hospitals* (Torrey, 1992). When NAMI families were surveyed, it was discovered that 40 percent of their relatives with mental illness had been jailed at one time or another because of symptoms of their

TABLE 37–1
Deming's 14 Points for Total Quality Management

1. Create constancy of purpose for service improvement
2. Adapt the new philosophy
3. Cease dependence on inspection to achieve quality
4. End practice of awarding business on price alone—make partners out of vendors
5. Constantly improve every process for planning, production, and service
6. Institute training and retraining on the job
7. Institute leadership for system improvement
8. Drive out fear
9. Break down barriers between staff areas
10. Eliminate slogans, exhortations, and targets of the workforce
11. Eliminate numerical quotas for the workforce and numerical goals for the management
12. Remove barriers to pride of workmanship
13. Institute a vigorous program of education and self-improvement for everyone
14. Put everyone to work on transformation

Note. Date adapted from *The Deming Management Method,* by M. K. Walton, 1986, New York: Dodd, Mead.

illnesses (Flynn, 1993). By publishing these documents, NAMI educates the public and, as a result, citizens are prompted to support better funding for mental health care.

A NAMI's publication, *In Our Own Voice: Living with Mental Illness,* is given by trained consumers of a recovery, educational program for other consumers, family members, friends, professionals, students of all academic levels, and lay audiences. This interactive presentation focuses on mental illness that includes a video, personal testimony, and rich discussions of consumers who discuss how they cope with their serious illness, while recovering and reclaiming a quality life.

Performance improvement places the responsibility for improving care to persons with mental illnesses directly to the provider of services. The provider of services ranges from the housekeeper, who ensures a safe, clean environment, to the professional nurse, who determines the needs for intervention for the client. No longer can either say it was not her job to worry about the client's experience. Each member of the team is expected to be concerned about the care delivered and suggest and implement changes to improve that care.

In 2000, the ANA identified standards of professional performance for psychiatric-mental health nursing. Standard I establishes that the psychiatric-mental health nurse must systematically evaluate the quality of care and effectiveness of practice. The rationale for this standard is that this specialty has its own body of knowledge derived from research and practices that provides the means and impetus to improve the care delivered. This standard will be measured by appropriate nursing activities based on each nurse's education, role, and work setting. Activities include identification of aspects of care that should be monitored such as consumer satisfaction, functional status, symptom management, health behaviors, and quality of life. Indicators should be monitored for effectiveness by using the nursing process and working with interdisciplinary teams. Quality of care results will be documented and used by the nurse to make changes in personal practice, team activities, and the mental health care system.

Client and family satisfaction with services should be one of the quality indicators included in every aspect of care. As health care has moved out of hospitals and into community agencies and the home, clients and families have assumed more and more responsibility for the treatment of mental illness. Because professionals have less contact with clients and their families have more, both parties must actually be included in treatment planning if they are to be important members of the mental health care team. Therefore, satisfaction with treatment options and services is essential information for nurses to obtain.

THE ROLE OF STRESS, COPING, AND ADAPTATION IN PSYCHIATRIC-MENTAL HEALTH NURSING PRACTICE

Stress is known to play a role in the development of some mental disorders. Chrousos and Gold (1992) reviewed literature on stress and stress system disorders by looking at original articles of controlled studies with sound methodologies from the basic and human sciences. Dysregulation of the stress system results in numerous disorders. If the system activity increased, the results ranged from panic disorder, anorexia nervosa, addictions to alcohol or drugs, and premenstrual disorders. Decreased activity in the stress system resulted in Cushing's disease, seasonal and atypical depressions, obesity, inflammatory disorders, and post-traumatic stress disorders. The authors concluded that dysregulation of the stress system can lead to "a number of health problems of enormous impact on society" (p. 1249).

Nurses have long focused on mediating the effect of stress. Emphasis on recognizing stress and its effects has led to a large body of stress-reduction techniques. Foa, Stein, and McFarlane (2006) and Killien (2004) discussed the phenomena of stress and coping and their relationships to health and illness. More rigorous study of nursing interventions for stress mediation and teaching of coping strategies should be the focus of nursing research in the future. The role of stress response on immune and genetic function has been a particular interest as identified by the National Institute of Nursing Research (2006) in its 10-year agenda for research funding.

The 2006–2010 Mission and Research Opportunities of the NINR include:

◆ Integration of biological and behavioral science for better health

◆ Implementing and adapting new technologies to ensure better health care

◆ Health promotion and disease prevention

◆ Eliminating health disparities

◆ Caregiving research

◆ Symptoms management of acute and chronic illness

◆ Self-management in health and illness

◆ End of life or palliative care

CAREGIVERS

The role of caregivers is often overlooked in mental health care. Contributions of caregivers in the daily care and support of individuals with psychiatric conditions is well documented, although infrequently discussed. Growing research indicates their impact on adherence to treatment, quality of life, and emotional support of loved ones (van Vliet, Schuurmans, Grypdonck, & Duijnstee, 2006). Of greater significance is the cumulative effect of caregiving on the caregiver. There is ample evidence of the long-term impact of caregiving on the caregiver and client when support is unavailable to reduce stress. Availability and quality of support often govern how individuals cope with caregiving. A recent study (*n* = 83) of caregivers of persons with serious mental illness demonstrated that family caregivers of persons with serious mental illness typically turn to spirituality for support, and religious beliefs may play a key role in caregiver adjustment. Implications from these findings suggest the importance of nurse-client and family psycho-education about mental illness and health promotion, collaborative relationships, and religious communities as a potential and powerful and culturally sensitive resource for supporting caregivers of persons with serious mental illness (Murray-Swank et al., 2006). The growing number of caregivers of persons with Alzheimer's disease is often overtaxing and overwhelming. Interventions, such psychoeducation about the disease process and the disease manifestations being exhibited, must be an integral part of treatment. Referrals to family and caregiver support groups are equally helpful. More nursing research is needed to identify the vast needs of caregivers that include establishing collaborative relationships and interventions to reduce stress and promote health across the life span.

Online health care, or eHealth, has arrived and transformed nurse-client interactions and health care delivery. It was inevitable to become an integral part of nursing and nursing curriculum (Barnard, Nash, & O'Brien, 2005). Booth (2006) submits that this is a revolutionary era in which new paradigms of client care continue to evolve. She advocates the necessity to address this revolution by developing curriculum that ensures that nursing curricula in relation to nursing informatics must be proactive to meet advance eHealth across practice settings (Booth, 2006).

THE IMPACT OF TECHNOLOGY IN PSYCHIATRIC-MENTAL HEALTH NURSING PRACTICE

Historically, caring is an essential activity of nursing. Some authors have dichotomized human caring and the use of technology. Hall and Allen (1985) stated that the disease model and the health model nurses use could not exist in the same profession. They went as far as to suggest that the discipline of nursing be split into two professions, one called "healthing" and the other still to be called "nursing," if these models cannot be reconciled. Watson (1988) warned of the tendency in nursing to dichotomize. Examples of dichotomies in nursing are research and practice, theory and practice, wellness and illness, and mind and body. When dichotomies are overused, common grounds for agreement are elusive.

We live in an age of technological advances, and this has influenced us in many ways. It behooves us to question the use of technology, but it is unreasonable to eliminate it because the use of that technology can improve the caring aspect of the nursing profession. Some issues that arise with the use of technology are ethical, and some are practical.

HEALTH INFORMATICS

Perhaps the most powerful technological influence on consumer health care decision making is the Internet. Today's client with a mental illness is likely to present with questions about information obtained from the Internet. They also surf the Internet to seek information and use chat rooms or listserves and other dialogues to share their concerns, learn about the quality of others' experiences with mental illness, and available treatment. The availability of vast health information supports consumers and challenges psychiatric nurses to understand digital care resources. Likewise, the Internet provides opportunities for the client to gain a greater understanding of mental illness and its appropriate treatment and helps them find providers who meet their needs. Lewis and Pesut (2001) stated that technological advances in informatics increase availability of health care information, "seamless networks of data, services, information, and connectively available on the Internet" (p. 7). Ultimately, the "information-enable consumer" is likely to revolutionize the health care delivery systems (Eminovic, Wyatt, Tarpey, Murray, & Ingrams, 2004).

NURSING INFORMATICS

Gorn (1983) defined informatics as computer science plus information science. Nursing informatics refers to the use of computer and information sciences to manage and process data, knowledge, and information in nursing practice and client care (Graves & Corcoran, 1989). Information is viewed as data, objective bits of facts, that are organized and interpreted. Informatics allows for the clustering and arranging of data so that information may be efficiently organized. Data can then be processed to yield pertinent information that can lead to meaning in clinical practice.

Online health care has arrived and will transform the nurse-client relationship. Clients will be able to meet their health care needs in nontraditional settings. Nontraditional settings are projected to include e-health websites, which clients will be able to download and receive health care by E-mail. Psychiatric nurses are key positions to explore evolving and emerging technology in consumer health informatics. New roles will require specialized educational preparation and will generate research opportunities (Yellowlees & Cook, 2006).

COMPUTERIZED DOCUMENTATION AND CONFIDENTIALITY

The use of computers for documentation in psychiatry, particularly of psychiatric services within general hospitals, has lagged behind that in the other areas because of concerns expressed about confidentiality. The danger of access to computerized information and the known potential for computer "hackers" to find passwords for entrance into records has been foremost in these arguments. Because mental illness has been stigmatized, access to information that a person has been treated for mental illness has led to loss of jobs, marriages, and custody of children. Much adverse publicity has accompanied the release of information on politicians or celebrities who have been treated for depression, suicide attempts, or drug- and alcohol-related disorders, so the real fear of discovery of mental illness has not been exaggerated.

CONTINUITY OF CARE AND COST-EFFECTIVE HEALTH CARE

There are many positive aspects to introducing computers into psychiatric-mental health nursing. The greatest benefit is continuity of seamless care from community-based programs to the hospital and back to the community. Many problems arise because of the lack of continuous quality care. Clients may find themselves being reassessed every time they move into a new setting, which may disturb their previous care and medication regimens. Sometimes services are duplicated—the community-based service may have drawn blood samples and taken radiographs and the client incurs the unnecessary expense of repeating these tests when hospitalized. This duplication not only leads to increased cost, it also affects the client's trust in the system. Links between services could be facilitated by the increased use of computers.

Quality improvement indicators can be tracked with computers. Continuous care issues that arise when the client transfers from the hospital to the community can be monitored so clients do not become lost to follow-up services. Linkages between systems can be facilitated through computer networks when clients and their families are included in the network. Nurses who have experience in collaborating with clients and their families can be instrumental in working out this linkage to ensure quality of services.

COMPUTER NETWORKS

Provider access to state-of-the-science information is possible through computer networks even in remote areas. Some of these, such as computer network on information about psychoactive drugs and practice guidelines, are already available. These networks can be helpful to clinicians in rural areas where specialists are unavailable; however, clinicians must not devalue their own experience and knowledge when employing an information system.

Computer networks for consumers and their families can be used to help clients make online health care decisions. People with various medical conditions such as those with human immunodeficiency virus (HIV) disease can be linked up early in the course of illness to discuss current treatment trends. Clients with mental illness are now sharing their experiences with others on the Internet in an effort to inspire and encourage others. Client and family advocacy groups provide an array of educational material about mental disorders, psychoactive agents, and client rights. Nurses can play a role in psychoeducation and learning from their clients' experiences by joining the computer networks and entering the interaction.

PROMOTION OF PSYCHIATRIC-MENTAL HEALTH CARE ACROSS THE LIFE SPAN

Another factor that will influence nursing practice in the future is the addition of new groups at risk for mental illness. Traditional groups have been those with acute and chronic mental disorders; new vulnerable populations are infants exposed to noxious substances (like cocaine) in utero, children and adolescents with behavior disorders and developmental disabilities, people with HIV disease and their families, substance abusers, women and children survivors of family violence, and older adults with cognitive disorders and psychiatric problems. Nurses have focused on the needs of populations at risk for health deviations and have worked with communities for social changes, which result in healthy citizens.

PREVENTION CONCEPTS

The NIMH developed a plan of prevention of mental disorders with a focus on current state of science, training of mental health care professionals in prevention, and future directions for prevention research. Shea (1991) submitted a report to the NIMH on the role of nursing in prevention research. In this report the author stated that, historically, nursing has been involved with integrating prevention of disease with the restoration of health, yet it was not identified by the NIMH for its strengths and potential contributions to the national prevention effort.

Concepts most associated with prevention are vulnerability, developmental processes that may lead to pathological outcomes, and epidemiological orientation (DHHS, 1999).

The interface between biology and behavior and health promotion and disease prevention is part of the 2006–2010 NINR research strategic initiatives (NINR, 2006). It parallels dramatic changes in mental health in almost 2 decades in which the decade of the brain has heralded research and initiatives to develop interventions that parallel alterations in complex processes such as dysregulation of neurotransmitters and neuroanatomical structures; the role of stress and genetics involved in schizophrenia, bipolar and depressive, anxiety and substance-related disorders. Psychiatric nurses continue to be poised to work with clients and families and develop pharmacological and nonpharmacological interventions that control symptoms and behaviors unique to psychiatric disorders and prevent disease and disability.

Vulnerability

Vulnerability refers to potential susceptibility of person, family, or group to a health deviation. In evaluating vulnerability, the environment and a person's interaction with it should be considered. For example, a person may have a high risk for developing depression because of characteristics of serotonin release or inhibition. However, if the environment interacts with the person so that loss is not experienced or appropriate interventions are provided when loss is expected, depression may not occur.

Developmental Stage

Nurses have long been concerned about human development across the life span. Developmental theories, models, and interventions have been developed and implemented with various populations with some success. One area of concern for nurses has centered on adolescence as a stressful period of development. This age group experiences dramatic change during puberty, including hormonal changes that greatly influence emotions and mood, establishes new roles with parents and peers, and deals with pressure to conform to peer pressure. Some problems associated with adolescence are drug and alcohol abuse, pregnancy, and violence. For more information on disorders and behaviors across the life span, see the life span issues section of other chapters in this text. Nurses have begun to develop and test strategies to prevent long-lasting problems related to adolescent behaviors. Psychiatric nurses subspecialize in working with children and adolescents—many more are needed as specialists in this area.

Epidemiological Orientation

Nursing and epidemiology were developed concurrently. Florence Nightingale first described modern nursing as focused on health and illness. In a paper issued at the 1893 World's Fair, Nightingale wrote, "Sick nursing and health nursing . . . nursing proper is . . . to help the client suffering from disease to live—just as health nursing is to keep or put the constitution of the healthy child or human being in such a state as to have no disease" (Nightingale, 1894, p. 446). Nightingale first employed statistical data to track health and illness, and nurses have followed her leadership into this practice. The discipline has used a biological, psychological, social, and cultural model of human beings that addresses the environment and the person-environment interaction as a source to define health and pathological states.

As psychiatric nursing as moves into the twenty-first century, it continues to be influenced by epidemiologic studies. Large epidemiologic studies provide invaluable data about the prevalence and coexistence of psychiatric disorders and vulnerable populations. Data obtained from randomized controlled trials offer effective treatment options for clients and their families with psychiatric disorders. Psychiatric nurses must collaborate with clients, families, mental health consumers, and other health care providers to develop and implement evidence-based mental health services.

CULTURAL COMPETENCE

The changing face of the American population must be reflected in interventions used to treat mental illness. ANA's *Position Statement on Cultural Diversity in Nursing Practice* (ANA, 1992) emphasized that all nurses must appreciate how various cultures define health and illness, delivery of care, and interactions with health care providers. Nursing models must reflect cultural sensitivity and competence and global mental health needs (Caffrey & Neander et al., 2005; Levine & Perpetua, 2006). Cross, Bazron, Dennis, and Isaacs (1989) define cultural competence as the synthesis and modification of knowledge concerning people and groups

into distinct standards, policies, practices, and attitudes. It also implies that the nurse has learned new patterns of behaviors, effectively implements them in appropriate cultural settings, and uses them to improve client outcomes. In addition, the culturally competent psychiatric-mental health nurses develop individualize treatment planning that is culturally appropriate and guide research, practice, and education (Owen & Khalil, 2007). Psychiatric nurses must develop culturally sensitive mental health care models to meet the challenges of an expanding diverse society. (See Chapter 7 for a detailed discussion on culture.)

PSYCHIATRIC NURSING'S ROLE IN MEETING NATIONAL CARE GOALS

The next sections include discussions on the national goals to improve health and the role of psychiatric mental-health nurses in achieving these goals.

HEALTHY PEOPLE 2010

"*Healthy People 2010* is about improving health—the health of each person, the health of communities, and the health of the Nation" (U.S. DHHS, 2000, p. 1). However, *Healthy People 2010* goals are described as a part of a greater, systematic approach to health improvement. The basis of goal achievement involves community partnerships that use a systematic approach to improve health, such as violence among teens. The leading health indicators that will be used to measure the health of the nation over the next 10 years (2010) reflect primary health concerns in the United States at the turn of the twenty-first century. Leading indicators were determined on the basis of their ability to motivate action, the availability of data to measure progress, and relevance to public health issues.

The leading health indicators are:

◆ Physical activity

◆ Overweight and obesity

◆ Tobacco use

◆ Substance abuse

◆ Responsible sexual behavior

◆ Mental health

◆ Injury and violence

◆ Quality of environment

◆ Immunization

◆ Access to health care

The *Healthy People 2010* document reflects the diversity of the American population and the challenges it faces to improve health in the person, community, state, and the nation. It also stresses the significance of interdisciplinary approaches to achieve health equity that involves health promotion, education, housing, labor, justice, transportation,

TABLE 37-2
Priority Areas for America: *Healthy People 2010*

Health Promotion

Health Protection

Preventive Services

Data System

Age-Related Objectives

The Nation's Health: Special Populations

Goals For The Nation

Note. Data from *Healthy People 2010* (DHHS Publication No. PHS), by the United States Department of Health and Human Services, 2000, Washington, DC: U.S. Government Printing Office.

agriculture, the environment, and data collection. Its greatest challenge to achieving these goals lies in reducing health disparities, empowering people to make informed health choices and decisions, and promoting safety, education, and access to health care in all communities. *Healthy People 2010* is also committed to ensuring equal access to health care that is comprehensive, culturally competent, community based regardless of age, race or ethnicity, gender, income, education, regional location, disability, or sexual orientation.

Twenty-eight priority areas have been identified in their order of importance to American health (Table 37–2). Included in these priorities are issues of interest to the psychiatric-mental health nurse, such as substance abuse, mental health and mental disorders, and injury and violence. Many of the other identified objectives have mental health implications as well.

Age-related objectives and objectives for special populations are also identified in *Healthy People 2010* (U.S. DHHS, 2000). Special populations are of particular interest to those in psychiatric-mental health nursing because they include cultural and ethnic minorities, people residing in poverty, and people with disabilities. The last two groups are known to have large numbers of people with mental problems who have poor access to health care and treatment.

What is the psychiatric-mental health nurse's responsibility in relation to the goals of *Healthy People 2010*? The focus of the nation's goals is health improvement, health protection, preventive services, and surveillance and data systems. We have both advanced-practice and generalist skills with which to respond to the goals and objectives for the nation's health. Nurses practicing in all areas of psychiatric-mental health should develop knowledge and skills needed to respond to people in stigmatized, impoverished, and isolated groups. As a professional group we must educate ourselves as to the

needs of citizens, then assume an active role in helping groups meet their goals for a healthy life.

Psychiatric-mental health nursing has already directed its energy toward developing knowledge, skills, and models of care that address the nation's goals. The ANA set forth goals for the development of new knowledge in relevant areas. More can be done to address the needs of people with serious, persistent mental illnesses. Outcomes of care must be assessed through rigorous methods, including comprehensive assessments of quality of life and client satisfaction.

The NINR (2006) has set forth an agenda for research that must be evaluated in light of the goals for the nation's health. Nurse scientists must rapidly move into areas of health promotion and disease prevention. Some of this is already established; examples include Pender's (1996) work on health promotion (Carreno & Vyhmeister et al., 2006). More must be done in the area of mental health in particular.

IDENTIFYING POPULATIONS AT RISK

One area of intensive effort is promotion of healthy, nonabusive environments for children. The school nurse should be involved not only with the school-age child but also children from early infancy and later. Avance is one such program in San Antonio, Texas, that combines childcare with parent education for families at risk for health deviations. The mothers tend to be young, single, uneducated, and impoverished. Mothers and their children are nurtured through intensive community efforts to help the family escape poverty and improve their quality of life.

Other examples may be drug awareness programs aimed at parents and children. These have had some success in reducing drug use in children. Community-based programs can best meet these needs for a comprehensive, holistic approach to health. The nurse must recognize the interaction among the environment, genetics, and behaviors. She must have the necessary skills to work effectively with the community to address these concerns.

Packaged health-promotion programs are not helpful in this situation. For example, cholesterol screening may be viewed as a waste of time in an area where poverty prevents adequate nutrition. Even if the nurse can show the need for such a program, if the community perceives greater needs, the nurse will fail. Experienced nurses have always valued addressing the community's concerns first and then educating the group to additional areas for improvement.

War-Related Trauma

Although the concept of war-related trauma has existed for years, veterans returning from wars in Afghanistan and Iraq are predicted to utilize a high rate of mental health services 12 months postwar (Hoge, Auchterlonie, & Milliken, 2006; Turner et al., 2005). An estimated one-third of combat veterans accessed mental health services within 2 months of returning home. Implications from these data suggest the intensity of mental health services required in the military.

In addition, these findings indicate growing evidence that the wars are burdening the overall health care system. Preliminary data was obtained from mass mental health screening for mental health and health problems among this population. The prevalence of PTSD among returning Iraq combat veterans was 9.8 percent compared to 4.7 percent in veterans returning from Afghanistan (Hoge et al., 2006). Implications for psychiatric nurses include the growing need for mental health screening, use of mental and health care services, and provision of client-centered treatment for war-related illnesses to reduce symptoms and disabilities. (See In The News box.)

CASE MANAGEMENT

Several models of nursing care delivery have been suggested to change the access, effectiveness, and choice of mental health care. Primary mental health care must be available to the population across the life span. Case management is one such approach. Thornicroft (1991) defined case management as an ongoing process that comprises the coordination, integration, and allocation of holistic care within allocated resources with one or more identified staff. Most clinical studies indicate that case management improves outcomes for clients (Burns et al., 2007; Meyers & Morrissey, 2007). Case management remains a viable treatment option for clients with serious persistent mental disorders.

Initially, the case management model has been used to coordinate and integrate vast services into a seamless program individualized to meet the needs of persons with serious, persistent mental disorders such as schizophrenia. Nehls (2001) noted that traditionally, case management services have extended to other mental disorders, including borderline personality disorder. She submitted that case management offers these clients a single caregiver who provides continuous holistic care and reduction in needed resources. Although these basic attributes remain an integral part of case management, the responsibilities of the case manager have grown. The growing responsibilities of the case manager have increased the need for different case management models (Mueser, Bond, Drake, & Resnick, 1998).

For the past two decades, case management has become a popular model of mental health delivery in vast practice settings. As case managers, psychiatric-mental health nurses provide a means of increasing access to care while maintaining seamless holistic mental health care services and reducing duplication of services. Nurses, by virtue of their education, are grounded in a tradition of holistic care. Professional nursing care is often limited by policies made by those people more concerned with immediate cost saving than prevention of problems. Professional nurses must assert themselves to provide adequate, safe, and appropriate care for each client.

The exact definition of case management remains unclear and complex and tends to parallel the organization's values and structure (Mueser et al, 1998; Nehls, 2001). Mueser et al. (1998) also described six models: broker case management, clinical case management, strengths case management, rehabilitation case management, assertive community treatment case management, and intensive case management. For purposes of this discussion four models will be discussed in this chapter: broker or expanded broker case management model (Moore, 1990); clinical case management model (Kanter, 1989); intensive case management (ICM) model (Surles, Blanch, Shern, & Donahue, 1992); and assertive community treatment (ACT) model (Essock et al., 2006; Stein, 1990). (See Chapter 33 for an in-depth discussion of home- and community-based mental health care.)

In the first model, the case manager focuses on determining which needs each client may have and then securing these from a variety of sources. The case manager may come from various disciplines or be trained on the job in the skills necessary to broker services.

The second type of case manager is a clinician who acts as the client's and family's source of support. A therapeutic relationship is developed and maintained as a basis for ongoing support. When the need for additional services is identified, the therapeutic case manager selects and oversees the provision of these services. Overall, assessment and management remain with the case manager. This type of case management model has the following characteristics:

- A higher level of professional education is required.
- It requires effort and skills to develop and maintain the therapeutic relationship.
- The relationship is expected to last over a long period.
- A clinician model with skills in areas including psychotherapy and psychoeducation.

The clinical case management model would be more effective with people who have serious and persistent mental illnesses. The trust level among client, family, and case manager will gradually increase and strengthen over time. Professional nurses are well prepared to distinguish between exacerbation of mental disorders and development of other illnesses. Emergence of new symptoms is often ignored or

THE MORE KNOW

In 2007, according to the Army Suicide Event Report (ASER) (2007), 2006 marks the highest rate of military suicides in 26 years, and more than a quarter of those soldiers who killed themselves did so while serving in Iraq and Afghanistan. Reportedly, ninety-nine U.S. soldiers killed themselves in 2006. More disheartening is high prevalence of PTSD (i.e., 50 percent) in soldiers and Marines who have been deployed to Iraq more than once. Few psychiatric-mental health professionals are trained to address the needs of individuals suffering from war-related trauma. Psychiatric nurses must respond to these needs by seeking special training and educational offerings that enable them to work with veterans at risk for PTSD to mitigate the alarming incidence of suicide in this vulnerable population.

overlooked by those who are less skilled working with these clients (Goff & Newcomer, 2007).

The third example is the ICM model. This model emerged out of the need to deal with clients who are high users of the most costly mental health resources, such as emergency room visits. Similar to the ACT model, the ICM employs a low client-to-clinician ratio and assertive outreach services in the client's natural community setting. The primary difference between the ICM and the ACT model is the use of an interdisciplinary or shared caseload in the latter (Surles et al., 1992).

The final concept is the ACT model. An interdisciplinary team delivers the services of the ACT model. Major distinctions between the former two case management models and ACT model include the following:

◆ Low client-to-clinician ratio (10:1 rather than 30:1)
◆ Community-based or outreach services rather than an office
◆ Interdisciplinary approach (shared caseloads rather than individual caseloads)
◆ 24-hour coverage
◆ Time-limited services

Major priorities of the ACT model are providing pragmatic support of daily living such as housing, laundry, and transportation (Mueser et al., 1998; Essock et al., 2006).

In brief, assertive community treatment seems to be more advantageous than clinical case management in reducing hospitalizations (Essock, Frisman, & Kontos, 1998). Meta-analytic studies indicate the effectiveness of assertive community treatment—clients had shorter lengths of stay and had better outcomes on housing, employment, and client satisfaction with services (Burns et al., 2007). Research findings indicate that assertive community treatment and clinical case management are effective treatment models for clients with serious and persistent mental illnesses.

Regardless of the case management model, psychiatric nurses can confidently use it to manage the care of their clients in the community, whether clients are in a homeless shelter or in the home of their family. It takes the combination of psychiatric-mental health and community health nurses to deliver holistic, comprehensive, and effective care to this population.

What nurses have not done systematically is study the effectiveness of nurses as case managers. This area of research is greatly needed if nurses are to be involved in care of persons with serious, persistent mental illness. All nurses in the psychiatric-mental health specialty can cite anecdotal information on the ineffectiveness of non-nurse case management models. We have seen people in the emergency centers who are exhibiting the effects of the broker-type case manager's failure to recognize dystonia or akathisia. We have seen people who are in acute pain from broken bones who are noted to have "delusions" of physical illness by their case managers. We have also seen emergency medical personnel who have failed to distinguish between delirium and dementia or have not recognized delirium tremens in psychiatric clients. These breakdowns in the system of care delivered to people with mental disorders must be eliminated and professional nurses should be in the forefront of these efforts.

TELEHEALTH

Mental health services in remote regions are often insufficiently staffed with few mental health care providers. Communication technology offers psychiatric mental health nurses opportunities to provide various services. One such model is teleconferencing. Teleconferencing enables mental health care providers to deliver services using technological advances. *Telehealth* refers to the use of digital equipment and other technological approaches, including teleconferencing and telephone services, that provide psychiatric-mental health nurses and consumers with clinical, consultative, and educational services in isolated areas of the country. Telehealth provides opportunities for nurses to perform and provide vast services, including the following (Frueh et al., 2000):

◆ diagnostic assessments such as mental status and cognitive examinations
◆ individual psychotherapy and pharmacotherapy
◆ consultation with client and family members
◆ discharge planning
◆ crisis intervention
◆ various forms of group therapy
◆ supportive employment interviews
◆ psychoeducation
◆ clinical supervision

Recent studies support the notion that telemental health is a useful, cost-effective, and quality option to perform psychiatric evaluations, consult with clients and providers in remote or rural areas, and a means of delivering quality mental health services. More quantitative and qualitative research is necessary on clinical outcomes, predictors of satisfaction, costs, and educational outcomes (Frueh et al., 2007).

Telehealth offers great hope to clients and families in remote regions. Psychiatric-mental health nurses can also use this mental health care delivery model to advance their own clinical expertise through clinical supervision.

PSYCHOEDUCATION AND ANTICIPATORY GUIDANCE

Anticipatory guidance and health care education are methods the professional nurse uses to reduce the risk of disease in vulnerable populations. Psychiatric-mental health nurses have thought of psychoeducation of clients and families during healthy periods as well as illness as one of their primary roles and responsibilities. Anticipatory guidance has been centered on stressful situational and developmental life events like natural disasters or childbirth and adolescence. Examples of anticipatory guidance are given in many chapters throughout this textbook in the section on life span issues. Psychoeducation is most often used for specific health issues such as coping with rape and sexual assault and medication or social skills training.

The profession can have a positive impact on the nation's health through efforts that provide anticipatory guidance and psychoeducation for populations at risk. More research on the issues of this specific type of intervention needed during which period in the life span for which high-risk group should be conducted. For example, when do we provide education about topics such as alcohol and drug use, responsible sexual behaviors, transitions during the life span, and psychopathology?

When prevention strategies fail, psychiatric-mental health nurses must be available to provide care to those experiencing addiction, teen pregnancy, and violence (both perpetrators and survivors). We must work with policy makers to address social problems that lead to increased failures in prevention for vulnerable groups.

PSYCHOACTIVE MEDICATION MANAGEMENT

Another set of knowledge and skills available through professional nurses is the management of clients who are taking psychoactive medication. Nurses have skills that enable them to help the client assume self-care responsibilities in terms of symptom management and adherence to medication regimen that will prevent exacerbation of illness (Gensichen et al., 2005). Nurses are also experienced in working with families, who assume care for two thirds of clients discharged from psychiatric hospitals. As more and more advanced-practice psychiatric nurses become primary care providers and prescribe psychoactive medications, they must be able to assess the client's physical, psychosocial, cultural, and spiritual needs. This holistic approach that involves medication management requires the advanced-practice psychiatric-mental health nurse to understand the complexity of neurobiological and physiological process that contribute to health and illness. See Chapter 29.

SUMMARY

◆ The crisis in psychiatric-mental health nursing needs to be addressed and resolved to ensure its survival. Trends that suggest changes are beginning to emerge.

◆ Psychiatric nursing continues to be an important specialty and offers great promise to clients and consumers with psychiatric disorders.

◆ Nurses in the specialty continue to provide holistic, client-centered, and culturally sensitive care in primary, secondary, and tertiary settings.

◆ The integration of neurobiology, psychological, sociological, spiritual, and cultural aspects of human beings into a holistic entity that cannot not be reduced to its parts.

◆ Advances in technology, particularly neuroimaging studies, offer a glimpse into the complexity of psychiatric disorders and target sites for pharmacologic and non-pharmacologic interventions.

◆ Leadership skills are an integral part of psychiatric nurses and must be developed and massaged to prepare current and future nurses entering this unique specialty.

◆ Information technology and data continue to be major drivers in the future of psychiatric nursing.

◆ Leaders must mentor inexperienced nurses and value experienced nurses to ensure we maintain a cadre of nurses to care for individuals at risk for and with psychiatric disorders.

◆ Quality and effective mental health care must be measured by data that demonstrate client satisfaction and positive clinical outcomes and ensures that environments of care provide safe and humane mental health services.

◆ Genetics continue to provide hope and opportunities for psychiatric nurses to identify high-risk groups and to implement interventions that reduce stress and genetic vulnerability to psychiatric conditions.

Some of these recommendations have been or are already being implemented. The effort that is required to effect such broad change is immense. Change is upon us, and such change brings out the best and the worst the profession has to offer. We have the strength of Florence Nightingale, Dorothea Dix, Clara Barton, Lillian Wald, Hildegarde Peplau, and other nurse heroes within our ranks. We must just step forward with a creative, innovative idea; take the risk of success or failure, but above all, engage in the struggle to take our rightful place in psychiatric-mental health care.

SUGGESTIONS FOR CLINICAL CONFERENCES

1. Ask several experienced psychiatric-mental health nurses from different practice settings to discuss changes in mental health care they have observed.

2. Have students attend a meeting with a mental health consumer or advocacy group and discuss their experience with other students.

3. Ask a nurse manager to talk about the role.

4. Ask students to explore various Internet and download resources for clients and their families.

5. Identify leadership in preceptor nurses.

6. Invite a nurse case manager who is using telemental health equipment to demonstrate its use in a remote area.

STUDY QUESTIONS

1. When the document *Healthy People 2010* was developed, the impact for psychiatric-mental health nurses included:
   a. integrating mental health into health care reform
   b. priority areas for research and practice

c. role transformation

d. essentials in mental health care

2. V. I., age 28, was diagnosed with bipolar disorder II 4 years ago. The case manager, a nurse, is concerned about V. I.'s lack of support from family members. To decrease V. I.'s isolation, the nurse refers the client to:

a. a singles club for young adults

b. a support group sponsored by the National Alliance for the Mentally Ill

c. a psychotherapist who specializes in young people with bipolar disorder

d. a church group for young adults

3. The nurse meets with V. I. every week to assess the effectiveness of the medication and to provide counseling as the need arises. Which type of case manager is this nurse?

a. Broker for services

b. Referral source

c. Therapeutic

d. Symptom

4. As members of a profession, nurses try to keep abreast of current trends in psychiatric nursing. To do this, nurses must:

a. register for a new course at the local college every year

b. join the professional organization and stay active at the local chapter

c. read the local and state newspapers daily

d. subscribe to at least three journals in the specialty

5. Martha, a psychiatric nurse, works with the local community center and provides parenting classes to pregnant adolescent girls. Which *Healthy People 2010* indicator does this address?

a. Mental health

b. Injury and violence

c. Access to health care

d. All of the above

6. The nurse is working with a young man diagnosed with bipolar disorder, current episode is depressed. Which of the following statements best described trends in mental health care for this client?

a. A focus symptom management, improved quality of life, and client satisfaction

b. Symptom management and increased hospitalization

c. Increased dependency on outpatient services, symptom management

d. Reduced dependency on family members and symptom management

7. The nurse is caring for the client with schizophrenia who was admitted to the acute inpatient unit several days ago. Which of the following statements reflects the nurse's understanding of client-centered care?

a. "I have your treatment plan and will review it with you."

b. "What is a good time for us to talk about your care, wishes, and preferences?"

c. "The treatment team expects you to follow these directions. What are your thoughts?"

d. "Because of your culture I know how important it is to include your family in this discussion."

8. The nurse is working with a client with major depression in his home using telemental health videoconferencing. Which of the following states indicates the client needs additional education about this technology?

a. "Can other people see me on camera?"

b. "What is the best time for us to meet next week?"

c. "I am going on vacation and will not be available next week."

d. "This has saved me so much money because I don't have to drive to the clinic."

RESOURCES

Please note that because Internet resources are of a time-sensitive nature and URL addresses may change or be deleted, searches should also be conducted by association or topic.

Internet Resources

Explore the Internet and NAMI's consumer advocacy efforts using the following websites:

http://www.nami.org/update/991217.html

http://www.ssa.gov/work/Resources

http://www.nami.org   National Alliance of the Mentally Ill

Support Groups and Organizations

http://www.jointcommission.org/NR/rdonlyres/5DD15D2A-09A0-4353-8290-C3C73A1E763F/0/FutureGoals.pdf   The Joint Commission. 2005–2010 Goals and Objectives.

http://www.addinfonetwork.com   The Attention Deficit Information Network, Inc. (AD-IN)

http://www.mentalhealth.org   KEN website provides quick access to state mental health resource guides, mental health resources, grant-funding opportunities E-mail: ken@mentalhealth.org

http://www.cms.hhs.gov/   Centers for Medicare & Medicaid Services (CMMS). U.S. federal agency which administers Medicare and Medicaid (Accessed May 17, 2006).

http://www.markle.org/resources/facct/index.php   Foundation for Accountability (FACCT) Documents (Accessed May 17, 2006).

National Alliance on Mental Illness
2107 Wilson Blvd., Suite 300
Arlington, VA 22201-3042
http://www.nami.org   (Accessed May 17, 2006)
HelpLine: 800-950-NAMI (6264)

The Mental Health Parity Act
CMMS Regulations and Guidance
www.cms.hhs.gov/HealthInsReformforConsume/04_TheMentalHealthParityAct.asp   (Accessed May 17, 2006)

http://www.ncqa.org/sohc2003/follow_up_after_hospitalization.htm National Committee for Quality of Assurance. State of Health Care 2003 Quality Report: Follow-Up after Hospitalization (Accessed 17, 2006).

REFERENCES

Advisory Commission on Consumer Protection and Quality in the Health Care Industry. (1997). *Consumer bill of rights and responsibilities: Report to the President of the United States.* Executive Order 13040.

Allen, M. H., Carpenter, D., Sheets, J. L., Miccio, S., & Ross, R. (2003). What do consumers say they want and need during a psychiatric emergency? *Journal of Psychiatric Practice, 9,* 39–58.

Allen, M. H., Currier, G. W., Carpenter, D., Ross, R. W., & Docherty, J. P. (2005). The expert consensus guideline series. Treatment of behavioral emergencies 2005. *Journal of Psychiatric Practice, 11*(Suppl 1), 5–108.

American Association of Colleges of Nursing. (1986). *Essentials of college and nursing education for professional nursing.* Washington, DC: Author.

American heritage dictionary of the English language (3rd ed.). (1992). New York: Houghton Mifflin.

American Nurses Association. (1992). *Position statement on cultural diversity in nursing practice.* Washington, DC: Author.

American Nurses Association. (1993). *The grassroots of lobbying book.* Washington, DC: Author.

American Nurses Association. (2000). *The scope and standards of psychiatric-mental health nursing practice.* Washington, DC: American Nurses Publishing.

Antai-Otong, D. (2007). Professional development: Leading through effective communication. In D. Antai-Otong (Ed.), *Nurse-client communication: A lifespan approach* (pp. 195–223). Sudbury, MA: Jones and Bartlett Publishers.

Aubry, T. D., Flynn, R. J., Gerber, G., & Dostaler, T. (2005). Identifying the core competencies of community support providers working with people with psychiatric disabilities. *Psychiatric Rehabilitation Journal, 28,* 346–353.

Barnard, A., Nash, R., & O'Brien, M. (2005). Information literacy: Developing lifelong skills through nursing education. *Journal of Nurse Educator, 44,* 505–510.

Baumann, A. E. (2007). Stigmatization, social distance and exclusion because of mental illness: The individual with mental illness as a 'stranger'. *International Reviews in Psychiatry, 19,* 131–135.

Bäuml, J., Froböse, T., Kraemer, S., Rentrop, M., & Pitschel-Walz, G. (2006). Psychoeducation: A basic psychotherapeutic intervention for patients with schizophrenia and their families. *Schizophrenia Bulletin, 32*(Suppl. 1), 1–9.

Billings, D. M., Skiba, D. J., & Connors, H. R. (2005). Best practices in Web-based courses: Generational differences across undergraduate and graduate nursing students. *Journal of Professional Nursing, 21,* 126–133.

Bishop, A., & Scudder, J. (1990). *The practical, moral, and personal sense of nursing: A phenomenological philosophy of practice.* New York: State University of New York Press.

Bodenheimer, T. (2001). The American health care system: The movement for improved quality in health care. In P. R. Lee & C. L. Estes (Eds.), *The nation's health* (6th ed., pp. 444–451). Sudbury, MA: Jones & Bartlett.

Bodenheimer, T. (2005). The political divide in health care: A liberal perspective. *Health Affairs (Millwood), 24,* 1426–1435.

Booth, R. G. (2006). Educating the future eHealth professional nurse. *International Journal of Nursing Education Scholarship, 3*(1), article 13. http://www.bepress.com/ijnes/vol3/iss1/art13/

Brimblecombe, N., Tingle, A., Tunmore, R., & Murrells, T. (2007). Implementing holistic practices in mental health nursing: A national consultation. *International Journal of Nursing Studies, 44,* 339–348.

Bradbury-Jones, C., Irvine, F., & Sambrooke, S. (2007). Empowerment of nursing students in the United Kingdom and Japan: A cross-cultural study. *Journal of Advanced Nursing, 59,* 379–387.

Burns, T., Catty, J., Dash, M., Roberts, C., Lockwood, A., & Marshall, M. (2007). Use of intensive case management to reduce time in hospital in people with severe mental illness: Systematic review and meta-regression. *British Medical Journal, 335,* 336. Retrieved August 31, 2007, from http://www.bmj.com/cgi/content/full/335/7615/336

Caffrey, R. A., Neander, W., Markle, D., & Stewart, B. (2005). Improving the cultural competence of nursing students: Results of integrating cultural content in the curriculum and an international immersion experience. *Journal of Nurse Education, 44,* 234–240.

Callahan, C. M., Boustani, M. A., Unverzagt, F. W., Austrom, M. G., Damush, T. M., Perkins, A. J., Fultz, B. A., & Hui, S. L., et al. (2006). Effectiveness of collaborative care for older adults with Alzheimer's disease in primary care: A randomized controlled trial. *Journal of the American Medical Association, 295,* 2148–2157.

Carreno, J., Vyhmeister, G., Grau, L., & Ivanovic, D. (2006). A health promotion programme in Adventist and non-Adventist women based on Pender's model: A pilot study. *Public Health, 120,* 346–355.

Chrousos, G. P., & Gold, P. W. (1992). The concepts of stress and stress system disorders: Overview of physical and behavioral homeostasis. *Journal of the American Medical Association, 267,* 1244–1252.

Cleary, M., Horsfall, J., & Hunt, G. F. (2003). Consumer feedback on nursing care and discharge planning. *Journal of Advanced Nursing, 42,* 269–277.

Cross, T., Bazron, B., Dennis, K., & Isaacs, M. (1989). *Towards a culturally competent system of care* (Vol. I). Washington, DC: CASSP Technical Assistance Center.

Deming, W. E. (1982). *Out of the crisis.* Cambridge, MA: Massachusetts Institute of Technology Center for Advanced Engineering Study.

Dobscha, S. K., Leibowitz, R. Q., Flores, J. A., Doak, M., & Gerrity, M. S. (2007). Primary care provider preferences for working with a collaborative support team. *Implementation Science, 2,* 16. Retrieved August 13, 2007, from http://www.implementationscience.com/content/2/1/16

Drake, R. E., Goldman, H. H., Leff, H. S., Lehman, A. F., Dixon, L., Mueser, K. T., et al. (2001). Implementing evidence-based practices in routine mental health service settings. *Psychiatric Services, 52,* 179–182.

Eminovic, N., Wyatt, J. C., Tarpey, A. M., Murray, G., & Ingrams, G. J. (2004). First evaluation of the NHS direct online clinical enquiry service: A nurse-led web chat triage service for the public. *Journal of Medical Internet Research, 6,* e17.

Essock, S. M., Frisman, L. K., Kontos, N. J. (1998). Cost-effectiveness of assertive community treatment teams. *American Journal of Orthopsychiatry, 68,* 179–190.

Essock, S. M., Mueser, K. T., Drake, R. E., Covell, N. H., McHugo, G. J., Frisman, L. K., Kontos, N. J., & Jackson, C. T., et al. (2006). Comparison of ACT and standard case management for delivering integrated treatment for co-occuring disorders. *Psychiatric Services, 57,* 185–196.

Flynn, L. M. (1993). Political impact of the family-consumer movement. *National Forum, 73,* 13–15.

Foa, E. B., Stein, D. J., & McFarlane A. C. (2006). Symptomatology and psychopathology of mental health problems after disaster. *Journal of Clinical Psychiatry, 67* Suppl 2, 15–25.

Frueh, B. C., Deitsch, S. E., Santos, A. B., Gold, P. B., Johnson, M. R., Meisler, N., et al. (2000). Procedural and methodological issues in telepsychiatry research and program development. *Psychiatric Services, 51,* 1522–1527.

Frueh, B. C., Monnier, J., Yim, E., Grubaugh, A. L., Hamner, M. B., & Knapp, R. G. (2007). A randomized trial of telepsychiatry for post-traumatic stress disorder. *Journal of Telemedine and Telecare, 13,* 142–147.

Gensichen, J., Torge, M., Peitz, M., Wendt-Hermanski, H., Beyer, M., Rosemann, T., Krauth, C., et al. (2005). Case management for the treatment of patients with major depression in general practices—rationale, design and conduct of a cluster randomized controlled trial—PRoMPT (PRimary care Monitoring for depressive Patient's Trial) [ISRCTN66386086]—study protocol. *BMC Public Health, 5:*101. Published online 2005 Octobers 5. doi: 10.1186/1471-2458-5-101.

Gilliam, T. R. (1988). Deming's 14 points and hospital quality: Responding to the consumer's demand for the best value health care. *Journal of Quality Assurance, 2,* 70–78.

Goff, D. C., & Newcomer, J. W. (2007). Integrating general health care in private community psychiatry practice. *Journal of Clinical Psychiatry, 68,* e19.

Gorn, S. (1983). Informatics (computer and computer science): Its ideology, methodology, and sociology. In F. Machlup & U. Mansfield (Eds.), *The study of information: Interdisciplinary messages* (pp. 121–140). New York: Wiley.

Gould, T. D., Dow, E. R., O'Donnell, K. C., Chen, G., & Manji, H. K. (2007). Targeting signal transduction pathways in the treatment of mood disorders: Recent insights into the relevance of the Wnt pathway. *CNS and Neurological Disorders Drug Targets, 6,* 193–204.

Gould, T. D., & Manji, H. K. (2005). The molecule medicine revolution and psychiatry: Bridging the gap between basic neuroscience research and clinical psychiatry. *Journal of Clinical Psychiatry, 65,* 598–604.

Graves, J. R., & Corcoran, S. (1989). An overview of nursing informatics. Image: *The Journal of Nursing Scholarship, 21,* 227–231.

Hall, B. A., & Allen, J. D. (1985, June). Sharpening nursing's focus by focusing on health. *Nursing and Health Care,* 315–320.

Hall, C. D., & Fabayo, A. O. (2006). Nursing students' adjustment to a new phenomenon. *Journal of the National Black Nurses Association, 17,* 24–29.

Hall, L. L. (1997). Health care quality. *NAMI Advocate, 19,* 8–9.

Hatfield, A. B. (1990). Incorporating the family's contribution to clinical training. In *Clinical training in serious mental illness* (DHHS Pub. No. ADM 90–1679). Washington, DC: U.S. Government Printing Office.

Henderson, V. A. (1991). *The nature of nursing: Reflections after 25 years.* New York: National League of Nursing.

Hoge, C. W., Auchterlonie, J. L., & Milliken, C. S. (2006). Mental health problems use of mental health services, and attrition from military service after returning from the deployment to Iraq or Afghanistan. *JAMA, 295,* 1023–1032.

Kanter, J. (1989). Clinical case management: Definition, principles, components. *Hospital and Community Psychiatry, 40,* 361–368.

Killien, M. G. (2004). Nurses' health: Work and family influences. *Nursing Clinics of North America, 39,* 19–35.

Levine, M. A., & Perpetua, E. M. (2006). International immersion programs in baccalaureate nursing education: Professor and student perspectives. *Journal of Cultural Diversity, 13,* 20–26.

Lewis, D., & Pesut, D. J. (2001). Emergence of consumer health care informatics. *Nursing Outlook, 48,* 7.

Mahoney, J. S., Marfurt, S., daCunha, M., & Engebretson, J. (2005). Design and evaluation of an online teaching strategy in an undergraduate psychiatric nursing course. *Archives of Psychiatric Nursing, 19,* 264–272.

Matsuzaki, S., & Tohyama, M. (2007). Molecular mechanism of schizophrenia with reference to disrupted-in-schizophrenia 1 (DISC1). *Neurochemistry International, 51,* 165–172.

McBride, A. B. (1990). Psychiatric nursing in the 1990s. *Archives of Psychiatric Nursing, 41,* 21–27.

McBride, A. B. (1999). Breakthroughs in nursing education: Looking back, looking forward. *Nursing Outlook, 47,* 114–119.

McCabe, S. (2000). Bringing psychiatric nursing into the twenty-first century. *Archives in Psychiatric Nursing, 14,* 109–116.

McCabe, S. (2002). The nature of psychiatric nursing: The intersection of paradigm, evolution, and history. *Archives in Psychiatric Nursing, 16*(2), 51–60.

Meyer, P. S., & Morrissey, J. P. (2007). A comparison of assertive community treatment and intensive case management for patients in rural areas. *Psychiatric Services, 58,* 121–127.

Moore, S. A. (1990). A social work practice model of case management: The case management grid. *Social Work, 35,* 444–448.

Mueser, T., Bond, G., Drake, R., & Resnick, S. (1998). Models of community for severe mental illness: A review of research on case management. *Schizophrenia Bulletin, 24,* 37–74.

Murray-Swant, A. B., Lucksted, A., Medoff, D. R., Yang, Y., Wohlheiter, K., & Dixon, L. B. (2006). Religiosity, psychosocial adjustment, and subjective burden of persons who care for those with mental illness. *Psychiatric Services, 57,* 361–365.

National League of Nursing. (1988). *Curriculum revolution: Mandate for change.* New York: Author.

National Institute of Nursing Research. (2006). The NINR strategic plan 2006–2010. http://www.ninr.nih.gov/NR/rdonlyres/9021E5EB-B2BA-47EA-B5DB-IE4DB11B1289/4894/NINR_StrategicPlanWebsite.pdf (Accessed March 24, 2007)

National League of Nursing. (1989). *Curriculum revolution: Reconceptualizing nursing education.* New York: Author.

Nehls, N. (2001). What is a case manager? The perspective of persons with borderline personality disorder. *Journal of the American Psychiatric Nurses Association, 7,* 4–12.

Nightingale, F. (1894). Sick nursing and health nursing. In J. S. Billingas & H. Hurd (Eds.), *Hospitals and dispensaries and nursing* (p. 446). Baltimore: Johns Hopkins University Press.

Olson, T. (2004). Spasm or transformation? Advanced practice psychiatric nursing education in the United States. *International Journal of Psychiatric Nursing Research, 10,* 1152–1163.

Owen, S., & Khalil, E. (2007). Addressing diversity in mental health care: A review of guidance documents. *International Journal of Nursing Studies, 44,* 467–478.

Pender, N. J. (1996). *Health promotion in nursing practice* (3rd ed.). Stamford, CT: Appleton & Lange.

Perraud, S., Delaney, K. R., Carlson-Sabelli, L., Johnson, M. E., Shephard, R. & Paun, O. (2006). Advanced practice psychiatric mental health nursing, finding our core: The therapeutic relationship in 21st century. *Perspectives in Psychiatric Care, 42,* 215–226.

Repique, R. J. (2007). Computers and information technologies in psychiatric nursing. *Perspectives in Psychiatric Care, 43,* 77–83.

Reverby, S. (1987). A caring dilemma: Womanhood and nursing in historical perspective. *Nursing Research, 36,* 5.

Schutzenhofer, K. K. (1992). Essentials of nursing in the year 2000. *Nursing Connections, 5,* 15–26.

Shea, C. A. (1991). *Nursing and prevention research.* Submitted to the Panel on Training in Prevention Research, National Institute of Mental Health National Conference on Prevention Research. Washington, DC: American Psychiatric Nursing Association.

Smeltzer, S. C. (2007). Improving the health and wellness of persons with disabilities: A call to action too important for nursing to ignore. *Nursing Outlook, 55,* 189–195.

Society for Education and Research in Psychiatric-Mental Health Nursing. (1994). *Position paper.* Pensacola, FL: Author.

Sperling, A. (1997). State and federal politics. *NAMI Advocate, 19,* 3–4.

Stein, L. I. (1990). Comments by Leon Stein. *Hospital and Community Psychiatry, 41,* 649–651.

Stewart, S. E., Rosario, M. C., Brown, T. A., Carter, A. S., Leckman, J. F., Sukhodolsky, D., et al. (2007). Principal components analysis of obsessive-compulsive disorder symptoms in children and adolescents. *Biological Psychiatry, 61,* 285–291.

Surles, R. S., Blanch, A. K., Shern, D. L., & Donahue, S. A. (1992). Case management as a strategy for systems change. *Health Affairs, 11,* 151–163.

Swanson, C. J., Bures, M., Johnson, M. P., Linden, A. M., Monn, J. A., & Schoepp, D. D. (2005). Metabotropic glutamate receptors as novel target agents for anxiety and stress disorders. *National Review of Drug Discoveries, 4,* 131–144.

Thornicroft, G. (1991). The concept of case management for long-term mental illness. *International Review of Psychiatry, 3,* 125–132.

Torrey, E. (1990). *Care of the seriously mentally ill: A rating of state programs.* Arlington, VA: National Alliance for the Mentally Ill.

Torrey, E. (1992). *Criminalizing the seriously mentally ill: The abuse of jails as mental hospitals.* Arlington, VA: National Alliance for the Mentally Ill.

Turner, M. A., Kiernan, M. D., McKechanie, A. G., Finch, P. J., McManus, F. B., & Neal, L. A. (2005). Acute military psychiatric casualties from the war in Iraq. *British Journal of Psychiatry, 186,* 476–479.

U.S. Department of Health and Human Services (DHHS). (1999). *Mental health: A report of the surgeon general—executive summary.* Rockville, MD: U.S. Department of Health and Human Services, Substance Abuse and Mental Health Services Administration, Center for Mental Health Services, National Institute of Health, National Institute of Mental Health.

U.S. Department of Health and Human Services (DHHS). (2000). *Healthy people 2010* (DHHS Publication No. PHS). Washington, DC: U.S. Government Printing Office.

U.S. Department of Health and Human Services. (2005). *The 2005 Surgeon General's call to action to improve the health and wellness of persons with disabilities: Calling you to action.* U.S. Department of Health and Human Services, Office of the Surgeon General. Retrieved August 11, 2007, from http://www.surgeongeneral.gov/library/disabilities/calltoaction/whatitmeanstoyou.pdf

van Vliet, M. J., Schuurmans, M. J., Grypdonck, M. H., & Duijnstee, M. S. (2006). Improper intake of medication by elders—insights on contributing factors: A review of the literature. *Research and Theory and Nursing Practice, 20,* 79–93.

Walton, M. K. (1986). *The Deming management method.* New York: Dodd, Mead.

Watson, J. (1988). A case study: Curriculum in transition. In *Curriculum revolution: Mandate for change.* New York: National League of Nursing.

Weich, S., Nazareth, I., Morgan, L., & King, M. (2007). Treatment of depression in primary care: Socio-economic status, clinical need and receipt of treatment. *British Journal of Psychiatry, 191,* 164–169.

Williamson, G. R., Webb, C., Abelson-Mitchell, N., & Cooper, S. (2006). Change on the horizon: Issues and concerns of neophyte advanced healthcare practitioners. *Journal of Clinical Nursing, 15,* 1091–1098.

Yellowlees, P. M., & Cook, J. N. (2006). Education about hallucinations using an Internet virtual reality system: A qualitative survey. *Academic Psychiatry, 30,* 534–539.

SUGGESTED READINGS

Institute of Medicine. (2001). *Crossing the quality chasm: A new health care system for the 21st century.* Washington, DC: National Academy Press.

Karp, D. A. (2000). *The burden of sympathy: How families cope with mental illness.* Oxford: Oxford University Press.

Spaniol, L., Zipple, A. M., Marsh, D. T., & Finley, L. Y. (2000). *The role of family in psychiatric rehabilitation.* Boston: Boston University Center for Psychiatric Rehabilitation.

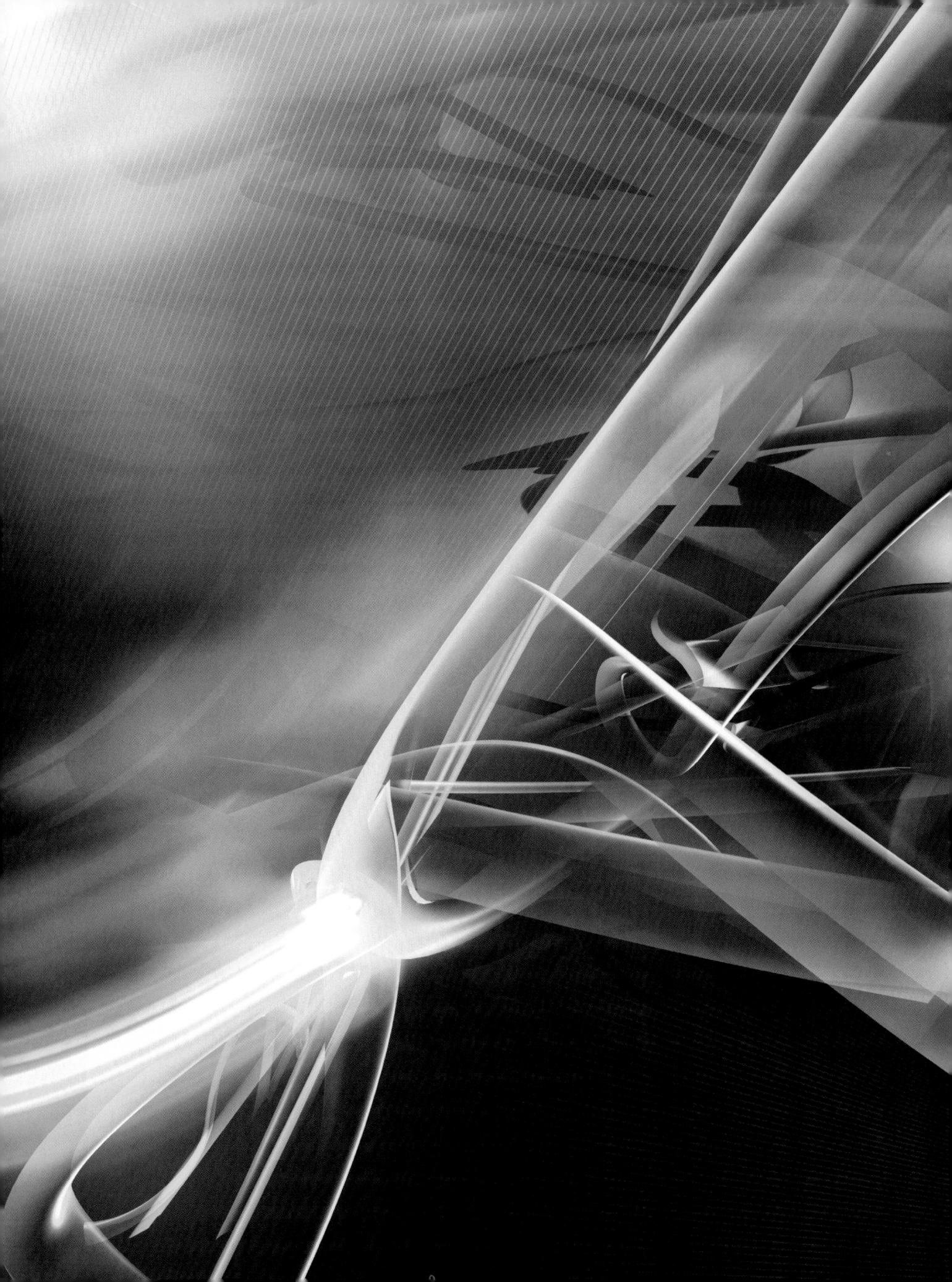

APPENDIX A

NANDA Diagnosis 2007–2008

Activity Intolerance

Risk for Activity Intolerance

Ineffective Airway Clearance

Latex Allergy Response

Risk for Latex Allergy Response

Anxiety

Death Anxiety

Risk for Aspiration

Risk for Impaired Parent/Child Attachment

Autonomic Dysreflexia

Risk for Autonomic Dysreflexia

Risk-Prone Health Behavior

Disturbed Body Image

Risk for Imbalanced Body Temperature

Bowel Incontinence

Effective Breastfeeding

Interrupted Breastfeeding

Ineffective Breathing Pattern

Decreased Cardiac Output

Caregiver Role Strain

Risk for Caregiver Role Strain

Readiness for Enhanced Comfort

Impaired Verbal Communication

Impaired Communication

Readiness for Enhanced Communication

Decisional Conflict

Parental Role Conflict

Acute Confusion

Chronic Confusion

Risk for Acute Confusion

Constipation

Perceived Constipation

Risk for Constipation

Contamination

Risk for Contamination

Compromised Family Coping

Defensive Coping

Disabled Family Coping

Ineffective Coping

Ineffective Community Coping

Readiness for Enhanced Coping

Readiness for Enhanced Community Coping

Readiness for Enhanced Family Coping

Risk for Sudden Infant Death Syndrome

Readiness for Enhanced Decision Making

Ineffective Denial

Impaired Dentition

Risk for Delayed Development

Diarrhea

Risk for Compromised Human Dignity

Moral Distress

Risk for Disuse Syndrome

Deficient Diversional Activity

From *Nursing Diagnosis: Definitions and Classifications, 2007–2008,* by North American Nursing Diagnosis Association, 2007. Philadelphia: Author. Copyright 2007 by North American Nursing Diagnosis Association.

Disturbed Energy Field

Impaired Environmental Interpretation Syndrome

Adult Failure to Thrive

Risk for Falls

Dysfunctional Family Processes: Alcoholism

Interrupted Family Processes

Readiness for Enhanced Family Processes

Fatigue

Fear

Readiness for Enhanced Fluid Balance

Deficient Fluid Volume

Excess Fluid Volume

Risk for Deficient Fluid Volume

Risk for Imbalanced Fluid Volume

Impaired Gas Exchange

Risk for Unstable Blood Glucose

Grieving

Complicated Grieving

Risk for Complicated Grieving

Delayed Growth and Development

Risk for Disproportionate Growth

Ineffective Health Maintenance

Health-Seeking Behaviors (Specify)

Impaired Home Maintenance

Readiness for Enhanced Hope

Hopelessness

Hyperthermia

Hypothermia

Disturbed Personal Identity

Readiness for Enhanced Immunization Status

Functional Urinary Incontinence

Overflow Urinary Incontinence

Reflex Urinary Incontinence

Stress Urinary Incontinence

Total Urinary Incontinence

Urge Urinary Incontinence

Risk for Urge Urinary Incontinence

Disorganized Infant Behavior

Risk for Disorganized Infant Behavior

Readiness for Enhanced Organized Infant Behavior

Ineffective Infant Feeding Pattern

Risk for Infection

Risk for Injury

Risk for Perioperative-Positioning Injury

Insomnia

Decreased Intracranial Adaptive Capacity

Deficient Knowledge

Readiness for Enhanced Knowledge

Sedentary Lifestyle

Risk for Impaired Liver Function

Risk for Loneliness

Impaired Memory

Impaired Bed Mobility

Impaired Physical Mobility

Impaired Wheelchair Mobility

Nausea

Unilateral Neglect

Noncompliance

Imbalanced Nutrition; Less Than Body Requirements

Imbalanced Nutrition: More Than Body Requirements

Readiness for Enhanced Nutrition

Risk for Imbalanced Nutrition: More Than Body Requirements

Impaired Oral Mucous Membrane

Acute Pain

Chronic Pain

Readiness for Enhanced Parenting

Impaired Parenting

Risk for Impaired Parenting

Risk for Peripheral Neurovascular Dysfunction

Risk for Poisoning

Post-Trauma Syndrome

Risk for Post-Trauma Syndrome

Readiness for Enhanced Power

Powerlessness

Risk for Powerlessness

Ineffective Protection

Rape-Trauma Syndrome

Rape-Trauma Syndrome; Compound Reaction

Rape-Trauma Syndrome; Silent Reaction

Impaired Religiosity

Readiness for Enhanced Religiosity

Risk for Impaired Religiosity

Relocation Stress Syndrome

Risk for Relocation Stress Syndrome

Ineffective Role Performance

Readiness for Enhanced Self-Care

Bathing/Hygiene Self-Care Deficit

Dressing/Grooming Self-Care Deficit

Feeding Self-Care Deficit

Toileting Self-Care Deficit

Readiness for Enhanced Self-Concept

Chronic Low Self-Esteem

Situational Low Self-Esteem

Risk for Situational Low Self-Esteem

Self-Mutilation

Risk for Self-Mutilation

Disturbed Sensory Perception (Specify: Visual, Auditory, Kinesthetic, Gustatory, Tactile, Olfactory)

Sexual Dysfunction

Ineffective Sexuality Pattern

Impaired Skin Integrity

Risk for Impaired Skin Integrity

Sleep Deprivation

Readiness for Enhanced Sleep

Impaired Social Interaction

Social Isolation

Chronic Sorrow

Spiritual Distress

Risk for Spiritual Distress

Readiness for Enhanced Spiritual Well-Being

Stress Overload

Risk for Suffocation

Risk for Suicide

Delayed Surgical Recovery

Impaired Swallowing

Effective Therapeutic Regimen Management

Ineffective Therapeutic Regimen Management

Ineffective Community Therapeutic Regimen Management

Ineffective Family Therapeutic Regimen Management

Readiness for Enhanced Therapeutic Regimen Management

Ineffective Thermoregulation

Disturbed Thought Processes

Impaired Tissue Integrity

Ineffective Tissue Perfusion (Specify Type: Renal, Cerebral, Cardiopulmonary, Gastrointestinal, Peripheral)

Impaired Transfer Ability

Disturbed Thought Processes

Impaired Transfer Ability

Risk for Trauma

Impaired Urinary Elimination

Readiness for Enhanced Urinary Elimination

Urinary Retention

Impaired Spontaneous Ventilation

Dysfunctional Ventilatory Weaning Response

Risk for Other-Directed Violence

Risk for Self-Directed Violence

Impaired Walking

Wandering

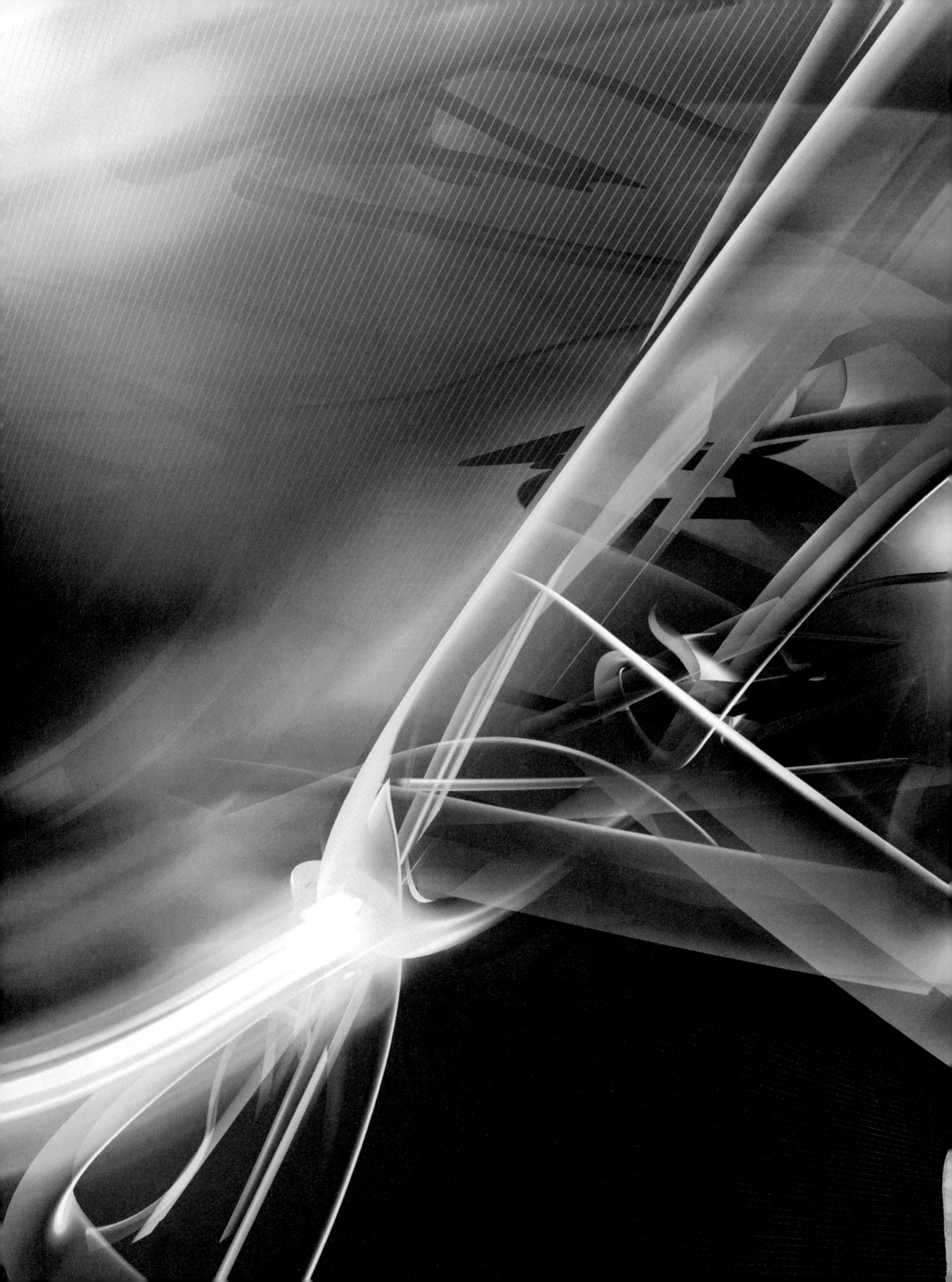

GLOSSARY

Abstinence   Avoidance of all substances with abuse potential. It denotes cessation of addictive behaviors, such as substance abuse/dependence.

Abulia   Functional errors of omission; failing to perform activities to meet basic human needs; inability to make decisions; lack of will or willpower.

Acalculia   Inability to do simple arithmetic calculations.

Acting out   Living out unresolved developmental issues or fantasies impulsively in out-of-control behavior.

Active listening   A dynamic process that requires using all senses to assess verbal and nonverbal messages.

Acute confusion   Refers to the cognitive phenomenon of delirium (rapid onset of a disturbance in consciousness and cognition) before the actual diagnosis is made.

Adaptation   Sustaining homeostasis; the ability to mobilize resources and adjust to demands of internal and external environments.

Addiction   A pattern of out-of-control or compulsive use of psychoactive substances in which use continues despite negative consequences; often used interchangeably with the terms chemical dependency or substance dependence.

Advanced sleep phase syndrome (ASPS)   A circadian rhythm disorder common in the older adult, with early bedtime and related early rising time, inability to remain asleep during the night, and the perception of being "out of sync" with the rest of the population. Associated with napping, which worsens the problem.

Advocacy   Defending a cause or pleading a case on another's behalf (Bloom & Asher, 1982); putting the interest of the client before the interest of the nurse.

Affect   The visible and overt manifestations of the person's feelings or mood. Examples of affect are appropriate or congruent with mood and thought content, blunted, flat, labile, restricted, or constricted.

After-care   Care that occurs after a person's discharge from the hospital.

Aggression   Hostile, injurious, or destructive behavior or outlook, particularly when caused by frustration.

Aggressive   Physical or verbal behavior that is forceful, hostile, or enacted to intimidate others.

Agitation   To give motion to or to disturb. It also refers to a state of increased mental and motor activity.

Akathisia   Subjective feelings of restlessness and an inability to sit still resulting from dopamine blockade by antipsychotics; part of the extrapyramidal side effects.

Akinesia   A condition characterized by the inability to make voluntary movements.

Al-Anon   A self-help group for spouses, parents, or significant others of alcoholics.

Alcoholics Anonymous   An international self-help organization whose purpose is to help alcoholics achieve and maintain sobriety.

Alexithymia   Refers to a lack of introceptive awareness, mistrust of self and others, cognitive dysfunction, and starvation-induced depression.

Alogia   Inability to speak owing to a mental condition or a symptom of dementia.

Alter   A distinct identity with its own enduring pattern of perceiving, relating to, and thinking about the world and the self.

Altered sensory perception   The physical and psychological changes that affect brain functioning, behavior patterns, and the five senses.

Alzheimer's disease (AD)   A condition characterized by progressive loss of memory, intellect, language, judgment, and impulse control. Neurofibrillary tangles and neuritic plaques are found in the cerebral cortex, particularly the hippocampus.

American Association of Sex Educators, Counselors, and Therapists (AASECT)   A multidisciplinary national organization of professionals dedicated to the study, education, and role of spokesperson for sexuality.

Amygdala   A nucleus in the limbic system or medial temporal lobe that affects neuroendocrine and behavioral functions. It also plays a role in behaviors, including eating, drinking, and sexuality, and the emotions linked to these behaviors. It plays a role in the emotional significance of events or memories and governs the level of hippocampal activity accordingly.

Analytic worldview   Worldview perspective that espouses and values specific details of time, calculation, individuality, and acquiring material objects as being important in life.

Anhedonia   The inability to experience pleasure from activities that usually produce pleasurable feelings.

Anima   The female aspect of the male personality.

Animus   The male aspect of the female personality.

Anomia   Inability to recall or recognize names of objects.

Anorexia nervosa (AN)   Self-induced starvation resulting from fear of fatness; not caused by true loss of appetite.

Antipsychotic   Psychotropic medications used to treat acute and chronic psychotic disorders; agitation and aggression. These agents are divided into second generation or atypical and conventional or typical agents.

Anxiety   An affect or emotion arising from stress or change accompanied by biological arousal, behavioral responses, and elements of apprehension, impending doom, and tension.

Anxiolytic   Drug used to reduce anxiety, synonymous to the term sedative. Examples include benzodiazepines such as diazepam, lorazepam, and clonazepam.

Aphasia   Loss of power of expression by speech or writing, or signs of loss of comprehension of spoken or written language owing to brain injury or pathology.

Apraxia   Loss of ability to carry out familiar, purposeful movements in the absence of paralysis or other motor or sensory impairments, especially the inability to make proper use of an object.

Apraxic agraphia   Inability to express oneself in writing due to apraxia.

Archetypes   Primordial images that serve as the building blocks of the collective unconscious.

Aromatherapy   The practice of using essential oils, the pure volatile aspects of aromatic plant products, for therapeutic purposes, including ameliorating anxiety, stress, and depression.

Asimultanagnosia   Inability to visually integrate the components of an ordinarily complex scene into a coherent whole.

Assault   A violent physical or verbal attack.

Assertive community treatment (ACT)   A model of mental health care that provides the client and family with many case management functions, including ongoing assessments, treatment planning, and monitoring of mental, physical, and social functioning. The precise approach varies, but an individual is generally designated as the broker of care or treatment coordinator. ACT programs are available 24 hours a day.

Assertiveness   Clearly communicating one's needs, desires, or beliefs directly and tactfully with self-confidence.

Attachment   A classic term for the primary tie between a child and her caregiver and a process seen as evolving, biologically adaptive, and critical to emotional and physiological development and survival.

Attachment system   A system that is instinctual or motivational and, like hunger and thirst, integrates the infant's memory processes, prompting the child to satisfy them by interacting with the caregiver.

Attachment theory   Theory based on the classic works of Bowlby and Ainsworth that define attachment or bonding as an evolutionary and biological process of eliciting and maintaining physical closeness between a child and a parent or primary caregiver. This theory also infers that the infant's relationships with early caregivers are responsible for influencing future interactions and relationships.

Aural comprehension   Understanding of stimuli perceived by the ear.

Autism   The presence of abnormal and impaired development in social and communication skills and severely restricted activity and interests.

Autonomy   The ability of individuals to make independent personal decisions and act on their own behalf, recognizing the inherent value of each individual.

Avoidant behavior   Constricted social interaction with unfamiliar people or in situations that activate intense anxiety reactions, resulting in excessive social impairment and impaired interactions with others.

Avolition   A marked decrease in motivation and attention.

Behavior management plans   A plan designed to reinforce positive and reduce negative behaviors through the use of visual cues, charts, communication tools, and reward systems.

Behavioral/cognitive model   Combines behavioral and cognitive therapies. That is, the behavioral model focuses on behaviors that present in the here and now, identification of maladaptive behaviors that will become targets for change, motivation for the behaviors, and reinforcers of the behaviors.

Beneficence   Doing good and avoiding doing harm.

Binge   A period of uncontrolled eating in which a large amount of food is consumed unrelated to physical hunger.

Binge use   Five or more drinks at the same time or within two hours of each other at least once in the past month (SAMHSA, 2004).

Bioethics   Ethics applied to health care.

Bipolar   The two extreme mood states of mania and depression illustrated in bipolar disorder.

Body dysmorphic disorder   A chronic and debilitating mental health condition characterized by a preoccupation with imagined defects in appearance (e.g., a "large" nose, "thinning" hair, facial "scarring").

Body image   One's physical perception and sense of identity, strengths, and limitations.

Body image disturbance   A distortion in the image of the body that is of near or actual delusional proportions; may include strong feelings of self-loathing projected onto the body, body parts, or perceived fat.

Body language   Nonverbal communication or transmission of messages by way of physical gestures.

Body mass index (BMI)   A mathematical formula that is highly correlated with body fat. It is weight in kilograms divided by height in meters squared (kg/m^2). In the United States and the United Kingdom, people with BMIs between 25 and 30 kg/m^2 are considered overweight and those with BMIs of more than 30 kg/m^2 are categorized as obese.

Boundary   Rules defining who and how members participate in a subsystem or a relationship. The clearer the boundary, the healthier the relationship.

Brain lesion   A condition in which an abnormality is noted in the brain, such as a tumor or hematoma. A potentially reversible dementia.

Bulimia nervosa (BN)   Binge eating followed by self-inflicted vomiting, laxative or diuretic abuse, or starvation.

Case management   A model of comprehensive and holistic health care delivery that concentrates the responsibility for all care given to a client in one person or agency.

Case manager   A collaborative director with the consumer in the management of her holistic care.

Cataplexy   Sudden loss of motor control while awake, usually occurring with strong emotions, associated with narcolepsy.

Catecholamine   Any of the sympathomimetic amines, such as epinephrine, dopamine, and norepinephrine. These biochemicals play critical roles in the stress response and are targets for psychotropic medications.

Catharsis   The healthy release of ideas that helps the client gain insight into conflicts and early developmental turmoil.

Character Learned personality traits that influence behavioral patterns.

Chemical dependency A pattern of out-of-control or compulsive use of psychoactive substances in which use continues despite negative consequences; a popular term often used interchangeably with the terms addiction or substance dependence.

Child maltreatment Actions and behaviors that result in serious physical injury, neglect, sexual abuse, or serious mental injury to a child.

Chorea The ceaseless occurrence of a wide variety of rapid, jerky, but well-coordinated movements performed involuntarily.

Choreiform Resembling chorea.

Chronic fatigue syndrome A chronic and debilitating disorder characterized by chronic fatigue, flu-like symptoms, muscle pain, headaches, and malaise lasting more than 24 hours.

Chronic insomnia Insomnia that lasts more than 3 weeks.

Chronobiology Field of science and medicine that explores the many bodily changes governed by the hours and the seasons; includes studies of cellular rhythms all the way to those of populations and ecosystems.

Circadian rhythms Biological cycles occurring over an approximate 24-hour period and influencing biochemical, biological, and behavioral processes.

Circumstantiality A thought and speech process in which an individual digresses into unnecessary details and inappropriate unrelated thoughts while trying to express a central idea.

Civil commitment The ability of the state to hospitalize a person without consent.

Clarifying technique Act of clearing or making a message understandable.

Classic conditioning A form of learning in which existing responses are attached to new stimuli by pairing of those stimuli with stimuli that naturally elicit the response; also referred to as respondent conditioning.

Client advocate A person who tries to ensure that the rights of all prospective research subjects and actual subjects are adequately protected.

Client-centered care An approach that conveys empathy and compassion, a willingness to understand the client's experience of illness and health, and respect for the client's preferences, wishes, expressed needs, and values.

Clinical practice guidelines Evidence-based statements that facilitate implementation of quality and client-centered health care established by syntheses of the evidence.

Closed system In systems theory, this refers to a limited exchange of energy and information about the environment. Boundaries are often rigid and impermeable.

Cognitive The mental process involved in obtaining knowledge, including the aspects of perceiving, thinking, reasoning, and remembering.

Cognitive behavioral therapy A psychotherapy that is based on the assumption that feelings, thoughts, and behaviors influence one's perception of self, others, and the future. Negative or distorted cognitions often play a role in mood and anxiety disorders. The aim of psychotherapy is to challenge distorted cognitions by modifying cognitions, beliefs, feelings, and behaviors.

Cognitive disorders Those conditions in which "the predominant disturbance is a clinically significant deficit in cognition or memory that represents a significant change from a previous level of functioning" (APA, 2000).

Cognitive enhancement therapy A behavioral intervention designed to improve cognition in individuals with schizophrenia who exhibit neurocognitive symptoms.

Cognitive processes Higher cortical mental processes, including perception, memory, abstraction, and reasoning, by which one acquires knowledge, solves problems, employs judgment, and makes plans.

Cognitive symptoms Dissimilar to positive and negative symptoms are discreet and denote poor executive functioning or deficits in attention, working memory, secondary (storage) memory, and semantic memory. Normally, cognitive symptoms are only detected when neuropsychological tests are performed. Cognitive deficits are associated with poor social and occupational functioning in persons with schizophrenia.

Cogwheeling Rigidity or rhythmic contractions noted on passive stretching of muscles, as occurs in Parkinson's disease.

Communication The act of transmitting feelings, attitudes, ideas, and behaviors from one person to another.

Communication/systems model Communication theory applied to group therapy that considers both the content of messages of the group members and the method of transmission of these messages. The systems model aspect of this type of group considers subgroups, boundaries, and communication within and between these groups in relation to the whole group.

Community mental health A treatment approach that provides various levels of mental health, wellness, and illness services to individuals living within various community settings.

Community mental health centers Treatment facilities located within the community that provide different specialized levels and varieties of mental health care as well as coordination of physical and mental health care to any person needing mental health treatment.

Community support systems (CSS) Integrative approaches to quality mental health care for consumers that combine various types of mental health at the primary, secondary, and tertiary levels of care.

Community worldview Worldview perspective that espouses and values the importance and needs of the community over the individual in the context of transcendence and meditation in life.

Competency The ability of a person to perform certain tasks; the ability to understand legal proceedings and assist in that process.

Complementary therapies Unconventional therapies that encompass a spectrum of practices and beliefs, including herbs, visual imagery, acupuncture, and massage therapy.

Compulsion Repetitive, ritualistic, unrealistic behaviors used to neutralize or prevent discomfort of stressful events, circumstances, or recurring thoughts, images, or impulses such as obsessions.

Conflict The opposition of mutually exclusive impulses, desires, or tendencies; controversy or disagreement.

Confrontation The act of pointing out contradictions or incongruencies among feelings, thoughts, and behaviors, specifically pointing out parts of the assessment or treatment process that are contradictory or confusing.

Congruent communication Messages that do not contradict each other. Normally, these messages promote clear and consistent boundaries and roles and effective problem solving.

Constructional praxis Inability to copy simple drawings or reproduce patterns of blocks or matchstick constructions.

Consultation Rendering of an expert opinion in response to a request.

Consumerism A movement seeking to protect the rights of those acquiring a service (in this instance, mental health care) by requiring standards of effectiveness and safety.

Containment A term for safety, food, shelter, and medical care issues in milieu therapy.

Content analysis The evaluation of themes and specifics about what was said during the group therapy session. Examples of content themes are sadness, loneliness, leisure time activities, and relationship issues.

Continuous quality improvement A method of ensuring the adequacy of care developed by Deming and adopted by health care systems.

Continuum of mental health care A model that is distinct from one area of treatment planning and encompasses a comprehensive or multisystem perspective mental health care delivery model.

Conversion disorders Unexplained physical manifestations or deficits affecting voluntary motor or sensory function that suggest a neurological or other underlying medical condition.

Co-occurring Psychiatric or physical disorder that occurs with a primary psychiatric disorder.

Coping An effort to reduce tension by minimizing, replacing, and resolving uncomfortable feelings such as anxiety, anger, frustration, and guilt.

Countertransference Refers to intense emotional reactions to the client stemming from the therapist's early childhood experiences.

Creutzfeldt-Jakob disease (CJD) A syndrome of motor, sensory, and mental disturbances. There is widespread degeneration and atrophy of the cerebral cortex, basal ganglia, and thalamus. Course of disease can run from months to years.

Crisis A turning point, or acute emotional turmoil, that stems from developmental, biological, situational, or psychosocial stressors that momentarily renders the person's normal coping mechanisms inadequate.

Crisis intervention Short-term, here-and-now focused intervention that alleviates the impact of crisis-generated stress, enhances coping and problem-solving skills, and mobilizes resources of affected clients.

Critical thinking Systematic and purposeful process of reasoning.

Critiquer of research findings A person who evaluates research findings and determines the usefulness of these findings to nursing practice.

Cues Internal and external response signals that, if noticed, predict when, where, and what response will occur.

Cultural competence Circular process whereby a person develops an understanding and valuing of different worldview perspectives and then enculturates the understanding and valuing into interactions with clients and other health care professionals.

Culturally bound factors Health ideas and behaviors that a person exhibits in relationship to his environment and everyday life functioning.

Culture A person, group, or community's internal and external daily expression of beliefs, values, and norms.

Culture of nursing The nursing profession's body of values, knowledge, beliefs, and practices, which form the bases of how individual nurses delineate their nursing roles and functions within health care environments.

Cycle of violence A dynamic described by some survivors of intimate partner abuse. The cycle begins with low levels of abuse, which build to an acutely abusive incident involving levels of violence higher than that of the abuse experienced on a regular basis. Following the acute violence, the perpetrator engages in actions designed to keep the relationship from ending, creating an "ideal" dynamic to keep the survivor involved. If there is no change in the abusive behaviors, the tension-building stage begins again, leading to another cycle of acute violence.

Cyclothymia A condition in which numerous periods of abnormally elevated, expansive, or irritable moods are experienced interspersed with periods of depressed mood. Neither mood state reaches the height nor depth to qualify as bipolar disorder.

Cytochrome P450 (CYP) enzymes Enzymes primarily located in the liver, which play a key role in the metabolism of most psychotropic medications.

Data collector A person who gathers information for a research study, such as obtaining information from research subjects.

Decade of the Brain Proclamation by the United States Congress that explains mental illness as a disease of the brain. It underscores the significance of technological advances in neurobiology and genetics and their impact on understanding mental illness.

Decerebrate A sign characterized by adduction and extension of the arms, pronated wrists, and flexed fingers. The legs are stiffly extended, with plantar flexion of the feet. This sign indicates upper brain stem damage and usually heralds neurological deterioration.

Declaration of sexual rights A document that identifies 11 human rights stating that sexuality is an integral part of the personality of every human being.

Decompensation The exacerbation of mental disorder symptomatology that affects a person's everyday functioning ability.

Decorticate A sign characterized by adduction and flexion of the arms, with wrists and fingers flexed on the chest. The legs are extended and internally rotated, with plantar flexion of the feet. Most often, it results from cerebrovascular accident or head injury. It is a sign of corticospinal damage and carries a more favorable prognosis than decerebrate posture.

Deep brain stimulation (DBS) A surgical procedure involving implantation of a medical device called a brain pacemaker used to treat various disabling neurological symptoms, such as Parkinson's disease and intractable or treatment-resistant depression.

De-escalation Verbal interventions that aim to defuse potentially and actual volatile situations using empathetic, calm, yet firm limit-setting approaches.

Defense mechanisms Unconscious, self-protective processes that seek to protect the ego from intense and overwhelming feelings of affect and impulses.

Defuse To reduce tension and harm in a potentially violent situation.

Deinstitutionalization The systematic process of moving mentally ill clients from long-term, inpatient institutions to less structured settings such as group homes and community mental health centers.

Delayed sleep phase syndrome (DSPS) A circadian rhythm disorder, common in adolescence, with late sleep onset and resultant desire to oversleep.

Delirium A medical syndrome characterized by acute onset and impairment in cognition, perception, and behavior. Also known as acute confusion.

Delirium tremens (DTs) The most serious form of alcohol withdrawal; can be potentially fatal; characteristic symptoms include profound confusion, disorientation, and autonomic arousal; also known as alcohol withdrawal delirium.

Delusion A fixed false belief unchanged by logic. False, rigid belief that is incongruent with the client's cultural background. Examples of delusions include thought insertion, paranoid, somatic, and jealousy.

Dementia A condition manifested in the insidious development of memory and intellectual deficits, disorientation, and decreased cognitive functioning.

Denial An assertion that an allegation is false despite evidence to the contrary.

Depersonalization A person's subjective sense of feeling unreal, strange, unfamiliar, or emotionally numb.

Depression A mental disorder marked by sustained alteration in mood in which there is loss of interest and pleasure, altered weight, altered concentration, and sleep disturbance.

Derealization A subjective sense that one's environment is unreal or unfamiliar.

Desensitization A cognitive-behavioral therapy technique developed by Joseph Wolpe that involves three steps: relaxation training, gradual or hierarchical exposure (using visual imagery or real situations) to an anxiety-provoking or fearful situation or object, and desensitization to the stimulus. This technique is useful in the treatment of phobias.

Dialectical behavior therapy (DBT) A psychosocial cognitive behavioral therapy approach used in the treatment of borderline personality disorder. It is an adaptation of behavioral therapy using skills training to help the client with borderline personality disorder and other impulsivity disorders effectively control or manage intense emotional states and associated self-harm or self-injurious behaviors.

Disaster A sudden, unexpected, and calamitous event that leads to great loss, damage, or destruction.

Disengagement Implies that family boundaries are rigid or impermeable and distant.

Disruptive To throw into disorder or confusion; to disturb a balance.

Dissociation An unconscious defense mechanism that refers to a detachment or alteration in one's sense of reality, psychogenic amnesia, and perception of self and environment; used by a person to protect self from being overwhelmed by anxiety, usually from a traumatic experience. Memory and feeling related to an event are sealed off from the conscious awareness.

Dissociative disorders A continuum of disorders experienced by individuals exposed to trauma, including depersonalization disorder, dissociative amnesia, dissociative fugue, and dissociative identity disorder. These disorders involve a disturbance in the organization of identity, memory, perception, or consciousness.

Distractibility The inability to maintain attention, shifting from one area or topic to another with minimal provocation, or attention being drawn too frequently to unimportant or irrelevant external stimuli.

Distributive justice The concept that resources should be distributed equitably across society or a collective group.

Dopaminergic pathway Nerve fibers in the mesocortical area that project to the cortex and hippocampus regions of the limbic system.

Double-bind messages Refers to transactions that involve a binder and a victim.

Drive Instinctual urges and impulses arising from biological and psychological needs.

Drug polymorphism Contextual chemical factors involved in individuals' genetic responses to pharmacologic agents.

Dual diagnosis Refers to the condition of a person who has been diagnosed with a mental disorder and substance use or abuse. The term *dual diagnosis* may also be used to describe a person who has a mental disorder and mental retardation or developmental disability diagnosis. May also be known as a co-occurring diagnosis.

Dyad A two-person relationship, such as husband-wife and father-child.

Dysarthria Imperfect articulation of speech caused by muscular weakness resulting from damage to the central or peripheral nervous system.

Dysphoria Marked feelings of sadness.

Dystonia Slow sustained muscle spasms of the trunk, neck, or limb; the result of dopamine blockade from antipsychotic medications.

Eating disorder (ED) A general term for abnormalities in behavior toward food, growing out of fear of fatness and pursuit of excessive thinness.

Echolalia Stereotyped repetition of another person's words or phrases.

Eclecticism Implies that the therapist uses two or more theories to develop an effective treatment to meet a client's needs.

Ecological worldview Worldview perspective that a person espouses, values, and accepts his role of interconnectedness and responsibility for the world.

Ego   The part of the mind that mediates between external reality and inner wishes and impulses.

Ego dystonic   Discomfort in the presence of a disordered mental state.

Ego function   Intrapsychic processes that enable people to mediate stress and adaptation using various defense mechanisms.

Ego syntonic   Personal comfort with symptoms that create discomfort in others.

Elder abuse   Abuse of a person over 60 years of age, which may include physical abuse but also sexual, emotional, or financial abuse and abandonment.

Electroconvulsive therapy   Electric current induction of seizures, primarily for treatment of mental disorders; used most frequently in depression.

Emotional lability   An affective disturbance characterized by excessive and inappropriate emotional response.

Empathy   Refers to putting oneself into the psychological frame of reference of another. It conveys an understanding of the client's situation without becoming emerged or overwhelmed by the experience.

Enculturates   A person's internalization and adoption of another worldview perspective into his existing worldview perspective.

Enculturation   Process by which a person accepts and internalizes another person's or group's worldview into or in place of his or her existing worldview.

Enmeshment   Implies over-involvement or lack of separateness of family members.

Entrepreneur   An individual who organizes, manages, and risks assumption of a business venture or enterprise.

Entropy   The tendency to increase randomness by the degradation of energy; the running-down of a system.

Enuresis   Bedwetting after having been toilet trained; generally resolves by school age.

Equifinality   The sameness of the end result starting from various points.

Equilibrium   The capacity of a system to use available resources to manage and reduce tension and stress.

Erogenous zone   Part of the body that is a source of pleasure, such as the lips, mouth, genitals, and anus.

Eros   The instinct or drive for love.

Ethnicity   Categorical determination of a group whose members have a common social and cultural heritage that is passed from generation to generation.

Ethnopsychopharmacology   The study of intensity and duration (e.g., absorption, distribution, metabolism, elimination) of psychotropic medications in different racial groups of individuals.

Euphoria   An exaggerated feeling of well-being or elation.

Evidence-based practice   Refers to interventions for which there is substantial empirical evidence that they improve client outcomes.

Evoked potential   A short train of large slow waves recorded from the scalp that reflects dendritic activity and is influenced by many variables—a useful indicator of brain activity in the processing of information.

Excessive sleeplessness (ES)   Defined as sleepiness that occurs regardless of the amount of sleep a person gets. Rest does not relieve ES.

Excitement phase   First phase of the human sexual response cycle, in which vasocongestion builds in the man and woman.

Executive function   Ability to set a goal, make decisions, and implement appropriate activities toward meeting that goal.

Existential/Gestalt model   Facilitates people's self-actualization processes by helping them become more aware of their full potential, their alternatives or choices, and their feelings and emotions. The primary goal in this model is to help individual members take responsibility for their emotions and behaviors through the process of support and feedback.

Exponential kinetics   A pharmacokinetic model in which a constant fraction of a drug is eliminated in a set unit of time.

Extended care   Long-term, more intensive care for someone who has been discharged from the hospital.

Extrapyramidal side effects (EPS)   Involuntary motor movements and muscle tone side effects that result primarily from dopamine blockade by antipsychotic medications.

Eye movement desensitization and reprocessing (EMDR)   Therapy technique that involves asking the client to imagine an anxiety-provoking or traumatic memory. This technique is used to treat posttraumatic stress disorder by processing a traumatic experience in a non-threatening manner.

Family   A dynamic system of people living together who are united by meaningful emotional bonds.

Family roles   Expected patterns or specific behaviors within a social context.

Family structure   The manner in which a family adapts and maintains itself.

Family therapy   A specialized intervention that is used to treat clients within a social context, rather than individually.

Feedback mechanism   A process that permits exchange of energy and matter across various boundaries.

Fetal alcohol syndrome (FAS)   A distinctive pattern of physical characteristics and developmental deficits seen in the offspring of women who consume alcohol during pregnancy.

Fibromyalgia syndrome   A nonspecific condition whose primary symptoms include diffuse musculoskeletal pain, fatigue, distress, and sleep disturbances.

Fidelity   Keeping promises and obligations.

Flight of ideas   Manifests as rapid thinking or ideas that have a common theme and that are likely to be seen in clients with major psychotic disorders such as a manic episode of bipolar disorder.

Focal neurological signs   Specific signs of neurological impairment, such as blurred vision or aphasia.

Focusing   The act of clarifying a perception or spotlighting a specific aspect of communication.

Foster care   An alternative living arrangement for underage persons who legally cannot or choose not to live with their biological families or guardians.

Free association   The client's spontaneous expression of thoughts.

Freebase cocaine   A purer form of cocaine produced by removing the water-soluble base; commonly referred to as "crack" or "rock" cocaine.

Frustration   A condition that emerges when a goal is blocked. The stronger the frustration, the greater the potential for aggression. It is the single most potent means of provoking aggression.

Functional family system   Open systems composed of individuals, couples, children, and communities who are able to adapt to change or crisis.

Gender   A psychosocial construct that changes over time and is distinct from sex, which is an individual's biological state of maleness or femaleness.

Gender dysphoria   An intense, persistent discomfort resulting from one's own perception of the inappropriateness of sex assignment made at birth.

Genetic vulnerability   The relationship between genetic and enzymatic defects and vulnerability to mental illness. Genetic function is influenced by prenatal and environmental factors that activate intricate biochemical processes and affect behavior. A number of researchers have attempted to explore the relationship between genetic factors and mental disorders using twin, adoption, and family studies.

Genogram   A family assessment tool that maps a pictorial illustration of family history (generations).

Genomics   The study of human genome sequencing and its contributions to disease and treatment.

G-proteins   Part of the cell's second messenger system in the plasma, involved in sending signals from regulatory chemicals such as hormones and neurotransmitters to target cells.

Grandiosity   An inflated appraisal of one's worth, power, knowledge, importance, or identity that may include delusional thinking.

Gratification   To be satisfied; receive pleasure from.

Grief   A normal profound response to loss.

Group home treatment   A structured living environment in which persons live with other individuals who are at various stages of their recovery process.

Group therapy   In mental health, a modality of treatment for more than one person that provides therapeutic outcomes for each individual.

Hallucination   False sensory perception of internal stimuli. Examples of hallucinations include auditory, visual, olfactory, and tactile.

Hardiness   A personality trait that enables people to maintain health and cope with stressful events.

Heavy drinking   Consuming five or more drinks on the same occasion on each of 5 or more days in the past month (SAMHSA, 2000).

Hippocampus   Located in the medial temporal lobe, it is an important site for the formation and storage of immediate and recent memories, and it is influenced by the amygdala's emotional rating of an event. This part of the brain is damaged by Alzheimer's disease.

Holding environment   A descriptive term for a therapeutic milieu that incorporates traditional milieu therapy variables. The term healing environment is sometimes used interchangeably with holding environment.

Homeostasis   A state of adaptation or ability to effectively manage internal and external environmental demands.

Hopelessness   A state of despondency and absolute loss of hope.

Hospice   End-of-life health care for clients.

Hostility   Overt antagonism, opposition, or resistance in thought or principle.

Human sexual response cycle   Encompasses four distinct stages in which the body responds to sexual arousal.

Hydrotherapy   Use of continuous baths and cold wet-sheet packs to produce a calming effect to control emotional and mental disturbances.

Hyperactivity   Excessively active; having too much energy to handle. An activity level that is out of proportion for the situation, setting, and person's developmental level.

Hyperphagia   Excessive amount of eating.

Hypersomnia   Excessive amount of sleep.

Hypochondriasis   Persistent preoccupation with fears of having, or the idea that one has, a serious disease based on the person's misinterpretation or exaggeration of bodily functions.

Hypomania   A clinical syndrome that indicates an elated mood state similar to but less severe than that described by the term mania or manic episode; it generally does not cause social or occupational impairment and has a duration of more than 4 days.

Hypothalamus   Together with the pituitary gland, thyroid gland, adrenal glands, gonads, and pancreas, the hypothalamus forms a major regulatory system and is involved in the biological aspects of behavior. The hypothalamus-pituitary-adrenal axis (HPA) is important in understanding certain mental disorders. The hypothalamus regulates autonomic, endocrine, and visceral integration and is surmised to be the foundation of the limbic system and the brain center for emotions and certain behaviors such as eating, drinking, aggression, and sexuality. Information in the hypothalamus is modulated by ascending sensory pathways, hormones, and descending pathways of the cerebral cortex.

Id   The sum total of biological instincts, including sexual and aggressive impulses.

Identified client   The client whose symptoms are the focus and serve as the reasons for seeking treatment.

Illusion   A misinterpretation of an external stimulus, such as mistaking a shadow for a person.

Impulsivity   The act of taking spontaneous actions without thinking about consequences. Closely related to disinhibition and central to conceptions of attention-deficit/hyperactivity disorder (ADHD) and personality disorders and the aggression spectrum or disruptive behavior disorders.

Inattention A failure to focus attention on those elements of the environment that are most relevant to the task at hand.

Incongruent communication Occurs when more than one message is sent and the messages contradict each other.

Inferiority complex An exaggeration of feelings of inadequacy and insecurity resulting in defensiveness and anxiety.

Infradian rhythms Biological variations with a frequency lower than circadian (i.e., rhythms that have longer, slower cycles than 24-hour circadian rhythms).

Insight The client's self-awareness and understanding of the meaning and reason for her behavior or motives.

Insight-oriented or process-oriented groups For individuals with high levels of cognitive functioning. Insight-oriented groups focus on the development of intellectual awareness, thinking patterns, and emotional factors influencing behavior.

Insomnia Inability to fall asleep, difficulty staying asleep, or early morning awakening.

Insulin-shock therapy Administration of large doses of insulin to induce marked hypoglycemia, which produces a coma or seizure.

Intensive case management A concept similar to ACT that has been shown to be cost-effective and efficacious in the treatment of serious mental illnesses.

Intergenerational transmission of violence The phenomenon in which violent behaviors are learned and repeated by subsequent generations of abusive families.

Internalized relationships Those relationships that are maintained as supportive or destructive to the psyche and that continue to affect the individual long after the experience.

Intimate partner violence Physical, sexual, or emotional and psychological abuse of men or women occurring in past or current intimate relationships, cohabiting or not, and including dating relationships.

Intracultural variations Alterations in cultural ideation and psychological or physical characteristics between persons from different racial and ethnic groups.

Intrapreneur An individual who expands the traditional role as direct health care provider to that of creator of quality-of-care products and services within an institution or organization.

Involvement Includes the basic milieu therapy concept of the client's responsibility to participate actively in treatment and other decision making.

Justice Treating all people fairly and equitably.

Kindling The electrophysiological process that over time produces an action potential after repetitive subthreshold stimulation or progressive sensitization of a neuron. This concept is thought to play a role in recurrent mood disorders.

Korsakoff's syndrome A psychosis, usually based on chronic alcoholism, that is accompanied by disturbance of orientation, susceptibility to external stimulation and suggestion, falsification of memory, and hallucinations.

Language A complex phenomenon and tool used to communicate.

Leadership The ability to show others the way by going in advance; to act as a guide for others.

Learning disability A condition that makes it difficult for a person to learn information in a usual manner.

Lethality Level of dangerousness or injury.

Lewy bodies Proteinaceous structures composed of a central core with radiating filaments, located in the substantia nigra in Parkinson's disease and in the cortex in diffuse Lewy body disease.

Liaison Facilitation of the relationships between the client, the client's illness, the consultee, the health care team, and the environment.

Libidinal object constancy Maintenance of the image of the primary caretaker in the growing infant's memory so that the figure remains in the mind even when the object is not immediately present and interactive.

Libido Urge or desire for sexual activity. Also, the basic driving force of personality in Freud's system; it includes sexual energy but is not restricted to it.

Life expectancy The age at which an individual born into a particular cohort may be expected to die.

Life span The maximum age that could be attained if an individual were able to avoid or be successfully treated for all illnesses and accidents.

Light therapy A biological intervention that increases exposure to artificial light whose intensity is equivalent to outdoor levels, more than 2,000 lux. The aim of therapy is to suppress melatonin secretion and produce phase shifts of melatonin production.

Linear kinetics A pharmacokinetic model in which a constant amount of drug is eliminated in a set unit of time.

Loose association Manifests as a flow of thoughts or ideas that are unrelated to each other and shift from one subject to another. It is often seen in clients with schizophrenia and other major psychotic disorders.

Malpractice Intentional professional misconduct that fails to comply with professional standards and results in injury.

Mania A disorder characterized by exalted feelings, delusions of grandeur, elevated mood, and psychomotor overactivity.

Marital schism Intense marital conflict in which a parent attempts to enlist a child as an ally against the other parent.

Marital skew Severe marital discord arising from acceptance of maladaptive behaviors in one partner by the other partner.

Maturational crisis Developmental stages marked by biological, psychosocial, and social transitions that generate predictable and characteristic disturbances in behavior and emotional responses.

Melatonin A metabolite of serotonin produced by the pineal gland. It is produced during darkness and is involved in the feedback loop that is regulated according to the degree of environmental light. Melatonin is implicated in the regulation of seasonal and circadian variance and in the body's adjustment to time zones; it is a biological marker for the effects of light therapy in seasonal affective disorder (SAD).

Memory A complex brain function that involves storing and retrieving information that is later recalled to consciousness.

Mental disorder or illness Any health condition that is identified by a change in thinking, mood, or behavior and that creates distress or problems with everyday functioning.

Mental health   A relative state of well-being that enables persons, couples, families, and communities to adaptively respond to external and internal stressors.

Mental health movement   A movement that began more than 25 years ago that focuses on humane treatment of the mentally ill, initially advocating their release from state institutions to community mental health centers.

Mental health team   An interdisciplinary group of mental health staff who collaborate to assess, intervene, and evaluate client responses to treatment.

Mental status examination (MSE)   The part of the clinical assessment that compiles nursing observations and impressions of the client during the interview. Data from this examination include general appearance, mood and affect, speech patterns, perception, thought content and processes, level of consciousness and cognition, impulsivity, ability to abstract, judgment and insight, and reliability. Also involves the assessment of functional status, risk of harm to self or others, and level of safety.

Metabolic pathways   Chemical sites (e.g., acetylation, debrisoquine-ds, mephenytoin) that are involved in the conversion of pharmacologic agents within a person's biological system.

Milieu   Environment, from French for middle space, or a safe place.

Milieu therapy   A treatment modality that uses the total physical and social environment as a therapeutic agent to provide psychosocial rehabilitation for psychiatric clients. Traditionally, milieu therapy includes key variables or components that are also defined here. The term is sometimes used interchangeably with the term therapeutic milieu.

Mixed state   A behavioral condition displayed for a period of at least 1 week in which both manic and major depressive mood states are exhibited every day. Symptoms are sufficiently severe to cause impairment in social and occupational functioning.

Modeling   A form of learning in which a person observes another person perform a desired response.

Mood   Refers to the client's sustained emotional state that reflects the client's perception of the world—depressed, sad, labile, elated, expansive, or anxious.

Moral treatment   Humane treatment of the mentally ill; for example, releasing clients from mechanical restraints and improving physical care. Phillippe Pinel, a French physician, and Benjamin Rush, an American physician, were instrumental in promoting this movement.

Morgan Russel scales   A widely used measure of outcome for anorexia nervosa that consists of two scores: an average outcome score and a general outcome score. The average outcome score is based on the outcome in five areas: nutritional status, menstrual function, mental state, sexual adjustment, and socioeconomic status.

Multi-infarct dementia (MID)   A probable irreversible dementia caused by many small strokes or by a large stroke.

Myoclonus   Shocklike contractions of a portion of a muscle, an entire muscle, or a group of muscles, restricted to one area of the body or appearing synchronously or asynchronously in several areas.

Narcolepsy   A rare disorder of chronic daytime sleepiness, cataplexy, and sleep paralysis. No amount of normal sleep ameliorates the disorder; individuals have disturbed nocturnal sleep, including vivid dreams, nightmares, or night terrors.

National Institute of Mental Health   A federally funded agency whose goals include developing and helping various states to identify and use the most effective methods for prevention, diagnosis, and intervention of mental illnesses through research funding, staff development, and education of mental health professionals to provide mental health treatment.

Negative symptoms   Schizophrenic symptoms associated with structural brain abnormalities. Most negative symptoms include blunted affect, inability to experience pleasure, apathy, a lack of feeling, and impaired attention.

Negentropy   The counterforce to entropy; the evolving of more complete organization, complexity, and ability to convert resources.

Neglect   The failure to provide for the individual's basic needs for subsistence, including food, housing, clothing, education, medical care, and emotional care. At its most extreme, neglect results in death, especially in older adults and in very young children.

Negligence   Unintentional injury that results from failure to act as a reasonable person would.

Neuritic plaques   A patch or flat area of neurons.

Neurobiology   Biology of the nervous system, particularly the brain.

Neuroendocrinology   The study of how the neural and endocrine systems work together to maintain homeostasis. Communication between these systems is involved in biological and behavioral responses. Major organs of the neuroendocrine system are the hypothalamus, pituitary, thyroid, and adrenal glands; the gonads; and the pancreas.

Neurofibrillary tangles   Tangles of the neurofibrils, the delicate threads running in every direction through the cytoplasm of the body of a nerve and extending into the axon and the dendrites of the cell.

Neuroleptic malignant syndrome (NMS)   A rare and potentially life-threatening syndrome primarily caused by antipsychotic medications and characterized by marked muscle rigidity, high fever, altered consciousness or delirium, tachycardia, hypoxia, hypertension, and diaphoresis.

Neuroscience   The science and study of the central nervous system.

Neurotransmitters   Biochemicals found in the central nervous system that are involved in the transmission of impulses across the synapses between neurons. Examples include serotonin, norepinephrine, and dopamine.

Neurovegetative   Refers to biological functions such as sleep pattern, eating pattern, energy level, sexual functioning, and bowel functioning.

Non–rapid eye movement (NREM) sleep   Four stages of sleep occur: Stage I is light sleep; in Stage II, eye movements are minimal or absent; in Stages III and IV, there is slow EEG wave activity, with difficulty in arousal.

Non-restorative sleep   Sleep associated with fatigue, difficulty awakening, poor concentration, and low productivity.

Nonverbal communication   Body language or transmission of messages without the use of words.

Normal pressure hydrocephalus (NPH) A condition in which the cerebral spinal fluid pressure reading is normal or high-normal, but excessive fluid exists in the ventricles of the brain.

Nurse-client relationship A dynamic, collaborative, therapeutic, interactive process between the nurse and the client.

Nursing diagnosis A statement of the client's nursing problem that includes both the adaptive or maladaptive health response and contributing stressors.

Nursing informatics The use of computers and information sciences to manage and process data, knowledge, and information in nursing practice and client care.

Nursing process An interactive, problem-solving process; a systematic and individualized problem-solving approach for administering nursing care that meets the client's needs comprehensively and effectively.

Object relations Internalized relationships recollected from early primary caregivers.

Obsession Intrusive, recurrent, and persistent thoughts, images, or feelings that generate intense anxiety. Anxiety is usually temporarily dampened by ritualistic behaviors, known as compulsions, such as excessive hand washing associated with intense fears of contamination.

Ocular apraxia Inability to voluntarily direct the gaze to a target of visual interest.

Off-label medication Denotes a prescribed medication to use for a purpose other than the parameters of the approved label.

Open communication Active and honest sharing of feelings, thoughts, and information. Confidentiality is unit based, and unhealthy secret-keeping is discouraged, but privacy is respected.

Open system In systems theory, a term used to imply that members or parts are interrelated and responsive to each other's needs.

Operant conditioning A type of learning in which responses are modified by their consequences.

Optic ataxia Inability to benefit from visual guidance in reaching for an object.

Orgasm phase Third phase of the human sexual response cycle, in which men and women experience rhythmic contractions followed by extreme pleasure.

Orientation One's sense of time, person, or place.

Overarousal To be excessively excited or stimulated.

Pain disorder Disorder whose major symptom is pain in one or more anatomic sites. It is the predominant focus of the clinical presentation and is of sufficient severity to necessitate clinical attention. It also produces significant distress that results in impaired occupational, interpersonal, and social performance.

Palliative care Combines the use of culturally competent, compassionate, therapeutic, and supportive therapies for persons who are diagnosed with a life-threatening disorder and for their families or significant others.

Paradoxical reaction A response to a drug that is opposite to what would be predicted by the drug's pharmacology.

Paraphasia Speech defect characterized by disorderly arrangements of spoken words.

Parasomnias Also called arousal disorders; include nightmares or night terrors, sleepwalking, and confusion with arousal.

Paresthesia Unnatural tactile sensations manifested by tingling, tickling, or creeping sensations that have no physical basis. This sensation often results from activation of the hypothalamic-pituitary-adrenal axis.

Parkinson's disease The chronic condition marked by rigidity and tremor with intention. Pathology in the substantia nigra.

Partial hospitalization/day treatment A specific time-defined, outpatient, active psychiatric treatment program that is grounded in therapeutic communication and structured clinical services.

Patterns A person's typical behavioral organization that resists change.

Pedophile An adult who is sexually attracted to children and who abuses them sexually.

Perpetrator A person who inflicts abuse or injury on another.

Persona A disguised or masked attitude useful in interacting with one's environment but frequently at variance with one's true identity.

Personal boundaries A mental idea of how one experiences and maintains a line of separation between oneself and the world.

Personal space A subjective definition of comfortable space between one person and another.

Personality Characteristic traits that are generally predictable in their influence on cognitive, affective, and behavioral patterns. Enduring patterns of perceiving, relating to, and thinking about the world and oneself.

Pharmacodynamics The study of biochemical and physiological actions and effects of drugs.

Pharmacogenetics The study of molecular genetic variation that explains individual drug responses and may help identify biological predictors of adverse effects.

Pharmacokinetics The study of a drug's absorption, distribution, metabolism, and excretion or elimination.

Pharmacology The scientific study of chemical formulations (drugs), including their sources, properties, uses, actions, and effects.

Phase advancing A response to a light stimulus that is intentionally presented hours before the expected onset of solar or wavelength of environmental light.

Phase delaying Refers to a response elicited by a light stimulus presented hours later than expected.

Phase-specific community-oriented intervention Intervention that targets specific symptoms during various stages of treatment within an intensive case management model, specifically for persons with first-episode psychosis.

Phobia An exaggerated or irrational fear of an event (e.g., a presentation) or of an object (e.g., a spider).

Phonemic Speech sounds that are the basic units of speech (e.g., "leviator" instead of "elevator," "grontologs" instead of "gerontology").

Physical abuse The intentional use of physical force against another person, including, but not limited to, pushing, slapping, biting, choking, punching, beating, and using a gun, knife, or other weapon.

Physical assault Attacks ranging from slapping and beating to rape, homicide, and the use of weapons such as knives, firearms, or bombs.

Physical restraint Any physical or mechanical device, material, or equipment that is attached to or placed adjacent to the client's body that cannot be removed easily by the client and limits freedom of movement or normal access to one's body.

Pick's disease (PD) A rare, fatal degenerative disease of the nervous system, occurring mostly in middle-aged women. Characterized by signs of severe frontal or temporal lobe dysfunction. Overall symptomatology is very similar to Alzheimer's disease.

Plateau phase Second phase of the human sexual response cycle, marked by vasocongestion and myotonia.

Play therapy An individualized intervention that offers children a symbolic way to express feelings, anxiety, aggressions, and self-doubt.

Positive symptoms Refer to schizophrenic symptoms with good premorbid functioning, acute onset, and positive response to typical and atypical antipsychotics. Common positive symptoms include hallucinations, delusions, disorganized thinking and speech, and gross behavioral disturbances. These symptoms are linked with dysregulation of biochemical processes.

Potentially reversible dementia A condition characterized by an acute onset, causing neurological symptoms and changes in level of consciousness. If treated in time, the condition may be reversed. See delirium.

Praxis The performance of an action; "doing."

Preoccupation Having recurrent thoughts or centering on a particular idea or thought with an intense emotional component.

Pressured speech Disturbance in verbal expression of thought characterized by an overproduction of rapid speech that is frequently loud, unsolicited by social interaction, and difficult to interrupt.

Primary appraisal Refers to initial responses to a stressor and the ultimate goal of prevailing over or effectively managing a given situation.

Primary prevention Refers to measures or interventions to counteract circumstances or conditions that are potentially harmful. Additionally, these measures generate coping skills and reduce vulnerability to illness and promote health.

Principal investigator A person who takes the major role in the development and conduct of a research study.

Probable irreversible dementia Progressive loss of intellectual functioning caused by permanent brain damage.

Process The manner in which clients talk about themselves and the way the group responds. Analysis of group process provides assessment of the therapy's effects on individual group members.

Program for Assertive Community Treatment (PACT) Refers to an intensive case management approach involving careful monitoring of clients, access to mobile mental health teams, and aggressive holistic client-centered treatment planning. PACT programs are available 24 hours a day.

Progressive relaxation A form of relaxation training that involves visualizing and sequentially relaxing specific muscle groups, starting with the scalp and moving to the tips of the toes. This technique involves teaching the client to tense and relax various muscle groups in an effort to reduce tension and stress.

Prosody The variations in stress, pitch, and rhythms of speech that convey meanings.

Prosopagnosia Inability to recognize faces.

Protein kinase C (PKC) A group of enzymes that activate other enzymes.

Pseudoaddiction A syndrome of behaviors resembling addiction that develops in chronic pain management; with adequate pain management, drug-seeking behaviors cease.

Pseudomutuality A transaction that infers a sense of relatedness and emotional connectedness; in reality, it represents shallow and empty relationships.

Psyche organizers Repetitive developmental experiences that guide the person's experience and expectations, resulting in the style of reaction that is typical of that person.

Psychiatric genetics The science of heritable factors related to psychiatric disorders.

Psychoanalysis A form of psychodynamic psychotherapy in which the therapist and client explore the client's conscious and unconscious conflicts and coping patterns.

Psychoeducational group Group that offers information to a large number of people, simultaneously, providing both information and emotional support. Persons who are motivated to learn about their illness or to develop self-awareness benefit from this type of group.

Psychological abuse Usually verbal abuse designed to control another through use of intimidation, degradation, or fear.

Psychological autopsy A standard procedure following a suicide in which team members present and discuss the case with other staff, with the intent of evaluating issues of quality of care and learning from the experience. It also offers an opportunity for staff to process their feelings and thoughts about the tragedy.

Psychomotor retardation A slowing of physical and emotional reactions, including speech, affect, and movement.

Psychoneuroimmunology The study of the role of the immune system in health and illness in the face of biological and psychosocial stress. This field is developing knowledge about the interconnectedness of the nervous system and the immune system.

Psychophysiologic insomnia (PI) Refers to complaints of difficulty attaining or maintaining sleep during a normal sleep period.

Psychophysiological disorder Denotes emotional states producing or exacerbating physical problems.

Psychosis A person's symptom state that includes the presence of reality misinterpretations, disorganized thinking, and lack of awareness regarding true and false reality.

Psychosocial assessment The data collection process that includes major elements such as psychosocial, biological, cultural, and spiritual data collections.

Psychosocial rehabilitation Health services whose goal is to restore the client's ability to function in the community through social interaction, independent living, and vocational enhancement.

Psychostimulants A class of medications that temporarily increases the functioning activity of the brain.

Psychosurgery Surgical or chemical alteration involving the severing of brain fibers with the purpose of modifying behavioral disturbance, thoughts, or mood.

Psychotherapy A global process in which people seek professional help to resolve problems, promote personal growth, and reduce or eliminate maladaptive responses.

Psychotropics Various pharmacologic agents, such as antidepressants and antipsychotic, antimanic, and antianxiety agents used to affect behavior, cognition, mood, and emotions.

Purge Self-induced vomiting or misuse of laxatives, diuretics, or enemas.

Qualitative research Research that focuses on the meaning of the experiences to individuals rather than on the generalizability of study results.

Quantitative research Research that focuses on gathering numerical data, with the intent of generalizing the findings of the study.

Race Taxonomy of a group's identity based on genetic factors that produce physical characteristics and distinguish the persons within that group from persons within another group.

Racing thoughts A rapid series of ideas that occur during manic episodes.

Rapid cycling A pattern of bipolar disorder characterized by at least four dictinct episodes of depression, mania, or mixed states each year.

Rapid eye movement (REM) sleep Sleep associated with relative paralysis of skeletal muscles, rapid eye movement, penile erection, and dreaming.

Rapport Harmony or accord between people.

Reality principle A perception of the environment that fairly matches what others perceive and that fosters adaptive responses toward productivity, enjoyment of life, and maintenance of homeostasis.

Reality testing The ability to logically and objectively evaluate and judge the world outside self.

Recovery Refers to a state of wellness or function characterized by symptom management and attaining an optimal level of function and quality of life. It is client-centered and based on principles of hope, healing, and optimism. In substance-use treatment, it refers to a state of physical and psychological health in which abstinence from dependency-producing drugs is complete and comfortable.

Reinforcement In classic conditioning, the process of following the conditioned stimuli with the unconditioned stimulus; in operant conditioning, the rewarding of desired responses.

Reinforcers Personal, complex, learned, and biochemical rewards that are used to modify maladaptive behavior. Reinforcers can be positive, negative, or punishing, and are personally determined.

Relapse Use of psychoactive substances after a maintained period of abstinence.

Relational resilience The family's ability to mobilize resources and confront psychosocial and biological stresses effectively using adaptive coping responses.

Relational worldview Worldview perspective that espouses and values the development of interactions, relationships, and spirituality as contextually important in life.

Repression An unconscious process that removes anxiety-producing thoughts, desires, or memories from conscious awareness.

Resilience The capacity to recover from or adapt to distress, overwhelming change, or potentially harmful risk factors.

Resolution phase Fourth phase of the human sexual response cycle, in which the body returns to an unaroused state.

Restless leg syndrome (RLS)/periodic limb movement disorder (PLMD) Motor movement during sleep characterized during the day by akathisia (inability to sit still) and a "deep uneasy" feeling in the legs, as well as aching, and "crazy legs," which is uncommon in the daytime, with an onset in the evening or at bedtime; associated with renal failure and iron deficiency anemia.

Restorative sleep Sleep that restores normal brain activity and equilibrium in the central nervous system and bodily processes.

Restraint A physical or chemical way to stop a client from being free to move in order to prevent injury.

Ruminations Repetitive or continuous thinking about a particular subject that then interferes with other thought processes.

Scapegoating A form of displacement that involves blaming a member for the actions of others.

Schemata Cognitive structures, or patterns, that consist of the person's beliefs, values, and assumptions.

Seasonal affective disorder (SAD) Recurrent depression that occurs during winter months and remits in the spring. Major symptoms include depressive mood, hypersomnia, tiredness, increased appetite, and cravings for carbohydrates.

Seclusion Placing and keeping a client in a bare room (free of sharp or dangerous objects) for the purpose of containing a clinical situation that may evolve or has evolved into an emergent situation.

Secondary appraisal Emerges with any form of perceived threat or harm if primary appraisals are ineffective or maladaptive. The rationale for secondary appraisal is to assess coping resources, options, and choices.

Secondary gain Attempting to earn the sympathy of others, receiving financial gain, or obtain other benefits by suffering from a disorder.

Secondary prevention Refers to measures or interventions used to curtail disease processes.

Sedatives Drugs that are virtually synonymous with anxiolytics; used to calm nervousness, irritability, or excitement; these agents depress the central nervous system and tend to cause lassitude and reduced mental activity.

Self-deprecatory ideas Negative thoughts about the self.

Self-destructive behavior Behavior that tends to harm or destroy the self.

Self-disclosure Exposing oneself to others; to make publicly known.

Self-efficacy Refers to the expectation that one can effectively cope with and master situations such as addictions, achieving desired outcomes through one's own personal efforts.

Self-mutilation or self-injurious behavior The act of self-induced pain or tissue destruction void of the intent to kill oneself.

Semantic paraphasia Substituting a similar word for an object (e.g., "staple" for "paper clip").

Semantic precision Use of words that are appropriate or significant to the meaning of the intended communication (e.g., substituting "machine" for "automobile").

Separation anxiety A common childhood and adolescent anxiety disorder whose symptoms involve panic or intense fear of losing one's primary caregivers.

Serious disabling mental disorder (SDMD) A term used to describe a person who has the diagnosis of schizophrenia, depressive disorder, and/or bipolar disorder.

Serotonin syndrome A condition characterized by serotonergic hyperstimulation that includes restlessness, hyperthermia, myoclonus, hypertension, hyperreflexia, diaphoresis, lethargy, confusion, and tremor and may cause death.

Sexual abuse Abusive sexual contact, completed or attempted, against the will of the other, or in circumstances in which the other is unable to understand, refuse, or communicate unwillingness to engage in the sexual activity.

Sexual assault Abusive sexual contact, completed or attempted, against the will of the other, or in circumstances in which the other is unable to understand, refuse, or communicate unwillingness to engage in the sexual activity.

Sexual attitude reassessment (SAR) An intensive 2-day workshop to assist participants in reevaluation of sexual attitudes.

Sexual desire One's internal psychological state of pleasure governed by sexual pleasure centers in the brain.

Sexual health Integration of the somatic, emotional, intellectual, and social aspects of sexual being in ways that are positively enriching and that enhance personality, communication, and love (WHO, 1975).

Sexual orientation Sexual preference for erotic partners of the same, opposite, or either sex. An individual may be heterosexual, homosexual, lesbian, bisexual, or asexual.

Shadow Carl Jung's term that refers to the unconscious.

Shaken baby syndrome A form of child abuse depicted by a compilation of signs and symptoms associated with the violent shaking of an infant or small child.

Shift work sleep disorder (SWSD) Develops in shift workers and is characterized by insomnia or excessive sleepiness unrelieved by sleep.

Short-term hospitalization Structured, inpatient treatment that provides clinical services, psychotherapy, counseling, and monitoring of physical, mental, and pharmacologic status.

Sick role Dependent, helpless, and ill behavior often associated with control and maintenance of maladaptive relationships.

Situational crisis An unexpected crisis that arises from several sources, including environmental, physical or personal, or psychosocial.

Sleep apnea Various disorders arising from respiratory obstruction or cessation; associated with decreased oxygenation, fragmented sleep, and increased risk for injury, particularly with coexisting medical disorders such as chronic obstructive pulmonary disease (COPD), congestive heart failure (CHF), coronary artery disease (CAD), and myocardial infarction (MI). Characterized by snoring, gasping, or absence of breathing.

Sleep cycles Composed of cycles of REM and NREM sleep, with REM sleep occurring every 1 to 2 hours in normal situations.

Sleep deprivation Chronic lack of sleep, but may occur acutely; inability to get the needed 8.3 hours of sleep nightly.

Sleep paralysis Associated with narcolepsy, inability to move or speak just after or before awakening; breathing is not affected.

Sleepiness to somnolence Hypersomnia, common in persons with shift work, jet lag, or sleep disorders; individuals are likely to fall asleep if there is no stimulating or stressful activity occurring. Characterized by sleepiness, fatigue, poor concentration and memory lapses, depression, motor vehicle accidents (MVA), or on-the-job injuries.

Sleep-wake cycle One of the body's biological rhythms normally determined by the day-night cycle.

Somatic preoccupation Excessive focus on one's own body functioning.

Somatization disorder A disorder whose primary symptoms are progressive and recurrent somatic complaints of pain or of sexual, gastrointestinal, or pseudoneurological manifestations. These symptoms produce significant distress and global disability.

Somatoform Refers to a group of psychiatric disorders whose symptoms are severe enough to cause global impairment or functioning. Typically, clients present with recurring, multiple, clinically significant somatic complaints. In addition, these complaints are colorful and exaggerated but lack specific factual information to support the diagnosis.

Speech The process of expressing ideas, thoughts, and feelings through language; use of words and language.

Spiritual assessment Process that involves gathering data concerning the client's belief system, affirmation coping mechanisms, and psychosocial resources.

Spirituality A dynamic phenomenon that enables a person to discover meaning and purpose in life, particularly during stressful life events.

Splitting The internal mechanism wherein the person is unable to evaluate, synthesize, and accept imperfections in others so that a significant other is viewed as all good or all bad, causing the phenomenon of setting persons up against each other.

Steady state The state whereby the amount of drug eliminated from the body equals the amount being absorbed.

Stress A stimulus or demand that has the potential to generate disruption in homeostasis or produce a reaction.

Stress debriefing A crisis intervention technique that relies on three therapeutic modalities: provide an opportunity to express one's feelings in the context of group support, facilitate normalization of reactions to an abnormal event, and learn about postdisaster reactions.

Substance abuse Repeated intentional use or misuse of a psychoactive substance; use is modified or discontinued with the occurrence of significant adverse consequences.

Substance dependence The accepted diagnostic term for a pattern of out-of-control or compulsive use of psychoactive substances in which use continues despite negative consequences; often used interchangeably with the terms addiction or chemical dependency.

Substance intoxication   Substance-specific physical, psychological, and cognitive effects produced as a result of ingesting a psychoactive substance.

Subsystem   A smaller system within larger systems.

Suicidal ideation   A thought or idea of suicide.

Suicidal intent   Refers to the degree to which the person intends to act on his suicidal ideations.

Suicidal threat   Verbalization of imminent self-destructive action, which, if carried out, has a high probability of leading to death.

Suicide   The act of killing oneself.

Superego   The part of the personality structure that evolves out of the ego and reflects early moral training and parental injunctions.

Switching   The process in which one alter is changed into another.

Synaptic transmission   The process of nerve impulse transmission through the generation of action potentials from one neuron to another.

Tangentiality   A speech pattern that illustrates an inability to respond completely in a focused manner. Individuals may begin to respond appropriately but progress to related topics, never completing the originally desired response.

Tardive dyskinesia   A chronic, progressive, and potentially fatal syndrome caused by prolonged dopamine blockade usually associated with high-potency antipsychotic medications. Major manifestations include choreiform movements of the face, tongue, and upper and lower extremities, such as tongue movement or protrusion, lip sucking, chewing, and smacking; other symptoms include puffing of cheeks and pelvic thrusting.

T-cells   Viral- and tumor-fighting lymphocytes (all called natural killer cells) of the immune system. They are referred to as "T" cells because they are processed by the thymus gland.

Telemental health   The use of technologies such as videoconferencing and home telemonitoring devices to provide mental health and psychiatric services.

Teratogenic   A substance or medication that can interfere with normal embryonic development and results in malformation.

Termination   The final phase of psychotherapy. This process involves exploring areas of accomplishment, goal attainment, and feelings generated by ending the relationship.

Tertiary prevention   Refers to measures that minimize relapse and chronic disability and restore the client to an optimal level of functioning.

Thanatos   The instinct toward death and self-destruction.

Theory   An organized and systematic set of statements related to significant questions in a discipline. Theories describe, explain, predict, or prescribe responses, events, situations, conditions, or relationships and consist of concepts that are related to each other.

Therapeutic alliance   A trusting relationship that helps the client explore interpersonal and intrapersonal conflicts and gain insight into maladaptive behaviors.

Therapeutic communication   A healing or curative dialogue between people.

Therapeutic factors   The standards for the conduct of group therapy. They include the following: imparting of information, instillation of hope, universality, altruism, corrective recapitulation of the primary family group member, development of socializing skills, imitative behavior, interpersonal learning, group cohesiveness, catharsis, and existential factors.

Therapeutic use of self   An intervention that involves self-awareness, empathy, acceptance, self-disclosure, and other means of facilitating a therapeutic relationship.

Thought content   Refers to what the client is actually thinking about, which may include preoccupations, obsessions, compulsions, suicidal or homicidal ideations, and delusions.

Thought disorder   Often found in individuals with schizophrenia, this term refers to impaired thought processes or disorganized thoughts during which time the client has difficulty organizing thoughts or connecting them logically. Manifestations of disorganized thoughts or thought disorder include incoherent speech, thought blocking, or using unintelligible words (neologisms).

Thought process   The client's form of thinking or organization; examples include flights of ideas, phobias, tangentiality, circumstantiality, and racing thoughts.

Threat   An expression of intent to cause harm, including verbal threats, threatening or intimidating body language, and written threats.

Time-out   A behavior modification method that involves restriction of a youth for a period of time to an assigned area from which the child is not physically restricted from leaving for the purpose of providing the child an opportunity to regain self-control.

Tolerance   A pharmacologic property of some abused substances in which increased amounts over time are required to achieve similar results as in earlier use.

Tort   Unintentional or intentional injury.

Traits   Personality structure that typifies a person's responses in various situations.

Transactional   Refers to a set of pattern interactions among family members.

Transcranial magetic stimulation (TMS)   A noninvasive and relatively safe stimulation of the dorsa lateral prefrontal area used to rapidly change magnetic fields to induce electrical current to flow in the brain. Its antidepressant properties may involve induction to get electrical current across the insulating tissues of the scalp and skull without discomfort. It has recently been indicated as an effective treatment for depression. Repetitive transcranial magnetic stimulation is known as rTMS.

Transference   Unconscious displacement or reenactment of feelings and attitudes from the client to the psychotherapist.

Transgendered   Arching term that describes transsexuals, whose sense of themselves clashes with their original biological sex; cross-dressers; and others whose appearance is at odds with traditional gender expectations.

Transsexual   An individual who is profoundly unhappy in the sex assignment made at birth and who seeks to change or has changed the body to be as much as possible like that of the opposite sex.

Trauma An overwhelming stressful event that has the potential to result in acute and chronic neurobiological changes and distress.

Triangulation A maladaptive triad transactional pattern.

Twin studies Researchers attempt to explore the relationship between genetic factors and mental disorders using these studies, which usually include monozygotic (single-ovum) and dizygotic (two-ova) twins. Twin studies are helpful in isolating genetic and environmental influences and determining preventive and precipitating factors.

Type A personality A constellation of personality traits, such as highly driven, time-conscious, and competitive behavior, associated with high risk for coronary artery disease.

Type B personality A constellation of personality traits opposite from Type A and manifested by "easy-going, laid-back, and reposed" behavior.

Untradian rhythms Biological variations with a frequency higher than circadian (i.e., rhythms that have shorter, faster cycles than 24-hour circadian rhythms). Biological rhythms refer to cyclic variations in biological and biochemical function, activity, and emotional state.

Utilizer of research findings A person who integrates research findings into clinical practice.

Vagus nerve stimulation (VNS) A surgical procedure involving subcutaneous implantation of a pace-maker-like generator, which sends electric pulses to the left vagus nerve. It is used to treat refractory depression and epilepsy. It is used as the last resort in clients who fail to respond to traditional antidepressant treatment.

Validation Affirmation of the client's individuality and right to be treated with respect and dignity.

Veracity Telling the truth; honesty.

Verbal memory Ability to remember speech.

Violence Verbal abuse or threatening behavior, damage to property, self-harm, and physical aggression.

Visual imagery A stress- or anxiety-reducing cognitive exercise that involves creating relaxing thoughts or visual images of a place of serenity and calmness.

Visual memory Ability to remember what is seen.

Visuospatial ability Refers to time and space.

Vulnerability The potential susceptibility of a person, family, or group to a health deviation.

Wernicke-Korsakoff syndrome A complication of Wernicke's encephalopathy characterized by profound memory impairment and an inability to learn new material.

Wernicke's encephalopathy A reversible delirium seen in alcoholics; it is associated with thiamine deficiency.

Withdrawal syndrome Substance-specific signs and symptoms precipitated by the abrupt cessation or reduction of a substance that produces tolerance and dependence after prolonged use.

Working or immediate memory The ability to sustain a limited amount of information for a few seconds while utilizing it for problem solving.

World Association for Sexology (WAS) An international association of sexologists, researchers, and policy makers who develop international policies related to sex.

Worldview perspective A person's belief regarding what he considers to be true and valued.

Zeitgeber A synchronizer or periodic environmental stimulus that is the dominant factor in determining a rhythm.

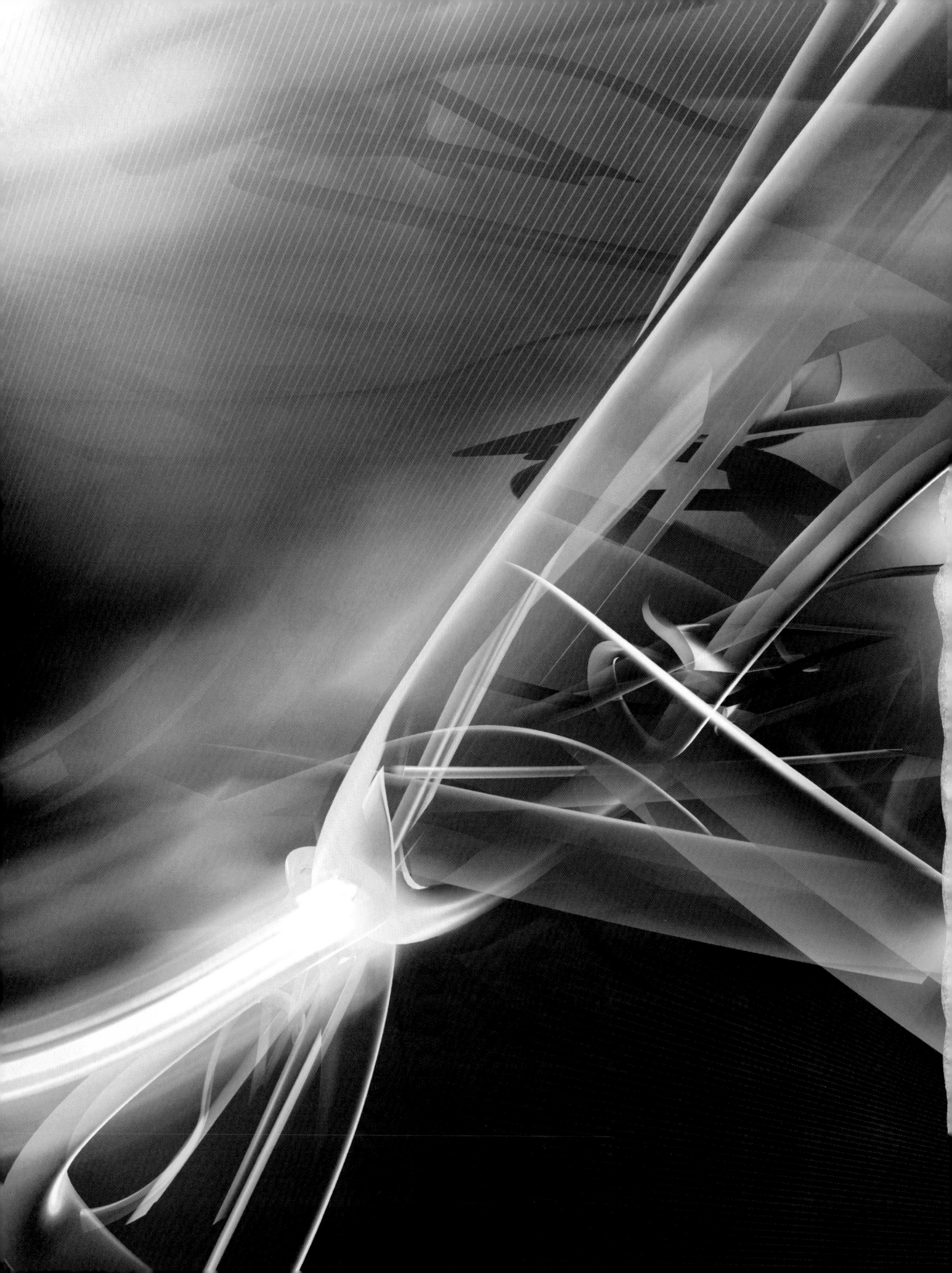

INDEX

Page numbers followed by f indicate figures; t, tables; b, boxes. Entries in italics indicate publication titles.

A

AASECT. *See* American Association of Sex Educators, Counselors, and Therapies
Abilify, 79
Absolute discharge, 206
Absolutist, 47t
Absorption, drug and, 884
Abstinence, 617, 623
Abuse. *See also* Abuse and violence
  of children and neurological damage, 86
  elder, 209–210
  reporting of, 209
  sexual disorder history and, 735
Abuse and violence
  across the life span, 771–774
  case studies, 759b, 763b, 766b, 778b
  clinical example, 762
  coping and adaptation, 770–771
  critical thinking, 764b
  nurse's role in, 776–777
  nurse's role in legal system, 777–778
  nursing care plan, 759–760b, 763–764b, 767–768b, 779–781b
  nursing process, 778–779, 781
  research abstract, 770b
  theories and perspectives of, 668–671
treatment modalities, 774–775
Acceptance, as quality, 113
Acetylcholine, 882
Acetylcholinesterase inhibitors, older adults and, 922–923
Acquired immune deficiency syndrome (AIDS), 99, 477
ACT. *See* Assertive community treatment
ACTH. *See* Adrenocorticotropic hormone
Acting out, 587
  conduct disorder, 423–424
  as defense mechanism, 35t
  defined, 411
Active listening, 149, 160
  barriers to, 160–161, 160t
Active metabolites, 885
Acupuncture, 16, 953
Acute confusion, 455, 460, 481
Acute psychiatric hospitalization, in abuse and violence, 775
Acute stress disorder, 202t, 323–324
AD. *See* Alzheimer's disease
ADA. *See* Americans with Disabilities Act
Adaptation
  anxiety disorder and, 299
  crisis and, 961, 963

  defined, 97, 297, 365
  depression, coping and, 234
  stress related disorder and, 368
  as tertiary prevention component, 100
Addiction, 617
  genetics and, 82–83
  substance-related disorder and, 620
ADHD. *See* Attention-deficit hyperactivity disorder
Adjustment disorder, clinical example, 109b
Adler, Alfred, 40
Admission criteria laws, 204–206
Adolescence
  abuse and violence, 772–773
  anxiety disorder and, 308, 311–316
  attention-deficit hyperactivity disorder in, 506–507
  bipolar disorder and, 278–279
  characteristics of depression in, 237t
  community mental health care, 1012
  coping and adaptation in, 111–112
  culture and, 181
  depressive disorder in, 236, 237t, 238
  dissociative disorders, 538–539
  eating disorder in, 684–685
  Erikson (social theory) and, 39t
  Freud and, 37t
  group therapy and, 835
  identity *vs.* role conflict and crisis in, 971–972
  individual psychotherapy in, 798
  maladaptive coping behavior in, 419t
  maturational crisis, 971–972
  medical-surgical setting and, 1031–1033
  milieu therapy and, 993, 994–995t
  overanxious disorder, 312
  personality disorder in, 425–427
  post-traumatic stress disorder, 312–314
  psychiatric nursing research and, 1083
  psychobiological disorder and, 376
  psychopharmacologic therapy and, 916–921
  psychosexual theory and, 38
  schizophrenia and other psychotic disorder in, 399
  separation anxiety disorder, 311–312
  sexual disorder in, 738–739
  sleep disorder in, 710
  social phobia, 312
  somatoform disorder and, 356
  substance-related disorder in, 643–644
  suicide risk in, 571–572
  Sullivan, Harry Stack, 41
Adolescents
  cognitive disorder in, 458
  electroconvulsive therapy in, 942–943
  life-span considerations of, 139–140, 141t
  manifestations of normal grief in, 245t
  psychiatry, 19t
  stages of psychosexual development, 37t

Cognitive theory(ies), 46–50, 233–234
Cognitive therapy, 9t, 47, 49
  clinical example, 795b
  individual psychotherapy and, 794–795, 797
Cogwheeling, 875
Collaborative process, 116
Collective counseling, group therapy and, 815
Committee on the Quality of Health Care in America and National Institute of Medicine, 22
Communication, 149
  causative factors, 150–153
  developing self-awareness of, 170–171
  developmental issues and, 152–153
  evaluation, 170
  neurobiological issues and, 151–152
  nonverbal, 155
  patterns, factors of, 157–160
  psychosocial issues and, 152
  sexual disorder and lack of, 734–735
  technologies and, 165–166
  theories of, 154–155
  transactional analysis and, 154
  types of, 155–157
  verbal, 156–157
Communication competency theory, 154
Communication/systems models, 813
  group therapy and, 822–823
Communication techniques, therapeutic. See Therapeutic communication
Communication theory, family therapy and, 855–856
Community and home settings
  anxiety disorder treatment in, 326–327
  attention-deficit hyperactivity disorder in, 508–509
Community-based care, 13
Community mental health
  across the life span, 1012–1013
  defined, 1005
  history of, 1007–1008
  levels of care in, 1009
  psychiatric-mental health nurse role in, 1008–1009
  special populations, 1012–1013
Community Mental Health Act Movement, 14t
Community mental health care
  case study, 1016b
  nurse's role in, 1015
  nursing care plan and, 1017–1019b
  nursing process and, 1016
Community mental health centers, 1005, 1009–1011
Community Mental Health Centers Act, 13, 197, 197t, 198
  amendments to, 20–21
Community Mental Health Movement, 12, 963
Community mental health settings, social factors in, 1013, 1015
Community services for children, development of, 19t
Community support systems (CSS), 1005, 1009
Community worldview, 177, 180–181
Comorbidity factors
  anxiety as, 278t, 316
  defined, 297

eating disorder in, 679–681
substance-related disorder and, 278t
Competency
  defined, 195
  vs. incompetency, 206
Complementary therapies, 15, 16, 953–954
  of anxiety disorder, 331–332
  sleep disorder and, 714
  substance-related disorder and, 650–651
Comprehensive Mental Health Act, 8t
Compulsion(s), 125, 130, 297
Concrete operational stage, 49, 50t
Conditional discharge, 206
Conditioning, 45
Conduct disorders, 423–424
Confidentiality, clients and, 208–209
Conflict, 495, 506
Confrontation, 789
  defined, 149
  therapeutic communication and, 164
Congruent communication, 849, 856
Consolidated Omnibus Budget Reconciliation Act (COBRA), 205
Consultation, 1047
Consultation process, psychiatric consultation-liaison nurse and, 1054–1060
Consumerism, 1093, 1103
Containment, 985, 988
Content analysis, 813
Continuum of mental health care, 985
Conversion disorder, 350–351
  diagnostic criteria for, 350t
Conversion disorders, 343
Convulsive therapies, 937–939
Co-occurrence, 495, 497
Coping. See also Adaptation; Coping and Adaptation
  adjustment disorder and, 109b
  agoraphobia and, 109b
  defined, 97, 100
  mechanisms, 108–109, 967–968
  temporomandibular disorder and, 104–105b
Coping and adaptation
  abuse and violence, 770–771
  depression and, 234
  life span, 109–115
Coronary heart disease, stress and, 371–372
Cortical degenerative syndromes, 471–476
Cortical structures, 879–880
Corticotropin-releasing hormone (CRH), 228
Counseling, substance-related disorder and, 659, 661
Countertransference, 789, 793
Couples/marital therapy, abuse and violence, 774
Cowles, Edward, 17
Creutzfeldt-Jakob disease (CJD), 455, 476–477
CRH. See Corticotropin-releasing hormone
Crisis Intervention: Theory and Methodology, 9t

Hand movement, as nonverbal communication, 156

Hans Seyle's stress syndrome and general syndrome adaptation syndrome, 12

Hardiness, 365, 368

Hazardous threats, 63, 108

HD. *See* Huntington's Disease

Health Insurance Portability and Accountability Act of 1996 (HIPAA), 209

Health Promoting Lifestyle Profile (HPLP), 159

Healthy family systems, 852–853

Healthy People 2010, 178, 1108–1109

Herbs, 16

Heterocyclics, 887, 890–892

High Level Wellness (1961), 61

Higher brain function, assessment of, 137, 139

HIPAA. *See* Health Insurance Portability and Accountability Act of 1996

Hippocampal abnormalities, 231f

Hippocampus, 77, 84, 879–880

Historical figures
  Aguilera, D., 9t
  Bailey, Harriet, 8t
  Caplan, G., 9t
  Leininger, Madeline, 8t
  Mellow, June, 8t
  Messick, J., 9t
  Muller, Theresa, 8t
  Nightingale, F., 8t
  Orlando, Ida, 8t
  Peplau, Hildegard, 8t
  Richards, Linda, 8t
  Tudor, Gwen, 8t

History, psychiatric-mental health care and. *See also* Psychiatric-mental health care

Histrionic personality disorder, 435–436

Holding environment, 985

Home and community settings. *See* Community and home settings

Home-based services, abuse and violence, 774–775

Homelessness, 1013

Homeostasis, 27, 299

Homophobia, sexual disorder and, 735–736

Hopelessness, 553
  suicide and, 562

Hopelessness Rating Scale for Depression, 253t

Horney, Karen, 12, 41
  social theory application to nursing, 41–42

Hospice, 1005, 1013

Hospital of St. Mary of Bethlehem, England, 6

Hospitalization, U.S. mental health laws and, 203–210

Hostility, 587, 589

HPA axis. *See* Hypothalamic-pituitary-adrenal axis; Hypothalamus-pituitary-adrenal axis

HPLP. *See* Health Promoting Lifestyle Profile

Human costs, substance-related disorder and, 626–627

Human genome, 875, 878

Human Genome Project, 14t

Human need theory, 60–61
  application to nursing, 61

Human sexual response cycle, 725, 730

Human sexuality, 730–733

Humor
  as defense mechanism, 36t
  as therapeutic communication technique, 162–163

Huntington's Disease (HD), 476

Hydrocephalus, normal pressure, 456, 464

Hydrotherapy, 935, 937

Hyperactivity, 495, 496

Hyperphagia, 225, 230

Hypersomnia, 225, 230, 701

Hypertension, stress and, 372

Hypnotics, 911–912

Hypochondriasis, 35t, 343, 352–353
  diagnostic criteria for, 353t

Hypoglycemic shock, 12

Hypomania, 267, 269

Hypothalamic-pituitary-adrenal (HPA) axis, 228, 229–231, 303

Hypothalamus, 52f, 77, 81, 85t, 230f

Hypothalamus-pituitary-adrenal (HPA) axis, 81

Hysteria. *See also* Somatization disorder
  explanations of, 11

I

Id, 31, 34

Identification, empathy process, 114

Identification phase, in nurse-client relationship, 167–168

Identified client, 849, 864

Identity, in ego development, 39t

Illicit substances, substance-related disorder and, 624–625

Illusion, 125, 130

Immature mechanism, 35t

Immune system studies, 58

Immunological disorders, stress and, 374

Impaired communication, 855–856

Implementation, in nursing process, 119, 144, 253, 257

Impulsivity, 139, 495, 496, 553, 562, 587, 589

Inattention, 495, 496

Incompetency, *vs.* competency, 206

Incongruent communication, 849, 855

Incorporation, empathy process, 114

Individual psychotherapy
  across the life span, 796–800
  case studies, 804–805b
  cultural considerations in, 791
  eating disorders and, 686
  historical perspectives of, 790–791
  nurse's role in, 800–801
  nursing process, 801–804
  theories and concepts of, 791–796

Individual therapy, abuse and violence, 774

Indolamines, 881–882

U

United States, nature and extent of substance use, 623–624
United States Mental Health Laws, 203–210
Untradian rhythms, 32, 59
Utilizer of research findings, 1075, 1081

V

Vagus nerve stimulation (VNS), 215, 249, 935, 938–939
Validation, 985, 989
Valium, 307
Valliant, G. E., 34
Valproic acid and derivatives, 898
Valproic acid (Depakene), children and adolescents, 920
Vascular dementia, 471
    DSM-IV-TR diagnostic criteria for, 473b
Venlafaxine (Effexor), 248t
Veracity, 195, 199
Verbal communication, 156–157
Veterans, group therapy and, 837

Violence, 587, 589
    legal and ethical issues and, 606
Visual imagery, 298, 330
Visual memory, 456, 472
Visuospatial ability, 126, 137
Vitaly Tarasoff v. the Regents of the University of California, 207
VNS. *See* Vagus nerve stimulation
Voice tone, as nonverbal communication, 156
Voluntary hospitalization, 204
Vulnerability, 1093

W

Walters, R. H., and Bandura, A., 44–45
War-related trauma, 1109–1110
Warren worldview perspective, 180t
WAS. *See* World Association for Sexology
Weissman, Myrna, 250
Wellbutrin, 247

Wellness-illness continuum, 61–63, 62t
  application to nursing, 62–63
  health recovery, 63
Wernicke-Korsakoff syndrome, 617, 634
Wernicke's encephalopathy, 617, 634
White House Conference on Children, 19t
Withdrawal syndrome, 617, 620
Women
  cultural positions and sexual disorder, 735
  depressive disorder in, 238
  risk factors for bipolar disorder, 269, 273
World Association for Sexology (WAS), 725, 727, 728
World War II period. *See* Twentieth century

Worldview prospective, 177, 179, 180t
Wyatt v. Stickney, 210

Y

Yalom, I., therapeutic factors of group therapy, 820t
York Retreat, 7

Z

Zeitgeber, 32, 59
Zoloft, 79, 88, 247